TEXTBOOK OF
ADULT EMERGENCY MEDICINE

Content Strategist: Jeremy Bowes
Content Development Specialist: Fiona Conn
Project Manager: Julie Taylor
Designer: Miles Hitchen
Illustration Manager: Jennifer Rose
Illustrator: Ethan Danielson

TEXTBOOK OF ADULT EMERGENCY MEDICINE

FOURTH EDITION

EDITED BY

Peter Cameron MBBS, MD, FACEM

Professor of Emergency Medicine, Department of Epidemiology and Preventive Medicine,
Monash University, Victoria, Australia;
The Alfred Hospital, Melbourne, Australia

George Jelinek MBBS, MD, DipDHM, FACEM

Director, Emergency Practice Innovation Centre, St Vincent's Hospital Melbourne, Australia;
Professorial Fellow, Faculty of Medicine, Dentistry and Health Sciences, The University of Melbourne, Melbourne, Australia

Anne-Maree Kelly MD, MBBS, MClinEd, FACEM, FCCP

Academic Head of Emergency Medicine and Director, Joseph Epstein Centre for Emergency Medicine Research,
Western Health, Melbourne, Australia;
Professorial Fellow, Faculty of Medicine, Dentistry and Health Sciences, The University of Melbourne, Melbourne, Australia;
Adjunct Professor, Faculty of Health, School of Public Health and Social Work, Queensland University of
Technology, Brisbane, Australia

Anthony Brown MBChB, FRCP, FRCSEd, FACEM, FCEM

Professor of Emergency Medicine, School of Medicine, University of Queensland, Queensland, Australia;
Senior Staff Specialist, Department of Emergency Medicine, Royal Brisbane and Women's Hospital, Brisbane, Australia

Mark Little MBBS, FACEM, MPH&TM, DTM&H, IDHA

Emergency Physician and Clinical Toxicologist, Cairns Hospital, Cairns, Queensland, Australia;
Associate Professor, School of Public Health & Tropical Medicine, Queensland Tropical Health Alliance,
James Cook University, Queensland, Australia

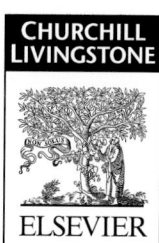

CHURCHILL LIVINGSTONE

ELSEVIER

Edinburgh • London • New York • Oxford • Philadelphia • St Louis • Sydney • Toronto 2015

CHURCHILL
LIVINGSTONE
ELSEVIER

First edition 2000
Second edition 2004
Third edition 2009
Fourth edition 2015
   Reprinted 2015 (third)

ISBN 978-0-7020-5335-1
Ebook ISBN 978-0-7020-5438-9

British Library Cataloguing in Publication Data
A catalogue record for this book is available from the British Library

Library of Congress Cataloging in Publication Data
A catalog record for this book is available from the Library of Congress

Notices

Knowledge and best practice in this field are constantly changing. As new research and experience broaden
our understanding, changes in research methods, professional practices, or medical treatment may become
necessary.

Practitioners and researchers must always rely on their own experience and knowledge in evaluating and
using any information, methods, compounds, or experiments described herein. In using such information or
methods they should be mindful of their own safety and the safety of others, including parties for whom they
have a professional responsibility.

With respect to any drug or pharmaceutical products identified, readers are advised to check the most
current information provided (i) on procedures featured or (ii) by the manufacturer of each product to be
administered, to verify the recommended dose or formula, the method and duration of administration, and
contraindications. It is the responsibility of practitioners, relying on their own experience and knowledge of
their patients, to make diagnoses, to determine dosages and the best treatment for each individual patient,
and to take all appropriate safety precautions.

To the fullest extent of the law, neither the Publisher nor the authors, contributors, or editors, assume any
liability for any injury and/or damage to persons or property as a matter of products liability, negligence or
otherwise, or from any use or operation of any methods, products, instructions, or ideas contained in the
material herein.

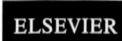 **ELSEVIER** your source for books,
journals and multimedia
in the health sciences

www.elsevierhealth.com

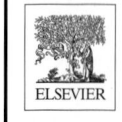 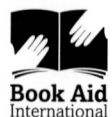 Working together
to grow libraries in
Book Aid developing countries
International

www.elsevier.com • www.bookaid.org

Printed in China

Last digit is the print number: 8   7   6   5   4

The
Publisher's
policy is to use
**paper manufactured
from sustainable forests**

Contents

CONTENTS

CONTENTS

CONTENTS

Preface to Fourth Edition

It is wonderful that this text is now being published as a fourth edition. As editors, we have had the privilege to coordinate, probe, push and arbitrate the many contributions and ensure the success of this comprehensive textbook. The hundreds of experts involved in developing this text have generously given their time and expertise and the result has been worth this effort!

It will be evident to readers of the previous editions that we have gradually increased the subject matter over time. This reflects the growing depth and breadth of emergency medicine and the increasing expectations of emergency medicine practitioners. As well as covering the mainstream clinical subjects including resuscitation, trauma, cardiac, respiratory, gastrointestinal, neurology, musculoskeletal, infectious disease, toxicology and psychiatry – we have also emphasized the other skills and knowledge that are needed by an advanced emergency medicine practitioner. Unlike other emergency medicine texts, there are major sections on administrative issues such as staffing, overcrowding, triage, patient safety and quality. In addition, difficult topics such as death and dying, the challenging patient, ethics, giving evidence and domestic violence are covered. There is also an overview of academic emergency medicine, the foundation of clinical emergency medicine into the future.

Most governing bodies overseeing training schemes around the developed world are now realizing that simply teaching a variety of clinical strategies to front line clinicians will not ensure high quality emergency medicine. Understanding the governance, organization and training is essential. Training schemes for emergency medicine internationally are now extending beyond the 2–3 years originally required in the USA, when emergency medicine first developed as a specialty, out to at least 4–5 years. In addition to basic Board exams, Fellowships are being added in critical care, pre-hospital, administration, toxicology, ultrasound, public health and other subspecialty interests, to underpin more comprehensive training. The Australasian approach has always been to have a much longer training scheme (minimum 7 years post-graduate) to allow broad clinical exposure and a less narrowly focused curriculum. This text reflects that approach, examining a broad spectrum of issues with which emergency physicians are expected to be familiar.

This is the first edition to be developed as both a print and an electronic version. This has the advantage that electronic material can be accessed without adding multiple extra pages and making the printed text unwieldy. It also allows us the advantage of adding features such as multiple choice questions and high quality pictures. A further important feature of the electronic version is that browsers searching for material on a topic will be able to access individual chapters through the Elsevier site, allowing clinicians to look for particular topics that are not covered well by other texts or articles. We believe, however, that clinicians will still require access to one major printed text with a consensus view on major topics.

There are many people to thank for the success of this book. More than 200 contributors have ensured a broad spectrum of opinions and consensus on a huge variety of topics. No doubt their partners, children and significant others will also have their opinions on the book and the time involved! Importantly, the outstanding support from people at Elsevier led by Fiona Conn as well as Jessica Hocking at Hamad Medical Corporation in Qatar have ensured that the operational aspects of the programme ran smoothly, for which we are all indebted. Thank you.

Peter Cameron
George Jelinek
Anne-Maree Kelly
Anthony Brown
Mark Little

Contributors

Jonathan Abrahams, MPH, BSc, Grad Dip(Population Health), Cert.(Emergency Management)
Emergency Risk Management and Humanitarian Response, World Health Organization, Geneva, Switzerland
Chapter 26.3 Medical issues in disasters

Nicholas Adams, MBBS
Emergency Physician, Emergency and Trauma Centre, The Alfred Hospital, Melbourne, Australia
Chapter 10.1 Acute kidney injury

Muhammad Shuaib Afzal, MBBS, CABMS (EM), MCEM
Emergency Physician, Hamad Medical Corporation, Qatar
Chapter 9.10 Needlestick injuries and related blood and body fluid exposures

Peter Aitken, MBBS, FACEM, EMDM, MClinEd
Clinical Director – Counter Disaster and Major Events, Qld Health, Brisbane, Australia
Associate Professor School of Public Health, Tropical Medicine and Rehabilitation Sciences, James Cook University, Townsville, Australia
Chapter 26.9 Public health and emergency medicine

Sam Alfred, MBBS, FACEM, Dip Tox
Emergency Physician and Clinical Toxicologist, Royal Adelaide Hospital, Adelaide, Australia
Chapter 29.17 Hydrofluoric acid

Peter Allely, MBBCh, BAO, FCEM, FACEM
Emergency Physician, Sir Charles Gairdner Hospital, Perth, Australia
Chapter 4.6 Pelvic injuries
Chapter 4.7 Hip injuries
Chapter 4.8 Femur injuries

Sylvia Andrew-Starkey, MBBS, FACEM
Emergency Department, Caboolture Hospital, Caboolture, Queensland, Australia
Chapter 20.1 Mental state assessment

Philip Aplin, MBBS, FACEM
Emergency Physician, Emergency Department, Flinders Medical Centre, Adelaide, Australia
Chapter 8.2 Stroke and transient ischaemic attacks

Michael W Ardagh, ONZM, PhD, MBChB, DCH, FACEM
Professor of Emergency Medicine, University of Otago, Christchurch, New Zealand
Chapter 25.5 Ethics in emergency medicine

Sean Arendse, FACEM, MBBS, BSc, AKC
Emergency Physician, Emergency and Trauma Centre, The Alfred Hospital, Melbourne, Australia
Chapter 9.10 Needlestick injuries and related blood and body fluid exposures
Chapter 10.3 Renal colic
Chapter 13.4 Haemophilia
Chapter 13.5 Blood and blood products

Jason Armstrong, FACEM, MBChB
Emergency Physician and Clinical Toxicologist, Sir Charles Gairdner Hospital, Perth;
Medical Director, Western Australia Poisons Information Centre, Perth, Australia
Chapter 29.9 Antidiabetic drugs

Richard H Ashby, AM, MBBS, BHA, FRACGP, FACEM, FIFEM, FRACMA
Chief Executive, Metro South Health, Brisbane, Australia
Chapter 27.4 Business planning

Michael R Augello, MBBS, FACEM
Emergency Physician, Emergency Department, St Vincent's Hospital, Fitzroy, Victoria; Honorary Fellow, Department of Medicine, St Vincent's Hospital, University of Melbourne, Melbourne, Australia
Chapter 7.14 Perianal conditions

Michael Baker, MBBS, FACEM(PEM), DipCh
Emergency Physician, Princess Margaret Hospital and Sir Charles Gairdner Hospital, Perth, Australia
Chapter 4.9 Knee injuries
Chapter 4.10 Tibia and fibula injuries
Chapter 4.11 Ankle joint injuries
Chapter 4.12 Foot injuries

Ashis Banerjee, MBBS, MRCS, LRCP, MS, FRCS(Eng), FRCS(Edin), FCEM, DTM&H
Consultant/Lead Clinician, Emergency Medicine, Chase Farm Hospital, London; Honorary Senior Lecturer, University College London Medical School, London; Honorary Senior Lecturer, University of Hertfordshire, Hatfield, UK
Chapter 7.10 Acute appendicitis

Simon Baston, RGN, RMN
Mental Health Liaison Nurse, Liaison Psychiatry, Accident and Emergency Department, Northern General Hospital, Sheffield, UK
Chapter 25.1 Mental health and the law: the Australasian and UK perspectives

Anthony J Bell, MBBS, FACEM, MBA
Director, Emergency Department, Queen Elizabeth II Jubilee Hospital, Brisbane; Associate Professor, School of Medicine, University of Queensland, Queensland, Australia
Chapter 22.3 Procedural sedation and analgesia

Stephen A Bernard, MD, FACEM, FCICM, FCCM
Senior Staff Specialist, The Intensive Care Unit, Alfred Hospital, Melbourne, Victoria, Australia
Chapter 1.1 Basic Life Support
Chapter 2.1 Airway and ventilation management
Chapter 2.7 Cerebral resuscitation after cardiac arrest
Chapter 26.1 Pre-hospital emergency medicine

xiii

CONTRIBUTORS

Shom Bhattacharjee, MBBS, FRACP
Consultant Physician and Rheumatologist, The
Alfred Hospital, Melbourne, Australia
Chapter 14.3 Polyarthritis

Peter Bosanac, MBBS, MMed (Psychiatry), MD,
FRANZCP
Director Clinical Services, St Vincent's Mental
Health, Melbourne, Australia
Chapter 20.3 Deliberate self-harm/suicide

David A Bradt, MD, MPH, DTM&H, FACEM,
FAFPHM, FAAEM
Center for Refugee and Disaster Response,
Johns Hopkins Medical Institutions,
Baltimore, USA
Chapter 26.3 Medical issues in disasters

George Braitberg, MBBS, FACEM, Grad Dip Epi
and Biostatistics
Professor of Emergency Medicine, Southern
Clinical School, Monash University and Director
of Emergency Medicine Monash Health,
Melbourne, Australia
Chapter 29.15 Cyanide

Crispijn van den Brand, MD
Emergency Physician, Medisch Centrum
Haaglanden, The Hague, The Netherlands
Chapter 4.1 Injuries of the shoulder
*Chapter 4.4 Fractures of the forearm and carpal
bones*

Victoria Brazil, MBBS, FACEM, MBA
Staff Specialist, Department of Emergency
Medicine, Royal Brisbane and Women's
Hospital, Brisbane, Australia
*Chapter 24.5 Postgraduate emergency
medicine teaching and simulation*

Richard J Brennan, MBBS, MPH, FACEM,
FIFEM
Director, Department of Emergency Risk
Management and Humanitarian Response,
World Health Organization, Geneva, Switzerland
Chapter 26.3 Medical issues in disasters

Edward Brentnall, MBBS, DipObstetrics(RCOG),
FACEM
Retired Emergency Physician Melbourne,
Victoria, Australia
*Chapter 25.3 Consent and competence – the
Australasian and UK perspectives*

Anthony Brown, MBChB, FRCP, FRCSEd, FACEM,
FCEM
Professor of Emergency Medicine, Discipline
of Anaesthesiology and Critical Care, School
of Medicine, University of Queensland,
Queensland; Senior Staff Specialist, Department

of Emergency Medicine, Royal Brisbane and
Women's Hospital, Brisbane, Australia
Chapter 2.8 Anaphylaxis
*Chapter 11.1 Diabetes mellitus and
hypoglycaemia: an overview*
*Chapter 11.2 Diabetic ketoacidosis and
hyperosmolar, hyperglycaemic state*
*Chapter 14.4 Musculoskeletal and soft-tissue
emergencies*
*Chapter 19.4 Abnormal vaginal bleeding in the
non-pregnant patient*
Chapter 22.2 Local anaesthesia

Sheila Bryan, MBBS, FACEM, BSc(Hons), CHPE,
Dip Ven, GDHSM, GCClinSim
Emergency Physician, Monash Health, Victoria,
Australia
*Chapter 19.2 Ectopic pregnancy and bleeding
in early pregnancy*
*Chapter 19.3 Bleeding after the first trimester
of pregnancy*
*Chapter 19.4 Abnormal vaginal bleeding in the
non-pregnant patient*
Chapter 19.5 Pelvic inflammatory disease

Nicholas Buckley, MD, FRACP
Professor of Medicine, Prince of Wales
Clinical School, The University of New South
Wales, Sydney; Senior Staff Specialist, New
South Wales Poisons Information Centre, The
Children's Hospital at Westmead, New South
Wales, Australia
Chapter 29.20 Carbon monoxide

Lyndal Bugeja, BA(Hons), PhD
Manager, Coroners Prevention Unit, Coroners
Court of Victoria, Melbourne; Adjunct Research
Fellow, Monash Injury Research Institute,
Monash University, Victoria, Australia
Chapter 21.3 Family violence

Simon Byrne, BA(Hons), MBBS, FRANZCP
Consultant Psychiatrist, Departments of
Psychiatry and Emergency Medicine, Sir
Charles Gairdner Hospital, Perth; Clinical Senior
Lecturer, University of Western Australia, Perth,
Australia
Chapter 20.4 Depression
Chapter 20.5 Psychosis
*Chapter 20.6 Pharmacological management of
the aroused patient*

Adam B Bystrzycki, MBBS, FACEM
Staff Specialist, Emergency Department, The
Alfred Hospital, Melbourne, Australia
Chapter 14.1 Rheumatological emergencies
Chapter 14.2 Monoarthritis
Chapter 14.3 Polyarthritis

Michael Cadogan, FACEM
Clinical Senior Lecturer (UWA), Staff Specialist
in Emergency Medicine, Department of
Emergency Medicine, Sir Charles Gairdner
Hospital, Perth, Australia
Chapter 4.6 Pelvic injuries
Chapter 4.7 Hip injuries
Chapter 4.8 Femur injuries
Chapter 4.9 Knee injuries
Chapter 4.10 Tibia and fibula injuries
Chapter 4.11 Ankle joint injuries
Chapter 4.12 Foot injuries
Chapter 19.6 Pelvic pain

Peter Cameron, MBBS, MD, FACEM
Professor of Emergency Medicine, Department
of Epidemiology and Preventive Medicine,
Monash University; The Alfred Hospital,
Melbourne, Australia
Introduction
Chapter 3.1 Trauma overview

Gregory Cham, MBBS, FRCSEd, FAMS
Senior Consultant, Department of Emergency
Medicine, Alexandra Hospital, Singapore
Chapter 6.8 Haemoptysis

Betty Shuk Han Chan, MBBS, PhD, FACEM
Emergency Physician and Clinical Toxicologist,
Prince of Wales Hospital, Sydney, New South
Wales; Clinical Toxicologist, New South Wales
Poisons Information Centre, The Children's
Hospital at Westmead, New South Wales,
Australia
Chapter 29.2 Cardiovascular drugs

Kim Chai Chan, MBBS, FRCSEd(A&E)
Senior Consultant, Department of Emergency
Medicine, Alexandra Hospital, JurongHealth,
Singapore
Chapter 7.2 Approach to abdominal pain

Rabind Charles, MBBS, FRCSEd(A&E)
Senior Consultant, Department of Emergency
Medicine, Alexandra Hospital, Singapore
Chapter 9.5 Skin and soft-tissue infections

Raymond Chi Hung Cheng, MBChB, MRCS,
FHKAM
Associate Consultant, Emergency and Trauma
Centre, Prince of Wales Hospital, Hong Kong
Chapter 4.2 Fractures of the humerus
Chapter 4.3 Dislocations of the elbow

Angela Chiew, BSc(Med)MBBS, FACEM
Emergency Physician and Clinical Toxicologist,
Prince of Wales Hospital, Randwick, New South
Wales, Australia
Chapter 29.2 Cardiovascular drugs

xiv

CONTRIBUTORS

Chi-Keong Ching, MBBS, MRCP, FAMS, FHRS
Director, Cardiac Pacing & Electrophysiology,
National Heart Centre Singapore; Assistant
Professor, Duke-National University of
Singapore Graduate Medical School, Singapore
Chapter 5.4 Arrhythmias

Matthew WG Chu, MBBS(Hons), FACEM
Senior Specialist, Emergency Medicine Director,
Medical Assessment Unit
Director of Prevocational Education and Training,
Canterbury Hospital, Sydney, Australia
Chapter 27.2 Emergency department layout

Flavia M Cicuttini, MBBS, PhD, MSc, DLSHTM,
FRACP, FAFPHM
Head, Musculoskeletal Unit, Head
Rheumatology Unit, The Alfred Hospital,
Melbourne; Department of Epidemiology
and Preventive Medicine, Monash University,
Victoria, Australia
Chapter 14.1 Rheumatological emergencies
Chapter 14.2 Monoarthritis
Chapter 14.3 Polyarthritis

James Collier, MBBS, FACEM
Co-Director, Emergency Medicine, Princess
Alexandra Hospital, Brisbane, Australia
*Chapter 27.5 Accreditation, specialist training
and recognition in Australasia*

Michael Coman, MBBS, FACEM
Department of Emergency Medicine, Monash
Medical Centre, Monash Health Melbourne,
Victoria, Australia
Chapter 5.10 Aortic dissection

Julie Considine, RN, RM, BN, Cert Acute Care
Nurs, Gdip Nurs, GCert Higher Ed, MN, PhD, FACN
Professor of Nursing, Deakin University/Director,
Eastern Health – Deakin University Nursing and
Midwifery Research Centre, Victoria, Australia
*Chapter 26.8 Rapid response systems and the
emergency department*
Chapter 27.1 Emergency department staffing

Geoffrey A Couser, FACEM, Grad Cert ULT
Associate Professor, School of Medicine,
University of Tasmania, Hobart, Tasmania;
Staff Specialist, Emergency Department, Royal
Hobart Hospital, Hobart, Tasmania, Australia
*Chapter 24.4 Undergraduate teaching in
emergency medicine*

Roslyn Crampton, MBBS, FACEM
Senior Staff Specialist, Emergency Medicine
and Forensic Medical Service, Westmead
Hospital, New South Wales, Australia
Chapter 21.2 Sexual assault

Stuart Dilley, MBBS, FACEM
Emergency Physician, St Vincent's Hospital,
Senior Fellow, Department of Medicine,
Dentistry and Health Sciences, University of
Melbourne, Melbourne, Australia
Chapter 6.8 Haemoptysis

Simon Dimmick, BPTHY, MBBS(Hons), FRANZCR
Department of Radiology, Royal North Shore
Hospital, St Leonards, Australia
Chapter 3.8 Radiology in major trauma

Jenny Dowd, MD, FRANZCOG
Obstetrician, Royal Women's Hospital,
Melbourne, Australia
*Chapter 19.3 Bleeding after the first trimester
of pregnancy*

Robert Dowsett, BM, BS, FACEM
Visiting Medical Officer, Clinical Toxicology,
Drug Health Service, Western Hospital, Victoria;
Visiting Medical Officer, New South Wales
Poisons Information Centre, The Children's
Hospital at Westmead, New South Wales; Senior
Lecturer, Faculty of Medicine, Dentistry and
Health Sciences, The University of Melbourne,
Melbourne, Australia
Chapter 29.16 Corrosive ingestion

Pieter van Driel, DEMT, FNVSHA
Emergency Physician, St Elisabeth Hospital,
Tilburg, Netherlands
Chapter 3.3 Spinal trauma

Dino Druda, BMedSci(Hons), MBBS, MRCP,
FACEM
Emergency Physician and Fellow in Clinical
Toxicology, Emergency Department, Austin
Health, Melbourne, Australia
Chapter 29.3 Antipsychotic drugs
Chapter 29.4 Antidepressant drugs

Martin Duffy, MBBS, MMed, FACEM
Senior Staff Specialist, Emergency Medicine,
St Vincent's Hospital, New South Wales,
Australia
*Chapter 6.5 Chronic obstructive pulmonary
disease*

Steven J Dunjey, MBBS, FACEM, DDU
Senior Consultant, Emergency Medicine, Royal
Perth Hospital, Australia
Chapter 23.2 CT scanning in emergency medicine

Rebecca Dunn, MBBS
Consultant Dermatologist, Department of
Dermatology, Royal Melbourne Hospital,
Parkville, Victoria, Australia
Chapter 15.1 Emergency dermatology

Linas Dziukas, MBBS, MD, FRACP, FACEM
Emergency Physician, The Alfred Hospital,
Melbourne, Australia
Chapter 10.1 Acute kidney injury

Robert Edwards, MBBS, FACEM
Senior Staff Specialist, Emergency Medicine;
Senior Staff Specialist, Department of Trauma,
Westmead Hospital, New South Wales; Clinical
Senior Lecturer Emergency Medicine, Western
Clinical School, Sydney Medical School, Sydney,
Australia
Chapter 29.14 Methaemoglobinaemia

Diana Egerton-Warburton, MBBS, FACEM,
M Clin Epi
Emergency Physician, Monash Medical Centre,
Monash Health; Adjunct Senior Lecturer,
Southern Clinical School, Monash University,
Melbourne, Australia
*Chapter 26.9 Public health and emergency
medicine*

Tor NO Ercleve, BSc, MBChB, FACEM
Consultant, Emergency Medicine, Sir Charles
Gairdner Hospital, Perth; Senior Clinical
Lecturer, Emergency Medicine, University
Western Australia, Crawley, Australia
Chapter 22.2 Local anaesthesia

Maisse Farhan, MBBS, MRCSEd, FCEM
Emergency Department, Western Health,
Melbourne, Australia
Chapter 5.9 Hypertension

Daniel M Fatovich, MBBS, FACEM, PhD
Professor of Emergency Medicine, Royal Perth
Hospital, University of Western Australia, Centre
for Clinical Research in Emergency Medicine,
Harry Perkins Institute of Medical Research,
Perth, Australia
Chapter 22.1 General pain management
*Chapter 28.6 Electric shock and lightning
injury*

Louise Finnel, MBChB, FACEM, PGDipClinEd
Emergency Physician, Emergency
Department, Middlemore Hospital, Auckland,
New Zealand
Chapter 7.11 Inflammatory bowel disease

Mark Fitzgerald, MBBS, FACEM
Director, Trauma Service, The Alfred Hospital,
Melbourne; Medical Adviser, Ambulance
Victoria, Melbourne; Professor, Department
of Surgery, Central Clinical School, Monash
University, Victoria, Australia
Chapter 3.6 Chest trauma

CONTRIBUTORS

Peter Freeman, MBChB, FCEM, FACEM
Director of Emergency Medicine, Department of Emergency Medicine, Rotorua Hospital, Rotorua, New Zealand
Chapter 4.5 Hand injuries

James K Galbraith, MBBS, FRANZCO, FRACS
Ophthalmology Department, The Royal Melbourne Hospital, Melbourne, Australia
Chapter 16.1 Ocular emergencies

Peter Garrett, MBBS, BSc(Hons), FCICM, FACEM, FCEM
Director, Critical Care, Noosa Hospital, Noosa; Senior Staff Specialist, Intensive Care, Sunshine Coast Health Service, Sunshine Coast, Queensland, Australia
Chapter 2.4 Shock overview
Chapter 27.7 Complaints

Alan Gault, MBChB, BAO, BAHSc, FACEM
Emergency Department, Sir Charles Gairdner Hospital, Perth, Australia
Chapter 12.1 Acid—base disorders

Michael J Gingold, BMedSc(Hon), MBBS(Hon), FRACP
Consultant, Department of Rheumatology, The Alfred Hospital, Melbourne, Australia
Chapter 14.1 Rheumatological emergencies
Chapter 14.2 Monoarthritis

Robert Gocentas, MBBS, DipClinEpi, FACEM
Emergency Department, The Alfred Hospital, Melbourne, Australia
Chapter 3.6 Chest trauma

E Shaun Goh, MBBS, MRCSEd, FAMS, FCEM, MSc
Consultant, Acute and Emergency Care Center, Khoo Teck Puat Hospital, Singapore; Chairman, Trauma Committee, Khoo Teck Puat Hospital, Singapore; Consultant, Unit for Prehospital Emergency Care, Singapore; Senior Clinical Lecturer, Yong Loo Lin School of Medicine, National University of Singapore, Singapore
Chapter 7.13 Rectal bleeding

Neil A Goldie, MBBS, FACEM
Director of Emergency Medicine, Dandenong Hospital, Monash Health, Victoria, Australia
Chapter 7.4 Hernia

Steve Goodacre, MBChB, MRCP, Dip IMC, FCEM, MSc, PhD
Professor of Emergency Medicine, University of Sheffield, School of Health and Related Research, Sheffield, UK
Chapter 5.1 Chest pain
Chapter 5.2 Acute coronary syndromes

Adrian Goudie, B Med Sci(Hons), MBBS, FACEM, DDU
Emergency Physician, Emergency Department, Fremantle Hospital, Fremantle, Australia
Chapter 23.1 Emergency department ultrasound

Colin A Graham, MBChB, MPH, MD, FRCPEd, FRCSEd, FRCSGlasg, FIMCRCSEd, FCCP, FCEM, FHKCEM, FHKAM(Emergency Medicine)
Professor of Emergency Medicine, Chinese University of Hong Kong; Honorary Consultant in Emergency Medicine, Prince of Wales Hospital, Shatin, Hong Kong; Editor-in-Chief, European Journal of Emergency Medicine, London, UK
Chapter 5.7 Heart valve emergencies
Chapter 5.8 Peripheral vascular disease
Chapter 7.6 Haematemesis and melaena

Andis Graudins, MBBS(Hons), PhD
Professor of Emergency Medicine and Clinical Toxicology Research, Monash University, Victoria; Principle Specialist in Emergency Medicine and Clinical Toxicology, Department of Emergency Medicine, Monash Health, Victoria; Visiting Consultant Clinical Toxicologist, New South Wales Poisons Information Centre, The Children's Hospital at Westmead, New South Wales, Australia
Chapter 29.6 Antihistamine and anticholinergic poisoning
Chapter 29.7 Paracetamol
Chapter 29.8 Salicylate
Chapter 29.17 Hydrofluoric acid

Tim Gray, MBBS, FACEM, Grad Cert Emerg Health
Senior Lecturer, Central Clinical School, Monash University, Victoria; Director of Education and Training, Adult Retrieval Victoria, Victoria, Australia
Chapter 3.11 Burns

Digby Green, BSc, MBChB, FACEM
Emergency Physician, Cairns Base Hospital, Cairns, Australia
Chapter 29.8 Salicylate

Tim Green, MBBS, FACEM
Director, Emergency Department, Royal Prince Alfred Hospital, Sydney; Clinical Senior Lecturer, Sydney Medical School, Sydney University, Sydney, Australia
Chapter 8.7 Weakness

Shaun Greene, MBChB, MSc, FACEM
Emergency Physician, Austin Hospital, Austin Health, Melbourne; Clinical Toxicologist, Victorian Poisons Information Service, Melbourne, Australia
Chapter 29.3 Antipsychotic drugs
Chapter 29.4 Antidepressant drugs

Naren Gunja, MBBS, MSc, FACEM, FACMT
Clinical Toxicologist, New South Wales Poisons Information Centre, The Children's Hospital at Westmead; Emergency Physician and Toxicologist, Emergency Department, Westmead Hospital, Sydney; Clinical Associate Professor, Discipline of Emergency Medicine, Sydney Medical School, Australia
Chapter 29.6 Antihistamine and anticholinergic poisoning

Barry Gunn, MBBS, FACEM
Emergency Physician, Department of Emergency Medicine, Sunshine Hospital, Melbourne, Australia
Chapter 5.9 Hypertension

Andrew Haig, MBBS, FACEM, DDU
Director of Emergency Medicine, The Mater Hospital, Brisbane, Australia
Chapter 23.1 Emergency department ultrasound

Richard D Hardern, MBChSCB, FRCP(Ed), FCEM
Consultant and Honorary Clinical Lecturer, Emergency Medicine, University Hospital of North Durham, Durham, UK
Chapter 11.2 Diabetic ketoacidosis and hyperosmolar, hyperglycaemic state

Jason Harney, MBBS, BMedSci, FACEM
Emergency Physician, Department of Emergency Medicine, Sunshine Hospital, Melbourne, Australia
Chapter 5.6 Pericarditis, cardiac tamponade and myocarditis

Roger Harris, MBBS, FACEM
Emergency Physician, Royal North Shore Hospital, University of Sydney, New South Wales, Australia
Chapter 3.8 Radiology in major trauma

James Hayes, MB, BS, FACEM
Staff Specialist, The Northern Hospital, Epping, Victoria, Australia
Chapter 5.6 Pericarditis, cardiac tamponade and myocarditis

Kenneth Heng, MBBS, FRCS (Edin)A&E, FCEM
Senior Consultant, Emergency Department, Tan Tock Seng Hospital, Singapore; Adjunct Assistant Professor, Yong Loo Lin School of Medicine, Singapore
Chapter 7.9 Pancreatitis

Ruth Hew, MBBS, BA, MSc(Clin Epi), FACEM
Emergency Physician, Sunshine Hospital, Melbourne, Australia
Chapter 8.4 Altered conscious state

Liz Hickson, BMed Sci, MBChB, MRCP, FCICM
Staff Specialist, Intensive Care Medicine, Royal
North Shore Hospital, Sydney, Australia
Chapter 2.3 Haemodynamic monitoring

Rosslyn Hing, MBBS, BSc(Med), FACEM
Emergency Physician, Royal Prince Alfred
Hospital, Sydney; Clinical Senior Lecturer,
Sydney Medical School, University of Sydney,
Sydney, Australia
Chapter 8.6 Syncope and vertigo

Weng Hoe Ho, MMed(A&E), MRCSEd(A&E),
MSc(DM)
Consultant, Emergency Medicine Department,
National University Hospital, Singapore
Chapter 6.1 Upper respiratory tract

Kerry A Hoggett, MBBS, GCert Clin Tox,
FACEM
Emergency Physician and Clinical Toxicologist,
Royal Perth Hospital, Perth, Australia
Chapter 29.13 Drugs of abuse

Anna Holdgate, MBBS, MMed, FACEM
Associate Professor, Department of Emergency
Medicine, Liverpool Hospital, Sydney; Associate
Professor, South West Clinical School, University
of New South Wales, Sydney, Australia
Chapter 2.5 Sepsis and septic shock

Anthony D Holley, BSc, MBBCh, Dip Paeds,
DipDHM, FACEM, FCICM
Senior Staff Specialist, Department of
Intensive Care Medicine, Royal Brisbane and
Women's Hospital, Brisbane; Senior Lecturer,
School of Medicine, University of Queensland,
Queensland, Australia
Chapter 2.6 Arterial blood gases

Craig Hore, MBBS, FACEM, FCICM, MHPol
Staff Specialist, Intensive Care Unit, Liverpool
Hospital, Liverpool, New South Wales; Staff
Specialist, Aeromedical Retrieval Service,
Ambulance Service of New South Wales, New
South Wales; Clinical Senior Lecturer, Faculty
of Medicine, University of New South Wales,
Australia
Chapter 2.3 Haemodynamic monitoring

Kevin KC Hung, MBChB, MPH, EMDM, MRCSEd,
FHKCEM, FHKAM(Emergency Medicine)
Assistant Professor, Collaborative Centre of
Oxford University and The Chinese University
of Hong Kong for Disaster and Medical
Humanitarian Response, The Chinese University
of Hong Kong, Hong Kong
Chapter 5.7 Heart valve emergencies

Jennie Hutton, MBChB, FACEM, MPH
Emergency Department, St Vincent's Hospital,
Melbourne, Australia
Chapter 20.3 Deliberate self-harm/suicide
*Chapter 26.9 Public health and emergency
medicine*

Sue Ieraci, MBBS, FACEM
Senior Staff Specialist Emergency Medicine,
Bankstown Hospital, New South Wales,
Australia
Chapter 27.1 Emergency department staffing

Geoffrey Isbister, BSc, MBBS, FACEM, MD
Senior Staff Specialist, Department of Clinical
Toxicology and Pharmacology, Calvary Mater
Newcastle, Newcastle, New South Wales;
Associate Professor, School of Medicine and
Public Health, University of Newcastle, Newcastle,
New South Wales; Consultant, New South Wales
Poison Information Centre, Sydney Children's
Hospital Network, New South Wales, Australia
Chapter 30.1 Snakebite
Chapter 30.3 Spider bite

Angela Jackson, RN RM, B Health Sc, Crit Care
Cert, MPH&TM, LLB, IDHA
Nurse Practitioner Candidate, Emergency,
Cairns Hospital, Queensland, Australia
*Chapter 26.5 Emergency care in a
humanitarian crisis*

Trevor Jackson, MBBS, FACEM
Emergency Physician, Cabrini Hospital,
Melbourne, Australia
Chapter 4.13 Osteomyelitis
Chapter 9.3 Septic arthritis

George Jelinek, MBBS, MD, DipDHM, FACEM
Director, Emergency Practice Innovation Centre,
St Vincent's Hospital Melbourne, Australia
Professorial Fellow, Faculty of Medicine,
Dentistry and Health Sciences, The University of
Melbourne, Melbourne, Australia
Chapter 20.1 Mental state assessment

Paul A Jennings, BN, MClinEpi, PhD, FPA
Deputy Head of Department and Director
of Research, Department of Community
Emergency Health and Paramedic Practice,
Monash University, Victoria, Australia
Chapter 26.1 Pre-hospital emergency medicine

Daryl A Jones, BSc(Hons), MBBS, MD, FRACP,
FCICM
Associate Professor Intensive Care Medicine,
Austin Health, Melbourne, Australia
*Chapter 26.8 Rapid response systems and the
emergency department*

Anthony P Joseph, RACOG, FACEM, MRCP(UK),
DipRACOG, Grad Cert Health Science (Med
Sonography)
Senior Staff Specialist, Emergency Department
and Director of Trauma (Emergency), Royal North
Shore Hospital, St Leonards, NSW Australia;
Associate Professor, Discipline of Emergency
Medicine, University of Sydney, Australia
Chapter 3.8 Radiology in major trauma

David V Kaufman, FRACS, FRANZCO
Ophthalmology Department, The Royal
Melbourne Hospital, Melbourne, Australia
Chapter 16.1 Ocular emergencies

Anne-Maree Kelly, MD, MBBS, MClinEd, FACEM,
FCCP
Academic Head of Emergency Medicine and
Director, Joseph Epstein Centre for Emergency
Medicine Research, Western Health, Melbourne;
Professorial Fellow, Faculty of Medicine,
Dentistry and Health Sciences, The University
of Melbourne, Melbourne; Adjunct Professor,
Faculty of Health, School of Public Health
and Social Work, Queensland University of
Technology, Brisbane, Australia
Chapter 4.1 Injuries of the shoulder
Chapter 5.2 Acute coronary syndromes
*Chapter 5.6 Pericarditis, cardiac tamponade
and myocarditis*
Chapter 6.2 Asthma
Chapter 6.6 Pneumothorax
Chapter 8.1 Headache
Chapter 24.2 Writing for publication

Marcus Kennedy, MBBS, FACEM, FRACGP,
DA(UK), DipIMC(RCSEd), MHlth ServMt
Clinical Adjunct Associate Professor, Monash
University; Director, Adult Retrieval Victoria,
Ambulance Victoria, Australia
Chapter 26.2 Retrieval

Diane King, MBBS, FACEM
Emergency Physician, Noarlunga Hospital,
South Australia
*Chapter 27.3 Quality assurance/quality
improvement*

Jonathan Knott, MBBS, PhD, FACEM
Head of Education and Research, Emergency
Department, The Royal Melbourne Hospital,
Melbourne, Australia
*Chapter 9.1 Approach to undifferentiated fever
in adults*

Ian Knox, MBBS, FACEM
Specialist in Emergency Medicine, The Wesley
Hospital, Toowong, Queensland, Australia
Chapter 21.2 Sexual assault

Zeff Koutsogiannis, MBBS, FACEM, GCert Clin Tox
Emergency Physician and Clinical Toxicologist
Austin Health, Victoria; Consultant for NSW and
Victoria Poisons Information Centres, Australia
Chapter 29.12 Iron

Win Sen Kuan, MBBS, MRCSEd(A&E), MCI, FAMS
Consultant, Emergency Medicine Department,
National University Health System, Singapore;
Assistant Professor, Department of Surgery,
National University of Singapore, Singapore
Chapter 7.7 Peptic ulcer disease and gastritis

Sashi Kumar, MBBS, DLO, FACEM
Senior Staff Specialist, Department of
Emergency Medicine, The Canberra Hospital,
Canberra; Department of Emergency Medicine,
Calvary Hospital, Canberra, Australia
Chapter 17.1 Dental emergencies
Chapter 18.1 Ear, nose and throat emergencies

Willem Landman, MBChC, FACEM, PGCertClinED
Emergency Department, North Shore Hospital,
Auckland, New Zealand
Chapter 7.3 Bowel obstruction

Francis Lee Chun Yue, MBBS, FRCSEd(A&E),
FAMS
Emergency Physicia, Acute & Emergency Care
Centre, Khoo Teck Puat Hospital, Alexandra
Health, Singapore
Chapter 7.13 Rectal bleeding

Marian Lee, MBBS, DCH, FACEM, MHA
Emergency Physician, Senior Staff Specialist,
Prince of Wales Hospital, Randwick, New South
Wales; Senior Conjoint Lecturer, University of
New South Wales, Prince of Wales Hospital
Clinical School, Australia
Chapter 5.9 Hypertension
Chapter 19.7 Pre-eclampsia and eclampsia

Wee Yee Lee, MBBS, FRCS Edin (A&E), FAMS (EM)
Senior Consultant, Emergency Department,
Changi General Hospital, Singapore
Chapter 6.2 Asthma

Julie Leung, MBBS, FACEM, GCertTox
Emergency Physician, Department of
Emergency Medicine, St Vincent's Hospital,
Sydney, New South Wales, Australia
*Chapter 6.5 Chronic obstructive pulmonary
disease*

David Lightfoot, BSc(Med), MBBS, FACEM
Emergency Physician, Department of
Emergency Medicine, Monash Medical Centre,
Victoria, Australia
*Chapter 5.3 Assessment and management of
acute pulmonary oedema*

Swee Han Lim, MBBS, FRCS Edin (A&E), FRCP
Edin, FAMS
Sr Consultant, Department of Emergency
Medicine, Singapore General Hospital; Clinical
Associate Professor, Yong Loo Lin School of
Medicine, National University of Singapore;
Adjunct Associate Professor, Duke-NUS
Graduate Medical School Singapore
Chapter 5.4 Arrhythmias

Mark Little, MBBS, FACEM, MPH&TM, DTM&H,
IDHA
Emergency Physician and Clinical Toxicologist,
Cairns Hospital, Cairns, Queensland
Associate Professor, School of Public Health
and Tropical Medicine, Queensland Tropical
Health Alliance, James Cook University,
Queensland, Australia
Chapter 13.2 Neutropaenia
Chapter 13.3 Thrombocytopaenia
*Chapter 26.5 Emergency care in a
humanitarian crisis*

Anita Liu, MBBS, FACEM
Emergency Department, Box Hill Hospital,
Victoria, Australia
Chapter 7.5 Gastroenteritis

John Loy, MBBS, BSc(Hons), FACEM
Staff Specialist, Emergency, Western Health,
Melbourne, Australia
Chapter 5.11 Aneurysms

William Lukin, MBBS, FACEM
Deputy Director, Emergency Department, Royal
Brisbane and Women's Hospital, Brisbane,
Australia
Chapter 21.1 Death and dying
*Chapter 21.6 End of life decision making and
palliative care*

Lewis Macken, MBBS, FACEM, FCICM
Senior Staff Specialist, Intensive Care Unit,
Royal North Shore Hospital, St Leonards,
Sydney, Australia
Chapter 3.4 Facial trauma

Andrew Maclean, MBBS, FACEM
Director, Emergency Services, Box Hill Hospital,
Victoria, Australia
Chapter 11.3 Thyroid and adrenal emergencies

John E Maguire, MBBS, DipObsRACOG, FACEM
Senior Staff Specialist in Emergency Medicine,
John Hunter Hospital, Newcastle, New South
Wales; Lecturer in Emergency Medicine, School
of Medicine and Public Health, University of
Newcastle, New South Wales, Australia
Chapter 1.2 Advanced Life Support

Amit Maini, BSc, MBBS, FACEM
Emergency Physician, Emergency and Trauma
Centre, The Alfred Hospital, Melbourne,
Australia
Chapter 3.7 Limb trauma

Shin-Yan Man, MBChB, MMedSc, FRCSEd,
FHKCEM, FHKAM
Associate Consultant, Accident and Emergency
Department, Prince of Wales Hospital, Shatin,
Hong Kong
*Chapter 6.4 Influenza and emerging respiratory
infections*

Sander Manders, MD, FACEM, FCEM
Medical Retrieval Consultant, Royal Darwin
Hospital, Darwin; Retrieval Consultant,
CareFlight, Darwin, Northern Territory, Australia
Chapter 9.11 Tropical infectious disease

Paul D Mark, MBBS, FACEM, Dip DHM, AFCHSE,
GAICD
Executive Director Clinical Services, Fiona
Stanley Hospital, Perth; Clinical Associate
Professor of Emergency Medicine, University of
Western Australia, Perth, Australia
Chapter 28.4 Radiation incidents

Suzanne Mason, MBBS, FRCS, FFAEM, MD
Reader in Emergency Medicine, Health Services
Research Section, School of Health and Related
Research, University of Sheffield, Sheffield, UK
*Chapter 25.1 Mental health and the law: the
Australasian and UK perspectives*

David McCoubrie, MBBS, FACEM
Consultant Emergency Physician and Clinical
Toxicologist, Royal Perth Hospital, Perth; VMO
Clinical Toxicologist, New South Wales Poison
Information Service, Children's Hospital at
Westmead, Sydney, Australia
Chapter 12.1 Acid–base disorders
Chapter 29.19 Ethanol and other 'toxic' alcohols

Biswadev Mitra, MBBS, MHSM, PhD, FACEM
Emergency Physician, Emergency and Trauma
Centre, The Alfred Hospital, Melbourne, Australia
Chapter 3.11 Burns
Chapter 3.12 Massive transfusion
Chapter 9.6 Hepatitis
Chapter 13.5 Blood and blood products
Chapter 25.4 Privacy and confidentiality

Mark Monaghan, MBBS, FACEM
Emergency Physician and Clinical Toxocologist,
Fremantle Hospital, Perth, Australia
*Chapter 20.6 Pharmacological management of
the aroused patient*
Chapter 29.5 Lithium

Vanessa Morgan, MBBS, FACD
Dermatology Department, The Royal Melbourne Hospital, Melbourne, Australia
Chapter 15.1 Emergency dermatology

Mark Morphett, MBBS, FACEM
Emergency Physician, Flinders Medical Centre, Adelaide, Australia
Chapter 8.2 Stroke and transient ischaemic attacks

Alfredo Mori, MBBS, CertPGHE DipEBHC (Oxon), FACEM
Staff Specialist, The Alfred Hospital Melbourne; Clinical Senior Lecturer, Monash University Medical School, Australia
Chapter 3.7 Limb trauma

David Mountain, BBS, FACEM
Associate Professor, Academic Emergency Medicine Department, University of Western Australia, Perth; Associate Professor, Emergency Department, Sir Charles Gairdner Hospital, Perth, Australia
Chapter 5.5 Pulmonary embolism
Chapter 28.5 Drowning

Lindsay Murray, MBBS, FACEM
Emergency Physician, Lismore Base Hospital, New South Wales, Australia
Chapter 13.1 Anaemia
Chapter 29.1 Approach to the poisoned patient
Chapter 29.10 Colchicine
Chapter 29.11 Theophylline

Sandra L Neate, MBBS, DipRACOG, DA, FACEM, Grad Cert Forensic Med
Emergency Physician and Medical Donation Specialist, Emergency Department, St Vincent's Hospital, Melbourne, Australia
Chapter 21.3 Family violence
Chapter 21.5 The challenging patient
Chapter 21.6 End of life decision making and palliative care
Chapter 21.7 Organ and tissue donation

Marcus Eng Hock Ong, MBBS, MPH
Senior Consultant, Department of Emergency Medicine, Singapore General Hospital; Associate Professor, Office of Clinical Sciences, Duke-National University of Singapore Graduate Medical School, Singapore
Chapter 5.4 Arrhythmias

Ken Ooi, MBBS, FACEM
Director of Emergency Medicine, The Queen Elizabeth Hospital, Woodville South, South Australia
Chapter 6.1 Upper respiratory tract

Shirley Ooi, MBBS, FRCSE (A&E), FAMS(EmergMed)
Clinical Associate Professor, Chief/Senior Consultant, Emergency Medicine Department, National University Hospital, Singapore
Chapter 7.7 Peptic ulcer disease and gastritis

Gerard O'Reilly, MBBS, FACEM, MPH, MBiostat
Emergency Physician, Emergency and Trauma Centre, The Alfred Hospital, Melbourne, Australia; Adjunct Senior Research Fellow, Department of Epidemiology and Preventive Medicine, Monash University, Victoria, Australia
Chapter 3.1 Trauma overview
Chapter 3.2 Neurotrauma
Chapter 3.11 Burns

Debbie Paltridge, BAppSc(Phty), MHSc (Ed)
Education Consultant, Health Education Innovative Solutions, Carindale, Queensland, Australia
Chapter 24.3 Principles of medical education

Robyn Parker, MBBS, FACEM
Emergency Physician, Maroondah Hospital, East Ringwood, Victoria; Emergency Physician, Health and Medical Investigation Team, Department of Justice, Melbourne, Australia
Chapter 25.2 The coroner: the Australasian and UK perspectives

John Pasco, MBBS, FACEM
Emergency Department, Werribee Mercy Hospital, Victoria, Australia
Chapter 12.2 Electrolyte disturbances

Sameer Pathan, MBBS, CABMS (EM), MCEM
Emergency Physician, Emergency Medicine Department, Hamad Medical Corporation, Doha, Qatar
Chapter 1.1 Basic Life Support

Peter Pereira, MBBS, FACEM
Emergency Physician, The Cairns Hospital, Queensland Tropical Health Alliance, Queensland; Clinical Associate Professor, School of Medicine and Dentistry, James Cook Unviersity, Queensland, Australia
Chapter 30.4 Marine injury, envenomation and poisoning

Georgina A Phillips, MBBS, FACEM
Emergency Physician, St Vincent's Hospital, Melbourne; Senior Lecturer and Honorary Fellow, Department of Medicine, The University of Melbourne, Australia
Chapter 21.5 The challenging patient
Chapter 25.1 Mental health and the law: the Australasian and UK perspectives

Grant Phillips, MNSc
Senior Clinician, St Vincent's Hospital Melbourne, Crisis Assessment and Treatment Team, Victoria, Australia
Chapter 20.3 Deliberate self-harm/suicide

David Pilcher, MBBS, MRCP, FRACP, FCICM
Intensivist, The Alfred Hospital, Melbourne; Director, ANZICS Adult Patient Database; Medical Advisor to Donate Life, Victoria, Australia
Chapter 21.7 Organ and tissue donation

Stephen Priestley, MBBS, FACEM
Director of Emergency Medicine, Sunshine Coast Hospital and Health Service, Queensland, Australia
Chapter 19.1 Emergency delivery and complications

Mark Putland, MBBS, Grad Cert Emerg Hth (Aeromed), FACEM
Co-Director Emergency Medicine Training, Emergency Medicine, Bendigo Health Care Group, Bendigo, Victoria; Emergency Physician, Epworth Hospital, Richmond, Victoria, Australia
Chapter 6.3 Community-acquired pneumonia

Timothy H Rainer, MD
Professor, Chinese University of Hong Kong; Director, Accident and Emergency Medicine Academic Unit; Consultant, Department of Accident and Emergency Medicine, Trauma and Emergency Centre, Prince of Wales Hospital, Shatin, Hong Kong
Chapter 4.2 Fractures of the humerus
Chapter 4.3 Dislocations of the elbow
Chapter 6.4 Influenza and emerging respiratory infections

Shammi Ramlakhan, MBBS, MBA, FRCSEd, FCEM
Consultant Emergency Physician, Sheffield Teaching Hospitals, Sheffield; Honorary Senior Lecturer, University of Sheffield, Sheffield; Honorary Consultant Paediatric Emergency Physician, Sheffield Children's Hospital, Sheffield, UK
Chapter 6.7 Pleural effusion

Kevin Reynard, MBChB, FRCP, FCEM
Consultant, Emergency Medicine, St James's University Hospital, Leeds, UK
Chapter 27.6 Specialist training and recognition in emergency medicine in the UK

Drew Richardson, MBBS(Hons), FACEM
Emergency Department, The Canberra Hospital, Garran, ACT, Australia
Chapter 26.4 Triage
Chapter 26.7 Overcrowding

James Rippey, MBBS, DDU, DCH, FACEM
Emergency Physician, Sir Charles Gairdner Hospital, Perth, Western Australia, Australia
Chapter 23.1 Emergency department ultrasound
Chapter 23.3 Magnetic resonance imaging in emergency medicine

Darren M Roberts, PhD, FRACP
School of Medicine, University of Queensland, Queensland, Australia
Chapter 29.18 Pesticides

Karen Robins-Browne, MBBS, FACEM
Emergency Physician, Austin Hospital, Melbourne, Australia
Chapter 6.3 Community-acquired pneumonia

Eileen M Rogan, MBBS, FACEM, PhD
Emergency Department Director, Canterbury Hospital; Staff Specialist, Emergency Department, Royal Prince Alfred Hospital, Sydney, New South Wales, Australia
Chapter 8.7 Weakness

Ian Rogers
Professor of Emergency Medicine, St John of God Murdoch Hospital, Murdoch, Western Australia; Professor of Emergency Medicine, Faculty of Medicine, University of Notre Dame, Fremantle, Australia
Chapter 28.1 Heat-related illness
Chapter 28.2 Hypothermia
Chapter 28.7 Altitude illness

Pamela Rosengarten, MBBS, FACEM
Associate Professor Emergency Medicine & Clinical Director Emergency Services, Peninsula Health, Victoria, Australia
Chapter 8.3 Subarachnoid haemorrhage

John M Ryan, FCEM, FRCSEd(A&E), FFSEM, Dip Sports Med
Professor, Emergency Department, St Vincent's University Hospital, Dublin, Ireland
Chapter 7.12 Acute liver failure

Eillyne Seow, MBBS, DIMC, FRCSEd, FRCP
Associate Professor, Emergency Department, Tan Tock Seng Hospital, Singapore
Chapter 7.2 Approach to abdominal pain
Chapter 7.9 Pancreatitis

Jamie Seymour, BSc, PhD
Associate Professor, Queensland Tropical Health Alliance, James Cook University, Queensland, Australia
Chapter 30.4 Marine injury, envenomation and poisoning

Andrew Singer, MBBS, FACEM, FIFEM
Principal Medical Adviser, Acute Care and Health Workforce Divisions, Australian Government Department of Health, Canberra; Adjunct Associate Professor, Medical School, Australian National University, Acton; Senior Specialist in Emergency and Retrieval Medicine, The Canberra Hospital, Garran, Australia
Chapter 9.2 Meningitis

David R Smart, BMedSci, MBBS(Hons), MD(UTas), FACEM, FIFEM, FACTM, FAICD, DipDHM, Cert DHM(ANZCA)
Medical Co-Director, Department of Diving and Hyperbaric Medicine, Royal Hobart Hospital, Hobart, Tasmania; Clinical Associate Professor, Faculty of Health Sciences, University of Tasmania, Hobart, Tasmania; Director, Department of Emergency Medicine, Calvary Health Care Tasmania, Lenah Valley, Tasmania, Australia
Chapter 2.2 Oxygen therapy
Chapter 28.3 Dysbarism

Jessamine Soderstrom, MBBS, FACEM, Cert Clin Toxicol
Emergency Physician, Clinical Toxicologist, Royal Perth Hospital, Perth; Clinical Senior Lecturer, University of Western Australia, Perth, Australia
Chapter 26.6 Emergency department observation wards

Swithin Song, MBBS, FRANZCR
Radiologist, Radiology Department, Royal Perth Hospital, Perth, Western Australia
Chapter 23.2 CT scanning in emergency medicine

David Spain, MBBS, FRACGP, FACEM
Clinical Medical Director, Emergency Department, Gold Coast University Hospital, Southport, Queensland, Australia
Chapter 20.2 Distinguishing medical from psychiatric causes of mental disorder presentations

Peter Sprivulis, MBBS, PhD
Professor Emergency Medicine, Fremantle Hospital, Fremantle, Australia
Chapter 27.8 Patient safety

Helen E Stergiou, BSc, MSC, MBBS, FACEM
Deputy Director, Emergency Services, Alfred Health, Melbourne, Australia
Chapter 9.6 Hepatitis

Jeremy Stevens, MBBS, FACEM
Consultant Emergency Physician, Emergency and Trauma Centre, The Alfred Hospital, Melbourne, Australia
Chapter 3.6 Chest trauma

Alan C Street, MBBS, FRACP
Deputy Director, Victorian Infectious Diseases Service, The Royal Melbourne Hospital, Melbourne, Australia
Chapter 9.7 HIV/AIDS

Varadarajulu Suresh, MBBS, FRCSEd, FCEM
Senior Consultant, Emergency Medicine, Hamad Medical Corporation, Doha, Qatar
Chapter 4.13 Osteomyelitis
Chapter 9.3 Septic arthritis

Gim Tan, MBBS, FACEM
Senior Emergency Physician, Emergency and Trauma Centre, The Alfred Hospital, Melbourne, Australia; Adjunct Lecturer, Monash University, Melbourne, Australia
Chapter 3.10 Wound care and repair

James Taylor, MBBS, FACEM
Emergency Department, Sandringham and District Memorial Hospital, Sandringham, Victoria, Australia
Chapter 19.6 Pelvic pain

David M Taylor, MBBS, MD, MPH, DRCOG, FACEM
Director of Emergency and General Medicine Research, Austin Health, Melbourne, Australia
Chapter 24.1 Research methodology

Jane Terris, MBChB, MSc, FRCP, FACEM, FCEM
Consultant Emergency Physician, Emergency Medicine, Guy's and St Thomas' NHS Foundation Trust, London, UK
Chapter 9.8 Sexually transmitted infections
Chapter 25.2 The coroner: the Australasian and UK perspectives
Chapter 25.3 Consent and competence – the Australasian and UK perspectives

Graeme Thomson, MBBS, MBA, FACEM
Director of Emergency Medicine, Angliss Hospital, Melbourne, Australia
Chapter 7.1 Dysphagia

Gino Toncich, MBBS, FACEM, MBA, Dip Anaes
Emergency Physician, The Royal Melbourne Hospital, Melbourne, Australia; Honorary Senior Lecturer, Medicine, Melbourne University, Melbourne, Australia
Chapter 10.2 The acute scrotum

Greg Treston, BMedSci, MBBS, DTMH, DIMCRCS, FACEM, FACRRM
Director of Emergency Medicine, Executive Director of Medical Stream, Bundaberg Hospital, Bundaberg Queensland, Australia
Chapter 22.3 Procedural sedation and analgesia

Steven Troupakis, MBBS, DipRACOG, FACEM
Emergency Physician, Monash Medical Centre, Monash Health, Victoria, Australia
Chapter 3.9 Trauma in pregnancy

Stacy Turner, MBChB, BSc Hons, MSc, FCEM, FACEM
Emergency Medicine Consultant, Emergency Department, Western Hospital, Footscray, Victoria, Australia
Chapter 7.8 Biliary tract disease

Hilary Tyler, MBChB, FACEM
Emergency Physician, Alice Springs Hospital, Australia
Chapter 26.9 Public health and emergency medicine

Anthony Tzannes, MBBS, FACEM
Emergency Physician, Western and Sunshine Hospitals, Western Health, Melbourne, Australia
Chapter 14.4 Musculoskeletal and soft-tissue emergencies

George Varigos, MBBS, PhD, FACD
Dermatology Department, The Royal Melbourne Hospital, Melbourne, Australia
Chapter 15.1 Emergency dermatology

John Vinen, MBBS, MHP, FACEM, FIFEM, FACBS
Director of Medical Services, Calvary Hospital, Canberra, Australian Capital Territory, Australia
Chapter 9.9 Antibiotics in the emergency department

Ioana Vlad, MD, FACEM
Emergency Consultant and Clinical Toxicology Fellow, Sir Charles Gairdner Hospital, Perth, Australia
Chapter 21.4 Alcohol-related illness

Abel Wakai, MD, FRCSI, FCEM
Consultant in Emergency Medicine, Beaumont Hospital, Dublin; Director, Emergency Care Research Unit (ECRU), Division of Population Health Sciences, Royal College of Surgeons in Ireland (RCSI), Dublin, Ireland
Chapter 7.12 Acute liver failure

Andrew Walby, MBBS, DipRACOG, FACEM
Staff Specialist, Department of Emergency Medicine, Western Hospital, Footscray, Victoria, Australia
Chapter 7.8 Biliary tract disease

Mark J Walland, MBBS, FRANZCO, FRACS
Royal Victorian Eye and Ear Hospital, Melbourne, Australia
Chapter 16.1 Ocular emergencies

Richard Waller, MBBS, BMedSc, FACEM
Consultant Emergency Physician, The Royal Melbourne Hospital, Melbourne; Consultant Emergency Physician, Cabrini Health, Malvern,Victoria, Australia
Chapter 3.10 Wound care and repair

Lee Wallis, MBChB, MD, FRCS, FCEM, FCEM, FIFEM
Professor of Emergency Medicine, University of Cape Town, Cape Town, South Africa
Chapter 3.2 Neurotrauma

Bryan G Walpole, MBBS, FRCS, FACEM, DTM&H
Consultant, Diving and Hyperbaric Medicine Unit, Royal Hobart Hospital, Hobart, Tasmania
Chapter 21.1 Death and dying

Carolyn Walsh, BPsych(Hons)
Coroners Court of Victoria, Melbourne, Australia
Chapter 21.3 Family violence

Ben White, LLB Hons, DPhil
Professor and Director, Health Law Research Centre, Queensland University of Technology, Queensland, Australia
Chapter 21.6 End of life decision making and palliative care

Julian White, MBBS, MD
Professor and Department Head, Toxinology Department, Women's and Children's Hospital, Adelaide, Australia
Chapter 30.2 Exotic snakebite

Garry J Wilkes, MBBS, FACEM
Director of Emergency Medicine, Calvary Hospital, Canberra, Australia; Assistant Professor, School of Nursing, Midwifery and Post Graduate Medicine, Edith Cowan University, Perth, Australia
Chapter 3.5 Abdominal trauma
Chapter 8.5 Seizures

Kim Yates, MBChB, MMedSci, PGCertClinEd, FACEM
Emergency Medicine Specialist, North Shore and Waitakere Hospitals, Auckland, New Zealand
Chapter 7.11 Inflammatory bowel disease
Chapter 7.3 Bowel obstruction

Anusch Yazdani, MBBS, FRANZCOG, CREI
Associate Professor, University of Queensland, Queensland; QFG Research Foundation, Brisbane, Australia
Chapter 19.6 Pelvic pain

Allen Yuen, MBBS(Hons), FRACEP, FACEM
Associate Professor, Monash University, Director of Emergency Medicine, Epworth Hospital, Richmond, Victoria, Senior Examiner ACEM, Australia
Chapter 25.4 Privacy and confidentiality
Chapter 27.5 Accreditation, specialist training and recognition in Australasia

Salomon Zalstein, MBBS, BMedSc, FACEM
Emergency Physician, Epworth Health, Richmond, Victoria, Australia
Chapter 9.4 Urinary tract infection

International Advisory Board

Joseph Lex MD
Associate Professor, Emergency Medicine,
Temple University, Philadelphia, USA

Suzanne Mason MBBS, FRCS, FFAEM, MD
Reader in Emergency Medicine, Health Services
Research Section, School of Health and Related
Research, University of Sheffield, Sheffield, UK

Colin A Graham MBChB, MPH, MD, FRCPEd,
FRCS(Ed), FRCS(Glasg), FIMCRCS(Ed), FCCP, FCEM,
FHKCEM, FHKAM(Emergency Medicine)
Professor of Emergency Medicine, Chinese
University of Hong Kong; Honorary Consultant in
Emergency Medicine, Prince of Wales Hospital,

Shatin, Hong Kong; Editor-in-Chief, European
Journal of Emergency Medicine, London, UK

Lee Wallis MBChB, MD, FRCS, FCEM, FCEM, FIFEM
Professor of Emergency Medicine, University of
Cape Town, Cape Town, South Africa

Silvio Aguilera MD, MBA
Medical Director, Vittal Socorro Medico Privado,
Buenos Aires; Ex-President of Argentine
Emergency Society, Argentina

Juliusz Jakubaszko MD PhD
Professor, Chair of Emergency Medicine at
Wroclaw University of Medicine, Wroclaw, Poland

Introduction

The specialty of emergency medicine has become a central pillar in the delivery of acute medical services in advanced economies across the globe. Although the systems of emergency care vary in maturity in different countries, there is consensus that having skilled and dedicated staff at the 'front door' of the hospital significantly improves outcomes and improves efficiency in the system.

Definition

Emergency medicine is defined by the International Federation for Emergency Medicine (IFEM) as 'a field of practice based on the knowledge and skills required for the prevention, diagnosis and management of acute and urgent aspects of illness and injury affecting patients of all age groups with a full spectrum of episodic undifferentiated physical and behavioural disorders; it further encompasses an understanding of the development of pre-hospital and in-hospital emergency medical systems and the skills necessary for this development'.

This definition is deliberately broad and encompasses both the pre-hospital and in-hospital domains of practice. It is important to note that, in many countries, elements of emergency medicine are practised under other specialties, such as anaesthesia, general practice and internal medicine. There is a strong belief among emergency physicians that, although there will always be a cross over between different specialty training, the emergency medical system will only be optimized by having a strong cadre of physicians trained specifically to provide emergency care available 24 hours every day.

The Franco-German model of emergency care has traditionally involved doctors in the pre-hospital sphere initiating resuscitation and assessment and then transporting the patient directly to inpatient services (without a formal emergency department). This model of care is becoming more difficult to sustain as inpatient services become more specialized and a greater emphasis is placed on early diagnosis, treatment and discharge. Many patients with potentially complex presentations can be fully 'packaged' within hours of arrival and discharged home. The idea of a consultant/professorial ward round the following day is difficult to justify. Triage from the roadside to an inpatient bed is predicated on accurate pre-hospital diagnosis. When patients are placed on the wrong pathway, there are dangers for the patient and inefficiencies in the system.

The development of emergency medicine

In many ways, emergency medicine is the foundation of modern medicine. Going back to ancient times, patients were forced to seek the help of a physician for emergencies, such as wound management, and painful conditions, such as renal colic. Approaches to some of these conditions were quite sophisticated, even in ancient Egyptian and Chinese societies. There was, however, little attention to systems of care and final outcomes were literally in the hands of the gods.

War – although a terrible thing – can have some positive influences. From Napoleonic times, it became evident that casualties could be better managed by triaging patients – identifying those most likely to live and attending to life-threatening injuries early. In the last century, the First and Second World Wars saw huge improvements in the organization of the emergency response to injured soldiers. However, it was not until the Vietnam/American war that we saw a huge change in the way medical services responded to war casualties. With helicopter transport and well-organized paramedics, scene times were reduced to minutes and times to definitive surgery were shortened. Surgeons returning from duty on the war front realized that civilian practice in major urban centres was lagging behind services offered on the front line and set about improving response to civilian trauma.

At the same time, major improvements in medical practice meant that access to technology and skills, delivered quickly, could save lives. Examples included cardiac arrest, trauma, and sepsis. Prior to the 1950s, there were few time-dependent treatments that actually changed the final outcome for most patients.

A further influence on the development of medical systems was the transfer of industrial processes from the factory to the hospital. The lessons learnt in industry showed that if processes could be standardized with clear pathways and reduced variation, quality could be improved and costs reduced. The idea of the friendly doctor who knew his/her patients and everything that happened to them became a thing of the past. Hospitals changed from a 'cottage industry' to a 'factory' model. Emergency Medicine, when it is performed well, ensures that patients are received, assessed and treated in a standardized fashion, 24 hours per day, 7 days per week. The necessity for emergency specialists to manage this system is clear. Putting patients on the wrong 'conveyor belt' of management because of poorly trained staff in the initial assessment period can have a devastating impact on outcome and lead to major inefficiencies in the hospital.

A final influence on the development of emergency medicine is the problem of worsening access to emergency care across the Western world. It is clear that demand for emergency care has risen at the same time that hospital bed numbers have been reduced. Governments have tried to make the best use of limited bedstock by reducing 'inappropriate' admissions and reducing length of stay. In good emergency medical systems, only those patients who are unable to be managed as outpatients will be admitted. In addition, patients will receive the right treatment from skilled practitioners at the earliest possible time. Realization of the importance of skilled practitioners to direct emergency patient management around the clock has led to a massive global investment in emergency medicine over the last 20 years.

Scope of practice

The fact that emergency physicians have general training which can act as a foundation for many subspecialties has led to a large variation in practice around the world – according to local needs and skills. There are core diagnostic and resuscitation skills that should be common to all emergency doctors. However, depending on practice location some physicians may become more expert in specific skills because of need. For example, in many underdeveloped countries, expertise in obstetrics is essential, including the ability to perform a caesarian section. Drugs and alcohol will be very important in some inner city emergency departments, whereas geriatrics may be more important in other locations. The basic skills of an emergency physician remain the same; identifying life/limb-threatening issues immediately, then prioritizing, diagnosing and treating other conditions before discharging home or admitting to an inpatient team. Finally, an emergency physician must coordinate the clinical team and the system to ensure optimal outcomes for the patient.

Emergency medicine now has a large number of subspecialties including toxicology, paediatrics, trauma, critical care, pre-hospital/disaster medicine, sports medicine, hyperbaric medicine, academic emergency medicine and many more. There are now 1–2 year fellowships available in most of these disciplines. It is important, however, that every emergency physician has a basic grounding in these subspecialties so that when confronted with the unexpected, they feel comfortable managing the situation. Having subspecialist skills is important in large departments with many specialists, so that there are expert resource people to develop the clinical service as a whole.

The future

Emergency medicine is a specialty that has developed as a result of the way modern medical treatments must be delivered. This is not static and is likely to change even more dramatically into the future. It is certain that the work pattern of an emergency specialist will be very different in 20 years time. Changes to diagnostics, therapeutic modalities, patient demographics and the work pattern of our medical colleagues will all impact on what emergency medicine practice entails. Patient expectations regarding service delivery are also changing.

There are potential threats to the quality of emergency medical care delivered, such as 'The 4-Hour rule' to push patients out of the emergency department within 4 hours (whether this is best for the patient or not). There are potential threats from other specialties, such as internal medicine physicians, wanting to undertake 'acute medicine' and replace emergency physicians. Overcrowding has made life difficult to practice good care in many emergency departments and government changes to funding arrangements have served to deny poor people access to emergency care. These potential threats and others may also represent further opportunities to streamline care and improve interaction with colleagues in acute management and demand advocacy on the part of emergency physicians. Despite these threats, there is an underlying strength in our specialty – the ability to provide the best care to undifferentiated emergency patients 24 hours per day, 7 days per week. If we focus on our core business, the specialty will continue to grow and remain a central pillar of the overall medical system.

Peter Cameron
George Jelinek
Anne-Maree Kelly
Anthony Brown
Mark Little

RESUSCITATION

Edited by *Anthony Brown*

1.1 Basic Life Support

Stephen A Bernard • Sameer Pathan

ESSENTIALS

1 A patient with sudden out-of-hospital cardiac arrest requires activation of the 'Chain of Survival', which includes an immediate call to emergency medical services and the initiation of cardiopulmonary resuscitation, with emphasis on chest compressions.

2 External chest compressions alone are equally as effective as chest compressions plus expired air ventilation for a patient in cardiac arrest of primary cardiac cause.

3 Early defibrillation should be regarded as part of Basic Life Support training as it is essential in ventricular fibrillation.

4 Early defibrillation can be provided using co-responders to ambulance services, such as firefighters.

5 Early defibrillation may also be readily delivered by untrained or minimally trained lay rescuers in public areas (known as public access defibrillation).

Introduction

Basic Life Support (BLS) aims to maintain respirations and circulation in the cardiac arrest victim. BLS involves a major focus on cardiopulmonary resuscitation (CPR) with minimal use of ancillary equipment. It includes chest compressions with or without rescue breathing and defibrillation with a manual or semi-automated external defibrillator (SAED). BLS can be successfully performed immediately by any rescuer with little or no training and, in the out-of-hospital cardiac arrest (OHCA), BLS has proven value in the survival of neurologically intact victims [1–3].

This chapter outlines an approach to BLS that can be delivered by any rescuer, while awaiting the arrival of emergency medical services (EMS) or medical expertise able to provide Advanced Life Support (ALS) (see Chapter 1.2).

Chain of Survival

The series of linked actions for a victim of sudden cardiac arrest is known as the 'Chain of Survival' [4]. The first steps are early recognition of those at risk of or in active cardiac arrest and an immediate call to activate help from the emergency medical services. This is followed by early commencement of CPR with an emphasis on chest compressions and rapid defibrillation, which significantly improves the chances of survival from ventricular fibrillation (VF) in OHCA [1–3]. Cardiopulmonary resuscitation plus defibrillation within 3–5 min of collapse following VF in OHCA can produce survival rates as high as 49–75% [5–7]. Each minute of delay before defibrillation reduces the probability of survival to hospital discharge by 10–12% [2,3]. The final links in the Chain of Survival are effective Advanced Life Support and a new focus (5th link) on integrated post-resuscitation care, targeted at optimizing and preserving cardiac and cerebral function [8–10].

Development of protocols

Any guidelines for BLS must be evidence based and consistent across a wide range of providers. Many countries have established national committees to advise community groups, ambulance services and the medical profession on appropriate BLS guidelines. Table 1.1.1 shows the national associations that made up the International Liaison Committee on Resuscitation (ILCOR) in 2010. The ILCOR group meets every 5 years to review the BLS and ALS guidelines and to evaluate the scientific evidence that may lead to changes. The next scheduled update is in 2015.

Revision of the BLS guidelines, 2010

The most recent revision of the BLS guidelines occurred in 2010 and followed a comprehensive evaluation of the scientific literature for each aspect of BLS. Evidence evaluation worksheets were developed and were then considered by ILCOR (available at http://circ.ahajournals.org/content/122/16_suppl_2/S606.full.pdf). The final recommendations were published in late 2010 [11].

Australian Resuscitation Council (ARC) and New Zealand Resuscitation Council (NZRC) BLS guidelines

Subsequently, each national committee endorsed the guidelines with minor regional

Table 1.1.1 Membership of the International Liaison Committee on Resuscitation (ILCOR) 2010
American Heart Association (AHA)
European Resuscitation Council (ERC)
Heart and Stroke Foundation of Canada (HSFC)
Resuscitation Council of Southern Africa (RCSA)
Australian and New Zealand Committee on Resuscitation (ANZCOR)
InterAmerican Heart Foundation (IAHF)
Resuscitation Council of Asia (RCA)

variations to take into account local practices. The recommendations of the Australian Resuscitation Council (ARC) combined with the New Zealand Resuscitation Council (NZRC) on BLS were co-published in 2010 (available at http://www.resus.org.au/policy/guidelines/ and http://www.nzrc.org.nz/ respectively) [12].

DRSABCD approach to Basic Life Support

A flowchart for the initial evaluation and provision of BLS for the collapsed patient is shown in Figure 1.1.1. This is based on a DRSABCD approach that includes Dangers?; Responsive?; Send for help; open Airway; normal Breathing? start CPR; and attach Defibrillator. This process therefore covers the recognition that a patient has collapsed and is unresponsive, with a safe approach checking for danger and immediately sending for help to activate the emergency medical response team. This is followed by opening the airway and briefly checking for abnormal or absent breathing, with rapid commencement of chest compressions with breaths if the pulse is absent. A defibrillator is attached as soon as it is available and prompts followed if it is automatic or semiautomatic.

Change to the adult BLS in 2010

A significant change to the adult BLS in the ILCOR 2010 resuscitation guidelines was the recommendation for a CAB (Compressions, Airway, Breathing) sequence instead of an ABC (Airway, Breathing, Compressions) sequence. This was aimed at minimizing any delay to initiate chest compressions, particularly when sudden collapse is witnessed and of likely cardiac origin. Thus, rescuers of adult cardiac arrest victims should begin resuscitation with 30 compressions followed by two breaths, rather than opening the airway and delivering breaths first (that wastes valuable time) [11]. ILCOR 2010 also mentions that, for unresponsive adults and children, the airway may be opened using the head tilt–chin lift manoeuvre when assessing breathing or giving ventilations.

Regional variations

There are, however, regional variations in the interpretation and incorporation of opening the airway within the BLS algorithm. In the European Resuscitation Council (ERC) and the Australian Resuscitation Council (ARC) with the New Zealand Resuscitation Council (NZRC) algorithm, opening the airway comes before assessment of breathing followed by compression if required. This effectively preserves the ABC sequence to avoid confusion, whereas the ILCOR 2010 guidelines and the American Heart Association (AHA) Resuscitation Guidelines 2010 recommend following a CAB sequence.

The ILCOR 2010 universal BLS algorithm with ARC and NZRC considerations is discussed in the remainder of this chapter.

Check for dangers

As the patient is being approached, the rescuer should immediately consider any dangers that may be associated with the collapse of the patient. For example, the patient may have been electrocuted and there is a substantial risk of death to the rescuer if the power source is not switched off prior to patient contact.

There may also be significant danger from injury from a passing vehicle in the case of a motor vehicle collision where a patient is unconscious, as well as the potential for fire. Therefore, unless the patient is entrapped, an unconscious patient should be carefully extricated from a vehicle prior to the arrival of emergency medical services, taking care to minimize movement of the spine. The risk of injury from fire or explosion is considered to exceed the risk of moving an unconscious patient prior to immobilization of the cervical spine with a collar.

Collapse in a confined space

A patient who has collapsed in a confined space raises the possibility of poisoning with a toxic gas such as carbon monoxide. Do not enter the scene until it is declared safe by emergency services, usually the fire brigade. Likewise, the potential for hazardous agent release must be considered if multiple victims are present, such as an organophosphate causing multiple collapses and cardiac arrest. In this setting, rescuers must not enter the area and should await the arrival of EMS with a specialist Hazmat team to declare the area safe.

Check for response and send for help

The patient who has collapsed is rapidly assessed to determine whether there is unconsciousness and absence of normal breathing, indicating possible cardiorespiratory arrest. This is assessed by a gentle 'shake and shout' and observation of the patient's response, rather than looking specifically for signs of life (that was deemed potentially confusing). Unresponsive patients should then be assessed for absent or inadequate breathing.

Lay rescuers should suspect cardiac arrest if the patient is unresponsive to 'shake and shout' and immediately telephone the EMS ('call first'). Lay rescuers should then follow the advice given by a dispatcher to provide BLS care. A trained rescuer or healthcare providers may check for unresponsiveness and abnormal breathing at the same time and then activate the EMS or cardiac arrest team.

Alternatively, healthcare rescuers may commence resuscitation focusing on the airway for approximately 2 minutes before calling the EMS ('CPR first'), when the collapse is due to suspected airway obstruction (choking) or inadequate ventilation (drowning, hanging, etc.).

Assessment of airway, breathing and circulation

Make an assessment of breathing if a patient has collapsed and is apparently unconscious [12]. Place the patient supine if face down. A trained lay rescuer or healthcare rescuer may open the airway using the head tilt–chin lift manoeuvre when assessing breathing or giving ventilations, taking care not to move the neck in a suspected trauma case.

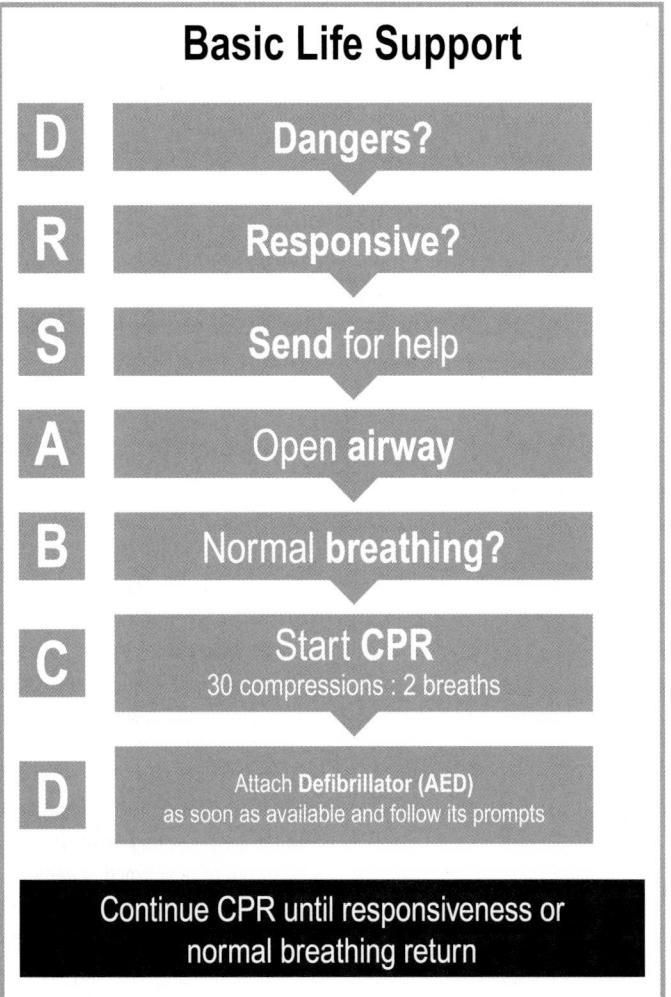

Basic Life Support

D Dangers?

R Responsive?

S Send for help

A Open airway

B Normal breathing?

C Start CPR
30 compressions : 2 breaths

D Attach Defibrillator (AED)
as soon as available and follow its prompts

Continue CPR until responsiveness or normal breathing return

Fig. 1.1.1 Australian Resuscitation Council and New Zealand Resuscitation Council Basic Life Support (BLS) flowchart. *(Reproduced with permission from Emergency Medicine Australasia 2011; 23:259–60.)*

Adequate respiration is assessed by visually inspecting the movement of the chest wall rise and listening for upper airway sounds. Occasional deep (agonal gasps) respirations may continue for a few minutes after the initial collapse in cases of cardiac arrest. These respirations are not considered to represent normal breathing.

Cardiopulmonary resuscitation

Cardiopulmonary resuscitation (CPR) is required if the patient is found to have inadequate or absent breathing on initial assessment. If the initial assessment of an unconscious patient reveals adequate respiration, turn the victim on his/her side and maintain in the semi-prone recovery position. Make constant checks to ensure continued respiration while awaiting the arrival of the EMS.

Current recommendations for the untrained lay rescuer is that he or she should not attempt to palpate for a pulse, as a pulse check is inaccurate in this setting [11]. A healthcare provider should take no more than 10 seconds to check for a pulse. If the rescuer does not definitely feel a pulse within 10 seconds, chest compressions should be started immediately.

The prior ABC sequence of BLS meant that chest compressions were often delayed while the rescuer opened the airway, positioned the patient, retrieved a barrier device or gave mouth-to-mouth expired air resuscitation (EAR) breaths as two initial 'rescue breaths'. These are difficult and challenging to an untrained lay rescuer and result in significant delay in starting chest compressions, or worse still, not attempting CPR at all. Therefore, in the CAB sequence of BLS, the assessment is limited

to checking for response and breathing and management starts with delivering 30 chest compressions.

Management

Chest compressions

All lay rescuers (trained or untrained) and healthcare rescuers should begin CPR if the victim is unresponsive and not breathing (ignoring occasional agonal gasps). Place the patient supine on a firm surface, such as a backboard, hard mattress or even the floor, to optimize the effectiveness of chest compressions. The emphasis is on delivering high-quality chest compressions: rescuers should push hard to a depth of at least 5 cm (or 2 inches) at a rate of at least 100 compressions per minute, allowing full chest recoil and minimizing interruptions in chest compressions [11]. Hence the maxim: '*push hard, push fast, allow complete recoil and minimize interruptions*'.

'Cardiac pump' or a 'thoracic pump' mechanism

There is still ongoing debate as to whether external chest compressions generate blood flow via a 'cardiac pump' mechanism or a 'thoracic pump' mechanism. Whatever the predominant mechanism of blood flow, owing to the relative rigidity of the chest wall, chest compressions result in around 20% of normal cardiac output in the adult.

Chest compressions with ventilation

Rescuers trained to provide ventilation should give two rescue breaths after each 30 compressions, for a compression–ventilation ratio of 30:2.

Chest compression only CPR

In untrained rescuers, 'compression-only' CPR is recommended where rescuers are unable or unwilling to perform mouth-to-mouth breaths ('standard' CPR). This 'compression-only' CPR technique is also recommended when EMS dispatchers are providing telephone advice to the untrained rescuer.

Healthcare professionals as well as lay rescuers are often uncomfortable doing mouth-to-mouth ventilations with an unknown victim of cardiac arrest. This should not, however, prevent them from carrying out 'Hands only' or 'Chest compression only' CPR. Compression only CPR by lay rescuers still improves survival over no CPR at all. In addition, there is growing evidence to support compression only CPR being as effective as conventional CPR, particularly when sudden collapse is witnessed and of likely cardiac origin [13–18].

Passive chest recoil

In support of 'Hands only' or 'Chest compression only' CPR is that if the airway is open, passive chest recoil during the relaxation phase of the chest compressions does also provide some air exchange. However, during prolonged CPR supplementary oxygen with assisted ventilation will be necessary. The precise interval during which the performance of compression only CPR is acceptable is currently unknown. Interestingly, no prospective adult cardiac arrest study has demonstrated that lay rescuer conventional CPR provides a better outcome than compression only CPR prior to EMS arrival.

Airway and breathing

It is reasonable to open the airway using the head tilt–chin lift manoeuvre when assessing breathing or giving ventilations in an unresponsive adult or child. Solid material in the oropharynx should be removed with a careful sweep of a finger if inspection of the airway reveals visible foreign material or vomitus in the upper airway. Take particular care not to cause pharyngeal trauma or propel material further down into the lower airway and not to be bitten!

Foreign body airway obstruction

If a victim suspected of a foreign body airway obstruction (FBAO) can cough, encourage him or her to cough and expel it out. If the cough is ineffective and the patient is conscious, give him/her up to 5 back blows with the heel of the hand and then up to 5 chest thrusts at the same compression point as in CPR, but sharper and slower. These techniques may be alternated, but make certain to call for EMS.

Airway obstruction manoeuvres A number of manoeuvres have been proposed to clear the airway if it is completely obstructed by a foreign body. In many countries, abdominal thrusts are still endorsed as the technique of choice (Heimlich manoeuvre). However, as this technique is associated with life-threatening complications, such as intra-abdominal injury, it is no longer recommended by the ARC or NZRC. Instead, the preferred technique for clearing an obstructed airway is by alternating back blows and/or chest thrusts.

Airway equipment

Simple airway equipment may be used as an adjunct to EAR, when cardiac arrest occurs in a medical facility. These include a simple face-mask, or bag/valve/mask ventilation, with or without an oropharyngeal Guedel airway. This equipment has the advantage of familiarity, decreases the risk of cross-infection, is aesthetically more appealing and may deliver additional oxygen, but does require prior training [19].

Whichever technique of assisted ventilation is used, the adequacy of the tidal volume is assessed by a rise of the victim's chest, delivered over one second. There is insufficient evidence to support or refute the use of a titrated oxygen concentration or constant 21% oxygen (room air), compared with 100% oxygen during adult cardiac arrest. Current guidelines during adult cardiac arrest therefore support the use of any of expired air ventilation, bag/valve/mask using air, or up to 100% oxygen if available [11].

Defibrillation

As soon as a defibrillator arrives, the electrode pads are attached to the victim and the device switched on. Self-adhesive defibrillation pads have practical benefits over paddles for routine monitoring and defibrillation. They are safe, effective and now preferred to standard defibrillation paddles but, in all cases, the safety of rescuers and other team members is still paramount on shock delivery.

Shock delivery

When using a semiautomatic external defibrillator, the rescuer follows the voice instruction 'stand clear' and 'press the button' when asked to deliver the shock, if this is indicated. When using a manual defibrillator, the healthcare rescuer must personally select the desired energy level and deliver a shock after recognizing a shockable rhythm (VF or pulseless VT).

Minimizing interruptions to chest compressions Irrespective of the resultant rhythm, chest compressions must be resumed immediately after each shock to minimize the 'no-flow' time; that is the time during which compressions are not delivered, for example during any rhythm analysis. Strategies to reduce the delay between stopping chest compressions and the delivery of a shock, the 'pre-shock pause', must also be kept to an absolute minimum to improve the chances of shock success [20,21]. Even a 5–10 second delay will reduce the chances of the shock being successful [22–24].

All modern defibrillators are now biphasic rather than monophasic and are more effective in terminating ventricular arrhythmias at lower energy levels [25,26]. However, there is still no randomized study that shows superiority in terms of neurological survival or survival to hospital discharge.

If a shock is not indicated, the rescuer should immediately resume CPR at a 30:2 compression–ventilation ratio and wait for EMS arrival or for the victim to start to recover.

Semiautomatic external defibrillator

The semiautomatic external defibrillator is now considered part of BLS. SAED devices are extremely accurate in diagnosing ventricular fibrillation or ventricular tachycardia. SAEDs are simple, safe and effective when used by either lay rescuers or healthcare professionals (in or out of hospital) [27]. A systematic review assessing the risk of SAED use to the rescuers reported 29 adverse events associated with defibrillation [28], but none have been published since 1997 [29].

Lay rescuer/non-medical personnel and public access SAED

SAEDs have been shown to be an effective part of the BLS programme in public places, such as airports [6], sport facilities, offices, aircraft [30,31], and in casinos [7], where minimally trained rescuers are on the scene quickly for a witnessed cardiac arrest. Lay rescuer AED programmes by police officers as first responders have achieved reported survival rates as high as 49–74% [32,33].

Recent data from national studies in Japan and the USA [34,35] showed that where an AED was available, victims were defibrillated sooner and had a better chance of survival.

Home access SAED

Finally, an SAED may be placed in the home of a patient who is at increased risk of sudden cardiac arrest, for use by a relative who might witness the event. However, a recent study that enrolled 7001 patients concluded that survival rates from sudden cardiac arrest at home were not increased, even when a defibrillator was available in the home [36].

Implantable cardioverter defibrillator and CPR

Patients at highest immediate risk of unexpected cardiac arrest may have an implantable cardioverter defibrillator (ICD) inserted which, on sensing a shockable rhythm, will discharge approximately 40 J through an internal pacing wire embedded in the right ventricle. Although most patients with an implanted defibrillator remain conscious during defibrillation, CPR should be commenced if the patient fails to respond to the ICD counter shocks and becomes unconscious. In such cases, any intermittent firing of the implanted defibrillator presents no additional risk to bystanders or medical personnel. However, wearing gloves and minimizing contact with the patient while the device is discharging is prudent.

Basic Life Support (BLS) summary

The five links in the 'Chain of Survival' BLS for a patient with sudden cardiac arrest include the following:

❶ Immediate *recognition* of the emergency and *activation* of help/the EMS system
❷ Early *CPR* with an emphasis on chest compressions
❸ Earliest use of *defibrillation*
❹ Effective *Advanced Life Support*
❺ Integrated *post-resuscitation care*.

Cardiac arrest may be presumed if the adult victim is unresponsive and not breathing normally (ignoring occasional gasps) without assessing for a pulse. A trained rescuer may open the airway using the head tilt–chin lift manoeuvre as part of the breathing assessment, but the lay/untrained rescuer should waste no time to initiate chest compressions. Rescuers should activate help/the EMS system and start chest compressions immediately. If a lone healthcare rescuer responds to suspected asphyxia or respiratory-related cardiac arrest (e.g. immersion or drowning), it is still reasonable for the healthcare rescuer to provide 2 minutes CPR before leaving the victim alone to activate EMS.

All rescuers, whether trained or not, should at least provide chest compressions to a victim of cardiac arrest, with a strong emphasis on delivering high quality chest compressions.

Trained rescuers should also provide 2 rescue breath ventilations after each 30 chest compressions at a ratio of 30:2, that is to deliver 5 cycles each 2 minutes. The compression rate should be at least 100 per minute and a depth of at least 5 cm (or 2 inches). All BLS guidelines encourage the use of an SAED by lay rescuers in cardiac arrest, maintaining chest compressions while charging the defibrillator to minimize any pre-shock pause.

Basic Life Support care should be continued until advanced help arrives, the victim starts to wake or the rescuer becomes exhausted and the situation is considered hopeless.

Controversies

- Chest compressions only versus compression plus ventilation CPR.
- The time interval before oxygenation should be added to compression only CPR.
- How external chest compressions cause blood to circulate.
- Use of room air, titrated or fixed volume oxygen delivery in cardiac arrest.
- Whether CPR should be initiated before defibrillation in an unwitnessed cardiac arrest due to VF or pulseless VT.

References

[1] Holmberg M, Holmberg S, Herlitz J. Factors modifying the effect of bystander cardiopulmonary resuscitation on survival in out-of-hospital cardiac arrest patients in Sweden. Eur Heart J 2001;22:511–9.

[2] Waalewijn RA, Tijssen JG, Koster RW. Bystander initiated actions in out-of-hospital cardiopulmonary resuscitation: results from the Amsterdam Resuscitation Study (ARREST). Resuscitation 2001;50:273–9.

[3] Valenzuela TD, Roe DJ, Cretin S, et al. Estimating effectiveness of cardiac arrest interventions: a logistic regression survival model. Circulation 1997;96:3308–13.

[4] Cummins RO, Ornato JP, Thies WH, Pepe PE. Improving survival from sudden cardiac arrest: The 'chain of survival' concept. A statement for health professionals from the advanced cardiac life-support subcommittee and the emergency cardiac care committee, AHA. Circulation 1991;83:1832–47.

[5] Stiell IG, Wells GA, Field BJ, et al. Improved out-of-hospital cardiac arrest survival through the inexpensive optimization of an existing defibrillation program: OPALS study phase II. Ontario Prehospital Advanced Life Support. J Am Med Assoc 1999;281:1175–81.

[6] Caffrey S. Feasibility of public access to defibrillation. Curr Opin Crit Care 2002;8:195–8.

[7] Valenzuela TD, Roe DJ, Nichol G, et al. Outcomes of rapid defibrillation by security officers after cardiac arrest in casinos. N Engl J Med 2000;343:1206–9.

[8] Nolan JP, Neumar RW, Adrie C, et al. Post-cardiac arrest syndrome: epidemiology, pathophysiology, treatment, and prognostication. A Scientific Statement from the International Liaison Committee on Resuscitation; the American Heart Association Emergency Cardiovascular Care Committee; the Council on Cardiovascular Surgery and Anesthesia; the Council on Cardiopulmonary,

Perioperative, and Critical Care; the Council on Clinical Cardiology; the Council on Stroke. Resuscitation 2008;79:350–79.

[9] Sunde K, Pytte M, Jacobsen D, et al. Implementation of a standardised treatment protocol for post resuscitation care after out-of-hospital cardiac arrest. Resuscitation 2007;73:29–39.

[10] Gaieski DF, Band RA, Abella BS, et al. Early goal-directed hemodynamic optimization combined with therapeutic hypothermia in comatose survivors of out-of-hospital cardiac arrest. Resuscitation 2009;80:418–24.

[11] ILCOR International Consensus on Cardiopulmonary Resuscitation and Emergency Cardiovascular Care Science with Treatment Recommendations. Resuscitation 2010; 81:e1–e332.

[12] Australian Resuscitation Council (ARC) New Zealand Resuscitation Council (NZRC). Basic life support. Emerg Med Australas 2011;23:244–60.

[13] Sayre MR, Berg RA, Cave DM, et al. Hands-only (compression-only) CPR: a call to action for bystander response to adults who experience out-of-hospital sudden cardiac arrest: a science advisory for the public from the American Heart Association Emergency Cardiovascular Care Committee. Circulation 2008;117:2162–7.

[14] Ong ME, Ng FS, Anushia P, et al. Comparison of chest compression only and standard cardiopulmonary resuscitation for out-of-hospital cardiac arrest in Singapore. Resuscitation 2008;78:119–26.

[15] Iwami T, Kawamura T, Hiraide A, et al. Effectiveness of bystander-initiated cardiac-only resuscitation for patients with out-of-hospital cardiac arrest. Circulation 2007;116:2900–7.

[16] SOS-KANTO Study Group. Cardiopulmonary resuscitation by bystanders with chest compression only (SOS-KANTO): an observational study. Lancet 2007;369:920–6.

[17] Bohm K, Rosenqvist M, Herlitz J, et al. Survival is similar after standard treatment and chest compression only in out-of-hospital bystander cardiopulmonary resuscitation. Circulation 2007;116:2908–12.

[18] Lam KK, Lau FL, et al. Effect of severe acute respiratory syndrome on bystander willingness to perform CPR – is compression-only preferred to standard CPR?. Prehosp Disaster Med 2007;22:325–9.

[19] Part 12: Education, implementation, and teams: 2010 International Consensus on Cardiopulmonary Resuscitation and Emergency Cardiovascular Care Science with Treatment Recommendations. Resuscitation 2010; 81:e288–e330.

[20] Jneid H, Fonarow GC, Cannon CP, et al. Sex differences in medical care and early death after acute myocardial infarction. Circulation 2008;118:2803–10.

[21] Khraim FM, Carey MG. Predictors of pre-hospital delay among patients with acute myocardial infarction. Patient Educ Couns 2009;75:155–61.

[22] Eftestol T, Sunde K, Steen PA. Effects of interrupting precordial compressions on the calculated probability of defibrillation success during out-of-hospital cardiac arrest. Circulation 2002;105:2270–3.

[23] Edelson DP, Abella BS, Kramer-Johansen J, et al. Effects of compression depth and pre-shock pauses predict defibrillation failure during cardiac arrest. Resuscitation 2006;71:137–45.

[24] Gundersen K, Kvaloy JT, et al. Development of the probability of return of spontaneous circulation in intervals without chest compressions during out-of-hospital cardiac arrest: an observational study. BMC Med 2009;7:6.

[25] van Alem AP, Chapman FW, et al. A prospective, randomised and blinded comparison of first shock success of monophasic and biphasic waveforms in out-of-hospital cardiac arrest. Resuscitation 2003;58:17–24.

[26] Morrison LJ, Dorian P, Long J, et al. Out-of-hospital cardiac arrest rectilinear biphasic to monophasic damped sine defibrillation waveforms with advanced life support intervention trial (ORBIT). Resuscitation 2005;66:149–57.

[27] Hallstrom AP, Ornato JP, Weisfeldt M, et al. Public-access defibrillation and survival after out-of-hospital cardiac arrest. N Engl J Med 2004;351:637–46.

[28] Hoke RS, Heinroth K, Trappe HJ, Werdan K. Is external defibrillation an electric threat for bystanders?. Resuscitation 2009;80:395–401.

[29] Dickinson CL, Hall CR, Soar J. Accidental shock to rescuer during successful defibrillation of ventricular fibrillation – a case of human involuntary automaticity. Resuscitation 2008;76:489.

[30] O'Rourke MF, Donaldson E, Geddes JS. An airline cardiac arrest program. Circulation 1997;96:2849–53.

[31] Page RL, Hamdan MH, McKenas DK. Defibrillation aboard a commercial aircraft. Circulation 1998;97:1429–30.

[32] White RD, Bunch TJ, Hankins DG. Evolution of a community-wide early defibrillation programme experience over 13 years using police/fire personnel and paramedics as responders. Resuscitation 2005;65: 279–83.

[33] Mosesso Jr VN, Davis EA, Auble TE, et al. Use of automated external defibrillators by police officers for treatment of out-of-hospital cardiac arrest. Ann Emerg Med 1998;32:200–7.

[34] Weisfeldt ML, Sitlani CM, Ornato JP, et al. Survival after application of automatic external defibrillators before arrival of the emergency medical system: evaluation in the resuscitation outcomes consortium population of 21 million. J Am Coll Cardiol 2010;55:1713–20.

[35] Kitamura T, Iwami T, Kawamura T, et al. Nationwide public-access defibrillation in Japan. N Engl J Med 2010;362: 994–1004.

[36] Bardy GH, Lee KL, Mark DB, et al. Home use of automated external defibrillators for sudden cardiac arrest. N Engl J Med 2008;358:1793–804.

1.2 Advanced Life Support

John E Maguire

ESSENTIALS

1 Follow the Advanced Life Support (ALS) resuscitation guidelines developed by, or based on, those of the International Liaison Committee on Resuscitation (ILCOR).

2 Perform cardiopulmonary resuscitation (CPR) without interruption for patients with no pulse, except when performing essential ALS interventions.

3 Defibrillate ventricular fibrillation (VF) and pulseless ventricular tachycardia (VT) until the rhythm has reverted to a stable, perfusing pattern.

4 Institute other ALS interventions as indicated.

5 Correct reversible causes of cardiac arrest – the '4 Hs and 4 Ts'.

6 Implement a comprehensive, structured post-resuscitation treatment protocol.

Introduction

A patient in cardiac arrest is the most time-critical medical crisis an emergency physician manages. The interventions of Basic Life Support (BLS) and Advanced Life Support (ALS) have the highest probability of success when applied immediately, become less effective with the passage of time and, after only a short interval without treatment, are ineffectual [1,2].

Larsen et al., in 1993, calculated the time intervals from collapse to the initiation of BLS, defibrillation and other ALS treatments and analysed their effect on survival from out-of-hospital cardiac arrest [3]. When all three interventions were immediately available, the survival rate was 67%. This figure declined by 2.3% per minute of delay to BLS, by a further 1.1% per minute of delay to defibrillation and by 2.1% per minute to other ALS interventions. Without treatment, the decline in survival rate is the sum of the three, or 5.5% per minute.

Chain of Survival

The importance of rapid treatment for cardiac arrest led to the development of a systems management approach, represented by the concept of a 'Chain of Survival', which has become the accepted model for emergency medical services (EMS) [4]. The Chain of Survival concept implies that more people survive sudden cardiac arrest when a cluster or sequence of events is activated as rapidly as possible. This Chain of Survival sequence includes:

- early access to the EMS system
- early BLS
- early defibrillation
- early advanced care.

All the links in the chain must connect, as weakness in any one reduces the probability of patient survival. ALS involves the continuation of BLS as necessary, but with the addition of manual defibrillation, advanced invasive airway and vascular access techniques and the administration of pharmacological agents.

Aetiology and incidence of cardiac arrest

The commonest cause of sudden cardiac arrest in adults is ischaemic heart disease [1,2]. Other causes include respiratory failure, drug overdose, metabolic derangements, trauma, hypovolaemia, immersion and hypothermia.

The population incidence of sudden cardiac death (within 24 hours of the onset of any symptoms) is estimated as 1.24:1000/year in the USA [5]. The incidence of cardiac arrest notified to ambulances in western metropolitan Melbourne, Australia in 1995 was approximately 0.72:1000/year [6]. Among 20 communities in developed nations worldwide a population average of 0.62:1000/year received attempted resuscitation after out-of-hospital cardiac arrest [5].

Advanced Life Support guidelines and algorithms

The most clinically relevant advance in ALS, over the last two decades, is the substantial simplification of the management of cardiac arrest by the development of widely accepted universal guidelines and algorithms that include scientifically proven therapies.

International Liaison Committee on Resuscitation (ILCOR)

The American Heart Association, in collaboration with ILCOR, convened the International Guidelines 2000 Conference on CPR and

Emergency Cardiac Care (ECC) in 2000. This was the first international assembly gathered specifically to produce international resuscitation guidelines and the International Guidelines 2000 for CPR and ECC were developed and then published [7]. These guidelines represented a consensus of expert individuals and resuscitation councils and organizations across many countries, cultures and disciplines. The underlying principle guiding decision making was that additions to existing guidelines had to pass a rigorous evidence-based review. Revisions or deletions occurred because of:

- lack of evidence to confirm effectiveness, and/or
- additional evidence to suggest harm or ineffectiveness, and/or
- evidence that superior therapies had become available [7].

The ILCOR member councils committed to holding an International Consensus Conference and releasing guidelines every 5 years to maintain and develop the level of scientific rigour and cooperation. The most recent conference was held in Dallas in February 2010 and the *Consensus on Science and Treatment Recommendations* (CoSTR) documents arising from that conference were published later that year [1].

Australasian guidelines and algorithms

Each ILCOR member body is expected to use the CoSTR documents to develop its own guidelines for local use. The Australian Resuscitation Council (ARC) and the New Zealand Resuscitation Council (NZRC) released joint Australasian guidelines in December 2010 [2]. These Australasian guidelines include an Adult Cardiorespiratory Arrest algorithm (Fig. 1.2.1) that is clear, concise and easy to memorize and adapt into poster format and is readily applied clinically. This algorithm provides the framework used throughout this chapter to discuss ALS interventions.

However, resuscitation knowledge is still incomplete and some ALS techniques currently in use are not supported by the highest levels of scientific rigour. Thus, strict adherence to any guideline should be informed by common sense. Individuals with specialist knowledge may modify practice according to the level of their expertise and the specific clinical situation or environment in which they practise.

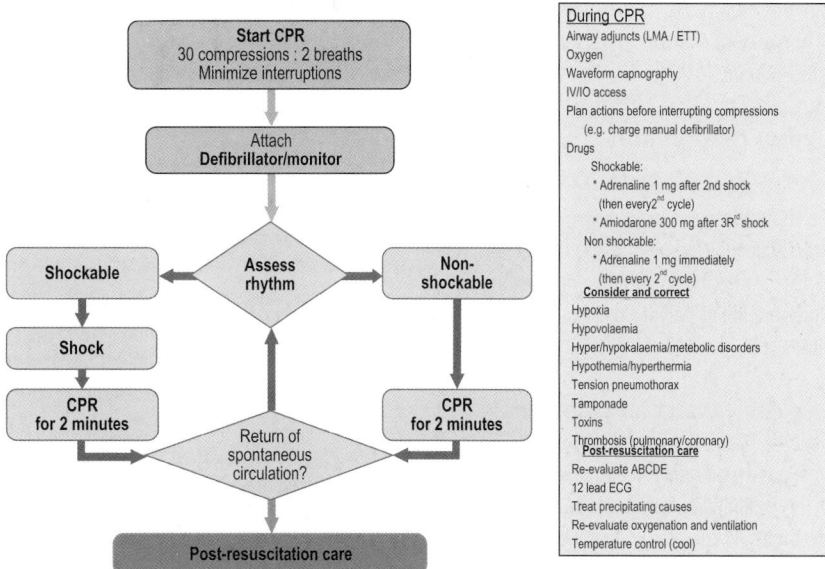

Fig. 1.2.1 Algorithm for management of adult cardiorespiratory arrest. *(Reproduced with permission of John Wiley & Sons, Inc., Emergency Medicine Australasia 2011;23:271–4.)*

Initiation of ALS

The Australasian guidelines and algorithm qualify the commencement of BLS with the statement 'if appropriate' [2]. This is because BLS is only a temporary and inefficient substitute for normal cardiorespiratory function. ALS interventions are almost always necessary to produce the return of spontaneous circulation (ROSC).

The purpose of BLS is to support the patient's cardiorespiratory status as effectively as possible until equipment – particularly a defibrillator – and drugs become available [1,2]. Electrical defibrillation is fundamental to successful treatment for VF and pulseless VT. However, the likelihood of defibrillation restoring a sustained, perfusing cardiac rhythm and of a favourable long-term outcome is greatest for as little as 90 seconds after the onset of cardiac arrest. The chances of survival to hospital discharge decline rapidly thereafter, so minimizing time to defibrillation is the priority in resuscitation from sudden cardiac arrest. There is some evidence indicating that a brief period (1.5–3 min) of CPR before defibrillation may improve survival in patients where the EMS response is greater than 4–5 minutes, but this is not strong enough to make a practice recommendation.

The point of entry into the ALS algorithm depends on the circumstances of the cardiac arrest. In situations where there are multiple rescuers, BLS should be initiated or continued while the defibrillator-monitor is being prepared. When a defibrillator-monitor is readily available it should be obtained and attached immediately and a single rescuer should do this without commencing BLS. Diagnosis must be swift and the defibrillator attached without delay when the patient is being monitored at the time of a cardiac arrest [1,2].

Attachment of the defibrillator-monitor and rhythm recognition

Automated external defibrillator

Apply the self-adhesive pads in the standard anteroapical positions for defibrillation (see below) when using an automated external defibrillator (AED). An internal microprocessor analyses the ECG signal and, if VF/VT is detected, the AED displays a warning and then either delivers a shock (automatic) or advises the operator to do so (semiautomatic) [1,2,8,9].

Manual external defibrillator

The critical decision for a rescuer, after applying the self-adhesive pads or paddles of a manual external defibrillator, is whether or not the cardiac rhythm is VF/VT [1,2]. Up to 70% of patients with an out-of-hospital cardiac arrest will be in VF/VT at the time of arrival of the EMS personnel and a defibrillator-monitor [8]. The vast majority of cardiac arrest survivors come from this group [1,2,4].

Rhythm recognition

Ventricular fibrillation
VF is a pulseless, chaotic, disorganized rhythm characterized by an undulating, irregular pattern that varies in amplitude and morphology, with a ventricular waveform of more than 150/minute [1,2].

Pulseless ventricular tachycardia
Pulseless VT is characterized by broad, bizarrely shaped ventricular complexes associated with no detectable cardiac output. The rate is more than 100/minute by definition and is usually in excess of 150 [1,2].

Asystole
Asystole is identified by the absence of any electrical cardiac activity on the monitor. Occasionally, it is incorrectly diagnosed ('apparent asystole') on the ECG monitor because:

- ECG lead may be disconnected or broken. Look for the presence of electrical artefact waves on the monitor during external chest compression, indicating that the ECG leads are connected and intact. A perfectly straight line suggests lead disconnection or breakage.
- Lead sensitivity may be inappropriate. Increase the sensitivity setting to maximum. The resulting increase in the size of electrical artefact will confirm that the sensitivity selection is functioning.
- VF has a predominant axis. Even coarse VF may cause minimal undulation in the baseline if the axis is at right angles to the selected monitor lead and thus resembles asystole. Select at least two leads in succession before asystole is diagnosed, preferably leads at right angles, such as II and aVL.

Pulseless electrical activity/electromechanical dissociation
The absence of a detectable cardiac output in the presence of a coordinated electrical rhythm is called pulseless electrical activity (PEA), also known as electromechanical dissociation (EMD) [1,2].

Defibrillation

The only proven effective treatment for VF and pulseless VT is electrical defibrillation [1,2,9]. The defibrillator must be brought immediately to the person in cardiac arrest and, if the rhythm is VF/VT, defibrillation delivered without delay.

Placement of pads or paddles
Pads or paddles are often identified as 'sternum' and 'apex', or 'anterior' and 'posterior', which is of no relevance for emergency transthoracic defibrillation. It simply allows detection by the pads/paddles of the correct orientation of certain perfusing cardiac rhythms prior to synchronized cardioversion [1,2,8–10].

Anteroapical pad or paddle position
There are two accepted positions for the defibrillation pads or paddles to optimize current delivery to the heart. The most common is the anteroapical position: one pad/paddle is placed to the right of the sternum just below the clavicle, and the other is centred lateral to the normal cardiac apex in the anterior or midaxillary line (V5–6 position).

Anteroposterior pad or paddle position
An alternative is the anteroposterior position: the anterior pad/paddle is placed over the praecordium or apex and the posterior pad/paddle is placed on the patient's back to the left or right of the spine at the level of the lower scapula, or even in the interscapular region.

Do *not* attempt defibrillation over ECG electrodes or medicated patches and avoid placing pads/paddles over significant breast tissue in females. Also the pads/paddles should be placed at least 8 cm away from the module and pulse generator, if the patient has an implanted pacemaker or a cardioverter–defibrillator, respectively. Arrange to check the function of any pacemaker or cardioverter–defibrillator as soon as practicable after successful defibrillation [1,2,8,9].

Waveform and energy of shocks
Two main types of waveform are available from cardiac defibrillators.

Biphasic waveforms
All modern defibrillators use biphasic waveforms with impedance compensation now considered the 'gold standard'. Biphasic (bidirectional) truncated transthoracic shock defibrillators are effective at lower energies and

result in fewer post-defibrillation ECG abnormalities [1,2,8–10].

Set the level at 200 J for all shocks when using a biphasic defibrillator in adults. Other energy levels may be used if the relevant clinical data for that defibrillator suggest an alternative energy level provides comparable success to the 'default' energy level of 200 J [1,2].

Monophasic sinusoidal waveform
Old defibrillators use a damped monophasic sinusoidal waveform, which is a single pulse lasting for 3–4 ms. Set the energy level at the maximum when using a monophasic defibrillator in adults, which is usually 360 J for all shocks [1,2].

Optimizing transthoracic impedance
A critical myocardial mass must be depolarized synchronously for defibrillation to be successful. This interrupts the fibrillation and allows recapture by a single pacemaker. The transthoracic impedance must be minimized to maximize the probability of success [1,2,8–10].

Reduction of transthoracic impedance
- Use pads/paddles of 10–13 cm in diameter for adults. Smaller paddles/pads allow too concentrated a discharge of energy that may cause focal myocardial damage [8,9]. Larger pads/paddles do not make good chest contact over their entire area and/or may allow current to be conducted through non-myocardial tissue [8,10].
- Use conductive pads or electrode paste/gel. This reduces impedance by 30% [8]. Take care to ensure that there is no electrical contact between the pads or paddles, either directly or through electrode paste, as this results in current arcing across the chest wall [8–10].
- Apply a pressure of 5–8 kg to the paddle when adhesive pads are not being used [1,2,8].
- Perform defibrillation when the chest is deflated, i.e. in expiration [10].

Current-based defibrillation
Conventional defibrillators are designed to deliver a specified amount of energy measured in joules. Depolarization of myocardial tissue is accomplished by the passage of electrical current through the heart; clinical studies have determined that the optimal current is 30–40 amps (A) [8,10]. The current delivered at

a fixed energy is inversely related to the transthoracic impedance, so a standard energy dose of 200 J delivers about 30 A to the average patient.

The current generated may be inadequate in patients with greater than average impedance, whereas patients with smaller transthoracic impedance may sustain myocardial damage from excessive current flow [8–10].

Some newer current-based defibrillators automatically measure transthoracic impedance and then predict and adjust the energy delivered to avoid an inappropriately high or low transmyocardial current. These devices have defibrillation success rates comparable to those of conventional defibrillators, while cumulatively delivering less energy. The reduced energy should result in less myocardial damage and may reduce post-defibrillation complications [8–10].

Automated external defibrillators (AED)

AEDs were first introduced in 1979 and have become standard equipment in EMS systems for use outside hospital, as well as in many areas within hospital.

AEDs are highly accurate, some models demonstrating 100% specificity and 90–92% sensitivity in correctly identifying coarse VF [9]. Their precision is less for fine VF and least for VT, but overall accuracy is comparable to that of an experienced cardiologist [8]. EMS systems equipped with AEDs are able to deliver the first shock up to 1 minute faster than when using a conventional defibrillator. Rates of survival to hospital discharge are equivalent to those achieved when more highly trained first responders use manual defibrillators [4].

The major advantage of AEDs over manual defibrillators is their simplicity, which reduces the time and expense of initial training and continuing education and increases the number of persons who can operate the device [4,8,9]. Members of the public have been trained to use AEDs in a variety of community settings and have demonstrated that they can retain skills for up to one year [4]. Encouraging results have been produced when AEDs have been placed with community responders, such as firefighters, police officers, casino staff, security guards at large public assemblies and public transport vehicle crews [4,8].

The Australasian College for Emergency Medicine recommends that all clinical staff in healthcare settings should have rapid access to an AED or a defibrillator with AED capability [11].

Delivering a shock

If the rhythm is assessed as shockable (VF or pulseless VT), the defibrillator should be charged while CPR continues. Then, after healthcare personnel are clear of the patient, a single shock is delivered [1,2]. Following this shock, CPR should be recommenced *immediately*, without delaying to assess or analyse either the pulse or the rhythm.

If the resuscitation team leader is uncertain whether the rhythm is shockable or non-shockable, no shock should be given.

Three stacked shocks

Previous ARC guidelines have recommended up to three stacked shocks as initial management when the arrest is witnessed and a defibrillator is immediately available. This is no longer included in the algorithm but can be considered if the delay before and between each shock will be less than 10 seconds, or during cardiac catheterization and/or early post-cardiac surgery.

The pads or paddles should remain on the chest wall and the defibrillator immediately recharged after each shock. The rhythm is checked while the defibrillator is recharging and the shock is repeated up to a total of three if VF/VT persists. Any delay over 10 seconds between shocks is unacceptable and should lead to abandonment of the stacked shocks and immediate commencement of CPR [2].

Technical problems

Whenever attempted defibrillation is not accompanied by skeletal muscle contraction, take care to ensure good contact and that the defibrillator is turned on, charged up, develops sufficient power and is not in synchronized mode [1,2,9]. The operational status of defibrillators should be checked regularly and a standby machine should be available at all times. The majority of defibrillator problems are due to operator error or faulty care and maintenance.

Complications of defibrillation

- Skin burns may occur, which are usually superficial and can be minimized by ensuring optimal contact between the defibrillator pad/paddle and the patient.
- Myocardial injury and post-defibrillation dysrhythmias may occur with cumulative high-energy shocks.
- Skeletal muscle injury or thoracic vertebral fractures are possible, albeit rare.

- Electrical injury to the healthcare provider may occur as a result of contact with the patient during defibrillation. These range from paraesthesia to deep partial-thickness burns and cardiac arrest. The defibrillator operator must ensure that all rescue personnel are clear of the patient before delivering a shock.
- Also ensure that the patient, rescuers and equipment are dry before defibrillation is ever attempted in wet conditions, such as outdoors or around a swimming pool area [1,2,8,9].

CPR 'Code Blue' process

Shockable rhythms

Immediate defibrillation is essential for VF/pulseless VT, although periods of well-performed CPR help maintain myocardial and cerebral viability and may improve the likelihood of success with subsequent shocks [1,2]. After delivering a single shock, CPR should be resumed immediately and continued for 2 minutes or until the patient becomes responsive or resumes normal breathing.

The rationale for this is that after one defibrillator shock there is typically a delay of several seconds before a diagnostic-quality ECG trace is obtained. Additionally, even when defibrillation is successful, there is temporary impairment of cardiac function from seconds to minutes, associated with a weak or impalpable pulse. Thus, waiting for a recognizable ECG rhythm or palpating for a pulse that may not be present even after successful defibrillation unnecessarily delays the recommencement of CPR. This is detrimental to the patient who does not yet have ROSC [1,2].

At the conclusion of this period of CPR, reassess the ECG rhythm and, when appropriate, the pulse. Give a single shock without delay if VF/pulseless VT persists [1,2].

Non-shockable rhythms

When PEA or asystole are present on ECG rhythm and/or pulse assessment, do not defibrillate as this may be deleterious. The prognosis for these conditions is much worse than for VF/VT and, unless there is potentially a reversible cause, the application of other ALS interventions (see below) is indicated, but seldom of value [1,2].

Cardiac pacing does *not* improve survival from asystole, either pre-hospital or in the emergency department (ED) setting [1,2].

RESUSCITATION

1

Algorithm loops

Either continuously or during each 2-minute CPR cycle of the algorithm, give attention to the following [1,2]:

- minimize interruption to CPR during ALS interventions by planning and confirming their utility before attempting them
- administer 100% oxygen when available
- attempt to secure an advanced airway/ventilation technique, but do not interrupt CPR for more than 20 seconds
- use waveform capnography to confirm airway placement and monitor the adequacy of CPR
- obtain vascular access
- administer adrenaline every second loop, i.e. every 4–5 minutes
- administer other drugs or electrolytes as indicated for individual circumstances
- correct potentially reversible conditions that may have precipitated the cardiac arrest and/or reduced the chances of successful resuscitation. These are listed in Figure 1.2.1 and are conveniently remembered under the headings of the '4Hs and 4Ts'.

'4Hs'

Hypoxaemia
Hypovolaemia
Hyper-/hypokalaemia/other metabolic disorders
Hypo-/hyperthermia.

'4Ts'

Tension pneumothorax
Tamponade
Toxins, poisons, drugs
Thrombosis: pulmonary or coronary.

Even the best-trained team will be unable to complete all of these management aspects within a single loop of the algorithm, but further opportunity will present if subsequent cycles are necessary [1,2].

Other ALS interventions

Not one ALS intervention other than defibrillation has been proven to improve patient outcome [1,2]. Some clinicians maintain that ALS has an incremental benefit compared to defibrillation alone [4], but although some data support this, it remains impossible to prove.

Advanced airway management

Endotracheal intubation is considered the technique of choice for airway management during cardiac arrest and is recommended in the Australasian guidelines [2]. However, no randomized controlled study exists that shows an improved outcome with endotracheal intubation compared to basic airway management [1,2]. Other alternative advanced airway devices studied during CPR include the laryngeal mask airway (LMA), and the oesophageal–tracheal combitube (Combitube). None is definitely superior to basic airway management during cardiac arrest in terms of consistently improved survival [1,2].

Endotracheal intubation

The optimal technique for airway management depends on the equipment available, the circumstances of the cardiac arrest and the training and experience of the resuscitation team [1,2]. A self-inflating bag/valve/mask system and/or an airway intubation device remain the mainstay of advanced airway and ventilation management in ALS.

When a sufficiently experienced person is available tracheal intubation should be performed, providing it does not interfere with or impede the CPR process. Laryngoscopy should be carried out during chest compressions with a strong recommendation that only a short interruption in chest compressions, not exceeding 20 seconds, should be permitted when the tracheal tube is inserted between the cords.

Once the tube has been inserted, correct placement must be verified by seeing the tube pass between the cords, clinical observation of chest rise/fall and auscultation and, importantly, an exhaled carbon dioxide detector, such as a waveform capnograph.

The main benefit of an advanced airway, such as endotracheal intubation, is that no interruption to chest compressions is then necessary for ventilations during CPR. Also, an endotracheal tube isolates and protects the airway, allows suction and facilitates ventilation [1,2].

Ventilation and oxygenation

Cardiac arrest and CPR cause an increase in dead space and a reduction in lung compliance that compromise gas exchange. Therefore, a fractional inspired oxygen concentration (F_1O_2) of 1.0 (100% oxygen delivery system) is essential in cardiac arrest to maximize oxygen delivery [1,2].

Minute volume

Carbon dioxide (CO_2) production and delivery to the pulmonary circulation are limited by the markedly reduced cardiac output achieved during CPR. As a consequence, a relatively low minute volume of 3.5–5.0 L is sufficient to achieve adequate CO_2 excretion and prevent hypercapnia. This situation will be altered if a CO_2-producing buffer, such as sodium bicarbonate, is administered. A small increase in minute ventilation is then required to prevent the development of a respiratory acidosis [1,2].

Ventilation rate and tidal volume

A ventilation rate of 8–10 per minute without pausing during chest compressions and a tidal volume of 400–500 mL (5–6 mL/kg) are sufficient to clear CO_2 during most cardiac arrest situations when an advanced airway is in place. This should cause a visible rise and fall of the patient's chest [1,2].

Vascular access and drug delivery

Intravenous route

The ideal route of drug delivery should combine rapid and easy vascular access with quick delivery to the central circulation. The intravenous (IV) route is preferred. This is most easily performed by inserting a cannula into a large vein in the upper limb or into the external jugular vein. Avoid lower limb veins because of their poor venous return from below the diaphragm during CPR, as well as immediate or inexperienced central line insertion which can have fatal consequences, such as pneumothorax or arterial laceration.

Drug delivery

Give a 20–30 mL IV fluid flush following any drug administered and/or raise the limb to facilitate delivery to the central circulation [1,2]. A central venous cannula delivers drugs rapidly to the central circulation and should be used when already in place. Otherwise, their insertion during CPR requires time and technical proficiency and interferes with defibrillation and the CPR process, which is unacceptable [1,2].

Intraosseous (IO) route

The intraosseous (IO) route is also acceptable for drug delivery in adults as well as children [1,2]. Suitable sites of insertion include above the medial malleolus or the proximal tibia. Practice is needed to perfect the technique, usually with a semiautomatic, hand-held drill device.

Intratracheal route

The intratracheal instillation of drugs is an alternative during CPR, especially when

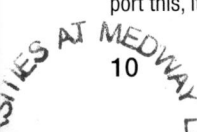

1.2 ADVANCED LIFE SUPPORT

tracheal intubation precedes venous access. Adrenaline, lignocaine and atropine may be safely administered through the endotracheal tube if there is a delay in achieving vascular access, although their efficacy is unproven (as it is for all ALS drugs by any route).

The ideal dose and dilution of drugs given by this route are unknown, but using 3–10 times the standard IV drug dose diluted in 10 mL of water or normal saline is recommended. The drug should be delivered via a catheter or quill placed beyond the tip of the endotracheal tube and followed by ventilations to aid dispersion [1,2].

Fluid therapy

Crystalloid solutions are used for the IV delivery of drugs during CPR. Glucose-containing solutions are avoided during CPR as they may contribute to post-arrest hyperglycaemia, which reduces or impairs cerebral recovery [1,2].

Drug therapy in ALS

Not one drug used in resuscitation has been shown to improve long-term survival in humans after cardiac arrest [1,2]. Despite this, a number of agents are employed based on theoretical, retrospective or anecdotal evidence of their efficacy [1,2].

Adrenaline (epinephrine)

The putative beneficial actions of adrenaline in cardiac arrest relate to its α-adrenergic effects, which result in an increased aortic blood pressure with increased perfusion of the cerebral and coronary vascular beds and reduced blood flow to splanchnic and limb vessels. Adrenaline is considered the 'standard' vasopressor in cardiac arrest [1,2].

Indications
- VF/pulseless VT when there is no ROSC after initial attempts at defibrillation. Give immediately after the second shock and then every second loop thereafter.
- Asystole and PEA as initial treatment and then during every second loop thereafter.

Adverse effects
- Tachyarrhythmias.
- Severe hypertension after ROSC.
- Tissue necrosis after extravasation.

Dosage
The standard adult dose is 1 mg IV every 4–5 minutes. Higher doses have not been shown to improve long-term outcome.

Amiodarone

Amiodarone has some benefit in refractory VF/VT in the setting of out-of-hospital cardiac arrest [1,2]. Additionally, studies show an improvement in defibrillation response when amiodarone is given in VF or haemodynamically unstable VT.

Indications
- Persistent VF/pulseless VT during the third loop following failed defibrillation and adrenaline administration.
- Prophylaxis of recurrent VF/VT.

Adverse effects
- Hypotension, bradycardia, heart block, QTc prolongation with proarrhythmic effects.

Dosage
The initial bolus of amiodarone is 300 mg or 5 mg/kg, followed by a further 150 mg if necessary.

Atropine

Atropine has no consistent benefits in cardiac arrest and is no longer recommended for routine use in asystole/PEA [1,2].

Calcium

Calcium is only indicated when the cardiac arrest is caused or exacerbated by the conditions listed below [1,2].

Indications
- Hyperkalaemia.
- Hypocalcaemia.
- Poisoning by calcium-channel blocking drugs.

Adverse effects
- Increase in myocardial and cerebral injury mediated by cell death.
- Tissue necrosis with extravasation.

Dosage
The initial dose is 5–10 mL of 10% calcium chloride, or 15–30 mL of 10% calcium gluconate (three times the volume of calcium chloride for the equivalent cation dose).

Lignocaine (lidocaine)

The antiarrhythmic properties of lignocaine in cardiac arrest are inconsistent [1,2]. Its continued use is based purely on familiarity and historical precedent. The role of lignocaine in the prophylaxis of VF/VT is also unclear and at best equivocal.

Indications
- VF/pulseless VT refractory to defibrillation and adrenaline, when amiodarone cannot be used.
- Prophylaxis of recurrent VF or VT.

Adverse effects
- Hypotension, bradycardia, heart block, asystole.
- Central nervous system (CNS) excitation with anxiety, tremor and convulsions, followed by CNS depression with coma.

Dosage
The initial dose is 1–1.5 mg/kg, with an additional bolus of 0.5 mg/kg after 5–10 minutes if indicated.

Magnesium

Magnesium is indicated when the cardiac arrest is caused or exacerbated by the conditions listed below [1,2]. There is no support for routine use at present.

Indications
- *Torsades de pointes* (polymorphic VT). This is often associated with a prolonged QT interval due to ischaemia, electrolyte disturbances and drugs.
- Hypokalaemia.
- Hypomagnesaemia.
- Digoxin toxicity.
- Cardiac arrest due to VF/VT refractory to defibrillation and adrenaline.

Adverse effects
- Muscle weakness and paralysis if excessive quantities administered.

Dosage
The initial dose is a 5 mmol bolus (1.25 g or 2.5 mL of a 49.3% solution) repeated if indicated and followed by an infusion of 20 mmol (5 g or 10 mL of a 49.3% solution) over 4 h.

Potassium

Potassium is only indicated when the cardiac arrest is caused or exacerbated by the condition listed below [1,2]. There is no support for its routine use in cardiac arrest.

Indication
- Hypokalaemia.

Adverse effects
- Hyperkalaemia with attendant dysrhythmias.
- Extravasation may cause tissue necrosis.

RESUSCITATION

11

Dosage

A bolus of 5 mmol of potassium is given IV.

Sodium bicarbonate

Sodium bicarbonate is only indicated when the cardiac arrest is caused or exacerbated by the conditions listed below [1,2]. There is no support for its routine use in cardiac arrest.

Indications

- Hyperkalaemia.
- Poisoning by tricyclic antidepressants.
- Severe metabolic acidosis.
- Protracted cardiac arrest beyond 15 minutes.

Adverse effects

- Metabolic alkalosis, hypernatraemia, hyperosmolality.
- Production of CO_2 causing paradoxical intracellular acidosis, which may in part be ameliorated by adequate ventilation in CPR.

Dosage

The initial dose is 1 mmol/kg (1 mL/kg of 8.4% sodium bicarbonate) over 2-3 minutes, then as guided by the arterial blood gases.

Vasopressin

Vasopressin is an alternative vasopressor to adrenaline. There is currently insufficient evidence to support or refute its use either alone or in combination with adrenaline in any cardiac arrest rhythm [1,2].

Consider administration for:

- Vasopressor effect as an alternative to adrenaline.

Adverse effects

- Cerebral oedema or haemorrhage after ROSC.
- Persistent vasoconstriction following ROSC, which may exacerbate myocardial ischaemia and interfere with left ventricular function.
- Procoagulant effect on platelets.

Dosage

The dose is a single IV bolus of 40 U administered once during the episode of cardiac arrest.

Haemodynamic monitoring during CPR

End-tidal CO_2 (ETCO$_2$)

Animal and clinical studies indicate that measuring ETCO$_2$ is effective and informative for determining progress during CPR, particularly if there is ROSC [1,2].

ETCO$_2$ typically falls to less than 10 mmHg at the onset of cardiac arrest. It can rise to between one-quarter and one-third of the normal level with effective CPR, and rises to normal or supranormal levels over the next minute following ROSC. The changes in ETCO$_2$ parallel similar proportionate increases in cardiac output.

Changes in ETCO$_2$

An ETCO$_2$ of less than 10 mmHg during attempted resuscitation from cardiac arrest is an indication of ineffective CPR. This may be as a result of inadequate ventilation due to airway obstruction or even oesophageal intubation; or due to a minimal cardiac output because of poor technique or underlying causes, such as hypovolaemia, pulmonary embolism or pericardial tamponade (part of the 4Hs and 4Ts). Conversely, a sharp rise in ETCO$_2$ may be the first indication of ROSC.

ETCO$_2$ may also have a prognostic value, as patients who are eventually successfully resuscitated have higher ETCO$_2$ values during CPR than those who never have ROSC. Exercise caution when interpreting ETCO$_2$ following the administration of adrenaline, as this causes a decrease in ETCO$_2$ which does not necessarily indicate a poorer prognosis, unless it simply reflects a prolonged resuscitation attempt.

Australasian guidelines advise that ETCO$_2$ monitoring is a safe and effective non-invasive indicator of cardiac output during CPR and is an early indicator of ROSC in an intubated patient.

Arterial blood gases

Arterial blood gas (ABG) monitoring during cardiac arrest is used as an indicator of oxygenation and the adequacy of ventilation, but is not an accurate measure of tissue acidosis [1,2]. An increase in $PaCO_2$ may indicate improved tissue perfusion during CPR or with ROSC, if ventilation is constant. The measurement of ABGs should never interfere with the overall performance of good CPR.

Post-resuscitation care

This is covered in detail elsewhere but is mentioned here as successful ROSC is only the first step in recovery from cardiac arrest [1,2]. The post-cardiac arrest syndrome comprising brain injury, myocardial dysfunction, a systemic ischaemia/reperfusion response and persistence of the causative pathology often complicate the post-resuscitation phase. Among patients surviving to ICU admission but subsequently dying in hospital, brain injury is the cause of death in 68% after out-of-hospital cardiac arrest and in 23% after in-hospital cardiac arrest.

Implementation of a comprehensive, structured post-resuscitation treatment protocol may improve survival in cardiac arrest victims after ROSC. The most important elements of such a protocol are summarized in the algorithm for adult ALS management (see Fig 1.2.1):

- consideration of therapeutic hypothermia (TH, whose efficacy is challenged), and/or correction of hyperpyrexia
- optimized airway management including advanced airway techniques in patients requiring continued ventilation
- maintenance of normocapnoea and an arterial oxygen saturation of 94–98%
- circulatory support to maintain tissue perfusion
- control of seizures
- control of blood glucose at $\leq$ 10 mmol/L but avoiding hypoglycaemia
- treatment of any underlying cause of the cardiac arrest, in particular coronary reperfusion for myocardial ischaemia.

When to discontinue ALS

The vast majority of patients who survive out-of-hospital cardiac arrest have ROSC before arrival at the ED. Only 33 of 5444 patients (0.6%) in 18 studies between 1981 and 1995, who were transported to an ED still in cardiac arrest after unsuccessful pre-hospital resuscitation survived to hospital discharge [12]. Twenty-four of the surviving patients arrived in the ED in VF and 11 of these had their initial cardiac arrest in the ambulance *en route* to hospital or had temporary ROSC before arrival. Thus, virtually every patient arriving in an ED still in asystole from out-of-hospital cardiac arrest will die without leaving hospital.

Ceasing CPR pre-hospital

A recommendation made in 1993 for out-of-hospital cardiac arrest in the normothermic patient was that resuscitation should cease if there was no ROSC after 25 minutes of ALS [13]. Two important exceptions to this guide are:

- cardiac arrest occurs in the presence of ambulance personnel
- patient has persistent VF.

These recommendations were applied and considered valid in a prospective study in that same year [14].

In-hospital cardiac arrest outcome

There are no early absolute predictors of futility in the resuscitation of patients with in-hospital cardiac arrest. Some variables are, however, associated with a greater or lesser chance of survival to discharge. Better outcomes are linked to ventricular tachyarrhythmias, the commencement of resuscitation within 5 minutes of collapse and ROSC within 15 minutes of CPR.

In-hospital cardiac arrest with a poor outcome

A poor outcome is linked to pre-existing conditions, such as cardiogenic shock, metastatic cancer, renal failure, sepsis and an acute cerebrovascular accident. Age alone is not an independent predictor of outcome, either in hospital or for out-of-hospital cardiac arrest [15,16].

Outcome of prolonged ALS

ALS resuscitation efforts lasting more than 30 minutes without ROSC at any stage are so uniformly unsuccessful that resuscitation should be abandoned; except in certain special circumstances, such as hypothermia, possibly some drug overdoses and following thrombolysis in suspected massive pulmonary embolism (PE) [16]. The return of spontaneous circulation at any time during the resuscitation process resets the clock time to zero [1,2,16].

Prognosis for survival after cardiac arrest

The best prospect of neurologically intact long-term survival after a cardiac arrest occurs when:

- victim is witnessed to collapse
- CPR is commenced immediately

- cardiac rhythm is VF or pulseless VT
- defibrillation is performed as soon as possible, ideally within 2–3 min of collapse [3,4].

Out-of-hospital cardiac arrest

Some variation in survival after an out-of-hospital cardiac arrest is due to differences in EMS systems, as well as differing research methodology and data reporting. A 1996 meta-analysis of 36 articles published between 1973 and 1992 from 41 EMS systems in six countries showed survival varied from 0 to 21%, with an overall mean survival of 8% [17].

In-hospital cardiac arrest

The prognosis for survival from in-hospital cardiac arrest is only marginally better, with survival to discharge averaging 13.8% of 12 961 patients in reports published between 1961 and 1984 [15]. However, in a further seven reports published between 1978 and 1989 this dropped to 11% of 1804 patients [16].

Controversies

- Acceptance of a universal algorithm.
- Lack of a demonstrated role for any drug used in ALS.
- A role for therapeutic hypothermia (TH).
- When ALS should not be started.
- When ALS should be ceased.

References

[1] International Liaison Committee on Resuscitation. International Consensus on Cardiopulmonary Resuscitation and Emergency Cardiac Care Science with Treatment Recommendations. Resuscitation 2010;81:e1–332.
[2] Australian Resuscitation Council and New Zealand Resuscitation Council. Australasian Adult Resuscitation Guidelines 2010 Emerg Med Australas 2011;23:244–316. <http://www.resus.org.au/ and http://www.nzrc.org.nz/> [Accessed Feb. 2013].
[3] Larsen MP, Eisenberg MS, Cummins RO, et al. Predicting survival from out-of-hospital cardiac arrest: a graphic model. Ann Emerg Med 1993;22:1652–8.
[4] Cummins RO, Ornato JP, Thies WH, Pepe PE. Improving survival from sudden cardiac arrest: the 'chain of survival' concept: a statement for health professionals from the Advanced Cardiac Life Support Subcommittee and the Emergency Cardiac Care Committee, American Heart Association. Circulation 1991;83:1832–47.
[5] Becker LB, Smith DW, Rhodes KV. Incidence of cardiac arrest: a neglected factor in evaluating survival rates. Ann Emerg Med 1993;22:86–91.
[6] Bernard S. Outcome from prehospital cardiac arrest in Melbourne Australia. Emerg Med (Fremantle) 1998;10:25–9.
[7] The American Heart Association in collaboration with the International Liaison Committee on Resuscitation. Guidelines For cardiopulmonary resuscitation and emergency cardiovascular care – an international consensus on science. Resuscitation 2000;46:1–447.
[8] Truong JH, Rosen P. Current concepts in electrical defibrillation. J Emerg Med 1997;15:331–8.
[9] Bossaert LL. Fibrillation and defibrillation of the heart. Br J Anaesth 1997;79:172–7.
[10] Kerber RE. Electrical treatment of cardiac arrhythmias: defibrillation and cardioversion. Ann Emerg Med 1993;22:296–301.
[11] Australasian College for Emergency Medicine. Statement on early access, defibrillation. ACEM 2005; S1:1. <http://www.acem.org.au/> (Accessed Mar. 2013).
[12] Brennan RJ, Luke C. Failed prehospital resuscitation following out-of-hospital cardiac arrest: are further efforts in the emergency department warranted?. Emerg Med (Fremantle) 1995;7:31–138.
[13] Bonnin MJ, Pepe PE, Timball KT, et al. Distinct criteria for termination of resuscitation in the out-of-hospital setting. J Am Med Assoc 1993;269:1457–62.
[14] Pepe PE, Brown CG, Bonnin MJ, et al. Prospective validation of criteria for on-scene termination of resuscitation efforts after out-of-hospital cardiac arrest. Ann Emerg Med 1993;22:884–5.
[15] McGrath RB. In-house cardiopulmonary resuscitation after a quarter of a century. Ann Emerg Med 1987;16:1365–8.
[16] Jastremski MS. In-hospital cardiac arrest. Ann Emerg Med 1993;22:113–7.
[17] Nichol G, Destsky AS, Stiell IG, et al. Effectiveness of emergency medical services for victims of out-of-hospital cardiac arrest: a meta-analysis. Ann Emerg Med 1995;27:700–10.

CRITICAL CARE

Edited by **Anthony Brown**

2.1 Airway and ventilation management

Stephen A Bernard

ESSENTIALS

1 Respiratory failure is a common presentation to the emergency department and ventilatory support may be required.

2 Non-invasive ventilation is appropriate for many patients with respiratory failure; endotracheal intubation and mechanical ventilation are used for cases where non-invasive ventilation is unsuccessful or contraindicated.

3 Endotracheal intubation performed in the emergency department almost always requires the use of sedative plus muscle relaxant drugs to facilitate endotracheal tube placement.

4 If visualization of the vocal cords at laryngoscopy is difficult, a 'Failed Intubation Drill' should be initiated immediately to avoid patient hypoxaemia.

5 Clinical checks to confirm correct endotracheal tube position are unreliable. Waveform or similar capnography must be used to confirm tracheal placement.

6 In patients with acute lung injury and decreased pulmonary compliance, mechanical ventilation should use low tidal volumes to avoid barotrauma.

Introduction

Assessment and management of the airway is the first step in the resuscitation of a critically ill patient in the emergency department (ED). Once the airway has been assessed and managed, evaluation of adequacy of ventilation follows. This chapter outlines the initial management of airway and ventilation in the ED.

Evaluation of the airway

Evaluation of the airway commences with a '*look, listen, feel*' approach to detect partial or complete airway obstruction. If airway compromise is suspected, initial basic airway manoeuvres include the jaw thrust, chin lift and head tilt (providing with the latter that there is no suspicion of cervical spine injury); and placement of an oropharyngeal airway (OPA) (see Chapter 1.1 on Basic Life Support).

Gentle direct inspection of the upper airway using a laryngoscope may be necessary to detect a foreign body, which can be removed using a Yankauer suction catheter for liquids/secretions and/or Magill's forceps for solid

material. Once the airway is cleared, supplemental oxygen by face-mask is commenced as consideration is given to the breathing status.

Evaluation of breathing

Evaluation of breathing also uses a '*look, listen, feel*' approach. Confirmation of adequate oxygenation initially uses a pulse oximeter. The adequacy of breathing may be confirmed with an arterial or venous blood gas analysis to confirm that the PCO_2 is in the normal range.

Conscious patients with a patent airway but who have hypoxia and/or hypercapnoea should then be considered for non-invasive ventilation (NIV) or endotracheal intubation (ETI) and mechanical ventilation.

Non-invasive ventilation

Many patients in respiratory failure with hypoxaemia and/or hypercapnoea may benefit from a trial of NIV [1]. The use of NIV involves administration of a controlled mixture of oxygen and air delivered at a set positive pressure via a tightly sealed face-mask. The pressure is generally maintained between 5 and 10 cm H_2O during both inspiration and expiration. This continuous positive airway pressure (CPAP) recruits lung alveoli that were previously closed, improving the ventilation/perfusion ratio and thus helping to correct hypoxaemia. There may also be a reduction in the work of breathing as a result of an increase in pulmonary compliance.

Inspiratory support (i.e. 5–20 cm H_2O above the baseline pressure) during NIV is known as bi-level NIV. This additional inspiratory support is thought to further reduce the work of breathing when there is poor lung compliance or increased airway resistance.

Contraindications to NIV include comatose or combative patients, poor tolerance of a tight-fitting face-mask, poor seal of the face-mask due to facial hair, and/or the lack of trained medical or nursing staff to institute and monitor the NIV.

Clinical indications for non-invasive ventilation in the ED

Patients who present with severe acute pulmonary oedema (APO) should receive CPAP to improve cardiac and pulmonary function, while medical therapy with nitrates and diuretics is initiated [2]. On the other hand, patients who present with an exacerbation of chronic obstructive pulmonary disease (COPD) may benefit from bi-level NIV rather than CPAP alone [3].

There is also some evidence to support the use of NIV in patients with respiratory failure due to other common ED conditions, such as community-acquired pneumonia [1], although the role of NIV in the management of asthma remains uncertain [4]. Thus, it is common ED practice to administer a trial of NIV in most awake patients with respiratory distress or respiratory failure, prior to any consideration of a requirement for ETI and mechanical ventilation.

Endotracheal intubation

Endotracheal intubation (ETI) is performed for any one or more of the following four major reasons: to create an airway; to maintain an airway; to protect an airway; and/or to provide for mechanical ventilation.

Thus, a patient in respiratory arrest requires immediate bag/valve/mask (BVM) ventilation with supplemental oxygen while preparation is made for ETI and mechanical ventilation to protect and maintain the airway and provide mechanical ventilation. Alternatively, a patient with a reduced conscious state and/or depression of the cough reflex requires ETI for airway maintenance and protection. Also, ETI may be indicated as part of general anaesthesia in the combative patient who needs imaging and/or a practical procedure. Finally, ETI will be required for mechanical ventilation in a patient with respiratory failure in whom NIV has been unsuccessful or is contraindicated.

Challenges to ETI in the emergency department

There are additional challenges to ETI in the ED compared to ETI in the operating theatre. There is often inadequate time for consultation with the patient and/or family and details of current medications, previous anaesthetics and/or allergies may not be available. Also, the status of the cervical spine in a patient with an altered conscious state following trauma is unknown, even if initial plain imaging appears normal. Finally, patients who present to the ED are generally not fasted and thus at a higher risk of aspiration of stomach contents during ETI.

Accreditation in ETI

Given these risks, accreditation by the hospital for a medical practitioner to undertake ETI in the ED is essential. Such accreditation should be based on gaining appropriate qualifications as well as considerable experience in both the operating theatre or in the emergency department, under the supervision of an experienced anaesthetist or airway operator. In addition to initial accreditation, on-going skills maintenance in airway techniques using simulation training should be required [5].

A number of possible techniques for ETI in the ED are reviewed below. The selection of the appropriate technique depends upon physician preference and the clinical setting. A checklist approach is now becoming standard.

Rapid sequence intubation

Unless the patient is deeply comatose but not in cardiac arrest, upper airway reflexes will generally be present and ETI will require the use of sedative and neuromuscular blocking drugs to facilitate laryngoscopy and the placement of the endotracheal tube. Rapid sequence intubation (RSI) involves the simultaneous administration of sedative drugs and a rapid-onset muscle relaxant at a predetermined dose and is the technique of choice when intubation is required in the ED.

Precautions and relative contraindications to RSI

Precautions and relative contraindications to the performance of RSI aim to avoid the technique in those judged to be difficult or impossible to intubate, including a patient with upper airway obstruction, distorted facial anatomy, micrognathia or an ankylosed neck. An alternative elective intubation technique in such cases may be awake intubation under local

anaesthesia or an awake surgical airway (see later) to avoid at all costs creating the situation of 'can't intubate, can't ventilate'.

Preparation for RSI

Careful preparation is essential prior to RSI. If time and patient status allow, seek a history of current medications, allergies and time of the last meal. Make a careful examination of the upper airway looking for anatomical features that may predict difficult intubation. A '4 × 4' checklist to ensure adequate preparation prior to RSI is shown in Box 2.1.1.

Pre-oxygenation The conscious patient should receive explanation and reassurance during the preparatory phase. Pre-oxygenation with 100% oxygen is essential to prevent oxygen desaturation during the procedure. Ideally, NIV with 100% oxygen for a 3-minute period should be administered. If this is not possible, then spontaneous breathing through a tight-fitting bag/valve/mask using 15 L/min oxygen is an alternative way to pre-oxygenate the patient. In addition, the application of nasal prongs with continuous oxygen flowing at 15 L/min can decrease the incidence of hypoxia during the RSI process [6].

Box 2.1.1 '4 × 4' check list for rapid sequence intubation

Monitoring
Blood pressure
Electrocardiogram
Pulse oximetry
Waveform end-tidal CO_2 detector

Drugs
Sedation (usually 2 drugs, i.e. fentanyl/propofol)
Muscle relaxant (suxamethonium or rocuronium)
Atropine

Preparation
Pre-oxygenation
IV running (fluid preload)
Laryngoscope × 2
Suction

Failed intubation equipment
Video-laryngoscope
Bougie
Intubation laryngeal mask airway
Cricothyroidotomy kit

If the patient has suspected spinal column injury, the neck must be immobilized in the anatomically neutral position. Reliable intravenous access as well as equipment for suctioning the airway must be available as well as a tipping trolley.

Monitoring during RSI

Monitoring required during RSI must include a continuous ECG trace and pulse oximetry. The blood pressure should be measured either non-invasively using an automated monitoring device each minute or invasively using an intra-arterial catheter. Waveform capnography for end-tidal carbon dioxide ($ETCO_2$) measurement following RSI must be calibrated and ready to use. In addition, a disposable calorimetric capnograph should be available in case the waveform capnograph fails.

Drugs used in RSI

The drugs required will depend on physician preference and the clinical situation. Common choices for induction include propofol at 1–2 mg/kg, a narcotic, such as fentanyl 1.0 μg/kg, a benzodiazepine, such as midazolam 0.05–0.1 mg/kg, followed by a rapid-onset depolarizing neuromuscular blocking drug, such as suxamethonium 1.5 mg/kg.

Contraindications to suxamethonium include known allergy, hyperkalaemia, burns, crush injury, spinal cord injury (not in the acute setting) or a history of malignant hyperthermia. Therefore, an alternative when suxamethonium is contraindicated is the rapid acting non-depolarizing drug rocuronium 1 mg/kg [7]. Details of the indications, dosages and side effects of all the commonly used drugs for RSI intubation are shown in Table 2.1.1.

Preparation of equipment and personnel prior to RSI

All drugs must be drawn up and checked in advance and the syringes clearly labelled. A spare laryngoscope must be available in case of failure of the first and the appropriate size of endotracheal tube (ETT) opened, lubricated and the cuff checked. Another ETT (one size smaller) should be immediately available. Finally, a bougie must be ready to hand. An ETT introducer (stylet) is preferred by some to provide a 'hockey-stick' J-shape to the end of the ETT.

At least two assistants will be required; one to assist the operator with the drugs and equipment and another to provide cricoid pressure following the administration of sedation and muscle relaxation drugs. If cricoid pressure is utilized, it must not allow distortion or impediment to the visualization of the vocal cords; if this occurs, it may be abandoned to improve and optimize the laryngoscopic view. A fourth person is required to provide in-line manual immobilization in the case of RSI for the trauma patient with possible spinal column injury. Additional equipment in case of difficult or failed intubation should be readily available, ideally kept together in the 'Airway Trolley' containing the items necessary for a failed intubation protocol as shown in Figure 2.1.1.

Endotracheal tube insertion

When all preparations are complete, including pre-oxygenation, the sedative drugs are administered as a bolus with gentle cricoid pressure applied via the cricoid ring cartilage. As consciousness is lost, the muscle relaxant is administered. Following fasciculations and the loss of muscle tone, firm cricoid pressure is applied and laryngoscopy performed. The patient is positioned in the 'sniffing the morning air' position with the neck flexed and the head extended, using a pillow under the head.

The laryngoscope is inserted and the vocal cords visualized. If the larynx is sighted, the endotracheal tube is placed directly through the vocal cords into the trachea, the cuff inflated and the ETT secured with tapes. Many brands of ETT now include a line marked proximal to the cuff which should be visible at the conclusion of laryngoscopy, thus avoiding placement of the ETT in the right main bronchus. Cricoid pressure should be maintained until the position of the tube is checked with the waveform capnograph and the ETT secured. The operator then indicates that the ETT is correctly placed and cricoid pressure may be released.

Ensuring optimal tracheal position

Clinical methods of ensuring optimal tracheal position include sighting the passage of the ETT through the vocal cords, misting of the ETT during exhalation and auscultation of breath sounds in both the lung fields. However, these clinical tests may be misleading and, in all cases, the ETT *must* be confirmed as placed in the trachea using waveform capnography, which is the gold standard for confirmation of tracheal placement in patients with a palpable pulse. However, during cardiac arrest there may be inadequate delivery of carbon dioxide to the lungs and hence a false-negative reading.

Table 2.1.1 Common intravenous drugs for rapid sequence intubation				
Drug	Dose	Action	Onset (min)	Duration (min)
Premedication agents				
Atropine	0.02 mg/kg	Vagal blockade	1	30
Lidocaine	1.5 mg/kg	Decreases ICP	1	30
Fentanyl	1.5–3 μg/kg	Sympatholytic	2	20
Induction agents				
Thiopentone	1–5 mg/kg	Sedation and reduces ICP	0.5	10
Propofol	1–2 mg/kg	Sedation	0.5	10
Midazolam	0.05–0.1 mg/kg	Sedation	2	10
Ketamine	1–2 mg/kg	Dissociative state	2	20
Muscle relaxants				
Suxamethonium	1.5 mg/kg	Depolarizing MR	0.5	5
Vecuronium	0.2 mg/kg	Non-depolarizing MR	2	40
Rocuronium	1.0 mg/kg	Non-depolarizing MR	1	30
Atracurium	0.5 mg/kg	Non-depolarizing MR	3	30
Pancuronium	0.1 mg/kg	Non-depolarizing MR	3	40

ICP: intracranial pressure; MR: muscle relaxant.

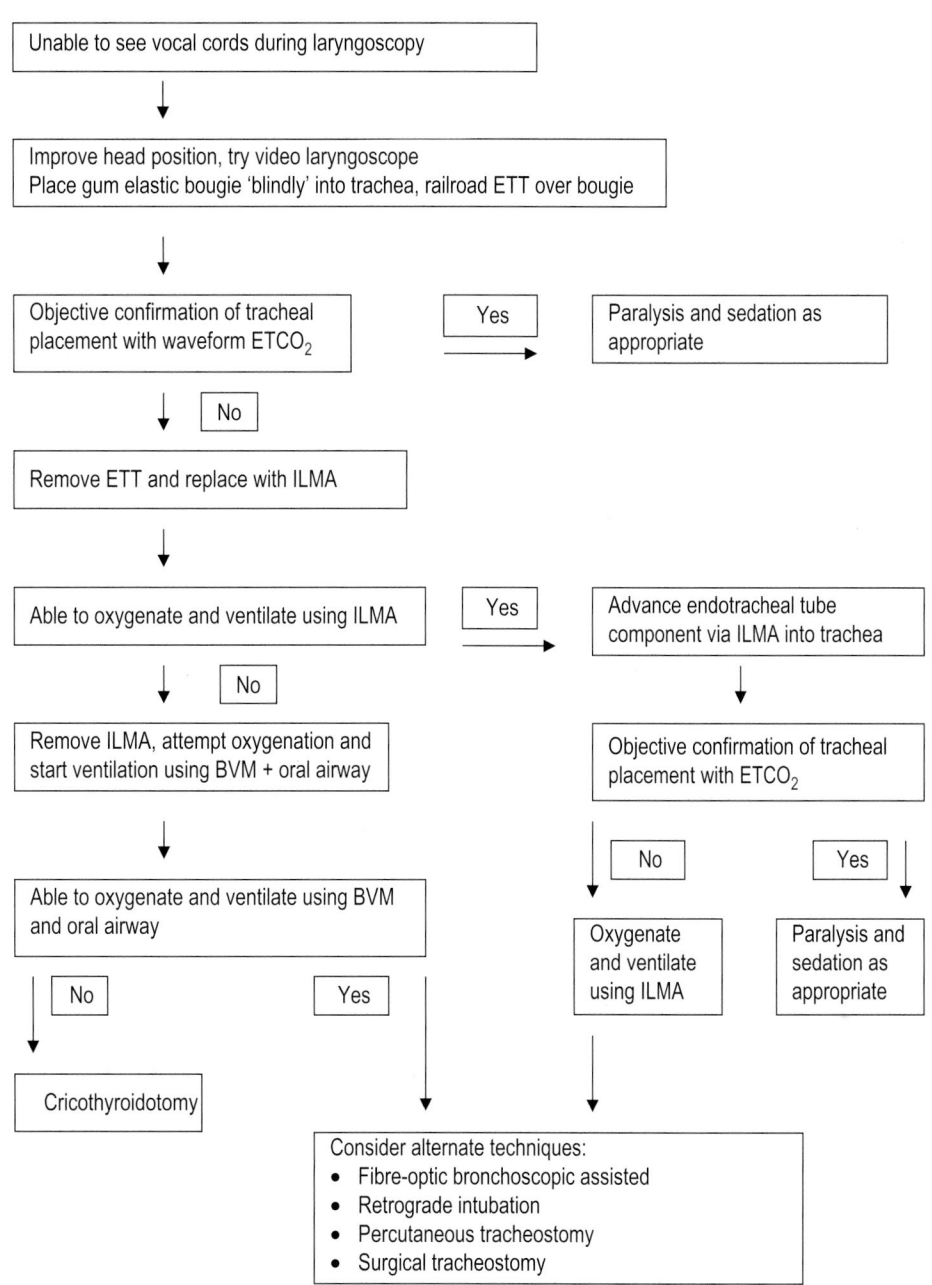

Fig. 2.1.1 **Algorithm** for failed intubation. ETT: endotracheal tube; BVM: bag/valve/mask; ILMA: intubating laryngeal mask airway; ETCO$_2$: end-tidal carbon dioxide.

In this setting, any doubt about correct airway placement should include removal of the ETT and ventilation using a supraglottic airway [8].

After placement of the ETI is confirmed, an orogastric or nasogastric tube should be inserted and a chest X-ray (CXR) performed to confirm correct positioning of the tip of the ETT in the trachea at least 1 cm proximal to the tracheal carina. The CXR also allows confirmation of correct placement of the orogastric or nasogastric tube in the stomach.

Maintenance of sedation and paralysis

As the drugs used for sedation and muscle relaxation wear off, further drugs for the maintenance of sedation and paralysis will be required. Appropriate monitoring of vital signs, pulse oximetry and waveform capnography with visual and audible alarms must be maintained at all times. Humidification of the inspired oxygen is desirable using a disposable heat and moisture exchange filter. When the

patient is placed on mechanical ventilation, the PaCO$_2$ should be checked to ensure adequate ventilation and to confirm correlation with the ETCO$_2$. The unconscious patient also requires eye care, pressure area care, temperature control and catheterization of the urinary bladder.

Complications of RSI

Hypotension following endotracheal intubation is common and must be addressed promptly. The causes include the vasodilator and/or negative inotropic effects of the sedative drug(s) given and/or the reduction in preload from positive-pressure ventilation decreasing venous return and cardiac output. Treatment consists of administration of a 10–20 mL/kg fluid bolus of crystalloid fluid, such as saline or Hartmann's and/or infusion of a vasopressor/inotrope, depending on the clinical setting.

Alternatively, in the setting of bronchospasm, hypotension may be due to gas trapping and dynamic hyperinflation from excessive ventilation, with the development of auto-PEEP (positive end-expiratory pressure), which is improved by immediate reduction in ventilation and allowing increased time for expiration. Importantly, hypotension can be due to the development of a tension pneumothorax occurring after the commencement of positive-pressure ventilation. On the other hand, hypertension usually indicates inadequate sedation and should be treated with supplemental sedation.

Intubation in a patient with severe head injury

The following additional measures need to be considered during intubation in patients with severe head injury. An assistant must hold the head in the neutral position due to the possibility of cervical spine instability, which increases the difficulty of visualizing the larynx. Laryngoscopy may raise intracranial pressure, although the benefit of pretreatment with lignocaine 1.5 mg/kg is uncertain in this setting [9]. In addition, thiopentone or propofol must be used cautiously in patients with severe head injury as profound hypotension due to unrecognized hypovolaemia may occur. In this setting, ketamine may be the preferred induction agent since this agent is more likely to maintain blood pressure compared with other sedating agents [10].

The technique of RSI is not recommended for a patient with a grossly abnormal upper airway and/or impending upper airway obstruction. In this setting, the larynx may then not be able to be visualized and ventilation of the now apnoeic patient may become impossible, leading to the 'can't intubate, can't ventilate' situation. An awake technique using local anaesthesia and/or a fibreoptic-assisted intubation should be performed in these patients (see later). Alternatively, an inhalational anaesthetic agent or a short-acting intravenous agent, such as propofol, can be used, as the sedative effects will rapidly reverse and spontaneous respirations resume if intubation and ventilation prove impossible.

Difficult intubation

Endotracheal intubation under direct vision may be easy or difficult, depending on the view of the larynx during laryngoscopy. This laryngeal view has been classified by Cormack and Lehane into grades 1–4 [11].

A Cormack and Lehane grade 1 laryngoscopy is a clear view of the entire laryngeal aperture. A grade 2 laryngoscopy is a view of only the posterior part of the larynx. In a grade 3 laryngoscopy, only the epiglottis is visualized and in grade 4 only the soft palate is seen. A difficult intubation is defined as a Cormack and Lehane grade 3 or 4 view at laryngoscopy.

Difficult intubation may be anticipated in the presence of pathological facial and upper airway disorders that may be congenital or acquired, such as maxillofacial and airway trauma, airway tumour or abscess or cervical spine immobility. There may also be anatomical reasons for a Cormack and Lehane grade 3–4 laryngoscopy, such as micrognathia or microstomia, poor mouth opening and/or a large tongue. A range of clinical tests have been proposed that help predict difficulty in visualization of the larynx, including relative size of the tongue to the pharynx, atlanto-occipital joint mobility and a thyromental distance <6 cm. However, these are not always clinically useful in the emergency setting. More recently, sonographic measurements of anterior neck soft tissue thickness at the level of hyoid bone and thyrohyoid membrane have been used to distinguish difficult and easy laryngoscopy [12].

Failed intubation drill

Attempts at blind placement of the ETT into the trachea when the larynx is not visualized are unlikely to be successful and may result in pharyngeal or laryngeal trauma making the situation even more difficult, with hypoxaemia. In this situation, a failed intubation drill must be immediately initiated [13]. A failed intubation algorithm suitable for use in the ED is shown in Figure 2.1.1.

The first step is to ensure that all medical and nursing staff present are made aware that the intubation is difficult and that a failed intubation drill is being initiated [14]. Second, depending on hospital resources, an urgent call for assistance from another physician with additional experience should be made.

Simple initial manoeuvres to improve visualization of the larynx include adding a second

pillow to flex the neck further (unless cervical spine injury is suspected), the use of a straight Mackintosh laryngoscope blade and 'backward/upward/rightward external pressure' (BURP) on the thyroid cartilage with abandonment of cricoid pressure if needed.

If the larynx still cannot be visualized, blind placement of a bougie and subsequent railroading of a well lubricated size 7.0 mm ETT over the bougie should be attempted [15]. Correct bougie airway placement is suggested by feeling the tracheal rings 'clicks' and by hold-up at around 30–40 cm as the bougie reaches distally in a mainstem bronchus. Absence of hold-up indicates likely oesophageal placement. Rotating the ETT through 90° in an anticlockwise direction may be helpful to facilitate passage along the bougie through the larynx.

If this initial step at ETI is unsuccessful, adequate oxygenation must be re-established and or maintained using a bag/mask with an OPA or a laryngeal mask airway (LMA) between attempts at intubation. If oxygenation is able to be maintained using bag/valve/mask ventilation, alternative approaches suitable for use in the ED should be considered. A summary of these approaches for a failed intubation is given in Figure 2.1.1. However, if oxygenation cannot be maintained during the drill, immediate cricothyroidotomy is indicated.

Laryngeal mask airway

The LMA is commonly used for airway management during elective general anaesthesia. During a failed intubation drill, the LMA may be superior to a bag/mask and oral airway for oxygenation and ventilation, even though there is still the potential risk of aspiration of the contents of the stomach into the airway as this remains unprotected. This risk may be decreased with the use of an LMA with a distal drainage tube (LMA ProSeal™) or an LMA incorporating an oesophageal vent that allows placement of an orogastric tube to provide access for suctioning the upper oesophagus (LMA Supreme™) [16].

Modified laryngeal mask airways

In addition to the provision of oxygenation and ventilation, there are a number of modified LMAs that may be useful to facilitate intubation during a failed intubation drill in the ED.

The intubating LMA is a modification of the standard LMA that incorporates a rigid curved outer airway tube with a metal handle and a special modified endotracheal tube specifically made to pass blindly through the LMA into the trachea (LMA Fastrach™). An LMA incorporating a video image of the larynx has been developed (LMA CTrach™), which may facilitate passage of a bougie through the LMA into the trachea. The LMA can then be removed and an ETT placed over the bougie. The latter has a higher success rate for first-time intubation compared with the LMA Fastrach [17].

Video-laryngoscope assisted intubation

There are an increasing number of laryngoscopes available that include a video image projected from the tip of the laryngoscope and displayed on a separate small screen or laryngoscopes with the screen fitted to the handle. These have the advantage of giving a superior view of the larynx and, although the first-pass success rate appears to be similar to traditional direct laryngoscopy [18]. Increasing familiarity may see this become the preferred method of laryngoscopy.

Fibreoptic bronchoscope-assisted intubation

A fibreoptic bronchoscope may assist in the intubation of the patient when RSI fails or is contraindicated. In particular, fibreoptic bronchoscope-assisted intubation (FBI) is the technique of choice in suspected traumatic injury to the larynx and in the obstructed airway, particularly with distorted anatomy, such as with an upper airway burn or tumour. The FBI may diagnose the severity of the laryngeal injury or pathology and the possible requirement for surgery. However, it requires considerable training and should only be performed by an experienced operator, usually in theatre. Equipment sterilization, maintenance and checking procedures must also be in place.

Technique of fibreoptic bronchoscope-assisted intubation

Topical anaesthetic is applied to the nasal passage using gauze soaked in 5 mL of lignocaine 2% with adrenaline 1:100 000 if the patient is aware. In addition, the upper airway

is anaesthetized with lignocaine 10% spray. A well-lubricated 7.0 mm ETT is introduced nasally and passed to the posterior pharynx. Then the bronchoscope is inserted through the ETT to visualize the vocal cords. The suction port of the bronchoscope is used to clear any secretions and also to administer further local anaesthesia into the airway.

The bronchoscope is advanced through the larynx and the ETT then railroaded over the bronchoscope and down the trachea. Further sedation to decrease the cough reflex will be required at this time. The bronchoscope is removed and the patient is then ventilated with oxygen and given additional sedation as needed.

If an LMA has been used during a failed intubation drill and is in place to provide ventilation, this may be utilized to guide the bronchoscope into the larynx. A guidewire may be passed via the bronchoscope into the trachea. The LMA is then removed and an ETT is replaced over the guidewire [19].

Limitations of fibreoptic bronchoscope-assisted intubation

The use of a fibreoptic bronchoscope in the ED is limited by several factors. The bronchoscope and light source must be immediately available for a failed intubation drill. The technique requires considerable additional practice for skills maintenance, yet its use is rare in routine ED practice. The larynx may be difficult to visualize in the presence of blood, vomitus or secretions. Finally, the equipment is expensive to purchase and maintain.

Other airway management techniques

Retrograde intubation

If the patient is able to be adequately oxygenated with a supraglottic airway, the technique of retrograde intubation may be used in the ED [20]. The cricothyroid membrane is punctured by a needle and a guidewire is passed and directed cephalad. The wire is then brought out through the mouth using Magill's forceps. The ETT may be passed over the wire and back into the larynx using the introducer of a cricothyroidotomy kit [21]. Alternatively, the wire may be passed inside the end of the ETT and then out through the 'Murphy eye'. Resistance may be felt when the ETT reaches the larynx and some anticlockwise rotation may be required to facilitate passage

into the larynx. When the level of the cricothyroid is reached, the guidewire is removed and the ETT passed further down the trachea. The technique of retrograde intubation takes time and experience to perform and is usually unsuitable in a critical airway emergency.

Blind nasotracheal intubation

Blind nasotracheal intubation (BNTI) is a traditional technique that may still occasionally be useful in the ED, either as the initial technique of choice or as part of a failed intubation drill once spontaneous respirations have resumed [22]. Contraindications include a fractured base of skull or maxillary fracture, a suspected laryngeal injury, coagulopathy and/or upper airway obstruction.

Technique of blind nasotracheal intubation

High-flow oxygen is administered by mask and the nasal passages are inspected to assess patency. The larger nasal passage is prepared as per the nasal fibreoptic intubation described above. Local anaesthetic may also be sprayed into the upper airway and intravenous sedation may be administered if required and clinically appropriate.

An ETT one size smaller than the predicted oral size is passed via the nose to the pharynx and advanced slowly towards the larynx with the operator listening for breath sounds. The head may need to be flexed, extended or rotated to facilitate entry into the larynx, the ETT rotated clockwise through 90° and/or a suction catheter used to guide the ETT. When the tube passes into the trachea, louder spontaneous respirations heard from the ETT or the onset of coughing down the tube, confirm successful placement. However, there are significant complications with BNTI including epistaxis, injuries to the turbinates, perforation of the posterior pharynx, laryngospasm and injury to the larynx.

Cricothyroidotomy

Cricothyroidotomy is an essential skill for all emergency physicians and must be considered immediately in the situation of 'can't intubate, can't ventilate'. There are several possible techniques for emergency cricothyroidotomy described below.

Guidewire cricothyroidotomy

Proprietary kits allow a cricothyroidotomy tube to be placed using a Seldinger technique. In this approach, the cricothyroid membrane is punctured with a needle mounted on a syringe; free aspiration of air confirms placement in the airway. A guidewire is passed through the needle caudad down the trachea. The needle is then removed and a dilator passed along the wire, then a 4.5–6 mm cricothyroidotomy tube is mounted on a guide and passed along the wire and into the trachea. The position of the cricothyroidotomy tube must be carefully checked as it is possible to misplace it anterior to the trachea. Note, if the cricothyroidotomy tube is uncuffed, interpretation of a capnograph waveform can be misleading as much of the exhaled gas passes into the upper airway and not out through the cricothyroidotomy tube during exhalation, resulting in a potentially false-negative end-tidal CO_2 trace.

Surgical cricothyroidotomy

Alternatively, a surgical cricothyroidotomy may be rapidly performed by making a small vertical incision over the cricothyroid membrane. Artery forceps are then used for blunt dissection to the cricothyroid membrane which is opened horizontally with the artery forceps. A bougie is passed through the opening into the trachea, then a size 6 mm cuffed ETT is 'railroaded' over the bougie. The ETT cuff is inflated, the bougie removed and bag/valve ventilation with oxygen commenced. This technique is faster to perform than a guidewire technique, although physicians with limited surgical experience may prefer the guidewire approach [23].

Longer-term placement of a larger (>6 mm) ETT through the cricothyroid membrane is unsatisfactory because of the possibility of stricture occurring at the level of the cricoid ring. Therefore, the cricothyroidotomy is subsequently converted to either oral endotracheal intubation or a tracheostomy when it is safe and convenient to do so.

Tracheostomy

Compared with cricothyroidotomy, a surgical tracheostomy is time-consuming and difficult to perform in the ED [24], but may be indicated in suspected direct laryngeal injury. Pre-tracheal dissection requires adequate lighting, instruments and diathermy, with distorted anatomy and bleeding making the technique more complex. Percutaneous dilatational tracheostomy is commonly performed in the ICU and can be rapidly performed by an experienced operator in the ED [25].

Mechanical ventilation

Once intubation has been achieved, the patient is connected to a mechanical ventilator to provide continued ventilatory support. Because ventilated patients can initially be managed for some time in the ED, it is important that recommendations for optimal mechanical ventilation are implemented in the ED.

Optimal mechanical ventilation

A tidal volume of 8 mL/kg and a respiratory rate of 10–14 breaths per minute are considered safe for most patients. In general, 5 cm of positive end-expiratory pressure (PEEP) is provided.

However, patients with acute lung injury may have reduced pulmonary compliance and elevated peak inspiratory and plateau pressures. These patients should receive a 'protective lung ventilation strategy' [26]. This involves limiting the tidal volume to 6 mL/kg, with the respiratory rate setting increased to 16–20 breaths per minute to prevent excessive hypercapnoea. If hypoxia persists (PaO_2 <60 mmHg), then additional PEEP is indicated. This may be titrated in steps of 2.5 mmHg towards a maximum of 22 mmHg [27]. It is important to measure peak and plateau pressures in such a patient to avoid excessive intrinsic lung pressures. The latter is undertaken by pausing ventilation at end-inspiration for 10 seconds and observing the pressure trace on the screen of the ventilator.

Permissive hypercapnoea

Patients with severe airways obstruction, such as asthma or COPD, should receive a standard tidal volume of 8 mL/kg, but at a decreased respiratory rate of 4 to 8 breaths per minute to allow sufficient time for adequate passive exhalation [28]. This slow respiratory rate reduces the risk of dynamic pulmonary hyperinflation and development of auto-PEEP leading to hypotension. Using this strategy, the $PaCO_2$ level will rise ('permissive hypercapnoea') as oxygenation is maintained.

Deliberate hyperventilation

In complete contrast, deliberate hyperventilation using a respiratory rate of 16–20 breaths per minute may be indicated to provide hypocapnoea in a patient who has been intubated and who has a severe metabolic acidosis, such as diabetic ketoacidosis. Also, hyperventilation in a patient with raised intracranial pressure to normocapnoea or slight hypocapnoea temporarily reduces the intracranial pressure while other treatments are being implemented.

Extubation in the emergency department

Increasingly, patients who are intubated pre-hospital by paramedics or by a physician in the ED may be considered for planned extubation in the ED, after investigation and treatment have excluded the requirement for mechanical ventilation in ICU. Examples include a patient with a drug overdose or those requiring brief general anaesthesia for a procedure.

In general, patients should be lightly sedated with a short-acting sedative, such as propofol, able to follow commands and able to cough adequately to tracheal suction. Ideally, a trial of spontaneous breathing with the ventilator set to a CPAP of 5 cm H_2O, with minimal inspiratory pressure support (i.e. 5–10 cm H_2O) with modest supplemental oxygen (i.e. <50% oxygen) is necessary. Also, the stomach should be emptied via an orogastric or nasogastric tube prior to extubation.

Controversies

- Training and skills maintenance of airway management techniques in the ED, including the use of standardized airway algorithms or pathways.
- The increasing role of video-laryngoscopy.
- Practising the failed intubation drill in the ED, including the role of simulation.
- The optimal surgical airway technique in the case of 'can't intubate–can't ventilate'.

References

[1] Boldrini R, Fasano L, Nava S. Noninvasive mechanical ventilation. Curr Opin Crit Care 2012;18:48–53.

[2] Nouira S, Boukef R, Bouida W, et al. Non-invasive pressure support ventilation and CPAP in cardiogenic pulmonary edema: a multicenter randomized study in the emergency department. Intens Care Med 2011;37:249–56.

[3] Brulotte CA, Lang ES. Acute exacerbations of chronic obstructive pulmonary disease in the emergency department. Emerg Med Clin N Am 2012;30:223–47.

[4] Lim WJ, Mohammed Akram R, Carson KV, et al. Non-invasive positive pressure ventilation for treatment of respiratory failure due to severe acute exacerbations of asthma. Cochrane Database Syst Rev 2012;12:CD004360.

[5] Okuda Y, Bond W, Bonfante G, et al. National growth in simulation training within emergency medicine residency programs, 2003–2008. Acad Emerg Med 2008;15:1113–6.

[6] Weingart SD, Levitan RM. Preoxygenation and prevention of desaturation during emergency airway management. Ann Emerg Med 2012;59:165–75.

[7] Herbstritt A, Amarakone K. Towards evidence-based emergency medicine: best BETs from the Manchester Royal Infirmary. BET 3: Is rocuronium as effective as succinylcholine at facilitating laryngoscopy during rapid sequence intubation? Emerg Med J 2012;29:256–8.

[8] Neumar RW, Otto CW, Link MS, et al. Part 8: Adult Advanced Life Support. 2010 American Heart Association Guidelines for Cardiopulmonary Resuscitation and Emergency Cardiac Care. Circulation 2010;122:S729–67.

[9] Robinson N, Clancy M. In patients with head injury undergoing rapid sequence intubation, does pretreatment with intravenous lignocaine/lidocaine lead to an improved neurological outcome? A review of the literature. Emerg Med J 2001;18:453–7.

[10] Sih K, Campbell SG, Tallon JM, et al. Ketamine in adult emergency medicine: controversies and recent advances. Ann Pharmacother 2011;45:1525–34.

[11] Cormack RS, Lehane J. Difficult intubation in obstetrics. Anaesthesia 1984;39:1105–11.

[12] Shiga T, Wajima Z, Inoue T, Sakamoto A. Predicting difficult intubation in apparently normal patients: a meta-analysis of bedside screening test performance. Anesthesiology 2005;103:429–37.

[13] Adhikari S, Zeger W, Schmier C, et al. Pilot study to determine the utility of point-of-care ultrasound in the assessment of difficult laryngoscopy. Acad Emerg Med 2011;18:754–8.

[14] Henderson JJ, Popat MT, Latto IP, et al. Difficult Airway Society. Difficult Airway Society guidelines for management of the unanticipated difficult intubation. Anaesthesia 2004;59:675–94.

[15] Heard AM, Green RJ, Eakins P. The formulation and introduction of a 'can't intubate, can't ventilate' algorithm into clinical practice. Anaesthesia 2009;64:601–8.

[16] Eschertzhuber S, Brimacombe J, Hohlrieder M, Keller C. The laryngeal mask airway Supreme – a single use laryngeal mask airway with an oesophageal vent. A randomised, cross-over study with the laryngeal mask airway ProSeal in paralysed, anaesthetised patients. Anaesthesia 2009;64:79–83.

[17] Liu EH, Goy RW, Lim Y, Chen FG. Success of tracheal intubation with intubating laryngeal mask airways: a randomized trial of the LMA Fastrach and LMA CTrach. Anesthesiology 2008;108:621–6.

[18] Mosier J, Chiu S, Patanwala AE, Sakles JC. A comparison of the GlideScope Video Laryngoscope to the C-MAC Video Laryngoscope for intubation in the emergency department. Ann Emerg Med 2013;61:414–20.

[19] Joffe AM, Arndt G, Willmann K. Wire-guided catheter exchange after failed direct laryngoscopy in critically ill adults. J Clin Anesth 2010;22:93–6.

[20] Dhara SS. Retrograde tracheal intubation. Anaesthesia 2009;64:1094–104.

[21] Slots P, Vegger PB, Bettger H, et al. Retrograde intubation with a Mini-Trach II kit. Acta Anaesthesiol Scand 2003;47:274–7.

[22] Dauphinee K. Nasotracheal intubation. Emerg Med Clin North Am 1988;6:715–23.

[23] Kanji H, Thirsk W, Dong S, et al. Emergency cricothyroidotomy: a randomized crossover trial comparing percutaneous techniques: classic needle first versus "incision first". Acad Emerg Med 2012;19:E1061–E1067.

[24] Dillon JK, Christensen B, Fairbanks T, et al. The emergent surgical airway: cricothyrotomy vs. tracheotomy. Int J Oral MaxillofacSurg 2013;42:204–8.

[25] Hamaekers AE, Henderson JJ. Equipment and strategies for emergency tracheal access in the adult patient. Anaesthesia 2011;66(Suppl 2):65–80.

[26] Petrucci N, De Feo C. Lung protective ventilation strategy for the acute respiratory distress syndrome. Cochrane Database Syst Rev 2013;2:CD003844.

[27] Briel M, Meade M, Mercat A, et al. Higher vs lower positive end-expiratory pressure in patients with acute lung injury and acute respiratory distress syndrome: systematic review and meta-analysis. J Am Med Assoc 2010;303:865–73.

[28] Oddo M, Feihl F, Schaller MD, Perret C. Management of mechanical ventilation in acute severe asthma: practical aspects. Intensive Care Med 2006;32:501–10.

2.2 Oxygen therapy

David R Smart

ESSENTIALS

1 Oxygen is the most commonly used drug in emergency medicine.

2 Oxygen-delivery systems may be divided into variable performance (delivering a variable concentration of oxygen) and fixed performance (delivering a fixed concentration of oxygen, including systems that deliver 100% oxygen).

3 Fixed-performance systems are essential where precise titration of oxygen dose is required, such as with chronic obstructive pulmonary disease (COPD) or where 100% oxygen is indicated.

4 Free-flowing circuits are least efficient at attempting to deliver 100% oxygen. A reservoir or demand system improves efficiency and a closed-circuit delivery system is most efficient.

5 There is increasing evidence for goal-directed oxygen therapy, which should be regarded as a drug prescribed in therapeutic doses titrated to SaO_2, rather than applied in a variable manner.

6 Titrated-dose oxygen therapy is required when treating patients with COPD, commencing with 24–28%. Response to therapy in these patients should be monitored with blood gases measurements.

7 Oxygen should never be abruptly withdrawn from patients in circumstances of suspected CO_2 narcosis.

8 Pulse oximetry provides valuable feedback regarding the appropriateness of oxygen dose provided to individual patients, but should not be used as a measure of ventilatory adequacy – this should be monitored by end-tidal CO_2 and conscious state.

Introduction

Oxygen was first discovered by Priestley in 1772 and was first used therapeutically by Beddoes in 1794. It now forms one of the cornerstones of medical therapy.

Oxygen (O_2) constitutes 21% of dry air by volume. It is essential to life. Cellular hypoxia results from a deficiency of oxygen, regardless of aetiology. Hypoxaemia is a state of reduced oxygen carriage in the blood. Hypoxia leads to anaerobic metabolism that is inefficient and may lead to death if not corrected. A major priority in acute medical management is correction of hypoxia, hence oxygen is the most frequently administered and important drug in emergency medicine. There are sound physiological reasons for the use of supplemental oxygen in the management of acutely ill and injured patients.

Uses of supplemental oxygen

- To correct defects in the delivery of inspired gas to the lungs. A clear airway is essential.
- Where there is inadequate oxygenation of blood due to defects in pulmonary gas exchange.
- To maximize oxygen saturation of the arterial blood (SaO_2) where there is

inadequate oxygen transport by the cardiovascular system.

- To maximize oxygen partial pressure and content in the blood in circumstances of increased or inefficient tissue oxygen demand.
- To provide 100% oxygen where clinically indicated.
- To titrate oxygen dose in patients with impaired ventilatory response to carbon dioxide.

Physiology of oxygen

Oxygen transport chain

Oxygen proceeds from inspired air to the mitochondria via a number of steps known as the oxygen transport chain. These steps include:

- ventilation
- pulmonary gas exchange
- oxygen carriage in the blood
- local tissue perfusion
- diffusion at tissue level
- tissue utilization of oxygen.

Ventilation

The normal partial pressure of inspired air oxygen (P_iO_2) is approximately 20 kPa (150 mmHg) at sea level. If there is a reduction in the fraction of inspired oxygen (F_iO_2), as occurs at altitude, hypoxia results. This is relevant in the transport of patients at 2400 m in commercial 'pressurized' aircraft, where ambient cabin pressures of 74.8 kPa (562 mmHg) results in a P_iO_2 of 14.4 kPa (108 mmHg).

Hypoxia can result from inadequate delivery of inspired gas to the lung. The many causes include airway obstruction, respiratory muscle weakness, neurological disorders interfering with respiratory drive (seizures, head injury), disruption to chest mechanics (chest injury) or extrinsic disease interfering with ventilation (intra-abdominal pathology). These processes interfere with the maintenance of an adequate alveolar oxygen partial pressure (P_AO_2), which is approximately 13.7 kPa (103 mmHg) in a healthy individual.

Alveolar gas equation An approximation of the alveolar gas equation permits rapid calculation of the alveolar oxygen partial pressures:

$$P_AO_2 = F_iO_2 \times (\text{barometric pressure} - 47) - PaCO_2/0.8$$

Pulmonary gas exchange

Oxygen diffuses across the alveoli and into pulmonary capillaries and carbon dioxide diffuses in the opposite direction. The process is passive, occurring down concentration gradients. Fick's law summarizes the process of diffusion of gases through tissues:

$$\dot{V}O_2 \propto A/T \times Sol/\sqrt{MW} \times (P_AO_2 - P_{pa}O_2)$$

where $\dot{V}O_2$ = rate of gas (oxygen) transfer, $\propto$ = proportional to, A = area of tissue, T = tissue thickness, Sol = solubility of the gas, MW = molecular weight, P_A = alveolar partial pressure, and P_{pa} = pulmonary artery partial pressure.

In healthy persons, oxygen rapidly passes from the alveoli to the blood and, after 0.25 seconds, pulmonary capillary blood is almost fully saturated with oxygen, resulting in a systemic arterial oxygen partial pressure (PaO_2) of approximately 13.3 kPa (100 mmHg). The difference between the P_AO_2 and the PaO_2 is known as the alveolar to arterial oxygen gradient (A–a gradient). It is usually small and increases with age.

Expected A–a gradient The expected A–a gradient when breathing air approximates to: Age (years) $\div$ 4 + 4.

An approximation of the actual value can be calculated as follows:

$$A-a\ O_2\ \text{gradient} = 140 - (PO_2 + PCO_2).$$

There is a defect in pulmonary gas exchange if the calculated value exceeds the expected value. The A–a O_2 gradient is increased if there is a barrier to diffusion, such as pulmonary fibrosis or oedema or a deficit in perfusion, such as a pulmonary embolism. An increased A–a gradient also reflects widespread ventilation–perfusion mismatch.

In circumstances of impaired diffusion in the lung, raising the F_iO_2 assists oxygen transfer by creating a greater pressure gradient from the alveoli to the pulmonary capillary. The increase in F_iO_2 may not be as helpful when lung perfusion is impaired as a result of increased intrapulmonary shunting.

Oxygen carriage in the blood

Four steps are required to deliver oxygen to the periphery:

- uptake of oxygen by haemoglobin (Hb)
- generation of a cardiac output to carry the oxygenated haemoglobin to the peripheral tissues
- dissociation of oxygen from haemoglobin into dissolved oxygen in plasma
- diffusion from blood to cells via plasma, extracellular fluid (ECF) and, finally, intracellular fluid (ICF).

Haemoglobin–oxygen (Hb–O_2) dissociation curve The haemoglobin–oxygen (Hb–O_2) dissociation curve is depicted in Figure 2.2.1, which also summarizes the factors that influence the position of the curve. If the curve is shifted to the left, this favours the affinity of haemoglobin for oxygen. These conditions are encountered when deoxygenated blood returns to the lung. A shift of the curve to the right favours unloading of oxygen and subsequent delivery to the tissues.

A number of advantages are conferred by the shape of the Hb–O_2 dissociation curve that favour uptake of oxygen in the lung and delivery to the tissues:

- Flat upper portion of the curve allows some reserve in the P_AO_2 required to keep the haemoglobin fully saturated; a reduction in P_AO_2 of 20% will have minimal effect on the oxygen loading of Hb
- Flat upper portion of the curve also ensures that a large difference remains between P_AO_2 and the pulmonary capillary oxygen partial pressure ($P_{pc}O_2$), even when much of the haemoglobin has been loaded with oxygen. This pressure difference favours maximal Hb–O_2 loading
- Lower part of the curve is steeper, which favours offloading of oxygen in peripheral tissues with only small falls in capillary PO_2. This maintains a higher driving pressure of oxygen, facilitating diffusion into cells

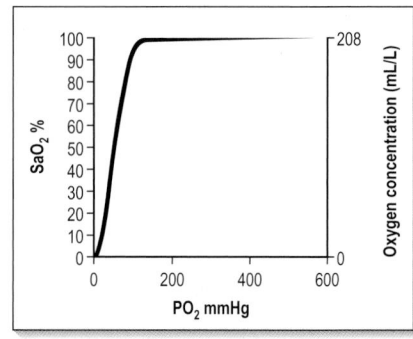

Fig. 2.2.1 The haemoglobin–oxygen dissociation curve.

- Right shift of the Hb–O_2 curve in circumstances of increased temperature, fall in pH, increased PCO_2 and increased erythrocyte 2,3 diphosphoglycerate (2,3-DPG) assists in further offloading of oxygen, even when the driving pressure has fallen and PO_2 has reached 5.3 kPa (40 mmHg), i.e. venous blood which is still 75% saturated with oxygen.

Oxygen is carried in the blood as dissolved gas and in combination with haemoglobin. At sea level (101.3 kPa), breathing air ($F_IO_2 = 0.21$), the amount of oxygen dissolved in plasma is small (0.03 mL oxygen per litre of blood for each 1 mmHg PaO_2). Hence at $P_aO_2 = 100$ mmHg, 3 mL of oxygen are dissolved in each litre of plasma. Dissolved oxygen is important because it is the first available oxygen to diffuse into the tissues. The dissolved component assumes greater significance in the hyperbaric environment, where at 284 kPa and $F_IO_2 = 1.0$ up to 60 mL oxygen can be carried dissolved per litre of blood.

Haemoglobin carries 1.34–1.39 mL oxygen per gram when fully saturated. Blood with a haemoglobin concentration of 150 g/L carries approximately 200 mL oxygen per litre.

Oxygen flux The total amount of oxygen delivered to the body per minute is known as oxygen flux.

$$\text{Oxygen flux} = (\text{oxyhaemoglobin} + \text{dissolved } O_2) \times \text{cardiac output}$$
$$= (1.39 \times Hb \times S_aO_2/100 + 0.03 \times PaO_2) \times Q$$

where Hb = haemoglobin concentration g/L; S_aO_2 = arterial oxygen saturation (percentage); PaO_2 = partial pressure of arterial oxygen (mmHg); Q = cardiac output (L/min).

A healthy individual breathing air transports approximately 1000 mL of oxygen per minute to the tissues, based on a cardiac output of 5 L/min; 30% or 300 mL/min of this oxygen is not available, because at least 2.7 kPa (20 mmHg) driving pressure is required to allow oxygen to enter the mitochondria. Therefore, approximately 700 mL/min are available for use by peripheral tissues. This provides a considerable reserve above the 250 mL/min consumed by a healthy resting adult.

In illness or injury, this reserve may be considerably eroded. Factors that reduce oxygen flux include a fall in cardiac output of any aetiology (including shock states), anaemia or a reduction in functional haemoglobin (carbon monoxide poisoning) and a drop in the S_aO_2. These situations are frequently encountered in the emergency department. Supplemental oxygen is required in addition to specific therapy, such as volume replacement, transfusion, and measures to improve cardiac output.

Local tissue perfusion and diffusion
Cellular hypoxia results if there is impairment of perfusion to local tissues. Oedema associated with medical illness or local injury increases the diffusion distance between blood and the cell, thus mandating a higher PaO_2 to ensure adequate tissue oxygen delivery.

Tissue utilization of oxygen
Increased oxygen flux is required if:

- tissue demands for oxygen are higher than normal or
- tissue utilization of oxygen is impaired.

Elevation of cardiac output increases oxygen flux in these circumstances but, frequently, this too is significantly impaired by the disease state.

Tissue demands for oxygen increase by 7% for each degree Celsius elevation in body temperature and considerably greater increases in demand occur in seizures, sepsis, severe dyspnoea, restlessness and shivering.

Tissue extraction of oxygen is impaired in sepsis and by poisons, such as carbon monoxide or cyanide. In all cases, oxygen therapy must be combined with general measures, such as reduction of fever and specific treatment of the primary disease process.

Oxygen delivery systems

Oxygen delivery systems are classified into three groups (Box 2.2.1):

- variable-performance systems
- fixed-performance systems
- 100% oxygen systems.

Definitions

Variable-performance oxygen delivery systems
These systems deliver a variable F_IO_2 to the patient which is altered by the inspiratory flow rate, the minute volume of the patient and the physical characteristics of the delivery system.

Fixed-performance oxygen delivery systems
These systems deliver a specified F_IO_2 to the patient that is not altered by changes in ventilatory pattern, volume or inspiratory flow rate.

Box 2.2.1 Oxygen delivery systems

Variable-performance systems
  Nasal cannulae
  Hudson mask ± reservoir
  T pieces and Y connectors

Fixed-performance systems
  Venturi mask
  Oxygen blenders

100% Oxygen systems
  Non-rebreathing circuits
    Free-flowing circuits
    Self-refilling circuits
    Soft reservoir bags
    Oxygen-powered resuscitators
  Partial-rebreathing circuits
  Closed circuit systems

One hundred per cent (100%) oxygen systems
This is a subgroup of fixed-performance systems wherein 100% oxygen is delivered to the patient.

General principles
The oxygen source in most Australasian emergency departments consists of a wall-mounted flow meter capable of delivering oxygen up to 15 L/min, with most available oxygen delivery systems connecting to this apparatus. A 15 L/min flow rate limits the delivery of high F_IO_2 to adults for the following reasons:

- The quietly breathing adult has a peak inspiratory flow rate (PIFR) of approximately 30–40 L/min, which exceeds the oxygen supply. Hence a free flowing system, such as a Hudson mask, must entrain air into the system in order to match the patient's PIFR, with a resultant reduction in F_IO_2 to a maximum of 0.6
- The quietly breathing adult has a respiratory minute volume of 4–8 L; in a child, this value is approximately 150 mL/kg. Oxygen is stored during expiration by incorporating a reservoir into the circuit for use during inspiration, with a considerable improvement in the economy of oxygen use. This system is limited by the patient's minute volume. If the minute volume exceeds 15 L, there is a danger of the patient asphyxiating due to insufficient gas supply and, if safety valves allow air into the system, the F_IO_2 falls.

CRITICAL CARE

2

Multiple-port oxygen supply outlets can overcome the above limitations of inspiratory flow rate and minute volume. The use of 'Y' connectors and 'T' pieces enable 30, 45 or 60 L per minute to be delivered to the patient to achieve an F_iO_2 of nearly 1.0, however, these systems can be untidy, using multiple hoses.

More efficient control of flow is achieved via higher output or dial-up flow meters. Extra source oxygen flow may cause variable-performance systems such as the Hudson mask to become fixed-performance systems. Hence the terms 'variable performance' and 'fixed performance' are loosely applied and are largely dependent on whether or not the gas flow delivered is sufficient to match the patient's ventilatory requirements.

An example of this is in paediatric oxygen delivery. A high F_iO_2 can be delivered using a standard 15 L/min oxygen source because the child's ventilatory requirements are smaller in proportion to the available oxygen supply.

The oxygen delivery systems available for use in emergency medicine, summarized in Box 2.2.1, can be further subdivided according to economy of oxygen use and whether or not the system can be used to ventilate the patient manually.

Variable-performance systems

The F_iO_2 delivered by these systems is summarized in Table 2.2.1. Options available for use in emergency medicine include:

- nasal cannulae
- face-masks with air inlets, with or without reservoirs
- T pieces and Y connectors.

Nasal cannulae

The system must be used at flow rates of 4 L/ min or less to avoid painful drying of the nasal mucosa, although a flow rate of 2 L/min or less is insufficient to create a nasopharyngeal reservoir during the expiration pause, ready for inspiration with the next breath.

The inspired oxygen concentration is a function of the patient's inspiratory flow rate and is usually in the vicinity of 22–28%. At flow rates of 2–4 L/min, the nasopharynx acts as a partial reservoir during the expiratory pause, resulting in an increased F_iO_2. The delivered F_iO_2 is then influenced by the pattern of breathing (mouth or nose) and the positioning of the nasal cannula.

Nasal cannulae provide a higher F_iO_2 in paediatric patients and nose breathers. They are less effective in dyspnoeic patients because of the greater amounts of air inspired through the mouth. They are frequently used in patients with *stable* COPD because of the absence of dead space that prevents CO_2 rebreathing. However, fluctuations in F_iO_2 make nasal cannulae less than ideal in the management of patients who rely on hypoxic respiratory drive and they are second choice after Venturi masks in the emergency management of these patients.

If nasal cannulae are used, there should be strict titration of flow rates to a target S_aO_2. Advantages for ward or home therapy include the ability to eat and drink, less noise than masks, and economy of oxygen use.

Face-masks (e.g. Hudson, Edinburgh, Medishield)

A small reservoir of oxygen is provided by these masks, but this has little effect on F_iO_2. The small increase in dead space created by the mask necessitates a flow rate greater than 6 L/ min to prevent rebreathing of CO_2. Two factors influence the F_iO_2 provided by this system:

- patient's inspiratory flow rate
- source oxygen supply flow rate.

At flow rates of 6–14 L/min, the delivered F_iO_2 varies from 0.35 to 0.6. This will be less in a dyspnoeic patient because of the higher inspiratory flow rate and greater in a child as the converse applies. If the PIFR increases, greater amounts of air will be entrained into the mask, diluting the oxygen. During expiration, the exhaled gas and excess oxygen are vented through the side perforations.

Attaching a reservoir bag to this mask improves the economy of oxygen use by storing these vented gases during the expiratory phase. This increases the delivered F_iO_2, but this may be at the expense of increased CO_2 rebreathing. Commercially available reservoir bags have a volume of 750 mL to 1 L, which is inadequate for a dyspnoeic patient. The author recommends a minimum flow rate of 12 L/min to avoid CO_2 retention.

Using a source oxygen supply of 15 L/min, the maximum F_iO_2 delivered via a Hudson mask to a quietly breathing adult is 0.6. By attaching another source of oxygen using a T piece or Y connector, the resultant flow rate of 30 L/min can deliver an F_iO_2 up to 0.8. With even greater flow rates, the mask may be converted into a fixed-performance system delivering an F_iO_2 of almost 1.0. Then the ability to deliver 100% oxygen is limited by the mask's 'fit'.

The Medishield mask is stated to be more efficient than the Hudson because dead space is reduced by bringing the oxygen supply closer to the mouth, allowing more effective entrainment during inspiration. An F_iO_2 of 0.75 may be obtained with a gas flow rate of 15 L/min.

T pieces and Y connectors

The term 'T piece' has been used to describe a number of different oxygen delivery systems, including the T piece for supplying humidified oxygen to patients with a tracheostomy and the 'Ayre's T piece' which is a Mapleson E circuit. The use of T pieces or Y connectors in emergency medicine is to supplement an existing oxygen supply with:

- extra oxygen
- nebulized medication
- humidification.

The disadvantage of the system is that several oxygen ports are necessary, which is untidy and may restrict the patient's mobility. There is loss of economy of oxygen use because of higher flow rates. T pieces allow a higher F_iO_2 to be delivered to severely dyspnoeic patients.

Fixed-performance systems

Two systems are available for use in emergency departments:

- high-flow Venturi masks
- oxygen blenders.

Table 2.2.1 Variable-performance oxygen delivery systems		
Apparatus	*Oxygen flow (L/min)*	*Oxygen concentration (%)*
Nasal catheters	1–4	24–40
Semi-rigid mask	6–15	35–60
Semi-rigid mask + double O_2 supply	15–30	Up to 80
Semi-rigid mask + reservoir bag	12–15	60–90

High-flow Venturi mask

Oxygen flow through a Venturi system results in air entrainment with delivery of a fixed concentration of oxygen to the patient. The masks deliver F_IO_2 values from 0.24, 0.28, 0.35, 0.40 and 0.50 to 0.60, using different colour-coded adaptors or by varying the position of a dial on the mask connector. Many studies have assessed their accuracy. The patient receives the stated F_IO_2 provided the total flow rate exceeds 60 L/min or is 30% higher than the patient's PIFR. As the patient's PIFR increases, the system's performance becomes variable.

In supplying an F_IO_2 of 0.24 using 6 L/min oxygen flow rate, the total flow rate delivered to the patient is 120 L/min. This falls to 30 L/min total flow for $F_IO_2 = 0.6$ using 15 L/min oxygen supply. This is just equal to the PIFR of a quietly breathing adult and unlikely to be sufficient to provide consistent performance in delivery of the stated F_IO_2. In severe dyspnoea, these masks may therefore not deliver the stated F_IO_2.

Increasing the oxygen flow rate above the manufacturer's recommendations will increase the total gas flow to the mask, while maintaining the stipulated F_IO_2. At very high-flow rates, however, turbulence is likely to reduce the performance of the system.

Venturi masks provide the best means of managing a patient with chronic obstructive pulmonary disease in the ED because they provide a predictable F_IO_2 and the air entrained is more humid than fresh oxygen (see below). The entrained gas mixture can be further heated and humidified to assist with sputum clearance. High gas flows minimize rebreathing of CO_2 and claustrophobia, but cause problems with sleeping due to noise.

Oxygen blenders

Air is blended with oxygen from a number of inlet ports to supply a fixed F_IO_2 to the patient. It is a high-flow system and fine-tuning of F_IO_2 from 0.21 to 1.0 is possible. The resultant mixture can then be channelled to the patient through systems such as continuous positive airways pressure or humidifiers. Lack of portability and high cost are disadvantages. Oxygen blenders are best suited to the resuscitation room and critical-care setting.

100% oxygen delivery systems

These systems vary in their economy of oxygen use and are summarized in Table 2.2.2. The least economical is the free-flowing system as it can only deliver 100% oxygen if the flow rate exceeds the patient's PIFR. Incorporating a reservoir and unidirectional valves into the circuit enables greater economy of oxygen use by storing oxygen during expiration ready for the inspiratory phase.

Devices incorporating a reservoir into the circuit are capable of delivering 100% oxygen only when the total oxygen flow equals or exceeds the patient's respiratory minute volume (RMV), plus there are no leaks in the system. The reservoir volume must exceed the patient's tidal volume, otherwise storage of oxygen is inefficient, fresh gas loss occurs when the reservoir is full, and there is the risk of asphyxia during inspiration.

A demand valve system delivers precisely the patient's minute volume without the added bulk and problems of a reservoir. It is able to cope with changes in RMV provided fresh gas flow always exceeds the patient's PIFR. Closed-circuit systems are the most economical in oxygen consumption. Carbon dioxide is absorbed by soda lime and low-flow fresh oxygen replaces that consumed during metabolism, which is approximately 250–1000 mL/min, which is considerably less than the patient's RMV.

Classification

One hundred per cent oxygen-delivery systems available for use in emergency medicine are summarized in Table 2.2.2.

Free-flowing circuits

Flow rates in excess of the patient's PIFR are required to provide 100% oxygen using a free-flowing system, which necessitates the use of multiple oxygen ports. The system may not deliver 100% oxygen, is wasteful of oxygen and may be untidy, restricting patient mobility for investigations. Sophisticated free-flowing systems using oxygen blenders and humidification are available, but restrict the ability to move the patient.

Soft reservoir circuits

These are non-rebreathing systems incorporating unidirectional valves to channel fresh

Table 2.2.2	Classification of 100% oxygen systems				
System	*Rebreathing of gases*	*Fresh gas flow to deliver 100% O₂*	*Use for spontaneous and/or manual ventilation*	*Comments*	
Free-flowing systems	Non-rebreathing	45–90 L/min	Spontaneous	High fresh gas flow prevents CO_2 rebreathing	
Soft reservoir bag circuit	Non-rebreathing	7–15 L/min	Spontaneous	Can increase to 15–30 L/min with Y connectors to maintain $F_IO_2 = 1.0$	
Self-refilling resuscitators (Laerdal, Air Viva)	Non-rebreathing	15 L/min	Spontaneous/manual	Manual ventilation possible with air if no oxygen available. $F_IO_2 < 1.0$ if minute volume exceeds O_2 flow	
Demand valve system (Oxy Viva III)	Non-rebreathing	Delivers up to 120 L/min for inspiration only Usual RMV = 7–15 L/min	Spontaneous/manual	Actual delivered volume of O_2 equals minute volume	
Mapleson circuits	Partial rebreathing	15–40 L/min	Spontaneous/manual	Fresh gas flow must be at least double minute volume to avoid CO_2 build-up	
Oxy resuscitator	Closed circuit rebreathing	0.5–2 L/min	Spontaneous/manual	Requires intermittent purging of reservoir to remove exhaled nitrogen from functional residual capacity	

oxygen to the patient and exhaled gas to the atmosphere. With one oxygen supply port the system delivers 100% oxygen, provided the patient's minute volume is less than 15 L/min. Higher flow first stage regulators or two oxygen supply ports enable delivery of up to 30 L/min. Fresh gas flow is titrated to the patient's minute volume by watching the reservoir bag, which should be fully distended at the start of inspiration and more than one-third full when inspiration is complete.

The reservoir bag has a minimum volume of 3 L and, for optimal performance, the patient's tidal volume should not exceed 2 L. A soft silicone mask is strapped to the head to ensure a firm but comfortable fit without leaks. The system cannot be used to ventilate patients manually and may be hazardous if the patient has an impaired conscious state owing to the risk of aspiration if they vomit and asphyxiation if there is a fall in fresh gas flow or a sudden rise in minute volume. Complications are avoided with clinical vigilance and the use of safety valves to entrain air if the oxygen supply ceases.

Self-refilling, non-rebreathing resuscitators (Air Viva and Laerdal systems)

Most Australasian emergency departments possess at least one type of self-refilling system. They can be used to ventilate a patient manually as well as allowing spontaneous ventilation. The Laerdal system has three sizes for adults, children and infants, whereas the Air Viva system has one size for adults only (Table 2.2.3).

Advantages

- Self-inflation and hence the ability to ventilate patients with air if oxygen supply is exhausted.
- Low-resistance unidirectional valves prevent rebreathing of CO_2.

Table 2.2.3 Self-refilling, non-rebreathing resuscitators		
	Self-refilling bag volume (mL)	Reservoir bag volume
Air Viva	1700	2300
Laerdal (Adult)	1600	2600
Laerdal (Child)	500	2600
Laerdal (Infant)	240	600

- Use in spontaneously ventilating patients and for manual ventilation.
- System is capable of delivering $F_iO_2 = 1.0$ provided fresh gas flow exceeds minute volume and the reservoir bag is attached. Without the reservoir bag, a maximum F_iO_2 of 0.6 is obtainable.
- A safety valve entrains air into the system to prevent asphyxiation if there is a sudden rise in minute volume, but this is at the expense of F_iO_2.
- Over-pressure relief valves are incorporated into the Laerdal paediatric and infant apparatus to prevent barotrauma in these patients.
- Addition of positive end-expiratory pressure (PEEP) to the system is possible by attaching a PEEP valve to the expiratory limb. Close apposition of the mask to the face or endotracheal intubation is required for this to be effective.

Disadvantages

- Reduction in F_iO_2 occurs when minute volume exceeds fresh gas flow. Dual oxygen supply ports can minimize this problem, especially in an extremely dyspnoeic patient.
- Unit is bulky and disconnections sometimes occur.
- There is less 'feel' during manual ventilation than with soft bag circuits. Inflation of the stomach is more likely during bag/mask ventilation, especially if there is airway obstruction or reduced pulmonary compliance.

Oxygen-powered resuscitators

Examples of this type of system include the Oxy Viva, Laerdal and DAN demand valve systems. High-pressure oxygen is fed to a demand valve which delivers high-flow oxygen to the patient. The system can be used in a spontaneously breathing patient and, for manual ventilation, by depressing a manual override button. Spontaneously ventilating patients initiate an oxygen flow of up to 120 L/min by generating a negative pressure of 0.3 kPa (2.25 mmHg) at the start of inspiration. Fresh gas flow is delivered at a pressure of up to 5.3 kPa (40 mmHg).

Advantages

- Portability, as it is easy to attach to an oxygen cylinder and take to the field. There are no bulky reservoir bags.

- Economy of oxygen use as the patient's minute volume is precisely delivered at sufficient flow rates to match the PIFR. Provided there are no leaks, the system delivers $F_iO_2 = 1.0$.

Disadvantages

- Increased work of breathing for spontaneous ventilation as negative pressure must be generated to initiate oxygen flow.
- System cannot function when fresh gas supply is exhausted.
- During manual ventilation, it is almost impossible to judge ventilatory volume except by observing the patient's chest. The safety over-pressure relief valve may not prevent barotrauma, especially in children.
- Lack of 'feel' during manual ventilation may lead to over-inflation of the stomach if there is airway obstruction or reduced pulmonary compliance.

Mapleson circuits

Mapleson circuits are still used in some emergency departments. Partial rebreathing of gases occurs with all of the circuits but CO_2 retention can be avoided if fresh gas flow exceeds minute volume by a ratio of 2–2.5:1.

The most commonly used versions are the Mapleson B and the Mapleson F, which are covered under paediatric considerations. Mapleson A, C, D and E circuits are not discussed further.

Advantages of the Mapleson B circuit

- Used for both spontaneous and manual ventilation. Its performance is similar in both circumstances.
- Soft bag has excellent 'feel' for manual ventilation and it is easy to monitor spontaneous ventilation by observing the filling and emptying of the reservoir bag.

Disadvantages

- Carbon dioxide build-up with lower oxygen flow rates. This can be avoided with higher flow rates or by intermittently purging the reservoir bag.
- System cannot function without a fresh gas supply.
- May be difficult to use when ventilating a patient manually using a mask.
- Valve assembly may occasionally 'stick'.

Closed-circuit systems

An example is the MD Oxyresuscitator. The circuit is the same as the Boyle's anaesthetic circle system. A soda lime canister absorbs exhaled CO_2 and a low-flow oxygen supply replaces oxygen consumed by metabolism at approximately 0.5–2 L/min. Considerable economy of oxygen use is thus achieved by rebreathing from the circuit.

Advantages

- Economy of oxygen use. More than 6 hours of oxygen can be provided by a 'C'-sized oxygen cylinder at 1 L/min. This markedly exceeds the endurance of the cylinder using other systems.
- Can be used for spontaneous or manual ventilation. A soft reservoir bag provides excellent 'feel' for ventilation.
- Pressure on the system is controlled by the operator during manual ventilation. This minimizes gastric distension.
- Portable and can easily be taken to the field.

Disadvantages

- Circuit ceases to function when fresh gas flow is exhausted.
- Exhaled nitrogen from the patient's early breaths may enter the circuit and reduce F_IO_2 below 1.0. This is prevented by intermittent purging of the reservoir.
- CO_2 may accumulate if the soda lime canister is old or stops functioning.
- Incorrect packing of the soda lime canister may result in inhalation of soda lime dust (which is extremely rare).
- Reservoir bag is remote from the patient mask and the system may be cumbersome to operate.

Helium and oxygen mixtures

Over the last decade, there has been interest in adding helium to oxygen (maximum 30% oxygen, also known as 'Heliox'). Heliox has a lower density than air with the potential to reduce airway resistance and hence the work of breathing when treating disease processes such as COPD and asthma.

Helium (He, MW = 4) is much lighter than nitrogen and therefore significantly lowers the density of the gas mix when combined with oxygen in the range of $F_IO_2 = 0.2$–0.4. This advantage is lost when $F_IO_2 > 0.4$. Despite

lower density, the viscosity of Heliox is not significantly lower than that of air. Its main theoretical advantage is if there is turbulent gas flow that is density dependent. This may occur with COPD where there is a combination of small and medium airways disease. Early studies also suggested that Heliox may enhance nebulizer particles in the lung; however, greater flow rates may be required to drive the nebulizer. Despite the potential advantages, the clinical evidence for use in COPD is not strong.

Cochrane reviews of the topic concluded that there is insufficient evidence to support the routine use of Heliox to treat COPD exacerbations or exacerbations of asthma. However, the review of adults and children with asthma did conclude that Heliox may improve pulmonary function when there is more severe obstruction. Most of the studies of Heliox for asthma have assessed it as a driver of nebulizer therapy rather than for continuous administration.

Of the two studies of Heliox therapy for COPD assessed in the Cochrane review, only one study included acutely decompensated patients in the ED. This study failed to show a benefit from Heliox when it was used to drive nebulized β-agonist therapy. Further randomized studies using Heliox are needed in asthma and COPD, both continuously and as a driver for nebulizer therapy, with hard endpoints such as physiological parameters, response to nebulized β-agonists, need for non-invasive ventilation or intubation and admission rates.

Measurement of oxygenation

Clinical assessment of oxygenation is unreliable and the time-honoured sign of cyanosis varies with the level of haemoglobin, skin pigmentation, perfusion and external light. Arterial blood gases and pulse oximetry provide an objective measurement of oxygenation and enable precise titration of oxygen therapy to the clinical situation.

Pulse oximetry

Pulse oximetry is the most frequently used indicator of oxygenation in emergency medicine as it is non-invasive. It is regarded as the 'fifth vital sign' and provides continuous real-time assessment of a patient's oxygenation and response to therapy. It has a proven role in emergency medicine and is an excellent clinical tool, provided the limitations are understood.

It is important to recognize that SaO_2 is not an adequate marker of ventilatory function and will not detect rising $PaCO_2$ in respiratory failure or a sedated patient until late, when conscious state becomes depressed or there is respiratory arrest. Hence all patients with potential respiratory compromise due to disease or sedative medication require careful monitoring of vital signs, conscious state and CO_2 via end-tidal CO_2 monitoring or arterial blood gases. Recent literature suggests a fall in SaO_2 may precede CO_2 accumulation during procedural sedation and analgesia in children.

A detailed knowledge of the haemoglobin–oxygen dissociation curve is required to interpret pulse oximetry, as well as the factors that influence readings obtained by this equipment. These factors are summarized in Table 2.2.4.

Paediatric considerations in oxygen therapy

The general principles of oxygen therapy and its indications apply equally well for children as for adults, but there are a number of important differences in relation to body size, psychology and oxygen toxicity.

Body size

Children are smaller than adults both anatomically and physiologically, so that any increase in equipment dead space will significantly increase CO_2 retention. Children are less able to tolerate increased resistance to ventilation, particularly if negative pressure must be generated to open valves in the apparatus.

Peak inspiratory flow rate and respiratory minute volume are lower; hence, a given oxygen supply flow rate will produce a higher F_IO_2 in a child than in an adult. A Hudson mask at 8 L/min may supply an F_IO_2 of 0.8 in a young child. Reservoir bags are not required to deliver F_IO_2 values near 1.0 to children weighing less than 15 kg as available supply flow rates (maximum 15 L/min) exceed the child's PIFR.

Appropriately sized equipment is essential: a range of sizes of oxygen masks, oximeter probes, laryngoscopes and endotracheal tubes must be available to manage children of different ages as serious barotrauma may result from the use of excessive volume during manual ventilation. Resuscitator bags are available with paediatric-sized reservoirs. The Laerdal system has both paediatric and infant sizes. These units also have a pressure relief

Table 2.2.4   Factors that influence pulse oximetry readings

Factor	Cause
Signal interference	High-intensity external light source
	Diathermy
	Shivering/movement of digit
Reduced light transmission	Dark-coloured nail polish
	Dirt (NB: melanin pigment/jaundice have no effect)
Reduction in plethysmographic volume	Peripheral vasoconstriction (shock, hypothermia)
Inaccurate readings due to abnormal haemoglobin	COHb causes overestimation as is not distinguished from O_2Hb
	Methaemoglobin >10% causes oximeter to read 85% saturation, regardless of true O_2 saturation
	Profound anaemia – insufficient haemoglobin for accurate signal
Falsely low readings	Intravenous dyes with absorption spectra near 660 nm, e.g. methylene blue
	Stagnation of blood flow

valve designed to prevent barotrauma. Pressure rapidly rises as the child's lung reaches full inflation.

Jackson–Rees (Mapleson F) circuit

A smaller Mapleson circuit, the Jackson–Rees (Mapleson F) circuit, is available to ventilate children, which can be used for both spontaneous and manual ventilation. Rebreathing of carbon dioxide does not occur provided the fresh gas flow is 2–3 times minute volume and the bag is separated from the patient by a tube of internal volume greater than the patient's tidal volume. The overall relationship between fresh gas flow, minute volume and $PaCO_2$ is complex.

The principal advantages over the Laerdal system are that the operator can observe bag movement in spontaneous respiration and has a better 'feel' for airway obstruction in manual ventilation. However, considerable skill and experience are required to use the system safely.

Psychological considerations

Gaining the trust and confidence of an ill child is an art learnt with experience. They frequently respond with fear when oxygen therapy is administered, so it is helpful to ask a parent to nurse the child during treatment. A tight-fitting mask is less important in a child because source flow rate more closely approximates PIFR. Parents may assist by holding the oxygen mask close to the child's face or by directing high-flow oxygen straight at the child's mouth using a tube only. A cupped hand with the oxygen tube held between middle and ring fingers can serve as a surrogate oxygen 'mask'.

Oxygen toxicity

Prolonged administration of oxygen at F_IO_2 >0.6 for longer than 24 hours may be toxic to infants. This toxicity may not become apparent during their acute stay in the emergency department, but the oxygen dose received there contributes to the cumulative toxicity. Appropriate monitoring using pulse oximetry ensures administration of the correct dose and minimizes the risk of toxicity. However, supplemental oxygen should never be withheld because of fear of toxicity.

Transfer of patients on oxygen therapy

Supplemental oxygen therapy is a vital part of transporting the ill patient and is especially important for air travel where lower ambient P_IO_2 may exacerbate hypoxia already present as a result of the patient's disease process. Patients with decompression illness or arterial gas embolism should not be transported at cabin pressures lower than 101.3 kPa (1 atmosphere absolute, ATA) because lower ambient pressure exacerbates their disease process by increasing bubble size. A number of factors must be considered for successful oxygen therapy during transport of a patient.

Knowledge of the oxygen delivery apparatus and its maximum rate of delivery are essential for estimating transport oxygen requirements. These estimates must take into account current oxygen consumption, duration of transport (including delays), oxygen required in the event of deterioration and a safety factor of at least 50%.

The sizes of oxygen cylinders available in Australasia, their filling pressures and approximate endurances are summarized in Table 2.2.5. The most economical circuit for prolonged transport with $F_IO_2 = 1.0$ is a closed circuit with a CO_2 absorber and the least economical is a free-flowing circuit.

Monitoring during transport should be of the same standard as that initiated in the emergency department. Pulse oximetry is an essential tool to detect hypoxia during transport and should include audible and visual alarms. Oxygen therapy can be titrated against SaO_2, which is particularly important in air travel where P_IO_2 varies with ascent and descent. All the usual clinical parameters must also be monitored.

Oxygen therapy in specific circumstances

Asthma

Hypoxia in asthma results from ventilation–perfusion mismatch created by bronchospasm, secretions and airway inflammation and oedema. Supplemental oxygen should be titrated to provide an SaO_2 >90% (preferably 94%) and must be continued during the interval between doses of inhaled bronchodilators.

Initial management should include a Hudson mask at 8 L/min flow rate, with SaO_2 monitored continuously by pulse oximetry. The oxygen dose should be rapidly increased up to 100% if the patient remains hypoxic. Bronchodilator therapy is administered proportionate to the severity of the attack, using oxygen to drive the nebulizer. Oxygen should not be withheld or administered in low doses for fear of respiratory depression. Hypercapnia is an indication of extreme airway obstruction and its presence mandates aggressive therapy and/or mechanical ventilation.

Mechanical ventilation in asthma

Mechanical ventilation requires an $F_IO_2 = 1.0$, high inspiratory flow rate (100 L/min), low tidal

Table 2.2.5 Oxygen cylinder sizes for patient transport

Cylinder size	Water capacity (kg)	Volume at 15 000 kPa 15°C (L)	Approximate endurance at		
			8 L/min	15 L/min	30 L/min
C	2.8	420	52 min	28 min	14 min
D	9.5	1387	173 min	92 min	46 min
E	23.8	3570	446 min	238 min	119 min
G	48	7200	900 min	480 min	240 min

volume (6–8 mL/kg), a prolonged I:E ratio of at least 1:3 and a low ventilation rate (6–10 breaths/min or less), to reduce the risks of progressive dynamic hyperinflation with the development of auto-PEEP (iPEEP) reducing venous return and hence preload, and of barotrauma with the development of a pneumothorax. Permissive hypercapnia is accepted with mechanical ventilation.

Occasionally, patients with asthma become hypoxic during nebulizer therapy because the oxygen flow rates driving the nebulizer (6–8 L/min) are lower than the flow rate required to maintain SaO_2 >90%. In these circumstances, extra oxygen is supplied to maintain SaO_2 via a T piece or Y connector during nebulizer therapy.

Chronic obstructive pulmonary disease

Most ED patients with COPD have a degree of acute respiratory failure that caused their emergency presentation. This may be due to infection, bronchospasm, retention of secretions, coexistent left ventricular failure, worsening right heart failure, pulmonary embolism, pneumothorax, sedation or reduction of regular therapy, such as inhaled or oral steroids. Clues to the degree of severity and chronicity of the COPD are obtained from the patient's history, past clinical records, emergency department blood gases and the response to initial oxygen therapy.

Clinical indicators of patients at risk of CO_2 retention include a housebound patient, FEV_1 <1 L, polycythaemia, a warm vasodilated periphery and cor pulmonale. In the acutely unwell patient, treatment may be required before the history can be obtained.

COPD groups
Patients with COPD fall into two groups as regards management, although this classification is still debated.

- Normal ventilatory response to CO_2 ('can't breathe' – the most common). Gas exchange and air flow into the lungs are impaired, but ventilatory drive is normal.
- Impaired ventilatory response to CO_2 ('won't breathe' – less common). Ventilation does not increase in response to hypercapnia and acidosis.

There is overlap between the advanced stages of illness. The aims of oxygen therapy are targeted to produce SaO_2 of 88–90% and to identify the second group of patients such that the oxygen dose can be titrated to achieve an acceptable clinical response without excessive elevation of $PaCO_2$. Serial arterial blood gas analysis is essential in their management.

The majority will have a normal ventilatory response to CO_2. Hypercapnia indicates that ventilatory failure is developing, with a danger of respiratory arrest if the patient's disease is severe and progressive. This can also result from uncontrolled oxygen therapy with failure to monitor the patient's clinical status and arterial blood gases. Any patient with impaired consciousness due to respiratory failure should be manually ventilated while being clinically assessed and treated.

Controlled titration of oxygen dose in COPD
Successful management of the cooperative patient with COPD necessitates controlled titration of oxygen dose. Variable-performance oxygen masks do not have a role in the emergency management of COPD, unless there is careful monitoring of SaO_2 and $ETCO_2$. A consistent initial approach to oxygen therapy for a conscious patient with advanced COPD is used as, at the time of presentation, their ventilatory response to CO_2 is unknown.

In most patients, the administration of 24–28% oxygen by Venturi mask will improve oxygenation, with a target SaO_2 of about 88–92%. It is also acceptable initially to titrate oxygen therapy to a target SaO_2 range. A recent Australian pre-hospital randomized clinical trial (RCT) showed lower mortality for patients with COPD if they received oxygen by nasal prongs titrated to SaO_2 range ≈88–92%. All nebulizer therapy was administered by air.

Below 90% saturation, the Hb–O_2 dissociation curve falls steeply and, unless a pulmonary shunt is present, even small increments in oxygen will make a positive difference. The patient's response to initial oxygen therapy (F_IO_2 = 0.24–0.28) will direct further oxygen dose changes and identify any patients not already known to be suffering chronic hypercapnia.

A repeat blood gas sample should be taken after 10 minutes of breathing F_IO_2 = 0.24–0.28. The $PaCO_2$ may rise slightly because of the 'Haldane effect'. If this rise is excessive (>1–1.3 kPa [8–10 mmHg]), it is consistent with an impaired ventilatory response to CO_2. The F_IO_2 should then be adjusted downwards in steps to achieve a satisfactory pulse oximetry reading that is compatible with an acceptable CO_2 level. In a patient with COPD, an acceptable range for SaO_2 is 88–92%.

Blood gas sampling in COPD
Blood gas samples taken during the initial assessment of these patients (breathing air or controlled oxygen) assists management. Venous samples are acceptable, provided they are used consistently to monitor trends. If the bicarbonate level is >30 mmol/L or is elevated by more than 4 mmol/L for each 1.3 kPa (10 mmHg) rise in $PaCO_2$ above normal (5.3 kPa, 40 mmHg), this provides strong evidence of chronic hypercapnia, provided there is no cause of a metabolic alkalosis.

Management in COPD
Patients with a normal ventilatory response to CO_2 will not exhibit a significant elevation of $PaCO_2$ in response to oxygen therapy. If hypoxaemia persists and the $PaCO_2$ remains stable, then the oxygen dose may be increased incrementally until the desired oxygen saturation is achieved. A lower than normal SaO_2 (≈88%) and PaO_2 (≈56 mmHg) may be acceptable provided the patient remains conscious and cooperative.

Non-invasive positive-pressure ventilation (NIPPV) is indicated if the patient remains hypoxic or becomes progressively more hypoxic and the elevation of $PaCO_2$ persists or worsens or their conscious state deteriorates. Intubation and ventilation may be required, which should be regarded as a last resort (and will not be covered). Supplemental oxygen should never be abruptly withdrawn from a patient with COPD as a catastrophic fall in PaO_2 will occur. All reductions in controlled oxygen dose should be in a stepwise manner, similar to incremental increases.

In the majority of cases, an acceptable balance between PaO_2 and $PaCO_2$ can be achieved, where both hypoxia and hypercarbia are reversed by specific therapy. Treating the cause of the ventilatory failure is a priority.

A pilot study showed that short-term administration of bronchodilators using oxygen-driven nebulizers in the acute management of chronically hypercapnic patients may be safe. Caution is advised, as some authors suggest that COPD is still poorly managed in the emergency department with respect to oxygen dose. Interestingly, the authors of that paper offered only limited practical advice on the titrated use of oxygen in the acute management of COPD and did not differentiate between COPD patients with an acute elevation of CO_2 and those with chronic elevation. The authors of the pre-hospital RCT were more specific, titrating to a target SaO_2.

Goal-directed oxygen therapy

The oxygen dose in the initial management of many medical conditions including myocardial infarction, asthma and even pneumonia has been questioned. A recent Cochrane review of oxygen therapy for myocardial infarction claimed oxygen may be harmful. This conclusion was based on a non-significant analysis, dominated by a 1976 trial (86% of the weighting). That trial contained many clinical deficiencies not reflective of modern practice (e.g. diagnostic criteria, no intravenous glyceryl trinitrate (GTN) or reperfusion therapy, not monitoring oxygen saturations and no blood gases and use of gas flow rates known to cause CO_2 accumulation). The authors correctly suggested that oxygen treatment for myocardial infarction should be further evaluated in a larger trial.

One recent trial suggested that high concentration oxygen therapy caused a greater rise in CO_2 in adults presenting with community-acquired pneumonia, compared with titrated dose oxygen. The study did not examine clinical outcomes. Another area of interest is oxygen dose for asthma. Perrins et al. using transcutaneous (tc) CO_2 monitoring demonstrated that high concentration oxygen therapy led to clinically significant increases in $P_{tc}CO_2$, compared to the titrated dose oxygen therapy. The high concentration group had 4.5 times greater gradient of increasing $P_{tc}CO_2$ and over twice the odds of requiring admission. Current trends in clinical evidence suggest that oxygen should be treated in the same way as any other drug, that is to provide the optimum dosage appropriately titrated to the clinical needs of the patient. Goal-directed oxygen therapy is no different in principle with available clinical monitoring systems to many other therapies for physiological disturbance.

Special delivery systems

Oxygen humidification

Humidification may be desirable when prolonged use (>6 h) of supplemental oxygen is required as oxygen is totally dry, possessing no water vapour. Humidification is particularly important in a patient ventilated with an endotracheal tube as the natural humidification that occurs in the nose, mouth and nasopharynx is bypassed. Patients with COPD and retained secretions benefit from humidification.

Additional heat is required to provide effective humidification by vaporization of water. Various systems are available to humidify inspired gas and, ideally, they should be able to deliver inspired gas to the trachea at 32–36°C with low resistance and at greater than 90% humidity. These devices should be simple to use and able to maintain temperature and humidity at varying gas flows and F_IO_2. There should also be safety alarms monitoring temperature and humidity.

Humidification of warmed inspired gas also enables heat transfer to hypothermic patients and is essential in treating the pulmonary complications of near drowning. Dry oxygen will exacerbate hypothermia. There are a number of commercial humidifiers available that provide humidification by heating coils with a large surface area for contact with inspired gas.

Continuous positive airways pressure

Continuous positive airways pressure (CPAP) has a role in the management of pulmonary oedema, pneumonia, bronchiolitis, respiratory tract burns and acute respiratory failure. Benefit to the patient is achieved as a result of increasing functional residual capacity and reduced pulmonary compliance. Hypoxaemia is reversed by reduction in intrapulmonary shunting and the work of breathing is reduced.

Circuit designs for CPAP

Circuit designs usually consist of a reservoir based on the Mapleson D circuit or a high-flow turbine system. Humidification can be added to the system and is considered essential for long-term use (>6 h). Use of an oxygen blender enables variable F_IO_2 to be administered. CPAP has a proven role in the emergency department in the acute management of cardiogenic pulmonary oedema. Reduced requirements for endotracheal intubation have been demonstrated when CPAP is used for severely ill patients. Complications of CPAP include aspiration and pulmonary barotrauma. It may elevate intracranial pressure and precipitate hypotension by reducing venous return to the thorax.

Hyperbaric oxygen treatment

Hyperbaric oxygen (HBO) treatment consists of administering oxygen at pressures greater than 1 ATA, usually in the range of 2.0–2.8 ATA. This requires a hyperbaric chamber which is pressurized with air while the patient breathes an $F_IO_2 = 1.0$ from various delivery systems for periods of 2–7 hours. The high P_IO_2 results in PaO_2 of up to 267 kPa (2000 mmHg) if 2.8 ATA treatment pressure is used. This is beneficial, as there is increased dissolved oxygen in the plasma (up to 300 mL oxygen may be carried to the periphery each minute in the dissolved form), which maintains oxygen flux even if haemoglobin is non-functional, for instance in carbon monoxide poisoning. Increased P_IO_2 enables more rapid elimination of toxic gases from the body, for example carbon monoxide or hydrogen sulphide.

Uses of hyperbaric oxygen

HBO treatment has a number of benefits in treating gas embolism and decompression illness (DCI). It provides extra oxygen to tissues rendered ischaemic by nitrogen bubbles and the increased pressure reduces bubble size and enhances nitrogen removal from the body. The increased PO_2 also creates a greater driving pressure of oxygen into ischaemic tissues in problem wounds and reduces swelling by vasoconstriction in crush injury. In addition, HBO treatment is used in anaerobic infections by virtue of being bacteriostatic to anaerobes, inhibiting clostridial α toxin and stimulating

Table 2.2.6 Indications for acute treatment with hyperbaric oxygen

Decompression illness Air or gas embolism Carbon monoxide poisoning
Gas gangrene and anaerobic fasciitis Necrotizing soft tissue infections
Acute crush injury with compartment syndrome
Acutely compromised skin flaps or grafts, due to injury or post-surgery

host defences via granulocyte function. Recognized indications for acute referral to a hyperbaric facility for HBO treatment are summarized in Table 2.2.6 (see Chapter 28.3).

Complications of oxygen therapy

These can be classified into three categories:

- equipment-related complications
- carbon dioxide narcosis
- oxygen toxicity.

Equipment-related complications

These are entirely preventable with careful supervision and monitoring. Tight-fitting masks may cause asphyxia if there is insufficient oxygen reservoir or flow and aspiration of vomitus may occur if the patient has depressed airway reflexes. Use of appropriate oxygen flow rates with rebreathing circuits prevents CO_2 accumulation.

Barotrauma can be prevented during mechanical ventilation by the use of appropriate volumes and pressures, although it can be difficult to avoid when there is reduced lung compliance, as in the moribund asthmatic. Knowledge of potential equipment complications enables prompt intervention should they arise. When investigating a sudden deterioration in the patient's condition, a thorough check of the equipment in use is mandatory.

Carbon dioxide narcosis

This can be prevented by controlled oxygen therapy titrating the F_iO_2 against SaO_2, arterial blood gases and conscious state (see above). An unconscious patient should be intubated and manually ventilated using high F_iO_2, preferably 100% oxygen. A patient with a deteriorating conscious state and respiration due to CO_2 narcosis should be vigorously stimulated and encouraged to breathe while F_iO_2 is reduced in a stepwise manner. Oxygen should never be suddenly withdrawn as this precipitates severe hypoxia. Reversible causes of respiratory failure should be treated and non-invasive ventilation instituted.

Oxygen toxicity

Oxygen is toxic in high doses which is a function of P_iO_2 and duration of exposure. Toxicity is thought to occur by the formation of free radicals and toxic lipid peroxides, inhibition of enzyme systems and direct toxic effects on cerebral metabolism. Toxicity is mainly restricted to the respiratory system and central nervous system (CNS), although it can affect other regions such as the eye. Premature infants develop retrolental fibroplasia after prolonged exposure to high F_iO_2. CNS oxygen toxicity manifested by neuromuscular irritability and seizures (Paul Bert effect) is restricted to hyperbaric exposures.

Pulmonary oxygen toxicity (Lorrain Smith effect) is of relevance to emergency medicine, although exposures of 0.6–1 ATA for more than 24 hours are required to produce demonstrable evidence of lung injury. Acute changes such as pulmonary oedema, haemorrhage and proteinaceous exudates are reversible on withdrawal of oxygen. Longer durations of high P_iO_2 may lead to permanent pulmonary fibrosis and emphysema. Physicians should be alert to acute symptoms of cough, dyspnoea and retrosternal pain, although these are non-specific symptoms of oxygen toxicity. A progressive reduction in vital capacity may be demonstrated. As with all drugs, oxygen dose should be monitored and carefully titrated against SaO_2 and clinical effect. However, oxygen therapy should never be withheld acutely because of fear of toxicity.

Controversies/emerging issues

- Is oxygen a drug with a therapeutic window?
- Is oxygen harmful in myocardial infarction?
- Should we monitor all patients with COPD and asthma using CO_2 measuring devices?
- What is the best device for monitoring CO_2 during emergency treatment?
- Goal-directed oxygen therapy titrated to target SaO_2 for specific disease processes will be the future best practice for oxygen therapy.

Further reading

Austin MA, Wills KE, Blizzard L, et al. Effect of high flow oxygen on mortality in chronic obstructive pulmonary disease patients in prehospital setting: randomised controlled trial. Br Med J 2010;341:c5462.

Cabello JB, Burls A, Emparanza JI, et al. Oxygen therapy for acute myocardial infarction. Cochrane Database Syst Rev 2010;6:CD007160.

Fracchia G, Torda TA. Performance of Venturi oxygen delivery devices. Anaes Intens Care 1980;8:426–30.

Gesell L. Hyperbaric oxygen therapy indications. USA Undersea Hyperbaric Med Soc 2011. Kensington, Maryland.

McKenzie DK, Frith PA, Burdon JGW, et al. The COPDX Plan: Australian and New Zealand Guidelines for the management of chronic obstructive pulmonary disease. Med J Austral 2003;178:S1–S39.

O'Driscoll R. Emergency oxygen use. Br Med J 2012;345:e6856.

Perrin K, Wijesinghe M, Healy B, et al. Randomised controlled trial of high concentration versus titrated oxygen therapy in severe exacerbations of asthma. Thorax 2011;66:937–41.

Rodrigo GJ, Pollack CV, Rodrigo C, Rowe BH. Heliox for non-intubated acute asthma patients. Cochrane Database Syst Rev 2006;4:CD002884.

Rodrigo G, Pollack C, Rodrigo C, et al. Heliox for treatment of exacerbations of chronic obstructive pulmonary disease. Cochrane Database Syst Rev 2001;1:CD003571.

Sivilotti M, Messenger D, van Vlymen J, et al. A comparative evaluation of capnometry versus pulse oximetry during procedural sedation and analgesia on room air. Can J Emerg Med 2010;12:397–404.

Smart DR, Mark PD. oxygen therapy in emergency medicine. Physiology and delivery systems. Emerg Med (Fremantle) 1992;4:163–78.

West JB. Respiratory physiology – the essentials, 9th ed. Baltimore: Lippincott, Williams & Wilkins; 2012.

CRITICAL CARE

2

2.3 Haemodynamic monitoring

Liz Hickson • Craig Hore

ESSENTIALS

1 Haemodynamic monitoring includes observation of the complex physiology of blood flow, with the aim of providing data that can be used to improve patient management and outcomes.

2 Numerous methods are available that should be considered in a stepwise fashion, from simple clinical assessment to highly technical, invasive procedures, such as the pulmonary artery catheter.

3 Effective use of haemodynamic monitoring devices requires an understanding of cardiovascular physiology.

4 Currently, there is a move away from simple blood pressure measurements towards targeting end-organ perfusion and the adequacy of cardiac output.

5 Use of any monitoring technology in the emergency department (ED) must consider the time associated with its introduction, the skill levels required and the clinical benefits that are provided.

6 No monitoring modality improves outcome unless it is linked to a treatment protocol.

7 The pulmonary artery (Swan–Ganz) catheter was for many years considered a 'gold standard' for haemodynamic monitoring, but evidence suggests no improvements in patient outcome. It should therefore not be used in the ED.

8 Less invasive devices have been developed in recent years. Their role in the ED is yet to be fully elucidated.

9 Further developments will likely result in greater use of less invasive methods for haemodynamic monitoring, with an increased ability to monitor at the microcirculation and/or cellular level, and better correlation between observed events and final diagnosis.

Introduction

Haemodynamics is concerned with the physiology of blood flow and the forces involved within the circulation. *Haemodynamic monitoring* involves studying this complex physiology using various forms of technology to understand these forces and put them into a clinical context that can be used to direct therapy. The utility of basic monitoring is universally accepted. However, the maxim that '*not everything that counts can be counted and not everything that can be counted counts*' (Albert Einstein, 1879–1955) should be borne in mind.

This is particularly salient in the emergency department (ED) where the pressure of work and the diversity of patients do not allow the unlimited use of complex and expensive monitoring systems.

This chapter provides an outline of current approaches to the various technologies available for haemodynamic monitoring and their applicability in the ED. Many methods are available which should be thought of in a stepwise progression from simple clinical assessment to invasive, highly technical methods using sophisticated devices.

Historical background

As recently as 100 years ago, only temperature, pulse and respirations were measured and used to manage patients. The technology for auscultatory blood pressure measurement was available, but did not come into regular use until the 1920s.

Intensive care as a medical/nursing specialty evolved in tandem with the electronic revolution of the 1960s. At the same time, increasingly sophisticated haemodynamic and laboratory techniques vastly improved diagnosis and provided a way further to evaluate therapy. Despite these major advances in the ability to monitor multiple physiological variables, there is little evidence to suggest that they have resulted in tangible improvements in patient outcome.

Practical use of monitoring

The practical use of any monitoring device must be appropriate to the individual clinical environment. Thus, it may be reasonable to insert a pulmonary artery Swan–Ganz catheter in the intensive care unit (ICU) where the necessary time can be taken, yet impractical and potentially unsafe in a busy ED. Another consideration is that haemodynamic monitoring should only be used when the clinical outcome may be influenced and potentially improved. Once irreversible cellular damage has occurred, no benefit occurs no matter how far therapy is maximized. Further, haemodynamic monitoring may not improve patient outcome unless linked to a clinical protocol or 'goal-directed therapy'.

Clinicians should only introduce monitoring equipment that will have a direct influence on their choice of therapy, as the use of invasive monitoring carries potential risks of harm to the patient. The injudicious use of physiologically based treatment protocols may lead to worse outcomes. All monitored variables must be evaluated and applied in a manner proven to lead to benefit, in terms of both the diagnosis and the management.

Overview of cardiovascular physiology

One possible reason that haemodynamic monitoring has not been associated with improvements in outcome is the inability to understand and manipulate patients' physiology effectively.

Circulatory model

Haemodynamic data are traditionally considered in the context of a circulatory model. This model varies, but usually consists of a non-pulsatile pump and a hydraulic circuit with discrete sites of flow resistance, alongside the Frank–Starling mechanism with its concepts of preload, contractility and afterload.

Cardiac output

Cardiac output (CO) is the volume of blood pumped by the heart per unit of time, usually expressed in litres per minute (L/min). The heart operates as a pump and ejects a bolus of blood known as the *stroke volume* (SV) with each cardiac cycle. CO is the product of SV and heart rate (HR).

A complex set of interrelated physiological variables determines the magnitude of CO, including the volume of blood in the heart (*preload*), the downstream resistance to the ejection of this blood (*afterload*) and the *contractility* of the heart muscle. However, it is the *metabolic requirements* of the body that are the most potent determinant of cardiac output.

Regulation of CO

The regulation of CO is therefore complex. A single measurement represents the summation of many interacting physiological processes. Basal CO is related to body size and varies from 4 to 7 L/min in adults. This value divided by the body surface area enables comparison between patients with different body sizes, giving the *cardiac index* (CI).

Bedside methods do not measure CO directly, meaning that the values obtained are only estimates. Assessment of CO is therefore not done routinely. Indeed, misuse of CO data may worsen outcomes. The International Consensus Conference on Haemodynamic Monitoring in Shock (2007) suggested that monitoring of CO is only of value if it guides therapies to improve outcome.

Cardiac index (CI)

CI measurement is valued over simple blood pressure recording as it describes the total volume of blood flow in the circulation per unit of time and hence serves as an indicator of oxygen delivery to the tissues. The CI is also useful for understanding and manipulating the pump activity of the heart.

Role of haemodynamic monitoring in the emergency department

The role of haemodynamic monitoring in the ED is even less well defined. Given the plethora of devices but the lack of a 'gold standard', there are insufficient data to recommend any one method over another.

Recent advances in the management of sepsis include haemodynamic optimization with early goal-directed therapy (EGDT) during the pre-intensive care period, especially in the ED. The latest Surviving Sepsis Campaign guidelines published in 2013 emphasized that resuscitation of a patient with severe sepsis should begin as soon as the diagnosis is made and not be delayed until ICU admission. The use of such an approach based on strict treatment protocols has been shown to reduce morbidity and mortality (see Chapter 2.5).

Early goal-directed therapy

Although widely accepted, the application of this strategy of early goal-directed therapy in clinical practice is far from common. Obstacles include a lack of skill to perform the initial procedures and difficulty in providing the required higher level of care due to ED staffing and patient flow constraints. However, with a potential patient stay in ED of up to 24 hours with finite critical care resources, approximately 15% of critical care is being provided in this setting already.

Clinical assessment

Current guidelines on haemodynamic monitoring recommend frequent measurement of blood pressure and physical examination variables, including signs of hypoperfusion, such as reduced urine output and abnormal mental status. Clinical examination is 'low risk' yet may yield much important information, but the sensitivity and specificity are low, even when individual elements are interpreted in isolation. Also, clinical assessment of the circulatory state may be misleading.

Nevertheless, clinical assessment still has an important role in the initial assessment of a critically ill patient. Paradoxically, the development of haemodynamic measuring devices was driven by the poor ability to assess the critically ill patient clinically, yet those patients managed simply by clinical assessment may do better than those managed with invasive, complex devices.

Key properties of an 'ideal' haemodynamic monitoring system include:

- measurement of variables that are clinically relevant

- measurements that are accurate and reproducible
- measurements that are continuous
- generation of data that are clinically interpretable and useful for guiding therapy
- operation that is simple and user-independent
- operation and utility that result in clinical benefit to the patient
- operation and utility that cause no harm to the patient
- operation and utility that are cost-effective.

Clinical markers of cardiac output

The underlying issue is not what a patient's CO *is*, but rather whether this CO is *effective* for that particular patient. Trends are more important than specific, single-point values in guiding therapy. An effective CO should need no compensation and therefore a patient should have warm toes simultaneously with a normal BP and HR. One of the advantages of *clinical endpoints* is that they remain the same whatever the phase of the illness.

Clinical endpoints

Clinical endpoints that are important in the management of septic shock were set out by the American College of Critical Care Medicine (ACCM) in 1999, and again in 2007 and 2012 by an International Consensus Conference. These are essentially markers of perfusion and include skin temperature, urine output and cerebral function.

In patients with heart failure, simple clinical assessment of perfusion and congestion can define profiles ('dry–warm'; 'wet–warm'; 'wet–cold'; 'dry–cold') that may be used to guide therapy and investigations. Further, in advanced heart failure, orthopnoea (≥ 2 pillows), jugular vein pulse (JVP) and a global assessment of perfusion ('cold' profile) help detect a reduced CI.

Physiological measurements and clinical endpoints should be viewed as complementary. Physiological measurements combined with clinical examination may provide a numeric target for a management strategy. Measurements also provide a universal language for information exchange.

Sound clinical evaluation in the ED in terms of markers of effective CO aid the early diagnosis and implementation of EGDT. Abnormal findings also suggest the need for more invasive haemodynamic monitoring and the need to involve the ICU team early in the patient's management.

Blood pressure monitoring

The pressure under which blood flows is related to the force generated by the heart and the resistance to flow in arteries. Measurement of mean arterial pressure (MAP) is a more reliable measure of blood pressure than either the systolic or diastolic pressures. It is least dependent on the site or method of measurement, least affected by measurement damping and it determines the actual tissue blood flow.

Traditionally, low blood pressure was used to reflect shock and haemodynamic instability. This approach is being challenged as more reliance is placed on concepts of global tissue hypoxia and the estimation of CO and its adequacy. While Ohm's law predicts a relationship between MAP and CO, MAP is a physiologically regulated variable and therefore can be a weak predictor of acute increases and decreases in CO.

Non-invasive blood pressure measurement

Non-invasive blood pressure (NIBP) measurements using a sphygmomanometer and palpation were first proposed in the late 1800s before Korotkoff introduced the auscultatory method in 1905. Originally, routine blood pressure measurements were not a regular part of clinical patient assessment. Today, non-invasive or indirect blood pressure measurement is the most common method used in the initial assessment of cardiovascular status.

Although there are significant differences between direct (i.e. invasive) and indirect measurements, non-invasive measurements should rightly form part of every patient's assessment and management in the ED.

Non-invasive blood pressure devices

Non-invasive measurement techniques use blood flow within a limb to measure pressure. Automated oscillometric devices are now the standard, with manual methods (using either palpation or auscultation) becoming increasingly obsolete in clinical ED practice.

The cuff width should be about 40% of the mid-circumference of the limb. Failure to use the appropriate size of cuff leads to inaccurate and misleading measurements. The cuff is inflated until all oscillations in cuff pressure cease, then the occluding pressure is gradually reduced and proprietary algorithms compute mean, systolic and diastolic pressures.

The 95% confidence limits in the normotensive range are ± 15 mmHg but, in states of hypotension and hypertension, oscillometry tends to over- and underestimate, respectively, the pressures. Complications are unusual, although repeated measurements could cause skin bruising, oedema and even ulceration.

Other non-invasive monitoring methods for cardiac output

The ideal device has yet to be developed for the non-invasive measurement of CO and other related variables in the ED. Devices that are available do not compare reliably with invasive methods and are not suited to all patient cohorts and/or may be too elaborate or time-consuming for a busy ED.

Ultrasonic cardiac output monitor (USCOM)

This device was developed in Australia and introduced for clinical use in 2001. It provides non-invasive transcutaneous estimation of CO based on continuous-wave Doppler ultrasound. An ultrasound transducer is used to obtain a Doppler flow profile (velocity–time graph) from either the aortic (suprasternal notch) or the pulmonary (left of sternum, below the second intercostal space) window. The transducer is manipulated to get the best flow profile and audible feedback. CO is calculated from the product of the velocity–time integral (VTI) and the cross-sectional area of the target valve.

The device performs well in terms of the time taken to become competent and the reproducibility of its readings. It appears to be a rapid and safe estimate of CO and may assist in the prompt starting of EGDT by emergency physicians, including pre-hospital and retrievals.

The correlation of USCOM with standard estimates of CO, such as by thermodilution using a pulmonary artery catheter, has been reported as good, although studies are conflicting. Concerns have also been raised that reliability is affected by patient pathology and the severity of illness.

More is needed to define clearly the utility of USCOM in the ED. The device can be used as part of the overall clinical assessment, but should not be used in isolation. It may be best at looking at responses to treatment, such as changes in CO associated with a fluid bolus.

Oesophageal Doppler

Estimation of CO using various Doppler-based techniques has been extensively studied. The main difficulties are an inability to obtain acceptable flow signals with the transthoracic approach and problems in the measurement of the cross-sectional area using flow. The transoesophageal approach (TOE) is more reliable than the transthoracic.

The oesophageal Doppler device requires minimal training and volume challenge protocols can be developed such that nursing staff may use them at the bedside. However, this technique is not well tolerated in the awake patient and thus has limited application in the ED.

Transthoracic echocardiography

Transthoracic echocardiography (TTE) is used to determine left ventricular size, thickness and performance. It can also help identify a patient who requires fluids. The use of TTE has increased as the technology and familiarity have improved, with a move towards training in TTE for most intensive care specialists. This would also seem a natural progression for ED physicians, given the uptake of ultrasonography in ED for other indications.

Treatment decisions

Effective treatment decisions can be based on the TTE screen and on subsequent assessment of left ventricular function. One widely used parameter is respiratory variation of the vena cava diameter for assessment of intravascular volume and fluid responsiveness in shock. This is quantified by measuring the decrease in the inferior vena cava (IVC) diameter with inspiration compared with expiration, expressed as the IVC caval index or the IVC collapsibility index (IVC–CI). Higher IVC–CI values have been correlated with lower right atrial (RA) filling pressures and lower values have been correlated with higher RA filling pressures.

The utility of the IVC caval index in the ED for assessment of volume responsiveness and for fluid management is unclear. One issue is its applicability in the spontaneously breathing patient, as using the IVC caval index for fluid responsiveness in mechanically ventilated ICU patients appears to be of more value. Further, other factors can affect IVC diameter and collapsibility including left and right ventricular function, pulmonary hypertension and tricuspid valve dysfunction, which need to be considered when interpreting the findings.

Left ventricular systolic function

The most common initial technique in the ICU for TTE assessment of left ventricular systolic function is simply looking at the amount of endocardial border excursion toward the centre of the left ventricle and at increasing wall thickness during contraction. Using these, at a minimum the systolic function of the left ventricle may be described as being normal, hyperdynamic or having moderate or severe dysfunction.

Other useful TTE information with signicant haemodynamic and therapeutic value includes valvular function, right ventricular function and evidence of pericardial tamponade, regional left ventricular hypokinesis, transient apical ballooning and left ventricular outflow tract (LVOT) obstruction. One major criticism as regards TTE for haemodynamic monitoring is that it cannot be done continuously. Other problems include the skill base needed and having to reassess variables after changes in patient management. Knowledge and skills are rapidly increasing and, with the development of hand-held and compact portable devices, TTE is becoming more common despite its usefulness for general haemodynamic monitoring in the ED remaining unclear.

Invasive devices

Invasive blood pressure measurement

Arterial cannulation allows continuous blood pressure measurement, beat-to-beat waveform display and repeated blood sampling. A cannula inserted into an artery is connected via fluid-filled, non-compliant tubing < 1 m in length to a linearly responsive pressure transducer. The system is then zeroed with reference to the phlebostatic axis (the midaxillary line in the fourth intercostal space). Modern transducers are pre-calibrated and therefore no further calibration is needed.

Sites and safety of arterial cannulation

The most common site for cannulation is the radial artery, as it is easy to access during placement and subsequent manipulations, the wrist has a dual arterial supply and there is a low complication rate. Temporary occlusion of the artery may occur and, in a small number of cases, this may be permanent. Other complications can include haematoma formation, bleeding, cellulitis and those associated with the catheter itself.

Alternative arterial cannulation sites are femoral, axillary and brachial, but all have similar complications. Arterial cannulation is a safe procedure if the optimal site for insertion is selected carefully for each patient. The preference in the ED is for the radial and femoral sites.

Use of invasive blood pressure monitoring

Invasive blood pressure monitoring should be used in all haemodynamically unstable patients and when vasopressor or vasodilator therapy is used. Relying on external NIBP monitoring to guide diagnosis and therapy does not provide sufficient diagnostic data, particularly in sepsis. Additional methods of haemodynamic monitoring may be considered in these patients, with early involvement of the intensive care department.

The remainder of this chapter discusses some of the supplementary methods available to assess important physiological measures that guide the management of the haemodynamically unstable patient.

Central venous pressure monitoring

Central venous access was first performed in Germany in the late 1920s, but the utility of the process was not really appreciated until the 1950s. This led to the development of cardiac angiography, central blood oxygenation determination and pressure recordings. The technique and clinical relevance of continuous central venous pressure (CVP) monitoring were first described in 1962, as it allowed direct determination of right heart function and assessment of intravascular volume status.

However, correlation with left heart function was found to be unpredictable and unreliable in the critically ill. Thus, the physiological meaning of the values obtained and their role in patient management are not clear. Problems result from errors in measurement and failure to understand the underlying pathophysiology involved.

Central venous access

Central venous access is obtained in the ED by inserting a catheter into a peripheral or central vein and is defined by the position of the catheter tip which should be positioned at the junction of the proximal superior vena cava and right atrium.

There is no ideal insertion site. Selection depends on the experience of the operator and patient factors, such as body habitus, disease or injury sustained and coagulation profile. The main routes used are the internal jugular, subclavian and femoral veins.

Indications for central venous access

Indications include fluid and electrolyte replacement; drug therapy where peripheral use is contraindicated, such as vasopressors; monitoring of the CVP to guide management; sampling of central venous blood to monitor central venous oxygen saturation ($ScvO_2$); venous access for insertion of a pulmonary artery catheter or transvenous pacemaker; and a lack of an accessible peripheral vein.

Complications of central venous access

Complications related to insertion are divided into early and late. Relevant early complications in the ED include pneumothorax, haemothorax, dysrhythmias and injury to surrounding structures, including arterial puncture, nerve and tracheal injury. Late complications include catheter-related sepsis, superior vena cava erosion with cardiac tamponade and venous thrombosis.

The CVP is often used as a marker of preload and is considered an estimate of right atrial pressure (RAP). The normal CVP in the spontaneously breathing supine patient is 0–5 mmHg, with 10 mmHg considered an upper limit of normal in those being mechanically ventilated. The CVP also correlates with left ventricular end-diastolic pressure (LVEDP) in a patient with normal heart and lungs. However, in disease states this relationship is frequently abnormal. Thus, the CVP can only be a rough guide to right ventricular preload, with emphasis on dynamic changes rather than absolute values.

Central venous oxygen saturation

Rivers et al. reported in 2001 that, in septic shock, early aggressive resuscitation guided by CVP, MAP and continuous $ScvO_2$ monitoring reduced 28-day mortality rates from 46.5% to 30.5%. $ScvO_2$ is measured in blood taken via the central venous catheter and reflects the balance between oxygen delivery and oxygen consumption. Oxygen extraction in health is normally about 25–30% and an $ScvO_2$ >65% reflects an optimal balance. $ScvO_2$ correlates well with mixed venous saturations (SvO_2) obtained via a pulmonary artery catheter.

Current guidelines recommend instituting goal-directed therapy in septic shock, especially when the $ScvO_2$ is below 70%. The $ScvO_2$ is also significant in postoperative surgical patients in the ICU, with levels <70% independently associated with a higher rate of complications and increased length of hospital stay.

Australasian Resuscitation in Sepsis Evaluation (ARISE)

Continuous measurement of $ScvO_2$ is possible in the ED where central venous catheterization is commonly performed and when the alternative of pulmonary artery insertion is impractical. The role of $ScvO_2$ and EGDT is being studied further in the current Australasian Resuscitation in Sepsis Evaluation (ARISE), a multicentre, unblinded, randomized, controlled trial of EGDT versus standard care in patients with severe sepsis presenting to the EDs of hospitals in Australia, New Zealand, Finland and Hong Kong. It will test the hypothesis that EGDT, compared to standard Australasian resuscitation practice, reduces 90-day all-cause mortality in patients presenting to the ED with severe sepsis.

Pulse contour techniques for cardiac output

The use of pulse contour techniques to obtain a continuous estimation of CO by analysis of the arterial waveform dates back over 100 years. Erlanger and Hooker first proposed a correlation between stroke volume and changes in arterial pressure and suggested there was a correlation between CO and the arterial pulse contour. Advances in computer technology have since led to the development of complex algorithms relating the arterial pulse contour and CO.

The appeal of arterial waveform monitoring is that it can now be performed using a minimally invasive technique, with several companies producing devices that take measurements from an arterial line. The PiCCO (Pulsion Medical Systems, Munich, Germany) is discussed as it is one of the most established of the commercially available systems.

PiCCO system of arterial waveform monitoring

The PiCCO system uses pulse contour analysis to provide a continuous display of CO according to a modified version of Wesseling's algorithm. The patient requires a central line, preferably sited in either the internal jugular or the subclavian vein so that the venous injectate port is placed in the central cardiopulmonary circulation. If the femoral vein is accessed the intrathoracic volumetric measurements may be overestimated, although the transpulmonary thermodilution CO measurement may still be reliable. An arterial catheter with a thermistor is also required, which needs to be placed in one of the larger arteries, such as the femoral or brachial-axillary access.

The PiCCO system combines the pulse contour method for continuous CO measurement and a transpulmonary thermodilution technique to offer complete haemodynamic monitoring. Transpulmonary thermodilution works on the principle that a known volume of thermal indicator (cold 0.9% NaCl) is injected into a central vein. The injectate rapidly disperses both volumetrically and thermally within the pulmonary and cardiac volumes. This volume of distribution is termed the intrathoracic volume. When the temperature signal reaches the arterial thermistor, a temperature difference is detected and a dissipation curve is generated. The Stewart–Hamilton equation is applied to this curve and the CO is calculated.

Transpulmonary thermodilution This transpulmonary thermodilution also gives measures of preload and volume responsiveness in terms of global end-diastolic blood volume (GEDV) as well as intrathoracic blood volume (ITBV). The extravascular lung water (EVLW) provides a measure of water content outside the pulmonary vasculature, including the interstitium and any alveolar fluid and may be useful as an indicator of pulmonary oedema. The technique of transpulmonary thermodilution appears to be comparable in accuracy to pulmonary artery thermodilution. Following calibration by thermodilution, the PiCCO then continually quantifies parameters such as:

- pulse-induced contour cardiac output (CO)
- arterial blood pressure
- heart rate
- stroke volume (SV)
- systemic vascular resistance (SVR)
- intrathoracic blood volume (ITBV)
- extravascular lung water (EVLW)
- cardiac function index (CFI).

Decision trees to guide the use of the last three parameters in the clinical setting have been devised. ITBV is used as an indicator of cardiac preload and may be helpful in guiding fluid therapy. It is derived from the GEDV and its clinical utility is likely to be equivalent. GEDV and ITBV may be of greatest clinical value when dynamic measures of volume responsiveness, such as stroke volume variation (SVV) and systolic pressure variation (SPV), cannot be used.

EVLW correlates with extravascular thermal volume in the lungs. The EVLW may also be used to guide fluid management, especially in those already known to have pulmonary oedema.

The cardiac function index is the ratio of CO to GEDV. It aids in evaluation of the contractile state of the heart and hence overall cardiac performance. It is a preload-independent variable and reflects the inotropic state of the heart. The CFI has the potential to become a routine parameter of cardiac performance, but it is a derived variable and its benefit over the individual components that comprise it (CO and GEDV) is not clear.

Advantages of the PiCCO system The main advantage of the PiCCO system is that it is less invasive than a pulmonary artery catheter, requiring only a central line and an arterial line which most critically ill patients already have. This, in turn, leads to fewer complications. The data collected are extensive and allow manipulation of haemodynamics using reliable parameters.

Contraindications to using the PiCCO include when access to the femoral artery is restricted, such as in burns. The PiCCO may also give inaccurate thermodilution measurements in the presence of intracardiac shunts, an aortic aneurysm, aortic stenosis, pneumonectomy, rapid changes in body temperature and during extracorporeal circulation. There can also be drift in measured values when there is a major change in vascular compliance.

The use of the PiCCO system in the ED is plausible. The technique is relatively non-invasive and uses access lines that are already used in the management of the critically ill. The device can aid both diagnosis and provide a monitoring tool for clinical decision making regarding fluid replacement. Further validation studies and technological advances will consolidate its potential.

Pulmonary artery Swan–Ganz catheter

The pulmonary artery catheter (PAC) or Swan–Ganz catheter was long considered the 'gold standard' method of monitoring unstable circulation, for example in patients with advanced heart failure. Since its introduction in the 1970s, it was assumed that the information provided improved patient outcome. However, various observational studies have now shown that its use does not improve outcomes and may even be associated with a worse outcome. Hence, the use of the PAC without targeting specific endpoints confers no benefit to the patient.

Disadvantages of pulmonary artery catheters

The insertion of a PAC is time-consuming and requires skill and experience. The technique also has significant complications (e.g. haematoma, arterial puncture, infection, pulmonary infarction, pulmonary artery perforation, arrhythmias, catheter knotting) and the data generated can be difficult to interpret. Current guidelines recommend that the PAC is not used routinely in the management of shock and, therefore, its use in the ED should *not* be considered.

Conclusion

The challenge in emergency medicine is to select those haemodynamic monitoring methods and technologies that are best suited to the clinical environment and which are able to influence positively both the diagnosis and the subsequent management to improve patient outcome. Currently, the best approach is to begin with sound clinical assessment and then to increase the invasiveness of monitoring in tandem with the patient's suspected diagnosis and response.

Future developments

- Interest in the microcirculation and metabolic assessment at a cellular level. Methods to assess these include near infrared spectroscopy (NIRS) and NADPH fluorescence, a novel method using fluorescence microscopy for real-time assessment of ATP release from individual cells. Both may have a role in the management of shock.
- NIRS appears the most advanced and promising modality with reported use in a number of settings including military, trauma, congestive cardiac failure and sepsis. It continuously and non-invasively measures peripheral tissue oxygen saturation (StO_2) utilizing oxygenation variables, such as deoxyhaemoglobin (HHb), oxyhaemoglobin (HbO_2) and total haemoglobin (HbT). How best to use this technology and the threshold StO_2 that should prompt intervention are not yet clear.
- Direct assessment of the microcirculation (e.g. sublingual) using orthogonal polarization spectral (OPS) or sidestream dark field (SDF) videomicroscopy.
- Non-invasive tonometry to reconstruct central aortic pressures from radial artery pressure waveforms.

Controversies

- Whether the PAC data are in fact of value, but interpretation of them is lacking, or whether the detailed haemodynamic data cannot ultimately be translated to the benefit of the patient.
- Whether any monitoring technology taken in isolation, rather than in an evidence-based protocol, influences patient outcome.
- The best haemodynamic monitoring devices to use and what physiological variables are important to measure.

Further reading

Antonelli M, Levy M, Andrews PJD, et al. Haemodynamic monitoring in shock and implications for management. International Consensus Conference, Paris, France, April 2006. Intens Care Med 2007; 33:575–90.

Connors AF, Speroff T, Dawson NV, et al. The effectiveness of right heart catheterization in the initial care of critically ill patients. SUPPORT Investigators. J Am Med Assoc 1996;276:889–97.

Corl K, Napoli AM, Gardiner F. Bedside sonographic measurement of the inferior vena cava caval index is a poor predictor of fluid responsiveness in emergency department patients. Emerg Med Australas 2012;24:534–9.

Darovic GO, editor. Haemodynamic monitoring, invasive and noninvasive: clinical application (3rd ed.). St Louis: WB Saunders; 2002.

Dellinger R, Levy M, Rhodes A, et al. Surviving Sepsis Campaign: International Guidelines for Management of Severe Sepsis and Septic Shock: 2012. Crit Care Med 2013;41:580–637.

Drazner MH, Hellkamp AS, Leier CV, et al. Value of clinician assessment of hemodynamics in advanced heart failure. The ESCAPE trial. Circulation: Heart Failure 2008;1:170–7.

Harvey S, Harrison DA, Singer M, et al. Assessment of the clinical effectiveness of pulmonary artery catheters in management of patients in intensive care (PAC-Man): a randomized controlled trial. Lancet 2005;366:472–7.

Litton E, Morgan M. The PiCCO monitor: a review. Anaes Intens Care 2012;40:393–409.

Morgan TJ. Haemodynamic monitoring Bersten AD, Soni N, editors. Oh's intensive care manual (6th ed.). Oxford: Butterworth–Heinemann; 2009.

Nelson M, Waldrop RD, Jones J, et al. Critical care provided in an urban emergency department. Am J Emerg Med 1998;16:56–9.

Nguyen HB, Rivers EP. The clinical practice of early goal-directed therapy in severe sepsis and septic shock. Adv Sepsis 2005;4:126–31.

Nohria A, Tsang SW, Fang JC, et al. Clinical assessment identifies hemodynamic profiles that predict outcomes in patients admitted with heart failure. J Am Coll Cardiol 2003;41:1797–804.

Pearse R, Dawson D, Fawcett J, et al. Changes in central venous saturation after major surgery, and association with outcome. Crit Care 2005;9:R694–9.

Rivers E, Nguyen B, Havstad S, et al. Early goal-directed therapy in the treatment of severe sepsis and septic shock. N Engl J Med 2001;345:1368–77.

Task Force of the American College of Critical Care Medicine SoCCM. Practice parameters for haemodynamic support of sepsis in adult patients with sepsis. Crit Care Med 1999; 27:639–60.

Vincent J-L, Rhodes A, Perel A, et al. Clinical review: update on hemodynamic monitoring – a consensus of 16. Crit Care 2011;15:229.

CRITICAL CARE

2

2.4 Shock overview

Peter Garrett

ESSENTIALS

1 Broad categories of shock include disorders of intravascular volume, vascular resistance, cardiac filling and the myocardial pump. Overlapping aetiologies are commonly encountered.

2 Hypotension is only one characteristic of shock, which should be considered a late and concerning finding.

3 Hypovolaemia and hence the need for volume resuscitation is a concern in every patient with shock.

4 Interventions in any form of shock are initially directed at the physiological deficit and act as a test of the underlying clinical hypothesis. Continuous reassessment is required.

5 Common errors in management are late diagnosis; inadequate control of the primary problem; inadequate fluid loading; delayed ventilatory assistance; and excessive reliance on inappropriate adjuncts. There is not sufficient evidence that any one of the investigated vasopressors is clearly superior over others.

6 Mortality following cardiogenic shock is improved by revascularization strategies and cardiothoracic surgical intervention. Thrombolysis alone is unproven, as is intra-aortic balloon counterpulsation.

7 Currently no adjunctive therapies are of benefit in septic shock over adequate fluid resuscitation, vasopressors and inotropes, timely and appropriate antibiotics and/or source control.

Introduction

Shock is a clinical syndrome where tissue perfusion, and hence oxygenation, is inadequate to maintain normal metabolic function of the cells and organ. Although the effects of inadequate perfusion are initially reversible, prolonged oxygen deprivation leads to generalized cellular hypoxia with disruption of critical biochemical processes, eventually resulting in cell membrane ion pump dysfunction, inadequate regulation of intracellular pH, intracellular oedema and cell death.

Shock is traditionally classified and managed according to the presumed aetiology, but a common approach in practice is to attend urgently to the cardiorespiratory physiological abnormalities, assess the response to adjust the working diagnosis with later attention to the underlying diagnosis.

Recognizing shock may be difficult, particularly at the extremes of age. Pre-existing disease and the use of medications modify the compensatory mechanisms that safeguard perfusion of vital organs. Consider the possibility of inadequate tissue perfusion ('shock') in any emergency presentation with symptoms, signs or laboratory findings of abnormal end-organ function. Early, aggressive and targeted treatment of shock is associated with an improved outcome.

Aetiology and epidemiology

Shock is due to malfunction of components of the cardiovascular system, not uncommonly with more than one contributing mechanism. If the aetiology is apparent, classification based on the mechanism, such as hypovolaemic, cardiogenic, septic, neurogenic or anaphylactic shock, will guide therapy.

When the aetiology is unclear or the shock fails to respond to therapy, the following physiologically based classification assists in decision making (see Boxes 2.4.1–2.4.4).

Box 2.4.1 Volume loss contributing to shock: 'hypovolaemic shock'

INTRAVASCULAR COMPARTMENT:

Blood Loss:

External bleeding
- trauma
- gastrointestinal tract bleeding

Internal (concealed) bleeding
- haemothorax
- haemoperitoneum (ruptured abdominal aortic aneurysm, ruptured ectopic pregnancy)
- retroperitoneum (ruptured abdominal aortic aneurysm, pelvic trauma)

Plasma Loss:
- Burns
- Sweating/dehydration
- Pancreatitis
- Ascites (peritonitis, liver disease)
- Toxic epidermal necrolysis (TEN), erythroderma, pemphigus

EXTRAVASCULAR LOSS:

Gastrointestinal tract
- Vomiting
- Diarrhoea
- Bowel obstruction

Renal tract
- Adrenal insufficiency (aldosterone deficiency)
- Diabetes mellitus (polyuria)
- Diabetes insipidus (polyuria)
- Diuretics
- Polyuric intrinsic renal disease

Reduced return to the heart – reduced preload – *hypovolaemia* (Box 2.4.1)
- Intravascular compartment
- Extravascular loss.

Reduced total peripheral resistance – reduced afterload – *distributive* (Box 2.4.2)
- Arterial vasodilatation
- Altered venous capacitance.

Box 2.4.2 Shock resulting from altered venous capacitance and/or reduced vascular tone: 'distributive shock'

Septic shock

Anaphylactic shock

Neurogenic shock

Vasoactive drugs (vasodilators, sedatives or toxins)

Adrenal insufficiency (cortisol deficiency)

Thyrotoxicosis/thyroid storm

Liver failure

Systemic inflammatory response features, e.g. pancreatitis, trauma, burns

Prolonged shock from any cause – 'decompensated shock'

Box 2.4.3 Inadequate filling due to extrinsic obstruction: 'obstructive shock'

Tension pneumothorax

Pericardial tamponade/other pericardial disease

Pulmonary hypertension (large pulmonary embolus, chronic pulmonary hypertension)

Atrial myxoma and left atrial mural thrombus

Obstruction to filling – obstructive (Box 2.4.3)

- Tension pneumothorax
- Pericardial tamponade
- Large pulmonary embolism/pulmonary hypertension
- Atrial myxoma.

Pump dysfunction – cardiogenic (Box 2.4.4)

- Reduced contractility – systolic dysfunction
- Impaired relaxation – diastolic dysfunction / RV infarction
- Abnormal cardiac rate or rhythm
- Forward flow failure – valvular dysfunction.

Box 2.4.4 Myocardial dysfunction resulting in shock: 'cardiogenic shock'

Reduced contractility (systolic dysfunction)

Ischaemia (acute myocardial infarction)

Myocarditis (infectious, hypersensitivity)

Myocardial contusion

Cardiomyopathy

Toxins/drugs (calcium channel blockers, doxorubicin)

Inadequate filling (due to intrinsic problem)

Diastolic dysfunction

Right ventricular infarction

Arrhythmia

Ventricular tachycardia

Atrial fibrillation (when cardiac output is dependent on atrial priming)

Bradycardia (heart block, drugs)

Failure of forward flow

Ruptured ventricular septum or free wall

Chordae tendinae rupture or papillary muscle dysfunction (post-MI)

Critical mitral or aortic stenosis

Mitral or aortic regurgitation

Prosthetic valve thrombus/dysfunction

No classification is exhaustive, and contributory causes may feature in more than one category.

Pathophysiology

Most organs and tissues are able to autoregulate or adjust their flow according to metabolic demand, as long as flow is adequate. This flow is dependent on a gradient between an area of higher pressure (mean arterial pressure, MAP) and the lower-pressure side of the venous system (represented by a central venous pressure, CVP).

The mean arterial pressure may fall if the cardiac output (CO) is reduced or if the total peripheral resistance (TPR) in the arterial tree falls:

$$MAP = CO \times TPR$$

Cardiac output is determined by the stroke volume (SV) and heart rate (HR). The heart is a relatively simple pump and hence preload (the volume of blood in the left ventricle at the end of filling or the amount of stretch of the left ventricle) determines SV until disease states intervene:

$$CO = SV \times HR$$

Relaxation of the arterial and venous tone by vasoactive mediators or lack of vasotonic mediators results in reduced resistance and increased capacitance and lower pressures in both the arterial and venous systems. Any injury to the endothelium will result in loss of volume, as well as failure of vascular autoregulation. Additionally, if there is a defective valve causing regurgitation of blood and repumping or a fixed narrow orifice, there is a failure in forward flow.

Compensatory mechanisms

Compensatory mechanisms are provoked by the combination of lowered pressure and inadequate perfusion of tissues and contribute to the symptoms and signs of shock. Neurohumeral stimulation produces increased circulating catecholamines, angiotensin, aldosterone and vasopressin manifesting clinically with anxiety, thirst, restlessness, tachycardia, diversion of blood from the skin bed and a reduction in urinary output and urinary sodium. Blood flow to the brain and heart is maintained at the expense of renal, splanchnic, skin and muscle blood flow [1]. Significant fluid shifts occur from the interstitium to the intravascular compartment, which may falsely maintain haematocrit.

Decompensated shock

The ultimate consequence of shock, if tissue perfusion is not returned by compensatory measures or resuscitation, is inadequate regeneration of adenosine triphosphate (ATP) causing failure of membrane ion pumps to maintain the function and structural integrity of the cell.

This cellular dysfunction manifests in the myocardium as systolic contractile dysfunction (also due in part to reduction in sensitivity to catecholamines and circulating myocardial depressant factors) and impaired ventricular relaxation (lusiotropy). This myocardial failure, along with failure of vascular beds despite the increased circulating catecholamines, contributes to what is described as 'decompensated shock'.

Clinical features

The clinical features in the initial diagnosis of shock are due to inadequate perfusion of tissues and resulting multiorgan dysfunction of the body's compensatory mechanisms. Clinicians should not wait for physical observations to trigger a preconceived BP limit before considering shock, but should actively look for signs of inadequate perfusion in any patient presenting with abnormal organ function:

- Mental state reflects reduced cerebral perfusion and may range from anxiety or confusion to coma.
- Patients may describe thirst, coldness or impending doom and have presyncopal symptoms including nausea, yawning and preferring to lie down.
- Retrospectively, the patient may have been a challenge to assess, the vital signs hard to elicit or variable and venepuncture or IV access difficult.
- Peripheral circulation reveals venoconstriction, with decreased peripheral temperature, pallor and mottling. Capillary return may be prolonged beyond 4 seconds, although peripheral mottling or central cyanosis are late signs. However, with vascular tone failure, such as spinal, anaphylactic, neurogenic shock and sepsis, the skin may initially be warm and dry and capillary refill indeterminate as a consequence of vasodilatation.
- Hypotension is a cardinal clinical sign, defined as a systolic blood pressure <90 mmHg or a reduction of >30 mmHg in a previously hypertensive patient. Shock can be present despite an elevated blood pressure and a low systolic blood pressure may not be associated with other signs of shock, or be physiological in young thin females.
- A low systolic blood pressure should be considered a highly significant, if not late, finding in shock. Mean arterial pressure is increasingly considered more relevant and accurate as a measured parameter [2]. Tachycardia is frequently present, but may be masked by drugs or advanced age.
- The trend with serial observations is more significant than absolute values. Bradycardia can occur in younger patients or following an inferior myocardial infarction (MI).
- Tachypnoea is regarded as a sensitive but non-specific predictor of deterioration and is part of the shock syndrome [3].
- Core temperature may be low, normal or elevated and will be affected by age, environment, volume status, coexisting disease, drug therapy and pre-hospital interventions.
- Oliguria.

Initial management of shock

A structured framework, such as that advocated by early management of severe trauma (EMST) (advanced trauma life support (ATLS)) or advanced cardiac life support (ACLS), promotes both a systematic survey and effective therapy to occur simultaneously. Treatments based on an initial working diagnosis are modified by the observed responses to therapy and/or the results of investigations. Frequent reassessment of status and adequacy of response is vital. Once shock is recognized as present this implies a high chance of death, thus urgent escalation to management by a multidisciplinary team in a monitored resuscitation area is indicated, with a designated team leader and communication being vital [4,5].

Primary survey

- Assess and support airway and ventilation. Give supplemental high-flow oxygen to ensure maximal arterial oxygen saturation. Consider tracheal intubation and mechanical ventilation in the significantly shocked patient for reasons over and above the standard indications of airway protection and intractable hypoxaemia: to divert needed cardiac output to other hypoperfused organs; reduce oxygen consumption from respiratory musculature; maximize arterial oxygenation; manage respiratory acidosis; facilitate invasive monitoring procedures; and guard against sudden catastrophic respiratory decompensation. The role of non-invasive ventilation is unproven in this setting. Positive-pressure ventilation and anaesthesia will have a significant effect in the setting of inadequate preload, so prior fluid resuscitation is vital (see Chapter 2.1).
- Circulation with haemorrhage control. Obtain and secure intravenous access in more than one site with short, large-bore peripheral cannulae, within the skill level of the operator. Central venous access is rarely required in an emergency and may increase delay and morbidity. Consider a supine/head-up position and elevation of the legs if tolerated [6].
- Draw blood for investigations, including immediate bedside glucose level and venous or arterial blood gases.
- Infuse fluid as the initial correction of shock with hypotension. Hypovolaemia and hence the need for volume resuscitation should be assumed in every patient with shock, until proven otherwise. Close observation of the response to fluid boluses will guide further boluses.
- The usual initial fluid is isotonic normal saline or Hartmann's (lactated Ringer's) solution.
- Use immediately available blood products (O-negative or group specific) warmed by a cartridge-warming device for haemorrhagic shock or where haemoglobin may fall to a point where oxygen carriage is compromised (7–9 g/dL, except in patients with acute haemorrhage or significant coronary artery disease).
- Add an effective vasopressor/inotrope, such as epinephrine (adrenaline) by infusion if, despite ongoing rapid fluid volume resuscitation, hypotension and inadequate perfusion persist (see 'Goal-directed' resuscitation). However, this may simply achieve an adequate blood pressure but at the expense of correct fluid volume replenishment.

Secondary survey

- Review vital signs and any available history obtained, followed by a directed physical examination. Cardiac rhythm and pulse oximetry (SaO$_2$) are monitored continuously.

All observations, including temperature, are recorded regularly.

- Perform a chest X-ray, ECG and other bedside emergency investigations, such as ultrasound, at this point, which may point to the aetiology (e.g. a ruptured aortic aneurysm or ectopic pregnancy, cardiac tamponade or right ventricular failure).
- Place an indwelling urinary catheter in all shocked patients.
- Anticipate complications and interventions and organize definitive care and disposal. Liaise with surgeons, radiologists and other specialists early. The complications of hypothermia, coagulopathy, hypoglycaemia, hypokalaemia and respiratory failure should be actively sought, prepared for and prevented. The need to move the patient to imaging or theatre should be anticipated and communicated to team members to allow for early preparation of the patient and monitoring set up.

Guidance for interventions and treatments

A key goal in the treatment of shock during and after the initial resuscitation is correction of the underlying problem. Methods used to guide resuscitation are discussed below.

Emergency department (ED) observations

The presence and progress of shock is detected in the ED by careful recording of vital signs and *frequent* and *repeated* clinical assessment.

- 'Vital signs' – pulse, respirations, blood pressure and temperature – are measured regularly and observed for absolute values, trend and adequacy of response to therapy. Accuracy and frequency of temperature measurement is facilitated by an indwelling catheter with temperature probe.
- ECG monitoring provides an assessment of heart rate and ST segment changes suggesting inadequate myocardial perfusion if calibrated.
- Continuous pulse oximetry provides assessment of hypoxaemia as the management of shock necessitates the adequate delivery of oxygen to tissues.
- Non-invasive oscillometric blood pressure (NIBP) measurement is convenient and set to frequent automated measurement. Accuracy is affected by cuff size, age,

movement, some disease states and extremes of hypotension or hypertension. Mean arterial pressure is more accurately and reliably measured than systolic [2,7].

- Urine output is the most apparent bedside monitor of the adequacy of end-organ perfusion. Levels below 0.5 mL/kg/h suggest underperfusion of the renal bed. Diuretics can both confuse and exacerbate the shock state.

ED investigations

- Bedside tests should include blood sugar to exclude hypoglycaemia, which will compromise resuscitation efforts.
- Arterial or venous blood gas measurements are available rapidly and contain information to assess the cause (e.g. haemoglobin level), guide the interventions required (hyperkalaemia correction, assisted ventilation) and monitor the adequacy of tissue perfusion by tracking lactate or base deficit changes with resuscitation.
- Lactate measurements are an objective marker of the presence and severity of shock. Normal levels are <2 mmol/L, with levels of >4 mmol/L associated with increased mortality. Lactate and base deficit (BD) are used to assess the adequacy of resuscitation and have been used to predict mortality, transfusion requirements, the need for ICU and the length of stay [8,9].
- Full blood count, coagulation profile, electrolytes, liver function tests and troponin, with a chest X-ray and electrocardiogram is usually enough to commence a working diagnosis of the aetiology of the shock.
- Bedside focused ultrasound (FAST) or formal trans-thoracic echocardiogram (TTE), if available, are now incorporated in many resuscitation algorithms. FAST is used to assess for free abdominal fluid and exclude pericardial tamponade. More advanced ultrasound allows assessment for intrathoracic free fluid, aortic or vena caval diameter and assessment of cardiac function: ventricular cavity dimensions (adequate filling); ventricular ejection fraction; regional wall motion abnormalities indicating ischaemia; and valvular dysfunction.

Invasive monitoring

Invasive monitoring in the ED may include:

- Intra-arterial blood pressure monitoring which gives more reliable arterial pressures

and detects hypotension earlier than intermittent non-invasive means [2].

- Systolic pressure variation or 'swing' of the arterial waveform baseline during respiration (usually with mechanical ventilation) is at least as sensitive as CVP or pulmonary artery (PA) wedge pressure as a marker of the need for more fluid [10].
- Stroke volume variation is the measured difference between the maximal and minimal systolic blood pressure values during one (mechanical) breath and 'delta down' is the component of this variation from apnoea to minimal SBP. A variation of greater than 5 mmHg suggests fluid responsiveness [11].
- Response and trends in CVP are followed after volume loading.
- End-tidal CO_2 in a ventilated patient may be compared to arterial $PaCO_2$. A difference of more than a few mmHg may suggest a shunt due to inadequate lung perfusion and has been used to track the adequacy of resuscitation [12].
- Central venous oxygen saturation can be measured using a specific central venous line (CVL) or aspirating blood. Lower levels than 65–75% suggest imbalance between oxygen delivery and consumption.
- Pulse contour analysis devices (e.g. Flowtrac, Edwards Lifesciences) use the arterial pulse wave contour and an algorithm to present cardiac output and other derived parameters which may be used to track responses in resuscitation.
- Pulmonary artery catheterization, peripheral invasive cardiac output monitors (PiCCO), gastric tonometry, sublingual capnometry, transoesophageal echocardiography, Doppler cardiac output studies and other more sophisticated investigations are best performed in an intensive care environment (see Chapter 2.3).

'Goal-directed' resuscitation

The concept of acheiving specific levels of cardiac output by manipulating haemoglobin concentration, inotropes, vasopressors, vasodilators and fluid volumes is promoted. Early hypotheses suffered from mathematical linkage error and balanced studies showed that 'supra-normal' cardiac outputs or oxygen delivery was *not* beneficial in undefined groups or trauma [13,14]. A seminal single centre study by Rivers in 2001 proposed that, in severe sepsis in the ED, a resuscitation algorithm guided by CVP,

MAP and central venous saturation 'goals' led to an improvement in survival. The commonest intervention change was an increase in fluid resuscitation volume [15].

Having clear clinical goals communicated during resuscitation does allow the team to focus together. These targets can be physiological, time or intervention based.

Interventions in shock

1. Fluid therapy

Choice of fluid

A sensible maxim is: 'Replace that which is lost, at the rate at which it is lost'.

- There is no evidence that any one fluid type is superior in undifferentiated shock, thus the commonest choice in the emergency situation remains 'isotonic' 0.9% normal saline. There is retrospective evidence that hypotonic fluids and glucose-containing fluid are detrimental in the critically ill [16]. Hartmann's (or similar strong ion 'balanced') solution reduces the risk of hyperchloraemic acidosis from normal saline use, but this appears to be clinically irrelevant [17].
  - The SAFE study investigators demonstrated that there was no difference in outcome, or any clinically significant measure, between those resuscitated with saline versus human albumin solution [18,19]. Hydroxyethyl starch has no clinical advantage over saline and has more complications [20]. The theoretical advantages of hypertonic saline have not been demonstrated [20].
- When blood is lost or diluted by large volumes of fluid, both oxygen carriage and coagulation activity must be maintained. Retrospective and prospective studies on transfusion triggers suggest that Hb levels of 70–90 g/L are appropriate in most patients and levels of 100 g/L are tolerated by patients with ischaemic heart disease [21,22]. Aiming for a higher target Hb (>100 g/L or HCt >0.4) may be sensible in those who are shocked due to active bleeding.
- Dilutional coagulopathy during resuscitation is sought for or proactively avoided by administering fresh frozen plasma (FFP). Clinical coagulopathy may be present before laboratory parameters alter.

Fluid administration

Aliquots of between 10 and 40 mL/kg (averaging 20 mL/kg) at free flow or 'stat' over minutes are recommended. If the heart is suspected of having abnormal compliance or being too 'full', a smaller bolus is given equally rapidly and the clinical response closely observed.

Cannulae sized 16 and 20 gauge may achieve flow rates of 1 L over 5 and 10 minutes, respectively [23]. In the emergency situation, hand-pump infusion lines or gravity or pressure bag-driven infusion will deliver volumes effectively. Volumetric infusion pumps or lines should not be used in resuscitation, as the maximum rate of infusion is inadequate and alarm features may delay infusion. Pressure infusion pumps can achieve high rates but at a significant risk of complications [24].

Route of fluid therapy

Large volumes can be delivered by any route, but central lines, smaller peripheral inserted catheters and intraosseous needles may require a driving pressure. The latter may fail unless carefully supervised. The antecubital, saphenous and femoral veins are reliably accessed with few complications. Consider ultrasound-guided access in difficult situations.

Titration targets

Defining a target for 'how much is enough' is problematic, as each shock scenario has a different aetiology, clinical features and monitoring requirements. Traditionally, the return of physiological variables towards normal and set perfusion targets are used (Table 2.4.1).

Decisions are made using multiple inputs preferably using the technique of fluid challenge and review of response to each challenge.

Complications of fluid therapy

- Hypothermia is likely after infusing large volumes of fluid and should be monitored for. Each ED should be proactive in including a warmed environment, warmed fluid and blanket stores and active warming devices. Consider using a commercial warming cartridge for all resuscitations anticipated above a certain volume and/or when a massive transfusion protocol is instituted.
- Coagulopathy may be due to dilution, sepsis, hypothermia or acidosis. Fresh frozen plasma will not resolve the latter causes. Hypocalcaemia is rarely an issue.
- Tissue oedema is common and usually clinically irrelevant, but may exacerbate limb and abdominal compartment syndromes.
- Pulmonary oedema is just as likely to be due to the inflammatory process accompanying significant shock as to excessive preload and is managed either by positive-pressure ventilation and/or diuresis if appropriate. Respiratory failure or the requirement for ventilation does not influence mortality in most ICU outcome studies. Conversely, renal failure and infarction of the myocardium, brain and gut are all major risk factors for death.
- Failure to recognize that ongoing fluid requirements are due to an unresolved primary process may cause later deterioration.

Table 2.4.1 Target physiological, perfusion and invasive parameters in the management of shock		
Traditional physiological targets	Perfusion targets	Invasive measurement targets
Return of systolic BP to >90 mmHg or to normal for that person	Urine output of >0.5 mL/kg/h	Stroke volume variation <5 mmHg
MAP >65 mmHg	Lactate <2 mmol/L	Cardiac index of >2.5 L/min/m^2
Pulse rate <100/min	Resolving base deficit	Pulmonary artery occlusion pressure >15 mmHg
CVP >10 mmHg	Central venous oximetry levels of 70–80%	Echocardiogram assessment of left ventricular end-diastolic volume and cardiac output
Sustained rise of CVP >7 mmHg in response to fluid	Capillary refill times <4 s	Mixed venous oximetry of 70–75%
Reduction in pressor/inotrope requirement	Clinical impression of improved skin perfusion and peripheral pulses	

- Dilutional or 'hyperchloraemic' acidosis is common but clinically insignificant.
- Anaphylaxis to synthetic colloids or blood products does occur and will complicate the management of shock.

2. Inotropes and vasopressors

Choice of inotrope

- Drugs described as vasopressors and inotropes overlap considerably in activity, thus traditional descriptions using receptor-based categories may confuse. Familiarity, institutional preference and awareness of both the clinical and side effects, desired and undesired, should influence individual choice (Table 2.4.2).
- A 'vasopressor' affects the venous or arterial vascular tone and should raise total peripheral resistance and hence mean arterial driving pressures as well as reducing venous capacitance and increasing preload/filling. Other vasoregulatory drugs affect the responsiveness of the vasculature to endogenous and infused vasopressors, including vasopressin and steroids.
- An 'inotrope' increases the velocity and force of myocardial muscle fibres and should result in increased contractility. This increased contractility, if combined with adequate preload/filling, will increase the stroke volume and hence cardiac output and raise the blood pressure. This will increase oxygen consumption, which may not be desirable, such as in myocardial ischaemia.
- Expert opinion-based recommendations guide the choice of vasopressor/inotrope

in septic shock [25], neurogenic shock and anaphylactic shock (see below). There is not sufficient evidence that any one of the investigated vasopressors is clearly superior over others [26,27].

- Dopamine appears inferior to other catecholamines in shock as it appears to increase the risk for arrhythmia [28]. It does not prevent or ameliorate the development of renal failure [29].
- Dobutamine was frequently recommended, but its deleterious effect on blood pressure means it is avoided in hypotension or used in combination with norepinephrine, or as guided by invasive monitoring.
- Dopexamine, levosimendan and the older phosphodiesterase inhibitors are rarely used in regular ED practice. They have not been convincingly shown to improve outcome in either undifferentiated or cardiogenic shock [30]. They can be used in specific and carefully monitored situations, such as shock with right ventricular (RV) failure or shock with excessive β-blockade.

Administration

- Norepinephrine, epinephrine (or salbutamol and isoprenaline) can be made up as 6 mg in 100 mL (or 3 mg in 50 mL) given by infusion pump into a central vein. The advantage of this particular dose dilution is that an infusion rate of 1 mL/h equates to 1 μg/min.

- Dobutamine and dopamine are presented as 250 mg and 200 mg ampoules and may be made up as weight (kg) × 6 mg in 100 mL or weight (kg) × 3 mg in 50 mL to give a dose dilution where an infusion rate of 1 mL/h equates to 1 μg/kg/min.

Route

- Vasopressors/inotropes may be administered into a large peripheral vein with fast-flowing crystalloid in an emergency. The clinical effect may be variable and thrombophlebitis can occur.
- Dedicated lines and lumina without side injection ports should be used to avoid inadvertent boluses.
- Placement of central venous lines (CVLs) or peripherally inserted central catheters (PICC) is performed under strict asepsis in an appropriate setting and may be required early in the ED for vasopressor/inotrope infusion.

Titration targets

- The use of vasopressors/inotropes without adequate preload is associated with a worse outcome [31,32], so volume infusion should *always* precede their use, unless there is unequivocal evidence that the heart is 'too full'. Even in cardiogenic shock, judicious boluses of fluid with close monitoring may result in improved cardiac output.
- Add an effective inotrope if, despite ongoing rapid fluid volume resuscitation, cardiac output markers such as MAP are low (see 'Goal-directed' resuscitation) and titrate

Table 2.4.2 Clinical effects of inotropes and vasopressors

Drug infused	Clinically observed		Measured		Calculated			
	Blood pressure (BP)	Heart rate (HR)	Cardiac contractility (stroke volume)	Cardiac output (CO)	Arterial vascular tone	Venous capacitance	Diastolic relaxation (lusitropy)	'Classical' receptor activity description
Adrenaline	++	++	++	++	+	+	+	β1 β2 α1 (α2)
Noradrenaline	++	0	+	+	+	++	−	β1, α1 (β2, α2)
Dopamine	+	++	+	+	+	+	−	β1 α1 dopA1
Dobutamine	−	+	++	++	−	−	0	β1 β2 (dopA1)
Metaraminol	++	0	0	0	+	++	0	α1
Isoprenaline	−	++	+	+	−	−	0	β1 β2
Levosimendan	+/−	+	++	++	0	0	+	Sensitizes troponin to Ca^{2+}
Vasopressin	+	0	0	0	++	+	0	V$_1$ V$_2$

rapidly upwards until an effect is noted. Wean the inotrope/vasopressor as further volume infusion allows or evidence develops that the heart is over-full. Reassess frequently to judge whether further fluid is needed.

- The upper level of the infusion is titrated to effect and only limited by the development of undesired side effects or a lack of therapeutic effect. Thus, any infusion is simply 'titrated to desired effect and monitored for undesired effect'.

Complications

- Side effects include excessive tachycardia, hypertension, tremor, anxiety and raised intracranial pressure (if monitored). Conversely, watch for disconnection or failure to infuse, when parameters unexpectedly fall.
- Epinephrine causes metabolic effects including hyperglycaemia, hypokalaemia and lactic acidosis (usually clinically irrelevant).
- Increased myocardial oxygen consumption can worsen myocardial ischaemia and precipitate cardiac arrhythmias.
- Peripheral digit and skin infarction described in the past is likely due to endothelial injury from prolonged shock or the underlying primary cause (e.g. meningococcus), with no evidence that it was due to a vasoconstrictor effect.
- Splanchnic or myocardial infarction also described is more likely to be due to inadequate resuscitation and hypotension rather than vasoconstriction, as these vessels are poorly reactive.
- 'Too large, too concentrated or too rapid' a bolus will cause severe hypertension and risks sequelae such as intracranial haemorrhage and myocardial damage.

3. Other interventions

- Corticosteroids in shock should be reserved for adrenal insufficiency or if the patient is already receiving corticosteroids. There is no evidence to support their routine use in anaphylactic shock (see Chapter 2.8).
- Corticosteroids such as hydrocortisone 200 mg per day may improve haemodynamic parameters in unresponsive septic shock, but two controlled multicentre trials found that corticosteroids have no effect on mortality [33,34]. Steroids are still

recommended in patients with bacterial meningitis in high-income countries to reduce hearing loss and neurological sequelae, but they do not reduce overall mortality [35]. Some spinal injury centres recommend high-dose methylprednisolone started within 8 h of injury given for 24–48 hours in spinal cord injury, but data are unconvincing [36].

- Military anti-shock trousers (MAST) or pneumatic anti-shock garments (PASG) increase morbidity and mortality and are no longer used [37].

Effects of shock on other interventions

- Hypoperfusion of tissues will affect the delivery of drugs, particularly orally and subcutaneously administered drugs, and affects the pharmacokinetics with a reduced clearance of drugs. Unpredictable delivery and efficacy may require dose changes or use of alternate routes. Carefully titrated intravenous doses given centrally are advisable.
- Sedative, analgesic and anaesthetic drugs, particularly thiopentone, midazolam, propofol and even ketamine (when the sympathetic ganglia are exhausted of catecholamine) have adverse effects on vascular tone and may worsen shock. These drugs also have a delayed circulation time and can appear not to be working, prompting inappropriate repeat dosing.
- Catecholamines are less effective in severe acidosis states, hence the theoretical but unproven use for sodium bicarbonate in severe, resistant metabolic acidosis.
- Endotracheal intubation and positive-pressure ventilation reduce venous return that may further reduce cardiac output and systolic blood pressure. Minimal initial tidal volume and positive end expiratory pressure (PEEP) settings ameliorate this effect. Physiological dead space may be increased by positive-pressure ventilation reducing lung perfusion, thus the arterial $PaCO_2$ may rise. 'Normalization' of $PaCO_2$ may then lead to an apparent worsening of compensated metabolic acidosis.
- Inotropes are arrhythmogenic and this complication is increased in the setting of hypokalaemia, acidosis and poorly perfused myocardium.

- The stress response and some inotropes cause or exacerbate hyperglycaemia.
- Infused fluids will eventually redistribute to all tissues and produce widespread oedema. An example is the burns victim who may have minimal airway burns, but after many litres of crystalloid may have a compromised oedematous airway.

Management of specific shock syndromes

The following shock syndromes are discussed briefly here and in other chapters:

- Hypovolaemia (absolute)
- Hypovolaemia (relative)
- Neurogenic shock (see Chapter 3.3)
- Anaphylactic shock (see Chapter 2.8)
- Hypoadrenal shock (see Chapter 11.3)
- Cardiogenic shock (see Chapter 5.2)
- Septic shock (see Chapter 2.5).

Absolute hypovolaemia

Clinical features

The history and examination may point to fluid loss from vessels, gut, kidneys or evaporation. Bleeding needs to be excluded in all hypovolaemia (see Box 2.4.1). In addition to those described previously, clinical features will include signs of reduced preload, with flat neck veins as a consequence of a low central venous pressure.

Relevant investigations

If hypovolaemia is due to bleeding, haemostasis is the most effective intervention by direct surgical or specialist intervention and may parallel resuscitation and precede investigations. If initial resuscitation allows, investigations, such as formal ultrasound, computed tomography (CT) with contrast angiography, may identify the site of bleeding. Radiographic intervention, such as angiography with embolization, may be life saving in severe pelvic trauma.

Therapy

- Initial resuscitation as described previously and ensure all efforts are made to avoid hypothermia.
- Passive leg elevation is more effective in hypovolaemic shock than the Trendelenburg (head lower than the pelvis body position) in increasing left ventricular end-diastolic

volume, stroke volume and cardiac output, but these effects are transient [6].

- External haemorrhage is controlled with firm, direct manual pressure. Tourniquets are associated with morbidity, but may be useful in the short term [38].
- Surgical consultation is required urgently. Efforts to return the systolic blood pressure to 'normal' in bleeding trauma patients may be counterproductive and occasionally harmful, particularly in penetrating truncal trauma. Surgical haemostasis must take priority and over-resuscitation should be avoided, adopting a 'minimal-volume' approach. Thus, patients with uncontrolled haemorrhage following penetrating truncal trauma, who are in close proximity to facilities capable of definitive care, should undergo minimal-volume or 'hypotense' fluid resuscitation pending prompt surgical intervention [39]. 'Minimal volume' is interpreted variously as fluid sufficient to keep the line open (TKVO) or small (250 mL) boluses titrated to a palpable radial pulse or conscious level, with the aim to 'keep the brain and heart perfused'. Any minimal-volume approach is contraindicated when traumatic brain injury is associated with hypotension, as cerebral perfusion pressure is dependent on maintaining the MAP.
- Infuse packed red cells in major blood loss where oxygen delivery is known to be impaired or Hb is less than 70 g/L. Recognition or anticipation of coagulopathy will need fresh frozen plasma and platelets as in a major transfusion protocol. Patients with lesser amounts of blood loss or controlled bleeding, or non-haemorrhagic hypovolaemic shock can be managed with warmed crystalloid [19].
- Hypertonic saline 3% or 7% was considered to improve outcome in a subgroup of patients with shock and traumatic brain injury, but this remains unproven. Despite this, hypertonic saline has been recommended as the initial fluid of choice in haemorrhaging battlefield casualties [40].
- There are no current definitive recommendations concerning the use of blood substitutes, such as modified haemoglobin or non-blood perfluorocarbons.
- Other causes of impaired preload or contractility, such as tension pneumothorax, cardiac tamponade and myocardial contusion, must be considered in the hypotensive trauma patient. Increasing

preload is still beneficial in these settings and all trauma patients should be assumed to be hypovolaemic until proven otherwise. Urgent bedside ultrasound is essential.

Relative hypovolaemia
This may be due to anaphylaxis, Addisonian crisis, neurogenic shock, septic shock or a drug or toxin effect.

Anaphylaxis
The mainstay of treatment in shock is the physiological antagonist epinephrine (adrenaline) plus oxygen and fluid, with the patient supine and the legs raised (see Chapter 2.8).

Adrenal shock
Hypotension due to hypoadrenalism is uncommon, but should be suspected in the acutely unwell patient with past or current steroid use or when hypotension occurs with relative polyuria or a relatively high urinary sodium >20 mmol/L (see Chapter 11.3).

Neurogenic shock
Neurogenic shock is manifested by the triad of hypotension, bradycardia and hypothermia in the setting of an acute spinal cord injury, related to the loss of sympathetic nerve tone. One in four patients with a complete cervical-cord injury may require haemodynamic support for their hypotension [41]. Other causes of hypovolaemia or shock in the trauma patient should still be actively sought, such as concealed bleeding, tension pneumothorax and cardiac tamponade (see Chapter 3.3).

Septic shock
Septic shock is sepsis accompanied by hypotension or hypoperfusion and can be underappreciated as the patient may have few signs of inadequate perfusion. Persistent hypotension and/or signs of organ hypoperfusion, despite ongoing rapid fluid resuscitation, are indications for early vasopressor/inotrope support. Vasopressin 0.04 units/min has no greater effect on survival [42]. A *post-hoc* analysis of the SAFE study suggests that albumin may have a survival advantage [19]. Hydrocortisone may improve unresponsive shock, as can high volume haemofiltration, but trials have found no overall effect on mortality [32–34] (see Chapter 2.5).

Drug effects
Multiple drugs or toxins cause hypotension by impairing vascular or cardiac muscle contractility

or permeability. Intervention with increased fluid or inotropes/pressors will manage hypotension. If the drug affects an inotrope/vasopressor receptor, either physiological antagonism or alternative receptor stimulation can overcome this effect. When the toxin is a metabolic or mitochondrial poison, the general principals of removal and support are used (see Chapter 29.2).

Cardiac causes of shock: cardiogenic shock
Cardiogenic shock is the inability of the heart to deliver sufficient blood to the tissues to meet resting metabolic demands and is clinically defined as a systolic blood pressure of <90 mmHg or MAP >30 mmHg below baseline for at least 30 minutes.

An alternative definition is a significant arteriovenous oxygen difference and a cardiac index of <2.2 L/min/m^2 where pulmonary capillary wedge pressure is >15 mmHg. Failure to respond to correction of hypoxaemia, hypovolaemia, arrhythmias and acidosis is a requirement for the diagnosis [43]. There is clinical evidence of poor tissue perfusion in the form of oliguria, cyanosis and altered mentation.

Aetiology
The most common cause of cardiogenic shock is myocardial infarction (MI) or ischaemia. Cardiogenic shock complicates 5–8% of patients with acute myocardial infarction and has a mortality as high as 56–74%. It is the commonest cause of in-hospital death post-infarction [43,44]. Only 10% of these patients develop cardiogenic shock in the ED, but this subgroup has a higher mortality [44].

Other cardiac causes of shock include valvular rupture or degeneration, critical stenosis, septal or free wall rupture and atrial myxoma. Cardiac tamponade or a large pulmonary embolus are better considered as obstructive causes of shock, as the myocardial pump is unaffected initially.

Older patients with anterior MI, previous MI, diabetes, angina or congestive heart failure are at greatest risk of cardiogenic shock. There is a higher prevalence in patients with multivessel disease (e.g. diabetes) and involving the left main coronary artery [45]. Patients with persistent occlusion of the left anterior descending artery are at the highest risk of developing shock [46]. Only aggressive revascularization within 12 hours of symptoms improves outcome in these patients.

Pathophysiology

Activation of the sympathetic nervous and renin–angiotensin systems contributes to an increase in myocardial oxygen demand which causes an increase in infarct size and further decreases contractility, cardiac output and coronary perfusion pressure. Systolic dysfunction results in an increase in end-systolic volumes and reductions in ejection fraction, stroke volume and cardiac output. Diastolic dysfunction is also present. Pulmonary oedema exacerbates hypoxia and systemic tissue hypoperfusion and selective vascular redistribution leads to organ failure and metabolic acidosis.

Clinical features

Clinical signs in cardiogenic shock in addition to those described previously include:

- Signs of excessive catecholamine outflow, such as tachycardia, pallor, poor capillary refill and evidence of low cardiac output with a decreased urine output and raised lactate.
- Blood pressure that may initially remain within normal limits as a result of compensatory mechanisms, which also produce tachycardia and narrowed pulse pressure.
- Classic signs of left heart failure with a third heart sound gallop rhythm and basal crackles from pulmonary oedema. A 'gallop' or additional heart sound suggests reduced ventricular compliance (fourth heart sound) and increased ventricular diastolic pressure (third heart sound).
- Raised jugular venous pressure (JVP), hepatic congestion and peripheral oedema of right ventricular failure may occur secondary to left heart failure or alone in right ventricular infarction usually associated with an inferior myocardial infarction. This can be inferred by ST elevation in a right-sided V4 chest lead (V_4R).
- Loud murmur or thrill in systole may be due to mitral regurgitation or critical aortic stenosis and, rarely, rupture of the ventricular septum.

Investigations in cardiogenic shock

- Twelve-lead ECG may define territory and need for reperfusion therapy. Adding leads V_4R and V_{7-9} are indicated to rule out right ventricular and posterior myocardial infarction, respectively.
- Troponin I (or T) levels.
- Chest X-ray to show pulmonary oedema and an enlarged cardiac silhouette.

Bedside echocardiography (TTE) should be performed in any patient who remains with undiagnosed shock, as an extension of the physical examination. Pericardial effusion or cardiac tamponade are excluded and global systolic function, filling and regional wall motion abnormalities assessed.

- Transoesophageal echocardiography (TOE) may additionally diagnose loculated cardiac tamponade, a haemodynamically significant pulmonary embolus and obscure valvular lesions.

ED therapy

- Initial care and monitoring should be provided as described earlier, with management of the myocardial infarct according to local reperfusion policy. When cardiogenic shock is recognized, immediate discussion regarding revascularization should be made with a referral centre, particularly if TTE does not show a mechanical cause of shock [47].
- Tracheal intubation and ventilation should be considered early for cardiac 'respite' and continuous positive airway pressure (CPAP) or non-invasive ventilation with bi-level positive airway pressure (BIPAP) in selected patients. Invasive blood pressure monitoring is recommended [47].
- Arrhythmias considered contributory to the presence of cardiogenic shock should be treated according to standard ACLS principles.
- Hypovolaemia must be sought and corrected in all patients with 250 mL aliquots of fluid given as a bolus and the response assessed. Volume loading to maintain higher right atrial filling pressures is important in inferior MI with right ventricular involvement, plus avoidance of drugs that reduce preload including nitrates, diuretics and excess opiates.
- Relevant targets should include evidence of perfusion, such as urine output, lactate and clinical signs of improved skin perfusion and resolution of pulmonary oedema. Coronary autoregulation occurs at a MAP of 60 mmHg.

- Persistence of the shock state following adequate fluid challenge in the presence of end-organ dysfunction is an indication for urgent revascularization. Intra-aortic balloon pump (IABP), extracorporeal membrane oxygenation (ECMO) and/or inotropic support may be considered as a bridge to this [45].
- Early revascularization by either percutaneous coronary intervention (PCI) or coronary artery bypass graft (CABG) is recommended for patients less than 75 years old with ST elevation or new left bundle branch block (LBBB) who develop cardiogenic shock within 36 hours of acute MI and who are suitable for revascularization that can be performed within 18 hours of shock onset [47]. Early transfer and revascularization confers a survival advantage in patients with MI plus cardiogenic shock [43–45,47].
- Initial therapy for patients who present to a facility without early primary PCI capability can include thrombolysis followed by urgent transfer [45,46].
- IABP does not appear to reduce 12 month all-cause mortality in patients undergoing early revascularisation for myocardial infarction complicated by cardiogenic shock [48]. Intra-aortic balloon counterpulsation increases aortic root diastolic pressure (and hence coronary perfusion) and duration of apparent systole (and hence MAP), with no increase in oxygen demand. Complications include leg ischaemia, arterial dissection, thromboembolism and thrombocytopenia [49,50].
- Use of inotropes and vasopressors in cardiogenic shock has not been shown to improve survival, but may be needed to maintain perfusion [47–49]. Dobutamine and levosimendan have inotropic and vasodilator effects, but are not recommended in hypotension. Norepinephrine (noradrenaline) is now the recommended inotrope/pressor [47], allowing the later introduction of a vasodilator. Dopamine was previously used, but the tachycardia limits its efficacy by increasing myocardial oxygen demand. There is no evidence for a reduction in mortality with the use of any of the newer inodilators, such as dopexamine, milrinone or levosimendan [30,49].

- ECMO is being increasingly used as support for refractory cardiogenic shock with reasonable outcomes described, but no definitive trial exists [49,51].
  - Vasodilators can be considered when blood pressure has been restored but fails to improve peripheral end-organ perfusion. Glyceryl trinitrate or angiotensin-converting enzyme inhibitors (ACEI) can be given if titrated carefully, although precipitate hypotension may occur.
- Consider referral for emergency cardiac transplantation in the younger patient.
- Overall, those patients with large infarctions, a resting tachycardia and signs of poor tissue perfusion should be identified early and managed aggressively with cardiology advice. There should be early discussion with a cardiac referral centre and, if the patient is unstable or unsuitable for transfer, an IABP can be considered with a lower threshold for thrombolysis if not contraindicated. Inotropes are a temporizing measure.

Pericardial tamponade

Pericardial (cardiac) tamponade causes a failure of filling of the right atrium as a result of increased pericardial pressure. The right ventricle, and subsequently the left ventricle, has limited stroke volume and cardiac output, so tachycardia and raised peripheral resistance are compensatory mechanisms (see Chapter 5.6).

The presence of pericardial tamponade should also be suspected when there is unexplained shock with blunt or penetrating chest trauma, pericarditis, anticoagulant use or iatrogenic misadventure, e.g. CVP insertion.

Volume loading will raise right-sided filling pressures and volumes and tachycardia should be preserved. Vasopressor support will maintain MAP until surgical pericardiotomy (traumatic cause) or pericardiocentesis under echo guidance are performed.

Conclusion

The aetiology of shock in patients presenting to the ED is varied. Interventions in all forms of shock are simple and initially directed at the physiological deficit and should be seen as a test of the clinical hypothesis. Continuous reappraisal is required. Hypovolaemia should be sought in all cases, although further specific management will depend on the underlying cause(s).

References

[1] Dutton RP. Current concepts in hemorrhagic shock. Anesthesiol Clin 2007;25:23–34. viii.

[2] Pickering TG, Hall JE, Appel LJ, et al. Recommendations for blood pressure measurement in humans and experimental animals. Part 1: blood pressure measurement in humans: a statement for professionals from the Subcommittee of Professional and Public Education of the American Heart Association Council on High Blood Pressure Research. Circulation 2005;111:697–716.

[3] Fieselmann JF, Hendryx MS, Helms CM, Wakefield DS. Respiratory rate predicts cardiopulmonary arrest for internal medicine inpatients. J Gen Intern Med 1993;8:354–60.

[4] American College of Surgeons Committee on Trauma Advanced Trauma Life Support. Student Course Manual, 9th ed. Chicago: ACS; 2012.

[5] Jones AE, Aborn LS, Kline JA. Severity of emergency department hypotension predicts adverse hospital outcome. Shock 2004;22:410–4.

[6] Terai C, Anada H, Matsushima S, et al. Effects of Trendelenburg versus passive leg-raising autotransfusion in humans. Intens Care Med 1996;22:613–4.

[7] Bur A, Herkner H, Vlcek M, et al. Factors influencing the accuracy of oscillometric blood pressure measurement in critically ill patients. Crit Care Med 2003;31:793–9.

[8] Bakker J, Coffernils M, Leon M, et al. Blood lactate levels are superior to oxygen derived variables in predicting outcome in human septic shock. Chest 1991;99:956–62.

[9] Davis JW, Parks JN, Kaups KL, et al. Admission base deficit predicts transfusion requirements and risk of complication. J Trauma 1996;41:769–74.

[10] Lamia B, ChemLa D, Richard C, Teboul JL. Clinical review: interpretation of arterial pressure wave in shock states. Crit Care 2005;9:601–6.

[11] Tavernier B, Makhotine O, Lebuffe G, et al. Pressure variation as a guide to fluid therapy in patients with sepsis-induced hypotension. Anesthesiology 1998;89:1313–21.

[12] Jin X, Weil MH, Tang W, et al. End-tidal carbon dioxide as a noninvasive indicator of cardiac index during circulatory shock. Crit Care Med 2000;28:2415–9.

[13] McKinley BA, Kozar RA, Cocanour CS, et al. Normal versus supranormal oxygen delivery goals in shock resuscitation: the response is the same. J Trauma 2002;53:825–32.

[14] Kern JW, Shoemaker WC. Meta-analysis of hemodynamic optimization in high-risk patients. Crit Care Med 2002;30:1686–92.

[15] Rivers E, Nguyen B, Havstad S, the Early Goal-Directed Therapy Collaborative Group. Early goal-directed therapy in the treatment of severe sepsis and septic shock. N Engl J Med 2001;345:1368–77.

[16] American Heart Association Guidelines for Cardiopulmonary Resuscitation and Emergency Cardiovascular Care 2005. Circulation 2005; 112.

[17] Waters JH, Gottlieb A, Schoenwald P, et al. Normal saline versus lactated Ringer's solution for intraoperative fluid management in patients undergoing abdominal aortic aneurysm repair: an outcome study. Anesth Analges 2001;93:817–22.

[18] Finfer S, Bellomo R, Boyce N, et al. A comparison of albumin and saline for fluid resuscitation in the intensive care unit. N Engl J Med 2004;350:2247.

[19] Bunn F, Trivedi D. Colloid solutions for fluid resuscitation. Cochrane Database Syst Rev 2012;7:CD001319.

[20] Myburgh JA, Finfer S, Bellomo R, et al. CHEST Investigators; Australian and New Zealand Intensive Care Society Clinical Trials Group. Hydroxyethyl starch or saline for fluid resuscitation in intensive care. N Engl J Med 2012;367:1901–11.

[21] Hebert PC, Wells G, Blajchman MA, et al. A multicenter, randomized, controlled clinical trial of transfusion requirements in critical care. N Engl J Med 1999;340:409–17.

[22] Australian and New Zealand Society of Blood Transfusion. Guidelines for the administration of blood component products, 2nd ed., 2011. < http://www.anzsbt.org.au/publications/documents/ANZSBT_Guidelines_Administration_Blood_Products_2ndEd_Dec_2011_Hyperlinks.pdf > (Accessed Mar. 2013).

[23] Becton Dickinson product information. Becton Dickinson Pty Ltd, Eight Mile Plains, QLD 4113.

[24] Mendenhall ML, Spain DA. Venous air embolism and pressure infusion devices. J Trauma 2007;63:246.

[25] Dellinger R, Levy M, Rhodes A, et al. Surviving sepsis campaign: international guidelines for management of severe sepsis and septic shock: 2012.Crit Care Med 2013;41:580–637.

[26] Myburgh JA. An appraisal of selection and use of catecholamines in septic shock – old becomes new again. Crit Care Resus 2006;3:353–60.

[27] Havel C, Arrich J, Losert H, et al. Vasopressors for hypotensive shock. Cochrane Database Syst Rev 2011;5:CD003709.

[28] Sakr Y, Reinhart K, Vincent JL, et al. Does dopamine administration in shock influence outcome? Results of the Sepsis Occurrence in Acutely Ill Patients (SOAP) study. Crit Care Med 2006;34:589.

[29] Bellomo R, Chapman M, Finfer S, et al. Low-dose dopamine in patients with early renal dysfunction: a placebo-controlled randomized trial. Australian and New Zealand Intensive Care Society (ANZICS) Clinical Trials Group. Lancet 2000;356:2139–43.

[30] Mebazaa A, Nieminen M, Packer M, et al. Levosimendan vs dobutamine for patients with acute decompensated heart failure: the SURVIVE Randomised Trial. J Am Med Assoc 2007;297:1883–91.

[31] Beale RJ, Hollenberg SM, Vincent JL, et al. Vasopressor and inotropic support in septic shock: an evidence-based review. Crit Care Med 2004;32:S455–65.

[32] Nordin AJ, Makisalo H, Hockerstedt KA. Failure of dobutamine to improve liver oxygenation during resuscitation with a crystalloid solution after experimental haemorrhagic shock. Eur J Surg 1996;162:973.

[33] Annane D, Sebille V, Charpenteir C, et al. Effect of treatment with low doses of hydrocortisone and fludrocortisone on mortality in patients with septic shock. J Am Med Assoc 2002;288:862–71.

[34] Lipiner-Friedman D, Sprung CL, Laterre PF, Corticus Study Group. Adrenal function in sepsis: the retrospective Corticus cohort study. Crit Care Med 2007;35:1012–8.

[35] Brouwer MC, McIntyre P, de Gans J, et al. Corticosteroids for acute bacterial meningitis. Cochrane Database Syst Rev 2010;9:CD004405.

[36] Bracken MB. Steroids for acute spinal cord injury. Cochrane Database Syst Rev 2012;1:CD001046.

[37] Roberts I, Blackhall K, Dickinson K. Medical anti-shock trousers (pneumatic anti-shock garments) for circulatory support in patients with trauma. Cochrane Database Syst Rev 1999;4:CD001856.

[38] Lee C, Porter KM, Hodgetts TJ. Tourniquet use in the civilian prehospital setting. Emerg Med J 2007;24:584–7.

[39] Bickell WH, Wall Jr MJ, Pepe PE, Martin RR. Immediate versus delayed fluid resuscitation for hypotensive patients with penetrating torso injuries. N Engl J Med 1994;331:1105–9.

[40] Alam HB, Rhee P. New developments in fluid resuscitation. Surg Clin N Am 2007;87:55–72. vi.

[41] Guly HR, Bouamra O, Lecky FE, on behalf of the Trauma Audit and Research Network. The incidence of neurogenic shock in patients with isolated spinal cord injury in the emergency department. Resuscitation 2007;76:57–62.

[42] Levy MM, Fink MP, Marshall JC, et al. 2001 SCCM/ESICM/ACCP/ATS/SIS International Sepsis Definitions Conference. Crit Care Med 2003; 31:1250–1256.

[43] Reynolds H, Hochman J. Cardiogenic shock: current concepts and improving outcomes. Circulation 2008;117:686–97.

[44] Webb JG, Sleeper LA, Buller CE, et al. Implications of the timing of onset of cardiogenic shock after acute myocardial infarction: a report from the SHOCK Trial Registry. Should we emergently revascularize occluded coronaries for cardiogenic shock? J Am Coll Cardiol 2000;36:1084.

[45] Goldberg RJ, Gore JM, Thompson CA, et al. Recent magnitude of and temporal trends (1994–1997) in the incidence and hospital death rates of cardiogenic shock complicating acute myocardial infarction: The second National Registry of Myocardial Infarction. Am Heart J 2001;141:65.

[46] Wong SC, Sanborn T, Sleeper LA, et al. Angiographic findings and clinical correlates in patients with cardiogenic shock complicating acute myocardial infarction: a report from the SHOCK Trial Registry. SHould we emergently revascularize Occluded Coronaries for cardiogenic shocK? J Am Coll Cardiol 2000;36:1077.

CRITICAL CARE

[47] Antman EM, et al. ACC/AHA Guidelines for management of patients with ST elevation MI: a report of the American College of Cardiology/American Heart Association Task Force on Practice Guidelines. Circulation 2004;110:e82–e29251.

[48] Thiele H, Zeymer U, Neumann F, et al. Intra-aortic balloon counterpulsation in acute myocardial infarction complicated by cardiogenic shock (IABP-SHOCK II). Lancet 2013;382:1638–45.

[49] Sayer GT, Baker JN, Parks KA. Heart rescue: the role of mechanical circulatory support in the management of severe refractory cardiogenic shock. Curr Opin Crit Care 2012;18:409–16.

[50] Prieto A, Eisenberg J, Thakar RK. Non-arrhythmic complications of acute myocardial infarction. Emerg Med Clin N Am 2001;19:397–415.

[51] Tsao NW, Shih CM, Yeh JS, et al. Extracorporeal membrane oxygenation assisted primary percutaneous coronary intervention may improve survival of acute myocardial infarction complicated by profound cardiogenic shock. J Crit Care 2012;27(530):e1–11.

2.5 Sepsis and septic shock

Anna Holdgate

ESSENTIALS

1 Early recognition and intervention in the emergency department (ED) reduces mortality in patients with sepsis and septic shock.

2 Appropriate broad-spectrum antibiotics should be administered within 1 hour of the recognition of sepsis.

3 Aggressive haemodynamic resuscitation with fluids, vasopressors and inotropes should begin as soon as possible.

4 Systemic blood pressure, serum lactate levels and urine output should be monitored closely to determine the effectiveness of treatment.

Introduction

Septic shock is the extreme end of the spectrum of septic syndromes. Globally, septic shock is associated with a mortality rate of up to 46%. In Australia and New Zealand, the reported mortality is substantially lower (27.6%) for septic patients admitted from the emergency department (ED) to intensive care (ICU) [1]. Each year more than 1500 septic patients are admitted to Australasian ICUs from the ED and this incidence has been steadily rising over the past decade [1]. Optimal, time-critical care of the septic patient in ED is crucial, as early intervention in several areas has been shown to reduce mortality.

Aetiology and pathophysiology

Approximately 95% of identified causative organisms are bacterial, with Gram-positive organisms (mostly *Staphylococcus aureus*, coagulase-negative staphylococci, enterococci and streptococci) now slightly more common than Gram-negative species (particularly *Escherichia coli*, *Klebsiella pneumoniae* and *Pseudomonas aeruginosa*). The remaining 5% are caused by fungi, mostly *Candida*, with the incidence of fungal sepsis increasing threefold in the last 20 years [2].

Pathogens are identified from blood or other tissue cultures in approximately 70% of patients. The primary sources of infection are respiratory, genitourinary, intra-abdominal, skin/other soft tissue and primary bacteraemia [3].

Pathogenic mechanisms

The pathogenic mechanisms in sepsis are initiated by a variety of host responses to the infecting organism. Pattern recognition receptors in the cell membrane (transmembrane toll-like receptors, TLRs) and in the cytoplasm (NOD-like receptors, NLRs) are responsible for initiating the immune response following recognition of an invading pathogen.

Inflammatory mediators

Inflammatory mediators, such as tumour necrosis factor α (TNF-α) and the interleukins, are produced by the host, resulting in activation of neutrophils, direct injury to the endothelium with increased vascular permeability and release of nitric oxide (NO) that results in vasodilatation. Modification of the coagulation cascade causes an increase in procoagulant factors and lower levels of the anticoagulant factors protein C, protein S and antithrombin III. These proinflammatory and procoagulant responses lead to reduced vascular resistance, relative hypovolaemia, loss of vasoregulatory control in microvascular beds, reduced myocardial contractility, acute lung injury and renal dysfunction.

These changes further impair oxygen delivery and consumption at a tissue level, resulting in tissue hypoxia and worsening organ dysfunction. Anaerobic metabolism causes a rising lactate when oxygen delivery cannot meet tissue oxygen demands. Central venous oxygen saturations ($S_{CV}O_2$) will generally be low (<70%) as the peripheral tissues extract a higher percentage of oxygen, resulting in less oxygen in venous blood returning to the central circulation [4,5].

The progression of sepsis to septic shock is associated with an inability to contain the infection, owing to (either or both) compromised patient immunity or characteristics of the infection itself, such as highly virulent organisms, a high burden of infection and antibiotic resistance.

Clinical features

Infection associated with systemic illness results in a spectrum of clinical syndromes based on clinical signs. Much broader definitions released in 2013 are now in use [6].

Clinical syndrome definitions

Systemic manifestations of infection

The systemic manifestations of infection have been vastly expanded and replace those features that were previously used to define the systemic inflammatory response syndrome (SIRS). These originally included two or more of the following:

- abnormal body temperature (>38°C or <36°C)
- tachycardia >90 bpm
- tachypnoea (respiratory rate >20/min or $PaCO_2$ <32 mmHg)
- abnormal white cell count (>12 000/μL or <4000/μL or >10% immature (band) cells).

Sepsis

Sepsis is defined as the presence (probable or documented) of infection together with systemic manifestations of infection (blood cultures do *not* need to be positive).

Severe sepsis

Severe sepsis is defined as sepsis plus sepsis-induced organ dysfunction or tissue hypoperfusion. Sepsis-induced tissue hypoperfusion is defined as infection-induced hypotension, elevated lactate, or oliguria. Sepsis-induced hypotension is defined as a systolic blood pressure (SBP) <90 mmHg or mean arterial pressure (MAP) <70 mmHg or a SBP decrease >40 mmHg, or less than two standard deviations below normal for age in the absence of other causes of hypotension.

Septic shock

Septic shock is defined as sepsis-induced hypotension persisting despite adequate fluid resuscitation.

History

Important components of the clinical history include the patient's immune status, prior infections and/or antibiotic use, co-morbid disease, such as diabetes or malignancy, travel or exposure history and an assessment of acute respiratory, abdominal or urinary symptoms, plus identification of potential sources for infection, such as recent procedures or prosthetic devices including stents and indwelling catheters.

Physical examination

Look for the systemic manifestations of infection, as well as for sites of infection, plus evidence of organ dysfunction, or hypoperfusion, such as an altered mental status, an episode of hypotension, tachycardia, tachypnoea from metabolic acidosis, hypoxia, pneumonia or acute respiratory distress syndrome (ARDS) or oliguria.

Include a top-to-toe assessment including the head and neck, oropharynx, skin, chest, abdomen, pelvis and perineum, back, limbs and joints.

A septic patient is relatively hypovolaemic due to peripheral vasodilatation in addition to fluid depletion from vomiting and third-space sequestration. The patient with severe sepsis may have warm peripheries and a bounding pulse early due to mediator-driven vasodilatation though, in the later stages, they are more usually hypothermic and peripherally shut down as a result of cardiovascular collapse and/or vasoconstriction.

Clinical investigations

Investigations are important in determining the nature of the condition as SIRS features occur in non-infectious conditions, such as post-trauma or surgery, burns, pancreatitis and other shock states, as well as confirming the aetiology and severity of the underlying infection.

Laboratory

Basic blood pathology helps identify potential causes, such as biliary obstruction, and will quantify end-organ dysfunction, such as renal failure, hypo-/hyperglycaemia and coagulopathy. Arterial blood gases should be measured early to assess both the adequacy of ventilation and the degree of lactic acidosis. A venous blood gas is equally useful for lactate estimation.

Source

A search for the underlying source should include two sets of paired blood cultures peripherally and a set from any indwelling line(s), urine microscopy and culture, chest X-ray, culture of any open wound and aspiration of any superficial collections.

In the absence of a clearly identified focus, abdominal computed tomography (CT) scanning and, particularly if there is an altered mental state, CT brain and lumbar puncture are usual, unless contraindicated by the patient's clinical status.

Risk stratification

Factors associated with an increased mortality include the initial lactate level, age and multiple co-morbidities. Elevated lactate levels are associated with a higher mortality independent of other signs of shock and organ dysfunction and are therefore useful in early risk stratification [7,8]. The elderly have a higher mortality, in part related to greater co-morbidity. However, age alone is an independent risk factor, as the elderly are more likely to present with seriously deranged physiological parameters. While fever is more commonly associated with sepsis, hypothermia is a worrying sign associated with a higher morbidity, particularly in the elderly [9].

Treatment

The principles of treatment in sepsis are haemodynamic resuscitation, supportive measures to maximize tissue oxygen delivery, early antibiotic therapy and source control (see also Chapter 2.4). The International Surviving Sepsis Campaign Consensus Guidelines were developed to promote a more uniform 'bundle of care' for the acute management of patients with sepsis, aimed at reducing mortality [10]. These guidelines incorporate the concept of early goal-directed therapy (EGDT), with specific targeted endpoints to guide sequential treatment.

The use of standardized ED guidelines focused on haemodynamic resuscitation and early, appropriate antibiotic therapy improves compliance with recommended treatment and reduces mortality [11,12].

Haemodynamic resuscitation and supportive care

Early goal-directed therapy

The components of EGDT are adequate volume replacement followed by vasopressor and inotropic therapy aimed at maintaining MAP ≥65 mmHg, urine output ≥0.5 mL/kg/h and, in some settings, $S_{cv}O_2$ ≥70% [10]. Whereas measurement of MAP and urine output is straightforward, measurement of $S_{cv}O_2$ requires either frequent blood gas sampling from a standard central venous catheter or continuous measurement using a commercial central venous catheter with a specialized fibreoptic module.

Fluid resuscitation

Fluid resuscitation begins with a minimum of 30 mL/kg of crystalloid, such as normal saline.

Patients who remain hypotensive, acidotic or oliguric usually warrant central venous pressure (CVP) and invasive arterial pressure monitoring to guide further therapy [10]. Fluid resuscitation should continue to a CVP of 8–12 mmHg in the absence of pulmonary oedema.

Vasopressor therapy

Vasopressor therapy is indicated concurrently with fluid resuscitation in the presence of profound hypotension or if fluid resuscitation fails to restore tissue perfusion (as indicated by normalization of MAP to at least 65 mmHg, lactate levels and urine output). Norepinephrine (noradrenaline) is commonly used first choice due to its potent α effects that increase blood pressure predominantly by direct vasoconstriction and more moderate β effects associated with some increase in heart rate and stroke volume. Thus, it is a preferred agent in patients with profound hypotension [10].

Epinephrine (adrenaline) can be used as an alternative vasopressor, although it may be associated with a higher incidence of arrhythmias, splanchnic ischaemia and metabolic effects than norepinephrine [13,14]. All vasopressor agents need to be administered via a central venous catheter and the infusion rate titrated to MAP measured by an intra-arterial catheter, urine output and cerebral perfusion.

Measurement of $S_{CV}O_2$

The measurement of $S_{CV}O_2$ is advocated as a further endpoint to assess tissue perfusion and guide ongoing therapy. In the seminal 2001 EGDT study by Rivers et al., red cell transfusion to a haemocrit $\geq$30% and dobutamine infusion to improve cardiac output were used in patients who failed to achieve $S_{CV}O_2$ $\geq$70% with fluids, vasopressors and ventilatory support [12].

Patients who received EGDT had a lower mortality than patients receiving 'standard' therapy. An alternative method of measuring improvement in tissue perfusion is to monitor the lactate level, aiming for a reduction of at least 10% which achieves a similar in-hospital mortality and does not require the insertion of an $S_{CV}O_2$-monitoring catheter [15].

Reported mortality rates for sepsis in Australasian patients are substantially lower than in the Rivers' study, hence the applicability of Rivers' EGDT in the Australasian setting is unclear [1]. International guidelines currently recommend the use of adjuvant dobutamine in patients with a low cardiac output despite fluids and vasopressors. Blood transfusion is recommended only to a target haemoglobin level of 7–9 g/dL, except in patients with acute haemorrhage or significant coronary artery disease [10].

Maximizing oxygen delivery

As sepsis is associated with increased oxygen consumption, oxygen delivery must be optimized at the beginning of resuscitation. Endotracheal intubation and mechanical ventilation with appropriate sedation and paralysis minimize oxygen consumption and should be considered early in patients with respiratory acidosis, hypoxia or persistent haemodynamic compromise. Low tidal volume ventilation (6 mL/kg) with peak inspiratory pressures maintained $\leq$30 cm H_2O are recommended to minimize further acute lung injury [10].

Antibiotic therapy

The early administration of appropriate antibiotic therapy in the ED is *essential* to the effective management of the septic patient. Time to appropriate antibiotic administration is one of the prime determinants of survival in severe sepsis. Patients with severe sepsis or septic shock who do not receive antibiotics within 1 hour have an increase in mortality of approximately 7.6% for each additional hour of delay [3,16]. Thus, a patient with severe sepsis should have appropriate cultures collected and antibiotics started within 1 hour of arrival. Collection of cultures or imaging studies must *not* delay the administration of antibiotics [10].

Choice of antibiotic

The choice of antibiotic depends on a number of criteria, including the likely source of infection, local bacterial sensitivities and patient factors, such as allergy, immunocompetence and renal function. The initial choice should be broad enough to cover a range of potential pathogens, as treatment with ineffective antibiotics is also associated with increased mortality [17,18]. Antibiotic therapy can be more specifically targeted once the causative organism and its sensitivities are known, but this is rarely appropriate in the ED [19]. Table 2.5.1 outlines one approach to initial antibiotic choice.

Empiric monotherapy with a third- or fourth-generation cephalosporin has been shown to be as effective as dual therapy with a β-lactam and an aminoglycoside. However, most of the evidence is derived from patients with febrile neutropaenia and only a few small studies have been conducted in immunocompetent patients with severe sepsis or septic shock. Many practitioners still prefer dual therapy on the basis that this may confer synergistic effects that enhance antibacterial activity and reduce the incidence of bacterial resistance [18]. These potential benefits must be weighed against the increased risk of nephrotoxicity and ototoxicity associated with the use of aminoglycosides [2].

Empirical treatment with glycopeptides, such as vancomycin, is recommended in patients with known methicillin resistant *S. aureus* (MRSA) colonization, severe penicillin hypersensitivity, high prevalence of community-associated MRSA (CA-MRSA), suspected line sepsis or in institutions with high levels of MRSA [2,18].

Empirical antifungal treatment with amphotericin or fluconazole is recommended in patients at high risk for invasive candidiasis, such as those who have been treated with prolonged broad-spectrum antibiotics, are immunosuppressed and have had *Candida* isolated from multiple sites [20].

Source control

Source control refers to physical measures to control or contain the focus of infection by drainage, debridement or anatomical repair. In principle, the removal of an infected nidus will help minimize the inflammatory response, but the size and site of the infective source will determine the feasibility and timing of source control. The focus in the ED is on identifying the likely source of infection and determining, in consultation with radiological, surgical and other specialties, the best method of drainage or containment.

Percutaneous drainage

Localized collections may be amenable to percutaneous drainage with or without radiological guidance. This is appropriate for renal, hepatic and other intra-abdominal abscesses and soft tissue collections. Immediate debridement of infected and necrotic tissue is mandatory for soft tissue infections, such as necrotizing fasciitis, but more deep-seated necrosis, such as pancreatitis, may require delayed debridement as early operative intervention in difficult-to-access areas is associated with significant morbidity [21,22].

Biliary tract obstruction with associated infection requires early decompression with percutaneous cholecystostomy or endoscopic

Table 2.5.1   Empirical initial intravenous antibiotic recommendations based on likely source of infection in a patient with severe sepsis

Source of infection	Antibiotic regimen [19]
Unknown	Di-/flucloxacillin 2 g 4–6-hourly
	PLUS
	Gentamicin 7 mg/kg daily (subsequent doses adjusted to renal function)
	If mild penicillin hypersensitivity, substitute di-/flucloxacillin with cephazolin 2 g 8-hourly
	If severe immediate penicillin hypersensitivity, substitute di-/flucloxacillin with vancomycin 1.5 g (25 mg/kg) 12-hourly
	If febrile neutropaenic, use ceftazidime 2 g 8-hourly or piperacillin + tazobactam 4.5 g 8-hourly. Add vancomycin 1.5 g (25 mg/kg) 12-hourly if shocked, high-risk MRSA incl. catheter-related
Biliary/gastrointestinal	Ampicillin 2 g 6-hourly (substitute with ceftriaxone for mild penicillin hypersensitivity and with vancomycin for severe penicillin hypersensitivity)
	PLUS
	Gentamicin 4–6 mg/kg daily (subsequent doses adjusted to renal function)
	PLUS
	Metronidazole 500 mg 12-hourly
Respiratory	Azithromycin 500 mg daily
	PLUS
	Ceftriaxone 1 g daily
	If severe immediate penicillin hypersensitivity, substitute ceftriaxone with moxifloxacin 400 mg daily
Urinary tract	Ampicillin 2 g 6-hourly
	PLUS
	Gentamicin 4–6 mg/kg daily (subsequent doses adjusted to renal function)
Skin	Di-/flucloxacillin 2 g 6-hourly.
	If severe immediate penicillin hypersensitivity, substitute with clindamycin 450 mg 8-hourly or lincomycin 600 mg 8-hourly.
	If high-risk MRSA, use vancomycin 1.5 g (25 mg/kg) 12-hourly

retrograde cholangiopancreatography (ERCP). Urinary sepsis with shock in association with ureteric obstruction should be managed by urgent percutaneous nephrostomy. Gastrointestinal perforation with leakage of luminal contents usually requires early surgical repair, except for contained perforations in diverticulitis.

Indwelling devices

The best approach for sepsis associated with indwelling devices is removal of the device, but this needs to be balanced against the risks of removal and the ongoing medical need [9,22]. An infected intravascular device can be exchanged by 'rewiring' over a guidewire, provided there are no signs of infection at the insertion site [23]. Alternatively, a combination of antibiotics and thrombolysis may be effective [22].

Other therapies

Patients who are on long-term steroids should receive 100 mg hydrocortisone IV as soon as possible in their ED care. Otherwise, the role of steroids remains controversial; intravenous hydrocortisone 200 mg per day is suggested in patients with unresponsive hypotension [10,24].

There is no evidence to support using activated protein C (APC) for treating patients with severe sepsis or septic shock. Additionally, APC is associated with a higher risk of bleeding [10].

Following initial stabilization, glycaemic control is indicated if the blood sugar level (BSL) is greater than 10 mmol/L, aiming for a BSL of 8–10 mmol/L. Aiming for tighter BSL targets has been shown to increase the risk of hypoglycaemia with no mortality benefit [25].

Pragmatically, most of these interventions are usually administered within the first 24 hours of care in an intensive care unit, rather than in the first few hours of ED management [10,26].

Controversies

- Efficacy of early goal-directed therapy has not been established in the Australasian environment where mortality rates are relatively lower than international figures. This is currently under investigation in the Australasian Resuscitation in Sepsis Evaluation Randomized Controlled Trial (ARISE-RCT).
- Routine measurement of central venous oxygen saturations as an endpoint for goal-directed therapy is currently not widely used in Australia or New Zealand. Measurement of lactate clearance may be an acceptable alternative.
- Use of dobutamine and liberal blood transfusion to attain designated endpoints of goal-directed therapy are not universally accepted. There is evidence in some critically ill patients that these strategies might be potentially harmful.

References

[1] ARISE: ANZICS APD management committee. The outcome of patients with sepsis and septic shock presenting to emergency departments in Australia and New Zealand. Crit Care Resus 2007;9:8–18.

[2] Bochud P-Y, Bonten M, Marchetti O, et al. Antimicrobial therapy for patients with severe sepsis and septic shock: An evidence-based review. Crit Care Med 2004;32:S495–512.

[3] Gaieski DF, Pines JM, Band RA, et al. Impact of time to antibiotics on survival in patients with severe sepsis or septic shock in whom early goal-directed therapy was initiated in the emergency department. Crit Care Med 2010;38:1045–53.

[4] Wiersinga WJ. Current insights in sepsis: from pathogenesis to new treatment targets. Curr Opin Crit Care 2011;17:480–6.

[5] Rivers E, McIntyre L, Morro D, Rivers K. Early and innovative interventions for severe sepsis and septic shock: taking advantage of a window of opportunity. Can Med Ass J 2005;173:1054–65.

[6] Dellinger R, Levy M, Rhodes A et al. Surviving sepsis campaign: international guidelines for management of severe sepsis and septic shock: 2012. Crit Care Med 2013;41:580–637.

[7] Mikkelsen ME, Miltiades AN, Gaieski DF, et al. Serum lactate is associated with mortality in severe sepsis independent of organ failure and shock. Crit Care Med 2009;37:1670–7.

[8] Shapiro N, Howell M, Talmor D, et al. Serum lactate as a predictor of mortality in emergency department patients with infection. Ann Emerg Med 2005;45:524–8.

[9] Tiruvoipati R, Ong K, Gangopadhyay H, et al. Hypothermia predicts mortality in critically ill elderly patients with sepsis. BMC Geriatrics 2010;10:70.

[10] Levy MM, Dellinger RP, Townsend SR, et al. The surviving sepsis campaign: results of an international guideline-based performance improvement program targeting severe sepsis. Intens Care Med 2010;36:222–31.

[11] Marti-Carvajal AJ, Sola I, Lathyris D, Cardona AF. Human recombinant activated protein C for severe sepsis. Cochrane Database Syst Rev 2012;3:CD004388.

[12] Rivers E, Nguyen B, Havstad S, et al. Early goal directed therapy in the treatment of severe sepsis and septic shock. N Engl J Med 2001;345:1368–77.

[13] Myburgh JA, Higgins A, Jovanoska A, et al. A comparison of epinephrine and norepinephrine in critically ill patients. Intens Care Med 2008;34:2226–34.

[14] De Backer D, Biston P, Devriendt J, et al. Comparison of dopamine and norepinephrine in the treatment of shock. N Engl J Med 2010;362:779–89.

[15] Jones AE, Shapiro NI, Trzeciak. Lactate clearance vs central venous oxygen saturation as goals of early sepsis therapy. J Am Med Assoc 2010;303:739–46.

[16] Kumar A, Roberts D, Wood K, et al. Duration of hypotension before initiation of effective antimicrobial therapy is the critical determinant of survival in human septic shock. Crit Care Med 2006;34:1589–96.

[17] MacArthur R, Miller M, Albertson T, et al. Adequacy of early empiric antibiotic treatment and survival in severe sepsis: experience from the MONARCS trial. Clin Infect Dis 2004;38:284–8.

[18] Kumar A. Optimizing antimicrobial therapy in sepsis and septic shock. Crit Care Clin 2009;25:733–51.

[19] Antibiotic guidelines. In: eTG complete [Internet]. Melbourne: Therapeutic Guidelines Limited; 2012. <http://www.tg.com.au> (Accessed Mar. 2013).

[20] Rex J, Walsh T, Sobel J, et al. Practice guidelines for the treatment of candidiasis. Clin Infect Dis 2000;30:662–78.

[21] Hsaio G, Chang C, Hsaio C, et al. Necrotizing soft tissue infections. Surgical or conservative treatment? Dermatol Surg 1998;24:247–8.

[22] Marshall J, Maier R, Jiminez M, Dellinger E. Source control in the management of severe sepsis and septic shock: an evidence-based review. Crit Care Med 2004;32:S513–26.

[23] Cook D, Randolph A, Kernerman P, et al. Central venous catheter replacement strategies: a systematic review of the literature. Crit Care Med 1997;25:1417–24.

[24] Annane D, Bellissant E, Bollaert P-E, et al. Corticosteroids in the treatment of severe sepsis and septic shock in adults: a systematic review. J Am Med Assoc 2009;301:236–7.

[25] Griesdale DEG, de Souza RJ, van Dam RM, et al. Intensive insulin therapy and mortality among critically ill patients: a meta-analysis including NICE-SUGAR data. Can Med Assoc J 2009;180:821–7.

[26] Osborn T, Nguyen H, Rivers E. Emergency medicine and the Surviving Sepsis Campaign: an internation approach to managing severe sepsis and septic shock. Ann Emerg Med 2005;46:228–31.

2.6 Arterial blood gases

Anthony D Holley

ESSENTIALS

1 The value of arterial blood gas analysis is almost entirely dependent on understanding and correctly interpreting the results in the clinical context.

2 When abnormalities are detected with arterial blood gas analysis, ensure the sample was obtained, transported and analysed appropriately.

3 An arterial blood gas result assists in the assessment of a patient's gas exchange, ventilatory control and acid–base balance.

4 Common sampling sites include the radial, femoral, brachial, dorsalis pedis or axillary artery. There is no evidence for superiority of any particular site.

5 The alveolar gas equation allows comparison of arterial and alveolar partial pressures of oxygen (PaO_2). A higher than expected value indicates a ventilation–perfusion defect (high A–a gradient).

6 Isolated hypoxaemia is referred to as type I respiratory failure; type II respiratory failure is characterized by a partial pressure carbon dioxide ($PaCO_2$) higher than 50 mmHg.

7 There are five potential pathophysiological mechanisms responsible for hypoxaemia, which include decreased inspired fractional oxygen, impaired diffusion, shunting, ventilation–perfusion (V/Q) mismatch and hypoventilaton.

8 Type II respiratory failure (hypercapnia) is due to inadequate alveolar ventilation, commonly secondary to poor central drive, neuromuscular disease or profound mechanical derangement of lungs or chest wall.

9 The primary acid–base disturbance is established by assessing the relationship between the direction of change in the pH and the direction of change in the $PaCO_2$.

10 When a metabolic acidosis is diagnosed, calculate the anion gap and delta ratio to narrow the differential diagnosis.

11 In the presence of a metabolic alkalosis, establish both an initiating and maintaining factor.

12 Venous pH, bicarbonate and base excess have sufficient agreement to be clinically interchangeable with arterial values in patients who are not shocked.

Introduction

Arterial blood gas analysis is an essential tool for diagnosing and managing the critically ill emergency department (ED) patient's respiratory status and acid–base balance (Table 2.6.1). Its usefulness is almost entirely dependent on the ability to understand and interpret the results correctly.

Technical aspects of arterial blood gas analysis

The technology for arterial blood gas analysis became available more than 50 years ago with the development of electrodes that allowed the measurement of partial pressures of oxygen (PaO_2) and carbon dioxide ($PaCO_2$) in arterial blood samples taken directly from the patient [1].

Blood gas analysers and applied physiology

Clarke's oxygen electrode constitutes a platinum probe suspended in an electrolyte

Table 2.6.1 Indications for arterial blood gas analysis

1. Determination of the partial pressures of gases reflective of gas exchange and ventilation
2. Monitoring gas exchange and ventilation in response to interventions or therapy
3. Identification of acid–base disorders
4. Monitoring of acid–base status in response to interventions or therapy
5. Identification of dyshaemoglobinaemias, e.g. carboxyhaemoglobin and methaemoglobin

solution and separated from the blood sample by a membrane permeable to oxygen. Oxygen molecules diffuse from blood through the membrane to the electrode where they are reduced to hydroxyl ions. The partial pressure of oxygen is directly proportional to the current measured from this reduction reaction [2].

A pH-sensitive glass probe maintained in a bicarbonate solution and protected by a carbon dioxide permeable membrane constitutes the Severinghaus carbon dioxide electrode. In this model, the measured $PaCO_2$ is proportional to the hydrogen ions produced, as CO_2 reacts with water to form hydrogen and bicarbonate ions [1].

The pH of arterial blood is measured directly by an electrode which then allows the blood gas analyser software to calculate the base excess (BE) and bicarbonate concentration.

The arterial oxygen saturation (SaO_2) may be calculated from the PaO_2. However, it may still be unreliable even if the haemoglobin–oxygen affinity shifts secondary to acid–base disturbances are accounted for in calculating SaO_2 from PaO_2. Most modern blood gas analysers now include a co-oximeter that is capable of measuring concentrations of saturated haemoglobin, reduced haemoglobin, carboxyhaemoglobin, and methaemoglobin [3]. Wavelengths of light corresponding to unique absorption spectra for each haemoglobin species allow for these measurements to be determined.

Temperature formulae and nomograms were previously applied to pH, $PaCO_2$ and PaO_2. However, modern automated blood gas analysers can report the pH, PaO_2 and $PaCO_2$ at either 37°C (the temperature at which the values are measured by the blood gas analyser) or at the patient's body temperature. Most machines report the values of pH, PCO_2 and PaO_2 at 37°C, regardless of the patient's actual temperature. The corrections are generally minimal and corrected values are no more clinically useful than 37°C values.

Collection and handling

Accurate results for arterial blood gases are dependent on appropriate collection and handling. Prepared syringes are pretreated with sodium or lithium heparin to prevent coagulation of the specimen. The presence of air bubbles in the sample syringe that exceed 1–2% of the blood volume can spuriously elevate PaO_2, but has little effect on pH and $PaCO_2$. Delaying the processing of a specimen beyond 20 minutes may result in a reduction in PaO_2 and pH, with a concomitant elevation in $PaCO_2$.

These changes reflect ongoing cellular metabolism which is more pronounced in the presence of a leucocytosis or thrombocytosis [4]. Erythrocytes in the arterial blood sample continue to undergo anaerobic glycolysis, generating lactic acid and thereby lowering the pH of the sample. Placing the specimen on ice immediately after drawing will improve its stability [5].

Arterial puncture technique

The most commonly accessed artery is the radial; other potential sites include the femoral, brachial, dorsalis pedis or axillary arteries [6]. Brachial artery puncture when performed properly is safe and reliable, with a minor complication rate of approximately 2% [7,8]. The radial artery is the most frequently accessed as it is convenient, accessible, and well tolerated. There is no evidence that any single site is superior.

Modified Allen test

The Allen test or modified Allen test may be performed in patients undergoing radial artery puncture to ensure that there is reliable collateral flow [9]. While the modified Allen test has been the most frequently used method clinically to assess the adequacy of ulnar artery collateral flow, it is controversial as to whether it can reliably predict ischaemic complications [10]. Its use is recommended as it is easily performed and, acknowledging its limitations, may be useful.

The patient's clenched fist is elevated with both the ulnar and radial arteries occluded. Subsequently, the hand is lowered, the fist released and occlusion of the ulna artery removed. Rapid colour return to the hand confirms that both the ulnar artery is patent and the superficial palmar arch is functional. The test is considered abnormal if there is a delay (>6 s) before the colour returns to the hand, in which case an alternate puncture site should be considered [11]. Ideally the non-dominant hand is selected when cannulating the radial artery.

Indwelling arterial catheter

An indwelling arterial catheter may be required in the ED for continuous blood pressure monitoring and/or regular blood gas sampling. A meticulous aseptic technique is needed during insertion and with catheter maintenance to decrease the risk of catheter-related infection. Complications of radial artery cannulation/puncture include haematoma (14.4%), local infection (0.72%), bleeding (0.5%), sepsis

(0.13%), pseudoaneurysm formation (0.09%) and permanent ischaemic injury secondary to embolization or thrombosis (0.09%) [12].

Interpretation

An arterial blood gas sample is useful in the evaluation of a patient's gas exchange, assessment of ventilatory function and determination of acid–base status. It is important that all measurements are evaluated in the context of the clinical history, the patient's examination findings and the normal values (Table 2.6.2).

Gas exchange

Respiration is the process whereby oxygen is delivered to metabolically active tissues and the carbon dioxide (CO_2) produced from this metabolism is subsequently removed. Respiratory failure occurs when the system can no longer effectively maintain this gas exchange resulting in organ dysfunction or death. If oxygenation is principally affected, this results in hypoxaemia; if ventilation is impaired, hypercapnia and respiratory acidosis may supervene. It is important to recognize that both processes frequently occur together.

Oxygenation of tissues is dependent on arterial oxygen content, delivery and consumption. Oxygen content may be expressed by the following equation:

$$Arterial\ oxygen\ content = Haemoglobin\ (g/dL)$$
$$\times Oxygen\ saturation\ (\%) \times 1.39$$
$$+ (PaO_2 \times 0.0031)$$

1.39 in the formula represents the amount of oxygen (mL) carried by haemoglobin (g) although some measurements give 1.34 or 1.36 mL as, under normal conditions, small amounts of Hb are in forms such as methaemoglobin that cannot combine with O_2.

Table 2.6.2 Normal arterial blood gas values on room air ($FiO_2 = 0.21$)	
Parameter	Reference range
pH	7.35–7.45
PaO_2	80–100 mmHg
$PaCO_2$	35–45 mmHg
HCO_3^-	22–26 mmol/L
Base excess	−2 to +2 mmol/L

FiO_2: fractional inspired oxygen.

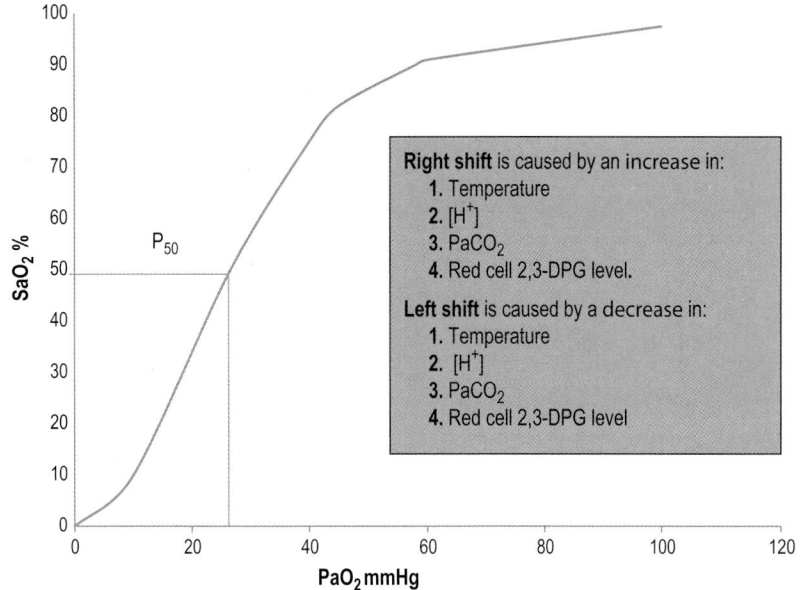

Fig. 2.6.1 Oxygen dissociation curve.

Thus, it is apparent that it is the oxygen saturation and not PaO_2 which is most important as regards oxygen delivery to the tissues.

Hypoxaemic respiratory failure is defined as a clinically significant decrease in PaO_2, usually considered to be a PaO_2 less than 60 mmHg. Although a definition based solely on an absolute PaO_2 value maybe an over simplification, it is useful when considered in the context of the oxygen–haemoglobin dissociation curve (Fig. 2.6.1). Importantly, when the PaO_2 declines below 60 mmHg, the haemoglobin oxygen saturation falls precipitously with any further decrease in PaO_2.

The position of the oxyhaemoglobin dissociation curve is modified by alterations in the partial pressure of carbon dioxide ($PaCO_2$), temperature and the presence of acidosis or red blood cell 2,3-diphosphoglycerate (2,3-DPG). The curve is displaced to the right by an increase in $PaCO_2$, a temperature rise, acidosis or an increase in 2,3-DPG concentration. This right shift facilitates more effective delivery of oxygen to peripheral tissues, which is beneficial in the presence of hypoxia. The P_{50} is used to reference the oxygen dissociation curve (see Fig. 2.6.1) [13]. It is the partial pressure of oxygen at which 50% of the haemoglobin is saturated with oxygen and specifies the position of the oxygen dissociation curve. Normally, a PaO_2 of 26.6 mmHg corresponds to 50% haemoglobin saturation. Modern arterial blood gas machines routinely report this value.

Alveolar–arterial oxygen gradient

The alveolar–arterial PO_2 gradient (A–a) PO_2 is determined to evaluate a patient's oxygenation. This gradient is defined by the difference between the partial pressure of O_2 in the alveoli (PAO_2) and the partial pressure of O_2 dissolved in the arterial blood plasma ($PAO_2 - PaO_2$). The partial pressure of O_2 in the alveoli (PAO_2) is established by using the alveolar gas equation:

$$P_AO_2 = FiO_2(P_{atm} - P_{H_2O}) - (PaCO_2)/R$$

where FiO_2 = fraction of inspired oxygen, P_{atm} = atmospheric pressure (760 mmHg at sea level, decreasing progressively with increasing altitude), P_{H_2O} = partial pressure of saturated vapour (47 mmHg at 37°C) and R = the respiratory quotient (≈ 0.8).

The normal reference range for the alveolar–arterial gradient is 5–15 mmHg, with increases encountered from cigarette smoking, increasing FiO_2 and advancing age. An approximate expected $P(A-a)O_2$ can be determined using the following formula:

$$P(A-a)O_2 = Age/4 + 4$$

Pathophysiology of hypoxaemic respiratory failure

There are five potential mechanisms responsible for hypoxaemia when determining the aetiology of a patient's respiratory failure which include decreased inspired fractional oxygen, impaired diffusion, shunting, ventilation–perfusion (V/Q) mismatch and hypoventilaton [14]. Isolated hypoxaemia is often referred to as type I respiratory failure, with type II respiratory failure characterized by a partial pressure of carbon dioxide ($PaCO_2$) higher than 50 mmHg [15].

Mechanisms responsible for hypoxaemia include:

Decreased inspired fraction of oxygen

This is not common in clinical practice, but may be encountered at high altitude or in environments where the gas mixture is oxygen depleted.

Impaired diffusion

Diffusion impairment secondary to thickening of the membrane between the capillary and alveolus is now accepted as a rare mechanism. Thickening of the blood–gas barrier is found in diseases such as diffuse interstitial fibrosis. Under normal resting conditions, oxygen diffusion at the alveolar–capillary barrier requires only a third of the circulatory time available for equilibration to be complete. Therefore, even in the presence of a moderate diffusion impairment, there is sufficient 'diffusion time' to compensate.

Severe impairments of diffusion become clinically significant, particularly during exercise, when blood flow rates are increased and the time for diffusion equilibration is restricted. Shunting or a V/Q mismatch are almost always found to coexist with a diffusion defect and are likely, quantitatively, to be far more significant as a cause of hypoxemia.

Shunt

Hypoxaemic respiratory failure may result from either extrapulmonary or intrapulmonary shunts, with a shunt defined as the movement of blood from the venous to arterial circulation without transiting ventilated lung tissue and thus not afforded the opportunity to be oxygenated.

The clinical feature suggestive of the presence of a shunt is the failure of partial pressure of oxygen (PaO_2) to rise despite inhalation of 100% oxygen (FiO_2 1.0). Extrapulmonary shunts are encountered in the setting of acquired or congenital cardiac abnormalities, where the ventricles or the atria communicate secondary to septal defects. When the pressure gradient favours blood bypassing the pulmonary circulation, a shunt is established.

Intrapulmonary shunts occur in severe pneumonia, atelectasis, pulmonary arteriovenous malformations or the hepatopulmonary syndrome (regional dilation of pulmonary capillaries). The situation where there is alveolar consolidation or collapse such that there is unventilated but perfused lung may also be considered an extreme V/Q mismatch [16]. This is distinguished from a shunt by virtue of the correction of PaO_2 in response to enhanced O_2 administration. The shunt fraction can be calculated with the following equation:

$$Q_S/Q_T = (Cc'O_2 - CaO_2)/(Cc'O_2 - CvO_2)$$

where Q_S = shunt flow, Q_T = total blood flow, $Cc'O_2$ = end capillary oxygen content derived from PAO_2, CaO_2 = arterial oxygen content, CvO_2 = mixed venous oxygen content.

A calculated shunt of less than 20% seldom requires support, whereas a calculated shunt greater than 30% usually needs significant cardiopulmonary intervention. However, the shunt equation is limited in clinical practice by the need for sampling mixed-venous blood and hence the presence of a pulmonary artery catheter.

Ventilation–perfusion (V/Q) mismatch

All the blood circulating through the lungs must perfuse individual ventilated lung units in order for effective gas exchange to occur. Theoretically, the ideal ratio of perfusion to ventilation (V/Q ratio) should numerically be one [17]. Under normal physiological conditions, perfusion is more pronounced at the lung bases as compared to the apices, while the converse is true for ventilation. Therefore, the usual overall V/Q ratio is approximately 0.8.

V/Q ratios demonstrate a wide spectrum of abnormalities: in some situations where alveolar units receive no ventilation, but are fully perfused, this results in a V/Q ratio of 0. This constitutes a shunt (as discussed above) and may be either cardiac or pulmonary in aetiology. Alternatively, the alveolar units may be fully ventilated, but receive no perfusion producing a V/Q ratio which trends to infinity [16]. A clinical example of this is a massive pulmonary embolus. Non-perfused alveolar units are referred to as physiological 'dead space'.

Table 2.6.3   Causes of hypoventilation resulting in type II respiratory failure

Mechanism	Disease
Airway induced	Foreign body
	Bronchospasm – asthma, anaphylaxis
	Chronic obstructive pulmonary disease
Central nervous system depression	Alcohol intoxication
	Opiate overdose
	Over-sedation
	High spinal/epidural anaesthesia
Hypoventilation secondary to neuromuscular disease	Myasthenia gravis
	Spinal cord injury/trauma
	Transverse myelitis
	Guillain–Barré syndrome
	Muscular dystrophy
Chest wall trauma	Pneumothorax
	Flail chest
Obesity with decreased alveolar ventilation	Obstructive sleep apnoea (OSA)

Clinically, derangements of V/Q matching are the most common cause of gas exchange impairment and are characterized by hypoxaemia, hypercapnia or a combination of both. The presence of an increased alveolar–arterial PO_2 gradient helps the emergency physician identify a V/Q abnormality.

Hypoventilation

The partial pressure of carbon dioxide in arterial blood ($PaCO_2$) is determined by the production of CO_2 (VCO_2) and alveolar ventilation (VA):

$$PaCO_2 = (VCO_2 \times K)/VA$$

where alveolar ventilation (VA) = (tidal volume (Tv) – dead space (VD)) × respiratory rate.

Type II respiratory failure is characterized by a $PaCO_2$ greater than 50 mmHg and is commonly encountered in clinical practice (Table 2.6.3).

The alveolar gas equation demonstrates how significant alveolar hypoventilation can result in a proportional decrease in alveolar oxygen pressure P_AO_2. When the respiratory quotient (R = 0.8) remains constant, an increase in $PaCO_2$ will be associated with a concomitant reduction in P_AO_2 which, in profound hypercapnia, may then result in hypoxaemia. If hypoventilation is the presumed mechanism of the

hypoxaemia, then the alveolar–arterial oxygen tension gradient (A–a) PO_2 should be calculated. This gradient will be normal when the hypoxaemia is entirely secondary to hypercapnia, but will be increased if there are other mechanisms, such as an impaired V/Q ratio or the presence of a shunt contributing to the hypoxaemia.

It is important when interpreting any blood gas that a standardized structured evaluation is undertaken to determine the aetiology of the respiratory failure (Table 2.6.4 and Fig. 2.6.2).

Acid–base balance

While this chapter principally addresses the respiratory aspects of arterial blood gas analysis, it is impossible to separate clinically the component information provided by arterial blood sampling (see Chapter 21.1). Under normal physiological conditions, humans maintain closely regulated acid–base homeostasis required for normal cellular activity. This homeostasis results from a complex series of interactions between the lungs and kidneys, moderated by a range of physiological buffers. The resultant blood hydrogen ion concentration (pH) is a function of the ratio of bicarbonate concentration and the partial pressure of CO_2 in arterial blood.

Table 2.6.4 Six-step approach to evaluate respiratory failure using arterial blood gases	
Step	**Parameter**
1	Confirm the presence of hypoxaemia by determining the PaO_2 <60 mmHg or SaO_2 <90%
2	Establish if there is an increased alveolar–arterial oxygen tension gradient ↑(A–a) PO_2
3	Determine if there is evidence for hypoventilation. If the $PaCO_2$ >50 mmHg, then alveolar hypoventilation is present
4	If there is hypoxaemia, a normal alveolar–arterial oxygen tension gradient (A–a) PO_2 and the $PaCO_2$ is not elevated, the patient is in a hypoxic environment, e.g. altitude
5	Determine if the hypoxaemia is entirely accounted for by hypoventilation, established by calculating the alveolar–arterial oxygen tension gradient (A–a) PO_2. If the gradient is normal (<15), hypoventilation alone is the cause, such as from central nervous system depression or respiratory muscular failure. Conversely, if the alveolar–arterial oxygen tension gradient (A–a) PO_2 is elevated, other conditions including pneumonia or acute respiratory distress syndrome are likely responsible
6	If the $PaCO_2$ is normal, hypoxaemia is present and there is an increased alveolar–arterial oxygen tension gradient (A–a) PO_2, the response to breathing an enhanced O_2 mixture discriminates between a ventilation/perfusion mismatch and a shunt

Acid–base disorders

Primary metabolic acid–base disorders and the secondary metabolic compensation for primary respiratory disturbances are reflected by changes in the serum bicarbonate concentration. Primary respiratory acid–base disorders and the secondary respiratory compensation for primary metabolic disturbances result in changes in the measured $PaCO_2$ (Table 2.6.5). Similarly to the evaluation of respiratory failure, evaluation of an acid–base abnormality requires a systematic approach:

Step 1: First determine if there is alkalaemia or acidaemia present, simply defined by the following: pH <7.35 = acidaemia, or pH >7.45 = alkalaemia.

Step 2: Then determine if the primary disturbance is respiratory or metabolic in origin, established by assessing the relationship between the direction of change in the pH and the direction of change in the $PaCO_2$.

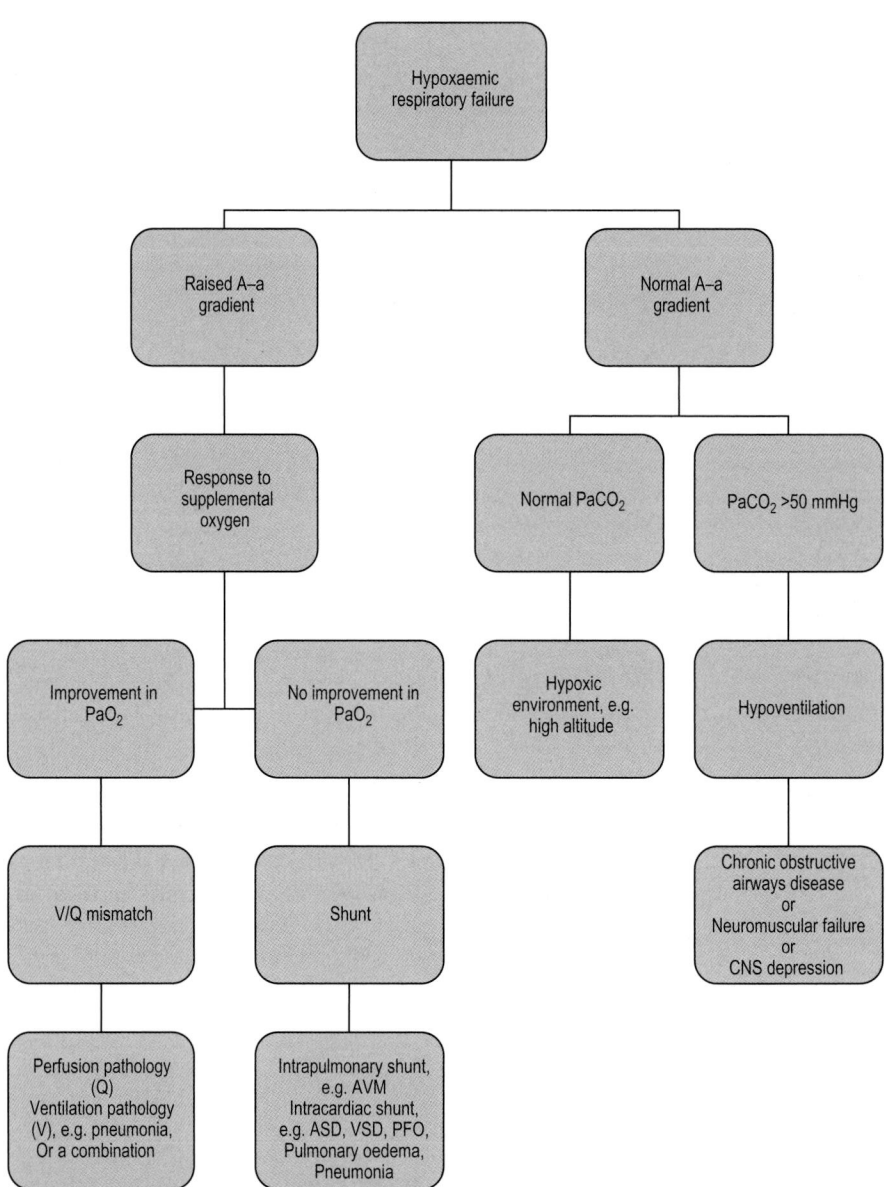

Fig. 2.6.2 Evaluating respiratory failure using arterial blood gases. CNS: central nervous system; AVM: arteriovenous malformation; ASD: atrial septal defect; VSD: ventricular septal defect; PFO: patent foramen ovale.

Table 2.6.5 Determining the primary acid–base disorder			
Primary disturbance	*pH*	*$PaCO_2$*	*Anticipated compensation*
Respiratory acidosis	↓	↑	↑ HCO_3^-
Respiratory alkalosis	↑	↓	↓ HCO_3^-
Metabolic acidosis	↓	↓	↓ $PaCO_2$
Metabolic alkalosis	↑	↑	↑ $PaCO_2$

Step 3: Then assess whether the primary disturbance has been compensated (Table 2.6.6), recognizing that compensation does not return the pH to normal. If the expected compensation is not present, it is likely that a mixed acid–base disorder exists [18,19].

Step 4: Calculate the anion gap in the presence of a metabolic acidosis, to allow for formulation of the differential diagnosis (high or normal anion gap):

$$\text{Anion gap} = [Na^+] - ([Cl^-] + [HCO_3^-]) = 12 \pm 2$$

Table 2.6.6 Predicting compensation for primary acid–base disorders

Primary disorder	Expected compensation
Metabolic acidosis	$PaCO_2 = (1.5 \times HCO_3^-) + 8$
Acute respiratory acidosis	For every 10 mmHg increase in PCO_2 the HCO_3^- should increase by 1 mmol/L
Chronic respiratory acidosis (3–5 days)	For every 10 mmHg increase in PCO_2 the HCO_3^- should increase by 3–4 mmol/L over 4 days
Metabolic alkalosis	$PaCO_2 = 0.8 \times HCO_3^- + 20$
Acute respiratory alkalosis	For every 10 mmHg decrease in PCO_2 the HCO_3^- should decrease by 1 mmol/L
Chronic respiratory alkalosis	For every 10 mmHg decrease in PCO_2 the HCO_3^- should decrease by 2 mmol/L

Table 2.6.7 Causes of a high anion gap metabolic acidosis

Mechanism	Clinical example
Lactic acidosis type A	Shock
	Hypoxia
Lactic acidosis type B1	Hepatic failure
	Sepsis
	Haematological malignancies
	Renal failure
	Thiamine deficiency
	Thyroid storm
Lactic acidosis type B2	Drug induced including:
	paracetamol
	biguanides
	cocaine
	diethyl ether
	adrenaline
	ethanol
	ethylene glycol
	isoniazid
	methanol
	antiretroviral therapy
	salbutamol
Lactic acidosis type B3	Rare inborn errors of metabolism, e.g. glucose-6 phosphate dehydrogenase deficiency
Ketoacidosis	Diabetic ketoacidosis
	Alcoholic ketoacidosis
	Starvation ketoacidosis

Table 2.6.8 Causes of normal anion gap metabolic acidosis

Mechanism	Clinical example
Renal bicarbonate loss	Tubulo-interstitial renal disease
	Renal tubular acidosis types 1, 2 and 4
Gastrointestinal bicarbonate loss	Diarrhoea
	Colostomy
	Ileostomy
	Enteric fistulas
	Use of ion-exchange resins
Drugs	Carbonic anhydrase inhibitors, e.g. acetazolamide
Endocrine	Hypoaldosteronism
	Hyperparathyroidism
Excess chloride	Rapid sodium chloride infusion

The differential diagnosis of a non-anion gap metabolic acidosis includes conditions characterized by bicarbonate loss, excess chloride or ingestions (Table 2.6.8).

If the anion gap is elevated (>12) and not explained by an obvious aetiology then, under appropriate clinical circumstances, a toxic ingestion, such as methanol or ethylene glycol, is considered. This is associated with a high osmolal gap, the difference between the measured serum osmolality and the calculated osmolality which, under normal physiological conditions, should be <10 mmol/L:

Osmolal gap = Measured − Calculated osmolality, where calculated osmolality (mmol/L)
= $2 \times$ [Na] + Glucose + Urea

Step 5: If an increased anion gap is present, then determine the delta ratio to establish whether a mixed acid–base disorder is present. This is deduced from assessing the relationship between the increased anion gap and the decrease in bicarbonate [21].

$$\text{Delta ratio} = \Delta \text{Anion gap} / \Delta [HCO_3^-]$$

$$= \frac{\text{Measured anion gap} - \text{Normal anion gap}}{\text{Normal} [HCO_3^-] - \text{Measured} [HCO_3^-]}$$

$$= \frac{\text{Measured anion gap} - 12}{(24 - [HCO_3^-])}$$

The magnitude of the delta ratio can range from <0.4 to >2 and allows for refinement of the differential diagnosis (Table 2.6.9).

A high anion gap acidosis is most commonly secondary to lactate or ketones (Table 2.6.7). Lactic acidosis was classified in 1976 into type A or B, based on the absence or presence of adequate tissue oxygenation [20]. Lactic acidosis is a common life-threatening form of metabolic acidosis in the critically ill.

Table 2.6.9	Delta ratio interpretation
Delta ratio	Interpretation
<0.4	Normal anion gap hyperchloraemic metabolic acidosis
<1	Combined high and normal anion gap acidosis
1–2	Isolated high anion gap metabolic acidosis
>2	Mixed high anion gap metabolic acidosis and metabolic alkalosis

Table 2.6.10	Causes of a metabolic alkalosis	
Mechanism	Clinical example	Saline responsive
Gastrointestinal hydrogen loss	Nasogastric suction	Yes
	Vomiting. Chloride-losing diarrhoea. Gastrocolic fistula. Villous adenoma.	
Renal hydrogen loss	Loop or thiazide diuretics. Post-chronic hypercapnia. Hypocalcaemia	Yes
	Bartter or Gitelman syndrome	
Transcellular hydrogen shift into cells	Hypokalaemia	Yes
Exogenous alkali	Administration of $NaHCO_3$, gluconate, acetate. Citrate load with massive blood transfusion. Excess antacids (milk alkali syndrome).	Yes
Contraction alkalosis	Loop or thiazide-type diuretics. Sweat losses in cystic fibrosis. Gastric losses in achlorhydria. Factitious diarrhoea (including laxative abuse).	Yes
Endocrine	Mineralocorticoid excess	No
	Primary aldosteronism	
	Cushing's syndrome	
	Exogenous steroids	
Miscellaneous	Barrter's	No
	Gitelman's syndrome	

Step 6: Identify the 'initiating factor' if the arterial blood gas reflects a primary metabolic alkalosis. This may include loss of hydrogen ions from the gastrointestinal system, transcellular hydrogen shifts, mineralocorticoid excess or addition of alkali. Furthermore, a 'maintenance' factor is also needed to preserve the metabolic alkalosis as, in the presence of an elevated serum bicarbonate, a patient with intact renal function will rapidly excrete excess bicarbonate in the urine. Therefore, for a metabolic alkalosis to persist, there must be a reduction in the renal ability to lose excess bicarbonate. In practice, this is usually secondary to hypovolaemia or reduced effective arterial blood volume (including heart failure and cirrhosis), chloride depletion, hypokalaemia, renal impairment or a combination of these factors (Table 2.6.10).

Venous blood gases

It is technically much easier and quicker to obtain a venous blood sample than an arterial one and, therefore, there is substantial interest in using venous blood as a surrogate for arterial blood gas analysis. In some situations, analysis of venous blood provides sufficiently reliable correlation with arterial blood to assist in clinical decision making.

The peripheral venous pH is approximately 0.02–0.04 pH units lower than the arterial pH, the venous serum HCO_3^- concentration is approximately 1–2 meq/L higher and the venous PCO_2 is approximately 3–8 mmHg higher [22]. There are currently insufficient data to determine if these relationships persist in a shocked patient or those with mixed acid–base disorders. In a patient who is not shocked, venous pH, bicarbonate and base excess have sufficient agreement to be clinically interchangeable for arterial values [23]. Agreement between arterial and venous PCO_2 is too unpredictable to be clinically reliable.

References

[1] Severinghaus JW. First electrodes for blood PO_2 and PCO_2 determination. J Appl Physiol 2004;97:1599–600.
[2] Clark Jr LC, Wolf R, Granger D, et al. Continuous recording of blood oxygen tensions by polarography. J Appl Physiol 1953;6:189–93.
[3] Barker SJ, Curry J, Redford D, Morgan S. Measurement of carboxyhemoglobin and methemoglobin by pulse oximetry: a human volunteer study. Anesthesiology 2006;105:892–7.
[4] Schmidt C, Muller-Plathe O. Stability of pO_2, pCO_2 and pH in heparinized whole blood samples: influence of storage temperature with regard to leukocyte count and syringe material. Eur J Clin Chem Clin Biochem 1992;30:767–73.
[5] Harsten A, Berg B, Inerot S, Muth L. Importance of correct handling of samples for the results of blood gas analysis. Acta Anaesthesiol Scand 1988;32:365–8.
[6] Scheer B, Perel A, Pfeiffer UJ. Clinical review: complications and risk factors of peripheral arterial catheters used for haemodynamic monitoring in anaesthesia and intensive care medicine. Crit Care 2002;6:199–204.
[7] Okeson GC, Wulbrecht PH. The safety of brachial artery puncture for arterial blood sampling. Chest 1998;114:748–51.
[8] Williams AJ. ABC of oxygen: assessing and interpreting arterial blood gases and acid–base balance. Br Med J 1998;317:1213–6.
[9] Kohonen M, Teerenhovi O, Terho T, et al. Is the Allen test reliable enough? Eur J Cardiothorac Surg 2007;32:902–5.
[10] Barone JE, Madlinger RV. Should an Allen test be performed before radial artery cannulation? J Trauma 2006;61:468–70.
[11] Puttarajappa C, Rajan DS. Images in clinical medicine. Allen's test. N Engl J Med 2010;363:e20.
[12] Clark VL, Kruse JA. Arterial catheterization. Crit Care Clin 1992;8:687–97.
[13] Morgan TJ. The oxyhaemoglobin dissociation curve in critical illness. Crit Care Resus 1999;1:93–100.
[14] West JB. Pulmonary pathophysiology: the essentials, 7th ed. Philadelphia: Lippincott Williams & Wilkins; 2008.
[15] Hanley ME, Bone RC. Acute respiratory failure. Pathophysiology, causes, and clinical manifestations. Postgrad Med 1986;79(166-9):72–6.
[16] Jones JG, Jones SE. Discriminating between the effect of shunt and reduced VA/Q on arterial oxygen saturation is particularly useful in clinical practice. J Clin Monit Comput 2000;16:337–50.
[17] West JB, Wagner PD. Pulmonary gas exchange. Am J Respir Crit Care Med 1998;157:S82–7.
[18] Carmody JB, Norwood VF. A clinical approach to paediatric acid–base disorders. Postgrad Med J 2012;88:143–51.
[19] Narins RG, Emmett M. Simple and mixed acid-base disorders: a practical approach. Medicine (Baltimore) 1980;59:161–87.
[20] Cohen RD, Woods HF. Lactic acidosis revisited. Diabetes 1983;32:181–91.
[21] Reddy P, Mooradian AD. Clinical utility of anion gap in deciphering acid–base disorders. Int J Clin Pract 2009;63:1516–25.
[22] Malatesha G, Singh NK, Bharija A, Rehani B, et al. Comparison of arterial and venous pH, bicarbonate, PCO_2 and PO_2 in initial emergency department assessment. Emerg Med J 2007;24:569–71.
[23] Kelly AM. Review article: can venous blood gas analysis replace arterial in emergency medical care. Emerg Med Australas 2010;22:493–8.

2.7 Cerebral resuscitation after cardiac arrest

Stephen A Bernard

ESSENTIALS

1 Anoxic neurological injury is common following out-of-hospital cardiac arrest (OHCA) and carries a high rate of morbidity and mortality.

2 Reperfusion of the ischaemic brain results in biochemical cascades that lead to further cell death, largely mediated by calcium influx into cells.

3 Therapeutic hypothermia (32–34°C) after resuscitation from cardiac arrest was considered an effective treatment for anoxic neurological injury and is recommended by the Australian Resuscitation Council (ARC) and New Zealand Resuscitation Council (NZRC). However the largest trial to date has shown no improvement in outcome in any measurable way, and has cast doubt on its efficacy.

4 There are currently no proven pharmacological interventions that improve neurological outcome after global cerebral ischaemia.

5 Hypotension is deleterious to the injured brain and should be promptly treated.

6 Recent laboratory and observational clinical evidence suggests that hyperoxia following resuscitation may be associated with worse outcomes.

Introduction

Out-of-hospital cardiac arrest (OHCA) is common and is a leading cause of death in patients with heart disease [1]. Prolonged OHCA causing global cerebral ischaemia may lead to permanent neurological injury, despite effective cardiopulmonary resuscitation with return of spontaneous circulation (ROSC). Many patients who are initially successfully resuscitated from OHCA remain comatose in the emergency department (ED) because of the anoxic neurological injury, which results in considerable morbidity and mortality following hospital admission. This chapter details the pathophysiology of anoxic neurological injury and current cerebral resuscitation therapies.

Definition

Cerebral resuscitation involves the use of pharmacological or other strategies to minimize injury to the brain following a prolonged ischaemic insult [2].

Pathophysiology of cerebral ischaemia

The brain is highly dependent on an adequate supply of oxygen and glucose for metabolism.

When cerebral oxygen delivery falls below 20 mL/100 g brain tissue/minute, aerobic metabolism changes to anaerobic glycolysis, with a marked decrease in the generation of adenosine triphosphate (ATP) [3].

After several minutes of cerebral ischaemia, the supply of ATP is exhausted and cellular metabolism ceases. The failure of the sodium/potassium transmembrane pump leads to a shift of sodium into the cell with subsequent cell swelling. In addition, hydrogen ions are generated with lactate ions and the resulting intracellular metabolic acidosis is toxic to intracellular enzyme systems. This acidosis is partly dependent on the concentration of glucose, with hyperglycaemia contributing to an increase in the intracellular acidosis.

Reperfusion injury

Additional injury occurs following resuscitation with reperfusion of the brain with oxygenated blood. The intracellular levels of glutamate, an excitatory neurotransmitter released from pre-synaptic terminals, increase dramatically during reperfusion. Glutamate activates calcium ion channel complexes which shift calcium from the extracellular fluid to the intracellular fluid [4]. The calcium influx into cells initiates

multiple biochemical cascades, leading to the production of so-called 'free-radicals' and the activation of degradative enzymes.

Free-radical production

Intracellular iron also plays an important role in free-radical production. Iron is usually maintained in the ferric state and is sequestered to intracellular proteins. During ischaemia, iron is reduced to the soluble ferrous form and reacts with peroxide, generating damaging hydroxyl free radicals.

There are also effects on leucocytes, endothelium and platelets. The generation of free radicals activates an upregulation of molecules that mediate leucocyte adhesion and extravasation of these into brain parenchyma. Also, microvessel occlusion with leucocyte–platelet complexes leads to increased cerebral ischaemia.

Ischaemia and reperfusion

Ischaemia and reperfusion are also a stimulus for nitric oxide (NO) synthase activation that generates NO, a potent mediator of injury. The NO may combine with superoxide to form peroxy-nitrite radicals, which are potent activators of lipid peroxidation. Other proposed actions of NO include DNA damage, increased glutamate release and microvascular vasodilatation.

Finally, some neurons that survive the initial anoxic insult proceed to 'programmed' cell death, known as apoptosis [5]. After reperfusion, this delayed neuronal death may occur at different rates, varying from 6 hours for neurons in the striatum to 7 days for hippocampal CA1 neurons. Apoptosis is characterized by cellular and nuclear shrinkage, chromatin condensation and DNA fragmentation.

Cerebral haemodynamics after reperfusion

Cerebral haemodynamics may remain abnormal for some hours after resuscitation and restoration of a spontaneous circulation [6]. In animal models, there is an initial hyperaemia after resuscitation, followed by decreased cerebral blood flow despite normal mean arterial blood pressure (MAP). Due to the inflammatory processes described above, cerebral metabolic rate for oxygen increases slightly. Thus, there may be a mismatch of cerebral oxygen delivery and demand for some hours following resuscitation from prolonged cardiac arrest. Cerebral oxygen delivery and/or demand are also adversely affected by arterial hypotension, hypoxaemia, raised intracranial pressure, fever and/or seizure activity.

Pharmacological interventions

There is considerable interest and research into pharmacological interventions that might decrease reperfusion injury, as much of the neurological injury seen following an ischaemic injury actually occurs after reperfusion. A number of drugs that showed promise in animal models of global cerebral ischaemia underwent randomized, controlled human trials. These included thiopentone [7], a corticosteroid [8], lidoflazine [9], nimodipine [10], magnesium [11], diazepam [11] and co-enzyme Q10 [12]. However, none of these have shown an improved neurological or overall outcome in clinical trials.

Therapeutic hypothermia

Therapeutic hypothermia (TH) was demonstrated to benefit patients who remain comatose after resuscitation from OHCA. It was thought that the TH decreased cerebral oxygen demand without decreasing cerebral oxygen supply. Also, that TH decreased the reperfusion injury by reducing the production of oxygen free radicals after reperfusion.

Two prospective, controlled, human studies suggested improved outcome using moderate TH in comatose survivors of pre-hospital cardiac arrest [13,14]. In an Australian study, 43 patients were randomized to TH (33°C for 12 hours) and 34 patients were maintained at normothermia [13]. Hypothermia was induced in the ED using surface cooling with ice-packs. At hospital discharge, 21/43 (49%) of the TH group had a good outcome compared with 9/34 (26%) in the control group ($p = 0.046$). Following multivariate analysis for differences at baseline, the odds ratio (OR) for good outcome in the hypothermic group was 5.25 (95% confidence

intervals [CI] 1.47 to 18.76: $p = 0.011$). There were no adverse effects of TH apparent, such as sepsis, lactic acidosis or coagulopathy.

A second clinical trial of TH after OHCA was conducted in Europe [14]. At 6 months post-arrest, 55% of the TH patients had a good outcome, compared with 39% of the normothermic controls (OR 1.4, 95% CI 1.08 to 1.81). The complication rate also did not differ between the two groups.

However, a much larger study of 939 unconscious survivors of OHCA of presumed cardiac origin in Europe and Australia failed to show a benefit of a targeted temperature of 33°C, as compared with a targeted temperature of 36°C [15].

Australian Resuscitation Council (ARC)/New Zealand Resuscitation Council (NZRC) recommendations

The original two trials form the basis of the recommendation by the Australian Resuscitation Council and New Zealand Resuscitation Council [16] that therapeutic hypothermia (32–34°C for 12–24 hours) should be induced in patients who remain comatose after OHCA, when the initial cardiac arrest rhythm is ventricular fibrillation (VF).

Techniques and timing of therapeutic hypothermia

Current research is focused on the techniques and timing of therapeutic hypothermia. Surface cooling in the clinical trials cited above had the significant limitation of a slow decrease in core temperature, with 0.9°C/h decrease in core temperature using ice packs and 0.5°C/h using forced cold air cooling.

Surface cooling

Proprietary cooling jackets have become available which circulate temperature-controlled water through a jacket applied to the patient. The core temperature is monitored and the machine adjusts the temperature of the water circulating through the jacket, thus 'overshooting' with inadvertent cooling should be avoidable. As surface cooling still has the drawback of a relatively slow heat exchange due to the poor perfusion of the skin in many post-arrest patients, other techniques have been tested.

Intravascular cooling

Intravascular cooling is now feasible using a catheter inserted into the femoral vein that

includes a saline-filled balloon for heating/cooling. A catheter balloon contains saline that is pumped via the balloon and back to the machine. This allows heating/cooling of blood in the inferior vena cava. This approach has been shown to be more effective at core temperature control compared with surface cooling, however, there is a significant cost to the catheter [17].

Another technique for rapid induction of TH is to administer rapidly a large volume (30–40 mL/kg) of ice-cold (4°C) intravenous fluid [18]. An infusion of 30 mL/kg lactated Ringer's solution at 4°C was studied in an ED in 22 patients resuscitated from OHCA and was found to be an effective and safe technique to induce mild hypothermia, with a decrease in the core temperature of 1.7°C over 25 minutes. In addition, there were improvements in mean arterial blood pressure, acid–base and renal function with no apparent complications, such as pulmonary oedema.

Pre-hospital cooling trials

A number of pre-hospital trials of large-volume, ice-cold crystalloid for the rapid induction of TH in patients resuscitated from OHCA have now been undertaken. Kim et al. randomized 125 patients who were comatose following resuscitation from OHCA to receive either standard care or intravenous cooling by paramedics using 2000 mL ice-cold (4°) saline [19]. Sixty-three patients received an infusion of 4°C normal saline before hospital arrival which resulted in a decrease in temperature of 1.2°C, whereas the 62 patients having standard care had an increase in temperature of 0.10°C.

Two randomized, controlled, clinical trials of paramedic cooling have now also been undertaken in Melbourne, Australia. In one, post-VF arrest patients were cooled using 2 L ice-cold crystalloid fluid immediately after resuscitation [20]. A total of 234 patients were assigned to either paramedic cooling (118 patients) or hospital cooling (116 patients). Patients allocated to paramedic cooling received a median of 1900 mL of ice-cold Hartmann's solution, which resulted in a mean decrease in core temperature of 0.8°C. In the paramedic-cooled group, 47.5% patients had a non-statistically favourable outcome at hospital discharge compared with 52.6% in the hospital-cooled group (RR 0.90, 95% confidence interval 0.70 to 1.17, $p = 0.43$).

In a parallel trial, 163 patients who had been resuscitated from cardiac arrest with an initial cardiac rhythm of asystole or pulseless electrical activity were randomized to either pre-hospital cooling using a rapid infusion of 2 L ice-cold Hartmann's solution (82 patients) or cooling after hospital admission (81 patients) [21]. Patients allocated to pre-hospital cooling received a median of 1500 mL of ice-cold fluid which resulted in a mean decrease in core temperature of 1.4°C compared with 0.2°C in hospital cooled patients ($p < 0.001$). The time to therapeutic hypothermia (<34°C) was 3.2 h in the pre-hospital cooled group, compared with 4.8 h in the hospital cooled group ($p = 0.0328$). Overall, there was no statistical difference in outcome at hospital discharge with a favourable outcome (discharge from hospital to home or rehabilitation) in 12% in the pre-hospital cooled patients, compared with 9% in the hospital-cooled patients ($p = 0.50$). In the patients with a cardiac cause of the arrest, there was a trend towards improved outcome in the paramedic-treated patients, with 8 of 47 patients (17%) who received pre-hospital cooling with a favourable outcome at hospital discharge, compared with 3 of 43 (7%) in the hospital-cooled group ($p = 0.146$).

Currently, there is a clinical trial comparing TH inducted by paramedics during CPR using a bolus of 30 mL/kg ice-saline [22]. It is hoped that an earlier bolus of cold fluid during CPR may lead to earlier TH and thus improved patient outcomes.

The negative findings of the European/Australian TH trial now cast doubt on this ubiquitous modality of care.

Hyperoxia compared with normoxia after resuscitation

A number of laboratory studies suggest that post-OHCA, the administration of 100% oxygen may be associated with increased neurological injury compared with an oxygen/air mix titrated to provide normoxia [23]. It is proposed that the excessive oxygen increases the degree of free-radical production in injured neurons. Clinical studies in neonates with hypoxic–ischaemic encephalopathy also support the proposal that hyperoxia causes additional neurological injury [24].

In a large, multicentre observational study, the association between the highest PaO_2 measured on the first day of admission to the intensive care unit and mortality was determined in 4459 patients following resuscitation from OHCA [25]. After multivariable analysis, each 100 mmHg increase in PaO_2 was associated with a 24% increase in in-hospital mortality risk (OR 1.24: 95% confidence interval 1.18 to 1.31).

While observational, these data support the concept that there may be a dose-dependent association between supranormal oxygen tension and risk of in-hospital mortality, suggesting that hyperoxia in the early post-resuscitation period may be harmful. Therefore, decreasing the fraction of inspired oxygen while carefully monitoring the patient with continuous pulse oximetry to avoid hypoxia should be considered. However, prospective, controlled trials are required to validate this finding.

Other interventions

Another strategy to improve neurological outcome following resuscitation from OHCA includes maintenance of adequate blood pressure using fluid therapy and/or vasopressors [15]. Although human studies have not established optimal targets for blood pressure or blood oxygenation, one study showed benefit in OHCA patients with goal-directed therapy that included aiming for a mean arterial pressure target >65 mmHg and a mixed venous oxygen target >70% [26].

Outcome prediction

The early prediction of outcome is important after a severe anoxic neurological injury. Once a poor prognosis is reliably established, then decisions concerning limitations of costly intensive care treatments may be made. Previously, the clinical examination at day three was regarded as an accurate predictor of expected outcome [27]. However, this time frame preceded the widespread use of TH and the possibility that decreased metabolism of sedative agents might mask neurological improvement. More recent recommendations suggest that prognostication should now occur at a minimum of 72 hours after rewarming from TH [28].

Investigations such as brain computed tomography (CT), magnetic resonance imaging (MRI) and/or electroencephalogram (EEG) are relatively insensitive and/or non-specific for the early prediction of neurological outcome. While absent somatosensory responses bilaterally reliably predict a poor outcome after anoxic brain injury in unsedated patients, this investigation is not available in most hospitals.

References

[1] Sasson C, Rogers MA, Dahl J, Kellermann AL. Predictors of survival from out-of-hospital cardiac arrest: a systematic review and meta-analysis. Circ Cardiovasc Qual Outcomes 2010;3:63–81.

[2] Schneider A, Böttiger BW, Popp E. Cerebral resuscitation after cardiocirculatory arrest. Anesth Analg 2009;108:971–9.

[3] Pundik S, Xu K, Sundararajan S. Reperfusion brain injury: focus on cellular bioenergetics. Neurology 2012;79:S44–51.

[4] Takata K, Takeda Y, Sato T, et al. Effects of hypothermia for a short period on histologic outcome and extracellular glutamate concentration during and after cardiac arrest in rats. Crit Care Med 2005;33:1340–5.

[5] Ferrer I. Apoptosis: future targets for neuroprotective strategies. Cerebrovasc Dis 2006;2:9–20.

[6] Oku K, Kuboyama K, Safar P, et al. Cerebral and systemic arteriovenous oxygen monitoring after cardiac arrest: inadequate cerebral oxygen delivery. Resuscitation 1994;27:141–52.

[7] The Brain Resuscitation Clinical Trial Study Group. Randomized clinical study of thiopentone loading in comatose survivors of cardiac arrest. N Eng J Med 1986;314:397–410.

[8] The Brain Resuscitation Clinical Trial Study Group. Glucocorticoid treatment does not improve neurologic recovery following cardiac arrest. J Am Med Assoc 1989;262:3427–30.

[9] Brain Resuscitation Clinical Trial II Study Group. A randomized clinical study of a calcium-entry blocker (lidoflazine) in the treatment of comatose survivors of cardiac arrest. N Eng J Med 1991;324:1225–31.

[10] Roine RO, Kaste M, Kinnamen A, et al. Nimodipine after resuscitation from out-of-hospital ventricular fibrillation: a placebo-controlled double-blind randomized trial. J Am Med Assoc 1990;264:3171–7.

[11] Longstreth Jr WT, Fahrenbruch CE, Olsufka M, et al. Randomized clinical trial of magnesium, diazepam, or both after out-of-hospital cardiac arrest. Neurology 2002;59:506–14.

[12] Damian MS, Ellenberg D, Gildemeister R, et al. Coenzyme Q10 combined with mild hypothermia after cardiac arrest: a preliminary study. Circulation 2004;110:3011–6.

[13] Bernard SA, Gray TW, Buist MD, et al. A randomised, controlled trial of induced hypothermia in comatose survivors of prehospital cardiac arrest. N Eng J Med 2002;346:557–63.

[14] The Hypothermia after Cardiac Arrest Study Group. Mild therapeutic hypothermia to improve the neurological outcome after cardiac arrest. N Eng J Med 2002;346:549–56.

[15] Nielsen N, Wetterslev J, Cronberg T, et al. Targeted temperature management at 33°C versus 36°C after cardiac arrest. NEJM 2013;369:2197–206.

[16] Australian Resuscitation Council; New Zealand Resuscitation Council. Post-resuscitation therapy in adult advanced life support. ARC and NZRC Guidelines 2010. Emerg Med Australas 2011; 23:292–296.

[17] Hinz J, Rosmus M, Popov A, et al. Effectiveness of an intravascular cooling method compared with a conventional cooling technique in neurologic patients. J Neurosurg Anesthesiol 2007;19:130–5.

[18] Bernard SA, Buist M, Monteiro O, Smith K. Induced hypothermia using large volume, ice-cold intravenous fluid in comatose survivors of out-of-hospital cardiac arrest: a preliminary report. Resuscitation 2003;56:9–13.

[19] Kim F, Olsufka M, Longstreth Jr WT, et al. Pilot randomized clinical trial of prehospital induction of mild hypothermia in out-of-hospital cardiac arrest patients with a rapid infusion of 4°C normal saline. Circulation 2007;115:3064–70.

[20] Bernard SA, Smith K, Cameron P, et al. Induction of therapeutic hypothermia by paramedics after resuscitation from out-of-hospital ventricular fibrillation cardiac arrest. A randomized controlled trial. Circulation 2010;122:737–42.

[21] Bernard SA, Smith K, Cameron P, et al. Induction of therapeutic hypothermia by paramedics after resuscitation from out-of-hospital non-ventricular fibrillation cardiac arrest. Crit Care Med 2012;40:747–53.

[22] Deasy C, Bernard SA, Cameron P, et al. Design of the RINSE Trial: The rapid infusion of cold normal saline by paramedics during CPR. BMC Emerg Med 2011;11:17.

[23] Pilcher J, Weatherall M, Shirtcliffe P, et al. The effect of hyperoxia following cardiac arrest – A systematic review and meta-analysis of animal trials. Resuscitation 2012;83:417–22.

[24] Saugstad OD. Resuscitation of newborn infants: from oxygen to room air. Lancet 2010;376:1970–1.

[25] Kilgannon JH, Jones AE, Parrillo JE, et al. Relationship between supranormal oxygen tension and outcome after resuscitation from cardiac arrest. Circulation 2011;123:2717–22.

[26] Gaieski DF, Band RA, Abella BS, et al. Early goal-directed hemodynamic optimization combined with therapeutic hypothermia in comatose survivors of out-of-hospital cardiac arrest. Resuscitation 2009;80:418–24.

[27] Wijdicks EF, Hijdra A, Young GB, et al. Quality Standards Subcommittee of the American Academy of Neurology. Practice parameter: prediction of outcome in comatose survivors after cardiopulmonary resuscitation (an evidence-based review): report of the Quality Standards Subcommittee of the American Academy of Neurology. Neurology 2006;67:203–10.

[28] Rossetti AO, Oddo M, Logroscino G, Kaplan PW. Prognostication after cardiac arrest and hypothermia: a prospective study. Ann Neurol 2010;67:301–7.

2.8 Anaphylaxis

Anthony Brown

ESSENTIALS

1 Anaphylaxis describes both IgE, immune-mediated reactions and non-allergic, non-immunologically triggered events. Co-morbidities, such as asthma, infection, exercise, alcohol or stress, and concurrent medications, such as β-blockers, angiotensin converting enzyme inhibitors and aspirin, increase the risk ('summation anaphylaxis').

2 Deaths occur by hypoxia from upper airway asphyxia or severe bronchospasm or by profound shock from vasodilatation and extravascular fluid shift.

3 Parenteral penicillin, hymenopteran stings and foods are the most common causes of IgE, immune-mediated fatalities. Radiocontrast media, aspirin and other non-steroidal anti-inflammatory drugs are the most common causes of non-allergic fatalities. Older patients with ischaemic heart disease or on treatment, such as a β-blockers, are at increased risk of death.

4 Oxygen, adrenaline (epinephrine) and fluids are first-line treatment.

5 The role of H_1 and H_2 antihistamines, steroids, glucagon and salbutamol is unclear and unproven. They should only be considered once cardiovascular stability has been achieved with first-line agents.

6 Discharge follows a period of observation from 4 to 6 h after full recovery. A written discharge plan with adrenaline autoinjector and referral to an allergist for all significant, recurrent, unavoidable or unknown stimulus reactions are essential. Patient education is important to successful, long-term care.

7 Two comprehensive practice guidelines recently released include the Joint Task Force on Practice Parameters (2010) in the USA and the World Allergy Organization (2011).

Introduction

Anaphylaxis represents the most catastrophic of the immediate-type generalized hypersensitivity reactions and remains the quintessential medical emergency. It usually occurs unheralded in otherwise healthy people following exposure to a trigger. It presents as a dynamic continuum from mild to severe, gradual in onset to fulminant and may involve multiple organ systems or cause isolated shock or wheeze. Prompt clinical recognition and treatment with oxygen, adrenaline and fluids to restore cardiorespiratory stability are essential to ensure a favourable outcome. Careful discharge planning, including allergy referral where appropriate, protects against further attacks of anaphylaxis.

Definition

The term 'anaphylaxis' was introduced by Richet and Portier in 1902, literally meaning 'against protection'. It is currently used to describe the rapid, generalized and often unheralded immunologically-mediated events that follow exposure to certain foreign substances in previously sensitized persons known as antigen-induced, or immune-mediated, allergic anaphylaxis.

An identical clinical syndrome known as non-allergic anaphylaxis follows non-immunological mechanisms, with the release of identical inflammatory mediators. Non-allergic anaphylaxis may occur on first exposure to an agent and does not require a period of sensitization. The term 'non-allergic anaphylaxis' is preferred by the World Allergy Organization (WAO) to the older one of an 'anaphylactoid reaction' [1]. This chapter will use the clinical term 'anaphylaxis' to describe *both* of these syndromes, despite their important aetiological differences.

Classification of anaphylaxis

Surprisingly, there is still no international agreement on the classification, diagnosis or severity grading of anaphylaxis [2]. One simple definition is that anaphylaxis is 'a serious, life-threatening generalized or systemic hypersensitivity reaction' [1]. Similarly, the National Institute of Allergy and Infectious Disease (NIAID) and the Food Allergy and Anaphylaxis Network (FAAN) recommend an equally brief, broad definition: 'Anaphylaxis is a serious allergic reaction that is rapid in onset and may cause death'. Their full definition is considerably longer yet more complete, aiming to capture over 95% of clinical cases within the three diagnostic criteria [3]. Criterion 1 aims to identify at least 80% of anaphylaxis cases, even if the allergic status of the patient and potential cause of the reaction may be unknown, as the majority of anaphylactic reactions include skin symptoms. Criterion

2 is to identify anaphylaxis in the absence of cutaneous features, such as in children with food allergy or insect sting allergy, but requires a known allergic history and possible exposure. Gastrointestinal symptoms are included. Criterion 3 aims to capture the rare patient with an acute hypotensive episode after exposure to a known allergen (Box 2.8.1) [3]. These inclusive definitions for anaphylaxis should be used by researchers unless and until refined by future prospective data [4].

Severity grading

No validated grading system exists that prospectively links the clinical features of anaphylaxis with severity, urgency, treatment or outcome. One system based on a retrospective multivariate analysis of over 1000 clinically diagnosed generalized hypersensitivity reactions defined three grades (Table 2.8.1) [5]. Generalized allergic reactions confined to the skin and subcutaneous tissues were considered as mild grade, but the moderate and severe grades with multisystem involvement that correlated with the need for adrenaline represent true anaphylaxis according to the NIAID/FAAN criteria. Again, this grading system should be used as a starting point by researchers for descriptive purposes, until prospective data in the future refine the criteria.

Aetiology

Important clinical categories of anaphylaxis include anaphylaxis related to medications, biologics and vaccines, as well as to insect stings, foods, anaesthesia, natural rubber latex exposure, exercise and idiopathic anaphylaxis (Box 2.8.2) [1,6]. Geographic variations are reported, such as sesame anaphylaxis in the Middle East and chickpea and rice reactions in Asia.

Drug-induced anaphylaxis

Penicillin is the most common cause of drug-induced anaphylaxis. Around 1:500 patient courses have an apparent allergic reaction, mostly urticaria alone [7]. True allergic cross-reactivity to cephalosporins only occurs in around 1–2% and is largely with the first-generation cephalosporins.

Aspirin and non-steroidal anti-inflammatory drugs (NSAIDs) are the next most common cause of drug-induced anaphylaxis. Reactions appear to be medication-specific, as there is no clinical cross-reactivity with structurally unrelated NSAIDs [6].

Valid tests for IgE-mediated reactions are unavailable for most drugs or biologics, with the exception of the penicillins.

Insect sting anaphylaxis

Reactions to stings from bees, wasps and ants of the order Hymenoptera are second only to drug-induced anaphylaxis and occur in up to 3% of the population (<1% of children). Fatalities are more common in adults often from shock. Non-anaphylactic toxic, large local or late serum sickness-like reactions also occur following a sting.

Food-induced anaphylaxis

This is most common in the young, particularly following peanuts, tree nuts, such as walnuts

Table 2.8.1	Severity grading system for generalized hypersensitivity reactions	
Grade	Defined by
1: Mild[1] (skin and subcutaneous tissues only)	Generalized erythema, urticaria, periorbital oedema or angio-oedema
2: Moderate[2] (features suggesting respiratory, cardiovascular or gastrointestinal involvement)	Dyspnoea, stridor, wheeze, nausea, vomiting, dizziness (presyncope), diaphoresis, chest or throat tightness, or abdominal pain
3: Severe[2] (hypoxia, hypotension, or neurological compromise)	Cyanosis or SpO_2 ≤92% at any stage, hypotension (SBP <90 mmHg in adults), confusion, collapse, LOC, or incontinence

SBP: systolic blood pressure; LOC: loss of consciousness; SpO_2: oxygen saturation on pulse oximetry.
[1]Mild reactions can be further subclassified into those with and those without angio-oedema.
[2]Only grades 2 and 3 constitute true anaphylaxis. Reproduced with permission from Brown SGA. Clinical features and severity grading of anaphylaxis. Journal of Allergy and Clinical Immunology 2004;114:371–6.

Box 2.8.1   Definition of anaphylaxis: clinical criteria for diagnosis

Anaphylaxis is highly likely when any one of the following three criteria are fulfilled:

1. Acute onset of an illness (minutes to several hours) with involvement of the skin, mucosal tissue or both (e.g. generalized hives, pruritus or flushing, swollen lips–tongue–uvula) and at least one of the following:
   - Respiratory compromise (e.g. dyspnoea, wheeze–bronchospasm, stridor, reduced PEF, hypoxaemia)
   - Reduced BP or associated symptoms of end-organ dysfunction (e.g. hypotonia (collapse), syncope, incontinence)
2. Two or more of the following that occur rapidly after exposure to a *likely allergen for that patient* (minutes to several hours):
   - Involvement of the skin-mucosal tissue (e.g. generalized hives, itch–flush, swollen lips–tongue–uvula)
   - Respiratory compromise (e.g. dyspnoea, wheeze–bronchospasm, stridor, reduced PEF, hypoxaemia)
   - Reduced BP or associated symptoms (e.g. hypotonia (collapse), syncope, incontinence)
   - Persistent gastrointestinal symptoms (e.g. crampy abdominal pain, vomiting)
3. Reduced BP after exposure to *known allergen for that patient* (minutes to several hours):
   - Infants and children: low systolic BP (age-specific) or greater than 30% decrease in systolic BP*
   - Adults: systolic BP of less than 90 mmHg or greater than 30% decrease from that person's baseline

PEF: peak expiratory flow; BP: blood pressure.
*Low systolic blood pressure for children is defined as less than 70 mmHg from 1 month to 1 year; less than (70 mmHg + [2 × age]) from 1 to 10 years; and less than 90 mmHg from 11 to 17 years. Reproduced with permission from Sampson HA, Munoz-Furlong A, Campbell RL, et al. Second symposium on the definition and management of anaphylaxis: summary report – Second National Institute of Allergy and Infectious Disease/Food Allergy and Anaphylaxis Network symposium. Journal of Allergy and Clinical Immunology 2006;117:391–7.

and pecans, shellfish, fin fish, cow's milk, soy and egg ingestion. Cross-reactivity with other foods is unpredictable or reactions may occur to additives, such as carmine, metabisulphite and tartrazine. Mislabelling and contamination during manufacturing or at home cause inadvertent exposure and associated factors such as exercise after food must be recognized (see later).

Although fatalities are rare and usually associated with pre-existing asthma, biphasic reactions are seen which, similar to all the other causes, means that the symptoms subside only to recur several hours later. Patient and carer education is paramount, with schools in particular prepared to respond with auto-injector adrenaline (epinephrine) in an emergency, such as the EpiPen or EpiPen Jr, or the Anapen or Anapen Jr.

Anaesthesia-related anaphylaxis

Perioperative anaphylaxis

Neuromuscular blocking agents and latex cause most cases, followed by antibiotics and induction drugs, but opioids, NSAIDs, colloids, blood products, radiocontrast dye, isosulphan or methylene blue, methylmethacrylate, chlorhexidine and protamine may be responsible for 'perioperative anaphylaxis'. The overall median annual incidence in France was 100:1 000 000 anaesthetics, of which 73% were IgE-mediated [8]. Other estimates range from 1:4000 to 1:25 000 anaesthetics, with up to 4% of reactions fatal.

General anaesthesia reactions are due to muscle relaxants in 60% of cases, with suxamethonium and rocuronium in the highest-risk group. Reactions to suxamethonium and other relaxants can occur in the absence of prior use suggesting cross-reactivity and rendering large-scale preoperative testing unfeasible.

Latex-induced anaphylaxis

Healthcare workers, children with spina bifida and genitourinary abnormalities who undergo multiple surgical procedures and occupational exposure are the highest-risk groups for natural rubber latex (NRL) allergy. Atopy and cross-reacting fruit allergy are also associated with an increased risk. Reactions may follow direct contact, parenteral contamination or aerosol transmission.

Patients at known high risk require treatment in a latex-free environment with special syringes and non-latex containing gloves, stethoscope, breathing-system, blood pressure cuff,

intravenous tubing and administration ports. Every emergency department (ED) must have the capacity to support an unexpected case of latex allergy, perhaps by sharing with the anaesthesia department access to a 'latex allergy resuscitation cart' containing relevant latex-free equipment. A clear patient warning should be posted in the ED at the time and staff access limited.

Exercise-induced anaphylaxis

Anaphylaxis occurs with a variety of physical activities, although up to 50% of exercise-induced reactions occur following the ingestion of a food or are associated with prior aspirin or NSAID use or high pollen levels. Mast cell degranulation appears to be triggered by cross-linking of allergen-specific IgE combined with neuropeptide release by adjacent nerve endings.

The severity of symptoms is generally influenced by the amount of food ingested, the vigour of the exercise and the lapse of time between the two, with more severe reactions occurring with exercise soon after food ingestion. Prophylactic medication is ineffective, unlike prophylactic salbutamol or sodium cromoglycate that prevent exercise-induced asthma.

Idiopathic anaphylaxis

This is defined as anaphylaxis in which no discernible causative allergen, inciting physical factor or disease state can be identified. The diagnosis is by exclusion, with the majority of cases seen in adults of whom 50% are atopic, although it does occur in children. Among other conditions, indolent systemic mastocytosis and hereditary or acquired angio-oedema require exclusion.

Co-factors 'summation anaphylaxis'

Many co-factors and co-morbidities or concurrent medications increase the risk of anaphylaxis, giving rise to the concept of 'summation anaphylaxis' [9]. These include asthma, severe atopy (which predisposes to some types of anaphylaxis, such as latex or exercise-induced), intercurrent infection, cardiac disease, exercise, alcohol, psychological stress, premenstrual status and drugs [1].

Summation anaphylaxis may also explain the unpredictable response of some individuals to recurrent antigen exposure.

Predisposing drugs

Drugs that predispose to or worsen anaphylactic reactions include β-adrenergic

blockers, NSAIDs and the angiotensin converting enzyme inhibitors (ACEIs). ACEIs, plus to a much lesser extent, angiotensin II receptor blockers (ARBs) together with the gliptins are associated in particular with non-histaminergic, bradykinin-related angioedema.

Epidemiology

The true incidence of anaphylaxis is unknown. Data are unreliable with the lack of a standard definition and are mostly derived from retrospective case collections from sources as diverse as the ED, perioperatively or the allergist–immunologist's office. Under-reporting is common as the diagnosis may have been missed or when there is spontaneous recovery, pre-hospital treatment or a fatality. However, despite this, all anaphylaxis data from Western countries show that the incidence is increasing [1,10].

Emergency department anaphylaxis

ED anaphylaxis presentations in adults have an annual incidence from 1:439 to 1:1100 ED cases, representing up to one adult presentation per 3400 population per year [11]. The annual incidence of paediatric anaphylaxis is around 1:1000 ED presentations, although generalized allergic reactions in children (that is, without multisystem involvement) are nearly 10 times more common than this [12].

The causative agent is suspected in 75% of ED anaphylaxis cases, recognized from a previous reaction or by close temporal association with symptom onset. The most frequent causes in adults are drug-related and hymenopteran stings whereas, in children, food-induced or drug-related predominate. Respiratory features appear more common in paediatric anaphylaxis and cardiovascular features in adults [12].

Fatal anaphylaxis

Deaths follow hypoxia from upper airway swelling with asphyxia, bronchospasm and mucus plugging and from shock related to vasodilatation, extravascular fluid shift and direct myocardial depression. Tachycardia is usual in shock, but bradycardia related to a neurocardiogenic, vagally-mediated mechanism (Bezold–Jarisch reflex) has occasionally been observed. This may respond to atropine if adrenaline fails (see under Management, second-line agents).

Fatalities are rare at less than one (0.33–0.64) per million population per year [10,13].

When they do happen, fatal reactions are rapid with a median time to cardiorespiratory arrest of just 5 min if iatrogenic, 15 min for venom and 30 min following foods, with no death occurring greater than 6 hours after contact with a trigger. Adrenaline was given in only 14% of cases prior to arrest and not at all in 38% of fatalities [13].

Fatal food-induced anaphylaxis in the UK included 43 of 48 patients having associated asthma usually with suboptimal daily inhaled steroid use, of which over half had only ever had a mild previous food reaction. This suggests that the severity of subsequent reactions cannot be predicted from the reaction history and that sound professional advice was often inadequate or absent [14].

Pathophysiology

Triggering events

Most cases of immune-mediated, allergic anaphylaxis are IgE- or occasionally IgG_4-mediated. Reaginic antibodies are released into the circulation by plasma cells derived from B lymphocytes, under the influence of helper T cells following previous exposure to an antigen (quite why this happens is unclear). These antibodies then bind to glycoprotein receptors on blood-borne basophils or tissue mast cells, sensitizing them. A huge variety of substances induce IgE antibody formation ranging from drugs, chemicals and biologic agents, foods, hymenopteran sting venom, insect saliva and other venoms, to latex and environmental allergens (see Box 2.8.2).

Non-IgE-dependent, non-allergic anaphylaxis

Non-IgE-dependent, non-allergic anaphylactic reactions are caused by mediator release triggered independently of reaginic antibodies, leading to complement activation, the direct pharmacological release of mediators or clotting/fibrinolysis system activation. Physical factors, medications, biologic agents and food additives may trigger these non-IgE reactions (see Box 2.8.2).

Cellular events

Tissue-based mast cells and circulating basophils release inflammatory mediators following the binding of multivalent allergen cross-linking the surface, high-affinity IgE Fc receptors (FcεRI) or from cell membrane perturbation. This, coupled with the mobilization of Ca^{2+} in the endoplasmic reticulum, leads to release of preformed granule-associated mediators by exocytosis, or to the *de novo* synthesis of eicosanoid lipid mediators from endogenous membrane arachidonic acid stores, and the activation of genes for various cytokines and chemokines [15,16].

Mast cell and basophil inflammatory mediators

The preformed mediators include histamine, serine proteases, such as tryptase, chymase and carboxypeptidase A, and proteoglycans, such as heparin and chondroitin sulphate E. Newly synthesized lipid mediators include prostaglandin D_2 and thromboxane A_2 via the cyclo-oxygenase pathway and the leukotrienes LTC_4, LTD_4 and LTE_4 via the 5-lipoxygenase pathway. The cytokines released include tumour necrosis factor alpha (TNF-α), various interleukins, such as IL-3, IL-5, IL-6, IL-10, IL-13 and IL-16, and granulocyte macrophage colony-stimulating factor (GM-CSF). Finally, chemokines include platelet activating factor, neutrophil chemotactic factor (IL-8) and eosinophil chemotactic factor, plus macrophage inflammatory protein 1α [16].

Modulation of mediator release

At the cellular level, mediator release is modulated by the steady-state resting intracellular cyclic AMP (cAMP) levels. Substances that elevate cAMP, such as adrenaline, inhibit mediator release, partly explaining adrenaline's essential role in treatment. Also, from knowledge of the complex array of mediators involved, it is self-evident why antihistamines cannot form the first line of therapy.

Box 2.8.2   Causes of anaphylaxis

IgE-DEPENDENT MECHANISMS:

Drugs, chemicals and biologic agents
penicillins, cephalosporins, sulphonamides, muscle relaxants, vaccines, insulin, thiamine, protamine, gamma globulin, cis-/carboplatinum and doxorubicin, monoclonal antibodies cetuximab/rituximab, antivenoms, formaldehyde, ethylene oxide, chlorhexidine, semen

Foods
peanuts, tree nuts, shellfish, fin fish, milk, egg, fruits, vegetables, sesame, flour

Hymenopteran sting venom, insect saliva, other venoms
bees, wasps, ants, hornets, ticks, triatomid 'kissing bugs', snakes, scorpions, jellyfish

Natural rubber latex

Environmental
pollen, horse dander, hydatid cyst rupture

NON-IgE-DEPENDENT MECHANISMS:

Physical factors
exercise, cold, heat, sunlight

Medications and biologic agents
opiates, aspirin and NSAID, ACEI, vancomycin, radiocontrast media, N-acetylcysteine, fluorescein

Food additives
metabisulphite, tartrazine

IDIOPATHIC
exclusion of all known causes including mastocytosis

NSAID: non-steroidal, anti-inflammatory drugs; ACEI: angiotensin converting enzyme inhibitors.
Note: Cross-reactivity is seen; both IgE-dependent and non-IgE-dependent reactions may occur with the same agent.
Several mechanisms may coexist such as exercise-induced following food.
Non-IgE-dependent mechanisms include complement activation, kinin production or potentiation and direct mediator release.
ACEI use is an important cause of unexplained angioedema, occurring in up to 1:200 patients on these drugs, and may develop at any interval after starting (most commonly early on).

Mediator pharmacology

Mediators act to induce vasodilatation, increase capillary permeability and glandular secretion, cause smooth muscle spasm, particularly bronchoconstriction and to attract new cells such as eosinophils, leucocytes and platelets. Positive feedback mechanisms amplify and perpetuate reactions recruiting further effector cells to release increasing amounts of mediators in a 'mast cell–leucocyte cytokine cascade' effect [17]. In addition, it appears that severe and/or fatal reactions also relate not only to the amount of mediators released, but also to the speed of their degradation, for instance in the case of reduced platelet activating factor (PAF) catabolism from lower levels of PAF acetylhydrolase [1,6].

Conversely, other anaphylactic reactions self-limit, with spontaneous recovery related to endogenous compensatory mechanisms including increased adrenaline, angiotensin II or endothelin 1 secretion [18].

Clinical features

Anaphylaxis is characteristically a disease of fit patients and is rarely seen or described in critically ill or shocked patients, other than asthmatics. The speed of onset relates to the mechanism of exposure and the severity of the reaction. Parenteral antigen exposure may cause life-threatening anaphylaxis within minutes, whereas symptoms can be delayed for some hours following oral or topical exposure.

Cutaneous and generalized allergic reactions

A premonitory aura, tingling or warm sensation, anxiety and feeling of impending doom precede generalized erythema, urticaria with pruritus and angioedema of the neck, face, lips and tongue. Rhinorrhoea, conjunctival injection and tearing are seen.

Eighty to 90% or more of patients with anaphylaxis have cutaneous features which assist in the prompt, early diagnosis [11,12,18]. However, alerting cutaneous features may be absent because of pre-hospital treatment or their spontaneous resolution, be subtle clinically and missed or the onset of other life-threatening systemic complications, such as laryngeal oedema or shock, may precede them.

Systemic reactions

The hallmark of anaphylaxis is the precipitate onset of multisystem involvement with respiratory, cardiovascular, gastrointestinal and or neurological system dysfunction (Box 2.8.3).

Respiratory manifestations

Throat tightness and cough precede mild to critical respiratory distress due to oropharyngeal or laryngeal oedema with dyspnoea, hoarseness, stridor even aphonia; or related to bronchospasm with tachypnoea and wheeze. Hypoxia with an oxygen saturation less than 92% on pulse oximetry and central cyanosis indicate severe anaphylaxis and the need for immediate treatment (see severity grading Table 2.8.1).

Cardiovascular and neurological manifestations

Light-headedness, sweating, incontinence, syncope or coma may precede or accompany cardiovascular collapse with tachycardia, hypotension and cardiac arrhythmias, which again, herald severe anaphylaxis. These arrhythmias can appear seemingly benign supraventricular rhythms, particularly in children, but may progress to an impalpable pulse requiring external cardiac massage (see severity grading Table 2.8.1).

Cardiac chest pain   Chest pain may occur due to coronary artery spasm from cardiac mast cell release of histamine, leukotrienes and platelet activating factor even in the absence of coronary artery disease, or exacerbating this when present or subclinical in the older patient [1,6,18].

Gastrointestinal manifestations

Difficult or painful swallowing, nausea, vomiting, diarrhoea and abdominal cramps occur in up to one-third of cases, but are usually overshadowed by the more immediately life-threatening features.

Differential diagnosis

The protean manifestations of anaphylaxis have a potentially vast differential diagnosis, although the rapidity of onset, accompanying cutaneous features and their relationship to a likely or known trigger suggests the true diagnosis in most cases. The following differential diagnoses should be considered.

Wheeze and difficulty breathing

Bronchial asthma, cardiogenic pulmonary oedema, foreign body inhalation, irritant chemical exposure and tension pneumothorax are distinguished by the history, co-morbidity and associated presenting features.

Light-headedness and syncope

An anxiety or vasovagal reaction should be considered where there is a history of exaggerated fear of an impending reaction or in

---

Box 2.8.3   Clinical features of anaphylaxis

Cutaneous
- Tingling or warmth, erythema (flushing), urticaria, pruritus (itch), angioedema
- Rhinorrhoea, conjunctival injection, lacrimation

Respiratory
- Throat tightness, cough, dyspnoea, hoarseness, stridor, aphonia
- Tachypnoea, wheeze, SpO_2 <92%,* cyanosis*

Cardiovascular/neurological
- Tachycardia (rarely bradycardia), hypotension,* chest pain,# arrhythmia,# cardiac arrest*
- Light-headedness, sweating, incontinence,* syncope,* confusion,* coma*

Gastrointestinal
- Odynophagia (difficult or painful swallowing), abdominal cramps, nausea, vomiting, diarrhoea

Miscellaneous
- Premonitory aura, anxiety, feeling of impending doom
- Pelvic cramps

SpO_2: oxygen saturation on pulse oximetry.
*: Indicative of a severe reaction (see Table 2.8.1 for grading system).
#: From cardiac mast cell-mediated coronary artery spasm (or adrenaline-related following treatment).

the context of a painful procedure, such as an injection or local anaesthetic infiltration with collapse. Bradycardia, sweating and pallor without urticaria, erythema or itch, associated with a brief prodrome and rapid response to the recumbent position favour a vasovagal reaction over anaphylactic shock.

Other forms of shock

Other types of distributive shock, such as septicaemia, spinal denervation, epidural or spinal block; hypovolaemic shock from haemorrhage or fluid loss; cardiogenic shock from primary myocardial dysfunction; and obstructive shock from cardiac tamponade or tension pneumothorax should all be apparent from the history and examination. Cutaneous and respiratory features other than tachypnoea are absent in these non-anaphylactic causes of shock.

Flushing

Scombroid poisoning following spoiled-fish ingestion, carcinoid syndrome, alcohol and systemic mastocytosis all produce flushing and require a careful history and investigation to differentiate.

Facial swelling or angioedema

Bacterial or viral infections usually have fever and/or pain and traumatic or anticoagulant-related bleeding causes recognizable bruising.

Angioedema in the absence of urticaria or itch can be caused by actual or functional C1 esterase inhibitor deficiency or be drug related.

C1 esterase inhibitor deficiency

This may be hereditary autosomal dominant, with a positive family history, the *absence* of pruritus or urticaria, prominent abdominal symptoms and a history of recurrent attacks related to minor stress. Alternatively, C1 esterase inhibitor deficiency may be acquired in lymphoproliferative and some connective tissue disorders. A rapid, inexpensive screening test for serum C4 should be performed and, if low, be followed by the more specific C1 esterase inhibitor assay to confirm the diagnosis. Management of a serious attack is with 20 units/kg C1 esterase inhibitor concentrate intravenously or with icatibant 30 mg subcutaneously, a bradykinin 2 receptor (B2R) antagonist.

Angiotensin converting enzyme inhibitor (ACEI) use

ACEI are the single most common cause of drug-related angioedema, usually within weeks of commencing the drug, but angioedema may occur months or years later and even after recently stopping them. The angioedema is non-histaminergic related to localized bradykinin effects, again without associated pruritus or urticaria. It does not respond to conventional treatment with adrenaline or antihistamines. A similar reaction is also seen with the gliptins.

Clinical investigations

The diagnosis of anaphylaxis is clinical. No immediate laboratory or radiological test confirms the process and must never delay immediate management. The measurement of electrolytes and renal function, blood glucose, chest X-ray and an ECG are indicated only if there is a slow response to treatment or when there is doubt about the diagnosis.

Disease progress may be monitored by pulse oximetry, haematocrit level, which may rise with fluid extravasation, and arterial blood gases to look for a respiratory or metabolic acidosis.

Laboratory testing

This is rarely performed or of immediate clinical relevance and should never delay management.

Mast cell tryptase

Ideally, three samples should be taken for mast cell tryptase (MCT) in liaison with the hospital laboratory. The first as soon as possible after resuscitation has commenced, the next at 1–2 h after the start of symptoms (but no longer than 6 h) and one at 24 h or in convalescence (for baseline tryptase levels) [19].

Despite initial promise, a serum MCT taken from 1 to 6 h after a suspected episode cannot solely be relied upon to diagnose anaphylaxis, as it is not consistently elevated above the reference range of 1–11.4 ng/mL, particularly following food allergy. Conversely, a mast cell tryptase assay may be elevated post-mortem in a non-anaphylactic death [6,19].

However, measuring change in levels 'delta tryptase', specific allelic subtypes such as mature *b* tryptase or using a multimarker approach to include PAF may improve the value of laboratory testing, providing this does not interfere with acute mangement.

Histamine

Histamine levels are impractical to measure as they are unstable and evanescent, only remaining elevated for 30–60 min maximum.

Management

Initial approach

Immediately stop any potential causative agent, such as an intravenous drug or infusion. Manage the patient in a monitored resuscitation area, including at least a pulse oximeter, non-invasive blood pressure device and ECG tracing. Call for immediate senior help.

Obtain a brief history of possible allergen exposure and perform a rapid assessment of the extent and severity of the reaction. Look particularly for signs of upper airway swelling, bronchospasm or circulatory shock.

The primary objective is to achieve stabilization of cardiorespiratory status by administration of oxygen, adrenaline (epinephrine) and fluids to the supine/recumbent patient. Antihistamines and steroids play no role until after this has been achieved and, even then, their value is debatable (Box 2.8.4) [3,6].

Oxygen and airway patency

Give oxygen by face-mask to all patients, aiming for an oxygen saturation above 92%. Place the patient supine, preferably with the legs elevated to optimize venous return. Elevate the head and torso if respiratory distress is prominent or worsened. Prepare for active airway intervention, including opening the difficult airway kit, if there are signs of impending airway obstruction or rapidly progressive respiratory failure.

Cyanosis and exhaustion indicate imminent respiratory arrest. Never give a sedative or muscle relaxant drug unless well trained in the management of the difficult airway, as endotracheal intubation and mechanical ventilation can be extremely challenging. Perform a surgical airway via the cricothyroid membrane as a last resort, before hypoxic cardiac arrest occurs.

Adrenaline (epinephrine)

Adrenaline is the drug of choice for acute anaphylaxis, whether allergic IgE-mediated or non-allergic. Give adrenaline in all but the most trivial cases and certainly if there is progressive airway swelling, bronchospasm or hypotension. Adrenaline has α-, β_1- and β_2-adrenergic effects to counteract the profound vasodilatation, mucosal oedema and bronchospasm. Equally important is that adrenaline triggers a rise in intracellular cyclic AMP inhibiting further mast cell and basophil mediator release [1,6].

CRITICAL CARE

Box 2.8.4   Treatment of anaphylaxis

Initial treatment

- Stop delivery of any potential causative agent
- Call for senior help
- Give adrenaline (epinephrine) 0.01 mg/kg intramuscular (IM) into upper lateral thigh, to maximum 0.5 mg, e.g. 0.3–0.5 mL of 1:1000 adrenaline (epinephrine) IM
  - may be repeated every 5–15 min
  - or use patient's EpiPen or Anapen if readily available – may be given through clothing
- Lay supine (or elevate legs) for shock
- Give high-flow oxygen
- Insert large-bore IV cannula (14 g or 16 g) and give crystalloid fluid bolus of 10–20 mL/kg

Deteriorating rapidly or failure to respond

- Start 1:100 000 adrenaline (epinephrine) infusion with 1 mL (1 mg) of 1:1000 adrenaline in 100 mL normal saline at 60–120 mL/h (10–20 μg/min) titrated to response:
  - *must* be on ECG monitor
  - give faster in cardiopulmonary collapse/arrest
- Consider assisted ventilation and endotracheal intubation by a skilled emergency doctor (may be technically challenging)

Adrenaline (epinephrine) dose

The dose of adrenaline is 0.01 mg/kg up to a maximum of 0.5 mg intramuscularly, repeated every 5–15 min as necessary. Give this as 0.01 mL/kg of 1:1000 aqueous adrenaline, or 0.3–0.5 mL (0.3–0.5 mg) into the upper outer thigh.

The adrenaline may be injected through clothing in an emergency, including when self-administered pre-hospital using an EpiPen or EpiPen Jr containing 300 μg and 150 μg respectively, or Anapen or Anapen Jr (same respective adrenaline doses).

Adrenaline (epinephrine) route

Intramuscular adrenaline

Intramuscular adrenaline is recommended when anaphylaxis is treated early, progressing slowly, venous access is difficult or delayed or in the unmonitored patient. The intramuscular route is superior to subcutaneous and the vastus lateralis muscle in the thigh is preferred to the deltoid muscle in the arm. Adrenaline IM is successful in the large majority of cases, particularly if given promptly [1].

Intravenous adrenaline Intravenous adrenaline is only necessary if there is rapidly progressive vascular collapse with shock, imminent airway obstruction or critical bronchospasm and/or impending cardiac arrest. The patient must have ECG monitoring and an experienced emergency physician in charge.

Administer the intravenous adrenaline slowly with extreme care, suitably diluted and titrated to response to avoid potentially lethal complications, such as myocardial ischaemia, cardiac arrhythmias and cerebrovascular accident [13,20,21].

Adrenaline (epinephrine) infusion

Although 1:10 000 adrenaline containing 100 μg/mL is readily available, for instance as 10 mL prefilled syringes, it is impossible to give this slowly enough at 10 μg/min, in the small initial quantities of 0.75–1.5 μg/kg (i.e. 50–100 μg) necessary.

Therefore, make up an infusion of adrenaline by putting 1 mg in 100 mL normal saline (that is 1:100 000 adrenaline with 10 μg/mL) and start at 60–120 mL/h via an infusion device, to deliver 10–20 μg/min and titrate to response. Be prepared to continue the infusion for anything up to 60 min after resolution of all the symptoms and signs of anaphylaxis, then wean over the next 30 min and stop, watching closely for any recurrence [22]. Patients with persistent symptoms (protracted anaphylaxis) require a maintenance infusion of 5–10 μg/min and admission to a monitored intensive care area.

Adrenaline (epinephrine) nebulizer

Nebulized adrenaline 5 mg, as 5 mL of undiluted 1:1000 adrenaline may be given particularly for upper airway oedema and bronchospasm, while parenteral adrenaline is being prepared as above.

Fluid replacement

Insert a large-bore intravenous cannula as soon as possible in patients showing signs of shock. Rapidly administer an initial fluid bolus of 10–20 mL/kg normal saline to counter the massive intravascular fluid shifts and peripheral vasodilatation that occur within minutes with anaphylactic shock. There are no outcome data favouring colloids over crystalloids.

Second-line agents

Once oxygen, adrenaline and fluids have been given to optimize the cardiorespiratory status and tissue oxygenation, the following drugs may be considered in a support role only, although evidence for their efficacy is lacking, being extrapolated from their use in urticaria or acute asthma [1].

H_1- and H_2-antihistamines

Reserve antihistamines for the symptomatic relief of skin symptoms, such as urticaria, mild angioedema and pruritus. There are no outcome data that support their use in anaphylaxis [23]. Antihistamines must never be relied upon as sole therapy in significant anaphylaxis. Side effects of sedation, confusion and vasodilatation with the H_1-antihistamines can be troublesome, particularly when given parenterally.

The combination of an H_2-antihistamine with an H_1-antihistamine is better at attenuating the cutaneous manifestations of a generalized allergic reaction than an H_1-antagonist given alone. Choose a non-sedating H_1-antihistamine, such as loratadine 10 mg daily, especially on discharge, if the patient wishes to continue working or driving a vehicle (see Discharge oral medication).

Corticosteroids

As with the antihistamines, there are no placebo-controlled trials to confirm the effectiveness of steroids in significant anaphylaxis, despite their many theoretical benefits on mediator release and tissue responsiveness, such as the downregulation of the late phase eosinophilic inflammatory response [24].

However, in view of their early safety, most clinicians give prednisone 1 mg/kg up to 50 mg orally or hydrocortisone 1.5–3 mg/kg IV, particularly in patients with airway involvement and bronchospasm, based on their important role in asthma. Side effects including sodium and potassium ion flux changes and anaphylaxis itself are more likely with the intravenous route for steroid delivery.

It is also possible that steroids prevent a biphasic reaction with recrudescence of symptoms following recovery but, again, supporting data are unconvincing (see Disposition). Steroids are, however, essential in the management of recurrent idiopathic anaphylaxis.

Glucagon, atropine and salbutamol

Patients taking β-blockers have more severe and/or treatment-refractory anaphylaxis. Give glucagon from 1 to 5 mg intravenously, followed by an infusion at 5–15 μg/min titrated to response, if adrenaline has been ineffective. Glucagon raises cyclic AMP by a non-adrenergic mechanism, but may cause nausea and vomiting.

As mentioned earlier, some patients with anaphylactic shock develop a bradycardia resistant to adrenaline, possibly mediated by a neurocardiogenic vagal reflex. Atropine 0.6 mg intravenously up to 0.02 mg/kg has been successful in this situation [20].

Finally, give nebulized salbutamol in addition to adrenaline for resistant bronchospasm, which has the advantage of familiarity.

Other vasopressors

Vasopressors, such as noradrenaline, metaraminol, phenylephrine and vasopressin, anecdotally have treated hypotension resistant to initial adrenaline and fluid therapy.

Methylene blue

Methylene blue, a competitive inhibitor of guanylate cyclase may counteract resistant, nitric oxide mediated vasodilatation particularly related to PAF but, in turn, it has caused anaphylaxis itself [6].

Pretreatment

There is no convincing justification for pretreatment. In particular, the practice of routine prophylactic corticosteroids and/or antihistamines to reduce the risk of serious iodinated contrast media reactions during radiological procedures is neither reliable nor supported by the literature and should be abandoned [25].

Disposition

Patients with systemic anaphylactic reactions, including all those who receive adrenaline, should be kept under observation for at least 4–6 h after apparent full recovery. Keep patients with reactive airways disease longer, as most deaths from anaphylaxis occur in this group [4]. Observation is safely performed in the ED if a suitable holding area exists and ECG monitoring is unnecessary [11,12].

Most anaphylactic reactions are uniphasic and respond rapidly and completely to treatment. Some patients develop protracted reactions with an incomplete response to adrenaline or deteriorate on attempted adrenaline weaning. Keep these patients with unstable vital signs monitored and admit to an intensive care area.

Biphasic anaphylaxis

Relapse after apparent complete resolution of all initial symptoms and signs is known as biphasic anaphylaxis, which is reported in 1–5% of cases or more (some consider up to 20%). It is unclear if more severe presenting features, delayed or inadequate doses of adrenaline or the non-use of steroids predispose to, or predict this biphasic response [26].

Discharge policy

Discharge the patient following observation and consider the need for take-home medication, self-injectable adrenaline and allergist–immunologist referral.

Discharge oral medication

There are no data to support the common practice of prescribing a 2- or 3-day discharge supply of combined H_1- and H_2-antihistamines plus oral steroids to prevent early relapse. However, consider loratadine 10 mg once daily, ranitidine 150 mg 12-hourly and prednisolone 50 mg once daily in adults with predominant cutaneous features following a generalized allergic reaction, or bronchospasm.

Self-injectable adrenaline (epinephrine)

As a guide, self-injectable adrenaline is prescribed for the patient with anaphylaxis after known allergen exposure outside of a medical setting, for patients with food allergy, particularly to nuts or peanuts, and for those in whom the reaction was severe and/or the cause unknown. The decision whether the emergency physician or general practitioner should initiate self-injectable adrenaline use or wait for specialist allergist–immunologist review with formulation of an individualized anaphylaxis action plan will depend on individual factors, such as local facilities and patient access to emergency services.

EpiPen and Anapen

The EpiPen and Anapen with 0.3 mg (300 μg) of adrenaline and the EpiPen Jr and Anapen Jr containing 0.15 mg (150 μg) are approved for self-administered intramuscular use. Up to two injectors are available at a time on the Pharmaceutical Benefits Scheme (PBS) Schedule on an Authority script for a patient after hospital or emergency department discharge for acute allergic anaphylaxis treated with adrenaline, or as a continuing supply for patients who have previously been issued with an Authority prescription [27].

When an EpiPen or an Anapen is dispensed in the ED, it is essential to explain and demonstrate exactly how to use the device and to educate both the patient and another caregiver, particularly with children. Teach the patient and carer how to recognize the symptoms and signs of anaphylaxis and encourage the actual use of the device, particularly if distant from a healthcare facility. As these devices differ in their administration technique, they should not be prescribed interchangeably. Tell recipients self-injectable adrenaline has a relatively short shelf-life of around 1–2 years, and how to look after it [28].

Allergist–immunologist referral

Disappointingly, few patients who suffer an episode of anaphylaxis are referred from the ED for specialist allergist–immunologist follow up. Refer anyone prescribed a self-injectable adrenaline (epinephrine) device, patients following a wasp or bee sting suitable for immunotherapy, suspected food-, drug-induced or exercise-induced anaphylaxis and patients with severe reactions without an obvious trigger [29].

Give the patient a letter detailing the nature and circumstances of the anaphylactic reaction, the treatment given and the suspected causative agent(s). Ask the patient also to write a brief diary of the events in the 6–12 h preceding the reaction, particularly when the cause is unclear. Ask them to include all foods ingested, drugs taken including non-proprietary, cosmetics used and activities performed outside as well as indoors. Later recall of these events at a specialist allergist–immunologist review will be flawed unless documented contemporaneously.

Drug and allergen avoidance

Patients at risk of recurrent anaphylaxis with hypertension or ischaemic heart disease should ideally be taken off β-blockers and care taken not to substitute an ACE inhibitor. Discuss this with the patient's other specialists to be certain the overall risk–benefit favours medication change.

Advise patients to reduce allergen exposure risk by destroying nearby wasp nests and removing allergenic foods in the house, plus to avoid insect sting with appropriate clothing and certain foods by checking the manufacturer's label [18].

IgE skin testing, *in vitro* testing and challenge testing

Skin or blood tests for specific IgE antibodies should only be done by those trained in their performance and interpretation, usually 3–4 weeks after the acute episode. Skin prick testing is the more sensitive and, when possible, standardized extracts should be used with correct technique. In addition, an experienced physician, such as a specialist allergist–immunologist, should supervise as occasional severe reactions occur. They are not appropriately performed by an emergency physician.

In vitro testing for allergen-specific IgE is less sensitive and depends on clinical correlation and the availability of specific assays. Over 500 different allergens are available for testing with the ImmunoCAP system (Thermo Fisher Scientific Inc, Waltham, Mass) or clinicians may use a radio-allergosorbent test (RAST) technique.

Finally, challenge testing may help diagnose non-allergic anaphylaxis. False-positive and false-negative reactions do occur but are much less likely than with skin prick or *in vitro* testing, but experienced specialist allergist–immunologist supervision is essential [18].

Controversies

- Exact mechanisms which underlie initial IgE antibody formation in response to a myriad of different substances and why this happens in one individual but not another.
- A single internationally agreed definition or grading system for anaphylaxis.
- Symptoms or signs which most reliably predict the risk of severe anaphylaxis.
- Utility of laboratory testing in confirming and quantifying the severity of an anaphylactic reaction.
- Most effective drug doses in acute treatment, particularly adrenaline.
- Predictors of biphasic reactions.
- Utility of discharge medications.

References

[1] Simons FER, Ardusso L, Bilò B, et al. World Allergy Organisation Guidelines for the assessment and management of anaphylaxis. J Allergy Clin Immunol 2011;127:593.

[2] Galli SJ. Pathogenesis and management of anaphylaxis: current status and future challenges. J Allergy Clin Immunol 2005;115:571–4.

[3] Sampson HA, Munoz-Furlong A, Campbell RL, et al, Second symposium on the definition and management of anaphylaxis: summary report – Second National Institute of Allergy and Infectious Disease/Food Allergy and Anaphylaxis Network symposium. J Allergy Clin Immunol 2006; 117:391–7.

[4] Sampson HA, Munoz-Furlong A, Bock SA, et al. Symposium on the definition and management of anaphylaxis: summary report. J Allergy Clin Immunol 2005; 115:584–91.

[5] Brown SGA. Clinical features and severity grading of anaphylaxis. J Allergy Clin Immunol 2004;114: 371–6.

[6] Lieberman P, Nicklas R, Oppenheimer J, et al. The diagnosis and management of anaphylaxis practice parameter: 2010 update. J Allergy Clin Immunol 2010;126:480.

[7] Sicherer SH, Leung DYM. Advances in allergic skin disease, anaphylaxis, and hypersensitivity reactions to food, drugs, and insects. J Allergy Clin Immunol 2005;116:153–63.

[8] Mertes P, Alla F, Tréchot P, et al. Anaphylaxis during anaesthesia in France: an 8-year national survey. J Allergy Clin Immunol 2011;128:366–73.

[9] Ring J, Brockow K, Behrendt H. History and classification of anaphylaxis. Novartis Found Symp 2004;257:6–16. (Discussion 16-24, 45-50, 276-85).

[10] Liew W, Williamson E, Tang M. Anaphylaxis fatalities and admissions in Australia. J Allergy Clin Immunol 2009;123:434–42.

[11] Brown AFT, McKinnon D, Chu K. Emergency department anaphylaxis: a review of 142 patients in a single year. J Allergy Clin Immunol 2001;108:861–6.

[12] Braganza SC, Acworth JP, McKinnon DRL, et al. Paediatric emergency department anaphylaxis: Different patterns from adults. Arch Dis Child 2006;91:159–63.

[13] Pumphrey RSH. Lessons for management of anaphylaxis from a study of fatal reactions. Clin Exp Allergy 2000;30:1144–50.

[14] Pumphrey RSH, Gowland MH. Further fatal allergic reactions to food in the United Kingdom, 1999–2006. J Allergy Clin Immunol 2007;119:1018–9.

[15] Chang TW, Shiung Y-Y. Anti-IgE as a mast cell-stabilizing therapeutic agent. J Allergy Clin Immunol 2006;117: 1203–12.

[16] Stone K, Prussin C, Metcalfe DD. IgE, mast cells, basophils, and eosinophils. J Allergy Clin Immunol 2010; 125:S73–80.

[17] Brown SGA, Mullins RJ, Gold MS. Anaphylaxis: diagnosis and management. Med J Austral 2006;185:283–9.

[18] Simons FER. Anaphylaxis: recent advances in assessment and treatment. J Allergy Clin Immunol 2009;124: 625–36.

[19] Association of Anaesthetists of Great Britain and Ireland. Suspected anaphylactic reactions associated with anaesthesia. Anaesthesia 2009; 64:199–211.

[20] Brown SGA, Blackman KE, Stenlake V, et al. Insect sting anaphylaxis: prospective evaluation and treatment with intravenous adrenaline and volume resuscitation. Emerg Med J 2004;21:149–54.

[21] Soar J, Perkins G, Abbas G, et al. European Resuscitation Council Guidelines for Resuscitation 2010 Section 8. Cardiac arrest in special circumstances: Electrolyte abnormalities, poisoning, drowning, accidental hypothermia, hyperthermia, asthma, anaphylaxis, cardiac surgery, trauma, pregnancy, electrocution. Resuscitation 2010;81:1400–33.

[22] Brown SGA. Anaphylaxis: clinical concepts and research priorities. Emerg Med Australas 2006;18:155–69.

[23] Sheikh A, Ten Broek V, Brown SGA, Simons E. H1-antihistamines for the treatment of anaphylaxis with and without shock. Cochrane Database Syst Rev 2007;1:CD006160.

[24] Choo K, Simons F, Sheikh A. Glucocorticoids for the treatment of anaphylaxis. Cochrane Database Sys Rev 2012;4:CD007596.

[25] Tramèr MR, von Elm E, Loubeyre P, et al. Pharmacological prevention of serious anaphylactic reactions due to iodinated contrast media: systematic review. Br Med J 2006;333:675–8.

[26] Lieberman P. Biphasic anaphylaxis: review of incidence, clinical predictors, and observation recommendations. Immunol Allergy Clin N Am 2007;27:309–26.

[27] Vale S, Smith J, Loh R. Safe use of adrenaline autoinjectors. Aust Prescr 2012;35:56–8.

[28] Australasian Society of Clinical Immunology and Allergy. Anaphylaxis Resources. <http://www.allergy.org.au/health-professionals/anaphylaxis-resources> (Accessed Mar. 2013).

[29] Leung D, Schatz M. Consultation and referral guidelines citing the evidence: how the allergist-immunologist can help. J Allergy Clin Immunol 2006;117:S495–523.

TRAUMA

Edited by **Peter Cameron**

3.1 Trauma overview

Peter Cameron • Gerard O'Reilly

ESSENTIALS

1 Trauma remains the leading cause of death in those from 1 to 44 years of age in the developed world. The burden of injury is especially high in the developing world.

2 Globally, road traffic crashes are the number one killer of young people.

3 Injuries cause 11% of disability-adjusted life years lost.

4 Improvements in trauma care systems have resulted in fewer patients dying from avoidable factors and less disability.

5 The key objective of a mature trauma system is to transfer 'the right patient to the right hospital in the shortest time'.

6 The initial management of trauma patients involves a team approach. A primary survey (ABCDE) is followed by a secondary survey involving head-to-toe examination.

7 Audit and feedback of trauma systems are essential to improve outcomes.

Epidemiology

Trauma is the leading cause of death from 1 to 44 years of age in developed countries. The burden of injury is especially high in developing countries, where systems of trauma care are generally non-existent [1,2]. Globally, road traffic crashes are the number one killer of young people [3]. Deaths from unintentional injury are much more common than suicide or homicide, even in the USA [1]. However, in the USA, homicide causes more deaths than suicide in the 15–24-year age group [1]; this differs from other developed countries. Suicide now causes more deaths than motor vehicle accidents (MVAs) in regions such as Australasia and the UK [4,5].

Morbidity due to injury affects a much larger group. The 2010 Global Burden of Disease Study showed that injuries cost the global population some 300 million years of health every year, causing 11% of disability-adjusted life years (DALYs) worldwide [3]. The economic and social costs are great as most victims are young and are major contributors to society through their work, family and organizational involvement.

The trauma system – background

In most developed countries, there have been significant reductions in mortality and morbidity due to injury as a result of a systematic approach to trauma care [6,7]. The majority of these reductions have resulted from prevention strategies, including seatbelt legislation, drink–driving legislation, improved road engineering, motor cycle and cycle helmet use and road safety and workplace injury awareness campaigns. Changes in both trauma system configuration and individual patient management have brought about improvements in the survival rate of those who are seriously injured, although the impact has not been as great as that of injury prevention.

Civilian interest in injury morbidity and mortality was initially most evident in the USA because of the high incidence of urban violence and road trauma and because of lessons learnt from the wars of the 20th century. Research into systems of trauma care began with epidemiological work by Trunkey and others examining trauma deaths [8]. These researchers developed the concept of a trimodal distribution of trauma deaths. Trunkey proposed that about 50% of deaths occurred within the first hour as a result of major blood vessel disruption or massive CNS/spinal cord injury. This could only be improved by prevention strategies. A second more important group (from the therapy perspective) accounted for about 30% of deaths and included patients with major truncal injury causing respiratory and circulatory compromise. The remaining 20% of patients were said to die much later from adult respiratory distress syndrome, multiple organ failure, sepsis and diffuse brain injury. Trunkey initially identified the second group as most likely to benefit from improvements in trauma system organization and it is a tribute to the effectiveness of such schemes that the number of patients dying from avoidable factors within the first few hours of injury has generally declined. In some systems, it is reported to be as low as 3% but, generally, is probably nearer to 10–15% [9,10]. Improvements in trauma system provision have resulted in a redistribution of the three groups proposed by Trunkey and it is now generally accepted that far fewer than 30% are included in the second group. In fact, more recent studies have shown that complications, such as multiple organ failure (MOF) and acute respiratory distress syndrome (ARDS), have decreased

to such an extent, with improved initial management, that, in mature trauma systems, even the third peak is now minimal, with the vast majority of deaths occurring in the first 1–2 hours from major head injury and massive organ disruption [11].

Trauma care systems have been developed to ensure a multidisciplinary approach and a continuum of care from the roadside through hospital care to rehabilitation. Identifying weakness in such a system is always difficult because of the delay between cause and effect. Inappropriate management does not usually lead to immediate death: for example, a period of hypoxia may result in organ failure many hours later. Another difficulty is the relatively low incidence of death. Although this is of course to be welcomed, it does make statistical analysis more difficult when the 'adverse event' occurs uncommonly. Careful audit of the entire trauma process and accurate measurement of 'input' (i.e. injury severity) and 'output' (i.e. death or quality of survival) is essential if the process of trauma care is to be reviewed.

The trauma system – pre-hospital

Whereas the initial work on trauma system development focused on the need for centres of expertise and trauma management, it is

now accepted that the pre-hospital phase is of critical importance. The linchpin of a mature trauma system is a highly skilled and resourced pre-hospital service following the key principle of 'the right patient to the right hospital in the shortest time' [12]. Timely triage of the injured patient to the closest most appropriate facility is essential. Specifically, high-risk patients should be taken to a hospital capable of managing critically ill trauma patients [12]. A diagrammatic representation of one integrated trauma system, at its inception in 1999, is provided in Figure 3.1.1 [13].

Criteria for identifying those patients who may require resuscitation at a tertiary level Trauma Centre or 'Major Trauma Service (MTS)' will depend on resources. In the most developed trauma systems, 'mechanism of injury' criteria are usually included in the pre-hospital triage tool. This ensures high sensitivity of the tool, but leads to considerable overtriage. In less-resourced settings, it may be appropriate to identify high-risk patients on the basis of abnormal vital signs and obvious major injury. The elements of a trauma system's triage tool may include most or all of the predictors of life-threatening injury listed in Table 3.1.1.

The appropriate application of pre-hospital triage guidelines relies upon adequate

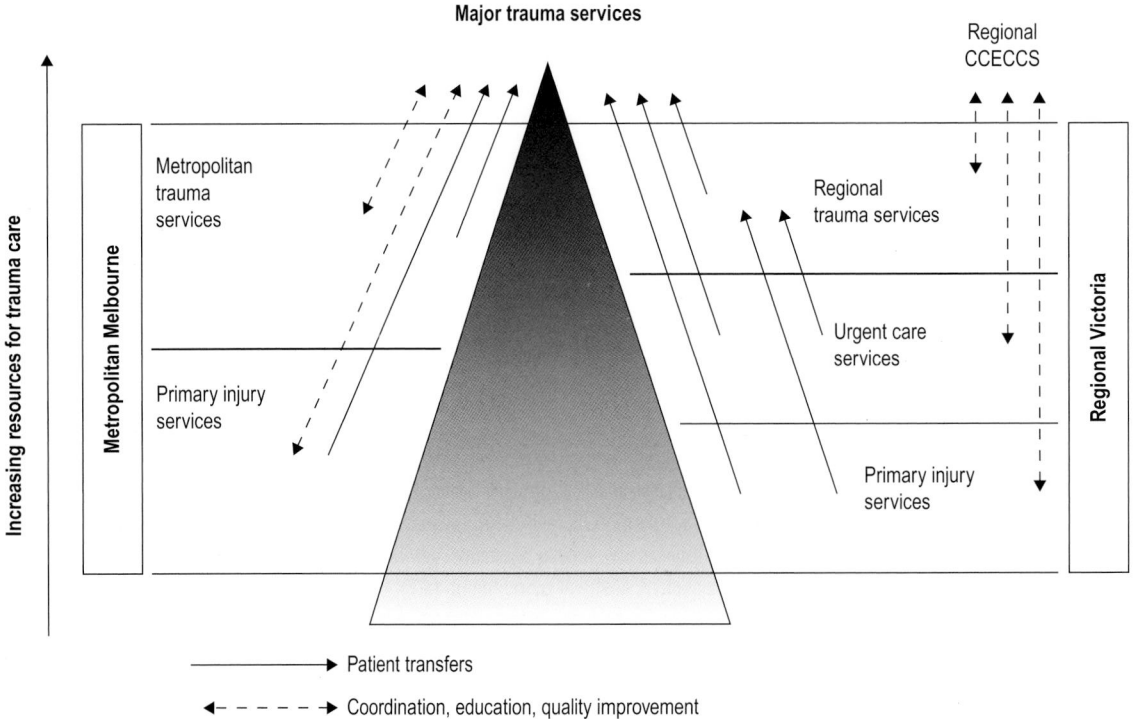

Fig. 3.1.1 Structure of the Integrated Victorian State Trauma System [13]. *(From Atkin C, Freedman I, Rosenfeld JV, et al. The evolution of an integrated state trauma system in Victoria, Australia. Injury 2005; 36:1277–87.)* CCECCS: Consultative Council on Emergency and Critical Care Services.

Table 3.1.1 Predictors of life-threatening injury appropriate for use in pre-hospital trauma triage

Mechanism	Ejection from vehicle High speed collision (>60 kph) Motorcycle/cyclist impact >30 kph Fall >5 m Vehicle rollover Fatality in same vehicle Explosion Pedestrian impact >30 kph Extrication >30 minutes
Injuries (any of the following)	Serious or suspected serious penetrating injuries: head, neck, chest, abdomen, pelvis, axilla, groin All significant blunt injuries as assessed by ambulance All injuries involving: evisceration, explosion, severe crush injury, any amputation, suspected spinal injury, serious burns, pelvic fracture
Vital signs	Respiratory rate <10 or >30 per minute Systolic blood pressure <100 mmHg (<75 mmHg for child) GCS <15 Oxygen saturation <90%
Treatment Patients who have undergone any of the following pre-hospital interventions	Intubation Any airway manoeuvre at any time Assisted ventilation Chest decompression Failure to control external bleeding >500 mL fluid Sedatives
Other criteria	All inter-hospital trauma transfers Significant co-morbidity Pregnancy

Box 3.1.1 Team roles

Team leader (emergency physician or trauma surgeon)
- Overview
- Resuscitation
- Assessment
- Communication
- Ambulance
- Referrals
- Investigations
- Task allocation
- Primary survey
- Secondary survey

Airway doctor (anaesthetist)
- Control of airway
- Inline immobilization of cervical spine
- Ventilation
- Gastric tube

Procedure doctor (emergency registrar/trauma registrar)
- Intravenous access/bloods
- Intercostal catheter
- Urinary catheter
- ABG/art line

Nurses
- Trauma nurse leader/scribe
- Airway nurse
- Circulation nurse

Radiographer

Orderly

TRAUMA

resourcing. In regions with developed trauma systems, pre-hospital staff are expected to provide a range of advanced life support interventions including patient intubation and chest decompression, thereby ensuring that further organ injury is limited during the pre-hospital phase. The pre-hospital care providers armed with these skills may be doctors (as in many European countries) or highly trained paramedics (as in the USA, Australia and the UK).

The trauma system – intrahospital

Preparation
Effective pre-hospital communication, usually by phone and/or radio, allows timely preparation for the arrival of a trauma patient. Proper communication includes trauma team notification, staff and trauma bay identification and the adoption of universal precautions (gloves, gowns, etc.).

Trauma team notification might occur by phone or paging system and ensures the gathering of the trauma team *prior* to the patient's arrival. Members of the trauma team may vary. An example of trauma team composition and roles in a Level 1 Trauma Centre is provided

in Box 3.1.1. Variations to this list may occur in different settings depending upon the availability of skilled staff and the nature of specific injuries or physiological status prior to the patient's arrival

Trauma team call-out criteria reflect the pre-hospital trauma triage criteria (see Table 3.1.1) and should be applied rigorously. Trauma team skill, functioning and leadership are essential to achieve the best patient outcome. The appropriate skill mix is reflected by the team membership listed in Box 3.1.1. Trauma team performance, including leadership and communication, will have an impact on patient outcome.

Initial management

The application of a consistent systematic approach to trauma resuscitation has been widely promulgated by training programmes, such as the Advanced Trauma Life Support (ATLS) [14]. The patient is brought directly to a prepared bay, the layout of which is illustrated in Figure 3.1.2. The principles of the initial identification and management of immediately

life-threatening injuries, with prioritization accorded to airway (including protection of cervical spine), breathing, circulation, (neurological) disability and exposure are applied to all injured patients. This is followed by a secondary survey involving a head-to-toe examination. In most departments, parallel processing of the patient will occur simultaneously with management of ABCDE problems.

Airway
It should be assumed that hypoxia is present in all patients who have sustained multiple injuries. Early expert airway intervention is essential. Every patient should receive initial supplemental oxygen via a well-fitting facemask. If the airway is clear and protected, the neck should be immobilized with a semi-rigid collar but, if airway manoeuvres are necessary, it is often better to use manual inline

RESUSCITATION BAY FLOOR PLAN

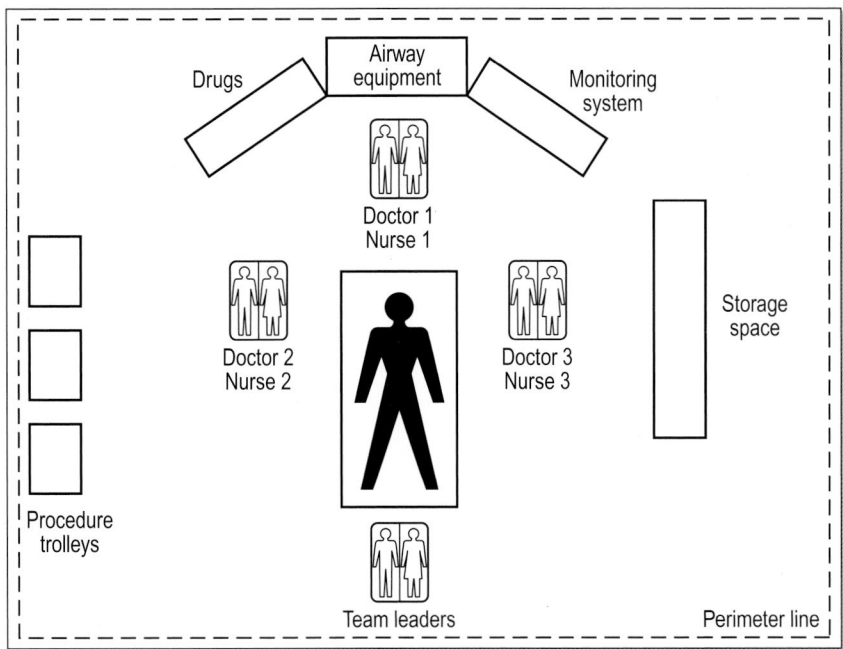

Fig. 3.1.2 The layout of a typical trauma resuscitation bay. *(Reproduced with permission from Myers CT, Brown AF, Dunjey SJ, et al. Trauma teams: order from chaos. Emerg Med 1993; 5:34.)*

immobilization without a collar, ensuring minimal neck movement with constant vigilance. The management of an obstructed airway in a trauma patient should be undertaken by an experienced senior clinician with significant anaesthetic experience. The first priority is to clear the upper airway by direct visualization, suction and removal of any foreign bodies. Insertion of an oropharyngeal or nasopharyngeal airway and the jaw-thrust manoeuvre are usually successful in clearing an upper airway obstruction. Insertion of a nasopharyngeal airway can be hazardous in patients with a fracture of the cribriform plate. The direction of insertion (backwards not upwards) is important. Chin lift is not recommended because it may cause additional movement of the cervical spine.

Early endotracheal intubation should be undertaken if the patient is apnoeic, has an unrelieved upper airway obstruction, has persistent internal bleeding from facial injuries, has respiratory insufficiency due to chest or head injuries or the potential for airway compromise (airway burns, facial instability, coma or seizures). Intubation may also be necessary for procedures such as computed tomography (CT) scanning or for the management of confused or disturbed patients. Any operator undertaking emergency intubation of

major trauma victims should be skilled in rapid sequence induction and prepared for a difficult intubation. He/she must also be equipped with the skills for dealing with a 'failed' intubation (see Chapter 2.1) with a variety of interventions, including surgical cricothyroidotomy.

Breathing

Once the airway is secure, the patient's breathing needs to be assessed. Particular attention is paid to optimizing oxygenation and maintaining normocapnia. During the primary survey, immediately life-threatening risks to breathing must be identified and dealt with. These injuries include tension pneumothorax, open pneumothorax, massive haemothorax, flail and pulmonary contusion. The specific features and management of these injuries is covered in Chapter 3.6.

Circulation

Shock is a clinical syndrome in which the perfusion of vital organs is inadequate to maintain function. Blood loss is the major cause of shock in the major trauma patient. Other less common causes of shock also need to be considered:

- Tension pneumothorax. This will cause rapid and severe disruption to the circulation.

- Cardiogenic shock. This may be pre-existing (e.g. acute myocardial infarction (AMI) causing accident, drugs causing reduced cardiac compensation and hypovolaemia) or secondary to injury, i.e. myocardial contusion, valvular/septal injury or pericardial tamponade.
- Neurogenic shock. This results from the loss of sympathetic tone. It may be caused by central brainstem injury and vasomotor instability or spinal cord injury and interruption of descending sympathetic tracts. It is characterized by bradycardia, but this may also occur in profound hypovolaemic states.
- Anaphylactic shock and septic shock may coexist with hypovolaemic shock.

The initial stages of hypovolaemia can be difficult to detect. Reliance on systolic blood pressure to identify shock is dangerous. All patients who have sustained an injury that could be associated with significant blood loss, however remote the possibility, must be carefully monitored. In the initial phase, measurement of the clinical parameters will give some information about vital organ perfusion. However, more invasive monitoring will be required if hypovolaemia is severe or sustained.

It is essential to gain good venous access at the earliest phase in resuscitation. This is usually via two large-bore peripheral cannulae. In the absence of accessible arm veins, central venous access may be indicated. The recommended site (subclavian, jugular or femoral) depends on a number of factors. The subclavian vein is reliable in terms of patency, while the ease of access to the femoral vein is offset by its potential futility in major truncal haemorrhage. The internal jugular veins can be difficult to access in the immobilized trauma patient. Cut-downs of the saphenous veins and cubital fossa may also be used.

At the initial stages, where the blood pressure is unchanged, patients with potential blood loss can usually be managed without blood transfusion, namely crystalloid. There has been no benefit demonstrated in using non-blood colloids over crystalloids in traumatic haemorrhage [15–17]. Similarly, for hypertonic crystalloid the available data are inconclusive [18].

Where there is hypotension and tachycardia, blood transfusion should commence immediately, initially using O-negative blood and changing to group-specific or cross-matched blood as it becomes available. Chapter 3.12

covers the role and details of massive transfusion therapy in the trauma patient. Conversely, until the source of haemorrhage has been identified and haemostasis achieved, vigorous over resuscitation with fluid may actually result in a worse outcome [19,20].

The essential point is that after securing the airway and optimizing oxygenation and ventilation, the most important determinant of outcome in the major trauma patient with haemorrhagic shock is the time to definitive haemostasis. There is certainly no point in delaying surgery 'to normalize the intravascular volume'. The major source of haemorrhage in the trauma patient must be identified early. The usual suspects are chest, abdomen, pelvis, long bone and/or external (e.g. scalp, major limb artery).

Disability

As the purpose of the primary survey is to identify immediate threats to life, the assessment for a head injury and its severity entails an examination of conscious state (Glasgow Coma Score) and neurological signs (pupils, limb weakness). If there is any risk of intracranial injury, a CT brain scan will be indicated immediately upon completion of the primary survey. Chapter 3.2 deals with the assessment and management of traumatic brain injury.

Exposure

Hypothermia is associated with worse outcomes in the major trauma patient [21]. Temperature control is now considered to be of critical importance in reducing the sequelae of major trauma (metabolic derangement, coagulopathy). The role of therapeutic hypothermia in isolated head injury remains controversial and is a subject of ongoing research. While maintaining normothermia, it is important to have fully exposed the patient, including a log roll with spinal immobilization, to enable a complete examination.

Next steps

By this stage, the trauma patient will have been received into a well-organized resuscitation area and the first life-saving procedures will have been initiated by an integrated and skilled team of doctors and nurses. Any immediately life-threatening conditions can be expected to have been identified and dealt with. Constant vigilance and reassessment are essential. Other occult injuries may be present in those patients identified with serious injuries.

While the trauma team leader continues to review the situation in the light of a constantly changing clinical scenario and, hopefully, the provision of more biomechanical data from the site of the incident, he or she should also be beginning to consider the next steps. The first of these is the calling in of other experts. Whereas it will have been clear that an airway doctor will be an essential part of the initial resuscitation team, it may be some minutes before it is known which other skills are required. Usually orthopaedic surgeons and neurosurgeons are near the top of the list. General surgery is not required as often as is commonly supposed [22], although general surgeons are often useful in coordinating ongoing care. Whichever specialty is required, the patient's emergency problems demand experience, therefore, 'if in doubt, refer'.

Radiographs are required at this stage. The initial films should be limited to those that will have a direct bearing on immediate management, including a chest AP view and a pelvis AP view.

Lateral X-ray of the cervical spine is no longer mandatory at this stage of assessment. Cervical immobilization is routine and it is not possible to exclude cervical injury with a lateral cervical spine X-ray. Therefore, a cervical X-ray does not alter initial management. Its utility at this stage would be to confirm an irretrievable injury, i.e. craniocervical dislocation.

Ideally, the resuscitation room should have an integrated X-ray facility but, if this is not available, portable films should be obtained. It is not appropriate to transfer a multiply injured unstable patient to a separate X-ray facility.

Other forms of imaging have become popular in localizing the source of haemorrhagic shock. The increasing availability of the focused assessment with sonography in trauma (FAST) has superseded diagnostic peritoneal lavage (DPL) as the bedside adjunct for detecting intraperitoneal haemorrhage.

Following the primary survey and investigations deemed necessary, the patient requires a secondary survey, the full head-to-toe examination for injuries not classified as immediately life-threatening.

Subsequent chapters deal with individual trauma problems, but it is essential that throughout the patient's stay in hospital a single clinician has overriding responsibility for his or her care. In the resuscitation area, this is the 'team leader', who may be from any trauma-related discipline. Handover to the clinician responsible for ongoing care must be comprehensive, timed and well documented.

Trauma audit

Trauma kills people in a variety of ways; hence no one department in a hospital will see a large number of deaths. Many trauma victims die before they reach hospital, some in the ED and others scattered through the inpatient specialties and in intensive care. Hence from any one clinician's perspective, trauma is not an outstanding problem. However, when looked at from a public health perspective, it is clearly a major issue, not least because some of the deaths are avoidable. Identifying these and the much more difficult-to-define group of patients who survive but whose outcome is not as good as expected is a major problem.

The most important variables to measure are the extent of the anatomical injury, the degree of physiological derangement that results, age and the previous well-being of the patient. All these have a direct effect on outcome and must therefore be measured before any comment can be made about the process of care. Outcome itself must also of course be measured. This is relatively easy in terms of mortality. However, disability is a much more difficult issue and, currently, there are no universally accepted measurement tools. The Glasgow Outcome Scale (GOSE) [23, 24], and the Short Form–36 (SF36) questions [25] are available tools that have been used. As 90% of major trauma patients survive their injury in a mature trauma system, it is important to measure disability and quality of life following major trauma when comparing outcomes [26].

Trauma audit was first formalized by Champion at the Washington Hospital Centre in the 1970s, using the Trauma Injury Severity Score (TRISS) methodology [27,28]. Most current trauma systems are now audited using some approach to examining risk-adjusted mortality. Injury severity adjustment, allowing intra- and intersystem comparison, usually requires measures of anatomical injury (e.g. Injury Severity Score), physiological effects (e.g. Revised Trauma Score) and age.

Trauma in developing countries

Globally, national governments are beginning to recognize the burgeoning human and economic cost of trauma, particularly road trauma. The public health achievements of the developed countries (seatbelts, helmets, alcohol and speed restrictions) are being implemented and, similarly, governments of developing countries are looking to implement trauma systems [29,30].

Research in developing countries reinforces the benefits of trauma systems previously described in countries with established emergency medical systems. For example, evidence indicates that people with life-threatening but potentially treatable injuries are up to six times more likely to die in a country with no organized trauma system than in one with an organized, resourced trauma system [31]. Trauma system development requires trauma outcome measurement [32,33]. As such, developing countries are likely to adopt trauma registries over the next several decades in an attempt to track the burden of trauma and the impact of system-wide interventions.

As developing countries embark upon trauma system development, it is becoming increasingly important to access standardized trauma care education through intensive short-courses. Advanced Trauma Life Support (ATLS) has been widely used. Other courses (such as Primary Trauma Care (PTC)) have also become popular in the developing world. Such courses are often less expensive and more flexible than ATLS.

Controversies

- The number of major trauma patients necessary for a hospital to maintain high-quality trauma care.
- The degree to which potential major trauma patients should be over-triaged to ensure that patients with major trauma are received at major trauma centres. There may be a greater risk in bypassing hospitals to take patients to a trauma centre, depending on distance

and injury type. There is also the issue of deskilling of personnel from non-trauma centres and what effect this has on overall system outcomes.

- The degree to which major trauma patients should be managed by protocol rather than clinical judgement. Clinicians are increasingly being asked to follow protocols in these critical situations. This prevents some adverse outcomes but may cause over-investigation and treatment.
- The role of hypotensive resuscitation in blunt trauma has not been defined. Where victims have prolonged delays to theatre or the bleeding is not surgically correctable, then hypotensive resuscitation may cause more complications.
- The role of controlled hypothermia in head-injured patients.

References

[1] Centre for Disease Control and Prevention, National Center for Injury Prevention and Control: WISQARS Atlanta. <http://www.cdc.gov/injury/wisqars/facts.html> [Accessed Dec. 2012].

[2] Australian Institute of Health and Welfare. <http://www.aihw.gov.au/deaths-faq/> [Accessed Dec. 2012].

[3] Murray CJL, Vos T, Lozano R, et al. Disability-adjusted life years (DALYs) for 291 diseases and injuries in 21 regions, 1990–2010: a systematic analysis for the Global Burden of Disease Study 2010. Lancet 2012;380:2197–223.

[4] Australian Bureau of Statistics. Causes of Death. <http://abs.gov.au/ausstats/>; 2010 [Accessed Dec. 2012].

[5] Injury and poisoning mortality in England and Wales. Office for National Statistics. <http://www.ons.gov.uk/ons/publications/> [Accessed Dec. 2012].

[6] Cameron PA, Gabbe B, Cooper DJ. A statewide system of trauma care in Victoria: effect on patient survival. Med J Aust 2008;189:546–50.

[7] Gabbe BJ, Simpson PM, Sutherland AM, et al. Improved functional outcomes for major trauma patients in a regionalized, inclusive trauma system. Ann Surg 2012;255:1009–15.

[8] Trunkey DD. Trauma. Sci Am 1983;249:28–35.

[9] Cales RH, Trunkey DD. Preventable trauma deaths. A review of trauma care systems development. J Am Med Assoc 1985;254:1059–63.

[10] Roy PD. The value of trauma centres: a methodologic review. Can J Surg 1987;30:17–22.

[11] Pang JM, Civil I, Ng A, et al. Is the trimodal pattern of death after trauma a dated concept in the 21st century? Trauma deaths in Auckland 2004. Injury 2008; 39:102–106.

[12] Eastman AB, Lewis FR, Champion HR, et al. Regional trauma system design: critical concepts. Am J Surg 1987;154: 79–87.

[13] Atkin C, Freedman I, Rosenfeld JV, et al. The evolution of an integrated state trauma system in Victoria, Australia. Injury 2005;36:1277–87.

[14] American College of Surgeons. ATLS (Advance Trauma Life Support) for Doctors Student Manual, 8th ed. Chicago: American College of Surgeons; 2008.

[15] Roberts I, Alderson P, Bunn F. Colloids versus crystalloids for fluid resuscitation in critically ill patients (Cochrane Review). In: The Cochrane Library (4); 2004.

[16] The SAFE Study Investigators. A comparison of albumin and saline for fluid resuscitation in the intensive care unit. N Engl J Med 2004;350:2247–56.

[17] The SAFE Study Investigators. Saline or albumin for fluid resuscitation in patients with traumatic brain injury. N Engl J Med 2007;357:874–84.

[18] Bunn F, Roberts I, Tasker R. Hypertonic versus near isotonic crystalloid for fluid resuscitation in critically ill patients (Cochrane Review). In: The Cochrane Library (3); 2004.

[19] Bickell WH, Wall MJ, Pepe PE, et al. Immediate versus delayed fluid resuscitation for hypertensive patients with penetrating torso injuries. N Engl J Med 1994;331:1105–9.

[20] Civil IDJ. Resuscitation following injury: an end or a means? Aust NZ J Surg 1993;63:921–6.

[21] Ireland S, Endacott R, Cameron P, et al. The incidence and significance of accidental hypothermia in major trauma: a prospective observational study. Resuscitation 2011;82:300–6.

[22] Cameron PA, Dziukas L, Hadj A. Patterns of injury from major trauma in Victoria. Aust NZ J Surg 1995;65:830–4.

[23] Jennett B, Bond M. Assessment of outcome after severe brain damage. Lancet 1975;1:480–4.

[24] Teasdale GM, Pettigrew LE, Wilson JT. Analysing outcome of severe head injury: a review and update on advancing the use of the Glasgow Outcome Scale. J Neurotrauma 1998;15:587–97.

[25] Garratt AM, Ruta DA, Abdulher MI. The SF36 Health Survey Questionnaire: an outcome measure suitable for routine use within the NHS? Br Med J 1993;306:1440–4.

[26] Willis CD, Gabbe BJ, Cameron PA. Measuring quality in trauma care. Injury 2007;38:527–37.

[27] Boyd CR, Tolson MA, Copes WS. Evaluating trauma care: the TRISS method. J Trauma 1987;27:370–8.

[28] Champion HW, Copes WS, Sacco WJ, et al. The major trauma outcome study: establishing national norms for trauma care. J Trauma 1990;30:1356–65.

[29] Mock C, Lormand JD, Goosen J, et al. Guidelines for essential trauma care. Geneva: World Health Organization; 2004. <http://whqlibdoc.who.int/publications/2004/9241546409.pdf>.

[30] Fitzgerald M, Dewan Y, O'Reilly G. India and the management of road crashes–towards a national trauma system. Ind J Surg 2006;68:237–43.

[31] Mock CN, Adzotor KE, Conklin E. Trauma outcomes in the rural developing world: comparison with an urban level 1 trauma center. J Trauma 1993;35:518–23.

[32] Mock C, Juillard C, Brundage S, et al. Guidelines for trauma quality improvement programmes. Geneva: World Health Organization; 2009. <http://whqlibdoc.who.int/publications/2009/9789241597746_eng.pdf>.

[33] O'Reilly GM, Cameron PA, Joshipura M. Global trauma registry mapping: A scoping review. Injury 2012;43:1148–53.

3.2 Neurotrauma

Gerard O'Reilly • Lee Wallis • Peter Cameron

ESSENTIALS

1 Neurotrauma is a major cause of death in trauma.

2 A detailed history of the mechanics of the trauma experienced is invaluable.

3 Secondary brain injury is a major and potentially preventable cause of mortality and long-term morbidity.

4 Cerebral cellular dysfunction secondary to trauma is a result of both primary and secondary mechanisms and involves sodium, calcium and potassium shifts across the cell membrane, the development of oxygen free radicals and lipid peroxidation.

5 There are two features of prime importance to resuscitation in patients suffering neurotrauma: maintenance of airway/ventilation and maintenance of cerebral perfusion pressure.

6 Inline stabilization of the cervical spine during rapid sequence induction and orotracheal intubation is the preferred method for gaining definitive airway control in the head-injured patient.

7 Current emergency department and neurosurgical practice involves the use of CT scanning to investigate mild, moderate and severe head injury.

Introduction

Neurotrauma is a common feature in the presentation of multisystem trauma, particularly when associated with motor vehicle accidents and falls. Over 50% of trauma deaths are associated with head injury. The implications for the health system are enormous, with an annual rate of admission to hospital wards associated with head trauma approaching 300 per 100 000 population [1] and twice this in the elderly [2]. The long-term sequelae of moderate and severe neurotrauma are a major health resource drain and the morbidities associated with mild brain injury are becoming clearer.

Advances in preventative strategies, trauma systems, resuscitative therapies and rehabilitation management have improved outcomes. However, neurotrauma remains a serious health issue, predominantly affecting the productive youth of society.

Pathogenesis

Primary brain injury occurs as a result of the forces and disruptive mechanics of the original incident: this can only be avoided through preventative measures, such as the use of bicycle helmets.

Secondary brain injury is due to a complex interaction of factors and typically occurs within 2–24 hours of injury [3]. A principal mechanism of secondary injury is cerebral hypoxia due to impaired oxygenation or impaired cerebral blood flow. Cerebral blood flow is dependent on cerebral perfusion pressure (CPP), mean arterial systemic blood pressure (MAP) and intracranial pressure (ICP).

$$CPP = MAP - ICP$$

Intracranial pressure may be raised as a result of the mass effect of the haemorrhage or by generalized cerebral oedema. Cerebral vasospasm further reduces cerebral blood flow in patients in whom significant subarachnoid haemorrhage has occurred.

Cellular dysfunction is a result of both primary and secondary mechanisms and involves sodium, calcium, magnesium and potassium shifts across the cell membrane, the development of oxygen free radicals, lipid peroxidation and glutamate hyperactivity. Excessive release of excitatory neurotransmitters and magnesium depletion also occur [4].

Classification of primary injury in neurotrauma

Primary injuries are classified as:

- skull fracture
- concussion
- contusion
- intracranial haematoma
- diffuse axonal injury
- penetrating injury.

Skull fracture

The significance of skull fracture is not related to the specific bony injury but rather the associated neurotrauma. Fractures in the region of the middle meningeal artery in particular may be associated with acute extradural haemorrhage. Fractures involving the skull base and cribriform plate may be associated with CSF leak and the risk of secondary infection. Depressed skull fractures may compress underlying structures, cause secondary brain injury and require surgical elevation. Injury to underlying structures may result in secondary epilepsy.

Concussion

Concussion is a transient alteration in cerebral function, usually associated with loss of consciousness and often followed by a rapid recovery. The proposed mechanism is a disturbance in the function of the reticular activating system. Post-concussive syndromes, including headache and mild cognitive disturbance, are common [5,6]. Symptoms, particularly headache, are usually short-lived but may persist. 'Second-impact syndrome' describes a greater risk of significant re-injury following an initial injury causing a simple concussion. It is likely to be due to diffuse cerebral swelling [7]. In animal models, concussion may be associated with modest short-term increases in intracranial pressure and disturbances in cerebral cellular function [8].

Contusion

Cerebral contusion is bruising of the brain substance associated with head trauma. The most common mechanism is blunt trauma. Forces involved are less than those required to cause major shearing injuries and often occur in the absence of skull fracture. Morbidity is related to the size and site of the contusion and coexistent injury. Larger contusions may be associated with haematoma formation, secondary oedema or seizure activity. The most common sites for contusions are the frontal and temporal lobes [9].

Intracranial haematoma

Extradural Extradural haematoma (EDH) is uncommon but classically associated with fracture of the temporal bone and injury to the underlying middle meningeal artery. Haemorrhage subsequently occurs, stripping the dura from the skull and expanding to cause a rise in intracranial pressure and eventually uncal herniation and death. Haemorrhage may be from vessels other than the middle meningeal artery (e.g. brisk arteriolar or venous bleeding). Signs will depend on the site of the haematoma.

Subdural Subdural haematomata (SDH) may have an acute, subacute or chronic course. It generally follows moderate head trauma with loss of consciousness. In the elderly, SDH may be associated with trivial injury and, in children, with shaking (abuse) injury. Haemorrhage occurs into the subdural space, slowly enlarging to cause a space-occupying collection whose functional implications will vary according to location. Acute subdural haemorrhage carries a high mortality (>50%), similar to acute EDH. Subacute and chronic SDH is associated with a degree of cerebral dysfunction, headache or other symptomatology and is associated with a significantly lower mortality (up to 20%) [10].

Intracerebral As with cerebral contusion, the most common sites of intracerebral haemorrhage associated with trauma are the temporal and posterior frontal lobes. Effects on function are variable, depending on the site. Intracerebral haemorrhage may progress from an initial contusion or be secondary to altered vascular characteristics. Symptom development and complications may be delayed as the size of the haemorrhage increases over time.

Subarachnoid and intraventricular haemorrhage Subarachnoid blood is relatively common after major head injury. Intraventricular haemorrhage may also be evident. As in non-traumatic settings, the presence of subarachnoid blood may lead to cerebral vasospasm and secondary ischaemic brain injury.

Diffuse axonal injury

Diffuse axonal injury (DAI) is the predominant mechanism of injury in neurotrauma, occurring in up to 50% of patients [11]. Shearing and rotational forces on the axonal network may result in major structural and functional disturbance at a microscopic level. Disturbance to important communicative pathways sometimes results in significant long-term morbidity, despite non-specific or minimal changes on computed tomography (CT) scanning. The exact pathogenesis of diffuse axonal injury is incompletely understood. Specific injury in the regions of the corpus callosum and midbrain has been proposed; however, DAI is believed to be the mechanism for persistent neurological deficits seen in head-traumatized individuals with normal CT scans [12].

Penetrating injury

Penetrating neurotrauma is characterized by high levels of morbidity and mortality. This is especially true of gunshot wounds. Exposure of cerebral tissue through large compound wounds or through basilar skull structures is associated with a dismal outlook. Penetrating injury in the periorbital and perinasal regions is associated with high risk of infection.

Epidemiology

Neurotrauma is surprisingly common. In some settings, more than 30% of the population have suffered from a trauma brain injury. In addition to being a major cause of death in trauma, neurotrauma leads to significant morbidity. More than 40% of those who have sustained a traumatic brain injury will have residual disability one year later [13].

Common causes include motor vehicle accidents (including vehicle versus pedestrian and bicycle collisions), falls, assault and firearms. In young males, alcohol is often involved.

Prevention

Primary prevention of neurotrauma depends on the cause. Most preventative strategies are directed at vehicular traffic and include speed-calming measures, in-car safety devices and bicycle helmets. Improving roadside lighting and enhancing pedestrian visibility contribute to reduction of injury in this group.

Prevention of secondary injury involves maintenance of cerebral perfusion and oxygenation and is addressed under clinical management.

Clinical features

Definition

Neurotrauma may be classified according to severity as minimal, mild, moderate or severe (Box 3.2.1) [14]. Such a classification allows for directed investigation and management, but there is clearly a continuum of injury within the spectrum of neurotrauma.

History

A detailed history of the mechanics of the trauma is essential. This should be followed

---

Box 3.2.1 Neurotrauma severity

Minimal
No loss of consciousness, and
Glasgow Coma Score (GCS) 15, and
Normal alertness and memory, and
No neurological deficit, and
No palpable depressed fracture or other sign of skull fracture

Mild
Brief (<5 minutes) loss of consciousness, or amnesia for event, or GCS 14, or
Impaired alertness or memory
No palpable depressed fracture or other sign of skull fracture

Moderate or potentially severe
Prolonged (>5 minutes) loss of consciousness, or
Persistent GCS <14, or
Focal neurological deficit, or
Post-traumatic seizure, or
Intracranial lesion on CT scan, or
Palpable depressed skull fracture

by consideration of time courses, pre-hospital care, pre-sedative and pre-relaxant neuromuscular function and episodes and duration of hypotension or other decompensation. A history of previous health problems, allergies, medications and social setting is desirable.

Primary survey

As with all trauma patients, the initial assessment and therapy must be directed at maintenance of airway, ventilation and circulatory adequacy along standard Advanced Trauma Life Support (ATLS) principles. Early assessment of neurological disturbance using the Glasgow coma score (GCS) or AVPU scale (Alert: GCS 14–15; response to Verbal stimuli: GCS 9–13; response to Painful stimuli: GCS 6–8; or Unresponsive: GCS 3–5) is important. Simultaneous protection of the cervical spine by immobilization is fundamental. This management should commence in the pre-hospital setting and the level of care be maintained.

The greatest risks to the patient with a moderate to severe head injury are hypoxic injury and deficient cerebral perfusion due to systemic hypotension.

Secondary survey

A full secondary survey, including log-roll, should follow.

Clinical assessment of the neurological status of head-injured patients commences with formal documentation of the GCS (Table 3.2.1). The maximum score is 15 and the minimum 3. Coma may be defined in terms of the GCS, in which patients have a total score of 8 or less:

- Fail to show eye opening in response to pain (eye-opening response = 1)

Table 3.2.1 Glasgow coma score	
Best motor response	
Obeys command	6
Localizes to pain	5
Withdraw to pain	4
Abnormal flexion to pain	3
Abnormal extension to pain	2
Nil	1
Best verbal response	
Orientated	5
Confused	4
Uses inappropriate words	3
Incomprehensible sounds	2
Nil	1
Eye opening	
Spontaneously	4
To verbal command	3
To pain	2
Nil	1

- Fail to obey commands (best motor response = 5)
- Make at best only incomprehensible sounds (best verbal response = 2).

Examination of pupillary responses, particularly in the unconscious patient, is important as an indicator of increasing intracranial pressure; a non-responsive dilated pupil indicating ipsilateral herniation. However, a more common cause of abnormal pupil reactions in head injury is the presence of direct ocular trauma.

A general neurological examination, including reflexes, should be performed; the degree to which cooperation is possible and lateralization of signs being particularly important to document. Consideration of the pre-injury mental state is important, particularly where drug or alcohol intoxication is possible.

Clinical investigations

Minimal–mild head injury

In head injury associated with loss of consciousness or amnesia and a GCS of 14–15, CT scanning will demonstrate a relevant positive scan (i.e. cerebral contusion, haematoma, oedema, pneumocephalus) in 7–12% and a subsequent craniotomy rate of 1–3% [15–18].

On the weight of research evidence, current ED investigation of *mild* head injury should include CT scanning in all patients in this group [14,19–22]. Certain high-risk groups (such as the intoxicated, the elderly (>65 years), anticoagulated or demented patients) warrant CT scanning even after *minimal* presumed or possible head injury.

Despite considerable research within the minimal–mild head injury group, reliable risk stratification has not been achieved. The Canadian Head Rules detail five high-risk criteria for neurosurgical intervention in patients with GCS 13–15 and mild head injury [23]. The NICE head injury rules were based in part on the Canadian rules [24]; the NEXUS II [25] investigators showed that development of a simple head injury CT rule that is both sensitive and specific is extremely difficult. There have been conflicting results as to which has the best predictive power in adults and children, however, each has its critics for over-scanning [26,27].

Cervical spine imaging is indicated if the patient has neck pain, neurological abnormality, altered conscious state, intoxication or significant distracting injury.

Moderate–severe head injury

Urgent CT scanning is the investigation of choice in moderate-to-severe neurotrauma (GCS of 3–13); however, other investigations and therapy may take priority in the patient with multisystem trauma, particularly in the presence of unresponsive haemorrhagic shock.

In the absence of a CT scan, consultation with a neurosurgeon or early transfer to an appropriate facility is essential.

Imaging of the cervical spine is indicated in all patients with moderate to severe neurotrauma. A significant proportion of patients with severe head injury will have cervical spine fractures.

Treatment

Minimal–mild head injury

All patients with mild head injury must be counselled appropriately and discharged with written advice in the care of a responsible adult. Specific advice must be provided regarding expected duration of symptoms, possible risks or delayed complications and reasons for re-presentation to the ED (Box 3.2.2). Information should also be given about the second-impact syndrome and exclusions from sporting activity.

Follow up by a local medical officer should be arranged and neuropsychological assessment may be warranted for high-risk groups. Patients should be cautioned about making major life, occupational and financial decisions until they are free of post-concussive symptoms.

In minimal and mild head injury, a normal CT scan and the absence of neurological abnormality are reasonable criteria for patient discharge [3]. It is essential to assess for ongoing post-traumatic amnesia (PTA), as this is frequently overlooked in the ED. A simple screen to use is the modified Westmead PTA scale [6]. In the presence of these criteria, the persistence of mild symptoms (e.g. mild headache, nausea, occasional vomiting) is common and patients should be advised accordingly. In adults, such symptoms may be treated with mild analgesics (paracetamol, aspirin) and antiemetics (metoclopramide, prochlorperazine) and the patient discharged when comfortable. Advising patients that there will be problems with post-concussive symptoms (including short-term memory and information processing) and providing them with written

Box 3.2.2 Patient advice

General advice following head injury

The patient should read and understand these instructions:

- Rest comfortably at home in the company of a responsible adult for the next 12–24 hours
- Resume normal activity after feeling recovered
- Drink clear fluids and consume a light diet only for the first 6–12 hours (a normal diet may be commenced as desired after that)
- Mild pain killers (such as paracetamol) may be taken for headache as directed by the doctor
- Following head injury, a small number of patients develop ongoing symptoms, such as recurrent mild headache, concentration difficulties, difficulty with complex tasks, mood disturbance, etc. If you notice such problems, consult your local doctor for appropriate referral
- Avoid exposure to activities that may create risk of further head injury within the next 2 weeks
- If you do not understand these instructions and advice, check with emergency department staff before your discharge or consult your local doctor
- If you require a certificate for work please make this clear to emergency department staff

Report immediately the following problems

- Persistent vomiting (more than twice)
- Persistent drowsiness–unable to be woken up completely
- Confusion or disorientation or slurred speech
- Increased headache (not relieved by standard doses of paracetamol)
- Localized weakness or altered sensation or incoordination
- Blurred or double vision
- Seizures, fits or convulsions
- Neck stiffness

---

material has been shown to improve outcomes at 3 months [6,28].

Currently there is no drug to treat the primary pathology in mild and minor head injury [29].

Moderate–severe head injury

Priority in the management of moderate to severe neurotrauma is given to maintenance of the airway and an adequate cerebral perfusion pressure. Hypotension (SBP <90) and hypoxia (PaO_2 <60 [8 kPa]) should be corrected immediately [30]. Control or modification of intracranial pressure has a place in the emergency management of neurotrauma. Avoidance of secondary brain injury and associated cerebral swelling is the mainstay of such therapy.

Intracranial pressure monitoring is generally indicated in patients with severe head injury (GCS <8) who remain comatose. Institutional variability exists in methods for measurement, as do specific indications for monitoring. Elevation of the head of the bed to 30° will reduce ICP modestly without altering CPP.

Mannitol (0.5–1.0 g/kg IV) may produce a short-term reduction in ICP. Mannitol causes an osmotic dehydration which is non-selective. Complications of mannitol therapy include fluid overload, hyperosmolality, hypovolaemia and rebound cerebral oedema. Mannitol may be used as a temporizing measure to enable a patient with a surgically remediable lesion to get to theatre.

Routine use of hyperventilation in head injury is contraindicated. Hypocarbia reduces cerebral blood flow (and ICP) through vasoconstriction which, if extreme, may reduce CPP to the point of exacerbation of secondary brain injury [31].

Anticonvulsant prophylaxis (phenytoin 15–18 mg/kg IV over 30–60 minutes) is indicated for the prevention of seizures within the first week after injury [32]. Seizures are managed acutely using standard therapies and guidelines (including benzodiazepines and phenytoin). The use of barbiturates, endotracheal intubation and mechanical ventilation may be indicated for status epilepticus or seizures that are refractory to therapy.

Antibiotic prophylaxis is indicated for compound fractures. Tetanus immunoprophylaxis is given as part of routine wound care. Steroid therapy has had varied support but is not recommended [33]; in 2005, the CRASH collaborators reported conclusively that intravenous corticosteroids should not be used in the treatment of head injury [34].

There has been considerable interest and experimental endeavour with regard to cerebral protection and salvage therapies. To date, no benefit has been demonstrated in the administration of aminosteroids, amino acids or monoamine antagonists in patients with head injury [35–37] and the role of calcium channel blockers remains unclear [38]. More recent research demonstrated worse outcomes for patients with diffuse traumatic brain injury who had a decompressive craniectomy [39]. The role of hypothermia is controversial; while animal studies have shown a benefit, prospective studies have shown either harm or no harm [40,41]. In summary, general supportive therapy, including the maintenance of thermoregulation, hydration, pressure care and nutrition are the mainstays of therapy.

Resuscitation in neurotrauma

There are two features of prime importance to resuscitation in patients suffering neurotrauma:

- maintenance of airway and ventilation
- maintenance of cerebral perfusion pressure.

With elevation of intracranial pressure and loss of autoregulation of cerebral circulation, relatively higher systemic blood pressures are required. The practice of minimal-volume resuscitation has no place in the patient with serious neurotrauma. Standard approaches to the management of hypovolaemia in head-injured patients should be adopted. The use of hypertonic solutions in resuscitation (including hypertonic saline) has been studied with variable conclusions [42]. But the only randomized controlled trial performed with hypertonic saline showed no improvement in outcome [43]. Albumin has also been shown to have detrimental effects in severe traumatic brain injury [44].

Indications for intubation and ventilation of the neurotrauma patient are inadequate ventilation or gas exchange (hypercarbia, hypoxia, apnoea); inability to maintain airway integrity (protective reflexes); a combative or agitated patient; and the need for transport where the status of the airway is potentially unstable (between hospitals, to CT, to angiography, etc.).

Disposition

In patients with minimal–mild head injury, recommendations with regard to a 'safe' period of observation, need for hospital admission or predictive value of injury mechanism are not consistent. Rural and isolated settings present logistic difficulties in the management of this group. Careful observation for a prolonged period is a reasonable alternative and early neurosurgical consultation, together with a low threshold to transfer to a neurosurgical centre, is prudent.

Patients with moderate to severe neurotrauma require hospital admission, preferably under the care of a neurosurgeon in a specialized neurosurgical unit or ICU. Rehabilitation and social readjustment is a focus of therapy from early in the clinical course.

Inter-hospital transfer of patients with significant neurotrauma requires the attendance of skilled transfer staff and the maintenance of level of care during transfer. Airway management must anticipate the potential for the patient to deteriorate *en route*. The presence of pneumocephalus precludes unpressurized (high) altitude flight. The use of teleradiology and neurosurgical consultation will be of value in the management of the remote head-injured patient.

Prognosis

The level of residual neurological impairment is a function of the severity of the degree of trauma and quality of care. A poor outcome is associated with prolonged pre-hospital time, delay of transfer to the appropriate facility, admission to an inappropriate facility and delay in definitive surgical treatment.

Overall mortality in severe head injury is of the order of 35%. A lower GCS at presentation is associated with a worse outcome. Approximately half the patients who remain comatose with GCS <9 for longer than 6 hours will die [12]. Acute subdural haematoma and diffuse axonal injury producing persistent coma are associated with the vast majority of neurotrauma deaths. Early neurological abnormalities are, however, not reliable prognostic factors and an initial period of maximally aggressive therapy is indicated in patients with closed neurotrauma.

Controversies

- Intracranial pressure monitoring has not been shown to improve outcome from major head injury.
- The role of CT scanning in minor head injury has become more widespread.

Although it is increasingly accepted that CT is indicated, the timing or urgency of the investigation is controversial. Further studies are required to define discriminators and high-risk markers as guides to the most rational application of this investigation.

- Consideration should be given to referral of patients with minor or worse head injury with persistent post-concussive symptoms for neuropyschological assessment in order to facilitate recovery and resumption of normal activities.

Acknowledgements

The chapter's authors for this edition would like to acknowledge the important contribution of authors for previous editions, including Dr Marcus Kennedy.

References

[1] Tennant A. Admission to hospital following head injury in England: incidence and socioeconomic associations. BMC Publ Hlth 2005;5:21–9.

[2] Jamieson LM, Roberts-Thomson KF. Hospitalised head injuries among older people in Australia 1998/1999 to 2004/2005. Injury Prevent 2007;13:243–7.

[3] Kay A, Teasdale MB. Head injury in the United Kingdom. World J Surg 2001;25:1210–20.

[4] Morris JA, Limbird TJ, MacKenzie E. Rehabilitation of the trauma patient. In: Moore EE, Mattox KL, Feliciano DV, editors. Trauma, 2nd ed. Norwalk: Appleton & Lange; 1991. p. 815.

[5] Lahaye PA, Gade GF, Becker DP. Injury to the cranium. In: Moore EE, Mattox KL, Feliciano DV, editors. Trauma, 2nd ed. Norwalk: Appleton & Lange; 1991. p. 247.

[6] Ponsford J, Willmott C, Rothwell A, et al. Factors influencing outcome following mild traumatic brain injury in adults. J Internatl Neurol Soc 2000;6:568–79.

[7] McCory P. Does second impact syndrome exist? Clin J Sport Med 2001;11:144–9.

[8] Goldman H, Hodgson V, Morehead M, et al. A rat model of closed head injury. J Neurotrauma 1990;8:129.

[9] Javid M. Head injuries. N Engl J Med 1974;291:890.

[10] Povlishock JT. Pathobiology of traumatically induced axonal injury in animals and man. Ann Emerg Med 1993;22:980.

[11] Meythaler JM, Peduzzi JD, Eleftheriou E, et al. Current concepts: Diffuse axonal injury-associated traumatic brain injury. Arch Phys Med Rehabil 2001;82:1461–71.

[12] Statham PF, Andrews PJ. Central nervous system trauma. Baillière's Clin Neurol 1996;5:501.

[13] Corrigan JD, Selassie AW, Orman JA. The epidemiology of traumatic brain injury. J Head Trauma Rehabil 2010;25:72–80.

[14] Stein S, Ross S. Minor head injury: a proposed strategy for emergency management. Ann Emerg Med 1993;22:1193–6.

[15] Shackford S, Waid S, Ross SE, et al. The clinical utility of computed tomographic scanning and neurological examination in the management of patients with minor head injuries. J Trauma 1992;33:385–94.

[16] Stein S, Ross SJ. Mild head injury: a plea for routine early CT scanning. Trauma 1992;33:11–13.

[17] Richards KA, Lukin WG, Jones P. Minor head injuries. (Royal Brisbane Hospital, personal communication. Unpublished data, 1997).

[18] Lenninger BE, Kreutzer JS, Hill MR. Comparison of minor and severe head injury emotional sequelae using the MMPI. Brain Injury 1991;5:199–205.

[19] Newcombe R, Merry G. The management of acute neurotrauma in rural and remote locations: a set of guidelines for the care of head and spinal injuries. J Clin Neurosci 1999;6:85–93.

[20] Victorian Road Trauma Committee. Report of the Consultative Committee on Road Traffic Fatalities. Victorian Institute of Forensic Pathology, Royal Australasian College of Surgeons, 1997.

[21] McAllister TW. Neuropsychiatric sequelae of head injuries. Psychiatr Clin N Am 1992;15:S395–413.

[22] Bullock R, Chesnut RM, Clifton G, et al. Guidelines for the management of severe head injury. Eur J Emerg Med 1996;2:109–27.

[23] Stiell I, Wells G, Vandenheem K, et al. The Canadian CT rule for patients with minor head injury. Lancet 2001;357:1391–6.

[24] National Institute for Clinical Excellence. Clinical Guideline 56. Head Injury: triage, assessment, investigation and early management of head injury in infants, children and adults. London: NICE; 2007. <http://publications.nice.org.uk/head-injury-cg56> [Accessed Jan. 2013].

[25] Mower W, Hoffman J, Herbert M, et al. Developing a clinical decision instrument to rule out intracranial injuries in patients with minor head trauma: methodology of the NEXUS II investigation. Ann Emerg Med 2002;40:504–14.

[26] Smits M, Dippel DW, De Hann GG, et al. External validation of the Canadian CT Head Rule and the New Orleans Criteria for CT scanning in patients with minor head injury. J Am Med Assoc 2005;294:1519–25.

[27] Dunning J, Daly JP, Malhotra R, et al. The implications of NICE guidelines on the management of children presenting with head injury. Arch Dis Child 2004;89:763–7.

[28] NSW Ministry of Health. Adult Trauma Clinical Practice Guidelines. Initial Management of Closed Head Injury in Adults, 2nd ed. North Sydney; 2011. <http://www.itim.nsw.gov.au/images/3/3d/Closed_Head_Injury_CPG_2nd_Ed_Full_document.pdf> [Accessed Jan. 2013].

[29] McCrory P. New treatments for concussion: The next millennium beckons. Clin J Sport Med 2001;11:190–3.

[30] Chesnut RM, Marshall LF, Klauber MR, et al. The role of secondary brain injury in determining outcome from severe head injury. J Trauma 1993;34:216–22.

[31] Fortune JB, Fenstel PJ, Graca L, et al. Effect of hyperventilation, mannitol and ventriculostomy drainage on cerebral blood flow after head injury. J Trauma Injury Infect Crit Care 1995;39:1091–9.

[32] Temkin NR, Dikmen SS, Wilensky AJ, et al. A randomised, double blind study of phenytoin for the prevention of post-traumatic seizures. N Engl J Med 1990;323:497–502.

[33] Clausen T, Bullock R. Medical treatment and neuroprotection in traumatic brain injury. Curr Pharm Design 2001;7:1517–32.

[34] Edwards P, Arango M, Balica L, et al. Final results of a randomised placebo controlled trial of intravenous corticosteroid in adults with head injury–outcomes at 6 months. Lancet 2005;365:1957–9.

[35] Marshall LF, Maas AIR, Bowers MS, et al. A multicenter trial on the efficacy of using tirilazad mesylate in cases of head injury. J Neurosurg 1998;89:519–25.

[36] Willis C, Lybrand S. Bellamy N. Excitatory amino acid inhibitors for traumatic brain injury. Cochrane Database Syst Rev 2003;1:CD003986.

[37] Forsyth RJ, Jayamoni B, Paine TC, Mascarenhas S. Monoaminergic agonists for acute traumatic brain injury. Cochrane Database Syst Rev 2006;4:CD003984.

[38] Langham J, Goldfrad C, Teasdale G, et al. Calcium channel blockers for acute traumatic brain injury. Cochrane Database Syst Rev 2003;4:CD000565.

[39] Cooper DJ, Rosenfeld J, Murray L, et al. Decompressive craniectomy in diffuse traumatic brain injury. N Engl J Med 2011;364:1493–502.

[40] Sydenham E, Roberts I, Alderson P. Hypothermia for traumatic head injury. Cochrane Database Syst Rev 2009;2:CD001048.

[41] Ireland S, Endacott R, Cameron P, et al. The incidence and significance of accidental hypothermia in major trauma – a prospective observational study. Resuscitation 2011;82:300–6.

[42] Vassar MJ, Fischer RP, O'Brien PE, et al. A multicenter trial for resuscitation of injured patients with 7.5% sodium chloride. The effect of added dextran 70. The Multicenter Group for the Study of Hypertonic Saline in Trauma Patients. Arch Surg 1993;128:1003–11.

[43] Cooper JD, Myles PS, McDermott FT, et al. Prehospital hypertonic saline resuscitation of patients with hypotension and severe traumatic brain injury. J Am Med Assoc 2004;291:1350–7.

[44] Myburgh J, Cooper J, Finfer S, et al. Saline or albumin for fluid resuscitation in patients with traumatic brain injury. N Engl J Med 2007;357:874–84.

3.3 Spinal trauma

Pieter van Driel

ESSENTIALS

1 Cervical spine injury can be confidently eliminated in conscious, clear-headed patients younger than 65 years, using clinical examination criteria (as described in NEXUS and Canadian C-spine rules) alone.

2 Physical examination alone does not assist in the diagnosis of unstable vertebral injury unless the deformity is gross.

3 A lack of neurological symptoms and signs does not eliminate spinal column injury or spinal cord at risk.

4 A patient can be ambulant and still have a major vertebral injury, even a potentially unstable one.

5 The natural history of spinal cord injury may lead to progressively increasing symptoms commencing some hours after the incident.

6 Magnetic resonance imaging is evolving as the imaging modality of choice in patients with neurological signs.

7 The likelihood of significant vertebral injury in unconscious trauma victims is 10%; 2% of all trauma victims with significant altered conscious state have a spinal cord injury.

8 Although spinal immobilization is a standard of care for protecting the spine, the use of these devices can have adverse clinical effects.

9 Methylprednisolone is not recommended in most Australian centres but, if given, it should be within 8 hours after spinal cord injury in order to improve both motor function and functional outcome.

Introduction

Spinal cord injury is one of the most disabling traumas, causing major and irreversible physical and psychological disability to the patient and permanently affecting their lifestyle. The emotional, social and economic consequences affect the individual, family, friends and society in general.

Approximately 2% of adult victims of blunt trauma suffer a spinal injury and this risk is tripled in patients with craniofacial injury [1].

Motor vehicle collisions, falls and sporting injuries – notably diving and water sports – are the major causes of acute spinal cord injury in Australia [2]. Road traffic accidents account for about half of all spinal injuries. Despite the work to minimize spinal injuries in contact sports, such as rugby, serious spinal cord injuries still occur [2]. Spinal injuries occur mostly in young people, but minor falls in the elderly or low-impact injuries in people with pre-existing bony pathology can also cause spinal cord damage. Spinal cord injury due to pathological vertebral fractures may be the first presentation of malignancy.

Observations from two studies [3,4] suggest that possibly preventable neurological deterioration may be due to one or more of the following:

- the injury not being recognized initially, e.g. not being specifically examined for, occult or masked by other injuries
- the onset of the secondary effects of the spinal cord injury involving oedema and/or ischaemia
- aggravation of the initial spinal cord lesion by inadequate oxygenation and/or hypotension
- aggravation of the initial spinal cord lesion by inadequate vertebral immobilization.

Pathophysiology

Level of vertebral injury

The level of neurological injury in patients who sustain spinal injuries is variously reported. In studies from Victoria and New South Wales [4,5], the distribution of the level of injuries was cervical 60%, thoracic 30%, lumbar 4% and sacral 2%.

Spinal cord injuries occur most commonly at the level of the 5th, 6th and 7th cervical vertebrae, largely because of the greater mobility of these regions. The C5–6 and C6–7 levels account for almost 50% of all subluxation injury patterns in blunt cervical spinal trauma [6].

Associated injuries

There are three noteworthy observations [3,5] from associated injuries in patients with spinal injury:

- Approximately 8–10% of patients with a vertebral fracture have a secondary fracture of another vertebra, often at a distant site. These secondary fractures are usually associated with the more violent mechanisms of injury, such as ejection or rollover. Secondary injuries are usually relatively minor and stable, e.g. fractures of the vertebral processes but, occasionally, they may be major and may also be associated with neurological damage. Therefore, when 'thinking spine', it is important to 'think whole spine' and, in particular, to attempt to avoid rotation of the vertebral column.
- Owing to the mechanism of injury, many patients with spinal injuries often have other associated injuries, including head, intrathoracic or intra-abdominal injuries, which may modify management priorities [5].
- Patients may complain of pain from other injuries and hence a back or neck injury may go unnoticed. Pain may often not be a significant feature despite severe vertebral column damage. Furthermore, spinal pain may take some time to become apparent

because of other pathological processes modifying pain, such as swelling and inflammation.

Spinal trauma might result in several injuries directly related to the spinal cord. Specific injuries, such as vertebral injuries, spinal shock, spinal cord injuries and their neurological symptoms, are described later in this chapter.

Autonomic nervous system effects of spinal cord damage

Autonomic nervous system effects are mentioned here as important pathophysiological mechanisms must be understood to deliver optimum care and treatment to patients with spinal cord injuries.

The whole of the sympathetic nervous system and the pelvic parasympathetic outflow is transmitted in the spinal cord. In an injury higher than the upper thoracic vertebrae, there is significant impairment of total body sympathetic and pelvic parasympathetic functions. The extent and severity of autonomic dysfunction is dependent on the segmental level(s) and the extent or completeness of the neurological insult.

Direct effects

Direct effects include manifestations related to the cardiovascular, gastrointestinal, urogenital and thermoregulatory systems.

Cardiovascular effects

In complete quadriplegia, sympathetic denervation causes relaxation of resting vasomotor tone, resulting in generalized systemic vasodilatation. It is recognized by dry extremities with variable warmth and colour during initial assessment. In males, there may be penile engorgement or priapism. Owing to the peripheral vasodilatation, there is a drop in total peripheral resistance, with consequent hypotension (neurogenic shock). Under normal circumstances, this would result in a baroreceptor response in order to achieve compensation. However, as the effector arm of the sympathetic nervous system is paralysed, the normal compensatory effects of tachycardia and vasoconstriction do not occur. The vagus nerve carrying parasympathetic supply to the heart is unopposed, with resultant bradycardia. The higher and more complete the spinal cord injury, the more extensive the autonomic dysfunction.

The usual symptoms and signs of the shock process in response to hypovolaemia cannot occur, as tachycardia and vasoconstriction are mediated by the sympathetic nervous system, which has been interrupted by the high spinal cord lesion.

Gastrointestinal effects

Following spinal cord injury, a paralytic ileus develops. This is usually self-limiting and recovers over 3–10 days. Paralysis of sphincters occurs at the lower end of the oesophagus and at the pylorus; as a consequence, passive aspiration of the stomach contents, especially of fluid, is a potential problem. Furthermore, owing to thoracic and abdominal wall muscle paralysis, the capacity to cough and hence clear the airway is diminished. In quadriplegia and high paraplegia, occult fluid aspiration due to passive regurgitation of retained gastric content may not be recognized. The airway therefore requires close observation and active protection. A nasogastric tube must be inserted and gastric contents drained.

Urinary effects

Urinary retention is partly the consequence of acute bladder denervation and, in the early post-injury phase, due to spinal shock. Catheter insertion is required to prevent overdistension of the bladder in order to optimize recovery. It also permits measurement of urinary output.

Thermoregulatory effects

Following cervical or upper thoracic spinal cord injury, the spinal patient effectively becomes poikilothermic. In a cold environment, they are unable to vasoconstrict to conserve heat or shiver to generate heat. The patient is already peripherally vasodilated which promotes loss of heat and lowering of body temperature. In the warm environment, although the patient is already peripherally vasodilated, the capacity to sweat is sympathetically controlled and therefore lost.

Pre-hospital issues

Extrication and immobilization

Emergency medical services (EMS) personnel are sent to see trauma patients in difficult circumstances. Patients, for instance, could be stuck in vehicles, (partially) submersed in water or found in small and inconvenient places. These circumstances often make it hard

initially to immobilize fully the (cervical) spine. Several devices have been developed to extricate a trauma patient from a crashed vehicle with maximum in-line protection of the spinal column.

Restlessness in patients, due to hypotension, hypoxia, drug abuse, anxiety or other causes, makes it even harder to immobilize fully the spine. Depending on local protocols, training and skills, EMS personnel should either be able to treat the cause of the restlessness or sedate these patients in order to immobilize the (cervical) spine.

Next to resuscitation interventions following the ABCDE approach, focus should be given to in-line immobilization of the total spine. Trauma patients should remain in immobilization devices until spinal trauma has been excluded and splinting of specific injuries can be effected. However, they do not need to be left in the devices applied by pre-hospital care providers: these are structured to provide rigid immobilization for initial stabilization and transport. Nor should they be left tied to spine boards or wrapped in extrication devices, as these are uncomfortable and can cause unwanted cutaneous pressure injuries. Tight webbing and wraps can interfere with respiratory excursion. In general, the pre-hospital devices are removed and replaced with more appropriate ones for the emergency department environment.

Immobilization of the spine

Immobilization of the spine continues to be a standard of care. However, the effectiveness of common techniques is largely unproven and there are side effects from unnecessary immobilization. The Cochrane Collaboration failed to infer a potential for good, in spite of the fact that splinting any suspected bony injury is universally considered standard management [7].

Although failure to detect and immobilize cervical spine injury in hospitalized patients is associated with a 7–10-fold risk of secondary neurological injury, it is unclear whether the secondary injuries occur in the out-of-hospital setting and can be prevented by spinal immobilization devices. Despite this, there is evidence that not immobilizing the cervical spine is not associated with an increase in neurological injury [8]. A benefit of applying a cervical collar can be to alert the medical team to the potential presence of spinal injury. The weight of opinion is in favour of splinting devices until spinal injury can be eliminated. Therefore, immobilization and the use of splinting devices remains commonplace in clinical practice.

Several types of devices exist and are used either alone or in combination. The common combination in out-of-hospital spine care comprises a cervical collar, spine board and associated padding to ensure a normal curvature of the spine. Other devices, such as extrication devices, not primarily designed as spinal immobilizers, have been used to splint the spine in special circumstances.

The various devices and techniques are variably effective and do not completely immobilize. However, they have generally been tested on uninjured subjects with normal muscular tone and posture.

As mentioned before, spinal immobilization can be harmful. Standard spinal immobilization applied to otherwise healthy subjects resulted in significant spinal pain in 100% of subjects [9]. Spinal immobilization can mask life-threatening injuries. Cervical collars have been shown to increase intracranial pressure. Spinal immobilization restricts pulmonary function in healthy adults and children. Prolonged immobilization of the cervical spine with rigid pre-hospital rescue collars and other immobilization devices may unnecessarily add to patient discomfort and the need for ongoing spinal nursing. Tissue perfusion in the sacral area is adversely affected within 30 minutes on a rigid spinal board [10]. This predisposes to pressure area problems and problematic decubitus ulceration. Therefore, upon arrival of the patient in the Emergency Department (ED), the pre-hospital devices should be removed as soon as possible (usually immediately after the primary survey) and replaced with more appropriate ones for the emergency department environment.

First treatment options

Primary survey

Patients presenting with a potential spinal cord injury are managed in keeping with the approach for any major trauma patient. Therefore, a standard approach of primary survey, resuscitation, secondary survey and definitive management is adopted.

Specific attention should be paid to the following issues important in the assessment and treatment of patients with (potential) spinal injury.

Airway

Assessment of the airway is vital in the management of suspected spinal cord injury, especially when the cervical spine is involved. Passive regurgitation and aspiration of fluid stomach contents may occur as a result of blunting or absence of cough, gag and vomiting responses. This is especially the case with higher cervical injuries. Therefore, the insertion of a nasogastric tube is of vital importance in minimizing the likelihood of aspiration. In quadriplegia and high paraplegia, unopposed vagal action owing to functional total or near-complete sympathectomy predisposes the patient to bradycardia on vagal stimulation of the pharynx. It is important that such patients have ECG monitoring and that atropine be immediately available to block these effects. Pretreatment with atropine prior to manipulation of the upper airway is a consideration.

Advanced airway management Early endotracheal intubation and assisted ventilation should be considered in patients with quadriplegia and high paraplegia. Regular assessment of respiratory status is undertaken and includes continuous pulse oximetry and frequent vital capacity measurement, in order to detect fatigue.

Blind nasal or endoscopic-assisted intubation under local anaesthetic is the preferred mode of non-emergency intubation. Additionally, every manipulation to the head and neck of the patient should be done with extreme caution to minimize further damage to the vulnerable spine.

The literature suggests that videolaryngoscopy results in less overall movement during intubation and it does not seem to have an impact on cord injury.

Since the rocuronium antagonist sugammadex has become widely available, rocuronium has become the muscle relaxant of first choice in many settings because of the beneficial side-effect profile. Suxamethonium is therefore used less often, but still acceptable for a rapid-sequence intubation in the emergency setting. The hyperkalaemia associated with denervation is a concern in injuries more than 10–12 hours old (see Chapter 2.1).

Breathing

Ventilation in patients with spinal cord injury may be affected by the level of cord injury, aspiration and primary lung injury. In the absence of major airway obstruction and flail chest, the presence of paradoxical breathing is considered highly suggestive of cervical spine injury. Paradoxical breathing occurs because of loss of motor tone and paralysis of thoracic muscles innervated by thoracic spinal segments. Diaphragmatic action results in a negative intrapleural pressure. As a consequence of chest wall paralysis, the tendency is for the soft tissues of the thorax to 'cave in', producing paradoxical chest wall movement. The diaphragm needs to undertake the full work of breathing, including overcoming added resistance to ventilation caused by paradoxical chest wall movement. In addition to standard respiratory status assessment, continuous pulse oximetry and assessment of vital capacity is necessary. Early intubation should be considered if vital capacity is inadequate or falling.

Ventilation may be reduced for several reasons:

- the diaphragm may simply fatigue and require assisted ventilation
- a progressively ascending spinal cord injury owing to either further primary damage or secondary ascending spinal cord oedema may encroach upon the third to fifth cervical segments
- the same segments may be involved with the initial injury and thus the diaphragm may itself be partially paralysed.
- the consequences of coexisting chest trauma must also be taken into consideration, as respiration may be embarrassed by the natural progression of thoracic cage, pulmonary or intrapleural injuries.

Circulation

Volume resuscitation in the resuscitative phase of the primary survey is undertaken in keeping with usual practices. With the exception of perhaps diving injuries, hypotensive trauma victims should be considered as intravascular volume depleted and bleeding until proved otherwise. Standard initial volumes of resuscitation fluid will not adversely affect the haemodynamic welfare. Owing to peripheral vasodilatation, spinal cord trauma patients are relatively intravascular volume depleted and, therefore, volume preloading is appropriate. However, unnecessary volume overloading in an attempt to raise systolic blood pressure substantially will lead to acute pulmonary oedema.

After resuscitation fluids have been administered, haemorrhage controlled, ongoing losses replaced and fluid required for oedema responses to injury considered, routine maintenance fluids are all that is needed.

Paralysis of the sympathetic nervous system and, hence, the compensatory mechanisms for intravascular volume depletion, necessitates a heightened suspicion of ongoing bleeding, the signs of which may be dramatic or subtle. Progressive hypotension is a key sign. Paradoxically, the heart rate may rise progressively from a bradycardia of 50–60 beats per minute to more normally acceptable rates. It is uncertain by which mechanism this pseudo or relative tachycardia of quadriplegia occurs. One thought is that with progressive hypotension and brainstem hypoperfusion, the vagal effects are switched off by the brainstem, thus allowing the heart rate to rise towards a more normal or denervated range. The skin may develop patchy or blotchy cyanosis. This is due to a sluggish peripheral circulation and hence locally elevated levels of deoxygenated or desaturated haemoglobin.

In cases of spinal cord injury, the impact of functional sympathectomy will depend upon the level and completeness of the neurological injury. Complete injuries above T1, and perhaps T4, can be expected to have clinically significant manifestations of neurogenic shock. The clinical signs are bradycardia due to unopposed vagal action, peripheral vasodilatation and cessation of sweating. Peripheral vasodilatation is responsible for variable cutaneous manifestations. Initially, flushing can be expected, however, the skin may be pale or cyanosed and its temperature elevated, reduced or within normal limits. The state of the above signs is dependent on perfusion pressure, adequacy of oxygenation and the ambient temperature.

Priapism in a trauma patient is due to penile vasodilatation and is regarded as a highly suggestive sign of spinal cord injury.

Circulatory status is best assessed by conscious state, urine output and venous pressure monitoring. In the early phases of management, close urine output monitoring is of major importance. Early insertion of the urinary catheter allows measurement of urine output, may assist in identifying occult renal tract injury and also prevents undesirable bladder overdistension.

Inotropic support is often unnecessary [5]. However, satisfactory cerebral perfusion is essential. In order to maintain cerebral perfusion, a mean arterial pressure (MAP) of at least 60 mmHg is recommended. In the patient with

a previously normal Mini Mental State examination, deterioration may suggest intracranial hypoperfusion due to either intracranial trauma or the neurogenic shock process. Chronotropic and vasoconstrictor agents are occasionally required. These are more likely to be necessary in older patients or those suffering from hypertension who are now relatively hypotensive despite volume loading. Chronotropic agents are occasionally required for patients prescribed β-blocker, peripheral and central vasodilator drugs. Likewise, patients with established cerebrovascular disease may require higher perfusion pressures than the resting pressure of the quadriplegic.

The degree of the physiological effects on the circulation will depend on the site and completeness of the injury. Spinal cord injury below the sympathetic outflow will have little effect on the circulation; complete spinal cord injury above the thoracic outflow will produce a total body sympathectomy. A complete spinal-cord injury in the mid-thoracic segments should result in preserved vasomotor function in the head, neck and upper limbs. Cardiac reflexes should also be relatively well preserved. Vasomotor tone to the abdominal cavity, pelvis and lower limbs will be paralysed. Likewise, incomplete lesions will have a varying affect depending on the site and completeness of the injury. Careful establishment of the segmental level and degree of spinal cord injury on secondary survey will assist in anticipating the likely extent of autonomic dysfunction.

The denervated lung is intolerant of volume overloading. Therefore, careful monitoring of fluid balance, including urine output and, in circumstances of low urine flow, central venous pressure, is required.

Disability

Spinal cord injury has an association with significant head trauma. In patients with altered conscious state due to head trauma, the early brief assessment of mental state and pupillary reflexes is important. All trauma victims with altered conscious state require spinal immobilization until spinal cord or unstable vertebral injury is excluded on physical examination and investigation.

In patients with injuries at or above T4, bilateral Horner's syndrome may be present, with relative pupillary constriction.

Exposure

As a spinal cord injury may be one of several injuries, the patient should be fully exposed and

then kept in a warming blanket in keeping with a routine approach to patients with multisystem trauma.

General management issues
The general management is in keeping with the approach to any victim of major trauma.

Analgesia and medications
Owing to the variable physiology of the peripheral circulation due to vascular tone denervation and sympathetic efferent interruption, the absorption of subcutaneous and intramuscular medications is unreliable. It is recommended that analgesia be provided by continuous intravenous infusion, with careful monitoring of vital signs. For similar reasons and where possible, all other medications are administered by the intravenous route.

Temperature
In complete quadriplegia, the patient has been rendered poikilothermic by the interruption of efferent sympathetic activity. Attention is directed to ensuring that the core temperature remains within the normal range. Such patients will demonstrate a core body temperature in keeping with changes in ambient temperature.

Clearing the spine

Clearing the cervical spine
Prolonged immobilization of the spine with rigid pre-hospital rescue collars and other rigid immobilization devices may unnecessarily add to patient discomfort, complications of the immobilization devices and the need for ongoing spinal nursing.

Although various algorithms exist for clearing the spine of significant injures and compliance with such clearing algorithms is high, none have been validated for clinical effectiveness. Most incorporate the elements of either the United States National Emergency X-Radiography Utilization Study (NEXUS) or the Canadian Cervical Spine Rules (Canadian C-Spine Rules [CCR]) thus restricting evidence-based decision rules to the cervical spine [11] (see Tables 3.8.7 and 3.8.8)).

It still is the emergency physician's responsibility to minimize exposure to radiation. The need for imaging of the cervical spine can be safely determined by applying both the criteria of NEXUS and the CCR. The application of both of these two clinical tests essentially clears the c-spine in a number of patients.

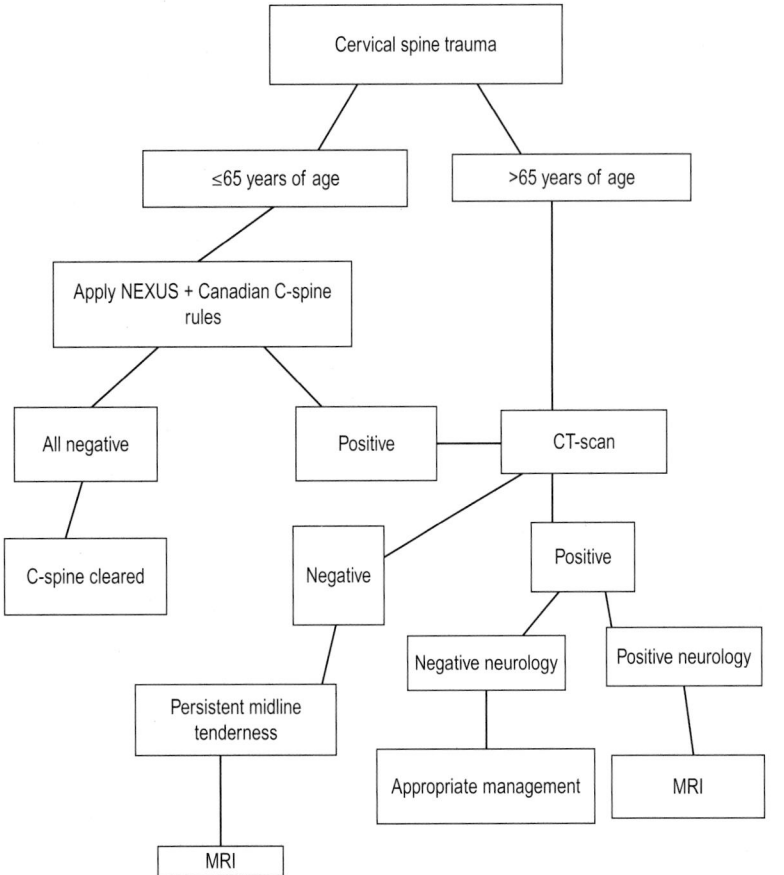

Fig. 3.3.1 Suggested radiological algorithm for cervical spine trauma.

The fundamental differences between the two tests are that the CCR incorporates the mechanism of injury, circumstances and examination findings of active movement of the cervical spine [12–14].

Following the (radiological) algorithm in Figure 3.3.1 is a safe way to approach the patient for cervical spine trauma.

Thoracic, lumbar and sacral spine clearance

There is little information available to provide evidence-based guidelines for clearing the thoracic, lumbar and sacral spine. The investigation and injury exclusion strategy is based on appropriate clinical reasoning (read the mechanism!) and an understanding of the effectiveness and limitations of medical imaging options, in both logistics and effectiveness. All patients with significant mechanisms of injury and pain or tenderness along the thoracic, lumbar and sacral spine should be imaged. Additionally, patients with multiple injuries and high-risk mechanisms should be routinely imaged.

Secondary survey, referral-disposition and definitive treatment

The secondary survey of spinal cord damage

The definitive diagnosis of a spinal cord injury is made from the findings on secondary survey. Two specific injury entities need to be considered: skeletal and neurological.

A head-to-toe clinical examination is conducted in keeping with the standard conventions used in examining any victim of major trauma. The following outlines the specific points of clinical examination pertinent to spinal injury.

Head and neck

An examination of the cervical spine is conducted maintaining immobilization. Palpation of the spine posteriorly may demonstrate generalized tenderness owing to diffuse muscular spasm. However, the point of maximal tenderness should be determined. In hyperextension injuries, the prevertebral and paravertebral muscles

are often contused. This is a helpful sign when evaluating hyperextension–hyperflexion injuries in patients who were in stationary vehicles hit from behind. Longitudinal pressure to the head increases cervical pain. Such patients should be considered to have a higher likelihood of a significant vertebral injury.

The neck should be examined for swelling and bruising. Deformity will be noted if there is a dislocation with significant displacement. It should be remembered that significant bony and soft tissue injury frequently occurs without any major findings on external examination.

As prolonged immobilization of the cervical spine with rigid pre-hospital rescue collars and other rigid immobilization devices may unnecessarily add to patient discomfort, complications from the application of splinting devices and the need for ongoing spinal nursing, it is important to determine whether immobilization devices can be removed early during the assessment and treatment phases of management. Reasons for lengthy periods of immobilization include times to definitive radiological assessment and waiting for windows of opportunity to ensure vertebral stability (see also Immobilization of the spine and Clearing the spine).

A re-examination of the upper airway is required. A prevertebral haematoma can cause obstruction; the gag reflex may be blunted; airway protection may be embarrassed owing to paralysis of muscles below the neck, resulting in inefficient gag and cough. The patient will have gastric stasis and is at considerable risk of fluid aspiration.

The torso

The patient should either be lifted or rolled on to the side using a formal spinal-lifting technique, so that the back can be examined. The spine is examined for alignment, swelling, bruising and abrasion. Deformity is generally not a feature, except in the presence of major dislocation or disruption.

The rise and fall of the chest is noted. Paradoxical movement is a sign of thoracic cage muscular paralysis and will be more pronounced the higher the segmental level of injury. Careful examination of the thorax, abdomen and pelvis is required. In both quadriplegia and high paraplegia, serious injury may be masked by the use of analgesia and anaesthesia. Significant vertebral injury to the thoracic and lumbar spines is associated with major injuries to the thoracic, abdominal and pelvic organs.

The abdomen is specifically assessed for an evolving paralytic ileus.

Neurological assessment

A thorough examination of the peripheral nervous system is required. It is strongly recommended that both motor and sensory examinations be undertaken in accordance with the following convention. Examine motor, sensory and reflex components independently. Examination begins at the head and then progresses across the shoulders. The upper limbs are then examined. The torso evaluation begins from just below the clavicles, extending inferiorly to the groin; each lower limb is then assessed. Finally, the saddle area and pelvic floor are assessed.

This approach reduces the likelihood of an incorrect diagnosis of paraplegia by finding a 'pseudo' neurological level of injury just below the clavicles when upper limbs have not been examined. It is therefore important that the upper limbs be assessed before examining the torso.

Motor function

Muscle power is assessed in terms of neurological segments and not muscle groups. Muscle power in each segment is graded from 0 to 5 as shown in Table 3.3.1.

It is often impossible to assess power grades in certain segments owing to the patient's injuries. The upper limbs are the most easily examined. The strength of a cough provides some information as to the state of thoracic and abdominal musculature.

In the emergency setting, the state of the pelvic muscles is determined through a rectal examination by assessing rectal tone and requesting the patient to tighten the sphincter on the examiner's gloved finger.

Table 3.3.1	Muscle power grading
Power grade	Clinical finding
Grade 0/5	No movement
Grade 1/5	Flicker
Grade 2/5	Movement present, but not a full range against gravity
Grade 3/5	Full range of movement against gravity with no added resistance
Grade 4/5	Full range of movement against gravity with added resistance but with reduced power
Grade 5/5	Normal power

Sensory function

Dorsal column sensation is assessed using a piece of cotton wool and testing for light touch. Spinothalamic sensation is assessed using a pin or sharp object. Although proprioception, vibration and temperature can be assessed, these are not essential and add little to the emergency examination. When testing with a sharp object, a hypodermic injection needle or a trocar stylet must not be used: these are engineered to stab the skin as painlessly as possible, therefore they cause trauma and are unreliable.

The general convention described below should be followed. Sensory examination begins on the face which, as it is supplied by the trigeminal nerve and bypasses the spinal cord, acts as a reference point. It is an important axiom based on anatomy that 'in the absence of head injury or local facial injury, sensation to the face is always normal in pure spinal cord injury' (the trigeminal nerve comes from above the spinal cord). It is recommended that examination of the head, neck and upper torso is performed as follows. Start by examining the C2 dermatome laterally on the neck behind the mandible and beneath the ear. Extend examination onto the top of the shoulder, thus assessing the C3, C4 and C5 dermatomes. In the upper limbs, examine the dermatomes in segmental order. This should include T2 on the upper medial aspect of the arm. Then carry on examining the torso in the mid-clavicular plane or at the outer border of the surface marking of the rectus sheath.

Reflexes

Reflexes are examined in keeping with usual examination practices. Superficial abdominal reflexes should be noted. The anal and bulbocavernosus reflexes are important in assessing sacral segments.

Corticosteroids–methylprednisolone

A Cochrane review from 2012 found that administration of methylprednisolone within 8 hours after injury gave a significant recovery of motor function [15].

Administration for an additional 24 hours (totalling 48 hours) may give an additional improvement of motor neurological function and functional outcome. On the other hand, the use of methylprednisolone is not without complications. It is contraindicated in patients with heavily contaminated open injuries, other heavily contaminated situations, such as perforated bowel and established sepsis. It has the risk of developing acute adrenal insufficiency in these patients, which needs recognition and prompt treatment to prevent further complications. It is relatively contraindicated in diabetes mellitus. Prophylactic measures, such as for acute peptic ulceration and monitoring of blood glucose, should be instituted.

The benefit of steroids in spinal cord injury is therefore considered questionable. Despite this, their use remains a treatment option and several centres prefer to use high-dose methylprednisolone in the early management of patients with neurological injury. In Australia, spinal cord injury is not listed as an indication for high-dose methylprednisolone. Therefore, the decision to use high-dose corticosteroids should be made in conjunction with the specialist services, either the major trauma service or spinal injuries service that will be managing continuing care. If used, treatment must be commenced within 8 hours from the time of injury. The total treatment period should be for 24 hours if treatment is commenced within 3 hours of injury and 48 hours if commenced between 3 and 8 hours.

A guideline for the use of methylprednisolone in acute spinal cord injury is presented in Figure 3.3.2.

Referral-disposition

Patients with a spinal cord injury should be referred to a centre with facilities for optimal management as soon as practicable. Specific treatments such as immobilization, specific therapy and transport considerations should be discussed with the continuing care provider or spinal injuries unit prior to transfer. If transport is delayed, it is appropriate that the spinal injuries unit be involved and contribute to the patient's initial management, especially in areas of specific management, as soon as possible, even if transfer is to be delayed by several days.

Specific conditions

Vertebral injury [2]

Cervical spine fractures

Cervical spine injuries may result from one or more combinations of the following mechanisms:

- hyperflexion
- hyperextension

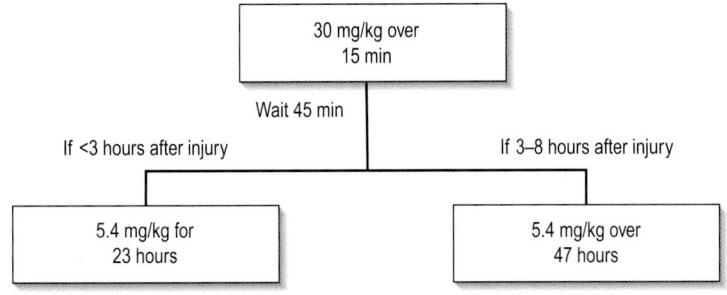

These doses may be approximated to the nearest 0.5 g. For example, a 70 kg patient requiring 24 hours of treatment would need:

Calculation
30 (mg/kg) x 70 (kg) = 2100 mg
followed by:
5.4 mg/kg/h x 70 (kg) = 8694 mg

Actual Dose
2g (1 x 2g or 2 x 1g or 4 x 500 mg vials)
followed by:
8.5g (4 x 2g + 1 x 500 mg or 8.5 x 1g or 17 x 500 mg vials) over 23 hours

Fig. 3.3.2 Methylprednisolone for acute spinal cord injury.

- flexion–rotation
- vertebral compression
- lateral flexion
- distraction.

Hyperflexion Hyperflexion produces the following injuries:

- a simple, stable wedge fracture
- a fracture with an anterior teardrop
- bilateral anterior subluxation
- clay shoveller's fracture
- bilateral facet dislocation.

Flexion injuries can cause a vertebral body fracture with an anteroinferior extrusion teardrop fracture. This is often associated with retropulsion of a vertebral body fracture fragment or fragments into the spinal canal.

The clay shoveller's fracture is a particular spinous process fracture produced by a sudden load on a flexed spine, with resulting avulsion of the C6, C7 or T1 spinous processes.

Hyperextension Anterior widening of disc spaces, prevertebral swelling, avulsion of a vertebral body by the anterior longitudinal ligament, subluxation and crowding of the spinous processes are features of the hyperextension injury. Encroachment on the canal by an extruded disc or a posterior osteophyte may occur in patients with osteoarthritis of the cervical spine.

Flexion–rotation This is responsible for unilateral facet dislocation or forward subluxation of the cervical spine.

Vertebral compression This is the mechanism responsible for burst fractures. The intervertebral disc is disrupted and driven into the vertebral body below. In addition, disc material may be extruded anteriorly into prevertebral tissues and posteriorly into the spinal canal. The vertebral body may be comminuted to varying degrees, with fragments being extruded anteriorly and posteriorly into the spinal canal.

Lateral flexion This may produce uncinate fractures, isolated pillar fractures, transverse process injuries and lateral vertebral compression.

Distraction These injuries may result in gross ligamentous and intervertebral disc disruption. The hangman's fracture may also occur by combined distraction and hyperextension mechanisms.

C1 – the atlas

Fractures of the atlas comprise 4% of cervical spine injuries. Mechanisms of injury generally involve hyperextension or compression. Around 15–20% of fractures may be associated with a C2 injury and 25% may be associated with a lower cervical injury. The Jefferson fracture is a blowout fracture of the ring. Other fractures include isolated injuries of the posterior arch, the anterior arch and the lateral mass.

C2 – the axis

Axis fractures comprise 6% of cervical spine injuries, with an association with concurrent C1 injury in the majority of cases.

Computed tomography (CT) scan images are examined for odontoid subluxation. Three types of odontoid fracture are described:

- Type 1 is an avulsion of the odontoid tip. It is generally a stable injury and accounts for 5–8% of odontoid fractures
- Type 2 injury is a fracture through the base of the dens and is generally unstable. It comprises 55–70% of odontoid injuries. In younger children, the epiphysis may be present and confused with a type 2 fracture
- Type 3 is a subdental fracture of the odontoid extending into the vertebral body. It comprises 30–35% of odontoid fractures.

Other fractures of the odontoid include avulsion fractures of the lower anterior margin of the body due to a hyperextension injury. A hangman's fracture is a bilateral neural arch fracture of C2. It is a hyperextension injury and is associated with prevertebral soft tissue swelling, anterior subluxation of C2 on C3 and avulsion of the anteroinferior corner of C2.

C3–C7

Fractures in this segment of the cervical spine are clearly picked up with CT scanning. Fractures are defined as unstable when:

- the anterior and all of the posterior elements are disrupted
- there is more than 3 mm overriding of the vertebral body above over the vertebral body below
- the angle between two adjoining vertebrae is greater than 11°
- the height of the anterior border of a vertebral body is less than two-thirds of the posterior border.

Fractures of the thoracic spine

Hyperflexion is the principal mechanism of injury to the thoracic spine, with resultant wedging of vertebral bodies. Owing to the rigidity of the thoracic cage and the associated costovertebral articulations, most thoracic spine injuries are stable. However, internal stabilization may be necessary where kyphosis is pronounced.

Thoracolumbar spine

Fractures of the thoracolumbar spine comprise 40% of all vertebral fractures responsible for neurological deficit. Most are flexion or hyperflexion-rotation injuries. Plain films may demonstrate facet joint disruption, evidence of interspinal ligament disruption, posterior bony fragments protruding into the spinal canal and burst fragments at the superior surface of the vertebral body. These fractures are generally unstable.

Lumbar spine

Injuries similar to those previously described do occur in the lumbar spine. Three specific injuries of the lumbar spine merit further discussion and are broadly considered posterior distraction injuries of the vertebral arch. They constitute a group known as seatbelt injuries, produced when a hyperflexion force is applied to a person wearing a lap-only type seatbelt. In unrestrained persons, a flexion injury generally flexes the spine around a point through the anterior spinal column, typically causing a wedge compression fracture of the body. In the restrained person, the point of flexion is moved forward to the anterior abdominal wall. This change in momentum forces converts the hyperflexion mechanism to one of distraction. These injuries are caused by deceleration from high speed, as seen in head-on road traffic accidents or aircraft crashes.

Plain film radiology remains the first-line imaging study. Suggestive findings include:

- a vacant or empty appearance of the vertebral body on the AP film
- discontinuity in the cortex of the pedicles or spinous processes on the AP view
- fracture, with or without dislocation in the lateral view, which may be subtle.

CT or magnetic resonance imaging (MRI) are of value in further delineating architectural disruption. However, the exact nature of the fracture complex may be difficult to delineate on axial images, as the fractures are often orientated parallel to the scanning plane. Three-dimensional reconstruction of multislice CT images has greatly improved spinal injury imaging.

These injuries are often associated with concurrent intra-abdominal visceral injuries.

Chance fractures

These are characterized by an oblique or horizontal splitting of the spinous process and neural arch, extending the superior posterior aspect of the vertebral body into and damaging the intervertebral disc.

Horizontal fissure fracture

This fracture is very similar to the chance fracture, with the exception of the fracture line, which extends horizontally through the vertebral body to its anterior aspect.

Smith fracture

This spares the posterior spinous process. The fracture line involves the superior articular processes, the arch and a small posterior fragment of the superior posterior aspect of the vertebral body. Although the spinous process is intact, the posterior ligaments are disrupted.

Spinal shock

Spinal shock is often confused with the neurogenic shock of sympathetic interruption. They are different entities. Complete separation of the spinal cord from the brain abolishes voluntary movement and sensory perception and causes changes in cord physiology and reflex activity. Acute cord confusion is a simple explanation of the resulting pathophysiology. Spinal shock is manifested by the transient cessation of cord activity in the normal cord below the injury. The cord distal to the injury is unable to function as one would expect from a newly created upper motor neuron lesion. Spinal shock may last for a few hours to several weeks, depending on the segmental level and extent of the cord injury. During this period, both somatic and autonomic reflexes below the injured segments disappear. Spinal shock has been attributed to the sudden loss of descending facilitatory impulses from higher centres. Recovery from spinal shock is heralded by the return of the Babinski response, followed by the perineal reflexes. In quadriplegia and high paraplegia, as the cord recovers from spinal shock, either recovery of function (depending on the degree of injury resolution at the injury site) occurs or, more commonly, spasticity develops. If the cord injury is at the conus medullaris or the cauda equina, unless recovery occurs, a lower motor neuron pattern with areflexia remains.

Spinal cord injuries

Spinal cord injuries should be divided into primary and secondary injuries, as the causes affect the choice of treatment. Primary spinal cord injuries refer to the injuries directly caused by the trauma mechanism and its damaging energy onto the spinal cord. Secondary spinal cord injuries are caused by other mechanisms often related to the initial trauma, i.e. hypotension, hypoxia, etc.

Primary spinal cord damage (Fig. 3.3.3)

Transverse spinal cord syndrome

The spinal cord is completely damaged transversely across one or more adjacent spinal segments. No motor or autonomic information can be transmitted below the damaged area and ascending sensory stimuli from below the damaged spinal segments are blocked. The manifestations are: total flaccid paralysis, total anaesthesia, total analgesia and, usually, areflexia below the injured segment.

The transverse cord syndrome can be incomplete, with partial paralysis, reduced sensation and pain sensibility below the injured part.

The term 'sacral sparing' implies that some sensibility with or without motor activity in the areas supplied by the sacral segments is preserved in an otherwise complete transverse cord syndrome. The presence of sacral sparing implies an incomplete injury, as some neurological transmission through the injured segments is preserved. It will be recalled that spinothalamic and corticospinal transmission to and from sacral segments are located in the outermost parts of the spinal cord and are, therefore, immediately adjacent to the origin of the spinal cord's blood supply.

Acute central cervical cord syndrome

The central part or grey matter of the spinal cord is injured. Transmission in the outer rim of the spinal cord is essentially intact but impaired. The signs of this injury are:

- motor function: there will be weakness in both upper and lower limbs, with weakness marked in the upper limbs
- sensation: there is sensory loss in both upper and lower limbs, which is more severe in the upper limbs
- reflexes are variable.

This is frequently caused by a hyperextension injury and is typically seen in older patients with cervical spondylosis. In this situation, the cord is compressed between posterior osteophytes and the intervertebral disc in front and the ligamentum flavum behind.

Acute anterior cervical cord syndrome

The anterior half of the spinal cord – the region supplied by the anterior spinal artery – is

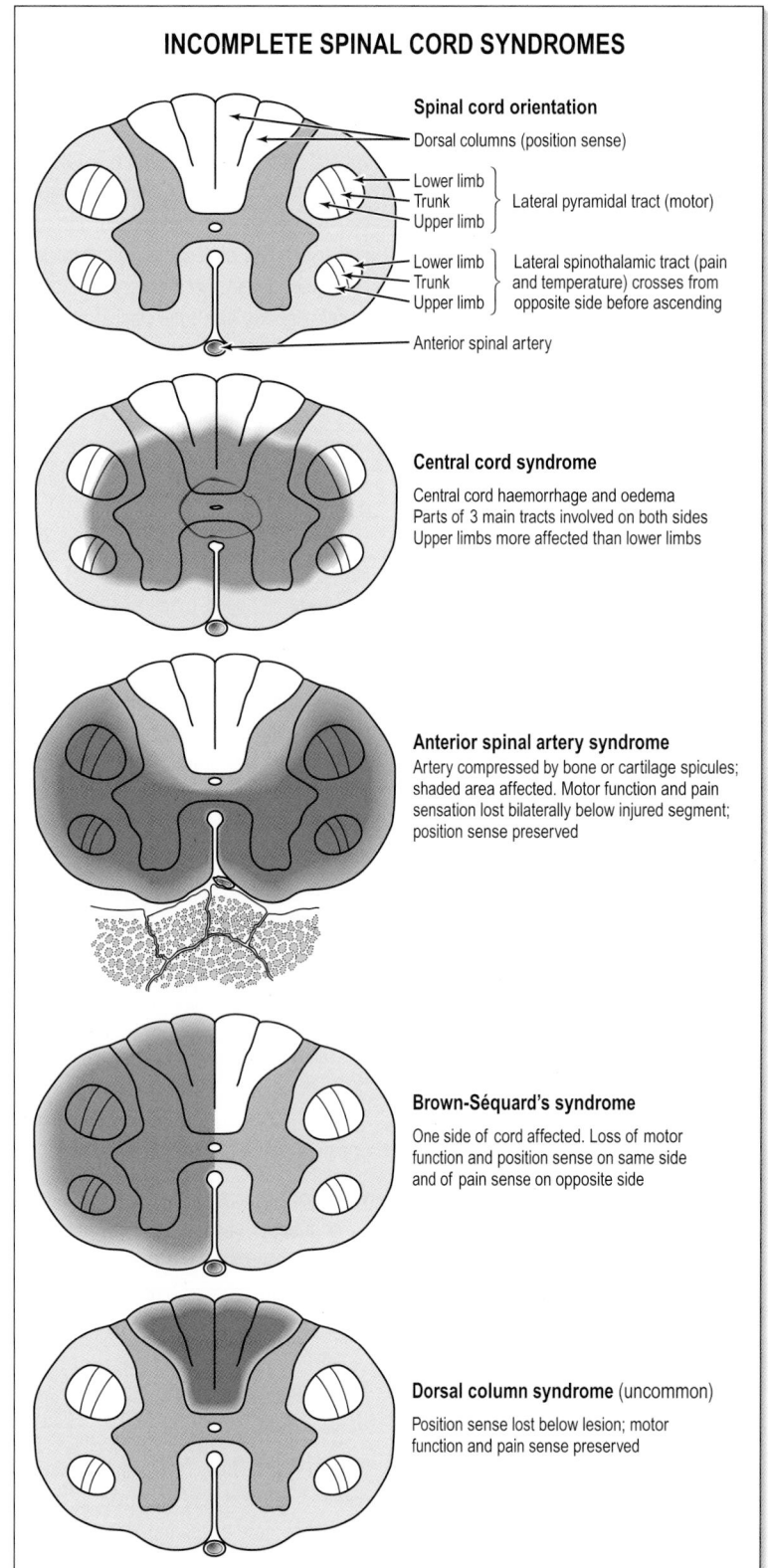

INCOMPLETE SPINAL CORD SYNDROMES

Spinal cord orientation

Dorsal columns (position sense)

Lower limb
Trunk
Upper limb } Lateral pyramidal tract (motor)

Lower limb
Trunk
Upper limb } Lateral spinothalamic tract (pain and temperature) crosses from opposite side before ascending

Anterior spinal artery

Central cord syndrome

Central cord haemorrhage and oedema
Parts of 3 main tracts involved on both sides
Upper limbs more affected than lower limbs

Anterior spinal artery syndrome

Artery compressed by bone or cartilage spicules; shaded area affected. Motor function and pain sensation lost bilaterally below injured segment; position sense preserved

Brown-Séquard's syndrome

One side of cord affected. Loss of motor function and position sense on same side and of pain sense on opposite side

Dorsal column syndrome (uncommon)

Position sense lost below lesion; motor function and pain sense preserved

Fig. 3.3.3 Spinal core and syndromes. *(From Clinical Symposia 1998; 34(2): 17. Comprehensive Management of Spinal Cord Injury, Plate 11. Redrawn with permission of Novartis Pty Ltd, Basel, Switzerland.)*

damaged (see Figs 3.3.3 and 3.3.5). There is motor loss or paralysis below the level of the injured segment(s). Spinothalamic transmission is impaired and thus there is analgesia with loss of temperature sensation and coarse touch. As the dorsal columns are relatively intact, there is some preservation of joint position, vibration sense and fine touch. In the context of an acute cord injury, the patient may not interpret dorsal column preservation in terms of joint position sense or light touch. Dorsal column function may be manifested as preservation of vague and poorly localized sensation in the extremities.

These injuries are frequently the result of flexion–rotation or vertical compression injuries.

Brown-Séquard's syndrome

This syndrome is a functional cord hemisection with dissociated sensory loss. One half of the cord is damaged. In a pure Brown-Séquard lesion, ipsilateral motor function is impaired, as are light touch, joint position sense and vibration. Contralateral spinothalamic sensation – that is, pain and temperature – is impaired, whereas ipsilateral sensation is relatively preserved. Reflexes are variable.

Posterior cord syndrome

This is an uncommon injury that causes contusion or disruption to the dorsal columns, leading to impaired or disrupted proprioception, vibration and fine touch sensation.

This syndrome is usually the result of penetrating trauma to the back or a hyperextension injury in association with fractures of the vertebral arch.

Spinal cord concussion

This diagnosis implies a temporary cessation of spinal cord neurological function. In this instance, there is a near full recovery of cord function within 48 hours. The patient will be first assessed as suffering from either a complete or an incomplete spinal cord injury and will then recover within the above period. The patient has suffered an injury to the spinal cord that has been enough temporarily to cease electrical activity in the injured spinal segment, with no, or very little, mechanical or anatomical injury to the cord, such as haemorrhage or contusion. It is the pattern of recovery over a day or two that allows the diagnosis to be made. Unfortunately, this constitutes less than 1% of all spinal cord injuries.

In all the incomplete spinal cord syndromes, the location of cord pressure or damage varies in terms of incompleteness and segmental level(s) of cord injury and so will the range of symptoms and signs.

Secondary spinal cord damage

It is often believed that most spinal cord damage occurs at the time of injury, but it may occur subsequent to the initial injury [6]. This secondary damage may be caused by:

- Inappropriate manual handling [4,5]. Subsequent mishandling causes significant movement at the site of the primary vertebral injury, leading to spinal cord damage. This can be prevented by careful handling of the patient. It is important to be aware of the possibility of a spinal cord injury and protect the spine until the diagnosis has been excluded. This involves standard cervical in-line immobilization, whole-spine immobilization using a spine board or a Jordan frame and 'log roll' for moving the patient.
- Hypoxia and hypotension. These aggravate the primary injury, causing progressive neurological deterioration by mechanisms similar to those that cause secondary brain damage in head injury.
- Acute response to injury. Intrinsic metabolic changes in the previously undamaged spinal cord at the region of the initial vertebral injury may also cause secondary deterioration due to oedema, haemorrhage and the release of metabolically active substances from damaged neurons. The culmination of the pathophysiological processes leads to cord ischaemia and oedema, thereby promoting further neurological damage. The oedema and haemorrhage tend to resolve within 10–14 days, with some improvement in neurological function. Resolving oedema results in local segmental recovery. However, residual ischaemic change in secondarily affected spinal cord adjacent to the primarily injured segments does occur, producing permanent neurological deficit.

Unconscious patients

As previously mentioned, the definitive diagnosis of spinal cord injury is a secondary survey consideration and hence identified primarily from symptoms and physical findings. There is no pathognomonic sign of a spinal cord injury in an unconscious patient. The following should alert the examiner to the possibility of a coexisting spinal cord injury in an unconscious trauma victim:

- paradoxical breathing or chest wall movement (diaphragmatic breathing) in the absence of a major airway obstruction, stove-in or large flail chest suggests a cervical cord injury
- priapism in the unconscious trauma victim suggests quadriplegia or high to mid-thoracic paraplegia
- preserved facial grimace in the absence of a response to painful stimuli in the limbs
- lower limb flaccidity in the presence of normal upper limb tone suggests paraplegia
- observed upper limb movement in the absence of lower limb movement suggests paraplegia
- the combination of the persistent bradycardia and hypotension despite volume challenge
- where this is accompanied by a flaccid rectal sphincter, there is an increased likelihood of spinal cord injury.

Special attention, again, should go to protection of the C-spine in this category of patients. As the golden standard of imaging, the cervical spine CT is highly sensitive and may reliably exclude unstable injuries in patients with obtunded or intubated blunt trauma [17].

Documentation conventions

Two of the pitfalls in the management of any neurological injury are terminology and documentation. The following convention is recommended.

Motor function is recorded either using segmental terminology in written format or on a muscle chart (Fig. 3.3.4). It will be impossible to chart every segment accurately, but motor power in the upper and lower limbs should be able to be confidently recorded. Power should be graded using the 0–5/5 system.

Sensation is recorded more descriptively. Normaesthesia, hyperaesthesia, hypoaesthesia and anaesthesia are the descriptors for dorsal column function and testing for light touch. Normalgesia, hyperalgesia, hypoalgesia and analgesia are used in describing pain perception. These are recorded on sensory charts or described according to the following two examples.

In a patient with a transverse spinal cord syndrome, incomplete below C6 and complete below T1, the sensation is described as:

- normaesthesia and normalgesia to C5
- hypoalgesia and hypoaesthesia below C5
- anaesthesia and analgesia below T1.

In a patient with an acute central cervical cord syndrome below C6, with total segmental paralysis in the C6–C8 segments and with some involvement of C5, the sensation might be described as:

- normaesthesia and normalgesia to C4
- hypoalgesia and hypoaesthesia below C4
- anaesthesia and analgesia below C5
- hypoalgesia and hypoaesthesia below T1.

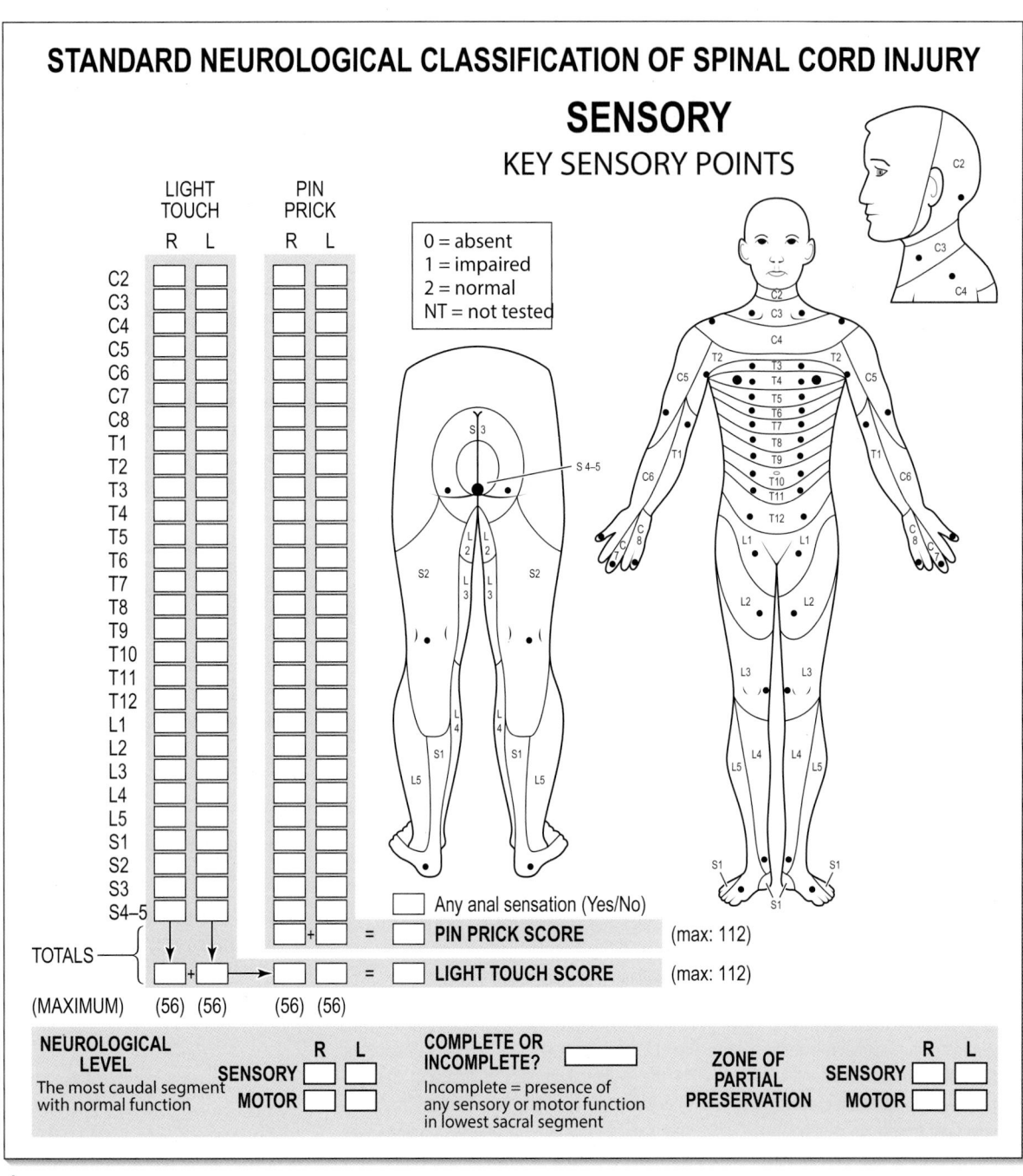

Fig. 3.3.4 (A–C) Documentation of neurological injury.

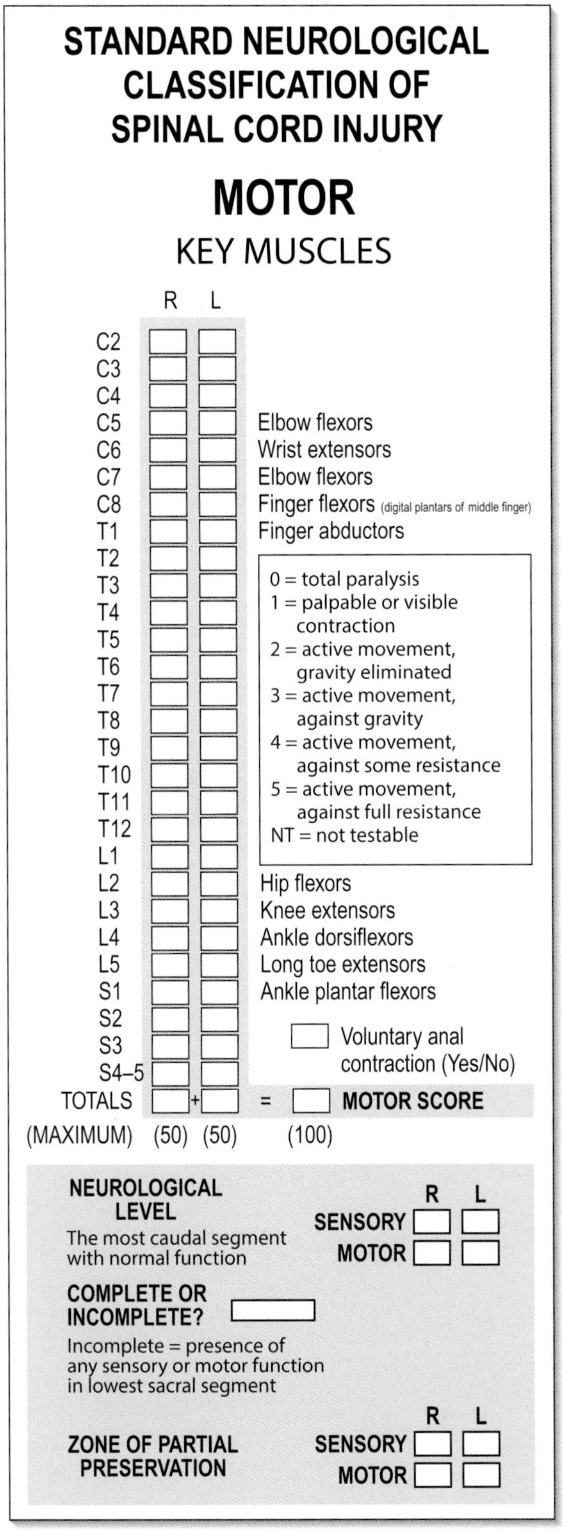

STANDARD NEUROLOGICAL CLASSIFICATION OF SPINAL CORD INJURY

MOTOR
KEY MUSCLES

R L

C2
C3
C4
C5 Elbow flexors
C6 Wrist extensors
C7 Elbow flexors
C8 Finger flexors (digital plantars of middle finger)
T1 Finger abductors
T2
T3
T4
T5
T6
T7
T8
T9
T10
T11
T12
L1
L2 Hip flexors
L3 Knee extensors
L4 Ankle dorsiflexors
L5 Long toe extensors
S1 Ankle plantar flexors
S2
S3
S4–5

0 = total paralysis
1 = palpable or visible contraction
2 = active movement, gravity eliminated
3 = active movement, against gravity
4 = active movement, against some resistance
5 = active movement, against full resistance
NT = not testable

Voluntary anal contraction (Yes/No)

TOTALS [ ] + [ ] = [ ] MOTOR SCORE
(MAXIMUM) (50) (50) (100)

NEUROLOGICAL LEVEL
The most caudal segment with normal function

R L
SENSORY [ ] [ ]
MOTOR [ ] [ ]

COMPLETE OR INCOMPLETE? [ ]
Incomplete = presence of any sensory or motor function in lowest sacral segment

R L
ZONE OF PARTIAL PRESERVATION
SENSORY [ ] [ ]
MOTOR [ ] [ ]

B

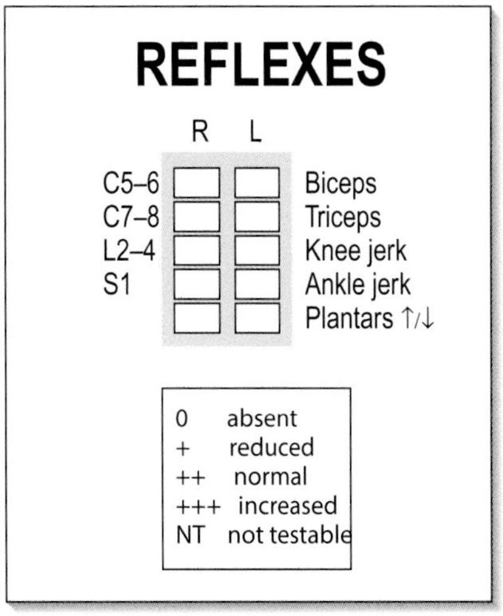

REFLEXES

R L
C5–6 Biceps
C7–8 Triceps
L2–4 Knee jerk
S1 Ankle jerk
  Plantars ↑/↓

0 absent
+ reduced
++ normal
+++ increased
NT not testable

C

Fig. 3.3.4 (A–C) (Continued)

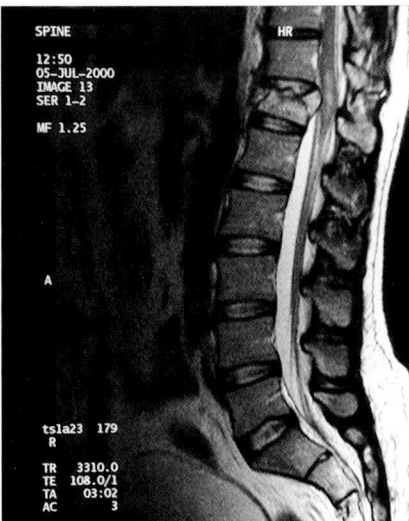

Fig. 3.3.5 MRI scan of acute central cord syndrome.

Controversies/emerging issues

- Recent research showed that patients with persistent midline cervical tenderness result in considerable healthcare costs [18]. With more and more understanding of the financial, social and psychological impact of spinal trauma, it is expected that more and more emphasis is going to be put on prevention, early detection and therapy in cases of (potential) spinal injury.

- Clinical decision rules for cervical spinal clearance will need further testing with CT scanning as the new standard diagnostic modality of first choice. It is therefore expected that these rules will change according to results found in future research.
- With the technical developments expected in the coming years, it is expected for MRI scanners to become more widely available, to be faster, to have higher diagnostic accuracy and to become cheaper. Also, since CT scanning has the disadvantage of the patient being exposed to radiation, it is expected that indications for MRI scanning of the spine will be broadened.

Acknowledgement

The author of this chapter in the previous edition of this textbook was Jeff Wassertheil. The text in this new edition is based on the original chapter for which Jeff Wassertheil must be acknowledged.

References

[1] Lowery DW, Wald MM, Browne BJ, et al. Epidemiology of cervical spine injury victims. Ann Emerg Med 2001;38:12–16.
[2] Rotem TR, Lawson JS, Wilson FW, et al. Severe spinal cord injuries related to rugby union and league football in New South Wales, 1984–1996. Med J Aust 1998;168:379–81.
[3] Selecki BR, Berry G, Kwok B, et al. Experience with spine injuries in NSW. Aust NZ J Surg 1986;56:567–76.
[4] Toscano J. Prevention of neurological deterioration before admission to a spinal cord injury unit. Paraplegia 1988;26:143–50.
[5] Superspeciality Service Subcommittee of the Australian Health Ministers Advisory Council Guidelines for acute spinal cord injury services. Australian Institute of Health, AGPS; 1990.
[6] Goldberg W, Mueller C, Panacek E, et al. Distribution and patterns of blunt cervical spine injury. Ann Emerg Med 2001;38:12–16.
[7] Kwan I, Bunn F, Roberts I, on behalf of the WHO Pre-hospital Trauma Care Steering Committee. Spinal immobilization for trauma patients. Cochrane Database System Rev 2001:2.
[8] Hauswald M, Ong G, Tandberg D, Omar Z. Out-of-hospital spinal immobilization: its effect on neurologic injury. Acad Emerg Med 1998;5:214–9.
[9] Chan D, Goldberg R, Tascone A, et al. The effect of spinal immobilization on healthy volunteers. Ann Emerg Med 1994;23:48–51.
[10] Keller BP, Lubbert PH, Keller E, Leenen LP. Tissue-interface pressures on three different support-surfaces for trauma patients. Injury 2005;36:946–8.
[11] Hoffman JR, Mower W, Wolfson AB, et al. Validity of a set of clinical criteria to rule out injury to the cervical spine in patients with blunt trauma. N Engl J Med 2000;343:94–9.
[12] Stiell IG, Wells GA, Vandemheen KL, et al. The Canadian C-Spine Rule for radiography in alert and stable trauma patients. J Am Med Assoc 2001;286:1841–8.
[13] Stiell IG, Clement CM, McKnight RD, et al. The Canadian C-Spine rule versus the NEXUS low-risk criteria in patients with trauma. N Engl J Med 2003;349:2510–8.
[14] Zoe A, Naher CG, Verhagen AP, et al. Accuracy of the Canadian C-spine rule and NEXUS to screen for the clinically important cervical spine injury in patients following blunt trauma: a systematic review. Can Med Assoc J 2012;184:E867–76.
[15] Bracken MB. Steroids for acute spinal cord injury. Cochrane Database Syst Rev 2012
[16] Brown D. Guidelines for the use of methylprednisolone in acute spinal cord injury. Melbourne: Victorian Spinal Cord Service Austin & Repatriation Medical Centre; 2000.
[17] Kirschner J, Sepaul RA. Does computed tomography rule out clinically significant cervical spine injuries in patients with obtunded or intubated blunt trauma. Ann Emerg Med 2012;60:737–8.
[18] Ackland HM, Wolfe R, Cameron PA, et al. Health resource utilisation costs in acute patients with persistent midline cervical tenderness following road trauma. Injury 2012;43:1908–16.

3.4 Facial trauma

Lewis Macken

ESSENTIALS

1 Facial trauma is a common problem in the emergency department (ED), usually as an isolated injury, often after an assault. It may also occur after multisystem injury.

2 Facial injuries that do not threaten the airway or risk life-threatening haemorrhage can usually be assessed and managed as part of the secondary survey.

3 Early diagnosis of facial injuries is important, as late diagnosis may lead to compromised function and an unsatisfactory cosmetic outcome.

4 CT scanning has replaced plain radiography for the delineation of facial fractures.

5 Visual assessment after facial trauma can be difficult, especially in the unconscious patient, but is an essential element of the clinical examination.

6 Penetrating trauma to the face is rarely fatal, but may result in significant morbidity. Attention to early airway intervention is vital after penetrating injuries, especially in patients with gunshot wounds to the face.

Introduction

Facial trauma is defined as injury to the facial soft tissues (including the ear) and bony skeleton. This covers a wide spectrum of injuries [1]. Patients with facial trauma are usually male, between the ages of 20 and 25 years and have usually sustained their injuries as a result of blunt trauma. Isolated facial injury after an assault accounts for most injuries, with motor vehicle injuries, contact sports and falls accounting for most of the remainder [2]. Up to 20% of patients with facial injuries as part of multisystem injury will have associated life-threatening injuries [3,4].

Management of blunt and penetrating trauma to the face can be challenging. Life-threatening facial injuries are those that result in airway compromise or ongoing haemorrhage. At the same time, attention must be given to preserving long-term cosmesis and the normal functions of sight, speech and mastication. After immediate resuscitation and stabilization, management of facial injuries requires a knowledge of anatomy, the injuries commonly associated with facial injury and an awareness of treatment methods for the differing injuries to the face [5,6]. Consultation should be sought when the injury threatens the restoration of normal function or appearance. Non-accidental injury should always be considered, as some studies report that over 20% of head, neck and facial injuries in women are the result of domestic violence [7].

History

The evaluation should commence with the history, with emphasis given to the mechanism of injury. The velocity of force directed to the face determines the degree of facial fracture [8]. Respiratory and haemodynamic observations and quantification of pre-hospital blood loss are important components of the history.

Examination

The physical examination involves evaluation of all facial areas by inspection, palpation and assessment of function. Inspection of the face may reveal deformity, loss of normal symmetry, changes in contour and localized areas of swelling. Skull-base fractures may be suggested by periorbital or postauricular bruising and the ears must be inspected to exclude haemotympanum or cerebrospinal fluid (CSF) otorrhoea. Gentle systematic palpation of the facial skeleton should follow, assessing for tenderness and feeling for asymmetry, bony margin irregularities, abnormal motion or crepitus. Specific attention should be given to the supraorbital and infraorbital margins, the zygomas, nasal bones, maxilla and mandible. Mobility associated with midfacial maxillary fractures is assessed by grasping the anterior maxilla with the thumb and index finger of one hand, while stabilizing the forehead at the nasal bridge with the other. Ophthalmological evaluation includes inspection for enophthalmos or exophthalmos and globe injury and assessment of pupillary responses, visual acuity, visual fields, extraocular movements and inquiry for diplopia. Although eye injury is an infrequent complication of blunt trauma, subjective impairment in visual acuity remains the most sensitive single predictor of eye injury [9] and examination that reveals the presence of an afferent pupillary defect or a non-reactive pupil is the most important factor in predicting the severity of eye injury [10]. The nose should be inspected for the presence of any septal deviation, haematoma (more common in children) or CSF rhinorrhoea. Oral examination is necessary to look for loose, broken or missing teeth, malocclusion of dentition, soft tissue lacerations and contusions. Examination of the mandible includes assessment of the temporomandibular joint in the open and closed positions.

Assessment of the function of facial structures is the final component of the examination of the face. Malocclusion, often identified by the presence of a new gap between the occlusal surfaces of the teeth when the patient closes his/her jaws, is a good indicator of maxillary or mandibular fracture. Similarly, pain on biting on a tongue depressor, loss of bite strength and limitation of jaw movement are strongly suggestive of a fracture; the patient should be asked if the bite has subjectively changed [11,12]. Motor function of the facial nerve should be assessed and all three branches of the trigeminal nerve should be evaluated. Commonly encountered symptoms and signs are hypoaesthesia or paraesthesia of the upper lip or upper alveolar margin, suggesting fracture of the maxilla causing injury to the alveolar branches of the infraorbital nerve. Sensory changes in the lower lip and lower alveolar margin suggest fracture through the mandibular canal, causing inferior alveolar nerve injury (a branch of the mandibular nerve) [11].

Radiographic examination

Computed tomography (CT) is the initial imaging modality of choice in evaluating patients with facial trauma. Although an orthopantomogram (OPG) view is very helpful in investigating a suspected fracture of the mandible, CT will be required for patients with clinically obvious complex facial injuries, especially of the upper and middle thirds of the face and for patients with multisystem injuries. CT and derived image reconstructions display soft tissue relations to the bony skeleton and the degree of skeletal distortion, displacement and comminution. CT assists with surgical planning and evidently allows other injured areas to be imaged at the same time for multitrauma patients.

Immediate management in the emergency department

It is important to prioritize injuries in the management of the patient with facial trauma because facial injuries that do not threaten the airway or risk life-threatening haemorrhage can usually be assessed and managed as part of the secondary survey. Proper attention should be given to potentially more significant head, chest and abdominal injuries before a non-life-threatening facial injury is thoroughly evaluated, no matter how impressive and disfiguring the facial injury appears. The association of facial injury with cervical spine or cord injury is questionable, especially if vehicular trauma was not the cause [13]. After blunt assault, the incidence of associated cervical spine injury is low, but is more likely if there is a fall after the assault [14]. Patients with clinically significant head injuries (especially Glasgow Coma Score [GCS] <9) are at greater risk of having cervical spine injuries than those with evidence of facial trauma [15–18]; intracranial injuries are more frequently associated with facial fractures than are cervical spine injuries [19].

Airway management

Asphyxia due to upper airway obstruction is the major cause of death from facial trauma.

The airway must be rapidly assessed, respiratory obstruction relieved and an adequate airway established. Managing these patients in the supine position is often risky and early semi-elective intubation may be required. Signs of partial airway obstruction include tachycardia, tachypnoea, restlessness, fighting to sit up, noisy respirations, stridor and supraclavicular and intercostal retractions. This may lead to complete obstruction. An unobstructed airway in the presence of facial trauma should be closely monitored because increasing oedema and persistent bleeding may later compromise airway patency.

Fractures of the mandible and maxilla with posterior or inferior displacement, together with displaced soft tissues, blood, secretions or other foreign material, may lead to airway embarrassment. Simple airway measures, such as chin lift and jaw thrust should be performed and the mouth immediately examined. Any loose foreign material, such as food, broken dentures or teeth or bone fragments, should be removed and blood clots suctioned. If anterior traction on the fractured mandible or on the mobile segment of the maxilla (performed by inserting two fingers behind the soft palate and lifting the middle third of the face forwards and upwards) fails to relieve posterior pharyngeal obstruction and does not establish unobstructed ventilation, a definitive airway must be placed. Distorted facial anatomy may make bag and mask ventilation difficult. Rapid-sequence orotracheal intubation can usually be performed. Awake fibreoptic intubation is an option, but the presence of persistent bleeding makes the procedure technically difficult. Standard drills for anticipated intubation difficulties should be at hand and equipment for performing a cricothyroidotomy and transtracheal jet ventilation should be available. A surgical airway may be life saving when anatomical disruption makes intubation difficult. A tracheostomy performed under local anaesthesia in the operating theatre is often the safest option in a stable patient with significant midfacial injuries in whom airway difficulties are expected [20].

Control of haemorrhage

Traumatic facial haemorrhage can be massive, difficult to manage and potentially life threatening in approximately 5% of patients with midfacial fractures [21]. Bleeding from midface trauma mainly originates from branches of the

external carotid artery (with branches of the internal carotid artery also supplying the nose). Most haemorrhage can be controlled with direct pressure, anterior nasal packs and double balloon catheters providing anterior and posterior nasopharyngeal tamponade (the placement of 12–14 G Foley catheters with 10 mL balloons inflated and taped under tension to the side of the face is an alternative) [22]. Care must be taken with nasal instrumentation: the incidence of associated skull-base fractures is more common with orbital wall or rim fractures than with more inferiorly located facial fractures. Also, a skull-base fracture is more likely in the presence of multiple facial fractures (the presence of three or more facial fractures is associated with an incidence of skull-base fracture of up to 33%) [23]. Attempts to clamp bleeding vessels in the emergency department (ED) should be avoided because of the associated risks of damaging important structures, such as the facial nerve, parotid duct or lacrimal apparatus. If simple measures fail to arrest the bleeding, operative reduction of the fractures, especially of the maxilla, and possible ligation of bleeding vessels should be undertaken, with angiography and selective embolization considered if other measures fail.

Disposition

After initial stabilization, immediate treatment of most facial injuries is mainly supportive. Fractures requiring operative management are often dealt with on a delayed basis, when soft tissue swelling is resolving. The need for antibiotics for patients with facial trauma depends on the mechanism of injury, the extent of the injury and the immune status of the patient. Systemic antibiotics are not required for most facial wounds. However, antibiotics should be given for bites and grossly contaminated wounds; wounds that extend into the oral cavity, nose and paranasal sinuses; wounds with exposed nasal or ear cartilage; crush wounds and wounds with considerable oedema; and for immunologically compromised patients. Specific antibiotic choices include amoxicillin–clavulanate or cephalexin. However, the evidence to support or refute the use of prophylactic antibiotics in facial trauma is weak. Tetanus immunity should be assessed.

Thorough documentation of injuries is important for medicolegal reasons, as facial injuries are frequently due to personal assault and so later litigation is often likely.

Specific injuries

Soft-tissue injuries

Soft-tissue injuries include abrasions, contusions, lacerations, avulsions and burns. The aim of treatment is to preserve appearance and function. The management of soft-tissue facial injuries involves consideration of how the wound should be repaired and whether it should be repaired in the ED. Possible reasons for delayed wound closure are more urgent coexisting injuries, severe crush injuries, the presence of a foreign body, severely contaminated wounds and an underlying fracture. In these cases, the wound should be irrigated, haemostasis achieved, covered with normal saline-soaked gauze and the patient referred to the appropriate specialty team.

Soft-tissue injuries that usually require repair in the operating theatre include ocular or significant eyelid injury; parotid gland or duct injury; facial nerve injury (injuries to the cheek between the tragus of the ear and a line drawn vertically through the pupil may be associated with damage to the facial nerve, parotid gland or duct); nasolacrimal apparatus injury; alveolar process wounds and significant tooth injuries; lacerations with significant tissue loss or contamination or requiring exact anatomical closure; or where difficulties with patient cooperation are expected. Careful consideration is required before areas of special concern are repaired in the ED, e.g. the lips and perioral area; tongue and oral cavity; nose; ears; periorbital structures; and eyebrows. The eyebrow should not be shaved. Subperichondrial haematomas of the ear require drainage within 7–10 days to avoid permanent cartilage injury (cauliflower ear) and to achieve best cosmetic results. For all wounds closed in the ED, careful attention must be given to thorough cleansing. This can be effectively achieved with pulsatile wound irrigation with normal saline and abrasions containing dirt or other foreign bodies must be scrubbed to prevent traumatic tattooing of the dermis. If the wound is gaping or if structures deeper than the skin and the subcutaneous layer are involved, then multiple-layer repair is usually advisable. This helps to prevent deep tissue space collections and may produce a better cosmetic result, with less scar depression or widening.

Visual assessment after facial trauma can be difficult, especially in the unconscious patient. Loss of vision after blunt facial trauma may be due to: direct injury to the globe; direct injury to the optic nerve (usually bony impingement); indirect injury to the optic nerve (deceleration injury); or due to raised local intraocular pressure (orbital compartment syndrome [OCS]) [24]. OCS is an uncommon ophthalmic emergency, but the diagnosis is clinical. Relief of the intraocular hypertension is time critical and usually requires a lateral canthotomy and inferior cantholysis [25].

Facial fractures

The facial skeleton is constructed to allow applied force to be dispersed via a series of small bone fractures, thereby protecting the skull and intracranial contents. The maxilla and mandible require three times the amount of applied force to cause a fracture as do the nasal bones [26]. Diagnosis of a facial fracture involves a combination of inspection, palpation and radiographic examination. Fractures other than undisplaced fractures of the nose, zygomatic arch or maxilla will usually require acute maxillofacial surgical review. All fractures should be managed initially with elevation of the patient's head, if associated injuries allow this, and the application of ice.

Mandible

The horseshoe shape of the mandible disperses applied force, which leads to fractures occurring at vulnerable sites regardless of the point of impact and a high incidence of multiple fractures. Common sites of fracture are the condylar neck and angle and the body at the level of the first or second molar [27]. Fractures of the mandibular body usually demonstrate point tenderness, malocclusion and abnormal range of motion and interference with normal mastication. The integrity of the dental arch must be assessed. The application of a soft cervical collar may offer symptomatic relief by providing mandibular support.

Antibiotics should be given when there is the suggestion of a compound fracture with extension into the oral cavity. Most fractures will require some form of internal fixation. Complications of mandibular fractures include chin paraesthesia or hypoaesthesia, delayed union, non-union, infection and malocclusion [28].

Zygomatic arch

Isolated fractures of the zygomatic arch are uncommon and are more commonly part of a more extensive zygomatic complex fracture. An isolated fracture may be evidenced by a depression over the arch, point tenderness and limited or painful mouth opening owing to impingement on the coronoid process of the mandible by the fractured arch. Surgical reduction is required for cosmetic reasons or to correct restricted mandibular range of motion.

Zygomatic complex

Blunt trauma to the zygoma more commonly results in fractures at the articulations of the zygomatic bones with the frontal bone, maxilla and zygomatic process of the temporal bone. Separation at the zygomaticofrontal suture, the zygomaticotemporal suture and at the zygomaticomaxillary suture or infraorbital rim produces the tripod or tripartite fracture. Frequently, the lateral wall of the maxillary sinus and the lateral and central portions of the orbital floor (not to be confused with the orbital blowout fracture) will also fracture as part of the zygomaticomaxillary complex fracture.

Clinical signs of a tripod fracture include flattening of the cheek initially (owing to depression of the fracture segment); this is best seen by standing behind and above the patient, but it is soon replaced by significant swelling. Other signs are hypo-/hyperaesthesia or paraesthesia in the distribution of the infraorbital nerve; asymmetry of the ocular levels; a palpable step defect of the inferior orbital margin; and circumorbital and subconjunctival ecchymoses [11]. Diplopia is often also present and 10–20% of these fractures are accompanied by an ocular injury [29].

Orbital fractures

Fracture of the orbital floor may occur as part of a zygomaticomaxillary fracture or as an isolated injury – the less common orbital blowout fracture. This is a fracture of the orbital floor without fracture of the orbital margin. An increase in intraorbital pressure, as delivered by a fist or a small ball, is transmitted to within the orbit and the relatively weak orbital floor is disrupted, with possible herniation of the contents into the maxillary sinus. Very rarely, a supraorbital rim fracture may be part of a frontal sinus fracture, or lateral orbital wall fracture may be associated with a fracture of the zygoma or a medial orbital wall fracture may occur with a nasoethmoidal fracture. Clinical examination in cases of fracture of the orbital floor may reveal enophthalmos, a difference in pupillary levels, diplopia and impairment of upward gaze and infraorbital hypo-/hyperaesthesia or paraesthesia [6]. An irregular edge to the orbital rim may be evident on palpation. The integrity and function of the eye should be documented to exclude associated injury. CT scanning is necessary to define these fractures fully. Orbital apex fractures are uncommon, but clinical or radiological signs of optic nerve compression (e.g. retro-bulbar haematoma or bone fragment impingement) necessitate urgent surgical referral [30]. All patients with orbital margin or floor fractures require referral. Complications of surgical treatment of orbital floor fractures include persistent diplopia, hypo-/hyperaesthesia or paraesthesia, ectropion and epiphora [31].

Maxillary fractures

Fractures of the maxilla include fractures of the alveolar ridge of the maxilla, fracture of the anterolateral wall of the maxillary sinus and the Le Fort fractures. Isolated maxillary fractures are rare.

In Paris in 1901, Le Fort described a classification of patterns of midface fractures, following cadaveric experiments [32]: Le Fort I (horizontal maxillary fracture) involves only the maxilla at the level of the nasal fossae; Le Fort II (pyramidal fracture) is the most common midface fracture and involves the maxilla, nasal bones and medial aspect of the orbit; Le Fort III (craniofacial dysjunction) separates the midfacial skeleton from the base of the cranium, with the fracture extending through the base of the nose and ethmoid region and across the orbits and zygomatic arches bilaterally.

Most midface fractures are combination injuries, with different Le Fort patterns on each side of the face. Le Fort II and III fractures may require urgent reduction in the ED to improve airway compromise and to arrest ongoing haemorrhage. Patients with such injuries may demonstrate mid-face mobility, and these fractures are associated with skull-base fractures, leading to CSF rhinorrhoea. All patients require a complete eye examination and these injuries necessitate referral.

Nasal fractures

These are common facial fractures. Diagnosis is largely clinical, plain X-rays are unreliable and usually unnecessary and the major concerns for the emergency physician are control of epistaxis and exclusion of a septal haematoma. Displaced fractures should be reduced within 7–10 days.

Nasoethmoidal fractures are more complicated and are caused by trauma to the bridge of the nose. Disruption of the medial canthal ligaments may produce rounding of the palpebral fissures or widening of the intercanthal distance (telecanthus) [11]. Persistent epistaxis and CSF rhinorrhoea may also be evident. Referral is necessary for these patients.

Temporomandibular joint dislocation

Dislocation of the temporomandibular joint may follow trauma to the face or may occur as a result of simply opening the mouth widely. Patients complain of inability to close the mouth and moderate discomfort. X-rays should be performed to confirm that no fracture is present and dislocation will be evidenced by the appearance of the condyle anterior to the articular eminence of the fossa. A directed history will exclude extrapyramidal dystonia mimicking a dislocation. Reassurance, sedation and firm downward pressure of the physician's thumbs on the patient's posterior teeth, with upward tilting of the symphysis, is usually successful in relocating the mandibular condyles. Post-reduction X-rays are not always necessary. Analgesia and a soft diet should be prescribed and the patient warned to avoid wide opening of the mouth in the short term [33].

Penetrating injuries to the face

Penetrating trauma to the face from gunshot, stab wounds and impaling foreign bodies is often dramatic at the time of presentation. Such isolated injury is rarely fatal, but may result in significant morbidity due to the combination of soft-tissue and bone defects. The wounding capability of penetrating projectiles (bullets and pellets) is proportional to the energy imparted to the tissue; therefore, the mass of the slug, its velocity and design and the density of the body tissue penetrated determine the amount of tissue destruction [34].

Early aggressive airway management is necessary in patients with gunshot wounds to the face, as respiratory decompensation may be rapid: approximately one-third of patients will require emergency airway intervention [35]. Shotgun and stab wounds are less likely to require an emergency airway, although the presence of a significant vascular injury or oedema remains a universal indication for airway intervention and patients with mandibular entry sites are more likely to require an emergency airway than those with midfacial entry sites. Orotracheal intubation can usually be achieved, with cricothyroidotomy the preferred alternative if necessary. Central nervous system injuries are common after gunshot injuries and CT scans of the head and cervical spine will be required [36].

Arterial injury is suggested by evidence of active bleeding and an expanding haematoma; angiography (carotid and vertebral arteries), which is required in approximately 35–40% of cases [35,36], should be performed when the bullet trajectory suggests proximity to major vessels or the skull base or where the knife or foreign body is in close proximity to a major vascular structure [36–38].

Peripheral nerve injuries, especially of the facial nerve and the mandibular branch of the trigeminal nerve, are also frequently present [36]. Careful eye examination is necessary because ocular trauma is the most common overall complication of penetrating facial trauma [39].

Antibiotics and tetanus prophylaxis are indicated and wounds are managed with conservative debridement, closed reduction of facial fractures and early repair of palatal injuries. Open facial fracture reduction is usually delayed [35].

Conclusion

Facial trauma is common in the ED, encompasses many types of injury and, after rapid exclusion of life-threatening complications, requires thorough patient evaluation to exclude other more urgent injuries. The aim of management of isolated facial injuries is the maintenance of normal function and appearance.

Controversies

- Consideration of an immediate surgical airway, rather than attempted oral intubation, in a patient with significant facial trauma and a compromised or deteriorating airway.
- The role of angiography and selective embolization in the management of patients with significant haemorrhage from blunt and penetrating trauma.
- Consideration of early intubation in the presence of midface fractures with ongoing haemorrhage in the supine patient with other system injuries.

References

[1] McKay M, Mayersak R. Facial trauma. In: Marx JA, Hockberger RS, Walls RM, editors. Rosen's emergency medicine – concepts and clinical practice, 7th ed. Philadelphia: Mosby Elsevier; 2010. p. 323–36.

[2] Hogg NJ, Stewart TC, Armstrong JE. Epidemiology of maxillofacial injuries at trauma hospitals in Ontario, Canada, between 1992 and 1997. J Trauma 2000;49:425–32.

[3] Tung T, Tseng WS, Chen CT. Acute life-threatening injuries in facial trauma patients: a review of 1025 patients. J Trauma 2000;49:420–4.

[4] Back CPN, McLean NR, Anderson PJ. The conservative management of facial fractures: indications and outcomes. J Plastic Reconstruct Aesthet Surg 2007;60:146–51.

[5] Bailitz J. Trauma to the face. In: Tintinalli JE, editor. Emergency medicine: a comprehensive study guide, 7th ed. New York: McGraw-Hill; 2010. p. 1730–8.

[6] Carithers JS, Koch BB. Evaluation and management of facial fractures. Am Fam Phys 1997;55:2675–82.

[7] Ochs HA, Neuenschwander MC, Dodson TB. Are head, neck and facial injuries markers of domestic violence? J Am Dent Assoc 1996;127:757–61.

[8] Rhee JS, Posey L, Yoganandan N. Experimental trauma to the malar eminence: fracture biomechanics and injury patterns. Otolaryngol Head Neck Surg 2001;125:351–5.

[9] Dutton GN, al-Qurainy I, Stassen LFA, et al. Ophthalmic consequences of mid-facial trauma. Eye 1992;6:86–9.

[10] Joseph E, Zak R, Smith S, et al. Predictors of blinding or serious eye injury in blunt injury. J Trauma 1992;33:19–24.

[11] Lynham AJ, Hirst JP, Cosson JA, et al. Emergency department management of maxillofacial trauma. Emerg Med Australas 2004;16:7–12.

[12] Alonso LL, Purcell TB. Accuracy of the tongue blade test in patients with suspected mandibular fracture. J Emerg Med 1995;13:297–304.

[13] Davidson JS, Birdsell DC. Cervical spine injury in patients with facial skeletal trauma. J Trauma 1989;29:1276–8.

[14] Kulvatunyou N, et al. Incidence and pattern of cervical spine injury in blunt assault: it is not how they are hit, but how they fall. J Trauma 2012;72:271–5.

[15] Hills MW, Deanne SA. Head injury and facial injury: is there an increased risk of cervical spine injury? J Trauma 1993;34:549–53.

[16] Williams J, Jehle D, Cottington E, Head Shufflebarger C. Facial, and clavicular trauma as a predictor of cervical spine injury. Ann Emerg Med 1992;21:719–22.

[17] Lalani Z, Bonanthaya KM. Cervical spine injury in maxillofacial trauma. Br J Oral Maxillofac Surg 1997;3:18–21.

[18] Adams C, Januszkiewicz J, Judson J. Changing patterns of severe craniomaxillofacial trauma in Auckland over 8 years. Aust NZ J Surg 2000;70:401–4.

[19] Sinclair D, Schwartz M, Gruss J. A retrospective review of the relationship between facial fractures, head injuries, and cervical spine injuries. J Emerg Med 1988;6:109–12.

[20] Taicher S, Givol N, Peleg M. Changing indications for tracheostomy in maxillofacial trauma. J Oral Maxillofac Surg 1996;54:292–5.

[21] Ardekian L, Samet N, Shoshani Y. Life-threatening bleeding following maxillofacial trauma. J Craniomaxillofac Surg 1993;21:336–8.

[22] Murakami WT, Davidson TM, Marshall LF. Fatal epistaxis in craniofacial trauma. J Trauma 1983;23:57–61.

[23] Slupchynskyj OS, Berkower AS, Byrne DW. Association of skull base and facial fractures. Laryngoscope 1992;102:1247–50.

[24] Perry M, Moutray T. Advanced Trauma Life Support (ATLS) and facial trauma: can one size fit all? Part 4: 'Can the patient see?' Timely diagnosis, dilemmas and pitfalls in the multiply injured, poorly responsive/unresponsive patient. Internatl J Oral Maxillofac Surg 2008;37:505–14.

[25] Lima V, et al. Orbital compartment syndrome: the ophthalmic surgical emergency. Surv Ophthalmol 2009;54:441–9.

[26] Luce EA, Tubb TD, Moore AM. Review of 1000 major facial fractures and associated injuries. Plastic Reconstruct Surg 1979;63:26–30.

[27] Dongas P, Hall GM. Mandibular fracture patterns in Tasmania, Australia. Aust Dent J 2002;47:131–7.

[28] Winstanley RP. The management of fractures of the mandible. Br J Oral Maxillofac Surg 1984;22:170–7.

[29] Larian B, Wong B, Crumley RL, et al. Facial trauma and ocular/orbital injury. J Craniomaxillofac Trauma 1999;5:15–24.

[30] Linnau KF, Hallam DK, Lomoschitz FM. Orbital apex injury: trauma at the junction between the face and the cranium. Eur J Radiol 2003;48:5–16.

[31] Whitaker LA, Yaremchuk MJ. Secondary reconstruction of posttraumatic orbital deformities. Ann Plastic Surg 1990;25:440–9.

[32] Le Fort R. Experimental study of fractures of the upper jaw. Rev Chirurg Paris 1901;23:208–27. 360–379. (Reprinted in Plastic Reconstruct Surg 1972; 50:497–506).

[33] Luyk NH, Larsen PE. The diagnosis and treatment of the dislocated mandible. Am J Emerg Med 1989;7:329–35.

[34] Kaufman Y, Cole P, Hollier L. Contemporary issues in facial gunshot wound management. J Craniofac Surg 2008;19:421–7.

[35] Kihitir T, Ivatury RR, Simon RJ. Early management of civilian gunshot wounds to the face. J Trauma 1993;35:569–75.

[36] Dolin J, Scalea T, Mannor L. The management of gunshot wounds to the face. J Trauma 1992;33:508–14.

[37] Hollier L, Grantcharova EP, Kattash M. Facial gunshot wounds: a 4-year experience. J Oral Maxillofac Surg 2001;59:277–82.

[38] Doctor VS, Farwell DG. Gunshot wounds to the head and neck. Curr Opin Otolaryngol Head Neck Surg 2007;15:213–8.

[39] Chen AY, Stewart MG, Raup G. Penetrating injuries of the face. Otolaryngol Head Neck Surg 1996;115:464–70.

3.5 Abdominal trauma

Garry J Wilkes

ESSENTIALS

1 One in 10 deaths from trauma is due to abdominal injuries.

2 Abdominal injuries are often occult, overshadowed by more apparent external and orthopaedic injuries and may be missed initially.

3 Detection of intra-abdominal injuries requires a high index of suspicion to avoid preventable morbidity and mortality.

4 CT scanning provides organ-specific diagnosis but requires sufficient stability for transfer from the resuscitation area.

5 Bedside investigations, such as focused assessment sonography in trauma (FAST) assist in the evaluation of suspected intra-abdominal trauma but have limitations.

6 Intra-abdominal trauma frequently coexists with other system trauma. Evaluation and disposition are greatly enhanced by early involvement of senior trauma surgeons.

Introduction

One in 10 deaths from trauma is due to abdominal injuries. These may be difficult to detect initially, as the abdominal cavity cannot be viewed with the naked eye, plain radiography is insensitive to intra-abdominal bleeding and solid organ injury and signs and symptoms of blood loss may be attributed to more obvious injuries. It is therefore not surprising that missed abdominal injuries are a major cause of preventable death in trauma patients. A high index of suspicion should be maintained for this important cause of morbidity and mortality.

A stepwise approach to the management of the multiply injured patient will address the possibility of significant intra-abdominal

Box 3.5.1 Risk factors for intra-abdominal injury in trauma patients

High-speed vehicular collisions

Pedestrian struck by vehicle

Fall from greater than standing height

Hypotension or history of hypotension (systolic BP <100 mmHg) at any time

Presence of significant chest or pelvic injuries

Significant injuries on physically opposing sides of the abdomen

Table 3.5.1 Organ injuries associated with blunt and penetrating trauma [1]

	Blunt trauma (%)	Stabbing (%)	Gunshot (%)
Spleen	40–55	–	–
Liver	35–45	40	30
Retroperitoneal haematoma	15	–	–
Small bowel	5–10	30	50
Diaphragm	–	20	–
Colon	–	15	40
Abdominal vascular structures	–	–	25

injury. The principles of initial management are to identify the presence or otherwise of such injury, the need for surgery and most appropriate timing of interventions. This process requires the presence of an experienced clinician at the earliest possible stage to direct and coordinate the trauma team. Ideally, the trauma surgeon should be present at the initial resuscitation.

The initial resuscitation, history, examination and specific investigations will be reviewed in turn.

Primary and secondary surveys

The abdomen does not normally form part of the primary survey. The unstable patient requiring continued fluid resuscitation without other sources of haemorrhage must be considered to have ongoing intra-abdominal bleeding. Specific points to remember are to expose the patient fully, including an examination of the back as well as the rectum and vagina.

History

The history and knowledge of the mechanism of injury will provide vital clues to the increased likelihood of significant intra-abdominal trauma (Box 3.5.1). Ambulance personnel will be able to provide valuable details of the incident. It is important to remember that trauma does not skip body regions and that significant intra-abdominal injuries frequently occur in the absence of external signs of abdominal trauma. Other important aspects of focused history are summarized by the acronym AMPLE: Allergies; Medications; Past medical history; Last ate and drank; Events associated with the trauma incident.

Abdominal examination

Penetrating injuries are overt and dramatic. Blunt trauma is more common and more difficult to assess on clinical grounds. Bruising and abrasions are associated with intra-abdominal pathology. The spleen and liver are the most commonly injured organs, with different patterns of injury seen in blunt and penetrating injuries (Table 3.5.1) [1]. Marks from lap-type seatbelts carry a high association with chance fractures (T12/L1), small bowel injury and pancreatic injury. Palpation of the abdomen may reveal local/generalized tenderness and evidence of peritonism, but is less reliable in detecting retroperitoneal injury and in the presence of altered sensorium. Auscultation is rarely useful; however, the absence of bowel sounds should increase the suspicion of intra-abdominal injury.

Rectal examination may demonstrate frank blood from injured bowel, a high-riding or mobile prostate from urethral rupture and may allow direct palpation of fractures or breaches of bowel wall integrity. Vaginal examination is important for similar reasons and may detect an unrecognized gravid uterus. The examination of the abdomen is not complete until the back, buttocks and perineum have been fully exposed.

Although unexplained hypotension suggests intra-abdominal haemorrhage, not all patients with significant blood loss will display the typical pattern of hypotension and tachycardia [2]. This is especially true of the younger patient. Less than one-third of patients with significant blood loss will have both hypotension and tachycardia [3]. More important are trends in pulse and blood pressure with time and in response to fluid resuscitation. Continuing falls in blood pressure and rises in pulse rate indicate ongoing haemorrhage which, if no other source is identified, must be assumed to be intra-abdominal. Abdominal distension does not occur until several litres of blood have been sequestered and can initially be confused with obesity.

Once the patient has been examined, a urinary catheter should be inserted, unless there is suspicion of a urethral injury. Blood at the urethral meatus, scrotal haematoma and a high-riding or mobile prostate are suggestive of urethral injury and a urological opinion should be sought before attempting to insert a catheter. In these circumstances, a suprapubic catheter may be preferable. Patients with a suspicion of abdominal injury also require a gastric catheter. Nasogastric catheterization is more comfortable for the patient than the oral route, but is contraindicated by evidence of basilar skull fracture. Gastric decompression may be both diagnostic and therapeutic. Penetration of the stomach or proximal small bowel will produce a bloodied aspiration. Aspiration of air will relieve gastric tamponade, which is occasionally an unrecognized cause of hypotension from impaired venous return. Urinary and gastric catheterization is mandatory prior to diagnostic peritoneal lavage (DPL).

A penetrating object, such as a knife protruding from the abdomen, should be left *in situ* unless it is an immediate threat to life. While tempting to remove such objects from stable patients in order to examine the patient and the wound tract, following this impulse can lead to disastrous consequences if the object is adjacent to or penetrates vascular structures. The sudden release of a tamponade may be rapidly fatal. The only place to remove a penetrating object is in an operating theatre, with staff on hand capable of dealing with all possible complications.

Box 3.5.2 Indications for laparotomy

Immediate
Evisceration
Gunshot wound
Stab wound with peritoneum breached
Haemodynamic instability despite correction of estimated blood loss from extra-abdominal sites
Frank peritonism (initially or on repeat examination)
Free gas on plain radiography
Ruptured diaphragm

Emergent
Positive trauma ultrasound
Positive DPL

Table 3.5.2 Comparison of abdominal CT, DPL and ultrasound for investigation of abdominal trauma

Abdominal CT	DPL	Ultrasound
Advantages		
Anatomical information	Rapid, cheap, sensitive	Rapid, portable, repeatable
Non-invasive	Minimal training	Non-invasive
Visualizes retroperitoneum	Ideal in unstable patients	Ideal in unstable patients
Also views chest, pelvis	Can be done in resus. room	Can be done in resus. room
		Also views chest, pelvis
Disadvantages		
Not suitable for unstable patients	Not organ specific	Requires specific training
Requires transport from resus. room	False negative	Operator dependent
Patient safety	Retroperitoneal injuries	False negative
Inaccessible while scanning	Hollow viscus injury	Retroperitoneal injuries
Time	Diaphragm injury	Hollow viscus injury
Cost	Iatrogenic injury	Diaphragm injury
False negative	Fluid and gas introduced	False positive
Hollow viscus injuries	during the procedure	Ascites
IV contrast reactions	interfere with subsequent imaging	

Investigations

The initial resuscitation of all trauma patients includes blood drawn for full blood count, urea and electrolytes, blood sugar determination, cross-matching, blood gases (if available) and a trauma radiology series. There is little place for plain radiology of the abdomen.

Gunshot wounds are unpredictable in their path, can produce secondary missiles and cavitation effects and all require laparotomy. Stab wounds that have penetrated the peritoneum may also require laparotomy and need immediate assessment by an experienced trauma surgeon. In cases where immediate laparotomy is indicated, the patient should be escorted to theatre with no further investigations (Box 3.5.2). Further investigations, such as trauma ultrasound or DPL, may assist in determining the need for or timing of laparotomy if other urgent procedures are also required. The final order is determined by the trauma team leader.

Unstable patients require surgical intervention as soon as possible. Stable patients can be investigated further, allowing better planning of further management. The difficulty arises in the common situation where there are multiple injuries and only a suspicion – not confirmation – of significant intra-abdominal pathology. Some patients are at risk of abdominal injury but cannot be assessed on clinical grounds. These include those with head, chest and spinal injuries, intoxicated or sedated patients and those who will be inaccessible while undergoing lengthy operations on other body regions. For these patients, it is important

to make a further assessment of the presence or otherwise of intra-abdominal injury. Additional investigations of benefit are ultrasound, DPL and computed tomography (CT).

Each has advantages and disadvantages (Table 3.5.2). They may also be consecutive and complementary, thereby minimizing the disadvantages of each individually. Areas poorly imaged

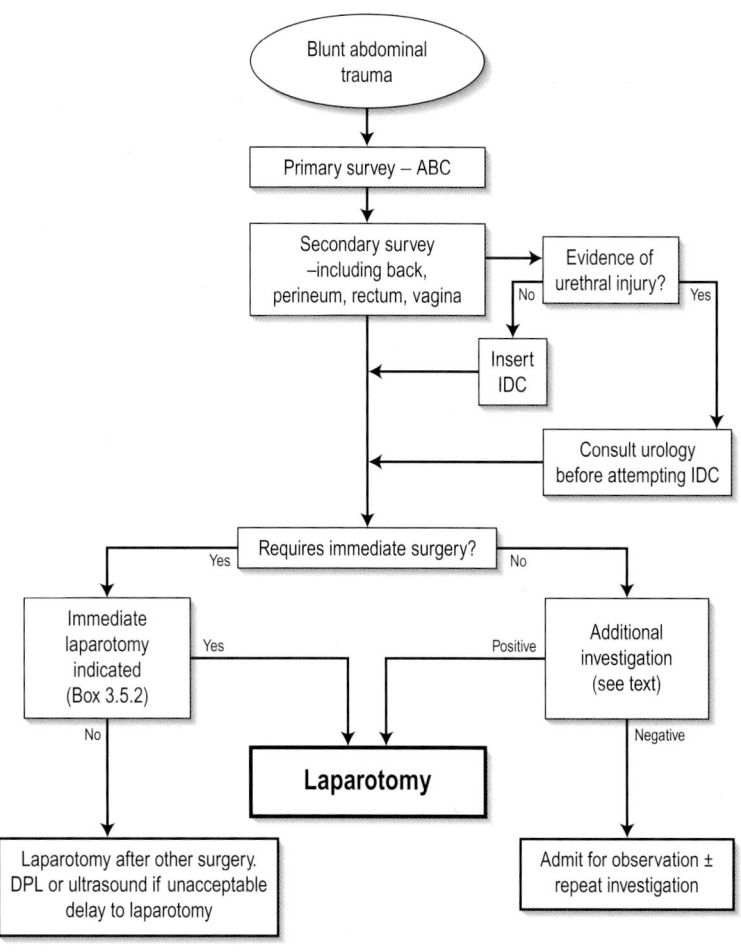

Fig. 3.5.1 Initial management of blunt abdominal trauma.

by all modalities are hollow organ injuries, such as small bowel rupture and vascular compromise. Serial clinical examination is essential to detect these injuries, even if investigation results are normal.

DPL was first described in 1965 and can be completed in less than 4 minutes by experienced operators [4,5]. However, DPL is of limited value when CT or FAST are available and the increasing availability of these modalities has largely resulted in this procedure no longer being used in trauma resususcitation.

Abdominal CT

Abdominal CT is non-invasive and provides precise anatomical details of intra-abdominal pathology. The major disadvantages are associated with the use of IV contrast and the need for the patient to be transported from the resuscitation area to the CT scanner, where they are not accessible during the procedure. Intravenous contrast may rarely produce allergic reactions and can precipitate or exacerbate renal impairment, particularly in higher doses and in the presence of renal hypoperfusion and hypofunction. Although modern machines complete scans in a single breath-hold, time is still required to load and unload the patient. Transport and transfer are times of maximum patient risk and minimum monitoring. Therefore, only stable patients are suitable for transfer for CT scanning. Unstable patients require further resuscitation or operative intervention if this is unsuccessful. The definition of stable is not agreed. The final decision can only be made by the most experienced physician available, although a systolic pressure of at least 90 mmHg and no requirement for additional fluids after correction of estimated losses would be minimum requirements.

Focused assessment sonography in trauma

Focused ultrasound is a skill practised by many clinicians involved in acute trauma management. Abdominal ultrasound is non-invasive, may be done at the bedside and can be repeated as needed. The technique can be easily learnt by clinicians and completed in less than 5 min without interfering with the function of a trauma resuscitation team [6]. Ultrasound combines the advantages of being rapid, accurate and non-invasive and can be performed at the bedside. It is at least as accurate as DPL and, in experienced hands, has similar results

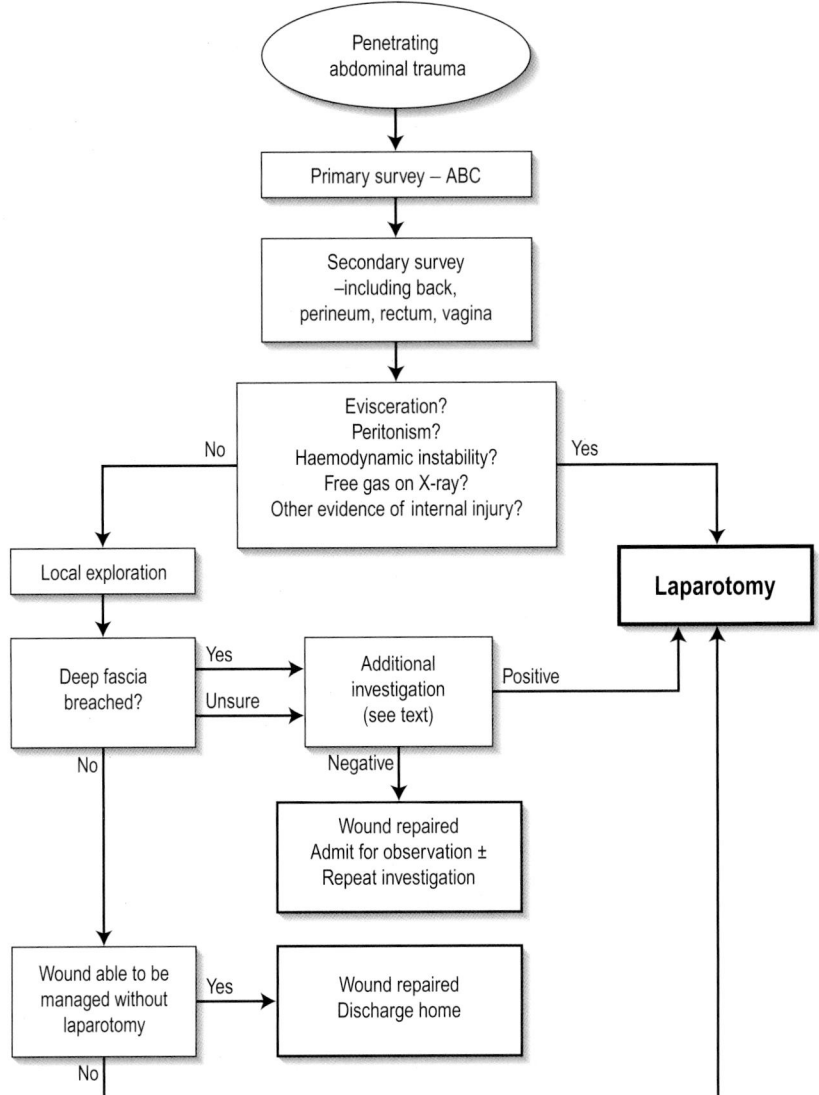

Fig. 3.5.2 Initial management of penetrating abdominal trauma.

to CT in determining the presence of intraperitoneal injury. As a decision-making tool for identifying the need for laparotomy in hypotensive patients (systolic BP <90), FAST has a sensitivity of 100%, specificity of 96% and negative predictive value (NPV) of 100% [7,8]. It is the bedside investigation of choice if an experienced operator is available.

Laparoscopy

Laparoscopy has been investigated in some centres, but the skills required and the time needed for a thorough examination limit the widespread usefulness of this modality in acute blunt trauma. However, it is useful in excluding peritoneal penetration in abdominal stab wounds.

Penetrating injuries

Penetrating injuries produce a different pattern of injury (see Table 3.5.1) and are managed in a different manner from blunt injuries (Figs 3.5.1 and 3.5.2). Cavitation effects and the potential for secondary missiles causing widespread injury mandate formal laparotomy in all cases. Stab wounds with haemodynamic compromise or other indications should also proceed to laparotomy without delay for other investigations. Local exploration of stab wounds by experienced surgeons in patients without evidence of internal injury may be useful, as up to one-third of wounds do not breach the peritoneum. Selected patients may then be managed conservatively.

Disposition

Disposition decisions may be difficult in the less seriously injured patient or those with suspected injury. Every patient suspected or at significant risk of intra-abdominal injury should be admitted for observation and serial examinations, ideally by the same individual. Injuries to the bowel wall or intestinal blood supply may not be evident on initial clinical examination or investigation and may take 24 h to declare themselves. A higher index of suspicion is required for patients who cannot be assessed clinically. Unconscious, intubated, head-injured and spinally-injured patients are all at increased risk of abdominal injuries and less able to declare them. Serial investigations and clinical vigilance are vital.

Future directions

The difficulty in managing abdominal trauma is determining the presence, location and details of intra-abdominal injury. Current imaging techniques have their disadvantages and limitations. The refinement of modalities, such as ultrasound and portable CT, will rapidly provide more detailed information at the bedside in the resuscitation area, without the need for invasive techniques. Non-operative management of injuries using radiological or minimally invasive surgical techniques continues to develop, thereby reducing the need for laparotomy.

Pharmacological agents such as Factor VIIa and transexamic acid have been assessed as adjuncts for haemorrhage reduction. Results are promising but more research is required.

Controversies

- Haemodynamic stability is not dictated by a single reading of pulse or blood pressure. The need for ongoing fluids in order to maintain adequate perfusion indicates instability even in the presence of normal vital signs.
- In the multiply injured patient, there is often difficulty in deciding whether to operate first on the head, chest, abdomen or limbs. All surgeons concerned must discuss the decision.
- Perhaps the most difficult decision is which is the most appropriate investigation in the otherwise stable patient? Each modality – CT, DPL and FAST – has inherent strengths and weaknesses.
- The role of newer pharmacological treatment, such as clotting factors, is promising and requires further evaluation. At present, the most important therapy is early surgery for injury with ongoing bleeding.
- Stopping bleeding early is achieved by 'damage control laparotomy'. This involves immediate attempts to stop the bleeding, either by ligation or tamponade with definitive surgery delayed until the patient is stabilized.

References

[1] American College of Surgeons Committee on Trauma. Advanced Trauma Life Support Student Course Manual, 9th ed. Chicago: ACS; 2012.
[2] Wilkes GJ, McSweeney PA. The diagnosis of traumatic intra-abdominal haemorrhage in patients with normal vital signs. Emerg Med 1996;8:19–23.
[3] Grant RT, Reeve EB. Clinical observations on air-raid casualties. Br Med J 1941;2:293–7.
[4] Root HD, Hauser CW, La Fave JW, et al. Diagnostic peritoneal lavage. Surgery 1965;57:633–7.
[5] Sugrue M, Seger M, Gunning K, et al. A modified combination technique for performing diagnostic peritoneal lavage. Aust NZ J Surg 1995;65:604–6.
[6] Shackford SR, Rogers FB, Osler TM, et al. Focused abdominal sonogram for trauma: the learning curve of nonradiologist clinicians in detecting hemoperitoneum. J Trauma 1999;46:553–62.
[7] Brohi K. Focused assessment with sonography for trauma (FAST). <http://www.trauma.org/index.php/main/article/214> [Accessed Nov. 2012].
[8] ACEM Policy on Credentialling for ED Ultrasonography: Trauma Examination and Suspected AAA. <http://acem.org.au/media/P22.pdf> [Accessed Nov. 2012].

3.6 Chest trauma

Mark Fitzgerald • Robert Gocentas • Jeremy Stevens

ESSENTIALS

1 Initial management priorities are oxygenation, ventilatory support if required, pleural and pericardial decompression when indicated, circulatory support, adequate analgesia and early imaging to identify evolving and potentially life-threatening injuries.

2 Less than 10% of blunt chest trauma patients require thoracic surgery.

3 Supine chest radiographs do not reliably exclude haemopneumothoraces, aortic transection, diaphragmatic disruption, cardiac tamponade or rib, sternal, thoracic spine and scapula fractures.

4 Multislice CT with IV contrast is the 'gold standard' screening and diagnostic tool for thoracic injuries. Sonography may demonstrate haemopneumothorax and cardiac tamponade.

5 Aseptic, percutaneous digital identification of the pleural space is the essential first step for pleural decompression. Drainage and insertion of a chest tube is a secondary priority. Needle thoracocentesis is an unreliable means of decompressing the chest of an unstable patient.

6 Pleural decompression and chest tube insertion during resuscitation is a procedure with a low complication rate.

7 There is a clear role for resuscitative thoracotomy in shocked patients with sonographic evidence of cardiac tamponade.

8 Non-invasive ventilation may avoid complications of mechanical ventilation in select patients with flail chest and pulmonary contusion.

Introduction

Incidence

Thoracic trauma is responsible for 25% of all trauma deaths and contributes to a further 25%. In Australasia and the UK, 90–95% of chest trauma is secondary to blunt injury.

Principles of initial management

The initial management priorities are oxygenation, ventilatory support if required, pleural and pericardial decompression when indicated, circulatory support, adequate analgesia and early imaging to diagnose evolving and potentially life-threatening injuries. The majority of chest trauma patients may be managed non-operatively. Only 10% of blunt thoracic trauma patients will require thoracotomy, the remainder requiring supportive care, including pleural decompression and drainage.

Supportive care, in particular resuscitation, is often suboptimal. Delayed or inadequate ventilatory resuscitation, inadequate shock management, insufficient monitoring of arterial blood gases, delay or failure to perform pleural decompression and drainage and delays in definitive diagnostic imaging remain identifiable problems that contribute to preventable morbidity and mortality [1,2].

Thoracic injuries evolve. Life-threatening injuries including flail chest, pulmonary contusion, thoracic aortic transection, pneumothorax, haemothorax, pericardial tamponade, respiratory insufficiency secondary to rib fractures and ruptured hemidiaphragm may not be apparent on initial presentation. These diagnoses need to be pursued and actively excluded. Supine chest radiographs do not reliably exclude these injuries. Multislice computed tomography (CT) with contrast is the 'gold standard' screening and diagnostic test for patients at high risk of potential life-threatening injuries [3]. However, life-saving procedures should be performed first (Table 3.6.1).

Oxygen

Hypoxia may be absent at the initial reception and resuscitation of chest trauma, but may develop as injuries evolve. Supplemental oxygen may be required for mild desaturation with the FiO_2 titrated to the clinical response. Higher FiO_2 can be achieved using positive airway pressure and invasive ventilation (CPAP, EPAP).

Increasing the normal I/E ratio may be beneficial in mechanically ventilated patients with severe hypoxia. The benefits of independent lung ventilation, inhaled nitric oxide, prone position, partial liquid ventilation and extracorporeal membrane oxygenation in the initial resuscitation setting are unproven strategies.

Support of pulmonary function

Pain, fatigue from increased work of breathing, disruption of lung mechanics and side effects of opiate analgesia may cause hypoventilation. The elderly as well as other patients with pre-existing poor chest wall compliance are particularly at risk of hypoventilation in the setting of chest wall injury.

Non-invasive ventilation

Patients with pulmonary contusions and high oxygen requirements do not necessarily require intubation but may be safely managed with non-invasive ventilation [4]. By avoiding mechanical ventilation, mortality from nosocomial infection is significantly reduced [5].

Mechanical ventilation

Contraindications to non-invasive ventilation in the trauma patient include the need for full spinal precautions, depressed conscious state and facial injury. Patients with pulmonary contusion and poor lung compliance require ventilation with low tidal volumes and low inspiratory pressures. This reduces barotrauma, secondary lung injury and mortality [6].

Fluid resuscitation

There is evidence that 'permissive hypotension' prior to surgical control of blood loss may

Table 3.6.1 Actions prior to CT

Situation	Response
Pneumothorax or haemothorax on initial supine chest X-ray	Insert chest drain on affected side
Spontaneously breathing patient with unilateral decreased air entry and normal chest X-ray, oxygenation and haemodynamic status	Await CT
Intubated and ventilated patient with unilateral decreased air entry and normal chest X-ray but hypoxic or hypotensive	Insert chest drain on affected side, then reassess
Intubated and ventilated patient with hypotension or hypoxia (no other apparent cause)	Insert bilateral chest drains

improve survival in hypotensive penetrating torso injury [7]. It may also reduce blood product requirements, coagulopathy and early postoperative mortality [8]. It is unclear whether these findings translate equally to hypotensive blunt trauma. Once haemorrhage has been controlled, fluid therapy to maximize cardiac output and oxygen delivery may reduce trauma mortality [9].

Conservative fluid resuscitation has been recommended to minimize extravascular lung water in patients with pulmonary contusion [10]. However, under-resuscitation and tissue hypoperfusion may compound organ dysfunction and secondary lung injury. The early use of invasive monitoring to guide fluid replacement may be required.

Analgesia

Adequate analgesia reduces hypoventilation secondary to pain and facilitates coughing and chest physiotherapy. It reduces complications of atelectasis, consolidation and respiratory failure and improves pulmonary function [11]. Oral analgesia is often sufficient for single rib fractures. Parenteral narcotic analgesia, intercostal nerve block or thoracic epidural analgesia is usually required for multiple rib fractures. Intercostal nerve block involves a number of injections to treat multiple rib fractures. This limits its usefulness compared to the other techniques.

Indications for emergency thoracotomy

Although more than 90% of chest trauma patients may be managed non-operatively, the following categories warrant surgical intervention [12]:

- cardiac tamponade
- acute deterioration – cardiac arrest in patients with penetrating truncal trauma
- vascular injury at the thoracic outlet
- traumatic loss of chest wall
- massive air leak from chest tube
- massive or continuing haemothorax
- mediastinal traversing penetrating injury
- endoscopic or radiographic demonstration of oesophageal injury
- endoscopic or radiographic demonstration of tracheal or bronchial injury
- radiographic evidence of great vessel injury
- thoracic penetration with industrial liquids (especially coal tar products).

Resuscitative thoracotomy

Left anterolateral thoracotomy as a resuscitative manoeuvre allows direct access to the heart and pericardial decompression for patients who have lost output following cardiac lacerations. Myocardial wounds can then be directly controlled. Right atrial catheterization facilitating IV fluid administration, pulmonary hilar clamping, cross-clamping of the descending aorta and open cardiac massage are adjunctive procedures performed if indicated.

Survival rates of better than 40% have been reported in some subgroups of penetrating trauma arrest, specifically precordial stab wounds. Survival was dependent on resuscitative thoracotomy performed within 10 minutes of arrest secondary to penetrating chest trauma and an organized cardiac electrical rhythm being present [13–16]. Left anterolateral thoracotomy allows pericardial decompression [17] in patients who have lost output following penetrating injury to the heart. Myocardial wounds can then be directly controlled. The role of resuscitative thoracotomy in blunt trauma arrest is more controversial, with a relatively low survival rate (<3%) [18].

Focused assessment with sonography in trauma (FAST) is an important triage tool in determining the presence of cardiac tamponade. Immediate use of ultrasonography can establish the diagnosis of haemopericardium and prompt repair of the injury may improve overall survival. Unresponsive hypotension with a systolic blood pressure of less than 70 mmHg and a FAST positive for pericardial tamponade is a consensus-based indication for immediate resuscitative thoracotomy. For patients with severe hypotension or *in extremis*, the treatment of choice is resuscitative thoracotomy, decompression of the pericardium and control of the cardiac injury [19].

Given the widespread availability of ultrasound, arguments about resuscitative thoracotomy for blunt trauma should include the important decision support provided by sonography. There is clearly a role for resuscitative thoracotomy in shocked patients with cardiac tamponade following blunt trauma. Procedural training and credentialing is recommended [19].

Thoracic injuries

Fractured ribs

Fractured ribs are a common sequela of focal trauma. Fractured ribs cause pain, which may then interfere with ventilation and coughing, causing ventilatory impairment and atelectasis. This impairment may not be manifest for hours and occasionally days after the injury.

Underlying structures are often injured concomitantly, particularly the lungs, pleura and intercostal vessels. Fractures of the lower left ribs are associated with splenic injury, the lower right with hepatic injury and the lower posterior ribs with renal injury. The first and second ribs are stronger and less easily injured and, when fractured, are usually indicative of significant force to the upper mediastinum. Although first and second rib fractures have been traditionally associated with thoracic aortic injury, the positive predictive value of this association has been questioned [20].

Rib fracture is essentially a diagnosis based on the clinical findings of local tenderness with or without deformity and crepitus. Up to 50% of fractured ribs are not apparent on the initial chest X-ray [21]. Reliance on the X-ray to diagnose fractured ribs inevitably results in under-diagnosis. This may lead to delays in diagnosis and therapy and an adverse outcome, particularly with elderly patients and those with coexisting airways disease.

The management of rib fractures centres on actively excluding associated injury as well as adequate pain relief including patient controlled administration of narcotics and local and regional anaesthetic blocks to allow breathing exercises, coughing and incentive spirometry. This in turn minimizes subsequent atelectasis and pulmonary sequelae.

Fractured sternum

This is a clinical diagnosis confirmed on CT scan or lateral chest X-ray. Associated intrathoracic injuries, specifically myocardial and other mediastinal injuries, need to be identified.

The possibility of underlying injury has been related to the mechanism of injury. For example, in North America, it is reported that up to 66% of patients with sternal fractures have intrathoracic injuries. It is believed that low seatbelt usage results in sternal fractures secondary to impact against the steering wheel. In Australasia, where seatbelt usage is high, sternal fracture is more often caused by the restraining belt. Therefore, comparatively lower deceleration forces are evident, resulting in a reduced association with underlying injury [22,23].

For isolated sternal fractures, admission for analgesia is usually required, although this may be only necessary for 1–2 days. Monitoring is not required unless the mechanism or subsequent investigations suggest underlying cardiac injury.

Vertebral column and spinal cord injury

Spinal stability must be determined prior to sitting the patient upright to improve ventilation and reduce VQ mismatch. Exclusion of thoracic spine fractures and spinal-cord injury forms part of the routine work-up of the chest trauma patient. Occult injuries are common and unstable injuries in ventilated patients require skilled nursing. Such injuries are easily overlooked.

Flail chest

Flail chest may occur where the continuity of the bony skeleton of the chest wall is disrupted in two places. It is characterized by paradoxical movement of the associated unanchored chest wall segment. Because of muscle spasm and splinting, this segment may not be apparent initially and may flail some time after the accident. Clinical features of a flail segment may also be masked by positive-pressure ventilation, which splints the chest wall internally.

Elderly patients have a less compliant chest wall and are at greater risk of developing a flail segment.

Flail chest is often associated with ventilatory insufficiency. Ventilatory disturbance is caused by hypoventilation of the affected hemithorax due to the mechanical disruption and associated pain, compounded by the underlying pulmonary contusion. Therapy centres on maintaining oxygenation, ventilation and euvolaemia. Adequate analgesia should be supplemented with intercostal nerve blocks or epidural analgesia. In general, patients with a significant flail, which impairs ventilation, will require respiratory support. Hypoxia may be managed with non-invasive ventilation. Mechanical ventilation is required if non-invasive ventilation is contraindicated or unsuccessful.

A small number of patients with severe wall instability may require operative fixation to facilitate the weaning of mechanical ventilation [24]. Operative reduction and internal fixation using malleable, absorbable splints for the flail segment is a new approach associated with a reduction in ventilator days [25].

Ruptured hemidiaphragm

Diaphragmatic rupture may be difficult to diagnose. High-velocity lateral torso trauma or thoracoabdominal crush injuries as well as lateral rib fractures, penetrating left upper quadrant wounds and fractured pelvis, are linked to an increased incidence of diaphragmatic disruption. There may be respiratory compromise, with diminished air entry in the involved hemithorax. Placement of a radiopaque nasogastric tube will facilitate the diagnosis of left hemidiaphragmatic disruption on chest X-ray. Although gross rupture may be apparent initially, the classic radiological findings of viscera in the thoracic cavity, the nasogastric tube coiled in the thoracic cavity or marked hemidiaphragm elevation are present only 50% of the time, with no intrathoracic pathology seen on 15% of occasions [26]. CT scan will display gross disruption but may miss small defects. Diagnostic yield may be better with magnetic resonance imaging (MRI) [27]. Smaller diaphragmatic injuries may evolve, with visceral herniation developing over time. Positive pressure ventilation may mask this. Thus, many diaphragmatic injuries present late. Occult diaphragmatic lacerations are associated with penetrating injuries of the thoracoabdominal region and should be actively excluded

by laparoscopy, thoracoscopy or open surgery. The treatment of diaphragmatic disruption is surgical repair.

Open pneumothorax

Open pneumothorax presents an immediate threat to life. An open chest wall defect disrupts the generation of a negative inspiratory pressure. If the opening is approximately two-thirds the diameter of the trachea, air will pass preferentially through the defect (a 'sucking' chest wound) and respiratory failure will occur [28].

Initial management includes covering the defect with a sterile dressing and taping it on three sides to achieve a flutter-valve effect, prior to placement of an intercostal catheter and sealing of the defect. Definitive surgical closure is required.

Pneumothorax

Simple pneumothorax is characterized by a visceral pleural rent and pleural air preventing expansion of the associated lung. Although small (<20%) pneumothoraces may be managed expectantly, larger ones mandate pleural decompression and drainage. There is no evidence that needle thoracotomy is a reliable means of pleural decompression (Fig. 3.6.1). The technique should be avoided during hospital trauma reception and resuscitation and used only as a technique of last resort. Blunt dissection and digital identification and decompression of the pleura using an aseptic technique should be the technique of first choice. Once successfully performed, it reduces the urgency of the situation and allows time for the subsequent placement of a chest tube [29].

Intercostal catheters with underwater seal or flutter-valve drainage should also be inserted for pneumothoraces if positive-pressure ventilation is anticipated or has been commenced. If small traumatic pneumothoraces are not drained, the patient should be followed closely with repeat chest X-rays. Intercostal catheters should be placed if the patient is to be air-transported to another facility. Clinicians should be aware of common problems with chest drain placement (Fig. 3.6.2).

Thoracic CT scanning will demonstrate pneumothoraces that may not be apparent on plain radiographs [30]. This should prompt consideration of intercostal catheter placement in ventilated patients. Small (occult) pneumothoraces in patients without major shunts may be managed expectantly [31].

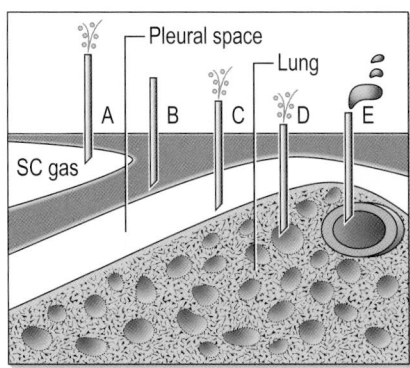

Fig. 3.6.1 Possible positions of needle thoracocentesis (NT). **(A)** False positive – as needle decompresses subcutaneous emphysema. **(B)** False negative – as needle does not reach pleural space. **(C)** Correct position of NT with decompression of tension pneumothorax. **(D)** False positive – with needle intrapulmonary in bulla or bronchial tree. If the tension pneumothorax is loculated due to pulmonary adhesions and missed by NT, a false-negative result may occur with intra-pulmonary placement. **(E)** True negative – with needle in a major vessel or the heart. This may be misinterpreted as a false positive for haemothorax. Only C will decompress a tension pneumothorax. A, B, D and E have all been associated with failure to decompress the pleural space and fatal outcomes. *(From Fitzgerald M, Mackenzie CF, Marasco S, Hoyle R, Kossman T. Pleural decompression and drainage during trauma reception and resuscitation. Injury 2008;39:9–20, with permission.)*

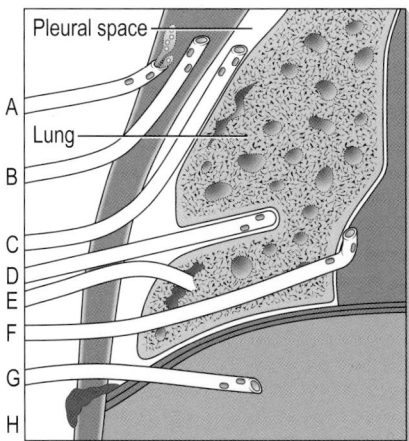

Fig. 3.6.2 Possible positions and complications of tube thoracostomy (TT). **(A)** Trauma to the intercostal neurovascular bundle. **(B)** Extrapleural placement. **(C)** Correct position in pleural space. **(D)** Intrafissural placement. **(E)** Intrapulmonary placement. **(F)** Mediastinal impingement or penetration. **(G)** Trans-diaphragmatic placement. **(H)** Infection. *(From Fitzgerald M, Mackenzie CF, Marasco S, Hoyle R, Kossman T. Pleural decompression and drainage during trauma reception and resuscitation. Injury 2008;39:9–20, with permission.)*

While ultrasound is superior to initial supine chest X-ray in the diagnosis of pneumothorax, it does not change the management of the patient as the majority of occult pneumothoraces are treated conservatively. Conversely, a negative ultrasound for pneumothorax may not sufficiently exclude the need for pleural decompression in the unstable patient [32].

Tension pneumothorax

Tension pneumothorax occurs with the formation of a 'one-way valve' from the lung through disrupted visceral pleura. Air collects under tension in the hemithorax, collapsing the lung and displacing the mediastinum, impairing ventilation and obstructing venous return. Tension pneumothorax is more commonly associated with positive-pressure ventilation. It is essentially a clinical diagnosis, characterized by tachypnoea, tracheal deviation away from the affected hemithorax, diminished ipsilateral breath sounds, diminished compliance, oxygen desaturation and hypotension.

If clinically suspected, the affected hemithorax should be immediately decompressed and an intercostal catheter subsequently inserted. There should be no attempt to delay chest decompression in an unstable patient in favour of a chest X-ray.

Intubated and ventilated thoracic trauma patients may demonstrate subcutaneous emphysema on initial chest X-ray without a pneumothorax being visible. This should prompt immediate chest tube placement, as this is a precursor of ipsilateral tension pneumothorax. The subcutaneous tissues in communication with the air leak offer less initial resistance and display air under pressure, prior to tension developing within the pleural space.

Haemothorax

Blood may accumulate within the pleural space after lung laceration or laceration of a chest-wall vessel and, less commonly, after mediastinal injury. It is indicated by diffuse opacification of a hemithorax on supine chest X-ray or blunting of the costophrenic angle on an upright film. Once digital pleural decompression has occurred the haemothorax is best drained via placement of a 32 Fr or larger intercostal catheter, positioned in the fifth or sixth intercostal space in the mid-axillary line on the affected side. The use of suction (20 cm H_2O) facilitates drainage.

Bleeding is usually self-limiting following drainage. Drainage of more than 1500 mL

following initial intercostal catheter insertion (massive hemothorax) or a loss of more than 200 mL/h for more than 2 h, are indications for thoracotomy [33]. Large blood losses frequently come from intercostal arteries.

Clamping the intercostal catheter in an attempt to tamponade bleeding and 'buy time' for an intubated and ventilated, unstable patient with a massive and ongoing hemithorax could be considered if delays to thoracotomy arise. However, this technique is yet to be prospectively validated.

Pulmonary contusion

Pulmonary contusion is characterized by the leakage of blood into the alveoli and pulmonary interstitium, culminating in consolidation and atelectasis. Associated hypoxia may be profound. The initial chest X-ray may not demonstrate the severity of injury. Pulmonary contusion may take some time to be radiologically apparent, with 21% of experimentally incurred contusions still not visible on chest X-ray 6 hours after injury [34].

CT scans provide the most sensitive test for gauging the extent of pulmonary contusion, although arterial blood gases provide the best measure of physiological derangement requiring intervention. Therapy is based on ensuring adequate oxygenation, ventilatory support and fluid restriction. Ventilation should involve low-volume, low-pressure techniques to reduce barotrauma and secondary injury.

Tracheobronchial injury

Injuries to the trachea and bronchi are rare, accounting for less than 1% of injuries after blunt chest trauma. Eighty per cent of injuries occur near the carina, with mediastinal and cervical emphysema resulting. A persistent air leak post-intercostal drain insertion should alert the clinician to the possibility of a tracheobronchial injury. Fibreoptic bronchoscopy is the investigative modality of choice. Persistent air leaks often require operative repair.

Myocardial contusion

Although myocardial contusion is common, significant sequelae are rare. Cardiac failure and hypotension are uncommonly associated with myocardial contusion. Although the ECG is used as a predictor of myocardial contusion, it is non-specific and poorly portrays the right ventricle – the area most commonly injured. Cardiac enzyme elevation does occur but is non-predictive. Echocardiography may demonstrate dyskinesis of the ventricular wall. Patients with hyperacute ECG changes or conduction defects should be admitted and monitored for dysrhythmias.

Myocardial laceration and cardiac tamponade

Precordial penetrating injury is associated with myocardial laceration. Bedside sonography is useful in demonstrating myocardial injury and pericardial collections. Patients presenting with signs of pericardial tamponade (hypotension, diminished heart sounds, jugular venous distension) require urgent surgical intervention.

Patients who acutely deteriorate into cardiac arrest yet who had signs of life *en route* to hospital or on arrival, require a resuscitative thoracotomy in the emergency department [35]. Outcome for blunt trauma patients without initial signs is very poor (<2%), but penetrating injury has a higher survival rate. This procedure should only be undertaken when there is some chance of survival because of the infection risks to personnel. Prolonged (>9 minutes) external cardiac massage is futile for these patients.

Tension pneumopericardium

Tension pneumopericardium, albeit much less common than tension pneumothorax, is thought to arise via a similar 'one-way valve' mechanism, particularly after the institution of positive-pressure ventilation. It is characterized by raised jugular/central venous pressure and hypotension and requires urgent pericardiocentesis [36].

Thoracic aortic transection

Eighty-five per cent of patients with transection of the thoracic aorta die before reaching hospital. Lateral as well as frontal impact motor vehicle crashes are associated with aortic transection [37]. High deceleration forces cause the aorta to accelerate and twist against fixation points – usually the ligamentum arteriosum just distal to the left subclavian artery. The associated shearing forces transect and tear the artery. Tears of the aorta are commonly fatal at the time of injury or immediately after, as the aorta usually tears completely and the injured rapidly bleed to death. However, it has been estimated that up to 15% of patients with thoracic aortic injuries survive to reach hospital and this is due to the outer concentric layers of the aorta remaining intact. Fifty per cent die

within the next 48 hours if not operated upon. Thus, early diagnosis and treatment of incomplete transection of the thoracic aortic injury is important.

Mediastinal widening on chest X-ray is 85% sensitive and 10% specific for aortic transection [38]. Associated fractures of the thoracic spine also cause mediastinal widening and make interpretation difficult. There is no thoracic skeletal injury that is a clinically useful predictor of acute thoracic aortic transection. Therefore, patients involved in high speed accidents require chest CT scans to exclude aortic injury.

Definitive treatment includes ensuring that the blood pressure is not elevated to reduce shearing and radiologically guided placement of a stent across the injured aorta [39–43].

Surgical repair of the injured thoracic aorta is uncommon and has a high mortality and morbidity. Published mortality rates of patients with thoracic aortic injury are: endovascular stent 9%, open surgical repair 19% and non-operative management without stent 46% [44].

Transoesophageal echocardiography has been used as a screening tool for aortic tears and is useful for patients in theatre or those unable to be moved to angiography [45,46].

Oesophageal perforation

Oesophageal rupture after blunt chest trauma is rare. The lower third of the oesophagus is

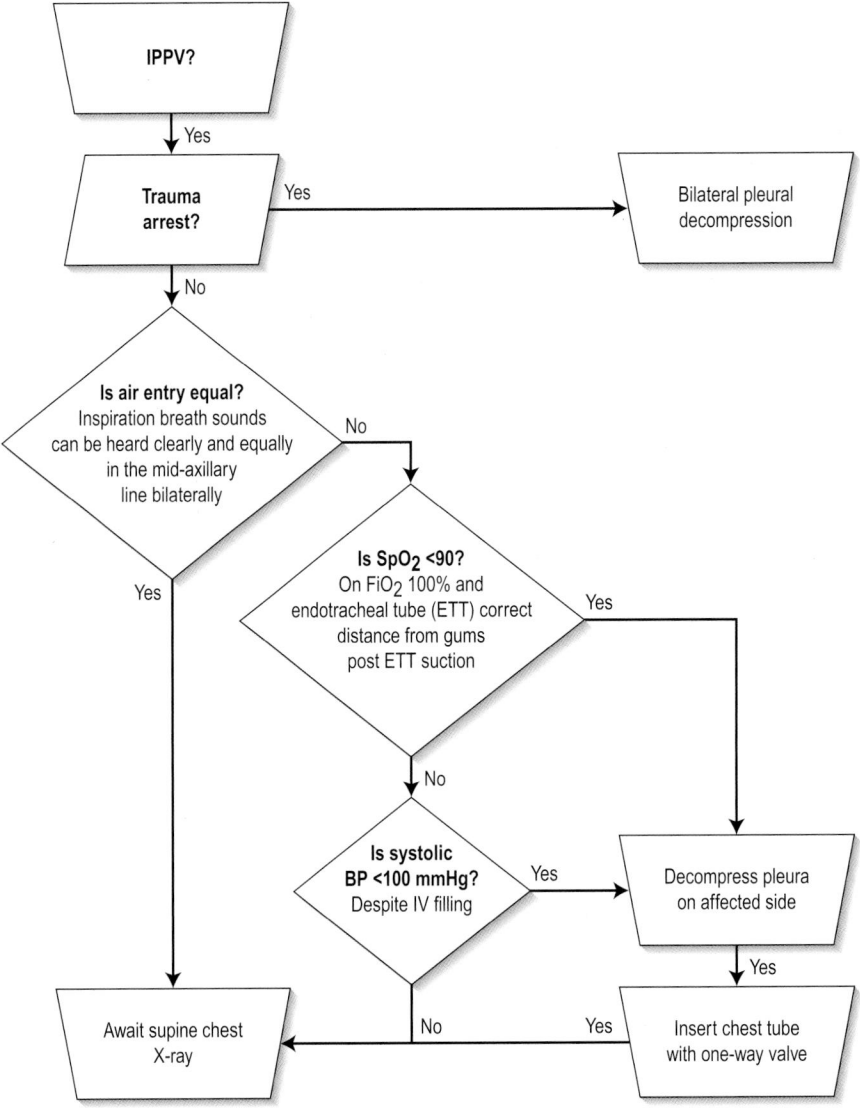

Fig. 3.6.3 Initial binary decision tree for pleural decompression. *(From Fitzgerald M, Mackenzie CF, Marasco S, Hoyle R, Kossman T. Pleural decompression and drainage during trauma reception and resuscitation. Injury 2008;39:9–20, with permission.)*

the commonest site of rupture, presumably secondary to a forced Valsalva manoeuvre. Mediastinitis is a subsequent development. Retrosternal pain is common and mediastinal air may be seen on chest X-ray. Gastrograffin swallow and CT scanning is the study of choice. Mortality is directly related to time to operative repair [47].

Gunshot injuries across the truncal midline more commonly involve mediastinal and spinal structures and therefore have a much greater mortality than unilateral injuries [48]. It is important to exclude oesophageal injury early with penetrating and transmediastinal wounds, as there is significant morbidity and mortality in those patients who survive to hospital [49].

Likely developments

Better systems of care, improved imaging and newer technologies will result in earlier diagnosis and treatment of injuries preventing subsequent evolution and deterioration.

There is a trend towards the increased use of non-invasive ventilation and operative rib fixation for flail chest. The role of ultrasound is evolving and there is increasing use of ultrasound in the assessment of chest trauma. Conservative management of occult pneumothoraces is likely to increase – more prospective studies are required to prove the safety of conservative management.

Conclusion

The significance and severity of chest trauma may not be obvious on initial examination as injuries evolve. Most seriously injured patients with blunt thoracic trauma require supportive care including chest decompression and drainage. Indications for immediate chest decompression are ventilatory or respiratory compromise (Fig. 3.6.3). Patients with underlying airway disease and elderly patients with diminished compliance are at particular risk. Delayed or inadequate ventilatory resuscitation, inadequate shock management, insufficient monitoring of arterial blood gases, delay or failure to perform pleural decompression and drainage and inadequate diagnostic imaging remain identifiable problems in emergency departments.

References

[1] McDermott F. Severe chest injuries: problems in Victoria. Issues and controversies in the early management of major trauma. Melbourne: Alfred Hospital and Monash University, Department of Surgery; 1994.
[2] Danne P, Brazenor G, Cade R, et al. The Major Trauma Management Study: an analysis of the efficacy of current trauma care. Aust NZ J Surg 1998;68:50–7.
[3] Mirvis SE. Imaging of acute thoracic injury: the advent of MDCT screening Semin Ultrasound. CT MRI 2005;26:305–31.
[4] Vidhani K, Kause J, Parr M. Should we follow ATLS guidelines for the management of traumatic pulmonary contusion: the role of non-invasive ventilatory support. 2002;52:265–8.
[5] Gurnduz M, Unugenc H, Ozalevli M, et al. A comparative study of continuous positive airway pressure (CPAP) and intermittent positive pressure ventilation (IPPV) in patients with flail chest. Emerg Med J 2005;22:325–9.
[6] ARDS Network Ventilation with lower tidal volumes for acute lung injury and the acute respiratory distress syndrome. N Engl J Med 2000;3:1301–8.
[7] Bickell WH, Wall Jnr MJ, Pepe PE, et al. Immediate versus delayed fluid resuscitation for hypotensive patients with penetrating torso injuries. N Engl J Med 1995;38:780–7.
[8] Morison CA, Carrick MH, Norman MA, et al. Hypotensive resuscitation strategy reduces transfusion requirements and severe post operative coagulopathy in trauma patient with haemorrhagic shock: preliminary results of a randomized controlled trial. J Trauma 2011;70:652–63.
[9] Bishol MH, Shoemaker WC, Appel PL, et al. Prospective, randomized trial of survivor values of cardiac index. J Trauma 1995;38:780–7.
[10] Richardson JD, Adam L, Flint LM. Selective management of flail chest and pulmonary contusion. Ann Surg 1982;196:481.
[11] Desai PM. Pain management and pulmonary dysfunction. Crit Care Clin 1999;15:151–66.
[12] Pickard LR, Mattox KL. Thoracic trauma and indications for thoracotomy. In: Mattox KL, Moore EE, Feliciano DV, editors. Trauma. Norwalk: Appleton & Lange; 1988. p. 315–20.
[13] Tyburski JG, Astra L, Wilson RF. Factors affecting prognosis with penetrating wounds of the heart. J Trauma Injury Infect Crit Care 2000;48:587–91.
[14] Battistella FD, Nugent W, Owings JT. Field triage of the pulseless trauma patient. Arch Surg 1999;134:742–6.
[15] Renz BM, Stout MJ. Rapid right atrial cannulation for fluid infusion during resuscitative emergency department thoracotomy. Am Surg 1994;60:946–9.
[16] Mattox KL, Feliciano DV. Role of external cardiac compression in truncal trauma. J Trauma 1982;22:934–6.
[17] Mulder DS, Barkun JS. Injuries to the trachea, bronchus and oesophagus. In: Moore EE, Mattox KL, Feliciano DV, editors. Trauma. Norwalk: Appleton & Lange, 1991, p. 345–55.
[18] Aihara R, Millham FH, Blansfield J, et al. Emergency room thoracotomy for penetrating chest injury: effect of an institutional protocol. J Trauma Injury Infect Crit Care 2001;50:1027–30.
[19] Fitzgerald M, Tan G, Gruen R, et al. Emergency physician credentialing for resuscitative thoracotomy for trauma. Emerg Med Australas 2010;22:332–6.
[20] Lee J, Harris JH, Duke JD, Williams JS. Noncorrelation between thoracic skeleton injuries and traumatic aortic tear. J Trauma 1997;43:400–4.
[21] Hehir MD, Hollands MJ, Deane SA. The accuracy of the first chest X-ray in the trauma patient. Aust NZ J Surg 1990;60:529–32.
[22] Brookes JG, Dunn RJ, Rogers IR. Sternal fractures: a retrospective analysis of 272 cases. J Trauma 1993;35:46–54.
[23] Hills MW, Delprado AM, Deane SA. Sternal fractures: associated injuries and management. J Trauma 1993;35:55–60.
[24] Lardinois D, Kreuger T, Dusmet M, et al. Pulmonary function testing after operative stabilization of the chest wall for flail chest. Eur J Cardiovasc Surg 2001;20:496–501.
[25] Marasco SF, Davies AR, Cooper J, et al. Prospective randomized controlled trial of operative rib fixation in traumatic flail chest. J Am Coll Surg 2013(12):01429. doi:pii: S1072-7515.
[26] Brasel KJ, Borgstrom DC, Meyer P. Predictors of outcome in blunt diaphragm rupture. J Trauma 1996;41:484–7.
[27] Mirvis SE. Diagnostic imaging of acute thoracic injury. Semin Ultrasound CT MRI 2004;25:156–79.
[28] American College of Surgeons Committee on Trauma. Advanced trauma life support student manual. Chicago: American College of Surgeons, 2004, p. 105.
[29] Fitzgerald M, Mackenzie CF, Marasco S. Pleural decompression and drainage during trauma reception and resuscitation. Injury 2008;39:9–20.
[30] Blostein P, Hodgman CG. Computed tomography of the chest in blunt thoracic trauma: results of a prospective study. J Trauma 1997;43:3–18.
[31] Mowery NT, Gunter OL, Collier BR, et al. Practice management guidelines for management of hemothorax and occult pneumothorax. J Trauma Injury Infect Crit Care 2011;70:510–8.
[32] Alrahji K, Woo M, Vaillancourt C. Test characteristics of ultrasonography for the detection of pneumothorax – a systematic review and meta-analysis. Chest 2012;141:703–8.
[33] American College of Surgeons Committee on Trauma. Advanced trauma life support student manual. Chicago: American College of Surgeons, 2004, p. 109.
[34] Cohn S. Pulmonary contusion: review of the clinical entity. J Trauma 1997;42:973–9.
[35] Jorden RC. Penetrating chest trauma. Emerg Med Clin N Am 1993;11:97–106.
[36] Fitzgerald MC, Foord K. Tension pneumopericardium following blunt trauma. Emerg Med 1993;5:74–7.
[37] Katyal D, McLellan B, Brenneman F, et al. Lateral impact motor vehicle collisions: a significant cause of traumatic rupture of the thoracic aorta. J Trauma 1997;45:769–72.
[38] Fabian T, Richardson JD, Croce MA, et al. Prospective study of blunt aortic injury: multicentre trial of the American Association for the Surgery of Trauma. Journal of Trauma 1997;42:374–83.
[39] Creasy JD, Chiles C, Routh WD, et al. Overview of traumatic injury of the thoracic aorta. Radiographics 1997;17:27–45.
[40] Andrassy J, Weidenhagen R, Meimarakis G. Stent versus open surgery for acute and chronic traumatic injury of the thoracic aorta: a single center experience. J Trauma 2006;60:765–72.
[41] Hoornweg LL, Maarten KD, Goslings CJ. Endovascular management of traumatic rupture of the thoracic aorta: a retrospective multicenter analysis of 28 consecutive cases in The Netherlands 2006. J Vasc Surg 2006;43:1096–102.
[42] Neschis DG, Moaine S, Gutta R. Twenty consecutive cases of endograft repair of traumatic aortic disruption: lessons learned. J Vasc Surg 2007;43:487–92.
[43] Reed AB, Thompson JK, Crafton CJ, et al. Timing of endovascular repair of blunt traumatic aortic transection. J Vasc Surg 2006;43:684–8.
[44] Lee WA, et al. Endovascular repair of traumatic thoracic aortic injury: clinical practice guidelines of the Society for Vascular Surgery. J Vasc Surg 2011;53:187–92.
[45] Cohn SM, Burns GA, Jaffe C, Milner KA. Exclusion of aortic tear in the unstable trauma patient: the utility of transoesophageal echocardiography. J Trauma 1995;39:1087–90.
[46] Ben-Menachem Y. Assessment of blunt aortic-brachiocephalic trauma: should angiography be supplanted by transoesophageal echocardiography? J Trauma 1997;42:969–72.
[47] Jackimczyk K. Blunt chest trauma. Emerg Med Clin N Am 1993;11:81–96.
[48] Hirshberg A, Or J, Stein M, Walker R. Transaxial gunshot injuries. J Trauma 1996;41:460–1.
[49] Patel M, Malinoski D, Zhou L, et al. Penetrating oesophageal injury: a contemporary analysis of the National Trauma Data Bank. Injury 2013;44:48–55.

3.7 Limb trauma

Amit Maini • Alfredo Mori

ESSENTIALS

1 Optimal trauma resuscitation and fracture management will reduce limb and life-threatening complications.

2 Skin under pressure over a fracture is an orthopaedic emergency.

3 Fracture management consists of reduction, immobilization and rehabilitation.

4 Specific limb trauma assessment is part of the secondary survey.

5 Early renal replacement therapy is potentially life saving in crush syndromes.

Introduction

Injuries to the limbs account for the most trauma-related presentations to emergency departments (EDs) and are a common source of disability in this patient group. These injuries span a spectrum, from seemingly trivial and benign, to limb and life threatening. Injuries may involve the soft tissues, bones, as well as the neurovascular structures and can occur as discrete injuries in isolation or in combination as is the case with more severe trauma.

The major consideration in managing extremity injury in a major trauma patient is to consider the treatment of the patient as a whole, rather than be distracted by any particular injury or fracture. A full primary survey should be performed on all patients, with simultaneous assessment and management of life-threatening injuries as the priority. Orthopaedic injuries should be picked up as part of the secondary survey, although bleeding from long bone fractures (especially open femoral fractures) may be categorized under the circulation component of the primary survey.

Specific complications of open fractures and crush injury include bleeding, crush syndrome and hyperkalaemia as well as sepsis. Early consideration should be given to these with respect to early haemorrhage control and early administration of appropriate antibiotics. Other complications include compartment syndrome, as well as fat embolus syndrome which will be considered later.

The only immediate threat to life from fractures is haemorrhagic shock. Limb trauma may pose a therapeutic challenge in trauma resuscitation by limiting available vascular access. Deformed or injured limbs should, as a rule, be avoided when placing intravenous cannulae and patients with multiple-injured limbs may require early central venous access. Estimates of blood loss, in addition to external scene and ED blood loss, include:

- 1200–1500 mL for femoral fracture
- 500–1000 mL for tibial fracture
- 500 mL for humeral fracture.

The immediate goal of management in the multitrauma patient is control of haemorrhage, followed by limb salvage. The overall aim of limb trauma care is a return to full pain-free function and good cosmesis. The function of the upper limb is to communicate a person's will to the external world and manipulate their surroundings. The function of the lower limbs is independent ambulation. Rehabilitation plays an essential part in recovery and must be considered early with regard to the role of splints from the outset of trauma care.

Fractures

A fracture is a soft-tissue injury with loss of bone continuity. The soft-tissue component is often underestimated. Tense or white skin over a closed fracture is an orthopaedic emergency requiring urgent reduction, even before imaging. Ischaemic skin over bone, such as in the area of the anterior

tibia, has a high rate of necrosis and a poor response to skin grafting. This may result in the disastrous complication of limb amputation.

All transferred patients should have splints removed and the underlying tissues carefully assessed. No splint should remain over skin for more than 8 hours without removal and reassessment. Discharged patients should have clear instructions for returning should there be an increase in pain, tightness under a plaster or splint or numbness and pain in the limb distal to the fracture. Planned early follow up is essential.

Fractures where the overlying skin is intact are closed. Open or compound fractures are defined by their being exposed to the environment. Compound fractures may be classified as follows:

- grade 1: wound <1 cm punctured from below (fracture fragment)
- grade 2: wound up to 5 cm long with no contamination, crush, skin loss or necrosis
- grade 3: large laceration with associated contamination or crush (closed after debridement). Periosteal stripping of bone (will require skin flap for closure)
- grade 4: total or subtotal amputation.

Patients at high risk of fracture complications from single limb trauma include the elderly, the immunocompromised, alcoholics (from repeated falls and poor follow up) and patients with peripheral vascular disease. High-risk mechanisms in limb injury from multiple trauma include falls from over 3 m, pedestrians, motorcyclists and high-speed motorists. Haemodynamically unstable patients, those with open fractures, with delayed (>6 hours) presentation times and the severely head injured also form a group of associated injuries at high risk of complications. Severely head-injured patients are prone to coagulopathy, further increasing fracture bleeding. Clinical assessment of limb trauma may be affected by poor feedback from a head-injured conscious state or sedation and intubation [1–5].

Associated injuries

Vascular injury

Arterial injury is a limb- and (potentially) life-threatening emergency. Ischaemic times of

4–6 hours may result in permanent damage to tissues. Peripheral circulation and distal pulses must always be assessed and sides compared. All splints in transferred patients should be removed and underlying tissues and distal circulation assessed. High-risk patients include those that have been transferred by air with air splints *in situ*, unconscious patients and shocked patients, as the shock state may mask local limb ischaemia.

There may be a role for hypotensive resuscitation in complete arterial injury, whereby a reduced, controlled perfusion pressure may leave intact a clot formed as a result of complete arterial laceration. Aggressive fluid resuscitation in these patients, where not otherwise indicated, or inadequate analgesia, may cause a rise in mean arterial pressure, dislodgement of the clot at the site of injury and resumption of arterial bleeding.

The presence of a distal pulse does not exclude arterial injury, which may be incomplete. Other signs to consider in this diagnosis include the presence of a dislocation, limb deformity or open fracture in that limb, brisk bleeding from an open wound, reduced pulses compared to the other side (either clinically or on Doppler) and an expanding wound haematoma. Delayed signs include a false aneurysm or the presence of a bruit on examination.

Sites at specific risk of arterial injury include:

- brachial artery in the upper limb
- popliteal artery around the knee and adductor canal of the medial distal femur
- deep femoral artery at the trochanter level of the femur
- the anterior tibial artery in the tibia.

Computed tomography (CT) angiography has largely replaced formal angiography as the investigation of choice and, if a vascular injury is suspected, early discussion with a vascular surgeon is recommended.

Nerve injury

Nerve injury in limb trauma may be a direct result of laceration by foreign bodies or fracture fragments. Nerves may be crushed, bruised or stretched. Ischaemia must be excluded as a cause for neurological deficits. Nerve injury from penetrating injury ideally should be explored in the operating theatre.

Nerve injuries may be classified into three major groups:

- Neuropraxia. This is a transient change in conduction. It usually follows crush or contusion or stretching of a nerve. There is usually some return of function within days and complete return of function within 8 weeks.
- Axonotmesis. Complete denervation with an intact nerve sheath, usually as a result of blunt trauma causing severe bruising and stretching. Regeneration takes place over months along the intact nerve sheath.
- Neurotmesis. Complete division of a nerve and its sheath. Spontaneous regeneration is not expected and surgical repair is required. This represents the most severe end of the spectrum and full recovery cannot be guaranteed.

The neurovascular status of the injured limb should be assessed and documented before and after any manipulation and relocation. Specific nerve injury presentations include:

- wrist drop from radial nerve injury of the middle or distal third of the humerus
- foot drop from peroneal nerve injury to the proximal fibula
- shoulder skin numbness from axillary nerve injury in shoulder dislocation
- lower limb numbness and weakness from sciatic nerve injury due to posterior dislocations of the hip
- hand numbness and weakness from median nerve injury in distal fractures of the wrist and dislocations of the carpal bones
- hand numbness and weakness from ulnar nerve injury in injuries to the medial forearm or humerus.

Presentation

History and examination

Injury history and pre-hospital care should be presented in the MIST format on arrival at hospital:

- Mechanism.
- Injuries identified or suspected. Specifically, attention to external blood loss, limb deformity (and correction) or amputation.
- Symptoms and signs: in particular vital signs, whether the patient mobilized at the scene, areas of limb weakness or numbness and pale or pulseless limbs.
- Treatments commenced and the responses to them: a note should be made of all splints placed and their type (hard, soft or anatomic).

The general history should also include patient's normal state of health, medications and allergies, hand dominance, tetanus prophylaxis and fasting state. The history should be presented at the same time as the primary survey commences. Only when this is completed may a meticulous secondary survey start to exclude and treat limb trauma. All splints should be removed for limb trauma assessment, especially in patients transferred between hospitals, given the often long intervals before definitive assessment and treatment.

The assessment of limbs for trauma includes:

- Looking for deformity, bruising, open fractures, bleeding, skin blistering (which denotes soft tissues under pressure) and white or pressured skin. Comparison should always be made with the other limb.
- Feeling for local pain, crepitus or deformity. All peripheral pulses should be examined for and their absence investigated further.
- Active (patient controlled) and passive (examiner controlled) movement. Joints with a full active range of movement are almost never dislocated. Full active movement of the elbow may exclude an elbow fracture and straight leg raising a major pelvic fracture. Passive movement should include an assessment of ligament stability, especially around the knee.
- Peripheral vascular assessment includes pulses and capillary refill.
- Peripheral neurological assessment includes motor power and sensation. The most accurate indicator of sensory function is two-point discrimination.
- Vascular injury should be suspected in elbow and knee dislocations, regardless of whether the peripheral vascular examination is normal after reduction. Abnormal peripheral vascular signs include absent or decreased distal pulses, prolonged capillary refill, pale peripheries unilaterally, ongoing wound bleeding or an expanding haematoma.

Investigations

Plain radiography

Plain X-rays are the investigation of choice in the diagnosis of limb fracture. They may be performed in the trauma bay where available or in the radiology area once the patient is stable for transfer.

Two views in two planes are required for accurate diagnosis and planning of reduction. The joints above and below the injury site should also be imaged.

Other indicators of injury that may alter management include the presence of air or foreign bodies around injury sites and joints and soft tissue swelling, such as the sail sign in distal humerus fractures. Joint injury may be indicated by soft tissue swelling and lipohaemarthroses (radiopaque effusions), which may indicate an underlying fracture.

Joints and fractures should be X-rayed again after reduction. Timed repeated X-rays may be used in injuries where there is doubt about the presence of a fracture (e.g. the scaphoid in peripheral wrist injuries).

The multitrauma patient may have over 30 X-rays as part of the diagnostic and specific radiological screen. Such large numbers of X-rays, or where there is any doubt about the presence of a fracture, should be reviewed in conjunction with a radiologist or other senior clinician.

Ultrasound

Ultrasound is now commonplace in trauma centres and many EDs and is increasingly being used in the pre-hospital setting. Also, many emergency physicians and registrars are becoming proficient in its use. Bedside ultrasonography is cheap, reliable, safe, non-invasive and easily repeatable. Its role in major trauma is to exclude traumatic cardiac tamponade and haemoperitoneum. Doppler scanning may be used to identify peripheral pulses.

The role of ultrasound in limb trauma is less well defined, but includes the diagnosis of muscle or tendon ruptures (the rotator cuff and the Achilles tendon, respectively) and soft-tissue foreign bodies or free fluid. Therapeutically, ultrasound may aid in peripheral and central line placement, as well as the accurate placement of peripheral nerve blocks in the patient with limb trauma.

Computed tomography (CT)

CT scans have a limited role in the acute management of fractures. Indications may include further imaging and quantification of tibial plateau fractures, particularly the posterior component of the tibial plateau, and carpal and tarsal injuries that may by difficult to assess on plain X-ray. CT has been used in the diagnosis of suspected femoral neck fractures in the elderly.

CT angiography (CTA)

Although historically, digital subtraction angiography (DSA) was the preferred method for assessing vascular integrity, it has now (for the most part) been superseded by CTA due to widespread availability, being relatively non-invasive, shorter image acquisition times, and all the while maintaining diagnostic accuracy [6].

CT angiography is indicated in:

- all dislocations or disruptions of the knee joint, as tears of the media of the popliteal artery may not be otherwise safely excluded
- all limb injuries with vascular compromise distally, in particular high velocity injuries such as firearm wounds.

Angiography

In cases where CT angiography is diagnostically inconclusive, traditional angiography may be employed to delineate further vascular integrity in those patients where arterial injury is suspected. It would also be the primary choice in patients with penetrating trauma where shrapnel might cause considerable image artefact, for instance in blast or gunshot injuries [6].

Angiograms may be performed in the trauma centre, in the angiography suite or in theatre and specialist staff, such as interventional radiologists, must be alerted early, as angiography suites may require some time to staff and prepare. In major trauma centres, this may take up to an hour in out-of-hours scenarios. This, and the preparation of a transfer team, should be the role of the trauma team leader.

Magnetic resonance imaging (MRI)

The indications for emergency MRI do not include limb trauma. Compartment syndromes may be identified using MRI, but this is of limited value in the acute setting. The role of MRI is usually limited to acute spinal injury with neurological deficits.

Bone scan

There is no place for bone scans in the early management of limb trauma. Bone scans are most reliable 3 days after injury in the diagnosis of occult fractures. They may also be used in the diagnosis and assessment of osteomyelitis as a complication of fractures.

Manometry

Pressure manometry is used specifically in the measurement of compartment pressures. Tools, such as the Stryker manometer or a peripheral cannula connected to a blood pressure or arterial line manometer, may be used repeatedly in the ED.

Management

Resuscitation and the primary survey take precedence in limb trauma. Splints and limb injuries may distract the team or clinician from this process. Limb trauma may impede or limit the placement of peripheral cannulae. In the primary survey, limb trauma assessment is limited to control of visible haemorrhage by external pressure. Open wounds should be covered with sterile dressings and fractures splinted in the initial phase of care.

All rings, bracelets and other constricting foreign bodies, such as clothing, should be removed from the affected limbs.

Tetanus prophylaxis should be provided. Severely contaminated wounds should receive tetanus immunoglobulin and urgent debridement in theatre.

There is very good evidence that early systemic antibiotics reduce infection rates in open fractures, with a number needed to treat (NNT) of 13 in a recent Cochrane Review [7]. Antibiotics are not a substitute for good wound care, which includes decontamination, irrigation and early surgical debridement. Crushed, penetrating and macerated injuries should receive antibiotic prophylaxis against *Staphylococcus aureus*, *Streptococcus pyogenes*, *Clostridium perfringens*, and aerobic Gram-negative bacteria. Recommended antibiotic combinations include flucloxacillin, gentamicin and metronidazole or cephalothin and metronidazole [8]. Cephazolin is also commonly used.

Gentamicin and benzylpenicillin are indicated in severely soiled wounds, severe tissue damage or devitalized tissue to cover against Gram negatives and *Clostridium perfringens*, respectively.

Compound wounds should be protected from secondary injury and decontamination by gentle washing with normal saline and a sterile moist dressing placed over the wound. A Polaroid photograph may be taken of the wound and placed over the dressing until definitive care is provided.

Pain, even in the sedated or intubated patient, may cause life-threatening arrhythmias or emergent hypertension, especially in the multitrauma patient. Analgesia may be pharmacological or non-pharmacological. Non-pharmacological measures include splinting and fracture reduction.

Pharmacological analgesia may be general or local. General agents include narcotics, which should be titrated to comfort and physiological response. The use of ketamine is increasingly widespread in the pre-hospital transport of injured patients and in reduction of fractures and dislocation in the ED. It should be used by experienced clinicians in monitored, selected patients. Some procedures, such as reduction of disrupted joints, or in the uncooperative, intoxicated or polytrauma patient, may require general intravenous anaesthesia and intubation.

Local nerve blocks may prove useful. Specifically, in splinted femoral shaft fractures, the femoral nerve block is very useful in reducing quadriceps muscle spasm.

The role of splints

Splinting is almost universal in limb trauma management, being used in every stage of care, from scene to long-term rehabilitation.

The role of splints includes communication, analgesia, haemorrhage control, tissue protection, immobilization, facilitating transport and, perhaps, reduction of fat embolism. All splinted areas should be treated as fractured till proved otherwise. All splints should be noted and removed when possible and a full inspection made of the whole limb. Pain relief is assisted by less movement of injured tissue. Splinted, reduced injuries have less local bleeding and oedema. Definitive bone apposition will reduce fracture bleeding. Injured tissues may be protected during transport until definitive assessment and care. Immobilized limbs are less painful and bleed less. Patient immobilization may facilitate safe and efficient transfer to definitive care. Fat embolism may be reduced, though the role of early splinting is controversial and based on poor historical evidence.

Splints may be classified by area (general splints, such as spine boards, or local, such as cervical spine collars) or type (anatomical, such as the unaffected leg, soft, rigid, air or slings).

All splints are foreign bodies, with consequent complications: they may be distracting to other injuries or cause local skin pressure and necrosis, compartment syndromes, loss of limb function and distal hypoperfusion. A limb cannot be adequately assessed while a splint is in place.

The definitive management of fractures and dislocations is reduction, immobilization and rehabilitation. Ideally, all deformed, injured limbs should be splinted to an anatomically neutral position. Early reduction offers pain relief by distracting fracture edges and pressure on local innervated tissue. It also facilitates patient transport. Pressure on the overlying skin and nearby neurovascular structures is also reduced. Limb deformities with overlying skin under pressure are true orthopaedic emergencies which should be reduced before imaging. Any suspect penetrating joint injury should be reviewed under anaesthesia for assessment and lavage.

Injured limbs should be immobilized in the pre-hospital setting in the anatomical or neutral position where possible. The joints above and below an injured area should be immobilized. Some specific injuries, such as femoral shaft fractures, will require traction immobilization to overcome local muscle spasm. Common devices include the Donway splint and variations of the Thomas splint. Once applied, all distal areas of splinted limbs should be neurovascularly reassessed.

Rehabilitation of limb trauma commences in the ED. Early movement of uninjured limbs should be encouraged. Supervised practice with crutches and the removal and care of slings will improve outpatient independence and reduce complications from these devices. Timed follow up of all fractures, complicated wounds and patient groups otherwise at risk of complications is essential. Patients should be discharged home from the ED when limb- and life-threatening injuries have been excluded, when they are safely ambulant, are tolerating food and drink, have adequate oral analgesia and have planned follow up arranged.

Compound fractures and contaminated wounds are time-critical emergencies. There is a paucity of evidence regarding the ideal time to theatre, but ethically, the sooner these injuries are definitively attended, the better the expected outcome. Time to theatre is related to infection rates and necrosis of overlying soft tissue.

Wound management

The role of wound irrigation agents in the acute setting is controversial. There is no evidence to support the use of full-strength povidone–iodine and, if used, it should be diluted to less than 1%. Povidone–iodine has been shown to delay wound healing and increase infection rates

in chronic wounds. Shaving of wounds should be avoided as it promotes local inflammation.

Gross contamination should be removed and the wound irrigated using normal saline. The efficacy of normal saline is related to the irrigation pressure. Pulsatile pressure at 7–10 psi (48–69 kPa) removes debris and bacteria without further dissemination of microorganisms in the tissue. This pressure may be produced with a 20 mL syringe and a 19 G needle with a splash guard. There is no evidence that high-pressure irrigation offers any benefit. Reviews of the techniques and materials used in wound irrigation recommend normal saline [9–11].

Tense haemarthroses (joint swelling from acute bleeding) should be assessed and drained. This may be diagnostic in revealing a lipohaemarthrosis (and thereby increase the suspicion of an underlying fracture), will facilitate joint assessment by increasing range of movement and is therapeutic in providing pain relief by reducing local joint pressure. A sterile field and an aseptic technique performed by experienced staff is essential to prevent iatrogenic septic arthritis.

Management of the mangled extremity

The mangled extremity, while often graphic in appearance, should not distract the trauma team from initiating rapid simultaneous assessment and management of life-threatening injuries in the multitrauma patient. A systematic approach in the ED will comprise restoration of anatomic alignment of the extremity, as well as evaluation for vascular and nerve injury.

The goals of management of the mangled extremity are:

- Control of ongoing haemorrhage using direct pressure. If this fails, then application of a tourniquet may be life saving as a temporizing measure to prevent further major bleeding until definitive haemostasis is achieved in the operating theatre [12,13].
- To achieve timely reperfusion of ischaemic tissues.
- Early reduction of long bone fractures using traction or splints. This may also improve perfusion by relieving potential impingement of vasculature [14].
- Providing adequate analgesia. Repeated, titrated doses of fentanyl may facilitate the humane manipulation of fractures. Ketamine

has also emerged as a safe, useful adjunct to analgesia for experienced providers in the setting of extremity trauma.

- Early communication with surgical specialists to expedite necessary early operative intervention.
- Assessment and careful documentation of extremity neurological status.

Hyperbaric oxygen therapy

The role of hyperbaric therapy (HBOT) in acute limb injuries is controversial and remains unresolved. Theoretically, it enhances oxygen delivery to areas affected acutely by hypoxia and at risk of such by cellular and tissue oedema. This may reduce the number of cells at risk from delayed ischaemia and necrosis from local oedema. Animal and human case studies have demonstrated benefit in crush injury, compartment syndrome and malunited or non-united fractures [42,43]. The US Hyperbaric Society lists crush injury and compartment syndrome as indications for hyperbaric therapy. A systematic review has demonstrated a possible benefit of HBOT in the management of acute, difficult to heal wounds [15]. Clinicians should be aware of the recommendations and practice in their region.

Disposition

The ED is a critical care area, not a final disposition. Patients will be discharged home, admitted to a general or trauma ward, taken to theatre or admitted to the intensive care unit. In the interim, some patients may require transfer for angiography, CT scanning or MRI. Patients who have been completely managed in the ED may be discharged home with a written care plan and timed follow up at their GP, an injury or fracture clinic, or the ED. Elderly patients with splints should be assessed for mobilization safety and appropriate aids provided by an expert team. Adequate oral analgesia should be prescribed for at least a week, with specific care taken to cover weekend and holiday periods. Non-steroidal anti inflammatories (NSAIDs) should be avoided, particularly in the elderly, as they offer no benefit and may cause harm. Sleep with injured limbs may be interrupted and difficult. Slings should be removed during rest periods and adequate replacements, such as cushions, planned for. Minor sedatives may be prescribed in some cases.

Patients with a plaster should have documented evaluation of the plaster, the affected limb(s) and use of any splints or walking aids, such as crutches. Upper limb slings should have cushioned supports where they come in contact with the neck, especially at the site of any securing knot. All injured limbs should be elevated for the first 48 hours, preferably in a splint such as a sling, or with specific instructions, such as elevation of the leg above the height of the hip when sitting or lying. Patients should be instructed to return if their injury becomes too painful to cope with, even with discharge analgesia, if the distal area becomes numb, painful to move or pale or blue in colour. All initial plasters should be reviewed at 24 hours and removed at 1 week or earlier should they become tight, wet or damaged, and the injury and the patient reassessed.

Operating theatre

Urgent transfer to the operating theatre specifically for limb injury is indicated in:

- uncontrollable haemorrhage
- severely contaminated wounds or open fractures
- limbs ischaemic for over 6–8 hours
- crushed limbs requiring amputation as a life-saving procedure
- infected limbs requiring amputation as a life-saving procedure.

In patients with complex polytrauma, patients *in extremis* with an otherwise high intra-operative mortality risk or in departments in which the surgical workload will overload theatre resources, damage control surgery may be indicated. In the 1970s, early fixation of fractures resulted in a dramatic fall in fat embolism syndrome and so became standard practice. Damage control orthopaedic surgery is the initial temporary fixation of fractures in patients in whom the overall burden of definitive surgery may be too great, with a definitive secondary procedure planned for a later date. The aims of damage control surgery are to control haemorrhage, contamination and wound swelling and reduce the potential risk of skin necrosis and fat embolism syndrome. The patient is then usually transferred to an intensive care unit for haemodynamic stabilization and correction of gross physiological derangements [16–18].

General or trauma ward

Patients transferred to a general or trauma unit ward should have the same documented

attention as discharged patients. Specific issues include fasting status, fluid requirements, mobilization restrictions, analgesia with particular stress on systemic analgesia for breakthrough pain or pain after wound care on the ward. Considerable care should be given to adequate sighting, labelling and communication of any procedures planned. Other general care issues include bladder and bowel care, pressure care and elevation of injured limbs in splints or on pillows.

Complications

Compartment syndrome

Acute limb compartment syndrome (ALCS) is a limb- and (occasionally) life-threatening complication of limb trauma. It is caused by bleeding or oedema in a closed muscle compartment surrounded by fascia, interosseous membrane and bone. The syndrome leads to muscle and nerve ischaemia and the release of potentially lethal potassium and hydrogen ions and myoglobin. Untreated compartment syndrome leads to muscle necrosis, limb amputation and, if severe in large compartments, acute renal failure and death.

Clinical suspicion, elevation with local ice packs, occasional compartment pressure measuring and surgical decompression with fasciotomy are the mainstay of treatment.

Clinically, the outstanding sign is ischaemic muscle pain. That is, pain that is difficult to control and greater than expected for the injury seen. This may be brought on by passive flexion or extension of the distal digits. Peripheral pulses are usually present and their loss is a very late sign as mean arterial pressure is usually adequately maintained. Affected muscle compartments are firm, tense and tender on palpation.

Causes of compartment syndrome include crush injuries, closed fractures, injections or infusions into compartments, reperfusion of arterial ischaemia, snakebite, electric shock, burns, exercise and hyperthermia. Splinting of suspected limbs and removal of any circumferential casts, splints or dressings is essential so as not to increase compartment pressure further.

Areas in which ALCS occurs most commonly are the leg (anterior, lateral, superficial and deep posterior compartments), thigh (quadriceps) and forearm (volar and dorsal compartments). Less commonly, it may also occur in the buttocks (gluteals), the hand (interosseous muscles) and the arm (biceps and triceps).

The investigation of choice is compartment pressure monitoring. The use of this modality is controversial, although some centres advocate continuous monitoring. Normal compartment pressure is 4–8 mmHg. The pressure mandating fasciotomy remains controversial, but most departments would agree on an orthopaedic review with a view to fasciotomy for any pressure above 40 mmHg. Compartment pressure may be monitored with commercial devices, such as the Stryker pressure monitor, or by insertion of an intra-arterial pressure monitor and cannula.

Patients who should have compartment pressure measured include all those with tense compartments whose contralateral limbs cannot be clinically compared, patients with distracting injuries, such as compound fractures, and severely intoxicated or intubated patients.

The definitive management of compartment syndrome is surgical decompression with fasciotomy [19–21].

Fat embolism syndrome

Fat embolism – the passage of fat from one area of the body to another via the vascular system – is a normal consequence of long bone fractures and was first described in 1862. Fat embolism syndrome (FES), the self-limiting, life-threatening multiorgan syndrome affecting the lungs, brain cardiovascular system and skin, is very rare, occurring in perhaps less than 1% of all long bone fractures. The exact incidence is difficult to measure given that FES may be subclinical or masked by other syndromes, such as acute respiratory distress syndrome (ARDS), and its investigative diagnosis is non-specific and inconsistent. It usually follows 6–48 hours after long bone fracture. Other causes include closed cardiac massage, severe burns, liver injury, bone marrow transplantation and liposuction.

Clinically, patients deteriorate with hypoxaemia, chest X-ray changes, skin petechiae and an altered conscious state. The respiratory syndrome is similar to ARDS. There may be petechiae on the skin and conjunctivae.

Investigations are useful only in the exclusion of other causes, such as ARDS, pulmonary contusion or pulmonary embolism. Some tomographic changes may be more specific for FES and these are thought to represent the fat emboli themselves and the systemic inflammatory response to them. Treatment is both prophylactic and supportive. General ICU management includes adequate oxygenation and ventilation, haemodynamic stability and prophylaxis for deep vein thrombosis (DVT) and stress-related upper gastrointestinal bleeding.

Studies support early fixation of fractures to prevent recurrent FES. There is controversy regarding the role of reaming with intramedullary nails for the fractures of long bones, such as the femur and tibia, as by the nature of this technique, relatively large amounts of fat are released into the systemic circulation [22–29].

Crush syndrome

Crush syndrome is a life-threatening systemic manifestation of muscle damage resulting from pressure or crushing. Crush syndrome was first described in the early 20th century following the Messina earthquake of 1906 and work in Germany in World War 1 and by Beals and Bywater in London in 1941. Following the Armenian earthquake of 1988, the International Society of Nephrology established the Renal Disaster Relief Task Force in direct response to the overwhelming demand for dialysis of crush injury survivors in these earthquakes. Specific protocols for the prevention and management of renal failure due to crush syndrome have been established.

Crush syndrome is a result of both external pressure on muscles and time. Crushed or compressed muscle cells may immediately burst due to overwhelming external compressive force, releasing potassium, hydrogen ions (causing hyperkalaemia and acidosis, respectively) and myoglobin, oxygen free radicals and phosphate ions (causing acute renal injury and death from renal failure). The release of the above may occur in cells not initially crushed but at risk of cell wall breakdown from local ischaemia, as in compartment syndrome, or cell membrane damage without disruption from external compressive force. The toxic metabolites, listed above, are initially usually restricted to the local tissue environment as venous return is impeded by the crush injury itself. Creatinine kinase (CK) is also released and may be a measure of myoglobin load, predicting renal injury and dialysis. Hence the release of crushed tissue from a compressive environment and the re-establishment of local blood flow may release all of the above systemically. Therefore, pre-hospital fluids may be able to pre-empt renal injury and death before a limb is released from crush injury.

Diagnosis is from the history of a crush injury. Apart from earthquake survivors, other groups at risk include trapped motor vehicle accident victims, IV drug users who collapse unconscious on a limb or limbs and elderly collapsed patients who remain unattended for some time (e.g. after a hip fracture). Other causes of rhabdomyolysis are the destruction of skeletal muscle, heat stroke, severe exertion, cocaine and amphetamine use, serotoninergic syndrome and snakebites.

As with compartment syndrome, clinically, patients may exhibit tense, hard, tender muscles, with overlying skin that may be bruised or blistered due to high interstitial pressure. They may be hypothermic and shocked due to prolonged exposure and inadequate fluid intake. The urine is dark (like machinery oil or black tea) and reflects the presence of myoglobin and other toxic haem proteins. The bedside investigation of choice is an ECG to exclude the consequences of life-threatening hyperkalaemia. Blood tests may initially only demonstrate hyperkalaemia but, in time, will reflect metabolic acidosis and worsening acute renal failure. The CK is often raised above 5000 in significant crush injury. A CK over 75 000 is predictive of acute renal failure and death.

Early deaths from crush syndrome are due to arrhythmias from hyperkalaemia and hypovolaemic shock. At 3–5 days after injury, death is from renal failure, coagulopathy and haemorrhage (DIC) and sepsis. Treatment is aimed at stabilizing the cardiac milieu against hyperkalaemia, aggressive volume therapy to prevent shock and renal failure, enhancing haem protein elimination and limiting haem protein cytotoxicity.

Trapped patients should have aggressive fluid loading with normal saline before extraction. They may also receive calcium gluconate or bicarbonate intravenously to counter ensuing hyperkalaemia. In severe crush injury, fluid requirements in addition to baseline needs average 12 L in the first 48 hours to prevent renal failure.

Once in the ED, patients should be monitored and, given the large fluid load expected intravenously and the brisk diuresis desired, have an arterial line placed and an indwelling catheter and a central line considered.

Once urine flow is established an alkaline–mannitol diuresis is recommended, aiming for 2 mL/kg/h output. Mannitol increases renal tubular blood flow, is a renal vasodilator and free-radical scavenger. It is also an osmotoic diuretic. It may have an effect on compartment pressures, though compartment syndrome should be treated by fasciotomy, as mentioned. Urine pH should be maintained at over 5, at which myoglobin is over 50% soluble and thus prevented from precipitating into the renal tubules. Bicarbonate at 50 mmol/h after the first 3 L of normal saline will help achieve this. Clinicians should be aware that, if safe to do so, intravenous potassium may be given in addition to bicarbonate to further alkalinize urine.

Acute renal failure has a high prevalence following crush syndrome and, ideally, renal replacement therapy (RRT) should be utilized in the early stages of management where possible, especially in the anuric patient with refractory hyperkalaemia and fluid overload. This is logistically challenging in the disaster/earthquake scenario, as was found in the January 2010 earthquake in Haiti [30].

Local management of affected limbs and assessment as outlined above is mandatory [30–41].

Immobilization

It is worth reminding clinicians that, by definition, an injured limb will result in some loss of function of that limb until fully recovered. Some patients may therefore require prolonged periods of immobilization, usually in hospital, but also in rehabilitation facilities or at home. The consequences of prolonged immobilization include pressure sores and skin breakdown, muscle atrophy and weakness (with an increased risk of falls subsequently), postural hypotension, dependent-lung atelectasis and secondary pneumonia, constipation, insomnia, social isolation and depression. Management plans that are well communicated and documented should prevent and manage many of these complications.

Controversies

- The type of fluid and technique for the irrigation of contaminated wounds.
- The role of limb compartment pressure monitoring, in particular continuous pressure monitoring.
- The role of early splinting in preventing fat embolism syndrome in long bone fractures.
- The role of hyperbaric therapy in the management of acute limb trauma.
- The timing of early fracture fixation and reduction to prevent fat embolism syndrome and skin necrosis.

References

[1] Deitch EA, Dayal SD. Intensive care unit management of the trauma patient. Crit Care Med 2006;34:2294–301.

[2] Sagraves SG, Toschlog EA, Rotondo MF. Damage control surgery – the intensivist's role. J Intensive Care Med 2006;21:5–16.

[3] Perron AD, Brady WJ. Evaluation and management of the high-risk orthopedic emergency. Emerg Med Clin N Am 2003;21:159–204.

[4] Tintinalli J, Stapczynski J, Ma J, et al. Emergency medicine: a comprehensive study guide, 7th ed. McGraw Hill; 2011.

[5] Marx J, Hockberger R, Walls R. Rosen's Emergency Medicine: concepts and clinical practice, 7th ed. Elsevier; 2009.

[6] Uyeda JW, Anderson SW, Sakai O, Soto JA. CT angiography in trauma. Radiol Clin N Am 2010;48:423–38.

[7] Gosselin RA, Roberts I, Gillespie WJ. Antibiotics for preventing infection in open limb fractures. Cochrane Database Syst Rev 2004:CD003764.

[8] Antibiotic Expert Group. Therapeutic guidelines: antibiotic. Version 14. Melbourne: Therapeutic Guidelines Limited; 2010.

[9] Crowley DJ, Kanakaris NK, Giannoudis PV. Irrigation of the wounds in open fractures. J Bone Joint Surg 2007;89B:580–5.

[10] Chatterjee JS. A critical review of irrigation techniques in acute wounds. Internatl Wound J 2005;2:258–65.

[11] Moreira ME, Markovchick VJ. Wound management. Emerg Med Clin N Am 2007;25:873–99.

[12] Kragh Jr JF, Walters TJ, Baer DG, et al. Survival with emergency tourniquet use to stop bleeding in major limb trauma. Ann Surg 2009;249:1–7.

[13] Beekley AC, Sebesta JA, Blackbourne LH, et al. 31st Combat Support Hospital Research Group. Prehospital tourniquet use in operation iraqi freedom: effect on hemorrhage control and outcomes. J Trauma 2008;64:S28–37. Discussion S37.

[14] Scalea TM, DuBose J, Moore EE, et al. Western Trauma Association critical decisions in trauma: management of the mangled extremity. J Trauma Acute Care Surg 2012;72:86–93.

[15] Eskes AM, Ubbink DT, Lubbers MJ, et al. Hyperbaric oxygen therapy: solution for difficult to heal acute wounds? Systematic review. World J Surg 2011;35:535–42.

[16] Noonburg GE. Management of extremity trauma and related infections occurring in the aquatic environment. J Am Acad Orthopaed Surg 2005;13:243–53.

[17] Okike K, Bhattacharyya T. Trends in the management of open fractures. A critical analysis. J Bone Joint Surg 2006;88A:2739–48.

[18] Houston M, Hendrickson RG. Decontamination. Crit Care Clin 2005;21:653–72.

[19] Salcido R, Lepre SJ. Compartment syndrome: wound care considerations. Adv Skin Wound Care 2007;20:559–65. Quiz 566–7.

[20] Gourgiotis S, Villias C, Germanos S, et al. Acute limb compartment syndrome: a review. J Surg Educ 2007;64:178–86.

[21] Rush Jr RM, Arrington ED, Hsu JR. Management of complex extremity injuries: tourniquets, compartment syndrome detection, fasciotomy and amputation care. Surg Clin N Am 2012;92:987–1007.

[22] Taviloglu K, Yanar H. Fat embolism syndrome. Surg Today 2007;37:5–8.

[23] Husebye EE, Lyberg T, Roise O. Bone marrow fat in the circulation: clinical entities and pathophysiological mechanisms. Injury 2006;37:S8–18.

[24] Habashi NM, Andrews PL, Scalea TM. Therapeutic aspects of fat embolism syndrome. Injury 2006;37:S68–73.

[25] White T, Petrisor BA, Bhandari M. Prevention of fat embolism syndrome. Injury 2006;37:S59–67.

[26] Giannoudis PV, Tzioupis C, Pape HC. Fat embolism: the reaming controversy. Injury 2006;37:S50–8.

[27] van den Brande FG, Hellemans S, De Schepper A, et al. Post-traumatic severe fat embolism syndrome with uncommon CT findings. Anaes Intens Care 2006;34:102–6.

[28] Pape HC, Krettek C. Management of fractures in the severely injured – influence of the principle of 'damage control orthopaedic surgery'. Unfallchirurgie 2003;106:87–96.

[29] Dunham CM, Bosse MJ, Clancy TV, et al. Practice management guidelines for the optimal timing of long-bone fracture stabilization in polytrauma patients: the EAST Practice Management Guidelines Work Group. J Trauma 2001;50:958–67.

[30] Bartal C, Zeller L, Miskin I, et al. Crush syndrome: saving more lives in disasters. Lessons learned from early-response phase in Haiti. Arch Int Med 2011;171:694–6.

[31] Buettner MF, Wolkenhauer D. Hyperbaric oxygen therapy in the treatment of open fractures and crush injuries. Emerg Med Clin N Am 2007;25:177–88.

[32] James T. Management of patients with acute crush injuries of the extremities. Internatl Anesthesiol Clin 2007;45:19–29.

[33] Vanholder R, van der Tol A, De Smet M, et al. Earthquakes and crush syndrome casualties: lessons learned from the Kashmir disaster. Kidney Internatl 2007;71:17–23.

[34] Sever MS, Vanholder R, Lameire N. Management of crush-related injuries after disasters. N Engl J Med 2006;354:1052–63.

[35] Gonzalez D. Crush syndrome. Crit Care Med 2005;33:S34–41.

[36] Garcia-Covarrubias L, McSwain NEJ, Van Meter K, Bell RM. Adjuvant hyperbaric oxygen therapy in the management of crush injury and traumatic ischemia: an evidence-based approach. Am Surg 2005;71:144–51.

[37] Greensmith JE. Hyperbaric oxygen therapy in extremity trauma. J Am Acad Orthopaed Surg 2004;12:376–84.

[38] Smith J, Greaves I. Crush injury and crush syndrome: a review. J Trauma 2003;54:S226–30.

[39] Better OS, Rubinstein I, Reis DN. Muscle crush compartment syndrome: fulminate local edema with threatening systemic effects. Kidney Internatl 2003;63:1155–7.

[40] Greaves I, Porter K, Smith JE. Consensus statement on the early management of crush injury and prevention of crush syndrome. J Roy Army Med Corps 2003;149:255–9.

[41] Eknoyan G. The Armenian earthquake of 1988: a milestone in the evolution of nephrology. Adv Renal Replacement Ther 2003;10:87–92.

[42] Butler J, Foex B. Best evidence topic report. Hyperbaric oxygen therapy in acute fracture management. Emerg Med J 2006;23:571–2.

[43] Bennett MH, Stanford R, Turner R. Hyperbaric oxygen therapy for promoting fracture healing and treating fracture non-union. Cochrane Database Syst Rev 2005:CD004712.

3.8 Radiology in major trauma

Anthony P Joseph • Roger Harris • Simon Dimmick

ESSENTIALS

1 The initial trauma series X-rays should include a chest X-ray (CXR) and pelvic X-ray (PXR). If there is suspicion or risk of cervical spine injury, a comuted tomography (CT) scan is required.

2 The trauma team should be mindful of the risks of radiation for both the patient and the team members.

3 Evaluation of facial trauma requires an adequate clinical and radiological examination.

4 CT of the cervical spine will identify most bony cervical spine abnormalities.

5 Injuries to the thoracolumbar spine should be evaluated by sagittal reconstruction of axial CT scans of the chest/abdomen/pelvis or by plain X-rays.

6 Injury to the carotid or vertebral arteries should be suspected clinically and investigated by CT angiography in the first instance and may require formal digital subtraction angiography for definitive diagnosis.

7 Chest CT is a useful screening test for mediastinal or large vessel injury.

8 Pelvic CT is invaluable for the classification of pelvic fractures and angiography/embolization should be part of the treatment algorithm for haemodynamically unstable patients with pelvic fractures.

Emergency department reception

The initial trauma X-rays usually consist of a supine chest and pelvic X-ray. A lateral cervical (Cx) spine X-ray provides limited information and an axial computed tomography (CT) scan of Cx spine from occiput to T4/5 with sagittal and coronal reconstructions will accurately rule in or out bony injury. Many trauma centres no longer perform a lateral Cx spine X-ray in the resuscitation room if a CT scan of the cervical spine is required.

Hazards of radiation

Exposure of both trauma team members and patients to ionizing radiation should be minimized and staff should wear protective lead gowns and thyroid shields. These garments have been shown to protect against ionizing radiation within recommended occupational limits [1].

The number of X-rays taken in the resuscitation area should be kept to a minimum. As radiation exposure decreases inversely with the square of the distance from the source, staff should position themselves at a maximum distance from X-ray equipment in use whenever possible. The use of permanent lead barriers should be considered.

Ionizing radiation in X-ray and CT examinations may directly or indirectly damage DNA which may not be corrected by cellular repair mechanisms. This damage to DNA has been associated with an increased risk of developing cancer. This risk has, in part, been estimated from similar radiation exposures experienced in World War II by atomic bomb survivors in Japan [2].

The radiation dose from various diagnostic imaging examinations may be calculated as an 'effective dose' for the purpose of comparison and quantification of risk. Effective dose, evaluated in millisieverts (mSv), refers to the radiation dose from an examination averaged over the entire body and accounts for the relative sensitivities of the different tissues exposed [1–4].

A single CT scan gives tissue doses in the range of 10–30 mSv. Tissue doses in the range 50–200 mSv have been shown to cause an increase in cancer risk among atomic bomb survivors and the risk is higher for lower age at exposure [5–7]. The United States Food and Drug Administration estimates that CT examination with an effective dose of 10 mSv may carry a 1:2000 lifetime risk of inducing fatal cancer [8]. Table 3.8.1 gives typical whole-body effective doses for selected radiological examinations.

Typical values cited for radiation dose should be considered as estimates, as they may vary with the size of the patient, the type of procedure and equipment and the operational technique used. This is particularly relevant for CT, where estimates of effective dose can vary widely.

The trauma series

The initial 'trauma series' of X-rays should consist of the lateral cervical spine, AP chest (CXR) and AP pelvic X-rays (PXR). The lateral cervical spine X-ray should be taken with a team member exerting gentle traction on the arms in order to pull down the shoulders and expose the lower cervical spine to the C7–T1 junction.

Systematic examination of this film includes assessment of Alignment, Bony structures, Cartilage and Soft tissue (ABCS) (Table 3.8.2, Fig. 3.8.1). Some trauma centres have abandoned the lateral cervical spine X-ray if the patient

Table 3.8.1 Whole-body effective doses (mSv)	
Examination	*Radiation dose (mSv)*
Annual background radiation	2.4
Chest X-ray [1]	0.02
Pelvic X-ray [1]	0.44
Skull X-ray [1]	0.07
Cervical spine X-ray	0.2
CT head [4]	1–2
CT chest [4]	5–7
CT abdomen/pelvis [4]	8

Table 3.8.2   Radiological examination of the lateral cervical spine

A	Alignment
B	Bony structures
C	Cartilage spaces
S	Soft tissue

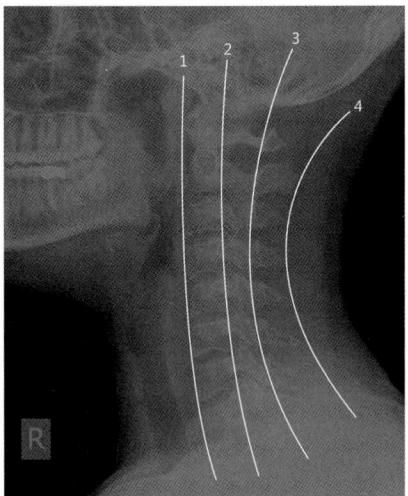

Fig. 3.8.1 Lateral cervical spine X-ray.
(1) Anterior vertebral line; (2) posterior vertebral line;
(3) spino-laminar line; (4) spinous process line.

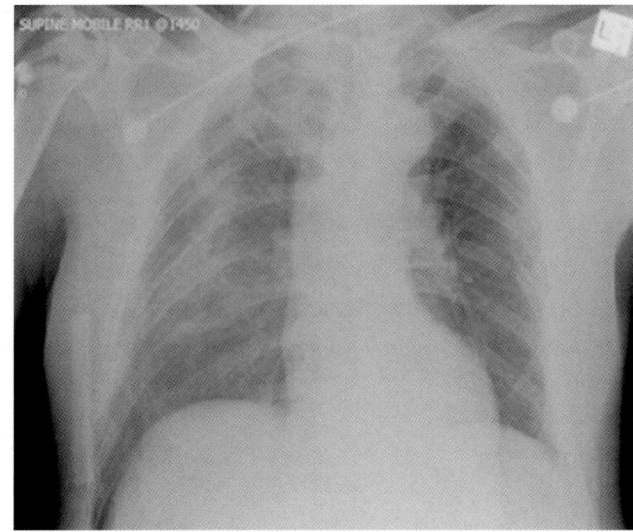

Fig. 3.8.2 Right-sided supine pneumothorax with tension.

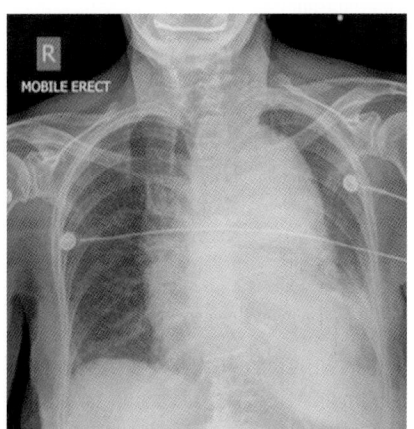

Fig. 3.8.3 Widened mediastinum secondary to aortic dissection and rupture.

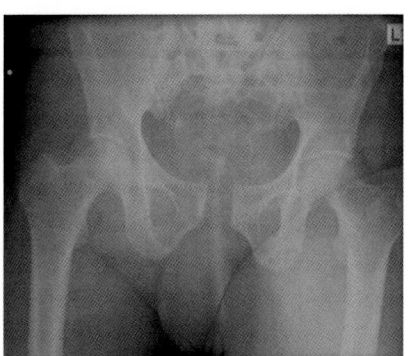

Fig. 3.8.4 Diastasis of the pubic symphysis.

requires a CT brain scan and will perform a CT of the cervical spine with axial images plus coronal and sagittal reformations. This approach gives more information than the lateral cervical spine film, which poorly visualizes both the occipitoatlantal junction and the cervicothoracic junction and is essentially a screening test. If a patient continues to have pain or tenderness, particularly in the midline of the cervical spine, a CT scan with sagittal and coronal reconstructions will be required.

The CXR performed is usually a supine (AP) rather than an erect (PA) film owing to the inability to sit the patient up until the spine is cleared. The CXR should include both clavicles, ribs, lungs, mediastinum and diaphragm. If there is adequate penetration, the thoracic spine may be seen. The mediastinum may be falsely enlarged owing to the AP projection and this should be taken into account. The CXR will exclude life-threatening injuries, such as massive haemothorax or pneumothorax, and may show signs of major vessel injury indicated by a widening of the mediastinum (Figs 3.8.2 and 3.8.3).

The pelvic X-ray will include all the bony pelvic components and the hip joints (Fig. 3.8.4).

Specific regional radiology

Head

Head trauma is responsible for 50–75% of the mortality associated with major trauma [9]. The spectrum of head injury ranges from mild concussion to diffuse axonal injury incompatible with life and includes all causes of intracranial haemorrhage.

A CT brain scan is the investigation of choice for all but minor head injuries (see Table 3.8.3 for CT indications in serious head injury). A non-contrast CT brain scan with bone windows is adequate for the detection of intracranial haematoma, cerebral oedema with or without midline shift and skull vault fractures.

The Canadian CT Head Rule [10] for patients with minor head injury also provides guidance for CT brain scanning in patients with minor head injury (GCS 13–15). The authors found that the presence of any of the high-risk factors (Table 3.8.4) was 100% sensitive for predicting the need for neurological intervention. They also found that the presence of medium-risk factors was 97.2% sensitive for detecting clinically important brain injury.

There are no indications for a skull X-ray in a trauma patient if a CT scanner is available, as it is extremely unreliable for the detection of either intra-or extracranial injuries.

If a compound or depressed fracture of the skull is suspected clinically, a CT brain scan should be performed. A compound depressed skull fracture is considered a neurosurgical emergency because of the increased risk of infection, such as meningitis or brain abscess (Fig. 3.8.5).

CT scan of the brain in children should be performed after careful consideration and explanation of the risks/benefits due to the exposure of the rapidly growing brain to a relatively high dose of radiation.

A magnetic resonance imaging (MRI) scan of the brain is not usually performed as first-line investigation in acute neurotrauma owing to the technical difficulties associated with the presence of patient monitoring and life support metallic equipment.

Classification of intracranial haemorrhage

Intracranial bleeding may be classified according to location. This includes: subdural, subarachnoid, extradural, intraventricular or parenchymal. These commonly coexist in the setting of trauma.

Epidural haematomas are commonly secondary to arterial bleeding due to a skull fracture with subsequent disruption of the middle meningeal artery. The haematoma is ovoid or lentiform in shape, does not cross cranial sutures but may cross the midline (Fig. 3.8.6).

Subdural haematomas usually occur as a result of venous bleeding. These haematomas are cresentic in shape, may involve a larger area when compared to an epidural haematoma, may cross cranial sutures but do not cross the midline (Fig. 3.8.7).

Subarachnoid haemorrhage may be due to disruption of small subarachnoid vessels or by direct extension from a parenchymal contusion/haematoma. Haemorrhage may be visualized in the sulci of the cerebral convexities or within the subarachnoid cisterns at the base of the skull (Fig. 3.8.8).

Table 3.8.3 Indications for a CT brain scan in significant head injury
Glasgow Coma Score (GCS) <9 after resuscitation
Neurological deterioration of 2 or more GCS points
Drowsiness or confusion (GCS 9–13) that persists for longer than 2 hours
Persistent headache or vomiting
Focal neurological signs (e.g. pupillary abnormalities or focal neurological signs)
Skull fracture known or suspected
Penetrating injury known or suspected
Age over 50 years with a suspicious mechanism of injury
Any head injury in a patient on anticoagulation therapy

Table 3.8.4 CT head rule is only required for patients with minor head injuries with any one of the following
High risk (for neurological intervention)
• GCS score <15 at 2 hours after injury
• Suspected open or depressed skull fracture
• Any sign of basal skull fracture (haemotympanum, 'racoon' eyes, cerebrospinal fluid otorrhoea/rhinorrhoea, Battle's sign)
• Vomiting ≥ two episodes
• Age ≥65 years
Medium risk (for brain injury on CT)
• Amnesia before impact >30 minutes
• Dangerous mechanism (pedestrian struck by motor vehicle, occupant ejected from motor vehicle, fall from height >3 feet or five stairs)
Minor head injury is defined as witnessed loss of consciousness, definite amnesia or witnessed disorientation in a patient with a GCS score of 13–15

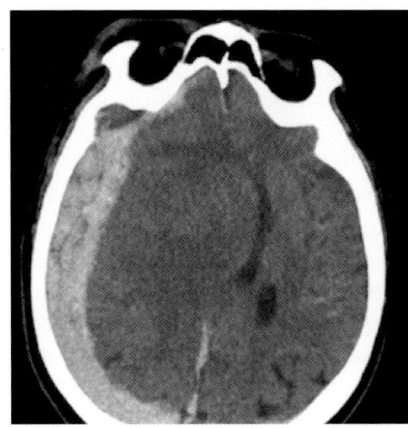

Fig. 3.8.7 Right cerebral convexity subdural haematoma.

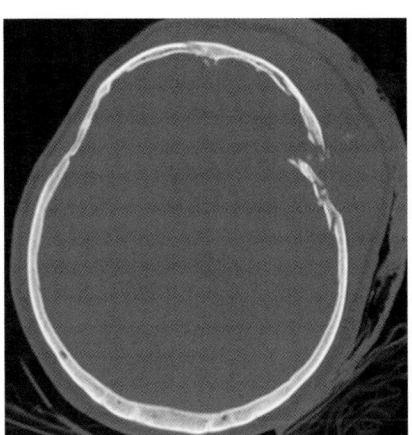

Fig. 3.8.5 CT brain with depressed skull fracture.

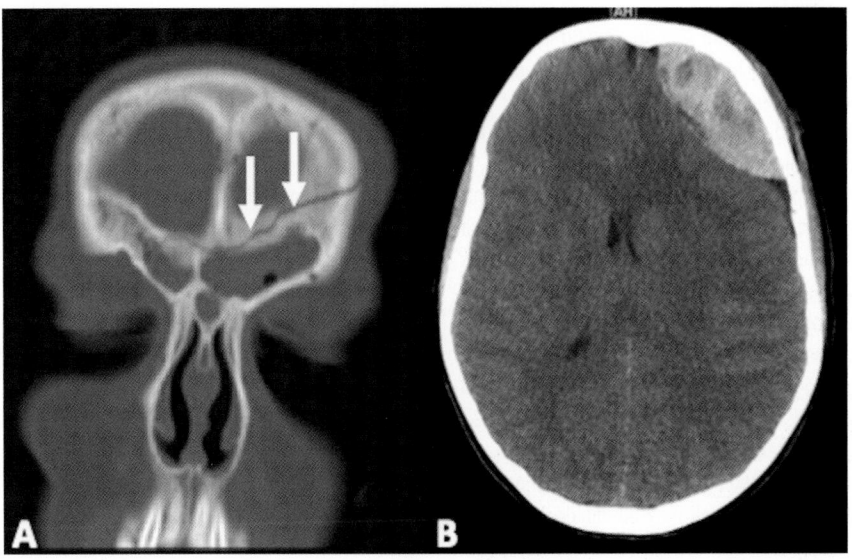

Fig. 3.8.6 (**A,B**) Left frontal extradural haematoma with an associated fracture (arrows).

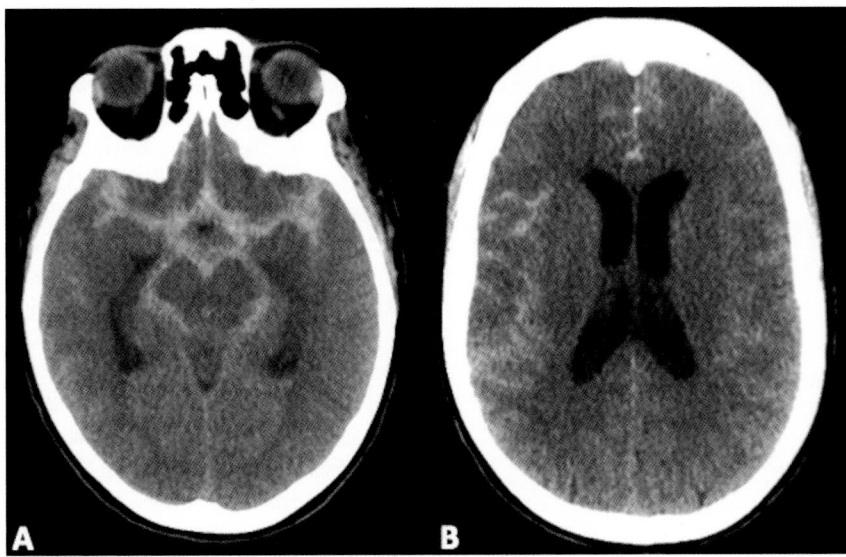

Fig. 3.8.8 Subarachnoid haemorrhage (**A**) within the basal cisterns and (**B**) within cerebral sulci.

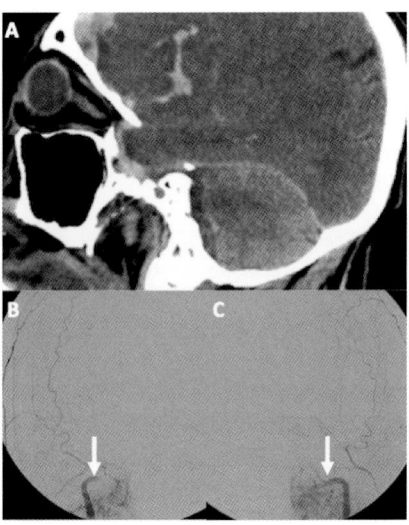

Fig. 3.8.10 Brain death. (**A**) Sagittal CT image demonstrating loss of supratentorial grey–white matter differentiation with preservation within the cerebellum ('white cerebellar sign'). This represents global supratentorial parenchymal infarction. (**B**) Right and (**C**) left common carotid cerebral angiograms demonstrate contrast filling of the external carotid vessels bilaterally but no intracranial filling of the ICA bilaterally. This represents brain death.

Intraventricular haemorrhage may be caused by tearing of subependymal veins on the surface of the ventricles or by direct extension from a parenchymal contusion/haematoma. These blood products tend to layer dependently on a CT scan with the patient imaged in a supine position, particularly within the occipital horns of the lateral ventricles.

Cerebral contusions represent foci of bleeding within the parenchyma of the brain. These may occur within superficial grey matter/subcortical white matter due to direct contact from bony protuberances of the calvarium or base of skull. Deeper parenchymal contusions are caused by disruption of intraparenchymal blood vessels. Cerebral contusions commonly increase in size and number within the first 24 hours post-trauma due to continued bleeding (Fig. 3.8.9). These haematomas also develop adjacent oedema which may increase the associated mass effect on the remainder of the intracranial structures.

Also noteworthy is the increased presentation of patients taking anticoagulation or antiplatelet therapy who fall and suffer head injuries. The bleeding as a result of the injury may progress over 24 hours and may occur in all of the above locations despite both pharmacological and neurosurgical attempts at reversal.

Diffuse axonal injury occurs due to acceleration–deceleration forces and is a shearing-type injury to the brain. It may be initially difficult to visualize on a non-contrast CT but can be identified as tiny foci of petechial haemorrhage at

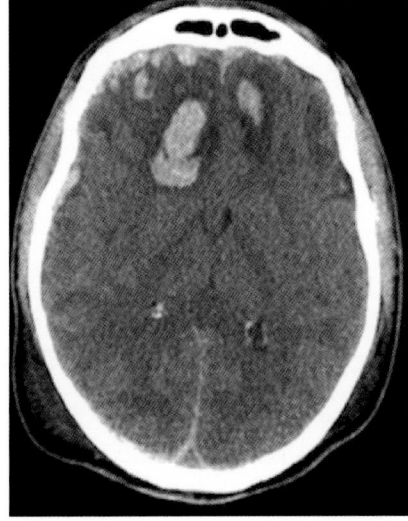

Fig. 3.8.9 Multiple bilateral frontal cerebral contusions.

the grey–white matter interface, within the corpus callosum or within the brainstem.

Non-contrast CT is also capable of identifying areas of acute established infarction. In the setting of trauma, this may be secondary to acute vascular injury or mass effect due to cerebral oedema (Fig. 3.8.10).

Fractures of the base of skull, including the temporal bones may occur in trauma. Findings on CT include opacification of the mastoid air cells, fluid in the middle ear cavity and pneumocephalus. Longitudinal temporal bone fractures occur after a blow to the side of the head and constitute 70–90% of temporal bone fractures. In comparison, transverse fractures

are secondary to a blow to the occiput or frontal region (E-Fig. 3.8.1).

Blunt cerebrovascular injury (BCVI)

Blunt injury to the carotid or vertebral vessels (BCVI) occurs in about 0.1% of all trauma patients in the USA. Many of these are diagnosed after the development of symptoms and signs due to central nervous system ischaemia with neurological morbidity of up to 80% and mortality approaching 40%. However, when asymptomatic patients are screened for BCVI, the incidence rises to 1% for all admitted blunt trauma patients and up to 2.7% for those with an injury severity score (ISS) >15 [11].

The Denver Modification of Screening criteria (Table 3.8.5) provides both risk factors as well as symptoms and signs for BCVI [11]. CT angiography is a valuable screening tool for the detection of these injuries; however, digital 4 vessel cerebral angiography (DFVCA) remains the diagnostic investigation of choice [12]. Table 3.8.6 shows a grading scale for BCVI as proposed by Biffi et al.[13].

[E-Figure 3.8.2 shows a dissection of the right vertebral artery due to blunt trauma in a patient with bilateral facet dislocation; E-Figure 3.8.3 demonstrates dissection of the right internal carotid artery with a large associated

Table 3.8.5 Denver modification of screening criteria for BCVI

Symptoms/signs of BCVI

Arterial haemorrhage
Cervical bruit
Expanding cervical haematoma
Focal neurological deficit
Neurological findings incongruous with CT scan findings
Ischaemic stroke on secondary CT scan

Risk factors for BCVI

High energy transfer mechanism with:
Le Fort 2 or 3 fractures
Cervical spine fracture patterns: subluxation, fractures extending into the foramen transversarium, fractures of C1–3
Basilar skull fractures with carotid canal involvement
Diffuse axonal injury with GCS <7
Near hanging with anoxic brain injury

Table 3.8.6 Grading scale for BCVI

Grade 1: intimal irregularity with <25% narrowing

Grade 2: dissection or intramural haematoma with >25% narrowing

Grade 3: pseudoaneurysm

Grade 4: occlusion of lumen

Grade 5: transection with extravasation

pseudoaneurysm; and E-Figure 3.8.4 shows a posterior inferior cerebellar artery infarct in a patient with a vertebral artery dissection.

CT is also capable of identifying injuries of the larynx (E-Fig. 3.8.5) which are usually due to a direct blow. Fractures of the thyroid or cricoid cartilage may be more difficult to visualize in younger patients who do not have calcification within their thyroid or cricoid cartilages.

Facial injury

Facial trauma may range from relatively trivial undisplaced nasal bone fractures to the life-threatening problems of airway protection and haemorrhage associated with midfacial (Le Fort) fractures. There may also be underlying cerebral injury associated with frontal bone fractures.

The commonest injury to the midface is the blowout fracture caused by a direct blow to the orbit, which results in a fracture of the orbital floor or the medial wall of the orbit in the region of the paper-thin lamina papyracea (E-Fig. 3.8.6). There may be tenderness over the fractured bone associated with diplopia due to entrapment of orbital contents or (less

commonly), visual disturbance due to globe or optic nerve injury. These fractures are best seen on CT scans with multiplanar reconstructions. Blowout fractures with entrapment of orbital contents require surgical elevation.

Mandibular fractures are usually obvious clinically because of pain, malocclusion and drooling. Mandibular fractures may be difficult to demonstrate on standard PA and oblique X-ray views. A panoramic view or orthopantomogram (OPG) is more useful, but CT of the mandible provides optimal demonstration of mandibular fractures, including those involving the mandibular neck, condyle and temporomandibular joint (TMJ) (E-Fig. 3.8.7).

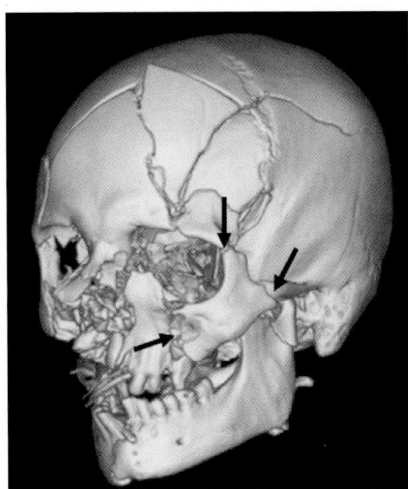

Fig. 3.8.11 Tripod fracture (arrows).

Dislocation of the TMJ is also optimally diagnosed on CT (E-Fig. 3.8.8).

Fractures of the zygoma are classified as (a) tripod fractures and (b) isolated fractures of the zygomatic arch. The tripod fracture or zygomaticomaxillary fracture separates the malar eminence of the zygoma from its frontal, temporal and maxillary attachments. Tripod fractures are usually caused by a significant force to the body of the zygoma or the malar eminence. The three fractures that constitute the tripod fracture are located in the inferior orbital margin, the lateral orbital margin or the zygomaticofrontal suture and the zygomatic arch. These fractures are best viewed on CT scans (Fig. 3.8.11).

The Le Fort fractures are caused by direct trauma to the midface. The Le Fort 1 fracture involves the maxilla at the level of the nasal floor and will allow mobility of the palate ('floating palate') (Fig. 3.8.12). Le Fort 2 passes through the nasal bones, as well as the medial, inferior and lateral walls of the maxillary antrum. The Le Fort 3 or 'craniofacial dysjunction/floating face' involves the nasal bones, the medial and lateral orbital walls and the zygomatic arch (E-Fig. 3.8.9).

Some facial fractures are unable to be classified owing to marked fragmentation of the bones and are termed as 'central facial smash' (Fig. 3.8.13). These fractures are best viewed by axial CT scans with multiplanar reformatting.

Frontal sinus fractures commonly occur as a result of direct force and are often compound,

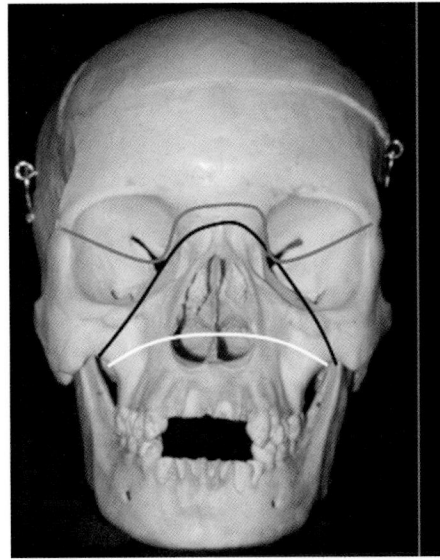
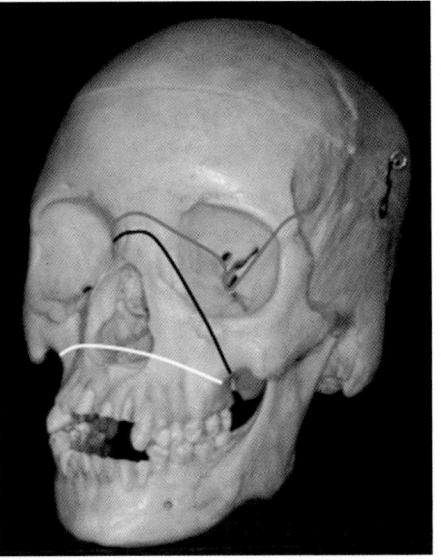

Fig. 3.8.12 Le Fort fracture classification. Le Fort 1, (white line), Le Fort 2 (black line) and Le Fort 3 (red line). (*Courtesy of Associate Professor Alf Nastri, Department of Maxillofacial Surgery, Royal Melbourne Hospital.*)

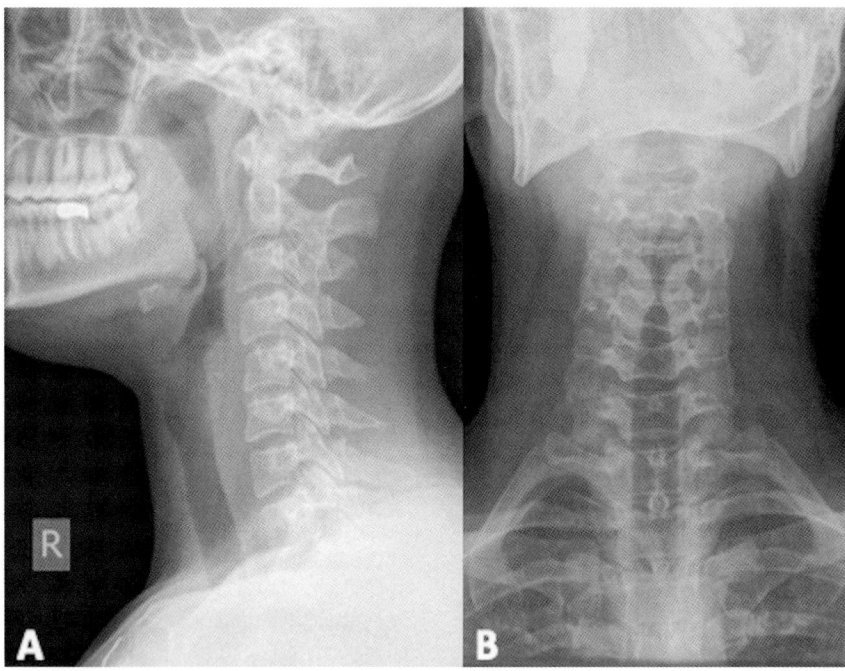

Fig. 3.8.13 (**A**) Lateral and (**B**) AP cervical spine X-rays.

Table 3.8.7 High-risk criteria for radiological clearance of the cervical spine in a multitrauma patient (NEXUS criteria)

Disturbed conscious state, e.g. head injury, intoxication for any reason
Any neurological motor or sensory signs
Midline cervical tenderness
Other major distracting injuries in a multitrauma patient

with the risk of associated intracranial infection. There may be an associated intracranial haematoma or cerebral contusion. A CT scan will best evaluate these fractures and determine the involvement of the posterior sinus wall. These fractures often require surgical exploration for debridement and repair.

Spinal Injury

Cervical spine

Cervical spine injuries can be classified into those with:

- fractures: stable or unstable
- fractures and no neurological deficit
- fractures associated with neurological deficit
- a small group of patients with cord injuries associated with contusion, haemorrhage or oedema without bony injury.

The bony Cx spine is best evaluated by axial CT scan with coronal and sagittal reconstructions. The cervical cord, discs and ligaments are best imaged by MRI scan. X-rays of the Cx spine do not provide the same detail and accuracy as a CT scan in detecting bony injuries.

The incidence of adult cervical spine injury after blunt trauma is 2–6% and any blunt trauma patient with physical findings of posterior midline neck tenderness, altered mental status or neurological deficit is considered at high risk for cervical spine injury. In this group of patients, one study [14] found a Cx spine injury in 9.5% of patients.

Cervical spine injury occurs in 5–10% of patients with traumatic brain injury, and with potentially devastating consequences for missing an injury in these patients. Plain X-rays miss 12–16% of Cx spine injuries while swimmer's views and/or oblique views identify more injuries but are frequently inadequate. A protocol at the Alfred Hospital in Melbourne [15] utilized multidetector CT (MDCT) with 1 mm cuts from C0–C3 and 3 mm cuts from C2–T4/5 with zero missed injuries. These authors also found that passive flexion/extension fluoroscopy in unconscious trauma patients was not sensitive for the detection of cervical instability and did not detect any injuries that had not been already seen in other imaging modalities.

MRI scan is invaluable for the detection of disco-ligamentous and cord injuries, however, its role in the routine clearance of the Cx spine in unconscious patients remains unclear. It is also problematic to transport critical care patients with metallic monitoring devices to the MRI scanner. There are also often delays to access the MRI scanner so that spinal precautions can be discontinued and the Cx collar removed. There are no prospective studies comparing modern MDCT and MRI for the evaluation of occult Cx spine injuries in unconscious patients and the use of either modality depends on clinician preference and level of suspicion with regard to the mechanism of injury. Of note, however, the Alfred Hospital investigators found three unstable Cx spine injuries detected by MRI scan which were not detected by MDCT [15].

There are also established criteria for identifying patients with a low risk for cervical spine injury who do not require imaging, as derived from the NEXUS Study (National Emergency X-Radiography Utilization Study) [16] (Table 3.8.7). The NEXUS study was a large validation study that identified 818 spinal injuries out of 34 000 patients and identified patients as low risk for cervical spine injury if all four high-risk clinical findings were absent. If the above criteria were met, there was no need for any imaging or further immobilization of the cervical spine. The results were 99.6% sensitive for clinically important cervical spine injuries. However, the specificity was only 12.9%.

The NEXUS study also found that cervical spine X-rays missed up to one-third of secondary spinal injuries where it was thought there was a single non-significant spinal injury and up to 25% of those missed injuries were non-contiguous with the original injury [17]. These findings have confirmed the use of CT in full evaluation of the cervical spine.

The Canadian C-Spine Rule for radiography in alert and stable trauma patients [18] may be more valuable clinically and is well validated in a prospective cohort study (Table 3.8.8). This rule demonstrated 100% sensitivity and 42.5% specificity for clinically important cervical spine injuries and there was good inter-observer agreement for each variable, with κ value >0.6 and a strong association with outcome (spinal injury) $p < 0.05$.

The above clinical decision rules should be applied with caution in the elderly, those with

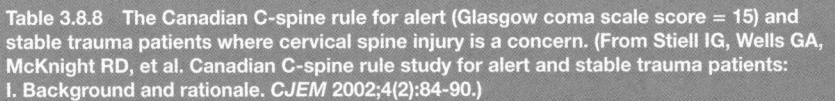

Table 3.8.8 The Canadian C-spine rule for alert (Glasgow coma scale score = 15) and stable trauma patients where cervical spine injury is a concern. (From Stiell IG, Wells GA, McKnight RD, et al. Canadian C-spine rule study for alert and stable trauma patients: I. Background and rationale. *CJEM* 2002;4(2):84–90.)

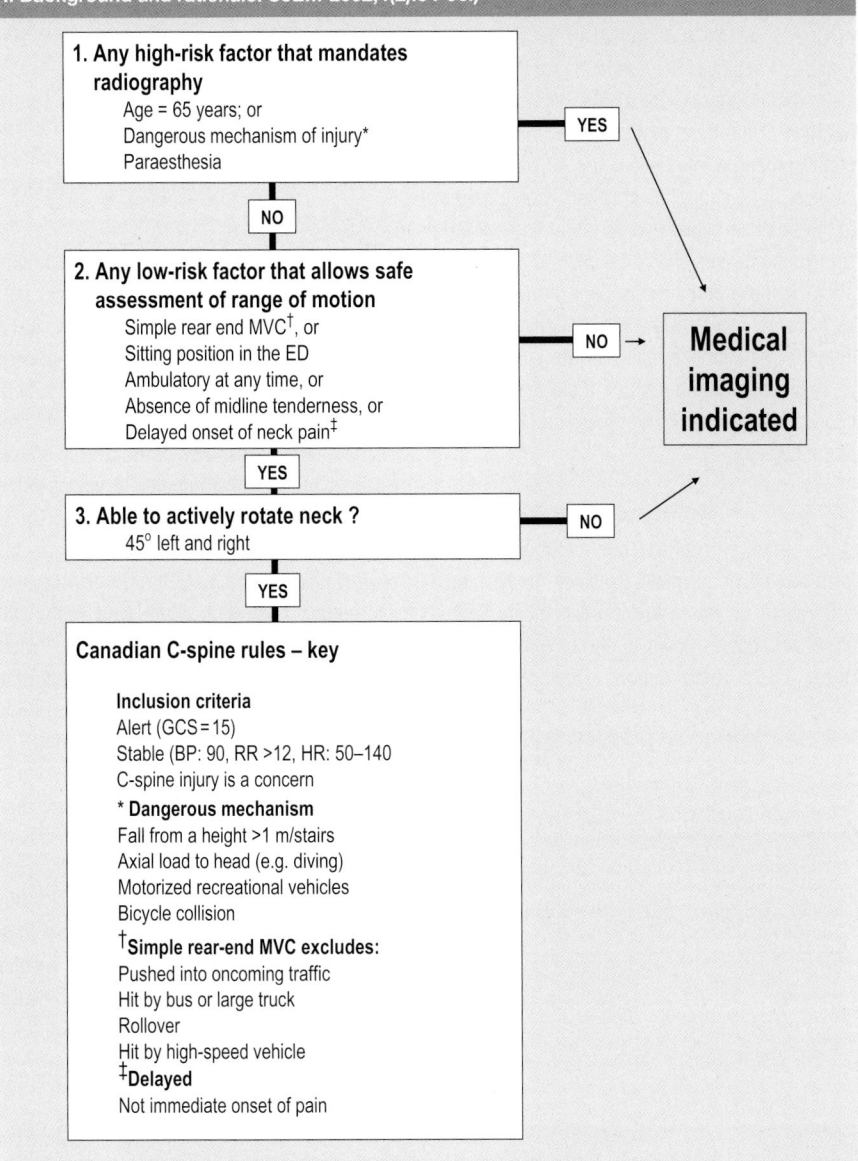

1. Any high-risk factor that mandates radiography
Age = 65 years; or
Dangerous mechanism of injury*
Paraesthesia

→ YES

NO

2. Any low-risk factor that allows safe assessment of range of motion
Simple rear end MVC[†], or
Sitting position in the ED
Ambulatory at any time, or
Absence of midline tenderness, or
Delayed onset of neck pain[‡]

→ NO →

YES

3. Able to actively rotate neck ?
45° left and right

→ NO

YES

Medical imaging indicated

Canadian C-spine rules – key

Inclusion criteria
Alert (GCS = 15)
Stable (BP: 90, RR >12, HR: 50–140)
C-spine injury is a concern

* Dangerous mechanism
Fall from a height >1 m/stairs
Axial load to head (e.g. diving)
Motorized recreational vehicles
Bicycle collision

[†]**Simple rear-end MVC excludes:**
Pushed into oncoming traffic
Hit by bus or large truck
Rollover
Hit by high-speed vehicle

[‡]**Delayed**
Not immediate onset of pain

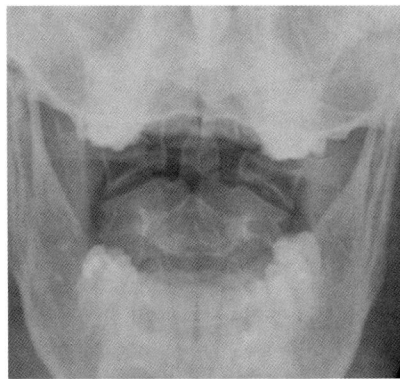

Fig. 3.8.14 PEG view.

line linking the tips of the spinous processes. In adults, up to 1.0 mm of anterior subluxation (and up to 3 mm in children) may be normal in a true lateral film taken at 1.8 m.

True pseudosubluxation is commonest in children up to the age of 8 years, but may be seen up to age 18 [19]. It commonly occurs between C2 and C3 and less commonly at the C3–4 and C4–5 levels. The key radiological feature is the preservation of the spinolaminar line in flexion/extension views of the lateral cervical spine [17].

The sagittal (AP) diameter of the spinal canal should be measured. At the C2 level, the lower limit radiographic measurement of the AP diameter of the spinal canal is 14 mm. At the C7 level, the lower limit of the AP canal diameter is 12 mm [20].

Bony canal All the cervical vertebrae should be systematically examined, including vertebral body, pedicles, facet joints, laminae and spinous processes and the interspinous distance.

The 'ring' of increased radiodensity formed by the odontoid process and the facet joints of C1–C2 is known as the 'Harris ring'. This ring should be intact anteriorly, superiorly and posteriorly, indicating an intact odontoid process and facet joints of C1–2. A type 2 fracture of the odontoid process through the body may be visible on the lateral cervical spine X-ray.

Cartilage All the spaces between adjacent vertebrae should be inspected for equality.

Soft tissue The prevertebral soft tissue should be inspected. A distance greater than 7 mm at C2 and 22 mm at C6 in the adult indicates the presence of a prevertebral haematoma [21]. If this is present, then a fracture or ligamentous disruption must be excluded. In

pre-existing spinal disease or the very young (<2 years). Owing to the relative immobility of the cervical spine or pre-existing spinal disease, such as ankylosing spondylitis, these patients may sustain cervical spine fractures even in the presence of a seemingly trivial injury.

If the cervical spine cannot be cleared clinically, then a radiological examination must be performed.

Cervical spine X-ray The trauma series for cervical spine clearance consists of lateral, anteroposterior and open-mouth odontoid process (peg) view (Figs 3.8.13 and 3.8.14). Plain

radiography of the Cx spine is now used infrequently in most trauma centres as it has been shown to have significantly less accuracy in detecting acute spinal fractures than is found in MDCT scans of the Cx spine from C0–T4/5.

The lateral view must be adequate (to the C7–T1 junction) and show appropriate *alignment* of the three lines (see Fig. 3.8.1). As well as alignment and adequacy, one should inspect the bones (for fractures), cartilage and soft tissues.

Inspection of *alignment and adequacy* on the lateral cervical spine X-ray should include the four lordotic lines: anterior and posterior vertebral lines, the spinolaminar line and the children, the upper prevertebral space may be larger than in adults owing to the presence of increased nasopharyngeal lymphoid tissue and it may also increase in infants during crying.

Atlanto-occipital and atlantoaxial bony injuries

Atlanto-occipital dislocation is usually associated with a fatal injury, whereas atlanto-occipital subluxation is radiologically subtle and the patients usually survive.

The diagnosis is made by recognizing an abnormal basion–axial interval and/or an abnormal basion–dental interval. Normally, neither should exceed 12 mm [22] and this is best seen on the lateral cervical spine X-ray or the sagittal CT scan of the cervical spine (Fig. 3.8.15).

The space between the odontoid and the anterior arch of C1 measured at its most inferior margin should not exceed 3 mm in adults and may be up to 5 mm in children. If this distance is exceeded, there may be a rupture of the transverse atlantal ligament of the dens. This distance may also increase atraumatically in patients with rheumatoid arthritis (due to ligamentous destruction by pannus) or in Down's syndrome.

Occipital condyle [23] and C1–C2 fractures are often missed on the lateral cervical spine X-ray, with the only indication of a fracture being an increase in soft-tissue swelling in this area. The initial lateral cervical spine X-ray

should be accompanied by an open-mouth (odontoid process) and an AP view.

The open-mouth (odontoid) view should be inspected for alignment of the lateral masses of C1–C2, which is abnormal in the Jefferson fracture, fracture of the odontoid process (types 1–3) and rotatory subluxation of C1 on C2. Rotation of the head can simulate pathological malalignment in this region. The AP view of the cervical spine should be checked for alignment of the articular pillars and vertebral bodies. The spinous processes should be centred and deviation of these from the midline may indicate a unilateral facet dislocation. Widening of the interspinous distance may indicate subluxation or dislocation. Fractures and dislocations may cause malalignment or compression of the vertebral bodies.

CT scan of cervical (Cx) spine

Many trauma centres now routinely perform limited or nil plain Cx spine X-rays and a CT scan of the entire cervical spine from occipital condyles down to and including T4–5 (Table 3.8.9). There is now a limited role for

Table 3.8.9   Imaging of patients with major trauma (based on Spinal Clearance Management Protocol, The Alfred Hospital, Melbourne, Australia)
Plain AP and lateral X-rays cervical spine
MSCT* 1 mm cuts C0–C3 (axial + sagittal and coronal reformats)
MSCT 3 mm cuts C2–T4/5 (axial + sagittal reformats)
*Multislice CT scans.

swimmer's and oblique views of the cervical spine, given the widespread use of CT scan (Fig. 3.8.16 [E-Fig. 3.8.10]).

Indications for MRI of the cervical spine include:

- patients with complete or incomplete neurological deficit
- deteriorating neurological status
- suspected ligamentous or intervertebral disc injury.

MRI will provide clear and concise images of all structures, particularly the spinal cord, intervertebral discs and soft tissues (E-Fig. 3.8.11). Bone structures and bone oedema are also demonstrated, but fine bony detail is best seen on a CT scan. A range of different MRI sequences may be utilized in trauma patients to identify a number of spinal pathologies (Table 3.8.10). There is a small group of patients who will be unsuitable for an MRI scan (Table 3.8.11). An MRI scan also provides information regarding spinal cord injury patterns, such as central cord syndrome, which have been previously unavailable with other imaging modalities (Fig. 3.8.17).

There are limited indications currently for dynamic flexion/extension films when looking for evidence of ligamentous instability, where there is ongoing pain or tenderness of the cervical spine in a patient who is neurologically intact and fully alert. The patient must be able to flex and extend his/her neck voluntarily and these X-rays should be supervised by the medical officer who ordered the investigation. However, as discussed previously, these films often fail to demonstrate the entire Cx spine [15].

Fig. 3.8.15 Atlanto-occipital dislocation.

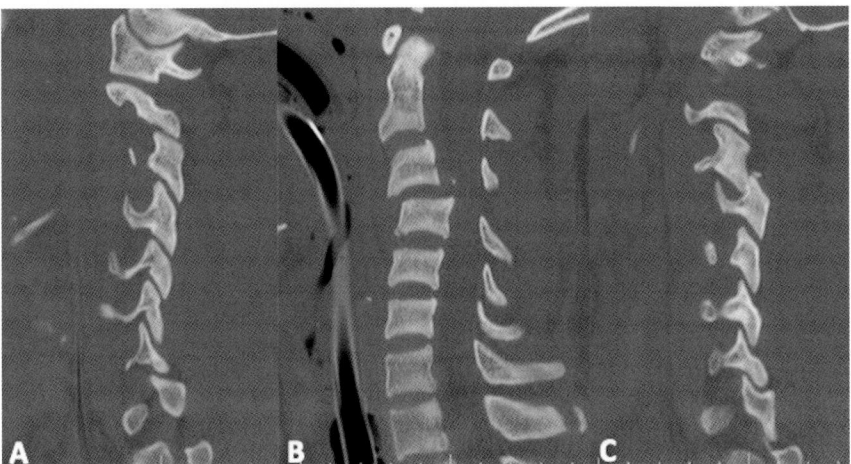

Fig. 3.8.16 Unilateral fracture dislocation. Sagittal CT image of the cervical spine. (**A**) Shows normal alignment of the left-sided cervical facet joints; (**B**) demonstrates a grade 1 anterolisthesis at C3/4 secondary to (**C**) a right-sided facet joint fracture dislocation.

In the unconscious patient, there is controversy as to the best approach for clearing the cervical spine, as there is a clear need to remove the rigid immobilization collar in order to prevent the development of scalp pressure areas. Prolonged use of rigid Cx collars causes pressure ulceration in 31% of unconscious trauma patients with the median length of stay increasing in this group of patients from 10 days, if they do not develop ulcers, to 23 days if they do develop pressure areas [15].

Dynamic flexion/extension X-rays in unconscious patients have a poor sensitivity for detecting cervical instability, have high rates of inadequacy, are not cost-effective and are potentially dangerous.

Trauma centres should have agreed guidelines, for clearing the cervical spine in unconscious patients, which involve multidetector CT. If there is any abnormality seen on CT (such as malalignment of the vertebrae or a high cervical fracture) an MRI is performed to exclude ligament, disc or atlanto-occipital/atlantoaxial disruption. Limited MRI of the Cx spine is highly sensitive for detection of ligament injury, disc and spinal cord oedema or haemorrhage which is often not apparent on MDCT of the Cx spine [15]. Also MRI does not expose the patient to ionizing radiation. The Alfred Hospital group [15] believes there may be a clinical advantage to include MRI scan in routine Cx spine clearance protocols for unconscious patients in whom clinical examination is not possible.

Thoracolumbar spine

The second most frequently injured area of the spinal column, after the cervical spine, is the thoracolumbar junction (T11–L2). Cord injuries in this region comprise about 20% of all spinal cord injuries [24]. The main reasons for the susceptibility of this vertebral region are the abrupt transition from the rigidly fixed thoracic spine to the more mobile lumbar spine and the fact that the spinal canal in the thoracic region is smaller in diameter than the cervical or lumbar spinal canals, which results in increased risk to the spinal cord.

An important concept used for interpreting thoracolumbar injuries is the 'three-column' theory described by Denis [25]. This is a widely accepted concept which divides a vertebra into three columns: the anterior column, which consists of the anterior longitudinal ligament and the anterior half of the vertebral body; the middle column, which includes the posterior half of the vertebral body and the posterior longitudinal ligament; and the posterior column, which includes all the bony and ligamentous structures posterior to the posterior longitudinal ligament. Fractures involving the anterior column are considered stable, whereas fractures involving the anterior and middle columns or all three columns are considered unstable.

It is also of note that injuries in the T1–T10 region comprise 16% of cord injuries and lumbosacral injuries, such as cauda equina lesions and comprise approximately 4% of spinal neurological injuries [24].

As it is often difficult to obtain satisfactory images of the upper thoracic spine, particularly the T1–T4 region, multislice CT with multiplanar reconstructions is currently the most effective method of establishing the extent of bony injury. It is the practice of many trauma centres to perform routinely a CT of the cervical spine to T4–5 with multiplanar reconstructions, and it has become routine to perform sagittal and coronal reconstruction of the thoracolumbar spine when a CT scan of the thorax/abdomen/pelvis is performed.

Classification of thoracolumbar spine injuries

- Stable fractures, which include transverse process fractures, spinous process fractures, pars interarticularis fractures and wedge compression fractures involving the anterior two-thirds only of the vertebral body.
- Unstable fractures/dislocations, which include compression fractures with middle and/or posterior column disruption, the 'Chance' fracture (E-Fig. 3.8.12), the burst fracture (E-Fig. 3.8.13) and flexion/distraction injuries.

Fractures in a fused thoracic spine (ankylosing spondylitis, diffuse interstitial spinal

Table 3.8.10   Spinal abnormalities seen on the MRI scan
Spinal cord injury (haemorrhage or oedema)
Disc herniation
Epidural haematoma
Epidural abscess
Occult bone fracture/dislocation
Ligamentous rupture
Facet joint – disruption or capsular injury
Nerve root avulsion and plexus injury (brachial or lumbosacral)

Table 3.8.11   Conditions unsuitable for MRI scan
Metallic components, e.g. bullets, aneurysm clips
Haemodynamically unstable patients
Patients requiring ventilation and extensive physiological monitoring

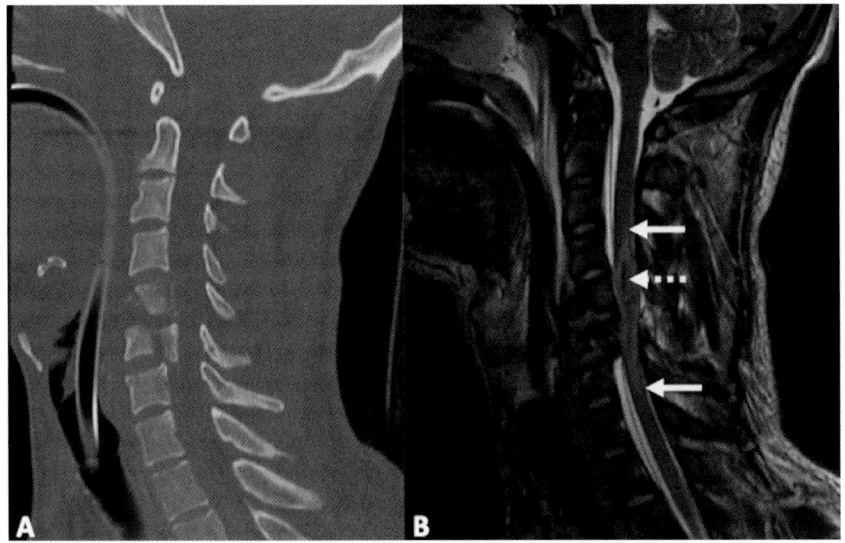

Fig. 3.8.17 Cord contusion. (**A**) Sagittal CT of the cervical spine shows fractures of the C5 and C6 verterbal bodies, with associated retropulsion. (**B**) Sagittal T2-weighted MRI demonstrates a cord contusion extending from C4 to C7 (solid arrows) and a focus of haemorrhage within the cord at C5 (dashed arrow).

hypertrophy (DISH) and advanced degenerative disc disease with bridging osteophytes) constitute a unique subset. Due to the rigidity of the spine, they are likened to a long bone fracture and may be called a 'carrot stick' fracture (E-Fig. 3.8.14). These injuries are typically a result of hyperextension, usually involve three columns and are therefore unstable. Cord damage is common in this type of fracture.

If a patient is unable to be examined clinically because of pain or tenderness of the thoracolumbar spine or is unconscious, this area must be imaged. If a CT scan of the chest and abdomen/pelvis is performed, then sagittal and coronal reconstructions of the thoracolumbar (TL) spine can be done.

If CT of the torso is not performed, then plain X-rays of the thoracolumbar spine should be taken, with limited CT of any areas difficult to visualize or where there is clinical suspicion.

The Chance fracture is an example of a distraction or seatbelt injury, with the lap belt as the axis of rotation and failure of the spinal column in its posterior ligamentous and bony elements. This fracture is directed in a horizontal plane through the entire bony column, including vertebral body, pedicles, laminae and spinous processes and is, by definition, unstable. This fracture may also be associated with injuries to the abdominal contents, e.g. pancreas or duodenum.

Fractures of the lower lumbar spine and sacrum may involve the cauda equina and associated sacral nerve roots. There may be bladder, bowel and sexual dysfunction, as well as variable motor and sensory deficit in the lower limbs. There is often significant neuralgia that is disabling and difficult to treat. Plain X-rays will give some indication of the severity of the bony injury, but a CT scan is required for definitive information if surgical fixation is required.

Coccygeal fractures are due to direct blows and are both treated and diagnosed clinically. Radiology is not usually necessary for diagnosis, which is best made by CT scanning. There may be an associated rectal injury that requires operative repair but, otherwise, analgesia only is required.

Chest trauma

The chest X-ray still has a key role in the investigation of multiple trauma involving the thorax. The combination of CXR and ultrasound may provide the simplest and fastest assessments of unstable patients and should usually precede MDCT, particularly in cases of low energy trauma [26–28]. The CT chest scan with IV contrast has become more accessible in recent years, and the use of both TOE (transoesophageal echo) and DSA (digital subtraction angiography) in assessing the mediastinal structures have become limited to situations where a CT cannot be done.

A study by Traub and colleagues [29] found that chest CT was more effective than X-rays in detecting lung contusions, pneumothoraces and mediastinal haematoma, as well as fractured ribs, scapula, sternum and vertebrae. The authors found that it was more likely than CXR to provide further diagnostic information in the presence of chest wall tenderness, reduced air entry and/or abnormal respiratory rate. However, the CXR can be done quickly and may provide urgent life-saving information regarding conditions, such as pneumothorax, haemothorax or malpositioned chest or endotracheal tubes [28].

The trauma room CXR should ideally be performed in the erect position with a nasogastric tube *in situ*. However, because it is often impossible to clear the cervical and/or thoracolumbar spine in the trauma room, the CXR is frequently taken in the supine position. This can create a number of difficulties in interpretation of the results. The AP projection of the X-ray beam will magnify the mediastinal structures and, when the patient is supine, the thoracic veins will passively distend and add to this appearance of mediastinal widening. Small pneumothoraces and haemothoraces are also difficult to detect on the supine CXR because the air distributes as a thin film anteriorly and blood as a thin homogeneous layer posteriorly. A haemothorax of 200–300 mL will normally be visible on a good-quality erect CXR, whereas it will usually require 800–1000 mL to produce the 'fuzzy' appearance of a haemothorax seen on the supine CXR [28].

Examination of the CXR will often begin with a review of the bones and soft tissues. The CXR is a poor diagnostic aid for rib fractures as it will miss up to 50% of anterior and lateral fractures [27,28], instead, the assessment should be directed more towards the complications of rib fractures, such as pneumothorax, haemothorax and lung contusion. It is also important to remember that the clavicles, glenohumeral joints and scapulae are visible on the CXR (E-Fig. 3.8.15). Fractures of these bones, along with fractures of the first and second ribs, are indicators of significant blunt thoracic trauma and should prompt a careful examination for underlying visceral and vascular injuries.

Sternal fractures may be seen on a lateral CXR but are best seen on CT. The significance of sternal fractures will largely direct the examination towards underlying mediastinal injuries. Brookes et al. [30], in a retrospective study, found a 2% incidence of sternal fractures associated with motor vehicle accidents. These patients had a very low incidence (1.5%) of cardiac arrhythmias due to cardiac muscle contusion requiring treatment and a mortality rate of less than 1%. The authors found that those at risk of cardiac arrhythmias requiring treatment were over 65 years of age and either had pre-existing ischaemic cardiac disease or were on digoxin treatment. They recommended that cardiac monitoring was not required unless the patient fulfilled the above criteria. They also found that the 12-lead ECG was not predictive for the development of arrhythmias requiring treatment.

In cases of penetrating chest trauma, a foreign body may be evident on the CXR. AP and lateral projections with appropriate skin markers will normally be required to help locate the position of the foreign object. In cases where the foreign object is embedded close to or in a pulsatile thoracic structure, the object may appear blurred on the film, indicating the proximity of the foreign body to the vessel.

Subcutaneous emphysema may be seen on the CXR and may result from injury to the lung, the tracheobronchial tree, the larynx, pharynx and oesophagus (Fig. 3.8.18). Subcutaneous

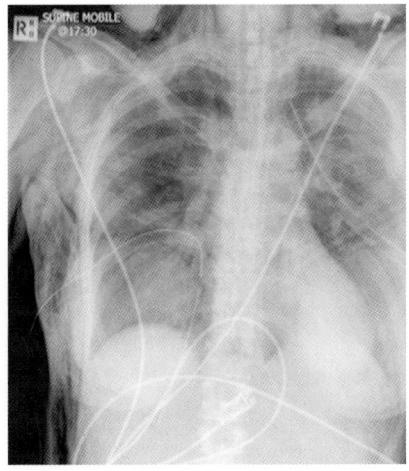

Fig. 3.8.18 Subcutaneous emphysema. Extensive subcutaneous emphysema is visualized overlying the chest wall bilaterally and in the supraclavicular regions.

Table 3.8.12   Chest X-ray signs of tracheal laceration
Subcutaneous emphysema/mediastinal emphysema/pneumothorax
Deviation of the endotracheal tube tip to the right relative to the tracheal lumen
Distension of the endotracheal tube balloon
Migration of the endotracheal tube balloon distally towards the tube tip

Table 3.8.13   Signs of diaphragmatic injury on CXR
Elevated hemidiaphragm
Abnormal or indistinct contour of the diaphragm
Collapse of the lower lung fields
Inhomogeneous mass in the relevant hemithorax
Displacement of the mediastinum away from the injury

Table 3.8.14   Signs of aortic disruption on chest X-ray [30]
Widened mediastinum >6 cm in erect PA film >8 cm in supine AP film
Deviation of the oesophagus/NG tube to the right of T4 spinous process
Obliteration of aortic knob
Opacification of the aortopulmonary window
Deviation of the trachea to the right of the T4 spinous process
Depression of the left main bronchus to below 40° from the horizontal
Increased right paratracheal stripe (>4 mm)
Increased left paravertebral stripe (>5 mm)
Left apical cap

emphysema should prompt a careful examination for evidence of a pneumothorax and pneumomediastinum. Subcutaneous emphysema and pneumothorax are common findings in traumatic injury to the lung and also occur in tracheobronchial injury.

In cases of suspected tracheal laceration, where the patient has been intubated, the appearance of the endotracheal tube on the CXR should be carefully examined. The normal position of the balloon is 2.5 cm proximal to the tip of the endotracheal tube (Table 3.8.12).

If a pneumothorax is suspected but not visible on the supine CXR, a CT scan is the definitive investigation.

In cases of penetrating chest trauma, the development of a detectable pneumothorax may be delayed and so it is recommended that check CXR be performed at 6 and 12 hours [29].

The lung parenchyma may become opacified by contusion, aspiration, pulmonary fat embolism and either cardiogenic or non-cardiogenic pulmonary oedema. Lung contusions will usually develop rapidly within 6 hours of an injury, whereas the changes of aspiration and pulmonary infarction are often delayed for 12–24 hours. Rib fractures are frequently associated with pulmonary contusions although, in paediatric patients and young adults, the ribs are more compliant and may bow in, causing a lung contusion without fracture.

Diaphragmatic injuries are more frequent in penetrating than in blunt trauma. In blunt trauma, however, 80% of diaphragmatic injuries occur on the left side because the liver and its ligamentous attachments protect the right side (Table 3.8.13).

If a nasogastric tube is *in situ*, it may be seen to pass down into the abdomen and back up into the chest contained within the herniated stomach. Lower rib fractures are often seen in association with injuries to the diaphragm.

Thoracic aortic injury

Ninety per cent of injuries occur in the region of the aortic isthmus, i.e. that part of the proximal descending aorta between the origin of the left subclavian artery and the site of attachment of the ligamentum arteriosum (1.5 cm in length). The ascending aorta is involved in only 5% of cases [31].

As previously described, the supine AP CXR magnifies the mediastinal silhouette. Superior mediastinal widening is a common finding in cases of both penetrating and blunt trauma to the great thoracic vessels. The mediastinal width is measured at the top of the aortic knob. A width greater than 8.0–8.5 cm in a supine film or 6 cm in an erect film is suggestive of a mediastinal haematoma.

The sensitivity of a widened mediastinum on CXR for the detection of thoracic aortic injuries has been estimated at 90% and the specificity 10%, but approximately 7% of patients with aortic rupture have a normal chest radiograph [32] (Table 3.8.14).

Injuries to the oesophagus may occur in association with both blunt and penetrating chest trauma. The predominant X-ray finding in oesophageal injury is pneumomediastinum and this may be associated with subcutaneous emphysema, pneumothorax, a left pleural effusion or a widened mediastinum.

Thoracic CT scan

Thoracic MDCT has become a common diagnostic aid in investigating the multitrauma patient with chest injuries. The increasing speed and greater clarity of the MDCT scan gives a reliable and rapid means of screening for most intrathoracic injuries. The strength of CT lies in its ability to distinguish mediastinal haematoma from other causes of mediastinal widening detected on initial chest radiographs, e.g. magnification, mediastinal fat and tortuous vessels [26,27].

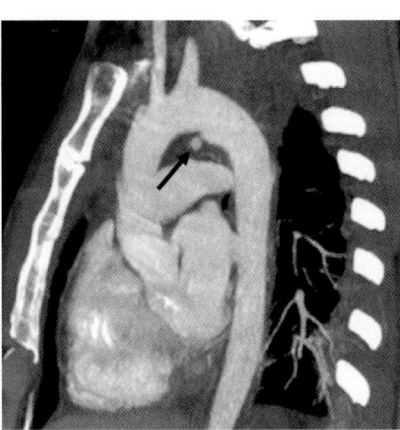

Fig. 3.8.19 Aortic transection with pseudoaneurysm formation (black arrow).

Chest CT is also a sensitive test for detecting pneumothorax, pneumomediastinum, pulmonary contusion and haemothorax and, with intravenous contrast, may demonstrate an intimal tear or pseudoaneurysm of the traumatized aorta (Fig. 3.8.19 [E-Figs 3.8.16–3.8.17]).

Mediastinal haematoma is an indirect sign of aortic injury and appears as a soft tissue density around mediastinal structures [26,27,32] or, in acute aortic dissection, a false lumen may be seen.

If mediastinal major vascular injury is initially suspected, a CT angiogram is the preferred screening investigation; however, DSA remains the gold standard. CT angiography with 2–3 mm slices using injections of 100–150 mL contrast may be reconstructed in multiple planes to produce detailed images of the aorta. Studies have shown that CT angiography is sensitive for traumatic aortic injury (83–100%) with a high negative predictive value (NPV) of 99–100% [32].

Angiography

Transfemoral angiography has been widely accepted as the gold standard for the diagnosis of major thoracic vascular injuries, particularly those involving the aorta and great vessels [32]. This investigation is not free from complications, although the morbidity and mortality are low. Significant complications, such as rupture at the site of injury during contrast injection, are rare, but have been reported [33].

Endoluminal repair of acute thoracic vascular injuries is now commonly undertaken. Formal angiography is therefore undertaken at the time of repair. Diagnostic information obtained on CT prior to repair is sufficient to confirm the diagnosis and provides images for surgical/endovascular planning.

Transoesophageal echocardiography (TOE)

TOE has many supporters of its value as both a screening and a diagnostic test in the investigation of suspected mediastinal haematoma. Some authors [34,35] suggest that TOE is more accurate than angiography in detecting aortic injuries, although it is acknowledged that interpretation is operator dependent.

The advantages of TOE are that it can be performed quickly in the resuscitation area, it is minimally invasive and it has a low rate of complications, such as aspiration and oesophageal perforation. It can demonstrate myocardial, pericardial and valvular injuries, which may not be demonstrated on MDCT. Disadvantages are that it may require sedation and intubation and may provide limited information about the distal ascending aorta, the aortic arch and the arch vessels [35]. Although the incidence of injury to the arch and major branch vessels is low, angiography is required when injury to these vessels is suspected.

Lung ultrasound

The use of ultrasound to detect evidence of pneumothorax has been reported for more than 20 years. It is easy to perform and safe. While the sensitivity of lung ultrasound in detecting pneumthoraces is significantly less than that of thoracic CT, it can be applied in conjunction with a plain CXR to provide timely information in the resuscitation room [36].

MRI is generally not practical for the diagnosis of traumatic aortic rupture.

Oral contrast studies

Oral contrast provides useful information in the investigation and diagnosis of oesophageal and diaphragmatic injuries. In cases of oesophageal perforation, Gastrografin is the preferred contrast medium, as it is less irritating than barium should there be a leak into the surrounding mediastinal tissues. A Gastrografin swallow is mandatory in the evaluation of suspected penetrating injuries of the oesophagus. If there is a risk of aspiration, Gastrografin should not be used as it produces a severe pneumonitis. In these circumstances, contrast designed for intravenous use can be administered orally in order to demonstrate oesophageal perforation.

A CT swallow study can also be performed. This would involve a non-contrast (control) study of the chest and upper abdomen, followed by a second study after the ingestion of oral contrast. In unconscious patients, a nasogastric tube is placed with its tip in the upper oesophagus and oral contrast is administered via this tube.

Flexible or rigid oesophagoscopy may also be used to exclude oesophageal perforation.

Abdomen/pelvis

Abdominal X-ray

The role of the plain abdominal X-ray (AXR) in the investigation of abdominal trauma is extremely limited. In cases of penetrating injuries, it may be useful in the detection and localization of foreign bodies and in the detection of free air under the diaphragm in hollow viscus rupture. An erect CXR may show free gas under the left hemidiaphragm more commonly than on the right. In cases of duodenal perforation, free retroperitoneal air may be seen as pockets of gas along the right psoas line (shadow) on a supine AXR. Importantly, all of these features will be better identified on an abdominal CT scan if it is available.

Abdominal CT scan

Abdominal CT is usually performed with both oral and intravenous contrast. However, as most multitrauma patients have delayed gastric emptying, the bulk of oral contrast tends to remain in the stomach and upper gastrointestinal tract. This phenomenon has led some authors to suggest that oral contrast is of little use in this setting [37]. The increased speed of the helical CT scanner has resulted in excellent resolution for the detection of vascular injuries involving the liver, spleen and kidneys after intravenous contrast. The American Association for the Surgery of Trauma (AAST) has developed a scoring system that grades the severity of injury to the solid intra-abdominal viscera including the spleen, liver, kidney, adrenal gland and the pancreas (Figs 3.8.20–22 [E-Figs 3.8.18-21], Tables 3.8.15–19) [38]. Scoring systems have also been developed for the hollow intra-abdominal viscera (see Table 3.8.18) [38].

In stable patients with possible intra-abdominal injuries, the abdominal CT has become the investigation of choice because, as well as being non-invasive, it reliably identifies intraperitoneal fluid, solid organ and hollow visceral injury, retroperitoneal injuries and spinal and pelvic fractures (E-Figs 3.8.22 and 3.8.23). The use of intravenous contrast will also give some indication of both renal perfusion and function, as contrast is excreted into

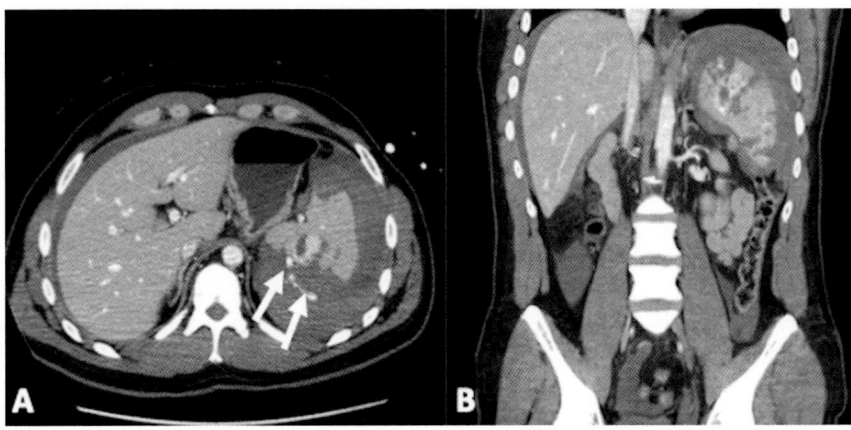

Fig. 3.8.20 Shattered spleen with active bleeding (arrows) and a large perisplenic haematoma – grade V.

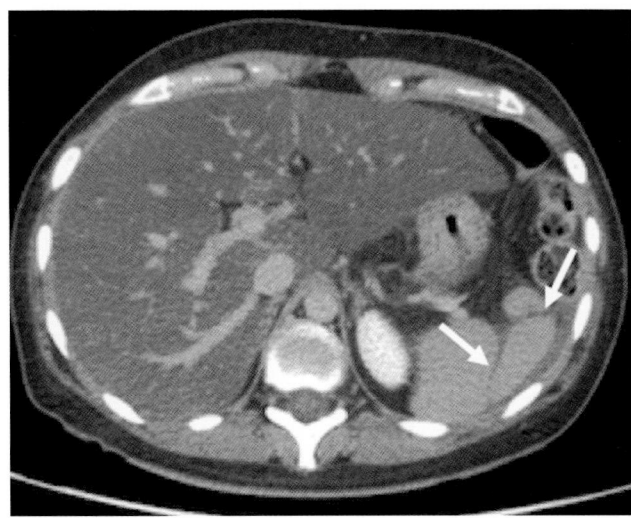

Fig. 3.8.21 Splenic lacerations (arrows) – grade III.

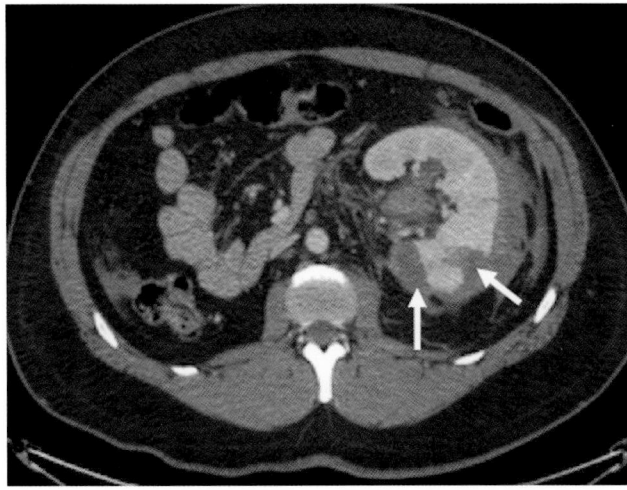

Fig. 3.8.22 Renal laceration (arrows) with surrounding perinephric haematoma – grade IV.

Table 3.8.15	Spleen injury scale (1994 revision)	
Grade	*Type of injury*	*Description of injury*
I	Haematoma	Subcapsular: <10% surface area
	Laceration	Capsular tear: <1 cm parenchymal depth
II	Haematoma	Subcapsular: 10–50% surface area; intraparenchymal, <5 cm in diameter
	Laceration	Capsular tear: 1–3 cm parenchymal depth that does not involve a trabecular vessel
III	Haematoma	Subcapsular: >50% surface area or expanding; ruptured subcapsular or parecymal hematoma; intraparenchymal hematoma ≥5 cm or expanding
	Laceration	>3 cm parenchymal depth or involving trabecular vessels
IV	Laceration	Laceration involving segmental or hilar vessels producing major devascularization (>25% of spleen)
V	Laceration	Completely shattered spleen
	Vascular	Hilar vascular injury which devascularizes spleen

the ureters and bladder. One of the main limitations of abdominal CT is that the investigation must be carried out in the radiology department and so is inappropriate for any unstable patient. Injuries that may be missed on abdominal CT include upper intestinal perforation as well as injury to the diaphragm, pancreas and bladder.

Focused assessment by sonography for trauma (FAST) examination

Since the introduction of the focused ultrasound examination for trauma in the early 1990s in North America and in the late 1990s in Australasia, there has been some debate regarding the sensitivity, specificity and accuracy of the examination compared to diagnostic peritoneal lavage (DPL). In those centres that use FAST on a regular basis, there has been a markedly reduced requirement for DPL. One of the criticisms of DPL has been its low specificity, resulting in an excessive non-therapeutic laparotomy rate of up to 30% in some centers [39,40]. The main utility of the FAST examination has been shown in the unstable trauma patient with intra-abdominal haemorrhage who requires urgent surgery and it has replaced DPL as the diagnostic modality of choice in these patients.

FAST requires the examination of four areas (Table 3.8.20). Its limitations include:

- it requires training
- it cannot differentiate between fluids (blood vs ascites vs urine)
- poor-quality images in obesity, subcutaneous emphysema and dilated bowel loops.

The FAST examination can be completed in 2–5 minutes, is non-invasive and is repeatable. It is very poor at detecting specific solid organ or hollow viscus intra-abdominal injuries but, if abdominal haemorrhage is ruled out and the patient is haemodynamically stable, then abdominal CT is indicated.

Many studies have reported a sensitivity of 80–100% and a specificity of 88–100% for the detection of intraperitoneal blood. It has also been consistently reported that FAST will not detect hollow viscus injuries, lacerations in the intra-abdominal solid organs, retroperitoneal or diaphragmatic injuries.

There is some evidence that FAST is of value in penetrating trauma. Boulanger et al. [41] found that the routine use of FAST in penetrating trauma was useful for the detection of

Table 3.8.16   Liver injury scale (1994 revision)

Grade	Type of injury	Description of injury
I	Haematoma	Subcapsular: <10% surface area
	Laceration	Capsular tear: <1 cm parenchymal depth
II	Haematoma	Subcapsular: 10 to 50% surface area; intraparenchymal <10 cm in diameter
	Laceration	Capsular tear 1–3 cm parenchymal depth, <10 cm in length
III	Haematoma	Subcapsular: >50% surface area of ruptured subcapsular or parenchymal hematoma; intraparenchymal hematoma >10 cm or expanding
	Laceration	>3 cm parenchymal depth
IV	Laceration	Parenchymal disruption involving 25 to 75% hepatic lobe or 1–3 Couinaud's segments
V	Laceration	Parenchymal disruption involving >75% of hepatic lobe or >3 Couinaud's segments within a single lobe
	Vascular	Juxtahepatic venous injuries; i.e. retrohepatic vena cava/central major hepatic veins
VI	Vascular	Hepatic avulsion

Table 3.8.17   Kidney injury scale

Grade	Type of injury	Description of injury
I	Contusion	Microscopic or gross haematuria, urological studies normal
	Haematoma	Subcapsular: non-expanding without parenchymal laceration
II	Haematoma	Non-expanding perirenal haematoma confined to renal retroperitoneum
	Laceration	<1.0 cm parenchymal depth of renal cortex without urinary extravasation
III	Laceration	<1.0 cm parenchymal depth of renal cortex without collecting system rupture or urinary extravasation
	Laceration	Parenchymal laceration extending through renal cortex, medulla and collecting system
IV	Vascular	Main renal artery or vein injury with contained haemorrhage
V	Laceration	Completely shattered kidney
	Vascular	Avulsion of renal hilum which devascularizes kidney

Table 3.8.18   Adrenal injury scale

Grade	Description of injury
I	Contusion
II	Laceration involving only cortex (<2 cm)
III	Laceration extending into medulla (≥2 cm)
IV	>50% parenchymal destruction
V	Total parenchymal destruction (including massive intraparenchymal haemorrhage) Avulsion from blood supply

Table 3.8.19   Pancreas injury scale

Grade	Type of injury	Description of Injury
I	Haematoma	Minor contusion without duct injury
	Laceration	Superficial laceration without duct injury
II	Haematoma	Major contusion without duct injury or tissue loss
	Laceration	Major laceration without duct injury or tissue loss
III	Laceration	Distal transection or parenchymal injury with duct injury
IV	Laceration	Proximal transection or parenchymal injury involving ampulla
V	Laceration	Massive disruption of pancreatic head

pericardial and peritoneal fluid. However, they cautioned that a negative FAST did not exclude hollow viscus or diaphragmatic injuries.

Many centres have introduced FAST into the algorithm for the routine assessment of victims of trauma. Over 10 years ago, Boulanger et al. [42] demonstrated in a prospective study that a FAST-based algorithm for blunt abdominal injury was more rapid, less expensive and as accurate as an algorithm that used CT or DPL only. Hence, there is a growing body of evidence showing that the only indication for DPL (when no FAST is available) is for suspected bowel perforation, which is usually diagnosed either by clinical examination or by CT.

Radiology in pelvic trauma

In addition to plain radiology, pelvic CT scanning and angiography are becoming increasingly important in the diagnostic and therapeutic work-up of pelvic trauma. The trauma room AP X-ray of the pelvis should include all the bony pelvic components as well as both hip joints and the proximal femora, including greater and lesser trochanters (Fig. 3.8.23).

Table 3.8.20   The FAST examination

1. The right upper quadrant (Morison's pouch)
2. The left upper quadrant (splenorenal recess)
3. The subxiphoid area (pericardium)
4. The suprapubic area (pouch of Douglas/ rectovesical pouch)

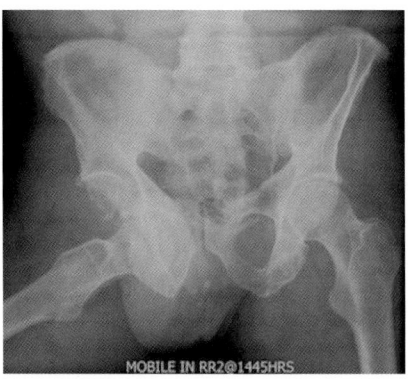

Fig. 3.8.23 Dislocated hip.

Most anterior pelvic fractures are seen on the AP film, but up to 30% of posterior fractures involving the sacrum and sacroiliac joints will not be seen on the plain radiology. These fractures will be best seen on a two-dimensional or reformatted 3D CT scan of the pelvis.

Acetabular fractures are often difficult to visualize on AP views and a CT scan of the pelvis may be required.

There are a number of radiological classifications of pelvic fractures that must be interpreted in association with the clinical impression of the fracture and the associated complications. The greater the AP disruption of the pelvic ring and hence the larger the pelvic cavity volume, the more there is potential for severe haemorrhagic shock and visceral damage.

A useful classification is that by Young and Resnik (Table 3.8.21) [43], which is a modification of the Pennel and Tile [44] classification of pelvic fractures. This classifies fractures by mechanism of injury into AP compression, lateral compression, vertical shear and a combination, and takes into consideration rotational and/or vertical instability of the pelvic ring (Fig. 3.8.24 [E-Figs 3.8.24 and 3.8.25]). If the pelvic ring is fractured anteriorly and posteriorly, stability is usually lost, with disruption of the posterior ligaments (sacroiliac, sacrotuberous and sacrospinous) and there will be widening of the sacroiliac joint(s) on the AP view. The classification provides a graded probability of bleeding related to the fracture, the development of haemorrhagic shock and associated organ damage.

Table 3.8.21 Young and Resnick classification of pelvic fractures

AP compression

Type 1: Disruption of the symphysis pubis with less than 2.5 cm diastasis; no significant posterior pelvic injury

Type 2: Disruption of the symphysis pubis of more than 2.5 cm with tearing of the anterior sacroiliac, sacrospinous and sacrotuberous ligaments

Type 3: Complete disruption of the pubic symphysis and posterior ligament complexes, with hemipelvic displacement

Lateral compression

Type 1: Posterior compression of the sacroiliac joint without ligament disruption; oblique pubic ramus fracture

Type 2: Rupture of the posterior sacroiliac ligament; pivotal internal rotation of the hemipelvis on the anterior SI joint with a crush injury of the sacrum and an oblique pubic ramus fracture

Type 3: Findings as in type 2 injury with evidence of an AP compression injury to the contralateral hemipelvis

Vertical shear

Complete ligament or bony disruption of a hemipelvis associated with hemipelvis displacement

This classification does not take into consideration isolated fractures outside the bony pelvic ring or acetabular fractures

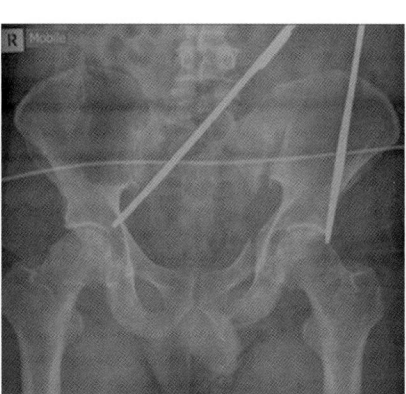

Fig. 3.8.24 Vertical shear injury of the pelvis. Unilateral fractures involving the left iliac wing and superior and inferior pubic rami.

CT scan of the pelvis

CT and plain X-rays are complementary modalities in the evaluation of pelvic fractures. Patients with pelvic fractures associated with haemodynamic instability are not suitable for placing in the CT scanner.

If the patient with pelvic fractures is haemodynamically unstable, it is important to ascertain whether or not there is intra-abdominal bleeding. If the FAST examination excludes intra-abdominal bleeding, then the patient should proceed to angiography and embolization if pelvic arterial bleeding is demonstrated [45] or, alternatively, to surgical fixation if the pelvic ring is widely disrupted. There are limitations for both treatment options as set out below.

In stable patients, CT is useful for demonstrating posterior fractures involving the sacrum and sacroiliac joints as well as sacroiliac joint diastasis. Reformatted 3D images are particularly useful for the assessment of acetabular and pubic bone fractures.

The speed and definition of MDCT scanners have meant that contrast-enhanced MDCT is a highly accurate, non-invasive way of identifying ongoing arterial bleeding, which will then require urgent interventional radiological (IVR) treatment.

Visceral angiography and embolization

In haemodynamically stable patients, solid visceral injuries may be treated conservatively. In haemodynamically unstable patients with solid intra-abdominal visceral injuries and active bleeding, either surgical or endovascular management could be considered in centres where both interventions are available. Embolization in trauma is the intentional and controlled occlusion of vessels to stop haemorrhage [46]. Embolization agents may be classified as temporary or permanent. Permanent agents include metallic coils, glue and embolization particles, while gelatin sponge (Gelfoam) is a temporary agent. Gelfoam is able to stop active bleeding, however, allows for recanalization of the embolized vessel. The spleen and kidneys are the most commonly embolized viscera post-trauma [E-Figs 3.8.27 and 3.8.28].

Pelvic angiography

Pelvic fractures that disrupt the posterior aspect of the pelvic ring have the potential to cause considerable arterial and/or venous injury. 'Open-book' or AP compression pelvic ring fractures are more likely to have venous rather than arterial bleeding and compression of the pelvic ring by external fixation should help to minimize this blood loss, although this practice has not been validated by prospective, randomized controlled trials.

There remains considerable controversy regarding the role of angiography and arterial embolization in pelvic trauma. Factors such as age >65, absence of long bone fractures and haemodynamic instability necessitating urgent angiography have been identified as predicting the likelihood of arterial bleeding in pelvic fractures [43]. Studies of the efficacy of angiographic embolization in select groups of haemodynamically unstable patients with pelvic fractures suggesting success rates for controlling bleeding in excess of 90% have led to a shift towards early radiographic intervention [47,48].

The femoral artery is catheterized and angiography of both internal iliac arteries performed. If arterial bleeding is identified, then the vessels can be selectively embolized (E-Fig. 3.8.26). There is a rich vascular supply to the pelvic viscera and major ischaemic complications are rare following pelvic embolization, but other problems, such as impotence, may occur.

Contrast studies

The main contrast studies used in pelvic fractures are the urethrogram and cystogram. Rupture of the membranous urethra may occur in association with pelvic fractures, particularly those involving distraction of the pubic symphysis or fractures involving both superior and inferior pubic rami. If there is clinical and radiological suspicion of potential urethral damage, an urethrogram should be performed. This is done by inserting a soft catheter into the urethral meatus and injecting contrast while screening with an image intensifier (Figs 3.8.25 and 3.8.26). The urethral passage, if patent, will be visualized and it may be possible to catheterize the urethra. If there is obstruction to the passage of dye or a false track is identified, a suprapubic catheter will be required. Further contrast is then injected into the bladder, then PA and oblique X-rays or CT scan can be performed to assess for extravasation of contrast suggesting bladder rupture.

Extremities

Missed injuries occur in about 2–6% of blunt trauma patients. One retrospective study [50] found that musculoskeletal injuries and spinal fractures featured highly (6%) among the injuries not found after the initial primary and secondary surveys. The musculoskeletal injuries comprised mainly fractures and a small number of soft tissue injuries. Among the factors contributing to the missed injuries were the presence of closed head injury and intoxication. In comparison, one study found the rate of abdominal missed injuries to be 2% [51].

A careful clinical examination of all joints and limbs looking for swelling, deformity and crepitus must be made in order to direct radiological investigation. Fractures, dislocations and ligamentous instability are more likely to be missed in the smaller, peripheral bones. As these injuries may be a source of ongoing disability due to late diagnosis, they may also be a potential source of litigation. Dislocations of joints, such as the anterior shoulder and elbow, should be readily obvious, but less so are posterior shoulder and lunate/perilunate dislocation in the wrist. AP and lateral X-rays should be taken of any joint considered abnormal on examination during the secondary survey. In the lower limb, posterior dislocation of the hip and knee joints may cause serious sciatic nerve and popliteal artery damage, respectively, and require urgent reduction. If the viability of the limb or skin is threatened, a dislocation (e.g. knee or ankle) should be immediately reduced on clinical grounds and X-ray performed after reduction to check for position and bony fractures.

Bony fractures in the upper limb commonly missed include medial or lateral epicondylar fractures and supracondylar fractures of the elbow in children. In the adult, fractures of the carpal bones, in particular the scaphoid and triquetrum, may be missed unless carefully looked for and these injuries may result in significant disability. Fractures and dislocations involving the metacarpals and phalanges are also easily missed in the multitrauma patient. The skier's (or gamekeeper's) thumb [52] is an acute sprain or rupture of the ulnar collateral ligament at the metacarpophalangeal joint caused by forceful abduction of the thumb. This injury may be missed unless the joint is specifically examined for stability and stress views taken if indicated.

In the lower limb, fractures of the tibial plateau and calcaneus, which may occur as a result of a fall, may be missed unless sought both clinically and radiologically. Appropriate AP and lateral X-rays should be taken of these areas. In the foot, loss of Boehler's angle (normal 25–40°) may indicate a depressed fracture of

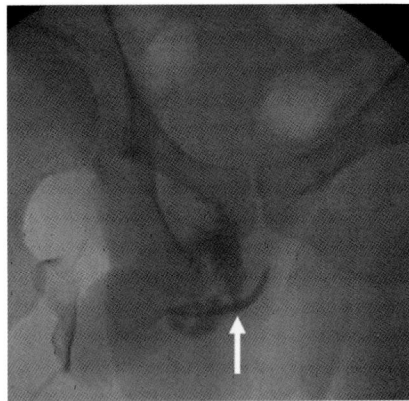

Fig. 3.8.26 Urethrogram in a patient with a fractured penis demonstrating active extravasation of contrast from the mid-penile urethra (arrow).

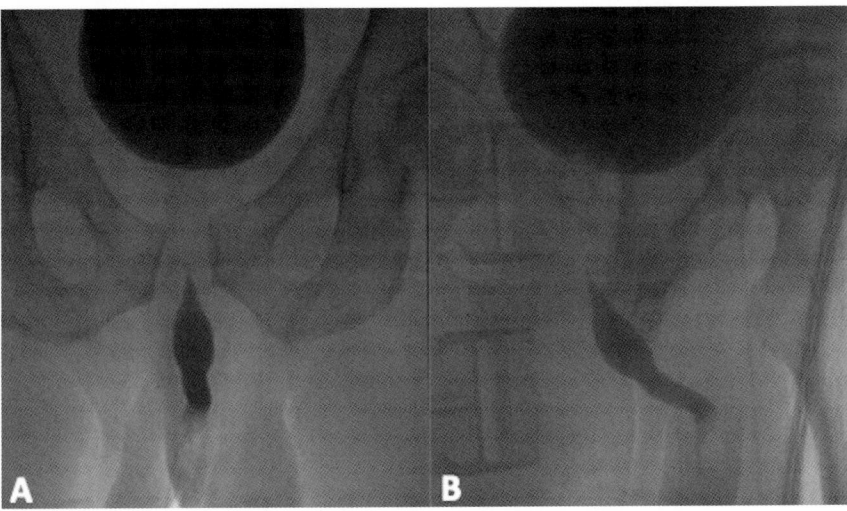

Fig. 3.8.25 Normal urethrogram in a patient with diastasis of the pubic symphysis.

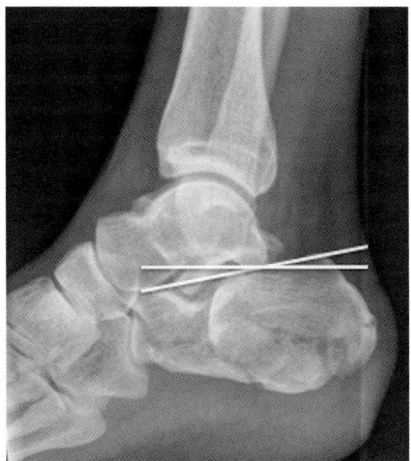

Fig. 3.8.27 Calcaneal fracture with loss of Bohler's angle.

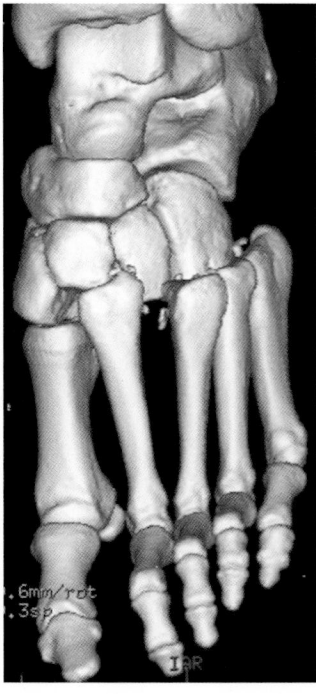

Fig. 3.8.28 Lisfranc injury and tarsometatarsal joint complex dislocation.

the subtalar part of the calcaneus (Fig. 3.8.27). Falls in general, and calcaneal fractures in particular, may be associated with fractures of the upper lumbar spine.

CT scans of complex fractures and dislocations may assist the orthopaedic surgeon in planning appropriate fixation (Fig. 3.8.28). Joints where this may be helpful include large joints, such as shoulder, hip and knee, e.g. tibial plateau fractures. Calcaneal fractures are often not clearly seen on plain X-rays and require a CT scan for a more accurate view. MRI is the investigation of choice for ligamentous or meniscal injuries in the knee.

Angiography is required when there is suspected or clinically obvious vascular compromise to either upper or lower limb. The axillary or brachial arteries may be damaged or transected in blunt or penetrating injuries to the upper limb. The brachial plexus can also be damaged in trauma around the shoulder joint and should be actively looked for in these injuries. The commonest serious vascular injury to the lower limb may be associated with posterior dislocation of the knee and intimal disruption of the popliteal artery. Angiography will give accurate information regarding the degree of arterial damage and the state of the collateral flow.

Conclusion

Radiology in the multitrauma patient requires judicious decision making and interpretation of X-rays and other specialized modalities, such as CT, MRI and ultrasonography. There is less reliance on plain X-rays and more emphasis on CT scans to rule in or out serious injury in the head, spine, chest, abdomen and pelvis. Radiation exposure should be considered for all CT scans, especially in younger trauma patients. Missed injuries that are not diagnosed in the first 24–48 hours often contribute significantly to patient morbidity and mortality. These injuries may involve the musculoskeletal system in the form of limb or spinal fractures and must be actively sought and excluded by appropriate clinical and radiological examination.

Controversies

- Clearance of the cervical spine in obtunded trauma patients can be made on the basis of fine cuts in a multislice CT scan. MRI may be indicated if there is strong clinical suspicion and the need to exclude a ligamentous injury.
- Dynamic flexion/extension X-rays of the Cx spine should only be performed on awake and cooperative patients, but they have low sensitivity and specificity for the detection of unstable spinal injuries.
- CT angiography and digital subtraction angiography are invaluable in the investigation of blunt cerebrovascular injury to the neck and should also be performed if there is cervical spine bony injury involving the foramen transversarium.
- Chest CT is the investigation of choice to exclude significant intrathoracic injury.
- The FAST examination will detect haemoperitoneum only but not hollow viscus perforation or solid organ haematoma.
- Pelvic angiography and embolization should be part of the resuscitation protocol in haemodynamically unstable patients with major pelvic fractures.

References

[1] Tan GA, Van Every B. Staff exposure to ionizing radiation in a major trauma centre. Aust NZ J Surg 2005;75:136–7.

[2] Shah DJ, Sachs RK, Wilson DJ. Radiation-induced cancer: a modern view. Br J Radiol 2012;85:e1166–e1173.

[3] Furlow B. Radiation dose in computed tomography. Radiol Technology 2010;81:437–50.

[4] Aldrich JE, Bilawich AM, Mayo JR. Radiation doses to patients receiving computed tomography examinations in British Columbia. Can Assoc Radiol J 2006;57:79–85.

[5] http://www.radiologyinfo.org/en/safety/index.cfm?pg= sfty_xray&bhcp=1

[6] Pierce DA, Shimizu Y, Preston DL, et al. Studies on the mortality of atomic bomb survivors. Report 12, Part 1, Cancer: 1950–1990. Radiat Rese 1996;146:1–27.

[7] Thompson DE, Mabuchi K, Ron E, et al. Cancer incidence in atomic bomb survivors. Part 11, Solid tumours: 1958–1987. Radiat Res 1994;137:S17–67.

[8] <http://www.pueblo.gsa.gov/cic_text/health/fullbody-ctscan/risks.htm>.

[9] Valadka AB, Narayan RK. Injury to the cranium. In: Feliciano DV, Moore EE, Mattox KL, editors. Trauma (3rd ed.). Stamford CT. Appleton and Lange, 1996, p. 267–78.

[10] Stiel IG, Wells GA, Vandemheen K, et al. The Canadian CT Head Rule for patients with minor head injury. Lancet 2001;357:1391–6.

[11] Bromberg WJ, Collier BC, Diebel LN, et al. Blunt cerebrovascular injury practice management guidelines: The Eastern Association for the Surgery of Trauma. J Trauma 2010;68:471–7.

[12] Emmett KP, Fabian TC, DiCicco JM, et al. Improving the screening criteria for blunt cerebrovascular injury: the appropriate role for computed tomography angiography. J Trauma 2011;70:1058–65.

[13] Biffi WL, Moore EE, Offner PJ, et al. Blunt carotid arterial injuries: implications of a new grading scale. J Trauma 1999;47:845–53.

[14] Griffen MM, Frykberg ER, Kerwin AJ, et al. Radiographic clearance of blunt cervical spine injury: plain radiograph or computed tomography scan? J Trauma Injury Infect Crit Care 2003;55:222–7.

[15] Cooper DJ, Ackland HM. Clearing the cervical spine in unconscious head injured patients – the evidence. Crit Care Resus 2005;7:181–4.

[16] Hoffman JR, Mower WR, Wolfson AB, et al. Validity of a set of clinical criteria to rule out injury to the cervical spine in patients with blunt trauma. National Emergency X-Radiography Utilisation Study Group. N Engl J Med 2000;343:94–9.

[17] Barrett TW, Mower WR, Zucker MI, et al. Injuries missed by limited computed tomographic imaging of patients with cervical spine injuries. Ann Emerg Med 2006;47:129–33.

[18] Stiell IG, Wells GA, Vandemheen K, et al. The Canadian C-spine rule for radiography in alert and stable trauma patients. J Am MedAssoc 2001;286:1841–8.

[19] Berquist TH. Cervical spine trauma. In: Kricum ME, editor. Imaging of sports injuries. Aspen Publications, 1992, p. 31–64.

[20] Lusted LB, Keats TE. The spine atlas of roentgenographic measurement, 2nd ed. Chicago: Yearbook Medical Publications, 1967, 101–103.

[21] Keene JG, Daffner RH. Spinal trauma. In: Rosen P, Doris PE, Barkin RM, editors. Diagnostic radiology in emergency medicine. St Louis: Mosby-Year Book, 1992, p. 210–70.

[22] Harris JH. The cervicocranium: its radiographic assessment. Radiology 2001;218:335–7.

[23] Noble EF. Smoker WRK. The forgotten condyle: The appearance, morphology, and classification of occipital condyle fractures. Am J Neuroradiol 1996;17:507–13.

[24] Satisky E, Votey S. Emergency department approach to acute thoracolumbar spine injury. J Emerg Med 1997;15:49–59.

[25] Denis F. The three column spine and its significance in the classification of acute thoracolumbar spinal injuries. Spine 1983;8:817–31.

[26] Mirka H, Ferda J, Baxa J. Multidetector computed tomography of chest trauma: Indications, technique and interpretation. Insights Imag 2012;3:433–49.

[27] Oikonomou A, Prassopoulos PCT. Imaging of blunt chest trauma. Insights Imag 2011;2:281–95.

[28] Ho M, Gutierrez F. Chest radiography in thoracic polytrauma. Am J Roentgenol 1992;200:599–612.

[29] Traub M, Stevenson M, McEvoy S, et al. The use of chest computed tomography versus chest X ray in patients with major blunt trauma. Injury 2007;38:43–7.

[30] Brookes JG, Dunn RJ, Roger IR. Sternal fractures: a retrospective analysis of 272 cases. J Trauma 1993;35:46.

[31] Sammett EJ. Aorta, trauma. <www.emedicine.com/radio/topic44.htm>; 2003.

[32] Creasy JD, Chiles C, Routh WD, et al. Overview of traumatic injury of the thoracic aorta. Radiographics 1997;17:27–45.

[33] Holtzman SR, Bettmann MA, Casciani T, et al. Expert Panel on Cardiovascular Imaging. Blunt chest trauma-suspected aortic injury. [online publication]. Reston (VA): American College of Radiology (ACR); 2005.

[34] Keaney PA, Wesley Smith D, Johnson SB, et al. Use of transoesophageal echocardiography in the evaluation of traumatic aortic injury. J Trauma 1993;34:696–703.

[35] Smith MD, Cassidy JM, Souther S, et al. Transoesophageal echocardiography in the diagnosis of traumatic rupture of the aorta. N Engl J Med 1995;332:356–62.

[36] Bouhemad B, Zhang M, Lu Q, Rouby J. Clinical review: Bedside lung ultrasound in critical care practice. Crit Care 2007;11:205.

[37] Tsang BD, Panacek EA, Brant WE, et al. Effect of oral contrast administration for abdominal computed tomography in the evaluation of acute blunt trauma. Ann Emerg Med 1997;30:7–13.

[38] Moore E, et al. Scaling system for organ specific injuries. <http://www.aast.org/Library/TraumaTools>.

[39] Henneman PL, Marx JA, Moore EE, et al. Diagnostic peritoneal lavage: accuracy in predicting necessary laparotomy following blunt and penetrating trauma. J Trauma 1990;30:1345.

[40] Hsu JM, Joseph AP, Tarlinton LJ, et al. The accuracy of focused assessment with sonography in trauma (FAST) in blunt trauma patients: experience of an Australian major trauma service. Injury 2007;38:71–5.

[41] Boulanger BR, Kearney PA, Tsuei B, et al. The routine use of sonography in penetrating torso injury is beneficial. J Trauma 2001;51:320–5.

[42] Boulanger BR, McLellan BA, Brenneman FD, et al. Prospective evidence of the superiority of a sonography-based algorithm in the assessment of blunt abdominal injury. J Trauma 1999;47:632–7.

[43] Gill Cryer H, Johnson E. Pelvic fractures. In: Feliciano DV, Moore EE, Mattox KJ, editors. Trauma (3rd ed.). Stamford: Appleton and Lange; 1996, p. 635–59.

[44] Pennel GF, Time M, Waddell JP, et al. Pelvic disruption: assessment and classification. Clin Orthoped 1980;151:12.

[45] Martin J, Heetveld, Harris I, et al. Management of unstable patients with pelvic fractures. Practice Guidelines, Liverpool Hospital NSW. <http://www.swsahs.nsw.gov.au/livTrauma>; 2003.

[46] Lopera JE. Embolisation in trauma: principles and techniques. Semin Intervent Radiol 2010;27:14–28.

[47] Velmahos GC, Toutouzas KG, Vassiliu P, et al. A prospective study of the safety and efficacy of angiographic embolization for pelvic and visceral injuries. J Trauma 2002;52:303–8.

[48] Miller PR, Moore PS, Mansell E, et al. External fixation or arteriogram in bleeding pelvic fracture: initial therapy guided by markers of arterial haemorrhage. J Trauma 2003;54:437–43.

[49] Fangio P, Asehnoune K, Edouard A, et al. The epidemiology of fractures and fracture-dislocations of the cervical spine. J Trauma 2005;58:978–84. discussion 984.

[50] Kremli MK. Missed musculoskeletal injuries in a University Hospital in Riyadh: types of missed injuries and responsible factors. Injury 1996;27:503–6.

[51] Sung C, Kim KH. Missed injuries in abdominal trauma. J Trauma 1996;41:276–8.

[52] Musharafieh RS, Bassim YR, Atiyeh BS. Ulnar collateral ligament injury in the emergency department. J Emerg Med 1997;15:193–6.

3.9 Trauma in pregnancy

Steven Troupakis

ESSENTIALS

1 Trauma in pregnancy is the most common cause of non-obstetric maternal death, with most deaths due to head injury and haemorrhagic shock.

2 Fetal death occurs far more often than maternal death and is dependent on the severity of the maternal injuries. Placental abruption and direct fetal trauma cause most deaths.

3 Common causes of trauma are motor vehicle collisions, falls and assaults.

4 Important sequelae are bruising, fractures, premature labour, placental abruption, disseminated intravascular coagulopathy, fetomaternal haemorrhage, intra-abdominal injuries, uterine rupture and haemorrhagic shock.

5 The physiological changes that occur with pregnancy, such as the relative hypervolaemia and the gravid uterus, can make clinical assessment of the patient difficult.

6 Continuous cardiotocographic monitoring for at least 4 hours is the best predictor of placental abruption and fetal distress.

7 Bedside ultrasound allows early evaluation for the presence of intraperitoneal fluid and the fetal heart.

8 Maternal resuscitation remains the best method of fetal resuscitation.

Introduction

Trauma during pregnancy presents a unique set of challenges for the emergency department (ED), as the anatomical and physiological changes that occur during pregnancy will influence the evaluation and management of the patient. An appreciation of these changes is important. Aggressive resuscitation of the mother remains the best treatment for the fetus. A multidisciplinary approach with early obstetric consultation will help improve the outcome of these patients.

Anatomical and physiological changes in pregnancy

Cardiovascular

Blood volume increases by about 50% by the end of the third trimester [1]. With relative hypervolaemia, the patient may lose up to 35% of her blood volume before signs of haemorrhagic shock appear. Maternal cardiac output increases by 30–50% above normal by the end of the second trimester. The resting heart rate increases by 15–20 beats/min by the end of the third trimester. Systolic and diastolic blood pressure fall by 10–15 mmHg during the second trimester, but rise again towards the end of the pregnancy. ECG changes may occur with the cephalic displacement of the heart, such as left axis deviation by 15°, T-wave inversion or flattening in leads III, V1 and V2 and Q waves in III and AVF [1]. After 20 weeks' gestation, supine positioning may cause inferior vena cava (IVC) obstruction by the gravid uterus, leading to a fall in cardiac output.

Haematological

A dilutional anaemia occurs with a fall in haematocrit (31–35% by the end of pregnancy). Pregnancy induces a leucocytosis, with levels up to $18\,000/mm^3$ in the third trimester. Coagulation factors increase (fibrinogen, factors VII, VIII, IX, X), increasing the risk of venous thrombosis. The buffering capacity of the blood is reduced [2].

Respiratory

The diaphragm is elevated by about 4 cm. Tidal volume and minute volume increase by 40%. A respiratory alkalosis results, with a fall in PCO_2 to 30 mmHg. The anteroposterior diameter of the chest is increased and the mediastinum is widened on chest X-ray.

Gastrointestinal

Cephalic displacement of intra-abdominal structures reduces gastro-oesophageal sphincter tone, combined with delayed gastric motility, there is an increased the risk of aspiration. The intestines are displaced to the upper part of the abdomen and may be shielded by the uterus. The peritoneum is stretched by the gravid uterus, which may make signs of peritonism less reliable [2]. Alkaline phosphatase levels may triple because of placental production.

Urinary

Dilatation of the renal pelvis and ureters occurs from the 10th week of gestation. The bladder becomes hyperaemic and is displaced into the abdomen from the 12th week, making it more susceptible to trauma.

Uterine

There is a massive increase in uterine size. Blood flow to the uterus increases from 60 to 600 mL/min by the end of the pregnancy.

Epidemiology

The incidence of trauma during pregnancy is approximately 6–7%, the causes being similar to those in the general population [1,3]. Blunt trauma is the commonest injury, with motor vehicle accidents, falls and assaults being the other common causes and in that order. Penetrating injuries are less common and usually the result of domestic violence. Stab wounds have a better prognosis for the fetus than do projectile wounds. Most trauma is of a minor nature, resulting in bruising, minor fractures and threatened premature labour. Maternal death from trauma is rare, but is the leading non-obstetric cause of death, with most fatalities due to head injuries and internal haemorrhage. Younger (age <20) and older (age >35) multiparous women at gestational ages of less than 28 weeks have a higher risk of adverse outcomes [4]. Women who are discharged undelivered continue to have delayed morbidity, with increased rates of placental abruption and low-birthweight infants. Fetal death occurs in about 1–2% of cases and is dependent on the gestational age and the pattern and severity of maternal injury. Most fetal deaths are due to placental abruption or direct trauma. High-speed (>80 km/h) and broadside motor vehicle accidents have a higher incidence of placental abruption and fetal and maternal death than do frontal collisions [5]. Similarly, ejection from a vehicle and motorcycle and pedestrian collisions are associated with poor fetal outcome [6]. Maternal hypotension and vaginal bleeding are associated with increased fetal loss. In one trauma series, pregnant patients with an injury severity score (ISS) >12 had a fetal death rate of 65%; those with an ISS <12 had no fetal deaths [7].

Specific injuries

Pelvic fracture

Pelvic fracture is often the result of a high-speed motor vehicle accident. Massive haemorrhage can occur from the uterus, as well as bladder, urethral and ureteric lacerations. Retroperitoneal haemorrhage occurs and may be difficult to diagnose. Direct fetal skull fractures can lead to fetal death. The majority of patients with a pelvic fracture can be delivered vaginally.

Placental abruption

Placental abruption complicates 1–5% of patients with minor trauma and between 20 and 50% of cases with major trauma [3,8]. The placenta separates from the underlying decidua because of shearing forces between the relatively inelastic placenta and the more elastic uterus. This leads to fetal hypoxia and death. Thromboplastin release may lead to the development of disseminated intravascular coagulopathy (DIC).

Uterine rupture

Uterine rupture is rare but leads to considerable haemorrhage and with 10% maternal mortality and almost 100% fetal mortality [3]. It usually occurs as a result of direct trauma to women with a uterine scar. It should be suspected when there is maternal shock, fetal death, difficulty defining a uterus, easily palpable fetal parts and intraperitoneal fluid on ultrasound.

Fetomaternal haemorrhage

Fetomaternal haemorrhage is the transplacental spread of fetal blood into the maternal circulation. It occurs in approximately 8–30% of trauma cases and may lead to Rhesus (Rh) sensitization of the mother, neonatal anaemia, fetal cardiac arrhythmias and fetal death [2]. The Kleihauer–Betke test is used to identify and quantify fetomaternal haemorrhage. This test relies on the principle that fetal cells are stable in acid (pH 3.2), whereas adult haemoglobin is eluted from maternal red cells. Microscopy will identify fetal red blood cells on blood smear. All Rh-negative pregnant trauma victims with a positive Kleihauer–Betke test should receive Rhesus immunoglobulin.

Presentation

History

Questions should be directed to determining the severity and type of trauma, as well as an obstetric history. In a motor vehicle accident, high speed, side collisions, ejection from the vehicle and improper use of seatbelts and lap belts alone are associated with a greater likelihood of serious injuries [3]. Direct trauma to the abdomen is more likely to cause fractures, splenic and hepatic injuries, whereas indirect trauma via shearing forces is more likely to cause placental abruption. Pelvic pain, uterine contractions and vaginal bleeding may indicate placental abruption. The gestational age (>22 weeks) is the main determinant for fetal viability. Lack of fetal movements may indicate fetal death.

Primary survey

The airway should be assessed and cleared. Intubation may be difficult because of aspiration risk, breast enlargement and cervical trauma.

Breathing should be assessed and the patient given supplemental oxygen to improve both maternal and fetal oxygenation. If the patient is more than 20 weeks pregnant, she should be placed on her side (preferably the left) to relieve any caval compression. If spinal immobilization is necessary, wedges can be placed underneath a spinal board or, alternatively, the uterus pushed to the left manually. The blood pressure and circulation can then be assessed, remembering that signs of shock may present late because of relative hypervolaemia.

A quick assessment of conscious level and any major neurological deficits should be made. The patient should be adequately exposed for a thorough examination, but protected from a drop in temperature.

Secondary survey

The sequence of the secondary survey is the same as in the non-pregnant patient, but with an obstetric examination included in the abdominal examination. The uterus should be assessed for fundal height, tenderness, contractions, fetal heart tone, fetal movements and position. Focused abdominal sonography for trauma (FAST) should be performed to assess for intraperitoneal haemorrhage. Bedside ultrasound can also be used to assess the fetal heart rate. The availability of FAST scans and CTs have caused diagnostic peritoneal lavage to fall out of routine use [9]. An obstetrician should perform the pelvic examination, looking for trauma to the genital tract, cervical dilation, fetal presentation and station relative to the ischial spines. Nitrazine paper can be used to test for the presence of amniotic fluid: it turns blue in the presence of the alkaline fluid. Rectal examination and urinalysis are essential.

Investigations

Blood tests

Routine blood tests, such as full blood count, electrolytes, coagulation studies, group and hold, should be performed looking for evidence of anaemia and DIC. A Kleihauer–Betke test will indicate the necessary dose of Rhesus immunoglobulin in Rh-negative patients.

X-rays

In severe trauma, it is necessary to take cervical spine, chest and pelvic films. The abdomen should be shielded and repetition of films avoided. There is negligible risk to the fetus when radiation exposure has been limited to less than 0.1 Gy and after 20 weeks' gestation radiation is unlikely to cause abnormalities [10]. A standard pelvic film delivers less than 0.01 Gy.

Ultrasonography

Ultrasonography is useful in determining gestational age, placental position and fetal well-being and estimating amniotic fluid volume [11]. Bedside FAST can be used to assess for free fluid in the peritoneum and in the pericardial and pleural cavities, especially in patients too unstable for CT. Ultrasonography will detect only 40–50% of placental abruptions [3].

Cardiotocography (CTG)

CTG monitoring beyond the 20th week of pregnancy has proved a sensitive way of diagnosing placental abruption early. It should be instituted early and continuously for at least 4 hours [2]. Fetal distress on CTG may be the earliest indicator of impending shock. Frequent uterine contractions and fetal distress are suggestive of placental abruption. In one study, no placental abruptions were missed if CTG monitoring remained normal for the first 4 hours [8].

Computed tomography

Computed tomography (CT) is an accurate and non-invasive way of assessing uterine and retroperitoneal structures, but it is time-consuming and involves a higher radiation dose than normal X-rays, with exposure for abdominal CT being between 0.05 and 0.1 Gy. Chest and head CT expose the fetus to far less radiation, especially if uterine shielding is used with radiation exposure of about 0.001 Gy [3,12].

Management

Maternal resuscitation is the best method of fetal resuscitation. If the injuries are severe, the patient should be in a resuscitation area with a multidisciplinary team approach to management and early surgical, anaesthetic and obstetrical consultation. Attention to adequate oxygenation, proper positioning and aggressive fluid replacement is important. Oximetry, ECG, blood pressure monitoring and cardiotocography should be started early. A nasogastric tube should be inserted to reduce the risk of aspiration, as should an indwelling catheter for urinalysis and to allow better assessment of the uterus. X-rays as indicated should be performed as well as a FAST scan and CT as necessary, to evaluate abdominal injuries. If the patient remains unstable with hypotension or continued bleeding, laparotomy is indicated. Ultrasound is particularly useful in the resuscitation phase to assess fetal heart rate and uterine bleeding.

If a thoracostomy is required, the entry point should be 1 or 2 intercostal spaces higher than normal to avoid the diaphragm and abdominal structures.

The presence of vaginal bleeding, abdominal tenderness or pain, hypotension, absent fetal heart sounds, fetal distress on CTG and amniotic fluid leakage requires an urgent obstetric opinion and possibly a caesarean section.

The use of leg veins for intravenous access should be avoided as the gravid uterus may affect venous return and compromise drug delivery. The uterine vasculature is very sensitive to catecholamines. If ionotropes are required, adrenaline and noradrenaline should be avoided. Ephedrine and dopamine at doses less than 5 μg/kg can be used to improve maternal BP without compromising uterine blood flow [1,3].

Premature labour can be treated with tocolytic agents, such as intravenous salbutamol. However, salbutamol causes maternal and fetal tachycardia, which may mask symptoms of hypovolaemia. Magnesium sulphate is recommended as an alternative tocolytic in abdominal trauma [3].

DIC may develop as a result of placental abruption, amniotic fluid embolism and fetal death. Clotting factors may need to be replaced.

Anti-D immunoglobulin should be administered to all Rhesus-negative mothers.

In general, penetrating injuries should be explored by laparotomy, especially if they involve the upper abdomen, where there is a high possibility of bowel perforation. Some authors argue that stab wounds over the uterus can be treated conservatively if there is no evidence of visceral injury, the entrance wound is below the fundus and the patient is stable [1].

Post-mortem caesarean section should be considered within the first 4 minutes of a maternal cardiac arrest. There have been many cases of fetal survival up to 20 minutes after maternal death. The fetuses that have the best chance of surviving neurologically intact are those delivered within 5 minutes of the arrest, who weigh more than 1000 g and are of more than 28 weeks' gestation [1,12].

Disposition

Patients who are haemodynamically unstable and who have extensive head or chest injuries will require surgical intervention and intensive-care support. Patients who are stable but show signs of fetal distress should undergo caesarean section. All patients with minor injuries who are more than 20 weeks pregnant should have CTG monitoring for at least 4 hours, preferably in a labour ward.

Prognosis

Most women who sustain trauma during pregnancy suffer few complications. There is greater maternal and fetal mortality in pregnant women with higher injury severity scores. Placental abruption can still occur as a result of minor trauma 24–48 hours after the accident, but 4 hours of CTG monitoring should detect this group of patients [2].

Prevention

Properly worn seatbelts reduce both maternal and fetal mortality. In one study of serious motor vehicle accidents, maternal mortality following ejection from the vehicle was 33%, compared to only 5% in those who were not ejected: fetal mortality was 47% and 11%, respectively [3]. A three-point seat bar system should be used, with the lap portion as low as possible, preferably over the thighs and with the shoulder portion passing between the breasts and above the gravid uterus.

Controversies

- The duration of CTG monitoring: most authors agree 4 hours should be enough to predict placental abruption, although some argue that 24–48 hours may be needed.
- Exploration of penetrating wounds to the abdomen: some authors argue for a conservative approach to a wound below the uterine fundus, whereas others argue that all such wounds should be explored.

References

[1] Muench MV, Canterino JC. Trauma in pregnancy. Obstet Gynecol Clin N Am 2007;34:555–83.
[2] Pearlman MD, Tintinalli JE, Lorenz RP. Blunt trauma during pregnancy. N Engl J Med 1990;323:1609–13.
[3] Hill CC. Trauma in the obstetric patient. Women Hlth 2009;5:269–85.
[4] El Kady D, Gilbert WM, Anderson J, et al. Trauma during pregnancy: an analysis of maternal and fetal outcomes in a large population. Am J Obstet Gynecol 2004;190:1661–8.
[5] Aitokallio-Tallberg A, Halmesmaki E. Motor vehicle accident during the second or third trimester of pregnancy. Acta Obstet Gynecol Scand 1997;76:313–7.
[6] Curet MJ, Schermer CR, Demarest GB, et al. Predictors of outcome in trauma during pregnancy: identification of patients who can be monitored for less than 6 hours. J Trauma 2000;49:18–25.
[7] Ali J, Yeo A, Gana TJ, McLellan BA. Predictors of fetal mortality in pregnant trauma patients. J Trauma 1997;42:782–5.
[8] Pearlman MD, Tintinalli JE, Lorenz RP. A prospective controlled study of outcome after trauma during pregnancy. Am J Obstet Gynecol 1990;162:1502–10.
[9] Oxford CM, Ludmir J. Trauma in pregnancy. Clin Obstet Gynaecol 2009;52:611–29.
[10] Goldman SM, Wagner LK. Radiological management of abdominal trauma in pregnancy. Am J Roentgenol 1996;166:763–7.
[11] Bode PJ, Niezen RA, Van Vugt AB, Schipper J. Abdominal ultrasound as a reliable indicator for conclusive laparotomy in blunt abdominal trauma. J Trauma 1993;34:27–31.
[12] Meroz Y, Elchalal U, Ginosar Y. Initial trauma management in advanced pregnancy. Anesthesiol Clin 2007;25:117–129.

TRAUMA

3

3.10 Wound care and repair

Gim Tan • Richard Waller

ESSENTIALS

1 Good cosmesis can be achieved in the emergency department with conservative treatment, thorough debridement and accurate apposition of everted skin edges.

2 Choose a suture that is monofilament, causes little tissue reactivity and retains tensile strength until the strength of the healing wound is equal to that of the suture.

3 Dirty, contaminated, open wounds should generally be cleansed, debrided and closed within 6 hours to minimize the chance of infection.

4 Suspected tendon injuries require examination of the full range of movement of joints distal to the wound while observing the tendon in the base of the wound for breaches. This is often done under anaesthesia.

5 The success of a tendon repair (as measured by function) relates in large part to the postoperative care and therapy, not simply to the suture and wound closure.

6 Appropriate splinting and elevation of limb wounds at risk of infection takes precedence over antibiotics in the postoperative prevention of infection.

7 If prophylactic antibiotics are used, they should be given intravenously prior to wound closure to achieve adequate concentrations in the tissues and haematomas that may collect. There is no need for antibiotics with simple lacerations not involving tendon, joint or nerves.

8 Wounds that breach body cavities, such as the peritoneum and joints, or involving flexor tendons, nerves and named arteries, should be referred to a specialist for consideration of repair and inpatient care.

9 Foreign bodies, such as clay, chemically impair wound healing.

10 Puncture wounds such as bites may be managed by either second-intention healing after thorough lavage or, better still, by excisional debridement, lavage, antibiotics and atraumatic closure, if less than 24 hours old (preferably less than 6 hours).

Introduction

Open wound injury comprises a significant component of emergency department (ED) workload. Data from the Victorian Injury Surveillance System [1] showed that 72% of all ED presentations for unintentional cutting and/or piercing injury that did not require admission were open wounds. In addition, open wounds may accompany other injuries, such as fractures. Of open wounds that occur in the home, 19% are in the paediatric age group (0–14 years), 62% occur in people under 35 and less than 10% in the over-65 s. Overall, 65% of patients are male.

Location data show that more than 53% of these wounds occur in the home [1], mostly during activity described as leisure. The three major causes are falls up to 1 m; contact with cutting or piercing objects; or having been struck or collided with. Most are unintentional and only 3% are due to an assault. Injuries to the face, head and neck comprise 12% and the upper extremity is involved in 62%. Eighty-eight per cent of all presentations are repaired in the ED and the patient is discharged home. Almost half are referred to GPs and specialists for review. It is those wounds suitable for ED repair that will be further discussed.

Clinical presentation

An initial general assessment of the patient is important as it defines the likely mode of repair and the injured structures and identifies factors for complications. The assessment includes the traditional history, examination and investigation of the patient.

It is important in the history to identify the time and mechanism of injury, the likely presence of foreign bodies and the patient's tetanus immunization status. Past medical history, allergies to agents, such as local anaesthetics, antibiotics, preparation solutions and tapes, and current medications, such as warfarin or cytotoxics, all have a bearing on management. For example, there is a greater risk of infection and poor wound healing in diabetic patients with extremity wounds of the lower limbs sustained in a crush injury. Other relevant general conditions, particularly in the setting of dirty wounds, such as bites, include prior mastectomy and other causes of chronic oedema of the affected region, prior splenectomy, liver dysfunction, immunosuppression or autoimmune disease, such as systemic lupus erythematosus (SLE). Smokers have impaired collagen production in healing wounds [2].

The general examination comprises a search for all injuries sustained and concurrent medical illness that may have a bearing on the results of repair, such as poor circulation in patients with peripheral vascular disease. The patient needs to be recumbent (beware of syncope) and any clothing that may obstruct a thorough examination removed. Constricting rings or other jewellery that encircle the injured body part should also be removed. A general examination is performed, followed by a local examination of the wound coupled with initial cleansing. Function and nerve or vessel injury are then examined for. A detailed examination of the depth of the wound, which usually requires good anaesthesia, is then performed. A surface wound caused by the entrance of a foreign body does not necessarily mean that the foreign body has remained in the vicinity. A decision is made regarding the requirement for further investigations which include radiographs for fractures and some foreign bodies or ultrasound for radiolucent foreign bodies.

An injury to a tendon in the base of the wound may only be apparent when the joints over which it acts are in a particular position, reflecting the position of the limb at the time of injury. At other positions, the tendon injury may slide out of view. Marked pain with use may be a clue to a partial tendon injury.

Any tendon injury or other factors, such as nerve damage, indicate the need for referral to a plastic surgeon.

Wound cleansing

To provide optimum conditions for healing without infection, it is essential to remove all contaminants, foreign bodies and devitalized tissue prior to wound closure.

Universal precautions, including eye protection (goggles or similar), clothing protection (gown) and gloves, must be taken for all wound care and repair. Gloves should be powder free to avoid adding starch as a foreign body to the wound, which will delay healing and produce granulomas [3]. One must be aware of the risk of latex allergy to both the glove wearer and the patient [3].

If necessary, hair can be removed by clipping 1–2 cm above the skin with scissors. Shaving the area with a razor damages the hair follicle and is associated with an increased infection rate. Scalp wounds closed without prior hair removal heal with no increase in infection [4].

The skin surface should be cleaned using sterile normal saline. This has the lowest toxicity and there is no benefit in using antiseptic [5].

Recent studies have shown that the use of tap water in the cleaning of simple lacerations is as effective as normal saline [6].

A wide variety of cleansing solutions is available (Table 3.10.1), with differing attributes.

Anaesthesia is necessary for wounds to be cleansed adequately. Extensive wounds, or particularly heavily contaminated wounds that need vigorous scrubbing, such as road debris tattooing, may require general anaesthesia.

Local anaesthetic may be given by local infiltration or as a regional nerve blockade. Needles introduced through the wound cause less pain, but may theoretically track bacteria into the tissues, although this has not been demonstrated to be a problem clinically. After anaesthesia, irrigation with a pressure of at least 8 psi (55 kPa) [7,8] is required to dislodge bacteria and reduce the incidence of infection. This can be achieved with a 19 G needle, a 25–50 mL syringe, a three-way tap and a flask of fluid, such as sterile saline (Fig. 3.10.1) [9]. High-pressure irrigation (>20 psi, 138 kPa) may cause tissue damage [10].

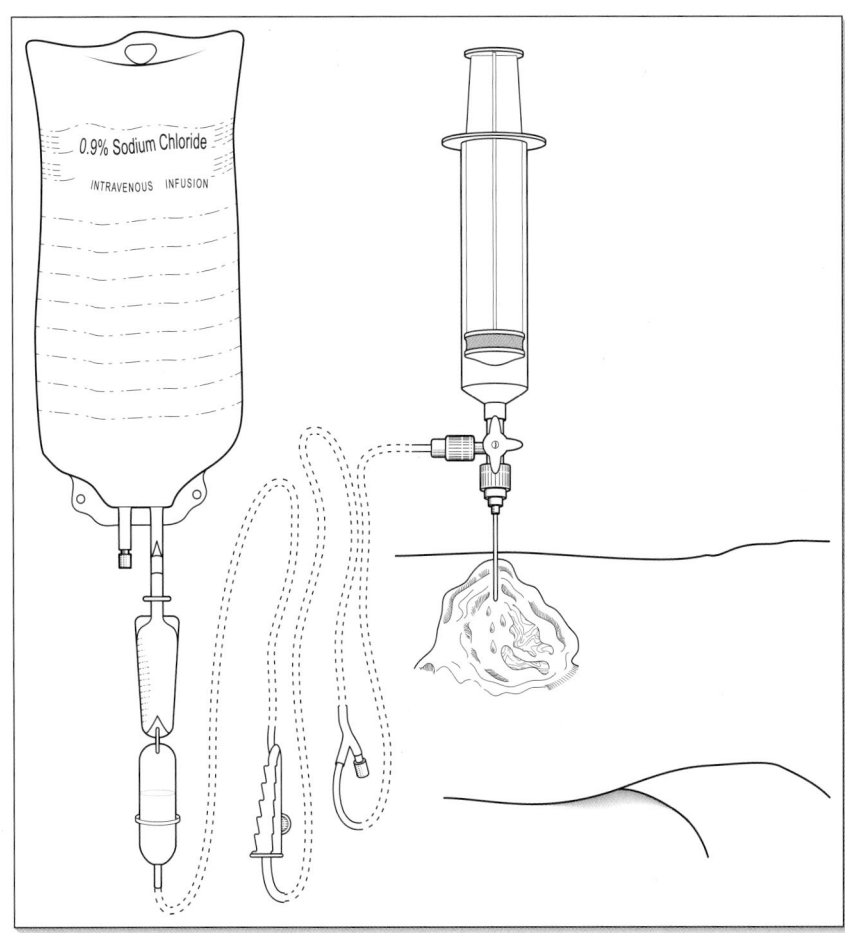

Fig. 3.10.1 Wound irrigation set-up comprising flask of fluid, IV tubing, three-way tap, syringe and 19 G needle designed to deliver fluid at a pressure of at least 8 psi (55 kPa). *(From an original drawing by Elaine Wheildon.)*

Table 3.10.1	Preparation solutions and their properties			
Solution	*Properties*	*Mechanism of action*	*Uses*	*Disadvantages*
Normal saline	Isotonic, non-toxic	Simple washing action	In wound for irrigation	No antiseptic action
Chlorhexidine 0.1% w/v – aqueous	Bacteriostatic	Antibacterial and washing action	Cleanse skin surrounding wound	Not near eyes (causes keratitis), perf. ear drum or meninges
Chlorhexidine 0.1% w/v + cetrimide 1% w/v	Bacteriostatic	Antibacterial and soap action, removes sebum, 'wetting' the skin	Cleanse skin surrounding wound	Not near mucous membranes, eyes (causes keratitis), perf. ear drum or meninges
H_2O_2 3%	Bactericidal to anaerobes	Forms superoxide radicals	Severely contaminated wounds with anaerobic type pathogens	Obstruction of wound surface capillaries and subsequent necrosis
Povidone–iodine 10% w/v	Bactericidal, fungicidal, viricidal, sporicidal	Releases free iodine	On surrounding skin, or in severely contaminated wounds (dilute 1% w/v)	Use on/in large wounds may cause acidosis due to iodine absorption

Radiopaque foreign bodies, such as gravel, metal, pencil lead and glass >2 mm in size [11], may be identified using X-rays. A radiopaque marker, such as a paperclip, can be placed at the wound to help identify the position of the foreign body [12]. This is not sensitive for plastic or wood, however [13], which may be detectable with ultrasound if larger than 2.5 mm. However, if there is gas due to an open wound, this will make ultrasound less sensitive.

Adequate debridement of devitalized tissue has always been a tenet of surgical practice. More recently, there has been a change in emphasis from radical to meticulous debridement. If the skin is devitalized, it should be removed using a scalpel blade. Viable tissue will bleed when cut and viable muscle will contract when stimulated. If viability is in doubt, it may be better to wait for demarcation over the following days, with regular close observation. Fat and fascia are relatively avascular and, if semiviable, in contaminated wounds, should be removed. Semiviable muscle can usually be preserved when well drained [13]. Nerves, major vessels and tendons should not be debrided in the ED. Lavage and debridement should be continued until the wound is clean. Organic material and anionic soils, such as clay, pose the greatest risk of infection if not removed. The highly charged clay particles directly affect leucocytes, preventing phagocytosis of bacteria. They also react chemically with antibiotics, limiting their action.

Once the wound is clean the decision to close immediately or later is made.

Guidelines for delayed closure may include:

- puncture wounds, such as with a tooth or a knife
- wounds unable to be adequately debrided
- contaminated wounds more than 6 hours old
- too much tension in the wound, particularly with crush injury.

In some cases, such as thoroughly lavaged puncture wounds, it may be prudent to allow healing by secondary intention. If in doubt, consult with a plastic surgeon. When repair in the ED may be delayed, it is prudent to have nursing staff perform a preliminary preparation of the wound along the lines shown in Table 3.10.2.

Antibiotics are only necessary in wounds involving joints, tendons, nerves, vessels, significant crush injury or if due to human or animal bites [14].

Table 3.10.2 Preliminary wound preparation procedure instructions for nurses
Explain the procedure to the patient
Identify any allergies, especially to iodine-like products and adhesive tapes
Medicate the patient prior to the irrigation, as needed, for pain control
Protect patient clothing from soiling by the irrigation solution or wound drainage
Position the patient so that irrigating solution can be collected in a basin, depending on the wound's location
Maintain a sterile field during the irrigation procedure as appropriate
Irrigate wound with appropriate solution, using a large irrigating syringe and set-up (see Fig. 3.10.1)
Instill the irrigation solution at 8 psi (55 kPa), reaching all areas
Avoid aspirating the solution back into the syringe
Cleanse from cleanest to dirtiest areas of the wound
Continue irrigating the wound until the prescribed volume is used or the solution returns clear
Position the patient after the irrigation to facilitate drainage
Cleanse and dry the area around the wound after the procedure
Dispose of soiled dressing and supplies appropriately
Lightly pack the wound with well wrung-out, saline soaked, lint-free, sterile gauze or an alginate dressing
Apply a sterile dressing as appropriate until repair is performed

Tetanus prophylaxis

The risk of tetanus is greatest in the very young and the very old, with an overall death rate of 1:10 in Australia [15], so prevention is all important. An average of 10 cases per year occur in Australia [13], usually in older adults who have not been immunized or who have allowed immunization to lapse. The anaerobic bacterium *Clostridium tetani* is present in soil and animal faeces. After incubation of 3–21 days after inoculation into a wound, the toxin produced by the bacteria causes severe muscle spasm and convulsions. Death occurs commonly as a result of respiratory failure. The types of wound at risk are listed in Table 3.10.3, but tetanus may occur after apparently trivial wounds.

Tetanus immunoglobulin is given into the opposite limb to the tetanus toxoid in patients with inadequate protection against tetanus (Table 3.10.4), providing passive protection.

Table 3.10.3 Wounds that are prone to tetanus
Compound fractures
Deep penetrating wounds
Wounds containing foreign bodies, e.g. wood splinters, thorns
Crush injuries or wounds with extensive tissue damage, e.g. burns
Wounds contaminated with soil or horse manure
Wound cleansing delayed more than 3–6 hours

Table 3.10.4 Tetanus vaccination schedule for acute wound management				
History of tetanus vaccination	(CDT) Td	Type of wound	DTP, DT(ADT)* or tetanus toxide as appropriate	Tetanus immunoglobulin
3 doses or more	If less than 5 years since last dose	All wounds	No	No
	If 5–10 years since last dose	Clean minor wounds	No	
		All other wounds	Yes	No
	If more than 10 years since last dose	All wounds	Yes	No
Uncertain or less than 3 doses		Clean minor wounds	Yes	No
		All other wounds	Yes	Yes

*DTP: diphtheria, tetanus, pertussis for children before 8th birthday; DT: child diphtheria tetanus (CDT) if pertussis is contraindicated; Td: adult diphtheria tetanus (ADT) for children after their 8th birthday.
Adapted from Lammers R. Foreign bodies in wounds. In: Singer AJ, Hollander JE, (eds). Lacerations and acute wounds: an evidence-based guide. Philadelphia: FA Davis; 2003: 147.

Wound-healing mechanisms

Wounds never gain more than 80% of the strength of intact skin [16].

There are three phases of healing. Days 1–5 are the initial lag phase (inflammatory), where there is no gain in the strength of the wound. Days 5–14 are a period of rapid increase in wound strength, associated with fibroplasia and epithelialization. The wound has only 7% of its final strength at day 5. Wound maturation progresses from day 14 onwards, with production, cross-linking and remodelling of collagen.

The surgical maxim that wounds heal from side to side is only partly true: if left to heal by itself the entire wound will contract around its margin prior to epithelialization. This has been termed secondary closure or healing by second intention. Allowing the wound to close without intervention relies on healing up from the base and from the edges and often results in unsightly scars. Primary closure involves the apposition of wound edges, preferably within 6 hours of injury, with sutures, staples, tissue adhesive glue, etc. After a delay of 6 hours or more the chance of a wound infection increases. Delayed primary closure is performed 4–5 days after injury, when it is clear there is no infection. This may be used for contaminated wounds that present more than 6 hours post-injury.

Factors that affect the rate of wound healing include:

- technical factors of the repair
- anatomic factors (intrinsic blood supply, etc.)
- drugs (steroids, cytotoxics, etc.)
- associated conditions and diseases (diabetes, vitamin C, zinc deficiency, etc.)
- the general nutritional state of the patient.

Suture types

Wounds may be closed with tape, staples, sutures or tissue adhesive.

Purpose-made commercial tapes reinforced with rayon provide an excellent means of closure. The adherence of tapes (Fig. 3.10.2) may be improved by the application of adhesive adjuncts, such as tincture of benzoin or gum mastic paint [17]. These adhesives must not be allowed to enter the wound [18] as they potentiate infection and cause intense pain. The

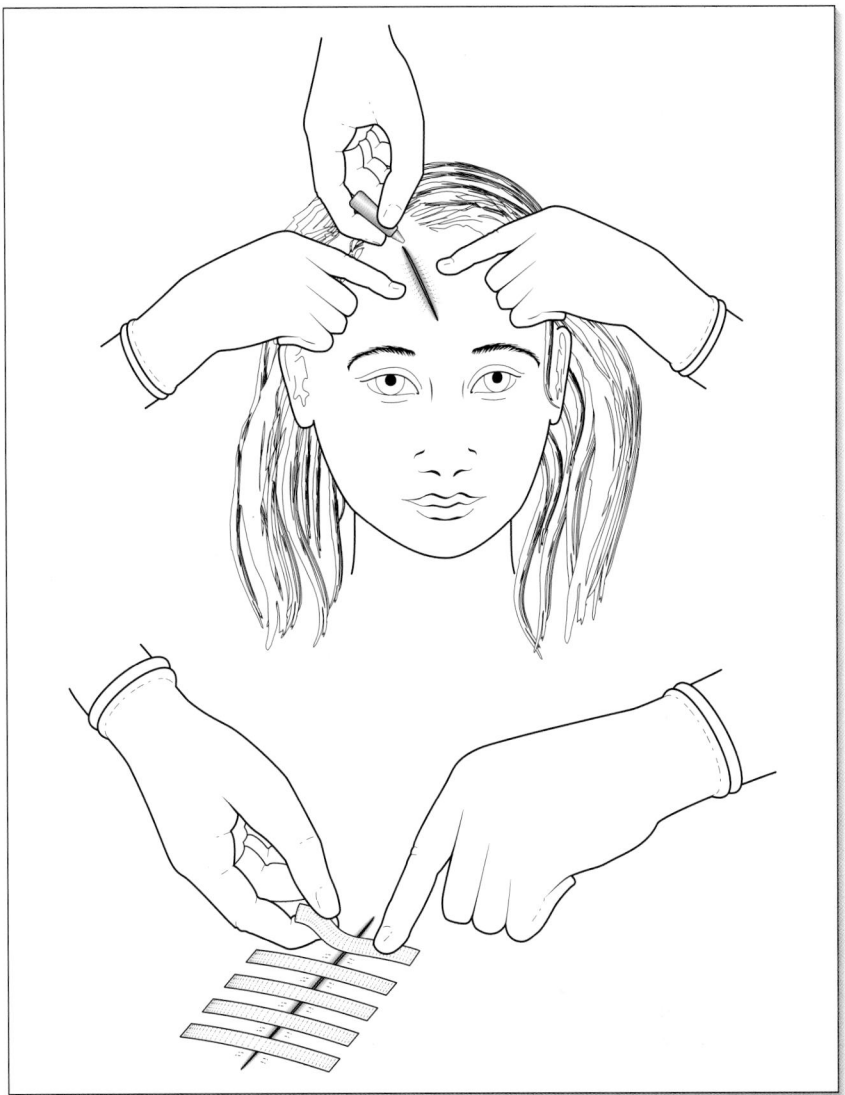

Fig. 3.10.2 Steristrips and glue are typically used for children in most simple split lacerations, thereby avoiding the use of needles. *(From an original drawing by Elaine Wheildon.)*

rates of infection with tapes and staples are lower than with conventional sutures [19].

Staples have the advantage of rapid insertion and wound closure, particularly for extensive wounds. They are applied using a staple gun and must be removed using the appropriate device, which may be a problem with follow-up arrangements.

From horsehair in World War II [20] to today's soluble monofilament plastics with prolonged tensile strength, necessity has seen the development of many different suture materials (Fig. 3.10.3) of different grades and using different types of needles. The ideal suture is monofilament, causes no tissue reaction, does not promote infection, is completely absorbed

and yet has a tensile strength and secure knots that last until tissue strength has equalled that of the suture. It should stretch to accommodate wound oedema, recoil to its original length and be inexpensive. However, as yet no such suture exists.

A key factor in choosing absorbable suture is the length of time over which it retains adequate strength. The inflammatory phase of healing lasts for 7 days. Catgut prolongs this phase and is removed by enzymatic action, whereas absorbable plastics simply hydrolyse. Braided sutures produce greater tissue reaction than monofilaments. Braided and catgut sutures should be avoided in contaminated wounds [21] as the interstices provide a

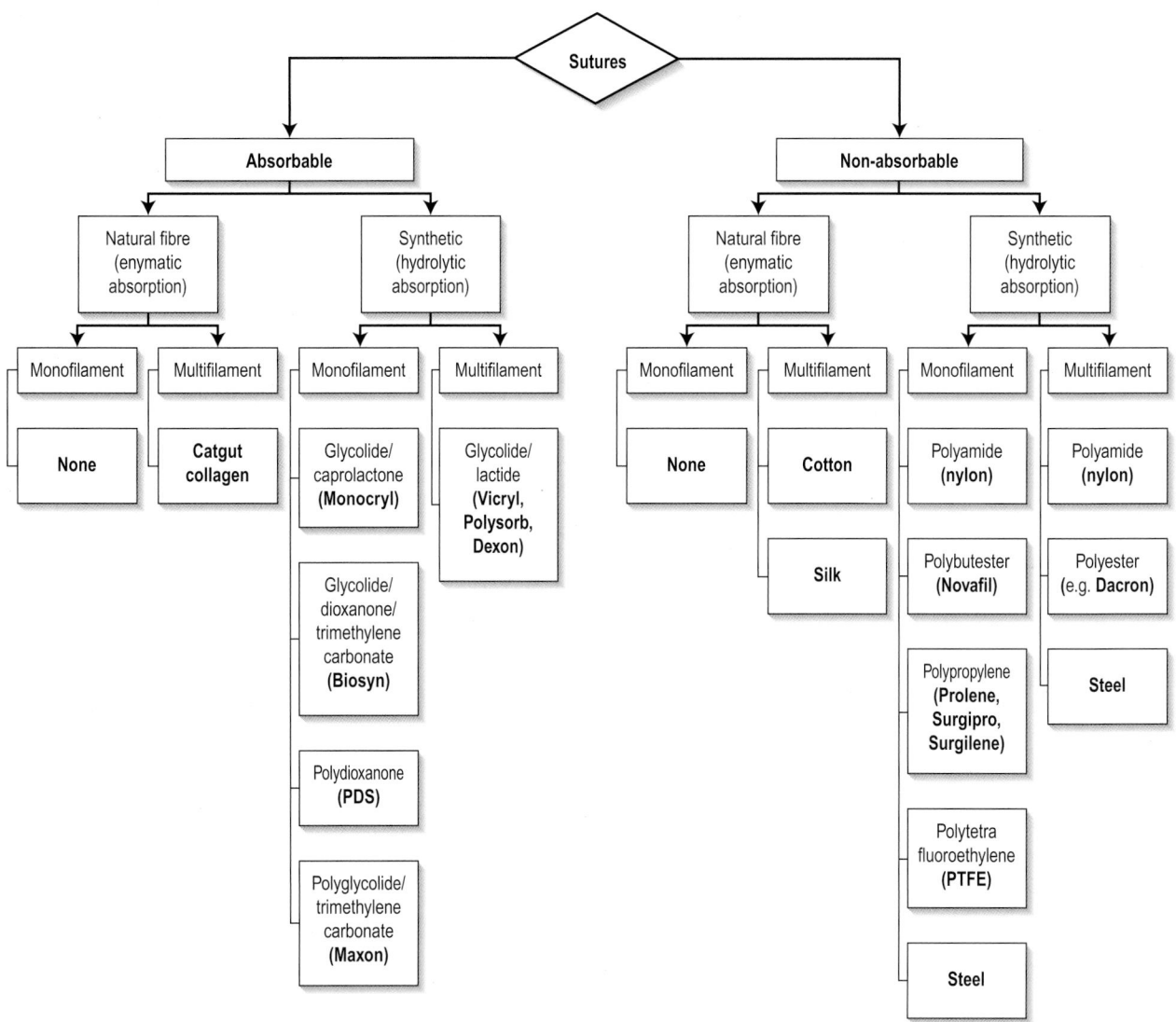

Fig. 3.10.3 A simple classification of suture types in current usage. *(Adapted from van Winkle W Jr, Hastings JC. Considerations in the choice of suture material for various tissues. Surg Gynecol Obstet 1972; 135:113–26.)*

haven for bacteria from phagocytes. Traditional absorbable sutures have included Vicryl and Dexon, both braided multifilament. Extensive studies have shown new monofilament absorbable sutures to have superior strength both initially and at 4 weeks: less interference with bacterial clearance; more secure knots requiring fewer throws; and lower drag forces through tissue, compared to the braided absorbable types [22].

Tissue adhesive agents such as Histoacryl (enbucrilate; B. Braun Surgical GmbH) – 'superglue' – have been developed particularly with the minor superficial paediatric wound in mind. The results can be excellent, provided good wound edge apposition is achieved prior to application of the glue on the surface (see Fig. 3.10.2).

In the future, biological tissue adhesive agents, such as fibrin sealant [20], for use in the wound may replace sutures as the means of wound closure. As yet these are experimental in sterile, surgically created wounds.

Needles

Early surgical needles had eyes like traditional sewing needles and caused tissue trauma as the bulk of folded-back thread and needle passed through the tissues. The first swaged needles were invented over 100 years ago and modern disposable swaged needles have largely replaced the reusable eyed needles. There are three parts to a needle: the swage, the body and the point (Fig. 3.10.4).

Advances in metallurgy have allowed the production of nickel stainless steel wire from which needles are cut. They may be straight or curved in arcs of varying degrees to produce portions of a circle, such as 90°, 135°, 180° and 225° parts. A compound curved needle comprises two different arcs, limiting the amount of supination necessary to pass it through tissue. Skin repair usually requires half-circle needles. The points of surgical needles may be tapered, cutting or a combination. Taper-point needles are generally round or oval bodied and are not suitable for skin as they are difficult to pass through the tightly bundled collagen fibres of the dermis. Their role is in repair of soft tissues, such as fascia, blood vessels and bowel, etc. Cutting needles

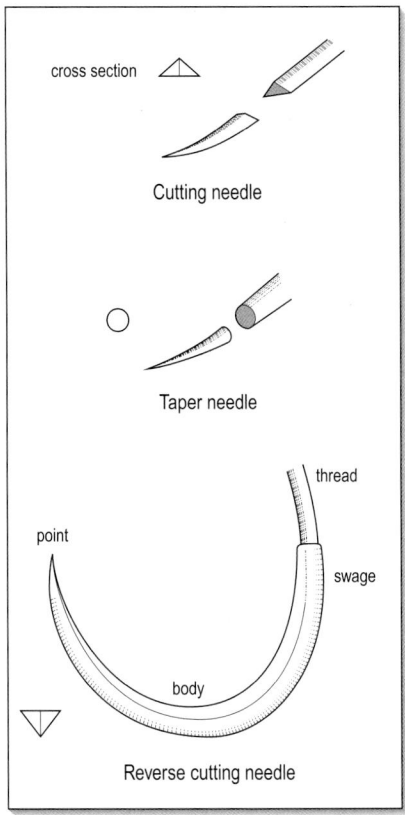

Fig. 3.10.4 Surgical needle characteristics and types. *(From an original drawing by Elaine Wheildon.)*

Table 3.10.5 Surgical instruments required for wound repair	
Contents of a typical simple suture tray	*Contents of a typical 'plastics' suture tray*
1 × Nelson Hegar needle holder 6.5 in	2 × Mosquito forceps curved
1 × Curved artery forceps	2 × Mosquito forceps straight
1 × Gillies dissectors	1 × Hegar needle holder 5.5 in
1 × McIndoe dissectors	1 × Gillies needle holder
2 × Small bowls	1 × Straight Mayo scissors
1 × Kidney dish autoplas 255 mm	1 × Curved Mayo scissors
1 × Fenestrated drape	1 × Vein straight scissors
1 × Huck towel	1 × Vein curved scissors
1 × McIndoe dissectors 1 × Adson dissectors	
1 × Gillies toothed dissectors	
2 × Skin hooks	
2 × Catspaw refractors	
1 × Bard–Parker handle no. 3	
1 × Bard–Parker handle no. 4	
1 × Vein hook Alcot	
1 × Rampley sponge holder	
3 × Gallipots	
1 × Kidney dish	
3 × Towel clips	
4 × Huck towel	

are for skin and have a triangular point with sharp cutting edges to facilitate tissue penetration. Conventional cutting needles have the apex of the triangle towards the concavity of the curved needle (see Fig. 3.10.4). Reverse cutting needles have the apex on the convexity of the needle. This style of needle and suture will not cut out when the needle is passed through tissue or once the knotted suture is resting against a block of tissue rather than a cut. Such needles are structurally stronger [23]. Combination cutting at the point and taper for the remainder of the body are for slightly denser tissues, such as tendon or aponeurosis. Needle holders are generally used with curved needles and straight needles are handheld. The risk of needle-stick injuries with handheld needles makes their use hazardous.

Basic suture technique

Prior to closure, prophylactic antibiotics (see Chapter 9.9) should be given intravenously if required. This ensures that any haematoma

that collects in the wound after or during closure will contain antibiotic.

Having prepared a sterile field with the contents of a suture tray (Table 3.10.5) laid out, the wound anaesthetized and cleaned and the sterile drapes placed around the wound, repair can begin. A very contaminated wound should be anaesthetized, lavaged and cleansed before re-preparing with antiseptic and draping for formal debridement, further lavage and repair.

One should choose the thinnest possible suture that will tolerate the tissue tensions and provide adequate strength. The needle holder must grasp the needle in the body, usually two-thirds of the length from the tip of the needle, rather than over the swage where the metal is relatively weak. Stretching the suture in the hands, supporting it at the needle swage, will remove its 'memory', making handling easier. The needle holder should be held in the palm of the hand and controlled with the index finger, using a supination/pronation action in the arc of the needle (Fig. 3.10.5). The placement of the first suture varies with the wound: in

a small linear wound, it may be convenient simply to suture from one end to the other. In longer wounds without good corresponding landmarks on either side, it is helpful to subdivide the wound serially, to ensure that one does not finish up with a 'dog-ear'. If an assistant is available, stretching the wound is helpful (Fig. 3.10.5). In more irregular complex wounds, it is helpful to approximate corresponding landmarks first: for example, the apex of a flap is best stitched first (Fig. 3.10.6).

After wound contraction has occurred, the wound edge has a natural tendency to inversion, resulting in a shallow crater. To prevent this, the edges must be everted at closure. To do this, the skin near the wound edge is depressed (Fig. 3.10.7) or lifted with a skin hook or forceps, so that the needle enters and exits perpendicularly to the skin in both running and interrupted sutures. The sutures so placed may be interrupted with separate tied closed loops or continuous loops passing through tissue, tied at either end. Vertical mattress sutures (Fig. 3.10.8) and horizontal mattress sutures (Fig. 3.10.9) are

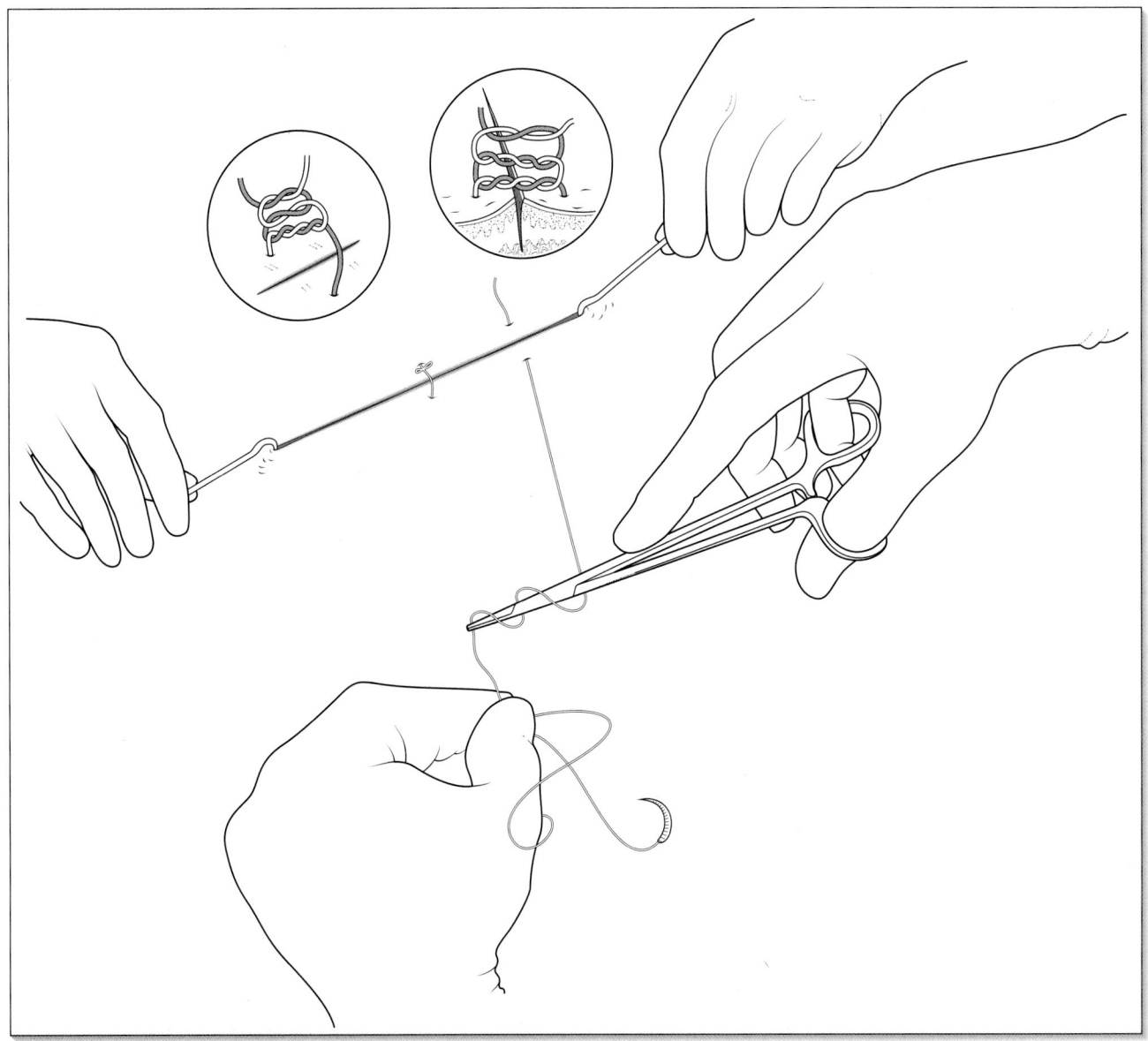

Fig. 3.10.5 The basic technique of how to hold a needle driver, put the wound on the stretch and suture a long wound in halves using surgical knots. For synthetic sutures, the reef knot with the third throw requires several twists, as illustrated, to prevent loosening. *(From an original drawing by Elaine Wheildon.)*

designed to evert wound edges that are difficult to maintain in eversion with simple sutures.

Knots are the weakest link in the suture, particularly for continuous sutures, where the failure of a knot will release the whole suture along the length of the wound. The knots may be tied with instruments or by hand. One must be careful, when using instrument ties, not to damage the suture by either crushing with the serrated jaws of a needle holder or tearing on the edges of the jaws. A reef knot with a snug third throw produces the best results for nylon or polypropylene. Synthetic monofilament sutures require several twists in the first and second throws to prevent unknotting (see Fig. 3.10.5). It is

important that the wound be closed without excessive tension on the sutures.

Interrupted sutures have the advantage of individual removal to allow drainage of an infected wound or, for cosmetic reasons, to limit the time a suture stays in while retaining some sutures for wound strength; however, there is a trade-off in the time it takes to close a wound using multiple knots. Sutures tied too tightly, exacerbated by oedema in the wound and from the trauma created by the needle's passage, will cause suture marks due to local ischaemia on the skin surface. An individual suture that is strangling tissue will continue to do so until it is cut. One way to avoid tissue

strangulation is to use a loop throw in an interrupted suture (Fig. 3.10.10) [16].

Studies have shown no increase in wound infection or reduction in wound strength with the use of continuous sutures [24], which may be placed rapidly in long linear wounds, distributing tension evenly. However, if one knot fails or the stitch is cut, they will loosen along the length of the wound. Continuous sutures may be percutaneous or intradermal (subcuticular). If intradermal, they should surface every 3 cm to facilitate removal [25].

Intradermal sutures are most appropriate for surgical wounds. Monofilament polypropylene has a very low surface coefficient of friction and

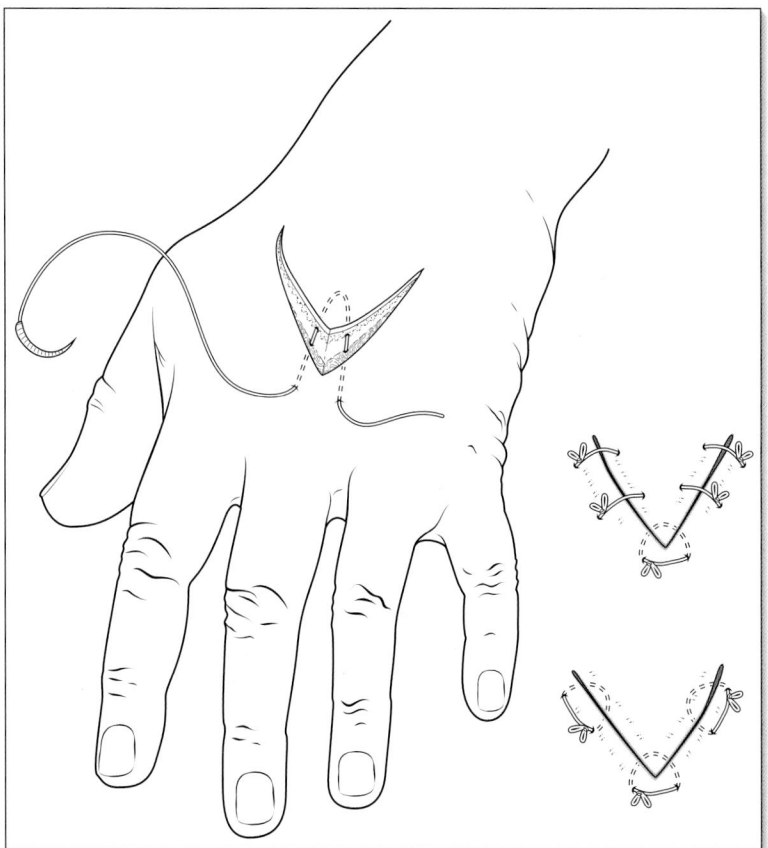

Fig. 3.10.6 Closure of a flap requires an initial suture of the apex, after which either simple or horizontal mattress sutures may be used. *(From an original drawing by Elaine Wheildon.)*

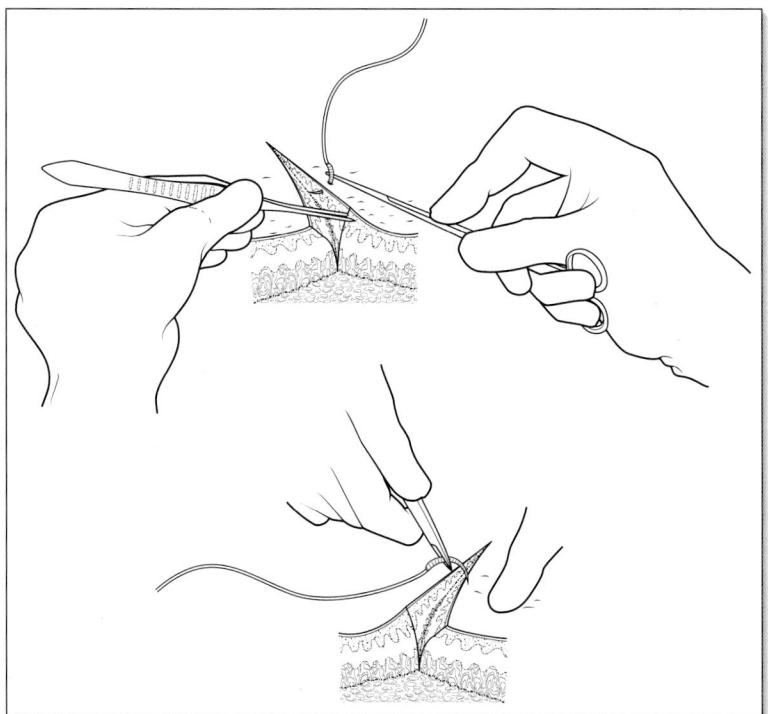

Fig. 3.10.7 Everting the wound edge using Gillies tissue forceps or digital pressure when placing a suture improves the cosmetic result. *(From an original drawing by Elaine Wheildon.)*

is thus easiest to remove in the setting of continuous percutaneous or subcuticular closure [26]. One should ensure that the suture glides easily through each segment and is not looped, otherwise removal may become very difficult. Recently, absorbable monofilament, such as glycolide caprolactone – Monocryl (Ethicon Inc.) – has supplanted polypropylene for continuous subcuticular suture as it does not have to be removed.

Historically, Halstead [27] considered it important to 'obliterate with the greatest care all of the dead spaces of a wound'. In 1974, it was demonstrated that suture closure of dead space increases the incidence of infection secondary to the foreign body (the suture) in the wound, thereby eliminating the benefits of dead space closure [28]. Some authors [16] stress the importance of using buried sutures to obtain wound edge eversion and dead space closure. Modern hydrolysable monofilament sutures allow this. The long-term maintenance of dermal edge apposition, either with or without deep sutures, is the key to obtaining the narrowest possible scar. Techniques have been developed to encourage this and to avoid leaving buried sutures, with their attendant risk of wound infection. To allow the removal of a deep space-obliterating suture without disrupting the wound some creative methods have been devised (Fig. 3.10.11) [29].

Wounds that slice obliquely through thick skin, such as on the back, can be trimmed with a scalpel blade perpendicular to the skin or sutured with a vertical mattress to prevent one bevelled edge sliding over the other. If necessary to prevent a wound edge step, adjustments in the height of the wound edges can be achieved by exiting the needle superficially on the high side and deeper on the low side, using either continuous or interrupted sutures [16].

Special sites and situations

Scalp lacerations may be closed using the 'hair braiding' technique [30,31], either on its own or combined with tissue adhesive. In this technique, four to five strands of hair from opposite sides are brought together, twisted once and tissue adhesive applied.

The face, particularly with dirty wounds, such as bites, requires early repair to achieve good cosmesis. Delay for up to 24 hours is acceptable, prior to definitive debridement and repair in the operating theatre, provided interim wound care is of a good standard. To enable adequate cleansing, local nerve blocks should be used.

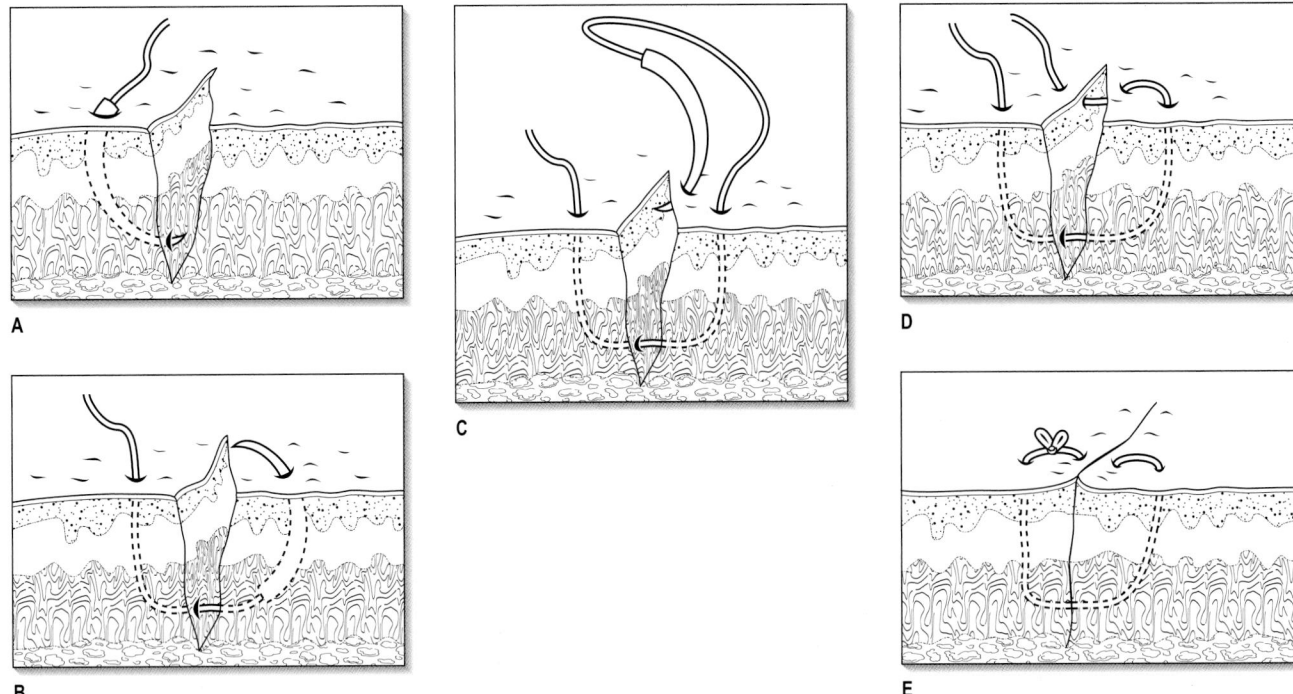

A

B

C

D

E

Fig. 3.10.8 **(A–E)** The vertical mattress suture technique is useful to evert wound edges with a natural tendency to roll inward despite correctly placed simple sutures. *(From an original drawing by Elaine Wheildon.)*

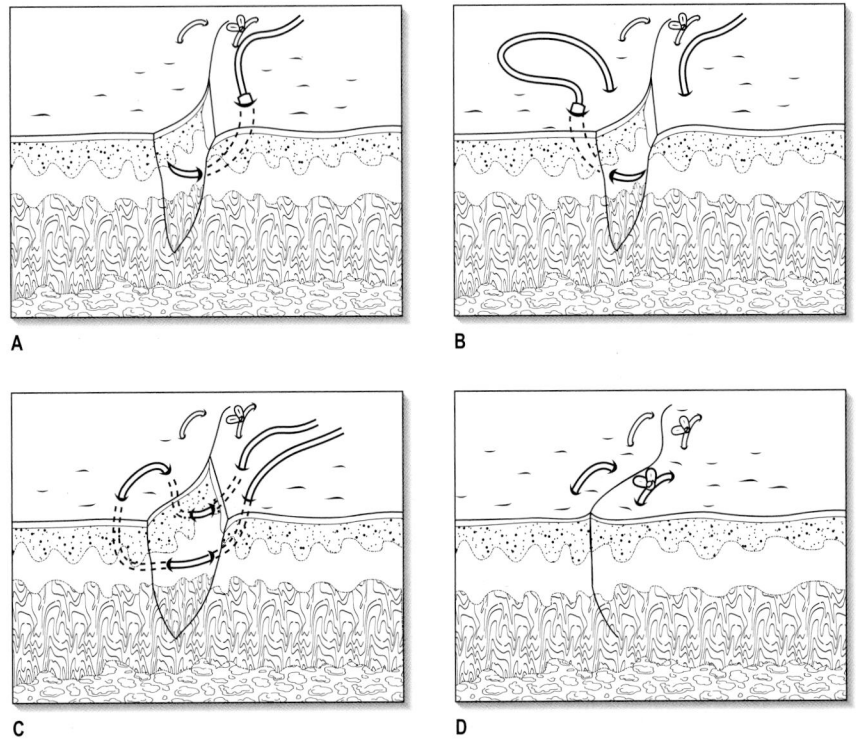

A

B

C

D

Fig. 3.10.9 **(A–D)** The horizontal mattress suture redistributes tension and everts wound edges. *(From an original drawing by Elaine Wheildon.)*

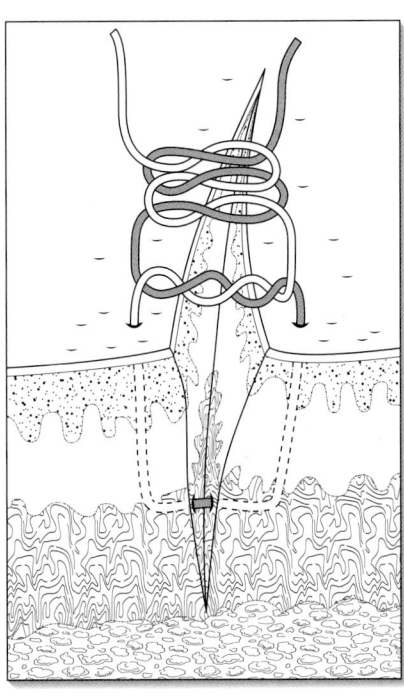

Fig. 3.10.10 The loop suture method of avoiding excessive tension on a stitch [16]. *(From an original drawing by Elaine Wheildon.)*

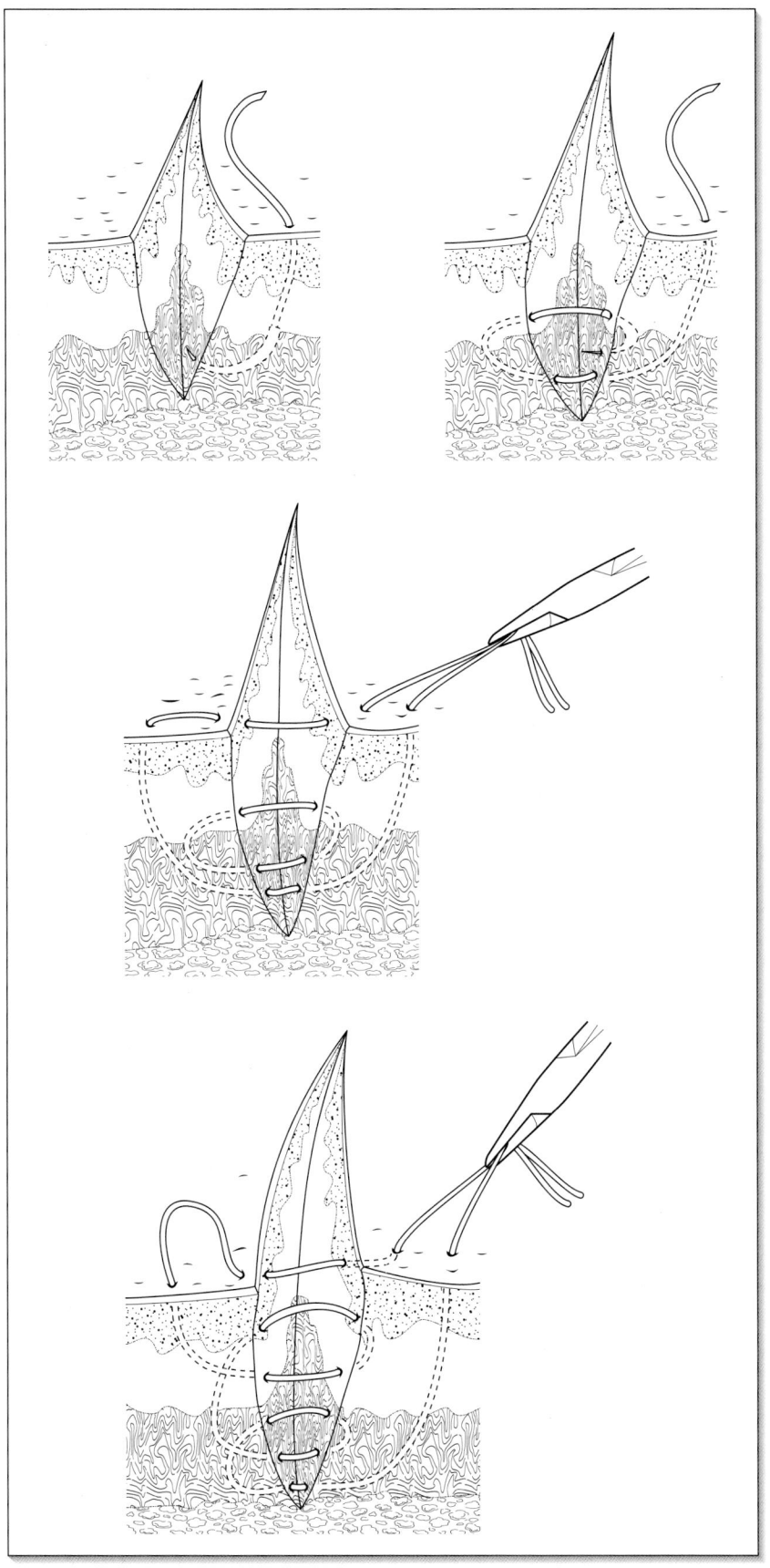

A field block is generally required for ears. Ear cartilage must be aligned and skin coverage achieved to prevent perichondritis.

Injuries involving the eyelid need a good examination of the underlying globe to exclude scleral and conjunctival lacerations; also, canaliculi may be torn. A lacerated canaliculus should be microsurgically repaired and stented within 24 hours. Accurate apposition of eyebrows and vermilion border is essential. Never shave an eyebrow.

Damaged facial muscle must be repaired in the interests of facial symmetry. In cheek injuries, the facial nerve and parotid duct must be checked for intactness. The nerves are generally deep in the cheek. Terminal repair of nerves medial to the midpupillary line is unnecessary.

Tattooing should be removed within 12 hours to avoid tissue fixation. Use a sterile brush and magnification and be meticulous. It is useful to have sterile toothbrushes available in the ED for this. After 12 hours, a formal dermabrasion and/or debridement may be needed.

Complications of facial wounds are numerous and provide some special problems (Table 3.10.6).

Fig. 3.10.11 A deep closure method utilizing a variable number of loops, adapted from a Mayo Clinic stitch [29]. *(From an original drawing by Elaine Wheildon.)*

Table 3.10.6	Complications of facial wounds
Complications	*Notes*
Infection with the brain	Potentially fatal owing to the valveless venous communication
AV fistulae	Due to profuse vascularity – uncommon
Scarring	Producing facial asymmetry and cosmetic implications
Deformity	Due to unrecognized fractures, such as of the nose or malar bone
Facial palsy	Due to damaged facial nerves
Epiphora damage	With tissue loss or scarring everting the lower lid, or canaliculus
Salivary fistula	After disruption of the parotid duct
Drooling	With tissue loss, scar contracture or local nerve damage
Corneal exposure	With tissue loss, scar contracture or local nerve damage

Special suture techniques

Techniques for relieving the tension in a wound include limited undermining and the use of horizontal mattress sutures (see Fig. 3.10.9). Very rarely should skin flaps be raised in acute trauma. These may be advancement (e.g. V–Y advancement), rotation or transposition in design. It is usually better to apply a split skin graft to heal the wound primarily and perform later scar revision or reconstruction. In some settings, V–Y flaps can be advanced or retreated, depending on the direction of tension (Fig. 3.10.12).

The 'dog-ear'

The term 'dog-ear' refers to a conical pucker of redundant skin that may collect at the end of a wound towards the end of closure (Fig. 3.10.13), particularly in wounds with an elliptical area of skin defect. In order to avoid a 'dog-ear', the wound should be sutured in halves, placing each new stitch between the previous ones (see Fig. 3.10.5). There are several ways to remove a dog-ear [32]:

- The direct overlap excision technique involves drawing the redundant skin from one side across the wound and excising along the line of the wound. Any remaining redundant skin is drawn across the wound from the other side and excised along the line of the wound (Fig. 3.10.13).

- Unilateral dog-ears are best removed by elevating the redundant skin with a skin hook in the centre, followed by incising along the edge of the fold and then allowing the created flap to fall back along the line of the sutures, where it is trimmed off. This results in a J-shaped repair (Fig. 3.10.13).
- An elliptical excision of the dog-ear in line with the closure can excise the defect (Fig. 3.10.13), but this also lengthens the wound.
- In very large dog-ears, a V–Y excision and closure will provide good closure.
- Thick dog-ears that are aligned perpendicularly to the original closure can be excised and closed in a T repair (Fig. 3.10.13).

Wound drainage

Fluid trapped within the closed wound predisposes to infection by:

- progressive loss of opsonins
- interfering with access of phagocytes to bacteria
- providing a nutrient medium for bacterial growth
- putting pressure on adjacent vasculature, compromising blood supply.

Fluid also prevents the apposition of healing tissues. The build-up of fluid can be prevented by immobilization, preventing shearing forces between tissue planes, firm but not tight dressings and drainage. The indications for drainage are:

- dead-space elimination to prevent fluid accumulation (with an active suction drain or a compressive dressing with a passive drain)
- removal of established fluid collections.

Suction drains are superior to passive drains which rely on gravity; however, blockage of drain holes and of the drain tube lumen can be a problem. There are many commercial closed suction systems on the market. A simple suction drain can be constructed from a 'butterfly' cannula and a vacuum blood specimen tube (Fig. 3.10.14) [7] by cutting off the syringe adapter and fenestrating the tubing prior to placement through a stab incision into the wound. The vacuum tube can be changed as necessary. Clamp the tube before changing it to prevent the ingress of contaminants into the wound via the drain. Patients with drains will need regular review, either in the ED or by the local doctor. Drains are generally removed at 48 hours unless they are draining copiously.

Dressings

It has long been recognized that the dressing and subsequent wound care are as important as the operative technique [33]. The depths of the wound must be moist for healing, but the skin surface must not become macerated.

The appropriate style of dressing for abrasions is still debated. The 'moist' versus 'dry' debate revolves around saline packs, sterile paraffin, solugel, seaweed preparations,

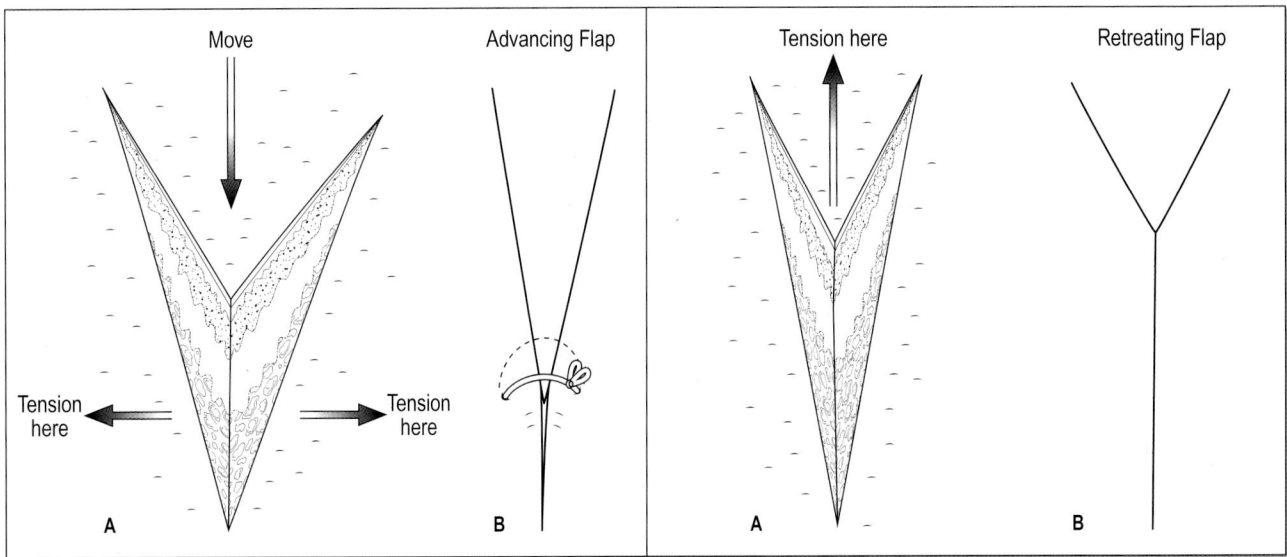

Fig. 3.10.12 The V–Y flap advancement or retreat is useful to redistribute and reduce tension across a wound. *(From an original drawing by Elaine Wheildon.)*

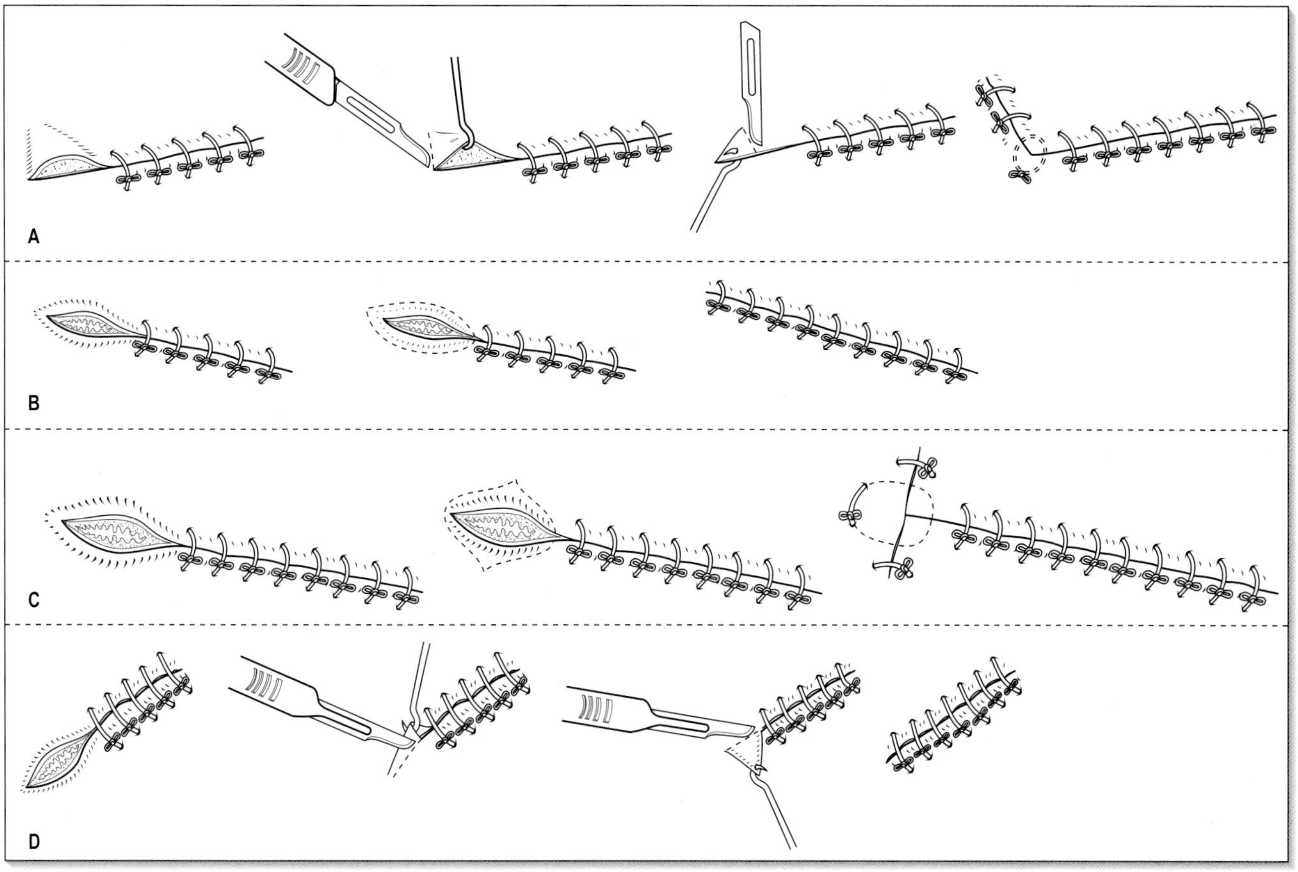

Fig. 3.10.13 Various methods of dealing with a dog-ear. (**A**) Hockey-stick or back-cut technique; (**B**) double elliptical incision technique; (**C**) perpendicular elliptical T-repair technique; (**D**) direct overlap excision technique. *(From an original drawing by Elaine Wheildon.)*

occlusive plastic film dressings and various foam preparations.

In covering the sutured wound, the dressing aims to keep the primarily apposed skin edges dry, wicking away any ooze, haemorrhage or exudate. It should only be changed if its capacity to absorb fluid is exceeded and, ideally, it should stay on until the time for suture removal. Where this is not possible, the wound may be bathed or showered 24 hours after closure, provided it is thoroughly dabbed dry and not immersed and soaked in water. In the case of scalp wounds, this allows showering and hair washing and avoids the problem of fixing a dressing to hairy skin. Wounds that are contaminated and at high risk of infection need review and re-dressing at 48 hours.

Immobilization

Wounds that traverse joints or which occur on highly mobile skin, such as in the hand, require immobilization. Splinting with plaster slabs is a cheap, traditional and reliable method. Apart

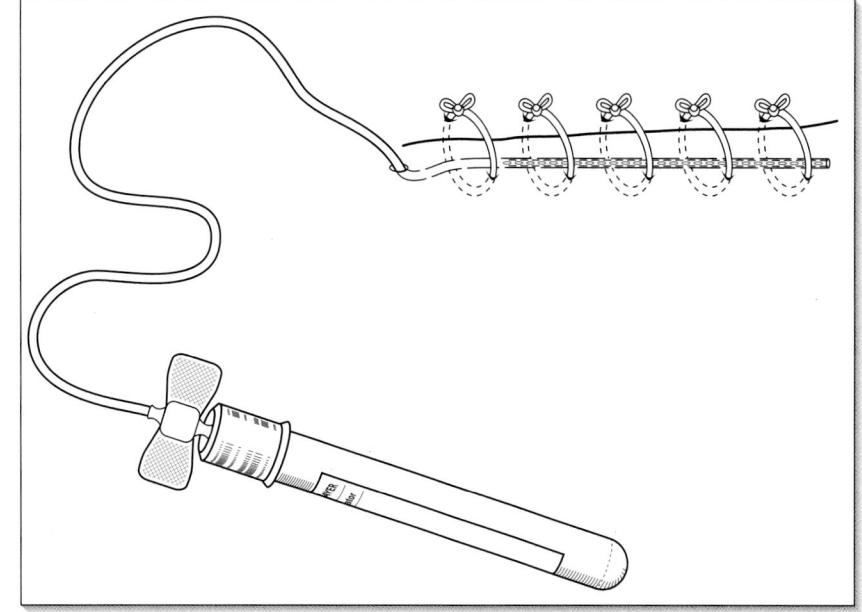

Fig. 3.10.14 A simple suction drain. *(From an original drawing by Elaine Wheildon.)*

Table 3.10.7 Guide to time for removal of sutures	
Location	*Days to removal*
Scalp	6–8
Face (incl. ear)	4–5
Chest/abdomen	8–10
Back	12–14
Arm/leg*	8–10
Hand*	8–10
Fingertip	10–12
Foot	12–14

*Add 2–3 days for lacerations crossing extensor surfaces of joints and if early motion is required for rehabilitation, e.g. post-flexor tendon repair. After Gusman D. Wound closure and special suture techniques. J Am Podiatr Med Assoc 1995; 85:2–10.

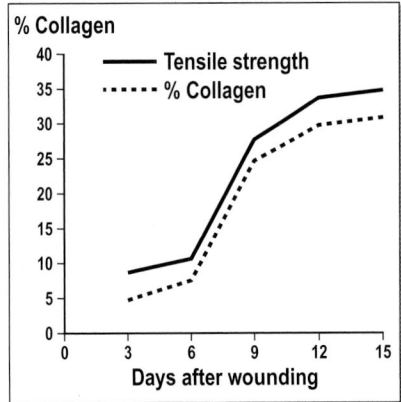

Fig. 3.10.15 The relationship between tensile strength and collagen deposition. *(From an original drawing by Elaine Wheildon.)*

Disposal/removal

Despite an apparently good cosmetic result at the time of suture removal (5–14 days) (Table 3.10.7), in head and neck wounds, there is evidence of a poor correlation with wound appearance 6–9 months later [34]. The degree to which different factors, such as wounding mechanism, wound repair technique and patient host factors, have a role remains to be determined. Keloid or hypertrophic scarring is more common in negroid and Asian races and in wounds located over the deltoid muscle or sternum.

All percutaneous stitches will cause needle marks if left *in situ* longer than 8 days, as epithelium migrates down the needle track. Removal too early predisposes to wound dehiscence (Fig. 3.10.15), however, the wound may be supported by skin tapes. If tapes were the primary method of closure they may be left on for at least 10 days or until they fall off, provided the skin is not sensitive to the adhesive, as evidenced by erythema or bulla formation.

Suture removal technique is also important. To avoid tissue trauma and additional scarring, stitches should be cut at the knots with iris scissors after gentle washing with saline to remove the eschar and the suture gently pulled through. So-called suture scissors are actually too big for the task.

Inelastic paper tape can be used to support a wound and help stop the scar from stretching until such time as the collagen is near maturation, beyond 3 months. Paper tape is also useful in the setting of keloid scarring in an attempt to provide pressure and encourage remodelling. In some cases, silicone gel pads and even pressure garments are required to control keloid scarring.

If the wound suppurates then the sutures will need to be removed, either partly or completely, to allow the egress of pus.

Likely developments over the next 5 to 10 years

There is a lot of work being done on knotless wound closure devices which will speed up suturing by eliminating the need for knot tying.

With surgical wounds, there are new developments with absorbable staples and fast setting cyanoacrylate.

Controversies

- Drainage will remove fluid and haematoma that potentiate infection, but the drain itself may predispose to infection. This is less the case with suction drains.
- Interrupted dermal sutures will close dead space, thereby reducing haematoma and wound infection, but may lead to infection in contaminated wounds. Their major role

is to reduce skin tension and they should be used in large clean wounds.
- The degree of debridement required for a dirty wound has moved from radical to conservative but meticulous, with an emphasis on preservation of viable skin to improve cosmesis.
- Povidone–iodine packs, which are tissue toxic, are used by some surgeons in the setting of open wounds over compound fractures while the patient awaits transfer to the operating theatre for definitive repair.
- Opinions as to the appropriate dressings for abrasions range from moist, such as plastic film, to dry, such as mercurochrome paint and dry gauze.

References

[1] Clark B, Cassell E, Ashby K, et al. Hazard, edn no. 52, Spring. Victorian Injury Surveillance and Applied Research System; 2002.
[2] Jorgensen LN, Kallenhave F, Christensen E, Siana JE. Less collagen production in smokers. Surgery 1998;123:450–5.
[3] Ellis H. Hazards from surgical gloves. Ann Roy Coll Surg Engl 1997;79:161–3.
[4] Howell JM, Morgan JA. Scalp laceration repair without prior hair removal. Am J Emerg Med 1988;6:7.
[5] Dire DJ, Welch AP. A comparison of wound irrigation solution used in the Emergency Department. Ann Emerg Med 1996;19:704.
[6] Bansal BC, Weike RA, Perkins SD, Abramo TJ. Tap water irrigation of lacerations. Am J Emerg Med 2002;20:469.
[7] Rodeheaver GT, Pettry D, Thacker JG, et al. Wound cleansing by high pressure irrigation. Surg Gynecol Obstetr 1975;141:357–62.
[8] Brown LL. Evaluation of wound irrigation by pulsatile jet and conventional methods. Ann Surg 1978;187:170.
[9] Gfeller RW, Crow DT. The emergency care of traumatic wounds: current recommendations. Vet Clin N Am 1994;24:1249–74.
[10] Wheeler CB, Rodeheaver GT, Tracker JG, et al. Side-effects of high pressure irrigation. Surg Gynecol Obstet 1976;143:775–8.
[11] Lammers R. Foreign bodies in wounds. In: Singer AJ, Hollander JE, editors. Lacerations and acute wounds: an evidence-based guide. Philadelphia: FA Davis, 2003, p. 147.
[12] Wyn T, Jones J, McNinch D, et al. Bedside fluoroscopy for the detection of foreign bodies. Acad Emerg Med 1995;2:979–82.
[13] Fackler MI, Breteau JP, Courbil CJ, et al. Open wound drainage versus wound excision in treating the modern assault rifle wound. Surgery 1989;105:576–84.
[14] Spicer WJ, Garland S, Christiansen K, et al. Skin and soft tissue infection: therapeutic guidelines antibiotic version 13. Melbourne: Therapeutic Guidelines Limited; 2006. 230–232.
[15] National Health and Medical Research Council. The Australian Immunisation Handbook, 9th ed. Canberra: NHMRC; 2008.
[16] Moy RL, Lee A, Zalka A. Commonly used suturing techniques in skin surgery. Am Fam Phys 1991;44:1625–34.
[17] Moy RL, Quan MB. An evaluation of wound closure tapes. J Dermatol Surg Oncol 1990;16:721–3.
[18] Panek P, Prusak MP, Bolt D. Potentiation of wound infection by adhesive adjuncts. Am Surg 1972;38:343–5.
[19] Edlich RF, Becker DG, Thacker JG, Rodeheaver GT. Scientific basis for selecting staple and tape skin closures. Clin Plast Surg 1990;17:571–8.
[20] Spotnitz WD, Falstrom MA, Rodeheaver GT. The role of sutures and fibrin sealant in wound healing. Surg Clin N Am 1997;77:651–69.

[21] Van Winkle W Jr., Hastings. JC. Considerations in the choice of suture material for various tissues. Surg Gynecol Obstet 1972;135:113–26.

[22] Rodeheaver GT, Beltran KA, Green CW, et al. Biomechanical and clinical performance of a new synthetic monofilament absorbable suture. J Long-Term Effects Med Implants 1996;6:181–98.

[23] Bendel LP, Trozzo LP. Tensile and bend relationships of several surgical needle materials. J Appl Biomat 1993;4:161–7.

[24] Mclean NR, Fyfe AH, Flint EF, et al. Comparison of skin closure using continuous and interrupted nylon sutures. Br J Surg 1980;67:633–5.

[25] Drake DB, Gear AL, Mazzarese PM, et al. Search for a scientific basis for continuous suture closure: a 30 year odyssey. J Emerg Med 1997;15:495–504.

[26] Pham S, Rodeheaver GT, Dang MC, et al. Ease of continuous dermal suture removal. J Emerg Med 1990;8:539–43.

[27] Halstead WS. The treatment of wounds with especial reference to the value of blood clot in the management of dead spaces. Bull Johns Hopkins Hosp 1990–91;2:255.

[28] De Holl D. Potentiation of infection by suture closure of dead space. Am J Surg 1974;127:716–20.

[29] Arnold PG. Space obliterating skin suture. Plast Reconstruct Surg 1997;100:1506–8.

[30] Aoki N, Oikawa A, Sakai T. Hair braiding closure for superficial wounds. Surg Neurol 1996;46:150.

[31] Hock M, Ooi SBS, Saw SM, Lim SHA. randomised controlled trial comparing the hair apposition technique with tissue glue to standard suturing in scalp lacerations (HAT) study. Ann Emerg Med 2002;40:19.

[32] Gusman D. Wound closure and special suture techniques. J Am Podiatr Med Assoc 1995;85:2–10.

[33] Ivy RH, et al. Manual of standard practice of plastic and maxillofacial surgery. Philadelphia: WB Saunders; 1943.

[34] Hollander JE, Blasko B. Poor correlation of short and long-term cosmetic appearance of lacerations. Acad Emerg Med 1995;2:983–7.

3.11 Burns

Tim Gray • Gerard O'Reilly • Biswadev Mitra

ESSENTIALS

1 Effective triage and advances in the treatment of severely burned patients, including fluid resuscitation, control of sepsis, early excision and use of skin substitutes have made previously lethal burns survivable.

2 Signs of impending or developed laryngeal oedema should prompt early intubation.

3 Burn resuscitation formulae should be considered as a guide only.

4 Meta-analysis of previous studies, suggests that resuscitation with colloid, as opposed to crystalloid, does not improve survival.

5 Extensive or complicated burns should be managed in a specialized burns unit.

6 Chemical burns, after decontamination and specific antidotes, are treated in a similar fashion to thermal burns.

Introduction

Advances in burn management over the last three decades have significantly reduced mortality and improved quality of life for victims. Appropriate fluid resuscitation, early debridement and the appropriate use of antibiotics have resulted in hypovolaemia and sepsis no longer being the major contributors to mortality in burns. Multiorgan failure is the most likely event leading to death, whereas age, burn surface area and inhalational injury are the major contributors to a poor outcome [1,3].

Pathophysiology

The skin is the largest organ of the body. Its most important functions are:

- to act as a vapour barrier to prevent water loss from the body

- to present the body's major barrier against infection
- temperature regulation.

The skin consists of two main layers. The epidermis is stratified squamous epithelium that acts as the major barrier to passive water loss from the body. The dermis contains the adnexal structures, namely sweat glands, hair follicles and sebaceous glands, as well as pain and pressure receptors and the cutaneous blood vessels, which play a major role in temperature regulation by controlling radiant heat loss (Fig. 3.11.1).

The adnexae are embryologic down-growths of the epidermis. Following burn injury, the epithelial cells of these structures undergo metaplastic change to stratified squamous epithelium, proliferate and gradually cover the wound. Thus, burns that partially or completely spare these structures will usually heal without

scarring. Deeper burns involve greater loss of adnexal cells, resulting in poorer epithelial coverage and hence greater scarring.

Burned skin undergoes coagulative necrosis with three distinct zones of injury. A central zone of coagulation, in which irreversible cell death occurs, is surrounded by a zone of stasis, in which vasoconstriction and intravascular coagulation contribute to local ischaemia. A zone of hyperaemia surrounds the wound. In the early stages of the burn, evolution of these zones results in a progressive deepening of the wound, which may be minimized by appropriate early treatment [4,5].

Classification

Burns may be classified according to their depth as superficial, partial thickness or full thickness.

Superficial burns involve only the epidermis. Pain and swelling usually subside within 48 hours and the superficial epidermis peels off within a few days. Healing occurs by proliferation of undamaged cells of the germinal layer of the epidermis and is usually complete within 7 days.

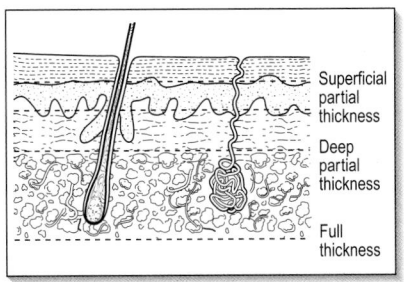

Fig. 3.11.1 Diagram of skin layers.

Partial thickness burns involve destruction of the epidermis and superficial dermis. They are characterized by blister formation and may be further classified into superficial and deep partial thickness. Healing is dependent on the amount of intact epithelium in the adnexae.

Superficial partial thickness burns are typically bright red with a moist surface, are exquisitely sensitive to stimulus and heal in 2–3 weeks, generally with minimal scarring. Deep partial-thickness burns are typically dark red or yellow-white and take longer than 3 weeks to heal, as few epithelial elements survive. Hypertrophic scarring usually occurs.

Full-thickness burns involve the epidermis and dermis, including the epidermal appendages. Clinically, they appear charred or pearly white in appearance and are usually insensate. Because loss of epidermal adnexae is complete, full-thickness burns only heal by scarring or skin grafting.

THERMAL BURNS

Presentation

History

History may be obtained from the patient, from witnesses and from fire or ambulance personnel. Details of the nature of the injury are important, especially the nature of the burning materials, duration of exposure, whether the patient was trapped in an enclosed space or lost consciousness or whether there was an associated fall, vehicular accident or blast injury.

A history of altered consciousness or confinement in a burning environment suggests the likelihood of carbon-monoxide poisoning. Past medical history, current medications, allergies and tetanus status should also be obtained.

Examination

The initial examination should be directed to identifying signs suggestive of airway burns as well as the presence of other injuries. Early haemodynamic compromise is rarely due to burn injury alone and should prompt a search for other causes.

Facial and oral burns, singed nasal hairs, carbonaceous sputum, tachypnoea and wheeze are clinical signs suggesting an increased risk of inhalation injury; however, in the absence of laryngeal oedema, inhalation injury may not become clinically evident for 12–24 hours [6,7].

Signs of laryngeal oedema, namely hoarseness, brassy cough or stridor, indicate the need for early endotracheal intubation as oedema formation may rapidly distort the anatomy, necessitating a surgical airway.

The adequacy of peripheral circulation should be assessed, particularly in the setting of circumferential limb burns.

Evaluation of burn area

The extent and depth of the burn must be assessed as accurately as possible. Representation of the burn area diagrammatically on a body chart aids assessment. The simplest method is the 'Rule of nines' where the adult body is divided into anatomical regions that represent 9% of the total body surface area.

In infants and young children, the Lund and Browder chart is used to correct for proportional variation at different ages: for instance, an infant's head is approximately 18% of the total body surface area, compared to 9% in an adult (Fig. 3.11.2).

Management

Pre-hospital

Pre-hospital care of the burned patient should be directed at stopping the burning process, assessing and stabilizing the airway, breathing and circulation and rapidly transferring the patient to hospital. Where possible, major burns should be triaged to a burn centre (Table 3.11.1) [8].

En route to hospital, recent burns should be covered with a clean dressing (e.g. Melolin), soaked in cool water or tea-tree/hydrogel dressing so as to limit the depth of burn by dissipation of heat. After this cooling process, or if it is not required, the burns can be covered with a clean dry dressing. Cling wrap is used for interhospital transfers. Prolonged exposure to cool water should be avoided and ice should never be applied directly to the wound as it may increase the depth of burn.

The patient should be kept warm, supplemental oxygen administered and, where prolonged transport times are anticipated, intravenous fluid therapy should be instituted.

Emergency department

Initial management

Supplemental oxygen should be administered and cardiac and oxygen saturation monitoring instituted.

Stabilization of the airway and treatment of life-threatening injuries take priority over management of the burn wound itself. Burns to the face, neck and airways result in massive fluid shifts from the circulating plasma into the interstitial space causing oedema and potentially resulting in rapid upper airway obstruction. Immediate intubation is indicated in apnoea or obstruction. Other indications for immediate intubation are the same as for any critically injured patients, including actual or impending cardiac arrest, impending respiratory failure and a decreased level of consciousness with inability to protect the airway.

Early intubation is indicated in burns to the face and neck where it is anticipated that oedema will make intubation difficult in the future or to facilitate initial pain and operative management. The nasal route is preferable in the presence of friable burnt oral tissue but requires a spontaneously breathing patient. The choice of an inducing agent is varied with thiopentone or propofol appropriate in haemodynamically stable patients. Succinylcholine may be used in the first 24 hours but, in later periods, has been associated with catastrophic potassium release leading to possible cardiac arrest and is best avoided [9]. Non-depolarizing muscle relaxants are preferred; however, the dose required may increase to 3–5 times normal. Uncut endotracheal tubes should be used and meticulously secured [10].

Airway patency alone does not guarantee adequate ventilation. Fumes and minute particles produced by the fire may cause bronchospasm, which can be treated by inhaled bronchodilators. Smoke particles also cause inflammation, hypersecretion and mucosal sloughing resulting in airway obstruction and atelectasis. Carbon monoxide (CO) poisoning should be suspected in anyone with a history of smoke exposure, an extended length of time in the fire or burns in an enclosed space. The features of CO poisoning include tachypnoea, tachycardia, vomiting, confusion and irritability to reduced conscious states and syncope. Oxygen saturation measured by pulse oximetry is not helpful in diagnosing CO toxicity, although recently developed oximetry devices display carboxyhaemoglobin levels. Blood

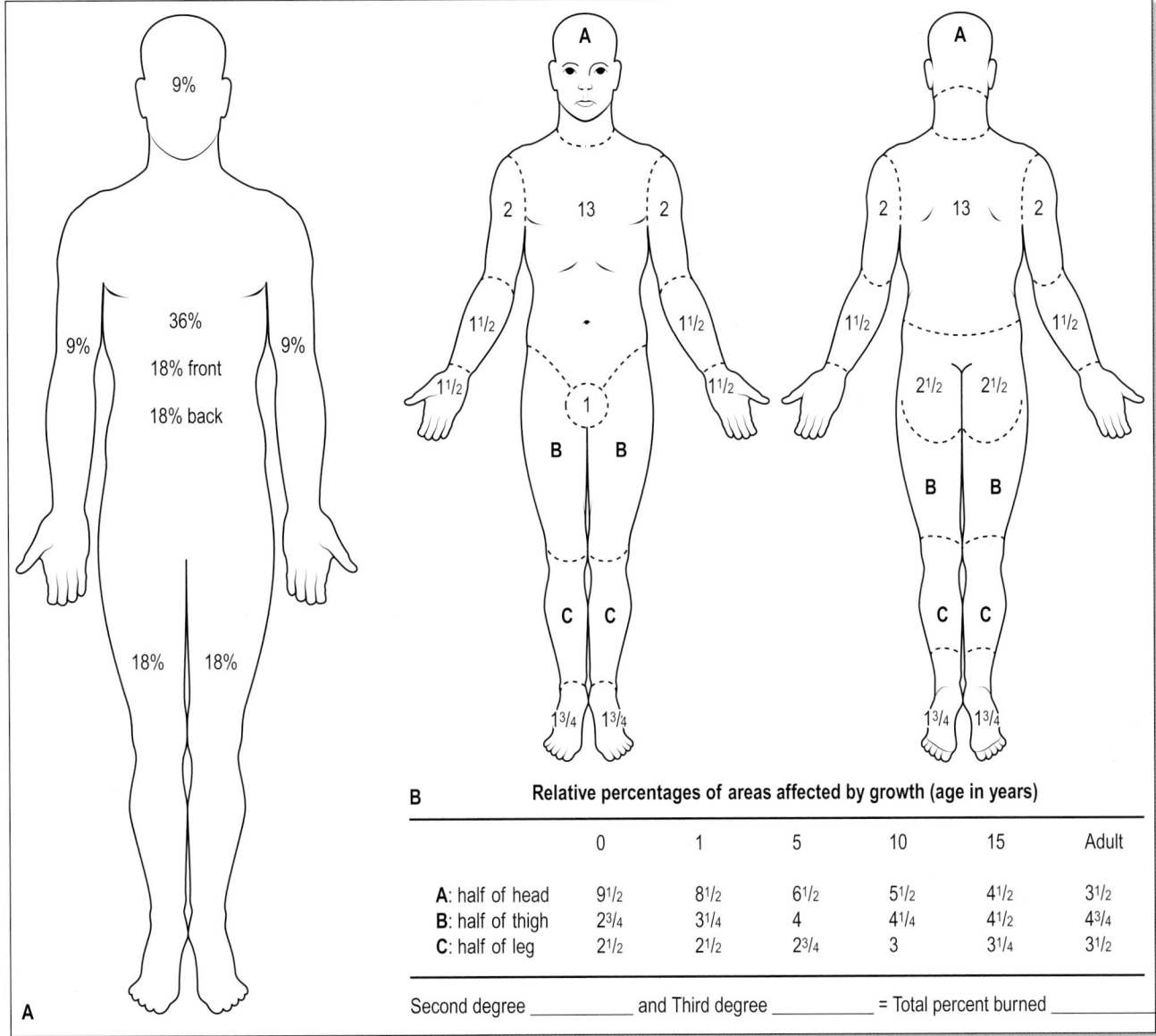

Relative percentages of areas affected by growth (age in years)

	0	1	5	10	15	Adult
A: half of head	$9\frac{1}{2}$	$8\frac{1}{2}$	$6\frac{1}{2}$	$5\frac{1}{2}$	$4\frac{1}{2}$	$3\frac{1}{2}$
B: half of thigh	$2\frac{3}{4}$	$3\frac{1}{4}$	4	$4\frac{1}{4}$	$4\frac{1}{2}$	$4\frac{3}{4}$
C: half of leg	$2\frac{1}{2}$	$2\frac{1}{2}$	$2\frac{3}{4}$	3	$3\frac{1}{4}$	$3\frac{1}{2}$

Second degree _____ and Third degree _____ = Total percent burned _____

Fig. 3.11.2 (A) 'Rule of nines' diagram. (B) Lund and Browder chart.

Table 3.11.1 Patients who fulfil the following criteria should be considered for transfer to a specialist burns unit

Partial-thickness burns >20% in all age groups, or >10% in the under 10 and over 50 age groups

Full-thickness burns >5% in any age group

Burns involving face, eyes, ears, hands, feet, genitalia, perineum or a major joint

Inhalation burns

Electrical burns, including lightning injury

Burns associated with other significant injuries

Smaller burns in patients with pre-existing disease that could complicate management

gases and carboxyhaemoglobin levels aid in diagnosis. An admission carboxyhaemoglobin level >15% suggests significant smoke inhalation [4]. The affinity of CO for haemoglobin is substantially more than oxygen with a slow dissociation half-life of 3–4 hours. Administration of high concentrations of O_2 can decrease the dissociation half-life to 50 minutes.

Cyanide poisoning can result from thermal decomposition of natural fibres, such as wool and silk, and manifests as persistent lactic acidosis with a high anion gap. Commercially available cyanide antidote kits contain amyl nitrite vials, sodium nitrite and sodium thiosulphate. The amyl nitrite is administered via

inhalation and is intended for use when intravenous access may not be available. Sodium nitrite is given intravenously. The second stage of antidote therapy is administration of sodium thiosulphate, which acts synergistically to counteract cyanide formation [11,12].

Ventilation difficulties through parenchymal damage from burns share a similar pathophysiology to the development of acute respiratory distress syndrome (ARDS). The onset is generally slow and may be an issue in delayed presentations. An exception is blast injury, which can cause lung contusions and alveolar trauma leading to ARDS. The most effective initial treatment is the application of positive end expiration pressure (PEEP). The mechanism by which PEEP improves oxygenation is linked to the increase in residual functional capacity (RFC) obtained both by increasing the volume of partially collapsed alveoli and by reopening totally collapsed alveoli.

Fluid Resuscitation [7]

Intravenous fluid resuscitation with crystalloid solution as outlined below should be started in any patient with burns of more than 20% total body surface area (TBSA). There are many formulae for the fluid resuscitation of burns victims. Although considerable debate continues, the general principles of fluid resuscitation are:

- In the first 24 hours, isotonic salt solution should be used to replace the large volumes lost to tissue oedema, with about half the fluid given in the first 8 hours after injury, coincident with the period of most rapid oedema formation.
- The administration of colloid is unnecessary for patients with burns of less than 40% TBSA and during the first 8 hours. Meta-analysis of previous studies suggests that resuscitation with colloid does not result in improved survival [13].
- Fluid resuscitation formulae are a guide only and the patient's haemodynamic status must be monitored by cardiovascular parameters and hourly urine volume measurement. Increased resuscitation fluid volume (per kg) is required in children weighing less than 30 kg, in high-voltage electrical injuries, if resuscitation is delayed and in the presence of inhalation injury.

The initial goal of fluid resuscitation is the restoration of cardiac output and tissue perfusion. Multiple formulae estimating the initial fluid requirement in patients with major burns have been proposed including the Brooke, modified Brooke, Parkland, Evans, MGH and Monafo regimens [14,15]. These formulae use the weight of the patient and the percentage of body surface area burnt to estimate fluid requirements. The percentage of body surface area burnt can be easily estimated using a Lund and Browder chart. Weight should be measured if possible or estimated from collateral history. The Parkland formula allows for 4 mL/kg/% TBSA burned over 24 hours, with half the total fluid requirement to be given in the first 8 hours. In children under 30 kg, the above fluid should be given in addition to calculated maintenance fluid [1].

Patients generally receive more fluid than the Parkland's formula dictates and this appears to be associated with better outcomes than historical data [16,17]. The proposed formula of (weight in kg × %TBSA) mL of fluid in the first 2 hours post-burns injury is approximately double that estimated by the Parkland formula and leads to maintenance of resuscitation endpoints without obvious adverse events [18]. This strategy has been currently adopted in the pre-hospital phase and needs to be followed by goal-directed management to maintain adequate resuscitation. Haemodynamic status may be difficult to evaluate in the severely burned patient. In patients with severe burns, the insertion of a central venous catheter allows the measurements of preload, tissue oxygenation via central venous oxygen levels, contractility and coronary perfusion pressure and may facilitate the measurement of afterload. Additional measures of tissue oxygenation are obtained by serial serum lactate measurements and monitoring urine output via an indwelling catheter. Inserting a urinary catheter with an electronic temperature probe will assist in monitoring core temperature.

Some strategies have been proposed to reduce the total volume of resuscitation fluid. These have included the use of colloid and hypertonic salt solutions. The generalized increase in capillary permeability that occurs with major burns results in the loss of plasma protein, particularly albumin, from the circulation. There is a coincident reduction in hepatic albumin production post-burn. Colloid administration helps maintain oncotic pressure, but does not reduce tissue oedema in the first 8 hours and has not been shown to improve clinical outcome compared to crystalloid [19,20]. There is currently inadequate evidence to support the routine use of colloids for burns resuscitation.

Hypertonic saline solution would appear to be useful in patients with limited cardiopulmonary reserve; however, there is considerable debate over the safety of this technique and, again, there is no evidence of outcome benefit compared to isotonic solution [6,7].

Subsequent management

Having stabilized the patient and initiated fluid resuscitation, a careful secondary survey should be performed, looking for associated injuries.

Adequate analgesia is an important facet of management. Small burns may be managed with a combination of cool compresses and oral analgesia; larger burns will require parenteral analgesia [8]. Opiates will generally be the first option; an infusion of ketamine can be useful for continuous analgesia where there are extensive burns.

Burns patients lose heat quickly. Wrapping the patient in blankets, foil or external warming devices may prevent hypothermia.

Simple initial management of the wound with cling-wrap is adequate in providing analgesia, protection from the environment and allowing visualization of pathological appearance (E-Fig. 3.11.1). Early definitive surgical therapy with excision and autologous skin grafting is currently widely practised for deep burns and constricting eschars [7,21,22]. Tangential escharectomies remove much of the necrotic tissue while leaving behind healthy tissue. Peripheries with circumferential burns are at a high risk of ischaemic necrosis and warrant urgent escharotomy. Such procedures can be undertaken in the emergency department where pulses are absent. In circumferential chest burns, escharotomy may be necessary to relieve chest wall restriction and improve ventilation. Routine fluorescein staining and examination of the eye in cases of facial burns result in early diagnosis and treatment of corneal burns.

Tetanus following burn injury has been previously reported [23,24]. A tetanus vaccine booster is recommended for all patients with no history of tetanus vaccination in the last 10 years. Tetanus immunoglobulin should be considered in wounds grossly contaminated with soil. Systemic prophylactic antibiotics are not indicated. While there have been some suggestions of antibiotics to prevent toxic shock syndrome, its incidence is low and does not warrant routine prophylaxis for all burnt patients [25]. Antibiotics should be considered in the immunocompromised on an individual basis.

There is strong evidence for the use of histamine2-receptor antagonists for stress ulcer prophylaxis and they are recommended in all patients with major burns [26].

A nasogastric tube should be inserted in patients with major burns to avoid gastric dilatation.

Burn shock

The pathophysiology of burn shock is complex and involves a combination of haemodynamic and local tissue factors.

The early post-burn period, i.e. within the first 8 hours, is marked by the rapid formation of tissue oedema, predominantly in the wound itself, but also in non-burned tissue. Factors contributing to this fluid accumulation are not fully understood, but include local release of inflammatory mediators, particularly prostaglandins and leukotrienes. These increase capillary permeability both locally and systemically, in addition to increasing regional blood flow. Increased interstitial osmotic pressure in burned tissue due to the release of osmotically active cellular components and partial degradation of collagen also contributes to tissue oedema [4,7,22]. The combination of tissue injury, shock and dilution of coagulation factors through exogenous fluid administration leads to coagulopathy in about a third of major burns patients [27].

Major evaporative loss from burned skin due to loss of epithelial integrity significantly adds to fluid losses. In addition to the fluid shifts, cardiac output may fall by 30–50% in major burns, possibly due to a circulating myocardial depressant factor [4].

Inhalation injury

The presence of inhalation injury has a considerable negative impact on prognosis in the burns patient [3]. Direct thermal trauma below the larynx is rare, except in the case of steam inhalation.

Pulmonary complications are largely due to inhalation of toxic products of combustion, particularly in house or vehicular fires. Smoke consists of a particulate fraction – predominantly carbon – and a gaseous fraction, which may include carbon dioxide, carbon monoxide, oxides of nitrogen and sulphur, hydrogen cyanide and PVC, depending on the materials being burnt. These agents adhere to the moist respiratory mucosa, forming corrosive compounds that cause inflammation, hypersecretion and mucosal sloughing, resulting in airway obstruction and atelectasis. Smoke inhalation also triggers the release of thromboxane, resulting in increased pulmonary artery pressures [3,6].

Disposition

Patients with major burns should be managed in a specialist burns unit as outlined in Table 3.11.1. The patient should be discussed with the receiving unit prior to transfer, so that appropriate measures may be undertaken to stabilize them. Plastic cling wrap applied directly over the burn provides a good non-adherent dressing that will reduce heat and fluid loss. As noted previously, silver sulphadiazine (SSD) cream should not be applied to these burns as it interferes with subsequent evaluation. At the burns centre, burns will be dressed with a silver-impregnated, non-adherent, occlusive dressing (e.g. Acticoat).

Current management of full- and deep partial-thickness burns involves early excision and autologous skin grafting. In extensive burns, excision and autologous grafting may need to be staged, allowing sufficient skin to regenerate.

Less extensive burns (i.e. not meeting the criteria for burns centre transfer) may be admitted to a general or plastic surgery service. Loose skin and broken blisters should always be debrided. Blisters may otherwise be initially left intact, although some would advocate that all blisters be deroofed. A moist silver-impregnated dressing (e.g. Acticoat) may then be applied to areas of epithelial loss.

Superficial or partial-thickness burns involving less than 10% TBSA may be suitable for outpatient management subject to the criteria in Table 3.11.1 and depending on the social and psychological status of the patient. The choice of dressings for outpatient management depends on the depth of the burn, the extent and size of blisters and the amount of exudate from the burn surface [4,7].

Superficial burns can also be covered with a moist ointment (e.g. paraffin-based Dermeze) or moist dressing (e.g. Burnaid, which contains melaleuca-derived local anaesthetic properties). Superficial partial-thickness burns involve loss of epithelium with considerable exudate and hence are prone to infection. After gentle cleansing and debridement of loose tissue, a moist, non-adherent dressing, such as Bactigras, should be applied. These patients will need to be reviewed the next day, at which time the dressing will be changed. A silver-impregnated occlusive dressing is also an option to minimize crusting and dressing adherence.

Epithelialization commences at 7–10 days, by which time the burn surface should be drying out. At this stage, the more convenient hydrocolloid or film dressings may be used until epithelialization is complete.

If healing is not well established by 10–14 days, the patient should be referred for specialist opinion, as excision and grafting may be required.

Chemical burns

A wide range of products available in both the industrial and domestic environments can lead to burns. Although the mechanism is different, chemical burns demonstrate a similar spectrum of injury to thermal burns. Superficial burns are associated with itching, burning or pain; partial-thickness burns are associated with tissue oedema and the formation of bullae; and full-thickness burns are associated with damage extending through the dermis. The extent of tissue damage in chemical burns is determined by the nature and concentration of the chemical, as well as the extent and duration of contact [28].

In addition to the burn itself, toxicity may occur as a result of systemic absorption.

The majority of chemical burns are caused by acids and alkalis. Acids cause coagulation, with the formation of a tough eschar that may limit further tissue damage. Alkalis cause liquefactive necrosis, allowing deeper penetration. Many other types of chemical cause burns, but distinguishing them by mechanism of action is not relevant to the clinician as their management, apart from a few exceptions, is similar.

General principles

Chemical agents continue to damage tissue until they are removed or inactivated. Therapy then is directed to decontamination and, where appropriate, the use of specific antidotes as well as recognition and treatment of systemic toxicity.

Adequate protection of medical personnel to prevent secondary contamination is essential. Copious irrigation is the cornerstone of therapy, but contaminated garments should be removed and dry chemical particles brushed away before irrigation commences. Adherent or oily compounds may need to be removed with mild soap and a scrubbing brush and nails, hair and intertriginous areas should be carefully checked.

The duration of irrigation depends on the agent. Alkali in particular may require prolonged lavage owing to its tissue penetration. The use of litmus paper to determine wound pH may guide the duration of irrigation in acid and alkali burns.

Other than decontamination and treatment of systemic toxicity, management is similar to that for thermal burns.

Disposition

Most patients with chemical burns can be treated on an outpatient basis. Indications for admission include:

- partial-thickness burns >15% TBSA
- all full-thickness burns
- burns involving hands, feet, eyes, ears or perineum
- evidence of or potential for systemic toxicity
- significant associated injuries or complicating medical conditions.

Specific chemicals

Hydrofluoric acid

Hydrofluoric acid is a relatively weak acid used in glass etching, electronics and oil-refining industries. It is also a component of many industrial and domestic rust removers. In strong solution it causes corrosion of tissue owing to the release of hydrogen ions; however, its major toxicity is caused by the dissociated fluoride ion that complexes calcium and magnesium to form insoluble salts. Cell destruction associated with severe pain results. In severe burns, hypocalcaemia and hypomagnesaemia may occur [28].

Contact with strong solution (>50%) causes immediate pain and tissue destruction; however, exposure to weaker solutions, particularly <20%, may cause little or no pain initially. Thus it may take up to 24 hours for the burn to become apparent. Once apparent, the burn causes excruciating pain that is difficult to control even with parenteral narcotics.

After irrigation, specific therapy is aimed at precipitation and hence neutralization of free fluoride ions. Methods depend on the severity and location of the burn. Calcium gluconate gel, made by mixing calcium gluconate with a water-soluble lubricant to make a 2.5–10% solution, should be applied directly to the affected area.

Relief of pain is the marker of adequate treatment. If pain is not relieved, or recurs, parenteral therapy is required. Generally, this consists of subcutaneous injection of calcium gluconate, aiming for 0.5 mL of 10% solution per square centimetre. Hand and digital burns pose a problem, as vascular compromise may occur if too much fluid is injected. Alternatives include intra-arterial injection of calcium gluconate or regional perfusion using Bier's technique.

References

[1] Wolf S, Rose J, Desai M, et al. Mortality determinants in massive paediatric burns. Ann Surg 1997;225:554–69.
[2] Miller S, Bessey P, Schurr M, et al. National Burn Repository 2005: a ten-year review. J Burn Care Res 2006;27:411–36.
[3] Fraser J, Mullany D, Traber D. Inhalational lung injury in patients with severe thermal burns. Contemp Crit Care 2007;4:1–12.
[4] Shaw A, Anderson J, Hayward A, Parkhouse N. Pathophysiological basis of burn management. Br J Hosp Med 1994;52:583–7.
[5] Singh V, Dengan L, Bhat S, Milner S. The pathogenesis of burn wound conversion. Ann Plast Surg 2007;59:109–15.
[6] Nguyen T, Gilpin D, Meyer N, Herndon D. Current treatment of severely burned patients. Ann Surg 1996;233:14–25.
[7] Monafo W. Initial management of burns. N Engl J Med 1996;335:1581–6.
[8] Reed J, Pomerantz W. Emergency management of paediatric burns. Paediatr Emerg Care 2005;21:118–29.
[9] Jeevendra M. Succinylcholine hyperkalaemia after burns. Anaesthesiology 1999;91:321–2.
[10] Gillies M, Krone S, Sim K. Use of cut endotracheal tubes should be avoided in the initial resuscitation of the burned patient. Emerg Med J 2003;20:109.
[11] Peddy S, Rigby M, Shaffner D. Acute cyanide poisoning. Pediatr Crit Care Med 2006;7:79–82.
[12] Megarbane B, Delahaye A, Goldgran-Toledano D, Baud F. Antidotal treatment of cyanide poisoning. J Chin Med Assoc 2003;66:193–203.
[13] Roberts I, Alderson P, Bunn F, et al. Colloids versus crystalloids for fluid resuscitation in critically ill patients. Cochrane Database Syst Rev 2004;18:CD000567.
[14] Yowler C, Fratianne R. Current status of burn resuscitation. Clin Plast Surg 2000;27:1–10.
[15] Warden G. Burns shock resuscitation. World J Surg 1992;16:16–23.
[16] Mitra B, Fitzgerald M, Cameron P, Cleland H. Fluid resuscitation in major burns. Aust NZ J Surg 2006;76:35–8.
[17] Freiburg C, Igneri P, Sartorelli K, Rogers F. Effects of differences in percent total body surface area estimation on fluid resuscitation of transferred burn patients. J Burn Care Res 2007;28:42–8.
[18] Mitra B, Fitzgerald M, Wasiak J, et al. The Alfred pre-hospital fluid formula for major burns. Burns 2011;37:1134–9.
[19] Ipaktchi K, Arbabi S. Advances in burn critical care. Crit Care Med 2006;34:239–44.
[20] Alderson P, Bunn F, Lefebvre C, et al. Human albumin solution for resuscitation and volume expansion in critically ill patients. Cochrane Database Syst Rev 2004;18:CD001208.
[21] McManus W, Mason A, Pruitt B. Excision of the burn wound in patients with large burns. Arch Surg 1989;124:718–20.
[22] Demling R. Improved survival after massive burns. J Trauma 1983;23:179–84.
[23] Karyoute S, Badran I. Tetanus following a burn injury. Burns 1988;14:241–3.
[24] Amy B, McManus W, Pruitt B. Tetanus following a major thermal injury. J Trauma 1985;25:654–5.
[25] Rashid A, Brown A, Khan K. On the use of prophylactic antibiotics in prevention of toxic shock syndrome. Burns 2005;31:981–5.
[26] Cook D, Reeve B, Guyatt G, et al. Stress ulcer prophylaxis in critically ill patients. Resolving discordant meta-analyses. J Am Med Assoc 1996;275:308–14.
[27] Mitra B, Wasiak J, Cameron P, et al. Early coagulopathy of major burns. Injury 2013;44:40–3.
[28] Bretolini J. Hydrofluoric acid: a review of toxicity. J Emerg Med 1992;10:163–8.

3.12 Massive transfusion

Biswadev Mitra

ESSENTIALS

1 Early prediction of massive transfusion and activation of massive transfusion guidelines can ease some of challenges of resuscitation.

2 Systems should be instituted for effective prenotification of patients at risk of massive transfusion and a team-based approach to resuscitation planned, with the emergency physician as the team leader.

3 Laboratory tests may require a considerable amount of time to provide results and are not always reliable in the setting of acidosis, hypothermia and ongoing bleeding.

4 It is recommended that massive transfusion guidelines are developed and followed in all centres expected to receive haemorrhaging patients.

5 Patients with coagulopathy in the setting of massive transfusion have been shown to be four times more likely to die than those without.

What is a massive transfusion?

A 70 kg male has an average circulating volume of 5 L of whole blood. Assuming a haematocrit of 0.40–0.50, this approximates to a red cell volume of just over 2–2.5 L. A leucocyte depleted unit of red blood cells, as distributed by the Australian Red Cross Blood Service, has a volume of 250–300 mL, with a haematocrit of 0.50–0.70. The traditional definition of massive transfusion of at least 10 units of packed red blood cells (PRBC) transfused in the first 24 hours was approximated from the total red cell volume in a 70 kg man. More recently, this definition has been challenged as being under-representative of patients during the acute resuscitative phase [1,2], as patients who die prior to receiving 10 units of red cells are excluded (mortality bias), as are patients whose transfusion requirements may not reach 10 units, while including patients who may not require transfusion during the acute resuscitative phase, but are transfused later secondary to surgical procedures or complications of management. Definitions using lower volumes of PRBCs in shorter times, such as at least 5 units in 4 hours or greater than 10 units in 6 hours, have also been used [3,4].

The definition of massive transfusion can be used to alert the clinician and blood bank to a massively haemorrhaging patient. A secondary use of the definition of 'massive'

transfusion lies in transfusion research for selecting patients for prospective or retrospective studies to establish the guidelines for massive transfusion and have little use in clinical practice. Some prospective studies on massive transfusion have appropriately selected the patients based on perceived need, rather than a predetermined definition [5,6]. However, most retrospective studies studying components of a massive transfusion guideline have used the traditional definition of massive transfusion as the inclusion criterion. For these guidelines to be useful, a clinician must anticipate the patients who are likely to suffer with a certain level of blood loss over a specified time frame.

The volume of red blood cells transfused is associated with increased mortality [7]. There are other clinical and ethical reasons to reduce the amount of blood transfusions during resuscitation. Blood is a scarce resource and there are significant costs associated with the administration of blood banks. Transfusion of blood has also been associated with multiple adverse effects. Independent of shock severity, blood transfusion is a risk factor for mortality. Blood transfusions are independently associated with increased incidence of acute respiratory distress syndrome (ARDS) and the volume of transfusion has a dose response with later development of multiorgan failure. Rarer risks associated with transfusions include minor

allergic reaction, blood-borne viral infections, bacterial infection, anaphylactic shock, clinically significant immunosuppression and graft-versus-host disease.

The adverse clinical risks of transfusion and the limited supply of blood have resulted in a trend in modern resuscitation protocols to limit the volume of blood transfused. Appropriate use of blood in the reception and resuscitation of the massively haemorrhaging patient can be achieved by the early definitive control of haemorrhage, restrictive transfusion practice in select patients, external warming and correction of coagulopathy.

Predicting massive transfusion

Massive transfusion (MT) post-injury is relatively infrequent, but presents major challenges to emergency departments (EDs) and blood banks. It is important to note that the most common indication for massive transfusion in the ED in non-trauma centres is for patients with gastrointestinal haemorrhage. In the hectic phase of reception and resuscitation of patients with critical bleeding, in addition to diagnosis and management of the underlying pathology, the complex processes of rapid checking and delivery of blood products, monitoring of accurate ratios and, later, goal-directed management of coagulopathy, must occur. Early prediction of MT and activation of MT protocols can ease some of these challenges, leading to the formulation of several predictive scoring tools (Table 3.12.1).

The primary utility of current predictors of MT is in mass casualties or combat, although in those scenarios it might result in directing limited resources away from patients with higher scores, just the opposite of its purpose in civilian trauma care. When used clinically, the primary benefit in scoring is the ability to select accurately patients who will undergo an MT due to the high specificity of the scores. This enables blood and products to be ready with minimal wastage. However, due to the current low sensitivity of the scores, a high clinical suspicion needs to be maintained for all patients and MT protocols promptly activated where clinically indicated.

Table 3.12.1 Examples of scores to predict massive transfusion

PWH score		ABC score		TASH score	
Criteria	Score	Criteria	Score	Criteria	Score
SBP ≥90 mm Hg	3	Penetrating mechanism	1	Hb <7 g/dL	8
GCS ≤8	1	SBP <90 mm Hg	1	Hb <9 g/dL	6
HR ≥120 b/min	1	HR >120 b/min	1	Hb <10 g/dL	4
Displaced pelvic fracture	1	Positive FAST	1	Hb <11 g/dL	3
CT scan or FAST positive	2			Hb <12 g/dL	2
BD >5 mmol/L	1			Base excess <−10	4
Hb <7 g/dL	10*			Base excess <−6	3
Hb 7.0–10 g/dL	1			Base excess <−2	1
				HR >120 b/min	2
				Free abdominal fluid	3
				Clinically unstable pelvic fracture	6
				Open or dislocated femur fracture	3
				Male gender	1
Maximum score	10	Maximum score	4	Maximum score	29
Cut-off	≥6	Cut-off	≥2	Cut-off	≥18

GCS: Glasgow coma scale; SBP: Systolic blood pressure; HR: Heart rate; BD; Base deficit.
*Maximum score.

Preparation

Systems should be instituted for effective prenotification of patients at risk of massive transfusion. Pre-hospital staff should be encouraged to contact receiving hospitals as early as possible. Upon notification, relevant staff should be informed. The most senior emergency physician should assume the role of team leader in all cases. Medical and nursing roles should be allocated for management of the airway, breathing and circulation, ensuring flexibility at the discretion of the team leader to reallocate according to patient needs. The role of transfusion specialists to monitor blood and blood-product administration has been reported, but has current limited availability. The blood bank, surgical, radiological and theatre staff should be notified. Allied health staff should be on standby to aid in the transport of blood products and equipment, transport of patient and cater to the needs of relatives.

Reception

On reception, the patient should be managed in a trauma or resuscitation cubicle with full physiological monitoring. The principles of reception of all critically ill patients apply and have been previously discussed. The team leader must prepare the team for specific procedures to assist in the diagnosis and management of the severely haemorrhaging patient. Where relevant, focused assessment with sonography for trauma (FAST) should be performed by staff trained and credentialled in its use. FAST screening in the haemodynamically unstable population has a higher sensitivity and specificity when compared with the stable population [8]. The likelihood ratio for presence of haemorrhage given a positive FAST is about 12.0. Where delays to the operating theatre are expected, preparation should be made for thoracotomy or laparotomy in the ED for appropriate indications.

History

History of haemorrhage should be obtained from the patient or collateral history from paramedics or family members if present. Essential items on history include:

- age, gender, mechanism of injury or bleeding
- history of external bleeding
- previous sources of bleeding, e.g. oesophageal varices, angiodysplasias
- bleeding disorders and coagulopathies:
  - pre-existent, e.g. associated with liver disease, use of antiplatelet and anticoagulants

- acquired, e.g. dilutional through massive fluid administration or pre-hospital blood cell transfusion
- pre-hospital management, including transfusions, fluid administration, use of procoagulant (or antiplatelet) medications
- if available, history of previous transfusions, blood typing and previous transfusion reactions
- family history, as well as the possible intake of medicinal herbs, including homeopathy, should be explored.

Consent for transfusions should be obtained as early as possible. If unable to obtain consent from patients, alternate sources, such as the next of kin, should be approached. However, transfusion in life-threatening situations should not be delayed where consent cannot be obtained.

Examination

Clinically assessed blood loss when the patient is awake using advanced trauma life support (ATLS) guidelines of shock classes is outdated and rarely useful in the clinical setting. Significant haemorrhage should be suspected when signs, such as tachycardia, hypotension, oliguria, deficient peripheral perfusion, venous collapse and pulmonary capillary bed collapse (increase of dead space with low end tidal (ET) CO_2 and hypercapnoea), are observed along with base deficit and increased lactate levels.

Observation of wound for clot formation can sometimes be enough to diagnose the coagulopathic sequelae of the massive haemorrhage. A thorough secondary survey will usually locate the source of the massive haemorrhage.

Investigations

Investigations should be initially directed at accurately determining the source of bleeding and then to facilitate transfusion management. In the setting of haemodynamic instability, investigations for accurate diagnosis may need to be delayed in preference of explorative surgery. Where available, radiological investigations, such as red cell scans or angiograms, may assist in diagnosis while facilitating management through embolization.

Laboratory tests may require a considerable amount of time to provide results and they are not always reliable when there is acidosis, hypothermia and ongoing bleeding. Blood samples should be taken to identify blood group and Rhesus status, perform cross-match compatibility tests, full blood examination (including platelet count), acid–base balance and lactate. Standard coagulation tests do not identify the pathophysiological mechanisms of haemorrhage. A prolonged activated partial thromboplastin time (aPTT) can be due to deficiency of intrinsic factors of coagulation, fibrinogen deficit, hypothermia, blood heparinization or increased fibrinolysis. Each requires a different approach and tests usually do not help to choose the appropriate therapy. Finally, common laboratory tests (international normalized ratio [INR] and aPTT) are carried out at 37°C without platelets and red blood cells; therefore, they are unable to determine the presence of coagulopathy associated with hypothermia and platelet dysfunction of fibrinolysis.

However, testing of coagulation status may have a prognostic value. A prolonged aPTT >1.8 normal value is related with significant haemorrhage and has been associated with an increase of >300% mortality rate in injured patients [9]. INR is a predictive factor independent of mortality in traumatized patients when it reaches >1.5–1.8.

Normal quantitative values do not ensure platelet function in patients with anaemia, hypothermia, hypocalcaemia or hypomagnesaemia. A decreased number of platelets is

a phenomenon with high personal variability and is not predictive of mortality in injured patients.

There has been renewed interest in the use of near-patient functional tests of coagulation, such as thromboelastometry for the diagnosis of coagulopathy. These devices (Rotational Thromboelastometry [ROTEM], Thromboelastography [TEG]) may be suitable for EDs. These tools are in routine use in some elective surgery settings, such as cardiac and liver transplant surgery. TEG and ROTEM are representative of a total coagulation process as well as thrombus formation and lysis. Blood samples are processed at the patient's temperature, including hypothermia in the dysfunction analysis. These procedures are easy to use and interpret and results are available within 15 minutes. Blood tests should be repeated every 30 minutes depending on the clinical condition.

Circulatory management

The goal of blood replacement is to maintain tissue perfusion and cellular oxygenation to avoid multiorganic failure from shock. In the setting of concomitant brain injury (traumatic and atraumatic) and the elderly, it is recommended that, during active bleeding, arterial pressure is kept at minimum safe values (mean arterial pressure 60–70 mmHg) to maintain perfusion of vital organs (kidney, heart and central nervous system). Patients with traumatic brain injury should maintain a cerebral perfusion pressure, despite increased intracranial pressure, by optimizing mean arterial pressure to ensure cerebral perfusion pressure at 60 mmHg. This may require the use of vasoconstrictors and inotropic drugs and may worsen bleeding if not first surgically controlled.

Permissive hypotension in the setting of blunt trauma resuscitation has been advocated recently, but level I evidence for the practice exists only in patients with penetrating truncal trauma. In other situations, the risks of reduced tissue perfusion must be weighed against potential benefits of preserving clot strength.

The specific goals of circulatory management are:

• surgical control of bleeding
• replacement of intravenous fluids (maintaining circulatory volume and oxygen transport)
• normothermia, acidosis and hypocalcaemia correction

• avoidance of hyperventilation and excessive positive end expiratory pressure (PEEP).

These goals are interactive and their correction should be simultaneously performed. The endpoint of resuscitation may be reached when vital signs are normal or even hyperdynamic as measured by cardiac output, arterial pressure, central venous pressure, haematocrit stable between 20 and 30% (according to patient's physical condition) and coagulation test results are normal.

Group O Rh-negative red blood cells may be used while awaiting results of the group. If the group O-Rh negative supply becomes compromised, the patient should be maintained with group O positive until such time as the patients' group can be determined. It is recommended to switch to the patient's specific group unless the patient's group cannot be determined. Group AB plasma may be used if necessary while awaiting results of the group. It is recommended that massive transfusion guidelines are developed at all centres expected to receive haemorrhaging patients and followed.

Massive transfusion guidelines

A guideline is defined as 'a systematically developed statement that assists in decision making about appropriate healthcare for specific clinical situations'. Due to the varied level of evidence on the management of the massively haemorrhaging patient, these guidelines remain largely variable across different regions. The following section discusses the key components that are likely to be uniform across most guidelines.

Fresh frozen plasma

Fresh frozen plasma (FFP) is a key component in massive transfusion protocols and most of the evidence has been gleaned for resuscitation post-trauma. The landmark study to suggest high dose fresh frozen plasma was in 2006, by Borgman et al. Combat casualties ($n = 246$) admitted to a combat hospital in Baghdad, Iraq who were given $\geq$ 10 units PRBCs (PRBCs or fresh whole blood) in the first 24 hours were divided into three groups and analysed according to low (1:12–1:5), intermediate (1:3.0–1:2.3) and high ratios (1:1.7–1:1.2) of FPP:PRBCs units. Overall mortality was 28%, but mortality in patients receiving a high ratio was significantly lower at 19%. This study was limited by being retrospective in design and included fresh whole blood which was viewed as 1:1:1 PRBCs:FFP:platelets (PLTs). Furthermore, the military setting was unlikely to be generalizable to a community setting with a high degree of penetrating trauma and pre-hospital care with short transit times involving standardized regimental care. There was a significantly higher incidence of thoracic trauma in the low ratio group with more severe injuries and lower initial haemoglobin levels in those who died early [10].

There have been multiple retrospective reviews to date on the topic, with similar weaknesses and with survival bias rarely controlled. Studies to date have provided inadequate evidence to support or refute the use of a high FFP:PRBC ratio in patients with severe trauma. It could be that the benefits accorded to the 1:1 strategy are solely due to survival. Specifically, those patients who survive injury are simply able to receive more plasma transfusions, as opposed to those who die from overwhelming injury from acute haemorrhagic shock immediately.

In the setting of massive haemorrhage, early treatment with thawed FFP is recommended with an initial dose of 10–15 mL/kg. Further doses should be guided by coagulation monitoring and the amount of other blood products administered. In patients with ongoing red blood cell requirement, best current evidence supports a ratio of 1:2 FFP:PRBC.

Platelets

The role of early platelet transfusion in the setting of haemorrhagic shock also continues to be debated. Platelets are obtained by two methods: (1) an apheresis machine separates anticoagulated blood into components with retention of the platelets and a portion of plasma to create a standard adult dose of platelets. The remaining elements may be returned to the donor. The platelet apheresis unit is then divided into four packs of equal volume to produce a paediatric platelet component. This is to reduce donor exposure for small paediatric transfusions and to minimize product wastage. (2) An adult dose of platelets derived from whole blood from ABO identical donors and resuspended in a nutrient additive solution to produce a platelet pooled leucocyte depleted component. Leucocyte depletion is performed during or soon after collection to remove most leucocytes.

In Australia, both apheresis and pooled platelets are irradiated before release from the Australian Red Cross Blood Service, unless other specific arrangements have been made with the receiving laboratory/institution. As with FFP, recent military reports have promoted routine administration of apheresis platelets to the injured patient. However, a similar survival bias has been suggested to explain the apparent benefit of early platelet administration.

Studies from more than two decades ago evaluating clotting factor and platelet counts in massively transfused patients concluded that a platelet count of 100 000/mm^3 is the threshold for diffuse bleeding and that thrombocytopaenia was not a clinically significant problem until transfusions exceeded 15–20 units of blood. Specifically, patients with a platelet count >50 000/mm^3 had only a 4% chance of developing diffuse bleeding. Although the classic threshold for platelet transfusion has been 50 000/mm^3, a higher target level of 100 000/mm^3 has been suggested for multiply injured patients and patients with massive haemorrhage. However, the relationship of platelet count to haemostasis and the contribution of platelets to formation of a stable clot in the injured patient remain largely unknown. Furthermore, platelet function, irrespective of number, is also of crucial importance. The complex relationship of thrombin generation to platelet activation requires dynamic evaluation of clot function. Accordingly, at this time, there is inadequate evidence to support an absolute trigger for platelet transfusions during resuscitation. Best evidence suggests a low threshold for transfusion, without specific defined levels.

Cryoprecipitate

The evidence for cryoprecipitate use during resuscitation remains similarly scant. It has been suggested that cryoprecipitate can rapidly increase the concentrations of fibrinogen and von Willebrand's factor, but the advantages of higher than normal concentrations remain speculative. Cryoprecipitate administration is recommended at a fibrinogen count of <1.0 g/L.

Calcium

Calcium in the extracellular plasma exists either in a free ionized state (45%) or bound to proteins and other molecules in a biologically inactive state (55%). The normal concentration of the ionized form ranges from 1.1 to 1.3 mmol/L and is influenced by the pH.

A 0.1 unit increase in pH decreases the ionized calcium concentration by approximately 0.05 mmol/L. The availability of ionized calcium is essential for the timely formation and stabilization of fibrin polymerization sites and a decrease in cytosolic calcium concentration precipitates a decrease in all platelet-related activities. In addition, contractility of the heart and systemic vascular resistance are compromised at low ionized calcium levels. Combining beneficial cardiovascular and coagulation effects, the level for ionized calcium concentration should therefore be maintained above 0.9 mmol/L [11]. Early hypocalcaemia following haemorrhage shows a significant correlation with the amount of infused colloids, but not with crystalloids, and may be attributable to colloid-induced haemodilution [12]. Also, hypocalcaemia develops during massive transfusion as a result of the citrate employed as an anticoagulant in blood products and is rare prior to the start of transfusion. The anticoagulant activity of Citrate is exerted by binding of ionized calcium causing hypocalcemia. This is most commonly seen with FFP and platelet transfusions because these products have high citrate concentrations. Citrate undergoes rapid hepatic metabolism and hypocalcaemia is generally transient during standard transfusion procedures. Citrate metabolism may be dramatically impaired by hypoperfusion states, hypothermia and in patients with hepatic insufficiency.

There are currently no evidence-based guidelines on calcium management during massive transfusion. It is recommended that ionized calcium levels be monitored during massive transfusion and that calcium chloride be administered during massive transfusion if ionized calcium levels are low or electrocardiographic changes suggest hypocalcaemia.

Synthetic agents

Pharmacological interventions that inhibit fibrinolysis (aprotonin, e-aminocaproic acid, tranexamic acid) or increase von Willebrand's factor release (desmopressin) have been used to decrease bleeding and reduce blood-product usage in selected settings. Agents that have shown promise in randomized controlled trials for the bleeding patient are recombinant activated factor VII (rFVIIa) and tranexamic acid.

Recombinant activated factor VII is approved for treatment of bleeding in haemophilia patients with inhibitors to factors VIII and IX. It has also been used during surgery to control haemorrhage and shown to be safe in these settings. To date, no effect of rFVIIa on mortality or thromboembolism has been demonstrated in the trauma population, but a significant reduction in blood usage and ARDS has been found. The use of rFVIIa should only be considered in the setting of continuing bleeding refractory to routine management [13].

Tranexamic acid (TXA) is an antifibrinolytic that inhibits both plasminogen activation and plasmin activity, thus preventing clot breakdown rather than promoting new clot formation. TXA (trans-4-(aminomethyl) cyclohexanecarboxylic acid) is a small molecule (molecular weight 157.2). It occupies the lysine-binding sites on plasminogen, thus preventing its binding to lysine residues on fibrin. This reduces plasminogen activation to plasmin. Similarly, blockade of lysine-binding sites on circulating plasmin prevents binding to fibrin and thus prevents clot breakdown. Tranexamic acid is 10 times more potent *in vitro* than an older drug of the same class, aminocaproic acid. At therapeutically relevant concentrations, TXA does not affect platelet count, aggregation or coagulation parameters. It is excreted largely unchanged in urine and has a half-life of about 2 hours in circulation.

CRASH-2 was a landmark study in the use of TXA for trauma [14]. The authors also reported a reduction in relative risk (RR) of death as a result of bleeding as 15% (4.9% vs 5.7%; RR, 0.85; CI, 0.76–0.96; $p = 0.0077$). Similarly, they reported an RR reduction in death as a result of bleeding on the day of randomization of 20% (2.8% vs 3.5%; RR, 0.80; CI, 0.68–0.93; $p = 0.0036$). Generalizability of the results of CRASH-2 to severely injured patients in mature trauma systems has been questioned. It is likely that patients most severely injured and those with acute traumatic coagulopathy were excluded from the study. Trauma mortality in mature trauma systems is also significantly lower than reported in CRASH-2. Together with advanced trauma reception, resuscitation, intensive care and rehabilitation in mature trauma systems, any additional benefits of TXA as a routine agent in this setting is debatable [15]. There may be some benefit in the pre-hospital phase where the management of acute traumatic coagulopathy is minimal and trials are underway to evaluate this question.

Prothrombin complex concentrates are indicated for bleeding in the setting of vitamin-K dependent oral anticoagulants (warfarin). There is no evidence for the routine use of desmopressin, but it may be considered in patients with refractory bleeding using antiplatelet agents. Antithrombin III should be avoided until further studies on its safety profile are conducted.

Acute traumatic coagulopathy

Acute traumatic coagulopathy (ATC) is a unique entity defined by coagulation disorders precipitated by tissue injury and shock. It has been shown that nearly 25% of major trauma patients arrive in the ED with a clinically significant coagulopathy. The existence of this early coagulopathy has been verified, with remarkably similar results, despite subtle differences in the definition of coagulopathy.

The key measures used in defining ATC are:

- Prothrombin time (PT): a measure of the extrinsic pathway of coagulation. PT measures function of factors I, II, V, VII and X. The reference range for PT is usually around 10–13 seconds. The prothrombin time is most commonly measured using blood plasma. Blood is drawn into a test tube containing liquid citrate, which acts as an anticoagulant by binding the calcium in a sample. The plasma is analysed at 37°C and excess of calcium is added (thereby reversing the effects of citrate), which enables the blood to clot again. Tissue factor (also known as factor III) is added and the time the sample takes to clot is measured optically. The prothrombin time was described by Quick in 1935 and the test is sometimes referred to as the 'Quick's test'.
- Prothrombin ratio (PTr): the prothrombin ratio is the prothrombin time for a patient, divided by the result for control plasma.
- International normalized ratio (INR): the result (in seconds) for a prothrombin time performed on a normal individual will vary according to the type of analytical system employed. This is due to the variations between different batches of manufacturer's tissue factor used in the reagent to perform the test. The INR was devised to standardize the results. Each manufacturer assigns an ISI value (International Sensitivity Index) for any tissue factor they manufacture. The ISI value indicates how a particular batch of tissue factor compares to an international reference tissue factor. The ISI is usually between 1.0 and 2.0. The INR is the ratio of a patient's prothrombin time to a normal (control) sample, raised to the power of the ISI value for the analytical system used.
- Activated partial thromboplastin time: the partial thromboplastin time (PTT) or activated partial thromboplastin time (aPTT or APTT) are all performance indicators of both the intrinsic and the common coagulation pathways. Blood samples are collected in tubes with oxalate or citrate to arrest coagulation by binding calcium. In order to activate the intrinsic pathway, phospholipid, an activator (such as silica, celite, kaolin, ellagic acid) and calcium (to reverse the anticoagulant effect of the oxalate) are mixed into the plasma sample. The time is measured until a thrombus forms. The test is termed 'partial' due to the absence of tissue factor from the reaction mixture.

Acute traumatic coagulopathy has been associated with the presence of both tissue injury and shock together. Its incidence appears to be very low when one of these two factors is present without the other. Patients with this acute coagulopathy from trauma have been shown to be four times more likely to die than those without. It should also be remembered that up to 30% of coagulopathic patients do not receive massive transfusions and therefore may not be amenable to massive transfusion guidelines. With no other guidelines to manage the acute coagulopathy that results secondary to tissue injury and shock, these patients potentially have delayed management of their coagulopathy.

Future directions

The varied nature of massive transfusion guidelines and the low level of evidence for its components have been barriers to adequately powered outcome studies. Future clinical trials are required to focus on improvements in the quality of supporting evidence for these agents.

The benefits of high volumes of fresh frozen plasma and the limitations of a relatively low level of evidence to guide this practice were highlighted above. Despite randomized controlled trials, the trials of rFVIIa and TXA suffered from deficiencies in design and the known difficulties of performing research in critical care environments. Uncertainties about these trials have led to a lack of consensus. Associated with the agents mentioned above, fibrinogen may be the key element of blood coagulation and is the first element to reach critically low levels. In addition to tissue injury, fibrin polymerization can be compromised by colloids, but it has been shown that this form of blood coagulation compromise can be reversed by the administration of fibrinogen. Fibrinogen quantity and function *in vitro* can be improved by multiple agents, including direct administration of fibrinogen concentrate and should be a key measure in future studies examining improvements in the management of the acutely haemorrhaging patient.

References

[1] Mitra B, Mori A, Cameron PA, et al. Massive blood transfusion and trauma resuscitation. Injury 2007;38:1023–9.

[2] Kashuk JL, Moore EE, Johnson JL, et al. Postinjury life threatening coagulopathy: is 1:1 fresh frozen plasma:packed red blood cells the answer? J Trauma 2008;65:261–70.

[3] Mitra B, Mori A, Cameron P, et al. Fresh frozen plasma (FFP) use during massive blood transfusion in trauma resuscitation. Injury 2010;41:35–9.

[4] Mitra B, Cameron PA, Gruen RL, et al. The definition of massive transfusion in trauma: a critical variable in examining evidence for resuscitation. Eur J Emerg Med 2011;18:137–42.

[5] Cotton BA, Au BK, Nunez TC, et al. Predefined massive transfusion protocols are associated with a reduction in organ failure and postinjury complications. J Trauma 2009;66:41–8. Discussion 48–9.

[6] Cotton B, Dossett L, Au B, et al. Room for (performance) improvement: provider-related factors associated with poor outcomes in massive transfusion. J Trauma 2009;67:1004–12.

[7] Marik PE, Corwin HL. Efficacy of red blood cell transfusion in the critically ill: a systematic review of the literature. Crit Care Med 2008;36:2667–74.

[8] Fitzgerald MC, Chan JY, Ross AW, et al. A synthetic haemoglobin-based oxygen carrier and the reversal of cardiac hypoxia secondary to severe anaemia following trauma. Med J Aust 2011;194:471–3.

[9] MacLeod JB, Lynn M, McKenney MG, et al. Early coagulopathy predicts mortality in trauma. J Trauma 2003;55:39–44.

[10] Borgman MA, Spinella PC, Perkins JG, et al. The ratio of blood products transfused affects mortality in patients receiving massive transfusions at a combat support hospital. J Trauma 2007;63:805–13.

[11] Dutton RP, Mackenzie CF, Scalea TM. Hypotensive resuscitation during active hemorrhage: impact on in-hospital mortality. J Trauma 2002;52:1141–6.

[12] Vivien B, Langeron O, Morell E, et al. Early hypocalcemia in severe trauma. Crit Care Med 2005;33:1946–52.

[13] Mitra B, Cameron PA, Parr M, Phillips P. Recombinant factor VIIa in trauma patients with the 'triad of death'. Injury 2012;43(9):1409–14.

[14] CRASH-2 trial collaborators Effects of tranexamic acid on death, vascular occlusive events, and blood transfusion in trauma patients with significant haemorrhage (CRASH-2): a randomised, placebo-controlled trial. Lancet 2010;376:23–32.

[15] Gruen RL, Mitra B. Tranexamic acid for trauma. Lancet 2011;377:1052–4.

ORTHOPAEDIC EMERGENCIES

Edited by **Anne-Maree Kelly and Anthony Brown**

4.1 Injuries of the shoulder

Crispijn van den Brand • Anne-Maree Kelly

ESSENTIALS

1 Most clavicular fractures heal despite displacement, therefore reduction is not necessary.

2 Injuries to the shoulder region may also involve injury to local neurovascular structures.

3 Acromioclavicular joint injuries and fractures of the scapula are usually treated conservatively.

4 Posterior sternoclavicular dislocations require reduction.

5 In dislocation of the shoulder, careful examination of the axillary (circumflex) nerve, brachial plexus and axillary artery is mandatory both before and after reduction.

6 In anterior dislocation of the shoulder, surgical repair of the capsule is recommended for recurrent dislocators and first-time dislocators who are young and engaged in high-risk sports.

Fractures of the clavicle

Fractures of the clavicle account for 2.6–5% of all fractures and usually result from a direct blow on the point of the shoulder, but may also be due to a fall on the outstretched hand. The most common site of fracture is the middle third of the clavicle, which accounts for 69–82% of clavicular fractures. Most other clavicular fractures are in the outer third.

There are varying degrees of displacement of the fracture ends, with overlapping fragments and shortening being common. Owing to the strategic location of the clavicle, injury to the pleura, axillary vessels and/or brachial plexus is possible but, fortunately, these complications are rare. They should be excluded by directed examination.

The clinical signs of clavicular fracture are a patient supporting the weight of their arm at the elbow coupled with local pain and tenderness, often accompanied by deformity.

In non-displaced or minimally displaced fractures, treatment consists of an elbow-supporting sling (e.g. broad arm sling) for 2–3 weeks. For comfort, this may be worn under clothes for the first few days. The sling may be discarded when local tenderness has subsided. Note that clinical union usually precedes radiological union by weeks. Early shoulder movement should be encouraged within the limits of pain and immobilization should be discontinued if clinical union has occurred, even if there is not yet radiological union. Non-union is rare.

Midshaft fractures with complete displacement, comminution or fractures in the elderly or women with osteoporosis have a higher rate of non-union and poorer functional outcome. Recent evidence suggests that this group may benefit from surgical stabilization with either plate-and-screw fixation or intramedullary devices.

Fractures of the outer third of the clavicle may involve the coracoclavicular ligaments. These fractures are generally displaced. If so, surgical management should be considered because these fractures have a high incidence of non-union (30%). Displaced fractures of the medial third of the clavicle are often associated with other serious injuries and warrant further examination. Early orthopaedic consultation is recommended for all (displaced) fractures of the medial and outer third of the clavicle.

Late complications of clavicular fractures include shoulder stiffness and a local lump at the site of fracture healing, which is rarely of cosmetic significance.

Acromioclavicular joint injuries

Acromioclavicular (AC) joint injuries usually result from a fall where the patient rolls onto his/her shoulder. The degree of the injury relates to the number of ligaments damaged; about two-thirds of AC injuries are incomplete and involve only part of the AC and coracoclavicular ligaments (CC) (types I and II).

AC dislocations are classified according to the Tossy/Rockwood classification system (Fig. 4.1.1):

- type I: partial tear of the AC ligament, CC ligament intact. Tenderness over the AC joint, no deformity
- type II: complete tear of AC ligament, partial tear of CC ligament. Radiographs show partial elevation of the distal clavicle
- type III: complete tear of AC and CC ligaments. Radiographs show substantial

elevation of distal clavicle and increased CC distance
- type IV: complete tear of AC and CC ligaments with dislocation of the distal clavicle posterior into or through the trapezius muscle
- type V: complete tear of AC and CC ligaments along with disruption of the muscular attachments of the distal clavicle
- type VI: complete disruption of AC and CC ligaments and muscular support. The distal clavicle is forced behind the tendons of the biceps and coracobrachialis.

On clinical examination of the standing patient, the outer end of the affected clavicle may be prominent and there will be local tenderness over the AC joint. The degree of damage can be ascertained by taking standing X-rays of both shoulders with the patient holding weights in both hands (stress X-rays) and by ultrasound. Stress X-rays may be normal in mild strains, but dynamic ultrasonographic techniques may better define the injury.

Treatment is with a broad arm sling. For minor injuries (Rockwood type I/II) 1–2 weeks is usually sufficient. For type II injuries, heavy lifting and contact sports should be avoided for 4–6 weeks to avoid conversion to a type

III injury. The treatment of type III injuries is controversial with some authors recommending conservative treatment and others surgery. Types IV to VI injuries are usually treated surgically.

Sternoclavicular subluxation and dislocation

Sternoclavicular dislocations are uncommon and usually due to a direct, high velocity blow to the medial clavicle or medial compression of the shoulder girdle. Subluxation is more common than dislocation, with the affected medial end of the clavicle displaced forwards and downwards. Dislocations may be anterior or, rarely, posterior. In the latter case, the great vessels or trachea may be damaged.

Clinical features include local tenderness and asymmetry of the medial ends of the clavicles. The diagnosis is essentially clinical. X-rays are difficult to interpret and are not necessary for subluxations. For dislocations, contrast enhanced CT scanning should be obtained.

Subluxations should be treated in a broad arm sling for 2–3 weeks. Anterior sternoclavicular joint instability should also be treated

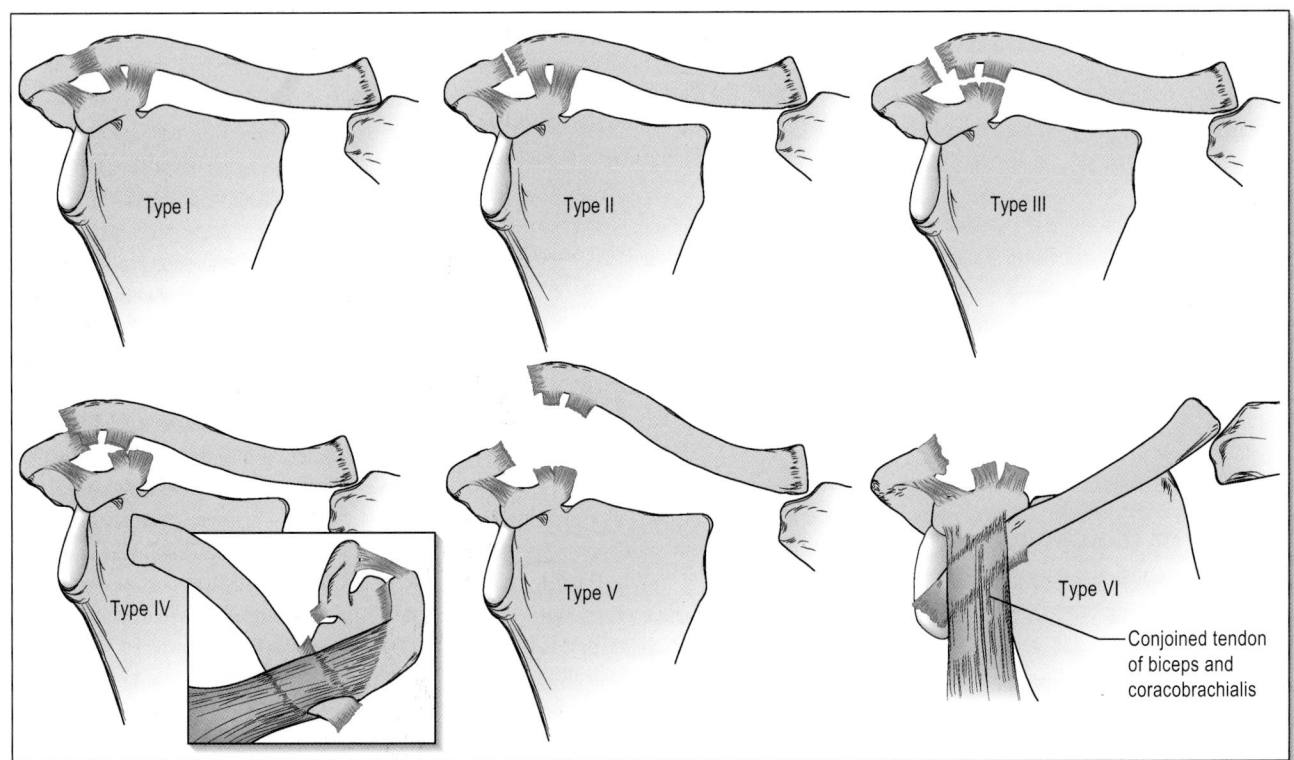

Conjoined tendon of biceps and coracobrachialis

Fig. 4.1.1 The Tossy/Rockwood classification system of AC dislocations.

conservatively; however, there is a significant risk of ongoing instability that is usually well tolerated and of little, if any, functional impact. For patients with posterior dislocation, expeditious diagnosis and treatment are important. Closed reduction, performed under general anaesthesia, is usually stable and the joint can then be managed in a brace or sling for 4–6 weeks. Operative stabilization is required if closed reduction is unsuccessful or there is persistent instability.

Fractures of the scapula

Fractures of the scapula are uncommon, accounting for less than 1% of all fractures. They typically occur after high-energy trauma. Up to 90% of patients have other associated injuries.

Fractures of the blade of the scapula are most common and are usually due to direct violence. Clinical features are local tenderness, sometimes with marked swelling. Healing is usually rapid, even in the presence of comminution and displacement, with an excellent functional outcome. Treatment is usually non-operative, with a broad arm sling and early mobilization. There is growing acceptance of surgical treatment for highly displaced fractures. However, there is no evidence comparing outcome for surgical versus non-surgical treatment.

Fractures of the scapula neck are often comminuted and may involve the glenoid. Swelling and bruising of the shoulder may be marked. Clinical examination and X-rays should ensure that the humeral head is enlocated. Computed tomography (CT) scans may be useful in defining the anatomy and the degree of involvement of the glenoid, including any steps in the articular surface. Surgery is often indicated for fractures involving the scapular neck or glenoid.

The 'floating shoulder' is an uncommon injury pattern. Although it is usually defined as an ipsilateral fracture of the clavicle and scapular neck, recent studies suggest that ligamentous disruption associated with a scapular neck fracture can give the functional equivalent of this injury pattern, with or without an associated clavicle fracture. Because the degree of ligament disruption is difficult to assess, indications for non-surgical and surgical management are not well defined. Minimally displaced fractures typically do well with conservative management. The degree of fracture displacement and ligament disruption that results in

poor outcome with conservative management is not well defined and the indications for surgery are controversial, as is choice of surgical technique. Options include fixation of the clavicular fracture, which often indirectly reduces the scapular fracture, or fixation of both fractures.

Supraspinatus tendon injuries

Rotator cuff tears most commonly affect the supraspinatus tendon and become more common with advancing age as degeneration weakens the cuff. Indeed, the presence of asymptomatic partial or complete tears identified on ultrasound or magnetic resonance imaging (MRI) may be as high as 40% in patients aged over 50.

Symptomatic injuries may follow minor trauma or the sudden application of traction to the arm. Many are acute or chronic in nature, rather than truly acute. This can be defined with ultrasound or MRI if required.

The clinical features of a strain include a painful arc of abduction centred at 90° of abduction, weakness in external rotation and tenderness under the acromion. If the tear is complete, no abduction at the glenohumeral joint will occur, although some abduction to 45–60% is possible by scapular rotation. In both partial and complete injuries, there is a full passive range of abduction. Another useful test to isolate the supraspinatus and test its integrity is the 'empty can' test. The patient abducts the arm to 30° with 30° of forward flexion and full internal rotation (i.e. thumb pointed down) and is then asked to forward flex the shoulder first without and then against resistance. Pain or weakness against resistance suggests supraspinatus injury.

The goals of emergency care for rotator cuff injuries are to provide pain relief and prevent further disability. For the acute symptoms, an arm sling can provide support but prolonged immobilization should be avoided. Treatment of supraspinatus tears is controversial, with no clear evidence guiding the choice of operative versus non-operative therapy or the components or duration of non-operative treatments. Most experts would still recommend a trial of non-operative therapy before considering surgery. An exception to this may be the patient with a previously asymptomatic shoulder who sustains trauma with resultant weakness (after the pain from the

injury subsides) in whom imaging studies indicate an acute full-thickness tear.

Dislocation of the shoulder

Dislocation of the shoulder results in the humeral head lying anterior, posterior or inferior to the glenoid. Of these, anterior dislocation is the most common.

Anterior dislocation

Anterior glenohumeral dislocation is most often due to a fall resulting in external rotation of the shoulder, for example, the body rotating internally over a fixed arm. It is most common in young adults, often being related to sports. There is inevitable damage to the joint capsule (stretching or tearing) and there may be associated damage to the subscapularis.

Anterior dislocations are associated with several fractures including Hill–Sachs deformities, (bony) Bankart lesions and greater tuberosity fractures. A Hill–Sachs deformity is an impression fracture of the humeral head caused by the glenoid and is present in 35–100% of all anterior dislocations. It is unclear if this is prognostically important. Bony Bankart lesions are caused by a disruption of the glenoid labrum with an avulsion of the glenoid. These occur in about 5% of patients. Another common fracture is of the greater tuberosity of the humerus. Other complications may include damage to the axillary (circumflex) nerve (resulting in inability to contract deltoid and numbness over the insertion of deltoid) and, rarely, the axillary vessels and the brachial plexus.

Clinical features include severe pain, reluctance to move the shoulder and the affected arm being supported at the elbow, often in slight abduction. The contour of the shoulder is 'flattened off' and there is a palpable gap just under the acromion where the humeral head usually lies. The displaced humeral head may be palpable anteriorly in the hollow behind the pectoral muscles.

Dislocation is confirmed by X-ray. The dislocation may be evident on the AP film but cannot be ruled out on a single view. Additional views (e.g. an axial lateral, translateral, tangential lateral) are required. These may reveal an associated fracture of the greater trochanter, but this does not influence initial management.

The principles of management are the provision of adequate analgesia as soon as possible, reduction of the dislocation and immobilization followed by physiotherapy. There are more than 20 described methods for the reduction of anterior dislocations, with reported success rates ranging from 60 to 100%. These include the FARES technique, the Spaso technique, the modified Kocher's manoeuvre, the Milch technique and scapular rotation techniques (www.youtube.com/watch?v=NXFPWxSTK5c). There is no high-quality evidence to assist in selecting the most effective method. That said, the Hippocratic method is not recommended as the traction involved may damage neurovascular structures. Gravitational traction (the Stimson technique), having the patient lie face down with a weight strapped to the limb, is occasionally successful and may be worthwhile if there will be a delay until reduction by another method. All reduction methods require adequate analgesia. Intra-articular local anaesthetic may also be useful. Sedation, in an appropriately controlled environment, may be of assistance in augmenting analgesia and providing a degree of muscle relaxation and amnesia, but is not required in most cases. Failure of reduction under analgesia/sedation is rare and mandates reduction under general anaesthesia.

If there is an associated fracture of the greater trochanter, it usually reduces when the shoulder is reduced. If it remains displaced, open reduction and internal fixation may be required.

Post-reduction X-rays confirm reduction and neurovascular status must be rechecked. Post-reduction care includes immobilization in a broad arm sling followed by physiotherapy. Available evidence suggests that there is no benefit from immobilization for more than 1 week. It was suggested that bracing in external rotation might reduce the incidence of recurrent dislocation but this has not been borne out in validation studies.

Primary surgery, usually by arthroscopic techniques, is recommended for patients having suffered recurrent dislocations and should be considered for first-time dislocators, especially those who are young, as surgery has been shown to significantly reduce the risk of recurrent dislocation.

Recurrence is rare in the elderly, but is common (64–68%) in young patients.

Reduction techniques (www.youtube.com/watch?v= NXFPWxSTK5c)

Most anterior glenohumeral dislocations can be reduced without anaesthesia or procedural sedation, although appropriate analgesia and a patient, gentle technique is required. Intra-articular lignocaine (lidocaine) has been shown to be a safe, effective alternative to procedural sedation for reduction of dislocated shoulders.

FARES technique

The patient may be in the supine or prone position. Hold the patient's wrist and apply traction to the affected limb in a neutral position. Move the limb anteriorly and posteriorly in small oscillating movements (about 5–10 cm) while continuing to apply traction slowly abducting the limb. Once the limb is abducted to 90°, externally rotate the limb at the shoulder, with ongoing traction and oscillating anterior/posterior movements. Continue slowly to abduct the limb past this position. Reduction is usually achieved once the limb is abducted to about 120°. Success rate of the order of 89% has been reported.

Spaso technique

The patient is placed in the supine position. The affected arm is held by the forearm or wrist and gently lifted vertically, applying traction. While maintaining vertical traction, the shoulder is then externally rotated, resulting in reduction. If necessary, countertraction by downward pressure over the shoulder joint may be applied. Success rate of the order of 75% has been reported.

Modified Kocher's manoeuvre

While applying traction to the arm by holding it at the elbow, the shoulder is slowly externally rotated, pausing if there is muscle spasm or resistance. External rotation to about 90° should be possible and reduction often occurs during this process. The elbow is then adducted until it starts to cross the chest and then internally rotated until the hand lies near the opposite shoulder.

Scapular rotation

This technique is traditionally performed with the patient prone, but can be performed on a seated patient. For both variations, the scapula is manipulated by adducting (medially displacing) the inferior tip using thumb pressure while stabilizing the superior aspect with the other hand.

Posterior dislocation

Posterior dislocation is frequently mentioned in medicolegal reports as it is easy to miss, especially in the unconscious patient. It may result from a fall on the outstretched or internally rotated hand or from a blow from the front. It is also associated with seizures and electrocution injuries, where it is not uncommonly bilateral. The dislocation is usually not apparent on an AP film, so additional views are required. Reduction is performed by traction on the limb in the position of 90° abduction, followed by external rotation. Aftercare is the same as for anterior dislocation.

Posterior dislocation is prone to recurrence. Good functional outcomes are associated with early detection and treatment, a small osseous defect and stability following closed reduction. Poor prognostic factors include late diagnosis, a large anterior defect in the humeral head, deformity or arthrosis of the humeral head, an associated fracture of the proximal part of the humerus and the need for an arthroplasty. The indications for surgery are controversial.

Inferior dislocation (luxatio erecta)

This type of dislocation is rare and usually obvious, as the arm is held in abduction. Neurovascular compromise is a significant risk requiring careful examination and prompt reduction. Reduction is by traction in abduction followed by swinging the arm into adduction. Aftercare is the same as for anterior dislocation.

Controversies

- The role of surgery for midshaft clavicular fractures.
- Optimal treatment for Rockwell type III AC joint disruptions.
- Surgical treatment of scapular fractures.
- Immobilization method after reduction of dislocation of the shoulder.
- The best technique for reduction of anterior dislocation of the shoulder.
- Surgery for first dislocations of the shoulder.

Further reading

Beitzel K, Cote MP, Apostolakos J, et al. Current concepts in the treatment of acromioclavicular joint dislocations. Arthroscopy 2013;29:387–97.

Bicos J, Nicholson GP. Treatment and results of sternoclavicular injuries. Clin J Sport Med 2003;22:359–70.

Canadian Orthopaedic Trauma Society. Non-operative treatment compared with plate fixation of displaced midshaft clavicular fractures. A multi-center randomized clinical trail. J Bone Joint Surg 2007;89A:1–10.

Cole PA, Gauger EM, Schroder LK. Management of scapular fractures. J Am Acad Orthop Surg 2012;20:130–41.

Dannenbuam J, Krueger CA, Johnson A. A review of techniques for anterior glenohumeral joint dislocations. J Spec Oper Med 2012;12:83–92.

Fitch RW, Kuhn JE. Intraarticular lidocaine versus intravenous
    procedural sedation with narcotics and benzodiazepines for
    reduction of the dislocated shoulder: a systematic review.
    Acad Emerg Med 2008;15:703–8.
Kuhn JE. Treating the initial anterior shoulder dislocation – an
    evidence-based medicine approach. Sports Med Arthrosc
    Rev 2006;14:192–8.

Oh LS, Wolf BR, Hall MP, et al. Indications for rotator cuff
    repair: a systematic review. Clin Orthopaed Relat Res
    2007;455:52–63.
Paterson WH, Throckmorton TW, Koester M, et al. Position and
    duration of immobilization after primary anterior shoulder
    dislocation: a systematic review and meta-analysis of the
    literature. J Bone Joint Surg Am 2010;92:2924–33.

Sayegh FE, Kenanisis EI, Papavasiliou KA, et al. Reduction
    of acute anterior dislocations: a prospective randomized
    study comparing a new technique with the Hippocratic
    and Kocher methods. J Bone J Surg Am 2009;91:
    2775–82.
Shoulder reduction techniques. <www.youtube.com/
    watch?v=NXFPWxSTK5c>.

4.2 Fractures of the humerus

Raymond Chi Hung Cheng • Timothy H Rainer

ESSENTIALS

1 Fractures of the proximal humerus occur primarily in the elderly, whereas distal humerus fractures occur more often in children.

2 Falls producing fractures in elderly patients are often precipitated by an underlying medical problem that should be sought and managed.

3 Most proximal humeral fractures do not require surgical intervention.

4 The aim of treatment is to minimize pain, to maximize the return of normal function as soon as possible and to achieve acceptable cosmesis.

5 Humeral shaft fractures, displaced distal humeral fractures and fractures associated with neurovascular compromise require early orthopaedic review.

6 Low-force fractures, especially in the elderly, suggest the presence of osteoporosis. 'At-risk' patients not already identified as having osteoporosis should be referred for bone density scans, vitamin D testing and treatment.

Introduction

The function of the upper limb depends on an intact shoulder girdle that is, in turn, affected by the integrity of muscles, tendons and ligaments, bones, joints, blood vessels and nerves. Fractures of the humerus severely limit efficient function of the upper limb and may be divided into proximal (proximal to the surgical neck), middle (shaft) and distal (supracondylar) segments.

Fractures of the proximal humerus

Patterns of injury

Fractures of the proximal humerus represent 5% of all fractures presenting to emergency departments (ED) and 25% of all humeral fractures. The fracture typically occurs as a result of an indirect mechanism in elderly, osteoporotic patients who fall on their outstretched hand with an extended elbow. The majority do not require surgical intervention and may initially be treated in the ED. A subset with a non-viable humeral head requires early surgical intervention and it is therefore important to identify this group. Fractures of the humerus may also occur in patients with multiple injuries or in the elderly with associated fractures of the neck of femur.

Clinical assessment

Patients typically present soon after injury holding their arm close to the chest wall. They complain of pain and exhibit swelling and tenderness of the shoulder and upper arm. Although crepitus and bruising may occur, the former should not be elicited because it causes excessive and unnecessary pain. Bruising is usually delayed, occurring several days after injury. It appears around the lower arm rather than at the fracture site as a result of gravity and blood tracking distally.

A neurovascular examination is essential as the axillary nerve, brachial plexus and/or axillary artery may be damaged. The axillary nerve is the most commonly injured and presents with altered sensation over the badge area (insertion of the deltoid) and reduced deltoid muscle contraction (which may be hard to assess because of pain). The axillary artery is the commonest vessel to be injured and may present with any combination of limb pain, pallor, paraesthesia, pulselessness and paralysis.

As these injuries frequently occur in elderly patients, careful attention must be paid to the reason for the fall, as an underlying acute medical condition may have precipitated the event and require management in its own right.

Clinical Investigations

Three radiographic views – anteroposterior, lateral and axillary – will allow most proximal humeral fractures to be correctly diagnosed.

Fracture classification

Although the majority of these fractures are easily managed in the ED, the challenge is to differentiate these from the minority that require orthopaedic intervention.

Neer classification system

In this system, fractures are classified first according to the number of the four anatomical sites (humeral head, humeral shaft, greater and lesser tuberosities) that were involved in the injury; second, according to the degree of fracture displacement, defined as 1 cm separation or >45° angulation (Figs 4.2.1 and 4.2.2).

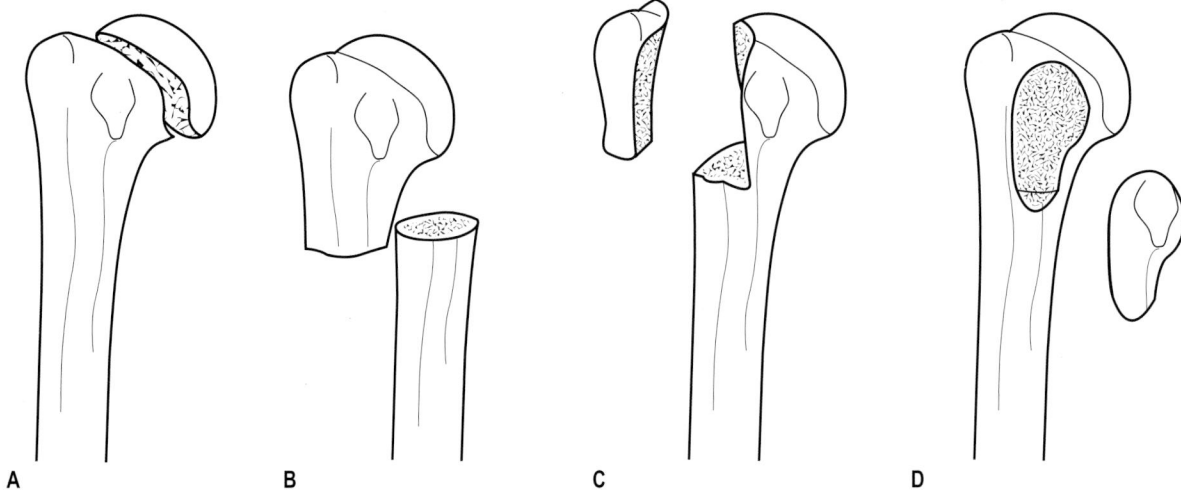

Fig. 4.2.1 Neer classification with two-part fractures of **(A)** the anatomical neck, **(B)** the surgical neck, **(C)** the greater tuberosity and **(D)** the lesser tuberosity.

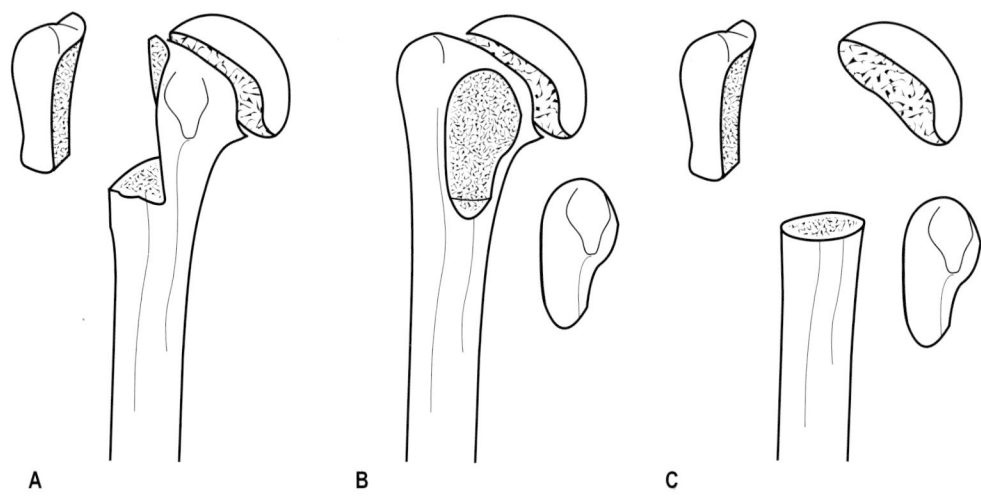

Fig. 4.2.2 Neer classification with three-part fractures of **(A)** the greater tuberosity and anatomical neck, **(B)** the lesser tuberosity and anatomical neck and **(C)** four-part fracture involving the anatomical neck, greater tuberosity and lesser tuberosity.

One-part fracture One-part fractures account for 80% of proximal humeral fractures. Any number of fracture lines may exist, but none are significantly displaced.

Two-part fracture Two-part fractures account for 10% of proximal humeral fractures and one fragment is significantly displaced or angulated. Two-part fractures of the humerus may involve the anatomical neck (see Fig. 4.2.1A), the surgical neck (see Fig. 4.2.1B), the greater tuberosity (see Fig. 4.2.1C) or the lesser tuberosity (see Fig. 4.2.1D).

Three- and four-part fractures Three- and four-part fractures account for the remaining 10% of proximal humeral fractures, with

two or three significantly displaced or angulated fragments (see Fig. 4.2.2A–C).

Treatment
One-part fractures and two-part fractures can be treated with a collar and cuff sling, adequate analgesia and follow up. Early mobilization is important and the prognosis is good.

Definitive management of the displaced fragment in two-part fractures may include open or closed reduction depending upon neurovascular injury, rotator cuff integrity, associated dislocations, likelihood of union and function. Early orthopaedic assessment is recommended.

For three- and four-part fractures, the consensus is for open reduction and internal

fixation. However, a review has suggested that there is little evidence that surgery is superior to the non-operative approach.

For displaced proximal humeral fractures, surgical management remains varied and controversial. A recent systematic review suggested that non-operative treatment of proximal humerus fractures has a high rate of radiological healing, good functional outcomes but a lower complication rate when compared with the operative approach. Small, randomized controlled trials suggest that external fixation may confer some benefit over closed manipulation and that conservative treatment is better than tension band osteosynthesis. Another study suggests that the decision should be made according to the viability of the humeral head. Locking plate technology may also provide better outcomes in patients with unstable displaced humeral fractures having a viable humeral head. Other small-scale studies suggest that some bandaging styles may be better than others and that early physiotherapy may improve functional outcome.

Special cases

Fracture of the anatomical neck and articular surface

Fractures at these sites are uncommon, but are important to recognize as they have a high incidence of compromised blood supply to the articular segment, may result in avascular necrosis and may require a humeral hemiarthroplasty.

Fracture dislocations

Fractures of the greater tuberosity accompany 15% of anterior glenohumeral dislocations and may be associated with rotator cuff tears. Although the fracture may be grossly displaced, reduction of the dislocated shoulder usually also reduces the fracture. In patients who require the full range of movement of their shoulders, surgical repair of the cuff may be required.

Fractures of the lesser tuberosity are associated with posterior glenohumeral dislocations.

Disposition

Most patients with undisplaced one- and two-part fractures may be discharged from the ED with a collar and cuff sling, analgesia, early mobilization and appropriate follow up. High-risk cases, including displaced three- and four-part fractures, all open fractures and the special proximal humeral fractures described above, require orthopaedic consultation and admission, as do those with medical problems requiring investigation or treatment.

Low-energy fractures, especially in the elderly, suggest the presence of osteoporosis. 'At-risk' patients not already identified as having osteoporosis should be referred for bone density scans, vitamin D testing and treatment.

Fractures of the shaft of humerus

Patterns of injury

Fractures of the humeral shaft commonly occur in the third decade (active young men) and in the seventh decade of life (osteoporotic elderly women). The commonest site is the middle third, which accounts for 60% of humeral fractures. The close proximity of the fracture to the radial nerve and brachial artery commonly leads to neurovascular deficits.

Direct blows tend to produce transverse fractures, whereas falls on the outstretched hand produce torsion forces and hence spiral fractures. Combinations of the two mechanisms may produce a butterfly segment. Pathological fractures are also common, most resulting from metastatic breast cancer.

The angle and degree of displacement of the fracture depends on the site of injury and its relationship to the action and attachment of muscles on either side of the injury (Fig. 4.2.3).

Clinical assessment

Patients typically present complaining of pain and supporting the forearm of the injured limb, flexed at the elbow, and held close to the chest wall. Examination of the limb reveals tenderness, swelling, shortening and possibly deformity. The skin should be assessed for tension or disruption and particular attention should be paid to the shoulder and elbow regions for associated fractures or dislocations. Initial and post-reduction assessments of the brachial artery and vein and ulnar, median and radial nerves are essential.

The commonest complication is radial nerve injury resulting either from the injury itself or reduction of the fracture and is evidenced by wrist drop and altered sensation in the first dorsal web space. A recent systemic review reported that radial nerve injury occurs in 11% of midshaft humerus fractures.

Clinical investigations

Two radiographic views – anteroposterior and lateral – will allow the correct diagnosis in most cases.

Treatment and disposition

Uncomplicated, closed fractures account for the majority of injuries and may be treated

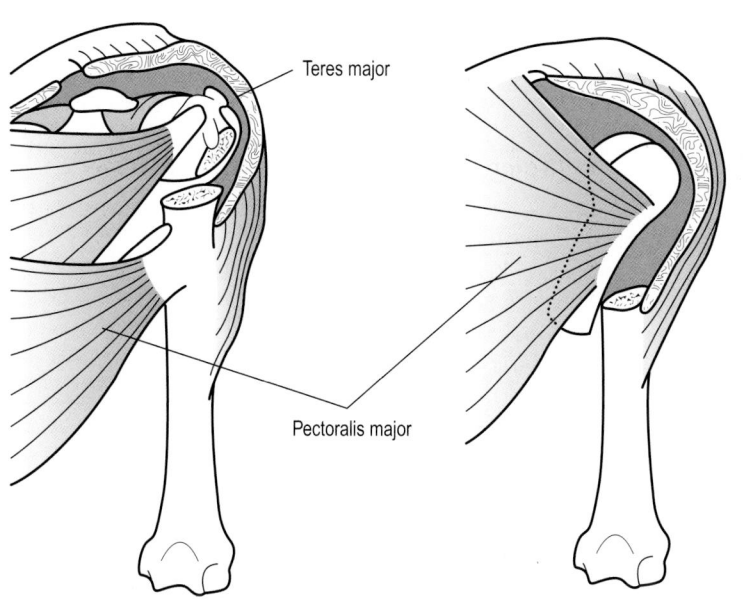
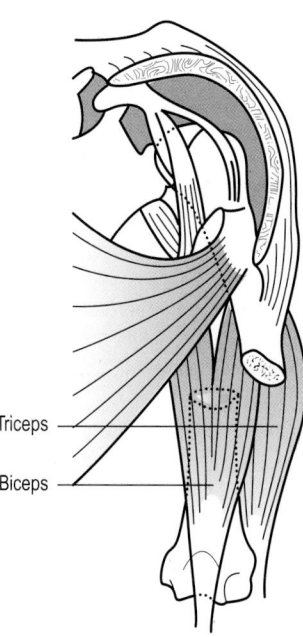

Fig. 4.2.3 Relationships between humeral fracture site and the actions of inserting muscles determine bony angulation and displacement.

conservatively by immobilization and analgesia. Immobilization can be by a hanging cast, U-shaped cast or with functional bracing and a broad arm or collar and cuff sling. The acceptable deformity is 20° anterior/posterior angulation and 30° valus/valgus deformity. The rate of fracture union is usually higher than 90%. Early specialist follow up is recommended.

Some authors prefer a functional humeral brace rather than U-shaped plaster for immobilization, as the former may permit greater functional use without affecting healing or fracture alignment. For oblique/spiral fractures, some orthopaedic surgeons prefer an operative approach for a better functional outcome.

Open fractures and complications affecting the vessels require surgical repair. Although the majority of radial nerve injuries are neuropraxia and recover without surgical intervention, each case should be considered individually by an orthopaedic surgeon with a view to possible operative exploration.

Fractures of the distal humerus

Classification and patterns of injury

Unlike in children, fractures of the distal humerus in adults are very uncommon and patterns of injury tend to reflect the anatomical two-column construction (condyles) of the humerus. Several classification methods have been used, such as the Riseborough and Radin, Mehne and Matta classifications, but the simplest and most commonly used are the AO/ASIF classifications. These classify injuries into three categories: type A are extra-articular fractures, type B are partial articular and type C are complete articular fractures. Practically, distal humeral fractures may be classified into supracondylar, intercondylar and other types. Supracondylar fractures lie transversely, whereas intercondylar T or Y fractures include an additional vertical extension between the condyles.

Mechanisms of injury usually involve a direct blow to the flexed or extended elbow. In the former, the olecranon is driven upwards, thereby either splitting the condyles apart producing a 'T' or a 'Y' pattern, or shearing off one condyle.

Clinical assessment

Patients typically present with a swollen, tender, deformed elbow. As very little subcutaneous or other tissue separates the bone from skin, any disruption of the skin should be carefully examined for the possibility of a compound fracture. Distal neurological and vascular injury must be assessed carefully, as the possibility of nerve injury has been reported to be as high as 12–20%.

Clinical investigations

Two radiographic views – anteroposterior and lateral – should be obtained. Some authors suggest that an internal oblique view may improve the diagnostic accuracy. Pain and inability to extend the elbow often result in poor-quality radiographs. Although high-quality radiographs are essential for operative planning, repeat films should not be attempted in the ED as they rarely provide the desired result. When there is any suspicion of severe injury, either from the history or from gross soft-tissue swelling, early computed tomography (CT) scanning should be considered to give better detail, especially of intra-articular fractures.

Undisplaced fractures may not be visible on radiography but may be suggested by posterior or anterior fat pad signs, which result from fat displaced by an underlying haemarthrosis. Ultrasonography, CT and magnetic resonance imaging may all improve diagnostic precision. They alter management and improve outcome in patients with occult fractures, mostly of the intra-articular type.

Treatment and disposition

Uncomplicated, undisplaced, closed fractures with minimal swelling should be immobilized for 3 weeks in 90° flexion with an above-elbow cast and a broad arm sling, followed by active mobilization.

Patients with severe swelling, compound fractures, displaced fractures or neurovascular compromise require orthopaedic intervention.

Controversies

- For humeral shaft fractures, it is unclear whether hanging plasters or functional braces are better than U-shaped plasters for fracture healing and position.
- Although the union rate of humeral shaft fracture treated with bracing method is high, the functional outcomes after brace treatment are still under investigation.
- Low-intensity pulsed ultrasound may be useful in the treatment of non-union. Whether it may enhance normal fracture healing is not known.
- The role of magnetic resonance imaging in the diagnosis of bone bruising and humeral fracture has not been studied.

Further reading

Camden P, Nade S. Fracture bracing the humerus. Injury 1992;23:245–8.

Diana JN, Ramsey ML. Decision making in complex fractures of the distal humerus: current concepts and potential pitfalls. Orthopaed J 1998;11:12–18.

Handol HHG, Madhok R. Interventions for treating proximal humeral fractures in adults. Cochrane Database Syst Rev 2003;4:CD000434.

Iyengar JJ, Devcic Z, Sproul RC, et al. Nonoperative treatment of proximal humerus fractures: a systematic review. J Orthopaed Trauma 2011;25:612–7.

Mulhall KJ, Ahmed A, Khan Y, Masterson E. Simultaneous hip and upper limb fracture in the elderly: incidence, features and management considerations. Injury 2002;33:29–31.

Ramachandran M, Birch R, Eastwood DM. Clinical outcome of nerve injuries associated with supracondylar fractures of the humerus in children, the experience of a specialist referral centre. J Bone Joint Surg 2006;88B:90–4.

Ring D, Chin K, Taghinia AH, Jupiter JB. Nonunion after functional brace treatment of diaphyseal humerus fractures. J Trauma 2007;62:1157–8.

Rommens PM, Heyvaert G. Conservative treatment of subcapital humerus fractures. Comparative study of the classical Desault bandage and the new Gilchrist bandage. Unfallchirurgie 1993;19:114–8.

Shao YC, Harwood P, Grotz MRW, et al. Radial nerve palsy associated with fractures of the shaft of the humerus: a systematic review. J Bone Joint Surg 2005;87B:1647–52.

Vallier HA. Treatment of proximal humerus fractures. J Orthopaed Trauma 2008;21:469–76.

Weber E, Matter P. Surgical treatment of proximal humerus fractures – an international multicenter study [In German]. Swiss Surg 1998;4:95–100.

Zyto K, Ahrengart L, Sperber A, Tornkvist H. Treatment of displaced proximal humeral fractures in elderly patients. J Bone Joint Surg 1999;79:412–7.

4.3 Dislocations of the elbow

Raymond Chi Hung Cheng • Timothy H Rainer

ESSENTIALS

1 Elbow dislocations are the third most common large joint dislocation.

2 Surgical intervention is rarely required for simple elbow dislocations.

3 Surgical intervention may be required when fractures of the radius, ulnar and humerus are associated with elbow dislocation or when neurovascular injury occurs.

4 The commonest neurovascular complication involves the ulnar nerve.

5 After reducing elbow dislocations, it is important to reassess joint stability and potential neurovascular complications.

Introduction

Elbow dislocation, along with glenohumeral and patellofemoral joint dislocations, is one of the three most common large joint dislocations. The elbow joint is a hinge-like articulation involving the distal humerus and proximal radius and ulna. Owing to its strong muscular and ligamentous supports, the joint is normally quite stable and rarely requires operative intervention, even for acute instability after dislocation.

Elbow dislocations can be classified as either anterior or posterior. Posterior dislocation is the most common type and can be further divided into posteromedial or posterolateral. It usually results from a fall on the outstretched hand with some degree of flexion or hyperextension at the elbow. The radius and ulna commonly dislocate together. Similarly, anterior dislocation can also be divided into anteromedial or anterolateral. This type is less common and is usually due to a direct blow to the dorsal side of the elbow.

Uncommonly, the radius or ulna alone may dislocate at the elbow. In such cases, there is always a fracture of the other bone. One common example is in Monteggia fractures, where anterior or posterior radio-humeral dislocation occurs alongside a fracture of the proximal one third of the ulna shaft (Fig. 4.3.1). A rarer example is a posterior ulna-humeral dislocation with fracture of the radial shaft. So, although elbow dislocations may appear to be isolated, it is essential to look for associated intra-articular or shaft fractures.

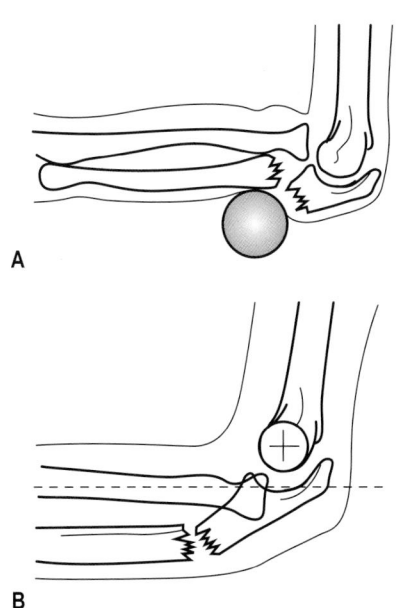

Fig. 4.3.1 Monteggia fracture dislocation. Fracture of the ulnar shaft may be associated with (A) anterior radio-humeral dislocation or (B) posterior radio-humeral dislocation.

Clinical assessment

History and examination

Patients typically present holding the lower arm at 45° to the upper arm and there is swelling, tenderness and deformity of the elbow joint. The three-point anatomical triangle of olecranon, medial and lateral epicondyles should be assessed for abnormal alignment, as this strongly suggests dislocation.

The commonest neurovascular injury involves the ulnar nerve, reported in 10–15% of elbow dislocations, but the median and radial nerves and the brachial artery may also be affected.

The differential diagnosis is a complex distal humerus fracture which, in a swollen elbow, may be hard to differentiate clinically from an elbow dislocation.

Clinical investigations

Anteroposterior and lateral radiographic views should be obtained and scrutinized for associated fractures of the coronoid process, radial head, capitellum and olecranon.

Magnetic resonance imaging (MRI) characterizes bony injury more accurately than radiography in children with elbow injuries, but its potential role for diagnosis and guiding management in adults has not been well evaluated. Duplex Doppler ultrasound can be use to identify early brachial artery injury.

Treatment

Simple dislocation can be reduced using a closed method. With adequate sedation, gentle traction and counter-traction, the joint relocates quite easily. Medial and posterolateral dislocations may also require sideways correction. Dislocation of the stable elbow joint produces severe soft-tissue injury and resultant instability, therefore, after reduction, signs and symptoms of compartment syndrome should be sought.

Joint instability should be tested by valgus and varus testing and by lateral pivot-shift test. The reduced elbow joint should move smoothly. Any crepitation or resistance, particularly during the mid-range, suggests incongruent reduction or soft tissue interposition, which is commonly associated with coronoid process or epicondylar fractures. Inability to fully flex or extend the elbow suggests a loose bone or cartilaginous fragment or a capsular tear.

Post-reduction films should be assessed, not only for correct joint relocation, but also for associated fractures. After successful reduction, the elbow should be placed in a posterior plaster slab in 90° of flexion. Cylinder casts are contraindicated because of the likelihood of severe soft-tissue swelling.

There is little evidence that surgical intervention improves outcome in patients with medial or lateral elbow instability after dislocation. A recent systematic review found that there is no difference in outcome between surgical repair of the ligament and plaster immobilization for simple elbow dislocation. Patients with functional treatment have a better range of movement, less pain, better functional scores, shorter disability and shorter treatment time when compared with plaster immobilization. The management of Monteggia fracture-dislocation is discussed in Chapter 4.4. Compound fracture dislocation should be reduced by the open method. Patients with irreducible dislocations, neurovascular complications, associated fractures or open dislocations require orthopaedic intervention.

Ulnar nerve injuries can occur both before and after closed reduction. The reported rate varies between 10 and 15%. Most of them are neuropraxia and will recover with conservative measures. The most sensitive sign and symptoms are numbness over the little fingers.

Disposition

Current practice is that most patients may be discharged from the emergency department with analgesia, pressure bandage for stable joints and plaster immobilization for unstable joints. A broad arm sling with appropriate follow up should be arranged after reduction.

A recent prospective, randomized study suggested that early mobilization is superior to plaster immobilization in terms of functional recovery, without any increased instability or a recurrence of dislocation for patients with uncomplicated posterior dislocations. The duration of immobilization should not be longer then 14 days to prevent joint stiffness. Patients with irreducible dislocations, neurovascular complications, associated fractures or open dislocations require admission.

Controversies

- There are no large-scale randomized studies comparing operative and non-operative management of elbow dislocation. It is therefore unclear whether one method may produce better outcomes than another.
- Early mobilization may be superior to prolonged plaster immobilization after reduction of uncomplicated posterior dislocations.
- The epidemiology of elbow injury, including dislocation in patients presenting to emergency departments, has not been well described and requires further studies.
- Roles for computed tomography and magnetic resonance imaging in evaluating acute elbow injury and influencing management require further study.

Further reading

Ergunes K, Yilik L, Ozsoyler I, et al. Traumatic brachial artery injuries. Texas Heart Inst J 2006;33:31–4.

Griffiths JF, Roebuck DJ, Cheng JCY, et al. Comparison of radiography and magnetic resonance imaging in the detection of injuries after paediatric elbow trauma. Am J Roentgenol 2001;176:53–60.

Haan JD, Schep NWL, Tuinebreijer WE, et al. Simple elbow dislocations: a systematic review of the literature. Arch Orthopaed Trauma Surg 2010;130:241–9.

Lam TP, Ng BKW, Ma RF. Cheng JCY. Monteggia fractures in children – a review of 30 cases. J Jap Pediatr Orthoped Assoc 2004;13:193–5.

McRae R. Practical fracture treatment. Edinburgh: Churchill Livingstone; 1994.

Partio EK, Hirvensalo E, Bostman O, Rokkanen P. A prospective controlled trial of the fracture of the humeral medial epicondyle – how to treat? Ann Chirurg Gynaecol 1996;85:67–71.

Rafai M, Largab A, Cohen D, Trafeh M. Pure posterior luxation of the elbow in adults: immobilization or early mobilization. A randomized prospective study of 50 cases. Chirurg Main 1999;18:272–8.

Reynders P, De Groote W, Rondia J, et al. Monteggia lesions in adults. A multi-centre Bota study. Acta Orthopaed Belg 1996;62:78–83.

Robert S, David R. Current concepts review: the ulnar nerve in elbow trauma. J Bone Joint Surg 2007;89A:1108–16.

Uehara DT, Chin HW. Injuries to the elbow and forearm. In: Tintinalli JE, Kelen GD, Stapczynski JS, editors. Emergency medicine. A comprehensive study guide. New York: McGraw-Hill, 2000, p. 1763–72.

Willet K. Upper limb injuries. In: Skinner D, Swain A, Peyton R, Robertson C, editors. Cambridge textbook of accident and emergency medicine. Cambridge: Cambridge University Press, 1997, p. 601–17.

4.4 Fractures of the forearm and carpal bones

Crispijn van den Brand

ESSENTIALS

1 Forearm fractures are among the most common fractures seen in the emergency department (ED).

2 When assessing the need for or success of reduction, the external appearance of the limb is a key feature.

3 Median nerve function must be assessed before and after reduction of all distal radial fractures.

4 Splinting or functional bracing may be sufficient for stable fractures. Early movement and load bearing aids functional recovery.

5 General indications for orthopaedic referral include fractures which are compound, unstable, associated with intra-articular or neurovascular injury and those that have failed reduction in the ED.

6 Displaced, isolated fractures of the ulna or radius may be associated with a dislocation of the radius or ulna respectively (Monteggia and Galeazzi fracture dislocations). These should be carefully sought, as there is high risk of long-term disability.

7 Significant or persistent symptoms with the absence of a visible fracture on plain X-ray may be due to an undetected fracture or significant soft-tissue injury. A high index of suspicion and early review are recommended. Further investigation with bone scintigraphy, CT or MRI may be indicated.

Radial head fractures

Clinical features

History

Radial head fractures occur frequently, usually as a result of a fall onto an outstretched hand or, less frequently, following a direct blow to the lateral side of the elbow. Radial head fractures present with pain and restricted movement at the elbow.

Examination

Usually, there is swelling and tenderness over the radial head. Sometimes, with more subtle injuries, rotating the forearm while palpating the radial head may be necessary to elicit tenderness. Elbow extension and forearm rotation are limited. Severely comminuted fractures may have proximal displacement of the radius,

which can be associated with disruption of the interosseous membrane and subluxation of the distal radioulnar joint (Essex–Lopresti fracture dislocation).

Clinical investigations

Imaging

Standard anteroposterior (AP) and lateral X-rays of the elbow are required. A radiocapitellar view may be necessary if the fracture is subtle. The presence of an anterior fat pad sign alone on X-ray is associated with an underlying radial head or neck fracture in up to 50% of patients. In this case, a fracture should be assumed to be present if there is an appropriate mechanism and local signs. A follow-up X-ray or computed tomography (CT) scan is indicated only in the presence or persistent pain, stiffness or locking.

Classification

Radial head fractures are usually classified according to the (modified) Mason classification (Fig. 4.4.1). About two-thirds of fractures are Mason type I.

The Mason classification is as follows:

- Mason type I, displaced less than 2 mm
- Mason type II, displacement more than 2 mm
- Mason type III, comminuted fractures of the entire radial head
- Mason type IV, radial head fracture with associated elbow dislocation.

Treatment

All non-displaced (type I) radial head fractures and those type II fractures without mechanical block may be managed with a bandage and sling. Mobilization should be started as early as possible. If there is severe pain, a posterior splint may be useful but should not be applied for more than 2 days. Prognosis is good, but full extension may not be possible for many months.

Displaced or complex radial head fractures (type II or III) may be treated in the acute setting with a sling or posterior splint. These patients should have early orthopaedic review (within days). The treatment of displaced or complex radial head fractures remains controversial and should be determined by an orthopaedic surgeon.

Mechanical block can be difficult to assess acutely due to pain. Intra-articular injection of bupivacaine may assist early assessment or assessment may be deferred until pain has settled. Surgical options include open reduction and internal fixation and excision of the radial head with or without implantation of a prosthesis.

Radial neck fractures with up to 20° tilts can be managed conservatively. More severe tilt can be reduced using intra-articular local anaesthesia. The forearm is pronated until the most prominent part of the radial head is felt. Then traction is applied to the forearm and pressure applied to the radial head. Open

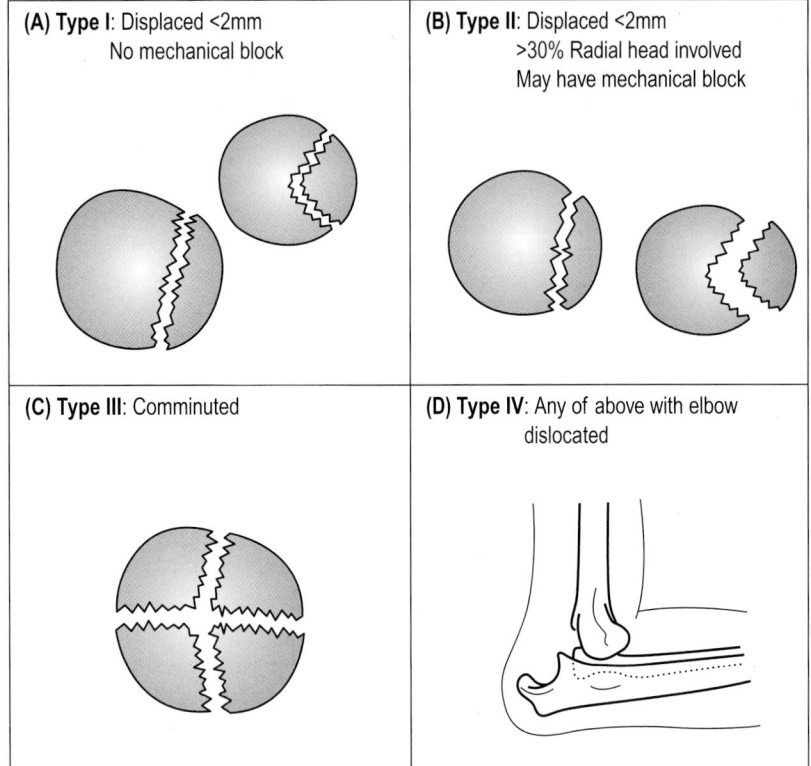

(A) **Type I**: Displaced <2mm
No mechanical block

(B) **Type II**: Displaced <2mm
>30% Radial head involved
May have mechanical block

(C) **Type III**: Comminuted

(D) **Type IV**: Any of above with elbow dislocated

Fig. 4.4.1 (A–D) Mason–Hotchkiss classification of radial head fractures.

reduction is indicated if closed methods fail or displacement is severe.

Complications

Neurovascular complications and compartment syndrome are uncommon. Most complications relate to disturbance of the relationships of the proximal radio-ulnar and radiocapitellar articular surfaces causing limitation of movement. This is uncommon with minor fractures.

Shaft fractures

Clinical features

History

This type of injury requires great force, typically from a motor-vehicle accident, a fall from a height or a direct blow. These fractures are commonly open and nearly always displaced.

Examination

The forearm is swollen and tender and may be angulated and rotated. Examination looking for an open wound, local neurovascular compromise, compartment syndrome or musculotendinous injury is required. Given the mechanism of injury, other injuries should also be sought.

Clinical investigations

Imaging

AP and lateral X-rays of the forearm, including the wrist and elbow joints, are needed. Displacement and angulation are easily determined, but torsional deformity may be subtle. Because the ulna and radius are rectangular in cross-section rather than circular, a change in bone width at the fracture site indicates rotation. The radial and ulnar styloid processes normally point in opposite directions to the bicipital tuberosity and coronoid process, respectively. A change in this alignment also suggests torsion.

Treatment

Adult forearm fractures are less stable than those in children and lack of remodelling limits tolerance to incomplete reduction. Undisplaced fractures may be managed with an above-elbow cast, but must be reviewed at 1 week for displacement and angulation. Most fractures, however, are displaced and require open reduction and internal fixation.

Complications

Early complications include wound infection, osteomyelitis, neurovascular injury and compartment syndrome. Later, non-union, malunion, reduced forearm rotation and reflex sympathetic dystrophy are possible complications.

Specific fracture types

Isolated fracture of the ulnar shaft

These fractures are due to a direct blow to the ulna, often when raised in defence; hence they are also known as 'nightstick' fractures. Patients present with localized pain and swelling. AP and lateral X-rays delineate the location of the fracture and degree of angulation. Look for associated dislocation of the radial head if displacement is present (Monteggia fracture dislocation).

Fractures displaced less than 50% of the ulna width heal well with a non-union rate of 0–4%. Traditional treatment involves fixing the forearm in mid-pronation with a plaster cast, extended above elbow if the middle or proximal thirds of the ulna are fractured. The cast is removed once union occurs, usually in about 8 weeks. Other proven options include a below-elbow plaster (BEPOP) for proximal fractures, early mobilization with bandage after 1–2 weeks in BEPOP or functional bracing after 3–5 days, which allows movement at wrist and elbow.

Fractures with more than 10° of angulation or displaced more than 50% of the diameter of the ulna require surgical intervention.

Monteggia fracture dislocation

This is a rare fracture of the proximal ulna with dislocation of the radial head. It occurs either through a fall onto the outstretched hand with hyperpronation or through a force applied to the posterior aspect of the proximal ulna. Patients present with pain, swelling and reduced elbow movement. The forearm may appear shortened and the radial head may be palpable in the antecubital fossa. Associated posterior interosseous nerve injury is common.

On X-ray the fracture is obvious, but the dislocation is commonly missed. Check that a line through the radial shaft bisects the capitellum on both views. There are four types of Monteggia fracture depending upon displacement of the radial head (Bado classification). Dislocation is anterior in 60% (Bado type I), but may be lateral or posterior.

All Monteggia fractures require open reduction and internal fixation. Common complications include malunion and non-union of the ulnar fracture and an unstable radial head.

AP view of wrist

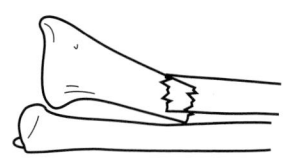

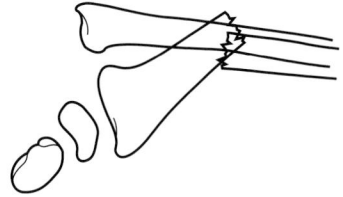

Fig. 4.4.2 The Galeazzi fracture dislocation.

Isolated radial shaft fracture

Isolated fractures of the proximal two-thirds of the radial shaft are uncommon and are usually displaced. Rare undisplaced fractures can be treated similarly to isolated ulnar shaft fractures. Displaced fractures require open reduction and internal fixation.

Galeazzi fracture dislocation

Fractures of the distal third of the radial shaft occur as a result of a fall onto the outstretched hand or a direct blow. There may be an associated subluxation or dislocation of the distal radioulnar joint (DRUJ), known as the Galeazzi fracture dislocation. Patients have pain and swelling at the radial fracture site. Those with a Galeazzi injury will also have pain and swelling at the DRUJ and a prominent ulnar head.

X-rays show the radial fracture, which is tilted ventrolaterally. Widening of the DRUJ space on the AP X-ray and dorsal displacement of the ulnar head on the lateral X-ray are seen (Fig. 4.4.2). An ulnar styloid fracture is seen in 60% of cases.

All Galeazzi fracture dislocations require surgical management. Complications include malunion or non-union of the radial fracture and subsequent instability of the DRUJ.

Fractures of the distal radius and ulna

Fractures of the distal radius and ulna are common, particularly in children and elderly women. Fractures in the latter group are indications for evaluation of bone-mineral density.

Clinical features

History and examination

Fractures usually occur after a fall onto the outstretched hand resulting in bending, shearing or impaction forces being applied to the distal metaphysis, or from a direct blow. Patients present with pain, tenderness and variable degrees of swelling and deformity. It is important to examine for associated injuries to carpal bones, radial and ulnar shafts, elbow and shoulder joints, for median nerve injury, vascular compromise and for extensor tendon injury.

Clinical investigations

Imaging

Anteroposterior and lateral X-rays of the wrist demonstrate most injuries. For patients with significant symptoms or signs and a normal X-ray, consider an occult undisplaced fracture or ligamentous injury.

Although this chapter uses eponymous names, it is important to be aware that orthopaedic circles have moved to more formal classification systems for distal radial fractures. Several have been proposed and are beyond the scope of this text. The author recommends being familiar with anatomical descriptions and fracture features associated with need for reduction, instability of reduction and indications for operative intervention.

Treatment

Management

Prompt attention to analgesia, splinting and elevation is essential while awaiting X-rays.

Reduction is indicated in the following circumstances to improve long-term function:

- visible deformity of the wrist
- loss of volar tilt of the distal radial articular surface beyond neutral
- loss of >5° of the radial inclination of the distal radius (normally approximately 20°)
- intra-articular step of >2 mm
- radial shortening >2–3 mm.

Greater deformity can be accepted in low-demand, elderly patients.

Anaesthetic options for reduction include haematoma block, Bier's block and procedural sedation. Reduction is traditionally maintained with an encircling plaster cast moulded to oppose displacement forces and extending from volar metacarpal crease to proximal forearm for 6 weeks. Displaced or comminuted fractures at high risk of swelling, especially

in the elderly or coagulopathic patients, are immobilized with non-encircling splints.

Factors associated with instability of the distal fragment and failure to maintain reduction include:

- intra-articular component (especially involving the distal radio-ulnar joint)
- shearing fractures (Barton-, Hutchinson's type)
- palmarly displaced fractures (Smith type)
- the magnitude of the initial displacement or comminution.

Weekly X-rays for 2–3 weeks with orthopaedic follow up are recommended for all displaced fractures, those with intra-articular extension and potentially unstable fractures.

Stable, undisplaced, extra-articular fractures can be managed more conservatively with splinting and referral to a family doctor for early mobilization after 4 weeks.

Indications for operative management are debated, but should be considered for:

- comminuted, displaced, intra-articular fractures
- open fractures
- associated carpal fractures
- associated neurovascular or tendon injury
- failed conservative treatment (failed reduction or unstable after reduction)
- bilateral fractures/impaired contralateral extremity.

Complications

Median nerve injury may occur acutely due to the injury, as a result of reduction or later due to pressure effects from the plaster. Median nerve function must be documented before and after reduction.

Loss of reduction may require delayed surgical intervention. Malunion with chronic wrist pain, arthritis and secondary radioulnar and radiocarpal instability are associated with intra-articular extension of the fracture.

Long-term complications include osteoarthritis, residual disability and complex regional pain syndrome (CRPS). The incidence of CRPS following distal radius fractures ranges in the literature from less than 1% to 22%. Prophylactic vitamin C may reduce the incidence of CRPS, the advised dose is 500 mg/day for 50 days.

Specific fractures

Colles' fracture

Colles' fracture is a metaphyseal bending fracture. The wrist has a classic 'dinner-fork' appearance, often with significant swelling of the soft tissues. This appearance is reflected in the radiographs (Fig. 4.4.3). There is often associated damage to the radio-ulnar fibrocartilage. There may be comminution, commonly dorsally, which can extend into the radiocarpal or radio-ulnar joints.

The aim of reduction is to restore radial length, volar tilt and radial angulation. A minimum of 0° tilt is acceptable if full reduction is not possible. Reduction is achieved by first disimpacting the fracture with traction in the line of the forearm. If this fails, traction in extension or hyperextension should be tried. Volar tilt is then restored with volar pressure over the dorsum of the distal fragment while traction is maintained. Lastly, correct radial tilt and radial displacement with ulnar pressure over the radial side of the distal fragment. Reduction is successful in 87%, but almost two-thirds lose reduction over 5 weeks, most of this occurring during cast immobilization.

The commonly accepted cast immobilization position is with the wrist joint in 15° palmar flexion, 10–15° ulnar deviation and slight pronation. However, some evidence suggests

AP view of wrist

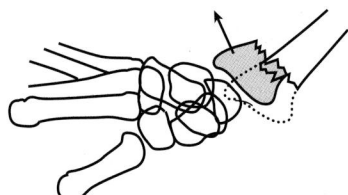

Lateral view of wrist

Fig. 4.4.3 Colles' fracture. A fracture of the distal radial metaphysis with six classic deformities. The lateral view shows dorsal angulation, dorsal displacement and impaction. The AP view reveals radial displacement, ulnar angulation and an ulnar styloid fracture.

better outcomes are achieved with the wrist in dorsiflexion and mid-supination. The cast must be carefully moulded over the dorsum of the distal fragment and the anteromedial forearm. Functional bracing allowing wrist movement has also shown good outcomes.

Smith's fracture
This metaphyseal bending fracture of the distal radius occurs through a direct blow or fall onto the back of the hand or a fall backward onto the outstretched hand in supination.

AP and lateral X-rays of the wrist show a 'reverse Colles' fracture' with a similar AP appearance, but with volar displacement and tilt on the lateral X-ray view.

Closed reduction to achieve anatomical radial length and volar tilt should be attempted. Traction is first applied to restore length, followed by dorsal pressure over the volar surface of the distal radius to reverse displacement and angulation. A full above-elbow cast is applied with the wrist in supination and dorsiflexion to prevent loss of reduction. However, most Smith's fractures are unstable and require operative management. Early orthopaedic follow up is mandatory.

Barton's fracture
Barton's fractures are dorsal or volar intra-articular fractures of the distal radial rim (Fig. 4.4.4). The mechanisms of injury are similar to those seen with Colles' and Smith's fractures, respectively. There is often significant soft-tissue injury and the carpus is usually dislocated or subluxed along with the distal

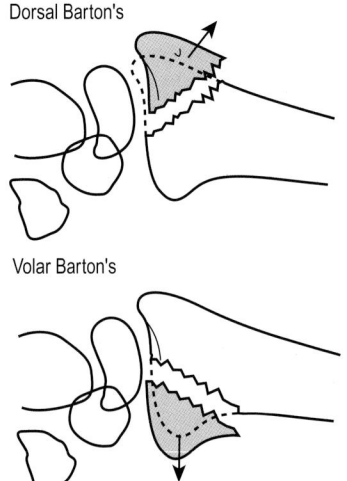

Dorsal Barton's

Volar Barton's

Fig. 4.4.4 Barton's fractures demonstrated on lateral views of the wrist.

AP view of wrist

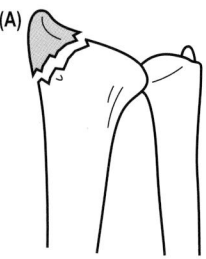

(A)

Fig. 4.4.5 Radial styloid (Hutchison's or chauffeur's) fracture.

fragment. These fractures are complicated by arthritis of the radiocarpal joints and carpal instability.

Minimally displaced fractures involving less than 50% of the joint surface and without carpal displacement may be reduced along the lines of a Colles' or Smith's fracture. Immobilization should occur with wrist flexed for dorsal Barton's and extended for volar Barton's. However, most fractures are unstable and potentially disabling, requiring early operative management, especially in younger patients. Early orthopaedic follow up is mandatory.

Radial styloid (Hutchison's or chauffeur's) fracture
This oblique intra-articular fracture of the radial styloid is caused by a direct blow or fall onto the hand. Displacement is associated with carpal instability and long-term arthritis. The fracture is seen best on AP X-rays of the wrist (Fig. 4.4.5). Undisplaced fractures can be treated with a cast for 4–6 weeks. Displaced fractures should be referred to an orthopaedic surgeon for anatomical reduction and fixation.

Ulnar styloid fracture
An isolated fracture can occur through forced radial deviation, dorsiflexion, rotation or a direct blow. Avulsion fractures involving the lesser portion of the ulnar styloid are not associated with significant instability of the distal radio-ulnar joint (DRUJ). In contrast, fractures involving the base of the ulnar styloid disrupt the major stabilizing ligaments of the distal ulna and the triangular fibrocartilage complex (TFCC) and may lead to subsequent DRUJ instability. Fractures should be treated with a splint or cast with the wrist in mid-supination and ulnar deviation, patients should be referred to an orthopaedic surgeon to assess DRUJ stability.

Carpal fractures and dislocations

Carpal fractures predominantly occur in young men. The bones in the proximal carpal row are more commonly involved, especially scaphoid fractures which account for 82–89% of all carpal fractures. Most other isolated carpal fractures are triquetral fractures. Management depends on the degree of displacement and damage and stability. Generally, undisplaced fractures with minimal comminution can be managed by cast immobilization. Given the importance of wrist function, early orthopaedic review should be sought for patients with displaced or comminuted fractures or where instability or an associated carpal dislocation is suspected.

Specific fractures

Scaphoid fracture

The most common mechanism of injury is a fall on the outstretched hand with the wrist in radial deviation. This mechanism also puts the distal radius and the scaphoid-lunatum (SL) ligament at risk. Clinical features include wrist pain and local swelling and tenderness over the scaphoid, palpated dorsally or via the anatomical snuffbox. Imaging with AP, lateral and scaphoid views will detect at most 70% of all scaphoid fractures.

Fractures of the scaphoid are classified by their location (proximal third, waist, distal third or tubercle) and by their stability. Stable fractures are undisplaced with little comminution and unstable fractures are displaced with considerable comminution. Stable fractures are generally treated with a below-elbow cast for 10–12 weeks. There is no evidence that cast immobilization with inclusion of the thumb leads to better outcome. Unstable fractures require surgical intervention. Complications include non-union and avascular necrosis of the proximal segment.

Some patients have clinical features suggestive of scaphoid fracture without confirmatory X-ray evidence. In the past, cast immobilization for 1–2 weeks followed by repeat X-ray was advocated. Although this is still advocated by some, it is not recommended. The additional sensitivity is low and scaphoid fractures are often missed. A number of alternative diagnostic approaches have been suggested, including bandaging with clinical review at

7–10 days followed by CT if clinical features persist, or early primary CT, magnetic resonance imaging (MRI) or bone scintigraphy. All of these imaging modalities have their advantages and shortcomings. Bone scintigraphy is recommended as a useful diagnostic modality to rule out occult scaphoid fractures. Bone scintigraphy can rule out scaphoid fracture with a sensitivity close to 100% but with the disadvantage of up to 25% false positives.

Dislocations of the wrist

Dislocations involving the wrist usually result from high-energy falls on the outstretched hand (such as from a height) that result in forced hyperextension. The distal row of carpal bones is commonly displaced dorsal to the proximal row as a result of a scaphoid fracture, a scapholunate dislocation or a perilunate dislocation. Trans-scaphoid perilunate fracture dislocation is slightly more common than perilunate dislocation.

Clinical features

Clinical features include mechanism of injury, wrist pain, swelling and tenderness and possibly reduced grip strength.

Clinical investigations

Imaging requires PA and lateral X-rays. The normal PA view should show two rows of carpal bones in a normal anatomic position with uniform joint spaces of no more than 1–2 mm. No overlap should be seen between the carpal bones or between the distal ulna and the radius. On the lateral film, a longitudinal axis should align the radius, the lunate, the capitate and the third metacarpal bone.

Radiographic features include:

- Lunate dislocation: on the usual PA image, the lunate has a triangular shape rather than its usual trapezoidal shape. On the lateral film, the lunate has a 'C-' or 'half-moon' shape. The rest of the carpal bones are in a normal anatomic position in relation to the radius.
- Perilunate dislocation: on the lateral film, the lunate is in a normal anatomical position with respect to the radius and with the rest of the carpal bones displaced dorsally. On the PA film, crowding is evident between the proximal and distal carpal bones.
- Scapholunate dislocation: on a PA radiograph, the scapholunate space is

greater than 4 mm (also known as the Terry-Thomas sign). The scaphoid rotates, producing the classic signet-ring sign. Associated carpal fractures, especially of the scaphoid, may be evident.

Treatment All wrist dislocations require orthopaedic consultation and prompt reduction.

Controversies

- Optimal management for Mason type II radial head fractures.
- Optimal immobilization for distal radial fractures.
- Operative versus non-operative management of distal radial fractures, particularly in the elderly.
- Vitamin C for prevention of CRPS following distal radius fractures.
- Optimal management strategy for suspected scaphoid fracture with normal initial X-rays.

Further reading

Connolly JF. Nonoperative fracture treatment Bucholz RW, Heckman JD, Court-Brown C, editors. Rockwood and Green's fractures in adults (6th ed.). Baltimore: Lippincott Williams & Wilkins; 2005.

Cruikshank J, Meakin A, Braedmore R, et al. Early computerized tomography accurately determines the presence or absence of scaphoid and other fractures. Emerg Med Australas 2007;19:223–8.

Hanel DP, Jones MD, Trumble TE. Wrist fractures. Orthopaed Clin N Am 2002;33:35–57.

Mackay D, Wood L, Rangan A. The treatment of isolated ulnar fractures in adults: a systematic review. Injury 2000;31:565–70.

Rhemrev SJ, Ootes D, Beeres FJP, et al. Current methods of diagnosis and treatment of scaphoid fractures. Internatl J Emerg Med 2011;4:4.

Ruch DS. Fractures of the distal radius and ulna. In: Bucholz RW, Heckman JD, Court-Brown C, editors. Rockwood and Green's fractures in adults (6th ed.). Baltimore: Lippincott Williams & Wilkins, 2005.

Sarmiento A, Latta L. The evolution of functional bracing for fractures. J Bone Joint Surg 2006;88B:141–8.

Uehara DT, Chin HW. Injuries to the elbow and forearm. In: Tintinalli JE, Kelen GD, Stapczynski JS, editors. Emergency medicine (5th ed.). New York: McGraw Hill, 2000.

Uehara DT, Chin HW. Wrist injuries. In: Tintinalli JE, Kelen GD, Stapczynski JS, editors. Emergency medicine (5th ed.). New York: McGraw Hill, 2000.

Van Glabbeek F, Van Riet R, Verstreken J. Current concepts in the treatment of radial head fractures in adults. A clinical and biomechanical approach. Acta Orthopaed Belg 2001;67:430–41.

Villarin Jr LA, Belk KE, Freid R. Emergency department evaluation and treatment of elbow and forearm injuries. Emerg Med Clin N Am 1999;17:843–58.

Zollinger PE, Tuinebreijer WE, Breederveld RS, et al. Can vitamin C prevent complex regional pain syndrome in patients with wrist fractures? A randomized, controlled, multicenter dose-response study. J Bone Joint Surg 2007;89A:1424–31.

ORTHOPAEDIC EMERGENCIES

4.5 Hand injuries

Peter Freeman

ESSENTIALS

1 Hand injuries are common and most carry a good prognosis if treated early and competently.

2 A comprehensive knowledge of hand anatomy and function is essential for appropriate initial management of the injured hand.

3 Aftercare and rehabilitation are essential for return to normal function.

Introduction

Hand injuries are common and up to 10% of emergency department (ED) attendances involve injury to the hand. Presentations may be due to wounds (≈35%), contusions (≈20%), fractures (≈20%), sprains (≈10%) or infections (≈5%). Males injure their hands more than females. The complex anatomy and tactile function of the hand mean that hand injuries can profoundly affect an individual. The importance of correct assessment and care of hand injuries cannot be overstated. Apart from the initial pain and trauma, occupational and psychological concerns play a major role in the aftermath of these injuries. Even a relatively minor fingertip injury can result in an individual being away from work for several days, with consequent loss of earnings and concerns for long-term function and appearance. It is therefore essential that initial assessment and management are appropriate. The role of ED management is as much about identifying cases that require specialist referral as it is about treating straightforward injuries.

Clinical features

History

Time taken eliciting a focused history of the mechanism of injury is essential in cases of hand injury. Key questions include:

- When did the injury occur?
- What was the position of the hand at the time?

- Was the hand injured with a sharp implement, such as glass, or crushed in a machine? Incised wounds caused by sharp implements tend to damage structures, such as nerves and tendons, whereas crush injuries may cause fractures and lacerations.
- Was there brisk bleeding and does any part of the hand feel numb? These symptoms are important as, in the fingers, the digital nerves lie adjacent to the arteries.
- What was the environment of the injury?
- Is it likely that the wound is contaminated or contains foreign material, such as glass?

Injury to the dominant hand should be noted as well as occupation and key leisure activities. It is also important to record medications and allergies to guide analgesia and antibiotic choice. Tetanus prophylaxis status should be determined.

Examination

The injured hand must be examined in a well-lit area. Temporary dressings may need to be soaked off if they have been allowed to dry out and become adherent. At triage, an initial moist dressing is preferred, with firm pressure and elevation if there is significant bleeding.

Hand and finger injuries are painful and suitable analgesia should be given prior to full examination. Local infiltration of local anaesthetic without adrenaline around a wound or as a digital nerve block will allow examination of all aspects except sensation, which must be tested and recorded prior to anaesthesia. A wrist block is useful when some or all of the

hand needs to be anaesthetized (Fig. 4.5.1). In this instance, longer-acting local anaesthetic is generally used to prolong the effect.

Testing sensation is achieved by point touch in the distribution of the three main nerves that supply the hand (Fig. 4.5.2). The median nerve supplies the palmar aspect of the thumb, index, middle and half of the ring finger, extending to supply the fingertip and nailbed. The ulnar nerve supplies both palmar and dorsal aspects of the other half of the ring finger and the little finger. The radial nerve supplies the radial dorsum of the hand, thumb, index, middle and radial aspects of the ring finger. If the patient is unable to describe sensation because they are too young or unconscious, it is useful to remember that the digital nerves also carry the sympathetic supply to the fingers and that division will cause a dry finger in the distribution of the digital nerve.

The hand examination should be holistic and not just concentrate on the obvious injury. Inspection of the hand will provide information about the perfusion of the tissues, local swelling and position of wounds. The resting position of the hand may be a clue to tendon injury, as the normal uninjured position is held with the fingers in increasing flexion from the index to the little finger (Fig. 4.5.3A). A pointing finger may indicate a flexor tendon injury (Fig. 4.5.3B). Testing for pinch grip is important if there is concern about the stability of the first metacarpal. Obvious bone or joint deformity should be recorded. The metacarpals and phalanges are all easily palpable subcutaneously and local tenderness may indicate underlying fracture.

Functional testing should be performed for all injured hands. Tendon integrity is tested by asking the patient to perform specific movements. Some tendon injuries may be obvious, however, two flexor tendons supply each finger and simply asking the patient to flex the finger will not exclude a divided flexor digitorum superficialis tendon. The profundus tendon flexes the distal interphalangeal joint and is tested by asking the patient to flex the tip of each finger in turn while the examiner holds the proximal interphalangeal joint in extension. The superficialis flexor tendon is tested by asking the patient to flex each finger individually,

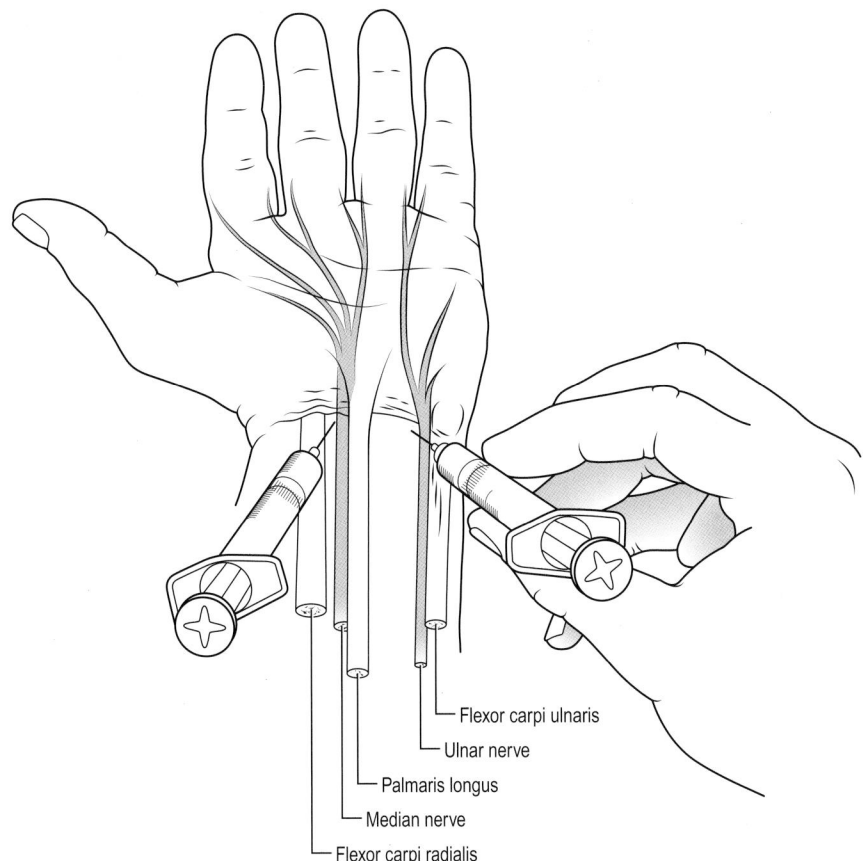

Fig. 4.5.1 Palmar wrist block. *(Reproduced with permission from American Society for the Surgery of the Hand. The Hand, 2nd edn. Boston: Churchill Livingstone; 1990.)*

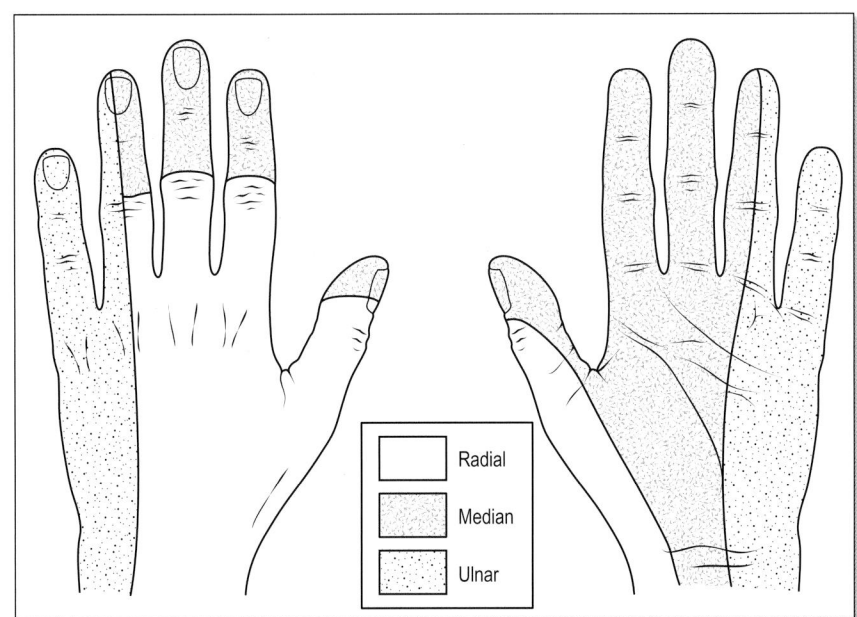

Fig. 4.5.2 The nerve supply to the hand.

while the examiner holds the other fingers straight. The extensor tendons to the fingers are tested by asking the patient to extend the fingers against resistance. It is important to remember that the broad interconnections between the extensor tendons make it possible to extend to near neutral in the presence of a divided tendon. Partial tendon injuries may still exist despite normal functioning of the fingers. A functioning hand should allow full extension of all fingers and comfortable flexion of the fingers into the palm.

Displaced fractures or dislocations may be apparent as deformity. More subtle rotational deformity will be detected by a finger crossing its neighbour when flexed.

Clinical investigations

Most information will be obtained from a focused history and examination. Radiology of the hand and fingers will be necessary if bone/joint deformity or tenderness is elicited. Even obvious dislocations should be X-rayed prior to correction as post-reduction X-rays may be overly reassuring despite significant soft-tissue damage. Glass is radiopaque to a varying degree and, if a wound is caused by glass, an X-ray should be done prior to closure. Organic foreign bodies and infections may be detected by ultrasound using a small-parts soft-tissue probe and this modality is becoming increasingly available in the ED. Ultrasound is also useful to establish tendon integrity but this is a more specialized examination.

Laboratory investigations are rarely of use in the injured hand unless there are signs of infection.

Magnetic resonance imaging (MRI) can be useful in selected injuries as it shows the soft tissues of the hand clearly, but it is relatively unavailable acutely and should be reserved for conditions where emergent treatment is dependent on the integrity of the soft structures in the hand which are not apparent on examination alone.

Treatment

Appropriate analgesia should be provided as previously described. Rings should be removed from injured fingers to prevent subsequent

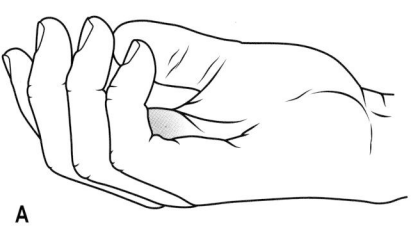
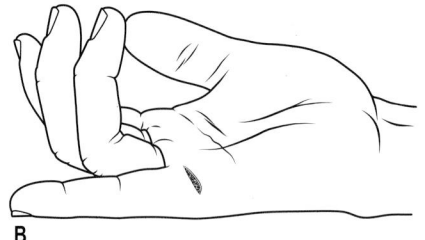

Fig. 4.5.3 (A) The normal resting hand. (B) The pointing finger. *(Reproduced with permission from American Society for the Surgery of the Hand. The Hand, 2nd edn. Boston: Churchill Livingstone; 1990.)*

compromise of circulation as the finger swells. Irrigating wounds with tap water does not increase the risk of infection and is economic. Simple hand and finger wounds can be treated along conventional lines with judicious use of local anaesthetic and skin approximation with fine (5.0) sutures or skin closures. Hand wounds generally heal well and a recent randomized controlled trial showed similar cosmetic and functional outcomes from either conservative treatment or suturing of small, uncomplicated hand wounds. Digital nerve block is useful for managing finger injuries. This technique involves infiltrating local anaesthetic around the digital nerve at the base of the finger or in the palm. Approaching the digital nerve from the dorsum of the finger is less painful but the palmar approach is more accurate as the digital nerves lie just deep to the palmar aponeurosis. A short, fine gauge (e.g. 30 gauge) needle is used with small amounts ($\approx$1 mL) of local anaesthetic for each nerve. Choice of anaesthetic will depend on the desired length of effect and consideration should be given to using long-acting agents for crush or bone injury when a prolonged analgesic effect is desirable. Studies have shown that the use of adrenaline with lignocaine is safe and also prolongs the anaesthetic effect.

Hand dressings can be held in place with a conforming crepe bandage to provide a degree of compression. Stable injuries to the fingers can be managed with 'buddy' strapping which allows for some joint movement. Elevation is essential after hand injury to reduce swelling. Minor injuries can be successfully managed in the ED, but more significant injuries usually require referral for surgical opinion.

Fingertip injuries

The fingertips have an excellent blood supply and will usually heal with good cosmetic and tactile function if basic wound care principles are followed. Fingertip injuries may involve skin, subcutaneous tissue, nail or terminal phalanx.

The most complex to manage is when the terminal phalanx is exposed and, in these cases, referral for surgical treatment is advised. If there is injury involving less than 50% of the nail and no bone is exposed conservative treatment is often the best option. Small tuft fractures of the underlying terminal phalanx are stable and will be supported by the dressing or nailbed repair.

Care of the fingertip will require haemostasis followed by a non-adherent dressing. There is good evidence that this kind of dressing promotes healing and re-epithelialization of the fingertip. Occlusive fingertip dressings are quick to apply, easily removed and comfortable for the patient. Most other dressings adhere to the wound and pull epithelial cells off when removed. Alternatives to conservative management include full-thickness skin grafts to the fingertips, advancement flaps and cross-finger flaps. These should be performed by surgeons trained in the specialist techniques and reserved for injuries involving large areas of tissue loss.

Major amputations of the fingertip or crush injuries may require terminalization of the finger. This should be fully discussed with the patient, who may be prepared to forgo finger length in exchange for early return of function. Patients requiring terminalization of a finger should be referred to a specialist hand service. Occasionally, patients will bring amputated pieces of the injured fingertip with them into the ED. Recently amputated fingers can be wrapped in moist gauze and then placed in a bag and packed with ice if re-implantation is being considered by specialist hand surgeons. If there is any doubt about the viability of fingertip tissue, the patient should be referred to a specialized hand service. No attempt should ever be made to resuture avascular tissue.

Digital nerve injuries

Nerve repairs distal to the distal interphalangeal joint are rarely required as the terminal branches are very fine. Any sensory loss with these distal injuries is minimal and improves with time. More proximal injuries can be repaired by hand or plastic surgeons using microsurgery. Good results are achieved with early repair of digital nerves when the ends can be approximated without tension using a fine (>8/0) suture. The return of protective sensation depends on the extent of damage, level of repair and axon regeneration.

Nailbed injuries

These injuries are frequently underestimated, often because of a reluctance to remove the nail. A displaced fracture or growth-plate slip of the terminal phalanx will usually be associated with nailbed disruption. Current practice is to leave a nail when the nail remains adherent to the underlying bed. Small painful subungual haematomas can be released using a hot paperclip or trephine burr. Often, damage to the nailbed results in spontaneous separation of the nail, followed by new nail growth which pushes any residual nail off. Assuming the nail root is intact, a new nail will grow back at a rate of 1 mm per week; thus full growth of a new nail takes approximately 80 days.

If required, removal of a displaced nail is achieved under digital nerve block using blunt dissection with a pair of fine forceps or scissors. The nail should be retained for use as a dressing later. Underlying fractures should be reduced with pressure and fracture haematoma irrigated away to achieve anatomical approximation of the bone ends. Fractures distal to the insertion of the profundus tendon are stable. Repair of the fragmented nailbed can be performed with fine (5/0 or 6/0) absorbable suture on an atraumatic needle. Care needs to be taken not to cut out with the needle as the nailbed is extremely friable. A prospective, randomized controlled trial has shown nailbed repair using tissue 'glue' provides similar cosmetic and function results to suture and is faster. Procedural haemostasis can be achieved with the prior application of a finger tourniquet or firm pressure over the digital arteries. Ideally, the nail is trimmed and reapplied as an organic splint and dressing.

Distal interphalangeal joint injuries

Acute flexion injuries of the terminal phalanx may either rupture the extensor tendon at the level of the distal interphalangeal joint (DIPJ) or avulse its insertion into the terminal phalanx. This produces an acute flexion deformity of the DIPJ, known as a mallet finger. An X-ray of the finger should be taken, as an intra-articular fracture involving more than one-third of the joint surface may require internal fixation. Small avulsion fractures and tendon ruptures are best treated by the application of a correctly fitting mallet finger splint, which should be retained for at least 8 weeks. Persisting mallet finger deformity after treatment or late presentations are best treated conservatively as the finger is still functional despite the mallet deformity and operative repair is usually less than satisfactory.

Hyperextension of the DIPJ can cause avulsion of the profundus tendon from the terminal phalanx and requires operative repair. In this injury, there is an inability to flex the DIPJ.

Simple dislocations of the DIPJ can be reduced in the ED and rarely cause long-term instability. However, prior radiography should be performed to differentiate dislocation from the more complicated intra-articular fractures. When associated with a palmar wound, copious irrigation is required prior to closure. Follow up is required and a course of antibiotics.

Middle phalangeal injuries

The middle phalanx takes the insertion of the flexor superficialis tendon slips through which passes the profundus tendon. Fracture of the middle phalanx can disrupt the fibrous tunnel of the profundus tendon and cause adhesions. These fractures need to be accurately reduced and may require internal fixation. They are usually unstable owing to the pull of the tendons. Palmar wounds at this level are likely to divide the profundus tendon or digital nerves and should be explored by a specialized hand service if these injuries are suspected on clinical grounds.

Proximal interphalangeal joint injuries

This is the joint that causes most long-term complications, owing to stiffness and joint contracture. It is also the most commonly dislocated joint in the hand. The proximal interphalangeal joint (PIPJ) is mechanically complex and is supported dorsally by the extensor apparatus and, on the palmar aspect, by the strong fibrous volar plate. Lateral stability is provided by the collateral ligaments. Rupture of either the extensor apparatus or the volar plate will result in joint instability and potential long-term disability. Tears in the extensor apparatus may result from relatively minor blunt trauma. Dislocations of the PIPJ invariably displace both structures. Hyperextension of the PIPJ, often from basketball or netball injuries, can result in an avulsion injury of the volar plate and a small fragment from the middle phalanx may be visible on lateral finger X-ray. Reduction of dislocations should be followed by extension splinting and early follow up. The boutonnière deformity (flexion of the PIPJ accompanied by hyperextension of the DIPJ) is a hand surgeon's nightmare and, ideally, should be prevented by careful attention to the extensor apparatus at the level of the PIPJ. These injuries should not be underestimated. Ultrasound can be used to aid in early diagnosis.

Proximal phalangeal injuries

Both flexor tendons pass along the palmar aspect of the proximal phalanx and, therefore, fractures of this bone tend to be unstable. Rotational deformity is particularly disabling and may not be noticeable with the finger held straight. These fractures usually require internal fixation. The lateral X-ray will often be the most useful in determining the degree of angulation or displacement. Wounds may damage digital nerves or either or both of the flexor tendons. Examination of the finger should detect these injuries and referral to a specialized hand service will be required.

Metacarpophalangeal joint injuries

Subluxation of the metacarpophalangeal (MCPJ) may occur in the older patient after a fall on the outstretched hand. The clinical appearances are subtle and the injury is easy to miss on X-ray. The clue is the inability of the finger to extend fully. In recent injuries, reduction is achieved by traction on the finger, although once the displacement is established, reduction becomes difficult even with open procedures.

MCPJ injuries caused by a fist and tooth impact (fight bite) are common and should be assumed to be infected. The extensor tendon may be divided and X-ray may show fracture of the metacarpal head. These injuries should be treated aggressively by joint irrigation, splinting and antibiotics.

Rupture of the ulnar collateral ligament (gamekeeper's or skier's thumb) results from an abduction injury of the thumb and, when complete, results in MCPJ instability. The ligament when completely ruptured may become folded back outside the adductor aponeurosis which prevents healing. X-rays may be taken to identify avulsion fractures of the base of the proximal phalanx. Stress X-ray views can demonstrate joint instability, but MRI will confirm injury. Treat suspected ulnar collateral ligament injuries in a thumb spica splint and refer for specialist assessment as early surgical repair gives the best outcome.

Metacarpal injuries

These injuries can be caused by punching, crush injury or falls onto the closed fist. The commonest injury is fracture of the neck of the fifth metacarpal, which is often treated conservatively. Correction of significant angulation (>45°) should be attempted but it is rare to achieve complete correction. Spiral fractures of the shaft of a metacarpal will result in shortening of the bone and loss of the contour of the knuckle. Angulation of index and middle finger metacarpal fractures should be corrected, but up to 20° of angulation in the ring and little fingers is acceptable. Conservative management of these fractures should involve splinting the hand in intrinsic plus position (Fig. 4.5.4) with the metacarpophalangeal joint flexed to 70%. The fingers must be splinted almost straight, with support extending to the fingertip. Abduction injuries of the thumb may cause a Bennett's fracture, which is an intra-articular

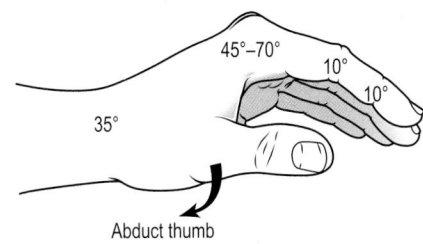

Fig. 4.5.4 Intrinsic plus – recovery position. *(Reproduced with permission from American Society for the Surgery of the Hand. The Hand, 2nd edn. Boston: Churchill Livingstone; 1990.)*

fracture of the base of the thumb metacarpal. Bennett fractures, when displaced, should be referred for specialist opinion.

Dorsal hand injuries

Wounds on the dorsum of the hand may divide the extensor tendons, which are relatively superficial. Complete division may be apparent by loss of full extension of a digit (extensor lag). Extensor tendons have extensive cross-insertions, so over 50% of the tendon can be divided without extensor lag. Visualization of the intact tendon gliding throughout its range of movement in a wound is the only safe way to exclude damage. Repair of these tendons is relatively straightforward as both ends of the tendon are usually visible within the wound. It should, however, only be performed by clinicians with appropriate training and experience. The extensor pollicis longus tendon can retract and, therefore, should be treated in a similar manner to divided flexor tendons and be referred for specialist repair.

Palmar hand injuries

Penetrating wounds on the palm of the hand are likely to divide flexor tendons or main digital nerves. These injuries should be detected by examination of the function of the individual fingers as mentioned previously. Briskly bleeding wounds proximal to an area of anaesthesia are a clue to digital nerve injury because of coexisting damage to both neurovascular structures. Neurovascular and flexor tendon damage will require referral for specialist repair.

Foreign bodies in the hand can be notoriously difficult to find and damage to other structures can result from injudicious exploration. The best results are achieved in a bloodless field with full anaesthesia. Nail-gun injuries require an X-ray prior to removal of the nail to establish its location with respect to bone and to see whether the nail has barbs that will make removal difficult. High-pressure grease or paint-gun injuries result in extensive tissue penetration and should not be underestimated. The extent of penetration may be seen on X-ray. Wide exposure and decompression of the tract will require the care of a specialist hand service.

Disposition

Many minor hand injuries can be well managed in an appropriately equipped ED ambulatory care area. No attempt should be made to operate surgically on a hand without experience, good instruments, adequate lighting and fine sutures. After treatment, the hand should be elevated in a high arm sling and suitable analgesia provided. More complex injuries will require access to a specialized plastic or orthopaedic hand service. When in doubt, early consultation is advisable.

Prognosis

Hand injuries recover best with early definitive treatment, as badly managed injuries can be very difficult to salvage at a later date. Stiffness and loss of function can be avoided if good surgical principles of wound management are adhered to. Appropriate initial splinting and guarded mobilization are the cornerstones of rehabilitation. The injured hand recovers best when splinting has been in a functional position. Whenever possible, the hand should be immobilized with the fingers straight and the MCPJ flexed to 70°. This can be achieved in even the most swollen hand by careful application of a volar plaster slab. Early referral for definitive surgery and subsequent rehabilitation will be essential for severe or complex injuries. An explanation to the patient of the need to prevent joint stiffness is important when the finger requires dressings for more than 3 weeks.

Prevention

Hand and finger injuries can be prevented. Strategies for prevention involve providing data for public awareness, identifying strategies (e.g. safety equipment, machinery modification) to prevent occupational injuries and lobbying officials to legislate for sensible measures to prevent injury.

Controversies

- Choice of wound dressings. There is good evidence that a sterile moist environment promotes re-epithelialization of fingertips. There is no doubt that dressings that adhere to wounds are uncomfortable to remove, damage new epithelial cells and delay healing.
- Solutions for wound irrigation. EDs have long used sterile solutions to cleanse wounds. In countries with clean drinking water, there is no evidence that using tap water results in more infected wounds and is certainly cost effective.
- Foreign body removal from the hand can range from being entirely straightforward to being excessively difficult and damaging. A judgement needs to be made on the likely ease of removal and the facilities available. The first attempt is usually the easiest. Wood and glass can be very difficult to find in the tissues without precise localization and a bloodless field. Ultrasound is increasingly being used to locate non-radiopaque foreign bodies which, if left, can predispose to infection.
- To suture or not? Injudicious suture of an acutely injured finger can compromise circulation and confer a secondary injury. Skin closures may be used to bring the skin edges together or, where there is gross swelling, dressings may be used to maintain the anatomy of the finger. Conservative non-suture management of small, uncomplicated hand and finger wounds is quick and safe.
- Use of antibiotics. Antibiotics have no role in the initial management of clean hand injuries. The exception to this is the grossly contaminated injury and those known to be caused by bites. Open fractures of the hand bones will need to be admitted for surgical debridement.

Further reading

Abraham M, Scott S. The emergent evaluation and treatment of hand and wrist injuries. Emerg Med Clin N Am 2010;28:789–809.

American Society for the Surgery of the Hand. The hand – primary care of common conditions, 2nd ed. Boston: Churchill Livingstone; 1990.

Angermann P, Lohmann M. Injuries to the hand and wrist. J Hand Surg 1993;18B:642–4.

de Boer P, Collinson PO. The use of silver sulphadiazine occlusive dressings for fingertip injuries. J Bone Joint Surg 1981;63B:545–7.

Harrison B, Holland P. Diagnosis and management of hand injuries in the ED. Emerg Med Pract 2005;7:2.

Quinn J, Cummings S, Callaham M, Sellers K. Suturing versus conservative management of lacerations of the hand (RCT). Br Med J 2002;325:299–300.

Strauss EJ, Weil WM, Jordan C, et al. A prospective, randomized, controlled trial of 2-octylcyanoacrylate versus suture repair for nail bed injuries. J Hand Surg 2008;33A:250–3.

Valente JH, Forti RJ, Freundlich LF, et al. Wound irrigation in children: saline solution or tap water? Ann Emerg Med 2003;41:609–16.

Wilhelmi BJ, Blackwell SJ, Miller JH, et al. Do not use epinephrine in digital blocks: myth or truth? Plast Reconstruct Surg 2001;107:393–7.

4.6 Pelvic injuries

Peter Allely • Michael Cadogan

ESSENTIALS

1 Pelvic fractures account for 3% of skeletal fractures.

2 Fractures are either stable or unstable. Unstable fractures are associated with considerable mechanical forces and result in concomitant injuries, with a significant overall mortality.

3 Understanding the mechanism of injury and recognizing the pelvic fracture pattern on X-ray provide insight into the potential for complications, such as associated haemorrhage or urogenital injuries.

4 Isolated stable pelvic fractures are usually treated conservatively.

Anatomy

The pelvic ring is formed by two innominate bones and the sacrum. The innominate bones are made up of the ileum, ischium and pubis and are joined anteriorly at the symphysis pubis and posteriorly at the left and right sacroiliac joints. The lateral surface of the innominate bone forms a socket, the acetabulum, contributed to by the ileum, ischium and pubis.

Stability of the pelvic ring is dependent on the strong posterior sacroiliac, sacrotuberous and sacrospinous ligaments. Disruption of the ring can result in significant trauma to the neurovascular and soft tissue structures it protects.

Classification of pelvic fractures

Pelvic fractures can be open or closed, major or minor, stable or unstable, depending on the degree of ring disruption and may be associated with haemodynamic compromise and/or hollow viscus or neurological injury.

Young and Resnik classification

The Young and Resnik pelvic fracture classification (also outlined in Chapter 3.8) classifies pelvic fractures by the mechanism of injury and the direction of the causative force. It does not include isolated fractures outside the bony pelvic ring or acetabular fractures, which are discussed later.

Most pelvic fractures result from lateral compression, anteroposterior compression or vertical shear forces. These injuries may be suggested by the history mechanism and are confirmed radiographically.

Lateral compression injuries

Lateral compression accounts for 50% of pelvic fractures and commonly occurs when a pedestrian or motor vehicle occupant is struck from the side. Most of these injuries are stable but, as a result of the considerable forces involved, there is a high potential for associated injury. This mechanism of injury can produce several fracture patterns involving anterior and posterior pathology.

Anteriorly, there is a transverse fracture of at least one set of pubic rami. These fractures may be unilateral or bilateral and can include disruption of the pubic symphysis. The posterior element of lateral compression fractures is important, but may be overlooked when concentrating on the anterior findings. However, it is critical in determining the functional stability of the pelvic ring and defining associated injuries.

Type 1 fractures Type 1 fractures are the most common and involve compression injury to the sacrum posteriorly and oblique pubic rami fractures anteriorly.

These injuries occur on the side of impact and are usually stable, involving impaction of

the cancellous bone of the sacrum without ligamentous disruption. X-rays confirm discontinuity of the sacral foramina posteriorly.

Type 2 fractures Type 2 fractures result from greater lateral compressive forces. The iliac wing is fractured posteriorly, with the fracture line often extending to involve part of the sacroiliac joint. This leaves part of the ileum firmly attached to the sacrum.

Anteriorly, there are associated fractures of the pubic rami. Stability is determined by the degree of sacroiliac joint disruption and mobility of the anterior hemi-pelvis involved. These fractures are usually stable to external rotation and vertical movement, but are more mobile to internal rotation.

Type 3 fractures Type 3 fractures usually occur when one hemi-pelvis is trapped against the ground and a lateral force rolls over the mobile hemi-pelvis. This produces a lateral compression injury to the side of primary impact and an unstable anteroposterior compressive injury to the contralateral sacroiliac joint.

Anteroposterior compression injuries

Anteroposterior compression injuries of the pelvis account for 25% of pelvic fractures. They result from anterior forces applied directly to the pelvis or indirectly via the lower extremities to produce an open-book type injury.

Type 1 injuries Type 1 injuries result from low-energy forces that stretch the ligamentous constraints of the pelvic ring. The pubic symphysis is disrupted anteriorly, but with less than 2.5 cm diastasis seen radiographically. These fractures are stable and there is usually no significant posterior pelvic injury.

Type 2 injuries Type 2 injuries classically cause an open-book fracture. They involve rupture of the anterior sacroiliac, sacrospinous and sacrotuberous ligaments posteriorly and disruption of the pubic symphysis anteriorly. There is widening of the anterior sacroiliac joint with diastasis of the pubic symphysis by more than 2.5 cm on radiology; occasionally, there is avulsion of the lateral border of the lower sacral segments.

Considerable force is involved to disrupt these ligaments and neurovascular injuries and complications are common. The pelvis is unstable to external rotation and external compression will 'spring' the pelvis, although this manoeuvre is no longer recommended diagnostically.

Type 3 injuries Type 3 injuries occur when an even greater force is applied and involves disruption of all the pelvic ligaments on the affected side. Rupture of the posterior sacroiliac ligaments leads to lateral displacement and disconnection of the affected hemi-pelvis from the sacrum. They are grossly unstable and associated with the highest rate of haemorrhage and neurological injury and haemorrhage (Fig. 4.6.1).

Vertical shear injury (Malgaigne fracture)
These injuries account for only 5% of pelvic fractures. They usually occur following a fall from a height or during a motor vehicle accident, when the victim reflexly extends their leg against the brake pedal before impact. These mechanisms force the hemi-pelvis in a vertical direction and result in complete ligamentous or bony disruption, with cephaloposterior hemi-pelvis displacement.

Anterior disruption occurs through the pubic symphysis or pubic rami. Posteriorly, dissociation usually occurs through the sacroiliac joint, but may occur vertically through the sacrum. These fractures are usually

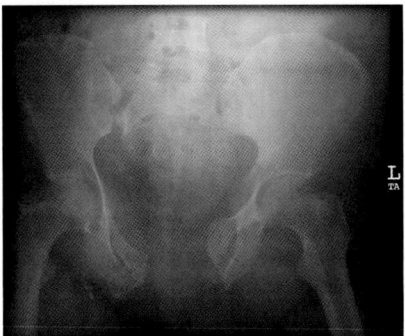

Fig. 4.6.1 'Open-book' pelvic fracture, with pubic symphysis diastasis and sacroiliac disruption, following an anteroposterior compression injury.

unilateral, but may be bilateral and are associated with significant bleeding and/or intra-abdominal injury.

Clinical assessment
A standard trauma management protocol is adhered to in managing the multitrauma patient, with usual attention being paid initially to the airway, breathing and circulation (ABCs) in the primary survey and resuscitation phases of care (see Chapter 3.1).

General examination
The back is examined to assess for external evidence of injury to the lumbar spine, sacroiliac regions and coccyx, with inspection and palpation. Abdominal, perineal, rectal and a vaginal examination are performed according to suspected injury. The rectal examination in the absence of overt urethral trauma includes observation for fresh blood and an assessment of anal sphincter tone and position of the prostate. A thorough perianal and lower limb neurovascular examination is performed.

Pelvic examination
The pelvis is briefly examined as part of the cardiovascular assessment in the ABC approach to trauma. The suprapubic, pelvic and urogenital regions are inspected for signs of bruising, abrasions, open wound and obvious deformity. In males, the urethral meatus is assessed for the presence of frank blood and the scrotum for bruising. Flank bruising may indicate retroperitoneal haemorrhage.

Pelvic compression or 'pelvic springing' has been in widespread use ostensibly as a means to assess for pelvic injury and to assess the stability of a fracture. It adds little to the assessment of a patient beyond gentle palpation. As it may dislodge clots in an injured pelvic venous plexus resulting in catastrophic bleeding, it is no longer recommended in anyone with haemodynamic compromise and/or an obvious pelvic fracture.

Radiology
The AP pelvic X-ray is an initial film that will usually rapidly alert clinicians to anterior fractures, such as pubic rami, diastasis and suggest complex hemi-pelvic injuries. Posterior fractures are difficult to visualize and further plain X-rays or usually a computed tomography (CT) scan are needed.

Injuries associated with pelvic fractures

Haemorrhage
Haemorrhage is the most serious complication of a pelvic fracture. It may result from bleeding at fracture sites, local venous or arterial tears and/or disruption of a major vessel. Catastrophic bleeding can result from disruption of the internal iliac arteries, their tributaries and accompanying veins as they pass over the anterior aspect of the sacroiliac joint.

Severe hypovolaemia due to persistent haemorrhage without major vessel disruption is a significant cause of mortality. Up to 4 L of blood may be lost into the retroperitoneal space before tamponade occurs. Anteroposterior type 3 injuries and vertical shear injuries disrupt the sacroiliac joint and are associated with significant haemorrhage.

Treatment to minimize or stop haemorrhage associated with a pelvic fracture includes the early application of a pelvic binder across the level of the greater trochanters. Treatment beyond that is complex and best led by a senior specialist team leader using a pre-agreed algorithm. This will vary between institutions and involve any combination of external fixation, interventional radiology with angiography and embolization, 'damage control' laparotomy with pelvic packing and/or open reduction with internal fixation.

Genitourinary and bladder injuries
Pelvic fractures are associated with injury to the lower urinary tract in up to 16% of cases. These are more prevalent in males who sustain a higher rate of urethral injury. Pelvic trauma may also result in bladder rupture. The bladder is normally protected by the pelvis and rupture usually indicates significant disruption of the pelvic ring.

Almost 90% of blunt trauma patients with bladder rupture have an associated pelvic fracture. Patients are usually hypotensive with frank haematuria, although gross haematuria is a non-specific sign of genitourinary trauma and does not necessarily indicate bladder rupture. Therefore, a retrograde urethrogram is performed to delineate any urethral trauma prior to performing retrograde cystography. However, this should be not performed before other emergent advanced imaging, such as CT scan of the abdomen and pelvis, as the contrast or spillage may obscure other important injuries.

Urethral and genital injuries

Urethral rupture is rare in females. Rupture of the urethra secondary to blunt trauma commonly occurs to the anterior bulbous urethra just distal to the urogenital diaphragm. It is associated with bilateral fractures of the pubic rami, pubic symphysis disruption and vertical shear injuries.

Suspect a urethral rupture in the adult male with a pelvic fracture, blood at the urethral meatus, perineal haematoma and urinary retention. A 'high-riding prostate' may be found on rectal examination, however, not all these signs may be present. A retrograde urethrogram is diagnostic and must be performed prior to urethral (Foley) catheterization when indicated clinically (see above).

Injury to the female genitalia is uncommon and often overlooked. Vaginal laceration is associated with a pelvic fracture in 4% of cases. These normally present with bleeding, but may be occult. A bimanual pelvic examination is necessary in women with a pelvic fracture, which may necessitate anaesthesia due to patient discomfort. Complications, such as abscess formation and sepsis, are severe, particularly if the injury is missed.

Management of the unstable pelvic fracture

The mainstay of pelvic fracture management in the emergency department (ED) is to identify and assess the degree of pelvic injury, to provide pain relief and to provide fluid resuscitation to minimize life-threatening haemorrhagic shock. Early identification of major pelvic trauma with mobilization of general surgical, orthopaedic, vascular, interventional radiology and intensive care specialties is essential, ideally using a pre-agreed algorithm approach.

Fluid resuscitation

Commence initial fluid resuscitation with intravenous crystalloid in the hypotensive patient with pelvic trauma using two large-bore peripheral intravenous cannulae, but rapidly change to blood and blood products if the hypotension is not immediately reversed. An average blood transfusion requirement for anteroposterior compression fractures is 15 units, for a vertical shear injury is 9 units and for lateral compression injuries is 3.5 units.

Therefore, activate a Major Transfusion Protocol (MTP) with blood and blood products, such as fresh frozen plasma (FFP) and platelets in a ratio that may approach 1:1:1 according to local protocol. Also give 1 g tranexamic acid IV in 100 mL normal saline over 10 min, followed by 1 g infusion over 8 h, providing these are commenced within a maximum of 3 h of injury.

Pelvic immobilization

Pelvic binder or sling

Immobilization of the pelvis with attempted reapproximation of bony fragments creates a tamponade effect that reduces the risk of haemorrhage prior to definitive treatment. This is best achieved using a proprietary radiolucent pelvic binder device with ratchet mechanism or pelvic sling to apply compression. Alternatively, simply brace the pelvis in a sheet, support it laterally with sandbags and internally rotate the hips with the lower legs splayed apart.

External fixation

External fixation is a rapid and simple procedure designed to immobilize and stabilize the anterior pelvis in the ED to reduce pelvic haemorrhage prior to definitive treatment. Three pins are placed through each iliac crest and are then clamped to an external frame to reduce the displaced pelvic ring injury.

The advantages of external fixation are that it is quick, effective and can proceed in the ED without delaying the continued management of the multiply injured patient. Disadvantages include a lack of support for the posterior component of the pelvic ring fracture, difficulty of placement in the obese patient and reduced pelvic surgical access in the event of laparotomy being required.

Embolization

Life-threatening arterial haemorrhage is estimated to occur in 5–20% of patients with blunt pelvic fracture. Emergency angiography is both diagnostic and therapeutic to control primary haemorrhage and (where available) has become the treatment of choice in patients with haemodynamic instability due to a pelvic fracture, particularly where a CT scan has shown an 'arterial blush' indicating ongoing bleeding.

Early recognition of these patients with organization of transfer to a hospital with angiography capabilities and mobilizing an interventional radiologist reduce mortality, but is a logistical challenge. The success of the procedure is operator dependent, time-consuming and does not address venous blood loss, which still requires appropriate replacement of blood and blood products and consideration of laparotomy with pelvic packing.

Laparotomy with pelvic packing

Continuing pelvic bleeding with haemodynamic instability when due to venous haemorrhage and/or when interventional radiology is unavailable or delayed may require laparotomy with pelvic packing, with continued blood and component therapy to prevent or treat coagulopathy paying attention to base deficit, coagulation profile and temperature; followed by admission for intensive-care monitoring. Surgical expertise is necessary to perform this temporizing procedure, prior to subsequent pack removal and definitive management that may include later open reduction with internal fixation.

Open pelvic fracture

Open pelvic fractures are rare and associated with increased morbidity and mortality of up to 40–50%. Open fractures with pelvic ring disruption lose any tamponade effect and can result in massive and fatal haemorrhage, as well as high risk of intra-abdominal injury and/or late sepsis.

Management

Control of haemorrhage is the priority in an open pelvic injury, with early surgery to avoid the increased risk of infection. Sterile gauze packed into the wound applies direct pressure tamponade. Urgent repair of associated open bowel and/or bladder injuries and to debride bleeding wounds is paramount, with stabilization of the pelvic fracture as the last step in treatment. The mortality remains high despite advances in imaging and aggressive treatment.

Acetabular fractures

Acetabular fractures account for 20% of pelvic fractures and are usually associated with lateral compression forces. They also occur with posterior forces applied distally through the femur. Their classification is complex.

Clinical features

Acetabular fractures are caused by direct impaction of the femoral head that may be associated with a central hip dislocation. These fractures are associated with sciatic and femoral nerve injury, depending on the position of the hip dislocation. A thorough neurovascular examination is mandatory.

ORTHOPAEDIC EMERGENCIES

4

In addition, these fractures are often associated with other pelvic injuries, knee injury, hip fractures and dislocations, which should all be looked for.

Management

Standard radiographs of the hip and pelvis may define the fracture, but a CT scan is necessary, particularly to show the anterior and posterior fragments and involvement of the ilioischial and iliopubic columns. All fractures are referred for inpatient orthopaedic management.

Stable fracture of the pelvis

Isolated pubic ramus fracture

These injuries are commonly seen in the elderly with direct trauma following a fall. The patient has difficulty in weight bearing and there is local pain and tenderness in the groin. These should be carefully looked for in any patient unable to bear weight with a suspected hip fracture, particularly when X-ray of the hip is normal.

Pain is usually reproduced with the FABER test. The ipsilateral foot is placed on the contralateral knee, forcing the ipsilateral hip to be Flexed, ABducted and Externally Rotated, which exacerbates the pain. Pelvic radiographs confirm the diagnosis.

Iliac wing fracture (Duverney fracture)

Direct lateral trauma may result in an isolated iliac wing fracture, known as the Duverney fracture. Patients complain of severe pain on weight bearing and walk with a waddling gait. Localized tenderness and bruising occur over the site of injury, associated with abdominal guarding, ileus and lower quadrant tenderness.

These fractures are usually minimally displaced, rarely comminuted and are readily visualized on AP pelvic X-ray.

Isolated avulsion fractures

These are often sustained by young adults following acute stress to the muscular and ligamentous insertions onto the bony pelvis. They include anterior superior iliac spine fracture, anterior inferior iliac spine fracture and the ischial tuberosity fracture.

Anterior superior iliac spine fracture

The anterior superior iliac spine may be fractured in jumping activities due to powerful contraction of the sartorius muscle and tensor fascia lata. Such injuries cause pain on weight bearing, with local tenderness and swelling at the fracture site. Active flexion and abduction of the thigh reproduces the pain. There is usually minimal displacement of the avulsed fracture on the AP film of the pelvis. Treatment is usually conservative, although operative management is possible for significant displacement.

Anterior inferior iliac spine fracture

Forceful contraction of the rectus femoris muscle in sports that involve sprinting or kicking (forceful hip extension) may avulse the anterior inferior iliac spine. These patients complain of a sharp pain in the groin and are unable actively to flex the hip. The fracture is usually evident on plain AP pelvic views, with the fragment being displaced distally. Conservative treatment is common.

Ischial tuberosity fracture

Fracture of the ischial tuberosity is rare and occurs with forceful contraction of the hamstrings, usually in young adults whose apophyses are not fully united. They are associated with hurdling and other jumping activities. Pain may be reproduced by local palpation and by active flexion of the hip with the knee extended. Plain X-rays of the pelvis reveal minimal displacement of the apophysis from the ischium. Conservative treatment is common.

Coccyx fracture

These fractures are more frequent in women and are caused by a fall onto the buttocks with both hips flexed. Patients have difficulty in mobilizing and have local pain, swelling, bruising and tenderness over the lower sacral region. X-ray confirmation is unnecessary if physical examination confirms an isolated injury.

Management of isolated stable fractures

Pubic ramus fractures, iliac wing fractures and avulsion fractures are treated conservatively with non-steroidal anti-inflammatory drugs (NSAIDs) and non-weight-bearing crutches for 10 days. Mobilization and physiotherapy allow resumption of normal activities in 3–4 weeks, followed by graduated return to high impact sporting activities. Coccygeal fractures require rest, analgesia and stool softeners. As sitting is painful, a doughnut-ring foam cushion is helpful.

Controversies

- Optimal multidisciplinary management in the ED of the hypotensive pelvic trauma patient; what protocol, who to call and when.
- The role of external pelvic fixation devices in the ED.
- The optimum timing of angiography and arterial embolization.

Further reading

Blackmore CC, Cummings P, Jurkovich G, et al. Predicting major hemorrhage in patients with pelvic fracture. J Trauma 2006;61:346–52.

Burgess AR, Eastridge BJ, Young JW, et al. Pelvic ring disruptions: effective classification system and treatment protocols. J Trauma 1990;30:848–56.

Dalal SA, Burgess AR, Siegel JH, et al. Pelvic fracture in multiple trauma: classification by mechanism is key to pattern of organ injury, resuscitative requirements, and outcome. J Trauma 1989;29:981–1002.

Fallon B, Wendt JC, Hawtrey CE. Urological injury and assessment in patients with fractured pelvis. J Urol 1984;131:712–4.

Gokcen EC, Burgess AR, Siegel JH, et al. Pelvic fracture mechanism of injury in vehicular trauma patients. J Trauma 1994;36:789–96.

Kellam JF. The role of external fixation in pelvic disruptions. Clin Orthopaed Relat Res 1989;241:66–82.

Mattox KL, Bickell W, Pepe PE, Mangelsdorff AD. Prospective randomized evaluation of antishock MAST in post-traumatic hypotension. J Trauma 1986;26:779–86.

Pennal GF, Tile M, Waddell JP, et al. Pelvic disruption: assessment and classification. Clin Orthopaed Relat Res 1980;151:12–21.

Rothenberger DA, Velasco R, Strate R, et al. Open pelvic fracture: a lethal injury. J Trauma 1978;18:184–7.

Sarin EL, Moore J, Moore E, et al. Pelvic fracture pattern does not always predict the need for urgent embolization. J Trauma 2005;58:973–7.

4.7 Hip injuries

Peter Allely • Michael Cadogan

ESSENTIALS

1 Trauma to the hip is a major cause of morbidity and mortality in the elderly, which has a large impact on healthcare and resources.

2 Hip injuries are frequently a pathological disease of the elderly. However, there is an increased incidence of hip fractures and dislocations in young people sustaining high-energy trauma.

3 Extracapsular neck of femur fractures are associated with significant haemorrhage.

4 Avascular necrosis (AVN) of the femoral head is a complication of intracapsular femoral neck fractures, as well as hip dislocation.

5 The hip joint is least stable when flexed and adducted and prone to dislocation. Posterior hip dislocations are an orthopaedic emergency, as they are associated with sciatic nerve injury and avascular necrosis.

6 Anterior hip dislocations are associated with femoral neurovascular injury and occult hip joint fractures.

Anatomy

The hip joint is a large ball and socket articulation encompassing the acetabulum and proximal femur. The hip joint provides a high degree of stability and mobility.

Blood supply

The head and intracapsular portion of the femoral neck receive the majority of their blood supply from the extracapsular trochanteric anastomosis arterial ring, with a minor supply arising from the foveal branch of the obturator artery, via the ligamentum teres to the femoral head.

Retinacular arteries from the extracapsular ring pass under the reflection of the hip capsule to supply the femoral neck and head in a retrograde manner. Intracapsular fractures disrupt this 'distal to proximal flow' and so may result in avascular necrosis of the femoral head.

Avascular necrosis

Avascular necrosis (AVN) following hip injury refers to ischaemic bone death within the femoral head due to compromise of its blood supply. Increased bone density of the femoral head is the radiographic feature of AVN, but this may take up to 6 months to become manifest.

AVN results primarily from the disruption of the trochanteric anastomosis in femoral neck fractures and is the commonest early complication of these fractures. Traumatic haemarthrosis, with or without a fracture, may also result in intracapsular tamponade. AVN occurs when the intracapsular pressure exceeds the diastolic blood pressure.

AVN is also seen following posterior dislocation and is related to the degree of trauma and the length of time the femoral head is out of the joint. Early management is thus an orthopaedic emergency, as reduction within 6 h results in an AVN rate of less than 10%.

In addition, chronic pancreatitis, alcohol abuse, sickle cell anaemia, vasculitis, irradiation, decompression illness (DCI) and the prolonged use of corticosteroids may all result in AVN.

Classification of hip fractures

Hip fractures are either intracapsular or extracapsular. Intracapsular fractures involve the femoral neck or head. Extracapsular fractures include intertrochanteric, trochanteric and subtrochanteric types and are four times more common than intracapsular fractures.

The incidence of hip fractures increases exponentially with age, with the fracture rate doubling for every decade over 50 years. Hip fractures occur most frequently in white postmenopausal women as 50% of 65-year-old women and 100% of women over the age of 85 have a bone mineral density below fracture threshold level (osteoporosis).

Intracapsular fractures

Femoral head

Femoral head fractures are uncommon and are usually associated with dislocations of the hip. They often occur in young patients, 75% of cases being associated with motor vehicle incidents.

Classification Fractures of the superior aspect of the femoral head are usually associated with anterior dislocation, whereas inferior femoral head fractures occur with posterior dislocation. Fractures may involve a single fragment (type 1) or comminution (type 2).

Clinical evaluation Symptoms and signs of femoral head injuries are usually those of the associated dislocation rather than the fracture itself. Femoral head fractures are not always picked up on initial X-rays. In the absence of abnormality on plain radiography, further imaging with a computed tomography (CT) scan should be performed in the presence of persistent pain following reduction of a hip dislocation.

Management Immediate orthopaedic referral is essential as prompt reduction of the dislocation and appropriate stabilization of the fracture reduce the risk of AVN, increasing the chances of a return to full mobility. The prognosis is related to the severity of the initial trauma, time to definitive reduction and the number of failed closed relocation attempts.

Complications AVN occurs in 15–20% of cases, post-traumatic arthritis in 40% and myositis ossificans in 2%.

Femoral neck fractures

Intracapsular fractures are four times more common in females than males. There are four main causes of this type of injury:

- elderly, with minimal trauma following a fall onto the greater trochanter (pathological fracture)
- elderly, with torsion or twisting injury prior to fall (pathological fracture)
- young person involved in high-energy trauma (excessive loading)
- repetitive stress or cyclical loading injuries (stress fracture).

Classification The Garden classification system is commonly used to describe intracapsular neck of femur fractures.

Garden I: incomplete, impacted or stress fractures that are stable. Trabeculae of the inferior neck are still intact and, although they may be angulated, they are still congruous.

Garden II: undisplaced fracture across the entire femoral neck. The weight-bearing trabeculae are interrupted, without displacement. These fractures are inherently unstable and must be fixed.

Garden III: complete femoral neck fracture with partial displacement. There is associated rotation of the femoral head, with non-congruity of the head and acetabular trabeculae.

Garden IV: complete subcapital fracture with total displacement of fracture fragments. There is no congruity between proximal and distal fragments, but the femoral head maintains a normal relationship with the acetabulum.

These fractures may be further simplified into non-displaced (Garden I and II) and displaced (Garden III and IV).

Clinical assessment and management

Non-displaced fractures Non-displaced fractures include stress fractures, Garden I and Garden II fractures. Stress fractures are usually the result of repetitive abnormal forces on normal bone in fit, active young people, such as military recruits or marathon runners, but may occur with repetitive normal stresses on abnormal bones, such as in rheumatoid arthritis or patients taking long-term steroids.

These present with pain that is gradual in onset and worse after activity, radiating from the groin to the medial aspect of the knee. Patients walk with a limp and often present late. Physical examination reveals no obvious deformity, although there is mild discomfort on passive movement at the extremes of motion and percussion tenderness over the greater trochanter.

Additional radiological examination with a bone scan and/or MRI is indicated when initial X-rays are normal but there is persistent pain. MRI is the investigation of choice, being more sensitive than bone scans in the first 24 hours. It is of similar accuracy to bone scans in fracture assessment at 72 hours.

Stress fractures and Garden I impacted fractures are considered stable and may be treated conservatively under close orthopaedic supervision. Garden II fractures, although non-displaced, are inherently unstable and must be fixed internally.

Displaced fractures Elderly patients with displaced fractures usually present with pain in the hip area and markedly reduced hip movement. The lower limb is shortened, abducted and externally rotated distal to the fracture, albeit less than with intertrochanteric fractures.

X-ray reveals the fracture and the degree of posterior comminution of the proximal fragment. Parenteral analgesia and a femoral nerve block reduce discomfort. Skin traction will also reduce pain and helps preserve femoral head vascularity.

Traumatic femoral neck fractures in the young adult are uncommon and usually involve normal bone. These fractures are outside of the Garden classification. They follow a large degree of force and have up to a 35% risk of AVN and up to a 57% risk of non-union.

Complications

Mortality Femoral neck fractures are associated with a mortality of 14–36% in the first year after injury, with the rate returning to the pre-fracture level after this. Mortality is increased threefold in those who were institutionalized prior to the fracture, with increased risk factors for mortality being male gender, older age, malnutrition, multiple medical problems and end-stage renal failure.

Morbidity AVN is the most common complication despite optimal treatment. Non-union, postoperative infection and osteomyelitis are also seen.

Extracapsular femur fractures

Intertrochanteric femur fractures

Fractures of the proximal femur that occur along a line between the greater and lesser trochanters are referred to as intertrochanteric. They are usually pathological, occur in the elderly and have a female preponderance.

Mechanism A simple fall with a direct force applied to the greater trochanter in the elderly is enough to cause an intertrochanteric femoral fracture. In young adults, they are associated with high-speed motor vehicle incidents or falls from a height.

Clinical assessment Patients sustaining an intertrochanteric fracture are unable to bear weight and have significant pain on hip movement. There is often a large haematoma overlying the greater trochanter, owing to the highly vascular bone that is fractured without any intracapsular containment. Examination reveals a markedly shortened, abducted, significantly externally rotated lower limb.

X-rays confirm the fracture in most cases. However, internal rotation of the hip on the AP view may obscure the fracture. The lateral view depicts the size, location and degree of comminution of the fracture fragments and determines stability.

Classification Numerous classification systems are available for intertrochanteric fractures, the simplest of which is by Evans. This divides intertrochanteric fractures into stable and unstable. However, for the emergency physician, an anatomical description of the fracture detailing the degree of comminution, subtrochanteric extension and the presence of displaced posterior fragments is adequate (Fig. 4.7.1).

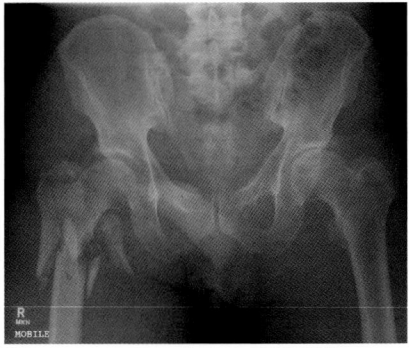

Fig. 4.7.1 Unstable comminuted intertrochanteric fracture with subtrochanteric extension.

Management A complete evaluation is essential to formulate an early treatment plan as intertrochanteric fractures occur most frequently in the elderly. Patients may lose up to 1.5 L of blood from a comminuted fracture and are often dehydrated, malnourished and in significant pain on arrival in the emergency department (ED). Parenteral analgesia and fluid resuscitation are important in preparation for theatre.

Skin traction or immobilization with sandbags prevents further soft-tissue damage and bony comminution and reduces blood loss. Full preoperative evaluation requires a search for associated injuries, such as rib fractures, distal radial fractures and vertebral compression fractures at the level of T12 and L1.

An ECG, bloods and chest X-ray help elucidate the cause of the fall and may indicate the need for associated medical treatment.

Treatment is with open reduction with internal fixation (ORIF) which produces better anatomical alignment, a shorter hospital stay and improved function with reduced mortality by comparison with conservative management.

Complications Survival is directly related to the patient's age and pre-existing medical factors.

Greater trochanteric fracture

Mechanism Isolated fractures of the greater trochanter are uncommon. They usually occur between 7 and 17 years of age and involve true epiphyseal separation secondary to indirect trauma. Forceful muscular contraction by the gluteus medius causes avulsion of the apophysis. The displaced, non-comminuted fragment may be separated by up to 6 cm.

Greater trochanteric fractures in adults are rare and usually result from direct trauma, causing a comminuted fracture whose fragments are rarely displaced and usually involve only part of the trochanter.

Clinical assessment Patients with a greater trochanter injury are tender to palpation over the area of avulsion or comminution, but bruising is uncommon. There is often an associated flexion deformity of the hip as a result of pain and muscle spasm and weight bearing causes a limp.

Management The prognosis is good after these fractures. Most are treated with bed rest for 3 days, followed by non-weight bearing

and crutches for 4 weeks. Open reduction and internal fixation are indicated for marked separation of the bony fragment.

Lesser trochanteric fracture

Isolated fractures of the lesser trochanter usually occur in children and young athletes, with 85% occurring before the age of 20.

Mechanism Lesser trochanter fractures are usually an apophyseal avulsion injury secondary to forceful contraction of iliopsoas.

Clinical assessment Patients complain of pain on flexion and internal rotation of the hip. Examination reveals tenderness in the femoral triangle. The patient is unable to flex the hip and raise the foot off the ground in a seated position (Ludloff sign specific for the iliopsoas muscle).

Radiology is often inconclusive, as there may not be complete separation of the bony fragment; comparison views may be required.

Management Ten days of bed rest and slow mobilization result in full recovery. Open reduction and internal fixation are not indicated, even with wide apophyseal separation.

Subtrochanteric femoral fractures

The subtrochanteric region of the femur lies between the lesser trochanter and a point 5 cm distally. Fractures in this region are termed subtrochanteric. They account for 11% of hip fractures and occur in the elderly with osteoporosis, bone metastases or end-stage renal failure. High-energy injuries in young adults with normal bone are less common.

Mechanism Ninety per cent of these fractures result from blunt trauma, either due to a simple fall in the elderly or following a high-speed motor vehicle accident (MVA) or fall from a height in young adults. In some countries, up to 10% are due to high-energy gunshot wounds.

Classification A variety of classification systems is available, but none is widely used. As with intertrochanteric fractures, it is best to describe the location, presence of comminution and the position of the lesser trochanter proximal or distal to the fracture line.

Clinical assessment A subtrochanteric fracture is usually isolated in the elderly.

However, as substantial force is required in young adults, the presence of other injuries must be sought. The limb distal to the fracture is usually held in abduction, flexion and external rotation. Haemorrhage from a comminuted subtrochanteric fracture may be up to 2 L. Assess the patient's circulatory status and commence fluid and blood.

Management The affected limb is immobilized in a splint following parenteral analgesia and a femoral nerve block. Suitable splints include proprietary splints, such as the Donway or Hare. Fluid resuscitation is started as required. The older, more laborious Thomas splint is now rarely used.

Orthopaedic referral is essential for open reduction and internal fixation of these fractures.

Complications There is up to a 20% mortality associated with these fractures within the first year in the elderly. They are associated with a higher rate of non-union and implant failure as subtrochanteric bone is cortical thus, unlike the cancellous bone involved in intertrochanteric fractures, these fractures often lack the vascularity for adequate new bone growth and repair. The further down the shaft of femur the fracture line is located, the greater the degree of non-union and implant failure.

Hip dislocation

The hip joint is inherently stable and considerable force is required to produce a dislocation. Associated injuries must always be sought. Hip dislocations are classified anatomically into anterior and posterior, depending on the final position of the femoral head relative to the acetabular rim.

Non-prosthetic hip dislocations are an orthopaedic emergency as the femoral head's blood supply is precarious and also due to the proximity of the sciatic nerve. Failure to reduce a hip dislocation within 6 hours dramatically increases the risk of AVN and sciatic nerve ischaemic damage.

Posterior hip dislocation

Mechanism

Posterior dislocations represent 85–90% of traumatic hip dislocations. Classically, a direct distal force applied to the flexed knee, with the hip in varying degrees of flexion as when seated in the front of a car, causes a posterior dislocation of the hip. The hip and knee are usually flexed to 90° and the hip adducted, which is the least stable position for the hip to be in.

The force applied by the dashboard in a head-on collision to a seated individual may produce an isolated posterior dislocation. The abducted and partially flexed hip in the same scenario is more stable and, if the force of impact is great enough, will result in a posterior dislocation with displaced acetabular fracture.

Clinical assessment

Examination of the affected limb reveals shortening, adduction, internal rotation and some degree of flexion. A single AP pelvis radiograph is usually adequate to confirm a posterior dislocation. However, as up to half of these dislocations are associated with an acetabular, femoral head or femur fracture, further radiological imaging is essential. Judet views, AP hip with internal rotation and AP and lateral femoral views have been used extensively in the past, but are now largely superseded by CT.

Neurological examination Neurological examination is essential in a posterior dislocation, particularly with marked internal rotation which may compress the sciatic nerve and its branches. This results in neurological deficit particularly in the peroneal nerve distribution. Associated injuries, such as ipsilateral knee ligament disruption with a posterior cruciate rupture, must be looked for as well.

Management

The orthopaedic team is consulted early. A thorough search for associated periarticular and distal limb injuries, neurological evaluation and adequate imaging are essential in the ED.

Closed reduction

Closed reduction of a posterior hip dislocation may be performed in the ED under procedural sedation, unless there is *immediate* access to an operating theatre (see Chapter 22.3).

Allis manoeuvre There are numerous methods of relocation, many requiring significant physical strength. The most common is the Allis manoeuvre, whereby the patient lies supine with assistants on either side stabilizing the pelvis by downward pressure on the anterior superior iliac spines. The operator applies longitudinal traction to the lower leg with the hip slightly flexed in the line of

the femur and knee in 90° of flexion. The leg is internally and externally rotated until the femoral head is rearticulated with the acetabulum. Lateral traction to the inside of the thigh may assist.

Other techniques include the lateral traction–countertraction method and the Whistler technique.

Complications

The risk of developing AVN is directly proportional to the length of time the hip remains dislocated and increases dramatically if the dislocation is not reduced within 6 hours of injury. Sciatic nerve neuropraxia may occur in 15% of cases but is usually relieved by reduction.

Permanent ischaemic changes with neurological deficit secondary to pressure necrosis have been reported in up to 3% of cases, usually in the peroneal nerve distribution. Missed knee injuries occur in up to 15% of cases as well as patellar, tibial plateau and posterior cruciate injuries.

Anterior hip dislocation

Anterior dislocations account for 10–15% of traumatic hip dislocations and are associated with femoral neurovascular injury and occult hip joint fracture. They usually result from a direct blow to the abducted and externally rotated hip. When the hip is in abduction, the femoral neck or greater trochanter impinges on the rim of the acetabulum. A direct force applied distally can lever the head out of the acetabulum and tear the anterior capsule of the hip.

Classification

Anterior dislocations may be superior or inferior. Type I or superior dislocations occur when the hip is extended at the time of injury. These are also known as iliac dislocations. Type II or inferior dislocations occur when the hip is flexed at injury and are also known as obturator dislocations.

They may be further subclassified as simple dislocation, associated femoral neck fracture or associated acetabular fracture.

Clinical assessment

The superior type of injury causes an extended, externally rotated and slightly abducted distal limb. The distal limb in the inferior type of dislocation is externally rotated, abducted and in flexion. The femoral head may be palpated around the anterior superior iliac spine in superior types and in the obturator foramen in inferior types.

A neurovascular examination is essential in anterior dislocation, particularly the superior type, where trauma to the femoral artery, vein and nerve is common. Hip and pelvis radiographs must be studied carefully for associated fractures of the acetabulum and femoral head. Further imaging with CT is indicated, particularly for persistent post-reduction pain.

Management

General examination looking for associated life-threatening injuries is essential as this type of hip dislocation is usually associated with high-energy trauma. Orthopaedic consultation is mandatory because of the high probability of vascular injury and the need for closed reduction under general anaesthesia.

Complications

Early complications in superior dislocations result from direct pressure on the femoral vessels with the potential for distal neurovascular compromise. Late complications include post-traumatic arthritis and AVN. Recurrent dislocation is common when anterior capsular healing is incomplete following inadequate immobilization after reduction.

Controversies

- Efficacy of applying skin traction and immobilization to reduce extracapsular femoral fractures in the ED.
- Early use of CT and MRI to evaluate the reduced non-prosthetic hip to limit (missed) associated morbidity.
- Whether the hip reduction should take place in the ED or in the operating theatre; it is essential to treat hip dislocations early.

Further reading

Dahners LE, Hundley JD. Reduction of posterior hip dislocations in the lateral position using traction–countertraction: safer for the surgeon? J Orthopaed Trauma 1999;13:373–4.

Garden RS. The structure and function of the proximal end of the femur. J Bone Joint Surg 1961;43B:576–89.

Hirasawa Y, Oda R, Nakatani K. Sciatic nerve paralysis in posterior dislocation of the hip. Clin Orthoped 1977;126:172–5.

Holmberg S, Conradi P, Kalen R, Thorgren KG. Mortality after cervical hip fracture: three thousand two patients followed for six years. Acta Orthopaed Scand 1986;57:8–11.

Jazayeri M. Posterior fracture dislocations of the hip joint with emphasis on the importance of hip tomography in their management. Orthoped Rev 1978;7:59–64.

Keller CS, Laros GS. Indications for open reduction of femoral neck fractures. Clin Orthoped 1980;152:131–7.

Walden PD, Hamer JR. Whistler technique used to reduce traumatic dislocation of the hip in the emergency department setting. J Emerg Med 1999;17:441–4.

4.8 Femur injuries

Peter Allely • Michael Cadogan

ESSENTIALS

1 Early femoral fracture reduction and immobilization in traction reduces mortality.

2 Haemorrhagic shock is a major complication, with a closed femoral fracture average blood loss of 1200 mL.

3 Femoral shaft fractures are associated with other significant injuries including those to the pelvis, hip, knee and/or multitrauma.

Femoral shaft fracture

Mechanism

Considerable force is required to break the adult femur in the absence of osteoporosis or metastatic disease with a bony secondary. The majority of femoral shaft injuries occur in young adults following road traffic incidents, falls from a height or a gunshot wound.

Classification

No universally accepted classification system exists for fermoral shaft fractures. A precise description of the fracture provides the orthopaedic specialist with an indication of the potential for blood loss and the urgency of definitive management.

Femoral fractures are either open or closed and may be transverse, oblique, spiral or segmental. They may occur within the proximal third, midshaft or distal third of the femur. The degree of fracture comminution, soft-tissue involvement and neurovascular status should also be described.

The majority of fractures occur in young adults with healthy bones and are transverse. Greater mechanical force usually results in comminution (Fig. 4.8.1). Minimal force with pathological bone tends to produce metaphyseal fractures with propagation into the shaft.

Stress fractures

Stress fractures of the femoral shaft are becoming increasingly common. They occur when repetitive mechanical forces are applied to the femur, such as in marathon running or

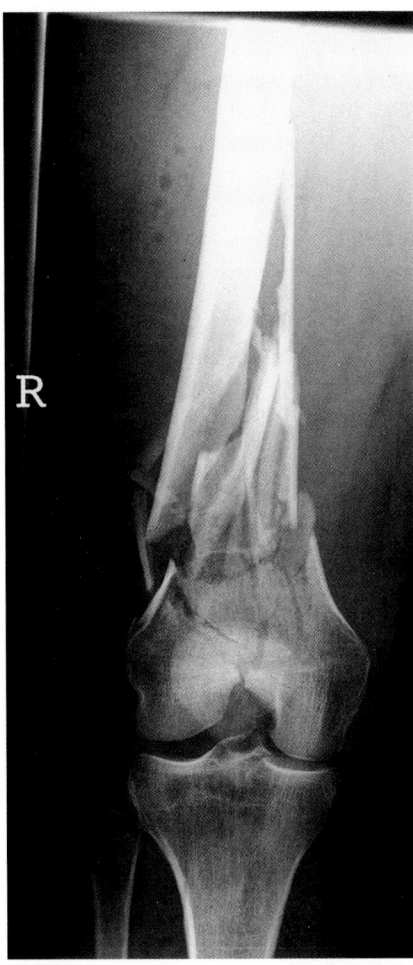

Fig. 4.8.1 Comminuted femoral fracture.

military recruits. They are associated with pain in the midthigh and apparently normal X-rays, although a bone scan will detect the fracture. Low-impact training, such as cycling, is used in rehabilitation. They are rarely displaced.

Clinical evaluation

The clinical diagnosis of femoral shaft fracture is usually straightforward. The thigh is shortened and externally rotated, with the hip held in slight abduction. Palpation reveals tenderness over the fracture site and extreme pain on attempted movement. Neurovascular injuries are rare, but the distal pulses, capillary refill and distal sensation must be carefully examined.

Vascular damage

Vascular damage is usually limited to rupture of the profunda femoris perforating branches in closed fractures. The resulting tense, swollen haematoma is limited to the thigh and is not associated with distal circulatory compromise. However, penetrating trauma from gunshot wound and open fractures may cause femoral artery disruption with distal circulatory compromise, so repeated vascular evaluations are important.

Any evidence of an expanding haematoma or diminished distal pulses requires further investigation with Doppler imaging or arteriography.

Associated injuries

Commonly associated injuries include fractures of the pelvis, the femoral head and neck, dislocation of the hip and soft-tissue disruption of the knee. Up to 50% of closed femur injuries are associated with meniscal and collateral ligament injuries in the knee, although it is usually impossible to evaluate reliably these injuries in the acute setting. Up to 1.5 L of blood may extravasate into the surrounding soft tissues.

Management

The treatment of any associated multitrauma to the head, neck, thoracic or pelvic injury should take priority. However, early reduction of a femoral fracture is an important part of haemorrhage control. Administration of analgesia, fluid resuscitation and fracture reduction and splinting are ideally performed prior to X-ray of the lower limb, unless this is immediately available.

Analgesia

Adequate pain relief is essential in the emergency department (ED). Intravenous opioid analgesia is necessary, and titrated to effect.

A femoral nerve block is an important adjunct that should be performed prior to fracture reduction and splinting (see Chapter 22.2).

Reduction and splinting

Early fracture reduction and splinting in traction decreases overall mortality and pain, limits blood loss and reduces the risk of fat embolism. Fractures are returned to near anatomical alignment using longitudinal traction following appropriate analgesia with the knee in extension.

Proprietary splints, such as the pneumatic Donway or Hare traction splint, have replaced the old skin traction (Thomas) splint in the ED.

Traction is an interim procedure prior to definitive management as it cannot hold a constant force of sufficient magnitude to maintain the length and alignment of an adult femur fracture.

Fluid resuscitation

Haemorrhagic shock is a major complication with an average blood loss from a closed femoral fracture of 1200 mL. All patients must be resuscitated with intravenous fluid and blood, kept fasted and an indwelling catheter inserted to monitor fluid balance.

Orthopaedic management

Early operative fixation, typically intramedullary nailing, is indicated in adults within 8 hours. Open fractures require immediate operative debridement with antibiotic cover such as flucloxacillin 2 g IV or cephazolin 2 g IV, followed by delayed intramedullary nailing.

Complications

Complications include fat embolus syndrome, haemorrhagic shock and adult respiratory distress syndrome, with a higher incidence in comminuted fractures. Long-term complications of shortening, malalignment and non-union may result in post-traumatic arthritis.

Early mobilization following intramedullary nailing greatly reduces complications associated with prolonged immobilization. Patients older than 60 years with closed femoral fractures have a complication rate of 54% and a mortality of 17%.

Controversies

- Arteriography, particularly in distal third femoral fractures following proximity penetrating trauma, even in the absence of initial vascular compromise.
- Diagnosis of stress fractures from repetitive exercise.

Further reading

Provost R, Morris J. Fatigue fracture of the femoral shaft. J Bone Joint Surg 1969;51A:487–98.

Russell RH. Fracture of the femur. A clinical study (abridged by Peltier LF). Clin Orthoped 1987;224:4–11.

Taylor M, Banerjee B, Alpar E. Injuries associated with a fractured shaft of the femur. Injury 1994;25:185–7.

Vanganess C, DeCampos J, Merritt P. Meniscal injury associated with femoral shaft fractures. An arthroscopic evaluation of incidence. J Bone Joint Surg 1993;75:207–9.

West H, Turkovich G, Donnell C. Immediate prediction of blood requirements in trauma victims. South Med J 1989;82: 186–9.

4.9 Knee injuries

Michael Baker • Michael Cadogan

ESSENTIALS

1 The knee is the most commonly injured joint in the body.

2 Knee injuries often occur in the young, usually associated with sport.

3 The mechanism of injury is an essential part of the history; examination should include the hip and ankle joint.

4 Anterior cruciate ligament disruption is associated with meniscal and collateral ligament injuries in 50% of cases.

5 Lateral tibial plateau fractures are associated with anterior cruciate and medial collateral ligament disruption, whereas medial tibial plateau fractures are associated with posterior cruciate and lateral collateral ligament disruption.

6 Knee dislocations require urgent reduction with assessment for a popliteal artery injury.

Anatomy

The knee is the largest, most complicated joint in the body. It is a synovial, complex hinge joint comprising the patellofemoral and tibiofemoral joints. Movement ranges from 10° of extension to 140° of hyperflexion, with up to 12° of rotation present through the full arc.

The ligaments of the knee are classified as extracapsular or intracapsular. The main extracapsular ligaments are the medial and lateral collaterals (MCL and LCL). The main intracapsular ligaments are the anterior and posterior cruciate ligaments (ACL and PCL), which are extrasynovial. The collateral ligaments provide lateral stability and stability in extension, whereas the cruciate ligaments provide knee stability in flexion.

Knee stability is further enhanced by muscular extensions, such as the vastus medialis giving patella stability, the fibrous extension of vastus lateralis and medialis (the patellar retinaculum) strengthening the knee anteriorly and the iliotibial tract strengthening the knee in slight flexion.

Clinical assessment

An exact history of the mechanism of injury, degree of force, presence of immediate swelling and the ability to bear weight straight after the injury are essential to guide the diagnosis of soft-tissue injuries. Injury may be due to direct or indirect trauma and may involve valgus or varus stress.

Knee physical examination

Always examine both legs with the patient undressed and lying supine on a trolley (not sitting). Visual inspection may reveal swelling, bruising, erythema, deformity and/or an associated wound.

Swelling appearing within the first few hours of trauma is usually associated with a haemarthrosis due to a vascular response to subchondral, bone or synovial injury. Swelling developing gradually over several hours to days is more likely due to a serous effusion from a synovial reaction.

Knee palpation

Start palpation away from the point of trauma to detect warmth, swelling, crepitus, muscle mass and neurovascular status and then to localize the areas of maximal tenderness to define the underlying pathology. Assess the insertion points of the quadriceps tendon, patellar tendon, collateral ligaments and the medial and lateral joint lines, as well as the bony structures of the knee joint.

Assess active and passive movements of the knee joint, noting the degree of flexion, extension and internal and external rotation. Always test for the ability to straight leg raise while supine, to assess for potential damage to the extensor mechanism of the knee.

Anterior and posterior drawer tests

Complete the examination with an assessment of the knee's functional stability. The stability of the anterior and posterior cruciate ligaments may be crudely determined with the anterior and posterior drawer tests. Ligamentous laxity decreases with age, so comparison with the opposite knee is more important than absolute laxity.

The patient must be supine with the hip flexed at 45°, the knee flexed at 90° and the hamstrings relaxed. The examiner sits on the patient's foot to stabilize the limb and attempts to demonstrate abnormal forward movement of the tibia on the femoral condyles (positive anterior drawer test) and/or abnormal backward movement of the tibia on the femoral condyles (positive posterior drawer test). However, the accuracy of the anterior drawer test, as defined by subsequent arthroscopy, is only 56% for rupture of the ACL, whereas posterior displacement of the tibia by more than

5 mm is indicative of PCL ruptures with a specificity of 85%.

Lachman's test

Lachman's test is a more sensitive manoeuvre in the acute setting for testing ACL integrity, with a sensitivity of 86% and specificity of 91% [1]. The operator supports the distal femur with one hand with the knee in 20–30° of flexion and uses the other hand to draw the tibia forwards on the femoral condyles. Increased anterior displacement of the proximal tibia compared to the unaffected limb indicates a positive test.

Collateral laxity

The collateral ligaments are assessed by applying a varus or valgus stress to the knee in 0° and 30° of flexion. The degree of ligamentous laxity is determined by the amount of movement produced between the tibia and fibula, compared to the normal side.

McMurray's test

McMurray's test is used to demonstrate a meniscal injury. The patient lies supine and the knee is passively flexed and extended. One hand is placed over the knee to feel for crepitus while the other hand rotates the tibia on the femur. Internal rotation tests the lateral meniscus and external rotation tests the medial meniscus. Pain and crepitus at the extremes of movement indicate a positive test.

Apley's test

Apley's test is also used to demonstrate a meniscal injury. This is performed with the patient lying prone with the knee flexed to 90°. The tibia is rotated on the femur with downward pressure on the heel. Meniscal tears are associated with pain on downward pressure at the extremes of movement, and relieved by the release of pressure.

Radiology

Clinical decision rules to determine the requirement for knee radiography aim to reduce emergency department (ED) radiographs, waiting times and costs. The most widely used is the Ottawa knee rule.

Ottawa knee rule

The Ottawa knee rule states an X-ray is indicated for acute knee injury in adults with any of the following:

- age >55 years
- tenderness at the head of the fibula

- isolated tenderness of the patella
- inability to flex knee to 90°
- inability to bear weight (take four steps) immediately and in the ED.

This rule has been validated in a number of studies, with a pooled sensitivity of 98.5% and specificity of 48.6% [2].

Standard knee X-rays

Standard knee X-ray evaluation includes AP and lateral views. The AP view assesses for the integrity of the medial and lateral joint spaces and the femoral tibial angle. It also shows the size, position and integrity of the patella.

Lateral view may identify a lipohaemarthrosis effusion, seen as a horizontal line demarcating darker, more radiolucent fat floating on lighter, more radiodense blood. This is indicative of an intra-articular fracture and is most helpful when the actual injury is hard to see, such as with an undisplaced condylar fracture, patellar or tibial spine fracture.

Oblique X-rays are helpful in elucidating a tibial plateau fracture. The tunnel view enhances the intercondylar region.

A skyline X-ray is taken to evaluate further the patella and patellofemoral joint, particularly following reduction of a patellar dislocation. It can identify undisplaced vertical fractures of the patella and subtle subluxation not seen on the conventional views.

Computed tomography

Computed tomography (CT) is important to define fractures, such as those of the tibial plateau. Magnetic resonance imaging (MRI) is reserved for evaluation of complex soft-tissue knee injuries, unless arthroscopy is preferred.

Fractures around the knee joint

Distal femur

Distal femoral fractures account for 4% of femoral fractures. They are usually associated with high-energy injuries secondary to a fall or a direct blow to the femur in a motor vehicle incident.

Classification

Distal femoral fractures are divided anatomically into supracondylar, intercondylar and isolated condylar fractures. Supracondylar fractures are extra-articular and occur immediately above the femoral condyles. Intercondylar fractures involve separation of the femoral condyles. Although the fracture line may extend through the supracondylar region, in general, these are treated as intra-articular fractures.

Isolated condylar fractures are uncommon and occur when a varus or valgus force is applied to a weight-bearing, extended knee. The tibial eminence is driven into the femoral intercondylar notch, creating an intra-articular fracture associated with significant ligamentous disruption.

Clinical assessment

Patients with an injury to the distal femur are in significant pain and unable to bear weight. Examination may reveal swelling, deformity, rotation and shortening. The joint is tender to palpate along the medial or lateral joint lines and an acute haemarthrosis secondary to associated ligamentous injury or intra-articular involvement is common.

Examine the whole lower limb to exclude ipsilateral hip dislocation, associated tibial fracture and quadriceps damage. Assess for any neurovascular deficit, including loss of sensation in the web space between the first and second toes due to deep peroneal nerve injury.

Anteroposterior and lateral X-rays of the femur and knee reveal the fracture and its degree of displacement or comminution. A pelvic X-ray is necessary to exclude an associated proximal femur fracture or hip dislocation.

Management

Administer adequate analgesia and apply a splint in the ED to prevent movement at the fracture site. Distal femoral fractures are a complex orthopaedic problem and long-term complications of malunion, quadriceps adhesion and osteoarthritis are common.

Early orthopaedic input is required in all cases. Fractures with joint incongruity or displacement require open reduction and internal fixation. Cast immobilization alone may be sufficient for undisplaced or impacted fractures without joint involvement, particularly in the elderly patient [3].

Tibial plateau fracture

The tibial plateaus are the superior articulating surfaces of the medial and lateral tibial condyles and are covered by hyaline cartilage and a fibrocartilaginous meniscus. Their integrity is vital for knee alignment, articulation and stability.

Mechanism

Tibial plateau fractures account for 1% of all skeletal fractures. They are most common in the elderly, often as a result of a simple fall. They occur when a valgus or varus deforming force is applied to the weight-bearing knee. Lateral tibial plateau fractures are twice as common as medial injuries, but both tibial plateaus are involved in 10–30% of cases.

Anterior fractures occur when the knee is in extension and posterior fractures when the knee is flexed. High-energy complicated fractures can also occur, often in the younger age group, and are associated with extensive ligamentous and soft-tissue injury.

Classification

Fracture classification is complex owing to the varying degrees of comminution, displacement and compression of the plateaus. The most widely used system is that of Schatzker, which divides the fractures into six different types [4]. Fracture types 1, 2 and 3 involve the lateral tibial plateau with increasing articular depression (Fig. 4.9.1). Type 4 involves the medial plateau. Fracture types 5 and 6 involve both tibial plateaus with increasing comminution and joint instability.

Segond fracture　A tibial plateau avulsion fracture at the site of lateral capsular ligament insertion is called a Segond fracture. It appears as an elliptical, vertical fragment of bone parallel to the lateral condyle just distal to the plateau. They are associated with excessive internal rotation and varus stress to the flexed knee and are usually associated with sporting

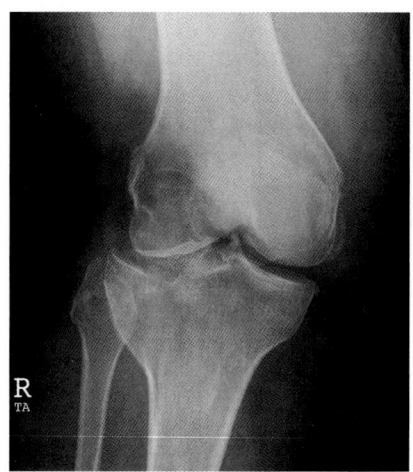

Fig. 4.9.1 Schatzker type 3 tibial plateau fracture.

injuries. They are an important marker of ACL disruption and/or medial meniscus injury and indicate severe rotatory instability.

Clinical assessment

Patients present with a painful, swollen knee and are usually unable to bear weight. Pain and haemarthrosis limit active and passive movements of the knee. Focal tenderness is palpated at the fracture site and over any associated collateral ligament tears.

Distal circulatory compromise may be secondary to compression of the popliteal artery by comminuted subcondylar fragments [5]. Peroneal nerve neurapraxia and paralysis may complicate displaced lateral condylar fractures, resulting in foot drop. Soft tissue injuries occur in up to 35% of injuries. Generally, lateral tibial plateau fractures are associated with ACL and MCL disruptions, whereas medial plateau fractures are associated with PCL and LCL disruptions.

Radiology

Most tibial plateau fractures are evident on standard knee X-rays, although oblique views may be required to elucidate a subtle fracture and to help classify a fracture. CT is important to evaluate further non-displaced and comminuted fractures and for operative planning. An MRI is preferred to quantify the degree of any associated ligamentous damage [6].

Management

Orthopaedic consultation is essential. Lateral fractures with <2 mm displacement and less than 5° of angulation may be treated conservatively with a cast or splint, but comminuted fractures with articular surface disruption require open reduction and internal fixation [7]. Other surgical indications include open injuries, fractures with vascular injury and a fracture associated with unstable ligamentous injury.

Common complications include undiagnosed neurovascular injury, compartment syndrome and osteoarthritis.

Fractures of the tibial spine and intercondylar eminence

The tibial spine separates the medial and lateral tibial condyles and is divided into anterior and posterior areas by the intercondylar eminence. These areas provide flat surfaces for the attachment of the ACL and PCL, respectively. The intercondylar eminence is divided into a medial and a lateral tubercle visible on anteroposterior X-rays, although nothing actually attaches to them.

Mechanism
Most tibial spine and intercondylar eminence fractures occur in children as the cruciate ligaments are stronger than the skeletal physeal plates [8]. Considerable force is required for these fractures to occur in an adult. The tibial spine is usually fractured during violent knee twisting movements.

The anterior tibial spine fractures 10 times more frequently than the posterior. Intercondylar eminence fractures are associated with severe hyperextension or hyperflexion injuries.

Clinical assessment
The patient complains of severe pain, immediate swelling of the knee and inability to bear weight. The knee is usually held in slight flexion and cannot be fully extended. Examination confirms the presence of an acute haemarthrosis and limited knee movement. An associated ACL disruption may be confirmed with a positive Lachman's or anterior drawer test, although pain may prevent these.

Radiology
AP and lateral X-rays plus tunnel or oblique views are used to confirm the diagnosis. MRI is preferred to quantify the degree of any associated ligamentous damage.

Management
Most injuries are treated conservatively, but refer a displaced fracture with marked ligamentous injury for open reduction and internal fixation.

Patellar fracture
The patella is the largest sesamoid bone in the body and lies within the quadriceps tendon. It improves the stability, strength and mechanical advantage of the extensor mechanism and offers some protection to the femur.

Mechanism
Patellar fractures account for 1% of skeletal injuries and occur predominantly in males between the ages of 20 and 50 years as a result of direct or indirect trauma. Direct trauma to the anterior aspect of the patella results in an incomplete, stellate, comminuted or vertical patellar fracture. These commonly occur in motor vehicle incidents when the knee strikes

the dashboard. There is usually little or no separation of the bony fragments as the medial and lateral quadriceps expansions remain intact.

Indirect trauma occurs when stumbling or falling forwards [9]. The combination of powerful quadriceps contraction proximally and the strong patellar insertion distally overcomes the intrinsic strength of the patella and leads to a transverse fracture. These fractures account for up to 80% of patellar fractures and occur mainly in the central and lower third of the patella. The extent of the fragment separation is dependent on the degree of quadriceps expansion tear.

Clinical assessment
Examination reveals pain, swelling and bruising over the patella. The ability to walk and extend the knee actively are dependent on the type of fracture and are important when considering surgical repair. Test for the ability to perform a straight leg raise while in a supine position in order to confirm the integrity of the knee extensor mechanism.

A patient with a non-displaced fracture may be ambulatory and able to demonstrate active knee extension against gravity. Patients with displaced transverse patellar fractures are unable to extend the knee actively.

Radiology
Patellar fracture is diagnosed by X-ray with additional skyline views. A fracture needs to be differentiated from a bipartite patella, which represents failure of the patella ossification centres to fuse, seen in 1–6% of the population. The bipartite patella has smooth borders that are well corticated, with minimal separation between fragments.

Management
Fractures with fragment displacement of more than 2 mm are associated with disruption of the extensor mechanism and require referral to an orthopaedic specialist for open reduction and internal fixation with tension band wiring.

Treat a non-displaced patella fracture conservatively with an intact extensor mechanism with a long-leg cast in full extension for 6 weeks.

Dislocations around the knee joint

Dislocation of the knee
Knee dislocations are rare and usually occur in males in their third decade. They are an

orthopaedic emergency that is associated with vascular damage and require urgent reduction.

Mechanism
Tibial femoral knee dislocation usually involves rupture of both cruciate ligaments and one collateral ligament. Such injuries are associated with high-velocity injuries, such as from a motorcycle incident. They are described with respect to the displacement of the tibia in relation to the femur. Anterior dislocations are the most common.

Clinical assessment
Spontaneous reduction prior to the emergency department is common, so a high index of suspicion and careful assessment are required. Examination usually reveals gross distortion of the knee, with the clinical deformity being easily palpable. Knee dislocations are associated with a high rate of peroneal artery (20–80%) and popliteal nerve injury, so a careful neurovascular assessment is essential.

Compression and distortion of the posteriorly placed popliteal artery and vein may cause distal vascular compromise, although 10% of vascular injuries are associated with normal pedal pulses. Peroneal nerve dysfunction is present in up to 50% of patients suffering knee dislocation, causing foot drop and sensory impairment of the dorsum of the foot and lateral border of the foot and leg.

Radiology
Immediate plain X-rays confirm the dislocation, but should not delay analgesia and reduction.

Management
Prompt consultation with the orthopaedic and vascular teams is essential, with early reduction under procedural sedation in the ED if necessary. Neurovascular status should then be reassessed and documented. The risk of developing a compartment syndrome and/or needing amputation is increased when reduction is not performed within 6 hours. Failed reduction secondary to buttonholing of the femoral condyle is uncommon and requires open reduction under general anaesthesia.

In the past, angiography was performed in all cases of knee joint dislocation. There is now a move towards serial examinations if the ankle brachial index (ABI) is >0.90 (the ratio of the systolic blood pressure [SBP] measured at the ankle to that measured at the brachial artery) and all distal pulses are equal and present [10].

Patella dislocation

Traumatic patellar dislocation is common and may become recurrent, with further patellar subluxation or dislocation. The majority of dislocations occur in the setting of patellofemoral dysplasia or malalignment syndromes secondary to hypoplastic vastus medialis, a shallow trochlear groove or genu valgum. Lateral dislocations are overwhelmingly the most common, usually caused by a direct blow to the anterior or medial surface of the patella. The medial retinaculum is disrupted by being stretched in subluxations and torn in a dislocation.

Clinical assessment

Patients complain of the knee suddenly 'giving way', accompanied by immediate pain and swelling. They are unable to bear weight or extend the knee. Palpation reveals an anterior defect, a laterally deviated patella, swelling and medial joint line tenderness. In a spontaneously reduced injury, the 'apprehension test', performed by applying gentle pressure on the medial border of the patella, may confirm the diagnosis.

Standard AP and lateral X-rays confirm the diagnosis and are important to exclude an associated osteochondral fracture. However, particularly in recurrent dislocations, X-ray can follow immediate reduction.

Management

Some dislocations reduce spontaneously or are reduced prior to arrival at the ED. Closed reduction is performed following suitable analgesia or procedural sedation. Apply anteromedial pressure to the lateral aspect of the patella with the thumbs while gently extending the knee. Immobilize the knee in an extension splint for 3–6 weeks after post-reduction X-rays, to allow the medial retinaculum time to heal.

Complications

Up to 50% of patients suffer symptoms of instability or anterior knee pain following traumatic dislocation. Recurrent dislocation occurs in over 15% of cases and may require surgical repair.

Proximal tibiofibular joint dislocation

Mechanism

The proximal tibiofibular joint is supported by a capsule anteriorly, the popliteus muscle posteriorly and the LCL superiorly. Tibiofibular joint dislocation is rare and only possible when the LCL support is relaxed with the knee in flexion. Thus, they occur mainly in violent athletic twisting injuries, such as during the shot put.

Clinical assessment

The patient holds the knee flexed at 20–30° and is able to bear weight with difficulty, with point tenderness over the fibula head. Common peroneal nerve neuropraxia is unusual.

Radiology

AP and lateral comparison views reveal the dislocation, which is usually anterolateral.

Management

Reduction is by firm pressure over the head of fibula towards the centre of the knee, under procedural sedation. Success is associated with a satisfying 'click'. Surgical intervention is rarely needed.

Soft-tissue knee injuries

Collateral ligaments

Medial and lateral ligament damage is often associated with sporting events. They are graded 1 to 3, indicating the degree of disruption to the ligamentous fibres:

- grade 1: stretching of the fibres only
- grade 2: partial tear, mild instability but firm endpoint on stress testing
- grade 3: complete disruption of fibres, clear instability with no endpoint on stress testing.

Medial collateral ligament

The medial collateral ligament (MCL) complex comprises a long superficial ligament with a distal point of insertion and a short deep ligament attached to, and stabilizing, the medial meniscus. The MCL provides medial stabilization to the knee joint in conjunction with the capsule and semimembranosus, resisting valgus laxity and medial rotational instability.

MCL injuries are the most common isolated knee ligament injury. They occur when an excessive valgus force is applied to the knee, usually by a direct blow to the lateral aspect. The greater the degree of the valgus deforming force, the greater the risk of an associated ACL disruption.

Lateral collateral ligament

The lateral collateral ligament (LCL) is the phylogenetically degenerate part of peroneus longus. It is a cord-like ligament running from the lateral epicondyle of the femur to the head of the fibula. It is separated from the lateral meniscus by the popliteal tendon. The LCL is the major lateral stabilizer of the knee, providing the main resistance to varus deforming forces, especially when the knee is extended.

LCL injuries are less common, but more debilitating, than MCL injuries. The lower incidence of LCL injuries is a result of the lateral ligament's mobility and the protective effect of the opposite leg. They result from a direct blow to the medial aspect of the knee. Associated injuries to the insertion of biceps femoris and to the common peroneal nerve at the fibular head must be excluded.

Clinical assessment

Examine for point tenderness at the site of injury, demonstrable laxity and a haemarthrosis. Gently stress the affected ligament complex to check for reproducible pain. Complete rupture of the ligament complex is associated with instability and stress testing causes the joint line to open up on the affected side.

Test the MCL in 0° and 30° of flexion. Apply pressure to the lateral joint line with one hand while the other hand creates a valgus stress by gently pushing the medial malleolus laterally. At 0°, the medial complex is reinforced by the ACL but, at 30°, testing is specific for MCL rupture.

Lateral instability is assessed with pressure applied to the medial joint line with one hand and by a varus stress performed by moving the lower leg medially.

Radiology

Standard X-rays can only reveal collateral ligament injury when there has been a bony avulsion. Calcification at the origin of the MCL occurs in chronic injuries (Pellegrini–Stieda). In complex cases, an MRI helps delineate the degree of ligamentous disruption and highlights associated injuries.

Management

The majority of isolated collateral ligament injuries are treated conservatively, provided damage to the ACL and PCL complexes has been excluded [11]. Discomfort is reduced by immobilizing the knee in a proprietary splint, such as a three-panel Velcro knee immobilizer, or by an elastic knee support, with ice massage and anti-inflammatory drugs.

Quadriceps strengthening exercises are essential to aid recovery and early return to movement using a hinged splint. Early orthopaedic opinion is sought for a grade 3 injury to consider surgical repair, as this is best done within 48 hours of injury.

Cruciate ligaments

The cruciate ligaments are the primary stabilizers of the knee in flexion and extension.

Anterior cruciate ligament

The anterior cruciate ligament (ACL) extends from the medial aspect of the lateral femoral condyle to the anterior inter-condylar area of the tibia. It prevents backward displacement of the femur on the tibial plateau and limits extension of the lateral condyle of the femur. It helps control the rotation of the knee in twisting and turning activities and is much more commonly injured than the PCL.

Mechanism The ACL is commonly injured during sporting activities, such as skiing and rugby, with patients readily able to define the causative mechanism. Injury results from direct trauma as the tibia is forcefully displaced anteriorly on the femur or the femur posteriorly on the tibia or by indirect injury when the flexed knee suffers a sudden twisting movement with the foot firmly planted on the ground.

Clinical assessment ACL injuries are classically associated with sudden severe pain and an audible 'pop', with an acute haemarthrosis and inability to bear weight. Immediate swelling of the knee indicates serious intra-articular pathology.

The anterior drawer test or Lachman's test is used to assess ACL integrity. ACL disruption is associated with meniscal and collateral ligament injuries in 50% of cases, with the most common combination involving the triad of ACL and MCL disruption with a lateral meniscal tear.

Radiology X-rays may show avulsion of the anterior tibial spine, although an MRI scan is necessary to determine ACL rupture with certainty, having over 90% sensitivity and specificity.

Management Arthroscopy is the gold standard in assessing the integrity of the ACL

and has the advantage of allowing simultaneous debridement and repair. The decision to undertake reconstruction is dependent on a number of factors including the patient's age, level of activity, the degree of instability, presence of other knee structures injured and the time post-injury (ideally within 2 weeks).

Both autograft and allograft materials have been utilized in the repair. However, meta-analysis shows insufficient evidence to determine superiority of surgical repair over conservative management as regards long-term function and joint stability [12].

Posterior cruciate ligament

The posterior cruciate ligament (PCL) extends from the lateral aspect of the medial femoral condyle to the posterior intercondylar area of the tibia. It prevents excessive forward displacement of the femur on the tibia and is essential in providing mechanical support when walking downhill or down stairs, as it is the only stabilizing structure in the flexed, weight-bearing knee.

Mechanism PCL rupture is normally caused by a posteriorly directed force on the proximal tibia, such as with falls onto the tibial tubercle, knee dislocation and dashboard injuries. It is less commonly associated with sporting injuries than ACL ruptures.

Clinical assessment Immediate pain and swelling are common with PCL rupture which, unlike the ACL, rarely causes any popping or tearing sensation. Stability is usually adequate to allow partial weight bearing. Isolated PCL ruptures result in posterior 'sag' of the tibia compared to the unaffected limb, with the posterior drawer test performed to assess PCL integrity. Associated MCL and ACL disruptions are common and must be actively sought.

Radiology X-rays may reveal avulsion of the posterior tibial spine but, as with ACL injuries, MRI demonstrates over 90% sensitivity and specificity for PCL rupture and may be more reliable than arthroscopic examination.

Management The treatment of isolated PCL rupture is largely non-operative and focuses initially on pain management and non-weight-bearing immobilization. When a PCL injury is combined with other ligamentous

injuries, operative intervention within 2 weeks is common.

Patellar tendon rupture

The patellar tendon is the final connection of the extensor mechanism from the inferior pole of the patella to the tibial tuberosity. Rupture usually occurs under the age of 40 years, often associated with a previous history of patellar tendonitis or steroid injections. Injury is associated with stressful sporting activity and occurs with forceful quadriceps contraction, with significant pain.

Examination

Examination reveals a palpable defect, which may be masked by significant swelling. Test the extensor mechanism by asking the patient to straight leg raise against gravity. This is impossible in a complete rupture and is painful and difficult in an incomplete injury. Comparison lateral X-ray views of both knees may reveal a high-riding patella.

MRI is indicated in complex cases to differentiate partial and complete tears. Partial tears are treated non-operatively with cast immobilization in extension for 6 weeks. Complete tears of the patellar tendon are referred to the orthopaedic specialist for surgical intervention.

Quadriceps tendon injury

The quadriceps tendon is a trilaminar junction of the quadriceps muscle. Rupture is commonest in the older age groups as the tendinous blood supply declines. Young persons usually suffer a muscular disruption. Rupture occurs three times more commonly than patellar tendon rupture, usually due to a direct blow to the knee or a hyperextension injury. It is associated with intense pain and the patient is unable to walk without assistance.

Examination

Examination reveals a tender, palpable defect more apparent on attempted knee extension. Swelling secondary to a haemarthrosis and bruising are usually present. The straight leg raise is impossible in complete rupture, whereas extension of the knee from a flexed position cannot be performed in a partial tear.

Comparison lateral knee X-rays may demonstrate a low-lying patella in the affected knee. In doubtful cases, MRI is indicated to distinguish between a partial and a complete rupture.

Management

A partial tear is treated non-operatively, but a complete rupture requires early surgical intervention for the best results.

Patellar and quadriceps tendonitis (jumper's knee)

Both these extensor tendons are susceptible to tendonitis secondary to repetitive overloading. Patellar tendonitis is more common than quadriceps tendonitis. Patients present with anterior knee pain with point tenderness over the inferior or superior pole of the patella, commonly in athletes who participate in running and jumping activities.

Inflammation and pain in patellar tendinitis at the insertion point of the patella tendon into the patella is six times more common than at the insertion to the tibial tuberosity. Patellar tendonitis may be associated with fragmentation of the inferior pole of the patella on X-ray.

Initial treatment includes rest, ice and anti-inflammatory medication. Longer-term recovery and prevention requires conditioning and training of the extensor musculature.

Meniscal injury

The menisci are semilunar fibrocartilaginous structures found on the medial and lateral sides of the superior aspect of the tibia. They enhance the fluidity of articulation between the femoral and tibial condyles and increase the stability of the tibiofemoral articulation.

The medial meniscus is immobile, being firmly attached to the deep portion of the medial collateral ligament and joint capsule. The lateral meniscus has a uniform thickness and a larger tibial area than the medial. It has no attachment to the LCL and is more mobile than the medial meniscus, making it twice as likely to be injured.

Mechanism

Meniscal injuries are usually associated with collateral or cruciate ligament injury, which should be sought when examining the acutely injured knee. Chronic degenerative processes account for only a small percentage of injuries. The menisci are uncommonly injured in isolation, but suspect an isolated meniscal injury in the young athlete sustaining a violent twisting or rotational injury to the weight-bearing knee.

Clinical assessment

The patient is able partially to bear weight following meniscal injury and usually complains of medial or lateral joint line pain. Delayed swelling, intermittent locking and a sensation of the knee 'giving way' with sudden loss of stability are clues to meniscal damage.

Examination usually confirms the presence of an effusion and joint line tenderness, especially in the extremes of flexion and extension. McMurray's test may be positive, but is not pathognomonic and, acutely, the pain prevents adequate hyperflexion for the test to be accurate.

The 'locked' knee is held in 30° of flexion, with a springy block to extension on examination and associated pain. A bucket-handle meniscal tear is classically associated with a true 'locked' knee. They are longitudinal tears, usually of the medial meniscus, and frequently associated with ACL disruption.

Radiology

Routine X-rays do not show any direct evidence of meniscal damage but are useful to exclude commonly associated bony injuries. MRI may determine both meniscal and ligamentous injuries in complex cases.

Management

Arthroscopy is used to evaluate and treat meniscal injuries, revealing the extent of damage and determining whether resection of the torn cartilage or meniscectomy are required. An acutely locked knee should be referred for urgent arthroscopy.

Controversies

- Evaluating and validating new clinical decision tools for radiography in acute knee injuries.
- Replacing cylindrical plaster cast treatment of patellar fractures and some soft-tissue injuries with three-panel Velcro knee immobilizer splints and hinged supports.
- Role of CT scan in condylar and tibial plateau knee injuries.
- Indications for MRI over arthroscopy in complex soft tissue knee injuries.

References

[1] Scholten R, Opstelten W, Van Der Plas C, et al. Accuracy of physical diagnositic tests for assessing ruptures of the anterior cruciate ligament: a meta-analysis. J Fam Pract 2003;52:689–94.

[2] Bachmann LM, Steurer J, Ter Riet G, et al. The accuracy of the Ottawa knee rule to rule out knee fractures: a systematic review. Ann Intern Med 2004;140:121–4.

[3] Crist B, Della Rocca G, Murtha Y. Treatment of acute distal femur fractures. Orthopedics 2008;31:681–90.

[4] Markhardt B, Gross J, Monu J. Schatzker classification of tibial plateau fractures: use of CT and MRI imaging improves classification. Radiographics 2009;29:585–97.

[5] Bandyk DF. Vascular injury associated with extremity trauma. Clin Orthoped 1995;318:117–24.

[6] Kode L, Lieberman JM, Motta AO, et al. Evaluation of tibial plateau fractures: efficacy of MR imaging compared with CT. Am J Roentgenol 1994;163:141.

[7] Fenton P, Porter K. Tibial plateau fractures: a review. J Trauma 2011;13:181–7.

[8] Kendall NS, Hsu SY, Chan KM. Fracture of the tibial spine in adults and children. J Bone Joint Surg 1992;74B:848.

[9] Scolaro J, Bernstein J, Jaimo A. Patellar fractures. Clin Orthop Relat Res 2011;469:1213–5.

[10] Nicandri G, Dunbar R, Wahl C. Are evidence-based protocols which identify vascular injury associated with knee dislocation underutilized? Knee Surg Sports Traumatol Arthrosc 2010;18:1005–12.

[11] Coen A, Chad J, Steinar J, et al. Injuries to the medial collateral ligament and associated medial structures of the knee. J Bone Joint Surg 2010;92A:1266–80.

[12] Linko E, Harilainen A, Malmivaaran A, Seitsalo S. Surgical versus conservative interventions for anterior cruciate ligament ruptures in adults. Cochrane Database Syst Rev 2005;18:CD001356.

Further reading

Roberts D, Stallard T. Emergency department evaluation and treatment of knee and leg injuries. Emerg Med Clin N Am 2000;18:67–84.

4.10 Tibia and fibula injuries

Michael Baker • Michael Cadogan

ESSENTIALS

1 Tibial shaft fractures are the commonest long bone fracture and the subcutaneous nature of the tibia leaves it vulnerable to open injury.

2 Neurovascular injury and compartment syndrome are a risk in tibial shaft fractures.

3 Proximal fibula fractures are associated with common peroneal (lateral popliteal) nerve injury.

4 Tibial tubercle injuries range from apophysitis to fracture.

Anatomy

The tibia is the weight-bearing strut of the lower leg. Proximally, the tibia articulates with the femoral condyles and distally, the bony extension provides medial stability to the ankle joint. Its shaft is triangular in cross-section and is subcutaneous anteromedially.

The fibula head is proximal and connects to the fibular shaft by the neck. Distally, the fibula is palpated subcutaneously as the lateral malleolus.

The tibia and fibula are connected by superior and inferior tibiofibular joints and a dense interosseous membrane. Distally, this union is strengthened by a syndesmosis, which enhances the stability of the ankle mortise.

Lower leg fascial compartments

The lower leg is divided into four compartments by bone and fascia. Each compartment contains a sensory nerve and muscles with specific functions. Increased pressure within a compartment is evaluated clinically by impaired function according to the functional anatomy.

Anterior compartment

The anterior compartment contains the tibialis anterior and the long toe extensor muscles (extensor hallucis longus and extensor digitorum longus) that dorsiflex the ankle and foot. The deep peroneal nerve supplies these muscles and the first web space of the foot. The anterior tibial artery is contained within the compartment down to the ankle, where it becomes the dorsalis pedis artery.

Lateral compartment

The lateral compartment contains the peroneus longus and peroneus brevis which evert the foot and the superficial peroneal nerve that supplies sensation to the dorsum of the foot.

Superficial posterior compartment

The superficial posterior compartment contains the gastrocnemius, plantaris and soleus muscles which plantarflex the ankle. The sural nerve lies in this compartment before piercing the fascia to supply the lateral side of the foot and distal calf.

Deep posterior compartment

The deep posterior compartment contains the tibialis posterior and long toe flexor muscles (flexor hallucis longus and flexor digitorum longus) which plantarflex the toes. The tibial nerve is within the compartment and supplies sensory function to the sole of the foot. The posterior tibial and peroneal arteries also lie in this compartment.

Fractures of the tibia

Tibial shaft fracture

Tibial shaft fractures are the most common long bone fracture and are usually easily recognized. They are also the commonest open fracture owing to the subcutaneous nature of the tibial shaft.

A considerable amount of direct or indirect energy is needed for the tibial shaft to fracture. Direct injuries may occur secondary to bending forces or a direct blow. Direct violence, such as

in a motor vehicle incident or when a pedestrian is struck, cause deformation at the site of contact, resulting in transverse or comminuted, usually open, fractures. High-energy injuries have an increased degree of displacement, comminution, soft tissue injury and fibular involvement. They are associated with marked vascular, interosseous and bony involvement and are unstable, with a high risk of compartment syndrome. Up to 15% are complicated by malunion or non-union.

Indirect torsional forces applied to the tibia produce a spiral fracture as the body rotates about a fixed foot. Such injuries are common in skiing incidents and have increasing degrees of comminution depending on the amount of energy applied.

Classification

The description of the fracture must be clear and concise in relation to the following (see also Table 4.10.1 for the AO classification of tibial shaft fractures) [1]:

- skin integrity: open or closed
- anatomical site: proximal, middle or distal third
- fracture type: transverse, oblique, spiral or comminuted
- angulation of the distal fragment in relation to the proximal fragment, expressed in degrees and direction (anterior, posterior, varus or valgus)
- degree of displacement and rotation
- involvement of the fibula
- any joint involvement.

Clinical assessment

Pain at the site of fracture is usually severe. The patient is unable to bear weight and inspection reveals swelling and deformity of the leg. The skin is checked for integrity and to identify areas of pressure caused by any displaced fragments. The neurovascular status of the lower leg and foot are assessed as a matter of urgency, including skin colour, capillary refill and the distal dorsalis pedis and posterior tibial pulses. Associated injuries of the ipsilateral femur, hip, knee, foot and pelvis must be excluded.

Nerve injury Contusion of the peroneal nerve may occur in high-energy injuries with

Table 4.10.1 AO classification of tibial shaft fractures		
Type A (simple)	1	Spiral
	2	Oblique (angle >30°)
	3	Transverse (angle <30°)
Type B (multifrag wedge)	1	Spiral wedge
	2	Bending wedge
	3	Fragmented wedge
Type C (multifrag complex)	1	Spiral wedge
	2	Segmental
	3	Irregular

proximal fibular fractures, although direct peroneal nerve injury can occur rarely in a closed tibial shaft fracture. The motor function of the deep peroneal nerve is tested by active ankle and toe dorsiflexion and the sensory function is tested in the first dorsal web space. The motor function of the superficial peroneal nerve is tested by active foot eversion and the sensory function is tested over the dorsal lateral aspect of the foot.

Radiology
AP and lateral views of the lower leg must include the entire tibia and fibula, from the knee to the ankle, to document tibial shaft fracture, identify associated fibula fracture, the fracture pattern and any degree of comminution and/or displacement (Fig. 4.10.1). X-ray the knee and ankle joint to look for associated joint involvement.

Management
Parenteral analgesia is the first priority, usually an intravenous opiate, followed by reduction of any displaced and/or compound fractures and immobilization in a long leg cast as early as possible.

Compartment syndrome
Emergency department (ED) documentation of the neurovascular status is essential to exclude acute neurovascular injury, as well as to detect actual or potential compartment syndrome. Development of a compartment syndrome may occur in up to 20% of closed injuries and can take up to 24 hours to appear. It is less common in compound injuries.

Increasing pain despite reduction and casting are an early indicator of compartment syndrome. This should be suspected if there is weakness of muscle action, pain on passive movement and diminished sensation over the distal sensory nerve territory. Pulses can

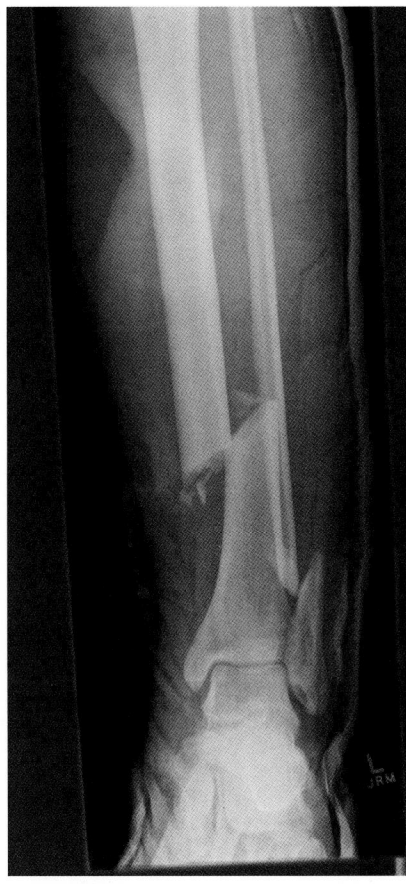

Fig. 4.10.1 Open, oblique, distal third tibial fracture with displaced varus deformity and fibula involvement.

still be present, so a strong pedal pulse does *not* exclude the presence of a compartment syndrome. The deep posterior compartment is most commonly affected, followed by isolated elevation of pressure in the anterior compartment.

Compartment pressures If there is concern, compartment pressures may be measured. A compartment syndrome can occur if the compartment pressure is >30 mmHg or within 30 mmHg of mean arterial pressure (MAP). Routine continuous pressure monitoring in tibial shaft fractures does not result in an improved outcome and is not recommended [2].

Open wounds
Open wounds are assessed for depth and associated soft tissue damage, then dressed to avoid further contamination. Reduce a displaced, rotated or angulated fracture in the ED under appropriate analgesia and procedural sedation (see Chapter 22.3). Reduction aims to stop local swelling, release the tension of

any skin 'tented' over a displaced fracture and relieve associated soft tissue damage. Exposed bone is returned under the skin after appropriate decontamination. Check the tetanus status and give parenteral antibiotics such as flu/dicloxacillin 2 g 6-hourly IV or cephazolin 2 g 8-hourly IV.

Immobilize the leg following reduction in 20° of knee flexion and request post-reduction X-rays to confirm the position. Re-check and document the neurovascular status of the lower leg and foot.

Definitive orthopaedic management
There are various options for definitive management including conservative, closed reduction, open reduction and internal fixation (ORIF) and intramedullary rods. No approach is superior, with a recent meta-analysis finding insufficient evidence to support any particular management option [3].

Non-operative management Non-operative management in an above-knee plaster of Paris (POP) cast is appropriate for a low-energy fracture without significant comminution, shortening or displacement. Conservative management may also be appropriate for fractures with >50% cortical contact, <5–10° of varus/valgus angulation, <10–15° of anterior or posterior bowing, <5–7° of rotation and no more than 10–15 mm of shortening [4].

Operative management Operative management is considered for patients with a high-energy displaced fracture, compound fracture or who have failed closed treatment. Intramedullary nailing results in shorter hospital stay, fewer outpatient visits and earlier return to work [5]. ORIF is also considered for displaced intra-articular fractures of the tibia involving the knee or ankle.

Tibial tubercle fracture
The tibial tubercle lies proximally on the anterior border of the shaft of the tibia. It is readily palpable beneath the infrapatellar bursa and receives the insertion of the patellar tendon. Fractures of the tubercle are uncommon and occur in adolescents, typically as a result of indirect injury sustained during sports involving jumping, such as sudden acceleration or deceleration of the extensor mechanism of the knee producing an avulsion fracture. Risk factors for this condition include Osgood–Schlatter's disease and osteogenesis imperfecta [6]. Similar to other tibial

fractures, up to 20% are complicated by compartment syndrome.

Three grades of injury are described by Watson–Jones. In type I injuries, the tubercle is hinged upwards without displacement; type II injuries involve avulsion of a small portion of the tubercle proximally; and type III injuries are intra-articular. The fragment is displaced and may be comminuted.

Examination reveals pain and tenderness over the anterior aspect of the knee and proximal tibia. There may be a haemarthrosis and loss of active extension, depending on the severity of the injury.

Plain X-rays confirm the diagnosis. The lateral tibial view reveals the avulsion fragment, its degree of displacement and comminution.

Management is dependent on the degree of displacement and the presence of joint involvement. Watson–Jones type I and II injuries are treated with cylindrical long leg casts until healed. Type III injuries require open reduction and internal fixation with tension band wiring and fixation screws [7].

Osgood–Schlatter's disease (traction apophysitis of the tibial tubercle)

The commonest differential diagnosis of tibial tuberosity fracture is Osgood–Schlatter's disease, that refers to traction apophysitis of the tibial tubercle caused by repeated microtrauma to the growing tubercle during adolescence. It is chronic and, unlike tubercle fractures, is not accompanied by a haemarthrosis. Active knee extension is possible, albeit painful.

Treatment is conservative with rest, ice, compression and non-steroidal anti-inflammatory drugs (NSAIDs), followed by graded return to sporting activities. This is a self-limiting condition with full recovery expected in 1–2 years, when the apophysis closes.

Tibial stress fractures

Tibial stress fractures are common, affecting the proximal third of the tibia in adolescents and the junction of middle and distal thirds of the tibia in runners. Clinically, there is point tenderness over an area of induration. X-rays may appear negative early or show periosteal reaction after 3–5 weeks. A bone scan or MRI can detect these injuries earlier.

The differential diagnosis includes 'shin splints' (see below), fascial hernias and exertional compartment syndrome. Management is conservative, reducing activity and impact on the tibia. Symptoms may persist for over 12 months.

Shin splints

Shin splints is also known as 'medial tibial stress syndrome' and is characterized by exercise-induced pain in the midsection of the leg, with tenderness along the posteromedial border of the middle and distal thirds of the tibia. The tenderness is usually more diffuse than the localized tenderness of a stress fracture. There may be periostitis near the origin of the soleus and flexor digitorum longus muscles. It is rare in children under 15 years of age.

Fractures of the fibula

Proximal fibula fractures may occur in isolation (uncommon) or in association with tibial and ankle injuries.

Associated tibial shaft fracture

Most fibula fractures are associated with a fracture of the tibial shaft and are managed as for tibial fractures. The pattern of the associated fibular fracture indicates the degree of energy imparted. Severe comminution of the fibula or tibiofibular diastasis implies disruption of the interosseous membrane and indicates an unstable fracture.

The fibula usually heals well with whatever treatment is selected for the tibia, with a better rate of union. Complications of fibula fractures associated with tibial shaft fractures are rare.

Isolated proximal fibula fractures

Isolated proximal fibula or fibula shaft fractures are less common. They are usually associated with a direct blow to the lateral aspect of the leg, causing local tenderness, swelling, bruising and difficulty walking. A neurovascular assessment is important as the common peroneal nerve passes around the neck of fibula and may be contused or disrupted in these isolated injuries. Rarely, thrombosis of the anterior tibial artery may occur.

Full-length AP and lateral X-rays of the tibia and fibula, including the ankle and knee joints, will confirm the fracture pattern.

Management

Non-displaced fractures associated with little pain are treated with ice, compression bandage, analgesia and non-weight-bearing crutches for 3 weeks. Weight bearing is progressive as tolerated. Mildly displaced fractures or those with significant pain may require a long leg cast for up to 6 weeks. A severely displaced fracture or one associated with peroneal nerve deficit, such as foot drop, requires orthopaedic consultation and consideration for fixation.

Maisonneuve fracture

A medial malleolus or distal tibial fracture associated with a proximal fibula fracture is termed a Maisonneuve fracture. These are unstable and occur when an external rotatory force is applied to the ankle, resulting in partial or complete disruption of the syndesmosis between the tibia and fibula. Palpation of the proximal fibula following a complex ankle injury is therefore essential to exclude this fracture. Refer all these fractures to the orthopaedic team for operative fixation.

Controversies

- Use and value of compartment pressure monitoring in the ED.
- Which clinical features or actual compartment pressure require active management.
- Indications for operative intervention in closed tibial shaft fractures.

References

[1] Muller ME, Nazarian S, Koch P. The AO classification of fractures. New York: Springer-Verlag; 1988.
[2] Harris I, Kadir A, Donald G. Continuous compartment pressure monitoring for tibia fractures: does it influence outcome? J Trauma 2006;60:1330–5.
[3] Littenberg B, Weinstein L, McCarren M, et al. Closed fractures of the tibial shaft. A meta-analysis of three methods of treatment. J Bone Joint Surg 1998;80A:174–83.
[4] Wheeless' Textbook of Orthopaedics. <http://www.wheelessonline.com/ortho/cast_treatment_of_tibial_fractures> [Accessed Feb. 2013].
[5] Hooper G, Keddell R, Penny I. Conservative management or closed nailing for tibial shaft fractures: a randomized prospective trial. J Bone Joint Surg 1991;73B:83–5.
[6] Frey S, Hosalker H, Cameron D, et al. Tibial tuberosity fractures in adolescents. J Child Orthop 2008;2:469–74.
[7] Balmat P, Vichard P, Pem R. The treatment of avulsion fractures of the tibial tuberosity in adolescent athletes. Sports Med 1990;9:311–6.

Further reading

Roberts D, Stallard T. Emergency department evaluation and treatment of knee and leg injuries. Emerg Med Clin N Am 2000;18:67–84.

ORTHOPAEDIC EMERGENCIES

4

4.11 Ankle joint injuries

Michael Baker • Michael Cadogan

ESSENTIALS

1 Ankle injuries are common and occur as isolated injuries or related to high-energy multitrauma.

2 Lateral malleolar fractures are the most common ankle fracture.

3 The Ottawa Ankle Rules (OAR) are used to determine the need for imaging of the ankle (or foot) in adults with an isolated acute ankle injury.

4 The Weber and Henderson (Potts) classifications are the most commonly used for describing ankle fractures.

5 Ankle sprains should be mobilized early.

6 The calf-squeeze test (Thompson or Simmond's test) is used to confirm the diagnosis of Achilles tendon rupture.

Anatomy

The ankle joint is a complex hinge joint that permits articulation between the tibia, fibula and talus, providing a stable but mobile support for the body. It helps absorb the forces of ambulation, maintain an upright posture and allows for uneven terrain.

The stability of the ankle joint relates to the bony architecture, joint capsule and the ligaments. The bones and ligaments are best visualized as a ring structure centring on the talus, which provides stability. This ring is made up of the tibial plafond, medial malleolus, the medial (deltoid) ligament, calcaneus, lateral collateral ligaments, lateral malleolus and the syndesmotic ligaments. The joint becomes unstable when more than one element of this ring structure is disrupted.

Bony mortise

The lateral malleolus of the distal fibula, the medial malleolus of the distal tibia and the distal tibial plafond form the bony mortise of the joint. This provides intrinsic stability constraining the wedge-shaped talus distally. The medial ligament of the ankle or deltoid ligament fans out from the tip of the medial malleolus to attach to the tuberosity of the navicular, the medial aspect of the talus and the sustentaculum tali of the calcaneus. The lateral ligament

comprises three discrete parts, the anterior and posterior talofibular ligaments and the calcaneofibular ligament.

Most ankle joint injuries are a result of abnormal movement of the talus within the mortise. Movement causes stress to the encompassing ring of structures of the ankle joint, with instability arising when disruption of the malleoli or their associated ligaments results in distraction of the talus within the mortise.

Clinical assessment

Injuries around the ankle include fractures to the ankle and adjacent tarsal bones, ligamentous sprains, dislocations and tendon ruptures. All these are considered when assessing the patient with an ankle injury.

History

Inability to bear weight and the presence of swelling immediately following an injury imply significant pathology. Additional essential information includes the circumstances of the injury, position of the foot at the time and the magnitude and direction of loading forces applied, particularly rotational. A history of inversion injury should prompt the examiner to assess also the base of the fifth metatarsal for an avulsion fracture by the insertion of peroneus brevis.

Examination

Give the patient analgesia, ice and elevate the affected limb. Examination of the ankle includes the entire lower leg and begins with a comparison between the injured and non-injured sides. Note the skin integrity and presence of bruising, swelling or deformity.

Palpate for point tenderness to localize ligament, bone or tendon injury, which should commence at a site away from the area of obvious injury. The entire length of the tibia and fibula as well as the base of the fifth metatarsal, calcaneus and Achilles tendon are examined. Palpation of the posterior aspects of the malleoli should commence 6–10 cm proximally and include both ends of the collateral ligament attachments. The anterior plafond and the medial and lateral aspects of the talar dome are then palpated in plantarflexion.

Then assess the range of active and passive movement at the ankle joint, including inversion, eversion, dorsiflexion and plantarflexion. A soft tissue injury is likely when there is a significant difference between the active and passive ranges of movement.

Finally, always check the foot for motor or sensory impairment, capillary return, the presence of dorsalis pedis and posterior tibial pulses and injury to the base of the fifth metatarsal.

Stress testing for ligamentous instability

Stress testing for ligamentous instability of the acutely injured ankle and/or an evaluation of weight-bearing ability should only proceed when clinical suspicion of a fracture is low. All require appropriate analgesia for evaluation.

The talar tilt test assesses the calcaneofibular ligament by applying a gentle inversion stress to the calcaneum.

The anterior and posterior drawer tests assess the anterior and posterior talofibular ligaments by gentle forward traction on the heel.

Radiology: Ottawa ankle rules

Standard radiography of the acutely injured ankle includes anteroposterior, lateral and mortise views. All patients with an obviously deformed fracture or dislocation should have immediate X-ray following analgesia.

The need for imaging of the ankle or midfoot in a patient with less obvious injury may be determined using the Ottawa ankle rules (OAR). When used on a competent patient, the OAR are more than 98% sensitive for detecting clinically relevant ankle fractures in adults [1,2] and 98% sensitive in children [3,4].

Ottawa ankle rules

These rules specify that an ankle X-ray series is only required if there is any pain in the malleolar region and any one of:

- bone tenderness over the posterior aspect or inferior tip of the distal 6 cm of the lateral malleolus
- bone tenderness over the posterior aspect or inferior tip of the distal 6 cm of the medial malleolus
- inability to bear weight for at least four steps, both immediately after the injury and at the time of emergency department (ED) evaluation.

The OAR also include indications for taking an additional foot X-ray series (see Foot injuries, Chapter 4.12).

Other imaging

Computed tomography (CT) is used to evaluate further complex fractures and magnetic resonance imaging (MRI) for difficult or recalcitrant ligamentous injuries.

Ankle fracture classification

Several classification systems are used to describe ankle fractures and dislocations, some more complicated than others.

Weber classification

The Weber classification system (1972) divides ankle fractures into three types, based on the level at which the fibula fractures. The more proximal the fibula fracture, the greater the associated syndesmosis disruption and potential for ankle instability.

Type A fractures involve the distal fibula below the level of the tibial plafond; type B involve an oblique or spiral fracture at the level of the syndesmosis; and type C occur when the fibula is fractured above the level of the syndesmosis (ankle joint).

The original Weber classification system does not take into account medial or posterior malleolar fractures. The AO system applies three subdivisions to each Weber fracture type

to account for these injuries and to define further ankle stability [5].

Henderson or Pott's classification

The Henderson or Pott's classification is a simple system based on radiographic findings:

- Unimalleolar fractures affecting the lateral or medial malleolus. The stability of these fractures is dependent on the integrity of contralateral ligaments and the inferior tibiofibular joint.
- Bimalleolar fractures affecting the medial and lateral malleoli, which are usually unstable.
- Trimalleolar fractures involving the medial, lateral and posterior tibial plafond, which are always unstable.

Fracture management

A grossly displaced fracture is reduced and splinted promptly in the ED, under procedural sedation, prior to imaging if distal ischaemia is identified and/or the skin integrity compromised (Fig. 4.11.1). These will require elevation and orthopaedic admission for operative management.

Non-displaced fractures

Non-displaced (<3 mm) unimalleolar Weber A fractures with an intact mortise joint (no talar shift) on X-ray are treated non-operatively in a below-knee plaster of Paris (POP) cast in a neutral position, that is, with the ankle at 90° with no inversion or eversion. Refer these injuries for orthopaedic follow up, with advice that fracture movement may occur and that operative intervention may still be required.

The management of an isolated non-displaced Weber B injury, with the fracture line at the level of the syndesmosis, is controversial. If the deltoid ligament is intact and there is no talar shift, a conservative approach results in good outcomes with low rates of subsequent surgical intervention [6].

Displaced fractures

Displaced and potentially unstable fractures require early orthopaedic consultation, including all bimalleolar and trimalleolar fractures, those unimalleolar fractures with contralateral ligamentous injuries and Weber C injuries. The majority of these injuries will require operative intervention (open reduction and internal fixation [ORIF]).

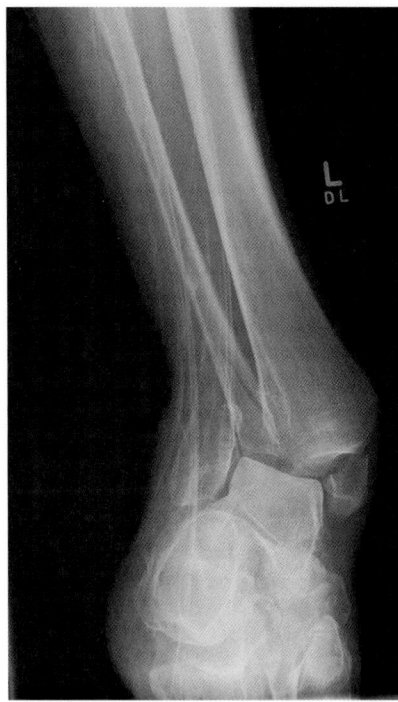

Fig. 4.11.1 Unstable bimalleolar ankle fracture.

Tibial plafond (pilon) fractures

Tibial plafond (pilon = hammer) fractures involve the distal tibial metaphysis and result from high-energy injuries directed through the talus into the distal tibia, with tibial plafond disruption. The frequency has increased with greater numbers of motor vehicle incidents and falls from heights. They are usually associated with other multiple injuries and often open, comminuted or associated with extensive soft tissue deformity.

Reduce and splint the fracture under appropriate analgesia and procedural sedation to decrease the potential for massive soft tissue swelling, with conversion of a closed fracture to an open one as a result of overlying skin necrosis. Treatment usually requires operative fixation.

Maisonneuve fracture

The Maisonneuve fracture is a fracture of the proximal end of the fibula associated with a medial malleolus fracture or disruption of the medial (deltoid) ligament, resulting from external rotation. The proximal fibula fracture is associated with disruption of the interosseous membrane from the tibiofibular syndesmosis up

203

to the proximal fibular head. It may be complicated by a common peroneal nerve injury. They are unstable and require operative fixation.

Ankle dislocations

Ankle dislocations are frequently associated with a fracture, but can occur in isolation and may be open or closed. They result from considerable energy, such as when force is directed against the plantarflexed foot, squeezing the talus out of the mortise. Posterior dislocations are the most common. All require orthopaedic advice for consideration of internal fixation and ligamentous repair.

Closed dislocations

Closed dislocations are associated with marked soft-tissue disruption and skin tethering, although neurovascular compromise is uncommon. These dislocations are reduced promptly in the ED to minimize associated soft-tissue injury, using gentle manipulation under appropriate analgesia and procedural sedation (just as for the grossly displaced fracture).

Despite the potential for ligamentous disruption, they usually have an excellent outcome following immobilization for 8 weeks.

Open dislocations

Open dislocations may be associated with disruption of the dorsalis pedis and posterior tibial vessels. They require surgical debridement in theatre, but again should initially be reduced and splinted with POP in the ED. Open injuries are associated with more long-term complications than closed, in particular traumatic arthritis and reduced mobility.

Soft-tissue injuries

Ligamentous injuries

Ankle sprains

Ankle sprains are one of the most common injuries presenting to the ED: 75% of injuries to the ankle are sprains and 90% of these affect the lateral ligament complex, predominantly the anterior talofibular ligament. Typically, injuries to the lateral ligament proceed from anterior to posterior as increasing force is applied.

Medial ligament disruption is more frequently associated with lateral malleolar fractures or Maisonneuve-type injuries involving the proximal fibula and syndesmosis disruption.

Lateral ligament injuries

Lateral ligament injuries are graded according to the degree of fibre disruption and reflect the progression of injury from anterior to posterior as well as subsequent stability of the ankle joint. However, an accurate assessment of joint stability is usually not possible in the ED setting due to pain limiting examination.

- Grade I: partial tear, usually of the anterior talofibular ligament. Patients are usually able to weight bear with minimal swelling and normal stress testing.
- Grade II: partial tear, usually extending to the calcaneofibular ligament. There is pain at rest, difficulty weight bearing, significant swelling and mild to moderate joint instability.
- Grade III: complete tear of two or more elements of the lateral ligament. Patients are unable to weight bear due to severe pain, with immediate swelling and marked joint instability.

Grade I and most grade II injuries are treated conservatively with rest, ice, compression, elevation and non-steroidal anti-inflammatory drugs for 48 hours. Early functional treatment is likely better than immobilization in the treatment of lateral ligament injuries [7].

Operative intervention for grade III lateral ligament injuries is controversial, with conservative and surgical therapy associated with similar clinical outcomes. Surgery may improve perceived stability and reduce pain and is more commonly undertaken in the athlete [8].

Conservative treatment includes cast immobilization for 6–8 weeks with orthopaedic follow up. Delayed surgical repair or reconstruction has similar results to early intervention.

Achilles tendon rupture

Achilles tendon rupture is traditionally associated with sedentary middle-aged individuals during a burst of unaccustomed strenuous physical activity, although young, fit athletes also sustain this condition.

Predisposing medical conditions when present include rheumatoid arthritis, systemic lupus erythematosus (SLE), chronic renal failure, gout, hyperparathyroidism and long-term steroid or fluoroquinolone use. The segment of the Achilles tendon particularly prone to rupture lies 2–6 cm proximal to the tendon's insertion into the calcaneus, as blood vessels that supply this area are prone to atrophy. The resultant reduction in collagen cross-linking leads to a reduced tensile strength in the tendon, with the majority of tears complete.

History

Rupture usually occurs while pushing off with a weight-bearing foot, but may occur with sudden dorsiflexion or direct trauma. The sensation of a direct blow to the back of the ankle and even an audible 'pop' are followed by difficulty in walking. The patient often states that they thought they had been hit or kicked from behind.

Examination

Examination reveals a visible and/or palpable deficit in the tendon, although swelling around the tendon sheath rapidly masks these signs. Some degree of plantarflexion of the ankle joint is preserved by the other long flexors of the ankle, foot and toes. This should therefore *not* be used to determine if the Achilles tendon is intact, although the patient cannot stand on tiptoe.

Calf-squeeze test (Thompson test or Simmond's test)

The calf-squeeze test (Thompson or Simmond's test) confirms the diagnosis of a rupture with a sensitivity of 96%. Perform this with the patient kneeling on a chair with the feet hanging free over the edge. Alternatively, it is often more comfortable for the patient to lie prone with the feet and ankles extended hanging freely beyond the end of the examination couch.

Demonstrate normal plantar flexion initially on the unaffected calf, by gently squeezing just distal to its maximal girth. Absence of plantarflexion in the affected limb is a positive test and confirms Achilles rupture. Ultrasound is useful if the diagnosis is in doubt and can demonstrate partial or full-thickness tears of the tendon, as well as measure the size of the defect.

Management

The choice of operative or non-operative treatment is controversial [9]. Surgery is more likely to be offered to younger patients, those who are diagnosed early and in those with a larger defect. Operative risks include fistula formation, skin necrosis and infection. However, the procedure has a lower rate of muscle atrophy, a lower re-rupture rate and allows earlier resumption of physical activity. Minimally invasive techniques have resulted in reduced infection rates and time to return to work.

Non-operative management includes applying a POP cast to the ankle in equinus (full plantar flexion) to bring the two ends of the ruptured tendon into apposition. One regimen involves a cast for 4 weeks in equinus, 4 weeks in partial plantarflexion and then 2 weeks in the neutral position. Complications of non-operative management include a higher re-rupture rate (requiring surgical intervention).

- Role of bracing, topical anti-inflammatories, laser and ultrasound therapy in the management of ankle sprains.
- Operative versus conservative management of Achilles tendon rupture.

Controversies

- Whether internal fixation results in an improved outcome compared to conservative management in Weber type B fractures.

References

[1] Stiell I, Greenberg G, McKnight R, et al. Decision rules for the use of radiography in acute ankle injury. Refinement and prospective validation. J Am Med Assoc 1993;269:1127–32.
[2] Bachmann L, Kolb E, Koller M, et al. Accuracy of Ottawa ankle rules to exclude fractures of the ankle and mid-foot: systematic review. Br Med J 2003;326:417–23.
[3] Libetta C, Burke D, Brennan P, et al. Validation of the Ottawa ankle rules in children. J Accident Emerg Med 1999;16:342–4.
[4] Plint A, Bulloch B, Osmond M, et al. Validation of the Ottawa ankle rules in children with ankle injuries. Acad Emerg Med 1999;6:1005–9.
[5] Muller ME, Nazarian S, Koch P. The AO classification of fractures. New York: Springer-Verlag; 1988.
[6] Martin A. Weber B ankle fracture: an unnecessary fracture clinic burden. Injury 2004;35:805–9.
[7] Jones M, Amendola A. Acute treatment of inversion ankle sprains: immobilization versus functional treatment. Clin Orthopaed Relat Res 2007;445:169–72.
[8] Pijnenburg A, Van Dijk C, Bossuyt P, et al. Treatment of ruptures of the lateral ankle ligaments: a meta-analysis. J Bone Joint Surg 2000;82A:761–73.
[9] Weatherall J, Mroczek K, Tejwani N. Acute Achilles tendon ruptures. Orthopedics 2010;33:758–64.

Further reading

Borrer R, Famo-Salek M, Totten V, et al. Managing ankle injuries in the emergency department. J Emerg Med 1999;17: 651–60.
Wedmore I, Charette J. Emergency department evaluation and treatment of ankle and foot injuries. Emerg Med Clin N Am 2000;18:85–113.

4.12 Foot injuries

Michael Baker • Michael Cadogan

ESSENTIALS

1 Most calcaneal fractures are intra-articular, associated with a Bohler's angle of less than 20° and are at risk of developing compartment syndrome.

2 Major talar fractures have a significant risk of subsequent avascular necrosis.

3 Navicular body fractures may require internal fixation.

4 Fractures of the base of the second metatarsal are pathognomic of Lisfranc injury (Fleck sign).

5 CT imaging is indicated in complicated talar, calcaneal, navicular as well as Lisfranc injuries.

Anatomy

The foot is composed of 28 bones with 57 articular surfaces. It may be divided into three anatomical regions: the hindfoot containing the talus and calcaneum; the midfoot containing the navicular, cuboid and cuneiforms; and the forefoot containing the metatarsals and phalanges.

The subtalar joint collectively describes the three articulations of the inferior aspect of the talus with the calcaneus. It allows inversion and eversion of the hindfoot. The midtarsal joints incorporate the talonavicular and calcaneocuboid joints that connect the hindfoot and midfoot and allow abduction and adduction of the forefoot. The five tarsometatarsal joints (Lisfranc joint complex) connect the midfoot and forefoot and form an arch, which gives stability to the foot.

Clinical assessment

History

Injury to the foot occurs as a result of direct or indirect trauma. Direct trauma is often associated with considerable soft-tissue swelling and fracture. Indirect trauma from a twisting injury usually results in minor avulsion-type injuries. Record any pain, swelling, loss of function, reduced sensation and deformity or associated ankle injury.

Examination

Inspect the area with the patient lying on a bed with both lower limbs exposed and compare to the unaffected limb to identify bruising, swelling, deformity, skin wounds, pallor or cyanosis.

Start gentle palpation over the entire foot away from the area of maximal pain. Point tenderness or crepitus may be elicited at the site of fracture. Specific areas to palpate include the Achilles tendon, calcaneus, base of the fifth metatarsal, the navicular and the area under the head of the second metatarsal.

Ask the patient to demonstrate active foot movements before performing gentle passive movements and compare with the other foot. Evaluate subtalar motion with the foot in a neutral position, with one hand on the lower leg and the other holding the heel. The heel is inverted and everted and should attain 25° of movement.

Midtarsal motion is assessed with one hand stabilizing the heel while the other hand grasps the forefoot at the bases of the metatarsals. The forefoot is pronated, supinated, adducted and abducted. Finally, forefoot motion is evaluated by individually flexing and extending the metatarsophalangeal (MTP) and interphalangeal (IP) joints.

Ask the patient to stand and walk if no obvious focus of the pain is found during the initial examination. Finally, assess the circulation by observing capillary refill, skin colour and the presence of the dorsalis pedis and posterior tibial pulses.

The posterior tibial pulse is palpable behind the medial malleolus, unless there is excessive swelling or damage to the artery. The dorsalis pedis is more variable, being too small to feel easily, or is absent in 12% of the population. Doppler may be needed to determine the presence of flow when there is doubt. Neurological assessment includes motor and sensory function.

Radiology

Standard imaging includes AP, lateral and 45° internal oblique projections. The lateral view visualizes the hindfoot and soft tissues, whereas the oblique and AP projections image the midfoot and forefoot. An axial calcaneal view should also be requested as clinically indicated to best visualize the hindfoot and may reveal a subtle calcaneal fracture.

Ottawa ankle and foot rules

The Ottawa ankle and foot rules provide indications for X-ray for suspected midfoot fractures [1]. All patients with obvious deformities should have X-rays. However, if clinical findings are more subtle, a foot X-ray is *only* required if there is pain in the midfoot region and any one of:

- bone tenderness over the navicular
- bone tenderness at the base of the fifth metatarsal
- inability to bear weight for at least four steps, both immediately after the injury and at the time of emergency department (ED) evaluation.

This clinical decision rule has a sensitivity approaching 100% and routine use has been predicted to reduce unnecessary X-rays by 30–40% [1]. These rules do not apply to suspected hindfoot or forefoot fractures.

Other imaging

A bone scan is indicated when a stress fracture is suspected and may become positive 2–3 weeks before conventional radiographs demonstrate a fracture. Computed tomography (CT) is used for imaging the calcaneum, subtalar joint and Lisfranc joint in more complex injuries or when a fracture is strongly suspected but plain X-rays are inconclusive.

Hindfoot injuries

Calcaneal fractures

The calcaneus is the largest bone in the foot and is the most commonly fractured tarsal bone. It forms the heel of the foot, provides vertical support for the body's weight and functions as a springboard for locomotion. The majority of fractures of the calcaneus occur as a result of direct axial compression during a fall from a height. Seven per cent are bilateral. Lower-extremity injuries are present in 25% of cases and vertebral compression fractures are found in 10%, so these regions must be examined as well.

Mechanism and classification

Patients usually present following a fall with direct trauma to the heel. Seventy-five per cent of calcaneal fractures are intra-articular. These fractures may be non-displaced, displaced or frequently comminuted owing to cancellous bone in the calcaneus and the magnitude of associated force (Fig. 4.12.1).

An isolated fracture of the anterior process of the calcaneus is commonly misdiagnosed as an ankle sprain [2]. It results from inversion causing an avulsion fracture or forced dorsiflexion producing compression against the cuboid.

Clinical assessment

The patient may be able to walk, but weight bearing on the heel is impossible. Examination reveals pain, swelling and tenderness over the heel, with bruising that may extend over the sole of the foot. Associated fractures are common, so examination of the vertebral column, pelvis, affected lower extremity and opposing calcaneus is essential.

Radiology

Standard X-rays usually reveal most comminuted calcaneal fractures, whereas more subtle fractures are visualized with the aid of specific axial (Harris) calcaneal views or on CT scan. The AP view demonstrates the anterosuperior

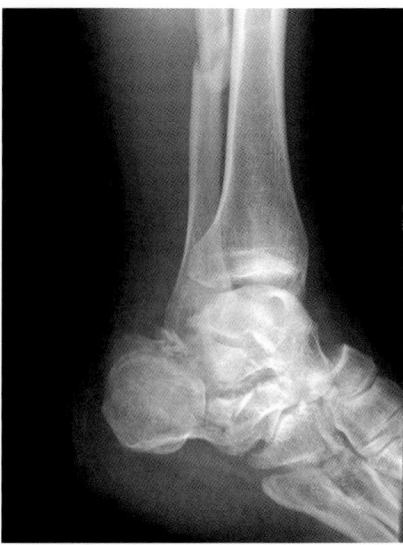

Fig. 4.12.1 Intra-articular comminuted calcaneal fracture.

calcaneus and calcaneocuboid joint. The lateral view may reveal compression fractures of the body and posterior facet.

Bohler's angle   Bohler's angle is formed by the intersection of a line drawn from the most cephalic point on the tuberosity to the highest point of the posterior facet, with the line from the latter to the most cephalic part of the posterior process of the calcaneus. It normally ranges from 20° to 40° measured on the lateral X-ray and a compression fracture is likely if Bohler's angle is less than 20° [3]. A CT scan is necessary to define complex fractures and is useful in preoperative planning.

Management

Calcaneal fractures are notoriously difficult to manage and frequently have a poor outcome, with up to 50% suffering chronic pain and functional disability. Intra-articular, displaced and comminuted fractures are prone to gross swelling of the foot with a risk of compartment syndrome. Admit patients with these fractures for elevation, further imaging, such as CT, and consideration of surgical intervention. Operative intervention may be indicated in younger patients and those with greater degrees of Bohler's angle disruption [4].

Extra-articular fractures and fractures of the anterior process of the calcaneus are usually non-displaced and are treated conservatively in a posterior non-weight-bearing cast for 6 weeks.

Talar fractures

The talus provides support for the body when standing and bears more weight per surface area than any other foot bone. It has no muscular attachments and is held in place by the malleoli and ligaments and comprises a head, neck and body.

The head has articulations with the navicular and calcaneus and the body articulates with the tibia, fibula and calcaneus. The neck joins the head and body and is extra-articular. The blood supply to the talus arises from an anastomotic ring from the peroneal, posterior and anterior tibial arteries and is tenuous and easily disrupted, leading to avascular necrosis.

Mechanism and classification

Major or minor talar fractures are the second most common tarsal fracture. Minor fractures are caused by inversion injuries to the plantar- or dorsiflexed foot, often from minimal trauma, and may present as an apparent ankle sprain. They include avulsion fractures, lateral process fractures commonly seen in snowboarders and posterior talar process fractures. A high index of suspicion is needed to identify these injuries and avoid long-term complications from a delay in diagnosis and treatment [2].

Talar dome fracture

Talar dome fracture is difficult to diagnose on plain films, although a large ankle joint effusion may be apparent. Request specific plain X-ray talar views, although a CT scan is frequently required to confirm the diagnosis. These fractures are important to diagnose as they involve the weight-bearing articular surface of the talus within the ankle joint and missed injury may result in chronic pain and osteoarthritis.

Talar neck fractures

Major talar fractures of the neck, body or head follow significant force, such as a motor vehicle incident, or involve axial loading in a fall from a height (when they are associated with calcaneal fracture). They are commonly accompanied by a subtalar dislocation.

Talar neck fractures account for 50% of major talar injuries and are related to extreme dorsiflexion injuries. The Hawkins classification is used to describe these fractures. Type I fractures are non-displaced with the fracture line entering the subtalar joint between the middle and posterior facets. The risk of avascular necrosis (AVN) with this injury is <10%. Type II fractures are identified by any degree

of displacement or subtalar subluxation and have a 30% incidence of AVN. Type III injuries involve displaced talar neck fracture with dislocation from both the subtalar and ankle joints. The incidence of AVN is up to 90%. Commonly associated injuries include vertebral compression, calcaneal and medial malleolar fractures.

Talar head fractures

Talar head fractures are uncommon and result from a compressive force applied to the plantarflexed foot and are associated with disruption of the talonavicular joint, navicular fractures and anterior malleolar fractures.

Clinical evaluation

Minor talar fractures are usually subtle. The patient presents following an inversion injury with mild swelling around the ankle joint and is able partially to bear weight. Active plantar- and dorsiflexion are possible, but inversion and eversion at the subtalar joint is painful. Major talar fractures are associated with large compressive forces and cause considerable swelling and tenderness dorsally.

Radiology

Standard X-rays of the foot reveal all but the most subtle avulsion fractures. A CT scan is required when there is clinical suspicion of talar fracture, but plain films are inconclusive and/or for preoperative planning.

Management

Major talar fractures have a significant risk of subsequent avascular necrosis. A displaced fracture, especially if associated with neurovascular or cutaneous compromise, should be reduced in the ED under appropriate analgesia and procedural sedation by grasping the hindfoot and midfoot and applying longitudinal traction in plantarflexion. Apply a plaster of Paris (POP) posterior splint with the ankle dorsiflexed at 90°. Refer major fractures to an orthopaedic specialist for open reduction and internal fixation.

Minor talar fractures are treated with a below-knee, non-weight-bearing posterior cast with orthopaedic follow up.

Subtalar dislocation

Subtalar dislocations are rare and follow considerable deforming forces. Such injuries involve the simultaneous dislocation of the talonavicular and talocalcaneal joints, with preservation of the tibiotalar joint.

Mechanism and classification

Subtalar dislocations are associated with motor vehicle incidents, but a number occur during sport, particularly basketball. They are described in terms of the final position of the foot in relation to the talus following dislocation. Medial dislocations account for 85% of these injuries and are caused by forceful foot inversion in plantarflexion. Ten per cent of subtalar dislocations are open and 50% are associated with proximally located injuries [5].

Clinical assessment

Subtalar dislocations are associated with obvious deformity, swelling and tension of the skin over the opposing joint margin. Neurovascular status is rarely compromised. Standard X-rays are difficult to interpret because of the distortion of the foot. The most helpful is the AP view, which confirms disruption of the talonavicular joint.

Management

Reduce a closed subtalar dislocation in the ED under appropriate analgesia and procedural sedation to minimize the chance of tented skin over the head of the talus becoming necrotic.

Closed reduction of a medial subtalar dislocation requires firm longitudinal traction applied to the foot, with countertraction on the leg with the knee flexed to relax the tension from the Achilles tendon on the calcaneum, thereby increasing the mobility of the hindfoot. The foot is initially inverted to accentuate the deformity and then everted with digital pressure over the head of the talus to reverse the deformity. Eighty per cent of dislocations can be reduced non-operatively. Following reduction, the ankle is placed in a posterior POP splint in 90° of dorsiflexion. Orthopaedic consultation is required.

Midfoot fractures

The midfoot comprises the navicular, cuboid and cuneiform bones. It is inherently stable and is rarely injured. However, midfoot fractures are associated with a delay in diagnosis owing to the difficulty in X-ray interpretation and poorly localized pain. The Ottawa ankle rules are accurate in determining which patients with midfoot pain require imaging [1].

Navicular fractures

The navicular is a curved bone with extensive articulations. It has a tenuous blood supply and, like the talus, is susceptible to avascular necrosis.

Mechanism and classification

The navicular is the most commonly injured midfoot bone, although the overall incidence is rare. Fractures may involve the dorsal surface, the tuberosity or the body. The dorsal avulsion fracture is the most common, due to an eversion injury and is associated with deltoid ligament or talonavicular capsular injury. Tuberosity fractures also result from eversion injuries with avulsion of the posterior tibial tendon insertion. Body fractures from axial loading are rare and are frequently comminuted.

Clinical evaluation

Point tenderness is elicited over the dorsum and medial aspect of the midfoot. Passive eversion and active inversion reproduce the pain. Standard X-rays usually reveal the fracture, but a CT scan may be required.

Management

Refer all intra-articular, displaced or comminuted fractures to the orthopaedic specialist, as they are frequently complicated by avascular necrosis. Treat dorsal avulsion and tuberosity fractures conservatively in a walking cast for 6 weeks. Navicular body fractures may require internal fixation.

Cuboid fractures

Isolated cuboid fractures are rare and are most commonly associated with Lisfranc-type injuries with lateral subluxation of the midtarsal joint, the so-called 'nutcracker' compression fracture of the cuboid between the calcaneus and lateral metatarsal heads, and fractures of the posterior malleolus. They are best visualized with an oblique foot X-ray.

Management

All cuboid fractures require orthopaedic consultation. Treatment ranges from weight-bearing POP casts for undisplaced fractures to operative fixation for displaced and comminuted fractures.

Cuneiform fractures

These fractures are extremely rare and usually occur from direct trauma. An associated Lisfranc injury should be excluded. Displaced fractures require orthopaedic intervention, but non-displaced fractures are treated conservatively in a cast.

Lisfranc fractures and dislocations

The Lisfranc joint complex includes the articulation of the first three metatarsal bases with their respective cuneiforms and articulation of the fourth and fifth metatarsal bases with the cuboid. The second metatarsal is the most important structure within this complex and holds the key to stability.

Mechanism and classification

Injury results from rotational forces applied to the fixed forefoot, axial loads and crush injury. Although commonly associated with vehicular crashes, Lisfranc injuries may also occur in sports that involve fixation of the forefoot, such as horse-riding and rowing.

There are three types classified by the direction of dislocation in the horizontal plane. Divergent dislocations usually involve medial and lateral splaying of the first and second metatarsals. In ipsilateral (homolateral) dislocations, all five metatarsals are displaced in the same direction, either medially or laterally. In isolated dislocations, one or more of the metatarsals is displaced away from the others.

Lisfranc dislocations

A Lisfranc dislocation is usually associated with fracture of the metatarsals, particularly the second metatarsal base and, in 40% of cases, with fracture of the midfoot [6]. Although vascular compromise is uncommon, significant haemorrhage can occur with disruption of the dorsalis pedis branch to the plantar arch as it passes between the first and second metatarsal bases.

Clinical assessment

Lisfranc injuries should be suspected when a midfoot fracture is present. They are associated with severe midfoot pain and inability to bear weight on the toes. Examination reveals deformity, swelling and bruising over the dorsum of the foot. Point tenderness over the joint, with pain on passive abduction and pronation, may also be present.

Radiology

Standard X-rays are sufficient to visualize most Lisfranc injuries. The AP view identifies Lisfranc fractures and oblique views determine their alignment. Lateral views delineate the soft tissues and identify the presence of dorsal or plantar displacement. Fracture of the base of the second metatarsal is pathognomic of a Lisfranc injury (fleck sign, indicating avulsion of the Lisfranc ligament), sometimes with diastasis between the first and second metatarsals. CT scan is frequently necessary to define the degree of disruption to the Lisfranc joint complex.

Management

Refer all Lisfranc injuries for orthopaedic consultation. Most are treated with closed reduction and screw and/or K-wire fixation, followed by non-weight-bearing for 12 weeks [7]. Despite aggressive management, chronic pain, reflex sympathetic dystrophy and degenerative arthritis are common.

Forefoot fractures and dislocations

Metatarsal shaft fractures

Metatarsal shaft fractures occur as a result of direct trauma or a rotational injury to the fixed forefoot. Metatarsal fractures are associated with difficulty in weight bearing and ill-defined tenderness and bruising over the plantar aspect of the foot. They are also commonly associated with Lisfranc injuries and phalangeal fractures. As the second and third metatarsals are relatively fixed, they are prone to stress fractures, typically occurring with repetitive trauma, such as long distance running.

Standard X-rays will detect most fractures and determine their alignment, angulation and displacement. Occult stress fractures may only be evident on CT or bone scan imaging.

Management

Undisplaced closed shaft fractures of the second to fifth metatarsals are treated in a below-knee walking cast for 3–4 weeks. Closed reduction and a non-weight-bearing cast for 6 weeks are necessary when these fractures have >3 mm of displacement or 10° of angulation [8].

Hallux (great toe) metatarsal

Injury to the great toe metatarsal requires more aggressive treatment because of its load-bearing function. Non-displaced fractures require 4–6 weeks in a non-weight-bearing cast, whereas displaced fractures require operative treatment. Orthopaedic consultation is required for multiple or displaced fractures and all fractures of the hallux metatarsal.

Metatarsal head and neck fractures

These fractures usually result from direct trauma and are often multiple. Treat a non-displaced fracture with a walking cast for 4–6 weeks. Displaced fractures require closed reduction to maintain the integrity of the transverse plantar arch.

Fractures of the base of the fifth metatarsal

These are the most common of the metatarsal fractures, with two distinct types. The commonest fracture is to the fifth metatarsal tuberosity, occuring when the plantarflexed foot suddenly inverts. It is caused by avulsion of the lateral band of the plantar aponeurosis and is transverse and usually extra-articular. Rarely, the fracture line extends into the cuboid–metatarsal articulation, but not into the joint between the fourth and fifth metatarsals.

Jones fracture

The second type of fracture is known as the Jones fracture and is defined as a transverse fracture through the diaphysis of the fifth metatarsal from 15 to 31 mm distal to the proximal end of the bone. This fracture is intra-articular as it involves the intermetatarsal articulation of the fourth and fifth metatarsals and is prone to non-union [7]. A Jones fracture occurs when a load is applied to the lateral aspect of the foot without inversion. Activities, such as jumping and dancing, are typically associated with such injury, which may also occur as a more distal 'stress-type' injury due to repetitive strain.

The patient has difficulty weight bearing with both types of fracture. There is point tenderness over the fifth metatarsal tuberosity and passive inversion is painful.

In children, the normal growth plate at the base of the fifth metatarsal should not be confused with an acute fracture. Fracture lines usually pass transversely through the base of the fifth metatarsal, whereas growth plates run in a longitudinal or oblique direction.

Management

Tuberosity fractures heal well regardless of size or degree of displacement and are treated symptomatically with either a compression bandage or, less commonly, a POP walking cast for 3 weeks [9]. A non-displaced Jones fracture that does not extend beyond the distal limit of the fourth/fifth intermetatarsal articulation is treated in a non-weight-bearing cast for 6 weeks. Jones fractures that are significantly displaced or extend distal to the intermetatarsal articulation should be considered for surgical fixation. There is a lower threshold to advise surgery in an athlete as it results in faster time to union and return to sport [10].

Metatarsophalangeal (MTP) dislocations

MTP dislocations are uncommon. The fifth MTP joint is most commonly dislocated laterally when the little toe is snagged on an object. First or hallux MTP joint dislocation is usually dorsal and follows violent hyperextension injury. They are usually obvious, with the metatarsal head palpable on the plantar surface. Other dislocations are more subtle.

Management

Most MTP joint dislocations are readily reduced with longitudinal traction under local anaesthesia. After reduction they are managed with a buddy strap.

First MTP joint dislocations are more difficult to reduce and may require open reduction if there is buttonholing of the joint capsule. If reduced, they are treated in a POP walking cast with a toe-plate extension for 3 weeks.

Phalangeal fractures and dislocations

Phalangeal fractures are common and usually occur with direct trauma, most often involving the proximal phalanx. They are associated with pain, deformity and difficulty walking.

Management

Non-displaced fractures heal well and are 'buddy strapped' to reduce pain and prevent displacement. Place gauze between the splinted toes to prevent skin maceration. Pain may be expected for up to 3 weeks until the fracture is stabilized by callus.

Reduce a displaced fracture with traction under digital nerve anaesthesia. Operative fixation may be indicated if the fracture is unstable, especially if it is intra-articular, is rotated or involves the hallux.

Interphalangeal dislocations are uncommon and usually involve the hallux. They are reduced with longitudinal traction under digital nerve anaesthesia. Those involving the great toe require a toe-plated walking cast for 3 weeks following reduction. All other interphalangeal dislocations are treated with a buddy strap once reduced.

Controversies

- Optimal use of nurse-initiated X-ray in lower limb injuries.
- Surgical versus conservative management of Jones fractures.
- Role of the bone scan, CT and MRI in foot injuries.

References

[1] Bachmann L, Kolb E, Koller M, et al. Accuracy of Ottawa ankle rules to exclude fractures of the ankle and midfoot: systematic review. Br Med J 2003;326:417–23.
[2] Judd DB, Kim DH. Foot fractures frequently misdiagnosed as ankle sprains. Am Fam Phys 2002;66:785–94.
[3] Chen M, Bohrer S, Kelly T, et al. Bohler's angle: a reappraisal. Ann Emerg Med 1991;20:122–4.
[4] Bajammal S, Tornetta P, Sanders D, et al. Displaced intra-articular calcaneal fractures. J Orthop Trauma 2005;19:360–4.
[5] Merchan E. Subtalar dislocations: long-term follow-up of 39 cases. Injury 1992;23:97–100.
[6] Vuori J, Aro H. Lisfranc joint injuries: trauma mechanisms and associated injuries. J Trauma 1993;35:40–5.
[7] Watson T, Shurnas P, Denker J. Treatment of Lisfranc joint injury: current concepts. J Am Acad Orthop Surg 2010;18:718–28.
[8] Armagan O, Shereff M. Injuries to the toes and metatarsals. Orthop Clin N Am 2001;32:1–10.
[9] Polzer H, Polzer S, Mutschler W, et al. Acute fractures to the proximal fifth metatarsal bone: development of classification and treatment recommendations based on the current evidence. Injury 2012;43:1626–32.
[10] Mologue T, Lundeen J, Clapper M, et al. Early screw fixation versus casting in the treatment of acute Jones fractures. Am J Sports Med 2005;33:970–5.

ORTHOPAEDIC EMERGENCIES

4

4.13 Osteomyelitis

Varadarajulu Suresh • Trevor Jackson

ESSENTIALS

1 *Staphylococcus aureus* is the most frequent pathogen in all age groups.

2 Surgery, trauma and diabetes predispose to chronic infection in adults.

3 Diagnosis may be difficult, relying on a combination of clinical features, imaging studies and microbiological cultures. Laboratory testing is often unhelpful.

4 Successful treatment requires appropriate parenteral antibiotics with complete surgical clearance of any necrotic bone.

Table 4.13.1 Bacterial causes of osteomyelitis

Age group	Typical bacteria
Children <2 years	*Staphylococcus aureus* including MRSA *Streptococcus* spp.
Older children	*Staphylococcus aureus* including MRSA
Adults	*Staphylococcus aureus*, *Streptococcus* spp. Gram-negative species
Unusual organisms	Anaerobic bacteria, *Brucella* spp., *Mycobacterium tuberculosis*, Fungi

MRSA: methicillin-resistant *Staphylococcus aureus*.

Introduction

Osteomyelitis is an inflammatory process of the bone secondary to infection usually with a pyogenic organism. It is an infrequent but important presentation to the emergency department (ED).

Aetiology, pathogenesis and pathology

Osteomyelitis predominantly occurs in children and the aged, via haematogenous spread in the former and associated with co-morbidity, such as trauma, surgery, vascular insufficiency and diabetes in the latter. Osteomyelitis may also be due to spread of infection from contiguous structures.

Common bacterial pathogens

Haematogenous spread in children typically affects the long bones whereas, in adults, it is most common in the spine [1]. Common bacterial pathogens are listed in Table 4.13.1 according to age group [2].

Pathology

Inoculation of bone by bacteria causes alterations in pH and capillary permeability which contribute to regional oedema, cytokine release, tissue breakdown, leucocyte recruitment and decreased oxygen tension. These processes increase local pressure leading to small vessel thrombosis and bone deterioration [3].

As the infection spreads into the medullary cavity, increased pressure causes extension into the cortex with subsequent spread into the subperiosteal space and, finally, to the periosteum and adjacent soft tissues, forming an abscess. Necrosis of cortical bone follows with the formation of bone fragments or sequestra harbouring bacteria. At this stage, the infection is considered as chronic osteomyelitis.

Rarely, infection also stimulates a layer of new bone deposition from stripping of the periosteum, known as an involucrum. Tracts may perforate the involucrum with an opening known as a cloaca. A tract reaching the skin surface is termed a sinus [4].

Epidemiology

Acute osteomyelitis affects 0.1–0.8% of the otherwise healthy adult population in the USA. Over the last decade, methicillin resistant *Staphylococcus aureus* (MRSA) strains have emerged, especially after surgery in hospital. A rising trend in infection rates related to increased surgical procedures has been noted.

In countries with limited medical resources, tuberculosis may be an important infection as well as brucellosis. Agricultural injuries, industrial incidents and traumatic wounds, where prompt and adequate debridement and repair are uncommon, as well as a lack of laboratory facilities plus effective antimicrobial agents, account for the increased incidence of osteomyelitis [2].

Clinical features

New onset of localized bone pain and fever is suspicious. Enquire about a history of injury including soft tissue, which may serve as a nidus of secondary bone infection. Enquire also about a history of diabetes, surgery or a compound injury. Intravenous drug abuse is associated with infection in unusual sites, such as the spine and clavicle. In the paediatric population, the onset may be insidious.

Risk factors

The risk factors for osteomyelitis are recent surgery including joint replacement, trauma including a puncture wound, other wound infections, peripheral vascular disease, diabetes especially in the presence of a diabetic foot ulcer, immune suppression such as chemotherapy, steroids, alcohol and intravenous drug abuse, sickle cell disease and iatrogenic such as a peripheral intravenous cannula or central line [1,2,5].

Examination

Patients may not appear toxic or unwell, but look for mild fever with warmth, tenderness and swelling at the site of pain. The elderly may present febrile, with non-traumatic back or neck pain and localized tenderness due to involvement of vertebral bodies. Joint movement may be restricted if osteomyelitis is periarticular or involves a joint space.

Diabetics may present with a painless foot ulcer due to associated neuropathy. The presence of a scar, ulcer or sinuses may signify chronic infection. Children can present with malaise, fatigue and irritability.

Investigations

Laboratory tests

Laboratory tests although useful are non-specific. The white cell count is unreliable in confirming or excluding osteomyelitis. An erythrocyte sedimentation rate (ESR) and C-reactive protein (CRP) will be elevated in acute infection, but are also elevated in conditions other than osteomyelitis.

Conversely, a normal ESR and CRP may occur particularly in chronic infection, however, when the clinical suspicion is low they are reassuring that no further urgent investigation is required [6].

Imaging studies

Plain X-rays

Plain radiographs help to suggest the correct diagnosis and exclude other differential diagnoses [7]. In pyogenic infection, the first changes in bone are periosteal elevation then focal lucency, bony resorption or radiodense, avascular areas known as sequestra.

Note that as X-ray changes are not seen until the infectious process has been present for 10 days to 2–3 weeks or more, they are of limited value in diagnosing early osteomyelitis.

Ultrasonography and bone scan

Musculoskeletal ultrasonography helps to localize the site and extent of infection and provides guidance for diagnostic aspiration or bone biopsy. As it is readily accessible, it may be performed without delay.

Nuclear medicine scans, though sensitive, lack specificity but are useful when magnetic resonance imaging (MRI) is contraindicated and or metalwork affects the computed tomography (CT) images.

CT and MRI

CT provides excellent images and identifies subtle changes, particularly in long bones; it is also used for spinal infection if MRI is not available.

MRI allows the earliest detection of osteomyelits usually within 3–5 days after the onset of infection and demonstrates the extent of involvement and activity of the disease. MRI is the investigation of choice in vertebral osteomyelitis and helps exclude extension to discitis or an epidural abscess.

Differential diagnosis

Arthrits, tumours such as a Ewing's sarcoma or osteoid osteoma, traumatic injury and gout all should be considered. Septic arthritis may coexist with osteomyelitis in joints, such as hip and shoulder.

Microbiology

Microbial cultures are essential to the diagnosis and treatment of osteomyelitis [5]. Positive culture from bone biopsy and histopathology are the key to the definitive diagnosis of osteomyelitis.

Blood cultures are positive in over 50% of infections, especially if spread is by the haematogenous route. However, a superficial wound culture does not contribute significantly to a diagnosis of osteomyelitis.

Chronic infections are more likely to have polymicrobial involvement including anaerobic, mycobacterial and fungal organisms. Specific cultures or microbiologic testing are needed for suspected pathogens. See Table 4.13.2 for criteria for the diagnosis, in order of decreasing diagnostic value [8].

Management

Hospitalization may be needed with multispecialty evaluation, imaging and treatment. Early admission under the orthopaedic team can shorten the length of hospital stay. Antibiotic therapy should be aimed at stopping disease progression as well as avoiding the development of resistance. Early surgical intervention helps confirm the infection, identify the aetiological agent and remove dead or devitalized tissue.

Treatment needs to be guided by the results of Gram stain and culture. All initial antibiotic regimens should include an anti-staphylococcal agent as this organism accounts for over 80% of cases. This should be with vancomycin if MRSA is suspected. Empiric antibiotic therapy for osteomyelitis is suggested in Table 4.13.3, but it is *essential* to seek expert microbiology advice on local organisms and their sensitivities [1,2,5].

Table 4.13.2 Criteria for diagnosis of osteomyelitis (in decreasing order of diagnostic utility) [8]

Bone biopsy with positive bacterial culture
Imaging studies demonstrating contiguous soft-tissue infection or bone destruction
Clinical signs of exposed bone, persistent sinus tract*
Chronic wound over a surgical site or fracture*
Laboratory evaluation – positive blood cultures, elevated ESR, CRP

*Chronic osteomyelitis; ESR: erythrocyte sedimentation rate; CRP: C-reactive protein.
Reproduced with permission from American Society of Plastic Surgeons. Evidence-based Clinical Practice Guideline: Chronic Wounds of the Lower Extremity. http://www.plasticsurgery.org/Documents/medical-professionals/health-policy/evidence-practice/Evidence-based-Clinical-Practice-Guideline-Chronic-Wounds-of-the-Lower-Extremity.pdf [Accessed Feb 2013].

Table 4.13.3 Empiric antibiotic therapy for osteomyelitis [1,2,5]

Risk factor	Likely infecting organism	Antibiotic regimen
Nil or MRSA unlikely	Staph. aureus	Di/flucloxacillin 2 g IV 6-hourly. Use lincomycin 600 mg IV 8-hourly if allergic to penicillin
Postoperative, with or without orthopaedic implant	Staph. aureus and coagulase-negative staphylococci	Vancomycin 1.5 g IV 12-hourly
Elderly, haematogenous spread	Staph. aureus including MRSA, Gram-negative bacteria	Vancomycin 1.5 g IV 12-hourly with piperacillin–tazobactam 4.5 g IV 6-hourly
Diabetes mellitus or vascular insufficiency	Polymicrobial: Staph. aureus and Streptococcus pyogenes plus coliforms and anaerobes	Vancomycin 1.5 g IV 12-hourly with piperacillin–tazobactam 4.5 g IV 6-hourly
IV drug use	Staph. aureus including MRSA and Pseudomonas aeruginosa	Vancomycin 1.5 g IV 12-hourly with piperacillin–tazobactam 4.5 g IV 6-hourly
Sickle cell anaemia	Salmonella, Gram-negative bacteria	Ceftriaxone 2 g IV daily

Note: essential to seek microbiology advice about local organisms and sensitivities.

Prognosis

The outcome for osteomyelitis depends on predisposing factors, underlying disease processes, the bone involved and treatment duration, although this may not be clear at the start of therapy. The duration of follow up is uncertain and the final outcome and morbidity may be influenced by the treatment and complicating factors.

Chronic osteomyelitis and sinus tracts will not be controlled by antibiotic therapy alone, and with surgery essential for eradication. A squamous cell carcinoma in a tract is a rare, long-term complication.

Prevention

The risk of osteomyelitis is reduced by eliminating sources of infection and by infection control measures prior to surgery. Prompt treatment of infections and effective surgical debridement of an injury may help avoid subsequent infection. Awareness of, and meticulous attention to infections and ulcers of the foot and sacrum in diabetics, particularly with neurological impairment, are imperative [2].

Controversies

- The optimum duration for parenteral antibiotics.
- Balance between parenteral and oral routes.
- Inpatient versus outpatient therapy.
- Role of surgery in complicated cases.

References

[1] Tintinalli JE, Stapczynski JS, Cline DM, et al. Tintinalli's emergency medicine: a comprehensive study guide, 7th ed. New York: McGraw Hill Medical, 2011.

[2] Longo DL, Fauci AS, Kasper DL, et al. Harrison's principles of internal medicine, 18th ed. New York: McGraw Hill Medical, 2011.

[3] Tsukayama DT. Pathophysiology of posttraumatic osteomyelitis. Clin Orthop Relat Res 1999;360:22–9.

[4] Resnick D, Niwayama G. Osteomyelitis, septic arthritis and soft tissue infection; mechanisms and situations. In: Resnick D, editor. Diagnosis of bone and joint disorders (3rd ed.). Philadelphia: WB Saunders, 1995, p. 2325–418.

[5] Hatzenbuehler J, Pulling TJ. Diagnosis and management of osteomyelitis. Am Fam Phys 2011;84:1027–33.

[6] Harris J, Caesar D, Davision C, et al. Review article: How useful are laboratory investigations in the emergency department evaluation of possible osteomyelitis? Emerg Med Australas 2011;23:317–30.

[7] Pineda C, Espinosa R, Pena A. Radiographic imaging in osteomyelitis: the role of plain radiography, computed tomography, ultrasonography, magnetic resonance imaging, and scintigraphy. Semin Plast Surg 2009;23:80–9.

[8] American Society of Plastic Surgeons. Evidence-based clinical practice guideline: chronic wounds of the lower extremity. <http://www.plasticsurgery.org/Documents/medical-professionals/health-policy/evidence-practice/Evidence-based-Clinical-Practice-Guideline-Chronic-Wounds-of-the-Lower-Extremity.pdf> [Accessed Feb. 2013].

CARDIOVASCULAR EMERGENCIES

Edited by **Anne-Maree Kelly**

5.1 Chest pain

Steve Goodacre

ESSENTIALS

1 Acute coronary syndrome (ACS) is common, life threatening and treatable, so identifying and treating ACS is fundamental to chest pain management.

2 Serious alternative causes, such as pulmonary embolus or aortic dissection, and extrathoracic causes, such as pancreatitis or peptic ulcer, should not be overlooked.

3 Anxiety-related chest pain is common, significantly impairs quality of life and is treatable, yet it is often ignored or dismissed.

4 Gastro-oesophageal pain should generally only be diagnosed in the emergency department after ACS has been ruled out.

5 A normal ECG does not rule out ACS.

6 Troponin predicts adverse outcome. Patients with a positive troponin may benefit from inpatient investigation and treatment. Patients with a negative troponin are unlikely to benefit from inpatient care, although this does not rule out coronary heart disease.

7 Cardiac biomarkers should be judged on the basis of their specificity and prognostic value, not just sensitivity.

8 CT coronary angiography can accurately identify coronary artery obstruction but its role in routine assessment has yet to be determined.

Introduction

Chest pain is one of the most common presenting complaints in emergency medicine. It is also associated with life-threatening pathology, so it is arguably the most important complaint faced by emergency clinicians. It is certainly one of the most challenging. Failure to diagnose and manage appropriately patients with acute chest pain is a frequent cause of avoidable mortality and morbidity and is a leading cause of malpractice litigation. It is therefore not surprising that physicians often err on the side of caution, yet this can also have adverse consequences for the patient and society. Patient anxieties following unnecessary investigation are often unrecognized but may severely affect quality of life, while over-investigation and unnecessary hospital admission for chest pain waste millions of healthcare dollars each year.

Epidemiology

The incidence of acute chest pain presenting to the emergency department appears to be increasing. Awareness of the importance of early treatment for myocardial infarction has led to public information campaigns that increase emergency department attendances with chest pain. Meanwhile, general practitioners are increasingly being bypassed in favour of an emergency ambulance response. These changes in health service use have coincided in many developed countries with a decrease in the incidence of coronary heart disease. It therefore seems likely that patients presenting to the emergency department with acute chest pain have decreasing prevalence of acute

Table 5.1.1   Causes of acute chest pain

Musculoskeletal	Muscular strain Epidemic myalgia Tietze's syndrome
Cardiac	Myocardial infarction Unstable angina Stable angina
Pericardial	Pneumomediastinum Pericarditis
Gastro-oesophageal	Gastro-oesophageal reflux Oesophageal spasm
Psychological	Anxiety/panic attacks Hyperventilation Cardiac neurosis
Pleuritic	Pulmonary embolus Pneumothorax Pleurisy Pneumonia
Neurological	Cervical/thoracic nerve root compression Herpes zoster
Abdominal	Peptic ulcer Biliary colic/cholecystitis Pancreatits
Mixed	Aortic dissection

coronary syndrome (ACS) and increasing prevalence of more benign conditions.

Differential diagnosis

The main differential diagnoses are outlined in Table 5.1.1. The most common causes of acute chest pain are ACS (unstable angina or myocardial infarction), musculoskeletal pain, anxiety, gastro-oesophageal pain and non-specific chest pain. The most serious causes (in terms of threat to life) are ACS, pulmonary embolism and aortic dissection. Since ACS is both common and life threatening, it is inevitably the primary focus of assessment.

ACS is discussed in detail in Chapter 5.2, pulmonary embolus in Chapter 5.5 and aortic dissection in Chapter 5.10.

Musculoskeletal chest pain may be related to a precipitating episode, such as chest wall injury or physical over-exertion. Alternatively, it may be caused by inflammation in chest wall structures. Tietze's syndrome (costochondritis) is most commonly seen in women and is characterized by tenderness of the costochondral cartilages. Epidemic myalgia (Bornholm disease) is due to inflammation of chest wall muscles and pleura occurring after viral infection, typically *Coxsackie B*. Herpes zoster produces severe pain along the distribution of a thoracic nerve and may be misdiagnosed as musculoskeletal pain if the patient presents before any rash or vesicles have developed.

Gastro-oesophageal pain occurs when gastric contents reflux into the oesophagus or when the oesophageal muscles spasm. Pneumomediastinum can occur spontaneously after vigorous exercise, vomiting or an asthma attack or may be associated with barotrauma from diving or inhalation during drug abuse. Pericarditis is most commonly caused by viral infection, but may be associated with systemic illness, such as uraemia or autoimmune disease, or follow myocardial infarction or cardiac surgery (Dressler syndrome).

Anxiety-related chest pain is a common and frequently unrecognized cause of acute chest pain. It may also coexist and be an important factor alongside other causes of chest pain. The patient with coronary heart disease and anxiety-related chest pain presents a particularly difficult diagnostic and management challenge. Anxiety may be related to a specific serious cause of chest pain and can be exacerbated by misguided efforts to provide reassurance through diagnostic testing. In extreme cases, this can lead to 'cardiac neurosis' in which the patient's anxieties about cardiac disease cause more severe disruption to their daily activities and quality of life than would be expected from the pathology that worries them.

Pleurisy is typically caused by a viral infection and produces pain that is worse on inspiration. It may be differentiated from pulmonary embolus by the presence of systemic features and the absence of breathlessness or risk factors for thromboembolism, although investigation for pulmonary embolism is often required. Pneumonia and pneumothorax can also cause pleuritic pain but should be evident on chest radiography.

There are a number of serious abdominal complaints that may present as chest pain. These include biliary colic (acute biliary pain), cholecystitis, peptic ulcer disease and pancreatitis. Failure to take a careful history and examine the abdomen may lead to delayed diagnosis.

Finally, a substantial proportion of patients will be labelled entirely appropriately as 'non-specific chest pain' after emergency department evaluation. These patients have pain that simply cannot be categorized into a clear diagnostic group. It is more honest to accept this than apply an inaccurate diagnostic label.

Clinical features

Clinical assessment is primarily aimed at identifying patients with a significant risk of serious pathology who require further investigation and possibly inpatient care. The most common serious pathology is ACS, so clinical assessment is often focused upon associated features. Other serious conditions, such as pulmonary embolism and aortic dissection, should not be neglected.

ACS is classically associated with chest pain that is crushing, gripping or squeezing in nature and radiates to the left arm, but presenting features in the emergency department may be much more variable, particularly in patients with no past history of coronary heart disease and a non-diagnostic ECG. Table 5.1.2 shows the likelihood ratios of clinical features that may help to diagnose ACS. It is notable that pain radiating to the right arm or to both arms is a powerful predictor of ACS. Pain described as 'burning' or 'like indigestion' can be associated with ACS, as can pain occurring on exertion. So the diagnoses of gastro-oesophageal reflux or stable angina should be made with great caution. Pain that is sharp or associated with inspiration or movement is less likely to be cardiac, but these findings alone do not exclude ACS. Risk factors for coronary heart disease should be routinely recorded, although they may have surprisingly little diagnostic value. This is perhaps because patients are aware of these risk factors and take them into account when deciding whether or not to seek help for episodes of chest pain. In this respect, social and cultural factors may have an important influence upon patient's interpretation of their symptoms and health-seeking behaviour.

Clinical examination is of limited diagnostic value and is mainly aimed at identifying non-cardiac causes of chest pain or complications of ACS, such as arrhythmia, heart failure or cardiogenic shock. Pain that can be reproduced by chest wall palpation is less likely to be cardiac, but this finding does not exclude the possibility of ACS. It is also important to determine specifically that chest wall palpation is reproducing the pain that led to presentation. Simply identifying chest wall tenderness has

Table 5.1.2 Likelihood ratios of clinical features useful for diagnosing acute myocardial infarction

Useful for ruling in myocardial infarction	
Radiation to the right arm or shoulder	4.7
Radiation to both arms or shoulders	4.1
Described as burning or like indigestion	2.8
Association with exertion	2.4
Radiation to left arm	2.3
Associated with diaphoresis	2.0
Associated with nausea or vomiting	1.9
Worse than previous angina or similar to previous myocardial infarction	1.8
Described as pressure	1.3
Useful for ruling out myocardial infarction	
Described as pleuritic	0.2
Described as positional	0.3
Described as sharp	0.3
Reproducible by palpation	0.3
Inframammary location	0.8
Not associated with exertion	0.8

Table 5.1.3 Likelihood ratios of ECG features useful for diagnosing acute myocardial infarction

New ST elevation >1 mm	5.7–53.9
New Q wave	5.3–24.8
Any ST-segment elevation	11.2
New conduction defect	6.3
New ST-segment depression	3.0–5.2
Any Q wave	3.9
Any ST-segment depression	3.2
T-wave peaking and/or inversion >1 mm	3.1
New T-wave inversion	2.4–2.8
Any conduction defect	2.7

little value – everyone has a tender chest wall if you press hard enough!

Clinical assessment should not just focus upon ACS, but should aim positively to identify other causes. Pulmonary embolism is diagnostically challenging. Suspicion should be raised by chest pain that is clearly pleuritic in nature, haemoptysis, associated breathlessness, features of deep vein thrombosis or risk factors for venous thromboembolism (immobilization, malignancy, recent trauma or surgery, pregnancy, intravenous drug abuse or previous thromboembolism). Clinical examination may reveal tachycardia, tachypnoea or features of deep vein thrombosis (see Chapter 5.5). Aortic dissection is characterized by severe pain radiating to the back with associated diaphoresis. Neurological symptoms or signs, sometimes transient, are common. Clinical examination may reveal discrepancy between blood pressure in right and left arms (see Chapter 5.10).

Clinical assessment of chest pain should always include examination of the abdomen to identify tenderness, guarding, rebound tenderness or a positive Murphy's sign.

Unnecessary investigation can be avoided if non-life-threatening pathology can be confidently diagnosed by clinical assessment. Pain that is reproduced by chest wall palpation in a patient at low risk of coronary heart disease and with no significant risk factors for pulmonary embolus can be confidently diagnosed as musculoskeletal. A positive diagnosis is particularly valuable for the patient who is primarily suffering from anxiety-related symptoms. In this case, pain is typically described as tightness around the chest and associated with a feeling of restricted breathing. Other features include palpitations (particularly awareness of the heartbeat), sweating, breathlessness, light-headedness, feelings of panic, or paraesthesia of the lips or fingertips.

Clinical investigations

The ECG is the most useful clinical investigation and should be performed on all patients presenting with acute non-traumatic chest pain. Table 5.1.3 shows the value of ECG features for diagnosing myocardial infarction. It is important to recognize that a normal ECG does not rule out myocardial infarction. ST-segment elevation or depression, new Q waves and new conduction defects are specific for acute myocardial infarction and predict adverse outcome. Patients with these features should be managed on a coronary care unit. Other changes associated with myocardial infarction are less helpful. T-wave changes are often non-specific and may be positional or due to

numerous other causes. ECG changes in pulmonary embolism are also non-specific.

A standard 12-lead ECG may be augmented by serial ECG recording or continuous ST-segment monitoring. These may detect evolving ECG changes or dynamic ST-segment changes. However, these techniques may also identify non-specific false-positive changes, such as minor T-wave inversions, especially if they are used inappropriately in patients with a low risk of coronary heart disease. ST-segment monitoring was developed for the high-risk coronary care population; in low risk emergency department patients with chest pain, it has a very low yield of significant findings.

Like clinical examination, the chest radiograph is mainly intended to identify non-cardiac causes for chest pain, such as a pneumothorax or fractured rib and complications of myocardial infarction, such as left ventricular failure. Although it is often routinely ordered, it is not usually helpful.

Cardiac biomarkers are key investigations in acute chest pain and are a source of much heated debate. They are also a progressively developing technology, so this chapter will focus upon the principles that should guide their use.

Three key features determine the clinical value of a cardiac biomarker. Sensitivity tells us how good the marker is at identifying patients with disease, and thus how useful it is for ruling out myocardial ischaemia. Specificity tells us how good the marker is at identifying patients without disease, and thus how useful it is for ruling in myocardial ischaemia (i.e. a specific test that is positive suggests that the patient is very likely to have ischaemia). The prognostic value (often expressed as a relative risk) tells us how good the marker is at predicting future adverse events, such as death, myocardial infarction or life-threatening arrhythmia.

Intuitively, clinicians tend to be most concerned about sensitivity. If a marker lacks sensitivity then it may miss cases of myocardial infarction leading to potentially catastrophic discharge home without appropriate treatment. However, sensitivity and specificity are often related and may be influenced by the threshold of the marker used to determine a positive test. The lower the threshold used for a positive test, the higher the sensitivity and the lower the specificity. Many evaluations of new markers deliberately optimize sensitivity by selecting a low threshold and sacrificing specificity. This may be an acceptable trade-off in a high-risk population, but emergency department patients with no past history of coronary heart disease and a non-diagnostic ECG typically have a low prevalence of myocardial infarction (<10%). In these circumstances, a test with low specificity will generate many false-positive results requiring hospital admission and investigation, as well as unnecessary anxiety for the patient.

Furthermore, it should be remembered that even a random process can be made to appear sensitive by setting a low diagnostic threshold so that most of the results generated are deemed positive. For example, rolling a pair of dice to diagnose myocardial infarction will have 97% sensitivity if all results, except double six, are deemed to be positive. This is, of course, an extreme example, but biomarkers with diagnostic value that is little better than rolling dice have been promoted by studies that report high sensitivity while hiding away poor specificity. Sensitivity should always be reported with a corresponding specificity.

The prognostic value of a marker is arguably even more useful than its diagnostic parameters, particularly if the marker can predict high-risk patients who will benefit from treatment. If a prognostically useful marker is positive, then we know the patient has the potential to benefit from intervention; if it is negative then we know that, even if further investigation is required to identify the exact cause of their chest pain, they are unlikely to benefit from hospital admission and treatment.

Prognostic considerations explain changes in the definition of myocardial infarction. The original World Health Organisation (WHO) definition of myocardial infarction was based upon creatine kinase, a cardiac marker with limited sensitivity and specificity and only weak evidence of an association with adverse prognosis. Subsequent definitions of myocardial infarction, from the American Heart Association and European Society of Cardiology, used troponin as the biomarker based on research showing elevated troponin levels were associated with increased risk of adverse outcome. Furthermore, research has shown that informing clinicians that their patient has an elevated troponin level can alter patient management and reduce the risk of major adverse cardiac events over the following year. This is important evidence that measuring troponin provides patient benefit by reducing adverse outcomes.

Creatine kinase is released by damaged myocardium, but is also released by muscles and the liver and is measurable in the blood in the absence of pathology. Its MB isoenzyme (CK-MB) is more cardiac-specific but shares the same problems. Substantial myocardial damage is required to produce an elevated CK-MB, but CK-MB may also be elevated in the absence of myocardial injury. Its role in diagnosis is generally limited to situations where troponin testing is unavailable or likely to be unreliable.

There are two troponin assays, troponin I and troponin T, with little to choose between them in terms of diagnostic or prognostic performance. The diagnosis of myocardial infarction is based upon elevation of the troponin level above the 99th percentile upper reference limit of a normal reference population. This value will vary between assays. The precision of the assay is described by the coefficient of variation (CV) at the 99th percentile. There have been several generations of troponin assays with newer assays having higher sensitivity and better precision. High-sensitivity troponin assays have optimal precision ($\leq$10% CV) at the 99th percentile and can detect myocardial infarction earlier after symptom onset than other assays. However, this appears to be at the cost of an increased number of low troponin rises that are of unclear diagnostic and prognostic significance.

Troponin elevation is not specific for myocardial infarction and low levels measured using a high sensitivity assay may not indicate significant pathology. Even substantial troponin elevations may not be due to ACS. Troponin can be elevated in pulmonary embolus, sepsis, renal failure, congestive cardiac failure and a number of other illnesses.

The use of troponin has tended to be limited by its lack of early sensitivity. It has been estimated that standard troponin assays take up to 12 hours after symptom onset to achieve optimal sensitivity, so if it is used too early after symptom onset it may produce a false-negative result. This has led to the widespread practice of delaying troponin measurement to at least 12 hours after symptom onset to achieve optimal sensitivity. This practice is problematic because most patients present a few hours after symptom onset, so enforcing a 12-hour delay will typically require hospital admission or use of observation facilities. If there is limited availability of such facilities, clinicians may feel under pressure to discharge the patient

without any testing. Thus, a strategy intended to increase patient safety may paradoxically put patients at risk when applied to the real world. Newer assays allow a 6-hour testing strategy and recently developed high-sensitivity assays appear to have good early sensitivity and may be able to rule out myocardial infarction within a few hours of presentation to hospital. However, as mentioned above, this may be at the cost of limited specificity resulting in the generation of troponin elevations that have little diagnostic or prognostic significance. Thus, the choice of testing strategy involves a trade-off between sensitivity and specificity. It is important to know the test used in your institution and its performance characteristics in order to decide on an appropriate serial testing strategy.

Awareness of the limited early sensitivity of standard troponin assays has led to research into alternative biomarkers that can detect myocardial infarction in the initial hours after symptom onset. These biomarkers often have poor specificity so any improvement in sensitivity achieved by combining troponin with another biomarker involves a trade-off in terms of reduced specificity. The development of high-sensitivity troponin assays is likely to undermine the need to develop and use alternative early biomarkers. Future evaluations of alternative early biomarkers will need to include comparison with high-sensitivity troponin.

The most extensively evaluated early biomarkers to date are myoglobin, heart-type fatty acid binding protein (HFABP) and ischaemia modified albumen (IMA). Table 5.1.4 shows the sensitivity and specificity of these biomarkers at presentation to hospital, compared to troponin. None of the alternative biomarkers have sufficient sensitivity to rule out myocardial infarction at presentation. Adding HFABP or myoglobin to a contemporary troponin assay at presentation increases sensitivity at the expense of specificity, but it is not clear whether either biomarker can improve the early sensitivity of a high-sensitivity troponin assay. IMA appears to have insufficient specificity to play any useful role in diagnosis.

Biomarkers are continually being developed and emergency physicians can expect to see headline-grabbing publications extolling their virtues. However, they should be wary before indiscriminately using new markers in their patients with chest pain. As described earlier, the emergency department population with

Table 5.1.4 Sensitivity and specificity of biomarkers for myocardial infarction at presentation to hospital

Biomarker	Sensitivity (%)	Specificity (%)
Troponin I*	77	93
Troponin T*	80	91
Roche high sensitivity troponin T	96	72
ADVIA Centaur Ultra high sensitivity troponin I	86	89
Abbot Architect high sensitivity troponin I	83	95
Quantitative heart-type fatty acid binding protein	81	80
Qualitative heart-type fatty acid binding protein	68	92
Myoglobin	62	83
Ischaemia modified albumen	77	39

*All assays combined, using 99th percentile as a diagnostic threshold.
The estimates are based on meta-analysis of data from heterogeneous studies and are therefore subject to substantial uncertainty. Goodacre S, Thokala P, Carroll C, Stevens J, Leaviss J, et al. Systematic review, meta-analysis and economic modelling of diagnostic strategies for suspected acute coronary syndrome. Health Technol Assess 2013;17(1) http://www.journalslibrary.nihr.ac.uk/hta/volume-17/issue-1 with permission.

chest pain are a heterogeneous population with a relatively low prevalence of ACS compared to the high-risk patients that usually comprise research study populations. Indiscriminate use of markers with limited specificity will lead to many false-positive results and consequent patient anxiety, unnecessary investigation and waste of resources.

Provocative cardiac testing, usually using an exercise treadmill, has been used in a number of emergency departments. Patients typically undergo a short period of observation and cardiac marker testing to rule out myocardial infarction before receiving an exercise treadmill test. Concerns about the safety of this procedure have been addressed by data from a number of centres, but it should be recognized that selection of low-risk patients plays a key role in ensuring safety.

Exercise treadmill testing has relatively poor sensitivity and specificity and cannot reliably rule in or rule out coronary artery disease. However, it is prognostically useful and predicts risk of adverse events over the months following attendance. It is therefore used to risk-stratify more than to diagnose. A patient with a negative treadmill test may have coronary artery disease but can be reassured that they are at low risk of adverse outcome. It is not clear whether the additional prognostic information provided by exercise treadmill testing justifies widespread use.

CT coronary angiography is developing an increasing role in the diagnostic evaluation of acute chest pain. Unlike exercise treadmill testing, CT coronary angiography detects coronary obstruction with a reasonable degree of accuracy. Sensitivity and specificity are both around 90% against a reference standard of invasive coronary angiography. However, coronary atheroma is a common finding and detecting atheroma, or even coronary obstruction, does not necessarily mean that this was the cause of the patient's chest pain. Studies of the prognostic value of CT coronary angiography in patients with suspected ACS have been limited by selection of patients with low rates of adverse outcome and have, as yet, failed to show worthwhile prognostic value. This means that, although CT coronary angiography is a promising diagnostic test for acute chest pain, evidence is lacking that its use improves patient outcomes and its role in routine assessment remains unclear.

The combination of observation and cardiac marker testing to rule out myocardial infarction, followed by provocative cardiac testing to risk-stratify or CT coronary angiography to diagnose coronary artery obstruction, has been adopted in many hospitals in the form of a chest pain unit or pathway. These have a number of potential benefits for patients and health services and some evidence to suggest that they reduce the probability of admission,

reduce the risk of discharge with ACS, improve patient satisfaction and quality of life and reduce health service costs. However, as an organizational intervention, the effect of the chest pain unit will depend upon local circumstances and may be influenced by staff attitudes, professional roles and local leadership. Furthermore, the presence of a chest pain unit may attract additional attendances with chest pain. Whether this represents identification of unmet demand or unnecessary work is a matter of opinion.

A number of clinical risk scores have been developed to risk-stratify patients with suspected ACS. The Goldman algorithm and acute cardiac ischaemia time insensitive predictive instrument (ACI-TIPI) were developed and validated on large cohorts of patients with chest pain in the 1980s and 1990s. The Goldman algorithm uses a series of questions about the patient's age, clinical history and ECG findings to categorize patients into a low (<7%) or high (>7%) risk of myocardial infarction, based on the WHO definition used at the time. ACI-TIPI can be incorporated into a computerized ECG. The user enters the patient's age, sex and whether chest or left arm pain is the primary symptom. The computer then uses these data and analysis of the ECG to generate a probability of acute cardiac ischaemia.

The thrombolysis in myocardial infarction (TIMI) score has been developed and validated as a predictor of adverse outcome in patients with diagnosed ACS (see Chapter 5.2). Studies have evaluated the TIMI score in emergency department patients with suspected ACS and shown that higher scores are associated with a higher risk of adverse outcome. This has led to the TIMI score being used to risk stratify patients with chest pain before a diagnosis of ACS has been confirmed. The ECG and cardiac biomarker components are the most powerful predictors among the elements of the TIMI score and a modified version of the TIMI score, with extra weighting for these elements, has been proposed for patients with acute chest pain. It is not clear whether either the original or modified TIMI score provides better prognostic information than that provided by ECG and biomarkers alone.

The Global Registry of Acute Coronary Events (GRACE) freedom-from-event score has recently been developed to predict adverse events in people with non-ST-elevation acute coronary syndrome and can identify up to 30% of the admitted population who are at low risk of death or any adverse in-hospital event. It is more complex to calculate than the TIMI score but bedside calculation can be easily facilitated by mobile technologies. The GRACE freedom-from-event score offers an alternative to the TIMI score for predicting adverse outcome but further validation in the wider chest pain population is required.

Treatment

Treatment of acute chest pain is directed at the specific cause. The treatment of ACS is outlined in Chapter 5.2, pulmonary embolus in Chapter 5.5 and aortic dissection in Chapter 5.10.

Musculoskeletal chest pain, whether due to muscular strain, chest wall injury, Tietze's syndrome or epidemic myalgia, should be treated with simple analgesia and the patient advised to see their general practitioner if the pain persists beyond a few weeks. It is also worth considering whether anxiety may be exacerbating the patient's symptoms.

Gastro-oesophageal pain can be treated acutely by antacids, although the diagnostic value of observing relief of pain with antacids (the so-called 'GI cocktail') is debatable. ACS can present as burning or indigestion-type pain and, pain being typically fluctuant, may ease coincidentally with administration of an antacid. Gastro-oesophageal pain should be diagnosed with caution and ideally only after ACS has been investigated and ruled out. In these circumstances, a course of treatment with a proton pump inhibitor is appropriate. Follow up will depend upon local practice along with the duration and severity of symptoms.

Anxiety-related symptoms range from simple chest wall muscular tension to panic attacks, hyperventilation syndrome and cardiac neurosis. Treatment should therefore be tailored to the patient's individual needs. In many cases, anxiety will be an understandable reaction to concerns about heart disease or other serious pathology. The first step is therefore to provide clear and unequivocal reassurance. If diagnostic uncertainty makes this impossible then it may still be possible to provide reassurance by highlighting the excellent prognosis of patients with chest pain whose tests are negative. Information leaflets have been shown to reduce anxiety after emergency department attendance with chest pain. Patients with more severe symptoms may

benefit from relaxation techniques, cognitive behavioural therapy or treatment with an antidepressant. These are best arranged through the patient's general practitioner.

Managing anxiety in the emergency department patient is often complicated by difficulties in satisfactorily ruling out serious physical illness. A diagnosis of anxiety may be considered likely, but until cardiac testing is complete (perhaps even involving coronary angiography), the treating physician may be reluctant to discuss treatment of anxiety with the patient. This is inappropriate. If the patient has significant anxiety-related symptoms then this will adversely affect their quality of life and should be addressed regardless of whether they ultimately also need treatment for cardiac disease.

Non-specific chest pain obviously presents a challenge. With no clear diagnosis it is difficult to advise an appropriate treatment. However, patients can be advised that, although no clear diagnosis can be made, about half such patients presenting to the emergency department have no further episodes of pain over the following month. Those who do suffer further episodes of pain are unlikely to be troubled. Treatment is therefore unlikely to be required.

Finally, an acute episode of chest pain provides an opportunity to identify and manage cardiac risk factors at a time when the patient is likely to be most receptive to lifestyle advice. Smokers should be advised to use the episode as a stimulus to stop smoking and referral to a smoking cessation service arranged. General dietary and exercise advice may also be helpful. Blood pressure, blood glucose and lipid profile may be requested as part of clinical assessment, although any abnormalities identified should preferably be referred to the patient's general practitioner, who will be best placed to provide overall cardiovascular risk assessment, intervention and long-term follow up.

Prognosis

Prognosis will also depend upon the underlying pathology and the prognoses of various causes of chest pain are discussed in the relevant chapters of this book. Patients with no obvious diagnosis after clinical assessment, ECG and troponin testing have an excellent prognosis. There is some evidence that patients who attend the emergency department with chest pain have a higher risk of adverse cardiac

events than the general population, even if cardiac disease is 'ruled out' at initial presentation, but this risk is not high enough to warrant active intervention beyond ensuring that any cardiac risk factors identified have been addressed.

Likely developments over the next 5–10 years

Chest pain is responsible for a substantial and growing number of emergency medical admissions in many countries. This is placing a major burden upon healthcare systems. The value of hospital admission for low risk ACS and pulmonary embolus is being questioned and it is likely that there will be increasing efforts to manage acute chest pain without admission to hospital. These efforts may be successful for younger patients with no co-morbidities and a single potentially serious cause for their chest pain, but may be difficult to implement among the growing population of older patients with co-morbidities or multiple potentially serious causes for their pain.

High-sensitivity troponin assays are increasingly replacing other contemporary assays. This will lead to more positive results and concerns that some of these may represent false-positive results with little prognostic value. Emergency physicians may therefore need to be more circumspect in their use of troponin and avoid measuring troponin in patients with a very low risk of ACS in whom an elevated high-sensitivity troponin measurement just above the diagnostic threshold is likely to cause confusion rather than provide a clear diagnosis.

Point-of-care troponin testing has been available for some time but widespread adoption has been limited by a number of factors, including lack of usability and difficulties converting reduced turnaround times into reduced length of hospital stay. The development of hand-held point-of-care machines using finger-stick capillary blood samples could improve the usability of point-of-care testing and extend use to the pre-hospital setting.

CT coronary angiography is likely to be more widely used in the assessment of acute chest pain. In the absence of randomized trial evidence of effectiveness, it will not be clear whether patients are benefitting from increased use. Both high sensitivity troponin assays and CT coronary angiography have the potential to increase the diagnostic yield of positive tests in the investigation of acute chest pain leading to over-burdening of cardiology services.

Chest pain management is likely to be influenced by changes in health service policy, which are, in turn, likely to depend upon local social, political and economic factors. These changes will be variable and may be unpredictable. On one hand, public awareness of the medical significance of chest pain and policies aimed at increasing rapid access to care may lead to increased numbers of patients presenting with chest pain. On the other hand, reorganization of services and attempts to control costs may result in an opposite effect. Specifically, development of primary angioplasty services may lead to centralization of chest pain services and patients bypassing facilities that do not provide primary angioplasty.

Controversies

- The role of clinical scores for acute coronary syndrome in the assessment of undifferentiated chest pain is unclear. The TIMI score was developed to predict future events in patients with acute coronary syndrome, but is often used for diagnostic assessment in patients with chest pain (i.e. estimating whether the patient has myocardial infarction at presentation). The GRACE freedom-from-event score may provide better prediction but needs

further validation in patients with undifferentiated chest pain.

- Although the development of high-sensitivity troponin assays has improved the early sensitivity of troponin for detecting myocardial infarction, it is still not clear when samples should be taken to optimize sensitivity without incurring excessive inconvenience for the patient and healthcare costs. Furthermore, high sensitivity assays appear to have lower specificity than other contemporary assays. It is not clear whether patients whose positive result is only detected by a high-sensitivity assay are at increased risk of adverse outcome.
- CT coronary angiography is being increasingly used in the evaluation of acute chest pain. It can accurately diagnose coronary artery obstruction, but it is not clear whether this provides useful prognostic information beyond that provided by the ECG and troponin measurement.

Further reading

Antman EM, Cohen M, Berninck PJ, et al. The TIMI risk score for unstable angina/non-ST elevation MI: a method for prognostication and therapeutic decision making. J Am Med Assoc 2000;284:835–42.

Arnold J, Goodacre S, Bath P, Price J. Randomised controlled trial of information sheets for patients with acute chest pain. Br Med J 2009;338:b541.

Brieger D, Fox KAA, FitzGerald G, et al. Predicting freedom from clinical events in non-ST-elevation acute coronary syndromes: the Global Registry of Acute Coronary Events. Heart 2009;95:888–94.

Cooper A, Calvert N, Skinner J, et al. Chest pain of recent onset: Assessment and diagnosis of recent onset chest pain or discomfort of suspected cardiac origin, Clinical Guideline 95. London: National Clinical Guideline Centre for Acute and Chronic Conditions, 2010.

Ebell MH, Flewelling D, Flynn CA. A systematic review of troponin T and I for diagnosing acute myocardial infarction. J Fam Pract 2000;49:550–6.

Goodacre S, Thokala P, Carroll C, et al. Systematic review, meta-analysis and economic modelling of diagnostic strategies for suspected acute coronary syndrome. Health Technol Assess 2013; 17. <http://www.hta.ac.uk/2269>.

Hulten EA, Carbonaro S, Petrillo SP, et al. Prognostic value of cardiac computed tomography angiography: a systematic review and meta-analysis. J Am Coll Cardiol 2011;57: 1237–47.

Keller T, Zeller T, Peetz D, et al. Sensitive troponin I assay in early diagnosis of acute myocardial infarction. N Engl J Med 2009;361:868–77.

Mills NL, Churchhouse AM, Lee KK, et al. Implementation of a sensitive troponin I assay and risk of recurrent myocardial infarction and death in patients with suspected acute coronary syndrome. J Am Med Assoc 2011;305:1210–6.

Mowatt G, Cummins E, Waugh N, et al. Systematic review of the clinical effectiveness and cost-effectiveness of 64-slice or higher computed tomography angiography as an alternative to invasive coronary angiography in the investigation of coronary artery disease. (Structured abstract). Health Technol Assess 2008;12:1–164.

Panju AA, Hemmelgarn BR, Guyatt GH, Simel DL. Is this patient having a myocardial infarction. J Am Med Assoc 1998;280:1256–63.

Reichlin T, Hochholzer W, Bassetti S, et al. Early diagnosis of myocardial infarction with sensitive cardiac troponin assays. N Engl J Med 2009;361:858–67.

Swap CT, Nagurney JT. Value and limitations of chest pain history in the evaluation of patients with suspected acute coronary syndromes. J Am Med Assoc 2005;294:2623–9.

Thygesen K, Alpert JS, White HD. Joint ESC/ACCF/AHA/WHF Task Force for the Redefinition of Myocardial Infarction. Universal definition of myocardial infarction. J Am Coll Cardiol 2007;50:2173–95.

Webster R, Norman P, Goodacre S, Thompson A. The prevalence and correlates of psychological outcomes in patients with acute non-cardiac chest pain: A systematic review. Emerg Med J 2012;29:267–73.

5.2 Acute coronary syndromes

Steve Goodacre • Anne-Maree Kelly

ESSENTIALS

1 Every patient with possible acute coronary syndrome (ACS) should receive a 12-lead ECG as soon as possible after arrival to identify whether they may benefit from reperfusion therapy. If interpretation is uncertain, then senior or specialist advice should be sought immediately.

2 Every patient with suspected ACS should be given aspirin, unless they have a strong contraindication.

3 Primary prevention of ACS involves overall cardiovascular risk assessment and is most appropriately undertaken in primary care.

4 The ECG can identify patients with ACS who are at high risk but cannot rule out ACS.

5 Primary angioplasty is more effective than fibrinolysis, but only if it can be delivered promptly by appropriately trained staff.

Introduction

Acute coronary syndrome (ACS) is the most common life-threatening condition in emergency medicine. Failure to identify and treat it promptly risks avoidable morbidity and mortality.

Aetiology, pathogenesis and pathology

ACS nearly always occurs as a consequence of atheroma in the coronary arteries, commonly known as coronary heart disease (CHD). Many people have coronary atheroma but are asymptomatic because it is not extensive enough to occlude coronary blood flow. Others have a degree of coronary occlusion that does not cause symptoms unless they exert themselves or if myocardial oxygen demand is increased by some other mechanism, such as anaemia. Cardiac chest pain that only occurs on exertion and is rapidly relieved by rest is known as stable angina and is not classified as an ACS.

ACS usually occurs when an atheromatous plaque ruptures or fissures. Haemorrhage may occur into the plaque or thrombus may accumulate over the fissure. The type of ACS that results depends on the extent of the rupture and degree of haemorrhage or thrombus formation. A gradually progressive occlusion will usually produce symptoms of unstable angina:

progressive symptoms of myocardial ischaemia occurring on less exertion or at rest. A rapidly progressive occlusion may lead to myocardial infarction (MI), with severe pain at rest and the potential for serious complications, such as arrhythmia, heart failure, cardiogenic shock or sudden cardiac death.

If coronary occlusion is minor or transient, the consequent myocardial ischaemia will not lead to myocardial damage. If coronary occlusion is severe or prolonged then myocardial necrosis will occur.

Not all coronary artery occlusion is due to coronary atheroma. Prinzmetal angina describes a syndrome in which myocardial ischaemia is associated with coronary artery spasm and is characterized by transient ST-segment elevation on the electrocardiograph (ECG). Coronary angiography may show minor atheroma or normal coronary arteries. Uncommonly, coronary artery spasm may be severe enough to cause myocardial necrosis and an associated biomarker elevation.

Other rare causes of coronary artery occlusion include Kawasaki's disease, in which occlusion is due to inflammation in the coronary artery and aortic dissection that involves the coronary arteries.

ACS may involve occlusion of one or more of the coronary arteries and the location of occlusion may determine the clinical presentation, ECG findings and likelihood of complications.

The most common site for MI is the anterior or anteroseptal region. It usually results from occlusion of the left anterior descending artery. It has a worse prognosis than other types of MI and complications are more common. Sudden cardiac death may result from total occlusion of the left anterior descending artery, giving a lesion in this location the grim sobriquet of 'widow-maker'. Lateral infarction is usually caused by occlusion of the circumflex artery or the diagonal branch of the left anterior descending artery. Inferior MI is usually caused by occlusion of the right coronary artery or the circumflex artery. It has a better prognosis than anterior infarction and ventricular dysfunction is less likely, although heart block due to involvement of the atrioventricular node is more common. Posterior infarction is usually due to occlusion of the right coronary artery or, less commonly, the circumflex artery in patients with dominance of the left coronary circulation. Posterior or inferior MI may result in right ventricular infarction leading to right ventricular failure.

ACS may be associated with a range of life-threatening complications, including arrhythmia, such as atrial fibrillation, ventricular tachycardia and ventricular fibrillation. Supraventricular tachycardias are not usually associated with ACS. Heart block may occur with infarcts affecting the nodal branch of the right coronary artery or septal infarcts. Infarction may lead to myocardial dysfunction, resulting in heart failure or cardiogenic shock. Uncommon complications include papillary muscle dysfunction and mitral regurgitation, ventricular septal defect or cardiac rupture. The probability of any of these complications increases with the severity of myocardial damage incurred.

Epidemiology

Coronary heart disease is the leading cause of death in the world. It is responsible for 6.8% of disability-adjusted life years (DALYs) lost through disease by men and 5.3% of DALYs lost by women. The global burden of CHD is expected to rise from 47 million DALYs in 1990 to 82 million in 2020. Most of this increased burden will be in developing countries. However, CHD mortality rates have dramatically decreased in many developed countries since the 1980s. Studies suggest that 50–75% of the fall in cardiac deaths can be attributed to population interventions, particularly those relating to smoking, hypertension and high cholesterol. The remaining 25–50% is due to treatments for patients with CHD, such as acute reperfusion therapies (including thrombolysis and percutaneous coronary intervention (PCI)), aspirin, angiotensin-converting enzyme inhibitors, statins and coronary artery bypass surgery.

The main risk factors for CHD are well established and include smoking, diabetes, hypertension, hyperlipidaemia and a family history of CHD at a young age, while obesity and lack of exercise may play a contributory role. Age and sex are also important. CHD prevalence increases with age and increases at an earlier age (40–50 years) in men than in women (over 60 years). Everyone over the age of 60 is effectively at risk of CHD. Conversely, a history of CHD presenting in a relative when they were aged over 60 should not be considered a significant risk factor.

Patients presenting to the emergency department (ED) with chest pain in general, and ACS specifically, show a diurnal variation with a peak of attendances during the morning, although many of these attendances relate to symptoms occurring overnight. Presentation is more common on a Monday, when cardiovascular mortality appears to be higher. Cardiovascular mortality also increases during the winter months, particularly in colder climates.

Prevention

Prevention of ACS is achieved principally by preventing underlying CHD, although secondary prevention of ACS in patients with established CHD can be attempted by ensuring appropriate treatment with daily low-dose aspirin, angiotensin-converting enzyme (ACE) inhibitor, β-blockers and lipid-lowering therapy.

Primary CHD prevention can take place by addressing the important coronary artery disease risk factors that are amenable to intervention. The most important modifiable risk factors at a population level are smoking, obesity and lack of exercise. These may be tackled by legislation and education and by economic and social policy. Diabetes, hypertension and

hyperlipidaemia can be addressed at an individual level. It is increasingly recognized that the importance of any one risk factor depends on the presence of other risk factors, so cardiovascular risk is most appropriately assessed by a comprehensive assessment involving all risk factors, along with age and sex. Screening programmes should be based on overall cardiovascular risk assessment, rather than individual risk factors. Similarly, the decision to prescribe treatments for risk factors, particularly lipid-lowering therapy, should be based on overall cardiovascular risk.

This has implications for emergency medicine. It may be tempting to use the patient's attendance at the ED to undertake opportunistic screening by, for example, measuring blood pressure, blood sugar or lipids, even though they will not influence management of the presenting complaint. This approach is inappropriate because it does not involve overall cardiovascular risk assessment. Furthermore, it may be considered unethical because the patient is effectively being screened (with potential implications for health insurance) without the opportunity to make an informed choice about whether they wish to receive screening. For these reasons, coronary risk assessment for primary prevention is best left to primary care physicians.

Although opportunistic screening in the ED is best avoided, opportunistic patient education about risk factors may be very salient, particularly if the patient has presented with symptoms that could be related to CHD. For example, an episode of chest pain, even if ultimately diagnosed as non-cardiac, may offer an ideal opportunity to promote smoking cessation.

Clinical features

Clinical assessment of suspected ACS is described in detail in Chapter 5.1. Chest pain is suggestive of MI if it radiates to either arm, both arms or shoulders; is described as burning, like indigestion, heavy, pressing or band-like; occurs on exertion; is associated with diaphoresis, nausea or vomiting; or is worse than previous angina or similar to previous MI. Chest pain is less likely to be MI if it is sharp, pleuritic, positional, reproduced by palpation, inframammary in location or not associated with exertion.

Clinical assessment of cardiac pain is required to determine whether it is due to

stable angina or ACS. Stable angina is characterized by pain that is predictable, precipitated by exertion, relieved promptly by rest or glyceryl trinitrate (GTN) and is not becoming more frequent or severe. Unstable angina is caused by a dynamic narrowing of the coronary artery and is characterized by pain that may be unpredictable, may occur at rest or minimal exertion, may not be immediately relieved by rest or GTN or may be increasing in frequency or severity.

Patients with stable angina do not typically present to the ED. They are often used to their symptoms and will not seek medical help unless something unexpected happens. If a patient presents with apparently stable angina, the diagnosis should be considered carefully. It should be remembered that pain precipitated by exertion is known to be predictive of MI in ED patients.

Clinical examination is generally unhelpful in making the diagnosis of ACS, which should be based on clinical history and investigations. However, clinical examination is essential to identify complications of ACS and to rule out differential diagnoses. Heart failure may be identified by poor peripheral circulation, tachycardia, pulmonary crepitations, elevated jugular venous pressure and a third heart sound on cardiac auscultation. The additional finding of hypotension may suggest cardiogenic shock. A systolic murmur raises the possibility of papillary muscle rupture or ventricular septal defect secondary to MI, although pre-existing aortic or mitral valve disease are much more common.

Differential diagnosis

Alternative diagnoses and their differentiation from ACS are described in Chapter 5.1. The most potentially serious alternative diagnoses are pulmonary embolus and aortic dissection. These should be considered in any patient with suspected ACS who is diaphoretic, tachycardic, tachypnoeic, hypotensive or reports associated neurological symptoms (transient or persistent) but does not have definite ECG features of ACS.

Clinical investigations

The 12-lead ECG is the essential investigation to identify ACS requiring emergency reperfusion. It should be performed as soon as possible after arrival in any patient with any suspicion of ACS. Pre-hospital ECGs can be obtained by some emergency medical services and in some settings is used to prioritize patients and guide triage to high-dependency areas/cardiac catheter laboratories.

The critical decision is to determine whether there is evidence of ST-elevation MI (STEMI) or MI with new bundle branch block. If there is any doubt, senior or specialist advice should be sought immediately. Repeat ECG recording may be helpful if a senior clinician feels there is insufficient certainty to allow for an immediate decision but a high suspicion of evolving MI persists.

Identifying new bundle branch block presents a challenge, especially if previous medical records are not immediately available. In the past, the Sgarbossa criteria have been suggested as indicative of increased likelihood of MI. These criteria are ST elevation of 1 mm or more that is concordant with (in the same direction as) the QRS complex; ST depression of 1 mm or more in leads V1, V2 or V3 and ST-segment elevation of 5 mm or more that is discordant with (in the opposite direction to) the QRS complex. Recent research has questioned their utility, reporting low sensitivity for diagnosing MI. Other research has suggested that the presence of concordant ST changes is closely correlated with acute coronary occlusion but that the discordant criteria and left bundle branch block (LBBB) without Sgarbossa criteria are not. These findings have yet to be validated. In the absence of clear decision-making criteria, decisions regarding acute reperfusion will depend on specialist clinical judgement.

Other ECG changes may be useful in diagnosing AMI and are described in Chapter 5.1 and Table 5.1.3. Q waves typically follow ST elevation but may appear as early as 4 hours after symptom onset. Their presence does not therefore preclude early reperfusion. Tall, upright T waves ('hyperacute' T waves) may be present in the very early stages of infarction. Deep (>3 mm) inverted T waves suggest a subendocardial MI which would be confirmed by biomarker elevation. Similarly, patients with significant (>1 mm) ST depression have an increased risk of adverse outcome and are likely to have a troponin rise. Unfortunately, despite an association with increased risk of adverse outcome, neither ST depression nor deep T-wave inversion is associated with benefit from acute reperfusion therapy.

Other T-wave changes, such as small inversions (<3 mm), flat T waves and biphasic T waves, are common and non-specific. They may suggest ACS, but may also occur in patients with hypertension, patients who are hyperventilating and in the normal population.

In addition to changes directly suggesting ACS, the ECG should be inspected for any concurrent pathology or evidence of complications. Cardiac rate and rhythm and P-wave presence and morphology should be evaluated for evidence of arrhythmia or heart block. Tall R waves or S waves suggest ventricular strain or hypertrophy that may contribute to or be a consequence of ACS.

A subtle sign that can indicate ischaemia or ventricular dysfunction is poor anterior R-wave progression. Normally, R waves progressively increase in size across leads V1 to V4. Small R waves across these leads suggest pathology.

Repeated 12-lead ECG recording or continuous ST-segment monitoring can help to identify transient or dynamic ECG changes. The development of significant (>1 mm) ST deviation provides clear evidence of ischaemia, identifies high-risk patients and may facilitate rapid identification of patients requiring reperfusion. T-wave changes, by contrast, are non-specific and often arise as a result of hyperventilation or changes in patient position during monitoring. The incidence of significant ST changes decreases and the incidence of false-positive T-wave changes increases in patients with a lower likelihood of significant ACS. Therefore, repeated ECG recording and ST-segment monitoring should be reserved for high-risk patients.

A normal or non-diagnostic ECG does not rule out ACS or necessarily stratify the patient to a very low-risk group. In fact, the majority of patients admitted with ACS do not have diagnostic ECG changes. Serial ECG recordings and ST-segment monitoring do not substantially increase the negative predictive value of the ECG or provide very useful prognostic data. Negative ECG recording therefore has limited value.

Biochemical markers are discussed in detail in Chapter 5.1. Their role is to identify patients with probable ACS and to rule out ACS if negative. However, it should be remembered that a negative cardiac marker, even if highly sensitive and performed at an optimal time after the worst symptoms, does not rule out CHD. Patients with negative markers require risk stratification and further cardiac testing if CHD is considered a likely diagnosis, although further cardiac testing does not necessarily have to be undertaken at the initial hospital attendance.

Biochemical markers (particularly troponin) have a valuable prognostic role. Any patient with an elevated troponin is at increased risk of adverse outcome and has the potential to benefit from hospital admission, although the prognostic importance of small elevations of a high sensitivity assay is uncertain. If ACS is the likely cause of a troponin elevation, then the patient should be admitted under the care of a cardiologist. As a general rule, the higher the troponin level the greater the risk of adverse outcome. Patients with minor troponin elevations may be managed conservatively and possibly without ECG monitoring. A recent paper has reported the rate of significant ventricular arrhythmia in patients with troponin rise without ischaemic ECG changes as 0% (95% CI 0–2.3%). Those with substantial troponin elevations should be managed in a coronary care unit and considered for early percutaneous coronary intervention, even if they have no significant ECG changes.

Criteria for diagnosis

The term ACS covers a spectrum of disorders, including unstable angina, non-ST-elevation MI (NSTEMI) and STEMI. The diagnostic definition of MI has been a matter of intense debate in recent years and a consensus has gradually emerged. In contrast, the challenge of defining a diagnosis of ACS per se has been largely overlooked.

The original World Health Organization (WHO) diagnosis of MI is outlined in Table 5.2.1. It required an elevation of creatine kinase to more than twice the upper limit of the normal range. With the development of troponins, it became apparent that this definition failed to include a substantial number of patients with prognostically significant myocardial damage, as evidenced by a troponin rise. Therefore, the American Heart Association and European Society of Cardiology (AHA/ESC) developed a

Table 5.2.1   WHO criteria for definite acute MI (1970)

1. Definite ECG, or
2. Symptoms typical or atypical or inadequately described, together with probable ECG or abnormal enzymes, or
3. Symptoms typical with abnormal enzymes with ischaemic or non-codable ECG, or ECG not available, or
4. Fatal case with necropsy findings or MI or recent coronary occlusion

Table 5.2.2   The AHA/ESC criteria for MI (2012)

Typical rise and fall of biochemical markers of myocardial necrosis with at least one of the following:
1. Symptoms of ischaemia
2. New or presumed new significant ST-segment–T-wave (ST–T) changes or new left bundle branch block (LBBB)
3. Development of pathological Q waves in the ECG
4. Imaging evidence of new loss of viable myocardium or new regional wall motion abnormality
5. Identification of an intracoronary thrombus by angiography or autopsy

new definition of MI, outlined in Table 5.2.2, which required a rise in serum troponin above the 99th percentile of the values for a reference control group.

The AHA/ESC definition has been widely adopted, despite a number of concerns and criticisms. Patients with ACS who fulfil this definition have a higher risk of adverse outcome than those who do not. However, patients with MI according to the AHA/ESC criteria alone have a lower risk of adverse outcome than those who fulfil both the AHA/ESC and WHO criteria. This has led to problems in maintaining consistent care over time and some experts have suggested identifying a threshold level for troponin (e.g. troponin T >1 ng/mL) above which clinically important MI should be diagnosed. This controversy is unlikely to be resolved in the near future, particularly as newer and more sensitive biochemical markers are developed. However, the most important issue to recognize is that any detectable troponin is associated with a potentially increased risk of adverse outcome and, the higher the troponin level, the higher that risk.

MI can be usefully defined as STEMI or NSTEMI on the basis of the ECG. If there is evidence of significant ST elevation on any ECG (>2 mm in two consecutive chest leads, or >1 mm in two consecutive limb leads) then the patient has STEMI. These patients are likely to benefit from early reperfusion therapy. Patients without these changes but with evidence of myonecrosis based on cardiac markers are defined as having NSTEMI and do not benefit from reperfusion with thrombolytics, although PCI may be beneficial. NSTEMI and ACS without criteria for MI may be categorized together as non-ST-elevation ACS.

AHA/ECS have introduced a classification system for MI based on underlying pathophysiological mechanisms. Of most relevance to emergency medicine practice are type 1 and type 2 MI. Type 1 MI is defined as spontaneous MI related to atherosclerotic plaque rupture, ulceration, fissuring, erosion or dissection with resulting intraluminal thrombus in one or more

of the coronary arteries leading to decreased myocardial blood flow or distal platelet emboli with ensuing myocyte necrosis. Type 2 MI is defined as instances of myocardial injury with necrosis where a condition other than coronary artery disease (CAD) contributes to an imbalance between myocardial oxygen supply and/or demand, e.g. coronary endothelial dysfunction, coronary artery spasm, coronary embolism, tachy-/brady-arrhythmias, anaemia, respiratory failure, hypotension and hypertension with or without left ventricular hypertrophy (LVH).

Treatment

Some treatments are indicated for all ACS, whereas others have specific application to STEMI, NSTEMI and other ACS.

Treatments for all ACS

Analgesia
Glyceryl trinitrate (GTN) and intravenous (IV) morphine are the analgesic agents of choice. Sublingual GTN may be appropriate if pain is mild to moderate, but severe pain usually requires titrated IV morphine. Doses of up to 20 mg, in small increments, are sometimes required. If IV morphine fails to control pain and the clinical condition is suitable, IV GTN by infusion at a rate titrated to effect (20–200 µg/min) is indicated. If this is insufficient to control pain and the patient is tachycardic, control of rate with small increments of IV β-blocker may be beneficial. It is important to note that ongoing severe pain, particularly in the absence of ECG changes, should raise concerns about an alternative diagnosis, such as aortic dissection.

Aspirin
Aspirin 300 mg should be administered unless already given (e.g. by emergency services or general practitioner) or contraindicated. The principal contraindication to aspirin is known allergy. A previous history of gastritis or

indigestion is not a contraindication to the use of aspirin in ACS.

Oxygen
Recent analyses have raised questions about the role of routine oxygen therapy in the treatment for ACS. There is also a lack of evidence of benefit. Until further research clarifies the risk–benefit of supplemental oxygen therapy, its routine use is not recommended. Oxygen therapy is indicated for patients with hypoxia (oxygen saturation <93%) and those with evidence of shock to correct tissue hypoxia.

STEMI

Reperfusion
Patients with STEMI who present within 12 hours of symptom onset should have a reperfusion strategy implemented emergently. Reperfusion can be obtained by fibrinolytic therapy, PCI, or rarely, with emergency coronary artery bypass grafting. The choice of reperfusion therapy will depend on time from symptom onset, availability of PCI, delay to fibrinolysis, contraindications to fibrinolysis, location and size of the infarct and the presence or absence of cardiogenic shock.

PCI is the best available treatment if provided promptly. It is generally accepted that a delay of 90 minutes between presentation and balloon inflation is the maximum desirable. If this is not possible, fibrinolysis should be used. For patients presenting very early (symptom duration less than 1 hour), fibrinolytic therapy is highly effective, so the maximum tolerable delay to PCI is 1 hour from presentation. For patients aged less than 75 years with cardiogenic shock, PCI markedly improves outcomes.

Fibrinolytic agents include streptokinase and tissue fibrin-specific agents, such as alteplase and tenecteplase. Available evidence suggests that fibrin-specific agents reduce mortality compared to streptokinase, despite an increased risk of intracranial bleeding. Note that streptokinase should not be given to patients who have been previously exposed to it (more than 5 days ago) due to antibody formation. There is also some evidence that it may be less effective in populations with high levels of exposure to streptococcal skin infections, such as Aboriginal and Torres Strait Islander peoples. Contraindications to fibrinolytic therapy are shown in Table 5.2.3. All patients receiving fibrinolyic therapy should

Table 5.2.3   Contraindications to fibrinolytic therapy in STEMI (ECS, 2011)

1. Absolute contraindications
   * Known bleeding diathesis (excluding menses)
   * Recent major trauma/surgery/head injury within the preceding 3 weeks
   * Suspected aortic dissection (including new neurological symptoms)
   * Previous intracranial haemorrhage or stroke of unknown origin at any time
   * Ischaemic stroke in the preceding 6 months
   * Central nervous system damage or neoplasm or atrioventricular malformation
   * Gastrointestinal bleeding within the past month
   * Non-compressible punctures in the last 24 hours (e.g. liver biopsy, lumbar puncture)

2. Relative contraindications
   * Current use of oral anticoagulants: the higher the INR, the higher the risk of bleeding
   * Traumatic or prolonged resuscitation (>10 minutes)
   * Active peptic ulcer disease
   * Refractory hypertension (systolic >180 mmHg, diastolic >110 mmHg)
   * Transient ischaemic attack in the preceding 6 months
   * Advanced liver disesae
   * Infective endocarditis
   * Pregnancy or within 1 week postpartum

be transferred to a PCI-capable centre for further assessment and treatment. In cases of failed fibrinolyisis or if there is evidence of re-occlusion/re-infarction (e.g. recurrent ST elevation), this transfer should be emergent.

Pre-hospital fibrinolysis should be considered when delay to PCI exceeds 90 minutes and transfer times to a fibrinolysis-capable facility exceed 30 minutes.

The evolution of primary PCI has resulted in some systems identifying STEMI prior to hospital arrival and bypassing the ED, instead taking the patient directly to the catheterization laboratory. Even in these systems, it is important that emergency physicians remain knowledgeable and skilled in the diagnosis and management of STEMI, as a substantial proportion of cases self-present to the ED and pre-hospital diagnosis can sometimes be inaccurate.

$P2Y_{12}$ receptor inhibitors

Patients undergoing primary PCI for reperfusion for STEMI should receive an antiplatelet agent. The choice of agent will depend on balancing the risk of recurrent ischaemic events and bleeding risk in individual patients. If clopidogrel is used it should be given as a high-dose clopidogrel regimen (600 mg oral bolus and 150 mg daily for 7 days, then 75 mg/day for at least 12 months). Potent oral antiplatelet agents (prasugrel and ticagrelor) are alternatives to clopidogrel for subgroups at high risk of recurrent ischaemic events (e.g. those with diabetes, stent thrombosis, recurrent events on clopidogrel or a high burden of disease on angiography). Prasugrel is contraindicated in patients with prior stroke/transient ischaemic attack. Neither prasugrel or ticagrelor should be used in patients with a previous haemorrhagic stroke or in patients with a moderate-to-severe liver disease. For patients undergoing fibrinolysis, 300 mg clopidogrel is recommended.

Antithrombin therapy

Antithrombin therapy should be used in conjunction with PCI and fibrin-specific fibrinolytic agents. The use of antithrombin therapy with Streptokinase is optional. Low molecular weight heparin (e.g. enoxaparin) or unfractionated heparin can be used. There are data suggesting that enoxaparin may provide benefit over unfractionated heparin and dosing and administration are easier leading to recommendations listing it as the preferred agent. If unfractionated heparin is used it should be administered according to local dosing and monitoring guidelines taking into account whether there is concomitant use of glycoprotein IIb/IIIa inhibitors (GP inhibitors) and whether PCI or fibrinolysis was the reperfusion strategy used.

Bivalirudin (a direct thrombin inhibitor) has shown similar efficacy to the heparins with less bleeding. Its place in the management of ACS is evolving.

Glycoprotein IIb/IIIa inhibitors

The role of GP inhibitors is evolving and data are conflicting and complex. Current recommendations are that the decision to use GP inhibitors is a specialist cardiologist decision and that there is no benefit in initiating it before the catheterization laboratory. An exception is that use before the catheterization laboratory may be considered in high-risk patients undergoing transfer for primary PCI in consultation with the receiving cardiologist. Abciximab is the preferred agent.

Non-STEMI

$P2Y_{12}$ receptor inhibitors

In addition to aspirin, patients should receive $P2Y_{12}$ receptor inhibitor agents, e.g. clopidogrel 300 mg loading dose and 75 mg/day. This should be withheld if emergency coronary bypass surgery is planned. There are limited data regarding newer antiplatelet agents (prasugrel and tricagrelor) in non-STEMI. In particular, data regarding prasugrel are limited to patients undergoing PCI. Both these agents have increased bleeding risk compared to clopidogrel. The decision to use them in preference to clopidogrel will require careful balancing of the bleeding risk and the risk of recurrent ischaemic events and is best left to the treating cardiologist.

Antithrombin therapy

Subcutaneous low molecular weight or unfractionated heparin should be given until angiography or for 48–72 hours. The dose of low molecular weight heparin should be reduced if there is renal impairment. The dose of heparin is as above.

Glycoprotein IIb/IIIa inhibitors

Current evidence supports selective use of GP inhibitors. Indications may include ongoing ischaemia despite antiplatelet and antithrombin therapy, diabetes and troponin elevation.

β-Blockers

Initiation of a β-blocker is recommended unless contraindicated.

Invasive management

Patients with NSTEMI should have early coronary angiography (ideally within 48 hours), unless they have severe co-morbidities.

Disposition

Disposition depends on the type of ACS. Patients with STEMI and NSTEMI require admission to hospital for further care. Those with STEMI should be admitted to a monitored bed in a cardiac care unit because of the small but significant risk of life-threatening arrhythmia. It has been the practice also to admit patients with NSTEMI to monitored beds, but this is being challenged on the basis that there are subgroups within this classification at very low risk of adverse events. Patients with ACS without ECG changes or cardiac marker elevations require a period of assessment in the ED/chest pain unit and disposition will depend on the risk identified during that process (see Chapter 5.1).

Complications

Arrhythmias and conduction disturbances (see Chapter 5.4)

Pericarditis (see Chapter 5.6)

Acute left ventricular failure and cardiogenic shock

Most MIs are accompanied by some degree of left ventricular failure, which may range in severity from asymptomatic to pulmonary oedema or cardiogenic shock. Mortality depends in part on the degree of left ventricular failure, with cardiogenic shock having a reported mortality of approximately 80%.

Management includes maintaining adequate oxygenation, correcting electrolyte imbalances and optimizing ventricular filling pressures. Patients with pulmonary oedema may require non-invasive ventilatory support (see Chapter 5.3), but this need not be routine as most cases respond to medical therapy. If there is hypotension or other evidence of inadequate perfusion in the presence of adequate intravascular volume, inotropes should be initiated early and aggressively. PCI has been shown markedly to improve outcome for patients with STEMI accompanied by cardiogenic shock. Left ventricular assist devices may bridge to recovery, cardiac surgery or transplantation in selected patients.

Thromboembolism

Thrombus can form on areas of hypokinetic myocardium due to relative stasis and the prothrombotic effects of local inflammatory changes. It is more common with large anterior infarctions with left ventricular aneurysm formation, where the incidence has been reported to be up to 10%. Echocardiography is used to confirm the presence of thrombus. Systemic anticoagulation is required to prevent embolic complications.

Mechanical defects

Mechanical defects may include:

- ventricular aneurysm formation with the attendant risk of thrombus formation and embolization
- acute mitral insufficiency secondary to papillary muscle dysfunction/rupture

- ventricular septal defect
- cardiac rupture, which may present as sudden death or acute pericardial tamponade.

Prognosis

The prognosis of ACS varies substantially between patients, depending on age, co-morbidities, risk factors, severity of coronary occlusion and myocardial necrosis and the presence of complications. Treatment of ACS should be guided by prognosis: the worse the prognosis, the greater the potential impact of treatment. Prognostic scoring therefore has an important role to play in the management of ACS.

The thrombolysis in myocardial infarction (TIMI) score has been developed and validated as a predictor of adverse outcome (mortality, life-threatening arrhythmia or subsequent myocardial infarction) in ACS. Patients are ascribed a score between zero (lowest risk) and seven (highest risk) by scoring one point for each factor listed in Table 5.2.4. Higher scores are associated with a higher risk of adverse outcome, as shown in Table 5.2.5. The TIMI

Table 5.2.4 Components of the TIMI score
Age ≥65 years
Previous coronary artery stenosis >50%
Three or more risk factors for coronary heart disease
ST-segment deviation
Aspirin use in the preceding 7 days
Two or more anginal events in last 24 hours
Elevated cardiac biomarkers

Table 5.2.5 TIMI score and risk of death or MI at 14 days	
TIMI score	Risk of death or MI at 14 days (%)
0 or 1	3
2	3
3	4
4	6
5	11
6 or 7	19

score is simple to calculate and applicable to a wide range of patients. It can be used to predict which patients will benefit from early invasive management. Patients with a TIMI score of 3 or more appear to benefit from early invasive treatment, whereas those with a TIMI score of 2 or less do not. Patients with a TIMI score of 3 or more with ACS should therefore be considered high risk and receive early coronary angiography.

An alternative to the TIMI score is the Global Registry of Acute Coronary Events (GRACE) score, which uses the components outlined in Table 5.2.6. Each component is weighted to give an estimate of the probability of in-hospital and 6-month death or MI. The weighting process makes the GRACE score a little more difficult to calculate in the clinical setting, but allows for a more precise estimate of prognosis. Both web-based calculators and apps for hand-held devices are readily available.

It is worth noting that ST-segment deviation on the ECG and elevated cardiac markers feature in both the TIMI and GRACE scores and are powerful predictors of adverse events following ACS.

Risk-stratification determines subsequent management of patients with ACS. Although this process is typically undertaken by cardiologists, it is worth emergency physicians understanding the process. If patients have a high risk of subsequent adverse events (e.g. 6-month mortality risk exceeding 3%), then early invasive coronary angiography is often recommended. It should also be considered for patients with unstable symptoms even if their estimated risk is lower. Patients whose symptoms are controlled and have a low risk of adverse events can be offered conservative treatment and cardiac testing for ischaemia, such as exercise treadmill testing. CT coronary angiography is

Table 5.2.6 Components of the GRACE score
Age
Heart rate
Systolic blood pressure
Creatinine
Killip class
Cardiac arrest at presentation
ST-segment deviation
Elevated cardiac markers

increasingly being offered as an alternative to testing for ischaemia and as a step in the diagnostic pathway between risk stratification and invasive coronary angiography.

Likely developments over the next 5–10 years

- Improved systems of care to facilitate early primary angioplasty or thrombolysis for STEMI. The exact model for reperfusion will depend upon geography, local services and health service policy. It is likely that widely dispersed rural populations will benefit more from pre-hospital thrombolysis, whereas primary angioplasty is more likely to be feasible in densely populated urban areas where specialist services are within reach of a large population. This will require integration across services (community, pre-hospital, hospital).
- New biochemical markers to assist in diagnosis of non-infarction ACS and better to diagnose and risk-stratify ACS. These markers may detect ischaemia in patients with unstable angina but no myocardial necrosis and thus be useful for risk stratification of troponin-negative patients.
- Innovative models of care allowing safe, outpatient management of selected patients with non-STEMI ACS, perhaps similar to those developed for pulmonary embolism. Whether this becomes a reality in the next 5–10 years will depend on the degree to which barriers to outpatient care can be overcome.
- Further advances in pharmacotherapy for ACS.
- Increased use of CT coronary angiography as an alternative to testing for ischaemia and as a step in the diagnostic pathway between risk stratification and invasive coronary angiography.

Controversies

- Primary angioplasty for STEMI is more effective than fibrinolysis, provided

it is rapidly available. It has been estimated that primary angioplasty is only more effective than fibrinolysis if the comparative delay between the provision of primary angioplasty and the provision of thrombolysis is less than 90 minutes. Systems of care to meet this target are in evolution.
- The potential de-skilling of ED staff by some systems that identify STEMI prior to hospital arrival and bypass the ED, instead taking the patient directly to the catheterization laboratory.
- The role of pre-hospital thrombolysis. Data from meta-analyses show that pre-hospital thrombolysis is more effective than in-hospital thrombolysis. However, the advantage is likely to be marginal in settings where the transport times to hospital are short and may not justify the resources, such as staff training and audit, required to support the service.
- Selective ECG monitoring of patients with ACS. ECG monitoring can be useful for facilitating rapid recognition of life-threatening arrhythmia in patients with ACS. However, if it is used indiscriminately in all patients with ACS, it will provide a very low yield of significant positive findings. This has led some to argue that ECG monitoring should only be used in selected high-risk patients and to develop risk-stratification rules to identify those who will benefit from monitoring.
- The development of high-sensitivity troponin assays has allowed early identification of NSTEMI and increased the diagnostic yield, but there are doubts about the prognostic importance of low troponin elevations and whether their detection leads to improved patient outcomes.
- The role of CT coronary angiography in the diagnostic assessment of ACS requires clarification. It can accurately identify coronary artery obstruction and has a potential role in the diagnostic

pathway between risk stratification with ECG and biomarkers and definitive investigation with invasive coronary angiography. Research is required to determine the exact role and to determine whether using CT coronary angiography leads to more selective and appropriate use of invasive coronary angiography.

Further reading

American College of Cardiology Foundation/American Heart Association Task Force on Practice Guidelines. 2012 ACCF/AHA focused update of the guidelines for the management of patients with unstable angina/non-ST-elevtaion myocardial infarction. J Am Coll Cardiol 2012; 60:645–81.

Antman E, Cohen M, Bernink P, et al. The TIMI risk score for unstable angina/non-ST elevation MI: a method for prognostication and decision-making. J Am Med Assoc 2000;284:835–42.

Aroney CN, Aylward P, Kelly A-M. Guidelines for the management of acute coronary syndromes. Med J Aust 2006;184:S1–30.

Braunwald E, Antman EM, Beasley JW, et al. ACC/AHA guidelines for the management of patients with unstable angina and non-ST-segment elevation myocardial infarction. J Am Coll Cardiol 2000;36:970–1062.

Camm J, Gray H, Antoniou S, et al. Unstable angina and NSTEMI: the early management of unstable angina and non-ST-segment-elevation myocardial infarction. Clinical Guideline 94. The National Clinical Guideline Centre: acute and chronic conditions, Royal College of Physicians, 2010.

Fox KAA, Birkhead J, Wilcox R, et al. British Cardiac Society Working Group on the Diagnosis of Myocardial Infarction. Heart 2004;90:603–9.

Fox KAA, Dabdous OH, Goldberg RJ, et al. Prediction of risk of death and myocardial infarction in the six months after presentation with acute coronary syndrome: prospective multinational observational study (GRACE). Br Med J 2006;333:1091–4.

Thygesen K, Alpert JS, White HD. Joint ESC/ACCF/AHA/WHF Task Force for the Redefinition of Myocardial Infarction. Universal definition of myocardial infarction. J Am Coll Cardiol 2007;50:2173–95.

Keeley EC, Boura JA, Grines CL. Primary angioplasty versus intravenous thrombolytic therapy for acute myocardial infarction: a quantitative review of 23 randomised trials. Lancet 2003;361:13–20.

McMahon R, Siow W, Bhindi R, et al. Left bundle branch block without concordant ST changes is rarely associated with acute coronary occlusion. Int J Cardiol 2013;167:1339–42.

Mukherjee D, Eagle KA. The use of antithrombotics for acute coronary syndromes in the emergency department: considerations and impact. Prog Cardiovasc Dis 2007;50:167–80.

Jain S, Ting HT, Bell M, et al. Utility of left bundle branch block as a diagnostic criterion for acute myocardial infarction. Am J Cardiol 2011;107:1111–16.

The task force on the management of ST-segment elevation acute myocardial infarction of the European Society of Cardiology (ESC). ESC guidelines for the management of acute myocardial infarction in patients presenting with ST-segment elevation. Eur Heart J 2012; 33:2569–619.

5.3 Assessment and management of acute pulmonary oedema

David Lightfoot

ESSENTIALS

1 Severe acute pulmonary oedema (APO) is associated with high morbidity and mortality.

2 APO is a pathophysiological state characterized by a maldistribution of fluid; most patients do not have fluid overload.

3 Diagnosis relies on a thorough history, focused physical exam and investigations including ECG and chest X-ray. Newer modalities, such as chest and heart ultrasound and biomarkers, may improve diagnostic accuracy.

4 Therapy is aimed at maintaining oxygenation and cardiac output and reversing the underlying pathophysiology. Reversible causes should be sought and corrected.

5 Hypotensive patients require ventilatory and inotropic support.

6 For most patients, the mainstays of therapy are oxygen, vasodilatation, usually with nitrates, and non-invasive ventilation (NIV).

7 NIV is safe and effective in APO. It has been shown to reduce rates of intubation, ICU admission and death.

Table 5.3.1 Causes of cardiogenic pulmonary oedema
Acute valvular dysfunction
Anaemia
Atrial fibrillation and other arrhythmias
Dietary, physical or emotional excess
Fluid overload – may be iatrogenic
Medication adverse effect
Medication non-compliance
Myocardial ischaemia/infarction
Myocarditis
Post-cardioversion
Pulmonary embolus
Severe hypertension
Worsening congestive cardiac failure

Introduction

Acute pulmonary oedema (APO) occurs mainly in elderly patients and, if severe, is associated with a very poor long-term prognosis (1-year mortality approaching 40%). It is a pathophysiological state characterized by fluid-filled alveolar spaces, with impaired alveolar gas exchange and reduced lung compliance. Acute dyspnoea, hypoxia and increased work of breathing are the resultant symptoms and signs. APO occurs when increased pulmonary capillary pressure, reduced plasma oncotic pressure or pulmonary capillary permeability changes lead to plasma leaving the capillaries and building up in the pulmonary interstitium. When this occurs at such a rate that lymphatic drainage from the lung cannot keep up, flooding of the alveoli results.

Aetiology and pathophysiology

The causes of APO can be divided into cardiogenic (the commonest cause in ED patients) and non-cardiogenic. In cardiogenic APO, an acute reduction in cardiac output associated with an increase in systemic vascular resistance (SVR) leads to back-pressure on the pulmonary vasculature, with resultant increased pulmonary capillary pressure. Once established, APO can lead to a downward spiral where decreasing oxygenation and increasing pulmonary vascular resistance (with its resultant increased right ventricular end-diastolic pressure) worsens left ventricular dysfunction and worsens pulmonary oedema. In most cases, the patient has a maldistribution of fluid rather than being fluid overloaded. They may, in fact, have a whole-body fluid deficit. This understanding has led to a change in the management of this condition, from the use of large doses of diuretics to a focus on vasodilators and non-invasive ventilation that reduce SVR and improve cardiac output. Some of the causes of cardiogenic pulmonary oedema are listed in Table 5.3.1.

In non-cardiogenic APO, the mechanism is thought to be increased pulmonary vascular permeability, brought about by an insult, leading to alveolar flooding. Injury to alveolar cells will also reduce their ability to clear this oedema fluid from the alveolar space (this may also play some role in cardiogenic APO). Some of the causes of non-cardiogenic pulmonary oedema are listed in Table 5.3.2.

Clinical assessment

History

As with all emergencies, clinical assessment and management should take place in parallel. There is usually a history of sudden-onset severe dyspnoea. A focused history concentrating on the recent occurrence of chest pain, a past history of ischaemic heart disease or congestive heart failure or an other causative factor is sought. Details of current medication and compliance are also important.

Examination

Patients are usually pale or cyanosed, sweaty (sometimes profusely) and frightened. They strive to maintain an upright position at all costs and may be unable to sit still. They may cough up pink or white frothy sputum, adding to their feeling of drowning. The respiratory

Table 5.3.2   Causes of non-cardiogenic pulmonary oedema
Airway obstruction
Aspiration
Asthma
Disseminated intravascular coagulopathy (DIC)
Eclampsia
Head injury, intracerebral haemorrhage, hyperbaric oxygen treatment, inhalation injury
Lung re-expansion, e.g. after treatment of a pneumothorax
Lung reperfusion
Near drowning/cold water immersion
Opiates and opiate antagonists (naloxone and naltrexone)
Pancreatitis
Pulmonary embolism (thrombus, fat, amniotic fluid, other)
Rapid ascent to high altitude
Renal/hepatic failure
SCUBA diving
Sepsis
Shock
Toxins
Trauma

rate is high, with use of the accessory muscles of respiration, and breathing is often noisy. Oxygen saturation is severely reduced, reflecting hypoxia. Most patients are hypertensive or normotensive. Hypotension indicates cardiogenic shock and a very poor prognosis. There may also be a raised jugular venous pressure (JVP), third heart sound or gallop rhythm and signs of right heart strain. Signs of chronic heart failure should also be sought, as well as murmurs that may hint at the cause. The chest may be dull to percussion and fine crepitations, which are often extensive, will be heard on auscultation. Importantly, there may be other adventitial lung sounds, including wheeze – so-called 'cardiac asthma'.

Clinical investigations

Electrocardiogram
An ECG is required, looking for acute ischaemia, especially evidence of ST-elevation myocardial infarction (STEMI), which should be immediately treated with appropriate reperfusion strategies.

Imaging
A chest X-ray will show cardiac size (usually enlarged) and help differentiate APO from airways disease. The chest X-ray findings of pulmonary oedema reflect the changes in fluid distribution. Initially, blood is diverted to the upper lobe veins, which become more prominent than normal. As the oedema worsens, interstitial oedema results in basilar and hilar infiltrates, which are hazy and more confluent than patchy, and interlobular oedema is seen as Kerley B lines. There is loss of vascular delineation. In severe APO, widespread changes representing alveolar oedema appear. There may also be pleural effusions if the interstitial pressure exceeds pleural pressure. Changes associated with the underlying cause can also be seen, e.g. cardiomegaly and pleural effusions in cardiogenic APO. It is important to note that the X-ray changes may not be bilateral and may mimic consolidation from other causes, e.g. pneumonia.

Ultrasound scanning (USS) in the emergency department (ED) can be a useful adjunct to physical examination. During ultrasound of the chest, homogeneous vertical comet tails or B-lines, which originate from the pleural line and continue to the bottom of the screen, characterize pulmonary oedema. These are ultrasound resonance artefacts generated by oedematous interlobular septa and are initially seen in the lung bases but, as oedema worsens, extend upwards to the apices. USS can be used to help differentiate the cause of a patient's dyspnoea. In acute lung injury or acute respiratory distress syndrome (ARDS), the B-lines are non-homogeneous with areas of sparing. In patients with airways disease, horizontal A-lines may be seen, with an absence of B-lines. The B-lines will resolve as pulmonary oedema improves and may be used to follow response to therapy. Findings of jugular venous distension on ultrasound exam are also consistent with APO. Ultrasound scanning of the heart (echocardiography) may also be useful in determining the cause of the APO (e.g. wall motion abnormalities in acute myocardial infarction, right ventricular strain in pulmonary embolus and acute valvular dysfunction).

Blood tests
Blood tests include haemoglobin, electrolytes, cardiac biomarkers or other cause specific bloods as indicated, e.g. lipase.

Brain or B-type natriuretic peptide (BNP) or N-terminal pro-brain natriuretic peptide (NT-proBNP) levels may be useful in distinguishing APO from other causes of acute dyspnoea. BNP is the active part of a hormone (pro-BNP) secreted by ventricular myocytes in response to stretch. Its physiological function is to oppose the effects of the activated renin–angiotensin–aldosterone system. NT-proBNP is the inactive part cleaved from pro-BNP and has a longer plasma half-life than BNP. Its levels are also age dependent meaning 'rule in' cut points must be age-qualified. Plasma levels rise during acute heart failure and APO. In the setting of acute dyspnoea, levels of BNP <100 pg/mL (or NT-proBNP <300 pg/mL) make a diagnosis of acute heart failure and APO less likely. Conversely, when the BNP levels are >500 pg/mL (or NT-proBNP >450 pg/mL (age <50), >900 pg/mL (age 50–75) and >1800 pg/mL (age >75)), acute heart failure is more likely. Unfortunately, intermediate levels are difficult to interpret and other diagnoses should be sought prior to making a diagnosis of APO. That said, it has been estimated that by combining the intermediate natriuretic peptide marker levels with historical and exam findings consistent with APO, a diagnostic probability of heart failure is around 75%. Diagnostic accuracy may also be improved by combining USS with NP levels or using predictive modelling. False-positive levels may result from such conditions as pulmonary embolism, sepsis and renal failure, as well as advancing age. Positive levels may also occur in patients with chronic heart failure, but with a different cause of their acute ED presentation of dyspnoea. In addition, false-negative results may occur in the early phases of APO, owing to the delay prior to secretion of natriuretic peptides, as well as in obese patients and those with valvular or pericardial heart disease. These aspects, as well as the relatively high cost of the test, have limited its uptake in EDs in some countries. Currently, its main utility in the Australasian context involves following levels as a guide to therapeutic response, often in chronic heart failure patients. There is potential for using natriuretic peptide level changes within an ED presentation to guide disposition decisions (including discharge of non-APO heart failure patients), but this has not yet been studied prospectively.

Oximetry
Oximetry (in some cases supplemented with arterial blood gases) will reflect severity and

help monitor the patient's response to therapy. Rarely, in more severe cases, invasive monitoring may be useful.

Treatment

In all patients with APO, management strategies should provide supportive care to maximize cardiac output and oxygenation, followed by treatment of the underlying cause.

Treatment of the patient with non-cardiogenic pulmonary oedema consists of removing the patient from the causative environment, supportive therapies aimed at maintaining oxygenation, including non-invasive and invasive ventilation in severe cases, and treating the underlying cause. These patients have lung injury and therefore low volume; low pressure lung protective ventilation regimens should be followed.

Most patients with APO in the ED have a cardiogenic aetiology. Therapy varies according to haemodynamic parameters.

Normotensive or hypertensive patients

The mainstays of treatment are reduction of preload and afterload with nitrates and optimization of oxygenation, often with non-invasive ventilatory support. The patient should be managed sitting up. This posture reduces ventilation–perfusion mismatch and helps with the work of breathing.

Nitrates

Nitrates are the mainstay of pharmacological therapy of APO. They act to increase cyclic guanosine monophosphate (cGMP) in smooth muscle cells, leading to relaxation. In lower doses, this predominantly causes venodilatation and preload reduction. At higher doses, the arterioles are also affected, leading to afterload and blood pressure reduction. In addition, coronary artery dilatation leads to increased coronary blood flow. Myocardial work and oxygen demands are reduced and oxygen delivery is improved. Nitrates are therefore the ideal agents for treating APO by reversing pathophysiological processes that underlie it. Their use is limited by their hypotensive effect and by the tachyphylaxis that occurs with prolonged use. Therefore, they should be titrated against the patient's haemodynamics and require careful monitoring. Nitrates are contraindicated in those patients who have taken sildenafil or similar agents within the previous 24 hours, owing to profound vasodilatation and hypotension. They should also be used with caution in patients with fixed cardiac output (e.g. those with severe aortic stenosis or hypertrophic obstructive cardiomyopathy). Although nitrates may also be used topically or sublingually, in the patient with APO, the IV route is preferred, as dosing can be titrated to effect and therapy ceased promptly if the patient becomes hypotensive. Topical or sublingual therapy is often used as a temporizing measure until IV access can be secured. The peak effect of IV nitrates occurs after 5 minutes.

The usual dosing regimen is to begin the infusion at 5–10 μg/min and increase the rate by 10–20 μg/min every 3 minutes, titrated to clinical effect and limited by falling blood pressure. If a patient has not responded to nitrate by a dose of 200 μg/min, they are unlikely to respond to further dose increases. Some studies have looked at using higher-dose bolus IV nitrates and have shown good efficacy and safety, with improved results over low-dose nitrates, frusemide and non-invasive ventilation. These studies, however, have limitations of small patient numbers, retrospectivity or non-randomization and these dosing regimens are not currently widely used.

Sodium nitroprusside

Sodium nitroprusside is a potent vasodilator with rapid action on both the venous and arterial systems. It has beneficial actions in APO by reducing both preload and afterload. It can lead to rapid improvements in haemodynamic parameters and cardiac output without the renal complications of other agents. Due to its swift and sometimes profound hypotensive action, invasive blood pressure monitoring is recommended. Rebound vasoconstriction can occur if the drug is stopped abruptly, so it should be slowly weaned. In addition, longer duration of use (>72 hours) has been associated with cyanide toxicity, especially in patients with renal or hepatic disease, in whom it should be used with extreme caution. Nitroprusside is a valid vasodilator alternative to nitrates and can be used when nitrates are contraindicated in non-hypotensive patients.

Angiotensin-converting enzyme inhibitors (ACEIs)

ACEIs have a clear role in the treatment of chronic heart failure. Their use in APO is more controversial. ACEIs effectively reduce afterload and, in cardiogenic pulmonary oedema, can also improve pulmonary capillary wedge pressure and cardiac output. In a small prospective study, when added to standard therapy, they produced a more rapid improvement in haemodynamic parameters and symptoms than placebo. Their use in pulmonary oedema was also associated with reduced intubation rates and ICU length of stay. Unfortunately, there are no large randomized trials looking at the use of ACEIs in APO patients.

ACEIs can also produce prolonged first dose hypotension and can worsen renal function, especially when used in combination with diuretics. Therefore, these agents should be used with caution, especially in patients who have renal impairment or are hypotensive. At present, it is not recommended they be initiated as first-line therapy in APO patients, but should be commenced, with appropriate monitoring of blood pressure and renal function, once the patient has stabilized.

Frusemide

Frusemide has been the first-line treatment for patients with APO for many years. Its usefulness is due to venodilatatory properties that lead to reduced preload, as well as to its diuretic properties. The venodilatation occurs about 15 minutes after IV dosing, well before diuresis begins. Frusemide can, however, lead to increased peripheral vascular resistance via reflex sympathetic and renin–angiotensin system actions. As mentioned above, fluid overload is not usually a contributing factor in acute heart failure and so diuresis is not a necessary endpoint of therapy. The obvious exception is in patients with APO of iatrogenic origin after IV fluid therapy.

Although it is an established therapy, there are no controlled studies that show benefit from the use of frusemide in APO. At least two studies have shown that nitrates are more beneficial than frusemide in relation to haemodynamic and clinical outcomes. High-dose frusemide has been associated with worsening renal function, ICU admissions and poor outcomes in patients with acute heart failure. Nevertheless, a single dose of frusemide at 1–1.5 mg/kg is still commonly recommended in the initial management of this illness.

Morphine

In the past, morphine has been one of the major drugs used in the treatment of APO. It can cause vasodilatation and decreased sympathetic activation; however, it has significant adverse effects including respiratory and central nervous system depression, hypotension and decreased cardiac output. A small prospective study and a number of large retrospective studies have shown an association between morphine use in APO patients and increased rates of intubation, ICU admission and death. As there is no evidence showing benefit from the use of morphine in the treatment of APO and there is an increasing body of literature associating it with harm, morphine should not be used routinely in the treatment of patients with APO. It may be considered for the relief of chest pain that is resistant to nitrate therapy in patients who do not have an altered conscious state, respiratory depression or hypotension. If it is used, it should be in small, titrated IV doses with close observation.

Aspirin

The most common cause of APO in patients presenting to ED is myocardial ischaemia/infarction. Aspirin has been shown to reduce the risk of death and myocardial infarction in patients with myocardial ischaemia. Although it does not directly treat APO, when the cause is thought to be myocardial ischaemia, aspirin should be given.

Ventilatory support

Patients with APO should be given high-flow supplemental oxygen using an oxygen delivery system that can meet their minute volume needs, such as a Venturi system. They are hypoxic and, uncorrected, this will worsen APO through direct pulmonary vascular constriction and reduced myocardial oxygen delivery. Prolonged supranormal oxygenation, however, should be avoided, especially in those patients with underlying airways or other chronic lung disease. In these patients, oxygen should be used judiciously and weaned as soon as the patient is improving, aiming for low normal oxygen saturations.

Patients with a severely reduced level of consciousness, agonal respirations or respiratory arrest require endotracheal intubation and mechanical ventilatory support. This should be accomplished using rapid-sequence intubation.

The introduction of non-invasive ventilation (NIV) using continuous positive airway pressure (CPAP) or bi-level positive airway pressure (Bi-PAP) has allowed many patients to avoid endotracheal intubation. Initial CPAP pressures of 5–10 cm H_2O are used and then titrated to

effect. When using Bi-PAP, expiratory pressures are usually begun at 3–5 cm H_2O, with the inspiratory pressure 5–8 cm higher. The benefits of these therapies are due to a number of effects. Oxygen concentration can be accurately controlled and higher percentages can be delivered than via a face-mask. By using CPAP, functional capacity is increased by alveolar recruitment, with a resultant increase in gas exchange area, improved pulmonary compliance and reduced work of breathing. The addition of inspiratory pressure support with Bi-PAP further reduces the work of breathing and may be more useful in hypercapnic or tiring patients. Cardiovascular effects result from positive intrathoracic pressures, with reduced venous return and reduced left ventricular transmural pressures. These preload and afterload effects improve cardiac output without increasing myocardial oxygen demand. In general, these therapies have few complications and are considered safe. Complications that have been reported include nasal bridge abrasions, patient intolerance, gastric distension and aspiration, pneumothorax and air embolism. The last three potentially serious adverse events are extremely rare and appear to occur in selected populations with other underlying disease processes (e.g. pneumothorax in patients with *Pneumocystis carinii* pneumonia).

A number of studies have compared CPAP and/or Bi-PAP both with each other and with conventional therapy in APO. Most studies have been small and a number of meta-analyses have analysed their combined data. When CPAP was compared to standard medical therapy, there were significant improvements in oxygenation, ventilation, respiratory rate and distress and heart rates, without significant adverse events. There were also significantly reduced rates of endotracheal intubation, intensive care unit length of stay and, more importantly, reduced mortality. There is also a clear reduction in the rate of intubation and ICU admission when using Bi-PAP compared to standard therapy. There also appears to be a trend towards a mortality benefit although, in most analyses, it does not reach significance. Bi-PAP is associated with a more rapid reduction in symptoms than CPAP and may be particularly useful in patients with coexisting airways disease and acute on chronic respiratory acidosis. In the earliest trials of Bi-PAP in APO, there appeared to be an unexplained increase in the rate of myocardial infarction among patients in the Bi-PAP groups. These trials involved very small

numbers and had methodological issues. Subsequent trials and meta-analyses have not shown an increase in myocardial infarct rates among the Bi-PAP groups.

When CPAP and Bi-PAP were compared with each other, there was no significant difference in intubation, myocardial infarction or death rates. As there is no convincing evidence of benefit of Bi-PAP over CPAP and no proven mortality benefit of Bi-PAP over standard therapy, CPAP is currently the NIV method of choice in APO, unless the patient has underlying airways disease or significant acute on chronic respiratory acidosis.

New pharmacological agents

Levosimendan comes from a class of drugs known as the calcium sensitizers and is currently only available in Australasia via the special access scheme. It binds to troponin-C and stabilizes the molecule in its pro-contraction state, prolonging contraction. This occurs without impairment of diastolic relaxation and without increasing calcium concentration (with its concomitant risk of arrhythmia and cell death). Cardiac output increases and pulmonary capillary wedge pressures decrease without significantly increased oxygen demand. It also causes vasodilatation (venous and arteriolar) via potassium channel opening, leading to reduced preload and afterload. Adverse effects include tachyarrhythmias, hypotension, hypokalaemia and headache. QTc may also increase. A large randomized trial failed to show a mortality benefit when levosimendan was compared with dobutamine in patients with acute decompensated heart failure requiring inotropic support. Adverse events including hypotension, atrial fibrillation and hypokalaemia were also increased in the levosimendan group. As yet, there are no trials examining its use in patients with acute pulmonary oedema.

Nesiritide is currently available in the USA and some other regions, but not in Australia. It is a recombinant brain natriuretic peptide and acts to cause arterial (including coronary) and venous vasodilation and to suppress the renin–angiotensin–aldosterone and sympathetic nervous systems. Although its mechanism of action would suggest a benefit in patients with APO, a recent large randomized controlled study failed to show any benefit over standard care in symptom control, rehospitalization rate or death and demonstrated problems with hypotension in patients with acute decompensated heart failure. Its use is limited to patients not responding to or with contraindications to other therapies.

Nicorandil is a hybrid vasodilator that causes combined preload and afterload reduction via activated K_{ATP} channels and a nitrate-like effect. It also has a cardioprotective effect by activating mitochondrial K_{ATP} channels. When given as a bolus to heart failure patients, it decreases pulmonary capillary wedge pressure and improves cardiac index. It has been associated with decreased in-hospital mortality and readmission rates of patients in acute heart failure. There are no prospective trials and it has not been specifically studied among APO patients.

Adenosine A1 receptor antagonists are a class of drugs that can improve diuresis by inhibiting sodium-induced tubuloglomerular feedback (with resultant fall in renal blood flow and glomerular filtration rate) seen with loop diuretics. Initial studies of the first drug in this class, rolofylline, showed encouraging improvements in dyspnoea without worsening renal function in acute heart failure patients. However, when compared with placebo in a recent large randomized trial, the drug did not show benefits and there were increased adverse events, particularly seizures. It has not been studied in APO patients.

Serelaxin. Relaxin is a hormone released during pregnancy with actions that include nitric oxide production and inhibition of endothelin and angiotensin II. It produces systemic and renal vasodilatation and increased vascular compliance. In the RELAX-AHF trial, serelaxin, a synthetic form of human relaxin, was compared to placebo in addition to standard therapy in patients with acute heart failure. Serelaxin was associated with improved dyspnoea and signs of cardiac failure with less diuretic use, as well as decreased intensive care unit and hospital length of stay. There was no mortality or decreased rehospitalization rate at 60 days. As with all the newer acute heart failure drugs, there is only a small body of evidence concerning this medication and none looking specifically at APO.

Endothelin receptor antagonists. Endothelin is a potent vasoconstrictor and modulator of the sympathetic nervous and renin–angiotensin–aldosterone systems. Tezosentan, an endothelin receptor antagonist, was shown to increase cardiac index, reduce pulmonary capillary wedge and pulmonary arterial pressures and reduce systemic vascular resistance in patients with moderate to severe heart failure. Unfortunately, in large randomized trials (VERITAS 1 and 2), when compared with placebo and added to standard care, it showed no benefit in terms of dyspnoea, worsening heart failure or death.

Hypotensive patients

In general, patients with APO who are hypotensive are at the most severe end of the disease spectrum, defined as cardiogenic shock. They require both ventilatory and haemodynamic support. Endotracheal intubation using rapid-sequence intubation and ventilation maximizes oxygen delivery and minimizes oxygen utilization. A positive end-expiratory pressure of 5–10 cm H_2O may be useful. These patients may have a fluid deficit and, therefore, cautious fluid bolus resuscitation should be titrated against haemodynamic parameters and clinical effect. Inotropic support is also required, with epinephrine (adrenaline) being the first-line agent. Cardiac output may be improved with dobutamine but can it lead to hypotension requiring the concomitant use of vasopressors. These drugs will increase cardiac output, but do so at the expense of increased myocardial oxygen demand and increased arrhythmogenicity. Invasive monitoring will be required in this group as it helps guide fluid and inotropic management. Some time may be bought by the use of invasive therapeutic manoeuvres, such as an intra-aortic balloon pump. This device reduces myocardial oxygen demand via afterload reduction and increases coronary flow through diastolic augmentation. Reversible causes should be treated, e.g. reperfusion for acute myocardial infarction or surgical correction of acute valvular dysfunction.

Controversies

- The use of natriuretic peptide levels as diagnostic aids. The potential use of changes in natriuretic peptide levels as a guide to patient disposition.
- The use of standard-dose infusions versus high-dose bolus nitrates.

- The optimal use and dosage of frusemide.
- The role of new agents, such as serelaxin and nicorandil.

Further reading

Adnet F, Le Toumelin P, Leberre A, et al. In-hospital and long-term prognosis of elderly patients requiring endotracheal intubation for life-threatening presentation of cardiogenic pulmonary edema. Crit Care Med 2001;19:891–5.

Coon JC, McGraw M, Murali S. Pharmacotherapy for acute heart failure syndromes. Am J Health-system Pharm 2011;68:21–35.

Cotter G, Metzkor E, Kaluski E, et al. Randomised trial of high-dose isosorbide dinitrate plus low-dose furosemide versus high-dose furosemide plus low-dose isosorbide dinitrate in severe pulmonary oedema. Lancet 1998;351:389–93.

Cotter G, Kaluski E, Moshkovitz Y, et al. Pulmonary edema: new insight on pathogenesis and treatment. Curr Opin Cardiol 2001;16:159–63.

Hamilton RJ, Carter WA, Gallagher EJ. Rapid improvement of acute pulmonary edema with sublingual captopril. Acad Emerg Med 1996;3:205–12.

Liteplo AS, Marill KA, Villen T, et al. Emergency thoracic ultrasound in the differentiation of the etiology of shortness or breath (ETUDES): sonographic B-Lines and N-terminal pro-brain-type natriuretic peptide in diagnosing congestive heart failure. Acad Emerg Med 2009;16:201–10.

Maisel A, Mueller C, Adams Jr K, et al. State of the art: using natriuretic peptide levels in clinical practice. Eur J Heart Fail 2008;10:824–39.

Mariani J, Macchia A, Belziti C, et al. Noninvasive ventilation in acute cardiogenic pulmonary edema: a meta-analysis of randomized controlled trials. J Cardiac Fail 2011;17:850–9.

Marti C, Cole R, Kalogeropoulos A, Georgiopoulou V, Butler J. Medical therapy for acute decompensated heart failure: what recent clinical trials have taught us about diuretics and vasodilators. Curr Heart Fail Rep 2012;9:1–7.

Massie BM, O'Connor CM, Metra M, et al. Rolofylline, an adenosine A1-receptor antagonist, in acute heart failure. N Engl J Med 2010;363:1419–28.

McMurray JJV, Teerlink JR, Cotter G, et al. Effects of tezosentan on symptoms and clinical outcomes in patients with acute heart failure: the VERITAS randomized controlled trials. J Am Med Assoc 2007;298:2009–19.Mebazaa A, Mieminen M, Packer M, et al. Levosimendan vs dobutamine for patients with acute decompensated heart failure. The SURVIVE randomized trial. J Am Med Assoc 2007;297:1883–91.

O'Connor CM, Starling RM, Hernandez AF, et al. Effect of nesiritide in patients with acute decompensated heart failure. N Engl J Med 2011;365:32–43.

Peacock WF, Hollander JE, Diercks DB, et al. Morphine and outcomes in decompensated heart failure: an ADHERE analysis. Emerg Med J 2008;25:205–9.

Reissig A, Copetti R, Kroegel C. Current role of emergency ultrasound of the chest. Crit Care Med 2011;39:839–45.

Sharon A, Shpirer I, Kaluski E. High-dose intravenous isosorbide dinitrate is safer and better than Bi-PAP ventilation combined with conventional treatment for severe pulmonary oedema. J Am Coll Cardiol 2000;36:832–7.

Steinhart B, Thorpe KE, Bayoumi AM, et al. Improving the diagnosis of acute heart failure using a validated prediction model. J Am Coll Cardiol 2009;54:1515–21.

Teerlink JR, Cotter G, Davison BA, et al. Serelaxin, a recombinant human relaxin-2, for treatment of acute heart failure (RELAX-AHF): a randomised, placebo-controlled trial. Lancet 2013; 381: 29–39.

Weng C-L, Zhao Y-T, Liu Q-H, et al. Meta-analysis: noninvasive ventilation in acute cardiogenic pulmonary edema. Ann Intern Med 2010;152:590–600.

CARDIOVASCULAR EMERGENCIES

5.4 Arrhythmias

Marcus Eng Hock Ong • Swee Han Lim • Chi-Keong Ching

ESSENTIALS

1 Cardiac arrhythmias require urgent attention, as some are life threatening and can lead to sudden death.

2 The most important initial evaluation is for haemodynamic stability. Patients who are haemodynamically stable should have a 12-lead electrocardiogram (ECG), whereas unstable patients require immediate intervention.

3 The patient's underlying medical condition is very helpful in making a correct diagnosis of the arrhythmia.

4 Bradyarrhythmias should always be evaluated in the light of the patient's presenting symptoms as well as the ECG abnormality.

5 Patients with wide complex tachycardia should be considered to have ventricular tachycardia unless proved otherwise.

Introduction

Arrhythmia is the term used to describe an abnormal heart rhythm. The most common arrhythmias are atrial or ventricular ectopic beats. Tachycardia occurs when the heart rate is >100 beats per minute (bpm) and bradycardia is defined as a rate of <60 bpm. The management of cardiac arrhythmias depends on the presentation of the patient, haemodynamic stability, underlying heart disease (if any) and the exact type of the arrhythmia. Patients with asymptomatic stable arrhythmias in the absence of underlying heart disease usually do not require emergency treatment. However, patients with symptomatic arrhythmias, especially when associated with underlying heart disease, require more urgent therapy. The key objective in a patient with haemodynamic instability is restoration of adequate cardiac output to maintain cerebral perfusion as well as a stable rhythm, using interventions least likely to cause harm.

Pathophysiology and pathogenesis

An understanding of cardiac arrhythmia requires knowledge of the normal conduction system (Fig. 5.4.1). In the normal heart, electrical impulses start from the sinoatrial (SA) node and conduct via the atria to the atrioventricular (AV) node. The electrical impulses then conduct down the bundle of His to the right and left bundle branches and, subsequently, via the Purkinje fibres to the ventricular myocardium.

Different mechanisms, such as re-entry, enhanced automaticity and triggered activity, can result in arrhythmias. Generally, arrhythmias are thought of as abnormal impulse generation or abnormal impulse conduction. Abnormal impulse generation in the SA node, as in sick sinus syndrome, can result in failure of impulse formation. Abnormal impulse conduction in the AV node can result in failure of electrical conduction from the atrium to the ventricles, resulting in various degrees of AV block. Ectopic impulses in the atria result in atrial ectopics or atrial tachycardia. Accessory pathways between the atrium and ventricle can result in supraventricular tachycardia. Abnormalities in ventricular conduction can result in bundle branch blocks or a variety of intraventricular conduction abnormalities. The most dangerous arrhythmias arise from the ventricles, as these, especially in the presence of underlying structural heart disease, may be associated with sudden death.

Re-entry

Re-entry occurs when a closed loop of conducting tissue transmits an electrical impulse around the loop and stimulates atrial or ventricular electrical activity with each pass around the circuit. Atrial and ventricular fibrillation and flutter are examples of micro re-entry, whereas paroxysmal supraventricular tachycardia is an example of macro re-entry.

Principles of assessment and management

Patients with arrhythmias may present with symptoms due to the arrhythmia or may be asymptomatic and have the arrhythmia noticed during routine examination or investigations. All patients should initially be managed in an area where cardiac and other physiological monitoring is available.

The urgency of treatment is dictated by the patient's clinical condition. For stable patients, the usual clinical process including history, physical examination and investigations (particularly ECG), is appropriate. For the unstable patient, urgent intervention is required, with restoration of a stable cardiac rhythm and cerebral perfusion being the priority. Clinical information, if promptly available, may be useful. For example, a patient with a history of renal failure or heart failure taking spironolactone should raise the suspicion that a wide complex tachycardia is due to hyperkalaemia.

Intravenous access should be obtained and blood drawn for investigations, such as full blood counts, electrolytes and cardiac markers (if indicated). A 12-lead ECG is essential and a chest X-ray may be helpful. Other specific investigations, such as serum digoxin level, thyroid function tests and theophylline levels, may sometimes be indicated, depending on the arrhythmia and the clinical context.

The management of arrhythmias should begin with attention to the airway, breathing and circulation. Management of cardiac arrest is discussed in Section 1.

BRADYARRHYTHMIAS

Bradycardia is defined as a heart rate of less than 60 bpm. It is important to take into account the patient's underlying clinical state when treating bradyarrhythmias. ECG

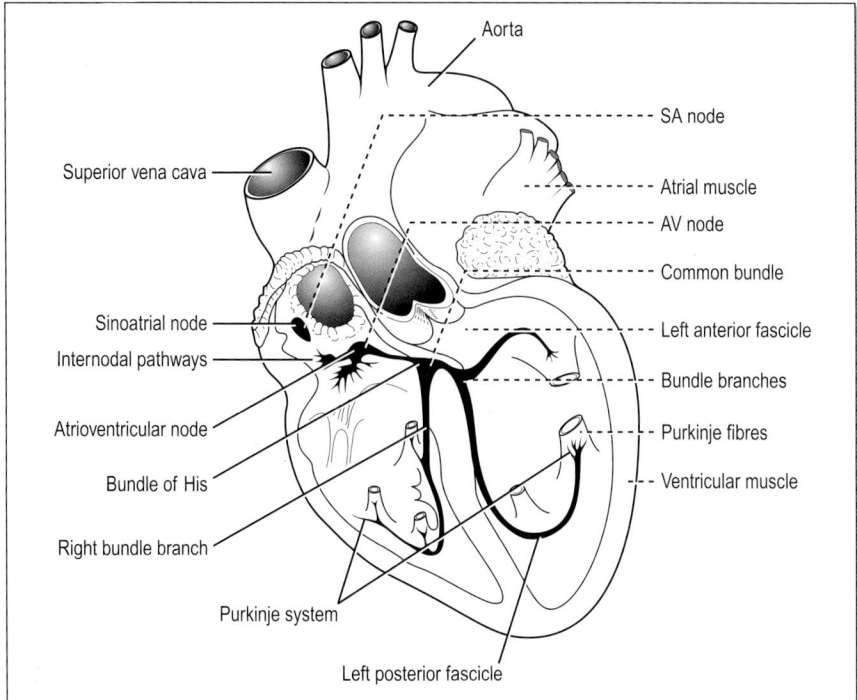

Fig. 5.4.1 Conducting system of the heart. *(Reproduced with permission from Ganong WF. A review of medical physiology, 17th edn. Connecticut: Appleton & Lange, 1995.)*

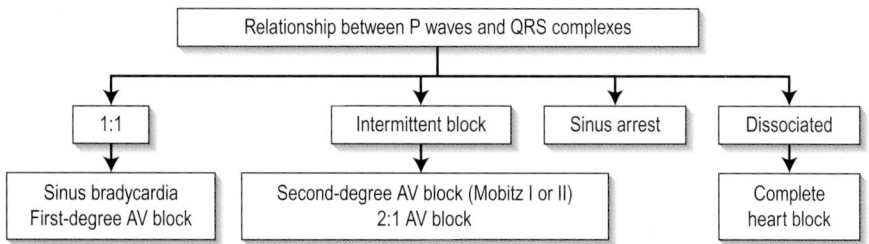

Fig. 5.4.2 Algorithm for ECG diagnosis of bradyarrhythmias.

diagnosis of bradyarrhythmias can be simplified by the algorithm in Figure 5.4.2. Note that denervated transplanted hearts will not respond to atropine and so, if treatment is required, pacing, catecholamine infusion or both should be used.

Sinus bradycardia

Physiological sinus bradycardia may be associated with good physical conditioning (e.g. marathon runners), drug effects (e.g. β-blockers, calcium antagonists) and vagal stimulation (e.g. vomiting). More serious causes include acute inferior myocardial infarction, raised intracranial pressure, hypothermia and hypothyroidism.

Clinical features
There are often no signs or symptoms. Symptoms may be related to the underlying cause.

Clinical investigations
ECG features are:

- atrial rate equal to ventricular rate
- normal PR interval
- normal P-wave morphology.

Treatment
Treat the underlying cause. If there is evidence of hypoperfusion, intravenous atropine 0.4–0.6 mg may be used while the cause is investigated. Physiological bradycardia does not require treatment. Disposition will depend on the cause.

Sick sinus syndrome (bradycardia–tachycardia syndrome)

This is most commonly found in elderly patients and results from fibrosis around the sinus node. It can also occur with congenital heart disease, rheumatic disorders, myocarditis, pericarditis, rheumatological disease, metastatic tumours, surgical damage, cardiomyopathies and ischaemic heart disease. It is a heterogeneous disorder that includes a wide variety of intermittent supraventricular tachycardias and bradyarrhythmias. Pathophysiologically, there is sinus bradycardia with intermittent failure of sinus node function, with the prolonged pause interrupted by a temporary escape rhythm. Drugs, such as β-blockers, digoxin and anti-arrhythmics, as well as conditions, such as abdominal pain, thyrotoxicosis and hyperkalaemia, can exacerbate the condition.

Clinical features
Typical features are syncope, light-headedness, palpitations, dyspnoea, chest pain, collapse and cerebrovascular accidents.

Clinical investigations
ECG features are:

- sinus bradycardia
- intermittent cessation of P-wave activity
- long pauses interrupted by escape rhythms
- resumption of sinus node activity.

Treatment
Unstable patients should be managed with atropine 0.4–0.6 mg IV as a bridge to pacing. If not effective, then consider adrenaline (epinephrine) infusion (2–10 μg/min) or dopamine (2–10 μg/kg/min) infusion if pacing is delayed. Transcutaneous pacing should be required if drugs are ineffective. Drug treatment for tachyarrhythmia risks aggravating pre-existing AV block or sinus arrest and should be avoided until pacemaker insertion. These patients eventually require a permanent pacemaker.

Heart block

First-degree AV block
In first-degree AV block, conduction of the atrial impulse to the ventricle is delayed. A P wave precedes each QRS complex, but the PR interval is more than 0.2 seconds. Causes

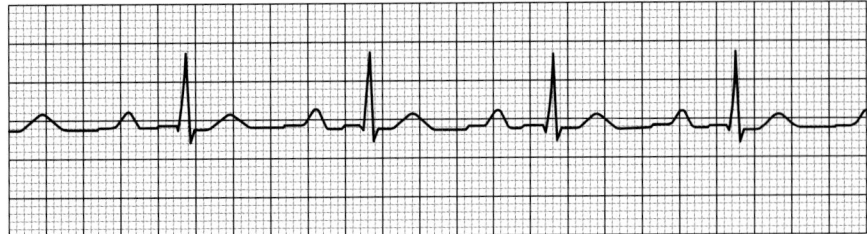

Fig. 5.4.3 Rhythm strip of first-degree AV block.

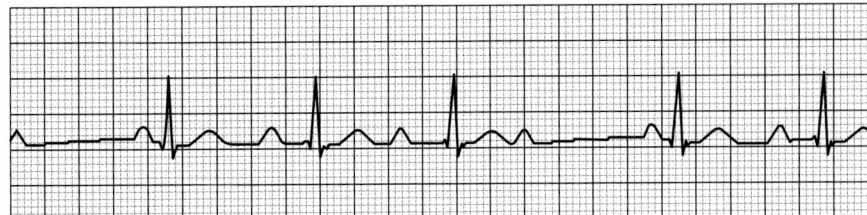

Fig. 5.4.4 Rhythm strip of second-degree AV block, Mobitz I.

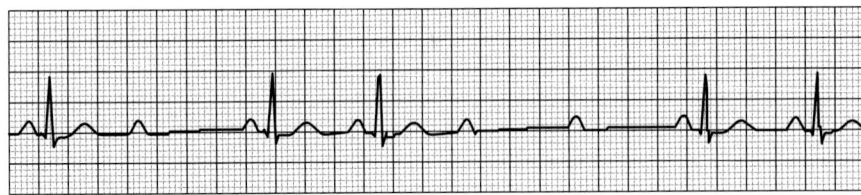

Fig. 5.4.5 Rhythm strip of second-degree AV block, Mobitz II.

include drug effects, vagal stimulation, inferior myocardial infarction and high vagal tone (especially in young patients). Rarely, it is a sign of myocarditis (e.g. rheumatic myocarditis), digoxin toxicity, idiopathic fibrosis or aortic valve disease.

There are no specific clinical features. ECG features (Fig. 5.4.3) are:

- every P wave is followed by a QRS
- PR interval is constant but >200 ms (five small squares on the ECG recorded at 25 mm/s).

Usually, no specific treatment is required. Unless associated with acute ischaemia, first-degree AV block is not itself an indication for hospital admission.

Second-degree AV block: Mobitz type I (Wenckebach)

In Mobitz type I AV block, conduction of the atrial impulses to the ventricles is intermittently blocked. This condition is due to impaired conduction in the AV node and so the atrial rate is greater than the ventricular rate. There

is a progressive increase in the PR interval until a dropped QRS complex occurs. After the dropped QRS, AV conduction recovers, resulting in a normal PR interval and then the progressive increase in PR interval starts again. Anatomically, this block is above the bundle of His in the AV node. It is thought to be due to an increased impulse conduction interval at the AV node.

Causes include inferior myocardial infarction, digoxin toxicity and high vagal tone. The condition is nearly always benign and asymptomatic but, in the setting of acute ischaemia, may progress to complete heart block.

There are no specific clinical features. ECG features (Fig. 5.4.4) are:

- progressive increase in PR intervals until a dropped QRS complex occurs
- grouped beating
- first PR after dropped QRS is shorter.

No treatment is required for stable patients. Atropine, dopamine/adrenaline infusion or cardiac pacing may be indicated in the haemodynamically unstable patient.

Second-degree Mobitz type II AV block

Mobitz type II AV block is due to intermittent failure of conduction of atrial impulses to the ventricles. The PR interval remains constant, but there is regular, intermittent failure of P-wave conduction. This is usually due to impaired conduction in the bundle of His or bundle branches (i.e. it is infranodal). Advanced second-degree block is the block of two or more consecutive P waves. This condition may be seen with acute coronary syndrome involving the left coronary artery or, less commonly, idiopathic fissure of the bundle branches.

Although it may be asymptomatic, Mobitz type II AV block is more likely to be associated with stroke, Stoke–Adams attacks (syncope), a slow ventricular rate and sudden death.

ECG features (Fig. 5.4.5) are:

- atrial rate > ventricular rate
- atrial rhythm is regular (Ps plot through)
- some P waves are not followed by a QRS (more Ps than QRS)
- PR interval may be within normal limits or prolonged, but is constant for each conducted QRS
- QRS complexes are dropped periodically. They may be narrow or widened.

If the patient is haemodynamically unstable, give atropine 0.4–0.6 mg IV. If not effective, consider adrenaline (2–10 µg/min) or dopamine (2–10 µg/kg/min) infusion. Occasionally, pacing may be needed. Patients with this condition should be admitted, as it can deteriorate to complete heart block.

Third-degree (complete) AV block

In third-degree or complete AV block, conduction of the atrial impulse to the ventricles is completely blocked. Subsidiary pacemakers arise. If they are within the bundle of His, QRS complexes are narrow (Fig. 5.4.6). In contrast, if the block is infranodal, subsidiary pacemakers usually arise in the left or right bundle branches and the QRS complexes are wide (Fig. 5.4.7). The commonest cause of complete heart block is myocardial fibrosis. It is also seen in up to 8% of inferior myocardial infarctions, where it is often transient. Complete heart block is also associated with sick sinus syndrome, Mobitz type II block and transient second-degree block with new bundle branch or fascicular block.

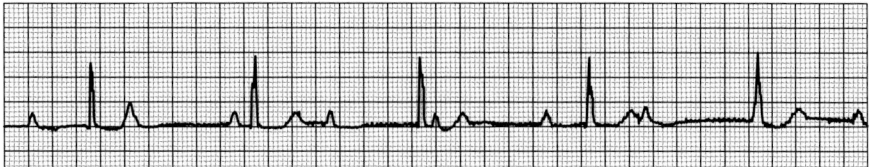

Fig. 5.4.6 Rhythm strip of narrow complex third-degree heart block.

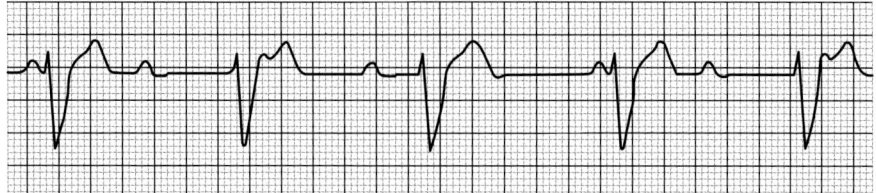

Fig. 5.4.7 Rhythm strip of third-degree heart block.

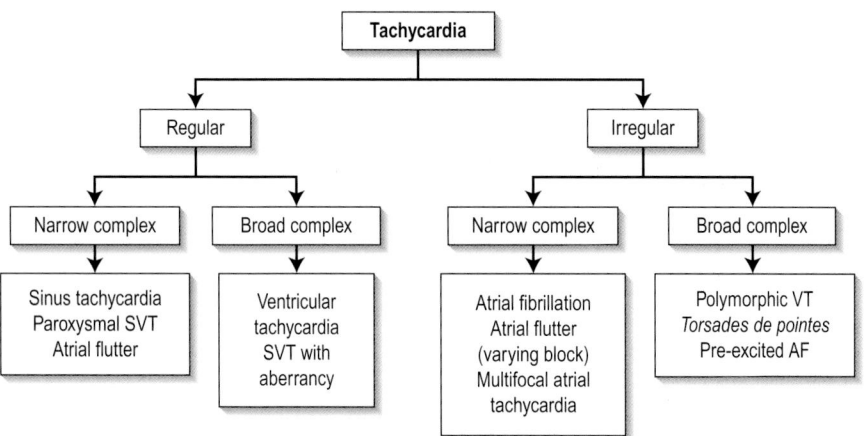

Fig. 5.4.8 Approach to tachyarrhythmias.

The patient may be asymptomatic, however, syncope or near syncope is common. Clinically, cannon 'a' waves may be seen in the neck veins and the first heart sound may vary in loudness.

ECG features are:

- complete dissociation of P waves and QRS complexes
- ventricular escape pacemaker is at 20–50 bpm
- QRS may be wide or narrow.

Haemodynamically compromised patients should have measures taken to increase ventricular rate to a level that results in adequate perfusion. Judicious use of atropine 0.4–0.6 mg IV may be helpful. If this is unsuccessful, dopamine or adrenaline infusions, titrated to effect, may be effective. In ischaemic tissue, adrenaline is preferred, as coronary perfusion is better maintained. External pacing may be required if these measures are ineffective. Admission is required and permanent pacing is often necessary.

Never treat third-degree heart block with ventricular escape beats using lignocaine or any agent that suppresses ventricular escape rhythms as this will suppress the already slow heart rate, resulting in reduced cardiac output.

TACHYARRHYTHMIAS

There is a wide range of tachyarrhythmias. Immediate diagnosis and management may be considered on the basis of the width of the QRS complex and the regularity of the rhythm (Fig. 5.4.8).

Broad complex tachycardias

The differential diagnosis of a regular broad complex tachycardia includes ventricular tachycardia (VT) or supraventricular tachycardia (SVT) with aberrant conduction. Considerable research has been undertaken in an attempt to define ECG criteria that can reliably distinguish SVT from VT. Although relatively high sensitivities for some criteria have been reported, the high prevalence of VT in emergency department (ED) patients with broad complex tachycardia (approximately 80% in some studies) lowers the predictive value of those criteria. Features that increase the chance of a broad complex tachycardia being VT are shown in Table 5.4.1. It is usually safest to treat a broad complex tachycardia as VT unless there is very strong evidence to the contrary. In the older patient with underlying ischaemic heart disease, syncope and hypotension, VT would be the most likely diagnosis.

Ventricular tachycardias

The proper identification of a ventricular arrhythmia is important in the evaluation of a patient. The management of ventricular arrhythmia depends on the correct identification of the rhythm, assessment of the risk–benefit ratio of antiarrhythmic drug therapy and an awareness of non-pharmacological modes of treatment. The presence or absence of heart disease and left ventricular function (ejection fraction) also influence the management approach. Risk increases with the severity of structural heart disease and left ventricular dysfunction.

Monomorphic ventricular tachycardia

Sustained VT is defined as a succession of ventricular impulses at a rate of >100 per minute and lasting more than 30 seconds or resulting in haemodynamic compromise. If the patient is haemodynamically stable, a 12-lead ECG should be recorded to characterize morphology.

Patients may be asymptomatic or complain of palpitations, dizziness or chest pain. Cannon 'a' waves may be seen in the neck veins. The patient may lose consciousness.

ECG features (Figs 5.4.9 and 5.4.10) are:

- AV dissociation
- fusion beats or capture beats
- wide QRS complexes >140 ms

Table 5.4.1 Features that increase the chance of broad complex tachycardia being diagnosed as VT

History	Clinical features	ECG features
Age >35 years	Cannon 'a' wave in JVP	AV dissociation
Smoker	Variable intensity of S1	Fusion beats
Ischaemic heart disease	Unchanged intensity of S2	Capture beats
Previous VT	QRS with >140 ms (<120 ms SVT)	Left axis variation >30° favours VT
Active angina	Concordance of QRS vectors in pericardial leads	QRS morphology in V1

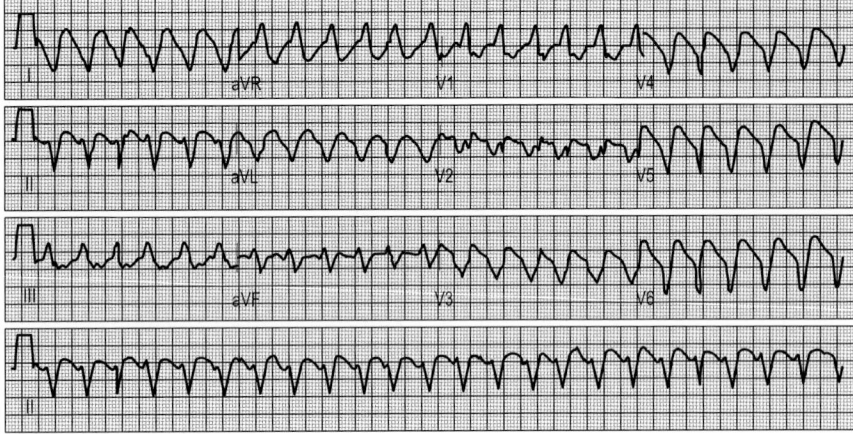

Fig. 5.4.9 Ventricular tachycardia (VT).

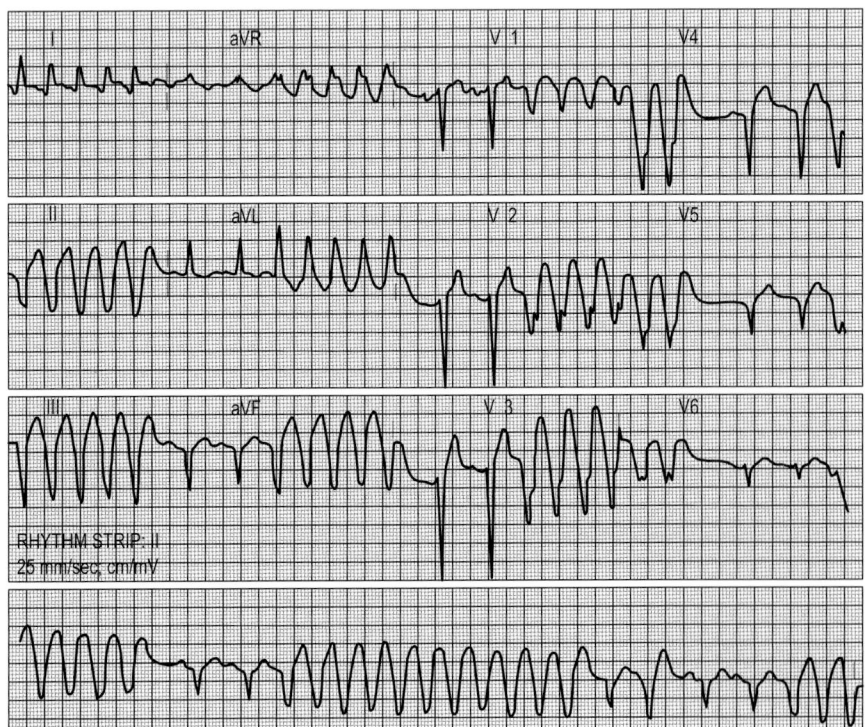

Fig. 5.4.10 Non-sustained VT.

- rate >100 bpm: commonly 150–200 bpm
- rhythm regular, although there is some beat-to-beat variability
- constant QRS axis, often with marked left axis deviation or northwest axis
- deep S wave with r/S ratio <1 in right bundle branch block (RBBB) morphology VT.

AV dissociation, captured beats or fusion beats, if present, are pathognomonic of VT. However, they are rarely seen because the rate of VT must be slow, usually <120 bpm for it to be easily visible.

Treatment VT should be managed according to current AHA/ACC guidelines. Management of pulseless VT is addressed in Section 1 of this book. All patients with VT require oxygen therapy and IV access, at which time blood for electrolyte and cardiac marker analysis is obtained. Electrolyte imbalances, particularly of potassium, should be corrected.

An unstable patient requires emergency cardioversion, with sedation as required. Caution is needed, especially as these patients usually have low blood pressure. The first recommended DC shock should be 100 J (synchronized). If this does not convert the rhythm, it can be increased to 150 J and then 200 J. This can be further increased to 360 J if required. The equivalent biphasic energy should be used for biphasic defibrillators (e.g. escalating 70 J, 120 J, 150 J, 170 J). Shock-resistant VT may respond after administration of amiodarone. Lignocaine, magnesium and procainamide are considered second-line adjuncts to cardioversion as there is less evidence to support their efficacy. Nifekalant can also be considered, where available. An infusion of either amiodarone or lignocaine should be commenced after cardioversion. If the blood pressure is low, consider the use of inotropic support, for example dopamine infusion.

Stable patients may be treated with:

- intravenous amiodarone 150 mg as a slow bolus over 10 minutes. This can be repeated a second time if conversion has not been achieved
- an alternative is IV procainamide 100 mg (where available) every 5 minutes to a maximum dose of 10–20 mg/kg body weight
- intravenous lignocaine 50–100 mg IV push at a rate not more than 50 mg/min. This can be repeated a second time if conversion is not achieved. It should be noted, however,

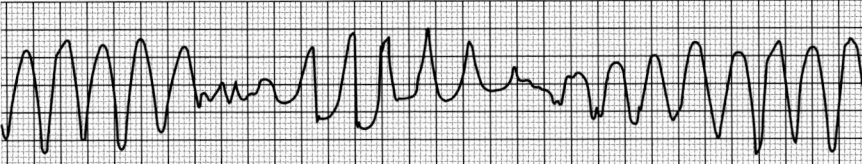

Fig. 5.4.11 Torsades de pointes.

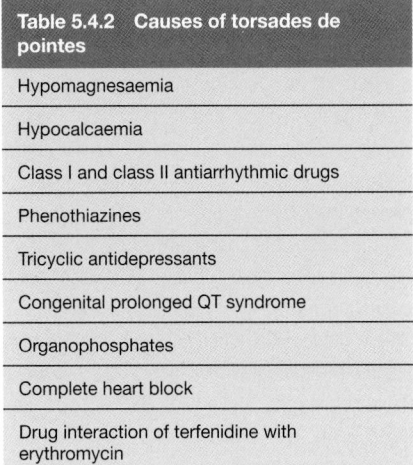

Table 5.4.2	Causes of torsades de pointes
Hypomagnesaemia
Hypocalcaemia
Class I and class II antiarrhythmic drugs
Phenothiazines
Tricyclic antidepressants
Congenital prolonged QT syndrome
Organophosphates
Complete heart block
Drug interaction of terfenidine with erythromycin

that lignocaine is relatively ineffective for terminating haemodynamically stable VT of unknown aetiology.

Sotolol 1 mg/kg is used as second-line agent. Following successful conversion, an infusion of the successful agent should be commenced for maintenance therapy. If pharmacological therapy is unsuccessful, cardioversion under sedation is indicated.

Polymorphic VT

VT with a continuously varying QRS morphology is called polymorphic VT. It is often associated with ischaemia and tends to be more electrically unstable than monomorphic VT.

Polymorphic VT includes a specific variant called torsades de pointes, which is associated with a prolonged QT. This is characterized by QRS peaks that twist around the baseline (Fig. 5.4.11) and this occurs in the presence of repolarization abnormalities. Causes are summarized in Table 5.4.2.

Syncope is the usual presenting symptom. ECG features include:

- regular or irregular fast, wide QRS complexes
- continuously varying QRS morphology.

Torsades de pointes may be sensitive to magnesium. A bolus of 2 g over 1–2 minutes followed by an infusion will usually cause reversion. Cardioversion is recommended if the patient is haemodynamically compromised, but torsades de pointes can be resistant. Accelerating the heart rate, thereby shortening ventricular repolarization (e.g. by overdrive pacing to a rate of 90–120 bpm or isoprenaline infusion titrated to similar effect) may be successful. Treatment of the underlying cause is essential as torsades de pointes is very difficult to control. Beta-blockers can also be considered for congenital prolonged QT syndrome.

Idiopathic ventricular tachycardia

Idiopathic ventricular tachycardia is a monomorphic VT that occurs in the absence of structural heart disease. It is often exercise dependent and is named according to its site of origin. The QRS morphology during tachycardia can indicate the site of origin.

Idiopathic ventricular tachycardia presents as one of two subclasses:

- left bundle branch block (LBBB) morphology: inferior axis VT due to right ventricular outflow tract ventricular tachycardia
- RBBB morphology: VT due to idiopathic left ventricular tachycardia.

Right ventricular outflow tract ventricular tachycardia

Right ventricular outflow tract ventricular tachycardia has a typical LBBB inferior axis morphology. The aetiology is believed to be cyclic-AMP (cAMP)-mediated triggered activity.

It typically occurs in young patients and is slightly more common in females. There is usually no evidence of underlying structural heart disease.

ECG features are:

- QRS is broad (>120 ms) with a left bundle branch inferior axis morphology

- AV dissociation is not usually seen as the tachycardia is often very rapid
- repetitive monomorphic forms may occur.

It is usually responsive to β-blockers as it is catecholamine sensitive. It is important to exclude underlying structural heart disease, especially arrhythmogenic right ventricular cardiomyopathy.

Idiopathic left ventricular tachycardia (ILVT)

Idiopathic left ventricular tachycardia is a fascicular ventricular tachycardia. The pathophysiology is a re-entrant phenomenon in the posterior fascicle of the left bundle branch.

It occurs in young patients without structural heart disease.

On ECG (Fig. 5.4.12), QRS morphology is broad and shows a right bundle branch block pattern with left axis deviation. The duration of the QRS complex is 100–140 ms with an RS interval <80 ms. For ischaemic VT the duration of the QRS complex is usually >140 ms and the RS interval >100 ms. ECG may also show capture beats or fusion beats.

The drug of choice is intravenous verapamil. Amiodarone and sotalol have been reported to be equally effective. Vagal manoeuvres and intravenous adenosine are ineffective in converting this arrhythmia. Lignocaine is not effective for ILVT.

Pre-excited atrial fibrillation

Pre-excited atrial fibrillation (Wolff–Parkinson–White (WPW) AF) is a differential diagnosis for an irregular, wide complex tachycardia.

The patient is usually young (age <50 years) with a previous history of palpitations, rapid heart rate, syncope or documented history of WPW.

ECG features (Fig. 5.4.13) are:

- rapid ventricular response (>180 bpm; this response rate is much too rapid for conduction down the AV node)
- broad and bizarre QRS complex, signifying conduction down the aberrant pathway
- occasionally, a narrow QRS can be seen, representing conduction through the AV node
- changing RR intervals; a QRS complex that changes frequently.

During sinus rhythm, the ECG of patients with WPW shows a PR interval <0.12 seconds, a slurred R-wave upstroke (δ wave) and a wide QRS >0.10 seconds (Fig. 5.4.14).

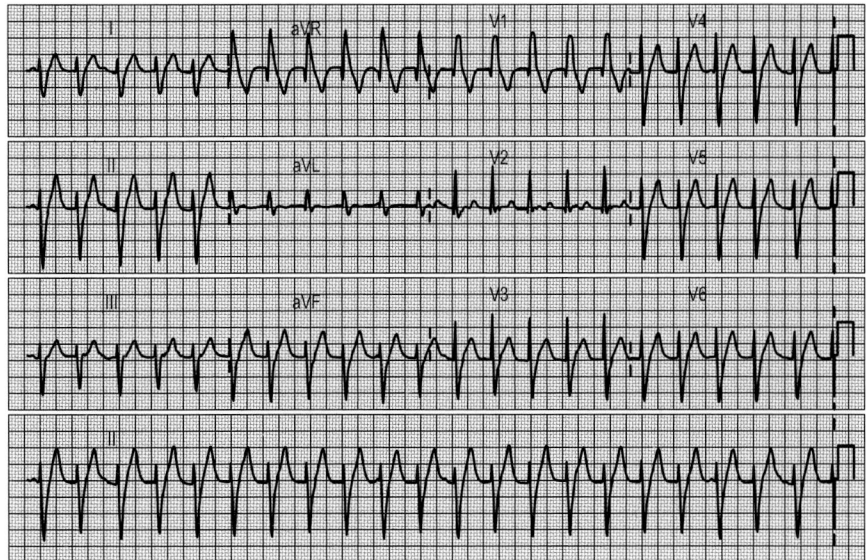

Fig. 5.4.12 Idiopathic left ventricular tachycardia (ILVT).

It is important to distinguish WPW AF from other wide complex tachyacardias. Certain subtypes of polymorphic VT, such as torsades de pointes, present with an undulating baseline. In contrast, WPW AF usually has a stable electrocardiographic baseline with no alteration in the polarity of the QRS complexes.

AF with aberrant conduction occurs when a patient with a pre-existing bundle branch block (or a rate-responsive bundle branch block) has a rapid ventricular response to AF. The ECG will show a wide complex tachycardia of irregular rate with stable beat-to-beat QRS configuration, contrasting with the variable beat-to-beat QRS configuration in WPW AF.

Haemodynamically unstable pre-excited AF is managed by immediate synchronized cardioversion. Haemodynamically stable pre-excited AF could be treated with:

- IV procainamide (30 mg/min, maximum dose 17 mg/kg). Because of the potential for severe hypotension with rapid IV administration, procainamide requires a slow rate of infusion. It may not reach therapeutic blood levels for 40–60 minutes.
- IV ibutilide, a class III antiarrhythmic agent, can also be used. Dosage is 1 mg (0.01 mg/kg for patients <60 kg) over 10 minutes, repeated once after 10 minutes if needed. It has a short half-life of 4 hours. Its dosing does not require adjustment for hepatic or renal function and it is safe in elderly patients. It acts rapidly, with a mean conversion time of approximately 20 minutes
- IV flecainide has been described as an alternative treatment.

Amiodarone administration modifies sinus and AV node properties with little, if any, effect on fast-channel tissues (i.e. accessory pathways) and it is not effective in treatment of WPW with AF.

Narrow complex tachycardias

Sinus tachycardia

Sinus tachycardia is defined as a heart rate >100 bpm. It not an arrhythmia *per se*, but rather an indication of an underlying disorder. Common causes include shock, hypoxia, cardiac failure, anaemia, drug effects, fever/infection, pain, anxiety, thyrotoxicosis and pregnancy.

Patients may complain of palpitations, but are often asymptomatic. Clinical features would be those of the underlying cause.

ECG features are:

- rate: 100–160 bpm
- rhythm: regular
- P waves: uniform and upright in appearance, one preceding each QRS complex
- PR interval: 0.12–0.20 s
- QRS: <0.10 s.

Management is focused on treatment of the underlying cause.

Paroxysmal supraventricular tachycardia

Paroxysmal supraventricular tachycardia (PSVT) originates from either an ectopic atrial focus or a re-entry circuit. Those caused by atrial flutter and fibrillation will be considered separately below.

Re-entry circuits are responsible for pre-excitation, which exists when the whole or part of the ventricular muscle is activated earlier than anticipated. The majority of re-entry circuits involve the AV node. Retrograde conduction may also involve an AV bypass tract. WPW syndrome is the most common of these. It is characterized by an electrically conductive muscle bridge (bundle of Kent) connecting atria and ventricle and bypassing the AV node. ECG when in sinus rhythm may show a PR interval of less than 0.12 s, a δ wave (slurred upstroke) and a wide QRS >0.10 s (see Fig. 5.4.14).

Patients may have palpitations, chest pain or syncope.

ECG features (Fig. 5.4.15) are:

- rate: 150–250 bpm
- rhythm: regular
- P waves: atrial P waves differ from sinus P waves
- P waves are usually identifiable at the lower end of the rate range but seldom identifiable at rates >200 bpm
- P waves may be lost in preceding T wave
- PR interval: usually not measurable because the P wave is difficult to distinguish from the preceding T wave. If measurable it is 0.12–0.20 s
- QRS: <0.10 s.

If the patient is haemodynamically unstable, cardioversion is indicated. Sedation is usually required. If the patient is mildly symptomatic but blood pressure is >100 mmHg, vagal manoeuvres may be tried. If vagal manoeuvres are unsuccessful or inappropriate, the choice of drug therapy lies between adenosine (escalating 6 mg, 12 mg and 18 mg rapid boluses into a large vein) or verapamil (continuous slow infusion of 1 mg/min to a maximum of 20 mg or 5 mg IV slowly, which may be repeated). Diltiazem infusion (2 mg/min to a maximum of 50 mg) is an alternative. There is scant evidence to show one

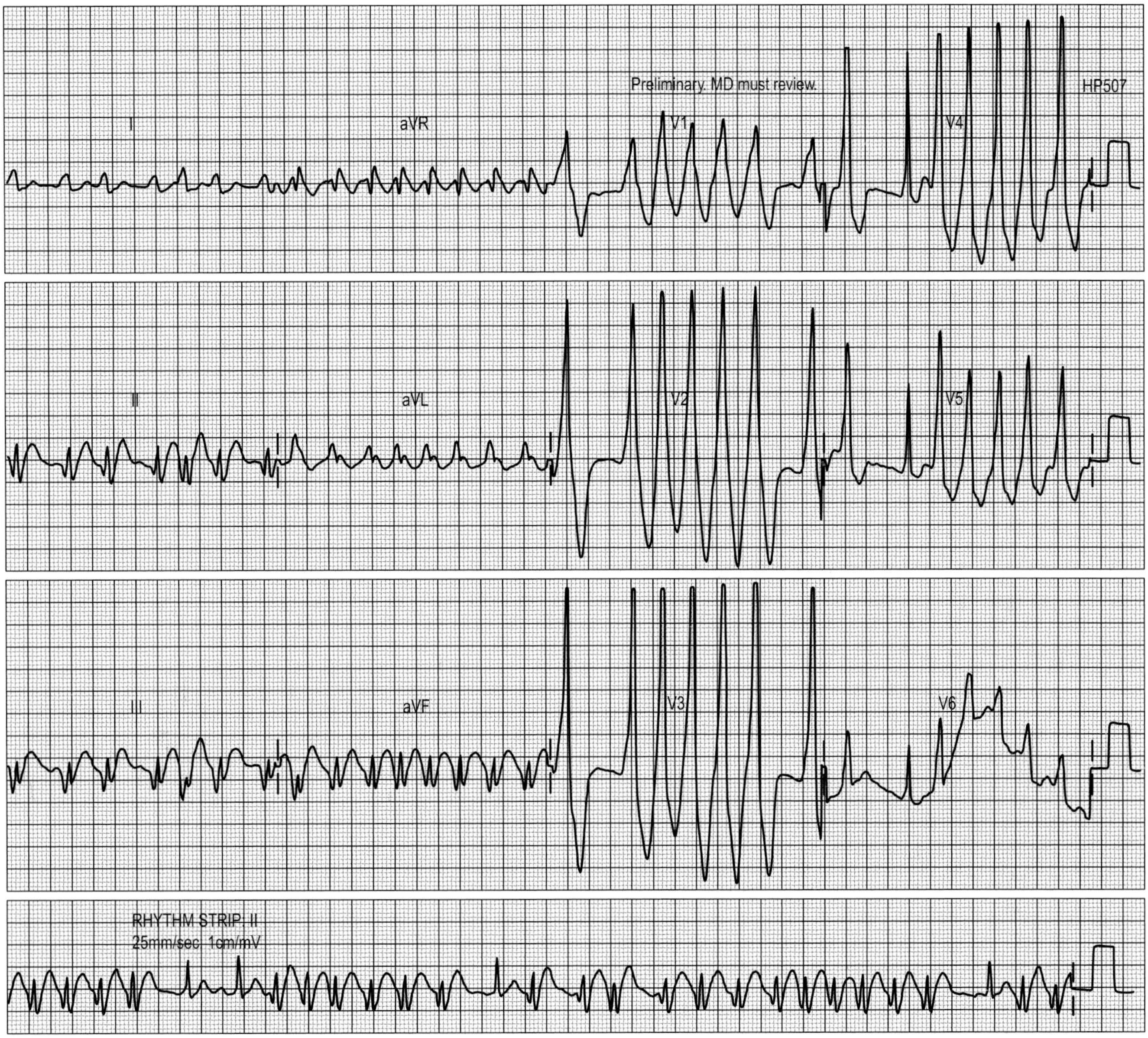

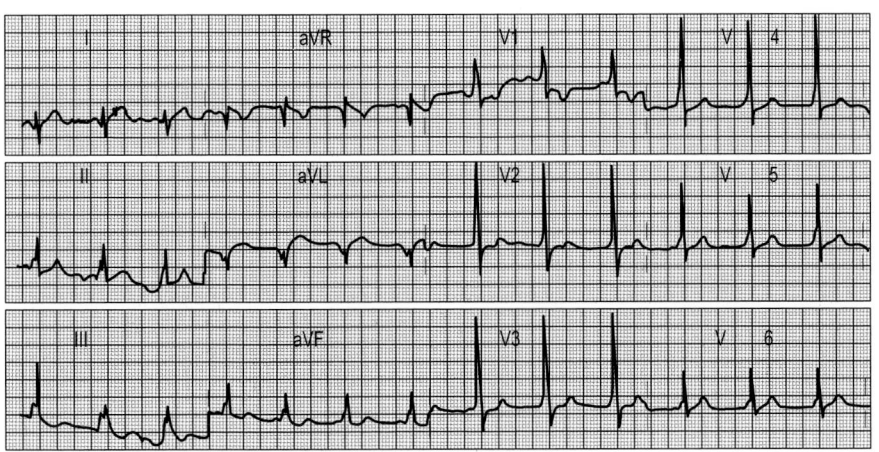

Preliminary. MD must review.
HP507
I
aVR
V1
V4
II
aVL
V2
V5
III
aVF
V3
V6
RHYTHM STRIP: II
25mm/sec; 1cm/mV

Fig. 5.4.13 Pre-excited atrial fibrillation.

I
aVR
V1
V 4
II
aVL
V2
V 5
III
aVF
V3
V 6

Fig. 5.4.14 Wolff–Parkinson–White syndrome: 12-lead ECG showing δ waves.

approach is more effective than the other. Both have adverse effects. With adenosine, patients experience a transient sense of impending doom, chest discomfort and shortness of breath that can be very distressing. With verapamil, hypotension may occur, hence the cautious administration. Concurrent use of β-blockers may potentiate this. Flecainide (2 mg/kg over 30–45 minutes) would be considered third-line therapy. Patients who are resistant to chemical cardioversion may require electrical cardioversion.

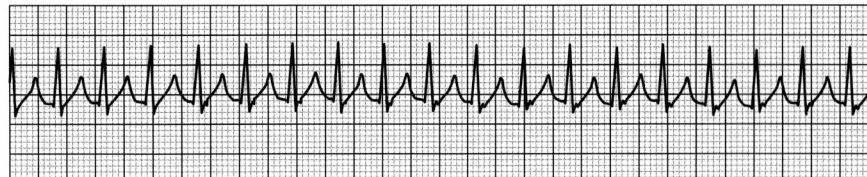

Fig. 5.4.15 Paroxysmal supraventricular tachycardia (PSVT).

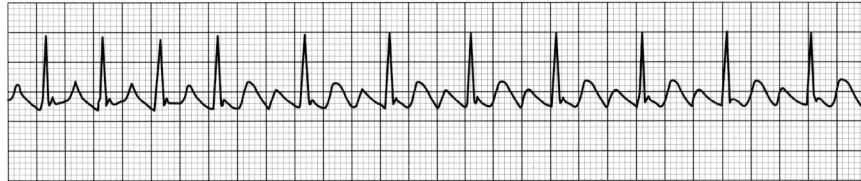

Fig. 5.4.16 Rhythm strip of atrial flutter.

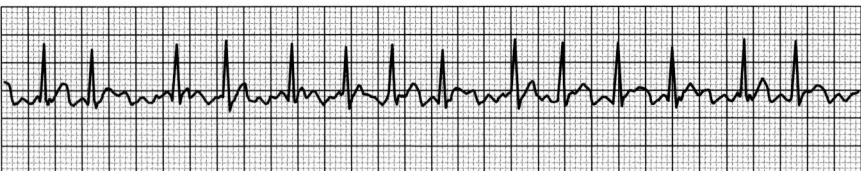

Fig. 5.4.17 Rhythm strip of atrial fibrillation.

Table 5.4.3 Causes of AF seen in the ED
Cardiac Ischaemic heart disease Pericarditis Hypertension Rheumatic heart disease Pre-excitation syndromes Cardiomyopathy Atrial septal defect Atrial myxoma Postoperative
Non-cardiac Electrolyte imbalances Sepsis Pulmonary embolism Drug and alcohol intoxication Chronic obstructive airways disease Thyrotoxicosis Lung cancer
Intrathoracic pathology

Atrial flutter

Atrial flutter rarely occurs in the absence of underlying heart disease. Causes include ischaemic heart disease, acute myocardial infarction, congestive cardiac failure, pulmonary embolism, myocarditis, chest trauma and digoxin toxicity.

Patients may have palpitations and chest pain or more commonly are asymptomatic.

ECG features (Fig. 5.4.16) are:

- rate: atrial rate 250–350/min, flutter rate usually about 300/min
- ventricular rate variable, usually 150/min with 2:1 AV block. Rarely 1:1 or higher-degree AV block (3:1, 4:1)
- rhythm: atrial rhythm regular; ventricular rhythm usually regular, but may be irregular
- P waves: sawtoothed 'flutter waves'. Best seen in II, III, and aVF
- PR interval: not measurable
- QRS: usually <0.10 s, but may be widened if flutter waves are buried in the QRS complex.

Treatment of the underlying illness is essential and will often result in spontaneous reversion. Haemodynamically unstable patients will usually respond to low-energy cardioversion (e.g. 50 J). Flecainide can be used for chemical reversion and verapamil for rate control, if required.

Atrial fibrillation

AF is the result of chaotic atrial depolarization from multiple areas of re-entry within the atria. Thus, there is a lack of coordinated atrial activity. AF is characterized by an irregularly irregular rhythm without discrete P waves and may be acute or chronic. Causes of AF seen in the ED are summarized in Table 5.4.3.

There are three variations of AF:

- AF
- AF with slow ventricular response
- AF with regular ventricular response.

Clinical features

Patients with acute episodes of AF often experience palpitations, dyspnoea, dizziness or angina. Those with chronic AF often have no specific symptoms, especially if their heart rate is <100 bpm. Clinically, the pulse is irregularly irregular and S1 varies in intensity.

Clinical investigations

Investigations will be guided by the clinical context. Patients with acute-onset AF should have electrolyte studies and thyroid function tests as well as consideration of cardiac marker levels in appropriate clinical contexts. All patients with AF should have echocardiography, if not recently performed. This can be done as an outpatient procedure for those successfully treated in the ED.

ECG features (Fig. 5.4.17) are:

- absent P waves
- chaotic irregular baseline – fibrillatory waves
- regularly irregular RR cycles – fast or slow AF
- wide QRS due to aberrance may occur intermittently (Ashman's phenomenon).

Treatment

Emergency management depends on the chronicity of the condition, the ventricular response rate, haemodynamic stability, the presence of underling structural heart disease and any associated conditions.

The aim of treatment for patients with chronic AF is rate control and treatment of any associated illness. In patients with acute-onset AF, the choice lies between cardioversion in the ED (electrical or pharmacological), rate control and anticoagulation with delayed elective electrical cardioversion or rate control alone. The choice will be governed by the duration of the episode, the age of the patient, known structural heart disease, co-morbidities and previous attempts at cardioversion. There is no evidence that a rhythm control strategy is superior to a rate control strategy. That said, a rhythm-control strategy may be preferred for younger patients, those who are symptomatic, those presenting for the first time with lone AF and those with AF secondary to a

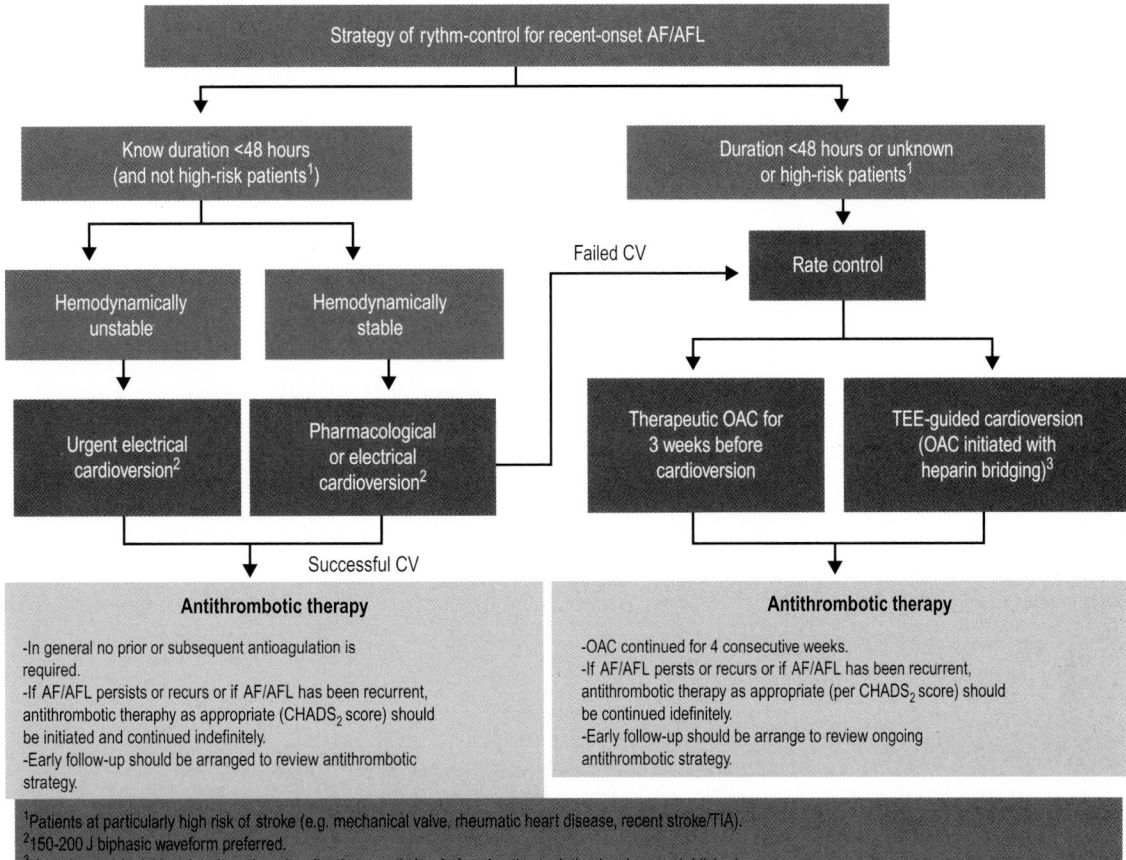

Fig. 5.4.18 Management algorithm for atrial fibrillation in ED. *(Reproduced with permission from Stiell IG, Macle L. CCS atrial fibrillation guidelines committee. Canadian cardiovascular society atrial fibrillation guidelines 2010: management of recent onset atrial fibrillation and flutter in the emergency department. Can J Cardiol 2011;27:38–46.)*

treatable/correctable precipitant. A rate-control strategy may be preferred for patients aged over 65, those with coronary artery disease, those with contraindications to antiarrhythmic drugs, those unsuitable for cardioversion and those with congestive heart failure.

Treatment of AF in the ED is summarized in Figure 5.4.18. Haemodynamically stable patients where onset of AF is within 48 hours may be treated with either pharmacological or electrical cardioversion. Where AF is of a longer duration, a delayed elective cardioversion or rate-control-only strategy is indicated. There is a case in otherwise well patients with very recent-onset paroxysmal AF in the absence of structural heart disease or other underlying condition for a period of observation as up to 90% will revert spontaneously – usually within 24 hours.

For pharmacological cardioversion in patients without structural heart disease, a class Ic agent, such as flecainide (2 mg/kg over 20–30 minutes) or propafenone, is recommended. Where structural heart disease is present, amiodarone (2–3 mg/kg over

5–10 minutes, repeated if necessary) is the drug of choice. Ibutilide, dofetilide, quinidine or procainamide (where available) may also be useful for cardioversion.

Rate control can be achieved with β-blockers (e.g. metoprolol 2.5–5 mg IV over 2 minutes, repeated if necessary to a maximum of 15 mg), verapamil (5–10 mg IV over 2–5 minutes), amiodarone or diltiazem.

In patients with life-threatening haemodynamic instability, emergency electrical cardioversion should be attempted, irrespective of the duration of the AF. In patients with WPW syndrome, flecainide may be used as an alternative to attempt pharmacological cardioversion. Atrioventricular node-blocking agents (such as diltiazem, verapamil or digoxin) should not be used.

In patients with known permanent AF where haemodynamic instability is caused mainly by a poorly controlled ventricular rate, a pharmacological rate-control strategy should be used. Beta-blockers or rate-limiting calcium antagonists are the agents of choice or, where these are contraindicated or ineffective, amiodarone should be used.

Multifocal atrial tachycardia

This rare arrhythmia is characterized by three or more atrial foci, a ventricular rate of more than 100 bpm and variable PP, PR and RR intervals. It is associated with chronic obstructive lung disease, hypoxia, electrolyte disturbance, pulmonary embolus and digoxin toxicity. Treatment is directed at improving the underlying condition. Specific treatment of the arrhythmia is rarely required and often not helpful.

UNIFASCICULAR BLOCKS

A unifascicular block is a conduction block that affects one of the major infranodal conduction pathways: right bundle branch block (RBBB), left anterior fascicular block (LAFB) or left posterior fascicular block (LPFB). Conduction blocks can be caused by ischaemia, cardiomyopathies, valvular disease, myocarditis, surgery, congenital disease and degenerative diseases (Lenegre or Lev disease).

Left anterior fascicular block

There are no specific clinical features.
ECG features are:

- left axis deviation
- normal QRS duration.

Usually no treatment needed. Treat the underlying cause.

Left posterior fascicular block

There are no specific clinical features.
ECG features are:

- right axis deviation
- normal QRS duration.

Usually no treatment needed. Treat the underlying cause.

Right bundle branch block

RBBB can be a normal variant. Other causes include pulmonary embolism, right ventricular hypertrophy, ischaemic heart disease, congenital heart disease and cor pulmonale.
Clinical features will be those of the underlying cause.

ECG features (Fig. 5.4.19) are:

- rSR pattern, most noted in V1 and V2
- broad S wave in left ventricular leads
- QRS >120 ms in complete RBBB and ≤120 ms with incomplete RBBB.

Treatment is of the underlying cause. If there is a new RBBB, the cause should be actively determined.

Left bundle branch block

LBBB is usually pathological. Causes include myocardial infarction, ischaemic heart disease, left ventricular hypertrophy, congenital heart disease and left ventricular strain.
Clinical features will be those of the underlying cause.
ECG features (Fig. 5.4.20) are:

- RR pattern, best seen in left ventricular leads V5 and V6
- QRS >120 ms.

Treatment is of the underlying cause. If there is a new LBBB in the setting of myocardial ischaemia, management should be as for acute myocardial infarction.

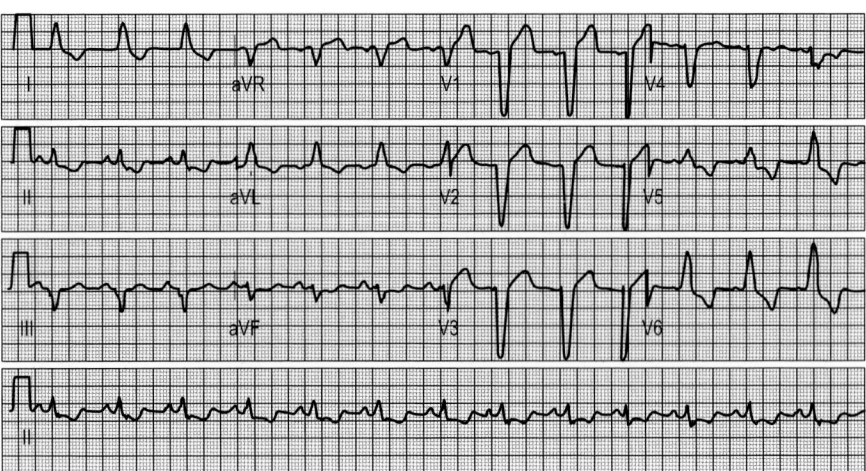

Fig. 5.4.20 Left bundle branch block.

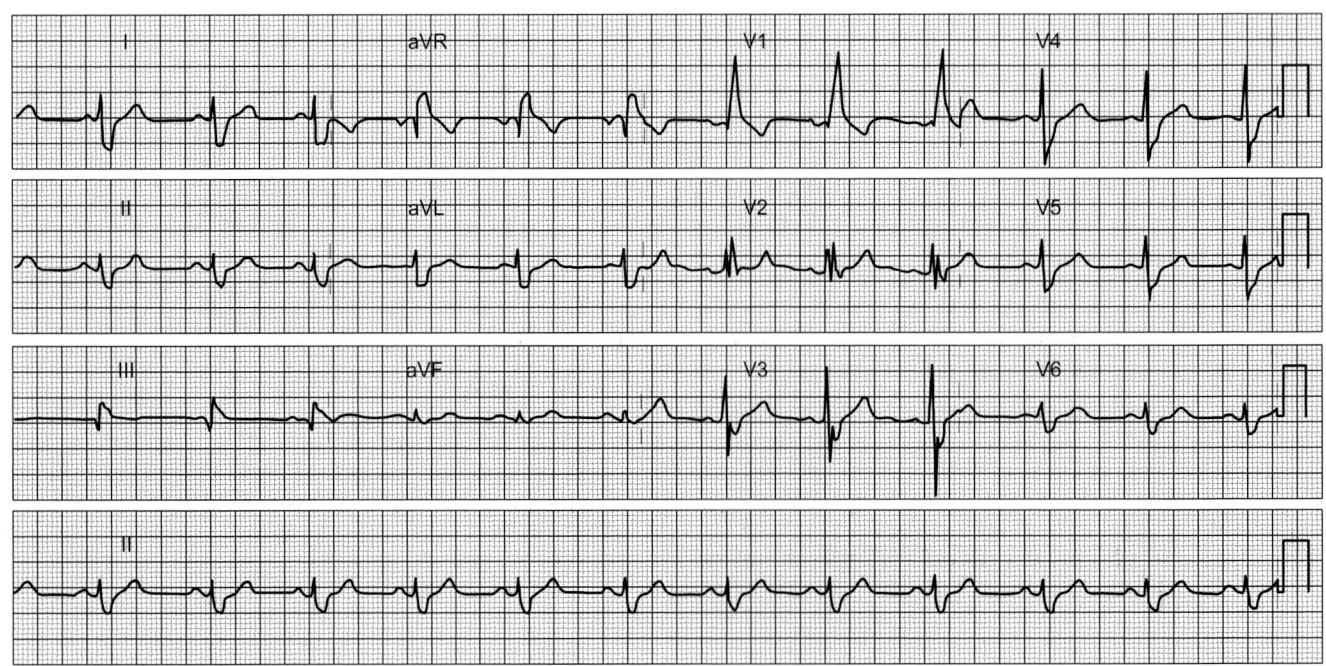

Fig. 5.4.19 Right bundle branch block.

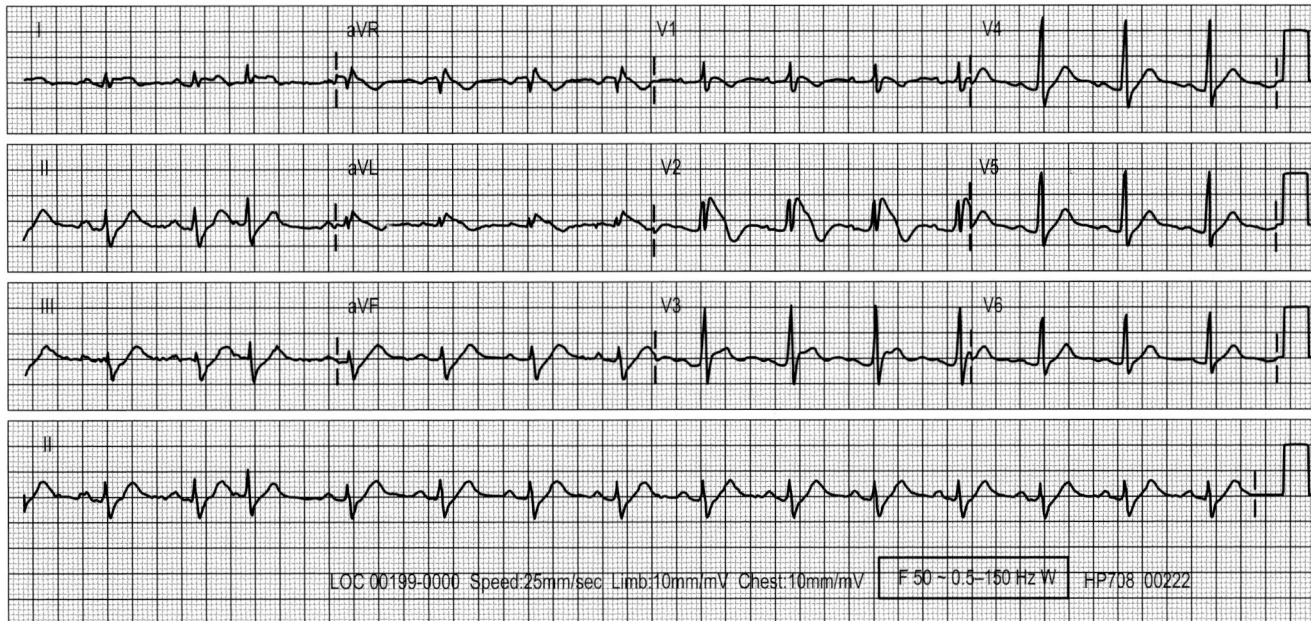

Fig. 5.4.21 Brugada syndrome.

LOC 00199-0000 Speed:25mm/sec Limb:10mm/mV Chest:10mm/mV   F 50 ~ 0.5–150 Hz W   HP708 00222

Combination blocks

A bifascicular block is a conduction block that affects two of the major infranodal conduction pathways. This may be an LBBB or a combination of RBBB and LAFB or LPFB. Trifascicular block is a combination of conduction blocks of all three fascicles. Examples include:

- RBBB and LAFB with first-degree AV block
- RBBB and LPFB with first-degree AV block
- LBBB with first-degree AV block
- alternating RBBB and LBBB.

Blocks may be permanent or transient. In the setting of an acute myocardial infarction, both bi- and trifascicular blocks may degenerate to complete heart block. Thus admission to a monitored bed is needed and pacemaker insertion considered.

OTHER DISTURBANCES OF CARDIAC RHYTHM AND CONDUCTION

Atrial ectopics

Atrial ectopics are mostly asymptomatic and may be precipitated by alcohol, nicotine and caffeine. They may be associated with AF, underlying heart disease or respiratory disease.

ECG features are:

- complexes are usually earlier than normal (premature)
- P-wave morphology different from sinus P. May be lost or deformed
- PR interval may be short or long
- QRS usually normal unless aberrantly conducted
- when early, may be blocked – blocked atrial ectopic.

Usually no treatment is necessary.

Junctional rhythm

A junctional rhythm is usually asymptomatic. ECG features are:

- rate is slower than sinus rhythm
- rhythm is regular
- no preceding P wave
- infrequently P wave may precede or be just after the QRS (the P waves are inverted in II, III, and aVF)
- QRS is usually narrow unless aberrantly conducted.

Usually no treatment needed.

Brugada syndrome

The Brugada syndrome is a syndrome with the ECG showing right bundle branch morphology and coved ST segment elevation in V1 and V2 with terminal T inversion (Fig. 5.4.21). The ECG pattern may be associated with sudden cardiac death from ventricular fibrillation. There may be a family history of sudden death. Occasionally, the ECG pattern is seen only during fever or after taking anti-arrhythmic drugs, especially class Ic antiarrhythmics, such as flecainide or propafenone. Patients with the Brugada pattern should be referred for further evaluation and risk stratification.

Controversies

- There is not much evidence for the use of many second-line antiarrhythmic drugs from randomized controlled trials.
- How safe is it to attempt immediate cardioversion for AF in the ED without formal echocardiography to exclude atrial thrombosis? Is 24 or 48 hours the safer cut-off duration?
- Is there a role for a period of observation for minimally symptomatic recent-onset paroxysmal AF?
- Is a slow-infusion calcium antagonist safer, more effective and more cost-effective than adenosine in converting supraventricular tachycardia?

Further reading

Atkins DC, Dorian P, Gonzalez ER, et al. Treatment of tachyarrythmias. Ann Emerg Med 2001;37 S91–110.

Blaauw Y, Crijns HJ. Atrial fibrillation: insights from clinical trials and novel treatment options. J Intern Med 2007;262:593–614.

Brugada P, Brugada J. Right bundle branch block, persistent ST segment elevation and sudden cardiac death: a distinct clinical and electrocardiographic syndrome. A multicenter report. J Am Coll Cardiol 1992;20:1391–6.

Gorgels AP, van den Dool A, Hofs A, et al. Comparison of procainamide and lidocaine in terminating sustained monomorphic ventricular tachycardia. Am J Cardiol 1996;78:43–6.

Morrison LJ, Deakin CD, Morley PT, Advanced Life Support Chapter Collaborators. Part 8: Advanced Life Support:

2010 international consensus on with treatment recommendations cardiopulmonary resuscitation and emergency cardiovascular care science. Circulation 2010;122:S345–421.

National Collaborating Centre for Chronic Conditions. National clinical guideline for management in primary and secondary care. In: Atrial Fibrillation. London (UK): Royal College of Physicians, 2006. <http://www.guideline.gov/summary/summary.aspx?ss=15&doc_id=9629&nbr=5149#s23> [Accessed Nov. 2007].

Sgarbossa EB, Pinski SL, Barbagelata A, et al. Electrocardiographic diagnosis of evolving acute myocardial infarction in the presence of left bundle-branch block. GUSTO-1 (Global Utilization of Streptokinase and Tissue Plasminogen Activator for Occluded Coronary Arteries) Investigators. N Engl J Med 1996;334:481–7.

Sgarbossa EB, Pinski SL, Wagner GS. Left bundle-branch block and the ECG in diagnosis of acute myocardial infarction. J Am Med Assoc 1999;282:1224–5.

Shah CP, Thakur RK, Xie B, et al. Clinical approach to wide complex tachycardias. Emerg Clin N Am 1998;16:331–59.

Stiell IG, Macle L, CCS atrial fibrillation guidelines committee. Canadian cardiovascular society atrial fibrillation guidelines 2010: management of recent onset atrial fibrillation and flutter in the emergency department. Can J Cardiol 2011;27:38–46.

Teo KK, Yusuf S, Furberg CD. Effects of prophylactic antiarrhythmic drug therapy in acute myocardial infarction. An overview of results from randomized controlled trials. J Am Med Assoc 1993;270:1589–95.

Tzivoni D, Banai S, Schuger C, et al. Treatment of torsade de pointes with magnesium sulfate. Circulation 1988;77:392–7.

5.5 Pulmonary embolism

David Mountain

ESSENTIALS

1 Venous thromboembolic (VTE) disease has protean clinical manifestations and is a continuum from deep venous thrombosis (DVT) to the main life-threatening complication of pulmonary embolus (PE).

2 Patients with a diagnosis of PE, left untreated, have a significant recurrence rate and mortality that is considerably reduced by anticoagulation.

3 Diagnostic and treatment decisions rely on good risk stratification preferably using validated scores, such as the PERC rule, Wells scores and PESI rules to avoid excessive investigation, unnecessary therapy and, for those diagnosed with PE, to guide management and disposition.

4 The investigative algorithm should include ECG, chest X-ray (CXR) and measures of oxygenation (plus other investigations for alternative diagnoses) to stratify risk, guide radiological testing and search for alternative causes. Which validated combinations of D-dimer, lower limb ultrasound, ventilation–perfusion scan (V/Q) (± *single-photon emission computed tomography [SPECT]*) scan and CT pulmonary angiogram (CTPA) (± CT venography (CTV)) are used to refine probability will depend on local resources.

5 The decision to treat is based on reaching a diagnostic threshold (more than 80% chance of PE) where PE morbidity/mortality is seen to outweigh the risks of anticoagulation.

6 The previous gold standard test of pulmonary angiography is rarely used and has been replaced mainly by CTPA. VQ with low intensity CT (VQ SPECT) is a viable alternative to CTPA.

7 In massive (clinically unstable) PE, transthoracic or, if available, transoesophageal echocardiography is the recommended initial investigation.

8 Low molecular weight heparin (LMWH) or Fondoparinux are recommended for therapy of PE because of logistic and outcome advantages. LMWH can safely be used on an outpatient basis in selected patients.

9 Thrombolysis (or embolectomy if thrombolysis is contraindicated) is indicated for haemodynamically unstable/shocked PE. Stable patients with evidence of right ventricular strain should be monitored vigilantly with thrombolysis initiated urgently if they deteriorate clinically.

Introduction

Pulmonary embolus (PE) is the third most common cardiovascular disease. Historical data suggest that, left untreated, it has high mortality. Treating PE with anticoagulation reduces the overall in-hospital mortality to 4–12%. Of these, most (4–9%) are due to co-morbidity and 1.5–5% directly to PE.

The diagnosis and management of PE is often difficult. It requires careful clinical assessment and methodical application of aids to diagnosis. It relies on the estimation of probabilities rather than any truly definitive test. At all times, the possibility of alternative serious conditions causing the clinical presentation should be considered. All patients being considered for any diagnostic test for PE (including D-dimer assay) should have a documented risk assessment to ensure that use of those tests is safe and appropriate (see diagnostic risk assessment below). In general, if the risk of PE is below 5% (e.g. most low-risk emergency patients), then an alternative diagnosis should be sought first and investigation for PE pursued only if no alternative disease can be found. Indeed, in this population, excessive aggressive radiological investigation may find more false-positive venous thromboembolism (VTE) than real PE or deep venous thrombosis (DVT). The threshold for diagnosis is around 70–80% probability of PE, at which point the benefits of treatment outweigh the risks of non-treatment. These probabilities may vary in individuals if the risks of PE are high (e.g. pre-existing severe lung/heart disease) or bleeding risks are excessive (e.g. high risk of falls, recent major non-compressible bleeding).

Most institutions now use computed tomographic pulmonary angiography (CTPA) and/or ventilation/perfusion (V/Q) scan where definitive diagnosis is necessary. Most diagnostic pathways also include an initial D-dimer assay and venous ultrasound (or CT venography) in cases where there is clinical doubt after imaging. Some centres may also use echocardiography for risk stratification after diagnosing PE and, if available, it should be used for unstable cases. Magnetic resonance imaging (MRI) has been investigated in some centres but is not routinely used (Fig. 5.5.1).

Aetiology, pathogenesis and pathology

Many risk factors and conditions are associated with PE, with major risks (e.g. cancer and surgery) clearly provocative. However, up to 30% of PEs, particularly those presenting to the emergency department (ED), are idiopathic. Most risk factors act via more than one of the processes in Virchow's triad, e.g. vessel wall injury, venous stasis or hypercoagulable states. The major risk factors associated with secondary (provoked) PE are:

- surgery or trauma (particularly affecting the pelvis, lower limb or CNS) (15–30%)
- malignant neoplasms (10–25%)
- systemic disease with immobilization (>24 hours bed rest), particularly heart disease and disabling strokes (5–15%) and
- a past history of DVT/PE (particularly unprovoked and recent).

Other provoking factors important individually, but not common overall, are hypercoagulable states (e.g. antithrombin 111 deficiency, antiphospholipid syndrome, protein C and S deficiencies and hyperhomocysteinaemia) and many others both congenital and acquired. Other associations include increasing age (particularly age over 60), indwelling venous devices, hormone replacement therapy or contraception, obesity, pregnancy, some vasculitic diseases with venous involvement, smoking, use of non-steroidal anti-inflammatory drugs and long-haul air travel.

Prevention

The greatest single preventable cause of DVT is surgery. Low-dose preventative anticoagulation should be routine with low molecular weight heparins making this safer and more effective for most groups. Venous stasis as a result of illness-related bed rest, serious cardiopulmonary disease and (to a much lesser degree) travel are important avoidable causes of PE and early mobilization techniques are important for the hospitalized. Low-dose anticoagulation has been demonstrated to improve outcomes in medical patients admitted for bed rest. This should be started as early as possible. There is a role for emergency physicians and nurses to identify DVT risk and start thromboprophylaxis in high-risk ED patients.

Clinical Features

History

The history is the most important clue to a diagnosis of PE. Virtually all patients with PE will present with a history of either recent onset dyspnoea (particularly if rapid or recurrently episodic), chest pain (of any type) or both (sensitivity 97%, specificity 10%). Syncope either with respiratory symptoms or signs (even if transient) or in patients at high risk of VTE, is often a marker for severe PE. Symptoms of DVT should be sought in all patients. Haemoptysis has some predictive value but is an uncommon clinical feature.

Other symptoms (e.g. clear musculoskeletal symptomatology) are less important in the diagnosis of PE, but often help to suggest or exclude other causes in low-risk cases. Associated risk factors, divided into major and minor as described below, increase the probability of PE and should be documented and incorporated into clinical risk assessment. No single symptom or sign has the sensitivity or specificity to either establish or exclude the diagnosis.

Examination

Physical signs confirming PE are rare. That said, some increase the likelihood of a diagnosis of PE. A persistent unexplained tachycardia at rest increases the concern for PE and is part of many prediction rules. Leg (or arm) signs of DVT, particularly a swollen, oedematous leg with pain in the venous distribution, or significant thrombophlebitis, significantly increase the PE risk and mandates imaging for a complete work-up. Other features include tachypnoea (50–80%), cough (10–20%), mild fever (<38.5°C), wheeze and pleural effusion. They are not discriminatory for PE. Occasionally, elevated jugular venous pressure (JVP), a loud cardiac S(P)2 heart sound and/or pulmonary systolic murmur may be found and are markers of right ventricular strain.

Risk assessment for the diagnosis of PE

The pre-test probability (PTP) calculation used to decide on investigation strategies is based on history, examination and investigations, including chest X-ray, arterial blood gas analysis or oximetry, ECG and investigations for alternative diagnoses depending on presentation. For non-experts, this estimate is best made using validated scoring systems. The best validated and most widely disseminated is the Wells rule (Table 5.5.1). This is usually followed by a D-dimer test if PE has not been excluded on initial clinical review, particularly in low- or intermediate-risk patients. Other validated risk assessments are the Geneva score, modified (dichotomous) Wells score and estimation by senior experienced/expert clinicians.

Recently, the PERC rule (available on line at http://www.mdcalc.com/perc-rule-for-pulmonary-embolism/) developed by Kline et al. has been used in EDs to exclude some low-risk patients from any further investigations, including D-dimer, by making them very low risk (<2% chance of PE). It is only safe when applied to patients thought to be low risk either by another rule, e.g. Wells, or by an experienced treating clinician.

Investigations

The initial screening tests for PE are discussed below.

245

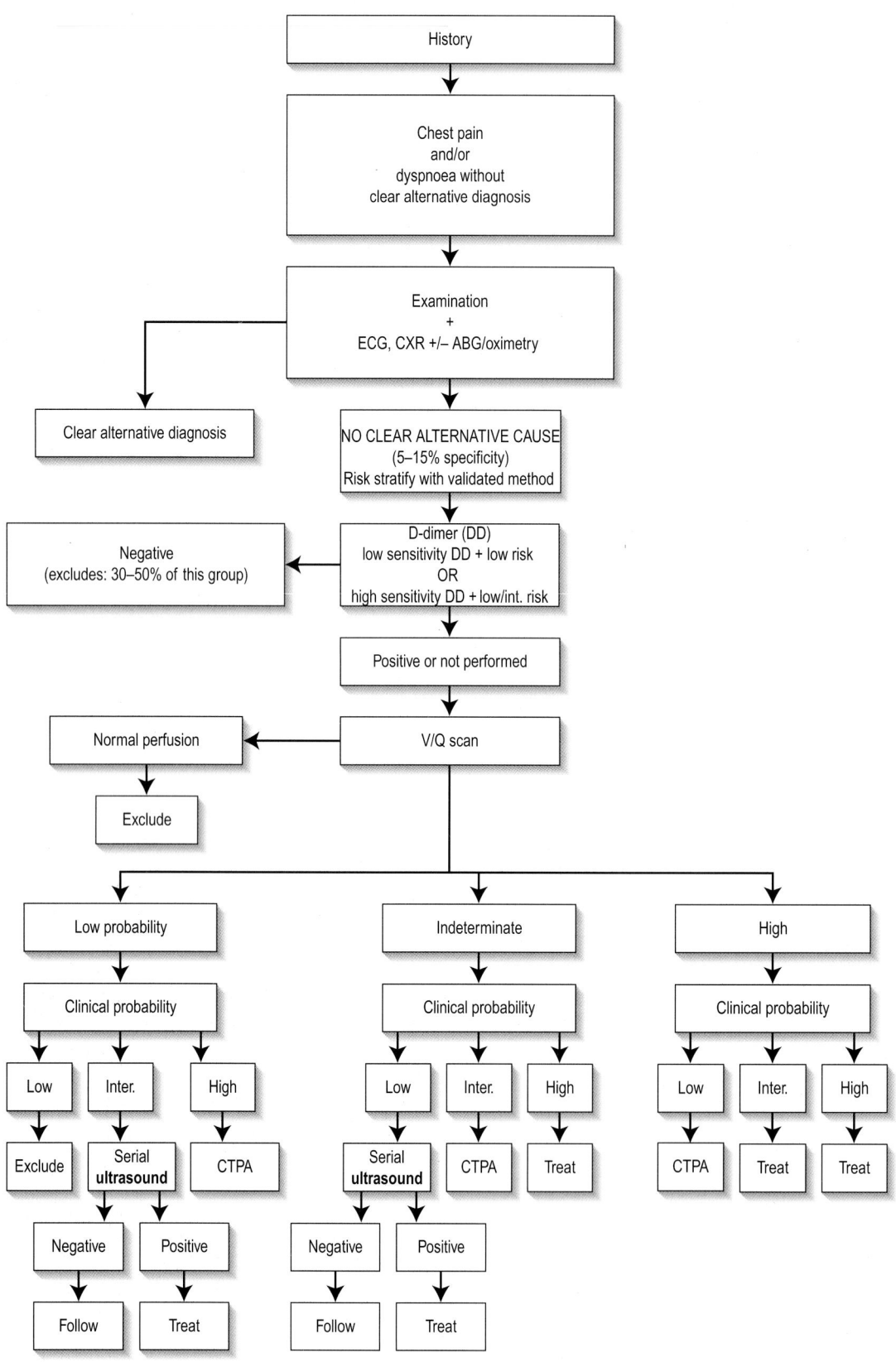

Hypoxaemic/haemodynamically unstable consider CT angiogram/TOE

Fig. 5.5.1 Investigation algorithm for pulmonary embolism using VQ scan as the primary imaging technique.

Table 5.5.1 Wells clinical criteria for PE[†]	
Clinical signs of DVT	3.0
Pulse rate >100 (at rest)	1.5
Immobilized ≥3 days	1.5
Surgery <4 weeks	1.5
Past history PE/DVT	1.5
Haemoptysis	1.0
Current/recent neoplasm	1.0
No alternative diagnosis more likely than PE	3.0*
Score	
Low	<2
Moderate	2–6
High	>6

*Including information from ECG, ABG, CXR and other tests for alternative diagnoses.
[†]A dichotomized (modified Wells) scale of ≤4 (low) or >4 (high) is also validated and allows lower sensitivity D-dimers to exclude more patients. On line version at http://www.mdcalc.com/wells-criteria-for-pulmonary-embolism-pe/

Chest X-ray

A normal chest X-ray (CXR) in the presence of significant hypoxia is suggestive of PE. However, the CXR is reportedly abnormal in 80–90% of patients diagnosed with PE. If definitely present, an enlarged descending pulmonary artery, pulmonary oligaemia or cut-off, a plump pulmonary artery and 'Hampton's hump' (a semicircular opacity with the base abutting the pleural surface) are all quite specific for PE (70–90%). However, these signs may be subtle (e.g. often identified in retrospect) and have poor sensitivity. Pleural effusion, plate atelectasis, enlarged heart shadow and non-specific consolidation are seen commonly but do not occur more often in PE patients than in other diagnoses. The main role of CXR is the identification of alternative diagnoses. It also assists in deciding which radiological test is best to use between non-SPECT V/Q and computed tomography pulmonary angiogram (CTPA).

ECG

At least 21 potential features on ECG have been postulated as suggesting PE, but they are insensitive and most lack specificity. The most significant are tachycardias (particularly atrial), right bundle branch block (including incomplete or transient patterns), right axis deviation (particularly S1–3), T-wave inversion (especially deep V1–3) and the S1-Q3-T3 pattern. The more features that are present on the ECG, the more suggestive it is for right ventricular strain. These changes have been associated with poorer outcome in PE, particularly the rare S1-Q3-T3 pattern.

Arterial blood gas analysis (ABG)

In recent years, the role of ABG in PE has been challenged. A PaO_2 <80 mmHg without other cause makes PE much more likely, however, 12% of patients with PE have PaO_2 >80 mmHg. An abnormal A–a gradient marginally increases PE risk, but 20% of patients with PE have normal A–a gradients. In most patients, oximetry is sufficient to exclude significant hypoxaemia (<92%) and little is gained from routine ABG.

D-dimer tests

D-dimer tests have been available since the 1980s. They are well validated in emergency practice and recommended by current guidelines. They have only been shown to have reasonable specificity when used in ED populations.

The D-dimer test is sensitive but nonspecific. Positive results occur with many other conditions. Their main role is to reduce the need for further investigations in a significant number of patients (20–60%). By identifying many low-risk patients who do not undergo further investigation, they increase the PE yield in the remaining investigated patients to over 5%, making further investigation of these patients worthwhile. D-dimers are only useful when negative, allowing PE to be excluded in low/intermediate-risk patients.

To be used safely and efficiently, it is important that the following steps are used:

- They should be used as part of a documented diagnostic process.
- Patients must be adequately stratified into either dichotomous low/high- or low/intermediate/high-risk groups, preferably using a validated scoring system. The test is only useful in low or low/intermediate risk-populations, depending on the test being used (see below).
- Patients with little chance of a negative D-dimer should not undergo this test (e.g. recent major surgery, advanced cancer or the shocked patient).
- Patients with prolonged symptoms (over a week) are much more likely to have false-negative tests and should not be tested.

- Other groups with low specificity (e.g. pregnant or older patients, etc.) should have a D-dimer if the avoidance of radiological imaging is deemed important enough to accept the delay for what will likely be a positive result.
- The test should not be used if PE is not a realistic part of the differential diagnosis.

Knowledge of the diagnostic performance of the D-dimer test being used is required to guide test application and interpretation. If a high-sensitivity test, such as VIDAS or one of the newer validated rapid latex tests, is available it is safe to use in low- and intermediate-ED risk groups (<30% chance of PE). Low-sensitivity tests, such as SimpliRed or most latex agglutination tests, are only appropriate for use in low-risk patients (<10% chance of PE).

Further investigation

If the D-dimer is positive and no alternative diagnosis has become clear, further investigation is indicated. Following screening tests, more definitive investigations, including CTPA or V/Q scan, in some cases supplemented by ultrasound (US) or CT venography, should be performed. V/Q or CTPA are the usual initial investigations. If both are available, the choice is driven by patient-related issues (discussed below with each modality) and local logistics. Pulmonary angiography (PA) is now rarely available as most radiology departments have replaced it with multislice scanners. In unstable patients, echocardiography is the preferred initial test, looking for severe right ventricular dilatation and overload. MRI scanning may be used occasionally for patients where V/Q and CTPA are contraindicated or unavailable.

Computed tomographic pulmonary angiography and venography (CTPA and CTV)

Multislice (16–128) CTPA is available in most centres and after-hours availability is generally better than V/Q scanning. CTPA is preferable to V/Q scan in most patients with pre-existing lung disease because of the likelihood of intermediate probability V/Q scans in these patients. CTPA appears accurate in diagnosing main, lobar and most segmental vessel emboli. Sensitivity for subsegmental emboli is low, but the prevalence (reported to be 6–30%) and clinical significance of these PE is not clear. CTPA with 32–256 slices increases sensitivity

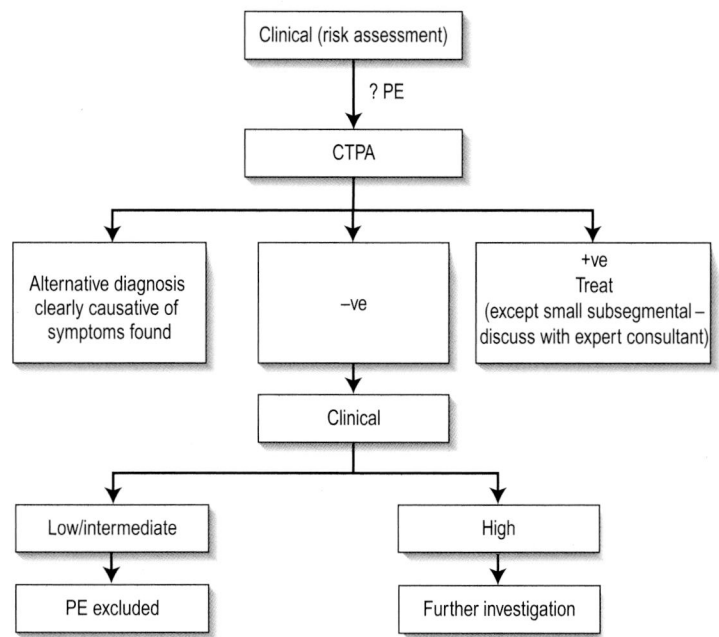

Fig. 5.5.2 Alternative algorithm.

for smaller PE, reported as over 90% in some studies and with good specificity (93–99%). However, the PIOPED2 study suggested sensitivity as low as 85% for PE, although when combined with CT venography (CTV), sensitivity improved to 90%. Large numbers of patients have been followed up after a negative CTPA, plus leg imaging if appropriate, with recurrent PE/death only seen in 1–2% and 0.2–0.5% respectively. This prognostic performance is similar to that reported for negative PA or normal V/Q scans.

Many centres now use CTPA alone to exclude significant PE. This is probably a safe strategy in all but high-risk patients without an alternative diagnosis. High-risk patients with negative CTPA should have leg imaging to exclude an embolic source (Fig. 5.5.2).

A major proposed advantage of CTPA is that other thoracic causes of chest pain may be identified. In some series, abnormal findings are seen in up to 60% of scans, with acute serious conditions in 20–30%. However, it is important to note that many of these findings may be incidental but then lead to prolonged further work-ups and additional radiation. Additionally, as scanners become quicker, data on right ventricular size, shape and function may help PE risk stratification.

In some centres, CTV, using the dye run-off from CTPA, images the venous system (legs to heart) instead of separate ultrasound testing.

Almost all the additional yield (3–5% additional PE/DVT diagnosed in some studies) is from leg veins. Radiation doses to gonadal areas from pelvic/abdominal scanning should be avoided.

CTPA has some significant problems in clinical practice. In some studies, up to 15% of scans are technically inadequate. It requires significant dye loads, so is unsuitable for patients with renal dysfunction or contrast/iodine allergies. The radiation dose is high. In males, scans are generally to radio-insensitive tissues but, in women with proliferative breast tissues, high radiation doses (2–4 Gy per breast) confer significant increased lifetime breast cancer risk. V/Q scanning and US of the legs should be preferred in all young (including pregnant) female patients. The dose of radiation to the fetus is minimal in both CTPA and V/Q scanning if proper precautions are taken.

Ventilation–perfusion scan (V/Q scan)

V/Q scanning is usually readily available, has a low complication rate, moderate radiation exposure and can be used in patients with renal dysfunction and dye allergies. Problems are that potentially unwell patients may spend a long time in often distant nuclear medicine departments and many centres do not provide 24/7 scanning. Additionally, critics complain that the majority of V/Q scans are non-diagnostic (>50% in the PIOPED study if not

risk stratified), requiring additional testing to rule PE in or out adequately. Because patients with obvious CXR abnormalities (e.g. major collapse, pleural effusions, etc.) or major lung disease almost always have indeterminate V/Q scans, they should have CTPA if available.

Two major studies (PIOPED and McMaster) have defined the probabilities of various V/Q scan results and their combination with clinical risk assessment. In most hospitals, scans were defined as normal, low, intermediate or high probability according to the number ± size of unperfused lung segments, matched against ventilation. Further management depends on combining clinical risk and V/Q results as discussed below:

- Normal/near-normal scan (14% of scans in PIOPED). This result excludes significant PE. In ED patients and if abnormal CXR is excluded, it is likely that more than 14% of scans will fall into this group.
- High probability (13% in PIOPED). A high-probability scan had a greater than 85% chance of PE. However, this means 15% of patients treated on the basis of a high-probability scan alone would be anticoagulated unnecessarily. The majority of the false positives in this group will be those who had a low pre-test probability. Therefore, patients assessed clinically as low risk with a high probability V/Q scan should have further investigations.
- Low/intermediate (42%/36% in PIOPED). The low- and intermediate-probability groups had around 10–15% and 35% chance, respectively, of PE. Patients with a low clinical risk assessment and a low-probability V/Q have <5% chance of PE. Most of these patients can be discharged if other major diagnoses are excluded. However, consideration of further imaging should occur in patients with critical cardiorespiratory problems, as they have high mortality from even small PE.

Much debate continues on how to manage patients with low clinical pre-test probability and intermediate V/Q. In PIOPED, this combination had rates of PE of 16%. However, studies have shown that with serial, or even single negative lower limb studies excluding DVT, recurrent PE or death rates are acceptably low. Patients with dichotomous risk versus V/Q results (low vs high) or intermediate/intermediate results need further alternative investigation with CTPA and/or leg vein imaging.

V/Q single-photon emission computed tomography (V/Q SPECT)

V/Q SPECT is a new technique combining V/Q scanning with computed tomographic scanning (circular arrays) allowing three-dimensional imaging of the lungs. This improves the clarity of images, gives better anatomical delineation of perfusion defects against known vascular domains and can be combined with low dose CT to look at patients with abnormal CXR or known abnormalities. This allows those units that have familiarity with this technique to give a definitive diagnosis or exclusion of PE in 95% of cases.

There is good evidence that V/Q SPECT gives better information and results than planar V/Q. On this basis, it would be an acceptable alternative to CTPA. Small numbers of outcomes studies suggest that there is good negative predictive value. To date, direct comparisons with CTPA have been limited so the true performance between the two tests is still unclear. Early evidence suggests that V/Q SPECT is probably slightly more sensitive but less specific. The specificity issues are probably reduced by combining V/Q SPECT with a low dose thorax CT to look for lung abnormalities that may explain poor perfusion, particularly in those with known lung disease or with abnormal CXR. Caution should be applied when the result is not concordant with the clinical picture (e.g. low-risk patient with multiple perfusion defects, etc.) and cross-over examinations to a CTPA/US may be advisable. The same is true for single subsegmental perfusion defects. V/Q SPECT is the preferred technique where CTPA is relatively contraindicated or where inadequate CTPA studies have occurred (10–25%). Further studies directly comparing V/Q SPECT with CTPA are awaited.

Magnetic resonance imaging

Magnetic resonance imaging (MRI) techniques are improving rapidly. Although sensitivity for central emboli is >90% with high specificity, its diagnostic performance is much poorer even for PE in large segmental vessels. There is little place currently for MRI in the acute setting unless CT/VQ are unavailable/contraindicated.

Echocardiography – transthoracic or transoesophageal (TTE/TOE)

Echocardiography is a rapid, accurate method of diagnosing massive PE in patients with instability. It helps exclude other causes of hypotension and raised venous pressure, such as cardiac tamponade and major valve or myocardial dysfunction. In massive PE, it can demonstrate right heart distension/dysfunction and sometimes central pulmonary artery or atrial clot. Importantly, it can be performed in resuscitation areas and used to see if initiation of thrombolytic treatment for unstable patients is indicated. It is insensitive for peripheral emboli and is not used to diagnose non-massive PE. However, in haemodynamically stable patients, echocardiography provides prognostic information. If right heart strain is seen, there is a much higher risk of poor outcomes (5–15% vs 0–2% mortality). If available, this information assists management decision making after diagnosis of PE.

Pulmonary angiography

Pulmonary angiography has been the 'gold standard' in diagnosing PE with very good sensitivity (98%) and specificity (97–100%) in all but the smallest PE. Because of significant technical, logistical and clinical difficulties and a 0.3% mortality and 3% complication rate, it is now rarely used.

Further investigation of isolated sub-segmental clots

Whenever isolated subsegmental clots are reported on imaging, further tests to exclude false positives are recommended. These include:

- leg imaging if not already performed
- an alternative imaging test to confirm the original result if available/feasible
- senior (treating consultant) review and case-by-case decisions, including the patient's wishes/preferences, on benefits of treatment vs risk of bleeding.

It is important to remember that false positives are common in patients with these isolated small subsegmental findings no matter what imaging is used.

Treatment

Risk stratification

Patients diagnosed with PE should be risk stratified for short-term/in-hospital prognosis. There are significant differences in both ongoing therapeutic options and the monitoring required for PE patients with different prognoses. Features that determine prognosis are overt haemodynamic instability (including syncope) or prolonged respiratory failure, investigations suggesting right ventricular overload/strain or severe V/Q mismatch and severe underlying co-morbidities.

Haemodynamic or respiratory instability should be clinically obvious, although the use of venous/arterial gases to expose unexpected lactic acidosis/hypoxia, if there is clinical concern, is reasonable. In patients without obvious instability, prognosis may be determined by considering:

- historical features, such as collapse/syncope/arrest or severe co-morbidity and age (>80)
- physical examination findings, such as borderline perfusion, BP, persistent tachycardia, signs of right ventricular failure/cor-pulmonale
- bedside and laboratory investigations, e.g. ECG (right ventricular strain patterns, particularly if multiple markers of strain), elevated troponin (particularly troponin T >0.1 ng/mL; 5–20% mortality), elevated BNP (>90 pg/mL) or proNT-BNP (>450 pg/mL), hypoxia on oximetry (persistently <94%) or by ABG on room air
- echocardiography, e.g. signs of right ventricular strain (5–15% mortality) or thrombus in transit (mortality 20–60%).

Other features that raise concerns for patients are a demonstration of a massive clot load (e.g. massive DVT, centrally located emboli), recurrent PE on adequate therapy and serious cardiopulmonary co-morbidity.

Prognostic scores

Combinations of various clinical features and/or investigations have been studied to try to define low-risk groups for possible early or immediate discharge. The two major systems are the PESI (http://www.mdcalc.com/pulmonary-embolism-severity-index-pesi/) and Geneva prognostic scores, both of which have been prospectively validated. The PESI score was also validated in a large randomized trial confirming safety in selecting patients with PE for home therapy.

General measures

Almost all patients with diagnosed PE need to have a combination of supportive care, including oxygen therapy, thromboprophylaxis, analgesia and careful observation for an initial period while early prognosis is determined and heparin or fondoparinux plus warfarin therapy are initiated (unless there is an absolute contraindication). Thought should be given to taking a thrombophilia screen before heparin is started when there is an unprovoked PE or if the PE is recurrent and thrombophilia has not been investigated previously.

Heparin therapy

Heparin therapy can be given either as intravenous unfractionated heparin (UFH) or low molecular weight heparin (LMWH). LMWH therapy has been shown to be at least as effective as UFH (clinically and by cost) and is probably safer than UFH for DVT and PE. The evidence for this in PE is weaker than for DVT, but the equivalence of the therapies is accepted by evidence-based care bodies such as the Cochrane Collaboration and NICE and most accept an overall benefit from LMWH compared to UFH. Dosing for enoxaparin is usually 1.5 mg/kg daily or 1 mg bd, but all LMWHs probably provide adequate therapy. Dosing must be reduced for those with poor renal function (reduced dose and frequency) and the morbidly obese (e.g. 100 kg maximum lean weight) to avoid accumulation or excessive dosing.

LMWH is particularly useful if early discharge from inpatient units or even home therapy is being contemplated. Home therapy is now widely used in North America in low-risk PE and, in well-selected cases, it seems to be safe. It is recommended in some current guidelines but relies on good risk stratification. Currently, the best validated way to predict low risk is the PESI score (see above).

Warfarin therapy

Warfarin should be started at the same time as initial heparin therapy and maintained for at least 3 months. Duration of treatment should probably be longer in those at high risk (e.g. cancer patients, unprovoked large PE, etc.). The risk of anticoagulation causing major bleeding may be as high as 10% over 6 months in very high-risk patients (2–4% in well-controlled patients), with 1–3% intracranial haemorrhage rates in some registries and mortality from bleeding of 0.1–1% pa. Risk scores for assessing who is at high risk of bleeding are not validated in the PE population and have limited evidence of discrimination. Clearly, elderly, frail, hypertensive, falling, recently bleeding, alcoholic or severely co-morbid patients are at much higher risk.

Caval interruption techniques

The use of caval interruption techniques should be considered in cases of recurrent PE despite coagulation, or where there is bleeding precluding anticoagulation. It has also been recommended for massive PE or massive leg DVT with PE. Fatal PE usually occurs as a result of further clot progressing along the inferior vena cava (IVC). Percutaneous IVC umbrellas may be inserted relatively easily and prevent further deterioration.

Patients at high risk of deterioration

Patients without cardiorespiratory instability but with features of RV strain or major PE, such as a history of syncope/collapse, ongoing hypoxia or tachycardia, elevated troponins or BNP, large clot loads, RV strain on echocardiography or clinician concern, should undergo close observation and/or continuous monitoring in a high-dependency or critical care area. There is a high rate of deterioration or death in these patients, with up to 25% requiring inotropes, intubation or thrombolysis for instability and mortality rates of up 10%. A management plan should have been decided upon before transfer out of the ED, preferably with criteria for initiation of thrombolysis/thrombectomy or catheter endarterectomy.

Unstable patients

Patients presenting with overt shock, rapidly deteriorating respiratory failure or a history of recovery from cardiorespiratory arrest should be resuscitated, stabilized and, in most cases, given thrombolysis (or alternative treatments if thrombolysis is contraindicated; see below). Severe hypoxaemia may require endotracheal intubation and ventilation. Haemodynamic instability requires gentle intravascular fluid loading with 250–500 mL boluses of crystalloids totalling no more than 1 L unless dehydration or hypovolaemia are clearly coexistent with PE. The reason for this is that, in massive PE, the right ventricle is already pressure overloaded and failing and excessive fluids will further overstretch a failing ventricle (Starling's law).

Persistent hypotension will require inotropic support. There is little evidence to support the use of norepinephrine (noradrenaline) over epinephrine (adrenaline) as the inotrope of choice. Patients requiring inotropes should not be treated with isoprenaline as this results in vasodilatation, reduced peripheral resistance and

increased cardiac output, without improving coronary perfusion.

Thrombolysis

The widespread use of thrombolytic therapy for coronary disease led to a reappraisal of thrombolytics in PE. There is definite evidence of reduced pulmonary artery pressures and improved right ventricular function after thrombolysis, which may persist following the acute episode. One small, randomized trial in shocked patients showed a clear mortality benefit for thrombolysis. In addition, some meta-analyses suggest that in the sickest patients with PE there is probably a mortality benefit. Very few clinicians would withhold thrombolytics for massive (hypotensive/unstable) PE. There is widespread use of thrombolytics in Europe for moderate-sized PE causing right ventricular strain, with some registry evidence of improved mortality or reduced complications. However, there is much less acceptance in the USA and Australia for this indication as the evidence is weak and thrombolysis is actively discouraged in haemodynamically stable, non-deteriorating patients.

Tissue plasminogen activator (rTPA) appears to be the easiest and quickest to give and to have the fewest side effects (excepting intracranial haemorrhage [ICH]) compared to urokinase and streptokinase. rTPA has been used as an infusion of 100 mg over 2 hours. Bolus reteplase (two doses of 10 units separated by half an hour) or tenectaplase (weight-based infusion) should be just as effective, although they have not been properly studied in PE and do not have TGA approval for this indication.

Thrombolysis is associated with a major bleeding episode in up to 20% of patients, with ICH rates as high as 4% and death from bleeding in 0.3–2%.

Embolectomy

Patients with persistent haemodynamic instability or hypoxia with major contraindications to thrombolysis should be considered for thoracotomy and/or embolectomy. Patients in this category are not necessarily at hospitals with facilities for cardiopulmonary bypass and, therefore, alternative therapies have been developed. The use of mechanical clot disruption (catheter embolectomy) for massive PE has been reported in case studies, but controlled studies are difficult to design because of the infrequency of the event and the emergency nature of massive PE. Unlike other surgical techniques, the expertise and equipment for this procedure are readily available in most, larger hospitals. Pulmonary embolectomy without cardiac bypass has been used as a last resort for haemodynamically unstable patients, with a reported survival of more than 50%. Following cardiac arrest, survival rates are much lower, although survivors have been reported.

There is no evidence that mechanical removal of clot results in better outcome than does thrombolysis; in fact, it could be worse. In the pre-arrest or arrested patient, the transfer to cardiopulmonary bypass may buy additional time. In general, hospitals should decide on thrombolysis versus thrombectomy as their preferred management of unstable PE to avoid confusion and unnecessary delays to management in shocked patients.

Prognosis

Prognosis is largely dependent on coexistent illness and the size and eventual position of the initial PE. Patients with cardiorespiratory arrest or shock have mortality rates of 25–50% even with thrombolysis/thrombectomy. Right ventricular strain in haemodynamically stable patients has a mortality rate of 5–15%. In addition, this group is at risk of developing chronic thromboembolism and persistent pulmonary hypertension. Patients without significant co-morbidity or signs of severity have very low rates of poor outcomes. Even with anticoagulation, hospital mortality may still be high (2.5–10%), although much of this mortality is due to co-morbidity. Recurrent PE occurs in about 25% of patients by 8 years.

Disposition

Patients with haemodynamic instability, recovery post-arrest, those with significant persistent hypoxia (<92%) and those with evidence of right ventricular strain should be admitted to an ICU or high-dependency unit. Most patients with stable PE can be admitted directly to the ward. Early discharge on LMWH (or Fondoparinux) should be considered for compliant patients with smaller PEs, good home circumstances and a low risk of complications.

Controversies

- Is multislice CTPA the new gold standard for PE, or does it overdiagnose small inconsequential clots?
- Whether V/Q SPECT is equivalent to or better than CTPA as an imaging technique in PE.
- Should all patients with PE have an echocardiogram (or equivalent investigation of right ventricular function) and, if positive, should they be monitored and/or considered for thrombolysis?
- Are BNP/troponins equivalent to echocardiography for diagnosing significant right ventricular strain?
- The role of thrombolysis: it is generally accepted for use in massive/shocked PE, but is still very controversial for submassive PE with right ventricular strain.

- In what situations should thrombectomy/mechanical embolectomy be preferred to thrombolysis?
- Can we better risk stratify patients with PE so that more can be discharged home from the ED or discharged early from hospital?

Further reading

Aujesky D, Roy P-M, Verschuren F, et al. Outpatient versus inpatient treatment for patients with acute pulmonary embolism: an international, open-label, randomised, non-inferiority trial. Lancet 2011;378:41–8.

Fletcher J, MacLellan D, Fisher C, et al. Prevention of venous thromboembolism: best practice guidelines for Australia and New Zealand, 3rd edn. Sydney: Health Education Management International (HEMI); 2005.

Goldhaber SZ, Visani L, De Rosa M. Acute pulmonary embolism: clinical outcomes in the International Cooperative Pulmonary Embolism Registry (ICOPER). Lancet 1999;353:1386–9.

Kearon C, Akl EA, Comerota AJ, et al. Antithrombotic therapy for VTE disease: antithrombotic therapy and prevention of thrombosis, 9th edn: American College of Chest Physicians Evidence-Based Clinical Practice Guidelines. Chest 2012;141(2 Suppl):e419S–e4194.

Kline JA, Hernandez-Nino J, Rose GA, et al. Surrogate markers for adverse outcomes in normotensive patients with pulmonary embolism. Crit Care Med 2006;34:2773–80.

Leblanc M, Paul N. V/Q SPECT and computed tomographic pulmonary angiography. Semin Nucl Med 2010;40:426–41.

Mountain D. Diagnosing pulmonary embolism: a question of too much choice?. Emerg Med 2003;15:250–62.

NICE. Venous thromboembolic diseases [Internet]. NICE. <http://www.nice.org.uk/> [Accessed Dec. 2012].

Roy PM, Colombet I, Durieux P, et al. Systematic review and meta-analysis of strategies for the diagnosis of suspected pulmonary embolism. Br Med J 2005;30:259.

Singh B, Mommer SK, Erwin PJ, et al. Pulmonary embolism rule-out criteria (PERC) in pulmonary embolism – revisited: a systematic review and meta-analysis. Emerg Med J 2012 Oct 20. Epub ahead of print.

Squizzato A, Donadini MP, Galli L, et al. Prognostic clinical prediction rules to identify a low-risk pulmonary embolism: a systematic review and meta-analysis. J Thromb Haemost 2012;10:1276–90.

CARDIOVASCULAR EMERGENCIES

5.6 Pericarditis, cardiac tamponade and myocarditis

Jason Harney • Anne-Maree Kelly • James Hayes

PERICARDITIS

ESSENTIALS

1 Myocarditis is often associated with the clinical condition pericarditis. This has important clinical implications.

2 Pericarditis is most commonly diagnosed on ECG findings, but may ultimately be a purely clinical diagnosis.

3 The majority of cases of pericarditis have a presumed viral aetiology and most run a benign course.

4 The correct identification of pericarditis as opposed to myocardial infarction is essential, as the administration of fibrinolytic agents in cases of pericarditis may result in life-threatening complications.

5 Longer-term follow up is important as a subacute or chronic course can develop, with further complications such as chronic constrictive pericarditis.

Introduction

Pericarditis may be acute, subacute or chronic. It is defined as inflammation of the pericardium. It should be noted, however, that the condition is better described as perimyocarditis. In the majority of cases, there are variable degrees of associated 'epimyocarditis', which has important clinical implications. The causes of pericarditis are listed in Table 5.6.1.

Clinical features

History

Idiopathic or viral types may have a history of a recent viral illness and the history should be directed towards the known causative pathologies. The pain is usually retrosternal, sometimes with radiation to the trapezius muscle ridges, but not generally to the arms. It may also be pleuritic in nature, and worse with movement and respiration. It is typically worse when lying supine and better when sitting up and leaning forward. True dyspnoea is not a feature unless there are secondary complications, such as cardiac tamponade or chronic constrictive pericarditis.

Dyspnoea may also be due to the underlying disease process causing pericarditis. Respiration may however be shallow because of pain.

Examination

With viral or idiopathic types, fever may be present. Sinus tachycardia is common. A pericardial friction rub may be heard, caused by rubbing between parietal and visceral pericardial layers or between parietal pericardium and lung pleura. A rub may therefore be heard even with the presence of a large effusion. It may be audible anywhere over the precordium, but is best heard with the diaphragm of the stethoscope over the lower left sternal edge, where the least amount of lung tissue intervenes between the pericardium and the chest wall, with the patient leaning forward in full expiration. The rub has a superficial scratching or 'Velcro-like' quality. Rubs may be difficult to detect, as they can be transient and migratory. The patient should be examined for any signs of a complicating cardiac tamponade. A search should also be made for any signs of an underlying causative condition.

Temperature above 38°C is uncommon and may indicate purulent (i.e. bacterial) pericarditis, a much more serious condition.

High-risk features

The following high-risk clinical features should raise suspicion of serious underlying pathology, such as tuberculosis or other bacterial infection, malignancy or autoimmune disease:

- fever
- true dyspnoea
- a subacute course
- significant effusion or tamponade
- failure to respond to aspirin or non-steroidal anti-inflammatory drugs (NSAIDs)
- patients on anticoagulant therapy
- immunosuppression
- recent trauma
- patients with suspected significant associated myocarditis indicated by arrhythmias, significantly elevated ST segments or significantly elevated troponin levels.

Clinical investigation

Blood tests

- Full blood count: leucocytosis is common. A markedly elevated white cell count should raise suspicion of a more serious cause, such as bacterial infection.
- Serum biochemistry: may identify underlying renal failure.
- Erythrocyte sedimentation rate or C-reactive protein provide confirmatory evidence of an inflammatory process and can be used to follow treatment.
- Cardiac biomarkers may be elevated because of the associated myocarditis.
- Other blood tests will be dictated by the clinical assessment and the degree of clinical suspicion for any given causative pathology.

Chest X-ray

Chest X-ray does not confirm the diagnosis of pericarditis but may rule out other causes of pleuritic chest pain. It may also find evidence

Table 5.6.1 Causes of acute pericarditis	
Idiopathic (about 25%)	Most of these are probably viral
Malignancy (about 25%)	Primary, e.g. sarcoma and mesotheliomas Secondary, e.g. haematological, breast, lung and melanoma
Infective	Viral, e.g. Coxsackie B, mumps, Epstein–Barr virus, influenza, HIV Bacterial, e.g. staphylococcal, streptococcal, Gram-negatives and TB Mycotic, e.g. histoplasmosis
Autoimmune/connective tissue	Rheumatoid arthritis, systemic lupus erythematosus (SLE), sarcoidosis, scleroderma, Stevens–Johnson syndrome, inflammatory bowel disease
Trauma	Blunt or penetrating Post-pericardiotomy syndrome Radiation injury
Myocardial infarction associated	Acute: days to weeks following transmural myocardial infarction Dressler's syndrome: weeks to months following myocardial infarction
Drugs	SLE-type syndromes, e.g. hydralazine Hypersensitivity syndromes, e.g. penicillin
Systemic illnesses	Uraemia Myxoedema
Other	Dissecting aneurysm

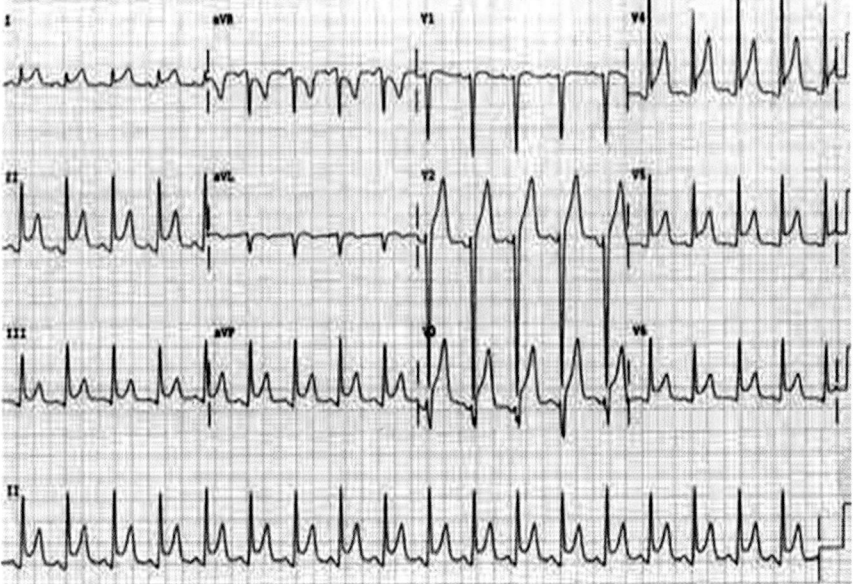

Fig. 5.6.1 Typical ECG in pericarditis.

of a complicating pericardial effusion or evidence of causative pathology, such as malignancy.

ECG

The ECG is the most important investigation and will show abnormalities in 90% of patients with acute pericarditis. ECG changes are the result of the associated epimyocarditis. The pericardium is electrically neutral and does not produce ECG changes. Therefore, in the occasional 'pure' case of pericarditis, the ECG will be normal. It may follow the typical evolution of changes, but in a sizeable minority will not.

The typical pattern follows four stages:

- Stage 1: hours to days:
  - diffuse concave upwards ST elevation. This may occur in all leads apart from AVR and often VI (Fig. 5.6.1)
  - PR-segment depression (reflecting subepicardial atrial injury). This may occur in all leads apart from AVR and V1. These two leads may in fact show PR-segment elevation.

- Stage 2: the PR and ST segments normalize, which can lead to a transiently normal ECG.
- Stage 3: days to weeks: T-wave inversion occurs.
- Stage 4: normalization of the ECG: over a period of up to 3 months, however, in some cases the T-wave changes may be permanent.

Atypical ECGs may include the following:

- a normal ECG in cases of 'pure' pericarditis (remembering that during stage 2 the ECG may also be transiently normal during a typical evolution)
- the PR-segment depression may occur in isolation, without any ST-segment elevation
- stages 1 and 2 without progression to stage 3
- localized as opposed to diffuse ECG changes.

Echocardiography

This may give indirect evidence for pericarditis by showing the presence of an effusion or a thickened pericardium. High-quality echocardiograms are able to distinguish bloody from serous effusions. Transoesophageal echocardiography (TOE) is better at measuring thickness of the pericardium than transthoracic echocardiography (TTE). A normal echocardiogram does not rule out a diagnosis of pericarditis.

Computed tomography (CT) scan/magnetic resonance imaging (MRI)

CT and MRI have the advantages of a larger field of view and excellent imaging of anatomy that is not possible with echocardiography. They also have high soft-tissue contrast. In most patients, they provide excellent images of the pericardium, including thickness, the presence of effusions and any pericardial lesions.

Pericardiocentesis and biopsy

Rarely required, pericardiocentesis and biopsy may be indicated in selected cases. Indications include suspected serious underlying pathology, such as a bacterial, tuberculous or neoplastic pericarditis, when cardiac tamponade is present or in chronic or recurrent cases for diagnostic purposes.

Criteria for diagnosis

Stage 1 ST-segment deviations are virtually diagnostic of acute pericarditis when typically

Table 5.6.2   Pericarditis vs AMI vs BER

ECG feature	Acute pericarditis	STEMI	BER
ST segment morphology	Concave upwards ST elevation	Convex upwards ST elevation	Concave upwards ST elevation
ST segment elevation	Usually <5 mm	If >5 mm, more suspicious	Usually <5 mm
ST segment changes distribution	Diffuse	Anatomic	Precordial only
Reciprocal changes	No, mild depressions only in AVR, V1	Deep reciprocal changes opposite ST elevated segments	No
Q waves	No (unless associated with infarction)	Yes	No
PR segments	PR-segment depressions (may be elevated in AVR and V1)	No	No
T-wave inversion	T-wave inversion after ST segments normalize	T waves may invert concurrently with elevation of ST segments	No
ST/T ratio	>0.25	N/A	<0.25
Usual pattern of evolution of changes	Days to weeks	Minutes to days	Stable over many years

AMI: acute myocardial infarction; BER: benign early repolarization; STEMI: ST-elevation myocardial infarction.

distributed among limb and precordial leads. However, a sizeable minority of ECGs will be atypical and, indeed, in some cases, may be normal. The diagnosis of pericarditis may therefore ultimately be a clinical one, based on the presence of typical pain and a rub heard on auscultation or the presence of an effusion on echocardiography. Cases where pain is typical but a rub is not heard present more difficulty and should be followed closely. If clinical suspicion is high, again, an echocardiogram finding of an effusion in the presence of typical pain would be highly suggestive. Convenient diagnoses, such as 'muscular', 'fibrositis', 'costochondritis' and 'viral' should be avoided until more important conditions, such as pericarditis, pulmonary embolus and pneumothorax, are excluded.

The most difficult clinical decision in the emergency department is differentiating between pericarditis, benign early repolarization (BER) and myocardial infarction. This is especially so when the decision to use fibrinolysis is being considered. Fibrinolytic therapy may result in life-threatening haemorrhagic cardiac tamponade in patients who have pericarditis. ECG features to assist in distinguishing between these diagnoses are summarized in Table 5.6.2.

Treatment

The symptoms of pericarditis are generally well controlled with NSAIDs. The role of corticosteroids has some controversy, as has the use of colchicine or immunoglobulins, with limited clinical studies and support for their use available. Rest is essential, as exercise may exacerbate an associated myocarditis. Complications, such as arrhythmias, are treated along conventional lines. If a significant effusion is suspected, this should be confirmed on echocardiography and signs of early cardiac tamponade sought. An underlying cause for the pericarditis should be sought and, if found, treatment directed at this, although the majority of cases will be viral. In high-risk patients, HIV should also be considered as a possible underlying aetiology.

Disposition

The clinical course really depends on the underlying pathology. Patients with pericarditis can usually be safely managed on an outpatient basis unless there are high-risk features, such as temperature >38°C, a subacute onset, immunosuppression, a history of recent trauma, oral anticoagulant therapy, myopericarditis, a large pericardial effusion and/or cardiac tamponade. A period of observation (e.g. in an emergency department short stay unit) may be prudent to ensure diagnostic accuracy and to detect early complications.

The viral and idiopathic groups commonly follow a benign and self-limiting course over 10–14 days. Patients with severe symptoms should be admitted; some may require narcotic analgesia. Those in whom the diagnosis remains uncertain, especially when other serious conditions, such as myocardial infarction, cannot be ruled out, should also be admitted. Follow up is also essential to monitor progress (particularly the development of features of myocarditis) and to identify the development of chronicity and constrictive pericarditis.

Controversies

- Whether all patients with pericarditis should be admitted. Although patients with typical pericarditis who do not have high-risk features are at low risk of adverse events, and clinical diagnosis is not always accurate.

NON-TRAUMATIC CARDIAC TAMPONADE

ESSENTIALS

1 Cardiac tamponade is a life-threatening condition.

2 The signs and symptoms of cardiac tamponade are non-specific and may be difficult to elicit. A high index of suspicion is therefore essential to ensure that the condition is not missed.

3 The 'gold standard' investigation is echocardiography, as it is the most sensitive and the most specific.

4 The urgency and type of treatment will depend on the rapidity, as well as the degree of accumulation of pericardial contents. It will also depend on the aetiology.

5 Needle pericardiocentesis is best reserved as a drainage procedure of last resort. The preferred methods are ultrasound guided drainage performed in the cardiac catheter laboratory or, more ideally, subxiphoid pericardiotomy performed in the operating theatre, if the clinical situation allows. In cases of myocardial rupture and aortic dissection, thoracotomy with drainage and definitive repair is the method of choice, rather than pericardiocentesis which can only be temporizing and, in some cases, may be harmful.

Introduction

Pericardial effusion is the accumulation of fluid (exudate, transudate, blood or chylus) within the pericardial cavity. Normally, this cavity contains up to 35 mL of fluid. More than this can be accommodated in the short term, up to about 200 mL. In the longer term, if it accumulates slowly, up to 2 L can be accommodated with little clinical consequence. However, above these values, the process of cardiac tamponade will occur, with lethal consequences if unrecognized.

Cardiac tamponade can be defined as an accumulation of pericardial fluid that inhibits the diastolic filling of the atria and ventricles and, if left unchecked, will lead to a clinical state of shock. It may be recognized by clinical signs in the late stages, but the diagnosis should be confirmed by echocardiography as these signs are non-specific. It is now recognized that the process of cardiac tamponade may occur before significant clinical signs develop. Echocardiography can diagnose this early 'compensated' stage of the process.

The best classification for cardiac tamponade is traumatic (dealt with elsewhere in this book) and non-traumatic (Fig. 5.6.2), as not only the aetiology but the clinical course and approach to management are very different.

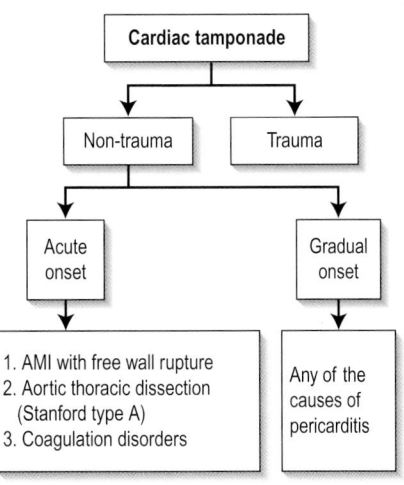

Fig. 5.6.2 Causes of pericardial effusion and cardiac tamponade.

Clinical features

History

The symptoms of cardiac tamponade are non-specific and their onset and course depend on whether the condition is acute or gradual. They are also inconsistent and sometimes difficult to elicit. A high index of suspicion for the condition must therefore be maintained, which requires thorough knowledge of the clinical settings in which tamponade can occur.

The commonest symptom of cardiac tamponade is dyspnoea (sensitivity 87–89%). Most other symptoms will relate to those of diminished cardiac output (e.g. faintness, dizziness, apprehension) or to the underlying disease process (e.g. pain of pericarditis).

Examination

Generally, signs are difficult to elicit and very non-specific. The classic signs are those of Beck's triad: hypotension, diminished heart sounds and elevated jugular venous pressure (JVP). It should be noted that cardiac tamponade may be present in the absence of an elevated JVP in conditions of significant hypovolaemia and that diminished heart sounds are a very non-specific and subjective finding. Furthermore, the absence of hypotension does not rule out cardiac tamponade; indeed, in some cases, hypertension may be present.

The most common clinical features are dyspnoea (sensitivity 87–89%), tachycardia (sensitivity 77%), pulsus paradoxus >10 mmHg (sensitivity 82%) and elevated JVP (sensitivity 76%). Loss of the apical impulse or, if present, an area of cardiac dullness extending beyond the apical impulse, may give a clinical clue to the presence of an effusion but not cardiac tamponade. In the later stages of cardiac tamponade, tachypnoea is common. If cardiac function is otherwise normal, the lung fields are typically 'clear'. There may be associated pleural effusions and signs of pericarditis (e.g. fever, pericardial rub). Pleuropericardial rubs may still be heard, even in the presence of a large effusion. There may be a degree of peripheral cyanosis, typically of the head, neck, chest and upper arms.

Differential diagnosis

The differential diagnosis of cardiac tamponade is given in Table 5.6.3.

Clinical investigations

Chest X-ray

The cardiac silhouette may be normal in cases of acute tamponade. At least 250 mL of fluid must be present within the pericardial cavity before an increase in the cardiac silhouette can

Table 5.6.3 The differential diagnosis of cardiac tamponade
Massive pulmonary embolism
Tension pneumothorax
Superior vena cava obstruction
Chronic constrictive pericarditis
Air embolism
Right ventricular infarct
Severe congestive cardiac failure/cardiogenic shock
Extrapericardial compression: haematoma, tumour

be appreciated. In subacute or chronic cases, cardiomegaly is common, but it is a non-specific finding and of limited practical use. Classically, the cardiac silhouette is globular or water-bottle shaped. The best indicators of a possible effusion are cardiomegaly where there has been a relatively acute increase in size, cardiomegaly with clear lung fields and the larger the cardiac silhouette the greater should be the index of suspicion.

ECG

This may provide clues to the presence of an effusion, with low voltages and electrical alternans but, again, will not indicate whether tamponade is occurring.

Bedside ultrasonography

Bedside ultrasonography performed in critical care areas is an excellent screening test if the tamponade is suspected and is reported to have sensitivity for detection of pericardial effusion of 75%. Although tamponade cannot be proven, presence of pericardial fluid provides supportive evidence for the diagnosis.

Echocardiography

Echocardiography is the current 'gold standard' investigation for the diagnosis of cardiac tamponade. It is the most specific and sensitive investigation for the detection of an effusion and of the process of tamponade. It can be performed rapidly and non-invasively (in the case of transthoracic echocardiography, TTE). In patients in whom a transthoracic study is difficult to perform or in whom the result is equivocal, then a transoesophageal (TOE) study

may be performed. This technique may detect occult loculated effusions missed by TTE and can even be performed in the intubated patient during CPR. Echocardiography can provide valuable information about associated cardiac function and abnormalities. It may also detect the process of tamponade before significant clinical signs develop.

It is important to remember that clinically significant tamponade is a clinical diagnosis and that 'echocardiographic signs of tamponade' are not in themselves an indication for acute intervention.

CT and MRI

CT and MRI are sensitive and specific for the detection of pericardial fluid and are good alternatives if echocardiography is not available. They are much less reliable in determining whether tamponade is occurring, giving only indirect clues. Neither is suitable in the critically ill patient.

Haemodynamic monitoring

In the ICU setting, pulmonary artery catheter findings of 'equalization' of the right heart diastolic pressures (i.e. right atrial, right ventricular end-diastolic, diastolic pulmonary artery and pulmonary artery wedge pressures) suggest the diagnosis of cardiac tamponade.

Treatment

The treatment of cardiac tamponade is drainage of the pericardial fluid. Medical management aims to improve the clinical condition while arrangements for drainage are being made.

General measures

Oxygenation should be optimized. Fluid loading may provide some minor 'temporizing' support of the cardiac output. Inotropic agents are usually ineffective. Institution of mechanical ventilation may cause a sudden drop in blood pressure as the positive intrathoracic pressure further impairs cardiac filling.

Definitive measures

Drainage procedures

Pericardiocentesis is best performed in the cardiac catheter laboratory under fluoroscopic or ultrasound guidance. Surgical drainage is required for purulent or recurrent effusions and

when tissue is required for diagnosis; a sub-xiphoid approach is preferred.

'Blind' needle pericardiocentesis should be considered a method of last resort. It is best reserved for the pre-arrest or just-arrested patient, as it can be technically difficult and has significant complications, especially when smaller volumes of fluid are involved. If it is to be carried out, it is best followed up with the insertion of an indwelling 'pigtail'-type catheter for ready aspiration should the patient's condition deteriorate. It must be remembered that CPR in the arrested patient will not be effective in cases of cardiac tamponade, when immediate needle drainage followed in many cases by thoracotomy will be required.

Thoracotomy without attempts at drainage should be performed when definitive surgical repair of the causative pathology is necessary. Examples in this category include trauma, rupture of the myocardium and dissecting thoracic aneurysm causing cardiac tamponade. Indeed, attempts at drainage before definitive repair in the case of dissecting aortic aneurysm may be positively detrimental.

Treatment must also be directed at the underlying pathology.

Disposition

Pericardial effusion may, with time, lead to cardiac tamponade. All cases of cardiac tamponade will lead to shock and death if left untreated, the rapidity of which will depend on the amount of fluid present, the rate at which it accumulated and the compliance of the pericardium.

Patients with clinically 'compensated' non-traumatic cardiac tamponade should be admitted to a high-dependency area for close observation while a definitive drainage procedure is planned and organized. In cases of decompensated tamponade, urgent drainage is required and the choice of management will depend on the aetiology, clinical urgency and expertise available.

Controversies

- The distinction between clinical and echocardiographic tamponade with the advent of more sensitive imaging.
- The type and timing of drainage procedures in the critically ill.

MYOCARDITIS

ESSENTIALS

1 Myocarditis is most commonly caused by viral infection; the majority of cases run a benign course with full recovery.

2 Occasionally, acute fulminating episodes occur, giving rise to arrhythmias, cardiac failure and death. Survivors of these episodes may, however, make a full recovery with supportive treatment.

3 Diagnosis is difficult and is usually made on clinical grounds.

4 Myocarditis may present in a similar manner to myocardial infarction, including similar chest pain, ECG changes and elevation of cardiac biomarkers.

5 Long-term follow up is important in patients who have had myocarditis, as some cases may progress to a chronic form with the development of dilated cardiomyopathy.

Table 5.6.4 Commoner causes of myocarditis	
Viral	Adenovirus Coxsackie B virus Cytomegalovirus Human herpes virus-6 HIV Influenza A Herpes simplex virus-1 Parvovirus Respiratory syncytial virus
Toxin or drug	Anthracyclines Trastuzumab Ethanol Clozapine Snake or scorpion bite Ionizing radiation
Immune mediated	Chagas' disease Sarcoidosis Scleroderma Systemic lupus erythematosus Alloantigen (heart transplant recipient) Kawasaki's disease
Bacteria	*Rickettsia* species *Leptospira* *Coxiella burnetti* *Corynebacterium diptheriae* *Mycoplasma pneumoniae*
Protozoa, fungi and parasites	Toxoplasma, *Cryptococcus* species

Introduction

Myocarditis is myocardial inflammation and injury in the absence of ischaemia. It is frequently associated with pericarditis, resulting in a myopericarditis.

Pathogenesis and pathophysiology

Myocarditis is caused by a wide range of viral, fungal, bacterial, protozoal and parasitic pathogens, toxins and drugs, as well as immune-mediated disease. The more common of these are shown in Table 5.6.4.

The exact mechanism by which viral myocarditis and its longer-term complications develop is unknown. It probably involves the interplay of several factors including direct damage due to the virus itself, damage in the acute and long term by the host's immune responses and a genetic predisposition in an individual.

Epidemiology

Given its highly variable clinical presentation, the real incidence of myocarditis is unknown. It accounts for up to one-third of cases of dilated cardiomyopathy.

Clinical features

The clinical spectrum of myocarditis is variable. It may manifest as any of the following:

- asymptomatic/subclinical
- fever with 'viral' illness, with minimal cardiac features
- acute myopericarditis
- unexplained arrhythmias, including conduction delays
- unexplained cardiac failure, ranging from mild to cardiogenic shock
- sudden, unexpected cardiac death
- delayed (years later) dilated cardiomyopathy.

History

Many cases are asymptomatic. There may be a history of an antecedent viral illness. After a delay of 10–14 days symptoms relating to cardiac involvement develop, such as arrhythmias causing palpitations or dizziness or cardiac failure causing shortness of breath. Pleuritic-type pain may be a feature owing to an associated pericarditis. Myocarditis may also present similarly to acute myocardial infarction, with chest pain, ischaemic ECG changes and elevated cardiac biomarkers. This presentation is more common in younger patients, with few cardiac risk factors, a preceding viral illness and subsequent normal coronary angiography.

Examination

On examination, a fever may be present, however, patients are often afebrile. Sinus tachycardia is often found and is said to be 'out of proportion' to the degree of fever. Other arrhythmias may also occur. A pericardial rub due to an associated pericarditis may be present. There may be signs of heart failure, ranging from mild to pulmonary oedema or cardiogenic shock.

Clinical investigations

A definitive diagnosis of acute viral myocarditis cannot be made in the ED and must, in the first instance, be presumptive. Presentation scenarios may include the young patient who presents with cardiac failure, shock or arrhythmias for which there is no obvious aetiology or young patients with features similar to acute coronary syndromes. Testing may provide supportive evidence for the diagnosis.

Blood tests

A number of blood tests can give supporting evidence to a diagnosis of myocarditis, but none are specific. These include elevation of the white cell count, elevation of the erythrocyte sedimentation rate (ESR) and/or C-reactive protein (CRP). Cardiac biomarkers may also be elevated. These parameters can be used to assess response to treatment.

257

Chest X-ray

This may show cardiomegaly with changes of congestive failure in severe cases, but again is non-specific. The chest X-ray may also be normal.

ECG

In most cases, the ECG will be abnormal, however, the changes are not specific for myocarditis. Sinus tachycardia is usually seen. The most common finding is non-specific ST-T-wave changes. Rhythm disturbances of any type may occur, including a significant proportion with conduction delays. Occasionally, ST elevation may occur that is indistinguishable from myocardial infarction.

Echocardiography

This can give supportive evidence but is not diagnostic. Global wall motion abnormalities are a characteristic finding but, in some cases, more regional abnormalities will be seen. An associated effusion may be found. Evidence of myocardial failure can be found with ventricular cavity dilation and reduced ejection fraction.

Cardiac MRI and ECG-gated multidetector CT (ECG-gated MDCT)

Cardiac MRI is being increasingly used to assist in the diagnosis of myocarditis. Regions of myocarditis are reported to correlate closely with regions of abnormal signal on MRI. It may also be used to identify target sites for biopsy.

ECG-gated MDCT is likely to show abnormal myocardial late hyperenhancement, either transmural or subepicardial.

Coronary angiography

Coronary angiography cannot diagnose myocarditis. It may need to be performed to exclude coronary artery disease.

Endomyocardial biopsy

This is currently the only way to make a definitive diagnosis. Despite flaws, it is still considered the gold standard, however, the following problems may be encountered:

- acute myocarditis may be patchy and diagnosis may be missed on a single specimen
- false-positive results are possible
- it may overestimate more minor cases of myocarditis.

There has long been debate about patient selection for endomyocardial biopsy, particularly after the negative results of the Myocarditis Treatment Trial. Patient selection remains controversial, even with case reports of treatment of myocarditis with interferon after polymerase chain reaction (PCR) detection of adenovirus and enterovirus on endomyocardial biopsy. Complications include venous injury, arrhythmias and cardiac perforation.

Treatment and disposition

Treatment consists of therapy for cardiac failure and supportive care, progressing to implantable defibrillators, aggressive mechanical assist devices as bridging therapy and, in severe cases, heart transplantation.

Supportive treatment should attend to airway, breathing and circulation. Oxygenation is important and, in cases of pulmonary oedema, ventilatory support (non-invasive or invasive) may be necessary. Analgesia will be required if pain is a significant feature. Strict bed rest is advised as exercise has been shown to increase the degree of myocyte necrosis. Diuretic therapy, vasodilators and inotropic support are used to optimize cardiac filling and increase cardiac output. Angiotensin-converting enzyme (ACE) inhibitors and angiotensin II receptor blockers should be initiated early. Complicating arrhythmias are treated along conventional lines. In patients who develop cardiogenic shock, intervention should be early and aggressive. The use of inotropes, extracorporeal membrane oxygenation (ECMO) or ventricular assist devices is recommended as a bridge to transplant or recovery. In severe refractory cases, cardiac transplantation may ultimately be required. Immunosuppression trials have to date been largely disappointing, with no randomized trial showing sustained clinical or mortality benefit. Preliminary data suggest that administration of interferon-β (INF-β) to patients with persistent depression of left ventricular ejection fraction (LVEF) and PCR-positive genome expression for enteroviral or adenoviral DNA may enhance viral clearance and improve LVEF. There have yet to be any multicentre trials conducted.

Survivors of myocarditis must be followed carefully for the possible future development of dilated cardiomyopathy. Patients should not undertake any competitive sport for 6 months after the onset of clinical myocarditis. Athletes may return to training if left ventricular function, wall motion and dimensions return to normal, arrhythmias are absent, serum markers of inflammation have resolved and the ECG has normalized.

All patients with suspected acute myocarditis should be admitted to the CCU/ICU.

Prognosis

Prognosis from acute myocarditis depends on severity of symptoms and signs, histological classification and biomarkers. Paradoxically, patients with more severe heart failure at

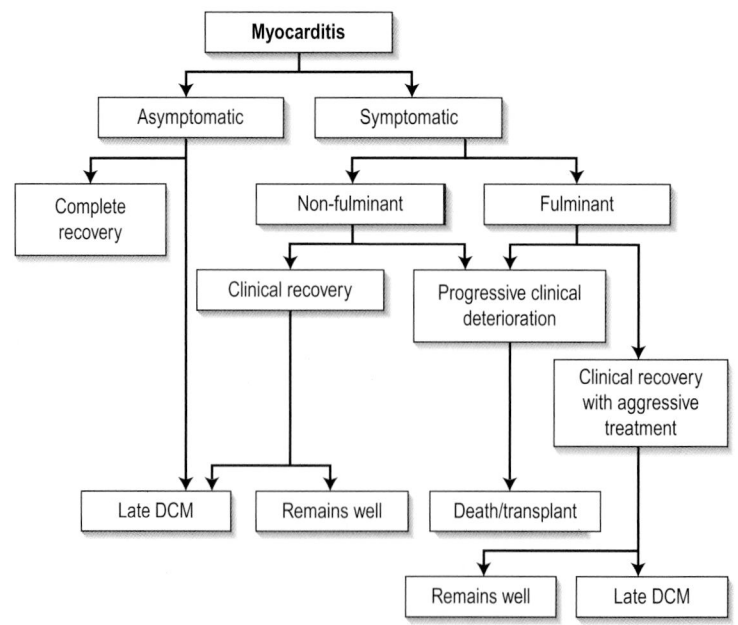

Fig. 5.6.3 Natural history of myocarditis.

presentation may have better overall survival. Clinical predictors of a fatal outcome include hypotension and elevated pulmonary wedge pressure. Biochemical markers associated with poorer outcome include serum Fas, Fas ligand, antimyosin autoantibodies and interleukin-10 (IL-10) levels. Increased tumour necrosis factor-α (receptor 1) expression and persistent viral genome expression for selected viruses have also recently been associated with progressive impairment/failure of recovery of LVEF.

Complications at presentation are usually the result of arrhythmias and heart failure; however, the majority of cases will run a benign course with a full recovery. Arrhythmias may include conduction delays with a potential for sudden death. Occasionally, an acute fulminant course may occur, with intractable arrhythmias or, more often, with acute heart failure rapidly progressing to cardiogenic shock and death. Survivors of this fulminant course will often make a complete recovery.

The whole spectrum of asymptomatic through to fulminant cases may progress to a chronic course. Myocarditis is thought to be the cause of up to one-third of cases of dilated cardiomyopathy. It may also explain some instances of recurrent unexplained arrhythmias and sudden unexpected cardiac death, especially in younger age groups. See Figure 5.6.3 for a summary of the natural history of myocarditis.

Controversies

- The role of interferon, immunoglobulin and corticosteroids in the management of viral myocarditis.
- Optimal diagnostic strategy, in particular the place of MRI.
- The role of endomyocardial biopsy in patients suspected of having autoimmune disease.

Further reading

Acker MA. Mechanical circulatory support for patients with acute fulminant myocarditis. Ann Thorac Surg 2001;71:S73–6.

Allen KB, Faber LP, Warren WH, Shaar CJ. Pericardial effusion: subxiphoid pericardiostomy versus percutaneous catheter drainage. Ann Thorac Surg 1999;67:437–40.

Ariyarijah V, Spodick DH. Acute pericarditis: diagnostic cues and common electrocardiographic manifestations. Cardiol Rev 2007;15:24–30.

Dambrin G, Laissy J, Serfaty J, et al. Diagnostic value of ECG-gated multidetector computed tomography in the early phase of suspected acute myocarditis. A preliminary comparative study with cardiac MRI. Eur Radiol 2007;17.2:331–8.

Ellis CR, Di Salvo T. Myocarditis: basic and clinical aspects. Cardiol Rev 2007;15:70–7.

Hayes JE. Cardiac tamponade. Emerg Med 1997;9:123–35.

Hoit BD. Pericardial disease and pericardial tamponade. Crit Care Med 2007;35:S355–64.

Imazio M, Spodick DH, et al. Controversial issues in the management of pericardial diseases. Circulation 2010;121:916–28.

Kim JS, Kim HH, Yoon T. Imaging of pericardial diseases. Clin Radiol 2007;62:626–31.

Little WC, Freeman GL. Pericardial disease. Circulation 2006;113:1622–32.

Lotrionte M, Biondi-Zoccai G. International collaborative systematic review of controlled clinical trials on pharmacologic treatments for acute pericarditis and its recurrences. Am Heart J 2010;160:662–70.

Magnani J, William Dec G. Myocarditis: current trends in diagnosis and management. Circulation 2006;113:876–90.

5.7 Heart valve emergencies

Kevin KC Hung • Colin A Graham

ESSENTIALS

1 Infective endocarditis is effectively a multiorgan disease and is an often missed diagnosis.

2 There has been a shift in the predominant organism in infective endocarditis from *Streptococcus viridans* to *Staphylococcus aureus* and nosocomial infections are becoming more common.

3 Degenerative heart disease and the presence of prosthetic valves are currently the high-risk factors for infective endocarditis in developed countries.

4 Antibiotic prophylaxis in patients with valvular or congenital heart disease is an important consideration in the appropriate clinical context.

5 The causes of acute deterioration in chronic valve lesions must be recognized and treated expeditiously to prevent life-threatening haemodynamic instability.

Introduction

Heart valve emergencies are a cause of sudden deterioration in cardiac function. The underlying cause depends on the valve involved.

Infective endocarditis

This is a commonly missed diagnosis. A high index of suspicion must be maintained, as delay in diagnosis will increase the mortality and morbidity.

Epidemiology

The incidence of infective endocarditis is 3–10 episodes/100 000 person-years, of which prosthetic valve endocarditis (PVE) accounts for 20–30%. The male to female ratio is $\geq$2:1 and it is more common in the fifth and sixth decades of life.

In the developing countries, rheumatic heart disease is the commonest risk factor for infective endocarditis. Despite a fall in the incidence of rheumatic fever in developed countries, the prevalence of infective endocarditis has not fallen. In the developed world, the risk factors include:

- Host-related factors:
  - poor oral hygiene
  - intravenous drug use (IVDU)
  - severe renal disease on haemodialysis
  - diabetes mellitus
  - mitral valve prolapse – particularly in the presence of valve incompetence or thickening of the valve leaflets
  - degenerative valve sclerosis associated with age (mitral valve most common, then aortic, tricuspid and pulmonary valves respectively)
- Procedure-related factors:
  - infected intravascular device
  - post-genitourinary procedure
  - post-gastrointestinal procedure
  - surgical wound infection.

Table 5.7.1 Bacterial pathogens associated with host categories

IVDU	*Staphylococcus aureus*; 80% of tricuspid valve involvement is due to this pathogen Streptococcal species *Pseudomonas aeruginosa* Fungi, especially *Candida* Multiple organisms
IVDU with HIV infection	Unusual organisms, such as *Salmonella*, *Listeria*, *Bartonella*
Insulin dependent diabetics	*Staph. aureus*
Prosthetic heart valves, within 2 months of valve surgery	*Staph. epidermidis* *Staph. aureus* *Enterococcus* species
Prosthetic valves, more than 2 months post valve surgery	*Staph. aureus* *Streptococcus viridans*
Pre-existing malignancy or procedures involving the genitourinary or gastrointestinal tracts	*Enterococcus* species

Table 5.7.2 Highest risk cardiac conditions for which prophylaxis with dental procedures is recommended

Antibiotic prophylaxis is recommended only for those with the highest risk of infective endocarditis
Prosthetic valve
Previous infective endocarditis
Congenital heart disease
Unrepaired cyanotic congenital heart disease
First 6 months of repaired congenital heart disease with prosthetic material
Residual defects with repaired congenital heart disease with prosthetic material

After Wilson W, Taubert KA, Gewitz M, et al. Circulation 2007; 116:1736-54. Epub 2007 Apr 19. Erratum in: Circulation 2007; 116:e376-7 with permission.

Pathology and pathogenesis

In infective endocarditis, the interactions between host and organism are complex. Platelet–fibrin deposits form at sites of endothelial damage, which is called non-bacterial thrombotic endocarditis. Invasion and multiplication by a virulent microbe leads to enlargement of these vegetations, which become infected. The consequences of this are the basis of the clinical complications of infective endocarditis. The vegetations can fragment and embolize, leading to distal foci of infection, called septic emboli. Obstruction of vessels by these fragments can also result in tissue ischaemia and infarction. Seeding from the fragments perpetuates the bacteraemia. Local destruction of the valve may produce intra-cardiac complications, such as rupture of the chordae tendineae, abscess of the valve annulus and conduction problems.

Staphylococcus aureus, entering through a breach in the skin, has surpassed *Streptococcus viridans* as the commonest bacterial pathogen in both native valve endocarditis (NVE) and prosthetic valve endocarditis. This change reflects better dental care and an increased incidence of nosocomial infections, although significant geographical variation exists. In proven *Staph. aureus* bacteraemia, the incidence of infective endocarditis is 13–25%. Overall, three major pathogens account for more than 80% of cases: *Staph. aureus*, *Streptococcus* species and *Enterococcus* species.

Nosocomial infective endocarditis is defined as endocarditis occurring after 72 hours of hospital admission or within 4–8 weeks of an invasive procedure performed in a hospital. Organisms responsible for nosocomial endocarditis are *Staphylococcus* species (>75%, mainly *Staph. aureus*) and *Enterococcus* species in genitourinary and gastrointestinal tract procedures. Organisms associated with particular host categories are shown in Table 5.7.1.

Fungal infections account for less than 10% of cases and are most common in IVDU, the immunocompromised and those with prosthetic valves. The Gram-negative HACEK group (*Haemophilus* species, *Actinobacillus actinomycetemcomitans*, *Cardiobacterium hominis*, *Eikenella corrodens*, *Kingella kingae*) are growing in importance and lead to large vegetations that may result in large vessel embolization or cardiac failure. Endocarditis caused by the HACEK group is often culture-negative, as these bacteria are fastidious.

Prevention

The decision to administer procedural prophylactic antibiotic to at-risk patients depends on the assessment of the risk of endocarditis in the abnormal valve coupled with the risk of bacteraemia of the procedure being undertaken. High-risk valve lesions are prosthetic valves, mitral valve prolapse with significant incompetence and acquired dysfunctional valves in indigenous patients (because of the high incidence of rheumatic heart disease). The indications for antibiotic prophylaxis have been significantly reduced in major infective endocarditis prophylaxis guidelines and many now recommend against prophylaxis for gastrointestinal or genitourinary tract procedures. Prophylaxis for dental procedures that involve manipulation of either gingival tissue or the periapical region of teeth or perforation of the oral mucosa is reasonable for those with highest risk of adverse outcomes from endocarditis (Table 5.7.2). These changes are due to the changes in the risk–benefit ratio of prophylactic treatment. It is believed that infective endocarditis is much more likely to result from frequent exposure to random bacteraemias associated with daily activities than from those listed procedures.

When indicated, single dose antibiotics 30–60 minutes before the procedure is now recommended. Current recommendations from the American Heart Association suggest:

- amoxicillin 2 g orally for adults (50 mg/kg for children) or
- cephalexin 2 g or clindamycin 600 mg or azithromycin 500 mg orally if allergic to penicillins.

Clinical features

Infective endocarditis should be considered a multisystem disease. The symptoms and signs are non-specific, compounding the difficulty of diagnosis. Symptoms usually occur within two months of the event responsible for the initiation of bacteraemia, although this may be difficult to identify. It is important to suspect infective endocarditis in patients with an unexplained fever and a predisposing factor.

The two most frequent systemic features are fever and malaise. Fever is present in 80–85% of cases; usually >38°C but rarely >39.4°C.

It can be absent in the severely debilitated, the elderly and those with cardiac failure, chronic renal failure, liver failure, recent antibiotic use and if the infection is by an organism with low virulence.

Malaise is reported in up to 95% of cases. Other symptoms are variable and non-specific and may include headache, confusion, cough, chest pain (more common in IVDU), dyspnoea, abdominal pain, anorexia, weight loss and myalgia.

Other clinical features include immunological phenomena as well as those related to the lesion itself and systemic embolization. Immunological phenomena include glomerulonephritis, Osler's nodes, Roth's spots and an elevated rheumatoid factor.

A new or changed incompetent murmur may be found on clinical examination of the heart. However, in 70–95% of cases, a murmur is already present; hence the discovery of an acute murmur is an uncommon but highly significant finding. The absence of a murmur does not exclude the diagnosis of infective endocarditis. A new murmur, or a change of murmur, is more likely in patients with a prosthetic valve or congestive cardiac failure.

Petechiae are commonly found in the palpebral conjunctivae and are also present in the mucosal membranes. Splinter haemorrhages under the fingernails, Osler's nodes (painful tender swellings of the fingertips or toe pads), Janeway lesions (small haemorrhages with a slightly nodular character on the palms and soles) and Roth's spots (oval retinal haemorrhages with a clear pale centre) are uncommon.

Complications

Congestive cardiac failure may occur and is usually a result of infection-induced valvular damage. Involvement of the aortic valve is more likely to cause congestive cardiac failure than mitral valve damage. The other cause is extension of the infective process beyond the valvular annulus. Involvement of the septum produces atrioventricular, fascicular and bundle branch blocks. Cardiac rupture and tamponade have been reported, but are rare. Pericarditis can result from extension into the sinus of Valsalva. Myocardial infarction can also occur as a result of infective embolism to the coronary arteries, but is rare.

Neurological manifestations, the result of embolic events from left-sided lesions, are present in approximately 15% of patients and are more likely if the pathogen is *Staph. aureus*. These include meningoencephalitis, focal deficits, transient ischaemic attacks and stroke. Embolic stroke is the most frequent event, but intracranial haemorrhage may occur as a result of rupture or leak of a mycotic aneurysm, septic arteritis or bleeding into an infarct. The mortality is high.

Systemic embolization occurs in 40% of cases and gives rise to the peripheral manifestations of infective endocarditis. The embolization usually precedes the diagnosis. Its incidence falls with the administration of appropriate antibiotics. They may involve any organ but skin, splenic, hepatic and renal emboli are most common. Notably, systemic emboli are absent in infective endocarditis of the tricuspid valve but multiple pulmonary abscesses are characteristically present.

Renal dysfunction may be due to altered renal haemodynamics, immune complex-mediated glomerulonephritis or nephrotoxicity from medications. Splenomegaly is present in 30% of cases. This is due to splenic abscesses arising from direct seeding from the bacteraemia or from an infective embolus. It leads to persistent fever, abdominal pain and diaphragmatic irritation. Tender hepatomegaly may also be present. Anaemia is common.

Complications are summarized in Table 5.7.3.

Diagnosis

The diagnosis of infective endocarditis requires an integration of data from various sources. This is due to the non-specific nature of the clinical manifestations. The Duke criteria for infective endocarditis are a useful diagnostic tool that has good specificity and a negative predictive value above 92%. These combine patient risk factors, isolates from blood cultures, the persistence of bacteraemia, echocardiographic findings and other clinical and laboratory data (Fig. 5.7.1).

Severely ill patients with obvious sepsis should be treated without delay according to the 'Surviving Sepsis' guidelines. However, infective endocarditis commonly presents in a more insidious way. When fever is persistent and unexplained, infective endocarditis must be considered, particularly in:

- patients with acquired or congenital valvular heart disease, pre-existing prosthetic valve, hypertrophic cardiomyopathy, congenital heart disease (patent ductus areteriosus [PDA], ventricular septal defect [VSD], coarctation of the aorta), intracardiac pacemakers, central venous lines or

Table 5.7.3 Complications of infective endocardititis	
Organ system	*Complications*
Cardiac	Congestive cardiac failure Valvular incompetence Arrhythmias Cardiac rupture/tamponade Pericarditis Myocardial infarction Cardiac fistulae
Renal	Immune-mediated glomerulonephritis
Neurological	Stroke or TIA Cerebral abscess Intracranial haemorrhage from aneurysm rupture Meningitis/encephalitis
Other	Mycotic aneurysm of any artery Emboli to any organ, e.g. spleen, liver, skin

TIA: transient ischaemia attack.

intra-arterial lines or a new or changed cardiac murmur
- patients with known bacteraemia. In *Staph. aureus* bacteraemia, the risk of infective endocarditis is higher if it is community acquired, there is no primary focus of infection, there is a metastatic complication and, in the context of an intravascular catheter being a possible focus of infection, if fever or bacteraemia is present for greater than 3 days, despite removal of the catheter
- cases with features of an embolic event, especially if recurrent
- young patients with unexpected stroke or subarachnoid haemorrhage
- patients with a history of IVDU, especially if there are pulmonary features, such as cough and pleuritic chest pain
- cases of persistent bacteraemia or fever despite treatment, congestive cardiac failure or new ECG features of atrioventricular heart block, fascicular block and bundle branch block.

Clinical investigations

Blood cultures

Blood cultures are crucial to the diagnosis of infective endocarditis. If no prior antibiotics have been given, blood cultures are positive in 95–100% of cases, often in the first two sets. The major causes of culture-negative infective endocarditis are prior use of antibiotics (62%) and fastidious organisms.

Clinical criteria for infective endocarditis require:
- Two major criteria, or
- One major and three minor criteria, or
- Five minor criteria

MAJOR CRITERIA:

- **Positive blood culture for infective endocarditis**
  Typical micro-organism consistent with IE from two separate blood cultures, as noted below:
    - viridans streptococci, *Streptococcus bovis*, or HACEK or
    - community-acquired *Staphylococcus aureus* or enterococci, in the absence of a primary focus

  or

  Micro-organisms consistent with IE from persistently positive blood cultures defined as:
    - Two positive cultures of blood samples drawn 12 hours apart, or
    - all of three or a majority of four separate cultures of blood (with first and last sample drawn 1 hour apart)

- **Evidence of endocardial involvement**
  Positive echocardiogram for IE defined as:
    - Oscillating intercardiac mass on valve or supporting structures, in the path of regurgitant jets, or on implanted material in the absence of an alternative anatomical explanation, or
    - abscess, or
    - new partial dehiscence of prosthetic valve

  or

  New valvular regurgitation (worsening or changing of pre-existing murmur not sufficient)

MINOR CRITERIA:

- **Predisposition:** predisposing heart condition or intravenous drug use
- **Fever:** temperature ≥38.0° C (100.4° F)
- **Vascular phenomena:** major arterial emboli, septic pulmonary infarcts, mycotic aneurysm, intracranial haemorrhage, conjunctival haemorrhages, and Janeway lesions
- **Immunological phenomena:** glomerulonephritis, Osler's nodes, Roth's spots and rheumatoid factor
- **Microbiological evidence:** positive blood culture but does not meet a major criterion as noted above or serological evidence of active infection with organism consistent with IE
- **Echocardiographic findings:** consistent with IE but do not meet a major criterion as noted above

---

Fig. 5.7.1 Duke criteria for the diagnosis of infective endocarditis. *(From Li JS, Sexton DJ, Mick N, et al. Proposed modifications to the Duke criteria for the diagnosis of infective endocarditis. Clin Infect Dis 2000; 30:633-8.)*

In the stable patient without evidence of complications, three sets of blood cultures should be collected from different vascular puncture sites at least 1 hour apart over a 24-hour period prior to the start of empirical antibiotics. Timing of venepuncture does not need to coincide with fever as bacteraemia is continuous. Both aerobic and anaerobic media should be used for each set. Arterial and venous blood samples are equally likely to be infected.

In unwell patients, empirical antibiotics should not be delayed and the timing between blood cultures can be truncated.

Full blood count
Anaemia (usually normochromic and normocytic) is demonstrated in most patients. There is a leucocytosis in acute infective endocarditis, but this may be absent in subacute cases. Thrombocytopaenia is rare.

Inflammatory markers
The erythrocyte sedimentation rate (ESR) is a non-specific test, however, it is raised in almost all patients to a magnitude of greater than 55 mm/h. A normal ESR makes infective endocarditis unlikely.

C-reactive protein (CRP) is also non-specific, but has been reported to be more sensitive than ESR. Procalcitonin levels are also raised in patients with infective endocarditis, although it may not be as sensitive as CRP.

Urinalysis
The urinalysis is abnormal in 50% of cases, with proteinuria and microscopic haematuria. Normal renal function may be maintained.

Echocardiography
Echocardiography provides morphological confirmation of the diagnosis by visualizing heart valves and vegetations, assessing haemodynamic impact and identifying complications (such as perivalvular involvement, and abscesses). Transthoracic echocardiography (TTE) is now recommended as the first-line imaging modality in suspected infective endocarditis and must be performed rapidly, as soon as infective endocarditis is suspected. In NVE, TTE has a specificity for vegetations of 98%, but a sensitivity of less than 60–70%. The reason for the low sensitivity is the technical problems in those with chest-wall deformity, chronic airway limitation and obesity. In PVE, sensitivity of TTE for vegetations is 15–35% and it is especially poor for mitral valve vegetations. However, it has the benefit of being non-invasive.

Transoesophageal echocardiography (TOE) is invasive and more difficult to obtain. It has a specificity of 85–98% and the sensitivity is 75–95% for vegetations. In particular, it is more likely to detect perivalvular lesions and abscesses. The indication for TTE in infective endocarditis is suspected NVE with no technical hindrance to imaging. If the result is negative and coupled with a low clinical suspicion, a subsequent TOE is not warranted. The indications for TOE in suspected infective endocarditis are:

- prosthetic valves/intracardiac device
- poor quality TTE
- negative TTE but high clinical suspicion of infective endocarditis.

In patients with positive TTE, subsequent TOE should be considered due to its better sensitivity and specificity, particularly for the diagnosis of abscesses and measurement of vegetation size.

Despite the virtues of TOE, a negative study does not exclude the diagnosis or the need to start treatment if clinical suspicion is high. The false-negative rate is 6–18%, which decreases to 4–13% with a repeat study. There are a number of limitations of echocardiography including that infectious vegetations cannot be distinguished from marantic lesions on native valves or thrombus on prosthetic valves and healed lesions cannot be easily separated from active ones. Entities that may mimic vegetations are thickened valves, ruptured chordae or valves, calcifications and nodules.

Treatment

Management involves the use of antibiotics to eradicate the pathogen and other interventions to deal with the intracardiac and distal complications of the infections. Cardiac surgery may be required, the timing of which is difficult to judge. Early specialist referral is critical, particularly if signs and symptoms of congestive heart failure are present.

Antibiotic therapy

In the emergency department, a microbiological diagnosis is not possible. Toxic patients must start empirical antibiotics after the collection of three sets of cultures at three separate vascular puncture sites. These do not need to be separated in time if patients are clearly septic.

Antibiotic penetration of vegetations is difficult as they are a mixture of fibrin, platelets and bacteria and it is hard to achieve local bactericidal drug levels. The principles of antibiotic therapy are to use antibiotics in combination, with empirical therapy determined by the most likely group of organisms in a given patient and to employ a long duration of therapy, usually 4–6 weeks. Antibiotic choice is tailored once the pathogen and its sensitivities are known. The choice of empirical antibiotics depends on local epidemiology, especially antibiotic resistance, and whether patients have received prior antibiotic therapy.

The current recommendations for empirical antibiotics in Australia are:

- for community-acquired NVE:
  - benzylpenicillin 1.8 g IV 4-hourly with
  - flucloxacillin 2 g IV 4-hourly with
  - gentamicin 4–6 mg/kg IV daily
- vancomycin (25 mg/kg up to 1 g IV 12-hourly) replaces penicillin in PVE, hospital-acquired infections or where there is penicillin sensitivity.

Surgery

Native valve endocarditis Patients with congestive cardiac failure, evidence of embolization to major organs and vegetations greater than 10 mm in size have been shown to have poor outcomes on medical management alone.

The indications for surgery in haemodynamically unstable patients are:

- cardiac failure, aortic incompetence or mitral incompetence
- complications including heart block, annular or aortic abscesses or the presence of perforating lesions, e.g. perforated valve leaflets
- virulent organisms resistant to treatment or
- fungal endocarditis.

The indications in haemodynamically stable patients are less clear, but early specialist support should be obtained.

Prosthetic valve endocarditis The indications for surgery include cardiac failure, valve dehiscence, valve dysfunction (increased stenosis or incompetence) and complications such as abscess formation.

Anticoagulation

Anticoagulation with aspirin or warfarin has not been shown to reduce the risk of embolic events and may contribute to an increased risk of bleeding, especially intracranial bleeding. They should be used with caution only where there is a clear indication for them distinct from endocarditis, e.g. presence of a prosthetic valve.

Prognosis

The overall mortality for native and prosthetic valve endocarditis is 20–25% at one year and 50% at 10 years. The major causes of death are congestive cardiac failure, haemodynamic deterioration and embolic complications. Nosocomial endocarditis has a higher inpatient mortality (24–50%) compared to community-acquired endocarditis (16–20%). In right-sided lesions in intravenous drug users, the mortality is 10%. The most important determinant of mortality is congestive cardiac failure.

Mortality is also related to the organism isolated. It is greater than 50% in *Pseudomonas aeruginosa*, Enterobacteriacae or fungal infection. *Staph. aureus* infection has a mortality of 25–47%.

The rate of relapse varies with the causative organism and occurs usually within two months

of stopping antibiotics. The rate of relapse in NVE is <2% for *Strep. viridans*, 11% for *Staph. aureus* and 8–20% for enterococci. In prosthetic valve endocarditis, the relapse rate is 10–15%.

Long term, approximately 50% of cases require heart valve replacement.

Acute aortic incompetence

Aetiology and pathophysiology

The causes of acute aortic valve incompetence are infective endocarditis, proximal aortic dissection, blunt chest trauma and spontaneous rupture of an abnormal valve.

The result is an acute and progressive volume overload within the left ventricle that has not had time to compensate. The consequently elevated left ventricular end-diastolic pressure is transmitted to the left atrium and pulmonary venous bed leading to pulmonary oedema. Cardiac output is diminished as the stroke volume is shared between forward and regurgitant flow into the left atrium. The compensatory mechanisms via the sympathetic nervous system result in positive inotropy and chronotropy. However, the rise in systemic peripheral vascular resistance impedes left ventricular outflow and worsens the regurgitation. Ventricular oxygen demand is also increased and myocardial ischaemia is a major risk even if coronary artery disease is not present.

Clinical features

Acute aortic incompetence is poorly tolerated. Severe congestive cardiac failure and hypotension are typical. Ischaemic chest pain may be reported. The diastolic murmur is soft and extends only to mid-diastole. The first heart sound is also of low intensity. The pulse pressure is large and tachycardia is almost always present.

Clinical investigations

The chest X-ray (CXR) may reveal the underlying cause. Pulmonary congestion is often present without cardiac enlargement. Echocardiography is diagnostic and provides useful data especially in the selection of timing for surgery. TTE/TOE is required if aortic root dissection is thought to be the cause and, in most emergency departments, urgent computed tomographic imaging will lead to a more rapid diagnosis and should be the key diagnostic tool. Cardiac catheterization can be considered before surgery, but is usually not performed in acutely unstable patients requiring emergency cardiac surgery for aortic dissection.

Treatment

Valve replacement is crucial to survival as severe left ventricular failure is the commonest cause of death. Medical treatment with an inotropic agent (dopamine or dobutamine) and concurrent vasodilatation (with nitrates or nitroprusside) can be used, but only serve as temporizing measures prior to surgery.

Intra-aortic balloon counterpulsation is contraindicated. Beta-blockers should be used with caution as the compensatory tachycardia will be prevented.

Acute deterioration in chronic aortic incompetence

Pathophysiology

In chronic aortic valve incompetence, the pathophysiology is dictated by the combination of pressure and volume overload. The initial stage of compensation is achieved by hypertrophy of the left ventricle. The left ventricular ejection fraction (LVEF) is never in the normal range even in the compensated stage. However, patients can be asymptomatic for decades. This is followed by the uncompensated stage where there is a significant reduction of the left ventricular ejection fraction, defined as an LVEF of 50% or less at rest. This results predominantly from volume overload. It is reversible initially, with full recovery of left ventricular function if aortic valve replacement is performed. The uncompensated phase eventually becomes irreversible with enlargement of the left ventricle. Symptoms become severe and surgery is less effective.

Decompensation can be the result of decreased myocardial contractility due to progressive left ventricular dilatation, myocardial ischaemia or excessive volume overload.

Apart from intrinsic abnormalities of the aortic valve, aortic root dilatation from various causes must be considered.

Clinical features

The clinical features are those of cardiac failure and angina. The patient is usually hypertensive. Clinical findings of severe disease are a wide pulse pressure, a displaced apical impulse, a diastolic murmur in the left 3rd–4th intercostal space, third heart sound and an Austin–Flint murmur.

Clinical investigations

The aim of investigations is to identify those who will need surgery. Serial investigations are usually performed. The most important is the assessment of ejection fraction and left ventricular systolic and diastolic volumes by echocardiogram. This also allows assessment of the aortic root and its size.

Treatment

Medical management

For symptomatic patients, medical management is aimed at improving left ventricular function as a temporizing measure prior to surgery. This is achieved by using vasodilators. The dose is titrated to the blood pressure, aiming to reduce it to a level tolerated by the patient. Medication options include nitrates, sodium nitroprusside and hydralazine. All of these reduce end-diastolic volume and increase forward flow. Nifedipine, in a single dose, does not consistently produce this result but may do so when used longer term.

Surgical management

Indications for aortic valve replacement are:

- symptomatic patient: angina or significant dyspnoea
- asymptomatic patients with ejection fraction ≤50%
- asymptomatic patients with severe left ventricular dilatation and left ventricular end systolic volume of >55 mm or LV end-diastolic volume >75 mm.

Prognosis

Patients with evidence of angina or cardiac failure have a poorer outcome. Mortality for those with angina is 10% per year and for those with cardiac failure, it approaches 20% per year.

Acute deterioration in critical aortic stenosis

Patients with severely stenosed aortic valves can remain asymptomatic for many years. Medical treatment can achieve a 5-year survival of 40% and a 10-year survival of 20%. The risk of sudden death in the asymptomatic patient is 2%, even when critical stenosis is present. With the development of syncope and angina, the survival falls to 2–3 years. When complicated by cardiac failure, 50% of patients will die within 18 months if there is no surgical intervention.

Pathophysiology

Aortic valve stenosis restricts left ventricular outflow and imposes a pressure load on the left ventricle. The latter is hypertrophied, with consequent poor compliance, and it is at risk of ischaemia and dysrhythmia. Cardiac function is delicately balanced between preload and afterload. Preload on the hypertrophied ventricle is elevated to support the stroke volume, but not high enough to lead to pulmonary congestion. Systemic vascular resistance is elevated but does not cause an increase in the oxygen demand that cannot be met. The increased demand during exercise causes abnormal distribution of flow leading to vulnerability of the subendocardium to ischaemia. The reserve margin is slim. A small and sudden alteration in any of these factors will precipitate pump failure.

Causes of aortic stenosis include:

- congenital bicuspid valve
- calcification of a normal valve, common in the elderly
- rheumatic heart disease, usually with associated mitral valve disease.

Pathophysiology of acute deterioration

Causes of acute deterioration include:

- acute fall in preload: hypovolaemia, excessive diuresis and vasodilatation
- atrial flutter or fibrillation: these are both uncommon and should raise suspicion of associated mitral valve disease
- acute afterload reduction: this leads to a reduction in coronary artery perfusion and places the hypertrophied left ventricle at risk of ischaemia. It does not improve the left ventricular stroke volume as the problem lies in the stenotic valve and not the systemic vascular resistance.

Clinical features

Patients with aortic stenosis may be asymptomatic for many years. Presentations to the emergency department may be for angina, syncope, left ventricular failure or hypotension. At worst, acute decompensation will result in acute pump failure, with shock and pulmonary oedema.

The murmur will have the expected features including aortic area location, systolic timing and radiation to the carotids. It will be less impressive and may be impossible to hear if cardiac output is poor. The most important finding consistent with critical stenosis is the paradoxical splitting of the second heart sound.

Clinical investigations

ECG, CXR and cardiac markers
Indications for these are dictated by the clinical presentation.

Echocardiogram
Echocardiography is the key diagnostic tool and allows assessment of transvalvular flow, transvalvular pressure gradients and the effective valve area.

Treatment
Medical therapy aims to relieve symptoms and optimize left ventricular function prior to definitive surgical management. Rapid reversal of the precipitant is essential.

Practice points
- Expedient treatment of atrial dysrhythmias may necessitate cardioversion. This helps by maximizing the contribution of atrial systole to left ventricular filling.
- Excessive reduction in preload will reduce stroke volume and hence cardiac output.
- Diuretics, digoxin and angiotensin converting enzyme (ACE) inhibitors should only be used with caution.
- Sodium nitrosprusside may be used for preload and afterload reduction, but only with invasive haemodynamic monitoring.
- Angina treatment requires cautious use of nitrates and β-blockers.
- Aortic valve replacement (AVR) is indicated for patients with severe aortic stenosis who are symptomatic or with left ventricular systolic dysfunction or an ejection fraction less than 0.5.
- Aortic balloon valvotomy may be a reasonable bridge to surgery in haemodynamically unstable patients who are at high risk of AVR or for palliation in whom AVR cannot be performed.
- Transcatheter aortic valve implantation (TAVI) is a relatively new procedure developed for patients with a poor prognosis

without treatment but who are at high risk if treated by open heart surgery. The procedure aims to implant a bioprosthetic aortic valve at the site of the native aortic valve with access achieved transluminally via the femoral artery or vein or using a minithoractomy (transapical) approach.

Acute deterioration in mitral stenosis

Pathophysiology
The adult mitral orifice is 4–6 cm^2. Symptom onset occurs when the valve orifice is less than 2.5 cm^2 and critical stenosis occurs when this is reduced to 1 cm^2. However, the patient may remain asymptomatic for many years. A pressure load is imposed on the left atrium, with consequent pulmonary congestion and pulmonary hypertension.

The predominant cause of mitral stenosis is rheumatic carditis. Other causes include atrial myxomas, severe annular calcification and ball valve thrombi. Congenital malformations are rare.

Pathophysiology of acute deterioration
Acute deterioration can be precipitated in two ways. When the heart rate is increased, the ventricular filling time in diastole is reduced. The atrial pressure rises and is transmitted retrogradely to the pulmonary bed, leading to acute dyspnoea and pulmonary oedema. Atrial fibrillation with a rapid ventricular response is a common example of this. Loss of atrial systole in atrial fibrillation leads to a 20% decrease in cardiac output, leading to major haemodynamic instability.

The second cause of acute deterioration is related to flow across the stenosed valve. When the flow is increased, the transvalvular pressure gradient is increased by a factor equal to the square of the flow rate. The left atrial pressure rises and can precipitate pulmonary congestion. Common clinical contexts in which the transvalvular flow is increased include sepsis, exercise, pregnancy, hypervolaemia and hyperthyroidism.

Clinical features
Patients may be asymptomatic for many years, but will have an abnormal physical examination. Symptomatic patients present with dyspnoea, fatigue, thromboembolic events, atrial

fibrillation or pulmonary congestion. The onset of symptoms is usually followed by a period of minimal disability that may last many years. Pulmonary congestion, pulmonary hypertension or systemic or pulmonary emboli herald rapid deterioration. Auscultatory findings include a loud first heart sound, an opening snap and a mid-diastolic murmur with presystolic accentuation.

Signs of critical stenosis are small pulse pressure, soft first heart sound, early opening snap, long diastolic murmur, diastolic thrill and evidence of pulmonary hypertension (right ventricular heave and loud P2). Acute pulmonary oedema may be present. Atrial fibrillation with a rapid ventricular rate is frequently the cause. Evidence of systemic embolization of a left atrial thrombus should be sought.

Clinical investigations

CXR and ECG
The CXR features are those of an enlarged left atrium, pulmonary congestion and pulmonary hypertension. The heart size is usually normal. Left atrial enlargement on the ECG is found in 90% of patients in sinus rhythm.

Echocardiogram
Echocardiography will confirm the diagnosis, exclude other causes of mitral valve obstruction, identify associated or coexisting structural heart disease, determine the severity of mitral stenosis and estimate pulmonary artery pressure.

Treatment
Medical management aims to reduce symptoms and prevent complications. It does not change the course of mitral valve deterioration, which requires surgery for definitive management. This is usually indicated when symptom severity is at NYHA functional class III.

Medical management for pulmonary oedema includes diuretics or long-acting nitrates (see Chapter 5.3). If atrial fibrillation with rapid ventricular response is a contributing factor, rate control is the first priority, either with drugs or with cardioversion (see Chapter 5.4). Anticoagulation is indicated for patients in atrial fibrillation.

Percutaneous mitral balloon valvotomy should be the first treatment to consider in patients with moderate or severe mitral stenosis in the absence of left atrial thrombus or moderate to severe mitral regurgitation. Mitral valve surgical commissurotomy or mitral valve replacement may be required for patients with unfavourable valve morphology or severe stenosis.

Prognosis

In asymptomatic or minimally symptomatic patients, average 10-year survival is greater than 80%. In those with significant symptoms, 10-year survival is 0–15%. In untreated patients, mortality is due to pulmonary congestion, right heart failure, systemic emboli, pulmonary emboli and infective endocarditis.

Acute mitral incompetence

Pathophysiology

Acute volume overload into the left atrium by the regurgitant stream is the crucial factor in acute mitral incompetence. The left atrium has a limited capacity to accommodate the excess volume and pulmonary oedema occurs. There is an associated rise in pulmonary vascular resistance and right ventricular failure may result. Cardiac output is reduced owing to a low stroke volume. The consequent elevation in the systemic vascular resistance impedes cardiac output. Tachycardia occurs but confers no benefit as the diastolic filling time is reduced.

Aetiology

The causes of acute mitral valve incompetence are:

- Infective endocarditis
- Papillary muscle disorder:
  - myocardial ischaemia or infarction
  - trauma
  - infiltrative disease
- Rupture of the chordae tendineae:
  - acute rheumatic fever
  - infective endocarditis
  - chest trauma
  - balloon valvotomy
  - myxomatous degeneration
  - spontaneous rupture
- Mitral leaflet disorder:
  - infective endocarditis
  - myxomatous degeneration
  - atrial myxoma
  - systemic lupus erythematosus
  - trauma.

Clinical features

Acute mitral valve incompetence is poorly tolerated and patients are always symptomatic.

There is reduced perfusion with concurrent acute pulmonary oedema. The blood pressure is variable and can be normal or low. The precordial findings do not correlate with the severity of the pathology; in fact a third heart sound may be the only finding. The apical mitral murmur is soft and occurs in early systole and does not become pansystolic. It radiates to the axilla and is commonly accompanied by a short apical diastolic murmur.

Clinical investigations

CXR and ECG

The CXR will show pulmonary oedema but not cardiomegaly. The ECG may show a recent infarct if this was the precipitant.

Echocardiogram

Echocardiography is diagnostic and provides valuable information on left ventricular function. It demonstrates the lesion and assesses its severity. In a patient with acute heart failure but with hyperdynamic systolic function of the left ventricle on TTE, suspicion for acute mitral valve incompetence is high. Both TTE and TOE may be required for adequate assessment.

Treatment

Surgery is urgently required. Medical treatment is usually only a temporizing step.

Medical treatment

Mortality in patients with severe left ventricular failure in this setting is high. Medical treatment is directed at the reduction of the regurgitant volume and hence diminishing the pulmonary congestion. It also aims to improve the forward output of the left ventricle. The modalities used depend on the blood pressure.

In normotensive patients, sodium nitroprusside may achieve all of the above objectives. In hypotensive patients, a combination of sodium nitroprusside and an inotrope, such as dobutamine, is required. Aortic ballon counterpulsation is often used to improve left ventricular ejection volume and further assist in the reduction of the regurgitant volume, but there is no clinical evidence to suggest that it improves outcomes.

In infective endocarditis, appropriate antibiotics are required.

Surgery

Valve repair should be considered before valve replacement due to the lower perioperative mortality, improved survival, better preservation of postoperative left ventricular function and lower long-term morbidity.

Acute deterioration in chronic mitral incompetence

Pathophysiology

In chronic mitral valve incompetence, the increased left ventricular end-diastolic volume leads to an increased left ventricular stroke volume and hence forward flow is preserved. The other factors that enable this are the increased preload on the left ventricle and the ability of the left ventricle to reduce afterload by backfilling into the left atrium. The result is enlargement of the left atrium and ventricle. In this compensated phase (which may last for years), the patient is asymptomatic.

In the decompensated phase, left ventricular systolic dysfunction occurs due to failure of contractility. This causes further left ventricular dilatation and increased left ventricular preload. A fall in cardiac output and pulmonary congestion may result. However, the factors are often still in favour of the left ventricle and the ejection fraction may be in the lower range of normal, i.e. 0.5–0.6.

Causes of chronic mitral incompetence include rheumatic carditis, ischaemic heart disease, mitral valve prolapse, collagen vascular disease and dilatation of the valvular annulus. Ischaemic causes have the worst prognosis as myocardial dysfunction is often coexistent.

Clinical features

Features of decompensation may be subtle. A history of reduced exercise tolerance is an important clue. Symptoms are those of pulmonary congestion and reduced cardiac output. Examination findings indicating severe disease include displacement of the apical impulse and evidence of pulmonary congestion. A third heart sound is commonly found and is not necessarily evidence of congestive heart failure.

Clinical investigations

CXR and ECG may provide useful information regarding cardiac size and heart rhythm. Echocardiography will confirm the diagnosis of mitral incompetence and document left ventricular and left atrial sizes. The integrity of the tricuspid valve is also important (E-Figs 5.7.1 and 5.7.2).

Treatment

Medical treatment

Atrial fibrillation is a common problem in chronic mitral valve incompetence, however, embolic risk is lower than for mitral stenosis with atrial fibrillation. AF is also an independent predictor of poor outcome after surgery. The ventricular rate requires control (see Chapter 5.4). Anticoagulation can be used as prophylaxis for embolic complications.

In functional mitral incompetence, preload reduction is beneficial if there is left ventricular dysfunction. Useful agents include ACE inhibitors and β-blockers, especially carvedilol, which is the only vasodilating β-blocker due to its additional α-1 blocking effects.

Surgical treatment

Surgical options include mitral valve repair, replacement with preservation of the mitral apparatus (papillary muscles and chordeae tendineae) or replacement with the removal of the apparatus (which has poorer outcomes). Surgery is indicated for:

- symptomatic patients in NYHA functional class II–IV with:
  - left ventricular ejection fraction ≥ 0.30 or
  - left ventricular end systolic dimension ≤ 55 mm
- asymptomatic patients with:
  - left ventricular ejection fraction between 0.30 and 0.60
  - left ventricular end systolic dimensions ≥ 40 mm

Prognosis

The risk of death is related to the degree of left ventricular decompensation.

Prosthetic valve complications

Prosthetic valve complications are common. As discussed, they are prone to infective endocarditis, so appropriate antibiotic prophylaxis is essential when indicated.

Antithrombotic therapy

Antithrombotic therapy is given to prevent embolic complications. The risk is greater for mitral compared to aortic prostheses regardless of the type. It is also highest in the first few

Table 5.7.4 Target INR values for prosthetic valves

Position	Valve	INR range
Aortic	Bileaflet or Medtronic Hall valve	2.0–3.0
	Starr–Edwards or other disc valves	2.5–3.5
Mitral	Any	2.5–3.5

months, as the prosthesis has not been fully endothelialized. Warfarin is the anticoagulant of choice. Newer antithrombotic agents, such as dabigatran, have not yet been trialled for patients with prosthetic valves.

Mechanical valves

Target INR values for mechanical valves are summarized in Table 5.7.4.

Aspirin in the dose range of 80–100 mg/day may be used in addition to warfarin in patients with an embolic event with the INR in the therapeutic range, known vascular disease or a susceptibility to hypercoagulability. This has been shown to reduce the risk of thromboembolism and cardiovascular mortality but does increase the risk of major haemorrhage. The data only refer to aspirin doses within this range.

Biological valves

The increased risk of thromboembolism is in the first 3 months, with the incidence at its greatest during the initial few days. After the 3-month period, the biological prosthetic valve can be regarded as a native valve.

Heparin therapy, followed later by warfarin, is started as soon as surgical bleeding is controlled. Warfarin therapy is stopped in two-thirds of the patients at 3 months. The remaining one-third stay on lifetime treatment with an INR in the range of 2.0–3.0. Patients requiring lifetime warfarin therapy include those with atrial fibrillation, a past history of thromboembolism, a risk of hypercoagulability and those with severe left ventricular dysfunction (LVEF <0.3).

Controversies

- Anticoagulation in infective endocarditis.
- Indications for and timing of surgery for haemodynamically stable patients with

infective endocarditis. The aim of early surgery would be to maximize salvage of the valvular apparatus and minimize the risk of endocardial complications.

- Use of intra-aortic balloon counterpulsation in patients with cardiogenic shock.

Further reading

Bonow RO, Carabello BA, Chatterjee K, et al. American College of Cardiology/American Heart Association Task Force on Practice Guidelines. 2008 focused update incorporated into the ACC/AHA 2006 guidelines for the management of patients with valvular heart disease: a report of the American College of Cardiology/American Heart Association Task Force on Practice Guidelines (Writing Committee to revise the 1998 guidelines for the management of patients with valvular heart disease). Endorsed by the Society of Cardiovascular Anesthesiologists, Society for Cardiovascular Angiography and Interventions, and Society of Thoracic Surgeons. J Am Coll Cardiol 2008;52:e1–142.

Habib G, Hoen B, Tornos P, et al. ESC Committee for Practice Guidelines. Guidelines on the prevention, diagnosis, and treatment of infective endocarditis (new version 2009): the Task Force on the Prevention, Diagnosis, and Treatment of Infective Endocarditis of the European Society of Cardiology (ESC). Endorsed by the European Society of Clinical Microbiology and Infectious Diseases (ESCMID) and the International Society of Chemotherapy (ISC) for Infection and Cancer. Eur Heart J 2009;30:2369–413.

Hill EE, Herijgers P, Herregods MC, Peetermans WE. Evolving trends in infective endocarditis. Clin Microbiol Infect 2006;12:5–12.

Hoen B. Epidemiology and antibiotic treatment of infective endocarditis: an update. Heart 2006;92:1694–700.

Karchmer AW. Infective endocarditis. In: Zipes DG, Libby P, Bonow R, editors. Braunwald's heart disease: a textbook of cardiovascular medicine, 7th edn. Philadelphia: Saunders, 2005.

Nishimura RA, Carabello BA, Faxon DP, et al. American College of Cardiology/American Heart Association Task Force. ACC/AHA 2008 guideline update on valvular heart disease: focused update on infective endocarditis: a report of the American College of Cardiology/American Heart Association Task Force on Practice Guidelines: endorsed by the Society of Cardiovascular Anesthesiologists, Society for Cardiovascular Angiography and Interventions, and Society of Thoracic Surgeons. Circulation 2008;118:887–96.

Prophylaxis Against Infective Endocarditis: NICE Clinical Guidelines, No. 64. Antimicrobial prophylaxis against infective endocarditis in adults and children undergoing interventional procedures. Centre for clinical practice at NICE (UK). London: National Institute for Health and Clinical Excellence (UK). <http://www.nice.org.uk/CG064>; 2008 [Accessed Nov. 2012].

Thiele H, Zeymer U, Neumann FJ, et al. IABP-SHOCK II Trial Investigators. Intraaortic balloon support for myocardial infarction with cardiogenic shock. N Engl J Med 2012;367:1287–96.

Vahanian A, Alfieri O, Andreotti F, et al. Guidelines on the management of valvular heart disease (version 2012): The Joint Task Force on the Management of Valvular Heart Disease of the European Society of Cardiology (ESC) and the European Association for Cardio-Thoracic Surgery (EACTS). Eur Heart J 2012;33:2451–96.

Wang A, Athan E, Paul A, et al. Contemporary clinical profile and outcome of prosthetic valve endocarditis. J Am Med Assoc 2007;297:1354–61.

5.8 Peripheral vascular disease

Colin A Graham

ESSENTIALS

1 The incidence of peripheral arterial and venous disease in the developed world continues to increase significantly with the continuing rise in the elderly population.

2 Claudication is the most important symptom of arterial disease in an extremity, although a well-developed collateral circulation will delay the onset of symptomatic extremity ischaemia.

3 Acute arterial occlusion is usually associated with a number of classic symptoms and signs. It is a time-critical emergency requiring urgent access to an experienced vascular surgeon.

4 If venous thrombosis is suspected, detailed assessment is essential. Unfortunately, the presence or absence of signs and symptoms of deep venous thrombosis (DVT) does not correlate well with the presence or absence of venous clot. Homan's sign is non-specific and unreliable.

5 Optimal assessment for DVT consists of defining a pre-test probability of disease and then performing appropriate non-invasive investigations in the first instance.

6 Compression ultrasonography is the investigation of choice for the diagnosis of DVT.

7 Anticoagulation is the recommended treatment for DVT above the level of the popliteal vein. Treatment of below-knee DVT remains controversial, but evidence suggests that these patients should also receive anticoagulation treatment to prevent complications.

8 Extensive iliofemoral thrombus or thrombus of the upper limb may require early surgical and/or thrombolytic treatment to minimize the risk of post-thrombotic syndrome.

Arterial disease

Extremity ischaemia may be acute, chronic or acute on chronic. The onset and severity of symptoms may be modified by the development of collateral circulation.

Chronic arterial ischaemia

Epidemiology, pathogenesis and pathology

The prevalence of peripheral arterial disease increases with age (most symptomatic patients are aged over 60) and is twice as high in men as in women between the ages of 50 and 70 years, but almost identical after the age of 70 at around 15–20%.

Peripheral arterial disease is usually due to atherosclerosis of the lower abdominal aorta or the iliac, femoral and/or popliteal arteries. In common with carotid and coronary artery disease, the disease processes that exacerbate peripheral arterial disease include diabetes mellitus, hypertension, smoking, hyperlipidaemia and previous limb surgery or trauma. A significant collateral circulation may develop. If so, it is made up of pre-existing pathways arising from the distributing branches of large and medium-sized arteries. It develops over time when there is an increase in the velocity of flow through them secondary to arterial occlusion developing in a main vascular pathway. Collateral flow can usually provide an adequate supply to the resting limb, but may be insufficient to meet additional requirements associated with moderate exercise.

Clinical features

Presentation may be acute or chronic. Symptoms consist of pain, ulceration or changes in appearance with swelling or discoloration. Lower limb ischaemia usually manifests as claudication – the most important symptom of extremity arterial occlusive disease. Chronic critical lower limb ischaemia is defined by either of the following two criteria:

- Recurring ischaemic rest pain persisting for more than 2 weeks and requiring regular analgesics. There should be an ankle systolic pressure of <50 mmHg, a toe systolic pressure of <30 mmHg, or both.
- Ulceration or gangrene of the foot or toes, with similar haemodynamic parameters.

The classic description of claudication is of pain in a functional muscle unit that occurs as a result of a consistent amount of exercise and is promptly relieved by rest. Limp may also be pronounced. The commonest site of occlusion leading to claudication is the superficial femoral artery, resulting in pain in the calf. This occurs on walking upstairs or slopes and is relieved by rest. Less commonly, aortoiliac disease produces symptoms of pain in the thigh or buttock. Night pain experienced in the foot, relieved by either dependency or, paradoxically, by walking around, implies a reduction in blood flow to a level below that required for normal resting tissue metabolism. Typically, rest pain tends to be distal to the metatarsals, severe, persistent and worsened by elevation.

Detailed examination of the peripheral vascular system is essential. Abnormalities tend to be related to changes in the peripheral arteries and tissue ischaemia. Distal pulses may be absent or diminished in amplitude and bruits (commonly femoral) may be present. Capillary return is usually reduced, atrophic changes are present and the foot is cool to the touch. Pallor may be apparent on exercise and is usually associated with pain. There may be pallor on elevation of the foot, with reactive hyperaemia on dependency: the more limited the elevation resulting in pallor, the greater the degree of stenosis (Buerger's test).

As ischaemia becomes more advanced, the skin becomes shiny and scaly, with associated atrophy of the subcutaneous tissues and muscle. In advanced stages of ischaemia, there may be red discoloration, caused by capillary blood stasis and high oxygen extraction. There may also be tissue necrosis and non-healing wounds or ulcers secondary to trauma, which may progress to gangrene.

Clinical investigations

Routine blood tests should be carried out to derive baselines for renal and hepatic function as well as to exclude anaemia, polycythaemia, hyperglycaemia, thrombocythaemia and hyperlipidaemia. In patients less than 50 years of age, a thrombophilia screen should be done and serum homocysteine levels measured.

The ankle–brachial pressure index (ABPI) should be measured to confirm the clinical diagnosis. This is calculated (for each leg) by dividing the highest systolic pressure recorded at the respective ankle by the highest systolic brachial pressure obtained in recordings from both arms. Resting ABPI is normally >1 and figures of <0.92 indicate arterial disease. Values between 0.5 and 0.9 may be associated with claudication and <0.5 with rest pain. Normal ABPI values may be recorded in diabetic patients, even though they have claudication, owing to the presence of medial arterial calcification and small vessel rather than large vessel disease.

Duplex ultrasound is initially used to assess the vascular tree non-invasively. Digital subtraction angiography (DSA) has now been superseded by computed tomography angiography (CTA) or magnetic resonance angiography (MRA) as they are both non-invasive and give a three-dimensional image of the disease extent. MRA is generally considered a first line investigation if available, with CTA being used if there is a contraindication to MRA; DSA is still required if intervention (e.g. angioplasty) is planned.

Treatment

In patients with chronic stable disease, treatment is focused on preventing progression of the disease. This is usually coordinated by the patient's primary care physician and consists of regular exercise, control of associated medical diseases and cessation of smoking. Specific measures should be taken to address hyperlipidaemia, diabetes mellitus and hypertension. A low dose antiplatelet agent (usually aspirin) should be given if there is no contraindication, but there is no benefit from warfarin therapy for this indication alone. Beta-blockers have been shown to be safe in patients with peripheral arterial disease.

In more advanced progressive disease, strategies to minimize other complications,

including lower limb ulcers and gangrene, should also be considered. Patients presenting to the emergency department (ED) at this stage or with debilitating symptoms merit early referral for vascular surgical assessment with a view to operative or radiological (endovascular) intervention.

Acute arterial ischaemia of the lower limb

Pathogenesis and pathology

Acute lower limb ischaemia, or 'limb-threatening' ischaemia, is associated with significant morbidity and mortality. Early recognition of the signs and symptoms is critical. Arterial occlusion will cause symptoms most obviously when there is inadequate collateral circulation. Causes may be embolic, thrombotic, traumatic or iatrogenic in nature, of which emboli are the most common. Most arterial emboli originate in thrombus formed in the heart (85%), the vast majority of these from left atrial thrombus related to chronic atrial fibrillation. Other uncommon causes include arterial thrombosis due to endothelial injury or alterations in the blood flow to the limb. Iatrogenic causes may be secondary to intra-arterial cannulation, recent cardiac catheterization or angiography or ischaemic limb anaesthesia (such as a Bier's block).

Clinical features

Sudden occlusion of a previously patent artery is a dramatic event. Unfortunately, recognition can be difficult, particularly in elderly people with chronic confusional states, and careful examination is therefore essential. Occlusion may be portrayed by one or more of the classic signs of pulselessness, pain, pallor, paraesthesia and paralysis (the '5 Ps'). However, none of the above, either alone or in combination, is sufficient to establish or exclude the diagnosis of an acute ischaemic limb. Loss of a palpable pulse in the symptomatic limb compared to the other side should raise significant concern.

The pain is a severe, constant ache which requires intravenous opiates for relief. The ischaemic periphery is pale, white or cadaveric in appearance and feels cold to touch. Progression occurs with blotchy areas of cyanosis and further discoloration. Pain, tense swelling and acute tenderness of a muscle belly are late findings. If these findings persist

for longer than 12 hours, irreversible ischaemia with gangrene is highly likely.

Clinical investigation

Doppler ultrasound should be used in all patients where there is concern about the arterial circulation of a limb. A handheld Doppler probe will confirm the presence or absence of a pulse and give some quantification of flow. Ultrasound may also be used to rapidly establish the level of arterial occlusion. Other investigations, including basic haematology and biochemical profiles, as well as electrocardiography and chest radiography, help to identify other diagnostic possibilities (e.g. low cardiac output state, polycythaemia, aortic dissection) and other contributing factors (such as atrial fibrillation) and establish fitness for urgent surgical intervention.

Differential diagnosis

It is important (but can be difficult) to differentiate between an embolic event and acute progression of a thrombus. The embolic event will tend to be sudden in onset and exhibit some combination of the '5 Ps'. *In-situ* progression of thrombus will occur in patients who have long-standing significant peripheral arterial disease and a well-developed collateral circulation. Other diagnoses that must be considered include aortic dissection and phlegmasia cerulea dolens. The latter is a massive iliofemoral deep venous thrombosis. The initial symptom may be an acutely swollen and painful leg. As the swelling continues, there may be secondary arterial insufficiency. Acute embolus, on the other hand, tends to produce pallor and a sharp demarcation, whereas with phlegmasia cerulea dolens there is a swollen cyanotic-appearing limb.

It is important to consider other medical causes that can mimic acute embolism of the upper or lower limb. These include neurological disorders (spinal subarachnoid haemorrhage) and low-output states, such as advanced sepsis, myocardial infarction or pulmonary embolus.

Treatment

The key to management is rapid diagnosis and access to definitive care. Irreversible changes begin to occur within 4–6 hours of symptom onset and revascularization is reported to be less effective after 8–12 hours of ischaemia. Intravenous heparin should be given immediately (in the absence of any contraindication) and other correctable aggravating factors (dehydration, sepsis, arrhythmias, myocardial infarction) should be considered and addressed appropriately.

Urgent surgical intervention is critical if an embolic event is thought to have occurred. Embolectomy using a Fogarty catheter, with or without a more definitive revascularization procedure, is the preferred option. Angiography is not necessary in such circumstances as it introduces unnecessary delay; it can be done intraoperatively if necessary.

In patients with acute limb ischaemia of less than 14 days duration due to thrombosis, intra-arterial thrombolytic therapy has been shown to have similar efficacy to surgical arterial reconstruction in two large randomized trials, both in terms of mortality and limb salvage. Intracranial haemorrhage does appear to be more common in the thrombolytic-treated group.

Patients with acute arterial ischaemia should be referred to an experienced vascular surgeon as early as possible; a multidisciplinary approach with vascular surgeons and interventional radiologists may give the best outcomes.

Acute arterial ischaemia of the upper limb

Epidemiology, pathology and pathogenesis

Symptomatic vascular disease of the upper limb is relatively rare compared to the lower limb. Presentation to the ED is usually due to coldness or colour changes in the upper limb or digits.

Acute arterial obstruction may arise secondary to emboli or from penetrating, blunt or iatrogenic trauma. Less commonly, acute occlusion may be associated with thoracic aortic dissection. Emboli affecting the upper limb most frequently involve the brachial artery. Radial and ulnar artery emboli tend to arise from atherosclerotic plaques, aneurysms of the subclavian and axillary arteries and from complications of thoracic outlet syndrome, rather than from a cardiac source. The diagnosis may be obvious (e.g. trauma) or suggested by the presenting history and clinical findings.

Acute occlusion of a digital artery results in profound ischaemia of the involved digit. Diagnosis is made on clinical grounds, with sudden onset of pain, pallor, coldness and numbness in the affected digit. A chest X-ray

may identify a cervical rib. Referral to a vascular surgeon is indicated for further investigations to identify the cause.

Clinical features

Examination of the limb, comparing with the other side, palpation of the pulses and assessment of capillary return, as well as detailed examination of the neck, may help localize the level of occlusion. Use of the hand-held Doppler and ultrasound may negate the need for preoperative angiography.

Management

When emboli are thought to be the cause (e.g. atrial fibrillation), embolectomy is the treatment of choice, usually under local anaesthesia. In some cases, thrombolysis may be considered. In the presence of acute ischaemic symptoms of the forearm and hand due to trauma, urgent operative repair is mandatory. In the case of injuries to the radial or ulnar arteries, if only one vessel is damaged and collateral flow is satisfactory, the injured vessel may be ligated.

Venous disease: lower limb

In contrast to arterial disease, chronic peripheral venous disease most commonly gives rise to cosmetic concerns (varicose veins) only. However, thrombosis in the deep venous system is a life-threatening emergency requiring urgent treatment.

It is important to understand that the venous drainage of the lower limb comprises superficial and deep systems connected by perforating veins. A complex system of valves and muscle pumps ensure that blood is carried up from the feet back to the heart. Venous pathology, such as valvular destruction, results in directional flow change and venous pooling.

Venous insufficiency and varicose veins

Primary varicose veins develop in the absence of deep venous thromboses (DVT). The main underlying physiological defect in varicose veins is venous valvular incompetence. Varicose veins may also arise secondary to venous outflow obstruction plus valvular incompetence or there may be primary venous outflow obstruction only.

Acute complications of varicose veins leading to ED attendance are uncommon. However,

the skin overlying varices can become thin and erosion can occur spontaneously or with minor trauma alone, resulting in bleeding. The essentials of treatment include elevation of the limb and gentle digital pressure on the site. Ligation of the offending vein may be necessary. Surgical treatment or injection of the varicosities is usually required as a later procedure.

Superficial venous thrombosis

Superficial venous thrombosis is a benign, self-limiting disease in most cases. Exclusion of DVT is usually required, although occasionally the diagnosis is obvious. Patients usually present with pain, tenderness and induration along the course of the vein, which may feel firm, cord-like and have associated erythema. There are usually no signs of impaired venous return. Underlying causes include varicose veins, surrounding cellulitis or a history of preceding trauma. In the upper limb, the commonest cause is intravenous cannulation.

Treatment depends on the extent, aetiology and symptoms. Superficial, mildly tender and well-localized thrombophlebitis may be treated with mild analgesics, usually oral non-steroidal anti-inflammatory agents (NSAIDs), topical NSAID creams, elastic supports and continued daily activity. More severe thrombophlebitis with marked pain, tenderness and erythema may require a period of rest and elevation of the limb. Antibiotics are not indicated. Anticoagulation is necessary only if the process extends into the deep venous system or approaches the saphenofemoral junction. The prognosis is usually good and there is no associated tendency for the development of deep venous thrombosis. The process may take 3–4 weeks to resolve. If associated with a varicose vein, superficial thrombophlebitis may recur unless the varix is excised.

Deep venous thrombosis

Deep venous thrombosis (DVT) is a condition characterized by active thrombosis in the deep venous system of one or both lower limbs. Depending upon the thrombus load and the level of extension of the thrombotic process, embolism proximally into the central pulmonary circulation can lead to sudden collapse and death. Early recognition and treatment is therefore essential. The diagnosis and management of acute DVT has changed in recent years, with a move towards structured assessment, non-invasive investigations and more aggressive treatment for patients with distal clots.

Clinical features

Symptoms and signs vary, with one-third having no clinical signs at all. A small number may have classic manifestations. Pain may be located in the calf and/or the thigh, ranging from a dull ache to a tight sensation, and is sometimes related to exercise. Examination findings include calf swelling, calf tenderness, tenderness over the popliteal or femoral veins and oedema, but may occasionally be entirely normal. Circumferential limb measurements may be helpful, but differences up to 1 cm occur naturally. Homan's sign is non-specific and unreliable. In addition, it is important to incorporate an objective assessment of risk factors for DVT.

One validated prediction model for assessment resulting in the generation of a pre-test probability of lower limb DVT has been developed and validated by Wells et al. (Table 5.8.1). A pre-test probability score of 2 or more means that DVT is 'likely' and compression ultrasonography should be performed. If the score is less than 2, then DVT is 'unlikely' and a D-dimer assay should be performed (see below).

Clinical investigation

If the derived pre-test probability of DVT is 'likely', compression ultrasonography is recommended. It is the imaging method of choice to diagnose DVT. Local protocols and expertise will determine whether this is done by a radiologist or an emergency physician. If necessary, patients who are haemodynamically stable and are otherwise fit for outpatient care can be given an injection of a low molecular weight heparin (LMWH) for the treatment of presumed DVT and allowed home, to return during office hours the following day for their compression ultrasound investigation. The overall sensitivity of ultrasound for any lower limb DVT is around 94–99%, with 89–96% specificity. A negative ultrasound result in the setting of persistent clinical suspicion or continuing symptoms of DVT warrants repeat testing at 5–7 days, but alternative diagnoses should also be actively sought. Venography is no longer recommended for the routine diagnosis of DVT.

If the pre-test probability of DVT is 'unlikely', a D-dimer assay is performed to determine the need for imaging to exclude DVT. D-dimers are degradation products of cross-linked fibrin blood clots, typical of those found in DVT. The level therefore rises in acute DVT, but it also rises in other acute conditions, such as infection and following trauma. Therefore, a positive test does not rule in DVT, but a negative test has a high negative predictive value for DVT and can therefore rule out disease. The combination of a low pre-test probability of disease and a negative D-dimer effectively excludes DVT and the patient can be safely discharged without the need for further investigation. However, D-dimer test characteristics vary greatly depending on whether the method used is an enzyme-linked immunosorbent assay (ELISA) or a variant of a whole blood latex agglutination study. Local expertise in the interpretation of these markers is essential in such circumstances. Local clinical protocols should therefore be followed to ensure that patients who are discharged are being appropriately and safely screened for DVT.

Differential diagnosis

The prevalence of DVT in patients with suggestive symptoms attending the ED ranges from 16 to 30%. Other alternative diagnoses include cellulitis, superficial thrombophlebitis, a ruptured Baker's cyst, chronic leg oedema, chronic venous insufficiency, postoperative swelling and arthritis.

Treatment

The standard treatment for established DVT is anticoagulation. If clinical assessment suggests that DVT is likely and there is any delay in confirming the diagnosis by compression ultrasonography, anticoagulation with LMWH should be instituted, provided there are no contraindications (e.g. active bleeding). The treatment of choice for DVT is now LMWH unless the patient has severe renal impairment, when unfractionated heparin should be used. LMWH has been shown to be superior to unfractionated heparin in terms of mortality, recurrence and bleeding events.

There is agreement that when a DVT is diagnosed in the popliteal vein and above, anticoagulation is indicated. In these circumstances, for most patients, LMWH can be administered on an outpatient basis.

Outpatient treatment is preferred by patients and appears to be cheaper. Hospital-based treatment is indicated if there is severe oedema of the whole of the lower limb or if there is thrombus above the groin. LMWH should be continued for several days while oral anticoagulation treatment is started. Warfarin remains the standard treatment and should be given along with the LMWH until the INR is above 2, with a target range between 2 and 3.

A recently approved alternative to LMWH and warfarin treatment is the direct Factor Xa inhibitor rivaroxaban. Oral rivaroxaban 15 mg is taken twice daily for the first 3 weeks after diagnosis, followed by 20 mg once daily for the duration of anticoagulation. It is contraindicated in severe hepatic and renal failure and doses should be reduced in moderate renal impairment. The anticoagulant activity of rivaroxaban is not reflected by the INR and there is no commonly available method of monitoring activity. The major benefit for patients is the removal of the need for injections and lack of requirement to monitor

Table 5.8.1 Well's criteria for DVT

Criterion	Score
Active cancer?	1
Bedridden recently >3 days or major surgery within 4 weeks?	1
Calf swelling >3 cm compared to the other leg?	1
Collateral (non-varicose) superficial veins present?	1
Entire leg swollen?	1
Localized tenderness along the deep venous system?	1
Pitting oedema, greater in the symptomatic leg?	1
Paralysis, paresis or recent plaster immobilization of the lower extremity	1
Previously documented DVT?	1
Alternative diagnosis to DVT as likely or more likely?	−2

anticoagulation status, in contrast to warfarin therapy which requires frequent monitoring and dose adjustment. The major problem with rivaroxaban is that if a bleeding complication does occur, unlike warfarin, there is no known method of reversing its anticoagulant activity.

Cancer patients may benefit from 3 to 6 months of LMWH treatment instead of warfarin therapy, but this should be guided by local protocols. Irrespective of the initial anticoagulation regimen employed, all patients require ongoing anticoagulation for 3–6 months, although the optimal duration continues to be debated. Patient care should be continued by referral to a haematologist or vascular physician according to local practice.

The use of below-knee graduated elastic compression stockings can reduce the incidence of post-phlebitic syndrome, but benefits are only evident after 2 years' use. Patients should be encouraged to use them after lower limb DVT.

For patients with an extensive iliofemoral thrombus, consideration should be given to thrombolysis, especially if there are haemodynamic changes suggestive of multiple pulmonary emboli. Thrombectomy may be indicated if the vital functions of the lower limb are threatened, with the aim of reducing the risk of post-thrombotic syndrome. Occlusive lower extremity venous thrombi respond poorly to systemic thrombolysis and the risks of bleeding may outweigh the justification of its use. Catheter-directed thrombolytic therapy, however, has been used to treat large symptomatic iliofemoral thrombi with some success.

Pregnant women with suspected DVT have not been extensively studied with respect to excluding DVT, so caution must be exercised when assessing these patients. In general, they should all undergo compression ultrasonography and there should be a low threshold for treatment with LMWH.

A dilemma arises when there is an isolated DVT below the level of the popliteal vein or when there is an equivocal finding in the infrapopliteal area and negative findings above. Options include withholding anticoagulation and following the patient with serial ultrasound studies or implementation of anticoagulation. In the setting of an infrapopliteal or calf-vein clot where anticoagulation is not commenced, repeat ultrasound at 5–7 days will determine with a high degree of sensitivity whether the clot has propagated above the knee. As the risk of pulmonary embolism from calf DVT is of

the order of 5% and given the safety of LMWH treatment, it is probably prudent to treat confirmed below-knee DVT and to investigate further equivocal cases with serial ultrasound studies. (See Chapter 5.5 for the diagnosis and management of pulmonary embolism.)

Venous disease: upper limb

Thrombosis of the subclavian and axillary veins is much less common than thrombosis of the lower extremity veins. It is usually associated with the presence of an indwelling venous catheter, active cancer or mechanical compression of the vein. It can follow upper extremity exertion such as weightlifting – the so-called 'effort thrombosis' – but this is very uncommon.

Clinical features

Patients present with swelling of the extremity, developing either rapidly or slowly over a period of weeks. Severe pain is uncommon: the usual symptoms are arm heaviness and discomfort exacerbated by activity and relieved by rest.

Clinical findings may include an increased prominence of hand and forearm veins, venous patterns over the shoulder and hemithorax, skin mottling or cyanosis and non-pitting oedema. There may be tenderness to palpation of the axillary vein within the axilla. The ipsilateral internal jugular vein is not usually enlarged. If it is, the possibility of a superior vena cava obstruction should be considered.

Clinical investigation

The diagnosis should be made by duplex ultrasound scanning, which has a high sensitivity and specificity for upper limb DVT.

Treatment

Standard treatment consists of anticoagulation with heparin to prevent progression of thrombosis. Traditionally, unfractionated heparin has been used, but there are increasing reports of successful management of upper limb DVT with LMWH. Rest, heat and elevation of the arm in a sling give good symptomatic relief. Catheter-directed thrombolytic therapy, anticoagulation and possibly venous angioplasty may be considered to restore vein patency and reduce the risk of re-thrombosis (although this is very low in the absence of other risk factors).

Thoracic outlet decompression should be considered if mechanical compression of the upper limb veins is diagnosed.

The use of long-term anticoagulation should only be considered if the patient has risk factors predisposing to recurrent thrombosis (e.g. thrombophilia).

Likely developments over the next 5–10 years

- The impact of statin therapy and other secondary prevention of vascular disease may lead to a reduction in the incidence of peripheral arterial disease in developed countries, while the increasing incidence of smoking and atherogenic dietary consumption in developing countries, along with the increasing age of the population, will lead to an increase in the incidence of arterial and cardiovascular disease in those countries.
- New developments in anticoagulant drug therapy are likely to change the management of venous disease further.
- In the future, all emergency physicians may be trained to diagnose or exclude DVT definitively by compression ultrasound to allow immediate treatment decisions to be made for patients with suspected DVT.

Controversies

- The evolving role of systemic or intra-arterial thrombolysis for acute arterial occlusion.
- Optimum drug regimens, costs and duration of anticoagulation therapy for DVT are still not clear.
- Anticoagulation for below-knee DVT.
- Investigative protocols and treatment algorithms for pregnant women have not been researched adequately, so the previous recommendations cannot be applied to pregnant women.

Further reading

Bauersachs R, Berkowitz SD, Brenner B, et al. EINSTEIN Investigators. Oral rivaroxaban for symptomatic venous thromboembolism. N Engl J Med 2010;363:2499–510.
Blinc A, Poredos P. Pharmacological prevention of atherothrombotic events in patients with peripheral arterial disease. Eur J Clin Invest 2007;37:157–64.

Cogo A, Lensing AWA, Koopman MMW, et al. Compression ultrasonography for diagnostic management of patients with clinically suspected deep vein thrombosis: prospective cohort study. Br Med J 1998;316:17–20.

Cohen AT, Dobromirski M. The use of rivaroxaban for short- and long-term treatment of venous thromboembolism. Thromb Haemost 2012;107:1035–43.

Marston WA, Davies SW, Armstrong B, et al. Natural history of limbs with arterial insufficiency and chronic ulceration treated without revascularization. J Vasc Surg 2006;44:108–14.

NICE Guidelines CG147. Lower limb peripheral arterial disease: full guideline. <http://guidance.nice.org.uk/CG147/Guidance/pdf/English> [Accessed Jan. 2013].

Ouriel K, Veith FJ, Sasahara AA. A comparison of recombinant urokinase with vascular surgery as initial treatment for acute arterial occlusion of the legs. Thrombolysis or Peripheral Arterial Surgery (TOPAS) Investigators. N Engl J Med 1998;338:1105.

Peach G, Griffin M, Jones KG, Thompson MM, Hinchliffe RJ. Diagnosis and management of peripheral arterial disease. Br Med J 2012;345:e5208.

Scottish Intercollegiate Guidelines Network (SIGN). Prevention and management of venous thromboembolism. Edinburgh: SIGN; SIGN Publication No. 122. <http://www.sign.ac.uk/guidelines/fulltext/122/index.html>; 2011 [Accessed Jan. 2013].

Tendera M, Aboyans V, Bartelink ML, et al. European Stroke Organisation. ESC Committee for Practice Guidelines. ESC

Guidelines on the diagnosis and treatment of peripheral artery diseases: Document covering atherosclerotic disease of extracranial carotid and vertebral, mesenteric, renal, upper and lower extremity arteries: the Task Force on the Diagnosis and Treatment of Peripheral Artery Diseases of the European Society of Cardiology (ESC). Eur Heart J 2011;32:2851–906.

Weaver FA, Comerota AJ, Youngblood M, et al. Surgical revascularization versus thrombolysis for nonembolic lower extremity native artery occlusions: results of a prospective randomized trial. The STILE Investigators. Surgery versus thrombolysis for ischemia of the lower extremity. J Vasc Surg 1996;24:513.

Wells PS, Owen C, Doucette S, et al. Does this patient have deep vein thrombosis? J Am Med Assoc 2006;295:199–207.

5.9 Humpertension

Barry Gunn • Maisse Farhan • Marian Lee

ESSENTIALS

1 Hypertension is defined as a systolic blood pressure ≥140 mmHg and/or a diastolic blood pressure ≥90 mmHg.

2 Hypertensive emergencies are more likely to complicate inadequately controlled hypertension, including those that are undiagnosed.

3 The exact mechanism for the acute rise in blood pressure in hypertensive crisis is not well understood.

4 The pathophysiological consequences of hypertensive crisis are fibrinoid necrosis in arterioles followed by endothelial damage, platelet and fibrin deposition, loss of autoregulatory function and microangiopathic haemolytic anaemia.

5 Management depends on the clinical syndrome, the presence of complications or coexisting conditions and the risks of intervention.

6 Hypertensive encephalopathy mandates urgent control of the blood pressure.

7 There is insufficient evidence to support aggressive blood pressure control in the setting of acute stroke.

Table 5.9.1	Spectrum of hypertension
Hypertension category	**Blood pressure range (mmHg)**
High normal	120–139/80–89
Grade I	140–159/90–99
Grade II	160–179/100–109
Grade III	>180/>110
Isolated systolic hypertension	>140/<90

Introduction

Normal blood pressure is defined as <120/<80 mmHg. Hypertension is defined as a systolic blood pressure ≥140 mmHg and/or a diastolic blood pressure ≥90 mmHg. The spectrum of hypertension is shown in Table 5.9.1.

Hypertensive crises are uncommon and occur in 1–2% of the hypertensive population. They are defined by a diastolic blood pressure >120 mmHg. However, some have argued that the absolute magnitude of the blood pressure is not important. Rather, the defining factor is the presence of end-organ dysfunction. The latter

is uncommon when the diastolic blood pressure is <130 mmHg.

Hypertensive crisis can be divided into two distinct clinical entities. Where the sudden rise in the systolic and diastolic blood pressure is associated with end-organ dysfunction, this is a hypertensive emergency and reduction of blood pressure within 1–2 hours is vital to outcome. A hypertensive urgency is when there is no evidence of end-organ dysfunction. The risk of decompensation is, however, high and blood pressure control within 24–48 hours is the goal. When a hypertensive crisis is present, it is

crucial that it is recognized early and appropriate management undertaken.

Epidemiology

The current prevalence of hypertension in the Australian population is 11% and hypertension is estimated to affect 1 billion people worldwide. Three per cent of the adult population develop hypertension each year. Hypertension is more common in males than in females and the risk of developing hypertension increases with age. Australian indigenous peoples and African-Americans have a predisposition to hypertension.

It is estimated that 30% of hypertensive patients are undiagnosed and 29% of patients with known hypertension are inadequately controlled.

Hypertensive emergencies

Aetiology and pathophysiology

Hypertensive emergencies can complicate both primary and secondary hypertension

Table 5.9.2   Causes of secondary hypertension

System	Specific pathology
Vascular	Aortic dissection
Renal disease (primary)	Renal artery stenosis Renal parenchymal disease IgA nephropathy
Endocrine	Thyrotoxicosis Cushing's syndrome Primary hyperaldosteronism Phaeochromocytoma Hyperparathyroidism
Drug-induced	Cocaine Amphetamines Selective serotonin reuptake inhibitors Monoamine oxidase inhibitors when taken with tyramine-containing foods
Drug withdrawal	Clonidine β-Blockers Angiotensin-converting enzyme inhibitors
Other	Autonomic hyperactivity

(Table 5.9.2), the former being more common. The majority of hypertensive emergencies occur in patients with pre-existing hypertension. The pathophysiology of hypertensive crisis remains incompletely understood. The actual magnitude of the blood pressure is not a dependable guide to the likelihood of end-organ damage.

The chronicity of the underlying pathology means that adaptive vascular mechanisms are present. Hence end-organ damage occurs at a higher pressure than in patients with recent-onset hypertension. For instance, a previously well patient with an acute rise in blood pressure as a result of acute glomerulonephritis will have end-organ dysfunction at a lower blood pressure than a patient with long-standing hypertension.

The actual precipitant of an acute increase in vascular tone is unknown, but the result is the release of humoral vasoconstrictors. The consequent increase in blood pressure leads to:

- Mechanical stress on endothelium, with local release of vasoconstrictors perpetuating hypertension, activation of platelets and the coagulation cascade and, ultimately, fibrinoid necrosis of small vessels.
- Natriuresis and consequent volume depletion results in activation of the renin–angiotensin–aldosterone system, thereby perpetuating vasoconstriction and increasing plasma volume. The consequent systemic vasoconstriction impairs target organ perfusion, culminating in ischaemia.

Clinical syndromes

The essential clinical features of hypertensive emergencies are symptom complexes reflecting the target organ concerned. Target organs of particular interest are the brain, heart, kidney and large arteries. Target organ dysfunction is uncommon at diastolic BP <130 mmHg.

The recognized hypertensive emergencies are:

- hypertensive encephalopathy
- hypertension with stroke
- acute pulmonary oedema
- acute myocardial ischaemia
- acute aortic dissection
- acute renal dysfunction
- pre-eclampsia (see Section 19).

Hypertensive encephalopathy

This is an acute organic brain syndrome resulting from a failure of cerebral vascular autoregulation. Autoregulation occurs between a mean arterial pressure (MAP) of 60 and 120 mmHg; cerebral blood flow is constant between this range. As blood pressure rises, there is compensatory vasoconstriction to prevent hyperperfusion. The upper limit of the compensatory mechanism is a MAP of 180 mmHg. When this point is reached, vasodilatation occurs, resulting in cerebral oedema (due to endothelial damage) and, less commonly, cerebral haemorrhage. The magnitude of the MAP at which hypertensive encephalopathy is manifested depends on the chronicity of the hypertension. In previously normotensive patients, this can occur at a BP of 160/100 mmHg, i.e. MAP of 120 mmHg. In patients with known hypertension, encephalopathy may not occur until the blood pressure is much higher, probably because of a shift in the cerebral autoregulation range.

The classic clinical triad is severe hypertension, altered level of consciousness (confusion, coma, seizures) and retinopathy (retinal haemorrhages, exudates, papilloedema). Symptoms may include headache of gradual onset and blurring of vision.

If unrecognized, cerebral haemorrhage, oedema and death result. Patients at higher risk include those with untreated or inadequately controlled hypertension, renal disease, thrombotic thrombocytopenic purpura, pre-eclampsia and eclampsia and those on medications, such as erythropoietin and certain immunotherapy treatments.

Accelerated malignant hypertension is an entity referring to severe hypertension with retinal changes, including flame haemorrhages and soft exudates but without encephalopathy. Papilloedema may or may not be present. It is found in patients with long-standing hypertension. Headache and blurred vision are common (85% and 55%, respectively).

Acute pulmonary oedema and myocardial ischaemia

An acute and severe rise in the blood pressure can cause an acute myocardial ischaemia syndrome and acute pulmonary oedema without obstructive coronary arteries disease. However, in patients who have pre-existing hypertension, coronary artery disease may already be present and the risk of myocardial dysfunction is increased. An acute blood pressure rise leads to increased mechanical stress on the left ventricular wall and, consequently, a rise in myocardial oxygen demand.

In patients presenting with symptoms and signs consistent with acute pulmonary oedema and myocardial ischaemia, the magnitude of the blood pressure will identify those with a hypertensive emergency.

Acute aortic dissection

This is the most rapidly deteriorating hypertensive emergency. It is also the most devastating and the mortality remains high. It should be suspected in the setting of hypertension associated with chest pain. This is discussed in detail in Chapter 5.10.

Acute renal failure

An acute and severe elevation in blood pressure may lead to deterioration in renal function, which is usually unsuspected. Acute and severe hypertension is more likely to be the result of renal disease than the cause of renal dysfunction, thus it is essential to look for evidence of underlying renal disease. Urinalysis may be abnormal. In acute severe hypertension, there is severe proteinuria, haematuria and cellular sediments. In chronic hypertension, mild proteinuria without haematuria is more usual.

Additionally, renal insufficiency may itself be the cause of the hypertensive emergency. This creates a vicious cycle of deterioration in renal function leading to an elevation of the blood pressure which, in turn, compounds the renal dysfunction. Risk groups include patients with chronic renal failure, especially those requiring dialysis, and patients who have had a renal transplant, especially if taking corticosteroids and cyclosporin.

Clinical features

History is focused on determining the cause of hypertension, whether it has been previously diagnosed and, if so, the type of treatment and compliance, a drug history and a search for symptoms of target organ dysfunction.

Examination concentrates on blood pressure measurement, a careful cardiovascular examination (peripheral pulses, cardiac failure, renal bruits), neurological examination and fundoscopy. The finding on fundoscopy of retinal haemorrhages, microaneurysms and exudates is associated with a high risk of subsequent stroke.

Clinical investigation

The objectives of investigations are to detect the presence of end-organ dysfunction as well as to identify the underlying cause of the hypertension.

Bedside tests

- ECG, particularly in the setting of chest pain and hypertension. ECG is abnormal in ~22% of asymptomatic patients with diastolic blood pressure >110 mmHg, although the clinical significance of this is unclear.
- Urinalysis: for haematuria and proteinuria.
- Urine drug screen: if sympathomimetic drugs are suspected.

Blood tests

- Full blood examination to detect anaemia and haemolysis.
- Renal function tests.
- Serum electrolytes may reveal a secondary cause for hypertension.

Imaging

- Chest X-ray: a routine chest X-ray is of little diagnostic value.
- Cerebral computed tomography (CT), if evidence of neurological impairment. This will rule out haemorrhagic stroke and may show the characteristic posterior leucoencephalopathy indicative of hypertensive encephalopathy.

Other investigations will be dictated by the clinical presentation.

Treatment

Management depends on the clinical syndrome, the presence of complications or coexisting conditions and the potential risks of intervention. The aim of treatment is to stop progressive deterioration of target organ function. The risk in treatment is iatrogenic target organ hypoperfusion from an overshoot in blood pressure reduction. In general, the aim is to reduce mean arterial pressure by no more than 25%, as a higher reduction risks organ hypoperfusion, especially in those with chronic underlying hypertension. The goal is to achieve this within 1–2 hours in order to halt progressive damage – the exception being aortic dissection, where blood pressure control within 5–10 minutes is desirable. If intravenous antihypertensive agents are used, this should take place in a resuscitation area with close blood pressure monitoring. Where control within a strictly defined range is required, intra-arterial blood pressure monitoring is preferable. Volume depletion is common secondary to pressure natriuresis. Volume replacement with normal saline to restore organ perfusion may prevent a precipitous fall in blood pressure and its consequences.

Large clinical trials looking at the optimum therapy in hypertensive emergencies are not available. Hence the specific treatments discussed below are largely not evidence-based but supported by consensus.

Hypertension and acute stroke

Management of hypertension is determined by the type of stroke. In ischaemic stroke, reduction in blood pressure is always at the risk of causing hypoperfusion of the peri-ischaemic area, which may result in an extension of the stroke. In ischaemic stroke, hypertension is usually transient and has not been shown adversely to affect the clinical course. In fact, there is some evidence that patients with

higher mean arterial pressures have better outcomes. In the absence of other end-organ dysfunction or intention to treat with thrombolysis, current American Heart Association guidelines recommend treatment if the systolic BP >220 mmHg and/or the diastolic BP >120 mmHg. Australian guidelines agree regarding the systolic cut-off but recommend treatment if the diastolic BP >110 mmHg. For patients suitable for thrombolysis, treatment is required to achieve systolic BP <180 mmHg or diastolic BP <105 mmHg. If there is evidence of other organ dysfunction, treatment should be tailored to reduce damage to that organ while balancing the risk of further cerebral ischaemia.

In haemorrhagic stroke/primary intracranial haemorrhage, hypertension is part of the reflex response to the resultant intracranial hypertension and is usually transient. The rationale for treatment of hypertension is that this would reduce further bleeding and hence haematoma expansion. This has not been proven for primary intracranial haemorrhage and evidence to support treatment of hypertension in this clinical scenario is lacking. It has been shown that isolated systolic BP <210 mmHg is not associated with intracranial haemorrhage expansion or neurological deterioration and that reduction of mean arterial pressure by 15% is not associated with neurological deterioration. Recommendations regarding treatment of intracranial haemorrhage-associated hypertension are largely based on consensus and vary around the world. As a general indication, recommendations in Australia are to treat if the systolic BP >180 mmHg or the diastolic BP >110 mmHg. The stated target blood pressure is 160/90 mmHg.

Myocardial ischaemia (see Chapter 5.2)

The aim is to reduce myocardial work and promote coronary blood flow and thus reduce ischaemia. The agent of choice is IV glyceryl trinitrate. Beta-blockers, especially metoprolol, may be a useful adjunct.

Acute pulmonary oedema (see Chapter 5.3)

Glyceryl trinitrate is preferred because of its vasodilatory effect on coronary arteries as well as preload and afterload reduction. Diuretics should be reserved for patients who are volume overloaded, as they may exacerbate pressure-induced natriuresis and increase stimulation of the renin–angiotensin system.

Hypertensive encephalopathy

The divide between the risks and benefits of treatment in hypertensive encephalopathy is small. The clinical manifestation may be reversible; however, the risks of treatment are ischaemia and infarction due to too rapid a fall in the mean arterial pressure. The consensus is a fall in mean arterial pressure by 20–25% or to a diastolic blood pressure of 100–110 mmHg, whichever value is greater, over 2–4 hours. Vigilant monitoring is essential as any deterioration of clinical status must result in reduction or cessation of the drug used, irrespective of the magnitude of the reduction in blood pressure.

Centrally acting drugs that can affect mental status are not used. The preferred agent is sodium nitroprusside (SNP). Possible alternatives are intravenous labetalol and glyceryl trinitrate. The dose range for sodium nitroprusside is 0.5–10 mg/kg/min. SNP requires normal hepatic and renal function for its metabolism and excretion and hence cannot be used in patients with renal or hepatic impairment. Labetolol, an α- and β-adrenergic blocker, is given as an infusion of 1–2 mg/min.

Aortic dissection (see Chapter 5.10)

Acute renal insufficiency

In patients with chronic renal failure, an acute elevation in blood pressure with subsequent worsening of renal function may require a combination of treatment targeting volume imbalance (e.g. by dialysis) as well as blood pressure (e.g. with sodium nitroprusside). Diuretic use should be judicious as, in the absence of hypervolaemia, it may be deleterious. In patients with *de novo* acute renal insufficiency, the management is complex and best done in consultation with a renal physician. Emergency ultrafiltration may be required in cases refractory to medical treatment.

Hypertensive urgency

Treatment

The appropriate management of hypertensive urgency relies on an accurate assessment of the presence or absence of end-organ dysfunction. In the asymptomatic patient, it can be difficult to determine whether the dysfunction is acute or pre-existing. Past history and laboratory results are extremely useful to provide a comparison. It may be that this decision cannot be made and treatment is started without a clear distinction between emergency and urgency. The importance of the clinical assessment in hypertensive urgency is to identify the subset of patients likely to progress to a hypertensive emergency. The features suggestive of this are a first presentation of severe hypertension, a history of poorly controlled hypertension, ischaemic heart disease or cerebrovascular disease.

As a general rule, treatment and hospital admission are required if the diastolic BP remains above 120 mmHg 30–60 minutes after resting. The treatment goal is a reduction in the mean arterial pressure by 20% over 24–48 hours using an oral antihypertensive agent.

A wide range of oral antihypertensive agents is available. Angiotensin-converting enzyme (ACE) inhibitors are a reasonable first-line selection in most patients. Note that the majority of patients are hypertensive due to poor or non-compliance with medications. In general, the disposition of the patient depends on the presence of significant co-morbidities, response to treatment and the availability and accessibility for outpatient follow up within 24 hours of discharge.

Prognosis and disposition

Prognosis depends on the success of treatment to halt deterioration of target organs.

All patients with hypertensive emergencies should be admitted to a suitable high dependency area. The high-risk patient with hypertensive urgency requires hospital admission for observation and blood pressure stabilization.

Developments in the next 5–10 years

- Better understanding of the precipitants of hypertensive emergencies.

Controversies

- Reduction of the elevated blood pressure in the acute phase of a stroke remains controversial. There is no consensus on the indication to treat or the timing of intervention. Each case should be considered individually, with careful consideration given to the risks and benefits of lowering the BP.

Further reading

Broderick J, Connolly S, Feldmann E, et al. Guidelines for the management of spontaneous intracerebral hemorrhage in adults. 2007 Update: Guidelines from the American Heart Association/American Stroke Association Stroke Council, High Blood Pressure Research Council, and the Quality of Care and Outcomes in Research Interdisciplinary Working Group. AHA/ASA Guideline. Stroke 2007;38:2001–23.

Cherney D, Straus S. Management of patients with hypertensive urgencies and emergencies – a systematic review of the literature. J Gen Intern Med 2002;17:937–45.

Feldstein C. Management of hypertensive crises. Am J Ther 2007;14:138–9.

Gray RO. Hypertension. In: Marx JA, editor. Rosen's emergency medicine: concepts and clinical practice (6th ed.). Philadelphia: Mosby, 2006, p. 1314–5.

Haas AR, Marik PE. Current diagnosis and management of hypertensive emergency. Semin Dial 2006;19:502–16.

Marik PE, Varon J. Hypertensive crisis: challenges and management. Chest 2007;131:1949–62.

National Heart Foundation Australia. Hypertension management guide for doctors. <http://www.heartfoundation.org.au/ Professional_Information/Clinical_Practice/Prevention. htm>; 2004 [Accessed Jan. 2012].

Shayne PH, Pitts SR. Severely increased blood pressure in the emergency department. Ann Emerg Med 2003;41:513.

Therapeutic Guidelines Ltd. Acute stroke treatment (revised November 2012) in: eTG complete <http://www.tg.com.au/ ip/complete/> [Accessed Dec. 2012].

Underwood M, Lobo BL, Finch C, et al. Overuse of antihypertensives in patients with acute ischaemic stroke. South Med J 2006;99:1230–3.

Varon J, Marik PE. Clinical review: the management of hypertensive crises. Crit Care 2003;7:374–84.

Vaughan CJ, Delanty N. Hypertensive emergencies. Lancet 2000;356:4411–17.

Waybill MM, Waybill PN. A practical approach to hypertension in the 21st century. J Vasc Intervent Radiol 2003;14:961–75.

5.10 Aortic dissection

Michael Coman

ESSENTIALS

1 Untreated aortic dissection has a mortality rate of approximately 1% per hour for the first 48 hours and 90% at 3 months. Early diagnosis and aggressive management improve mortality rates to 20–40%.

2 Aortic dissection is a clinical diagnosis confirmed through focused investigation. A high index of suspicion is required.

3 Both false-negative and false-positive diagnoses of aortic dissection result in increased morbidity and mortality.

4 If available, transoesophageal echocardiography in the unstable patient and CT aortography in the stable patient are the preferred imaging modalities for patients suspected of suffering aortic dissection.

5 Therapy aimed at reducing blood pressure and the force of ventricular contraction should commence as soon as the diagnosis is suspected.

6 Proximal dissections require emergency surgery. Uncomplicated distal dissections are generally treated medically, while complicated distal dissections are usually managed with endoluminal stenting or surgery.

Table 5.10.1 Predisposing factors for aortic dissection

Major associations
Hypertension
Congenital cardiovascular disorders
Aortic stenosis
  Bicuspid aortic valve
  Coarctation of the aorta
Connective tissue disorders
  Marfan's syndrome
Ehlers–Danlos syndrome

Other associations
Iatrogenic (post-cardiac surgery or balloon angioplasty for coarctation)
Cocaine
Pregnancy
Inflammatory diseases
  Giant-cell arteritis

CARDIOVASCULAR EMERGENCIES

Introduction

Aortic dissection is an uncommon yet potentially lethal condition. A high index of suspicion is required to diagnose it owing to the broad range of presenting signs and symptoms. Investigations must be carefully chosen and rapidly performed to confirm the diagnosis. Treatment should be commenced as soon as the diagnosis is suspected as, untreated, the mortality rate is approximately 1% per hour for the first 48 hours.

Aortic dissection is one of a group of similar conditions that constitute the acute aortic syndrome. Acute aortic syndrome describes several related life-threatening aortic pathologies, including aortic dissection, intramural haematoma, penetrating aortic ulcer and traumatic aortic transection with incomplete rupture. These conditions all progress to the same pathophysiological endpoint: separation of the aortic intima from the outer aortic layers, with predictable and often devastating consequences. There is considerable overlap in the signs, symptoms and principles of management of the conditions that constitute acute aortic syndrome.

Epidemiology, pathophysiology and classification

The incidence of aortic dissection is 3 patients/100 000 population/year. One-third to one-half of all cases are diagnosed at autopsy. Although the overall incidence is low, aortic dissection is the most common catastrophe of the aorta, being two to three times more common than rupture of the abdominal aorta.

Most cases occur in males, particularly between the ages of 50 and 70. Proximal dissections involving the aortic arch have a peak incidence 10 years earlier than distal dissections. Risk factors are shown in Table 5.10.1. Hypertension is the single most important risk factor. The diagnosis of aortic dissection must be considered in any patient with a history of hypertension who presents with sudden severe chest, back or abdominal pain.

Arterial hypertension and degeneration of the aortic media are the two key elements of aortic dissection. Dissection occurs when blood is forced along a low-resistance tissue plane within the wall of the aorta created by a diseased and weakened media.

Two pathophysiological processes have been proposed to initiate the dissection. The traditional explanation requires a breach in the intima (an intimal tear) to initiate the dissection process. The tear occurs at sites where hydrodynamic and torsional forces on the aorta are greatest, most commonly a few centimetres above the aortic valve (60–65%) or just beyond the insertion of the ligamentum arteriosum (30–35%). A column of high-pressure aortic blood gains access to the media and dissects through the weakened tissue plane, creating a false lumen. The dissection can extend in an antegrade or retrograde direction. The alternative mechanism suggests that diseased or unsupported vasa vasorum within the media rupture, creating an intramural haematoma. The haematoma dissects through the media as it expands, subjecting the unsupported media to increased shearing forces during diastolic recoil of the aorta. Eventually – but not necessarily – this may lead to a tear in the intima. In this mechanism, the intimal tear is a consequence of the dissection, not an initiating factor. An intimal tear is not identified in 12% of autopsies, suggesting that it is not a mandatory precursor for aortic dissection.

Regardless of the primary process producing dissection, the sequelae are identical. As the dissection extends, any structures caught in its path may be affected. Branch vessels of the aorta may be distorted or occluded, resulting in

277

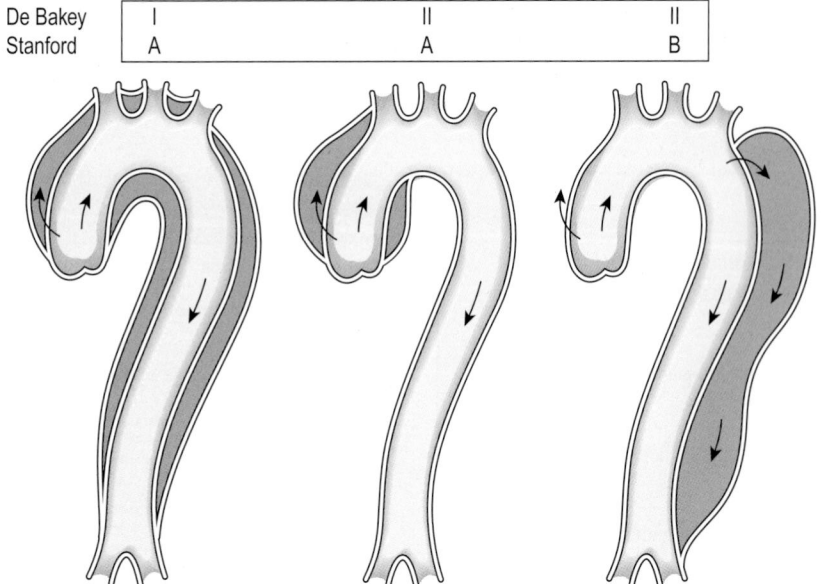

De Bakey I | II | II
Stanford A | A | B

Fig. 5.10.1 Anatomical classification of aortic dissection. *(Reproduced with permission from Erbel R, Alfonso F, Boileau C, et al. Diagnosis and management of aortic dissection. Eur Heart J 2001; 22:1642–81.)*

signs and symptoms of ischaemia to the organs they supply. Proximal dissection may produce acute aortic valve incompetence and continued proximal extension may enter the pericardial sac, tamponading the heart. The false lumen created by the dissection may also partially or completely obstruct the true lumen. It may end in a blind sac or rupture back into the true lumen at any point. The false lumen may also rupture outwards through the adventitia. If this occurs, rapid exsanguination will occur if the haematoma is not contained. Common sites of external rupture are into the left pleural cavity or mediastinum.

Once dissection begins, propagation is dependent on the blood pressure and the gradient of the arterial blood pressure wave, which is a function of the velocity of left ventricular contraction. This explains why urgent pharmacological treatment is aimed at lowering arterial blood pressure and reducing the ventricular contractile force.

Classification

The Stanford and De Bakey systems are two commonly used, anatomically based classification systems. Both describe the site of the dissection, providing information that assists management.

The Stanford system divides aortic dissection into two types (Fig. 5.10.1). Type A (65–70% of cases) involves the ascending aorta, with or without the descending aorta. The presence or absence of an intimal tear, the site of the tear and the extent of distal extension are not considered in this classification. Type B dissections (30–35%) involve the descending aorta only which, by definition, begins distal to the origin of the left subclavian artery. The Stanford system is simple, easy to remember and has become the primary classification system referred to in the literature.

The De Bakey classification system divides aortic dissection into three types (see Fig. 5.10.1). Type I involves both the ascending and the descending aorta. Type II involves the ascending aorta only. Type III involves the descending aorta only and is subdivided into type IIIa, which is confined to the thoracic aorta, and type IIIb, which extends into the abdominal aorta.

Aortic dissection is classified as acute if symptoms are present for fewer than 14 days, chronic if longer than 14 days.

Clinical features

History

Pain is the most common presenting symptom, occurring in 74–95% of patients. Pain is classically described as severe, unremitting, tearing or ripping in nature and maximal at onset. It may be migratory, reflecting proximal or distal extension of the tear. The site of the pain may reflect the site of the dissection, with involvement of the ascending aorta typically producing anterior chest pain. Interscapular pain can occur with involvement of the descending aorta and, as distal dissection continues, the pain may migrate to the lower back or abdomen.

Other symptoms of aortic dissection are related to the effects of major aortic side branch occlusion. Almost 20% of dissections present with coma, confusion or stroke. This may signify carotid artery involvement or may reflect end-organ hypoperfusion due to hypovolaemic shock from external rupture of the aorta or cardiogenic shock caused by pericardial tamponade. Neurological symptoms often fluctuate. Lower limb paraplegia or paraesthesia (2–8%) may occur as spinal arteries are separated from the aortic lumen. Syncope (18% type A and 3% type B) may suggest rupture into the pericardial sac.

Symptoms may also be due to local compression from a contained rupture. These are uncommon, but may include superior vena cava syndrome, dysphonia, dyspnoea, dysphagia, upper airway obstruction and Horner's syndrome.

A history of risk factors for aortic dissection should also be obtained (see Table 5.10.1).

Examination

There is no single examination finding that will confirm the diagnosis. It is common for patients to be acutely distressed, apprehensive and for their pain to be resistant to narcotic analgesia.

Patients usually present with a tachycardia owing to a combination of pain, anxiety and possibly shock. Hypertension is seen in 50–78% of patients, especially those suffering type B dissection. This may reflect an underlying history of hypertension or an acute response to pain and anxiety. Hypotension is an ominous sign, suggesting free rupture of the aorta or pericardial tamponade. Evidence of side branch occlusion may include stroke, limb ischaemia or neurological dysfunction, pulse deficits or a difference of 15 mmHg or more in manually taken blood pressures between the upper limbs.

Evidence of proximal extension to involve the aortic valve or pericardium may produce acute aortic incompetence, possibly with signs of acute left ventricular failure. A diastolic murmur indicative of acute aortic incompetence is a common finding in proximal dissection (50–68%). Pericardial tamponade may manifest with Beck's triad: hypotension, muffled heart sounds and raised jugular venous pressure. Pulsus

Table 5.10.2 Radiographic features suggesting dissection
Widening of the superior mediastinum (52–75%)
Dilatation of the aortic arch (31–47%)
Change in the configuration of the aorta on successive CXR (47%)
Obliteration of the aortic knob
Double density of the aorta (suggesting true and false lumina)
Localized prominence along the aortic contour (38%)
Disparity of calibre between the descending and the ascending aorta (34–67%)
Displacement of the trachea or nasogastric tube to the right
Distortion of the left main stem bronchus
Calcium sign (>6 mm between the intimal calcium and the shadow of the outer aortic wall: 7–17%)
Pleural effusion, more common on the left (15–20%)
Cardiomegaly (21%)

paradoxus may be present or a pericardial friction rub may be heard. Involvement of the renal arteries may result in oliguria or anuria.

Aortic rupture may present with shock or clinical signs of a haemothorax, usually left-sided.

Serial examination is important, as signs may change as the dissection progresses.

Clinical investigations

Specific investigations are required to confirm or exclude aortic dissection. There are, however, a number of initial investigations that may identify an alternative diagnosis or serve to increase the clinical suspicion of aortic dissection. Routine haematological or biochemical investigations are of little value in the immediate diagnosis of aortic dissection and, at best, provide baseline renal function and haemoglobin level.

Electrocardiography

An electrocardiogram (ECG) should be performed on all patients with suspected aortic dissection, as acute myocardial infarction (AMI) is a major differential diagnosis. Ten to 40% of patients with aortic dissection will have ECG evidence suggestive of acute ischaemia. Seven per cent of dissections involve the coronary arteries, yet only 0.9–2.4% of patients will have ECG changes in keeping with AMI. Total coronary artery occlusion is less common than partial occlusion and the right coronary artery is more commonly involved than the left. The ECG may display voltage criteria for left ventricular

hypertrophy, reflecting a long-standing history of hypertension.

Chest X-ray

A number of chest X-ray (CXR) abnormalities have been described in patients with aortic dissection (Table 5.10.2). The sensitivity and specificity of each individual finding is poor and, for this reason, no single finding should be used for predictive purposes. Many findings are subtle and are best seen on a good-quality erect PA film. In reality, the clinical condition of the patient may only allow a supine, mobile AP film. Retrospective audits of plain radiographs of patients known to have aortic dissection reveal abnormalities suggesting the diagnosis in 72–90% of cases; however, attempts to prospectively identify aortic dissection in blinded studies yield less reliable results (sensitivity of 81% and specificity of 82–89%).

Up to 20% of radiographs are normal in patients suffering dissection. At best, the CXR may increase the clinical suspicion of aortic dissection or identify alternative pathology. A normal-appearing CXR must never be used to exclude aortic dissection.

Specific investigations

All patients in whom aortic dissection is suspected must have a diagnostic test performed without delay. Options include computed tomography (CT), echocardiography, aortography and magnetic resonance imaging (MRI). The aim is to determine safely and rapidly whether a dissection is present, its site,

the structures involved and the presence of complications. The most appropriate investigation will depend on patient and institutional factors, including patient stability, test availability and access. Each emergency department should have a prearranged imaging strategy for the diagnosis of suspected aortic dissection.

Computed tomography

This is usually the imaging modality of choice to confirm the diagnosis of acute aortic dissection, assuming that the patient is suitable for transfer to the scanner. Arterial phase scanning with intravenous contrast creates a CT aortogram. Images are rapidly obtained and can be reconstructed in multiple planes. Motion artefact is reduced through the rapid data acquisition capabilities of modern scanners. Increased availability, after-hours reporting via teleradiology and the trend to position scanners in close proximity to emergency departments have increased the utility of CT.

CT is the preferred study in stable patients with a low-to-moderate index of suspicion for aortic dissection, as it is effective in identifying alternative pathologies. Diagnosis is based on the demonstration of an intimal flap, shown as a low-attenuation linear structure within the aortic lumen. Secondary findings of aortic dissection include internal displacement of luminal calcification and delayed contrast enhancement of the false lumen. Sensitivity and specificity for diagnosing arch vessel involvement is high (93% and 98%, respectively). CT can also identify complications of aortic dissection including pericardial, mediastinal and pleural blood. Disadvantages include the requirement for intravenous contrast and patient transport.

Recent advances in multislice CT, including CT coronary angiography, raise the possibility of diagnostic testing for both aortic dissection and coronary artery disease in one test, albeit with higher contrast and radiation loads. There are currently insufficient data to determine the safety or utility of this approach.

Echocardiography

Transoesophageal echocardiography (TOE) has emerged as an excellent diagnostic investigation for aortic dissection in centres where it is available. Ideal for critically ill patients, TOE can be rapidly and safely performed at the bedside and is highly sensitive and specific

Table 5.10.3 Sensitivity and specificity of diagnostic investigations

Investigation	Sensitivity (%)	Specificity (%)
CT	83–100	90–100
TTE	78–100: type A 31–55: type B 59–85: all	63–96
TOE	97–99	97–100
Aortography	81–91	94
MRI	95–100	95–100

Table 5.10.4 Differential diagnosis of aortic dissection

Cardiovascular
  Acute coronary syndrome with or without ST-segment elevation
  Shock
  Acute pulmonary oedema
  Acute valvular dysfunction
  Pericarditis
  Acute extremity ischaemia

Pulmonary
  Pulmonary embolus
  Pneumothorax

Gastrointestinal
  Pancreatitis
  Peptic ulcer disease (including perforation)
  Oesophageal spasm/reflux
  Ischaemic bowel

Neurological
  Stroke/transient ischaemic attack
  Spinal cord compression

Renal
  Renal colic

(Table 5.10.3). In addition, TOE can give a functional assessment of the aortic valve and the left ventricle and can identify other complications of aortic dissection, including the involvement of coronary arteries and the presence of pericardial blood.

Disadvantages of TOE include limited availability outside major centres and the requirement for a skilled and available operator. TOE is invasive and patients may require sedation and airway protection to perform the test. It is contraindicated in patients with known oesophageal pathology, including varices, strictures or tumours.

The diagnosis is confirmed by demonstrating the intimal flap separating the true and false lumina. The true lumen can be distinguished from the false lumen as it is usually smaller, expands during systole (compared to compression of the false lumen during systole) and is less commonly thrombosed. Central displacement of luminal calcium may confirm the presence of aortic dissection in situations where the false lumen has thrombosed.

Transthoracic echocardiography (TTE) is no longer considered a useful screening test in view of its low sensitivity and specificity (see Table 5.10.3). TTE is particularly poor at imaging the transverse arch and the descending aorta, owing to interference from the airway.

Aortography
Formerly the gold standard investigation for aortic dissection, aortography is now rarely performed owing to the development and refinement of less invasive, more sensitive and rapid alternatives.

Magnetic resonance imaging
MRI is highly sensitive and specific, providing excellent visualization of the site and extent of dissection and complications including side branch involvement. The major disadvantages relate to patient safety and ease of access. Studies are lengthy, patient accessibility is poor during the study and remote monitoring is required. MRI equipment is frequently located at a distance from resuscitation facilities. For these reasons, MRI is not suitable for unstable or potentially unstable patients despite the comprehensive information it can provide and is best reserved for surveillance or for ongoing evaluation of aortic dissection.

Biomarkers
The use of biomarkers, particularly the D-dimer, for early detection of aortic dissection and as part of a 'rule out' algorithm are attracting interest. A 2010 meta-analysis of the usefulness of D-dimer to diagnose acute aortic dissection could not conclude that it can be used as a 'rule-out' test and prospective trials are required to further assess the utility of D-dimer in diagnosis of aortic dissection. There remains no widely accepted strategy for biomarker-assisted diagnosis of acute aortic dissection, as no single biomarker has been validated and combination biomarker arrays are yet to be investigated.

Differential diagnosis
The diagnosis of aortic dissection is rarely straightforward and there is a long list of differential diagnoses (Table 5.10.4) owing to the wide range of presenting symptoms and signs. With the advent of thrombolysis for acute embolic stroke, care must be taken to consider aortic dissection as a stroke mimic prior to the administration of thrombolytic agents. This would be one reason why CT perfusion protocols for acute stroke image from the aortic arch, allowing aortic dissection to be identified.

Treatment
Initial management for all types of aortic dissection focuses on resuscitation, stabilization, prevention of ongoing dissection by management of haemodynamic parameters and facilitation of definitive care, if required.

Treatment must be started as soon as the diagnosis is suspected. Unstable patients require immediate resuscitation. Diagnostic investigations and management of life-threatening complications may need to take place simultaneously. Measures to minimize progression of the dissection need to be instituted rapidly and early surgical referral is mandatory. Early diagnosis, control of blood pressure and heart rate, and early surgical repair are all associated with improved survival.

Patients with aortic dissection are usually in severe pain and require large doses of titrated IV narcotic analgesia, which should not be delayed or withheld. A secondary benefit from the relief of pain is a reduction in blood pressure and heart rate.

Pharmcological control of pulsatile load
Pharmacological treatment is aimed at decreasing the pulsatile load ($\Delta p/\Delta t$) delivered by the left ventricle to the column of blood within the false lumen. This minimizes the likelihood of ongoing dissection. The pulsatile load is determined by the systolic blood pressure and the velocity of blood ejected from the heart. Importantly, blood pressure must be lowered without increasing the velocity of ventricular contraction, which can occur if afterload is reduced prior to blocking the reflex tachycardia and increased contractile velocity of the heart that afterload reduction produces.

If there is no contraindication, β-blockade is the ideal first-line agent owing to its negative inotropic and chronotropic effects on the heart. Esmolol, a short-acting β-blocker (half-life 9 minutes), which can be given by peripheral IV infusion and titrated to heart rate and blood pressure, is effective. A loading infusion of 0.5 mg/kg may be given by hand-held syringe over 1 minute. Following this, a maintenance infusion ranging from 50 to 200 µg/kg/min is commenced.

If esmolol is unavailable, or experience in its use is limited, titrated IV boluses of metoprolol are equally effective. A heart rate of 60–80 bpm and a systolic blood pressure of 100–120 mmHg are commonly quoted target ranges, but these figures are not defined by controlled trials. Intra-arterial monitoring is necessary for optimal blood pressure management.

If further blood pressure reduction is required following β-blockade, a vasodilator may be added. Sodium nitroprusside reduces afterload via systemic vasodilatation. Delivered by IV infusion, it is effective, has a rapid onset and short duration of action and can be readily titrated to effect. The usual infusion range is 0.5–10 mg/kg/min. Owing to the possibility of cyanide toxicity, the infusion should not continue for more than 24 hours.

An alternative agent to reduce blood pressure is glyceryl trinitrate (GTN), a drug more commonly and confidently used by most clinicians. Delivered by peripheral IV infusion, GTN reduces both preload and afterload by relaxing vascular smooth muscle. Reflex tachycardia is a common side effect and must be prevented by prior β-blockade. The infusion range is 5–50 µg/min and it can be rapidly titrated to clinical effect.

Treatment of type A aortic dissection

Open surgical repair of the aorta is the treatment of choice for acute proximal (type A) aortic dissection. The aim is to prevent rupture of the false lumen, re-establish blood flow to regions affected by occluded side branches, correct any associated acute aortic valve incompetence and prevent pericardial tamponade. Usual practice is to excise the section of the aorta containing the intimal tear and replace this with a prosthetic interposition graft. Operative mortality ranges from 5 to 21%. Without surgery, up to 90% of patients with acute type A dissection will die within 3 months. With surgery, there is a 56–87% 5-year survival.

Treatment of type B aortic dissection

Type B aortic dissection is classified as either complicated (30%) or uncomplicated (70%). Complicated aortic dissection refers to the presence of events carrying a high risk for death, including compromised lower body

Table 5.10.5 Indications for surgical repair/endoluminal stenting of type B aortic dissection
Leaking or ruptured aorta
End-organ ischaemia
Extension of dissection despite appropriate medical therapy
Refractory pain
Severe uncontrollable hypertension

perfusion or end-organ ischaemia, aortic rupture or impending rupture, progression of dissection, uncontrollable hypertension or refractory pain (Table 5.10.5).

Medical management has been generally accepted as the standard of care for uncomplicated type B aortic dissection. Tight blood pressure and heart rate control can produce survival rates of 80% over a 1-year period. Endoluminal stenting has not been shown to improve 2-year survival from uncomplicated type B aortic dissection when compared to medical management.

Complicated type B aortic dissection was historically managed by open surgical repair of the aorta, often in the setting of failed medical therapy. The mortality rates of open surgical repair were vey high, between 21 and 33.9%. The advent of less invasive endovascular stent deployment across the primary tear site has significantly improved mortality and morbidity from complicated type B aortic dissection. In-hospital mortality has fallen to 10% and major morbidity (renal failure and stroke) has halved from 40 to 20% when compared to open surgical repair.

All patients are discharged on lifelong β-blockers, regardless of initial medical or surgical treatment, or whether the patient is hypertensive or normotensive. Serial MRI examinations are necessary for long-term surveillance of the aorta.

Prognosis

A dramatic improvement in survival has been observed over the past 30 years owing to advances in medical and surgical management. One-year survival rates of 52–69% for type A and 70% for type B aortic dissection have been reported.

Eighty-six per cent of deaths from aortic dissection are due to aortic rupture, 70% of those

rupturing into the pericardial sac. Multiorgan failure is a significant cause of death following medical or surgical therapy.

Disposition

Those patients who do not require emergency surgery require admission to an intensive care area for monitoring and aggressive therapy aimed at minimizing propagation of their dissection. Patients in peripheral or regional centres will require transfer to a specialist cardiothoracic unit after their condition has been stabilized.

Controversies

- The role of intravascular ultrasound in diagnosis. Sensitivities and specificities of close to 100% have been reported but its practicality in the emergency department is unproven.
- Appropriate investigation. Lack of utility of CXR as a screening test. Choice of investigative modalities is governed by availability of testing modalities and stability of patient.
- The role of biomarkers.
- Preventative therapy in Marfan's syndrome. Routine β-blockade is advocated. Elective grafting of the aortic valve and ascending aorta is being advocated in some patients considered at high risk.

Further reading

Ahmad F, Cheshire N, Hamady M. Acute aortic syndrome: pathology and therapeutic strategies. Postgrad Med J 2006;82:305–12.

Bogdan Y, Hines GL. Management of acute complicated and uncomplicated type B dissection of the aorta. Cardiol Rev 2010;18:234–9.

Bourland MD. Rosen P, Barkin RM, editors. Emergency medicine: concepts and clinical practice. Chicago: Mosby, 1992, p. 1384–90.

Erbel R, Alfonso F, Boileau C, et al. Diagnosis and management of aortic dissection. Eur Heart J 2001;22:1642–81.

Gysi J, Schaffner T, Mohacsi P, et al. Early and late outcome of operated and non-operated acute dissection of the descending aorta. Eur J Cardiothorac Surg 1997;11:1163–9.

Jagannah AS, Sos TA, Lockart SH, et al. Aortic dissection: a statistical analysis of the usefulness of chest pain radiographic findings. Am J Radiol 1986;147:1123–6.

Kouchoukos NT, Dougenis D. Medical progress: surgery of the thoracic aorta. N Engl J Med 1997;336:1876–88.

Meszaros I, Morocz J, Szlavi J, et al. Epidemiology and clinicopathology of aortic dissection. A population-based longitudinal study over 27 years. Chest 2000;117:1271–8.

Nienaber CA, Rousseau H, Eggebrecht H, et al. Randomised comparison of strategies for type B aortic dissection: the

CARDIOVASCULAR EMERGENCIES

5

INvestigation of STEnt Grafts in Aortic Dissection (INSTEAD) trial. Circulation 2009;120:2519–28.

Ranasinghe MD, Bonser RS. Biomarkers in acute aortic dissection and other aortic syndromes. J Am Coll Cardiol 2010;56:1535–41.

Richards KA. Emergency department recognition and management of dissecting thoracic aneurysm. Emerg Med 1995;7:99–105.

Shimony A, Filion KB, Mottillo S, et al. Meta-analysis of usefulness of D-dimer to diagnose acute aortic dissection. Am J Cardiol 2011;107:1227–34.

Spittel PC, Spittel JA, Joyce JW, et al. Clinical features and differential diagnosis of aortic dissection: experience with 236 cases. Mayo Clin Proc 1993;68:642–51.

Trimarchi S, Nienaber CA, Rampoldi V, et al. Role and results of surgery in acute type B aortic dissection: insights from the

International Registry of Acute Aortic Dissection (IRAD). Circulation 2006;114:1357–64.

Zappa MJ, Harwood-Nuss A. Recognition and management of acute aortic dissection and thoracic aortic aneurysm. Emerg Med Rep 1993;14:1–8.

5.11 Aneurysms

John Loy

ESSENTIALS

1 Abdominal aortic aneurysms (AAA) are generally slow-growing and asymptomatic.

2 Screening programmes aim to detect their presence prior to rupture and promote early elective repair once size ≥5.5 cm.

3 Abdominal pain/back pain and hypotension should prompt a rapid search for abdominal aortic aneurysm in the ≥65 age group.

4 Rupture is an acute surgical emergency and requires minimal delay to operative intervention. Bedside ultrasound has assisted in rapid identification of aneurysms.

5 The mortality after rupture is very high – approximately 80% of those who reach hospital and 50% of those undergoing emergency surgery.

6 Emergency endovascular repair of abdominal aortic rupture is effective and may be preferable to traditional open repair in selected patients.

7 Symptomatic aneurysms of any size should be considered emergent.

8 Limited fluid resuscitation (hypotensive resuscitation) for abdominal aortic rupture has demonstrated improved outcome if the patient can tolerate such measures preoperatively.

9 Patients with femoral/popliteal aneurysms tend to present with complication from thrombosis/embolism rather than rupture. There is an association of lower limb aneurysms with abdominal aortic aneurysms.

10 The primary risk of central arterial aneurysms (aortic/iliac/pulmonary/visceral) is rupture which has a high risk of sudden death.

Abdominal aortic aneurysm

Introduction

An abdominal aortic aneurysm (AAA) is a permanent pathological dilation of the aorta >1.5 times the expected diameter. It involves all three layers of the vessel wall. For the infrarenal aorta in most adults, this is 3 cm which is the trigger for annual follow up once an AAA has been identified. AAAs are estimated to expand at 4–5 mm per year. Elective surgical repair is offered for AAAs discovered to be 5.5 cm or larger to prevent death from rupture.

They may unfortunately rupture without evidence of growth during the past year and therefore should be viewed as somewhat unpredictable.

The distal aorta is subject to the greatest arterial pressure changes and therefore biomechanical stress. Hence the majority of AAA are found below the renal arteries (90–95%). The remainder may involve the proximal renal arteries or even visceral branches of the aorta. They can also descend into the iliac vessels.

Most aneurysms are asymptomatic until a complication arises. These complications can be rupture, symptomatic expansion, thrombosis or embolism. The majority of ruptures are initially into the retroperitoneal space where it may be temporarily contained. Intraperitoneal rupture can be primary or follow a retroperitoneal event and has a higher mortality rate.

Rarely, an AAA will be complicated by chronic rupture, formation of a false or inflammatory aneurysm or an arteriovenous or aortoenteric fistula, atheroembolism, small bowel obstruction or ureteric obstruction.

Epidemiology

Five to 10% of men aged 65–79 years of age have an AAA and the prevalence increases by 6% per decade in men. AAA is more common in men, with a three- to fourfold higher prevalence than women.

The risk of aneurysm rupture has been shown to be proportional to aneurysm size, with aneurysms measuring less than 5.4 cm having an annual rupture rate of approximately 1–2% whereas those greater than 7.0 cm have an annual rupture rate of 32.5%.

Risk factors for AAA are age over 55 years, male, smoking, positive first-degree relative family history, chronic obstructive pulmonary disease, Marfan's syndrome and Ehlers–Danlos syndrome.

Aetiology/pathophysiology

Traditionally, arterial aneurysms were considered to be a consequence of atherosclerotic disease and intimal atherosclerosis does accompany AAA. Current thinking regarding aetiology is broadening and recent data are suggesting a causative role for matrix metalloproteinases.

This overall pathophysiology is multifactorial:

- There is proteolytic degradation of the aortic wall connective tissue. Matrix metalloproteinases along with other proteases derived from macrophages/aortic smooth muscle cells are secreted into the extracellular matrix. This enhanced enzyme activity may lead to the breakdown of the structural matrix proteins, such as collagen and elastin. Macrophages and lymphocytes are demonstrated to be present on histological analysis. This supports a theory of cytokine release and then structural protein degradation.

- There is an autoimmune process as IgG complexes have been located in the dilated aorta wall.
- Biomechanical wall stress is a component and the elastin–collagen ratio falls in the distal aorta. Diminished elastin is associated with aortic dilatation and the collagen degradation predisposes to rupture.
- Genetics play a role as there is familial clustering.

Prevention/screening

Screening may reduce the risk in high-risk groups and current regimens suggest one-time ultrasound screening for all men >65 years of age and for those 55 years of age with a positive family history.

Surveillance imaging at 12-monthly intervals is recommended for AAA 3.5–4.4 cm in diameter. For those 4.5–5.4 cm, 6-monthly surveillance imaging is indicated.

With regard to women in high-risk groups, one off ultrasound is suggested for those >65 years of age, although routine screening has insufficient evidence to support it currently.

Clinical features

History

The patient is usually male and over 65 years of age complaining of pain in the abdomen/back which may radiate into the flanks or down into the groin. There may be associated collapse or dizziness associated with rupture. Occasionally, neurological signs develop due to spinal cord ischaemia (T10–T12).

Examination

An AAA is felt as a pulsatile mass in the epigastrium above the level of the umbilicus. Generally, in thin patients, an AAA >5 cm can be found clinically. Physical examination can be insensitive in detecting aneurysms due to obesity, abdominal bloating, pain and when the aneurysm is less than 5 cm size.

Other physical examination findings may relate to consequences of bleeding, tachycardia, hypotension, postural drop in blood pressure, peritonism or pallor. Examination of the lower limb arterial pulses may reveal associated femoral/popliteal aneurysms or arterial insufficiency.

Of note, a contained retroperitoneal rupture may provide an unremarkable physical examination. The classical combination of abdominal pain, hypotension and a pulsatile abdominal mass is found in slightly less than 50% of patients with ruptured AAA. A high degree of clinical suspicion is advocated for patients over the age of 65 years of age with unexplained back/flank pain and syncope/hypotension.

Differential diagnosis

Symptomatic expansion or rupture may mimic other conditions, such as perforated viscus, intra-abdominal sepsis, renal colic, musculoskeletal back pain or myocardial infarction. Therefore, a high degree of suspicion is needed in patients over 65 years old.

Clinical investigations

This is directed by the initial index of suspicion and need to minimize delay. A patient with a known AAA who presents with abdominal pain and hypotension suggestive of rupture should not have surgery delayed by further investigations. A patient with a suspected AAA from history in whom a tender pulsatile abdominal mass consistent with an aneurysm is found, along with hypotension should also go directly to theatre.

Imaging

Bedside ultrasound is the test of first choice in those presenting with a history suggestive of aneurysm rupture and no prior aneurysm was known. Ultrasonography can detect AAA presence with sensitivity and specificity >95%, but can be limited by obesity, intraluminal gas and operator experience. A leak may not be identified on ultrasound and the exact anatomical mapping of the aneurysm may require further imaging in stable asymptomatic patients.

Other imaging modalities, e.g. computed tomography (CT), magnetic resonance imaging (MRI) or MR angiography (MRA), are mainly used for operative planning in stable patients. These modalities can also identify proximal aortic dilatation and renal artery involvement.

Other Investigations

Full blood count may reveal leucocytosis and pre-existing relative anaemia. Clinical

biochemistry, especially for renal function and glucose, is indicated. Cross-match of blood anticipating major transfusion (6–10 units) is essential. A coagulation screen may assist in identifying the risk of intraoperative disseminated intravascular coaglation (DIC). C-reactive protein and erythrocyte sedimentation rate (CRP/ESR) may be helpful if infective AAA suspected.

ECG should be performed to rule out myocardial infarction.

Treatment

Rapid surgical intervention is the definitive treatment of ruptured abdominal aortic aneurysm, so early notification of the vascular surgery team is essential.

Fluid resuscitation should be carefully chosen as large volume resuscitation (>3.5 L fluid) has reportedly worsened outcome. Currently, minimal fluid resuscitation aiming for a systolic BP 70–80 mmHg is the suggested approach in the preoperative phase. This approach should be tempered by maintaining vital organ perfusion. Lower limits have been suggested (50–70 mmHg) but this may not be practical in a majority of centres and there are significant institutional variations on acceptance of such lower limits. If they can be instituted quickly and do not delay surgery, intra-arterial pressure and urine output monitoring may assist in optimizing resuscitation endpoints.

Surgery

Emergency endovascular AAA repair (eEVAR) versus open repair Endovascular AAA repair (EVAR) is the most effective option for repair, aortoiliac anatomy permitting, otherwise traditional open repair is performed. eEVAR is less invasive, reduces surgical stress and can be achieved using locoregional anaesthesia. Intraoperative calibration angiography can be used to assess the anatomical suitability of aneurysms for eEVAR and reduce the preoperative delay. Approximately 50% of AAA are suitable for EVAR. A Cochrane review of endovascular repair for ruptured AAA (2007) concluded that no benefit has yet been established. However, reduction in mortality rates, reduction in ICU stay and reduction in blood loss are encouraging for EVAR.

Thirty-day mortality for open repair is around 50% compared to approximately 20% for EVAR in some studies. These data should be interpreted with caution as most studies of EVAR are observational and uncontrolled, so selection bias may have influenced results.

Some patients may be candidates for eEVAR who would not benefit from open surgical repair. This is a delicate time-critical decision process which involves the specialist surgeon/anaesthetist/interventional radiologist and patient/family representative.

Repair of symptomatic unruptured AAA is directed towards EVAR, anatomy permitting.

Prognosis

Rupture of abdominal aortic aneurysm leads to early death in over 80% of those affected. This includes 20–65% of those who undergo surgical repair. There are emerging data to suggest that long-term survival (>4 years) is similar between repair methods.

The conventional open surgical approach carries the significant risks of major open surgery and anaesthesia, haemorrhage, aortic clamping and lower torso ischaemic–perfusion injury.

After endovascular AAA repair, long-term surveillance is essential to monitor for endoleaks and stent integrity in order to reduce the small but significant incidence of late aneurysm rupture.

Thoracic aortic aneurysm (see Section 5.10)

Cerebral aneurysms (see Sections 8.2 and 8.3)

Visceral aneurysms

Introduction

The increased utilization of diagnostic imaging studies has led to increased identification of visceral aneurysms, which may involve the splenic, hepatic, coeliac, superior mesenteric, renal, gastroduodenal and other arteries.

Visceral aneurysms result from abnormal haemodynamics, atherosclerosis or infectious causes. Most are asymptomatic and are detected incidentally on imaging studies. However, they should be considered in any patient with abdominal pain, intra-abdominal bleeding or gastrointestinal bleeding. The diagnosis can be confirmed with CT, ultrasound (US), MRI or angiography. Up to 25% visceral aneurysms may be complicated by rupture and the mortality rate after rupture is between 25 and 70%.

Treatment should be considered in all patients with symptoms related to the aneurysm, if the aneurysm is greater than 2 cm in diameter, if the patient is pregnant or if there is demonstrated growth of the aneurysm. The

type of treatment depends on the clinical condition, the artery involved and the surgeon's preference. Options include open surgical ligation, prosthetic or venous graft reconstruction, percutaneous transcatheter metal coil embolization, endovascular stent–graft placement or even organ removal.

Splenic artery aneurysm

Splenic artery aneurysms (SAA) account for 60% of all visceral arterial aneurysms. They are the only aneurysms that are more common in women, with a female-to-male ratio of 4:1. Multiple aneurysms are present in about 20–30% of patients. The more common causes are atherosclerosis and portal hypertension. Splenic artery aneurysms are usually an incidental discovery on abdominal X-rays as signet ring calcifications in the left upper quadrant, especially in elderly patients. Most are less than 2 cm in diameter. Symptoms include left upper quadrant or epigastric pain radiating to the left shoulder or subscapular area. Only 2% of splenic artery aneurysms result in rupture. Of those that rupture, >95% occur in young women during the third trimester of pregnancy, with reported 35–75% maternal and 95% fetal mortality rates. Symptomatic SAAs require immediate operative intervention, particularly in pregnant women or women of childbearing age. In asymptomatic patients, treatment is controversial but should be considered if the diameter of the aneurysm is larger than 2 cm. Ruptured SAA is usually treated by splenectomy.

Hepatic artery aneurysm

Hepatic artery aneurysm constitutes 20% of visceral artery aneurysms and most commonly occurs in elderly males. More than 50% present with right upper quadrant/epigastric abdominal pain radiating to the back. Rupture into the biliary tract may result in the classic triad of acute biliary pain, haemobilia and jaundice. Erosion of the aneurysm into the stomach or duodenum may lead to haematemesis or melaena. Extrinsic compression of the biliary duct may cause obstructive jaundice. Because of the high mortality rate associated with rupture, surgical resection or transarterial catheter occlusion is warranted.

Superior mesenteric aneurysm

Superior mesenteric artery aneurysms are the third most common visceral aneurysm (8%). More than 90% are symptomatic, presenting with upper abdominal pain, gastrointestinal bleeding or acute mesenteric ischaemia from

thromboembolism. Around 50% have a pulsatile mass on physical examination.

Peripheral aneurysms

Peripheral aneurysms can occur in isolation or they may be found in association with other large vessel aneurysms (aorta). The most common site is the popliteal artery and, when symptoms are present, they generally reflect claudication, ischaemia or chronic embolization rather than rupture.

Popliteal artery aneurysm

A true popliteal aneurysm involves all layers of the vessel wall. They can be fusiform or saccular. An aneurysm is present once the size has exceeded 1.5 times the upper limit of normal (usually >1.7 cm in an adult). The pathogenesis is very similar to that described for aortic aneurysm. Growth is not quite as predictable as some popliteal aneurysms remain stagnant rather than expanding.

Clinical presentation may range from an asymptomatic individual with a pulsatile mass found in the popliteal fossa to acute limb threatening ischaemia. Bilateral popliteal aneurysms may be apparent.

Duplex ultrasonography is the first-line imaging modality when diagnosis is suspected clinically. This can be supplemented by CT or MR angiography.

Limb-threatening ischaemia is time critical and investigations should be under direction of the vascular surgeon who may opt for surgery over further emergent imaging.

Heparin infusion is utilized in patients with evidence of acute thrombosis, distal embolization or acute ischaemia.

Elective repair of popliteal aneurysms is generally offered once size is ≥2 cm.

Femoral artery aneurysm

Femoral artery aneurysms are less common then popliteal. They are, however, more prone to rupture. An aneurysm is present once size is ≥2.5 cm.

Upper limb aneurysms

Upper limb aneurysms are rare, usually the result of trauma and may involve the subclavian, axillary, brachial, radial and ulnar artery. The risks are of limb ischaemia and thromboembolic complications (including retrograde thromboembolism in the vertebral/carotid circulation). Brachial plexus compression may also occur due to growth of subclavian aneurysms.

Future developments

- Annual comprehensive screening programmes for abdominal aortic aneurysms do not currently exist; however, one-off screening in men ≥65 years of age is advocated for the initial detection of an aneurysm.
- The potential for macrolide antibiotics to be used as disease modification agents after the identification of an abdominal aortic aneurysm (animal studies suggest possible benefit).
- The nomination of the optimal blood pressure target for minimal fluid resuscitation in the ruptured abdominal aortic aneurysm.
- Extension of endovascular repair techniques and efficiency of delivery in time-critical emergency presentations.

Controversies

- The clinical decision not to proceed to emergency surgery with very high-risk cases of ruptured abdominal aortic aneurysms (refractory hypotension/cardiac arrest/age >80/requirement for massive blood transfusion).
- The long-term outcome with EVAR and subsequent risk of re-intervention/complications.
- The safe disposition of the stable patient with symptomatic but non-ruptured small AAA after imaging has been completed.
- Ultrasound credentialing for emergency clinicians who perform examinations to identify AAA and rupture.

Further reading

Basnyat PS, Biffin AH, Moseley LG, et al. Mortality from ruptured aortic aneurysm in Wales. Br J Surg 1999;86:765–70.

Brimacombe J, Berry A. Haemodynamic management in ruptured abdominal aortic aneurysm. Postgrad Med J 1994;70:252–6.

Chaikof EL, Brewster DC, Dalman RL, et al. Society for Vascular Surgery. The care of patients with an abdominal aortic aneurysm: the Society for Vascular Surgery practice guidelines. J Vasc Surg 2009;50:S2–49.

Cosford PA, Leng GC, Thomas J. Screening for abdominal aortic aneurysm. Cochrane Database Syst Rev 2007;2:CD002945.

Dillon M, Cardwell C, Blair PH, et al. Endovascular treatment for ruptured abdominal aortic aneurysm. Cochrane Database Syst Rev 2007;1:CD0056291.

Gorham TJ, Taylor J, Raptis S. Endovascular treatment of abdominal aortic aneurysm. Br J Surg 2004;91:815–27.

Johnston KW. Ruptured aortic aneurysm: six year follow up results of a multi-center prospective study. Canadian Society for Vascular Surgery Aneurysm Study Group. J Vasc Surg 1994;19:888–900.

Roberts K, Revell M, Youssef H, et al. Hypotensive resuscitation in patients with ruptured abdominal aortic aneurysm. Eur J Vasc Endovasc Surg 2006;31:339–44.

Ten Bosch JA, Teijink JA, Willigendael EM, Prins MH. Endovascular aneurysm repair is superior to open surgery for ruptured abdominal aortic aneurysms in EVAR-suitable patients. J Vasc Surg 2010;52:13–18.

Walker D. Vascular abdominal emergencies. Emerg Med Clin N Am 1996;14:584–91.

CARDIOVASCULAR EMERGENCIES

RESPIRATORY EMERGENCIES

Edited by **Anne-Maree Kelly**

6.1 Upper respiratory tract

Weng Hoe Ho • Ken Ooi

ESSENTIALS

1 Airway management and the ABCs take precedence over the history, examination and specific treatment of upper airway obstruction.

2 Direct laryngoscopy can be an important technique for both investigation and management of upper airway obstruction.

3 The Heimlich manoeuvre (abdominal thrust) is a useful first aid technique in foreign body upper airway obstruction, although scientifically unproven.

4 Acute viral respiratory infections are a frequent reason for seeking medical attention. Over-prescribing of antibiotics continues to be a major problem.

5 Bacterial infections and collections are uncommon but may compromise the upper airway.

6 A high index of suspicion is needed to diagnose blunt trauma injuries to the larynx and trachea.

7 Cervical spine injuries frequently accompany significant blunt laryngeal injuries.

Introduction

The upper respiratory tract extends from the mouth and nose to the carina. It comprises a relatively small area anatomically, but is of vital importance. The majority of presentations are not life threatening, however, those that are require immediate evaluation or treatment.

Emergent conditions are those likely to compromise the airway. Protection and maintenance of airway, breathing and circulation (the ABCs) take precedence over history taking, detailed examination or investigations. Possible causes of airway obstruction are listed in Table 6.1.1.

Non-urgent presentations include rash or facial swelling not involving the airway, sore throat in a non-toxic patient and complaints that have been present for days or weeks with no recent deterioration. Pharyngitis and tonsillitis are common causes for presentation in both paediatric and adult emergency practice.

Triage and initial evaluation

Initial evaluation should be aimed at differentiating those patients needing urgent management to prevent significant morbidity and mortality from those needing less urgent treatment. Triage must be based on the chief complaint and on vital signs since the same clinical presentation may result from a range of pathologies. For example, stridor can be due to trauma, infection, drug reactions or anatomical abnormalities, such as tracheomalacia.

Symptoms and signs of airway obstruction include dyspnoea, stridor, altered voice, dysphonia and dysphagia. Evidence of increased work of breathing includes subcostal, intercostal and suprasternal retraction, flaring of the nasal alar as well as exhaustion and altered mental state. The presence of these signs may

Table 6.1.1 Causes of upper airway obstruction

Altered conscious state

Head injury
Cerebrovascular accident
Drugs and toxins
Metabolic – hypoglycaemia, hyponatraemia, etc.

Foreign bodies

Infections

Tonsillitis
Peritonsillar abscess (quinsy)
Epiglottitis
Ludwig's angina
Other abscesses and infections

Trauma

Blunt or penetrating trauma resulting in oedema or haematoma formation
Uncontrolled haemorrhage
Thermal injuries
Inhalation burns

Neoplasms

Larynx, trachea, thyroid

Allergic reactions

Anaphylaxis
Angioedema

Anatomical

Tracheomalacia – congenital or acquired (secondary to prolonged intubation)
Other congenital malformations

Acute on chronic causes

Patients with chronic narrowing of the airway (e.g. due to tracheomalacia) may present worsening obstruction with an acute upper respiratory tract illness or injury

---

onset. It is essential that the adequacy of the airway is assessed first. Any emergency interventions that are required to maintain the airway should be instituted before obtaining a detailed history and examination. This may range from relieving the obstruction to providing an alternative airway.

Pathology

Obstruction may be physiological with the patient unable to maintain and protect an adequate airway due to a decreased conscious state. Despite the plethora of possible causes, the initial treatment of securing the airway is the same regardless of the cause. Mechanical obstruction may be due to pathology within the lumen (aspirated foreign body), in the wall (angio-oedema, tracheomalacia) or by extrinsic compression (Ludwig's angina, haematoma, external burns). Obstruction may be due to a combination of physiological and mechanical causes. A summary of potential causes of upper airway obstruction is provided in Table 6.1.1.

Clinical investigations

Investigations are secondary to the assessment of and/or provision of an adequate airway. Once the airway has been assessed as secure, the choice of investigations is directed by the history and examination.

Endoscopy

Direct laryngoscopy by an experienced operator is the single most important manoeuvre in patients with acute upper airway obstruction. It

may concurrently form part of the assessment, investigation or treatment. By visualizing the laryngopharynx and upper larynx, the cause of the obstruction can be seen. Any foreign bodies may be removed or, if necessary, a definitive airway, such as an endotracheal tube, introduced. In the case of the stable patient with an incomplete obstruction, this should only be attempted when there are full facilities available for intubation and provision of a surgical airway. It may be more appropriately deferred until expert airway assistance is available.

Bronchoscopy may be required to assess the trachea and distal upper airway but it is not part of the initial resuscitation. In the stable patient, it is more appropriate to transfer the patient to the operating suite or ICU for this procedure.

Blood tests

Some blood tests may be useful in guiding further management. These include full blood count, arterial blood gases and blood cultures. Those required will be guided by the clinical presentation. Initial treatment in the emergency department should not await their results.

Imaging

Neck X-rays

A lateral soft tissue X-ray of the neck is sometimes helpful once the patient has been stabilized. Metallic or bony foreign bodies, food boluses or soft tissue masses may be seen. A number of subtle radiological signs have been described for epiglottitis (Table 6.1.2).

---

vary with age and accompanying conditions. Cyanosis is a late sign.

Further examination will be directed by the presenting complaint and initial findings and includes:

- general appearance – facial symmetry, demeanour
- vital signs – temperature, heart rate, respiratory rate, blood pressure and pulse oximetry
- head and face – rash, swelling, mucous membranes, lymphadenopathy
- oropharynx – mucous membranes, dental hygiene, tongue, tonsils, uvula.

Upper-airway obstruction

Upper-airway obstruction may be acute and life threatening or may have a more gradual

Table 6.1.2 Radiological findings in adult epiglottitis

The 'thumb' sign	Oedema of the normally leaf-like epiglottis resulting in a round shadow resembling an adult thumb. The width of the epiglottis should be less than one-third the anteroposterior width of C4. In adults with epiglottitis, the width of the epiglottis is usually >9 mm
The vallecula sign	Progressive epiglottic oedema resulting in narrowing of the vallecula. This normally well-defined air pocket between the base of the tongue and the epiglottis may be partially or completely obliterated
Swelling of the aryepiglottic folds	
Swelling of the arytenoids	
Loss of the vallecular air space	
Prevertebral soft tissue swelling	The width of the prevertebral soft tissue should be less than half the anteroposterior width of C4
Hypopharyngeal airway widening	The ratio of the width of the hypopharyngeal airway to the anteroposterior width of C4 should be less than 1.5

Computed tomography In the patient with a mechanical obstruction, a computed tomography (CT) scan of the neck and upper thorax may be helpful in diagnosing the cause of the obstruction as well as the extent of any local involvement. It may aid in planning further management, especially if surgical intervention is indicated, for example for a retrothyroid goitre or head and neck neoplasm.

Treatment

Management initially consists of securing the airway. This is discussed in more detail elsewhere in this book, but simple interventions include chin lift or jaw thrust and an oropharyngeal airway. More sophisticated procedures, such as the laryngeal mask or endotracheal tube insertion or surgical airway, may be required.

A surgical airway is rarely necessary in the emergency department, although it is important that equipment is available and that the techniques have been practised. These include needle insufflation and cricothyrostomy. A number of commercial kits, such as the Mini-trach II and the Melker Emergency Cricothyroidotomy Catheter Set, are available. Further management will depend on the underlying cause.

Further treatment will be dictated by the underlying pathology.

Foreign body airway obstruction

Foreign body aspiration is often associated with an altered conscious state, for example in alcohol or drug intoxication, cerebrovascular accident (CVA) or dementia. Elderly patients with dentures are at increased risk.

Laryngeal foreign bodies are almost always symptomatic and are more likely to cause complete obstruction than foreign bodies below the epiglottis. Foreign bodies in the oesophagus are an uncommon cause of airway obstruction but, if lodged in the area of the cricoid cartilage or the tracheal bifurcation, they can compress the airway causing partial airway obstruction. Oesophageal foreign bodies may also become dislodged into the upper airway.

Treatment

In the management of incomplete airway obstruction with adequate gas exchange, care should be taken not to convert partial obstruction into complete obstruction by overzealous intervention.

Awake laryngoscopy can be performed to visualize the foreign body and remove it. The management of complete airway obstruction depends on the conscious level of the patient.

In conscious patients, the Heimlich manoeuvre (or abdominal thrust) is one recommended technique for dislodgement of a foreign body. The rescuer stands behind the patient placing clenched fists over the patient's upper abdomen well clear of the xiphisternum. A short sharp upward thrust is made to force the diaphragm up and expel the foreign body. There is a risk of injury to internal organs and thus should only be done by rescuers who have been trained in the technique. Chest thrusts may be more effective in obese patients if the rescuer is unable to encircle the patient's abdomen. Chest thrusts may also be used in children or in pregnant women. Patients who are asymptomatic after uncomplicated removal of a foreign body should be observed for a time in the emergency department and if they remain well may be discharged home.

In the unconscious patient direct laryngoscopy should be performed before bag/valve/mask ventilation. This prevents the foreign body from being moved from a supraglottic to an intraglottic position. If no foreign body is visualized, the patient should be intubated and ventilated. If the patient cannot be ventilated due to airway resistance, the endotracheal tube should be advanced maximally. This aims to convert a complete tracheal obstruction to a main stem bronchus obstruction. The foreign body can then be removed in the operating theatre.

Blunt trauma

Laryngotracheal trauma is rare, comprising 0.3% of all trauma presenting to emergency departments. The upper airway is relatively protected against trauma since the larynx is mobile and the trachea is compressible and because the head and mandible act as shields. Blunt trauma may be difficult to diagnose as external examination may be normal and there may be distracting head or chest injuries.

Mechanisms of injury

'Clothes-line injuries' involve cyclists or other riders hitting fences or cables. Direct trauma from assaults, sporting equipment or industrial accidents also occurs. Suicide attempts by hanging may cause traumatic injuries to the neck as well as airway obstruction due to the ligature. 'Dashboard injuries' occur when seatbelts are not worn, with sudden deceleration resulting in hyperextension of the neck and compression of the larynx between the dashboard and cervical spine.

Pathology

The most common laryngeal injury is a vertical fracture through the thyroid cartilage. Fractures of the hyoid bone and cricoid cartilage also occur and may be found in cases of manual or ligature strangulation. The cricothryoid ligament and the vocal cords may be ruptured and the arytenoids dislocated. Complete cricotracheal transection may occur. Up to 50% of patients sustaining significant blunt airway trauma have a concurrent cervical spine injury.

Clinical features

Tracheal or laryngeal injury should be suspected if aphonia, hoarseness, stridor, dysphagia or dyspnoea occur. Patients may present with complete obstruction or may deteriorate rapidly after arrival. There may be minimal external evidence of injury or the larynx may be deformed or tender and there may be subcutaneous emphysema. It is important to check for associated head, chest and cervical spine injuries.

Clinical investigations

Endoscopy

Both laryngoscopy and bronchoscopy may be required. This should be performed in the operating theatre, as urgent surgical intervention may be indicated.

Imaging

Plain X-ray X-rays should only be considered if the patient is stable with adequate ventilation. Lateral soft-tissue X-rays of the neck may provide information about airway patency, subcutaneous or soft-tissue emphysema and fractures of the hyoid and larynx. Elevation of the hyoid bone indicates cricotracheal separation. Plain X-rays may also confirm the presence of a foreign body. Cervical spine X-rays should be considered due to the association between upper airway injuries and cervical spine injuries. Chest

Table 6.1.3	Grading of blunt laryngeal injury
Grade	Endoscopic and radiological findings
I	Minor laryngeal haematoma without detectable fracture
II	Oedema, haematoma or minor mucosal disruption without exposed cartilage, or non-displaced fractures on CT
III	Massive oedema, tears, exposed cartilage, immobile cords

X-rays may show signs of trauma and subcutaneous or mediastinal emphysema.

CT CT of the neck is useful in assessing the extent of injuries to larynx, oesophagus, cervical spine and adjacent structures but should only be considered once the patient is stabilized.

A classification system for severity of blunt upper airway injury based on endoscopic and radiological findings has been developed (Table 6.1.3).

Treatment
Airway management with protection of the cervical spine is essential. Fibreoptic bronchoscopic intubation is preferable to minimize complications, such as laryngeal disruption, laryngotracheal separation or creating a false tracheal lumen. Cricothyrostomy is relatively contraindicated due to the altered anatomy. Emergency tracheostomy may even be required, ideally performed in the operating theatre. Early ENT involvement is important and indications for surgical exploration include airway obstruction requiring tracheostomy, uncontrolled subcutaneous emphysema, extensive mucosal lacerations with exposed cartilage as identified on bronchoscopic or laryngoscopic examination, vocal cord paralysis and grossly deformed, multiple or displaced fractures of the larynx, thyroid cartilage or cricoid cartilage.

Prognosis
Mortality rates depend on the location of the injury, ranging from 11% for isolated fractures of the thyroid cartilage to 50% for injuries involving the cricoid cartilage, bronchi or intrathoracic trachea. Asphyxiation is the most common cause of death in blunt laryngeal trauma.

Penetrating trauma
Mechanism
Penetrating injuries may be secondary to assault or to sporting or industrial accidents. Other causes include eroding head and neck malignancies or post-radiotherapy. A focused history is mandatory.

Clinical features
Penetration of the airway should be suspected if there is difficulty breathing, hoarseness or change in voice, stridor, pain on speaking, subcutaneous emphysema, haemoptysis or bubbling from the wound. Penetrating airway injury is often associated with great vessel or pulmonary injuries. Uncontrolled haemorrhage may lead to exsanguination as well as compromising the airway and requires prompt surgical intervention.

Clinical investigation
As for blunt trauma (see above).

Treatment
Airway management with protection of the cervical spine is essential. Airway management is as for blunt trauma (see above). Early involvement of relevant surgical specialties is a priority.

Thermal injury
Pathology and pathophysiology
Burns may affect the airway by way of facial and perioral swelling, laryngeal oedema or constricting circumferential neck burns. Smoke inhalation occurs in about 25% of burn victims and may cause bronchospasm, retrosternal pain and impaired gas exchange.

Clinical features
External examination may show evidence of burns. Carbonaceous material in the mouth, nares or pharynx suggests the possibility of upper airway thermal injury. If the patient presents with stridor or hoarseness, early intubation is essential because of the danger of increasing airway oedema and rapid progression to airway obstruction. Smoke inhalation may be associated with carbon monoxide poisoning and, in the setting of domestic or industrial fires, cyanide poisoning should also be considered.

Clinical investigations
Endoscopy
Endoscopy includes both laryngoscopy and bronchoscopy, performed in the operating theatre, as urgent surgical intervention may be required.

Imaging
Chest X-ray may show evidence of burn-associated acute respiratory distress syndrome (ARDS).

Infections
Introduction
Infections may involve the upper respiratory tract directly or adjacent structures. They range from the common and trivial to the rare and potentially life threatening. Croup and epiglottitis usually occur in children, but may be seen in adults. Acute respiratory infections are the most frequent reason for seeking medical attention in the USA and are associated with up to 75% of total antibiotic prescriptions there each year. Unnecessary antibiotic use can cause a number of adverse effects including allergic reactions, gastrointestinal upset, yeast infections, drug interactions, an increased risk of subsequent infection with drug resistant *Streptococcus pneumoniae* and added costs of over-treatment.

Non-specific upper airway infections
Upper airway infections are generally diagnosed clinically. Symptom complexes where the predominant complaint is of sore throat are labelled pharyngitis or tonsillitis and, where the predominant symptom is cough, bronchitis. Acute respiratory symptoms in the absence of a predominant sign are typically diagnosed as 'upper-respiratory-tract infections'.

Each of these syndromes may be caused by a multitude of different viruses and only occasionally by bacteria. Most cases resolve spontaneously within 1–2 weeks. Bacterial rhinosinusitis complicates about 2% of cases and should be suspected when symptoms have lasted at least 7 days and include purulent nasal discharge and other localizing features. High-risk patients for developing bacterial rhinosinusitis or bacterial pneumonia include infants, the elderly and the chronically ill. Treatment should be symptomatic only. Antibiotic treatment does not enhance illness resolution nor alter the rates of complications.

Pharyngitis/tonsillitis

Sore throat is one of the top 10 presenting complaints to emergency departments in the USA. The differential diagnosis is large and includes a number of important conditions (Table 6.1.4).

Pharyngitis has a wide range of causative viral and bacterial agents, most of which produce a self-limited infection with no significant sequelae. Group A beta-haemolytic streptococcus (*Strep. pyogenes*) (GABHS) is responsible for 5–15% of cases of pharyngitis in adults and, rarely, can trigger post-infectious syndromes of post-streptococcal glomerulonephritis and acute rheumatic fever.

Clinical investigations

Clinical diagnosis of streptococcal pharyngitis is unreliable. Clinical prediction rules have been developed to help identify patients in whom evaluation with a throat culture or rapid antigen-detection test (RADT) is warranted. The most reliable clinical predictors for GABHS are the Centor criteria. One point each is allocated for the features of tonsillar exudate, tender anterior cervical lymphadenopathy or lymphadenitis, absence of cough and history of fever >38°C. One point is deducted for age >45 years. For a score of 0–1, no further testing or antibiotics is recommended. For scores of 2–3, further testing is recommended with antibiotics only given to patients with positive RADT or

cultures. For a score of 4, empirical antibiotic treatment and/or further testing are advised.

Rapid antigen tests have sensitivities ranging between 65 and 97%. Throat cultures take 2–3 days and may give false-positive results from asymptomatic carriers with concurrent non-GABHS pharyngitis. Serological testing is not useful in the acute treatment of pharyngitis but is useful in the diagnosis of rheumatic fever.

The Infectious Diseases Society of America recommends throat cultures for children and adolescents with appropriate clinical criteria (fever, tonsillar exudates, tender cervical lymphadenopathy, absence of cough) but negative rapid antigen test. Adults with a negative RADT will not require cultures due to a lower incidence of GABHS pharyngitis and lower risk of rheumatic fever. Testing is not recommended for patients with clinical features suggestive of a viral aetiology (e.g. cough, oral ulcers, rhinorrhoea and hoarseness).

Neisseria gonorrhoeae is an uncommon cause of pharyngitis and may be asymptomatic. It is seen in persons who practice receptive oral sex. *N. gonorrhoeae* pharyngitis is important to diagnose correctly both for appropriate treatment and because of the need to trace and treat contacts.

HIV is an unusual cause of pharyngitis but should be considered in high-risk populations. The acute retroviral syndrome may present with an Epstein–Barr virus mononucleosis-like syndrome.

Treatment

Timely use of appropriate antibiotics prevents the development of acute rheumatic fever, decreases the duration of symptoms and decreases the incidence of suppurative complications, such as otitis media and peritonsillar abscesses. However, empirical antibiotic treatment on the basis of symptoms alone results in overuse of antibiotics, increased costs and an increased rate of side effects from antibiotics. Antibiotics have not been shown to decrease the incidence of post-streptococcal glomerulonephritis, which is related to the subtype of streptococcus.

First-line antibiotics include oral penicillin V, amoxicillin, cephalexin, clindamycin or clarithromycin for 10 days or a single dose of intramuscular penicillin G.

For uncomplicated pharyngeal gonorrhoea, ceftriaxone 125 mg IM as a single dose is the recommended treatment. Consideration should be given to concomitant treatment for Chlamydia if this has not been ruled out.

Most patients with pharyngitis are managed as outpatients. Airway compromise is rare as the nasal passages provide an adequate airway. Some patients who are toxic or dehydrated may need admission for IV hydration and antibiotics. Penicillin or amoxicillin remain the drugs of choice for streptococcal pharyngitis. Regarding adjuvant corticosteroid therapy, a recent Cochrane review of patients with pharyngitis treated with antibiotics concluded that those with adjuvant corticosteroid therapy were three times more likely to experience complete resolution of their sore throat symptoms by 24 hours compared to those taking placebo. In addition, corticosteroids improved the time to onset of symptom relief and the time to complete resolution of symptoms. Adverse events, relapse rates and recurrence rates were not different for corticosteroid compared to placebo groups.

Quinsy/peritonsillar abscess

Epidemiology and pathology

Peritonsillar infections occur between the palatine tonsil, its capsule and the pharyngeal muscles. Peritonsillar cellulitis may progress to abscess formation. Cellulitis responds to antibiotics alone, but differentiating between the cellulitis and abscess and identifying those who require drainage may be difficult. Peritonsillar abscesses occur most commonly in males between 20 and 40 years of age.

Clinical features, investigations and complications

Symptoms include progressively worsening sore throat (usually unilateral), fever and dysphagia. On examination, the patient may have a muffled 'hot potato' voice, trismus, drooling, a swollen red tonsil with or without purulent exudate and contralateral deviation of the uvula.

Clinical features do not always differentiate between quinsy and peritonsillar cellulitis. In such situations, imaging (e.g. CT), needle aspiration or trial of IV antibiotics help to differentiate between them.

Complications include airway obstruction and lateral extension into the parapharyngeal space.

Treatment

Antibiotic therapy should include cover for GABHS, *Staphylococcus aureus*, *Haemophilus influenzae* and respiratory anaerobic species (*Fusobacterium*, *Peptostreptococcus* and *Bacteroides*). Appropriate antibiotics include

---

Table 6.1.4 Differential diagnosis of sore throat in the adult

Infective pharyngitis
  Bacterial: Group A beta-haemolytic streptococcus most common pathogen. Diphtheria should be considered in patients with membranous pharyngitis
  Viral: including Epstein–Barr virus and herpes simplex virus

Traumatic pharyngitis (exposure to irritant gases)

Non-specific upper respiratory tract infection

Quinsy (peritonsillar abscess)

Epiglottitis

Ludwig's angina

Parapharyngeal and retropharyngeal abscesses

Gastro-oesophageal reflux

Oropharyngeal or laryngeal tumour

---

penicillin V or clindamycin for patients allergic to penicillin.

Needle aspiration in experienced hands can be useful but has a 12% false-negative rate and carries the risk of damaging the carotid artery. Formal surgical drainage or tonsillectomy may be necessary.

Ludwig's angina

Peripharyngeal 'space' infections have become rare in the post-antibiotic era but, of these, Ludwig's angina or cellulitis of the submandibular space remains the most common. It was first described by Wilhelm Fredrick von Ludwig in 1836 and, at that time, was usually fatal because of rapid compromise to the airway. With prompt treatment, including IV antibiotics, the mortality rate has declined to less than 5%.

Pathogenesis and pathology

Ludwig's angina is classically bilateral. Infection may spread rapidly into adjacent spaces including the pharyngomaxillary and retropharyngeal areas and the mediastinum. Ludwig's angina is related to dental caries involving the mandibular molars or it may be associated with peritonsillar abscess, trauma to the floor of the mouth or mandible and recent dental work.

Cultures are usually polymicrobial and include viridans streptococci (40.9%), *Staph. aureus* (27.3%), *Staph. epidermidis* (22.7%) and anaerobes (40%), such as *Bacteroides* species.

Clinical features

Clinical features include toothache, halitosis, neck pain, swelling, fever, dysphagia and trismus.

Treatment and disposition

Treatment necessitates admission and careful airway management. This may include endotracheal intubation as abrupt obstruction can occur. Surgical drainage is indicated if the infection is suppurative or fluctuant.

The antibiotics of choice are high-dose penicillin plus metronidazole or clindamycin which should be administered IV.

Other abscesses

Parapharyngeal abscesses

Parapharyngeal abscess involves the lateral or pharyngomaxillary space. Presentation and treatment are similar to Ludwig's angina, from which they may develop. As well as the complications of Ludwig's angina, including airway obstruction and spread to contiguous areas,

there is the added risk of internal jugular vein thrombosis and erosion of the carotid artery which has a mortality of 20–40%.

Retropharyngeal abscess

Retropharyngeal abscesses are more common in children below 5 years of age. In adults, they often result from foreign bodies or trauma. Presenting symptoms and signs include fever, odynophagia, neck swelling, drooling, torticollis, cervical lymphadenopathy, dyspnoea and stridor.

Lateral neck X-rays show widening of the prevertebral soft tissues and sometimes a fluid level. CT of the neck may help in determining the extent and in differentiating an abscess from cellulitis. Magnetic resonance imaging (MRI), if available, is more sensitive than CT in assessing soft-tissue infections of the head and neck but demonstrates cortical bone poorly. Treatment requires admission, airway management, IV antibiotics and may include surgical drainage.

Epiglottitis

Epidemiology and pathology

Epiglottitis is becoming an adult disease although, in adults, there is significantly less risk to the airway than in children. The incidence of adult epiglottitis has remained relatively stable at 1–4 cases per 100 000 per year with a mortality of 7%. This may change over the next 10–20 years as vaccinated children grow into adolescents and adults.

Acute adult epiglottitis is often referred to as supraglottitis because inflammation is not confined to the epiglottis, but also affects other structures, such as the pharynx, uvula, base of tongue, aryepiglottic folds and false vocal cords.

H. influenzae has been isolated in 12–17% of cases and the high rate of negative blood cultures may reflect viral infections or prior treatment with antibiotics in cases that present late. *Strep. pneumoniae*, *H. parainfluenzae* and herpes simplex have also been isolated. Epiglottitis may also occur following mechanical injury, such as ingestion of caustic material, smoke inhalation and following illicit drug use (smoking heroin).

Clinical features

Sore throat and odynophagia are the most common presenting symptoms. Other symptoms include fever and muffled voice. Drooling and stridor are infrequent. Factors shown to

be associated with an increased risk of airway obstruction include stridor, dyspnoea, preferred upright posture and short duration of symptoms.

Clinical investigations

A number of X-ray changes have been described in epiglottitis which are listed in Table 6.1.2.

Treatment

Antimicrobial therapy should provide cover against *H. influenzae* B, *Strep. pneumoniae*, beta-haemolytic streptococci and *Staph. aureus*. Third generation cephalosporins (ceftriaxone or cefotaxime) and antistaphylococcal agents active against methicillin-resistant *Staph. aureus* (MRSA) (e.g. clindamycin) should be used.

The role of steroids and nebulized or parenteral adrenaline (epinephrine) in airway management is controversial. Most adults can be treated conservatively without the need for an artificial airway.

Controversies

- Reaching a uniform approach to the use of antibiotics in adult pharyngitis.
- The role of intubation, steroids and nebulized or parenteral adrenaline (epinephrine) in adult epiglottitis.

Further reading

Burgess CA, Dale OT. An evidence based review of the assessment and management of penetrating neck trauma. Clin Otolaryngol 2012;37:44–52.

Fuhrman GM, Stieg FH. Blunt laryngeal trauma: classification and management protocol. J Trauma 1990;30:87–92.

Hayward G, Thompson MJ, Perera R, et al. Corticosteroids as standalone or add-on treatment for sore throat. Cochrane Database Syst Rev 2012;10:CD008268.

Michael RW. Clinical practice. Streptococcal pharyngitis. N Engl J Med 2011;364:648–55.

Murphy MF, Zane RD. Distorted airways and acute upper airway obstruction. In: Walls RM, Murphy MF, editors. Manual of emergency airway management (4th ed.). Philadelphia: Lippincott Williams & Wilkins, 2012, p. 377.

Powell J, Wilson JA. An evidence-based review of peritonsillar abscess. Clin Otolaryngol 2012;37:136–45.

Shulman ST, Bisno AL, et al.Clinical practice guideline for the diagnosis and management of group A streptococcal pharyngitis: 2012 update by the Infectious Diseases Society of America. Clin Infect Dis 2012;55:e86–102.

Sobol SE, Zapata S. Epiglottitis and croup. Otolaryngol Clin N Am 2008;41:551.

Toon MH, Maybauer MO, et al. Management of acute smoke inhalation injury. Crit Care Resusc 2010;12:53.

Walls RM. Foreign body in the adult airway. In: Walls RM, Murphy MF, editors. Manual of emergency airway management (4th ed.). Philadelphia: Lippincott Williams & Wilkins, 2012, p. 418.

6.2 Asthma

Anne-Maree Kelly • Wee Yee Lee

ESSENTIALS

1 Asthma is a major health problem worldwide, resulting in significant morbidity and mortality.

2 Asthma is characterized by episodic bronchoconstriction and wheeze in response to a variety of stimuli.

3 Features suggesting an increased risk of life-threatening asthma include a previous life-threatening attack, previous intensive care admission with ventilation, requiring three or more classes of asthma medication, heavy use of β-agonists, repeated emergency department attendances in the last year and having required a course of oral corticosteroids within the previous 6 months. Behavioural and psychosocial factors have also been implicated in life-threatening asthma including non-compliance with treatment or follow up, obesity and psychiatric illness.

4 Attacks vary in severity from mild to life threatening and may develop over minutes.

5 Clinical features supported by bedside pulmonary function tests and pulse oximetry are reliable guides to the severity of attacks.

6 Oxygen, β_2-adrenergic agents and corticosteroids are the mainstays of therapy.

7 Hospital admission is essential if pretreatment PEFR or FEV_1 is less than 25% of predicted or post-treatment levels are less than 40% of predicted.

Introduction

Asthma is a major health problem worldwide, resulting in significant morbidity and mortality. The prevalence of asthma varies significantly between regions across the world. In Australasia, New Zealand and the UK, it is thought to affect about 20% of children and 10% of adults. Sufferers tend to present to emergency departments when their usual treatment plan fails to control symptoms adequately. The respiratory compromise caused can range from mild to severe and life threatening. For these patients, the main role of the emergency care is therapeutic. Other reasons for patients with asthma to attend emergency departments (EDs) include having run out of medication, having symptoms after a period of being symptom and medication free and a desire for a 'second opinion' about the management of their asthma. For this smaller group, the primary role is one of educating about the disease, of planning an approach to the current level of asthma symptoms and of

referral to appropriate health professionals, e.g. respiratory physicians or general practitioners.

Epidemiology

Asthma is a major health problem in many countries, resulting in significant morbidity and mortality. Data from the Global Initiative for Asthma suggest that more than 300 million people in the world are currently affected by asthma. The cost in terms of long-term medications and lost school and work days is difficult to quantify, but would run to millions of dollars annually. Australasia, the UK and North America have a greater prevalence of asthma than the Middle East and some Asian countries. There is also considerable geographical variation in severity, with Australasia reporting the highest proportion of severe disease. The reason for this geographical variation is unclear, but may relate in part to ethnicity, rural versus metropolitan environment and air pollution. A number of epidemiological studies suggest that the

prevalence and severity of asthma is slowly increasing worldwide.

Aetiology, pathophysiology and pathology

Asthma is characterized by hyperreactive airways and inflammation leading to episodic, reversible bronchoconstriction in response to a variety of stimuli. It is a complex immunologically-mediated disease. There is strong evidence that it is inherited, although no single gene is directly implicated. A polygenic basis is likely to account for asthma's wide clinical spectrum.

Studies suggest that asthma sufferers may have abnormal immunological systems, innately hypersensistive airways and abnormal airway repair mechanisms. Environmental factors interact with this system to produce clinical disease.

Triggers of the immunological response (e.g. an extrinsic allergen, viral respiratory tract infection, pollutants, occupational exposures, emotion, exercise and drugs, such as aspirin and β-blockers) result in an exaggerated inflammatory response with activation of cell types including mast cells, eosinophils, basophils, Th-2 cells and natural killer cells. This leads to the release of primary mediators, including histamine and eosinophilic and neutrophilic chemotactic factors and secondary mediators, including leukotrienes, prostaglandins, platelet-activating factor, interleukins and cytokines. These result in bronchoconstriction via direct and cholinergic reflex actions, increased vascular permeability (resulting in oedema) and increased mucous secretions.

Studies suggest that airway remodelling occurs in asthma sufferers resulting in airways that are more hypersensitive than previously. It is postulated that this structural remodelling results in loss of lung function and loss of complete reversibility.

Pathophysiologically the effects of acute asthma are:

- increased physiological dead space
- respiratory muscle fatigue
- intrinsic positive end-expiratory pressure secondary to hyperventilation with air trapping.

Table 6.2.1 Categorization of asthma severity based on clinical features

Severity category	Features	Respiratory function
Life threatening	Exhaustion, confusion, coma, cyanosis Silent chest Inability to speak Poor respiratory effort Dysrhythmia, bradycardia Hypotension	FEV_1/PEFR inappropriate SpO_2 <90% despite supplemental oxygen
Severe	Laboured respiration Tachycardia, heart rate ≥110 Tachypnoea, respiratory rate ≥25/min Unable to complete a sentence in one breath (i.e. words, short phrases only)	FEV_1/PEFR unable or <40% predicted SpO_2 <90% on air PEFR <200 L/min
Moderate	Dyspnoeic at rest Able to speak in short sentences Chest tightness Wheeze Partial or short-term relief with usual therapy Nocturnal symptoms No features of severe asthma	FEV_1/PEFR 40–60% predicted PEFR 200–300 L/min
Mild	Exertional symptoms Able to speak normally Good response to usual therapy	FEV1/PEFR >60% predicted PEFR >300 L/min

Modified from Guidelines for Emergency Management of Adult Asthma, Canadian Association of Emergency Physicians, British Guideline on the Management of Asthma (SIGN) and Asthma Management Handbook (NAC) with permission.

Clinical assessment

The aims of clinical assessment are confirmation of the diagnosis, assessment of severity and identification of complications.

History

Asthma is characterized by episodic shortness of breath, often accompanied by wheeze, chest tightness and cough. Symptoms may be worse at night, which is thought to be due to variations in bronchomotor tone and bronchial reactivity. Attacks may progress slowly over days or rapidly over minutes. Atypical presentation includes cough and decreased exercise tolerance.

Features suggesting an increased risk of life-threatening asthma include a previous life-threatening attack, previous intensive care admission with ventilation, requiring three or more classes of asthma medication, heavy use of β-agonists, repeated emergency department attendances in the last year and having required a course of oral corticosteroids within the previous 6 months. Behavioural and psychosocial factors have also been implicated in life-threatening asthma including non-compliance with medications, monitoring or follow up, self-discharge from hospital, frequent GP contact, psychiatric illness, denial, drug or alcohol abuse, obesity, learning difficulties, employment or income problems and domestic, marital or legal stressors. These should be sought in order to assess risk more accurately and plan management.

Examination

Physical findings vary with the severity of the attack and may range from mild wheeze and dyspnoea to respiratory failure. Findings indicative of more severe disease include an inability to speak normally, use of the accessory muscles of respiration, a quiet or silent chest on auscultation, restlessness or altered level of consciousness, oxygen saturation on room air of <93% and cyanosis. Clinical features are a good guide to the severity of attacks. Features of the major severity categories are summarized in Table 6.2.1. Pulsus paradoxus has been abandoned as an indicator of severity.

Clinical investigations

Mild to moderate asthma

For mild and moderate asthma, investigations should be limited to pulmonary function tests (PEFR or FEV_1). A chest X-ray is only indicated if examination of the chest suggests pneumothorax or pneumonia. Arterial blood gases are not useful in this group of patients.

Severe asthma

Assessment should include an assessment of PEFR if possible.

Chest X-ray

For severe asthma, a chest X-ray is necessary as localizing signs in the chest may be hard to detect.

Blood gas analysis

Blood gas analysis may be useful if the oxygen saturation is less than 92% on room air at presentation, if improvement is not occurring as expected and if the patient appears to be tiring. For those with severe asthma, arterial blood gases may show:

- respiratory alkalosis and mild-to-moderate hypoxia (reflecting an increase in respiratory rate in an attempt to maintain oxygenation) or
- hypoxia and respiratory acidosis as the $PaCO_2$ rises with fatigue and air trapping.

Blood gas analysis may also be helpful if intubation is being considered because of worsening respiratory failure. That said, their impact taken early in management is minimal and they should never be considered 'routine'. There is increasing evidence that venous blood gases can accurately screen for arterial hypercarbia. Given the accuracy of pulse oximetry, venous blood gas analysis may be adequate for detecting acidosis and hypercarbia, avoiding significant discomfort for patients.

Blood tests

Full blood examination is usually not useful, as a mild-to-moderate leucocytosis may be present in the absence of infection. Electrolyte measurements may show a mild hypokalaemia, particularly if frequent doses of β-agonists have been taken.

Treatment

The emergency management of acute asthma varies according to severity, as defined by the clinical parameters above. The principles are to ensure adequate oxygenation, reverse bronchospasm and minimize the inflammatory response.

Mild asthma

Mild attacks are managed using inhaled $β_2$-adrenergic agonists, such as salbutamol, by metered dose inhaler (MDI) or spacer, the commencement of inhaled corticosteroids if the patient is not already taking them and education about the disease and the proposed management and follow-up plan.

Moderate asthma

Patients with moderate attacks may require oxygen therapy titrated to achieve oxygen saturation in excess of 92%. The mainstays of therapy are inhaled β_2-adrenergic agents (by MDI with a spacer or nebulizer) and systemic corticosteroids. The dosage of salbutamol is 5–10 mg by nebulizer or eight puffs by MDI and spacer, every 15 minutes for three doses. Corticosteroids are equally effective given by the oral or intravenous routes. The usual dose is 50 mg prednisolone orally or 250 mg hydrocortisone intravenously. Reassessment, including repeat pulmonary function tests, should occur at least 1 hour after the last dose of β_2-agonist. This will guide further therapy and disposition decision making.

Patients with PEFR >70% best or predicted 1 hour after initial treatment may be discharged from the emergency department unless there are concerns about compliance or social circumstances, the patient has a history of brittle or near fatal asthma, discharge would occur overnight or the patient is pregnant. This group are likely to benefit from a longer period of observation and treatment, e.g. in an emergency observation or short stay unit. Those who fail to respond quickly usually require extended treatment. In these patients, the addition of ipratropium bromide (0.5 mg 4–6 hourly) may be considered, particularly in those taking long-acting β-agonists, in whom a degree of tolerance to bronchodilation with short-acting β_2-agonists can occur.

For patients who are discharged, oral corticosteroids at a dose of 0.5–1 mg/kg/day, in addition to inhaled steroids at standard doses, should be continued for at least 5 days or until recovery. Oral steroids may then be withdrawn; tapering of dose is unnecessary.

Severe asthma

Patients should be managed in an area with close physiological monitoring.

Oxygen

Severe attacks require supplemental oxygen to achieve oxygen saturation in excess of 92%. Because of high respiratory rates, it is important to ensure adequate gas flow by the use of either a reservoir-type mask or a Venturi delivery system. High oxygen concentrations may be necessary.

Specific therapy

Patients should receive β_2-agonist by nebulizer at the doses described above, plus oral or intravenous corticosteroids (e.g. prednisolone 50 mg daily orally or hydrocortisone 100 mg 6-hourly IV). Metered dose inhalers with spacers can be used in patients with exacerbations that are not life threatening. Continuous nebulization may be more effective than intermittent bolus nebulization in patients with poor response to initial therapy. There is no evidence of any difference in efficacy between salbutamol and terbutaline. Nebulized adrenaline (epinephrine) does not have significant benefit over selective agents. The addition of nebulized ipratropium (500 μg 2-hourly) is recommended. If patients fail to respond, an intravenous β_2-agonist (e.g. salbutamol as a bolus of 250 μg followed by an infusion at 5–10 μg/kg/hour) and/or ventilatory support should be considered.

Ventilatory support

If ventilatory support is required for patients with an acceptable conscious state and airway protective mechanisms, non-invasive ventilation may be suitable. If the patient is unsuitable for or does not improve with non-invasive ventilation, endotracheal intubation and mechanical ventilation will be needed. Ketamine, which has been shown to be an effective bronchodilator, is the induction agent of choice. Care must be taken with ventilation, as severe air trapping can result in markedly raised intrathoracic pressure with cardiovascular compromise. A slow ventilation rate of 6–8 breaths/min with low volume ventilation and prolonged expiratory periods is recommended. To reduce the risk of barotrauma, permissive hypercapnia is allowed as long as adequate oxygenation is achieved.

Other agents

Magnesium

Magnesium can be administered IV or by nebulizer. It is postulated to have both bronchodilatory and anti-inflammatory effects.

With respect to IV magnesium, a Cochrane review suggests that there is no benefit from its use (in addition to standard therapy) in mild or moderate asthma, but that for severe asthma (FEV_1 <25% predicted) the addition of magnesium resulted in highly significant increases in FEV_1 and reduced admission rates. No serious adverse reactions were noted in any of the studies.

The current recommendation is that a single dose of IV magnesium sulphate (1.2–2 g over 20 minutes) be considered in patients with:

- acute severe asthma who do not have a good response to inhaled therapy or
- life-threatening asthma.

Aminophylline Although pooled studies and meta-analyses fail to show benefit in adults, there is anecdotal evidence that selected, rare patients who fail to respond to the above treatment may benefit from IV aminophylline (5 mg/kg loading dose over 20 minutes, followed by 0.3–0.6 mg/kg/h). It should not be used without specialist input and should be used with particular care in patients already taking oral xanthines at admission.

Leukotriene receptor antagonists There is insufficient evidence to make a recommendation about the use of these agents in acute asthma.

Antibiotics

Routine prescription of antibiotics is not indicated.

Non-invasive ventilation (NIV)

In acute asthma, NIV has been shown to reduce airways resistance, bronchodilate, counter atelectasis, reduce the work of respiration and reduce the cardiovascular impact of changes in intrapleural and intrathoracic pressures caused by asthma. It does not, when used alone, improve gas exchange. An unrandomized study of continuous positive airway pressure (CPAP) in combination with pressure support ventilation in patients with severe asthma found rapid correction of pH and improvement in ventilation at lower pressures than were necessary with mechanical ventilation. Other small studies also suggest that NIV may reduce the need for intubation in selected patients and result in faster improvement. NIV also appears to be associated with a lower risk of adverse events than endotracheal intubation. There are currently no guidelines governing the use of NIV in asthma, however, in suitable patients, a trial of NIV under closely supervised conditions would seem reasonable.

Heliox

Heliox is a blend of 70% helium and 30% oxygen. It has been postulated that it may have advantages in asthma because of its better gas flow dynamics. Small studies have had conflicting results and Cochrane review concluded that the existing evidence did not support the use of heliox in patients with acute severe asthma in the ED.

Ketamine

A potential benefit from cautious subinduction doses of ketamine in severe asthma has been suggested. The postulated mechanisms of action of ketamine in asthma are sympathomimetic effects, direct relaxant effects on bronchial smooth muscle, antagonism of histamine and acetylcholine and a membrane-stabilizing effect. There is only one randomized trial investigating the role of ketamine in acute asthma. It showed that, in doses with an acceptable incidence of dysphoria, ketamine did not confer benefit. For intubated patients, there is some preliminary evidence that ketamine infusion (bolus 1 mg/kg, followed by 1 mg/kg/h) may improve blood gas parameters. No outcome benefit has yet been demonstrated.

Anti-IgE therapy

Anti-IgE therapy (e.g. omalizumab) is used for severe chronic allergic asthma. Its role is the reduction of exacerbations. It has no role in acute management.

Disposition

Patients with mild disease can usually be discharged after treatment and the formulation of a treatment plan. For patients with moderate and severe asthma, bedside pulmonary function tests can be a useful guide to disposition decisions. Those with post-treatment PEFR >70% predicted/best after initial treatment can be discharged on appropriate therapy (see above). Those with PEFR 40–70% predicted/best require an extended period of observation and treatment (e.g. in an emergency observation unit) after which many will be suitable for discharge. Patients with life-threatening asthma or post-treatment PEFR <40% best/predicted require hospital admission. In addition, other factors should be considered in estimating the safety of discharge. These include history of a previous near-death episode, recent ED visits, frequent admissions to hospital, current or recent steroid use, sudden attacks, poor understanding or compliance, poor home circumstances and limited access to transport back to hospital in case of deterioration.

Indications for admission to an intensive care or high dependency unit include:

- deteriorating PEFR
- persisting or worsening hypoxia
- hypercapnia
- acidosis
- exhaustion/deteriorating respiratory effort
- drowsiness, confusion, altered conscious state
- requirement for ventilatory assistance
- respiratory arrest.

All discharged patients should have an asthma action plan to cover the following 24–48 hours, with particular emphasis on what to do if their condition worsens. They should also have a scheduled review, either in the hospital or with a general practitioner within that time. Discharge medications are as described above.

Controversies

- The role of intravenous and nebulized magnesium in severe asthma.
- The role of non-invasive continuous positive airway pressure as an alternative to intubation and mechanical ventilation.

Further reading

Beveridge RC, Grunfeld AF, Hodder RV. Guidelines for the emergency management of asthma in adults. CAEP/CTS Asthma Advisory Committee. Can Med Assoc J 1996;155:25–37.

Fernandez MM, Villagra A, Blanch L. Non-invasive mechanical ventilation in status asthmaticus. Intens Care Med 2001;27:486–92.

Haney S, Hancox RJ. Overcoming beta-agonist tolerance: high dose salbutamol and ipratropium bromide. Two randomized controlled trials. Resp Res 2007;8:19.

Holgate ST. Pathophysiology of asthma: what has our current understanding taught us about new therapeutic approaches? J Allergy Clin Immunol 2011;128:495–505. <http://www.brit-thoracic.org.uk/Portals/0/Guidelines/AsthmaGuidelines/sign101%20Jan%202012.pdf>.

Kelly AM, Kerr D, Powell CVE, et al. Is severity assessment after one hour of treatment better for predicting the need for admission in acute asthma? Resp Med 2004;98:777–81.

Kelly AM. Can venous blood gas analysis replace arterial in emergency medical care: a review. Emerg Med Australas 2010;22:493–8.

Murphy DM, O'Byrne PM. Recent advances in the pathophysiology of asthma. Chest 2010;137:1417–26.

National Asthma Council Australia Asthma Management Handbook. Melbourne: National Asthma Council Australia; 2006.

Parameswaran K, Belda J, Rowe BH. Addition of intravenous aminophylline to beta2-agonists in adults with acute asthma. Cochrane Database Syst Rev 2000;4:CD002742.

Rodrigo G, Pollack C, Rodrigo C, et al. Heliox for nonintubated acute asthma patients. Cochrane Database Syst Rev 2006;4:CD002884.

Rowe BH, Bretzlaff J, Bourdon C, et al. Magnesium sulfate for treating exacerbations of acute asthma in the emergency department. Cochrane Database Syst Rev 2000;1:CD001490.

Scottish Intercollegiate Guidelines Network. British guideline on the management of asthma. 2008; updated 2012 <http://www.sign.ac.uk/pdf/sign101.pdf>.[Accessed Dec. 2012].

RESPIRATORY EMERGENCIES

6

6.3 Community-acquired pneumonia

Mark Putland • Karen Robins-Browne

ESSENTIALS

1 The term community-acquired pneumonia refers to a syndrome of acute lower respiratory tract infection with a new infiltrate on chest X-ray in a patient who has not been hospitalized in the past 14 days.

2 The new scoring systems, SMART-COP and CORB, allow identification of patients at high risk of need for intensive care while the previously established Pneumonia Severity Index and CURB-65 were predominantly able to identify low-risk cases that could be treated at home.

3 *Streptococcus pneumoniae* is the most common causative agent. Others vary with demographics, severity and epidemics. Antibiotic susceptibilities vary widely around the world. Knowledge of local organisms, susceptibilities and outbreaks will allow for better empiric prescribing.

4 Beta-lactams and macrolides are the mainstay of antibiotic treatment. Respiratory fluoroquinolones have a role but cost and emerging resistance may limit it.

5 Use of locally adapted, structured guidelines for management of community-acquired pneumonia is associated with improvement in mortality.

Introduction

Community-acquired pneumonia (CAP) represents a spectrum of disease from mild and self-limiting to severe and life threatening. The great majority of cases are treated in the community with oral antibiotics, many without radiological confirmation. In the emergency department, CAP is generally not a great diagnostic challenge but rather represents a challenge of separating the serious cases that require inpatient treatment and supportive care from the mild cases that can be managed with minimal expense to the community and minimal inconvenience to the patient at home. Infrequently, CAP presents with the need for urgent, life-saving interventions and critical care.

The chest X-ray (CXR) remains the gold standard diagnostic test for pneumonia. Ancillary tests including urinary antigen test (UAT), sputum and blood cultures, inflammatory markers, renal and liver function tests and blood counts have roles in selected cases. A rational approach to the use of pathology testing is required to avoid excess healthcare cost and to prevent inappropriate decisions based on spurious or misleading results.

Antibiotic management of CAP has changed little for some decades, although respiratory fluoroquinolones, such as moxifloxacin and levofloxacin, have a role. In some patients, the emergence of drug resistant *Streptococcus pneumoniae* (DRSP) and community-acquired methicillin resistant *Staphylococcus aureus* (CA-MRSA) present new challenges in management.

Recent years have seen the publication of comprehensive evidence-based guidelines from the British Thoracic Society (BTS) and the Infectious Diseases Society of America and American Thoracic Society (IDSA/ATS) as well as similar documents from Japan, Sweden, Canada and other countries. The Australian Therapeutic Guidelines continue to provide up-to-date antibiotic guidelines for the Australian setting. There is mounting evidence that the use of a structured, guideline-based approach to CAP management improves mortality and that such guidelines should be adapted to local conditions.

Epidemiology

Rates of pneumonia are difficult to estimate due to issues of case definition and the fact that the majority of cases occur unstudied in the community. However, data from around the world suggest that the incidence is around 5–11/1000/year in 16–59 year olds and over 30/1000/year in those over 75 years old. Incidence of CAP requiring hospitalization in the UK is less than 5/1000/year and comprises probably less than 50% of CAP cases. On the other hand, CAP accounts for 8–10% of ICU medical admissions.

Rates of admission to ICU vary enormously around the world and probably represent resource availability and usage more than differences in disease severity. New Zealand studies report 1–3% of cases needing ICU while, in the UK, it is around 5% and, in Australia, 10%. Much higher percentages are reported from the USA.

The mortality rate of CAP treated in the community is thought to be very low: probably <1%. Mortality among hospitalized patients varies depending on health service but is around 5–10%. Mortality among patients admitted to ICU with CAP is much higher but the statistics are much more varied, again depending on ICU admission criteria. Mortality obviously varies with severity of disease (see the section below on severity assessment) and also with organism. *Staph. aureus*, Gram-negative bacilli (especially *Pseudomonas*), *Burkholderia pseudomallei* and *Legionella* spp. all carry a higher than baseline mortality while *Mycoplasma* and the *Chlamydophila* spp. have lower mortality.

Influenza and pneumonia (ICD codes J10-J18) account for 2.3% of all deaths in Australia and are a contributing cause in 13.3%.

Clinical features

Pneumonia should be suspected in patients with:

- fever
- new cough
- rigors
- change in sputum colour
- pleuritic chest pain
- dyspnoea.

Many patients with these features, however, will not have pneumonia and certain groups of patients (particularly the elderly) may have pneumonia with few or none of these features.

Table 6.3.1 Clinical features associated with specific organisms

Streptococcus pneumoniae
- Increasing age
- High fever
- High acuity
- Pleurisy

Bacteraemic pneumococcal pneumonia
- Female
- Diabetic
- Alcoholic
- COPD
- Dry cough

Legionella
- Young and previously healthy patient
- Smoker
- Multisystem illness (LFT abnormality, elevated CK, GIT upset, neurological disturbance)
- More severe illness

Mycoplasma
- Young and previously healthy patient
- Antibiotic use prior to presenting to hospital
- Isolated respiratory illness

Staph. aureus
- IVDU
- Severe illness
- History of influenza

Gram-negative rods
- Alcoholic
- Nursing home resident

A normal chest examination makes pneumonia less likely but does not rule it out. The classically described progression of chest examination findings is from crackles and reduced air entry in the first days, to dull percussion note and bronchial breathing which persists until resolution begins at around day 7–10 when crackles return. Fever is said to be persistent until a 'crisis' followed by resolution. The actual clinical reality may bear little resemblance to this. The presence of classical findings in the chest may precede radiological abnormality by several hours, particularly in pneumococcal pneumonia.

Much has been made of the role of the clinical syndrome as a predictor of aetiology but the evidence shows this to be unreliable. Previously 'typical' and 'atypical' pneumonia have been differentiated clinically but there is now a general consensus that these terms should be abandoned as they are misleading. The term 'atypical organism', however, has persisted as an umbrella term for the *Chlamydophila* spp., the *Legionella* spp. and *Mycoplasma*. With these caveats in mind, there

are certain associations that should be considered (Table 6.3.1).

The term 'community-acquired pneumonia', as opposed to hospital-acquired pneumonia, is generally defined as pneumonia occurring in a patient who has not been an inpatient in hospital in the last 10 or 14 days. Patients with AIDS, cystic fibrosis, current chemotherapy or active haematological malignancy presenting with pneumonia should be considered to be presenting with a complication of their underlying condition rather than with CAP. The question of how to classify patients with pneumonia presenting from nursing homes remains unresolved. Nursing home status carries an increased mortality risk and an increased risk of both aspiration pneumonitis and of infection with *Staph. aureus* and aerobic Gram-negative bacilli.

Pathogenesis and aetiology

Most cases of CAP result from aspiration of flora from the upper respiratory tract, although *Legionella* spp. and *Mycobacterium tuberculosis* may be aspirated directly in aerosolized droplets suspended in the atmosphere. Haematogenous spread to the lung also occurs, for example from right-sided endocarditis.

Large volume aspiration of gastrointestinal and upper respiratory tract contents is normally prevented by a coordinated swallow and intact gag and cough reflexes; however, microaspiration occurs routinely in normal individuals during sleep. Aspirated matter is generally quickly cleared by the mucocilliary escalator and by periodic coughing.

Pathogens lodging on the lower respiratory mucosa meet with a fine layer of mucus, rich in secreted IgA that acts to prevent their adhesion and to activate other arms of the immune system. These defences may still be breached by the common organisms. Derangement of the defences allows 'opportunistic' organisms to cause infection, such as the Gram-negative rods, anaerobes, *Staphylococcus* and fungi.

Estimates of the rates of occurrence of various organisms implicated in CAP are difficult for several reasons. Isolation of a causative organism occurs in only around 40–70% of cases in hospital-based studies, less so in community-based ones and much less commonly in actual clinical practice (particularly in CAP treated in the community). The most common organism isolated in all settings and in all classes of CAP, *Streptococcus pneumoniae*

(*Strep. pneumoniae* or *pneumococcus*), is one of the easiest to isolate whereas *Chlamydophila pneumoniae* and *psitacii* (formerly *Chlamydia pneumoniae* and *psittaci*) and the *Legionella* spp. present much greater difficulty, potentially skewing the data in favour of pneumococcus. There is a great deal of heterogeneity in the pneumonia studies with regard to underlying patient characteristics, setting, case definition, degree of diagnostic investigation and timing with relation to epidemics, which further complicates interpretation of the data.

Streptococcus pneumoniae

This encapsulated bacterium has previously been isolated from around 30% of cases of CAP in the community, hospital wards and ICU (50–60% of cases where a cause is found) and more commonly when highly sensitive methods are used for its detection. Recent studies have found lower rates, around 15% (or one-third of cases where a cause is found), which may be due to changing living conditions or pneumococcal vaccination programmes. In about 25% of cases, bacteraemia is identified and, in a few of these, there are other foci of invasive disease (such as meningitis).

Traditionally, this organism has been extremely sensitive to penicillin; however, DRSP is emerging around the world. Sensitivity is generally described by minimum concentration of antibiotic required to inhibit growth *in vitro* (MIC). MIC <0.1 mg/L represents a sensitive organism, MIC 0.1–1 mg/L represents intermediate sensitivity and MIC ≥2 mg/L, higher level resistance. In Australia, approximately 12–20% of isolates express intermediate sensitivity to penicillin but only around 1% have high level resistance. There is considerable local variation in resistance pattern. Invasive strains (isolated from blood or CSF) tend to be more susceptible; 5% are intermediate or highly resistant in Australia. Rates in the UK are lower where less than 3% of pneumococcal bacteraemias are of intermediate or high penicillin resistance while, in Asia, resistance is much more common with 23% of isolates exhibiting intermediate sensitivity and 29% high level resistance, again with marked local variation. Blood levels achieved by giving 1 g amoxycillin orally 8-hourly or 1.2 g benzyl penicillin IV 6-hourly are sufficient to treat the sensitive and intermediate sensitivity strains. In fact, it is only strains with an MIC >4 mg/L that present a significant likelihood of treatment failure at these doses.

Macrolide resistance ranges from 15% in the UK to 92% in Vietnam. Again, invasive strains are less commonly resistant than non-invasive ones.

Multiple drug resistance is a problem with around 17% of Australian isolates demonstrating diminished sensitivity to two or more classes of antibiotic. While respiratory fluoroquinolone resistance remains rare in Australia and the UK, in countries where levofloxacin or moxifloxacin have been more extensively used resistance is already becoming a problem.

Mycoplasma pneumoniae

These organisms are not strictly bacteria. They lack a cell wall and so are innately insensitive to beta-lactams but are treated by macrolides, tetracyclines and fluoroquinolones. They are fastidious *in vitro* and so diagnosis is generally by serological or complement fixation testing. Pneumonia due to *Mycoplasma* is most common in 5–20 year olds and is rare in the elderly and in the tropical north of Australia. A four-yearly cycle of winter epidemics (with the number of reports varying by a factor of 6–7) is well demonstrated in the UK and surveillance data from Australia suggests that the same phenomenon occurs. *Mycoplasma* accounts for perhaps 10–15% of cases of CAP. The disease is usually mild and probably self-limiting in adults, although patients with sickle cell disease or cold agglutinin disease are at risk of severe complications.

Legionella species

These aerobic Gram-negative bacilli are fastidious in culture. They occur in sources of lukewarm water, probably hosted by fresh water amoebae and are killed by temperatures above 60°C. *Legionella pneumophila* serogroup 1, *L. pneumophila* indeterminate serogroup and *L. longbeachiae* account for approximately equal shares of legionellosis in Australia. The genus causes a small percentage of cases of mild and moderate CAP (<5%) but is over-represented among severe cases causing 17.8% of cases in UK intensive care units. Outbreaks occur due to contaminated water in air conditioning cooling towers and water supplies and are a significant public health issue. The disease tends to be severe and is often a multisystem illness. Patients on long-term oral steroids are more susceptible but it is less common among the elderly.

Staphylococcus aureus

Staph. aureus, a Gram-positive coccus, is a commensal on the skin and in the oro- and nasopharynx and may reach the lung by aspiration or by haematogenous spread. It is over-represented in severe disease accounting for 25% of ICU pneumonia in the UK and is associated with a high mortality. It is almost universally resistant to penicillin but most cases are sensitive to flucloxacillin and dicloxacillin. CA-MRSA is an emerging problem. *Staphylococcal* pneumonia classically occurs following influenza and complicates two-thirds of cases of influenza pneumonia in the ICU.

Mycobacterium tuberculosis

A comprehensive review of TB pathogenesis and treatment is beyond the scope of this chapter. The classical pattern of disease is for inhalation of the bacillus to lead to a chronic inflammatory reaction, usually in the right lower lobe, producing a walled off granuloma containing surviving organisms and giant macrophages which gradually becomes calcified. At some time in the future, often in the context of immunocompromise due to steroids, malignancy, HIV, malnutrition or old age, the disease reactivates and lobar pneumonia develops (typically in the right upper lobe). The disease is usually subacute in onset and relentless without treatment. The patient often suffers chronic cough, weight loss, fevers and fatigue. That said, TB presents in many and varied ways and a high index of suspicion should be maintained. The patient with pulmonary TB and a productive cough presents a significant infection control and public health risk and respiratory isolation must be initiated while the diagnosis is confirmed.

Other important organisms

Non-typable *Haemophilus influenzae* is a rare cause of mild CAP and is uncommon in young patients. Although it is associated with exacerbations of chronic obstructive pulmonary disease (COPD), it is no more common as a cause of CAP in COPD patients than in the general population. It does, however, become more common with increasing severity of pneumonia and increasing age. Less than 25% of isolates are beta-lactamase producing, others are susceptible to aminopenicillins (and somewhat less so, to benzyl-penicillin). *Moraxella catarrhalis* has similar antibiotic susceptibilities and is less common than *Haemophilus*. Second-generation cephalosporins, tetracyclines or the combination of amoxycillin and clavulanate is adequate if amoxycillin alone fails.

Chlamydophila (formerly *Chlamydia*) *pneumoniae* causes a mild illness and there is some doubt about its role as a pathogen at all. It is sensitive to macrolides and tetracyclines.

Burkholderia pseudomallei occurs in the soil in the tropical north of Australia and in South-East Asia. Infection with it (melioidosis) typically causes a severe pneumonia, although any organ may be affected. Fifty per cent of cases are bacteraemic which is associated with 50% mortality. It makes up 25% of cases of bacteraemic pneumonia in tropical Australia (4% of all pneumonia presentations to hospital and 18% of cases where a cause is found). It is a problem mainly during the monsoon season and risk factors include diabetes mellitus, renal failure, chronic lung disease, alcoholism, long-term steroid use and excess kava intake. It is somewhat sensitive to third-generation cephalosporins, although better treated with ceftazidime or carbapenems. It is intrinsically resistant to aminoglycosides. The Gram-negative rod *Acinetobacter baumanii* occurs in a similar area, time of year and group of people and also causes severe pneumonia. It is much less common but the case fatality rate is similar. It is generally treated with aminoglycosides. Expert consultation should be sought.

Influenza A and B are common causes of pneumonia in adults. Disease may be mild, moderate or severe. Co-infection with *Staph. aureus* is a well-described complication. Clinical and radiological differentiation from bacterial pneumonia is unreliable and diagnosis is made usually with viral studies on nasopharyngeal or bronchial aspirates or on serological testing after convalescence.

Anaerobic organisms are generally aspirated in patients with poor dentition. Edentulous patients are thus protected and these organisms are actually rare in aspiration pneumonia among nursing home patients.

The Gram-negative rods are a varied group of opportunistic agents which all carry a high risk of severe pneumonia and mortality. They are more common in nosocomial pneumonia than CAP. They include *Pseudomonas aeruginosa*, *Serratia spp.* and *Klebsiella pneumoniae*. Emergence of antibiotic resistance during treatment is a particular problem with *Pseudomonas* and antibiotics from two classes should be used concurrently if infection is proven or highly likely.

Associations between particular risk factors and particular organisms in CAP patients are weak and it is important to remember that routine questioning about risk factors is likely to be misleading. For example, despite the well-known association between *Chlamydophila psittaci* and sick parrots, 80% of patients with psittacosis have no history of bird contact. Stronger associations are those between *Staph. aureus* and influenza, between *Staph. aureus* and intravenous drug use (IVDU) and between *Legionella* and travel. Workers in the animal handling and slaughtering industries are at risk of infection with *Coxiella burnetii* (Q fever). Awareness of any local epidemics is important, particularly outbreaks of *Mycoplasma* or legionellosis.

Prevention

Prevention of pneumonia in the first world centres on vaccination for influenza and pneumococcus. In developing regions, the provision of adequate nutrition and housing is more important. Legionellosis is avoided by appropriate design and maintenance of air-conditioning and water supply systems in large buildings.

It is worth noting that aspiration pneumonia is not prevented by the use of nasogastric or PEG feeding tubes.

Differential diagnosis

The clinical syndrome of pneumonia is non-specific and the differential diagnosis is broad. CXR findings of lobar infiltrate, however, narrow the possibilities significantly. Underlying malignancy should always be considered, especially in older patients with a history of smoking. Pulmonary embolus (PE) is less likely in the presence of a lobar infiltrate but this should be differentiated from the wedge-shaped opacification of a pulmonary infarction due to PE. Bi-basal pneumonia can be very difficult to distinguish from left ventricular failure, especially in the elderly patient in whom clinical signs and white cell count can be unreliable. CXR changes may be pre-existing, such as in localized fibrosis from radiotherapy or when there has been a recent pneumonia with opacification yet to resolve. Aspiration pneumonitis should be differentiated from pneumonia as antibiotic therapy is less likely to be of benefit. The main indicators are on history (neurological deficit, loss of consciousness, choking while eating or vomiting in the patient with diminished airway reflexes), although most episodes go unwitnessed.

Complications

Pleural effusion and empyema

Pleural effusion is a fairly common occurrence in hospitalized patients with CAP, occurring in 36–57% of admitted patients. Effusion detectable on CXR is an indicator of severity, especially if bilateral. Persistent fever raises the likelihood of an effusion. The majority of effusions resolve with antibiotic treatment but empyema requires drainage. As effusion and empyema are radiologically indistinguishable, any significant effusion should be aspirated. Cloudy fluid, WCC >100 000/mm^3, glucose <2.2 mmol/L, pH <7.2, or organisms on Gram stain indicate empyema and the need for drainage. Aspiration will also provide a specimen for aetiological diagnosis, although the yield is not high.

Abscess

Lung abscess is a rare complication, most common in the alcoholic, debilitated or aspiration pneumonia patient. Some will respond to antibiotics but drainage is often required. *Staph. aureus*, anaerobes and Gram-negatives are more likely culprits and polymicrobial infection is common. Tuberculosis should be considered in any patient with a cavitating lesion.

Severe sepsis syndromes

Severe sepsis syndromes are a relatively common occurrence in CAP. Approximately 40% of hospitalized patients develop non-pulmonary organ dysfunction, with 28% having evidence of it at presentation. Septic shock develops in 4–5% of cases and is manifest at presentation in just under half of these. The Pneumonia Severity Index (see below) correlates with the likelihood of severe sepsis and the SMART-COP score (see below) predicts the need for inotropic and respiratory support.

Respiratory failure

Respiratory failure is a common reason for ICU admission in CAP. In patients with moderate to severe disease, a widened A–a gradient can be detected with PCO$_2$ being depressed as the patient increases minute volume to compensate for failure of gas exchange. As severity increases, the PCO$_2$ will return to normal as the patient tires and PO$_2$ will fall. Type II respiratory failure generally occurs late.

Renal failure

Renal failure may occur in any case of severe CAP, but is particularly associated with legionellosis. Multiorgan failure may occur as a result of severe sepsis.

Clinical investigations

Imaging

Chest X-ray

Presence of a new infiltrate on CXR remains central to the diagnosis of pneumonia. Diagnosis without CXR is shown to be unreliable, although a normal chest examination makes the diagnosis unlikely.

CXR has proven to be an unreliable indicator of aetiology, however, some clues may be found. *Mycoplasma* is less likely in the presence of homogeneous shadowing but is suggested by lymphadenopathy. Multilobar infiltrates and pleural effusions make bacteraemic streptococcal pneumonia more likely, while a multilobar infiltrate with pneumatocoeles, cavitation and pneumothorax is suggestive of *Staph. aureus*. *Klebsiella* tends towards the right upper lobe but the described association between this agent and a bulging horizontal fissure is unsupported by evidence.

Tuberculosis should always be considered in cases of upper lobe infiltrate, especially in the presence of a Ghon focus or calcified nodule, usually found in the right lower lobe.

Clues to severity may be found on the CXR (see below).

The role of the repeat CXR is unclear. The rate of improvement is quite variable. It is slower with increasing age, presence of co-morbidity, multilobar infiltrates and *Strep.* (especially bacteraemic) or *Legionella* as pathogens. *Legionella*, in fact, is characterized by worsening radiological appearance after admission. The role of a convalescent film is likewise unclear. Rates of underlying lung cancer vary and most cases are diagnosed on the acute film. Smokers over 50 years of age are particularly at risk and routine convalescent imaging should be considered in this group.

Computed tomography

Computed tomography (CT) currently has a limited role in diagnosis of pneumonia due to cost, radiation dose and lack of a clear benefit over plain CXR. In some cases, a diagnosis may be made on CT when another diagnosis is being excluded (e.g. CTPA for exclusion of pulmonary embolus).

General pathology

The roles of non-microbiological pathological testing in CAP are to help confirm the diagnosis, to assess severity, to identify complications and to screen for underlying or co-morbid conditions. The majority of previously well young people with non-severe pneumonia are unlikely to benefit from routine tests.

Full blood count

The full blood count is routine in the patient requiring hospitalization with pneumonia. Anaemia, thrombocytopaenia, severe leucocytosis and leucopaenia are all markers of severity (see below). Polycythaemia may indicate dehydration or underlying chronic hypoxia. A white cell count over 15 000 cells/mm^3 is suggestive of bacterial cause (especially *Strep. pneumoniae*) but is insensitive and non-specific.

Urea and electrolytes

Urea, electrolytes and creatinine are also routinely measured in the hospitalized patient. Hyponatraemia (Na <130 mmol/L) and elevated urea ($\geq$11 mmol/L) are proven markers of severe pneumonia. Acute renal impairment is a relatively common complication of severe pneumonia, while chronic renal failure is a risk factor for severe disease.

Liver function tests

Liver function tests frequently demonstrate some abnormality, although this may not change management. Chronic liver disease is a risk factor for severe pneumonia. Hypoalbuminaemia is a marker of severity.

Blood gas testing

Measurement of arterial blood gases has been common practice in patients hospitalized with pneumonia. Recent evidence demonstrates that a venous blood gas is acceptable for assessment of acid–base status and may be a valid screening tool for hypercapnoea. Transcutaneous oxygen saturation measurement (SpO$_2$) is, likewise, an acceptable screening tool for hypoxia, although it becomes inaccurate when SpO$_2$ is <90%.

Inflammatory markers

Measurement of C-reactive protein (CRP) remains contentious. The recent British Thoracic Society guidelines update concluded that 'there is no clear consensus in the literature about value of CRP in differentiating between infective causes. There is no value of CRP in severity assessment'. At best, CRP may have a role in differentiation between exacerbation of COPD and pneumonia or non-infective causes and pneumonia in uncertain cases.

Serum procalcitonin, D-dimer, serum cortisol and other novel biomarkers have been found to correlate with severity of pneumonia but their discriminatory value and role, if any, remain undefined.

Testing for aetiology/ microbiology

As discussed above, achieving an aetiological diagnosis in CAP is difficult, even in the research setting in tertiary referral centres.

Advantages of doing so include the opportunity to tailor therapy, to detect outbreaks such as Legionnaire's disease, influenza or *Mycoplasma* and to identify resistant organisms. An emerging concern in recent years is that of bioterrorism which may be identified early due to reporting of aetiological diagnoses. A further consideration is the paucity of published data on the aetiology of pneumonia, particularly from Australia and New Zealand. Current knowledge depends heavily upon laboratory reports to surveillance authorities and 'accumulated knowledge' rather than scientific studies.

Disadvantages of an aggressive diagnostic approach are the cost compared to the low yield, the risk of inappropriate changes to therapy based on false-positive results from contaminants, the long lag time to get a result (particularly from culture and paired serology), the potential to delay treatment while specimens are obtained and the exposure of the patient to added unpleasant and invasive procedures (such as multiple venepunctures for blood culture). Moreover, it is uncommon for therapy to be streamlined even with microbiological diagnosis. The only randomized controlled trial comparing empiric to directed therapy found no benefit to a pathogen directed approach, although there was a small mortality benefit found in the ICU subgroup.

Sputum

Sputum can be collected for microscopy and for culture. The two should be considered separately as they are very different tests and are likely to be valuable in different settings. The value of sputum collection has been debated, however. Unfortunately, many patients are unable to produce sputum and waiting for them to do so may cause significant delays to antibiotic treatment.

Microscopy (generally with Gram stain, although Zeil-Neilsen stain for acid-fast bacilli should be requested if tuberculosis is suspected) can potentially provide useful guidance for empiric prescribing as well as an indication of whether the specimen is of sufficient quality for culture to be useful.

Sputum culture has a higher sensitivity than Gram stain and provides more definite identification, typing and sensitivity data; however, results are not available when treatment is started and colonization may be hard to distinguish from infection, particularly if Gram stain was negative or not performed. Special culture is indicated if *Legionella* or *M. tuberculosis* is to be identified.

Sensitivity of both microscopy and culture decline if antibiotic therapy has already started and, even under ideal conditions, neither is highly sensitive or specific.

Likewise, tuberculosis requires both special stains and culture media as well as prolonged culture time. Provision of good clinical details to the lab including suspected organism, timing of specimen and use of antibiotics is essential.

Blood culture

Blood cultures have traditionally been recommended for all patients admitted to hospital with suspected pneumonia. More recently, the performance of blood cultures in admitted pneumonia patients has been linked to hospital accreditation in the USA. The most common non-contaminant organism isolated is pneumococcus, which is generally covered by empiric treatment and yields are generally low (around 7% overall and 25% at most in pneumococcal pneumonia). Contaminants are found with similar frequency. Pneumococcal pneumonia with and without bacteraemia have been shown to have a similar prognosis. That said, a positive result (other than coagulase negative staphylococci) is highly specific for microbiological aetiology.

A rational approach is to limit blood culture use to cases where yield is higher, the likelihood of a resistant or non-pneumococcal organism is higher, the consequences of inappropriate prescription are greatest or where there is concern about a significant outbreak or epidemic.

Independent predictors of a positive blood culture in CAP include coexistent liver disease, systolic blood pressure <90 mmHg, temperature <35°C or $\geq$40°C, pulse $\geq$125/min, urea $\geq$11 mmol/L, Na <130 mmol/L, WBC <5000 cells/mm^3 or >20 000 cells/mm^3 and lack of prior antibiotic therapy. A prediction rule has been developed based on these variables with presence of two or more predictors associated with a 16% rate of positive blood culture. These indicators are also markers of severity and it is patients with severe pneumonia who are most at risk of adverse outcome if initial antibiotics are not sufficient. A positive pneumococcal urinary antigen test (UAT, see below) is associated with a higher yield from blood culture and may be an indication for performing blood culture to monitor community resistance rates.

Current British Thoracic Society guidelines indicate that blood cultures have little role in non-severe pneumonia and the IDSA/ATS guidelines recommend blood cultures for ICU patients and those with cavitation, leucopaenia, alcoholism, chronic liver disease, asplenia, a positive pneumococcal UAT or a pleural effusion.

Urinary antigen testing

The two commonly available urinary antigen tests (UAT) are the legionella and pneumococcal UAT. Both are fast and simple to perform and minimally affected by the use of antibiotics. The pneumococcal UAT is 50–80% sensitive and >90% specific. False positives occur in children with chronic respiratory illness and colonization with pneumococcus and in adults who have had CAP in the last 3 months. The legionella UAT is probably highly sensitive and specific for *L. pneumophila* serogroup 1, is positive from day 1 and remains so for up to 3 weeks.

The precise role of these tests remains uncertain, however. CAP is assumed to be pneumococcal by default and so a positive test provides little helpful information while a negative test is of little predictive value. As discussed above, the UAT might be used as a triage tool to identify patients who will have a higher yield from blood cultures. The legionella UAT identifies only *Legionella pneumophila* serogroup 1 which accounts for less than half of cases in Australia. It is, as yet, unclear whether a positive legionella UAT justifies streamlining to macrolide monotherapy in sick inpatients or whether it obligates upgrading from oral to IV macrolide. A positive legionella UAT is associated with ICU admission, perhaps because the higher antigen load present in cases with a positive test represents a greater infective burden. A negative legionella UAT, however, does not rule out legionellosis as other species and serogroups are not detected.

Other tests

Serology has little to offer the emergency management of CAP but has a public health role if an outbreak of viral or 'atypical' pneumonia is suspected. If symptoms have been ongoing for more than 7 days then a high titre of *Mycoplasma* or *Legionella* IgM is diagnostic but otherwise paired serology weeks apart are required, with the diagnosis coming only after treatment is completed.

Influenza rapid point-of-care testing has a low sensitivity (50–70%) and cross-reacts with adenovirus. A positive test is highly specific and may be an indication for treatment with antivirals, where available, and may be useful in outbreak detection, although it is unlikely to be superior to physician judgement in this role. Influenza direct fluorescent antibody testing is more reliable but takes 2 hours and requires special laboratory skills. It is used for identification of specific strains of influenza (e.g. avian influenza, H5N1 and 'swine flu', H1N1).

Severity assessment

A key clinical problem in assessment of a patient with suspected CAP is assessment of severity. The great majority of CAP cases are mild and would be self-limiting, although antibiotic treatment shortens the illness. However, a significant minority of cases cause an acutely debilitating illness and a small minority are life threatening. Attempts at formalizing the process of severity assessment with severity scoring systems have focused on two aims: identifying those who can safely be managed at home, thus reducing unnecessary admissions and unplanned readmissions, and identifying those who are likely to need ICU care with the aim of reducing mortality and complications from delayed recognition of severe disease while avoiding overuse of ICU. A number of scoring systems have been developed and validated, including the Pneumonia Severity Index (PSI), the British Thoracic Society's BTS, modified BTS, CRB, CURB and CURB-65 scores, the American Thoracic Society's ATS, modified ATS (m-ATS) and revised ATS (r-ATS) scores, the Spanish SEPAR score and the Australian scores SMART-COP and CORB.

Proven markers of severity

The following have all been defined as markers of severity in various studies:

- Demographic factors:
  - increasing age
  - residence in a nursing home or being bedridden
  - male sex
- Co-morbidity:
  - congestive cardiac failure, diabetes mellitus, coronary artery disease, chronic lung disease, liver disease, cerebrovascular disease, chronic renal failure and neoplastic disease
- Examination findings:
  - respiratory rate >30/min or <6/min
  - confusion (Abbreviated Mental Test Score <8 or new disorientation to time, place or person)
  - systolic BP <90 mmHg, diastolic BP <60 mmHg or septic shock requiring aggressive fluid resuscitation or vasopressors
  - temperature <35°C or ≥40°C
  - heart rate ≥125/min
- Haematological:
  - haematocrit <30%
  - white cell count <4000 cells/mm^3 or >20 000 cells/mm^3
  - platelets <100 000 cells/mm^3
- Biochemical:
  - urea elevated (cut-offs vary)
  - sodium <130 mmol/L
  - glucose >14 mmol/L
  - arterial pH <7.35
  - hypoxia (PaO$_2$ <60 mmHg, SpO$_2$ <92%, PaO$_2$:FiO$_2$ <250 mmHg)
  - albumin <3.5 g/dL
- Radiological features:
  - bilateral or multilobar involvement
  - effusions, especial bilateral
  - worsening radiological changes after admission in the ICU patient
- Microbiological:
  - positive blood culture (not available at time of initial assessment)
  - *Strep. pneumoniae*, Gram-negative bacilli, *Staph. aureus* and *Ps. Aeruginosa*.

SMART-COP

The SMART-COP score was derived and validated in temperate Australia as part of the ACAPS study and has since been validated in tropical Australia. It has been shown to predict the need for intensive respiratory or vasopressor support (IRVS) during the initial assessment in the emergency department with high sensitivity and negative predictive value (NPV). The score has eight components which have different weighting

Table 6.3.2   Calculating the SMART-COP score

S	Systolic BP <90 mmHg		2 points
M	Multilobar CXR involvement		1 point
A	Albumin <3.5 g/dL		1 point
R	Respiratory rate (age adjusted)	1 point	
		≤50 years	≥25 br/min
		≥50 years	≥30 br/min
T	Tachycardia ≥125 bpm		1 point
C	Confusion (new)		1 point
O	Oxygen low (age adjusted)		2 points
		≤50 years	PaO_2 <70 mmHg; SpO_2 ≤93% on air; PaO_2:FiO_2 <333 mmHg
		≥50 years	PaO_2 <60 mmHg; SpO_2 ≤90% on air; PaO_2:FiO_2 <250 mmHg
P	Arterial pH <7.35		2 points

Table 6.3.3   Interpreting the SMART-COP score

0–2 points	Low risk of needing IRVS
2–4 points	Moderate (1 in 8) risk of needing IRVS
5–6 points	High (1 in 3) risk of needing IRVS
≥7 points	Very high (2 in 3) risk of needing IRVS
In primary care, albumin, arterial pH and PaO_2 may be omitted and the results interpreted as follows:	
0 points	Very low risk
1 point	Low (1 in 20) risk
2 points	Moderate (1 in 10) risk
3 points	High (1 in 6) risk
≥4 points	High (1 in 3) risk

and some of the criteria are age adjusted (Table 6.3.2). Patients are then risk stratified into five risk groups ranging from very low risk to very high risk of requiring IRVS (Table 6.3.3). The score can be modified for primary care physicians without access to blood tests and is then called SMRT-CO.

Importantly, immunosuppressed patients were excluded from all derivation and validation studies of SMART-COP so the score should be used with caution in this patient population.

CORB

CORB is another Australian derived and validated study which predicts need for intensive care in patients with CAP. It has four components which are equally weighted scoring one point each:

- confusion: new onset or worsening impairment
- oxygenation: O_2 saturation <90% or PaO_2 <60 mmHg
- respiratory rate: ≥30/min
- blood pressure: SBP <90 mmHg or DBP <60 mmHg.

A score of ≥2 equates to severe pneumonia. CORB has the advantage of being easy to remember and all variables being available at the patient's bedside. However, it was a single centre derivation and validation study potentially limiting its external validity.

It has been shown to be less sensitive and have a lower negative predictive value than SMART-COP.

Pneumonia Severity Index (PSI)

The PSI was derived by retrospective chart review and validated both retrospectively and prospectively in separate groups of patients in the late 1980s and early 1990s. In all, over 54 000 patients and 275 hospitals from across the USA and Canada were involved in the study. The rule is a two-step process with low-risk patients identified on clinical grounds alone in the first step and then all other patients being further differentiated on the basis of age and 19 dichotomized and weighted clinical and investigation features into four further groups (Tables 6.3.4 and 6.3.5)

Despite its rigorous derivation and validation, the PSI is complex to remember or calculate and is heavily weighted toward elderly patients. A young patient, compensating well early in an illness, might be significantly hypoxic and still be stratified into the lowest risk group. Social factors and the presence of unusual co-morbidities are not accounted for and are often cited by clinicians as reasons for admission in patients with otherwise clinically mild pneumonia. Moreover, the PSI has subsequently been used to stratify patients not only for discharge and admission but for ICU care and for antibiotic regimen, purposes for which it was not originally intended and for which it has not been validated.

Studies have found that the PSI is poorly adhered to by clinicians, likely due to its complexity. In its favour, the variables used by the PSI are all available at the end of a typical work-up, particularly as there are data supporting the substitution of venous pH for arterial pH.

Finally, the PSI was derived and validated in adult patients with no recent hospitalization who did not have HIV. Use of the PSI in immunocompromised patients has been investigated in one study and was found to perform well in patients with HIV, solid organ transplant or treatment with immunosuppressive drugs and poorly in patients with haematological malignancy, on chemotherapy or after chest radiotherapy or bone marrow transplantation.

The CURB-65 score

The British Thoracic Society (BTS) currently recommends use of this score for stratification of CAP patients. The system stratifies patients

Table 6.3.4   Calculating the PSI

Step 1

The patient is **Class I** and needs no further investigation if they are ≤50 years old and have none of the following:

History

    Neoplastic disease
    Liver disease
    Renal disease
    Congestive cardiac failure
    Cerebrovascular disease

Examination

    Acutely altered mental state
    Respiratory rate ≥30/min
    Systolic BP <90 mmHg
    Temperature <35°C or ≥40°C
    Pulse rate ≥125/min

Step 2

If the above is not satisfied, then the PSI score needs to be calculated as follows:

Factor	Score
Demographic	
Age	Age in years
Sex	−10 if female
Nursing home (not hostel) resident	+10
Coexisting illness	
Neoplastic disease	+30
Liver disease	+20
Congestive cardiac failure	+10
Cerebrovascular disease	+10
Chronic renal disease	+10
Signs on examination	
Acutely altered mental state	+20
Respiratory rate ≥30/min	+20
Systolic blood pressure <90 mmHg	+20
Temperature <35°C or ≥40°C	+15
Pulse rate ≥125/min	+10
Investigations	
Arterial pH <7.35	+30
Serum urea ≥11 mmol/L	+20
Serum sodium <130 mmol/L	+20
Serum glucose ≥14 mmol/L	+10
Haematocrit <30%	+10
PaO_2 <60 mmHg or SpO_2 <90%	+10
Pleural effusion on CXR	+10

After Fine MJ, et al.: A prediction rule to identify low-risk patients with community-acquired pneumonia. N Engl J Med 1997; 336:243-50.

Table 6.3.5   Mortality and PSI class

Score	Class	30-Day mortality (%)
N/A	I	0.1
1–70	II	0.6
71–90	III	0.9
91–130	IV	9.3
>130	V	27

on the basis of a 0–5 scale with one point scored for each of:

- confusion of new onset (AMTS <8 or new disorientation to time, place or person)
- urea >7 mmol/L
- respiratory rate ≥30/min
- blood pressure <90 mmHg (systolic) or ≤60 mmHg (diastolic)
- age ≥65 years.

Scores are correlated with risk of death and site of care is suggested (Table 6.3.6).

The CURB-65 score has been validated in thousands of patients from the UK and other countries and is the result of a process of refinement of a series of other validated scoring systems. It has the significant advantage of simplicity and has been shown to perform as well as a previous two-stage BTS score. It is easy to remember and quick to calculate. It is worth noting, for community practitioners, that the CRB-65 score (CURB-65 without the urea measurement) performs similarly and that patients with a CRB-65 score of 0 are generally safely managed in the community while those with a score of 1 or more should be assessed at hospital.

The CURB-65 score has been compared with the PSI as well as the various ATS scores in a number of studies. All perform similarly well with the PSI generally gaining some increase in sensitivity and specificity for death and ICU admission at the expense of greater complexity. All are strong at identifying well patients who can be safely treated at home as long as clinical judgement is brought to bear as discussed above. However, all are fairly poor at identifying patients at high risk of death and should be used cautiously in this context.

No scoring system has been proven to be superior to clinical assessment of an experienced clinician. All scoring systems should be used in conjunction with clinical judgement. Scoring systems using age as a predictor should be applied with caution in young patients. Patients requiring supplemental oxygen cannot be discharged regardless of their score. A patient who is vomiting, homeless or unreliable should not be discharged on oral antibiotics from the ED and some underlying conditions may warrant admission for relatively mild pneumonia such as advanced neuromuscular disease and general frailty.

Identification of patients likely to require ICU care is not possible with the PSI or CURB-65, although CORB and SMART-COP do perform well in this regard. No scoring system is a substitute for regular review by an experienced clinician.

Treatment

Site of care

As discussed above, the PSI and the CURB-65 score are both useful for identifying patients who

Score	Risk of death or ICU admission (%)	Comments
0	0.7	Low risk. Non-severe pneumonia. May be suitable for treatment at home
1	3.2	
2	13	Increased risk of death. Consider for short inpatient or hospital supervised outpatient treatment
3	17	High risk of death. Treat as inpatients with severe pneumonia. Consider use of ICU
4	41.5	
5	57	

Table 6.3.6 Mortality and the CURB-65 score

are well enough to be discharged home as long as oxygenation, psychosocial factors and the overall clinical picture are considered. Typically, cases with of PSI class I or CURB-65 score of 0 can be treated at home with confidence and cases with PSI class II or CURB-65 score of 1 are probably safe to discharge as well.

Cases of intermediate severity (PSI ≥III or CURB-65 score ≥2) are likely to benefit from a short period of supervised hospital treatment to ensure that antibiotics are given effectively and to monitor for any deterioration. Emergency observation units or short stay units are ideal for this purpose. Alternatively a 'hospital in the home' service may be appropriate, particularly if it incorporates early medical review.

Decision to admit to ICU can be aided by SMART-COP (≥3) or CORB (≥2) scores.

General supportive care

For the patient being discharged to the community, general advice regarding rest, analgesia for chest wall pain and maintenance of adequate hydration and nutrition are appropriate. Physiotherapy is of no proven benefit. All discharged patients should undergo scheduled medical review within 24–48 hours in case of deterioration.

For the admitted patient, similar measures will be required. Hydration may need to be supplemented with intravenous fluids and, in severe or prolonged illness, nutritional support will be required. Oxygen should be provided to maintain SpO_2 >95% (PaO_2 >60 mmHg). A lower SpO_2/PaO_2 may be desirable in patients with severe COAD.

The role of non-invasive ventilatory support (NIV) in respiratory failure due to pneumonia is controversial. In patients with underlying COPD, it is almost certainly of benefit. In other patients, it has been shown to raise SpO_2 and decrease heart rate but deterioration requiring intubation is common and patients intubated

after a failure of a prolonged trial of NIV fair worse than those intubated early. At best, it is probably a temporizing measure if intubation is not immediately possible or if it is not immediately clear that intubation is appropriate.

Invasive ventilation should be low volume (6 mL/kg of ideal body weight) even if hypercapnoea results. Severe sepsis syndrome and septic shock should be recognized and treated early and aggressively.

The use of structured guidelines for CAP management, covering a range of interventions, has been shown to reduce hospital mortality. The particular guidelines used seem less important than that the guidelines are locally appropriate (taking into account local patient demographics, co-morbidity spectrum, social issues, organism prevalence and antibiotic resistance patterns). There is wide local variation noted in antibiotic resistance rates, both between countries and within them.

Antibiotic treatment

Initial therapy in CAP is almost always empiric with antibiotics selected to cover the likely organisms. *Strep. pneumoniae* is treated generally with a beta-lactam. The 'atypical' organisms are covered with a macrolide, although a tetracycline is acceptable if oral therapy is being used. These also provide cover against *Legionella spp.* Doxycycline and macrolides also provide some cover against *Strep. pneumoniae* but, due to high levels of resistance, should only be used as monotherapy in patients with mild pneumonia. A beta-lactam should be added if treatment fails. Addition of specific coverage for Gram-negative coliforms, *Staph. aureus*, *Pseudomonas aeruginosa*, *Burkholderia pseudomallei* and *Acinetobacter baumanii* are added when severity or the clinical or epidemiological picture warrant. Monotherapy with a fluoroquinolone is an alternative to the combination of beta-lactam and macrolide in

mild pneumonia or in patients with immediate hypersensitivity to beta-lactams, but emerging resistance is a problem.

Drug resistant *Strep. pneumoniae* is a growing problem around the world, particularly in Asia, but it remains an uncommon cause of pneumonia in Australia and the UK. Macrolide resistance is common *in vitro* but the significance of this has been questioned. Modern macrolides are concentrated at the site of infection and, until recently, few cases of treatment failure with macrolide monotherapy had been reported. Recently, macrolide resistance among pneumococci has been recognized as a significant clinical problem.

Community-acquired MRSA is another looming problem, although it has mainly been reported from skin and soft-tissue infections rather than CAP. It tends to be less broadly resistant than hospital-acquired MRSA. Ominously, the genes for drug resistance in CA-MRSA tend to be associated with the gene for panton-valentine leukocidin, which is associated with necrotizing pneumonia, respiratory failure and shock.

As discussed above, the clinical and radiological pictures are often unhelpful in assessing microbiological aetiology of CAP. In the absence of a positive UAT or sputum Gram stain, it is unlikely that initial treatment decisions will be made on data other than the clinical picture and knowledge of local pathogens. With increasing severity of pneumonia, antibiotic coverage is generally broadened for two reasons: organisms other than *Strep. pneumoniae* become more likely and there is more to be lost by failure to cover the causative agent in the first instance.

Despite widespread dissemination of antibiotic guidelines, overprescribing of broad-spectrum antibiotics remains a problem. Pneumonia guidelines are often generalized to non-pneumonic lower respiratory tract infections, such as bronchitis and exacerbations of COPD, and severe pneumonia tends to be over-diagnosed. Overprescription of broad-spectrum antibiotics contributes to many adverse outcomes including: increases in antibiotic-associated enteropathy and *C. difficile* infection; increases in other side effects, such as anaphylaxis; increased healthcare costs; and increased spread of resistant organisms.

SMART-COP and CORB have been recommended by the *Australian Therapeutic Guidelines: Antibiotic* as tools for selection of antibiotic coverage. It is to be noted that this is not directly supported by the available evidence, although it is in line with the principles discussed above.

Mild pneumonia

Oral therapy is preferred in patients well enough to be treated at home who are able to tolerate oral medications and are likely to be adherent to a treatment regimen. Given the known spectrum of pathogens as described above, whether to use a beta-lactam alone or in combination with dedicated 'atypical cover' is debated. A Cochrane review has found no benefit in addition of 'atypical cover', although most of the studies examined compared fluoroquinolone monotherapy to beta-lactam monotherapy. In the UK, where the four-yearly cycle of *Mycoplasma* epidemics is well described, amoxycillin as a single agent is recommended with erythromycin as an alternative, if tolerated, unless a *Mycoplasma* outbreak is known to be occurring. In the USA, the practice of using macrolide monotherapy is well established but it can fail against DRSP. Australian guidelines recommend monotherapy with amoxycillin unless there is specific concern about atypical organisms.

The combination of a macrolide with amoxycillin has always been shown to be effective against DRSP and the combination increases the likelihood of covering *H. influenzae* adequately. Cefuroxime is an alternative to amoxycillin as it has a similar spectrum including moderate activity against *Haemophilus*. Monotherapy with a fluoroquinolone, such as moxifloxacin, is an alternative for mild pneumonia and is useful if immediate hypersensitivity to penicillins is suspected, however, these drugs remain expensive and treatment failure due to resistance is starting to be reported in parts of the world. There is concern that use of these agents will increase resistance to important reserve agents, such as ciprofloxacin.

In cases where a single dose of IV antibiotic is to be given before discharge from the ED, benzyl penicillin is preferred to amoxycillin for its narrower spectrum of activity. Amoxycillin is preferred for oral treatment as oral phenoxymethyl penicillin is unlikely to reach adequate levels to cover intermediate resistant DRSP and is of no value against *H. influenzae*.

Patients who prefer to be treated at home, but who are unlikely to be adherent to oral therapy, can be treated with IM procaine penicillin 1.5 g daily for 5 days which can be supplemented by a supervised daily dose of oral azithromycin.

Moderate pneumonia

For patients requiring hospitalization, the combination of benzyl penicillin or amoxycillin and a macrolide remains most appropriate. The beta-lactam should be given intravenously to guarantee sufficient blood levels to treat intermediate sensitivity *Strep. pneumoniae*. If non-immediate penicillin hypersensitivity is thought to be a problem, a third-generation cephalosporin should be used intravenously instead and, in cases of immediate hypersensitivity to penicillin, a fluoroquinolone is indicated.

Sputum specimen should be sent for Gram stain if this service is available and, if Gram-negative bacilli are seen, gentamicin can be added or a third-generation cephalosporin substituted for penicillin/amoxycillin.

Severe pneumonia

Although *Strep. pneumoniae* remains the most common pathogen, there is an overrepresentation of *Staph. aureus*, *Legionella spp.* and Gram-negative organisms in severe cases. Moreover, it is of greater importance in this group that initial therapy is adequate. Therefore, empiric cover needs to be broader than for the less severe cases. The most commonly recommended approach is to use a combination of a third-generation cephalosporin with an intravenous macrolide. Alternatively, the combination of benzyl penicillin, an aminoglycoside and an intravenous macrolide has also been recommended, although head-to-head studies demonstrating equivalence of this to the former, more established regimen are lacking. Staphylococcal pneumonia should always be considered in this group (see below).

Staphylococcal pneumonia

In all severe cases of pneumonia, a sputum specimen should be examined if possible, but this should not delay therapy. If Gram-positive cocci in clusters are seen or if the clinical or radiological picture is suggestive of staphylococcal pneumonia, treatment should be instituted with flucloxacillin/dicloxacillin. It is important to be aware of local rates of CA-MRSA. In most settings, this remains a rare cause of CAP and it is not necessary to treat with vancomycin in the first instance in cases of moderate illness. In severely ill patients, CA-MRSA cover with vancomycin, co-trimoxazole or clindamycin should be used until susceptibilities are known.

Aspiration pneumonia

Most cases of aspiration do not result in any significant respiratory compromise and, of those that do, the majority are not infective pneumonia but non-infective chemical pneumonitis. Unfortunately, the two are very difficult to distinguish. Treatment recommendations vary and hard evidence is limited. If antibiotic therapy is to be used, a beta-lactam and metronidazole is an appropriate combination in most cases. In patients without teeth, anaerobic cover is probably not required while, in certain patients (nursing home residents and alcoholics), Gram-negative cover with a third generation cephalosporin should be considered.

Pneumonia in tropical areas

Patients in certain tropical areas are prone to infection with *Burkholderia pseudomallei* and *Acinetobacter baumanii* while 'atypicals', such as *Mycoplasma* and *Legionella*, are much less common. Mild pneumonia can generally be treated safely with a beta-lactam alone. In moderate cases, if risk factors for these infections are present (see above), a third-generation cephalosporin (for *Burkholderia*) and gentamicin (for *Acinetobacter*) should be used. In severe pneumonia in these regions, especially during the monsoon, all patients should be treated with a carbapenem and macrolide.

Likely developments over the next 5–10 years

- Novel biomarkers will continue to be proposed as diagnostic or severity predicting agents. Critical appraisal of evidence for their use will be required to avoid increasing cost of treatment without increasing benefit.
- Clinician performed bedside ultrasound has an emerging role for diagnosis and assessment of complications, however, expertise in its use it not yet widespread.
- Drug-resistant organisms will become an increasing problem, particularly multidrug resistant pneumococcus.
- Increasing rates of HIV, increasing numbers of patients on long-term immunosuppression after organ transplant and on long-term chemotherapy and an ageing population is likely to alter the spectrum of CAP with increasing frequency of opportunistic infection.
- Better transportation systems and increased movement of people around the world, coupled with an increasing population of immunocompromised patients is likely to contribute to resurgence in tuberculosis in the developed world with multidrug resistant strains becoming a particular problem.

- The emergency department short stay unit and or hospital in the home programmes may develop an increasingly important role in the management of mild–moderate pneumonia, in order to balance cost and risk-management concerns.

Controversies

- Optimal antibiotic therapy for mild pneumonia is not defined, particularly with regard to the need to treat for atypical organisms, such as *Mycoplasma* and *Chlamydophila spp.* Dual therapy (with a beta-lactam plus either a macrolide or tetracycline) is not standard worldwide. Monotherapy may offer similar success rates with less side effects and antimicrobial resistance problems.
- The value of an aggressive approach to aetiological investigation, given the expense. Pathogen-directed therapy has not shown to have a mortality benefit over empiric treatment.

- The use of SMART-COP, CORB and other risk stratification tools versus clinician judgement to guide empiric antibiotic therapy and site of care.
- Antibiotics are commonly prescribed for aspiration episodes despite the fact that most of them do not involve infection. A reliable way of predicting cases that require antibiotics is not available.
- Systemic corticosteroids have been investigated for pneumonia and found to lead to a slightly shorter duration of hospital stay and more rapid resolution of inflammatory markers and cytokine elevation. Significant improvements in patient orientated outcomes have not been found.

Acknowledgements

The authors acknowledge the assistance of Professor RM Robins-Browne, Department of Immunology and Microbiology, University of Melbourne for advice on microbiological detail.

Further reading

Buising KL, Thursky KA, Black JF, et al. Identifying severe community-acquired pneumonia in the emergency department: a simple clinical prediction tool. Emerg Med Australas 2007;19:418–26.

Charles PG, Whitby M, Fuller AJ, et al. The etiology of community-acquired pneumonia in Australia: why penicillin plus doxycycline or a macrolide is the most appropriate therapy. Clin Infect Dis 2008;46:1513–21.

Charles PG, Wolfe R, Whitby M, et al. SMART-COP: a tool for predicting the need for intensive respiratory or vasopressor support in community-acquired pneumonia. Clin Infect Dis 2008;47:375–84.

Community Acquired Pneumonia. In: eTG complete. (CD-ROM) Melbourne: Therapeutic Guidelines Ltd; 2006 (updated June 21, 2006, March, 2007).

Elliott JH, Anstey NM, Jacups SP, et al. Community-acquired pneumonia in northern Australia: low mortality in a tropical region using locally-developed treatment guidelines. Internatl J Infect Dis 2005;9:15–20.

Fine MJ, Auble TE, Yealy DM, et al. A prediction rule to identify low-risk patients with community-acquired pneumonia. N Engl J Med 1997;336:243–50.

Kennedy M, Bates DW, Wright SB, et al. Do emergency department blood cultures change practice in patients with pneumonia? Ann Emerg Med 2005;46:393–400.

Shefet D, Robesnshtok E, Paul M, Leibovici L. Empiric antibiotic coverage of atypical pathogens for community acquired pneumonia in hospitalized adults. Cochrane Database Syst Rev 2005;18:CD004418.

6.4 Influenza and emerging respiratory infections

Shin-Yan Man • Timothy H Rainer

ESSENTIALS

1 Influenza causes up to 500 000 deaths per year.

2 Influenza is difficult to differentiate clinically from the common cold.

3 Avian influenza is a potential pandemic threat with a mortality of 60%.

4 Antiviral medication is unlikely to be effective.

5 Organizational preparedness to manage pandemic influenza is vital.

6 Staff safety and morale are paramount in the fight against emerging and existing infectious diseases.

Introduction

Influenza, commonly known as 'flu', is an infectious disease that primarily affects the respiratory system of birds and mammals, including humans, swine, horses and dogs. It is caused by an RNA virus of the family Orthomyxoviridae. Every year, seasonal epidemics of influenza predictably cause between 250 000 and 500 000 deaths worldwide, primarily affecting the elderly, the immuno-compromised and the undernourished. The global community is familiar with flu, its regularity and its effects and so is generally unperturbed by its consequences. Of greater concern is the potential for a pandemic that could cause millions of fatalities. Lessons from pandemics of history and the emergence of two recent infections (namely sudden acute respiratory syndrome [SARS] and avian flu), coupled with the potential for huge economic effects, have focused interest on pandemic flu. Preparedness involves both individual case management and departmental organization. This chapter will summarize important aspects of the disease and epidemiological classification and describe the clinical features, diagnosis and management. There is also a brief summary of principles and practice at a managerial/organizational level which are important to implement if staff are to be safely protected during a pandemic. These principles nevertheless need to be part of day-to-day activity and applied before a pandemic arises.

History

Symptoms compatible with human influenza were first described by Hippocrates in 412BC. The term 'influenza' is thought to originate from 15th century Italy. The term *influenza di freddo*, meaning 'influence of the cold' was coined to describe the illness. In some senses this confuses influenza with the common 'cold', which is not helpful as the aetiological agents causing them and their associated mortality are distinctly different. However, in practice, it is often difficult to differentiate the two conditions clinically.

The first recorded pandemic attributed to influenza A was in 1580AD, which began in Asia and spread to Europe via Africa. In fact, many of the world's emerging infections appear to have originated in Asia. This may in part be due to the close proximity of human and animal populations, coupled with poor hygiene and climatic conditions. Since the 16th century, there have been six recorded pandemics, including the 'Asiatic' flu (H2N2) in 1890; another in 1900 (H3N8); the most famous and devastating outbreak, the Spanish flu (H1N1) which killed an estimated 40–100 million people in 1918; a fourth in 1957 (H2N2); the Hong Kong flu (H3N2) of 1968 which caused a million deaths; and, most recently, the 'swine flu' (new H1N1) emerged in Mexico in 2009. The SARS outbreak in 2003 was not caused by an influenza virus but rather by a coronavirus, a virus which causes the common cold. Nevertheless, within several weeks, it had affected at least 8437 cases in over 30 countries worldwide, with 10% mortality. Travel advisories were issued by the WHO, hospitals and schools were closed, small companies collapsed and economies failed. Although the disease originated in the community, it appeared that health workers faced the greatest threat. Avian influenza A (H5N1) also emerged in Asia in 2003. Although the illness has an overall mortality of 60%, there is no evidence of efficient or sustained human-to-human transmission so, at the time of writing, the number of cases is relatively few and a pandemic remains a potential threat rather than a present reality. In the spring of 2009, a new H1N1 virus emerged in Mexico, known as 'swine flu'. It has a new combination

of genes to which most people have little or no protection.

Epidemiology and pathology

Epidemiological definitions

It is important to understand the definitions of, and hence the differences between, endemic, epidemic and pandemic disease. Endemic means within people. A disease is endemic when the infection is maintained within the population without the need for external input and is usually in a steady state, e.g. chicken pox. Epidemic is when a disease/infection appears as new cases in a given population, during a given period, at a rate that exceeds what is expected based on recent experience and is not in a steady state but is increasing, e.g. rabies or SARS. A pandemic is an epidemic that spreads across a large region and increases massively. Generally speaking, three conditions need to be met for a pandemic. First, the emerging disease is new to the population. Second, the agent infects humans, causing serious illness. Third, the agent spreads easily and sustainably.

Epidemic and pandemic spread

Again, generally speaking, three factors contribute to the global spread of infectious disease: wind patterns, migratory birds and air travel. The last certainly contributed to the spread of SARS.

Influenza viruses are found in many different animals and wild birds are the primary source of influenza A viruses. The range of symptoms in birds varies greatly depending on the viral strain. Some of the H5 and H7 virus subtypes are known to cause highly pathogenic forms of disease leading to widespread disease and death among wild and domestic birds. Pigs can be infected with both human and avian viruses and the circulation of H5 and H7 virus in poultry allows the virus to mutate into a highly pathogenic form that may infect humans.

New viral strains are constantly being produced in two ways: antigenic drift and antigenic shift. Antigenic drift is a minor change in the antigenicity of haemagglutinin or neuraminidase by mutation, which enables the virus to evade immune recognition, causing most seasonal epidemics. Antigenic shift is a major change through genetic reassortment between different subtypes of influenza A during animal

Table 6.4.1 Stages of an influenza pandemic
Interpandemic period
No new influenza subtypes detected in humans
No new influenza subtypes detected in humans but an animal variant threatens human disease
Pandemic alert period
Human infections – new subtype; no human-to-human spread
Small clusters with limited human-to-human transmission
Large clusters but human-to-human spread still localized
Pandemic period
Increased and sustained transmission in general population

co-infection, which produces an entirely new antigen, e.g. the new H1N1 in 2009.

Human influenza epidemics typically occur during the winter months, where the cold and dry weather enables the virus to survive longer outside the body. There are two peak flu seasons each year because of different winter times in the northern and southern hemispheres and this explains why the there are two different vaccine formulations every year. The stages of an influenza epidemic are shown in Table 6.4.1.

Microbiological classification

The influenza viruses are classified into three types (A, B, C) based on their core proteins. Unlike influenza C, types A and B will cause epidemics. Influenza A is more virulent than the other two types and causes the most severe disease. Type A viruses are further divided into subtypes or strains based on two surface proteins, namely haemagglutinin (H) and the neuraminidase (N). There are 17 different haemaglutinin subtypes and 10 different neuraminidase subtypes. Haemagglutinin binds to the sialic acid receptors at the cell surface and mediates viral attachment and entry into the host cell. The specificity of this binding partly explains the species barrier between avian and human influenza viruses. Neuraminidase cleaves the binding between the host cells and viral particles which, in turn, facilitates the spread of the virus. Both haemagglutinin and neuraminidase are targets for antiviral drugs. Influenza B is not divided into subtypes. Current subtypes of influenza A affecting the human population include H1N1 and H3N2. The new influenza A, often called '2009 H1N1' has now mostly replaced the previous circulating H1N1 virus.

307

Incubation period and infectivity

The incubation period is typically 2 days (range 1–4 days) and transmission may be by one of three main modes:

- large droplet spread by coughs and sneezes. This is the main route of transmission
- contact, either direct or indirect, with respiratory secretions
- transmission through droplet nuclei, i.e. airborne spread.

Sneezing, coughing and even talking can produce droplets of a wide variety of particle sizes that can facilitate droplet or droplet nuclei infection. An infected person can be infectious from the day before they develop symptoms until 5–7 days afterwards. The infection is easily confused with other viral respiratory infections, such as the common cold, although influenza is usually a more serious illness. Infected persons with minimal symptoms may still shed the virus and be infectious. Primary infection in young children is usually symptomatic, although up to 50% may be asymptomatic. Viral shedding occurs for approximately 3–5 days in adults, up to 3 weeks in young children and for more than 3 weeks in severely immunocompromised persons. The amount of viral shedding correlates with the severity of illness and temperature elevation. Pre-existing antibodies against related influenza strains are partially protective, i.e. a higher infective inoculum is required with a lower likelihood of clinical illness.

Survival of the influenza virus outside the body varies with temperature and humidity. It generally survives 24–48 hours on hard, non-porous surfaces, 8–12 hours on cloth/paper/tissue and 5 minutes on hands. Survival of the virus is enhanced under conditions of low humidity and in the cold. Most influenza strains can easily be inactivated by disinfectants and detergents.

Clinical features

Influenza viruses can cause disease in all age groups, but the mortality and complication rates are higher in the elderly, young children and any persons who have chronic medical conditions.

The clinical manifestations of influenza are diverse, ranging from none to severe infection, including respiratory failure and death. Uncomplicated influenza illness is characterized by the abrupt onset of constitutional and respiratory symptoms and signs: fever, myalgia, headache, malaise, non-productive cough, sore throat and rhinitis. Gastrointestinal symptoms are more commonly seen in children than in adults. In children, otitis media, nausea and vomiting are also commonly reported.

Symptoms typically resolve after a limited number of days in the majority of cases, although cough and malaise can persist for more than 2 weeks. In some people, influenza can exacerbate underlying medical conditions (particularly pulmonary or cardiac disease), leading to secondary bacterial pneumonia, primary influenza viral pneumonia or co-infections with other viral or bacterial pathogens. Influenza infection has also been associated with encephalopathy, transverse myelitis, Reye's syndrome, myositis, myocarditis and pericarditis.

There are no pathognomonic signs and symptoms for influenza and it is difficult to distinguish influenza from other respiratory infectious disease. However, patients with symptoms of upper respiratory tract infections during an influenza outbreak are likely to have the infection. Some key similarities and differentiating features between influenza and the common cold are shown in Table 6.4.2.

Case definition in pandemic influenza outbreaks

It is important to realize that the World Health Organization case definitions are primarily designed for public health surveillance and disease reporting and not for early identification of disease. Emergency department staff will frequently have to make decisions based on the early presentation of illness when aspects of illness do not meet all the criteria for case definitions.

Case definitions are subcategorized into probable and confirmed cases. In view of the time required for laboratory confirmation of pandemic influenza infection, the probable case definition will be the working definition for operational considerations.

Persons are considered probable pandemic influenza cases when the following conditions are fulfilled:

- Abrupt onset of fever ≥38°C (except in persons aged ≥60 years, see below), and
- Non-productive cough, and either:
  - a positive epidemiological link (travel to a country with pandemic influenza or contact history with an infected person), or
  - a positive rapid test kit result, if available.
- Fever may often be absent in persons aged ≥60 years and in immunocompromised patients, such as diabetics and patients on steroids or other immunosuppressants. Therefore, in the absence of fever, any of the following symptoms, in addition to non-productive cough, should raise a high index of suspicion for persons in this category:
  - malaise
  - chills
  - headache
  - myalgia.

Persons are considered confirmed pandemic influenza cases when there is laboratory confirmation of infection with pandemic influenza.

Clinical investigations

Blood tests

Full blood count may show a leucocytosis in patients with pulmonary involvement. Lymphopaenia has been noted in severe H5N1 infection.

Imaging

A chest X-ray should be performed to exclude pulmonary involvement in high-risk patients. A thoracic computed tomography (CT) scan or bronchoscopic examination may be required later, depending on clinical progress.

Microbiology

Laboratory confirmation tests can help in the diagnosis and management of a patient who presents with symptoms of respiratory illness, although they are not necessarily done on all patients. Tests will be required to determine the cause when there is a respiratory illness outbreak. Although the commercially available rapid diagnostic test kits can detect influenza viruses

Table 6.4.2 Features differentiating influenza and the common cold	
Influenza	*Cold*
Flu virus	Corona virus
Fever, sore throat	Fever, sore throat
No runny nose	Runny nose
Myalgia, malaise, headache	Myalgia, malaise, headache
Pneumonia	No pneumonia
Days, severe	24 Hours, mild
High mortality	Low mortality

from throat swabs and nasopharyngeal aspirate specimens within 15 minutes, they cannot distinguish human from avian influenza virus or their subtypes. The sensitivities and specificities of most rapid tests range from 50 to 70% and 90 to 95% respectively. Therefore, false-negative results are more likely to occur when disease prevalence is high in the community. Case selection for testing will depend on disease severity and advice from public health departments and local infectious disease physicians.

Collecting clinical specimens for viral culture remains crucial to identifying the circulating influenza subtypes and strains. The information obtained helps to guide clinical decisions regarding influenza treatment, chemoprophylaxis and vaccine formulation. Public health departments arrange collection of data from a range of clinical settings, primarily from community health facilities.

Treatment

Management decisions are based primarily on the disease severity and the identification of 'at-risk' patients. Patients with mild disease and a low risk of developing disease complications can be managed in the community with symptomatic treatment. However, patients in the high-risk group or with severe illnesses should be managed in hospital. Antibacterial agents are used, in selected cases, for preventing or treating secondary bacterial pneumonia.

General measures

Patients with flu should rest, keep well hydrated and take antipyretics (e.g. paracetamol for fever and muscle aches). Antibiotics are not indicated unless there is clear evidence of a secondary bacterial infection in a previously healthy individual or if there is a very high probability of bacterial illness in a patient with a strong history of proven secondary bacterial infection.

Seriously infected patients may require respiratory support and intensive care management.

Antiviral agents

Antiviral agents are a second line of defence in the prevention and treatment of influenza. The administration of antiviral agents before infection or during the early stage of the disease may help prevent the infection, reduce the duration of illness by approximately 24 hours and reduce the disease complication rate.

There are two classes of antiviral agent: M2 inhibitors (adamantanes) and neuraminidase inhibitors. Adamantanes are less expensive antiviral drugs active against influenza A, but there is a high incidence of drug resistance. Neuraminidase inhibitors (oseltamivir and zanamivir) are newer, more expensive agents. They inhibit viral neuraminidase and have activity against both influenza A and B infection. They have also been shown to be effective in treating animals infected with H5N1. They are currently considered the drugs of choice in treating influenza. Antiviral medications should be started within 2 days of symptoms onset and should be prescribed for 5 days. However, they might still be beneficial in hospitalized patients with severe disease when given after 48 hours of the onset of illness. The major adverse effect of oseltamivir is nausea, which occurs in 10% of patients. Rare cases of transient neuropsychiatric events (self-injury or delirium) have been reported in Japan. Zanamivir is not recommended for persons with underlying airways disease.

The following points should be borne in mind when considering prescribing neuraminidases. They inhibit the spread of virus in the respiratory tract and, therefore, for better clinical response, they should be given early in the course of the disease and should not be delayed by waiting for laboratory confirmation. Usually, viral reproduction precedes symptoms and so neuraminidases tend to be prophylactic rather than therapeutic. They have no proven effect on mortality. Moreover, these antivirals are not equally effective against different subtypes of influenza virus and, therefore, it is difficult to predict their usefulness in future pandemics.

A word of caution

Although both the Center for Disease Control (US) and World Health Organization recommend oseltamivir (Tamiflu) as an effective antiviral agent in the treatment of influenza, and the Federal Drug Agency (USA) and the European Medicine Agency approve the drug for the treatment and prevention of influenza, there has long been a body of concern regarding the efficacy of such therapies. There are huge financial incentives for pharmaceutical companies and their investors in marketing such a product and debatable transparency about original data and results from some of the studies. Such factors have been a stimulus for the British Medical Journal's open data campaign.

Prognosis

Most people infected with influenza will recover within 1–2 weeks, but people with chronic medical conditions are at risk of developing life-threatening complications, e.g. pneumonia, or have their underlying medical problem worsened. According to the World Health Organization:

Every winter, tens of millions of people get the flu. Most are only ill and out of work for a week, yet the elderly are at a higher risk of death from the illness. We know the worldwide death toll exceeds a few hundred thousand people a year, but even in developed countries the numbers are uncertain, because medical authorities don't usually verify who actually died of influenza and who died of a flu-like illness.

Prevention

Although epidemics occur every year, their severity, duration and impact on society cannot be accurately predicted. Yearly vaccination remains the best effective method for preventing influenza and reducing the impact of epidemics. The seasonal flu vaccine protects against three most common influenza viruses (trivalent) among people today: influenza B viruses, influenza A (H1N1) viruses and influenza A (H3N2) viruses. Provided there is a good match between vaccine antigens and circulating viruses, influenza vaccines can offer approximately 70–90% protection against clinical disease in healthy adults, reduce hospital admissions among the elderly by 25–39% and reduce the overall mortality by 39–75%. Influenza vaccination is therefore useful in reducing both the healthcare costs and productivity losses associated with influenza epidemics. The frequent changes in the viral surface antigens make the annual reformulation of vaccines necessary to match the circulating viruses. Annual 'flu' vaccination is highly recommended for children, the elderly, patients with chronic medical illness, nursing home residents, healthcare workers and pregnant women. Influenza vaccines should not be used in people with allergy to egg proteins.

Avian influenza

A highly pathogenic strain of H5N1, also known as 'avian influenza', normally only infects birds, but it has been reported to cause disease in humans. It was first noted in Hong Kong in 1997, when 18 people were infected, of whom six died. The virus then disappeared until 2003, when it reappeared in the human population. By May 2006, a total of 218 patients had been infected, of whom 124 had died, a mortality rate of 57%.

Unlike the mild disease seen in normal seasonal influenza, the disease caused by H5N1 has a poor prognosis and a high fatality rate. This virus is now considered endemic in some parts of Indonesia, Vietnam, Cambodia, China, Thailand and Lao People's Democratic Republic. At present, there is no evidence to suggest efficient human-to-human transmission of avian influenza virus. Most infected patients have had direct contact with poultry. However, the constantly changing avian virus may eventually develop an efficient human transmission mechanism to start a pandemic. Vaccines against H5N1 are under development in several countries. They are, however, not commercially available to the general public. Neuraminidase inhibitors could be used for both chemoprophylaxis and as therapeutic agent, but there is limited evidence to support this.

No one is certain about the timing, scale and impact of the next pandemic. Strategic actions should be aimed at strengthening national, hospital and departmental preparedness, reducing the emergence of a novel virus, improving the warning system, delaying the international spread of disease and expediting vaccine development.

Organizational issues

Emergency departments and hospitals need to develop their own guidelines for an outbreak and regularly practise upgrading their systems. Such guidelines should cover:

- clinical characteristics of pandemic flu and its initial management
- alert criteria and their respective responses
- isolation and transfer to designated flu hospitals/health centres
- physical infrastructure and equipment in order to receive, manage and arrange for

the appropriate disposition of potentially infected patients
- staff personal protection and hygiene
- education and training, audits, exercises, surveillance, prophylaxis and stock piling.

Infection control in the emergency department

All emergency departments should have basic infection control measures. These routine measures should include the following:

- screening of all patients at the entrance of the ED
- separate pathways for potential patients with and without fever or contact history
- isolation of all such patients screened as infectious in a separate area, preferably with its own separate negative-pressure ventilation system
- use of personal protective equipment (surgical mask, hospital scrubs) when attending to patients who are potentially infectious
- hand-washing or use of alcohol rubs before and after attending to any patient
- special isolation facilities for high-risk patients who require inpatient care
- screening surveillance. This provides an early warning of an impending infectious disease outbreak and may also serve as a regular reminder to staff on the need to remain vigilant for such outbreaks.

Likely development over the next 5–10 years

An influenza pandemic is a global challenge which can potentially cause millions of deaths over a short period of time. Despite the tremendous effort that has been put into attempting to control the disease in the past, new outbreaks with new influenza strains, such as avian flu and swine flu, still appear. Future research is likely to focus on the development of new and more effective antiviral agents, on improving the technology for newer, faster and cheaper vaccine production and continuing research into the pathogenesis and epidemiology of influenza in order to enhance understanding of the disease and its management.

Controversies

- The therapeutic value of antiviral medication is unclear. Pharmaceutical companies and investors stand to make huge gains from promoting their potential value.
- The degree of personal protection equipment required to protect healthcare workers is unclear.

Further reading

British Infection Society. British Thoracic Society. Health Protection Agency. Pandemic flu: clinical management of patients with an influenza-like illness during an influenza pandemic. Provisional guidelines from the British Infection Society, British Thoracic Society, and Health Protection Agency in collaboration with the Department of Health. Thorax 2007;62:1–46.

Center for Disease Control. The influenza viruses. <http://www.cdc.gov/flu/about/fluviruses.htm> [Accessed Jan. 2008].

Center for Disease Control. Avian influenza: Current H5N1 situation. <http://www.cdc.gov/flu/avian/outbreaks/currents.htm>.

Center for Disease Control. How the flu virus can change: "drift" and "shift". <http://www.cdc.gov/flu/about/viruses/change.htm>.

Center for Disease Control. Influenza symptoms and the role of laboratory diagnostics. <http://www.cdc.gov/flu/professionals/diagnosis/labrolesprocedures.htm>.

Center for Disease Control. Key facts about seasonal flu vaccine. <http://www.cdc.gov/flu/protect/keyfacts.htm>.

Center for Disease Control. Rapid diagnostic testing for influenza. <http://www.cdc.gov/flu/professionals/diagnosis/rapidclin.htm>.

Center for Disease Control. Types of influenza viruses. <http://www.cdc.gov/flu/about/viruses/types.htm>.

Center for Disease Control. 2011–2012 influenza antiviral medication: a summary for clinicians. <http://www.cdc.gov/flu/professionals/antivirals/summary-clinicians.htm>.

Sandman PM, Lanard J. Bird flu: communicating the risk. Perspect Health Mag 2005;10:1–6.

Tamiflu campaign. <http://www.bmj.com/tamiflu> [Accessed Dec. 2012].

Wong SS, Yuen KY. Avian influenza virus infections in humans. Chest 2006;29:156–68.

World Health Organization. Epidemic and pandemic alert and response. Influenza. <http://www.who.int/csr/disease/influenza/en/> [Accessed Jan. 2008].

6.5 Chronic obstructive pulmonary disease

Julie Leung • Martin Duffy

ESSENTIALS

1 Chronic obstructive pulmonary disease (COPD) is characterized by airflow limitation that is not fully reversible.

2 The majority of exacerbations of COPD are due to infection, but other important precipitants need to be excluded.

3 It is prudent to control oxygen flow rate to achieve an arterial oxygen saturation of approximately 88–92% to ensure correction of hypoxia while avoiding the complication of hyperoxic hypercapnia.

4 The use of non-invasive ventilation in acute respiratory failure is associated with reduced mortality, reduced rates of intubation and reduction in treatment failure.

5 Bronchodilators and systemic steroids are recommended for acute exacerbations.

Introduction

Chronic obstructive pulmonary disease (COPD) is a major public health problem causing chronic morbidity and mortality throughout the world. It is characterized by airflow limitation that is not fully reversible, is usually progressive and is associated with an abnormal inflammatory response of the lung to noxious particles or gases. An acute exacerbation of COPD is a heterogeneous event believed to be caused by complex interactions between the host, respiratory viruses, airway bacteria and environmental pollution. It is clinically characterized by a change in the patient's baseline dyspnoea, cough and/or sputum that is beyond normal day-to-day variations, is acute in onset and may warrant a change in regular medication. COPD is a complex chronic systemic inflammatory disorder with multiple extrapulmonary manifestations and acute exacerbations that may include life-threatening respiratory failure.

Aetiology, genetics, pathogenesis and pathology

The most important factor leading to the development of COPD is cigarette smoking. Less common factors include genetic disorders, such as α_1-antitrypsin deficiency, occupational exposures and exposure to air pollution. An imbalance of matrix metalloproteases and anti-metalloproteases appears to play a significant role. However, why one patient with risk factors develops COPD and another with similar risk factors does not, remains unclear. For instance, only 10–15% of smokers develop clinically significant COPD and almost two-thirds of those homozygous for α_1-antitrypsin deficiency have well-preserved pulmonary function.

The airflow limitation seen in COPD is due to a variable combination of luminal obstruction with mucus hypersecretion, disruption of alveolar attachments and mucosal and peribronchial inflammation and fibrosis (obliterative bronchiolitis).

Epidemiology

Projections from the Global Burden of Disease Study suggest that COPD will be the fifth leading cause of disability-adjusted life-years lost worldwide by the year 2020. More than half a million Australians are estimated to have moderate to severe disease and, as the population ages, the burden of COPD is likely to increase. COPD ranks sixth among the common causes of death in Australian men and women. In the New Zealand population it ranks fifth.

Clinical features

History

Most patients with COPD experience a slow, steady deterioration in their respiratory function. Most emergency department (ED) presentations are the result of a superimposed acute exacerbation. As the disease becomes more severe, the frequency of exacerbations also increases.

It is important to have a good understanding of the patient's baseline function. Questioning to determine this should include the following:

Background

- When did the patient first develop symptoms?
- When was the diagnosis first made?
- The presence of risk factors
- Is the patient a smoker: past or present?
- Maintenance therapy: short- and long-acting bronchodilators, inhaled glucocorticoids
- Use of oral steroids
- Normal level of activity
- Home monitoring, e.g. PEFRs
- Use of home oxygen therapy
- Record of hospitalizations, including ICU admissions.

Acute deterioration

- Fever
- Increased cough and sputum production
- Chest pain suggestive of pulmonary embolus or pneumothorax
- Coexisting illnesses, e.g. ischaemic heart disease, congestive heart failure, diabetes
- Inhaler technique and compliance with medications
- Intercurrent use of inappropriate medications, e.g. β-blockers, sedatives.

Examination

Presentations are heterogeneous, ranging from the thin, barrel-chested patient with obvious dyspnoea, tachypnoea and pursed lip breathing, but no cyanosis, to the overweight, oedematous cyanosed patient suffering from chronic cough and sputum production. Features of cor pulmonale may be present in later stages.

There is insufficient evidence to assess the value of physical examination for diagnosing COPD. Clinical features strongly suggestive of airflow obstruction, with specificities of 98–99%, are the presence of wheezes, a barrel chest, reduced cardiac dullness and a subxiphoid cardiac impulse. Unfortunately, the sensitivities of these features are extremely poor (8–15%), limiting their clinical usefulness.

The goal of the initial evaluation of a patient presenting with an acute exacerbation of COPD is to determine the severity of the attack, as well as to search for and treat any precipitating factors and complications.

Important precipitants and complications to search for include:

Precipitants of acute respiratory failure

- Infection – acute bronchitis, pneumonia
- Bronchospasm
- Sputum retention
- Air pollution
- Pneumothoraces and bullae
- Pulmonary embolism
- Trauma, e.g. rib fractures, pulmonary contusion
- Reduced respiratory drive, e.g. inappropriate sedative use
- Reduced respiratory muscle strength, e.g. metabolic or neuromuscular cause
- Increased metabolic demands – sepsis, fever
- Left ventricular failure.

Complications of COPD

- Pulmonary hypertension
- Right ventricular failure
- Secondary polycythaemia
- Loss of weight
- Medication adverse effects, e.g. complications secondary to long-term steroid use; tachyarrhythmias with β-agonists.

Classification of severity

The Global Initiative on Chronic Obstructive Lung Disease classifies COPD into four stages of severity, based on spirometry:

- Stage I: mild COPD – characterized by mild airflow limitation (FEV_1/FVC <0.70; FEV_1 >80% predicted); the individual is usually unaware that his or her lung function is abnormal
- Stage II: moderate COPD – characterized by worsening airflow limitation (FEV_1/FVC <0.70; 50% <FEV_1 <80% predicted); patients typically seek medical attention because of chronic respiratory symptoms or an exacerbation of their disease
- Stage III: severe COPD – characterized by further worsening of airflow limitation (FEV_1/FVC <0.70; 30% < FEV_1 <50% predicted), greater shortness of breath, reduced exercise capacity, fatigue and repeated exacerbations that almost always have an impact on patients' quality of life
- Stage IV: very severe COPD – characterized by severe airflow limitation (FEV_1/FVC <0.70; FEV_1 <30% predicted or FEV_1 <50% predicted plus the presence of chronic respiratory failure); quality of life is very appreciably impaired and exacerbations may be life threatening.

The BODE Index, which includes assessment of weight (body mass index), airway obstruction (FEV_1), dyspnoea and exercise capacity, has been used to assess the risk of death and as a predictor of hospitalization, although its limited ability to do so has prompted the development of an updated BODE Index (scores adjusted to reflect more accurately prognostic weight) and the new ADO Index (incorporating age). Importantly, the above measures do not significantly affect the immediate management of COPD patients presenting acutely to the ED.

Clinical investigations

The following investigations may be used during the evaluation of a patient with COPD, but not all will be necessary in every situation. It is important to use tests that will have an impact on management decisions.

Tests performed at the bedside

- Pulse oximetry: provides invaluable 'real-time' non-invasive evaluation of oxygenation, assisting with the initial assessment of the patient and allowing observation of trends in response to therapy. The goal of oxygen therapy is a saturation of 88–92%. Oximetry does not provide information about carbon dioxide status and is inaccurate in the presence of poor peripheral circulation.
- Spirometry: provides confirmation of obstruction – FEV_1 <80% of predicted and FEV_1/FVC <0.7. In the acute situation, spirometry may not be able to be performed by the patient and is often inaccurate. It is no longer recommended by some.
- Electrocardiography (ECG): may detect arrhythmias, such as multifocal atrial tachycardia or atrial fibrillation, or demonstrate evidence of intercurrent ischaemic heart disease. ECG evidence of pulmonary hypertension and right ventricular hypertrophy may be present, but is often insensitive and non-specific.

Tests that have results available within minutes include:

- Arterial blood gases (ABG): provide information regarding acute versus chronic respiratory failure and, using serial tests, may be used to monitor improvement or deterioration. Acute hypercarbia can be distinguished from chronic hypercarbia by consideration of HCO_3 levels and pH. In the acute setting, an acidotic pH value in a patient with chronic carbon dioxide retention signifies superimposed acute decompensation. Although this information is useful, ABGs play little part in clinical decisions, such as the requirement for assisted ventilation or intubation.
- Venous blood gases: pH and HCO_3 readings closely agree with arterial results (95% limits of agreement −0.1–0.08 and −3.5–3.5 respectively). PCO_2 values vary markedly and cannot be adjusted with a simple correction factor. There is growing evidence that venous pCO_2 can be used as screening test for arterial hypercarbia. A recent systematic review reported that venous pCO_2 <45 mmHg has 100% sensitivity and negative predictive value for prediction of arterial hypercarbia.
- Chest radiograph (CXR): in the acute setting, CXR provides valuable information regarding the presence of coexisting illnesses which may be life threatening and require specific interventions, e.g. pneumothorax, pneumonia, pleural effusions and heart failure. Studies have demonstrated that up to 23% of admitted patients may have a change in their management related to their CXR findings. Features of chronic airflow limitation may include hyperinflation, flattened diaphragms, bullae, increased retrosternal airspace, reduced vascular markings and a small heart.
- Point-of-care tests: for diagnosis of infective acute exacerbations of COPD to guide treatment with antibiotics. These

can be used to rapidly diagnose influenza, pneumococcal infections, *Legionella* and respiratory syncytial virus infections. This may avoid the unnecessary use of broad-spectrum antibiotics and reduce the emergence of antibiotic-resistant organisms. However, they may not necessarily lead to better patient outcomes or financial savings and, presently, are not used commonly in Australasian EDs.

Other tests

Other useful tests are:

- Full blood examination: may reveal evidence of secondary polycythaemia or a raised white cell count due to infection, long-term steroid use or the hyperadrenergic stress response of the acutely ill patient.
- Electrolytes: note potassium levels, hyponatraemia, glucose.
- Sputum culture: 50% of exacerbations of COPD may be due to bacteria, with *Haemophilus influenzae*, *Streptococcus pneumoniae* and *Moraxella catarrhalis* the predominant pathogens. Exacerbations complicated by pneumonia have similar pathogens. Patients with more compromised lung function have a higher frequency of infections with *Pseudomonas aeruginosa* and other Gram-negative bacteria than those less severely affected. Colonization of the respiratory tract can make interpretation of results difficult.
- Viral cultures and detection assays: 20% of acute exacerbations are due to viruses, such as rhinoviruses, influenzae, parainfluenzae and coronaviruses. However, viral studies are usually not performed in the ED as they are expensive, have varying sensitivities and specificities and rarely alter management.
- Theophylline level: this is rarely required. Note: a patient may be toxic despite having a measured level within the therapeutic range.
- Plasma brain natriuretic peptide (BNP) level: adds to the current clinical and laboratory evaluation of patients with COPD presenting with worsening dyspnoea, although not widely available in Australia. A plasma BNP level <100 pg/mL argues against heart failure as a contributing factor in the clinical deterioration. A plasma level >500 pg/mL points to decompensation of heart failure but does not exclude concomitant COPD exacerbation. Plasma BNP levels

ranging from 100 to 500 pg/mL need to be interpreted in conjunction with clinical findings.

- Respiratory function tests: demonstrate largely irreversible airflow obstruction with elevated lung volumes; reduced carbon monoxide uptake implies emphysema.
- High-resolution chest CT: demonstrates air trapping and is thus useful in the diagnosis of emphysema, but is of questionable value in the ED setting given the limited availability and as yet undetermined advance on other diagnostic modalities available for the assessment of most patients with COPD. CT pulmonary angiograms are useful for investigating possible pulmonary embolism, especially when the chest X-ray is abnormal.
- Cardiac studies: cardiac biomarkers, echocardiography and gated nuclear scans may be required to determine the role of cardiac ischaemia and ventricular dysfunction in the clinical picture.

Treatment

The overall goals of treatment in COPD are to confirm the diagnosis and assess severity; optimize function (including use of long-acting bronchodilators to provide sustained relief of symptoms in moderate-to-severe COPD and the use of inhaled glucocorticoids in those who have severe COPD with frequent exacerbations); prevent deterioration; develop a support network and self-management plan; and manage exacerbations.

The following is a summary of the therapeutic modalities used to treat an acute exacerbation of COPD. The timing and level of intervention depends on the disease severity. It is important to remember that management decisions for the patient in extremis are solely clinical – no further investigation is necessary to determine whether immediate intubation is required.

Oxygen therapy

Hypoxaemia must be corrected. Oxygen therapy for most patients with COPD will not produce clinically significant carbon dioxide retention, a multifactorial condition caused by changes in pulmonary blood flow, worsening ventilation/ perfusion mismatching and increasing dead space ventilation; not simply hypoventilation from loss of hypoxic drive. However, it is recommended that oxygen delivery be controlled, with

a target SpO_2 range of 88–92%, corresponding to an arterial oxygen tension of 60–70 mmHg. There is an increased risk of morbidity and mortality in patients with hypercapnic respiratory failure when the arterial oxygen tension is increased above this level (>93–95%). The degree of hypoxaemia at presentation rather than the initial degree of hypercapnia is a better predictor of hyperoxic hypercapnia.

For the mildly unwell patient, an oxygen saturation of 90% may be achieved with the use of nasal prongs at 2 L/min. For patients with more severe disease, the use of a Venturi mask with an appropriate fractional inspired oxygen concentration is more appropriate. In most cases, these devices are of the fixed-performance type, i.e. the FiO_2 is independent of patient factors. However, in the severely dyspnoeic patient, peak inspiratory flow rate may exceed the peak flow rate of the device, leading to fluctuations in FiO_2. To avoid this, a circuit with a large reservoir will be necessary. Persisting hypoxia (SpO_2 <85%) necessitates a search for complicating factors, such as pneumonia, pulmonary oedema, pulmonary embolus or pneumothorax, as well as consideration of ventilatory assistance.

Ventilatory assistance

Ventilatory assistance may be non-invasive (NIV) or invasive.

Non-invasive ventilation

Non-invasive ventilation (NIV) has become the first-line intervention in the management of acute respiratory failure in patients with COPD. Continuous positive airway pressure (CPAP) and bi-level positive airway pressure (BiPAP) are the two main modes of non-invasive positive-pressure ventilation.

The presence of dynamic hyperinflation and the development of intrinsic positive end-expiratory pressure (PEEPi) during an acute deterioration lead to an increased work of breathing. The application of CPAP or external PEEP at levels to overcome PEEPi, has been shown to reduce respiratory work. This has resulted in patients reporting less dyspnoea and laboratory evidence of better gas exchange.

BiPAP involves the use of both inspiratory and expiratory pressure support ventilation and has also proved an effective form of NIV in acute respiratory failure. Initiation of ventilation triggers the inspiratory positive airway pressure, which is limited to a predetermined level, usually 10–20 cm H_2O. Expiratory positive airway pressure of approximately 5 cm H_2O is predetermined and persists throughout expiration. The whole process thus reduces the work of breathing.

Numerous studies, using either a face-mask or nasal mask and varying combinations of the above airway pressure manipulations, have shown significant reductions in the need for intubation. A Cochrane review of 14 randomized controlled studies of patients admitted to hospital with acute respiratory failure secondary to an acute exacerbation of COPD concluded that non-invasive positive-pressure ventilation in addition to usual medical care resulted in reduced mortality (NNT 10, 95% CI 7–20), reduced need for intubation (NNT 4, 95% CI 4–5) and a reduction in treatment failure (NNT 5, 95% CI 4–6). In addition, NIV was associated with rapid improvement in acidosis and respiratory rate within 1 hour of initiation. Complications associated with treatment and length of hospital stay were also reduced. Clinical practice guidelines from ACP-ASIM/ACCP and the Thoracic Society of Australia and New Zealand/Australian Lung Foundation (COPD-X plan) and evidence-based management guidelines from the Global Initiative for Chronic Obstructive Lung Disease (GOLD) recommend that NIV should be considered early in the course of respiratory failure, before severe acidosis ensues.

Indications for NIV include moderate to severe dyspnoea with use of accessory muscles and paradoxical abdominal motion, moderate to severe acidosis and/or hypercapnia ($PaCO_2$ >45 mmHg) and respiratory rate >25 breaths per minute. Contraindications include respiratory arrest, cardiovascular instability (hypotension, arrhythmias, myocardial infarction), change in mental status or an uncooperative patient, high aspiration risk, viscous or copious secretions, recent facial or gastro-oesophageal surgery, craniofacial trauma and burns. However, there are no definite clinical predictors to identify which patients with respiratory failure will benefit from NIV. Patients who have a pH <7.30 and >7.25 appear to receive the greatest benefit. The chance of COPD patients with acute respiratory failure having a second episode of acute respiratory failure after an initial (first 48 hours) successful response to NIV is about 20%.

The concurrent delivery of nebulized $β_2$-agonists with NIV is an important therapeutic issue. Theoretical concerns of reduced drug delivery because of the rates of fresh gas flow required to run effectively CPAP circuits have been confirmed. However, these concerns were not of clinical significance in a group of stable asthmatic patients. Extrapolation to COPD patients with acute respiratory failure should be made with caution, but its use may be appropriate given the favourable effects of CPAP on respiratory mechanics and subsequent drug delivery.

Invasive ventilation

Endotracheal intubation with positive-pressure ventilation is used in patients who fail non-invasive ventilatory assistance or who have indications for intubation present at the outset, e.g. unprotected airway or respiratory arrest. The goal of mechanical ventilation is to prevent excessive work of breathing while maintaining a work of breathing that is sufficient to prevent respiratory muscle atrophy. The major problems with positive-pressure ventilation in this patient population are the risk of barotrauma and the production of PEEPi. Commonly recommended ventilation strategies include using tidal volumes of approximately 5–7 mL/kg, using a reduced respiratory rate and using an inspiratory:expiratory ratio of 1:3. Most patients also usually require a bolus of intravenous fluids to counter the effects of positive-pressure ventilation on venous return and cardiac output. Patients who need mechanical ventilation have an inpatient mortality of 17–30%.

Bronchodilators

Bronchodilators are used in the management of acute exacerbation of COPD (AECOPD) because of the possibility of a small reversible component to the airflow obstruction. In the ED setting, these drugs are usually given by nebulizer, though there is little evidence to support this route over metered-dose inhalers, particularly when used in conjunction with a spacer device. It is common practice to use the anticholinergic agents and $β_2$-agonists in combination.

Anticholinergic agents

A systematic review of randomized controlled trials comparing anticholinergic bronchodilators versus $β_2$-sympathomimetic agents for acute exacerbations of COPD found no significant difference in the degree of bronchodilation between the two agents and the combination of the two did not appear to increase the effect on FEV_1 more than either agent used alone. However, the duration of action of short-acting anticholinergics is greater than that of short-acting β-agonists. They also have a lower adverse effect profile.

The most commonly used agent in Australasia is ipratropium bromide. The usual dose is 500 µg by nebulizer every 4–6 hours. Doses as frequent as every 20 minutes are used in clinical practice, albeit with little supporting evidence.

Tiotropium bromide is a long-acting anticholinergic agent that is used once daily and has been shown to produce significant improvements in lung function, symptoms and quality of life, as well as reducing exacerbations in chronic stable COPD. However, its role in the immediate management of a patient presenting with an AECOPD is yet to be established.

$β_2$-Agonists

Salbutamol is commonly used as a first-line agent in Australasia. The usual dose is 5 mg via nebulizer, repeated as necessary. An equivalent alternative is 8–10 puffs of 100 µg salbutamol by metered-dose inhaler and spacer. Nebulized salbutamol is often used continuously in the severely ill patient. Occasionally, in the patient with a severe exacerbation, the intravenous route may be required, though evidence for this practice is lacking. Common side effects include tachycardia, tremor and a reduction in potassium levels.

Long-acting $β_2$-agonists (e.g. salmeterol, eformoterol) cause prolonged bronchodilatation for at least 12 hours and can thus be administered twice daily. They have been shown to produce statistically significant benefits in lung function, quality of life, use of 'reliever' short-acting bronchodilators and acute exacerbations. As with tiotropium, their role in the immediate management of a patient presenting with an AECOPD is not yet known.

Theophylline

Rarely used in the acute setting because of significant side effects and questionable efficacy.

Corticosteroids

Systemic corticosteroids have been shown to hasten recovery, reduce hospital stay and reduce early treatment failure in patients with acute exacerbations of COPD. It would be necessary to treat 10 patients (95% CI 7–16) to avoid one treatment failure. Maximal improvement is usually gained within 2 weeks of therapy; prolonging treatment thereafter does not result in further benefit and long-term systemic corticosteroid use in COPD is not recommended.

For acute exacerbations, the optimal initial dose and course duration is yet to be determined, but prednisolone 30–50 mg/day for 7–10 days is currently recommended. Evidence suggests that oral administration is just as effective as parenteral administration of steroids, except in conditions that preclude the oral route, such as vomiting. In these cases, 100–200 mg hydrocortisone may be administered IV. Short courses have been found to cause one extra adverse effect for every five people treated (95% CI 4–9) and the complications of long-term use are myriad. The potential role of hypothalamo-pituitary–adrenal axis suppression complicating patient presentations needs to be remembered.

The effects of inhaled corticosteroids (beclomethasone, budesonide, fluticasone, ciclesonide) on the course of an acute exacerbation of COPD are uncertain.

Antibiotics

Bacteria play a role in approximately 50% of exacerbations of COPD. In 30% of patients no clear cause can be found. Antibiotics have only been shown to have consistently beneficial effects in patients admitted to ICU. Further research is needed to determine the clinical signs and biomarkers that identify patients who may benefit. In the meantime, features suggesting an infective precipitant, such as the presence of increased dyspnoea, increased sputum purulence, increased sputum volume, fever or leucocytosis, are reasonable triggers for commencing antibiotic therapy. Patients with more severe exacerbations are more likely to benefit from antibiotic treatment than those with less severe exacerbations.

Drugs should cover *H. influenzae*, *S. pneumoniae* and *Moraxella catarrhalis*, depending on local sensitivities. A β-lactamase-resistant drug (e.g. ampicillin with clavulanic acid or doxycycline) is often required. The use of fluoroquinolones has increased, but they are expensive and have not been shown to be more effective than traditional antibiotics. The presence of an altered mental state, inability to swallow safely or a chest X-ray suggesting pneumonia may require the administration of intravenous antibiotics. The antibiotic treatment of pneumonia in COPD patients should follow the recommendations for initial treatment of community-acquired pneumonia. However, the results of recent sputum cultures may affect the final antibiotic regimen.

Heliox

There is currently little evidence to support the use of a helium–oxygen mixture in acute exacerbations of COPD. Theoretically, the low density of heliox mixtures may reduce airway resistance and hence the work of breathing.

Chest physiotherapy

Chest physiotherapy, in the form of mechanical percussion in an attempt to improve mucus clearance, has been shown to be ineffective.

Other therapies

- Monitor fluid balance and nutrition
- Correction of electrolyte abnormalities
- Consider subcutaneous heparin for deep vein thrombosis prophylaxis
- Identify and treat associated conditions.

Longer-term measures

- Smoking cessation
- Vaccinations (pneumococcal, influenza, Hib)
- Exercise training
- Home oxygen therapy
- Long-term NIV
- Homecare plans
- Other medications – statins, roflumilast, proton pump inhibitors, angiotensin-converting enzyme inhibitors
- Lung volume reduction surgery
- Transplantation.

Prognosis

Acute exacerbations of COPD often require hospital admission for treatment of respiratory failure. Hospital mortality for such patients is about 10%, reaching 40% by 1 year after discharge and is higher for patients aged over 65. Whether the patient requires admission will depend on the severity of the present exacerbation, how easily correctable the precipitating factor is and how well the patient responds to therapy.

Indications for hospitalization of patients with COPD include a marked increase in intensity of symptoms, inadequate response to initial medical management, inability to walk between rooms when previously mobile, inability to eat or sleep because of dyspnoea, inability to manage at home even with homecare resources, presence of high risk co-morbidity conditions, altered mental status suggestive of hypercapnia, worsening hypoxaemia or cor pulmonale, newly occurring arrhythmia or diagnostic uncertainty.

Indications for ICU admission of patients with exacerbation of COPD include severe dyspnoea that responds inadequately to initial emergency therapy, changes in mental status (confusion, lethargy, coma), persistent or worsening hypoxaemia despite supplemental oxygen, worsening hypercapnia ($PaCO_2 > 70$ mmHg) or severe or worsening respiratory acidosis, requirement for assisted mechanical ventilation and haemodynamic instability requiring vasopressors. The appropriateness of ICU admission is often questioned. Premorbid and diagnostic data have not been shown to be predictive of outcome. Variables associated with intermediate-term mortality are those which reflect the underlying severity of the acute illness–post-arrest, low Glasgow coma scale, cardiac dysrhythmia, high acute physiological score (APACHE II or CAPS) on ICU admission, and low bicarbonate (less than 20 mmol/L) on ICU admission.

A decision to discharge the patient from the ED requires the presence of good home conditions, social supports and the organization of appropriate follow up.

Controversies

- COPD should be considered a chronic syndrome of different disorders with distinct pathophysiological processes and treatment responses. Patients are heterogeneous, with different phenotypes requiring individualized treatment. The present GOLD definitions/classifications/guidelines are poorly generalizable and the present evidence base is inadequate for informing decisions in most patients with COPD.
- The role of prophylactic macrolide antibiotics. These appear to have anti-inflammatory and immune-modulating effects, leading to a reduced number of acute exacerbations and decreased rate of decline in lung function. Unfortunately, adverse effects include ototoxicity, cardiac toxicity and drug–drug interactions, making their role unclear at this stage.
- The role of matrix metalloprotease inhibitors.

Further reading

Beasley R, Weatherall M, Travers J, Shirtcliffe P. Time to define the disorders of the syndrome of COPD. Lancet 2009;374:670–2.

Broekhuizen BD, Sachs AP, Oostvogels R, et al. The diagnostic value of history and physical examination for COPD in suspected or known cases: a systematic review. Fam Pract 2009;26:260–8.

Global Initiative for Chronic Obstructive Lung Disease (GOLD). URL: <http://www.goldcopd.com>; 2011 [Accessed Dec. 2012].

Lim BL, Kelly AM. A meta-analysis on the utility of peripheral venous blood gas analyses in exacerbations of chronic obstructive pulmonary disease in the emergency department. Eur J Emerg Med 2010;17:246–8.

McCrory DC, Brown CD. Anti-cholinergic bronchodilators versus beta2-sympathomimetic agents for acute exacerbations of chronic obstructive pulmonary disease. Cochrane Database Syst Rev 2003:CD003900.

McKenzie D, Abramson M, Crockett AJ, et al., on behalf of The Australian Lung Foundation. The COPD-X Plan: Australian

and New Zealand Guidelines for the management of chronic obstructive pulmonary disease V2.30, 2011.

Messer B, Griffiths J, Baudouin SV. The prognostic variables predictive of mortality in patients with an exacerbation of COPD admitted to the ICU: an integrative review. Q J Med 2012;105:115–26.

Moons KGM, Kessels AG, Held U. Expansion of the prognostic assessment of patients with chronic obstructive pulmonary disease: the updated BODE index and the ADO index. Lancet 2009;374:704–11.

Ram FSF, Picot J, Wedzicha JA. Non-invasive positive pressure ventilation for treatment of respiratory failure due to

exacerbations of chronic obstructive pulmonary disease. Cochrane Database Syst Rev 2004;3:CD004104.

Vollenweider DJ, Jarrett H, Steurer-Stey CA, et al. Antibiotics for exacerbations of chronic obstructive pulmonary disease. Cochrane Database System Rev 2012;12:CD010257.

Walters JAE, Gibson PG, Wood-Baker R, et al. Systemic corticosteroids for acute exacerbations of chronic obstructive pulmonary disease. Cochrane Database Syst Rev 2009;1:CD001288.

Wenzel RP, Fowler III AA, Edmond MB. Antibiotic prevention of acute exacerbations of COPD. N Engl J Med 2012;367: 340–7.

6.6 Pneumothorax

Anne-Maree Kelly

ESSENTIALS

1 Pneumothorax can occur spontaneously, as a result of trauma, or iatrogenically. Spontaneous pneumothorax has been further subdivided into primary and secondary (related to underlying lung pathology). The utility of this distinction, as understanding of the pathology of pneumothorax evolves, is being challenged.

2 Clinical features are unreliable indicators of pneumothorax size.

3 The diagnostic test of choice is a chest X-ray.

4 Treatment options include observation, aspiration, thoracostomy and primary or delayed surgery. The evidence base to guide choice of therapy is weak. In determining management strategy, pneumothorax size is less important than the degree of clinical compromise.

5 Tension pneumothorax is rarely seen, particularly after spontaneous pneumothorax. It is, however, a life-threatening problem and must be managed immediately. It is a clinical, not a radiological, diagnosis.

Introduction

Pneumothorax is the presence of free air in the interpleural space which may occur spontaneously, as a result of trauma or iatrogenically.

The most common form of pneumothorax is spontaneous. By definition, primary spontaneous pneumothoraces arise in otherwise healthy people without lung disease and without any apparent precipitating event. The reported incidence is 18–28/100 000 per year for men and 1.2–6/100 000 per year for women. Many patients do not seek medical advice for several days, with 46% waiting more than 2 days before presentation, despite symptoms, in one study.

Secondary spontaneous pneumothorax occurs as the result of underlying lung disease.

The consequences of pneumothorax in this group are greater and the management potentially more complex.

Aetiology, genetics, pathogenesis and pathology

Despite the absence of underlying pulmonary disease in primary spontaneous pneumothorax, subpleural blebs and bullae are found in up to 90% of cases at thoracoscopy or on computed tomography (CT) scanning. Autofluorescent studies have revealed adjacent areas of pleural porosities. Small airways obstruction may characterize pneumothorax, usually associated with influx of inflammatory cells. Primary

spontaneous pneumothorax is more common in tall, thin males aged 20–40 years who smoke. There is no association with exertion.

Secondary spontaneous pneumothorax has a peak incidence at 60–65 years. It has a higher morbidity and mortality than primary spontaneous pneumothorax. Although chronic obstructive airways disease and asthma are the most common underlying conditions in developed countries, secondary pneumothorax may also be due to bacterial or tuberculous pneumonia, HIV with active *Pneumocystis* pneumonia, cancer, honeycomb lung disorders and cystic fibrosis. Secondary pneumothorax has also been seen in association with those who abuse amphetamine, cocaine, Ecstasy, marijuana and nitrous oxide. Rarely, secondary pneumothorax can occur in women with pelvic endometriosis who may develop pneumothoraces (predominantly right-sided) within 72 hours of menstruation.

Iatrogenic pneumothorax may result from central line placement, intercostal blocks, thoracocentesis, lung biopsy, bronchoscopy and high pressures from artificial ventilation. Traumatic pneumothorax occurs in up to 15–20% of patients who sustain blunt chest trauma and is usually secondary to fractured ribs. It may also be the result of penetrating wounds or barotrauma.

In most cases of pneumothorax, the air leak seals spontaneously. In a subset of those where a leak continues, a ball-valve effect can occur, with the development of tension pneumothorax. The trachea and mediastinal structures are pushed away from the collapsed lung and venous return to the heart may become obstructed. The result is severe respiratory compromise and hypotension. Emergent decompression is required. Tension is rare as a complication of primary spontaneous pneumothorax.

Clinical features

History

Symptoms of primary spontaneous pneumothorax often begin suddenly when the patient is at rest, but can be associated with deep inspiration, hyperventilation or coughing. It may also be precipitated by changes in atmospheric pressure that occur with flying and diving. Chest pain on the side of the pneumothorax is the most common presenting symptom (90% of cases). It can be sharp and pleuritic or dull and may radiate to the back or neck. Dyspnoea occurs in up to 80% of patients but is generally not severe. Some patients, however, may be relatively asymptomatic or become asymptomatic after 24 hours. Many patients do not seek medical advice for several days, with up to 50% waiting more than 2 days despite symptoms.

Clinical symptoms are usually more severe in secondary spontaneous pneumothorax. In particular, there is usually dyspnoea out of proportion to the size of the pneumothorax. These patients are more likely to be hypoxic, in part related to underlying lung pathology. Those with pneumothorax and pneumomediastinum related to drug abuse may also have neck pain, sore throat and dysphagia.

Examination

The physical signs of pneumothorax can be subtle. The classic signs are reduced or absent breath sounds, reduced chest expansion and hyper-resonance to percussion on the affected side. Less common findings include subcutaneous emphysema, unilateral enlargement of the chest, inferior liver displacement and Hamman's crunch (a noise heard with each heartbeat due to mediastinal emphysema). Patients who develop tension pneumothorax have evidence of air hunger, cyanosis, distended neck veins, tachycardia, hypotension and, classically, as a late sign, tracheal deviation away from the affected side.

Differential diagnosis

The differential diagnosis includes costochondritis, pneumonia, pleurisy, pulmonary embolus, exacerbation of bronchospastic disease and myocardial ischaemia.

Clinical investigation

No investigations are indicated for patients with suspected tension pneumothorax and cardiorespiratory compromise. It is a clinical, not a radiological diagnosis, and requires immediate treatment.

Imaging

X-ray

In stable patients with a suspected pneumothorax, erect PA chest X-ray has long been the primary investigation for pneumothorax. The characteristic feature is displacement of the pleural line, i.e. a gap between the line of the visceral and parietal pleura. Other findings may include hyperlucency, lack of pulmonary markings and an air fluid level in the costophrenic angle. Associated pneumomediastinum is seen in 1.5% of pneumothoraces. Although traditionally expiratory chest X-rays have been used for the detection of pneumothoraces, there is evidence that they do not increase detection of clinically relevant pneumothoraces. Large bullae or lung cysts may mimic a pneumothorax. If there is doubt about the presence of a pneumothorax or its differentiation from bullous disease, a CT scan is recommended.

On a supine chest X-ray (usually used in trauma patients), the only clue to a pneumothorax may be a deep sulcus sign on the affected side, an unusually distinct cardiac apex or increased hyperlucency of the upper abdominal quadrants. Supine X-rays are less sensitive than erect PA chest X-ray. If there is uncertainty, a CT scan will clarify.

Digital imaging has supplanted film-based studies in many hospitals. This has provided some challenges in the detection of pneumothorax as there are differences between the characteristics (screen size, pixel count, contrast and luminescence) of ward-based modules and those used by radiologists for reporting. This may affect the sensitivity of digital images for the detection of pneumothorax. Digital imaging also makes estimation of size using previously available methods difficult.

CT scan

CT scanning is the gold standard for detection of and size estimation of pneumothorax. It can also discriminate large bullae from pneumothoraces and identify dystrophic lung changes (primarily pulmonary blebs) in the affected and contralateral lung. The role of these findings in predicting recurrence and in defining which patients benefit from surgery remains to be determined.

Ultrasound

Specific features on ultrasound are diagnostic of pneumothorax. These include the absence of lung sliding and comet tail artefacts. While useful in trauma, ultrasound has yet to achieve wide usage.

Size estimation

Current therapeutic guidelines divide pneumothoraces into small and large, although the details of the definitions vary. The British Thoracic Society and *Therapeutic Guidelines (Australia): Respiratory* define 'small' as the presence of a visible rim of <2 cm between the lung margin and the chest wall on X-ray with the measurement taken at the level of the hilum. A 2 cm rim is said to approximate 50% collapse. The American College of Respiratory Physicians defines small pneumothoraces as those with less than 3 cm apical interpleural distance (Fig. 6.6.1).

Blood gas analysis

The patient's oxygenation is a key determinant of choice of management. Pulse oximetry is acceptable in most patients, but arterial blood gas analysis may be necessary in sicker patients (oxygen saturation <92% on room air or respiratory distress).

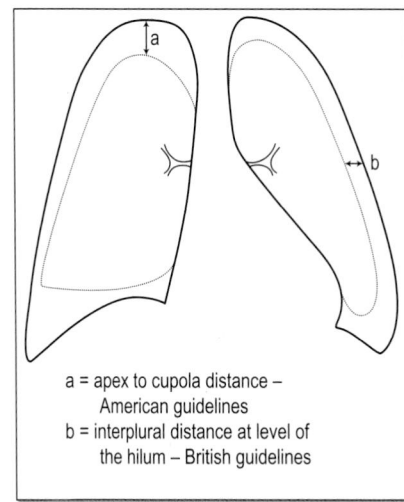

a = apex to cupola distance – American guidelines
b = interplural distance at level of the hilum – British guidelines

Fig. 6.6.1 Size of pneumothorax. *(Reproduced from MacDuff A, Arnold A, Harvey J on behalf of the BTS Pleural Disease Guideline Group, Thorax 2010; 65(Suppl 2):ii18–ii31, with permission from BMJ Publishing Group Ltd.)*

Treatment

The evidence base to guide choice of treatment for pneumothoraces is not strong. Important factors to consider in determining the appropriate treatment are:

- Type of pneumothorax: primary or secondary. Secondary pneumothoraces respond less well to interventions and require treatment of the underlying condition.
- Clinical evidence of respiratory compromise, in particular significant breathlessness.
- Size. Pneumothoraces resolve at a rate of approximately 1.25–2.2% of the volume of hemithorax per day.
- Age. Evidence suggests that aspiration is less successful in patients aged over 50.
- Cause of pneumothorax. Most iatrogenic pneumothoraces can be treated conservatively or by aspiration. Traumatic pneumothoraces may require continuous catheter drainage because of associated chest wall or lung injuries.

General measures

Patients should initially receive supplemental oxygen, particularly if hypoxic. This increases the rate of pleural air absorption considerably, by reducing the partial pressure of nitrogen and increasing the gradient for nitrogen absorption. It is useful for both pneumothorax and pneumomediastinum.

Emergency drainage

Patients who present in severe respiratory insufficiency or shock should be treated with immediate decompression. This involves the prompt placement of a large intravenous (e.g. 14 G) cannula or small-bore catheter by the Seldinger technique in the second intercostal space, midclavicular line (or the fifth intercostal space midaxillary line) with free drainage to air or drainage to a Heimlich valve. Definitive therapy is then required.

Minimal symptoms

Evidence supports conservative management of patients with minimal symptoms. While this has been usual practice for small pneumothoraces, available data also support this approach in selected patients with asymptomatic large pneumothorax with success rates of up to 90% reported. It has also been shown that, for small pneumothoraces, recurrence in those managed conservatively is less than in patients treated with intercostal tube drainage. These patients can be treated as outpatients provided they have easy access to medical care should their symptoms worsen.

The rate of resolution/reabsorption of primary spontaneous pneumothoraces was previously estimated as 1.25–2.2% of the volume of hemithorax per day, with significant between- and within-patient variations. Based on these data, a prudent follow-up strategy would be to repeat X-rays the next day (to detect deterioration) and weekly until resolution. The patient needs to be given clear, specific written instructions about what to do if their symptoms worsen or their condition deteriorates.

Symptomatic pneumothorax

The presence of significant breathlessness is the main indicator for intervention (needle aspiration or catheter drainage).

Simple aspiration

Simple aspiration can be performed as needle aspiration or, more commonly, via a small bore catheter (<14 F) inserted using the Seldinger technique. The aim of this treatment is to convert a larger pneumothorax into one that can safely be managed conservatively. A reasonable definition of success is reduction to a rim of <2 cm measured at the hilum without re-accumulation over 4–6 hours and resolution of significant breathlessness. For primary spontaneous pneumothorax, successful re-expansion of the lung after simple aspiration is of the order of 50–83%. Available data suggest that rates for secondary pneumothoraces are lower. Meta-analyses have confirmed that aspiration has similar effectiveness to catheter drainage, with some studies also reporting reduction in admission rate and hospital length of stay.

Successful aspiration has been shown to depend on age (under 50 years: 70–81%; over 50 years: 19–31%) and the volume of the pneumothorax (<3 L aspirated: 89% success; >3 L: no success). The latter probably represents the presence of a persistent air leak.

Following successful aspiration, including confirmation that the pneumothorax has not re-accumulated, further management as an outpatient is appropriate provided that the patient has clear instruction on the recognition of deterioration and ready access to medical care should this occur.

Few complications are reported to result from the use of aspiration and all are minor: vasovagal reactions, local subcutaneous emphysema and occasional problems with catheter kinking, blockage or dislodgement.

Catheter drainage

Catheter drainage is required if simple aspiration fails, if an emergency decompression for tension pneumothorax has been performed or if there is a significant coexisting haemothorax, e.g in trauma. There is evidence to suggest that small bore catheters (<14 F) have similar effectiveness to large bore catheters and are less painful. They also allow insertion using a Seldinger technique which is easier than open insertion techniques and obviates some of the complications seen previously with trocar-based techniques. Catheters may be inserted by an anterior, axillary or posteroapical approach. For practical and cosmetic reasons, an axillary approach is favoured.

Primary success rates of 66–97% have been reported. Reported duration of hospital admission ranges from 7 to 9 days; longer for secondary pneumothoraces. There is no evidence that the addition of suction improves outcome. Indeed, the addition of suction early after chest drain insertion may precipitate re-expansion pulmonary oedema, especially in larger primary spontaneous pneumothoraces that have been present for a few days.

The use of small bore catheters also promotes a stepwise pathway of care, being able to be used for aspiration and, in the event that fails, easily converted to Heimlich valve or underwater seal drainage (Fig. 6.6.2). Suction should not be routinely employed. While most patients undergoing catheter drainage are admitted to hospital, some studies are reporting safe and successful management of selected patients as outpatients using small bore catheters and Heimlich valves.

Potential disadvantages of intercostal catheters range from chest and abdominal visceral trauma from sharp trocars (now not favoured for insertion) to practical management issues such as the bulkiness of the underwater seal bottle system that must be kept upright. Available data suggest that, with traditional placement approaches, the rate of aberrant placement is 4–9% and empyema risk has been estimated at 1%. Other potential complications include bronchopleural fistulae, arteriovenous fistulae, perforation of the internal mammary artery, pulmonary or mediastinal blood vessels, focal lung infections, re-expansion pulmonary oedema and lung infarction. There are insufficient data to quantify the risk of these complications.

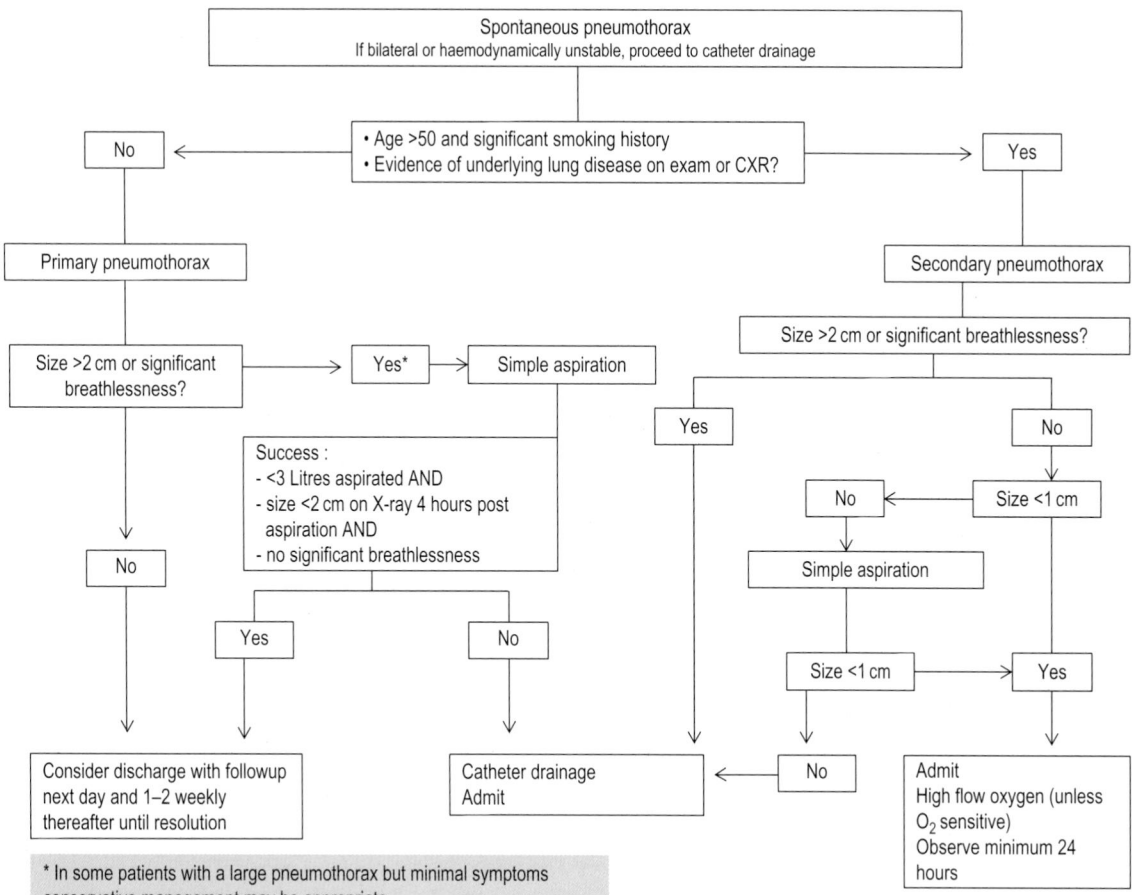

Fig. 6.6.2. Management algorithm for spontaneous pneumothorax. *(Adapted from MacDuff A, Arnold A, Harvey J on behalf of the BTS Pleural Disease Guideline Group. Thorax 2010; 65(Suppl 2):ii18–ii31, with permission from BMJ Publishing Group Ltd.)*

Surgery

Approximately 10% of patients require surgical intervention. Indications for surgical referral include persistent air leak after 2–7 days, recurrent pneumothoraces, airline pilots, frequent plane travellers and divers, contralateral or bilateral pneumothoraces and pregnancy. There are two main surgical approaches: open thoracotomy and pleurectomy and video-assisted thoracoscopic surgery (VATS). Open thoracotomy with pleurectomy has the lowest recurrence rate (≈1%) while VATS is better tolerated but with a higher recurrence rate (≈5%). Medical pleurodesis may be indicated in patients unfit for surgery.

Prognosis

Recurrence after the first pneumothorax is up to 50% for primary and secondary pneumothoraces. Half of these occur within 4 months and the risk does not drop substantially until 1 year from the index pneumothorax. This rate increases to 60–70% for subsequent recurrences.

Other issues

As pneumothoraces will increase in size at altitude owing to changes in atmospheric pressure, flying with a pneumothorax is potentially dangerous. Current guidelines suggest that the pneumothorax should be fully resolved for at least 1 week before flying. Owing to the theoretical risk that higher barometric pressures associated with scuba diving may precipitate recurrence, patients having suffered a primary or secondary pneumothorax are advised not to dive in future, unless they have undergone bilateral definitive surgery and have normal chest CT scan postoperatively.

Controversies

- The role of CT to identify pulmonary dystrophia with a view to predicting recurrence, in defining which patients benefit from surgery and in defining the role of preventative surgery on an unaffected lung.

- If patients fail conservative therapy, should they have an intercostal catheter placed or be referred for thoracoscopy?
- The place of primary VATS (without prior aspiration or intercostal catheter placement) in stable patients with recurrent pneumothorax.
- Given the high recurrence rate, the role of surgery or pleurodesis after first spontaneous pneumothorax.

Further reading

Baumann MH, Strange C, Heffner JE, et al. Management of spontaneous pneumothorax: an American College of Chest Physicians Delphi consensus statement. Chest 2001;119:590–602.

Kelly AM. Management of primary spontaneous pneumothorax: is the best evidence clearer fifteen years on? Emerg Med Australas 2007;19:303–8.

MacDuff A, Arnold T, Harvey J. Standards of Care Committee, British Thoracic Society. BTS guidelines for the management of spontaneous pneumothorax Pleural Diseases Group. Thorax 2010;62:(Suppl 2)18–31.

Therapeutic Guidelines: Respiratory Revision 4. Melbourne: Therapeutic Guidelines Limited; 2009. <http://online.tg.org.au/ip> [Accessed Oct. 2012].

6.7 Pleural effusion

Shammi Ramlakhan • Suzanne Mason

ESSENTIALS

1 In the vast majority of patients, a posteroanterior and lateral chest X-ray will confirm and localize an effusion. Lateral decubitus films, ultrasound and computed tomography (CT) scanning are more sensitive in diagnosing and localizing small effusions.

2 Pleural fluid analysis is the principal method of determing the underlying cause of an effusion. Ultrasound-guided pleural fluid aspiration is the preferred method for obtaining a suitable sample. The key to management is the differentiation of transudates from exudates.

3 Pleural biopsy improves the diagnostic yield in the presence of tuberculosis and malignancy to 80% and 90%, respectively when combined with pleural fluid analysis.

4 Treatment is dependent on the underlying disease. Large pleural effusions with cardiorespiratory compromise should be aspirated to provide symptomatic relief.

5 Transudates respond to treatment of the underlying condition. Exudates usually require further investigative procedures and specific local treatments.

Introduction

A pleural effusion is an accumulation of fluid in the pleural space caused by a disruption of the homoeostatic forces that control normal flow. Massive pleural effusions may produce significant cardiorespiratory compromise requiring urgent attention in the emergency department. However, many are asymptomatic or produce minimal disturbance. In this latter group, the role of the emergency department care is assessment to ascertain the aetiology of the effusion, as this dictates the most appropriate treatment. Information regarding the likely cause can be obtained by a thorough history and physical examination. Important adjuvant investigations include chest X-ray, examination of pleural fluid and biopsies obtained during thoracocentesis. Bronchoscopy and thoracoscopy have a role to play in the small group of patients in whom the above procedures fail to establish a cause, but their use is beyond the scope of initial emergency department assessment and stabilization.

Aetiology, pathogenesis and pathology

Pathology and pathogenesis

The pleural cavity is normally a small space bordered by the visceral and parietal pleura, both of which are composed of mesothelial lining cells. In normal conditions, it contains approximately 0.25 mL/kg of low protein liquid. The pleura act as semipermeable membranes and fluid movement is determined principally by capillary pressure, plasma oncotic pressure and capillary permeability, governed by Starling's law. The parietal pleura appears to be the more important pleural surface for pleural liquid turnover in the normal physiological state. Current evidence suggests that most pleural fluid drainage occurs via pleurolymphatic communications or stomas, augmented by respiratory muscle action and intrinsic lymphatic vessel contractility. Overall absorptive capacity can exceed production by a factor of 10–20, allowing maintenance of pleural fluid volume in most cases. Pleural effusions occur due to one of the following:

- disturbances in the hydrostatic–osmotic pressure gradients, resulting in a transudate
- pleural inflammation with loss of semipermeable membrane function, resulting in a protein-rich exudate
- lymphatic obstruction (usually producing a transudate).

Transudates are ultrafiltrates of plasma and arise as a result of a relatively small number of conditions. Exudates are produced by a wider variety of inflammatory conditions and often require more extensive investigation.

Aetiology

Table 6.7.1 lists the causes of transudative and exudative pleural effusions. The commonest causes are congestive cardiac failure, pneumonia, malignancy and pulmonary embolus.

Classification

Pleural effusions are classified according to their aetiology as transudates or exudates. Light first proposed the criteria to differentiate the two. This involved measurement of both serum and pleural markers. An exudate is present if any of the following are present:

- pleural fluid-LDH level divided by serum LDH level >0.6
- pleural fluid-LDH level >two-thirds upper limit of normal for serum LDH level
- pleural fluid protein level divided by serum protein level >0.5.

If the fluid is found to be an exudate, then further tests are required to determine the underlying cause of disease.

Clinical features

History

History will often identify the cause of a pleural effusion. Features suggestive of the common causes (congestive heart failure, pneumonia, malignancy and pulmonary embolism) should be sought. Specific questioning regarding previous occupational exposures, drug treatments, radiation therapy, trauma, tuberculosis exposure and collagen vascular disease may be revealing. Pleural effusions rarely cause symptoms other than dyspnoea, although a mild non-productive cough is sometimes described. A more severe or productive cough suggests underlying pneumonia or endobronchial pathology. Chest pain in association with an effusion may indicate malignancy, pulmonary embolus or pleural inflammation. Unusually, a chest wall swelling may be due to metastatic cancer or an expanding empyema.

Table 6.7.1   Causes of transudative and exudative pleural effusions

Effusion always transudative Congestive cardiac failure Cirrhosis Nephrotic syndrome Peritoneal dialysis Hypoalbuminaemia Urinothorax Atelectasis Constrictive pericarditis Superior vena caval obstruction CSF leaks (trauma, surgery, VP shunts) Glycinothorax	**Malignancy** Carcinoma Lymphoma Mesothelioma Leukaemia Chylothorax
'Classic' exudates that can be transudates Malignancy Pulmonary embolism Sarcoidosis Hypothyroidism	**Other inflammatory disorders** Pancreatitis Benign asbestos pleural effusion Pulmonary embolisn Radiation therapy Uraemic pleurisy Sarcoidosis Post-cardiac injury syndrome Haemothorax Post-myocardial infarction ARDS Trapped lung

Exudates
Infectious
    Bacterial pneumonia
    Tuberculosis
    Parasites
    Fungal disease
    Atypical pneumonia
    Nocardia, actinomyces
    Subphrenic abscess
    Hepatic abscess
    Splenic abscess
    Hepatitis
    Spontaneous oesophageal rupture
	Increased negative intrapleural pressure
	Atelectasis
	Cholesterol effusion

Iatrogenic Drug-induced (amiodarone, phenytoin, nitrofurantoin, β-bockers, dantrolene sodium, methysergide maleate, procarbazine HCl, methotrexate, medications causing drug-induced lupus syndrome: procainamide HCl, hydralazine HCl, quinidine) Oesophageal perforation Oesophageal sclerotherapy Central venous catheter migration Enteral feeding Post-coronary artery bypass graft	**Connective tissue disease** Lupus pleuritis Rheumatoid pleurisy Mixed connective tissue disease Churg–Strauss syndrome Wegener's granulomatosis Familial Mediterranean fever **Endocrine dysfunction** Hypothyroidism Ovarian hyperstimulation syndrome Postpartum **Lymphatic abnormalities** Malignancy Yellow nail syndrome Lymphangiomyomatosis **Movement of fluid from the abdomen to pleural space** Pancreatitis Pancreatic pseudocyst Meig's syndrome Carcinoma Chylous ascites Urinothorax

Patients may have myriad associated systemic symptoms due to the underlying pathological process, such as fever, weight loss, abdominal and joint pain.

Physical examination

Effusions smaller than 300 mL may be undetectable clinically. However, mild hypoxaemia is common and often associated with dyspnoea, which can be due to distortions of the diaphragm or altered chest wall mechanics during respiration. The physical signs of pleural effusion are reduced or asymmetric chest wall expansion, stony dullness to percussion, reduced or absent breath sounds, crackles, pleural rub, diminished or absent vocal resonance and tactile fremitus on the affected side. In large unilateral effusions (greater than 1 L), tracheal displacement toward the unaffected side may be detected. Tracheal deviation to the affected side suggests an obstructing endobronchial lesion. In addition, signs of underlying disease should be sought.

Clinical investigations

Investigation and initial management of pleural effusion is shown in Figure 6.7.1.

Imaging

In the majority of patients, a posteroanterior (PA) and lateral chest X-ray will provide the required information to confirm and localize an effusion (Figs 6.7.2 and 6.7.3). The classic radiological features of effusion are of a gravity-dependent homogeneous opacity within the pleural cavity with a concave lateral air–fluid interface (meniscus sign). Effusions larger than 75 mL can obliterate the posterior sulcus on lateral films and 175 mL are needed to blunt the lateral costophrenic angles on erect films (Fig. 6.7.3). Occasionally, the collection may be subpulmonary. Signs suggestive of this include apparent elevation of the diaphragm, abnormal diaphragmatic contour (lateral displacement of the apex on PA film, sharp angulation of apparent anterior diaphragm on lateral film) and more than a 2 cm space between the gastric bubble and the apparent left diaphragm. Very small and/or isolated effusions may not be seen on standard views. Lateral or lateral decubitus films are often helpful where a fluid level at least 1 cm deep indicates that the effusion is probably accessible by thoracocentesis and contains at least 200 mL of fluid. If the fluid does not form a uniform level, this may indicate the presence of a loculated effusion, which requires more careful management. Chest ultrasound and computed tomography (CT) are more sensitive in diagnosing and localizing small effusions. Contrast enhanced CT can also be helpful in the differential diagnosis of pleural effusions.

The chest X-ray can also provide other diagnostic clues to the aetiology of the effusion. Large effusions with lack of mediastinal shift usually indicate a bronchial obstruction, infiltration of the lung with tumour, mesothelioma or a fixed mediastinum (due to tumour or fibrosis). Bilateral effusions with an enlarged heart shadow are usually due to congestive cardiac failure. Pleural plaques and calcification may indicate asbestos exposure and findings consistent with pneumonia or malignancy may indicate a cause for the associated effusion.

Thoracocentesis

If the diagnosis is known (e.g. congestive heart failure with recurrent effusions), further investigations need only be performed to aid management of the underlying problem. When the diagnosis is still uncertain, the most useful investigation is diagnostic thoracocentesis. A variety of techniques have been reported, but the common underlying principle is the advancement of a needle, trocar or cannula into the pleural space under strict aseptic conditions and the withdrawal of a volume of fluid for analysis. Ultrasound-guided aspiration is recommended as this reduces both the failure and complication rates. Fluid should be procured for biochemical, microbiological and cytological analysis in order to classify the effusion as outlined above and indicate an

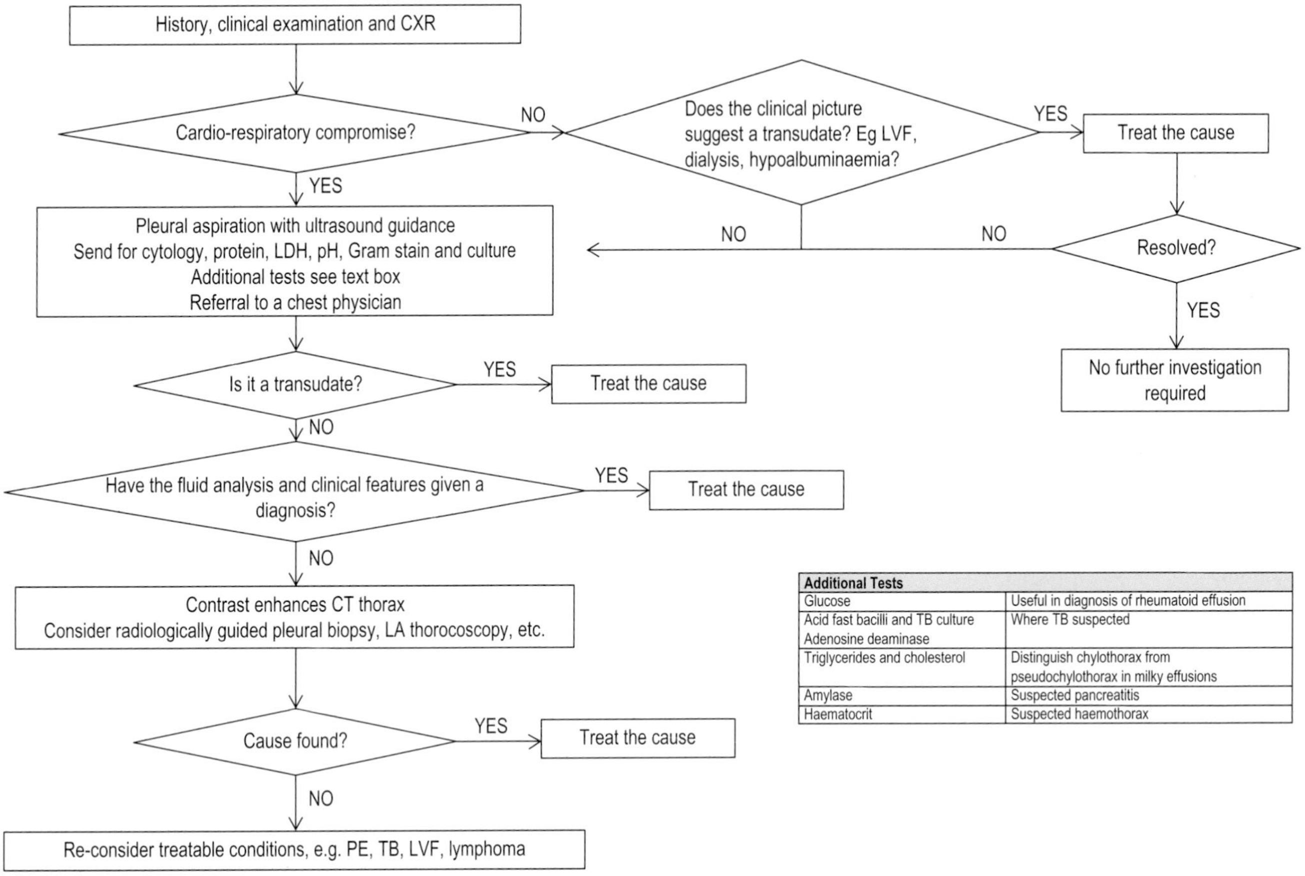

```
┌─────────────────────────────────────────┐
│   History, clinical examination and CXR   │
└─────────────────────────────────────────┘
                    │
                    ▼
        ◇ Cardio-respiratory compromise? ◇ ──NO──▶ ◇ Does the clinical picture
                    │                                   suggest a transudate? Eg LVF,
                  YES                                   dialysis, hypoalbuminaemia? ◇ ──YES──▶ ┌──────────────┐
                    │                                           │                              │ Treat the cause│
                    ▼                                          NO                              └──────────────┘
┌─────────────────────────────────────────┐                    │                                      │
│ Pleural aspiration with ultrasound guidance│◀──NO──────NO──── ◇ Resolved? ◇                          │
│ Send for cytology, protein, LDH, pH, Gram │                                                          │
│ stain and culture                          │                          YES                            │
│ Additional tests see text box              │                           │                             │
│ Referral to a chest physician              │                           ▼                             │
└─────────────────────────────────────────┘              ┌──────────────────────────┐                │
                    │                                      │  No further investigation  │                │
                    ▼                                      │         required           │                │
        ◇ Is it a transudate? ◇ ──YES──▶ ┌──────────────┐ └──────────────────────────┘                │
                    │                      │Treat the cause│
                   NO                      └──────────────┘
                    │
                    ▼
  ◇ Have the fluid analysis and clinical features given a
         diagnosis? ◇ ──YES──▶ ┌──────────────┐
                    │            │Treat the cause│
                   NO           └──────────────┘
                    │
                    ▼
┌─────────────────────────────────────────┐
│ Contrast enhances CT thorax                │
│ Consider radiologically guided pleural     │
│ biopsy, LA thorocoscopy, etc.              │
└─────────────────────────────────────────┘
                    │
                    ▼
        ◇ Cause found? ◇ ──YES──▶ ┌──────────────┐
                    │              │Treat the cause│
                   NO             └──────────────┘
                    │
                    ▼
┌─────────────────────────────────────────┐
│ Re-consider treatable conditions, e.g. PE, │
│ TB, LVF, lymphoma                          │
└─────────────────────────────────────────┘
```

Additional Tests	
Glucose	Useful in diagnosis of rheumatoid effusion
Acid fast bacilli and TB culture Adenosine deaminase	Where TB suspected
Triglycerides and cholesterol	Distinguish chylothorax from pseudochylothorax in milky effusions
Amylase	Suspected pancreatitis
Haematocrit	Suspected haemothorax

Fig. 6.7.1 Diagnostic algorithm for the investigation of a unilateral pleural effusion in adults. *(Modified from Hooper C, Lee YCG, Maskell N. Investigation of a unilateral pleural effusion in adults: British Thoracic Society pleural disease guideline 2010. Thorax 2010; 65(Suppl 2). ii4–17 with permission.)*

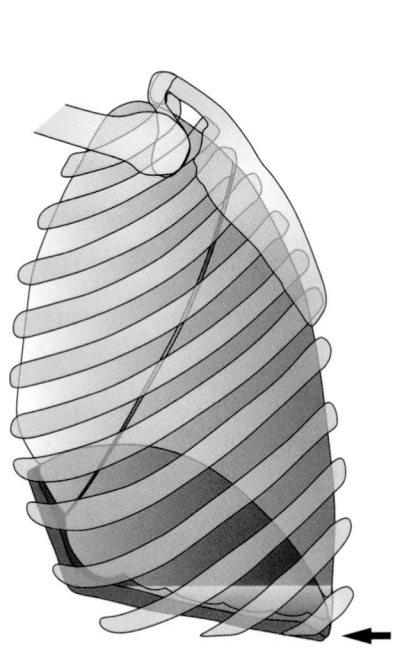

Fig. 6.7.2 Small pleural effusion detected on lateral chest X-ray (arrow indicates the effusion).

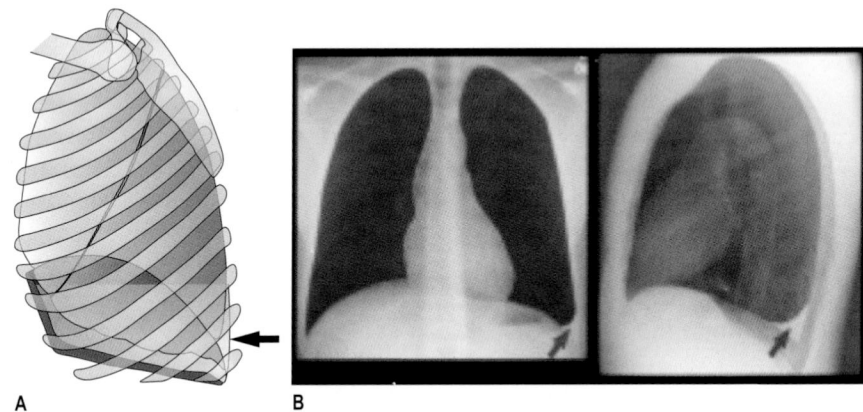

Fig. 6.7.3 Larger pleural effusion (A). This can be visible on both the lateral and PA chest views (B) (arrow indicates the effusion).

underlying cause (see Fig. 6.7.1). The gross appearance of the pleural fluid can be helpful in diagnosis (Table 6.7.2).

With respect to exudates, microscopy, Gram stain and cytology should be performed. About 60% of cultures of infected pleural effusion are positive and this yield is increased with direct inoculation into blood culture bottles. The diagnostic yield in malignant disease ranges from 50 to 90% with 50 mL of fluid sufficient for cytology. Pleural fluid pH may also be helpful in diagnosis. In parapneumonic effusions, a pH <7.2 indicates the need for urgent drainage, whereas a pH >7.3 suggests that treatment

Table 6.7.2 Gross appearance of pleural fluid

Appearance of fluid	Test indicated	Interpretation of result
Bloody	Haematocrit	<1% non-sigificant 1–20% malignancy, pulmonary embolus, trauma >50% haemothorax
Cloudy, milky or turbid	Centrifugation Triglyceride level	Turbid supernatant – high lipid levels >110 mg/dL chylothorax >50 mg/dL need lipoprotein analysis Chylomicrons chylothorax <50 mg/dL and cholesterol >250 mg/dL pseudochylothorax
Putrid odour	Gram stain and culture	Possible anaerobic infection
Food particles	GI imaging	Oesophageal rupture
Ammoniacal odour	Renal function and imaging	Urinothorax

Modified from Light RW. Pleural effusion. N Engl J Med 2002;346:1971–7.

with systemic antibiotics should be sufficient. In malignant effusions, a pleural pH <7.3 indicates more extensive pleural involvement and shorter survival times. A low pleural fluid pH also correlates well with glucose levels. Glucose <0.5 times serum is suggestive of bacterial infection, malignancy or rheumatoid arthritis. An elevated amylase in the pleural fluid suggests oesophageal rupture, effusion associated with pancreatitis or malignancy. Pleural fluid antinuclear antibody and rheumatoid factor tests should be ordered when collagen vascular diseases are suspected.

There are no absolute contraindications to thoracocentesis, but relative contraindications include a bleeding diathesis or anticoagulation, small fluid volumes (<1 cm on lateral decubitus film), mechanical ventilation and cutaneous disease over the proposed puncture site. The puncture location is chosen based on clinical examination and chest X-ray findings, preferably with ultrasound guidance.

Additional techniques

Two other procedures deserve consideration when thoracocentesis is not diagnostic. Percutaneous pleural biopsy involves obtaining a closed biopsy of the parietal pleura using an imaging-guided cutting needle. It is relatively easy to perform and improves the diagnostic yield in the presence of tuberculosis and malignancy to 80 and 90%, respectively when combined with pleural fluid analysis. The second is thoracoscopy, which involves pleural biopsy under direct visualization

through a thoracoscope. Thoracoscopy has a very high yield for diagnosing both benign and malignant pleural disease and can be performed under local anaesthetic. It is usually employed only after other diagnostic procedures have proved non-diagnostic and malignancy is suspected.

Treatment and prognosis

If a pleural effusion is causing respiratory distress, then it should be drained regardless of whether it is a transudate or an exudate (see Fig. 6.7.1). Drainage of a relatively small volume of fluid (500 mL) can cause significant relief from symptoms. All patients undergoing this procedure should be well oxygenated, with oxygen saturations monitored and kept above 90%, as thoracocentesis may increase ventilation–perfusion mismatches. Removal of large volumes (usually >1500 mL) may produce re-expansion pulmonary oedema, so large effusions should be drained in stages, with at least 12 hours between procedures.

Transudates should be managed by treating the underlying disease. Large-bore tube thoracostomy should generally be employed for empyema and traumatic haemothorax, although the former may be managed by imaging-guided small bore drainage. Empyemas tend to loculate early, in which case frequent (every 6–8 h) saline flushing or fibrinolytic (streptokinase, alteplase or urokinase) may be instilled to dissolve the fibrin membranes. Should this fail, surgical drainage or

decortication should be performed. Systemic organism-specific antibiotic therapy should also be instituted.

Malignant effusions can be managed by thoracostomy and tetracycline pleurodesis, thoracoscopy and talc poudrage or pleuroperitoneal shunt. Chylothoraces should be treated by pleuroperitoneal shunting, as long-term drainage may result in malnutrition and altered immunocompetence.

Prognosis depends on the underlying cause. Patients with parapneumonic effusions have higher morbidity and mortality than those with pneumonia only. Malignant pleural effusions are associated with a mean survival of less than a year.

Complications

Pleural effusions can produce significant respiratory distress which is alleviated only through drainage. Other complications are those of the underlying pathological process, such as fever and toxicity in the case of parapneumonic effusions.

There are recognized complications associated with thoracocentesis, such as pain at the puncture site, cutaneous or internal bleeding, pneumothorax, empyema and splenic or hepatic puncture. Pneumothorax complicates around 12% of thoracocenteses but this may not always require active treatment. Risk factors include chronic obstructive or fibrotic pulmonary disease, previous chest irradiation, using larger (>20 G) thoracocentesis needles, multiple passes to obtain fluid and aspiration of air during the procedure.

Disposition

The requirement for inpatient investigation and management will depend on the degree of respiratory compromise, the presence of coexisting or underlying disease and the patient's wishes and social circumstances. In many cases, pleural effusions in the otherwise stable patient may be investigated and managed on an outpatient basis.

Further reading

Davies HE, Davies RJO, Davies CWH. Management of pleural infection in adults: British Thoracic Society pleural disease guideline 2010. Thorax 2010;65(Suppl. 2):ii41–53.

Havelock T, Teoh R, Laws D, Gleeson F. Pleural procedures and thoracic ultrasound: British Thoracic Society pleural disease guideline 2010. Thorax 2010;65(Suppl. 2):i61–76.

Hooper C, Lee YCG, Maskell N. Investigation of a unilateral pleural effusion in adults: British Thoracic Society pleural disease guideline 2010. Thorax 2010;65(Suppl 2):ii4–17.

Light RW. Clinical practice. Pleural effusion. N Engl J Med 2002;346:1971–7.

Porcel JM, Light RW. Diagnostic approach to pleural effusion in adults. Am Fam Phys 2006;73:1211–20.

Roberts ME, Neville E, Berrisford RG, et al. Management of a malignant pleural effusion: British Thoracic Society pleural disease guideline 2010. Thorax 2010;65(Suppl. 2): ii32–40.

Wong CL, Holroyd-Leduc J, Straus SE. Does this patient have a pleural effusion? J Am Med Assoc 2009;301:309–17.

6.8 Haemoptysis

Gregory Cham • Stuart Dilley

ESSENTIALS

1 The majority of patients are stable and can be managed and investigated as outpatients.

2 It is difficult to predict which patient may develop life-threatening haemoptysis.

3 It is essential to differentiate between haemoptysis, haematemesis and bleeding from the upper airway.

4 The priorities in massive haemoptysis are the maintenance of ventilation, oxygenation, circulatory support and the identification of the source of bleeding.

5 Chest X-ray is normal in 20–30% of patients with haemoptysis.

6 Bronchoscopy is the investigation of choice if haemoptysis is thought to be due to a lesion in the bronchial tree.

7 In 30% of cases, no cause for haemoptysis will be found.

Introduction

Haemoptysis is the expectoration of blood from the lungs or tracheobronchial tree. Most patients who present with haemoptysis describe small amounts of blood mixed with sputum or saliva. The majority of patients are stable and can be managed as outpatients. Rarely, patients present with massive haemoptysis where respiratory and circulatory systems are severely compromised and death by asphyxiation or exsanguination can be quite rapid. These patients require urgent skilful management of airway and circulatory systems. A small blood clot may compromise ventilation by obstructing an airway just as effectively as a massive bleed that floods an entire lung.

Aetiology

The causes of haemoptysis are summarized in Table 6.8.1. In approximately 30% of cases no cause will be found.

Clinical features

Patients may have difficulty in differentiating between haemoptysis and haematemesis. Bronchial blood is usually coughed out, bright red, frothy and alkaline, while gastrointestinal blood is usually darker, may be mixed with food particles and is acidic. Haemoptysis also needs to be differentiated from nasopharyngeal bleeding, particularly posterior epistaxis.

History and examination should be tailored to elicit information relevant to the common causes of haemoptysis as listed above. Pallor could be secondary to anaemia. Clubbing of the fingers suggests carcinoma of the lung, bronchiectasis, lung abscess or, rarely, cyanotic congenital heart disease. Telangectasia over

Table 6.8.1 Causes of haemotypsis	
Pulmonary	*Extrapulmonary*
Pneumonia	Oral, pharyngeal or gastrointestinal blood
Bronchitis	Heart failure
Neoplasm	Mitral stenosis
Bronchiectasis	Coagulopathies
Lung abscess	Pulmonary embolism
Tuberculosis	Thoracic aortic aneurysm
Trauma	Cocaine
Iatrogenic	
Foreign body	
Connective tissue disorder	
Arteriovenous malformation	
Pulmonary infarction	
Cystic fibrosis	

the skin and mucosa could indicate the presence of hereditary haemorrhagic telangectasia. Spider naevi could suggest the presence of liver cirrhosis and haematemesis. Uraemia could suggest an underlying connective tissue disease. Examination of the heart may reveal the presence of pulmonary hypertension, valvular heart disease or heart failure.

Resuscitation should take precedence in cases of severe bleeding and respiratory compromise. Most patients do not have respiratory or circulatory compromise.

Differential diagnosis

Haemoptysis can be confused with bleeding from the upper airway, nasopharynx or haematemesis. Bleeding may be a complication of excessive anticoagulation.

Clinical investigations

The patient should be isolated during the course of assessment and investigations if pulmonary tuberculosis or other virulent airborne organisms are considered likely.

Chest X-ray

Between 20 and 30% of patients with haemoptysis will have normal chest X-rays. Abnormalities in the X-ray could reflect preexisting chronic lung disease or infiltrates resulting from pulmonary haemorrhage rather than identifying a definitive cause for bleeding. Evidence of pneumonia, abscess formation, tuberculosis, bronchiectasis or tumours may be seen. The presence of cavitation could indicate mycobacterial infection, lung abscess and bronchiectasis.

Computerized tomography

Computerized tomography (CT) of the chest may occasionally provide additional information not evident on the chest X-ray and is particularly useful in cases of bronchocarcinoma and bronchiectasis to further delineate anatomy. CT pulmonary angiography is indicated if the diagnosis is thought to be pulmonary embolism or pulmonary arteriovenous malformation.

Other imaging

Ventilation–perfusion scan is an alternative to computerized tomography in selected patients with suspected pulmonary embolism. Pulmonary and bronchial angiography may be useful if bleeding is ongoing and no source is found by other means.

Bronchoscopy

Bronchoscopy is the investigation of choice in cases where an abnormality of the bronchial tree is suspected. It allows direct visualization of the bronchial tree and the source of bleeding. In the case of massive haemoptysis, bronchoscopy should be performed early. It should also be performed on those patients diagnosed with pneumonia or bronchitis who continue to bleed or who do not respond to antibiotic therapy. In addition to direct visualization of the bronchial tree, bronchoscopy facilitates the collection of sputum and cytological samples for further analysis.

Rigid bronchoscopy allows for more complete removal of blood and better ventilation in the case of massive haemoptysis. It does not visualize upper lobe airways well and the procedure requires sedation or anaesthesia. The fibreoptic bronchoscope is more flexible and thinner and can be used to visualize areas of the bronchial tree not seen by the rigid bronchoscope. It cannot cope with the large volumes of blood that need suctioning in massive haemoptysis, but it can be passed down the lumen of the rigid bronchoscope once the majority of blood has been removed.

Sputum

Observe universal precautions when pulmonary tuberculosis or other virulent airborne pathogen is considered. When the origin of haemoptysis is thought to be infective or neoplastic, sputum should be collected for bacteriological and cytological assessment, including Zeihl–Neelsen staining for acid-fast bacilli.

Other

Haemoglobin, platelet count and clotting studies should be undertaken. A raised white cell count may indicate the presence of infection. Assessment of oxygenation by pulse oximetry or arterial blood gas analysis is particularly important for a patient with respiratory distress and massive bleeding. Blood group and cross-matching may be needed in the case of massive haemoptysis. Urea and electrolytes provide an assessment of underlying kidney function.

Nasoendoscopy, biopsy, CT or magnetic resonance imaging (MRI) may be indicated if the source of bleeding is from the upper airway, e.g. nasal polyps, laryngeal carcinoma or pharyngeal tumours.

Treatment

In most cases, haemoptysis is mild, transient and is usually due to an infective process. Malignant disease also needs to be excluded. Patients can usually be discharged on antibiotics if appropriate and have follow up of sputum studies, repeat chest X-rays and other studies as outpatients. Those with more serious respiratory compromise, pulmonary emboli or carcinoma should be managed accordingly.

Massive haemoptysis

Massive haemoptysis has been arbitrarily defined as expectoration of a large amount of blood, the volume of blood is not universally agreed upon, nor easily quantifiable. A more useful definition of massive haemoptysis is 'the volume that is life threatening by virtue of airway obstruction or blood loss'. Exsanguinating haemoptysis of more than 150 mL per hour and a loss of more than 1000 mL per day have a mortality of 75%.

Massive haemoptysis is rare, accounting for less than 2% of all cases of haemoptysis, but has a high mortality of up to 80% in some studies. It is alarming to the patient and clinically challenging. Opinions vary as to the most appropriate course of management; an indication of the paucity of evidence-based literature on this topic.

Massive haemoptysis is usually due to tuberculosis, bronchiectasis or infections, including fungal infections and lung malignancies. Haemoptysis arises from the systemic pressure in bronchial arteries in 90% of cases with only 5% arising from the low pressure pulmonary circulation.

The general principles of 'ABCs' apply as in all serious illness. The immediate threat to the patient is asphyxia or exsanguination. Provide supplemental oxygen. Patients may rapidly become severely hypoxic, restless and uncooperative and immediate intubation may be necessary. The airway should be vigorously suctioned and supplemental oxygen administered. Blood should be taken for full blood count, group and cross-matching and arterial blood gases. Gain intravenous access and provide volume resuscitation with intravenous fluids, blood and blood products. Coagulation, electrolytes and acid–base abnormalities should be corrected. A chest X-ray to locate the site of bleeding is helpful.

Although it is customary to nurse the patient with the suspected bleeding lung dependent to prevent aspiration into the normal lung, some have argued that this may increase the rate of bleeding. The Trendelenburg position is also recommended to aid drainage of blood from the thorax.

Early consultation with respiratory and/or cardiothoracic specialties is essential. This may include an early decision to transfer the patient to a hospital that has the facilities to intervene.

The need to secure an airway provides a dilemma. A large bore endotracheal tube (ETT) will permit ventilation but may not protect the lungs. However, it will allow the passage of a fibreoptic bronchoscope and large bore suction catheter both to visualize the bronchial tree and remove blood. In extreme circumstances, the ETT may be advanced into the right main-stem bronchus to protect the right lung if bleeding appears to be left sided, but this may lead to occlusion of the right upper lobe bronchus. The ETT can be used to guide a balloon occlusion catheter into the right main-stem bronchus to tamponade the right lung if bleeding appears to be right sided, although the ETT will then need to be replaced so that ventilator circuit connections can be made. Blindly advancing the ETT into the left main bronchus is a more difficult procedure. A bronchoscope may be directed into the left main bronchus and facilitate intubation over the bronchoscope with an ETT to protect the left lung if bleeding is right sided. Balloon catheters may also be more accurately placed under bronchoscopic guidance.

Double lumen endotracheal tubes provide protection for the normal lung and a chance to suction or tamponade the bleeding lung. However, they may not be readily available and take considerably more skill to insert than standard single-lumen endotracheal tubes. High rates of misplacement have been reported. They are also too narrow to allow the passage of a fibreoptic bronchoscope and hence limit further assessment of the bleeding source. They are perhaps best reserved for use after bronchoscopy has been performed.

Urgent bronchoscopy should be performed in unstable patients with massive haemoptysis to localize the bleeding segment, provide toilet and allow for various bronchoscopic techniques to arrest local haemorrhage. Bronchoscopy can facilitate the passage of a balloon-tip catheter into the bleeding bronchus to tamponade or isolate the bleeding source.

Angiography may also help identify the source of bleeding. However, there is significant anatomical variability in terms of number of bronchial arteries and their origins and bleeding is not usually fast enough to show extravasation of contrast. Radiologically guided bronchial artery embolization is a useful procedure, halting bleeding in most patients. Twenty per cent of patients will rebleed within 6 months and 50% will have significant bleeds in the longer term. However, this procedure may be an adequate temporizing measure to allow thoracotomy to be performed semi-electively. Significant complications, such as spinal cord injury and arterial perforation or dissection, although rare, have been reported.

The place of surgical treatment of massive haemoptysis is controversial. Some authors advocate early surgical resection of the bleeding site and adjacent lung. It may be difficult to identify the source of the bleeding and most surgeons prefer to operate on a stable patient whose bleeding has ceased. Additionally, some patients will not have the pulmonary reserve to cope with a partial or full lobectomy. Other authors suggest a more conservative approach, including airway management, suction, endobronchial balloon tamponade, antibiotics, iced saline lavage, topical adrenaline (epinephrine) and bronchial artery embolization and report mortality rates of 0–25%. They suggest surgery should be reserved for patients who continue to suffer massive haemoptysis despite these measures.

Other agents, such as tranexamic acid and vasopressin, have been tried with mixed results. Vasoconstriction may, however, hamper attempts at bronchial artery embolization. Direct instillation of antifungal agents in cases of massive haemoptysis due to mycetoma has shown greater promise than the use of systemic antifungal agents.

Controversies

- What is the appropriate positioning for the patient with massive haemoptysis?
- Should CT scan or bronchoscopy be the investigation of choice following chest X-ray?
- What method of endotracheal or endobronchial intubation is most appropriate for acute massive haemoptysis in the emergency department?
- Should rigid or flexible bronchoscopy be used to assess massive haemoptysis?
- Conservative versus operative management of massive haemoptysis.

Further reading

Dweik R, Stoller J. Role of bronchoscopy in massive hemoptysis. Clin Chest Med 1999;20:89–105.

Goldman J. Hemoptysis: emergency assessment and management. Emerg Med Clin N Am 1989;7:325–38.

Haponik E, Fein A, Chin R. Managing life-threatening hemoptysis. Has anything really changed?. Chest 2000;118:1431–5.

Jean-Baptiste E. Management of hemoptysis in the emergency department. Hosp Phys 2005;41:53–9.

Jones D, Davies R. Massive haemoptysis: medical management will usually arrest the bleeding. Br Med J 1990;300: 889–90.

Lordan J, Gascoigne A, Corris P. The pulmonary physician in critical care, illustrative case 7: assessment and management of massive haemoptysis. Thorax 2003;58:814–9.

Marshall T, Flower C, Jackson J. Review: the role of radiology in the investigation and management of patients with haemoptysis. Clin Radiol 1996;51:391–400.

Patel U, Pattison CW, Raphael M. Management of massive haemoptysis. Br J Hosp Med 1994;52:74–8.

Rudzinski JP, del Castillo J. Massive hemoptysis. Ann Emerg Med 1987;16:561–4.

Sakr L, Dutau H. Massive hemoptysis: an update on the role of bronchoscopy in diagnosis and management. Respiration 2010;80:38–58.

DIGESTIVE EMERGENCIES

Edited by *Anne-Maree Kelly*

7.1 Dysphagia

Graeme Thomson

ESSENTIALS

1 Dysphagia is a diagnostic challenge and a broad differential diagnosis should be considered. A carefully taken history will reveal the likely cause in most cases.

2 Dysphagia due to a new-onset pharyngeal or oesophageal disorder will increase the amount of food in the pharynx and may be complicated by aspiration. An assessment of that risk should be made before allowing the patient to take oral fluids or food. Care should be taken to ensure that a patient with known dysphagia who presents to the emergency department is not given inappropriately thin fluids.

3 Patients with moderate to long-term dysphagia may have significant fluid and electrolyte abnormalities and severe nutritional disturbances.

4 Emergency department investigations should be directed to the detection of high-grade obstructions and lesions causing significant risks from airway compromise, haemorrhage or sepsis.

5 Dysphagia is very rarely caused by a psychological disorder. There is nearly always a physical cause.

Introduction

Dysphagia is a broad term encompassing the many forms of difficulty with deglutition (swallowing). The main issues are to determine the likely cause, to identify those patients at risk of significant complications, to treat those causes that are amenable to acute intervention and to refer appropriately for further investigations and treatment.

Dysphagia may be associated with odynophagia (pain on swallowing). Globus is a related term that means the sensation of a lump in the throat. This is rarely of psychological origin. Since the advent of sophisticated investigative techniques, it has been recognized that, in the great majority of cases, there is an identifiable physical cause.

Aetiology

Problems may occur with any of the three stages of swallowing: oral, pharyngeal or oesophageal. Oral and pharyngeal causes may be grouped as transfer dysphagia and oesophageal problems may be referred to as transport dysphagia. Passage of food may be obstructed by a physical barrier, such as a tumour, or a disorder of muscle coordination, such as a neurological deficit.

In addition to diseases, several drugs are recognized as inducing dysphagia. They include tetracyclines, non-steroidal anti-inflammatory drugs, ascorbic acid, quinidine, ferrous sulphate and potassium chloride.

Clinical features

Symptoms may appear suddenly or develop insidiously. If insidious, there may be an acute precipitating event leading to presentation, often complete or partial obstruction owing to the impaction of a food bolus in the oesophagus. This may present as pain, a feeling of a lump in the neck or central chest, severe retching or drooling and an inability to swallow saliva. Patients may report increasing difficulty swallowing solids and then fluids but, in some cases, there may be no previous history of dysphagia.

Where a neurological disorder is causing difficulty initiating swallowing, there may be other neurological deficits. The voice may have changed. Regurgitation of food from the mouth or nose, coughing or frank aspiration may be evident when the patient eats. It should be assumed that patients with recent cerebrovascular events or bulbar dysfunction have dysphagia until formal assessment of swallowing and airway protection can be undertaken.

Examination should focus on testing cranial nerve function plus careful examination of the mouth, neck, chest and abdomen. Hydration status and nutritional status should be evaluated.

Perforation may be suspected if there is a history of ingestion of a corrosive substance or sharp object or if pain is a prominent feature. There may be evidence of surgical emphysema in the neck. If presentation is delayed there may be signs of sepsis.

Clinical investigations

Investigations are directed by the history and likely aetiology. For oropharyngeal and upper oesophageal lesions, a lateral X-ray of the soft tissues of the neck may reveal a lesion impinging on the oesophagus. An impacted dense bone or other solid foreign body may also be seen. For suspected mid- and lower-oesophageal lesions, frontal and lateral chest radiographs may reveal a fluid level, a mediastinal tumour, tuberculous lesions or an aneurysm of the thoracic aorta. Oesophageal perforation may also be detected. If food bolus obstruction is suspected a Gastrografin swallow may reveal the site and degree of obstruction.

Computed tomography (CT) scanning and endoscopy may also be indicated but, in most cases, they can be deferred and performed on a semi-elective basis. A video-fluorographic swallowing study is the best semi-elective investigation. It may reveal structural abnormalities as well as disorders of muscular coordination. Manometry is less reliable.

Laboratory investigations are guided by likely aetiology and complications, but should include basic biochemistry and full blood examination looking for electrolyte disturbances and anaemia.

Treatment

Definitive treatment depends on the underlying cause and will rarely be completed in the emergency department (ED). The degree of oesophageal obstruction, the acuity of onset and the presence of complications dictate the need for emergency treatment. Patients with high-grade obstruction should have oral fluids and food withheld and should be given intravenous fluids if the obstruction persists for more than a few hours.

For food bolus obstruction, intravenous glucagon may relax the oesophageal muscles enough to allow a bolus to pass through. This is less likely to be successful if the bolus is a piece of meat. An initial dose of 1 mg may be followed by a 2 mg dose if necessary. Complications are rare, but include allergy, nausea and hypotension. Phaeochromocytoma is a contraindication to the use of glucagon. Sublingual glyceryl trinitrate may be used as an alternative to glucagon, but hypotension is more likely. After glucagon, a gas-producing substance may be given in an attempt to dilate the oesophagus. Aerated drinks are adequate for this purpose. This technique should be used with great caution because a patient with upper oesophageal obstruction will be at greater risk of aspiration if given a foaming substance. This approach should be avoided if there is any suspicion of perforation. Endoscopic removal will be required in many cases, but this is usually attempted after a period of expectant treatment.

Bones or similar foreign bodies impacted in the pharynx can often be removed in the ED. Topical anaesthetic sprays may suppress the pharyngeal reflexes adequately to allow direct or indirect laryngoscopy and removal with forceps. Removal may immediately relieve the dysphagia, but symptoms due to local oedema or abrasions may persist.

Oesophageal or pharyngeal perforation is a serious complication requiring cover with broad-spectrum antibiotics and urgent surgical referral.

Odynophagia may be relieved by parenteral or topical analgesia. Oral administration of a viscous preparation of lignocaine will ease the pain caused by luminal inflammatory disorders. The maximum recommended dose is 300 mg and should be reduced in the elderly, who may be more affected by systemic absorption.

If a patient with known chronic dysphagia presents to the emergency department for an unrelated reason, care should be taken to avoid giving food or fluids that may be aspirated. Water is associated with a high aspiration risk.

Disposition

Appropriate disposition depends on the likely aetiology and the presence of complications. Admission is indicated for patients at risk of airway compromise, severe haemorrhage, sepsis or those with high-grade oesophageal obstruction. It will also be indicated when dysphagia is part of a broader disease process.

If a food bolus has passed spontaneously, the patient should be referred for semi-elective endoscopy.

Controversies

- Choice between flexible and rigid endoscopy for removal of a food bolus. In many departments, referral patterns will be fixed; however, if there is a choice, rigid endoscopy is preferred for removal of an upper oesophageal bolus and flexible endoscopy for boluses impacted more distally. Overall, flexible endoscopy has a lower complication rate.
- Observation unit management. There may be arguments for a period of observation of 12 hours or more before referral for endoscopy, as the majority of food bolus obstructions will resolve spontaneously.

Further reading

Glauser J, Lilja GP, Greenfeld B, et al. Intravenous glucagon in the management of oesophageal food obstruction. J Am Coll Emerg Phys 1979;8:228–31.

Gmeiner D, von Rahden BH, Meco C, et al. Flexible versus rigid endoscopy for treatment of foreign body impaction in the oesophagus. Surg Endosc 2007;21:2026–29.

Mendelson MH. Dysphagia tintinalli. In: JE, Kelen GD, Stapczynski JS, editors. Emergency medicine: a comprehensive study guide. New York: McGraw Hill, 2004, p. 509–10.

Mohammed SH, Hegedus V. Dislodgement of impacted oesophageal foreign bodies with carbonated beverages. Clin Radiol 1986;37:589–92.

Palmer JB, Drennan JC, Baba M. Evaluation and treatment of swallowing impairments. Am Fam Phys 2000;61:2453–62.

Sodeman TC, Harewood GC, Baron TH. Assessment of the predictors of response to glucagon in the setting of acute oesophageal food bolus obstruction. Dysphagia 2004;19:18–21.

Speech Pathology Australia. Dysphagia: General Position Paper. The Speech Pathology Association of Australia Limited; 2004.

Tsikoudas A, Kochillas X, Kelleher R, et al. The management of acute oesophageal obstruction from food bolus: can we be more conservative?. Eur Arch Otorhinolaryngol 2005;262:528–30.

7.2 Approach to abdominal pain

Kim Chai Chan • Eillyne Seow

ESSENTIALS

1 Abdominal pain accounts for 5–10% of all emergency department visits. A significant proportion of these patients will require hospital admission.

2 Abdominal pain most frequently arises from pathologies in the gastrointestinal and the genitourinary systems; however, it may also result from cardiovascular, pulmonary, metabolic, infective and toxic causes.

3 Special consideration should be given to four subgroups of patients: the elderly, the immunocompromised (including those with HIV infection), women of childbearing age and children. These patients require careful assessment to avoid missed diagnoses and poor outcomes.

4 In up to 25–40% of patients, the exact cause of the abdominal pain may not be determined in the emergency department. After ruling out life-threatening causes and with relief of symptoms, most of these patients may be discharged with appropriate advice.

5 Patients with abdominal pain should be given adequate analgesia (including the use of opioids). Adequate analgesia can aid diagnosis and does not conceal signs of an acute abdomen.

6 In selected patients where indicated, judicious use of imaging, laboratory or bedside tests may aid in the diagnoses and disposition of patients presenting with abdominal pain. The clinician ordering the investigations should be aware of their accuracy and limitations and interpret the results in the correct clinical context.

Introduction

The assessment of patients with abdominal pain is challenging because:

- the contact time with the patient is relatively short and diagnosis may be difficult, especially early in the disease process
- the presentation may be atypical, especially for the very young, the immunocompromised and the elderly
- the degree of pain may not be commensurate with the severity of the disease
- the absence of abnormal vital signs cannot rule out a serious underlying condition
- the absence of physical findings of an acute abdomen does not rule out a surgical abdomen, e.g. serious conditions, such as ischaemic colitis, may have very non-specific physical findings and
- a large number of potential differential diagnoses may need to be considered.

The emergency department (ED) approach to acute abdominal pain emphasizes disposition over diagnosis. It is more important to recognize an acute abdomen than to identify the exact cause of the pain.

Epidemiology, pathophysiology and differential diagnosis

It has been estimated that abdominal pain accounts for approximately 5–10% of all ED visits. A significant proportion (18–42%) of these patients will require admission. The elderly (aged 60 and over) are over-represented in the admitted patient group. In one study of elderly patients presenting with abdominal pain, at least 50% were hospitalized and about 30–40% eventually required surgery. Up to 40% of patients were initially misdiagnosed and the overall mortality was about 10%.

Abdominal pain may result from:

- Visceral pain: this pain is poorly localized and may be colicky, intermittent and recurrent in nature. Stimulation of nociceptors investing the visceral peritoneum causes visceral pain. For example, when hollow organs are distended or when capsules covering solid organs are stretched. Visceral pain localizes to the abdominal region that correlates with the embryonic segments of the viscera:
  - foregut structures (stomach, duodenum, liver, biliary tract, pancreas) localize to the upper abdomen
  - midgut structures (small bowel, proximal colon, appendix) localize to the periumbilical region and
  - hindgut structures (distal colon, genitourinary tract) localize to the lower abdomen.
- Somatic pain: this pain is well localized and is often constant and intense. Somatic pain results from local irritation of the parietal peritoneum. It is localized more specifically to the area of pathology. Differential diagnosis of pain by location is shown in Table 7.2.1. It is, however, important to recognize that the area of pain does not always correspond to the supposed anatomical location of the underlying pathology, e.g. acute appendicitis may present as suprapubic or flank pain.
- Referred pain: pain felt at a distance from the site of origin. It is thought that referred pain occurs because afferent pain fibres from areas of high sensory input (e.g. the skin) enter the spinal cord at the same level as nociceptive fibres from an area of low sensory input (e.g. the viscera). The brain, being more used to pain signals from the skin, wrongly interprets the pain signal from the viscera as that from the dermatome.

Both visceral and somatic pain may manifest as referred pain. Some examples are:

- shoulder pain due to diaphragmatic irritation
- pain at the tip of the scapula due to gallbladder pathology
- epigastric pain due to acute myocardial infarction.

Causes of diffuse abdominal pain

Generalized diffuse pain that is poorly localized may be due to benign causes (e.g. gastroenteritis, constipation and menstrual cramps) or from life-threatening conditions (Table 7.2.2).

Table 7.2.1 Differential diagnosis of pain by location (list is not exhaustive)

Right upper quadrant	Epigastrium	Left upper quadrant
Hepatobiliary pathology Duodenal ulcer, duodenitis Renal colic, pyelonephritis Retrocaecal appendicitis Pneumonia, pulmonary embolism	Gastritis, peptic ulcer Hepatobiliary pathology Pancreatitis Aortic aneurysm Early appendicitis Myocardial infarction	Gastritis, peptic ulcer Renal colic, pyelonephritis Splenic pathology Pancreatitis Pneumonia
Right lumbar or flank	**Midline or periumbilical**	**Left lumbar or flank**
Renal colic, pyelonephritis Aortic aneurysm Psoas abscess Appendicitis	Visceral pain from midgut structures Early appendicitis Aortic aneurysm	Renal colic, pyelonephritis Aortic aneurysm Psoas abscess
Right lower quadrant	**Suprapubic**	**Left lower quadrant**
Appendicitis Ectopic pregnancy, tubo-ovarian pathology, endometriosis, pelvic inflammatory disease Urinary tract infection, ureteric colic Diverticulitis Hernia Aortic aneurysm Testicular torsion, epididymo-orchitis	Cystitis, bladder pathology Urinary tract infection Prostatitis Ectopic pregnancy, tubo-ovarian pathology, endometriosis, pelvic inflammatory disease	Similar to causes for right lower quadrant pain except for appendicitis (very rarely left sided)
Pain radiating to the back		
Perforated peptic ulcer Acute pancreatitis Abdominal aortic aneurysm, aortic dissection		

Note: Pain from inflammatory bowel disease, diverticulitis, colitis, gastroenteritis, volvulus, intestinal obstruction, adhesions, ischaemic colitis and constipation may localize to any part of the abdomen.

Table 7.2.2 Some potentially life-threatening causes of generalized, diffuse abdominal pain

Haemoperitoneum from any cause, e.g. ruptured abdominal aortic aneurysm, ruptured ectopic pregnancy, trauma

Mesenteric ischaemia

Perforated viscus

Peritonitis (any cause)

Pancreatitis

Bowel obstruction

Diverticulitis

Inflammatory bowel disease

Metabolic disorders (e.g. diabetic ketoacidosis), sickle cell crisis, typhoid fever

Adapted from Gray-Eurom K, Deitte L. Imaging in the adult patient with non-traumatic abdominal pain. Emerg Med Pract 2007;9:2 with permission.

Extra-abdominal causes of abdominal pain

There are a number of extra-abdominal causes for abdominal pain that must be considered along with abdominal causes (Table 7.2.3).

Table 7.2.3 Extra-abdominal causes of abdominal pain

Thoracic
Myocardial infarction/unstable angina
Pneumonia
Pulmonary embolism
Herniated thoracic disc (neuralgia)

Genitourinary
Testicular torsion

Systemic
Diabetic ketoacidosis
Alcoholic ketoacidosis
Uraemia
Sickle cell disease
Systemic lupus erythematosus
Vasculitis
Hyperthyroidism
Porphyria
Glaucoma

Toxic
Methanol poisoning
Heavy metal poisoning
Scorpion bite
Black widow spider bite

Abdominal wall
Muscle spasm
Muscle haematoma
Herpes zoster

Infections
Strep pharyngitis (more often in children)
Mononucleosis

Adapted from Purcell TB. Nonsurgical and extraperitoneal causes of abdominal pain. Emerg Med Clin N Am 1989;7:721 with permission.

Clinical features

Vital signs and general condition

During triage, a rapid assessment is made by looking at the patient's general condition as well as vital signs. Obviously ill patients, those in severe pain or with abnormal vital signs should be given priority. However, it is not possible to rule out life-threatening causes of abdominal pain by the absence of abnormal vital signs. It has been estimated that up to 7% of patients with normal vital signs may have an underlying life-threatening process and this percentage increases in the elderly. Tachycardia may be absent in patients with autonomic dysfunction, in the elderly and in patients on medications that may blunt the cardiac response to illness or volume loss. Similarly, the elderly, the immunocompromised or those in severe septic shock may sometimes not mount a febrile response. Even in the immunocompetent, fever may not always accompany acute inflammatory conditions.

History

An accurate, focused history often provides the best clue to the possible aetiology of abdominal pain. Clinical impression derived from the history will direct decisions regarding further diagnostic work-up.

DIGESTIVE EMERGENCIES

Patient demographics and background history

- Age and gender: the likelihood of certain conditions is higher in patients of a specific age and gender (Table 7.2.4). For women of childbearing age, it is important to ascertain the presence or absence of pregnancy.
- Background history: key questions in the background history are:
  - previous abdominal surgery
  - use of tobacco, alcohol or recreational drugs
  - chronic illness, e.g. diabetes mellitus, hypertension, coronary artery disease, human immunodeficiency virus infection, systemic lupus erythematosus
  - vascular, thrombotic and embolic risks, e.g. atrial fibrillation, vasculitis, peripheral vascular disease
  - medication history, e.g. use of non-steroidal anti-inflammatory drugs, pain medications, antibiotics, steroids, and anticoagulants
  - history of recent trauma.

Pain attributes

The nature and time course of pain are key clues to diagnosis. The following attributes should be noted:

- Onset and progress of abdominal pain over time (Table 7.2.5): acute vascular events and rupture of hollow viscus typically presents with maximal pain at the onset. Ureteric and biliary colic also often presents with severe pain in the early stages. This is in contrast to pain from inflammatory processes, such as acute appendicitis, which tends to progress and 'mature' over hours.
- Location of pain (see Table 7.2.1), migration of pain, radiation of pain: location of pain helps to identify the area of pathology, although occasionally this may be misleading, especially if the pain is referred. Migration of pain over time gives a clue to possible underlying aetiology, e.g. pain from appendicitis typically starts at the umbilicus or epigastrium and later localizes to the right iliac fossa.
- Radiation of pain may suggest specific conditions (see Table 7.2.1), e.g. pain from acute pancreatitis and perforated peptic ulcers often radiates to the back.
- Severity of pain: severity of pain experienced is dependent on a number of factors in addition to the underlying

Table 7.2.4 Common causes of abdominal pain according to age group and gender		
Causes	*Age group*	*Gender*
Biliary tract disease	Peak age 35–50; rare in those <20	Female:male 3:1
Ruptured ectopic pregnancy	Childbearing ages	Female
Appendicitis	All ages and both genders, peak at young adulthood; higher risk of perforation in the elderly, women, and children	
Mesenteric ischaemia	Elderly, those with vascular, thrombotic or embolic risks	
Abdominal aortic aneurysm	Increased with advancing age	Men more common
Diverticulitis	Increased with advancing age	Men more common

Table 7.2.5 Temporal characteristics of abdominal pain
Sudden maximal pain at or near onset
Perforated peptic ulcer Ruptured abdominal aortic aneurysm Ruptured ectopic pregnancy, ruptured ovarian cyst Ovarian/testicular torsion Mesenteric infarction Pulmonary embolism Acute myocardial infarction
Progression to maximal pain within minutes
Acute pancreatitis Renal and ureteric colic Biliary colic Strangulated hernia Volvulus Intussusception
Gradual onset (increased pain over hours)
Appendicitis Strangulated hernia Inflammatory bowel disease Chronic pancreatitis Salpingitis/prostatitis Cystitis

From White MJ, Counselman FL. 2005 Troubleshooting acute abdominal pain. Emedmag 2002. http://www.emedmag.com/html/pre/cov/covers/011502.asp with permission.

pathology. Severity of pain is not always commensurate with the severity of the underlying illness. The elderly in particular often have a diminished sense of pain. Nonetheless, patients in severe pain should be assessed early and given pain relief. Pain scores may be used to record and monitor progress.
- Character of pain: colicky abdominal pain usually results from obstruction of a hollow viscus. Constant non-colicky pain usually denotes an inflammatory or vascular process.
- Precipitating and relieving factors: pain from peritonitis worsens with movement, deep breathing, coughing or sneezing. Pain from peptic ulcer disease classically increases with hunger and decreases with food, antacid or milk. Pain from biliary colic tends to occur after full or fatty meals. Pain from acute pancreatitis classically worsens with supine posture and is relieved by sitting up.
- Recurrent episodes of abdominal pain: this suggests chronic recurrent conditions, e.g. peptic ulcer, biliary colic, renal colic or diverticulitis. Mesenteric ischaemia and testicular torsion may also present with recurrent episodes.

Associated symptoms

Patients with abdominal pain often have other associated symptoms that may give a clue to the possible cause. These include:

- Constitutional symptoms, e.g. fever, chills, rigors, weight loss or arthralgia.
- Gastrointestinal tract symptoms, e.g. anorexia, nausea, vomiting, diarrhoea or constipation. Nausea and vomiting are non-specific and may result from intra- and extra-abdominal causes. However, feculent vomitus is highly indicative of intestinal obstruction. Vomiting of fresh or altered blood, as well as the passage of black tarry stools, indicates gastrointestinal haemorrhage. Failure to pass stools and flatus over a 24–48-hour period suggests possible intestinal obstruction.
- Genitourinary tract symptoms, e.g. dysuria, frequency, urgency or haematuria, suggest urinary tract pathologies. A purulent discharge from the vagina suggests possible pelvic inflammatory disease.

Table 7.2.6 lists some of the historical high-yield questions in abdominal pain.

Table 7.2.6 High-yield historical questions
1. How old are you? Advanced age means increased risk
2. Which came first – pain or vomiting? Pain first is more likely to be caused by surgical disease
3. How long have you had the pain? Pain for less than 48 hours is more likely to be caused by surgical disease
4. Have you ever had abdominal surgery? Consider adhesion or obstruction in patients with previous abdominal surgery
5. Is the pain constant or intermittent? Constant pain is more likely to be caused by surgical disease
6. Have you had this before? A report of no prior episode is more likely to be caused by surgical disease
7. Do you have a history of cancer, diverticulosis, pancreatitis, kidney failure, gallstones, or inflammatory bowel disease? All are suggestive of more serious disease
8. Do you have human immunodeficiency virus (HIV)? Consider occult infection or drug-related pancreatitis
9. How much alcohol do you drink per day? Consider pancreatitis, hepatitis, cirrhosis
10. Are you pregnant? Test for pregnancy; consider ectopic pregnancy
11. Are you taking antibiotics or steroids? These may mask infection
12. Did the pain start centrally and migrate to the right lower quadrant? High specificity for appendicitis
13. Do you have a history of vascular or heart disease, hypertension or atrial fibrillation? Consider mesenteric ischaemia and abdominal aneurysm

Adapted from Colucciello SA, Lukens TW, Morgan DL. Assessing abdominal pain in adults: a rational, cost-effective, and evidence-based strategy. Emerg Med Pract 1999;1:1 with permission.

Physical examination

A systematic, directed and thorough physical examination can help strengthen the clinical impression formed from the history or to uncover unexpected abnormalities. Physical findings help to rule in, but not rule out, the underlying diagnosis.

General

Consider the general condition and the vital signs of the patient. Patients who look drowsy or unwell or have abnormal vital signs need urgent attention. The posture of the patient may give a clue to the possible underlying disease. Patients with renal colic typically roll about in pain, whereas those with peritonitis lie still as movements aggravate the pain. Inspect for pallor, jaundice, hydration status, enlarged lymph nodes and signs of chronic liver or renal disease.

The abdomen

This is carried out with the patient lying supine and the abdomen exposed from the costal margins to the pubic symphysis. Ideally, the patient should be fairly relaxed, comfortable and cooperative. It is almost impossible to perform an abdominal examination in an uncooperative patient thrashing about in pain. Adequate pain relief should be given before examination if necessary. There is strong evidence that analgesia does not mask physical signs. Abdominal examination in an obtunded patient is unreliable and other assessment modalities such as imaging have to be considered.

- Inspection: look for movement with respiration, shape (e.g. distended or scaphoid), the presence of any surgical scars and external lesions (e.g. bruises, distended veins, hernias). Sometimes, markedly enlarged organs (especially the liver or spleen) or distended bowel may be seen.

- Palpation and percussion: palpation is usually the most informative part of the abdominal examination. Start with the abdominal region away from the area of pain. Perform light, followed by deep palpation systematically over all quadrants of the abdomen. Look for tenderness, guarding, rebound and masses. The area of abdominal tenderness helps to localize the pathology. The presence of involuntary guarding (or rigidity) and rebound indicates peritoneal irritation. Findings of abnormal abdominal masses may help point to the possible diagnosis. Finally, palpate and percuss for hepatosplenomegaly, palpate bimanually for renal masses and examine for costovertebral angle tenderness. Percussion for shifting dullness may be performed in patients with suspected ascites.

- Auscultation: this is performed to look for abnormal or absent bowel sounds and for vascular bruits. In gastric outlet obstruction, a succussion splash may be heard in the upper abdomen when the patient is shaken from side to side. Auscultation is the least rewarding aspect of physical examination as findings from auscultation have been found to be neither sensitive nor specific. However, high-pitched, tinkling or absent bowel sounds have been found to be associated with acute small bowel obstruction, especially in the presence of abdominal distension. Abnormal bowel sounds in the elderly may indicate serious underlying disease.

- Specific abdominal signs (Table 7.2.7): distinctive signs have been described that are associated with specific diagnoses. Some of these signs have not been studied and their sensitivity and specificity remain unknown.

Rectal examination

This is useful in cases of gastrointestinal haemorrhage, perianal or perirectal diseases, stool impaction, prostatic pathologies and rectal foreign bodies. Contrary to classic teaching, rectal examination does not provide additional input in suspected cases of appendicitis.

Examination of hernia orifices

All hernias should be examined for signs of strangulation. Hernias are most commonly present in the inguinal or femoral area, along the midline or arising from old surgical scars. Rarely, they may be present in the paramedian, lumbar or gluteal areas.

Table 7.2.7 Specific abdominal signs

Sign	Description	Association
Murphy's sign	Inability of patient to perform deep inspiration due to pain on palpation of right hypochondrium	Acute cholecystitis (sensitivity 97%; specificity 50%)
Kehr's sign	Severe left shoulder tip pain, especially when the patient is lying supine	Haemoperitoneum, e.g. from ruptured spleen or ectopic pregnancy
Cullen's sign	Ecchymoses around the periumbilical area	Retroperitoneal haemorrhage (haemorrhagic pancreatitis, abdominal aortic aneurysm rupture)
Grey–Turner's sign	Ecchymoses of the flanks	Retroperitoneal haemorrhage (haemorrhagic pancreatitis, abdominal aortic aneurysm rupture)
McBurney's sign	Tenderness localized to a point at two-thirds distance on a line drawn from the umbilicus to the right anterior superior iliac spine	Appendicitis
Iliopsoas sign	Extension of right hip causes abdominal pain	Appendicitis (sensitivity 16%; specificity 95%)
Obturator's sign	Internal rotation of the flexed right hip causes abdominal pain	Appendicitis
Rovsing's sign	Right lower quadrant (RLQ) pain with palpation of the left lower quadrant	Appendicitis
Heel-drop sign	RLQ pain on dropping heels on the ground after standing tiptoes; alternatively RLQ pain from forcefully banging the patient's heel with the examiner's hand	Appendicitis (sensitivity 93%)
Cough test	Post-tussive abdominal pain	Peritonitis (sensitivity up to 95%)

From White MJ, Counselman FL. Troubleshooting acute abdominal pain Emedmag, 2005. http://www.emedmag.com/html/pre/cov/covers/011502.asp with permission.

Examination of genitalia

In women, examination of the pelvic organs may yield important clues to possible gynaecological or obstetric causes of abdominal pain. Testicular pathology needs to be considered in male patients with lower abdominal pain.

Limitations of the abdominal examination

A significant proportion of patients with serious intra-abdominal conditions, such as ruptured aortic abdominal aneurysm and mesenteric ischaemia, may present with non-specific abdominal findings. The area of tenderness does not always correlate to the anatomical location of the disease. For example, up to 20% of patients with surgically proven appendicitis have no right lower quadrant tenderness. Signs of peritonism may not always be present, especially in the elderly and the immunocompromised.

Although involuntary guarding or rigidity increase the likelihood of peritonitis, rebound tenderness has been shown to have no predictive value.

Examination of extra-abdominal systems

Besides the abdomen, extra-abdominal systems, especially the cardiovascular and respiratory systems, should also be examined. Directed examination of extra-abdominal systems is important because:

- the cause of the abdominal pain may be extra-abdominal (see Table 7.2.3)
- it may provide clues to the possible intra-abdominal pathology, e.g. the presence of atrial fibrillation or peripheral vascular disease suggests possible mesenteric ischaemia
- there may be complications from the abdominal condition, e.g. associated chest infection.

Serial examination

Physical signs may often be non-specific in the early phases of the disease. Serial examinations over a period of hours can help to distinguish a surgical from a non-surgical abdomen and improve the diagnostic yield.

Clinical investigations

Although the history and physical examination may give a clue to the possible underlying pathology, many patients with abdominal pain do not present 'classically'. Where indicated, judicious use of investigations may assist in determining diagnosis and disposition. An investigation should be ordered to answer

focused clinical questions. It is also important to be aware of the test's accuracy and limitations. Results should be interpreted in the correct clinical context. Negative test results may not fully rule out serious pathologies in patients with high pre-test probabilities. Further observation, reassessment and admission may need to be considered.

Bedside tests

- Urine pregnancy tests: bedside urine tests are rapid and accurate. Most are able to detect β-hCG to a level as low as 25 mU/mL of urine. It has been estimated that up to 1% of ectopic pregnancies are associated with β-hCG values lower than this.
- Urine analysis: this provides useful early information for patients with suspected urinary tract infection and ureteric colic. However, it is important to interpret urine analysis results in the context of the patient's clinical presentation. About 30% of patients with acute appendicitis may present with blood and leucocytes in their urine and about 30% of patients with ruptured aortic abdominal aneurysm may have haematuria. Conversely, up to one-third of patients with urolithiasis may be negative for haematuria.
- Electrocardiogram (ECG): acute coronary events may manifest as abdominal

symptoms, e.g. epigastric pain, nausea and vomiting. ECG should be performed in cases where there is suspicion of acute coronary syndrome, especially in patients with cardiovascular risks or in the elderly. ECG may also suggest the possible cause of the abdominal pain in some cases, e.g. mesenteric ischaemia from atrial fibrillation, abdominal pain and vomiting from digoxin toxicity.

- Capillary blood sugar: patients with diabetic ketoacidosis may present with symptoms and signs mimicking an acute abdomen. Capillary blood sugar should be performed in all patients with known diabetes mellitus or in cases where there is clinical suspicion.

Laboratory tests

Most laboratory tests do not aid in differentiating surgical from non-surgical causes of abdominal pain.

- Full blood count: this laboratory study does not add value to the assessment of patients with abdominal pain. A normal white count (including normal absolute neutrophil count) may lead to a false sense of security even though it does not rule out a surgical cause of pain. Ten to 60% of patients with surgically proven appendicitis have a normal initial white cell count and only about 50% of patients with severe intra-abdominal pathology have an elevated white cell count. On the other hand, an elevated white cell count may lead to further investigations which may not add to the information already gleaned from the history and physical examination.
- Amylase and lipase: these tests are most useful in patients with suspected pancreatitis. Serum lipase has been found to be more accurate than serum amylase. Both lipase and amylase may be normal in patients with computed tomography (CT) proven pancreatitis, especially in those with recurrent disease.
- Liver function test: this should only be ordered selectively in cases where there is suspicion of hepatobiliary disease or when urine tests detect the presence of urobilinogen.
- C-reactive protein (CRP): this has been found to be about 62% sensitive and 66% specific for appendicitis. The sensitivity improved in patients with more than 12

hours of symptoms and appendicitis is rare in those with two normal CRPs performed 12 hours apart.

Imaging

Plain X-rays

The value of plain radiographs in the evaluation of patients with abdominal pain is limited. However, there is still a place for plain X-rays as a first-line investigation in patients with suspected bowel obstruction, bowel perforation and foreign body. A three-view series comprising upright chest, supine and upright abdominal radiographs is recommended. X-ray findings for bowel obstruction and perforation are fairly specific but not sensitive, i.e. they help to establish, but not exclude, these diagnoses.

Ultrasound

Ultrasound does not involve ionizing radiation, is rapid, non-invasive and may be performed at the bedside. This makes it the ideal evaluation tool in unstable patients or those who are pregnant. Selective use of focused ultrasound in the appropriate clinical context maximizes its diagnostic sensitivity. However, ultrasound is operator dependent and appropriate training is necessary to ensure competence. The sensitivity of ultrasound may also be reduced by technical limitations (e.g. obesity, bowel gas, subcutaneous emphysema). Focused bedside emergency ultrasound examination has significantly affected the diagnosis and management of the following life-threatening conditions:

- Haemoperitoneum from abdominal trauma: the focused abdominal sonogram for trauma (FAST) examination is now considered to be an essential evaluation in unstable patients who have sustained abdominal trauma. The presence of free intraperitoneal fluid implies the development of haemoperitoneum. FAST is highly specific (99%), although its overall sensitivity is about 66% compared to CT. FAST is almost 100% sensitive in the hypotensive patient. The sensitivity of FAST improves with serial examination.
- Abdominal aortic aneurysm (AAA): ultrasound is a useful screening tool for the presence of AAA (defined as an aortic diameter >3 cm), especially when the patient is not suitable for transfer to a CT facility. Ultrasound cannot reliably identify rupture, but the detection of an AAA in

a hypotensive patient with symptoms suggestive of rupture (abdominal pain, backache or flank pain) is an indication for urgent intervention.

- Ectopic pregnancy: in a patient with a positive pregnancy test, an empty uterus (especially in the presence of free intraperitoneal fluid) implies ectopic pregnancy until proven otherwise. Other ultrasound findings include detection of an adnexal mass, an extrauterine gestational sac, extrauterine blood clots and interstitial ectopic pregnancy. On the other hand, identification of intrauterine pregnancy essentially reduces the risk of an ectopic pregnancy to <1:5000 (1:50 for women undergoing assisted reproduction). Transvaginal ultrasound is more sensitive than transabdominal ultrasound in detecting early intrauterine pregnancy. Repeat examination in a stable patient may be needed if the study is inconclusive.

Ultrasound may also be used for evaluating patients in the following conditions that may not be immediately life threatening:

- Assessment of suspected gallbladder disease: ultrasound is the recommended imaging study of first choice for suspected gallbladder disease. Discretion should be applied to avoid over-interpretation, e.g. the presence of gallstones does not confirm choleolithiasis as the cause of the abdominal pain.
- Tubo-ovarian pathologies: ultrasound is the first-line investigation for patients with suspected pelvic inflammatory disease or tubo-ovarian pathology. Transvaginal ultrasound provides detailed visualization of the pelvic organs and trans-abdominal ultrasound provides a complementary global view.
- Ureteric colic: ultrasound combined with abdominal radiographs may be used to screen patients with suspected ureteric colic. The diagnostic sensitivity for nephrolithiasis is about 63–85%, fairly similar to that for intravenous urography, which has a sensitivity of 64–90%. The advantages of ultrasound are the radiation dose involved is much lower and the use of radiocontrast is avoided.
- Detection of free peritoneal fluid in non-traumatic abdominal pain: in the appropriate clinical context, this may suggest the

presence of ascites, intraperitoneal haemorrhage, pus or leakage of gut content.

- Appendicitis: ultrasound may be used to evaluate for the presence of appendicitis if there are contraindications to the use of CT (e.g. pregnancy) or if CT is unavailable. Ultrasound is not as sensitive as CT and helps to rule in but not rule out this diagnosis.

Computed tomography

With the advent of helical and multidetector scanning technology, CT has become the imaging modality of choice for evaluation of abdominal pain in the non-obstetric patient. It has a high degree of accuracy, establishing diagnoses in more than 95% of cases in one study. In the elderly, CT resulted in changes to the management and disposition of a significant proportion of patients.

CT allows for detailed visualization of intra-, extra- and retroperitoneal structures. It identifies the exact site of disease, as well as its impact on the surrounding structures, thereby guiding further management. CT may be performed with or without intravenous and oral contrast agents. In the emergency setting, CT is useful for:

- assessment in abdominal trauma
- detection of inflammatory lesions (e.g. appendicitis, pancreatitis, diverticulitis, abscesses)
- detection of neoplastic lesions
- evaluation of vascular pathology (e.g. aortic aneurysm, aortic dissection, mesenteric ischaemia)
- detection of intra-abdominal and retroperitoneal bleed or abscesses
- detection of pneumoperitoneum, obstruction of hollow organs and abnormal calcifications, e.g. ureteric calculi
- assessment of the kidneys and urinary tracts.

The main limitations to CT are that the patient must be stable enough for transport to the scanning facility, ionizing radiation is involved, it may miss up to 20% of gallstones because the stones may be of the same radiographic density as bile and it may miss up to 10–17% of traumatic small bowel perforations.

The sensitivity of CT is not 100% for most conditions. Clinical decisions should not be based on CT results alone. If initial CT findings are negative but clinical suspicion is high,

further observation, evaluation or even repeat scans may be needed.

In the patient with very high suspicion for conditions that require immediate surgical intervention (e.g. unstable patient with obvious peritonitis), use of CT may result in delay in definitive treatment. For the patient in whom the clinical suspicion for serious abdominal pathology is very low, urgent CT scan is likely to have a low yield and the cost and potential side effects of CT outweigh its benefits. In one study for ED patients with suspected urgent abdominal conditions, a diagnostic strategy with initial ultrasound examination, followed by CT when ultrasound findings were negative or inconclusive, resulted in the best CT sensitivity. This strategy also reduced CT use by up to 51%.

Magnetic resonance imaging (MRI)

With the introduction of high-speed techniques, MRI protocols for patients with acute abdominal pain can now be reduced to below 15 minutes.

MRI does not involve ionizing radiation and offers better soft tissue visualization than CT. The high intrinsic contrast resolution of images rendered by MRI may allow for contrast-free scanning in certain cases. Compared to CT, MRI is able to provide increased information for hepatobiliary disease, pancreatitis and mesenteric ischaemia. MRI has also demonstrated promising accuracy for diagnosis of appendicitis, diverticulitis, small bowel obstruction and abdominal and pelvic venous thrombosis.

Currently, the evidence for use of MRI in ED patients presenting with acute abdominal pain is still relatively limited; it is most frequently used in selected pregnant patients in whom ultrasound findings are non-diagnostic.

MRI is significantly more costly than CT, takes longer to perform and may have limited availability in some centres. MRI is contraindicated in patients with claustrophobia or implanted metallic devices.

Imaging for the pregnant patient

Ultrasound is currently still the most common initial imaging modality used to evaluate the pregnant patient presenting with acute abdominal pain, although MRI is now playing an increasingly important role. Both imaging techniques do not involve ionizing radiation and have not been shown to cause any ill effects to the fetus. The routine use of gadolinium-based MR contrast agents is currently not

recommended as these agents pass through the placenta into fetal circulation and their effects on the fetus remain unknown.

CT is a valuable imaging tool in evaluation of abdominal pain in the pregnant patient, as it remains one of the most reliable imaging modality in the diagnoses of many acute abdominal conditions. The ionizing radiation doses involved in CT studies are below the doses that would lead to developmental or neurological deficits. However, radiation levels should still be kept as low as reasonably achievable as there are no known radiation limits for fetal stochastic effects, e.g. carcinogenesis.

Iodine-based CT contrast agents are also known to cross the placenta into fetal circulation. Small studies have indicated that single dose exposure to CT contrast agents does not lead to fetal teratogenesis or hypothyroidism. Similar to MR contrast agents, intravenous CT contrast agents should be avoided unless the accuracy of the imaging study is dependent on their use.

Pitfalls

The elderly

In elderly patients presenting with abdominal pain, conditions requiring surgical intervention (e.g. cholangitis, intestinal obstruction), serious vascular pathologies (e.g. AAA, aortic dissection, mesenteric ischaemia) and intra-abdominal neoplasms are more common (Table 7.2.8). Unfortunately, abdominal pain is frequently misdiagnosed in the elderly because:

- the elderly often present atypically or with non-specific complaints, e.g. poor appetite, lethargy, constipation, vomiting, loose stools, falls
- pain perception in the elderly may be blunted
- vital signs may be normal in spite of serious underlying illness
- signs of peritonism may not be present in cases of a surgical abdomen and other physical findings may be non-specific or subtle
- laboratory tests, such as full blood count, may be normal.

Adverse outcomes in the elderly are more common as a result of missed or delayed diagnosis than in younger patients. This is because the elderly tend to seek treatment late in the disease process and complications tend to be more common, they have reduced physiological reserve and often more co-morbidities. It has been estimated that with each decade of life, diagnostic accuracy decreases while mortality increases, such that for the octogenarian diagnostic accuracy is about 30%, although the corresponding mortality rate is 70 times that of patients under 30. Therefore, geriatric patients with abdominal pain need to be carefully evaluated and the threshold for imaging studies, surgical consultation and admission should be lowered.

The immunocompromised

Inflammatory responses are suppressed in the immunocompromised and abdominal signs from peritoneal irritation may be absent. Patients with human immunodeficiency virus (HIV) infection may develop unusual conditions, such as opportunistic viral or bacterial enterocolitis (e.g. cytomegalovirus or *Mycobacterium avium intrecellulare* enterocolitis), AIDS-related cholangiopathy, lymphoma or drug-induced pancreatitis. Patients on peritoneal dialysis or with advanced liver cirrhosis are at risk of developing spontaneous bacterial peritonitis.

Women of childbearing age

It is important to determine whether these patients are pregnant. Menstrual history, compliance with contraception, history of tubal ligation or claims of sexual abstinence cannot reliably exclude the possibility of pregnancy.

If the patient is pregnant, the possibility of ectopic pregnancy should be considered. In addition, pelvic conditions (e.g. pelvic inflammatory disease, ovarian pathology, pregnancy-related complications, such as threatened or missed abortion) and urinary tract infections are relatively common.

For patients in the second or third trimester of pregnancy, the gravid uterus may displace structures in the lower abdomen away from their usual position, e.g. the appendix may migrate to a higher position in the right hypochondrium or the right flank, changing symptoms and signs. Clinical signs of peritonism may be obscured due to loss of abdominal wall musculature elasticity.

Dangerous mimics (Table 7.2.9)

Misdiagnosed patients are most commonly given the labels of gastroenteritis, constipation, gastritis, urinary tract infection or pelvic inflammatory disease.

Diagnosis versus disposition

In the ED management of patients presenting with abdominal pain, empirical management of acute conditions and proper disposition are more important than diagnostic accuracy. When the diagnosis is based only on clinical findings and basic laboratory investigations, overall diagnostic accuracy is about 50% (as high as 80% in young adults and as low as 30% in the elderly). Fortunately, the rate of inappropriate discharge from the ED is low (about 1% across all age groups), albeit slightly higher in the elderly (about 4%).

Treatment

Resuscitation

Prompt resuscitation should take precedence over diagnosis in unstable patients. Patients may be in shock as a result of blood loss, fluid loss, sepsis or from concurrent cardiovascular events. Appropriate fluid therapy and inotropic support should be instituted early to prevent further deterioration and end-organ dysfunction.

Symptom relief

Pain relief should be instituted as early as possible for patients presenting with abdominal pain. This may require intravenous opiates

Table 7.2.8 Disease spectrum in those less than 50 years old vs those over 50

Confirmed cause of acute abdominal pain	Acute abdominal pain in patient <50 (n = 6317) (%)	Acute abdominal pain in patient ≥50 (n = 2406) (%)
Biliary tract disease	6	21
Non-specific abdominal pain	40	16
Appendicitis	32	15
Bowel obstruction	2	12
Pancreatitis	2	7
Diverticular disease	<0.1	6
Cancer	<0.1	4
Hernia	<0.1	3
Vascular	<0.1	2

Adapted from deDombal FT. Acute abdominal pain in the elderly. J Clin Gastroenterol 1994;29:331–5 with permission.

Table 7.2.9 Dangerous mimics

True diagnosis	Initial misdiagnosis
Appendicitis	Gastroenteritis, pelvic inflammatory disease (PID), urinary tract infection (UTI)
Ruptured abdominal aortic aneurysm	Renal colic, diverticulitis, lumbar strain
Ectopic pregnancy	PID, UTI, corpus luteum cyst
Diverticulitis	Constipation, gastroenteritis, non-specific abdominal pain
Perforated viscus	Peptic ulcer disease, pancreatitis, non-specific abdominal pain
Bowel obstruction	Constipation, gastroenteritis, non-specific abdominal pain
Mesenteric ischaemia	Constipation, gastroenteritis, ileus, small bowel obstruction
Incarcerated or strangulated hernia	Ileus, small bowel obstruction
Shock or sepsis from perforation, bleed and abdominal infection in the elderly	Urosepsis or pneumonia (in elderly)

From Colucciello SA, Lukens TW, Morgan DL. Assessing abdominal pain in adults: a rational, cost-effective, and evidence-based strategy. Emerg Med Pract 1999;1:1 with permission.

titrated to response. Specific treatment (e.g. non-steroidal anti-inflammatory agents in renal colic) should be used when available. The previously widely held dogma that opiates mask signs of serious pathology (in particular peritonism) has been disproved in many studies. In fact, the use of opioids in abdominal pain is not only safe, but actually aids diagnosis by facilitating physical examination and relaxing the abdominal musculature. The dosage used should be titrated to the patient's response.

Antibiotics
Antibiotics are indicated in suspected intra-abdominal sepsis. The antibiotics used should cover Gram-negative aerobes as well as anaerobes. Additional coverage for Gram-positive aerobes is required in patients with spontaneous bacterial peritonitis. See chapters on specific conditions for more details.

Surgical review
Early involvement of surgeons should be the rule in cases of suspected surgical abdomen. Early surgical intervention is crucial in improving outcome for urgent conditions, e.g. ruptured abdominal aortic aneurysm, ruptured ectopic pregnancy, intraperitoneal haemorrhage and bowel perforation.

Disposition

Admission
The following patients need to be admitted:

- patients with specific diagnoses that require inpatient management
- patients who are ill, unstable or with altered mentation
- the elderly or the immunocompromised in whom diagnoses are unclear
- patients in whom potentially serious conditions cannot be excluded
- patients in whom symptoms (e.g. pain, vomiting) cannot be ameliorated
- patients who are unable to follow discharge instructions or who have poor social support.

In addition, the admission threshold should be lowered for patients returning to the ED for the same complaints, especially where the cause of the abdominal pain had not been fully elucidated.

Observation
Patients who do not meet admission criteria but have persistent pain may be observed over a period of hours, in the ED or an observation unit if appropriate. Serial examination over a period of hours has been found to improve diagnostic accuracy.

The main aims of observing the patient with abdominal pain are to improve diagnostic yield with serial examination, to monitor progress after treatment, to detect the development of signs of acute abdomen and for further diagnostic work-up if indicated.

Discharge advice
It is important to give discharge advice, as some conditions develop over time. The patient should be advised to return if:

- pain is persistent (>24 hours) or worsening
- they develop incessant vomiting or are unable to retain fluids
- vague pain has become localized, e.g. to the right iliac fossa
- they develop high fever or chills, or feel increasingly ill, weak or unwell
- they develop fainting episodes
- abdominal distension develops
- there is blood in the stools or vomitus
- they develop new medical problems requiring urgent consultation.

Non-specific abdominal pain

A large proportion of stable patients with abdominal pain will not have a definitive diagnosis on discharge from the ED. In patients under 50 years of age, non-specific abdominal pain may be as high as 40%. This figure is lower in the elderly, at about 15% (see Table 7.2.8).

Most younger patients may be safely discharged from the ED once their symptoms have resolved with treatment and a period of observation. They should be clearly informed that the cause of their pain has not been determined and appropriate discharge advice, including to return to the ED if symptoms recur or worsen, should be given. Referral to a specialist for further evaluation may be indicated.

Non-specific abdominal pain in younger patients tends to have a benign course. However, about 10% of the elderly labelled with it are subsequently found to have an underlying malignancy. It is also important to rule out extra-abdominal causes in the elderly.

Developments in the next 5–10 years
Early recognition of acute mesenteric ischaemia greatly improves patient outcome as timely angiographic or surgical intervention is required. However, clinical diagnosis of acute mesenteric ischaemia, especially in the early stages, remains challenging. Diagnosis currently relies heavily on imaging. The search for accurate serum and urine biomarkers has shown promise and may alter the management of this subset of patients presenting to the ED with acute abdominal pain.

Controversies

- Clinical scoring systems for abdominal pain. Various clinical scoring systems, e.g. the Alvarado score for acute appendicitis, have been proposed. These systems may involve relatively simple algorithms or may be 'computer-based'. They help to ensure a more systematic approach to the evaluation of a patient, but none has been shown prospectively to improve on the physician's judgement.
- Use of CT with intravenous contrast has been shown to increase the accuracy of CT evaluation for patients with acute abdominal pain. However, the role of oral contrast media has been more controversial. Current literature suggests that the use of enteral contrast media does not significantly improve CT accuracy for ED patients presenting with non-traumatic, non-operation related acute abdominal pain. Instead, its use may lead to increased ED length of stay.

Further reading
Bugliosi TF, Meloy TD, Vukov LF. Acute abdominal pain in the elderly. Ann Emerg Med 1990;19:1383–6.
Colucciello SA, Lukens TW, Morgan DL. Assessing abdominal pain in adult: a rational, cost-effective, and evidence-based strategy. Emerg Med Pract 1999;1:1.
de Dombal FT. Acute abdominal pain in the elderly. J Clin Gastroenterol 1994;19:331–5.
Gray-Eurom K, Deitte L. Imaging in the adult patient with non-traumatic abdominal pain. Emerg Med Pract 2007;9:2.
Katz DS, Klein MA, Ganson G, Hines JJ. Imaging of abdominal pain in pregnancy. Radiol Clin N Am 2012;50:149–71.
Laméris W, van Randen A, van Es HW, OPTIMA study group. Imaging strategies for detection of urgent conditions in patients with acute abdominal pain: diagnostic accuracy study. Br Med J 2009;338:b2431.
Marco CA, Schoenfeld CN, Keyl PM. Abdominal pain in geriatric emergency patients: variables associated with adverse outcomes. Acad Emerg Med 1998;5:1163–8.
Stoker J, van Randen A, Laméris W, Boermeester MA. Imaging patients with acute abdominal pain. Radiology 2009;253:31–46.
Woodfield CA, Lazarus E, Chen KC, Mayo-Smith WW. Abdominal pain in pregnancy: diagnoses and imaging unique to pregnancy – review. Am J Roentgenol 2010;194(Suppl):WS14–30.

DIGESTIVE EMERGENCIES

7.3 Bowel obstruction

Willem Landman • Kim Yates

ESSENTIALS

1 Small bowel obstruction is most often caused by adhesions. Large bowel obstruction more commonly results from neoplasms.

2 The common clinical features of bowel obstruction are paroxysms of poorly localized abdominal pain, constipation/obstipation, abdominal distension, nausea, vomiting and hyperactive or high-pitched bowel sounds. Examination for hernias is essential.

3 In most cases, the clinical findings are diagnostic for bowel obstruction. The presence of dilated loops of bowel with multiple air–fluid levels on abdominal X-ray can confirm the diagnosis of bowel obstruction. In cases where clinical suspicion is high and plain radiography is negative, a non-contrast CT scan is recommended.

4 Initial treatment consists of correction of dehydration and electrolyte abnormalities, decompression, analgesia and further assessment (particularly to identify strangulating bowel obstruction).

5 Strangulating bowel obstruction is an indication for urgent surgery.

Pathology and pathophysiology

Bowel obstruction is the interruption of the normal peristaltic progression of intestinal contents. Mechanical bowel obstruction can be caused by lesions outside or within the bowel wall or within the lumen itself. It may be partial or complete, strangulating or non-strangulating. Common causes of small bowel obstruction (SBO) include adhesions, hernias and neoplasms. Less common causes include inflammatory bowel disease, gallstones, foreign bodies, strictures, radiation, diverticulitis, endometriosis and abscesses. Common causes of large bowel obstruction (LBO) include neoplasm, diverticulitis and volvulus. Faecal impaction, inflammatory bowel disease, strictures and extraintestinal tumours are less common causes.

Paralytic ileus may mimic obstruction but there is no mechanical cause; rather, it is associated with abnormal propulsive motility. Paralytic ileus can be caused by a wide range of conditions. Metabolic causes include hypokalaemia (most common), hyponatraemia, hypomagnesaemia and hypoalbuminaemia. Drugs, such as tricyclic antidepressants, opiates, antihistamines, β-adrenergic agonists and quinidine, have also been implicated. Acute colonic pseudo-obstruction (Ogilvie syndrome) is characterized by acute large bowel dilatation without mechanical obstruction due to diffuse incoordination and reduction of colonic peristalsis. Its causes include a postoperative state, cardiorespiratory disease, trauma, infection, medications, such as opiates and antidepressants, and neurological disease.

The pathophysiology of mechanical bowel obstruction relates to rising intraluminal pressure, mucosal injury, bacterial overgrowth and inflammatory response. Bowel proximal to the obstruction distends with gas, fluid and electrolytes, then hypersecretion escalates, bowel absorptive ability decreases and progressive systemic volume losses occur. Vomiting ensues more quickly the more proximal the bowel obstruction is and worsens the dehydration and electrolyte disturbances.

If obstruction persists, then the intraluminal pressure rises and local vascular compromise can occur, especially venous stasis. As pressures rise and blood flow diminishes, the bowel can strangulate and necrosis may follow with consequent perforation and sepsis. A closed-loop obstruction implies both proximal and distal obstruction (e.g. strangulating hernia or volvulus) and, typically, leads to vascular compromise more quickly and therefore a higher risk of strangulation, necrosis and perforation.

Clinical features

History

In early bowel obstruction, abdominal pain is poorly localized and colicky, but later may become more constant and, if severe, suggests ischaemia or peritonitis. Pain from SBO tends to be more severe earlier and cramps tend to be more frequent compared to LBO where dull, lower abdominal cramps are more common. Vomiting is more common in SBO and is a late symptom in LBO. Faeculent vomiting or distension suggests a more distal SBO or a LBO. Obstipation was thought typical, but the passage of flatus and stool may continue.

The gastrointestinal and surgical history helps differentiate causes of mechanical obstruction and drug history and systems enquiry may identify potential causes of non-mechanical obstruction.

Examination

Classical examination findings are abdominal distension and absent, reduced or 'tinkling' bowel sounds. Abdominal tenderness, if present, is usually mild. A mass may or may not be palpable. The presence of fever, tachycardia, guarding or peritonism suggests strangulating obstruction; however, vascular compromise can occur in their absence. Signs of dehydration are often present. Abdominal distension is more commonly present in LBO or distal SBO. On auscultation, rushes or high-pitched tinkles may be heard, but are not absolute indicators of obstruction. Surgical scars suggest adhesions as a cause of obstruction and examination for hernias is essential. Rectal examination may be normal in SBO, but the presence of faecal impaction, blood or a mass may assist with diagnosis of cause. Pelvic examination may be useful if abscesses or inflammation are suspected.

A focused medical examination should also be performed to exclude causes of paralytic ileus and pseudo-obstruction and to assess anaesthetic risk.

Clinical investigations

Laboratory tests

Laboratory tests are of limited value for diagnosing bowel obstruction but help in assessment of severity and guiding resuscitation. Of all laboratory tests, only lactate and interleukin (IL)-6 levels appear to have significant predictive value for strangulating obstruction. If both are raised, the positive predictive value is 95% and the negative predictive value 97%. Haematocrit may be raised if dehydration is present. Electrolyte abnormalities, such as hyponatraemia, hypokalaemia and impaired renal function, are common. Serum amylase may be mildly raised in SBO. Blood gas analysis may show metabolic alkalosis if vomiting is severe, metabolic acidosis if shock, dehydration or ketosis is present. A blood or urine pregnancy test, where appropriate, and urine microscopy are important in excluding other causes of abdominal pain.

Imaging studies

The ideal study would define the grade of obstruction (complete, high grade, low grade), the level of the obstruction and the cause of the obstruction as well as any associated complications.

The presence of dilated loops of bowel with multiple air–fluid levels on abdominal X-rays is highly suggestive of bowel obstruction; however, the overall sensitivity of plain radiography is 30–70% and specificity is around 50% (E-Figs 7.3.1 and 7.3.2). X-rays may appear normal with closed loop or strangulated obstructions. Abdominal computed tomography (CT) is particularly useful in cases where plain radiology is non-diagnostic. The overall sensitivity and specificity of CT is around 95%. With a typical clinical picture for obstruction plain radiology and CT have similar sensitivities. On the other hand, ileus and pseudo-obstruction have a similar X-ray appearance to mechanical obstruction. CT can determine the level and cause of obstruction, as well as emergent causes of obstruction, such as volvulus and strangulation. For these reasons and its ability to do tumour staging, it is the modality of choice to facilitate decision making.

In the assessment of acute obstruction in adults, magnetic resonance imaging has improved sensitivity, specificity and accuracy compared to CT; however, limited availability, long scan times and the need for extensive oral preparation mean it is of limited use in the ED setting unless minimizing radiation exposure is paramount.

Bedside ultrasonography by a trained examiner looking for dilated small bowel has a similar sensitivity and a greater specificity than plain radiology, but is not widely used and is subject to significant operator dependency. It may have particular utility in unstable and pregnant patients.

Endoscopy

Careful sigmoidoscopy is safe in LBO and therapeutic in sigmoid volvulus when used to place a rectal tube. In some centres, endoscopy is performed acutely to decompress LBO by inserting drainage tubes or self-expanding metal stents.

Treatment and prognosis

General measures

Most patients with bowel obstruction are dehydrated, so treatment with crystalloid intravenous fluid is required and electrolyte disturbances should be corrected. Urinary catheterization and monitoring of urine output, vital signs and electrolytes should guide ongoing fluid and electrolyte therapy. Nasogastric decompression is customary, but evidence of benefit in patients without significant vomiting is weak. Analgesia is often required, with titrated increments of IV opiates the most appropriate option. Antibiotics are prescribed by some to counter bacterial translocation, but evidence of their effectiveness is sparse.

Patients with bowel obstruction associated with haemodynamic compromise, shock or sepsis require combined, ongoing management by surgical and intensive care teams. Patients with suspected strangulating bowel obstruction or perforation should have urgent surgery. Stable patients and those with partial bowel obstruction can be started on conservative therapy and monitored closely as inpatients for signs of deterioration.

Conservative therapy

Ongoing intravenous fluid therapy, electrolyte management and bowel rest are the mainstay interventions. Monitoring of vital signs, urine output and clinical state should continue and deterioration or failure to improve are indications for surgical therapy.

Where bowel obstruction due to malignancy is inoperable, octreotide appears superior to hyoscinebutyl bromide in relieving symptoms and, although corticosteroids are commonly advocated, evidence for their effectiveness is less clear.

In patients with acute colonic pseudo-obstruction unresponsive to conservative therapy, IV neostigmine 2 mg has initiated rapid colonic decompression.

A non-strangulating sigmoid volvulus can be temporarily decompressed by a rectal tube inserted via sigmoidoscope.

Endoscopic placement of self-expanding metallic stents can relieve malignant LBO, either prior to elective surgical resection or as definitive palliative therapy if the malignancy is inoperable. Reported complications of metallic stents include perforation, stent migration and reobstruction.

Surgical therapy

Bowel obstruction due to hernias and complete SBO usually requires surgery. Strangulating bowel obstruction is an indication for urgent surgery and should be suspected in the presence of severe pain and localized tenderness. Additional suggestive features include a fever, shock, mass, hernia, acidosis, marked leucocytosis, raised lactate, sepsis and confirmatory CT findings. It can, however, occur without these features. Broad-spectrum parenteral antibiotics are indicated preoperatively and if sepsis is suspected.

Mortality escalates dramatically the longer surgery is delayed in strangulating bowel obstruction or perforation ($\approx$30% compared to 3–5% in non-strangulating bowel obstruction), so prompt surgery is vital. The surgical approach adopted will depend on the suspected pathology and operative findings. Some centres use laparoscopy to treat SBO with variable success rates (33–87%). Higher success rates have been reported in those with a history of appendicectomy only, or with band adhesions. In LBO, decompressive stomas followed by a definitive operation at a later date are sometimes useful in very sick patients; however, right-sided lesions can often be resected at laparotomy with a primary anastomosis, avoiding a stoma completely. One-stage resection/anastomosis is possible with left-sided lesions, but there is a higher risk of contamination in unprepared bowel and higher mortality rates.

Controversies

- Diagnosis of strangulating bowel obstruction. Clinical features and plain radiography may not be helpful. Of all blood tests, lactate and IL-6 levels appear most predictive. CT findings are helpful and multidetector CT may be most useful.

- Tube decompression therapy in SBO. Both short nasogastric and long nasointestinal tubes have been used in adhesive SBO, but long tubes have not shown a definite advantage.

- Non-operative therapy. Some surgeons prefer early surgery because of the difficulty of diagnosing strangulating bowel obstruction. In adhesive partial SBO, without signs of strangulation, a 48-hour trial of non-operative therapy with frequent reassessment appears safe. With inoperable malignant

obstruction, octreotide may be more effective than corticosteroids in relieving symptoms.

Further reading

Atri M, McGregor C, McInnes M, et al. Multidetector helical CT in the evaluation of acute small bowel obstruction: comparison of non-enhanced (no oral, rectal or IV contrast) and IV enhanced CT. Eur J Radiol 2009;71:135–40.

Batke M, Cappell MS. Adynamic ileus and acute colonic pseudo-obstruction. Med Clin N Am 2008;92:649–70.

Feuer DJ, Broadley KE. Corticosteroids for the resolution of malignant bowel obstruction in advanced gynaecological and gastrointestinal cancer. Cochrane Database Syst Rev 2009:CD001219.

Hayden GE, Sprouse KL. Bowel obstruction and hernia. Emerg Med Clin N Am 2011;29:319–45.

Jang TB, Schindler D, Kaji AH. Bedside ultrasonography for the detection of small bowel obstruction in the emergency department. Emerg Med J 2011;28:676–8.

Lameris W, van Randen A, van Es HW, et al. Imaging strategies for detection of urgent conditions in patients with acute abdominal pain: diagnostic accuracy study. Br Med J 2009;338:b2431.

Markogiannakis H, Messaris E, Dardamanis D, et al. Acute mechanical bowel obstruction: clinical presentation, etiology, management and outcome. World J Gastroenterol 2007;13:432–7.

McKenzie S, Evers BM. Small intestine. In: Townsend CM, Beauchamp RD, Evers BM, Mattox KL, editors. Sabiston textbook of surgery: the biological basis of modern surgical practice (19th ed.). Philadelphia: Elsevier Saunders, 2012.

Mercadante S, Casuccio A, Mangione S. Medical treatment for inoperable malignant bowel obstruction: a qualitative systematic review. J Pain Symptom Manage 2007;33:217–23.

Stoker J, van Randen A, Lameris W, Boermeester MA. Imaging patients with acute abdominal pain. Radiology 2009;253: 31–46.

Suri S, Gupta S, Sudhakar PJ, et al. Comparative evaluation of plain films, ultrasound and CT in the diagnosis of intestinal obstruction. Acta Radiol 1999;40:422–8.

Turnage RH, Heldman M. Intestinal obstruction. In: Sleisenger MH, Feldman M, Friedman LS, editors. Sleisinger & Fordtran's gastrointestinal and Liver disease: pathophysiology, diagnosis, management (9th ed.). Philadelphia: Saunders Elsevier, 2010, p. 2105–22.

7.4 Hernia

Neil A Goldie

ESSENTIALS

1 A diagnosis of symptomatic hernia mandates early surgical repair to avoid life-threatening complications.

2 Hernia may present as a reducible lump or may incarcerate, strangulate and/or present as bowel obstruction.

3 Femoral herniae are often misdiagnosed and are associated with high morbidity when complicated.

4 All herniae presenting with a complication should undergo surgical repair promptly.

Introduction

A hernia is defined as a protrusion of a viscus or part of a viscus through a weakness in the wall of the containing cavity. It has an aperture, coverings (usually peritoneum and abdominal wall layers) and contents, which may be any intra-abdominal organ but are usually omentum or small bowel. Surgical treatment requires reduction of the contents and closure of the aperture, with reinforcement to prevent recurrence.

There are a number of described sites for herniae. This chapter will focus on the more common of these, but the principles of assessment and treatment apply to herniae at other sites.

Aetiology, pathology and clinical features

Inguinal hernia

Inguinal herniae are extremely common and account for 75% of all abdominal wall herniae. There is a lifetime risk of occurrence of 27% for men and 3% for women and an annual incidence of 130 per 100 000 population. Up to 9% of hernia repairs are performed urgently. Emergency repairs are more common in the elderly and carry greater morbidity than elective repair.

As their name implies, direct inguinal herniae bulge directly through the posterior wall of the inguinal canal. They are caused by weak

abdominal musculature, are common in the elderly and frequently bilateral. They have a large neck and hence seldom become irreducible or strangulate until they are of considerable size.

For indirect inguinal herniae, the hernial sac comes through the internal inguinal ring, travels the length of the inguinal canal and emerges from the external inguinal ring. Thus, it usually lies above and medial to the symphysis pubis. Later, the internal inguinal ring may stretch and the hernial sac and its contents may descend to and fill the scrotum, occasionally becoming very large. As the internal inguinal ring is usually narrow, irreducibility is common. Indirect inguinal herniae occur throughout life (E-Fig. 7.4.1).

Direct and indirect inguinal herniae may be distinguishable by simple clinical tests. When an indirect hernia is reduced, finger pressure over the site of the internal ring may hold it reduced; however, a direct inguinal hernia will flop out again unless several fingers or the side of the hand props up the entire length of the inguinal canal.

Femoral hernia

Femoral herniae appear lateral and inferior to the symphysis pubis. They are formed by the peritoneal sac and contents, which occupy the potential space of the femoral canal, medial to the femoral vein. They are proportionately more common in women and rarely large. Symptoms usually occur early and complications are common.

Both femoral canal areas should be closely examined in any patient presenting with abdominal pain or signs of bowel obstruction, as femoral herniae are frequently overlooked, especially in patients who are elderly and obese. Diagnosis of a femoral hernia mandates early surgery. Morbidity from emergency femoral hernia repair increases with the presence of small bowel obstruction. Mortality with emergency surgery can be as high as 5%.

Umbilical hernia

Umbilical and periumbilical herniae protrude through and around the umbilicus. They are very common in the newborn, but most resolve by 4 years of age. As they have a broad neck, emergency complications are uncommon. They can be difficult to diagnose in very obese people. If complicated, they can present resembling abdominal wall cellulitis.

Epigastric hernia

Epigastric herniae appear in the midline above the umbilicus. A small extraperitoneal piece of fat may be stuck in this hernia, causing pain.

Other herniae

Obturator hernia

Rarely, viscera may pass through a defect in the obturator foramen and present as a small bowel obstruction. This occurs most commonly in elderly emaciated women with chronic disease. Diagnosis of this internal hernia and the hernia of the foramen of Winslow is seldom made preoperatively.

Spigelian hernia

Spigelian herniae are rare and are due to a defect in the anterolateral abdominal wall musculature. They usually present as a reducible lump in the elderly male, lateral to the rectus muscle in the lower half of the abdomen. Complications are rare.

Incisional hernia

These may occur at the site of any previous abdominal wound, such as appendicectomy or laparotomy. The wound area becomes weak, allowing the protrusion of a viscus or part of a viscus.

Sportsman's (athlete's) hernia

This is a term used for those who present with the painful symptoms of a hernia in the groin following exertion. It is defined as an occult hernia caused by weakness or a tear of the posterior inguinal wall without a clinically recognizable hernia. Generally, by the time of diagnosis, non-operative treatment options have failed and surgery often results in a return to sport. Ultrasound can be a useful diagnostic medium to detect herniae which are intermittently symptomatic but without clinical signs.

Complications

In the early stages, herniae are usually reducible, producing only intermittent pain in the groin, but reducible herniae may become irreducible (incarcerated). Incarcerated herniae may lead to a bowel obstruction. Strangulation and interruption of the blood supply to the contents of the hernia (usually small bowel) may supervene. In this case, there will be increasing local pain, tenderness, warmth and overlying erythema. This is accompanied by signs of bowel obstruction and a leucocytosis.

Rarely, only part of the bowel wall is caught in a hernial constricting ring. Bowel wall necrosis ensues that is not circumferential; this is termed a Richter's hernia. In this case, there may be signs of strangulation without signs of obstruction.

Very rarely, neglected herniae can fistulate, with bowel contents appearing at the abdominal wall or through the hernial orifices.

Treatment

Reduction

It may be possible to reduce a hernia that initially appears irreducible in the emergency department, but caution must be exercised. If the skin over the hernia is already inflamed and pain is severe, the contents may be compromised and urgent surgical exploration is required. Reduction of the contents in this circumstance can be dangerous, as false reassurance can occur followed by the later development of peritonitis due to intra-abdominal perforation of the hernia contents.

As a general rule, if the hernia has been irreducible for less than 4 hours, vital signs are normal and there are no symptoms of bowel obstruction, reduction of an incarcerated hernia

may be attempted. This is achieved by giving adequate analgesia to relax the patient and applying gentle pressure manipulating the hernia site for several minutes. Elevating the foot of the bed may be helpful. Successful reduction relieves pain, may prevent strangulation and reduces the urgency for surgical intervention. Notwithstanding, all herniae that have undergone a complication require surgical consultation with view to definitive treatment at the time of presentation.

Surgical repair

Inguinal hernia repair is a very common operation in general surgery. Rates of repair range from 10 per 10 000 population in the UK to 28 per 10 000 in the USA.

Timely repair of herniae reduces the incidence of complications and avoids the greater risk associated with emergency surgery. Until the introduction of synthetic mesh, inguinal hernia repair had changed little for over 100 years. Mesh is used to reinforce the repaired defect and can be placed by an open method or laparoscopically. Laparoscopic transabdominal preperitoneal hernia repair takes longer than open surgery and has a more serious complication rate with regard to visceral injuries, but is being increasingly performed as it reduces postoperative pain and significantly reduces time off work. It is also much more operator dependent, is more difficult to learn and has higher overall hospital costs.

Patients requiring emergency surgery for bowel obstruction or strangulation should be prepared with adequate fluid resuscitation and analgesia.

Controversies

- The diagnosis and management of 'sportsman's hernia'.
- The role of laparoscopy in hernia repair.

Further reading

Brittenden J, Heys SD, Eremerin O. Femoral hernia: mortality and morbidity following elective and emergency repair. J Roy Coll Surg Edinburgh 1991;36:86–8.
Camary VL. Femoral hernia: intestinal obstruction is an unrecognized source of morbidity and mortality. Br J Surg 1993;80:230–2.
Chung L, O'Dwyer PJ. Treatment of asymptomatic inguinal hernias. Surgeon 2007;5:95–100. Quiz 100, 121.
Devsine M, Grimson R, Soroff HS. Benefits of a clinic for the treatment of external abdominal wall hernias. Am J Surg 1987;153:387–91.

Farber AJ, Wilckens JH. Sports hernia: diagnosis and therapeutic approach. J Am Acad Orthop Surg 2007;15:507–14.

Fredberg U, Kissmeyer-Nielsen P. The sportsman's hernia–fact or fiction? Scand J Med Sci Sports 1996;6:201–4.

Lo CY, Lorentz TG, Lau PW. Obturator hernia presenting as small bowel obstruction. Am J Surg 1994;167:396–8.

McCormack K, Scott NW, Go PM, et al. Laparoscopic techniques versus open techniques for inguinal hernia repair. Cochrane Database Syst Rev 2003;1:CD001785.

Primatesta P, Goldacre MJ. Inguinal hernia repair: incidence of elective and emergency surgery, readmission and mortality. Internatl J Epidemiol 1996;25:835–9.

Reuben B, Neumayer L. Surgical management of inguinal hernia. Adv Surg 2006;40:299–317.

Spangen L. Spigelian hernia. World J Surg 1989;13:573–80.

Swan KG, Wolcott M. The athletic hernia: a systematic review. Clin Orthop Relat Res 2007;455:78–87.

7.5 Gastroenteritis

Anita Liu

ESSENTIALS

1 Gastroenteritis is usually a benign, self-limiting disease that can be diagnosed clinically, warrants no specific investigation and settles spontaneously with symptomatic treatment and oral fluid therapy.

2 The cardinal clinical feature of gastroenteritis is diarrhoea, which may be accompanied by varying degrees of nausea and vomiting, abdominal cramping and pain, lethargy and fever.

3 The clinical examination is directed at confirming the diagnosis of gastroenteritis, excluding alternative diagnoses and determining the degree of dehydration.

4 A wide variety of viruses, bacteria and protozoa may cause gastroenteritis. In developed countries, common viral agents include rotavirus and norovirus. Common bacteria include *Campylobacter jejuni*, *Staphylococcus aureus*, *Escherichia coli*, *Shigella dysenteriae* and *Salmonella enteriditis*. Common protozoa include *Giardia lamblia*.

5 The principles of treatment of gastroenteritis are to replace the fluid losses orally or intravenously, minimize the patient's symptoms by the use of antiemetic therapy and, in some circumstances, administer specific antimicrobial agents.

6 Introduction of rotavirus vaccine in Australia in 2007 has lead to reduction of both rotavirus and non-rotavirus gastroenteritis.

Introduction

Gastroenteritis is a common clinical syndrome. It poses one of the world's major clinical and public health problems and, in developing countries with poor-quality drinking water and low levels of sanitation, it is a major cause of morbidity and mortality, especially among children and the elderly.

Gastroenteritis is caused by infection of the gastrointestinal tract by various viruses, bacteria and protozoa. Transmission is most commonly by the faecal–oral route. The syndrome consists of diarrhoea, abdominal cramping or pain, nausea and vomiting, lethargy, malaise and fever. Each of these features may be present to a varying degree and may last from 1 day to more than 3 weeks.

In developed countries, even though serious morbidity and mortality are low, gastroenteritis may be an extremely painful and unpleasant event causing disruption to daily life and significant loss of working and school days. Patients often seek emergency medical care because of the acuteness of onset of symptoms, the frequency of the diarrhoea, the severity of abdominal pain and cramps or because of concerns regarding dehydration.

Pathogenesis and pathology

Microorganisms of all descriptions are constantly entering the gastrointestinal tract through the mouth. Extremely few of these progress to cause clinical illness. The natural defences of the gastrointestinal tract against infection include gastric acid secretion, normal bowel flora, bile salt production, bowel motility, mucosal lymphoid tissue and secreted immunoglobulin A. People with disturbances in any of these defences are more prone to a clinical infection. For example, patients with achlorhydria, bowel stasis or blind loops, immunodeficiency states or recent antibiotic therapy that has disturbed bowel flora are prone to gastroenteritis. Some organisms, such as rotavirus, occur principally in children, as previous infection confers immunity.

Microbiology

A wide variety of viruses, bacteria and protozoa may cause gastroenteritis and the list is continually growing. Viral agents include rotavirus, enteric adenovirus, astrovirus, calicivirus, norovirus, coronavirus and cytomegalovirus. Bacteria include *Campylobacter jejuni*, *Staphylococcus aureus*, *Bacillus cereus*, *Escherichia coli*, *Vibrio cholerae*, *Shigella dysenteriae*, *Salmonella enteriditis*, *Yersinia enterocolitica*, *Clostridium perfringens* and *C. difficile*. Protozoa include *Giardia lamblia*, *Cryptosporidium parvum* and *Entamoeba histolytica*.

Microorganisms cause gastroenteritis by a number of mechanisms. They may release preformed toxins prior to ingestion, multiply and produce toxins within the gastrointestinal lumen, directly invade the bowel wall or use a combination of toxins and invasion.

Staphylococcus aureus and *Bacillus cereus* produce a variety of toxins in stored food that are subsequently ingested. These toxins are absorbed and, within hours, act on the central nervous system to produce an illness characterized predominantly by vomiting and mild diarrhoea.

Invasive bacteria are characterized by *Salmonella*, which invades the mucosa (primarily of the distal ileum) producing cell damage and excessive secretion. *Shigella* likewise invades the mucosa but also produces toxins that have cytotoxic, neurotoxic and enterotoxic effects.

The many strains of *E. coli* have been divided into five groups, depending on the pathology of the diseases they cause. These are enteropathogenic, enterotoxigenic, enteroinvasive, enteroaggregative and enterohaemorrhagic. Enterohaemorrhagic *E. coli* is associated with haemorrhagic colitis and the haemolytic–uraemic syndrome, whereas enterotoxigenic *E. coli* is associated with traveller's diarrhoea. The protozoan *Giardia lamblia* adheres to the jejunum and upper ileum, causing mucosal inflammation, inhibition of disaccharidase activity and overgrowth of luminal bacteria.

Rotavirus is estimated to be the cause of 50% of gastroenteritis admission in Australia prior to the introduction of rotavirus vaccine. Rotavirus vaccine was introduced into the funded Australian National Immunization Programme in July 2007. Comparison study of gastroenteritis prior to the vaccine introduction against the 30 months following the vaccine introduction shows marked reduction in emergency department (ED) encounters, as well as hospitalization for rotavirus and non-rotavirus gastroenteritis. There also appears to be an indirect population protective effect of the vaccine as older children who were ineligible for the rotavirus vaccine have also demonstrated reduced hospitalization and positive rotavirus test.

Epidemiology

In Australia, the estimated incidence of gastroenteritis is 17.2 million cases per year. Thirty-two per cent of these cases are food borne, which is equivalent to 0.3 episodes per person per year. Altogether, food-borne gastroenteritis causes 15000 hospitalizations and 80 deaths annually. The economic impact on the healthcare system is estimated at $30 million per year.

Norovirus, enteropathogenic *E. coli*, *Campylobacter* and *Salmonella* are the leading causes of gastroenteritis in Australia.

Gastroenteritis may occur in many settings. It may be a sporadic isolated event, a small outbreak either within a family or other close living group, such as in a geriatric residential facility, or part of a larger community epidemic. It may occur in a traveller, either while still overseas or on their return home. It is important to be aware of the circumstances and context in which the illness occurs, as these will often dictate the course of investigation or management.

Clinical Features

History

The clinical history and examination are directed at confirming the diagnosis of gastroenteritis, excluding other diagnoses and determining the degree of dehydration.

The principal clinical manifestation of gastroenteritis is diarrhoea. There is a lack of standardized definition of gastroenteritis. The World Health Organization syndromic definition of gastroenteritis is 'three or more abnormally loose or fluid stools over 24 hours'. The diarrhoea of gastroenteritis is often watery and profuse in the early stages of the illness and may last for up to 3 weeks. It is important to determine the frequency, volume and characteristics of the stool. Some organisms, such as enterohaemorrhagic *E. coli*, *Shigella*, *Salmonella*, *Campylobacter* and *Entamoeba histolytica*, may cause acute and bloody diarrhoea, whereas others, such as *Giardia*, may cause loose, pale, greasy stools.

Abdominal pain is common and is most often described as a diffuse intermittent colicky pain situated centrally in the abdomen. It may occur just prior to, and be partially relieved by, a bowel action. Severe pain is often caused by *Campylobacter*, *Yersinia* and *E. coli*. Abdominal pain is also the hallmark of many other forms of intra- and extra-abdominal pathology. Diagnoses other than gastroenteritis should be seriously considered if the pain is well localized, constant and severe or radiates to the back or shoulder.

Vomiting may be present, particularly early in the illness, and can be variable in severity and persistence. The amount of vomiting and the ability to keep down clear fluids should be determined, as this will dictate the management of dehydration. Severe vomiting often occurs with organisms that produce preformed toxin, although it does not usually persist for longer than 24 hours. Anorexia, nausea and lethargy are common. Fever and systemic symptoms, such as headache, are prominent with organisms that invade the bowel wall and enter the systemic circulation, such as *Yersinia*. Lethargy may be related to the dehydration or merely the strain of constant and persistent diarrhoea from any aetiology.

Specific inquiry regarding fluid status is essential. The aim should be to determine the amount of fluids that have been taken orally and kept down over the course of the illness, along with the estimated urine output. It is also important to ascertain pre-existing or intercurrent illness, such as diabetes or immunosuppression, which may alter management.

Physical examination

Suitable infection control procedures should be instituted prior to the examination to prevent spread to the examining doctor and hence to other patients. Where possible, the patient should be in an isolation cubicle. Hand hygiene procedures before and after the consultation, the use of gloves and prompt disposal of soiled clothing and linen are important.

A careful clinical examination should be performed, concentrating on the abdomen and the circulatory state of the patient. The vital signs, temperature and urinalysis should be obtained.

In mild to moderate gastroenteritis, the clinical examination is often unremarkable. There may be some general abdominal tenderness, active bowel sounds and facial pallor, but little else. In more severe disease, the abdominal tenderness may be pronounced and signs of dehydration present. Of note, uncomplicated gastroenteritis is extremely unlikely if the abdominal examination reveals localized tenderness or signs of peritoneal irritation.

Fluid losses through diarrhoea, vomiting and fever, together with poor oral fluid intake, can lead to clinically apparent dehydration. This may be manifest as tachycardia, tachypnoea, reduced tissue turgor, delayed capillary return, reduced urine output and, in its more severe stages, hypotension, impaired conscious state and death.

Extra-abdominal signs of a primary gastroenteritis can occur. *Campylobacter* has been associated with reactive arthritis and Guillain–Barré syndrome. The clinical features, course and complications for various causative agents are summarized in Table 7.5.1.

Table 7.5.1 Pathogen-specific syndromes

Causative agent	Incubation period	Duration of illness	Predominant symptoms	Foods commonly implicated
Bacteria				
Campylobacter jejuni	1–10 days (usually 2–5 days)	2–5 days occasionally >10 days	Sudden onset of diarrhoea, abdominal pain, nausea, vomiting	Raw or undercooked poultry, raw milk, raw or undercooked meat, untreated water
E. coli enterohaemorrhagic	2–10 days	5–10 days	Severe colic, mild to profuse bloody diarrhoea can lead to haemolytic uraemic syndrome	Many raw foods (especially minced beef), unpasteurized milk, contaminated water
E. coli enteropathogenic, enterotoxigenic, enteroinvasive	12–72 h (enterotoxigenic)	3–14 days	Severe colic, watery to profuse diarrhoea, sometimes bloody	Many raw foods, food contaminated by faecal matter, contaminated water
Salmonella serovars (non-typhoid)	6–72 h	3–5 days	Abdominal pain, diarrhoea, chills, fever, malaise	Raw or undercooked meat and chicken, raw or undercooked eggs and egg products
Shigella spp.	12–96 h	4–7 days	Malaise, fever, vomiting, diarrhoea (blood and mucus)	Foods contaminated by infected food handlers and untreated water contaminated by human faeces
Yersinia enterocolitica	3–7 days	1–21 days	Acute diarrhoea sometimes bloody, fever, vomiting	Raw meat, especially pork, raw or undercooked poultry, milk and milk products
Vibrio cholerae	A few hours to 5 days	3–4 days	Asymptomatic to profuse painless watery diarrhoea, dehydration	Raw seafood, contaminated water
Vibrio parahaemolyticus	4–30 h (usually 12–24 h)	1–7 days	Abdominal pain, diarrhoea, vomiting and sometimes fever Illness of moderate severity	Raw and lightly cooked fish, shellfish, other seafoods
Viruses				
Norovirus (and other viral gastroenteritis)	24–48 h	12–60 h	Severe vomiting, diarrhoea	Oysters, clams, foods contaminated by infected food handlers and untreated water contaminated by human faeces
Rotaviruses	24–72 h	Up to 7 days	Malaise, headache, fever, vomiting, diarrhoea	Foods contaminated by infected food handlers and untreated water contaminated by human faeces
Parasites				
Cryptosporidium	1–12 days	4–21 days	Profuse watery diarrhoea, abdominal pain	Foods contaminated by infected food handlers and untreated water contaminated by human faeces
Giardia lamblia	1–3 weeks	1–2 weeks to months	Loose pale greasy stools, abdominal pain	Foods contaminated by infected food handlers and untreated water contaminated by human faeces
Entamoeba histolytica	2–4 weeks	Weeks to months	Colic, mucous or bloody diarrhoea	Foods contaminated by infected food handlers and untreated water contaminated by human faeces
Toxin-producing bacteria				
B. cereus (toxin in food)	1–6 h (vomiting) or 6–24 h (diarrhoea)	<24 h	Two known toxins causing nausea and vomiting or diarrhoea and cramps	Cereals, rice, meat products, soups, vegetables
C. perfringens (toxin in gut)	6–24 h	24 h	Sudden onset colic, diarrhoea	Meats, poultry, stews, gravies, (often inadequately reheated or held warm)
Staphylococcus aureus (toxin in food)	30 min–8 h	24 h	Acute vomiting, and cramps, may lead to collapse	Cold foods (much handled during preparation) milk products, salted meats

Adapted from Guidelines for the Control of Infectious Diseases – The Blue Book. Communicable Diseases Section, Public Health Group, Victorian Government Department of Human Services; 2005. (Reproduced with the kind permission of the Communicable Diseases Section, Public Health Group, Victorian Government Department of Human Services.)

Diarrhoea in certain circumstances

Traveller's diarrhoea

Millions of travellers each year are affected by diarrhoea. Southeast Asia, the Middle East, the Mediterranean basin, Central and South America are areas of frequent occurrence. The incidence of diarrhoea in travellers to these areas is as high as 30–50%. Bacteria are the most common cause of traveller's diarrhoea. Pathogens include enterotoxigenic *E. coli*, enteroaggregative E. *coli*, *Salmonella*, *Shigella* and *Campylobacter*. Protozoans, such as *Giardia*, *Cryptosporidium* and *Entamoeba histolytica*, account for 10% of cases. Rotavirus and norovirus are the principal viral pathogens, but account for less than 10% of traveller's diarrhoea. Many cases do not become symptomatic until after return home. Antibiotic prophylaxis for traveller's diarrhoea, although effective, is not usually recommended as, in most instances, the illness will be self-limiting.

The immunocompromised patient

Patients with impaired immune (AIDS, IgA deficiency, immunosuppressive therapy following organ transplantation and long-term corticosteroid usage) are not only more susceptible to the common causes of gastroenteritis, but are also vulnerable to the less common organisms, such as *Cryptosporidium*, *Microsporidium*, *Isospora* and *Cytomegalovirus*. Infections are often more severe, have a higher incidence of complications and may be more resistant to conventional therapy. Isolation of the causative organism and determination of antibiotic sensitivity are essential to guide management.

Hospital-acquired diarrhoea

Clostridium difficile is the most common cause of antibiotic-associated and nosocomial diarrhoea.

It may range from a mild disease to life-threatening pseudomembranous colitis and can follow treatment with almost any antibiotic but particularly cephalosporins and clindamycin. Methods of laboratory detection include stool culture, polymerase chain reaction (PCR), cell-culture cytotoxicity assay and enzyme immunoassays. Patients should be treated empirically with oral metronidazole, reserving oral vancomycin for severe disease or subsequent recurrences.

Differential diagnosis

Many pathological conditions, especially early in their course, may present with a clinical picture similar to that of gastroenteritis. Appendicitis, mesenteric adenitis, small bowel ischaemia and inflammatory bowel disease can all present in a similar fashion. Conversely, *Campylobacter* may cause severe abdominal pain with little diarrhoea and may be misdiagnosed as appendicitis or inflammatory bowel disease. Medical conditions, such as toxic ingestions, diabetic ketoacidosis, hepatitis and pancreatitis, may also present with vomiting, abdominal pain, tenderness and 'loose' stools.

Clinical investigations

In most circumstances, no investigations are necessary in order to make the diagnosis of gastroenteritis or to manage the patient effectively.

Identification of the infective agent may be useful when there is an outbreak of gastroenteritis to ensure that adequate public health measures are instituted, in an attempt to limit spread of the disease. Additionally, in a patient who has a persistent illness or clinical features of a specific illness (such as *Campylobacter*, *Giardia* or *Salmonella*), identification of the organism may be helpful in directing antimicrobial therapy or identifying a carrier state. Although the history and examination may give clues as to the aetiological agent, they are unreliable as many similarities exist between the clinical syndromes produced by each organism. Laboratory identification is the only accurate method.

The infective agent may be identified by microscopy and culture of faeces, looking specifically for pathogenic bacteria, cysts, ova or parasites. A fresh specimen of faeces will assist in detection. Occasionally, multiple specimens

are required, especially for organisms which may shed into the faeces only sporadically.

Rotavirus infection is detected by looking for rotavirus antigen in the stool by electron microscopy, PCR, enzyme-linked immunosorbent assay (ELISA) or latex agglutination.

If a patient is dehydrated or systemically unwell, a full blood examination, serum electrolyte determination and serum glucose are warranted. In rare cases, where there are signs suggestive of septicaemia or severe systemic illness, blood cultures and liver function tests may be indicated.

Abdominal X-rays are only useful if it is necessary to exclude a bowel obstruction or free intra-abdominal gas.

Treatment

The principles of treatment for gastroenteritis are to replace fluid and electrolyte losses, minimize symptoms if possible and, in selected cases, administer specific antimicrobial therapy. Clear fluids for 24 hours are often recommended, with the rationale that keeping the stomach empty will minimize vomiting. If the patient wishes to eat, it is allowed. Strictly withholding feeding, especially from children, is not necessary.

Replacement of fluid losses may be achieved enterally, either by mouth or via a nasogastric tube or intravenously. The method selected will depend on the cooperation of the patient, the degree of dehydration, the rate at which rehydration is desired and the presence of other diseases, such as diabetes.

Specific oral rehydration solutions are the most appropriate for oral or nasogastric use. There are a number of commercial preparations available through pharmacies without prescription. These consist of a balanced formula of glucose, sodium and potassium salts and, in worldwide trials, have been shown to be extremely effective and safe, even when used in the most primitive of conditions. Although many commonly available fluids may be used and will probably be effective in mild disease, fluids that contain large amounts of glucose, such as degassed lemonade or undiluted fruit juice, should not be encouraged in adults and are contraindicated in children. These fluids are hyperosmolar and deficient in electrolytes, thus promoting further fluid losses. Glucose-containing electrolyte solutions use the gut's co-transport system for glucose and sodium, thereby facilitating the absorption of water

as well. Milk and other lactose-containing products should be avoided during the acute phase of the illness, as viral or bacterial enteropathogens often result in transient lactose malabsorption. Caffeine-containing products should also be avoided as caffeine increases cyclic AMP levels, thereby promoting the secretion of fluid and worsening diarrhoea.

Intravenous rehydration is necessary in patients who are in shock or who are becoming progressively dehydrated despite oral or nasogastric fluids. Resuscitation should be commenced with normal saline at a rate which accounts for ongoing losses, as well as replacing the estimated fluid deficit. In severely dehydrated patients, one or two 20 mL/kg boluses of normal saline may be necessary. Patients should also be encouraged to take oral fluids, unless vomiting is prohibitive. As soon as an adequate intake is achieved, the intravenous fluids can be scaled back and ceased.

Close monitoring of the serum electrolytes is necessary during intravenous rehydration. In particular, it is important to monitor serum sodium, as the exclusive use of normal saline for rehydration can lead to hypernatraemia. Potassium should be added to the fluid as determined by the serum potassium, remembering that low serum potassium in this circumstance is indicative of low total body potassium.

In adults, parenterally administered antiemetic drugs, such as metoclopramide, prochlorperazine or ondansetron, may be useful in the management of severe vomiting. In children, an unacceptably high incidence of dystonic reactions precludes the use of prochlorperazine and metoclopramide. There is growing evidence that oral ondansetron is useful for those children who fail initial oral rehydration therapy and can avoid the need for intravenous fluids. Data in adults are lacking. While antimotility agents, such as loperamide, have been shown to reduce the number of diarrhoeal stools and the duration of the illness, they have significant side effects and should only be used if it is essential.

Even though many bacteria that cause gastroenteritis respond to antibiotics, they are rarely indicated. In the majority of these cases, the illness will be short-lived and mild. Many isolates of *Campylobacter jejuni*, *Shigella* and *Salmonella* are resistant to many antibiotics. Choice of antibiotics should be based on antibiotic sensitivity patterns and local therapeutic guidelines. Antibiotics may be indicated

Table 7.5.2   Antibiotic treatment regimens
Giardia lamblia
Tinidazole 2 g (child: 50 mg/kg up to 2 g) orally, as a single dose OR Metronidazole 2 g (child: 30 mg/kg up to 2 g) orally, daily for 3 days
Amoebiasis
Tinidazole 2 g (child: 50 mg/kg up to 2 g) orally, daily for 3 days OR Metronidazole 600 mg (child: 15 mg/kg up to 600 mg) orally, 8-hourly for 7–10 days. PLUS Paromycin 500 mg (child: 10 mg/kg up to 500 mg) orally 8-hourly for 7 days (to eradicate cysts and prevent relapse)
Shigellosis
Ciprofloxacin 500 mg (child 12.5 mg/kg up to 500 mg) orally, 12-hourly for 5 days OR Norfloxacin 400 mg (child: 10 mg/kg up to 400 mg) orally, 12-hourly for 5 days OR Co-trimoxazole 160/800 mg (child: 4/20 mg/kg up to 160/800 mg) orally, 12-hourly for 5 days
Campylobacter
Azithromycin 500 mg (child: 10 mg/kg up to 500 mg) orally, daily for 3 days OR Ciprofloxacin 500 mg (child 12.5 mg/kg up to 500 mg) orally, 12-hourly for 3 days OR Norfloxacin 400 mg (child: 10 mg/kg up to 400 mg) orally, 12-hourly for 5 days
Clostridium difficile
Metronidazole 400 mg (child: 10 mg/kg up to 400 mg) orally, 8-hourly for 10 days (and cease implicated antibiotic) For severe disease: vancomycin 125 mg (child: 3 mg/kg up to 125 mg) orally 6-hourly for 10 days
After eTG complete [Internet] Melbourne: Therapeutic Guidelines Limited; 2013 July with permission.

- The reliability of clinical examination in determining the degree of dehydration.
- The role of ondansetron in facilitation of oral rehydration.
- The circumstances in which the empirical use of antibiotics may be appropriate.

in *Giardia* infections, *Shigella* causing severe disease, *Salmonella* in infants, the immunosuppressed or the elderly, *Campylobacter* in food handlers and in traveller's diarrhoea. Antibiotics are contraindicated in uncomplicated *Salmonella* infections as they may prolong the carrier state. Recommended antibiotic regimens are summarized in Table 7.5.2.

Controversies

- The role of faecal microscopy and culture.
- The public health role of EDs in monitoring and reporting the prevalence of gastroenteritis in the community.

Further reading

Aranda-Michel J, Giannella RA. Acute diarrhea: a practical review. Am J Med 1999;106:670–6.

Buttery JP, Lambert SB, Grimwood K, et al. Reduction in rotavirus-associated acute gastroenteritis following introduction of rotavirus vaccine into Australia's National Childhood Vaccine Schedule. Paediatr Infect Dis J 2011;30:S25–9.

Carter B, Fedorowicz Z. Antiemetic treatment of acute gastroenteritis in children: an updated Cochrane systematic review with meta-analysis and mixed treatment comparison in a Bayesian framework. Br Med J 2012;2:e000622, p. ii.

Centers for Disease Control and Prevention. Health information for international travel. Atlanta: CDC; 2005.

Cheng AC, Ferguson JK, Richards MJ, et al. Australasian Society for Infectious Disease guidelines for the diagnosis and treatment of *Clostridium difficile* infection. Med J Aust 2011;194:353–8.

Cheng AC, McDonald JR, Thielman NM. Infectious diarrhea in developed and developing countries. J Clin Gastroenterol 2005;39:1–17.

Galati JC, Harsley S, Richmond P, et al. The burden of rotavirus-related illness among young children on the Australian health care system. Aust NZ J Publ Hlth 2006;30:416–21.

Guerrant RL, Van Gilder T, Steiner S, et al. Practice guidelines for the management of infectious diarrhea. Clin Infect Dis 2001;32:331–50.

Horan TC, Andrus M, Dudeck MA. CDC/NHSN surveillance definition of healthcare-associated infection and criteria for specific types of infections in the acute care setting. Am J Infect Control 2008;36:309–32.

Roslund G, Hepps TS, McQuillen KK. The role of oral ondansetron in children with vomiting as a result of acute gastritis/gastroenteritis who have failed oral rehydration therapy: a randomized controlled trial. Ann Emerg Med 2008;52: 22–9.

7.6 Haematemesis and melaena

Colin A Graham

ESSENTIALS

1 Resuscitation is the priority, with particular attention to restoring perfusion of vital organs by replacing intravascular volume.

2 Upper gastrointestinal endoscopy is the key investigation and frequently allows definitive therapy. It should be performed at the earliest opportunity.

Introduction

Upper gastrointestinal bleeding (UGIB) is a common medical emergency with significant morbidity and mortality. Over the last two decades, there have been advances in drug therapy for peptic ulcer disease and varices, improvements in endoscopic techniques, interventional radiology and surgical management, in addition to advances in resuscitation and supportive care. Mortality for patients presenting with UGIB remains around 6–10%, although there is some evidence that mortality has declined in the UK and the USA. Fewer patients (approximately 2%) now require emergency surgery. Patients with UGIB are increasingly elderly and have more co-morbidity than in the past, which may explain the slow improvement in mortality despite the many technical advances in management, particularly endoscopy. Patients now rarely die of exsanguination, but more commonly of multiple organ failure secondary to pre-existing co-morbidities.

Definitions, epidemiology and pathogenesis

Upper gastrointestinal bleeding is defined as any bleeding within the gastrointestinal (GI) tract proximal to the ligament of Treitz. Any bleeding arising distal to that is a lower GI bleed. Haematemesis is the vomiting of bright red blood. 'Coffee-ground vomiting' is the vomiting of digested blood clot, whereas melaena is the passage of black, tarry stools as a result of bacterial degradation of

haemoglobin within the gut. Melaena usually represents a source of UGIB, but it can rarely occur due to a lower gastrointestinal source of bleeding. Haematochezia is the passage of bright red blood per rectum and, in the context of UGIB, represents a briskly bleeding source of haemorrhage. Melaena of itself is not associated with poorer outcomes in UGIB, but haematochezia due to an upper GI source is associated with double the risk of death.

Peptic ulceration remains the most common cause of UGIB despite the recognition and treatment of *Helicobacter pylori* infection as a primary cause of peptic ulcer disease (accounting for 36% of cases in a recent UK audit). The pathogenesis of peptic ulcer disease is complex but is closely related to a variety of risk factors, including *Helicobacter pylori* infection, use of non-steroidal anti-inflammatory drugs (NSAIDs) including aspirin, smoking and alcohol use.

Gastroduodenal erosions and oesophagitis make up a further 15% of cases. Oesophagogastric varices, resulting from portal hypertension, are the source of 11% of episodes of UGIB and up to 20% in patients less than 60 years old. Mallory–Weiss tears, the result of repeated vomiting, reportedly account for less than 5% of cases (although patients with a typical history often do not undergo endoscopy) and usually do not require specific treatment. The remaining causes (all <2%) include vascular lesions, such as angiodysplasia, Dieulafoy's lesion and aortoenteric fistula.

Prevention

The development of peptic ulcer disease is closely related to management of the risk factors. The effective identification and eradication of *H. pylori* has led to a significant reduction in the incidence of peptic ulcer disease as the cause of UGIB.

There is little doubt that restricting the prescription of NSAIDs in the elderly (the highest risk group for development of UGIB from NSAIDs and the age group with the highest risk of mortality from UGIB) would prevent a significant number of episodes of UGIB. This

is particularly relevant to emergency medicine practice, where NSAIDs are often prescribed as analgesia for musculoskeletal conditions. Care should be taken to prescribe the safest drugs (ibuprofen has the lowest risk profile) for the shortest possible time at the lowest effective dose. If patients are assessed at high risk for possible UGIB, NSAIDs should be avoided or, if unavoidable, a proton pump inhibitor (PPI) or high dose famotidine (40 mg twice daily) should be prescribed with the NSAID to maximize gastric mucosal protection.

Clinical features

It is usually necessary to determine whether the blood loss is from a gastrointestinal source. Blood from the nose or oropharynx can be swallowed, resulting in haematemesis and/or melaena. If bleeding is thought to be from the upper GI tract, then a number of diagnoses need to be considered (see below).

Some historical clues and caveats must be considered:

- A history of epigastric pain or dyspepsia suggests peptic ulcer disease. However, peptic ulcer disease may be painless, particularly in the elderly and in those taking NSAIDs and corticosteroids.
- A positive history of gastric or duodenal ulcer disease or reflux oesophagitis is associated with an approximately 50% chance of finding the same diagnosis at endoscopy.
- The risk of UGIB in patients taking NSAIDs is double that of patients not taking NSAIDs and is still higher than baseline in patients taking PPIs as gastric protection.
- The classic history of nausea and repeated vomiting prior to bleeding occurs in approximately one-third of cases of Mallory–Weiss tear.
- UGIB with a history of alcohol abuse and the stigmata of portal hypertension is suggestive of varices. However, up to 40% of patients with cirrhosis who present with GI bleeding are bleeding from causes other than varices (commonly from gastric erosions).

- Conditions associated with stress ulcers include burns, major trauma, head injury, sepsis and hypotension.
- Patients with chronic renal failure have a high incidence of angiodysplasia, peptic ulcer disease and oesophagitis.
- A history of aortic surgery and gastrointestinal bleeding raises the possibility of an aortoenteric fistula, even if the initial bleeding episode is not significant (the first bleed is often the so-called 'herald bleed').
- Clinical evidence of a coagulopathy should be sought, as this will influence subsequent investigation, treatment and prognosis.
- Stool examination, by rectal examination if required, is essential. As previously described, stool colour has prognostic significance. Testing for occult blood further increases the sensitivity of this examination as kits, such as the Hematest, are able to detect as little as 6 mg of haemoglobin per gram of stool. A positive test is dependent on the time of onset of bleeding in relation to gastrointestinal transit time. False positives may be produced by certain bacterial and vegetable peroxidases, such as bananas and horseradish. False negatives may result from ferrous salts.

Clues to the speed or acuity of blood loss include:

- The most likely diagnosis. Varices produce large amounts of dark (venous) blood; aortoenteric fistulae produce massive bright red haematemesis and haematochezia, with profound circulatory collapse.
- Signs of haemodynamic instability and response to initial resuscitation. If there is a poor response, there is likely to be significant haemorrhage.
- The character of the vomitus. Ongoing haematemesis is associated with large blood loss; 'coffee-ground' altered vomiting or clear fluid is often associated with a slower rate of bleeding.
- The colour of the stool (see above).
- The nasogastric aspirate if a tube is already in the stomach (commonly 'old age home' residents receiving enteral nutrition). Note that the practice of inserting a nasogastric tube in the emergency department (ED) to assess the aspirate is no longer recommended, as the absence of blood does not exclude significant bleeding.

The key message is that if there is haemodynamic instability or other evidence of significant ongoing UGIB, fluid resuscitation should continue but arrangements should be made to expedite emergency upper gastrointestinal endoscopy. The accuracy of diagnosis is not important at this stage, but the identification of major ongoing bleeding is.

Severity scores

Over the last decade, several scoring systems have been introduced to assist in the assessment of the severity of UGIB. The best known of these is the Rockall score, which requires endoscopic elements for completion, and the Glasgow–Blatchford score, which utilizes clinical criteria only. The Rockall score appears to be better at determining prognosis, whereas the Glasgow–Blatchford score is very sensitive and can be used to identify patients who may be suitable for outpatient care.

Clinical investigations

Blood tests

Blood should be drawn for full blood count, coagulation studies (INR/PT, APTT and fibrinogen), electrolytes, urea, creatinine, glucose level, liver function tests and urgent cross-matching. The initial haemoglobin is of limited value, as 24–48 hours are required for the intravascular volume to equilibrate. Thrombocytopaenia and leucocytosis are associated with increasing morbidity and mortality. UGIB may also result in an elevation of the urea level (relative to the creatinine), as there is a combination of an increased protein load in the gut and intravascular hypovolaemia. Blood should be taken for blood gas analysis to assess acid–base balance in those with significant bleeds. Venous blood gas analysis is appropriate unless coexisting respiratory failure is suspected. Similarly, a serum lactate level can help to identify patients with clinically occult hypoperfusion who are at high risk of significant haemorrhage.

Imaging

A chest X-ray may be indicated where aspiration is suspected, in the elderly or in patients with cardiopulmonary co-morbidities. It should also be performed if perforation is suspected, however, perforation associated with significant UGIB is rare.

Endoscopy

Although clinical and historical features can point towards the most likely diagnosis, they are not specific. The Rockall score (without the endoscopic components) and the Glasgow–Blatchford score can help predict the need for endoscopy. There is no empirical therapy that effectively treats all causes of UGIB. As a result, a specific endoscopic diagnosis almost always needs to be made. Exceptions may include those with a classic history suggestive of a Mallory–Weiss tear with no ongoing UGIB symptoms and stable haemoglobin and haemodynamic status and the very elderly with major co-morbidity and poor health status (e.g. patients with advanced dementia). Most centres rely on endoscopy to:

- Provide information on the source of bleeding with a high degree of specificity (90–95%).
- Allow prediction of the likelihood of re-bleeding and mortality, according to the nature and location of the lesion and stigmata of recent haemorrhage. These factors help in deciding the level of patient monitoring or whether they may be treated as an outpatient.
- Provide therapy. Endoscopy facilitates haemostasis through sclerotherapy, coagulation techniques and banding of varices and allows histological or microbiological diagnosis. In high-risk peptic ulcers, endoscopic therapy has been shown to decrease re-bleeding by 75% and mortality by 40%.
- Diagnose with safety (morbidity <0.01%). Safety is further maximized if endoscopy is delayed until the patient is haemodynamically stable and the airway patent and protected.

Endoscopy should be performed within 24 hours of presentation. Urgent endoscopy should be performed in patients with active or recurrent bleeding, bright red blood on haematemesis, large bleeds (>2 units of blood required) and when variceal bleeding is suspected. However, there is no evidence that early endoscopy (<12 hours) is associated with reduced mortality, although it is associated with a reduced length of hospital stay. Pro-motility agents, such as erythromycin, promote gastric emptying pre-endoscopy, but have not been shown to have any benefits on mortality, need for surgery or length of stay. They are now not routinely recommended in the ED prior to endoscopy.

DIGESTIVE EMERGENCIES

Treatment

Resuscitation

Continuous ECG monitoring, non-invasive blood pressure monitoring and pulse oximetry should be instituted, with frequent clinical reassessment. Urine output should also be measured and recorded hourly. Invasive arterial and central venous pressure monitoring may be necessary in massive bleeds, intubated patients and those with co-morbidities.

Oxygen should be administered to patients who are hypoxaemic (oxygen saturation <92%) or have evidence of significant ongoing bleeding. Massive ongoing bleeding may compromise the airway to the extent that endotracheal intubation may be required to secure and protect it. Intubation in these circumstances can be both difficult and hazardous and high-volume effective suction is essential. The extent of bleeding is often underestimated and, under these conditions, doses of induction agents should be dramatically reduced from normal levels.

The intravascular volume should then be optimized. The presence of shock (in most studies this was defined as a systolic blood pressure <100 mmHg) places the patient at high risk for re-bleeding, requirement for surgery and death. Note that, in the elderly, patients with autonomic neuropathies (frequently found in diabetics) and those taking β-blockers or calcium channel antagonists, the vital signs, including postural hypotension, may not be a reliable indicator of the degree of blood loss. Propranolol is a commonly used (and effective) prophylaxis for the prevention of variceal bleeding in cirrhotic patients and this may blunt the haemodynamic responses of patients with acute massive variceal bleeding.

Intravascular volume should initially be replaced with isotonic crystalloid (saline or Hartmann's) or colloid. There is no evidence of superiority for either class of intravenous fluid in UGIB. Blood should be given promptly if there is persistent haemodynamic instability despite 2 L of crystalloid or colloid, if the initial haemoglobin level is <7 mg/dL, if there is a significant risk of re-bleeding and in those patients with co-morbidities making them unable to tolerate periods of anaemia (e.g. chronic obstructive pulmonary disease, coronary artery disease). The thresholds for transfusion have recently been questioned, as early transfusion has been associated with increased mortality in UGIB. However, a higher haemoglobin level (>10 mg/dL) is generally accepted as desirable if there is a history of severe underlying cardiorespiratory disease (e.g. ischaemic heart disease).

Correction of coagulopathy

Transfusion of fresh frozen plasma and platelets should be considered early to prevent and treat coagulopathy associated with massive haemorrhage. Fresh frozen plasma should be given when the prothrombin time is 3 seconds greater than the control or when large transfusions are required. In all patients requiring massive transfusion, attempts should be made to avoid hypothermia by using blood warmers, heating blankets and overhead heaters.

Endoscopy

Although endoscopy is diagnostic for UGIB, it is also therapeutic in the majority of cases and should be performed within 24 hours of admission. It should be carried out without delay when patients remain unstable despite initial fluid and blood product resuscitation. Although many guidelines stress the need for 'haemodynamic stability' prior to endoscopy, in cases where this is difficult to achieve, consideration must be given to achieving haemostasis by endoscopic means as part of the ongoing resuscitation process.

Specific therapy

Peptic ulcer disease

Bleeding ceases spontaneously in 80% of cases and the mortality rate is approximately 5–6%, significantly less than with variceal bleeding.

Drug therapy

Haemostasis is known to be a pH-dependent process, so it has been hypothesized that medications that inhibit acid secretion will also reduce the rates of re-bleeding, need for surgery and mortality. The two main drug classes are the histamine (H_2) antagonists and the proton pump inhibitors.

H_2 antagonists Most data relating to the benefit of H_2 antagonists in acute upper GI bleeds are unconvincing. A large meta-analysis in 2002 reported that H_2 antagonists had only modest effects on bleeding gastric ulcers, reducing re-bleeding by 7.2%, surgery by 6.7% and death by 3.2%. There were no effects on bleeding duodenal ulcers. H_2 antagonists are not recommended in the contemporary management of UGIB.

Proton pump inhibitors The PPIs are the most common class of drugs used for peptic disease based on their profound and persistent acid suppression. Current guidelines recommend that PPIs should be given intravenously in high doses after endoscopy to promote ulcer healing and prevent re-bleeding, particularly in patients with high-risk stigmata at endoscopy. High dose oral PPIs may also be used when intravenous administration is not possible and is also effective. Oral doses of PPIs should be at least four times the standard oral dose. Reversible risk factors, such as *H. pylori* and NSAIDs, should be eliminated where possible. PPIs can be given prior to endoscopy and this recommendation is controversial. Randomized trial data do not show any effect on mortality or emergency surgery but do suggest that ulcer healing may be accelerated.

Somatostatin/octreotide Studies have found conflicting results in the use of somatostatin and octreotide in peptic ulcer disease. A meta-analysis suggested that there may be a reduction in re-bleeding and the need for surgery in patients with bleeding ulcers, but there was no effect on mortality. Somatostatin and octreotide are no longer recommended in the acute management of peptic ulcer disease.

Endoscopy

Endoscopic therapy is the core of all modern management of UGIB. The ongoing development of new endoscopic techniques for haemostasis means that endoscopy has almost completely replaced surgery as the definitive therapy. Combination therapy using submucosal adrenaline injections combined with cautery or mechanical clips is the best option for ulcers requiring endoscopic treatment.

Surgery

Surgery is required in <2% of patients. It is indicated for continuous or recurrent active bleeding, especially in patients aged over 60, in whom early surgery produces significant benefits in terms of mortality. Other indications include massive blood transfusion, refractory shock and failure to respond to endoscopic therapy. Salvage surgery is associated with poor outcomes and therefore early surgical consultation should be considered, particularly for patients aged over 60 years, those with significant co-morbidities, those with evidence of active bleeding (active bright red haematemesis, haematochezia), when there is a significant risk of re-bleeding or when there is continuing haemodynamic instability. Transarterial embolization appears to offer selected patients a good alternative to open surgery when bleeding is not manageable by conventional endoscopic means, although it is rarely used at present. Success rates of up to 69% have been reported, which is comparable to the results of open surgery.

Gastro-oesophageal varices

Although haemorrhage from gastro-oesophageal varices accounts for 2–15% of all UGIB, it represents a significant therapeutic challenge. Bleeding ceases spontaneously in only 20–30%, yet as bleeding is often more severe and recurrent, mortality approaches 25–40% for each episode of variceal haemorrhage. Factors influencing mortality include the stage and rate of deterioration of the underlying liver disease, the presence of co-morbidities, variceal size and specific endoscopic criteria. Patients with known severe varices should be considered for early transfer to a specialist hepatology centre with expertise in dealing with acute massive variceal bleeding.

Drug therapy

Drugs should be used when endoscopic expertise is not available, if massive bleeding prevents immediate sclerotherapy, or as an adjunct to further treatment if continued variceal haemorrhage is suspected. However, it must be emphasized that endoscopic haemostasis procedures are still the mainstay of treatment for varices and endoscopy is required for all cases despite drug therapy.

Somatostatin, octreotide, vasopressin and terlipressin have all been used in this situation. Somatostatin and octreotide therapy produces dramatic reductions in splanchnic arterial blood flow and portal venous pressure, while preserving cardiac output and systemic blood pressure. Treatment results in the control of bleeding in 74–92% of cases, with endoscopic evidence of cessation of bleeding in 68% of patients within 15 minutes. Vasopressin increases peripheral vascular resistance and mean arterial pressure, with reduced cardiac output and coronary blood flow; it is therefore contraindicated in patients with coronary artery disease. Vasopressin results in the control of bleeding in 50–75% of cases. Terlipressin is a synthetic analogue of vasopressin. It can be given by bolus IV injection and has been shown to have a 34% relative risk reduction in mortality from acute variceal haemorrhage and a much lower incidence of side effects than vasopressin. A systematic review in the recent NICE guidelines supports the use of terlipressin as soon as variceal bleeding is suspected or confirmed. Where available, terlipressin (2 mg IV bolus) is therefore recommended for patients with known or highly suspected oesophagogastric varices with UGIB.

There is evidence that patients with oesophageal varices who have chronic liver disease have higher survival rates if given broad-spectrum antibiotics on admission. Intravenous antibiotics should be started early and local advice should be sought on the most appropriate antibiotic for the region where the patient lives. In the absence of local guidance, intravenous cephalosporins or quinolones are a reasonable initial choice.

Endoscopy

Endoscopy is essential to confirm the diagnosis of variceal haemorrhage, as in up to 81% of patients with known varices an alternative bleeding site is found. Endoscopy is also therapeutic in many cases. Endoscopic variceal ligation (EVL) has been shown to be more effective than endoscopic sclerotherapy in the control of variceal haemorrhage, with significantly fewer complications, less re-bleeding and lower mortality; it also requires fewer treatment sessions. Control of bleeding can be achieved subsequently in up to 95% of cases, with a reduction in the risk of re-bleeding. Therefore, EVL should be considered first-line therapy in the control of bleeding from oesophageal varices. Sclerotherapy remains an option if EVL is technically impossible due to massive bleeding at the time of endoscopy.

It is very difficult to perform EVL on gastric varices, so injections of cyanoacrylate are recommended. This should be combined with drug therapy.

Balloon tamponade

Compression of fundal and distal oesophageal varices by balloon tamponade results in control of bleeding in 70–90% of cases. Balloon tamponade may be used as a temporary means of controlling bleeding that is refractory to medical or endoscopic treatment or when bleeding is too massive for endoscopy to be performed successfully.

Because of the problems of pooling of secretions in the oesophagus (thereby increasing the risk of pulmonary aspiration), the standard Sengstaken–Blakemore tube has been modified to incorporate an oesophageal aspiration channel. Further modifications have been made with the Linton–Nachlas tube, which incorporates a single large (600 mL) gastric balloon for the tamponade of gastric varices. The principal use for balloon tamponade now is to act as a bridge to facilitate transfer to a specialist hepatology or endoscopy centre for ongoing care. Endoscopy at the earliest opportunity remains the treatment of choice for UGIB.

There are a number of problems with balloon tamponade:

- It can only be used for a maximum of 48–72 hours. As up to 50% of patients re-bleed when the tube is deflated, further definitive procedures (EVL, sclerotherapy, surgery) need to be performed.
- There is a significant (25–30%) risk of complications, particularly pulmonary aspiration and oesophageal perforation.
- Balloon tamponade requires skilled staff and monitoring in an intensive-care setting for the initial insertion and maintenance of balloon position and function.
- Owing to the risks of pulmonary aspiration, endotracheal intubation should be considered in all patients requiring balloon tamponade.

Transjugular intrahepatic portosystemic stent

Transjugular intrahepatic portosystemic stent-shunt (TIPSS) involves the insertion of a stent under radiological guidance via the jugular vein, forming a portosystemic shunt between the hepatic and portal veins. This technique is effective, achieving control of bleeding in up to 90% of patients and is less invasive and faster to perform (range 30 minutes to 3 hours) than other surgical shunt procedures. However, it requires an experienced operator and often results in complications similar to those seen after other portosystemic shunts, particularly encephalopathy and deteriorating liver function.

The main role of TIPSS, therefore, appears to be in patients who continue to bleed in spite of EVL or sclerotherapy and who do not have hepatic encephalopathy, preterminal liver failure, portal vein thrombosis, intrahepatic sepsis or significant cardiac disease. TIPSS then acts as a bridging procedure until other definitive surgical procedures can be performed (such as liver transplantation, shunt surgery or, rarely, oesophageal transection).

Surgery

Since the advent of EVL and sclerotherapy, the role of surgery in the control of acute variceal bleeding has decreased and it is now largely confined to the small number of patients who continue to bleed despite endoscopic intervention. Shunt surgery and oesophageal transection have been shown to reduce bleeding. However, these techniques require specialist surgical skills and have not been shown to improve survival.

Disposition

The primary decision in most cases is whether the patient is to be admitted to the general ward or to an intensive care (ICU) or high-dependency unit (HDU). Ideally, patients with UGIB should be admitted under the joint care of a gastroenterologist and a surgeon in a specific gastrointestinal bleeding unit.

The main indications for ICU/HDU admission include:

- known or suspected variceal bleeding
- haemodynamic instability
- significant co-morbidities, including cardiac, renal, pulmonary or hepatic dysfunction.

The threshold for ICU/HDU admission should be lowered in patients over 60 years of age, owing to the high incidence of co-morbidities and poor physiological compensatory reserve. Lower-risk patients may be admitted to the general ward. The usual length of stay is 2–3 days, as the major risk of re-bleeding is during the first 24–48 hours.

Evidence for outpatient management of upper GI bleeding are less clear. Most UGIB ceases spontaneously and most patients compensate well, not requiring transfusion or surgery. Some authors have suggested outpatient management for selected patients. To minimize the risk of adverse events if the patient is managed as an outpatient, early endoscopy has been advocated. Early discharge is then suggested for those who are found to have clean-based ulcers or non-bleeding Mallory–Weiss tears. In the UK, patients with a score of zero on the Glasgow–Blatchford scoring system have been managed as outpatients, without adverse events. It would be interesting to see the approach used in this single centre study validated elsewhere to determine its applicability in other settings.

Likely developments over the next 5–10 years

- There is likely to be a continuing increase in the incidence of UGIB as the population ages, and particularly variceal bleeding, as the incidence of liver disease rises in most developed countries, particularly in those aged less than 60 years old.
- Further studies on doses, route of administration and duration of therapy for PPIs after UGIB, before and after endoscopy, will help to clarify the optimum treatment.
- Improvements in delivery of critical care may help to improve survival in patients with UGIB by improving care of co-morbid conditions.
- Capsule endoscopy in the emergency department, to rule out active bleeding and allow outpatient-based care, will be further studied and evaluated.
- Clinical risk evaluation tools facilitating outpatient management will be further validated in different settings and possibly become part of routine clinical practice.

Controversies

- The optimum dose, route of administration, timing and duration of therapy for PPIs after UGIB has not been clarified and requires further study.
- Despite improvements in re-bleeding rates and a reduction in the requirement for surgical intervention, mortality rates have not improved, probably because of increasingly elderly populations and more co-morbidity.
- Increasing co-morbidities and the increasingly elderly population may require more intensive critical care

to improve survival, rather than further improvements in endoscopic haemostasis.
- The pressure to manage more patients safely in the outpatient setting means that there is a need to validate and further refine scoring systems to evaluate risk or adverse outcomes in UGIB, both with and without early endoscopy.

Further reading

Acute upper GI bleeding: NICE guideline. NICE clinical guideline 141; 2012. <http://guidance.nice.org.uk/CG141/Guidance> [Accessed Jan. 2013].

Barkun AN, Bardou M, Kuipers EJ, et al. International consensus recommendations on the management of patients with nonvariceal upper gastrointestinal bleeding. Ann Intern Med 2010;152:101–13.

Blatchford O, Murray WR, Blatchford M. A risk score to predict need for treatment for upper-gastrointestinal haemorrhage. Lancet 2000;356:1318–21.

Hearnshaw SA, Logan RF, Lowe D, et al. Acute upper gastrointestinal bleeding in the UK: patient characteristics, diagnoses and outcomes in the 2007 UK audit. Gut 2011;60:1327–35.

Hearnshaw SA, Logan RF, Palmer KR, et al. Outcomes following early red blood cell transfusion in acute upper gastrointestinal bleeding. Aliment Pharmacol Ther 2010;32:215–24.

Hwang JH, Fisher DA, Ben-Menachem T, et al. The role of endoscopy in the management of acute non-variceal upper GI bleeding. Gastrointest Endosc 2012;75:1132–8.

Imperale TF, Birgisson S. Somatostatin or octreotide compares with H₂-antagonists and placebo in the management of acute non-variceal upper gastrointestinal haemorrhage: a meta-analysis. Ann Intern Med 1997;127:1062–71.

Jairath V, Kahan BC, Logan RF, et al. Outcomes following acute nonvariceal upper gastrointestinal bleeding in relation to time to endoscopy: results from a nationwide study. Endoscopy 2012;44:723–30.

Jairath V, Kahan BC, Logan RF, et al. National audit of the use of surgery and radiological embolization after failed endoscopic haemostasis for non-variceal upper gastrointestinal bleeding. Br J Surg 2012;99:1672–80.

Jairath V, Kahan BC, Logan RF, et al. Red blood cell transfusion practice in patients presenting with acute upper gastrointestinal bleeding: a survey of 815 UK clinicians. Transfusion 2011;51:1940–8.

Palamidessi N, Sinert R, Falzon L, Zehtabchi S. Nasogastric aspiration and lavage in emergency department patients with hematochezia or melena without hematemesis. Acad Emerg Med 2010;17:126–32.

Restellini S, Kherad O, Jairath V, et al. Red blood cell transfusion is associated with increased rebleeding in patients with nonvariceal upper gastrointestinal bleeding. Aliment Pharmacol Ther 2013;37:316–22.

Rockall TA, Logan RF, Devlin HB, Northfield TC. Risk assessment after acute upper gastrointestinal haemorrhage. Gut 1996;38:316–21.

Stanley AJ, Ashley D, Dalton HR, et al. Outpatient management of patients with low-risk upper-gastrointestinal haemorrhage: multicentre validation and prospective evaluation. Lancet 2009;373:42–7.

Sung JJ, Tsoi KK, Ma TK, et al. Causes of mortality in patients with peptic ulcer bleeding: a prospective cohort study of 10,428 cases. Am J Gastroenterol 2010;105:84–9.

7.7 Peptic ulcer disease and gastritis

Win Sen Kuan • Shirley Ooi

ESSENTIALS

1 *Helicobacter pylori* is responsible for 70–90% of peptic ulcers, with non-steroidal anti-inflammatory drugs accounting for most of the remainder.

2 Emergency presentations of peptic ulcer disease vary from mild indigestion to severe life-threatening complications.

3 Endoscopy is the investigation of choice for definitive diagnosis.

4 Most patients can be managed medically with a combination of anti-secretory drugs and antibiotics as indicated.

5 Surgical treatment may be indicated for complications, such as haemorrhage, perforation and obstruction.

6 A 'negative' erect chest X-ray does not exclude ulcer perforation.

Introduction

Peptic (gastroduodenal) ulcers are defects in the gastrointestinal mucosa that extend through the muscularis mucosa. The term 'gastritis' is used to denote inflammation associated with mucosal injury. Gastropathy is defined as epithelial cell damage and regeneration without associated inflammation.

The discovery of the organism *Helicobacter pylori* (*H. pylori*) has resulted in a dramatic change in our understanding of the aetiology and pathophysiology of peptic ulcer disease. What was once a chronic disease prone to relapse and recurrence has now become eminently treatable and curable.

Patients presenting to emergency departments may do so with 'classic' ulcer symptoms, undifferentiated abdominal or chest pain or, more dramatically, with life-threatening complications, such as perforation or haemorrhage.

Aetiology, genetics, pathogenesis and pathology

Aetiology

Peptic ulcer disease is associated with two major factors: *H. pylori* infection and the consumption of non-steroidal anti-inflammatory drugs (NSAIDs). Smoking is also an important contributory element but does not appear to be a risk factor for *H. pylori* recurrence or ulcer relapse following eradication of *H. pylori*.

Gastritis is usually due to infectious agents (such as *H. pylori*), autoimmune and hypersensitivity reactions. In contrast, gastropathy is usually caused by irritants, such as drugs (e.g. NSAIDs and alcohol), bile reflux, hypovolaemia, ischaemia or chronic congestion.

Genetics

There seems to be a distinct familial aggregation of peptic ulcer disease in pre-*H. pylori* studies, suggesting a polygenic inheritance of peptic ulcer disease. It remains uncertain if genetic factors predispose to *H. pylori* infection or whether the genetic factors function independently.

Pathogenesis and pathology

H. pylori disrupts the mucous layer of the gastroduodenal tissue, adheres to the gastric epithelium and releases enzymes and toxins. This causes the underlying mucosa to be susceptible to acid damage and incites inflammatory response by the host.

NSAIDs cause ulcers by inhibiting the production of prostaglandins in the stomach and duodenum. The decreased synthesis of prostaglandins leads to increased amounts of gastric acid being generated, decreased bicarbonate and glutathione production and reduced blood flow to the gastric mucosa. NSAIDs are more commonly associated with gastric ulceration.

Epidemiology

H. pylori infects about 50% of the world's population. There are significant regional differences in the prevalence of peptic ulcer disease not explained by *H. pylori* alone, purportedly due to dietary variations. Populations with poor hygiene and low socioeconomic status are predisposed to higher prevalence of *H. pylori* infection.

The vast majority of patients harbouring *H. pylori* are asymptomatic. Although decreasing in incidence in developed regions, *H. pylori* is the major cause of peptic ulceration or, at least, a major cofactor in its development. *H. pylori* has been isolated from 20 to 50% of patients with dyspeptic symptoms. More importantly, 90–95% of patients with duodenal ulcers and 70% of those with gastric ulcers are infected with the organism. Eradication of *H. pylori* has been shown to markedly reduce the recurrence rate for ulceration. At least 50% of patients taking NSAIDs will have endoscopic evidence of erythema, erosions or ulcers, even if asymptomatic.

There are several risk factors that influence gastrointestinal toxicity due to NSAIDs, the most important being a prior history of clinical ulcer disease or ulcer complications. Other risk factors are the dose and duration of therapy with NSAIDs, age above 75 years and cardiovascular disease. The risk of peptic ulcer disease is highest on commencement of NSAIDs. Combined therapy of NSAIDs with corticosteroids, anticoagulants, other NSAIDs or low-dose aspirin dramatically increases the risk of ulcer complications.

Some NSAIDs are more likely to produce ulcers than others. In general, shorter-acting agents, such as ibuprofen and diclofenac, are less likely to lead to ulcers than longer-acting agents. Even though cyclooxygenase (COX)-2 selective inhibitors (coxibs) have shown a reduction in the risk of peptic ulcers and their complications compared to traditional NSAIDs, this risk is increased compared with placebo.

Studies have shown that the combination of a proton pump inhibitor (PPI) with a coxib decreases the incidence of peptic ulcers. However, there is no evidence that coxibs have advantages over other NSAIDs for patients with unhealed ulcers. Coxibs appear to inhibit healing of peptic ulcers.

The interaction between NSAIDs and *H. pylori* is controversial and complex but evidence from two meta-analyses of case-controlled trials identified synergism between *H. pylori* and NSAIDs in producing peptic ulcer and ulcer bleeding. Traditional risk factors, such as smoking, alcohol and stress, may increase the risk of ulceration and delay healing, but their relative importance as aetiological agents has fallen considerably with the discovery of *H. pylori*. Other causes of peptic ulceration, such as Zollinger–Ellison syndrome, are rare.

Clinical features

History
Peptic ulcers may present with a wide variety of symptoms or may be completely asymptomatic until complications, such as haemorrhage or perforation, occur. 'Indigestion' is the most common symptom in patients found to have peptic ulcer disease. Patients classically describe a burning or gnawing pain in the epigastrium that may radiate into the chest or straight through to the back. This may be associated with belching, early satiety, nausea and vomiting. Food may either exacerbate or relieve the pain. The pain is classically both fluctuating and periodic, with bouts of discomfort of variable severity interspersed with symptom-free periods.

The symptoms 'indigestion' or 'dyspepsia', however, have relatively poor sensitivity and specificity for diagnosing the various peptic syndromes. Less than 25% of patients with dyspepsia have peptic ulcer disease proven by gastroscopy and 20–60% of patients presenting with complications of ulcer disease report no antecedent symptoms.

Other presentations include chest or abdominal pain that need to be differentiated from conditions such as myocardial ischaemia, biliary tract disease, pancreatitis and other abdominal emergencies.

Patients also present with the two most common complications of ulcer disease, namely acute gastrointestinal haemorrhage or acute perforation. The former gives symptoms of melaena with or without haematemesis, and the latter presents with sudden, severe abdominal pain.

Examination
In uncomplicated peptic ulcer disease, abdominal findings may be limited to epigastric tenderness without peritoneal signs. If perforation has occurred, patients experience severe pain and look unwell. Abdominal findings include generalized tenderness, widespread peritonism and so-called 'board-like' rigidity. Those with gastrointestinal bleeding will usually have melaena on per rectal examination.

Differential diagnosis

The differential diagnosis of upper abdominal pain is broad. Functional (idiopathic, non-ulcer) dyspepsia is the commonest (up to 60%) and the diagnosis is one of exclusion. Other important differential diagnoses include gastric, oesophageal or pancreatic cancer, pancreatitis, biliary tract disease, gastro-oesophageal reflux disease, ischaemic bowel disease and metabolic diseases, such as hypercalcaemia and hyperkalaemia.

Clinical investigations

The extent of investigations depends greatly on the patient's presentation and the degree of severity of symptoms. There are no blood tests that can reliably predict the presence of peptic ulcer disease. Pathology investigations are aimed primarily at eliminating alternative diagnoses or identifying the complications of peptic ulceration.

Full blood examination
Anaemia is most likely to represent chronic rather than acute blood loss, unless bleeding is particularly heavy and hence clinically obvious. A microcytic, hypochromic anaemia suggests chronic blood loss with iron deficiency and can be confirmed with iron studies. Unexplained anaemia warrants a detailed evaluation and may raise concern for an underlying malignancy.

Blood cross-match
Patients with active bleeding may need replacement with blood products. Several units of blood may be required.

Clotting studies
These are indicated in patients taking anticoagulants and those with massive bleeding and/or a history of liver disease or alcoholism.

Liver function tests/amylase/lipase
Biliary tract disease and pancreatitis are important differential diagnoses in patients presenting with upper abdominal pain. Pancreatitis may also be the consequence of ulcer penetration through the posterior wall of the stomach.

Radiology
Radiological imaging has a very limited place in the diagnosis of uncomplicated peptic ulcer disease. However, an erect chest X-ray (CXR) is an important investigation when perforation is being considered. Gas is usually visible under the diaphragm, but its absence does not rule out perforation with sensitivity of erect CXR for detection of pneumoperitoneum ranging from 70 to 80%. Upright lateral CXR has been shown to be more sensitive than posterior-anterior CXR in detecting pneumoperitoneum. Lateral decubitus abdominal X-rays may be needed to demonstrate free gas in those unable to sit erect. Computed tomography (CT) scans of the abdomen are regarded as the criterion standard in detecting small pneumoperitonea.

Contrast studies are no longer considered first-line investigations in the assessment of patients with dyspeptic symptoms. Abdominal X-ray and ultrasound studies are useful to exclude alternative diagnoses, as indicated.

Criteria for diagnosis

Endoscopy
Endoscopy is the investigation of choice. It allows direct visualization of the mucosa of the oesophagus, stomach and proximal duodenum. It provides a definitive diagnosis which forms the basis of drug therapy and allows biopsies to be taken to exclude malignant disease and to isolate *H. pylori*. Endoscopic intervention may also be therapeutic in some cases of upper gastrointestinal haemorrhage (E-Fig. 7.7.1).

H. pylori status
Currently, there are a number of tests available, both invasive (endoscopic) and non-invasive, though their exact role in the emergency department (ED) setting has not been defined. It should be remembered that the majority of

patients infected with *H. pylori* do not in fact have peptic ulcer disease and that the identification of *H. pylori* infection often bears little relation to presenting symptoms. Non-invasive tests can only make a diagnosis of *H. pylori* infection, not of peptic ulcer disease. A negative test in a patient not taking NSAIDs makes the likelihood of peptic ulcer disease low.

The invasive tests for *H. pylori* include haematoxylin and eosin staining of mucosal biopsies and rapid urease tests (e.g. CLO test). The non-invasive tests include urea breath tests and IgG serology. Urea breath tests are highly sensitive and specific for the presence of *H. pylori*. They are most useful in assessing *H. pylori* eradication without the need for further gastroscopy. The urea breath test should be done early as an important limitation is its decreased sensitivity with prolonged antisecretory therapy.

A number of IgG serology tests are available with varying specificities and sensitivities. They are inexpensive, non-invasive and well suited to primary care and, potentially, emergency medicine practice. Large studies have found uniformly high sensitivity (90–100%), but variable specificity (76–96%); the accuracy has ranged from 83 to 98%.

Treatment

The treatment of peptic ulcer disease depends on the underlying cause and clinical presentation. Traditional management of patients with dyspeptic symptoms requires the exclusion of other diseases, the removal of known precipitants, such as NSAIDs, alcohol and cigarettes, the institution of simple treatment measures aimed at symptomatic relief and referral for further investigation and management.

Cost-effectiveness analysis and consensus statements support the treatment of *H. pylori*-positive dyspeptic patients with antimicrobial and antisecretory therapy, followed by endoscopic study only in those with persistent symptoms, so it would also be reasonable to begin symptomatic therapy, order serological testing for *H. pylori* and refer for early follow-up with a primary care provider for initiation of antibacterial therapy if the test results are positive.

The choice of approach is open to debate. Early treatment prior to endoscopy may cure some patients without the need for expensive invasive procedures. However, this plan of action may hinder subsequent *H. pylori*

isolation and delay definitive diagnosis, including the diagnosis of malignant disease.

It should be noted that the prevalence of *H. pylori* is lower in patients with complicated duodenal ulcers (those complicated by bleeding or perforation) than in those with uncomplicated disease. Patients with *H. pylori*-negative ulcers appear to have a significantly worse outcome, especially if treated empirically for infection. Thus, documenting infection is important prior to initiating antimicrobial therapy.

For patients with mild symptoms of recent onset, empirical treatment with antacids and/or histamine receptor antagonists aimed at symptomatic relief is reasonable. Review of the literature concluded that for patients with non-ulcer dyspepsia, H_2-receptor blockers were significantly more effective than placebo at reducing symptoms, whereas proton pump inhibitors and bismuth salts were only marginally so. Antacids and sucralfate were not statistically superior to placebo.

Given the poor correlation between dyspeptic symptoms and gastro-oesophageal disease, gastroscopy should be considered, particularly if symptoms are not controlled or promptly recur. Early endoscopy has been advocated in patients above 45 years of age presenting with alarm symptoms, such as dysphagia, recurrent vomiting, weight loss or bleeding.

Antacids

'Antacids' containing combinations of calcium, magnesium, local anaesthetics and alginates are useful in providing symptomatic relief for patients with relatively mild symptoms. In many instances, patients have already tried these agents prior to presentation. Relief of symptoms with antacids are, however, not a diagnostic indicator.

Histamine-receptor antagonists

The H_2-receptor antagonists, such as cimetidine, ranitidine, famotidine and nizatidine, all have similar efficacies with regard to ulcer healing. All are well absorbed orally, but their absorption may be reduced when used with antacids but not by food. Eighty to 90% of duodenal ulcers will be healed in 4–8 weeks and 70% of gastric ulcers within 8 weeks. Relapse rates of 80% over the course of 1 year are to be expected if *H. pylori* eradication is not also undertaken in appropriate cases. H_2 antagonists are also useful in the treatment of gastro-oesophageal reflux disease and management of dyspepsia. Due to renal excretion,

dosage adjustments must be made in patients with renal dysfunction.

Proton pump inhibitors

The PPIs, omeprazole, lansoprazole, rabeprazole, pantoprazole, dexlansoprazole and esomeprazole, effectively block acid secretion by irreversibly binding to and inhibiting the $H^+/K^+ATPase$ pump of the gastric parietal cells, thereby inhibiting the cells' proton pump. Acidic compartments within the stimulated parietal cell are essential for activation of a PPI. Thus, PPIs work poorly in fasting patients or those with simultaneous dosing with other antisecretory agents (H_2-receptor antagonists, anticholinergic agents or somatostatin). PPIs are most effective when taken with or shortly before meals. Compared to H_2-receptor antagonists, these agents result in more rapid ulcer healing and pain relief over 2–4 weeks, although differences at 8 weeks are not significant. Again, relapse rates are high, particularly if *H. pylori* is present and eradication therapy is not used.

Cytoprotectants

Cytoprotective agents include colloidal bismuth subcitrate (De-Nol) and sucralfate. Both act by binding to or chelating with proteins in the base of the ulcer. Bismuth compounds also suppress *H. pylori*. A 6–8-week course is recommended and relapse rates are high. Bismuth compounds lead to the formation of black stools that may be confused with melaena. The primary concern with bismuth is bismuth intoxication. Sucralfate should not be taken with antacids as it requires an acid environment to achieve its optimal effects. Sucralfate has minimal adverse effects other than possible aluminium toxicity.

Prostaglandin analogues

Misoprostol (a synthetic analogue of PGE_1) interferes with histamine-dependent gastric acid secretion as well as being cytoprotective. It is particularly useful in the prevention of NSAID-induced ulcers, although it is probably no better than the other agents in actually treating such ulcers.

Misoprostol significantly reduces the risk of endoscopic ulcers. Standard doses of H_2-blockers were effective at reducing the risk of duodenal but not gastric ulcers. Double-dose H_2-blockers and proton pump inhibitors were effective at reducing the risk of both duodenal and gastric ulcers and were better tolerated than misoprostol.

H. pylori eradication

All patients with duodenal ulcers associated with *H. pylori* infection should undergo therapy to eradicate the organism. This recommendation is based on overwhelming data showing that cure of *H. pylori* infection reduces ulcer recurrence and complications, such as bleeding. A number of eradication therapies have been postulated, all with very high eradication (>80%) and low relapse rates (<5%). The development of resistance to metronidazole has resulted in amoxicillin and clarithromycin being recommended as the antibiotics of choice. These are usually combined with a proton pump inhibitor or colloidal bismuth subcitrate for 1 week. Several single-prescription packages are now available. It is generally accepted that acid suppression therapy be continued for 6–8 weeks after cessation of antibiotic therapy.

H. pylori eradication therapy in patients with non-ulcer dyspepsia may have a small yet statistically significant effect on symptoms.

Treatment of NSAID-induced ulcers

The American College of Gastroenterology issued a guideline in 2009 for the prevention of NSAID-related ulcer complications. It recommends that all patients who are to commence long-term NSAID therapy should first be tested for *H. pylori*. Those tested positive for *H. pylori* should discontinue NSAID use where clinically feasible and undergo *H. pylori* eradication therapy. Patients who are at moderate risk of peptic ulcer complications and high risk of cardiovascular disease should avoid NSAIDs or COX-2 inhibitors entirely and receive alternative therapy. Treatment of NSAID-induced ulcers should consist of a 4–8 week course of an H_2-receptor antagonist or PPI.

Surgical management

With the success of medical treatment for peptic ulcer disease, surgical intervention has been restricted to the management of complications rather than of the primary disease.

Complications

There are four major complications of peptic ulcer:

- haemorrhage
- perforation
- penetration and
- obstruction.

Haemorrhage

Peptic ulceration is a common cause of upper GI bleeding, occurring in 10–20% of ulcer patients and accounting for approximately 50% of all upper GI bleeds. Urgent endoscopy is usually indicated. Surgical intervention may be required in a small proportion of patients. A meta-analysis concluded that the use of acid-reducing agents was associated with a statistically significant decrease in re-bleeding, but not mortality. Assessment and management of haematemesis and melaena is discussed in detail in Chapter 7.6.

Perforation

Perforation occurs in approximately 5% of ulcers, with duodenal, antral and gastric body ulcers accounting for 60%, 20% and 20% of perforations, respectively. One-third to one-half of perforated ulcers are associated with NSAID use; these usually occur in elderly patients. Chemical peritonitis develops suddenly, with acute severe generalized abdominal pain. Examination reveals a sick patient with a rigid, quiet abdomen and rebound tenderness. Delay in presentation and treatment, which may occur in the elderly and debilitated, sees the rapid development of bacterial peritonitis and subsequent sepsis and shock. The overall mortality rate is about 5%.

Rapid diagnosis is essential as the prognosis is excellent if treated within the first 6 hours, but deteriorates to probable death after more than a 12-hour delay. Diagnosis should be confirmed with an erect chest X-ray, bearing in mind its sensitivity of 70–80%. If free air is found, no other diagnostic studies are necessary. If there is diagnostic uncertainty, CT or ultrasound can be useful to detect small amounts of free air or fluid.

Vigorous fluid resuscitation should be instituted and renal function (via urine output) should be closely monitored. Initial empiric antibiotic therapy consisting of a combination of beta-lactam/beta-lactamase inhibitor (e.g. ampicillin–sulbactam) or third-generation cephalosporin (e.g. ceftriaxone) and metronidazole should be given, along with adequate analgesia. Cardiac and respiratory support may be needed in some cases.

As the standard of care, patients with perforation should undergo surgery for decontamination and repair (e.g. Graham patch) after resuscitation. Non-operative management, including intravenous fluids, nasogastric suction, antibiotics and antisecretory drugs, may be successful in some patients in whom the leak seals quickly in response to medical management. It may also be considered in patients who have severe co-morbidities precluding surgery and those with delayed presentations. There is some evidence that an initial period of non-operative treatment with careful observation is safe in younger patients (age under 60 years), but this is not regarded as standard practice.

Penetration

Posterior ulcers may perforate the gastric or duodenal wall and continue to erode into adjacent structures, most commonly the pancreas, without free perforation and leakage of luminal contents into the peritoneal cavity. Patients may describe their pain as becoming more severe and constant, radiating to the back and no longer eased by antacids and food. There is also loss of cyclicity of pain with meals. The serum amylase level may be mildly raised but clinical pancreatitis is not common. Endoscopy may reveal ulceration, but 'penetration' is difficult to confirm.

Gastric outlet obstruction

This is the least frequent complication and may occur in up to 2% of patients with ulcer disease. It may arise acutely secondary to inflammation and oedema of the pylorus or duodenal bulb or, more commonly, as a consequence of scarring due to chronic disease.

Prognosis

The prognosis for peptic ulcer disease is excellent when the underlying cause is identified and treated. The mortality rate is approximately 1 death per 100 000 cases, which is a modest decrease from a few decades ago, contributed mainly by an improved mortality rate from bleeding peptic ulcers using intravenous PPIs after endoscopic therapy.

Poor prognostic factors for peptic ulcer perforation include shock at the time of admission, presence of renal impairment, delayed presentation for more than 12 hours, age over 70 years, liver cirrhosis, immunocompromised state and perforated gastric ulcer (twice the mortality of perforated duodenal ulcer).

Disposition

Patients without complications can usually be managed as outpatients.

Likely developments over the next 5–10 years

- Vaccination for *H. pylori* infection will benefit populations in unfavourable socioeconomic environments.
- Future research should focus on understanding of the pathophysiology and treatment of non-*H. pylori* and non-NSAID associated peptic ulcers.

Controversies

- Elimination of *H. pylori* in all infected individuals or only in symptomatic patients.

- Conservative versus surgical management of perforated ulcer.
- Concomitant use of PPI and clopidogrel.

Further reading

Chan FK, Ching JY, Hung LC, et al. Clopidogrel versus aspirin and esomeprazole to prevent recurrent ulcer bleeding. N Engl J Med 2005;352:238.

Chan FK, Wong VW, Suen BY, et al. Combination of a cyclo-oxygenase-2 inhibitor and a proton-pump inhibitor for prevention of recurrent ulcer bleeding in patients at very high risk: a double-blind, randomised trial. Lancet 2007;369:1621.

Chey WD, Wong BC. American College of Gastroenterology guideline on the management of *Helicobacter pylori* infection. Am J Gastroenterol 2007;102:1808.

Hooper L, Brown TJ, Elliott R, et al. The effectiveness of five strategies for the prevention of gastrointestinal toxicity induced by NSAIDs: systematic review. Br Med J 2004;329:948.

Huang J, Sridhar S, Hunt R. Role of *Helicobacter pylori* infection and NSAIDs in peptic ulcer disease: a meta-analysis. Lancet 2002;359:14.

Lanza FL, Chan FK, Quigley EM. Guidelines for prevention of NSAID-related ulcer complications. Am J Gastroenterol 2009;104:728.

Papatheodoridis GV, Sougioultzis S, Archimandritis AJ. Effects of *Helicobacter pylori* and nonsteroidal anti-inflammatory drugs on peptic ulcer disease: a systematic review. Clin Gastroenterol Hepatol 2006;4:130.

Rahman MM, Islam MS, Flora S, et al. Mortality in perforated peptic ulcer patients after selective management of stratified poor risk cases. World J Surg 2007;31:2341.

Sachs G, Scott DR. *Helicobacter pylori*: eradication or preservation. F1000 Med Rep 2012;4:7.

Tan HJ. Controversy of proton pump inhibitor and clopidogrel interaction: a review. J Dig Dis 2010;11:334.

Wang YR, Richter JE, Dempsey DT. Trends and outcomes of hospitalizations for peptic ulcer disease in the United States, 1993 to 2006. Ann Surg 2010;251:51.

Zullo A, Hassan C, Campo SM, et al. Bleeding peptic ulcer in the elderly: risk factors and prevention strategies. Drugs Aging 2007;24:815.

7.8 Biliary tract disease

Stacy Turner • Andrew Walby

ESSENTIALS

1 More than 95% of biliary tract disease is attributable to gallstones.

2 Most patients with gallbladder disease present with abdominal pain.

3 Investigations are directed to confirming the diagnosis and detecting the presence of complications.

4 The management of acute biliary pain (biliary colic) is supportive and discharge is often possible.

5 The management of cholecystitis and other complications of gallbladder disease is both supportive and surgical.

6 Acalculous cholecystitis occurs in the absence of gallstones.

7 Antibiotics are indicated for the treatment of cholangitis and for a subset of patients with cholecystitis.

8 Ultrasound is the imaging test of choice for most biliary tract disease.

Introduction

Biliary tract disease is common and the vast majority of disease is related to gallstones. Stones may cause acute or chronic cholecystitis, acute biliary pain (biliary colic), pancreatitis, cholangitis or obstructive jaundice. Acute biliary pain is the most common presentation, caused by a gallstone impacting in the cystic duct. The second most common presentation is acute cholecystitis, caused by distension of the gallbladder with subsequent necrosis and ischaemia of the mucosal wall. Other diseases of the biliary tree include tumours and acalculous cholecystitis, which occurs in the absence of gallstones and often complicates critical illness.

Gallbladder disease is diagnosed by a combination of clinical features, laboratory investigations and imaging.

Gallstones and acute biliary pain

Aetiology, genetics, pathogenesis and pathology

Most biliary pathology is secondary to gallstones. Eighty per cent of gallstones in the Western world are composed primarily of cholesterol, but stones may also be formed from bile pigment (due to haemolysis) or may be of mixed origin. These components precipitate out to form crystals when bile is concentrated in the gallbladder. The crystals, if trapped in the gallbladder mucus, can grow, producing gallbladder sludge then stones. Symptoms occur when the gallbladder contracts, often after a meal, resulting in occlusion of the cystic duct by a stone, causing visceral pain (biliary colic). On relaxation of the gallbladder, the stone falls back into the gallbladder and symptoms subside. More prolonged gallbladder outlet obstruction leads to acute cholecystitis. Gallbladder distension and increased intraluminal pressure lead to inflammation, ischaemia and subsequent necrosis of the mucosal wall. Infection is not thought to play an initial part in the development of acute cholecystitis, but secondary infection may occur in up to 50% of cases. The main difference between acute cholecystitis and biliary colic is the inflammatory component, leading to ongoing pain, fever, localized peritonism and raised white cell count (WCC). Secondary bacterial infection is usually caused by aerobic bowel flora (such as *Escherichia coli*, *Klebsiella* species and, less commonly, *Enterococcus faecalis*). Anaerobes are found infrequently, usually in the presence of obstruction.

Cholangitis requires the presence of two factors: biliary obstruction and infection.

Epidemiology

Around 10–15% of Western adults have gallstones (cholelithiasis). Stones are less common in African and Asian populations. In young adults, four times more females are affected than males, but the disparity narrows with age. The lifetime risk of gallstones is 35% in women and 20% in men. In women, the risk is increased further during and after pregnancy and with oral contraceptive use. This is likely to be due to endogenous sex hormones that enhance cholesterol secretion and increase bile cholesterol saturation.

Other risk factors for the development of gallstones include increasing age, diabetes, obesity, rapid weight loss, drugs (most notably exogenous oestrogens, octreotide, clofibrate and ceftriaxone), genetic predisposition, diseases of the terminal ileum and abnormal lipid profile.

Two-thirds of gallstones are asymptomatic. Gallstones may be present for decades before symptoms develop. Asymptomatic patients become symptomatic at a rate of 1–4% per year but the risk decreases with time. Risk factors for stones becoming symptomatic are smoking, pregnancy and obesity. Stones may cause acute or chronic cholecystitis, acute biliary pain (biliary colic), pancreatitis or obstructive jaundice. Biliary colic is the most common presentation (56%), followed by acute cholecystitis (36%), obstructive pancreatitis and cholangitis. Less common presentations include empyema, perforation, fistula formation, gallstone ileus, hydrops or mucocele of the gallbladder and carcinoma of the gallbladder.

Prevention

Many of the risk factors for gallstones, such as age and gender, are fixed. There is limited evidence to support preventative strategies but maintaining a healthy weight and following a low-fat, high-fibre diet may reduce the risk. Those on long-term statins also appear to be protected from gallstones. Ursodeoxycholic acid is useful in preventing high-risk patients (e.g. morbidly obese patients undergoing rapid weight loss following bariatric surgery) from developing gallstones. However, ursodeoxycholic acid has no effect on reduction of symptoms once stones have formed.

Clinical features

History

The pain of biliary colic characteristically starts suddenly in the epigastrium or right upper quadrant (RUQ) and may radiate round to the interscapular region of the back. Despite the use of the term biliary colic, pain is usually constant. Pain develops in the hours after a meal, most commonly starting at night, waking the patient from sleep and usually lasting from 1 to 5 hours, subsiding spontaneously or with analgesics. Ongoing pain suggests cholecystitis. Nausea and vomiting are often present. Complaints of fevers and chills may be indicative of either cholecystitis or cholangitis. Rigors are suggestive of cholangitis.

Examination

RUQ tenderness is the most common examination finding. Patients with biliary colic have relatively normal vital signs. Significant fever is uncommon.

Jaundice is usually absent. Its presence suggests cholangitis or obstruction of the common bile duct (CBD). The presence of pain, jaundice and high fever with rigors (Charcot's triad) is indicative of cholangitis.

Differential diagnosis

The differential diagnosis of RUQ pain includes:

- peptic ulcer disease, including perforation
- acute pancreatitis
- coronary ischaemia, especially involving the inferior myocardial surface
- appendicitis, especially retrocaecal or in pregnancy
- renal disease, including renal colic and pyelonephritis
- colonic pathology, such as irritable bowel syndrome
- hepatic pathology, especially hepatitis
- right lower lobe pneumonia.

Clinical investigations

Investigations in biliary pain are aimed at confirming the diagnosis, establishing the presence of gallstones and the detection of complications.

Imaging

Ultrasound is the investigation of choice and can be used to confirm the presence of gallstones, measure the thickness of the gallbladder wall and the diameter of the CBD and detect the presence of any local fluid collection. On ultrasonography, gallstones appear as echogenic foci that cast an acoustic shadow, are usually mobile and gravitationally dependent. Ultrasound has high sensitivity and specificity (84% and 99%, respectively) for the detection of gallstones, is non-invasive and requires little preparation of the patient. However, ultrasound is not as good at visualizing stones in the CBD, identifying about half. Also, it is operator dependent, but bedside ultrasound examination has satisfactory diagnostic capability.

Abdominal X-ray. In the majority of cases, plain radiographs are not helpful in the diagnosis of gallbladder disease. On occasion, they may be useful to rule out other potential diagnoses but only 10% of biliary calculi are visible on plain radiographs.

Computed tomography (CT) should not be used as a first-line test. It is not sensitive for detecting gallstones, but is useful in diagnosing acute cholecystitis and in patients with complicated disease. CT may better demonstrate dilatation of the bile duct and pneumobilia, gangrene and perforation. In non-specific abdominal pain, it can detect acute cholecystitis and identify extrabiliary disorders.

Blood tests

In acute biliary pain, blood tests are non-specific. Bilirubin and alkaline phosphatase levels should be normal. In acute cholecystitis, mild derangement may be seen in around 25% of cases. Amylase/lipase assays are useful to evaluate the presence of pancreatitis. Amylase may also be elevated mildly in cholecystitis. Full blood examination shows a leucocytosis and left shift in the majority of cases of cholecystitis and cholangitis; however, up to 40% of patients do not have a leucocytosis at the time of presentation.

Complications

Complications of gallstone disease include:

- cholecystitis
- obstructive jaundice
- cholangitis and Gram-negative septicaemia

- gallstone ileus
- perforation: the elderly and diabetics are at particular risk of rapid necrosis and perforation
- pancreatitis.

Treatment

General measures

The management of biliary colic focuses on pain control which can be achieved with oral analgesics, titrated intravenous opioids or parenteral non-steroidal anti-inflammatory drugs (NSAIDs). The choice will, in part, be guided by pain severity. NSAIDs may provide equivalent analgesia to opioids, with fewer side effects. There is also some evidence that NSAIDs may help reduce progression of acute biliary pain to cholecystitis due to the inhibition of prostaglandin release from the gallbladder wall. Those with prolonged attacks should also receive intravenous fluids, especially if there is associated vomiting. Keeping the patient starved may prevent the release of cholecystokinin, thus reducing gallbladder contraction.

Antibiotics

Antibiotics are indicated for the treatment of cholangitis, but it is not clear whether antibiotics are required routinely for treatment of uncomplicated cholecystitis as complication rates may not be affected. That said, if there are clinical, laboratory of radiological findings suggesting infection, antibiotics should be given. Choice of antibiotic should be guided by local policy.

Definitive care

Cholecystectomy is the definitive treatment of choice for symptomatic stones. It provides symptomatic relief in up to 99% of patients. Minimally invasive surgery (either laparoscopic or using a small-incision technique) is preferred to the classical open operation technique as recovery is more rapid. Laparoscopic technique and the small-incision operation are equivalent. Early cholecystectomy (immediate or within 7 days) is the preferred approach for biliary colic or acute cholecystitis requiring hospital admission. Early cholecystectomy for biliary colic appears to decrease morbidity during the waiting period, conversion rate to open removal of the gallbladder and operating time and hospital stay.

Dissolution methods and lithotripsy are of limited utility due to restricted indications for their use and gallstone recurrence in approximately 50% of cases at 5 years.

Prophylactic cholecystectomy is not recommended in asymptomatic patients as the risks of the procedure outweigh the potential benefits.

Endoscopic retrograde cholangiopancreatography (ERCP) is indicated for the treatment of biliary obstruction.

Disposition

In the absence of cholecystitis or other complications, many patients with biliary colic can be discharged for outpatient surgical follow up if pain settles and if an early operative route is not being pursued. Most patients with complications such as acute cholecystitis, cholangitis or pancreatitis, require hospital admission. Admission may also be indicated in some cases because of recurrent severe pain.

Acute cholecystitis

Epidemiology

Distribution parallels that of cholelithiasis. Acute cholecystitis develops in 1–3% of patients with symptomatic stones.

Clinical features

RUQ pain and fever are the most common features. Usually, patients have experienced previous episodes of biliary pain. Nausea and vomiting are often present. Local peritonism and Murphy's sign (pain on inspiration during palpation of the right subcostal region) may be present but are not specific. A distended, tender gallbladder is not usually evident: the RUQ mass palpated in approximately 20% of patients represents omentum overlying the inflamed gallbladder. Approximately 20% of patients are jaundiced. The presence of hyperbilirubinaemia suggests CBD obstruction. Neutrophilia may be present.

Clinical investigations

Blood tests

No single test or combination of tests is sufficiently sensitive or specific to rule in or rule out the diagnosis. A leucocytosis is usually present. Elevated bilirubin and alkaline phosphatase concentrations are not common in uncomplicated cholecystitis, since biliary obstruction is limited to the gallbladder. If present, they should raise concerns about complications, such as cholangitis, choledocholithiasis or the Mirizzi syndrome (a gallstone impacted in the distal cystic duct or Hartmann's pouch causing extrinsic compression of the CBD).

Ultrasound

Findings on ultrasound are often diagnostic, showing cholelithiasis with concomitant gallbladder wall thickening (5 mm or greater), pericholecystic fluid or a positive ultrasonographic Murphy's sign.

Complications

Complications include bacterial superinfection leading to cholangitis or sepsis, gallbladder perforation leading to local abscess formation or diffuse peritonitis, biliary enteric (cholecystenteric) fistula, with a risk of gallstone-induced intestinal obstruction (gallstone ileus) and deterioration in pre-existing medical illness.

Treatment

General measures and antibiotics

Treatment requires hospital admission and includes supportive care (in particular analgesia), antibiotics and cholecystectomy. It is recommended that antibiotics be given if infection is suspected on the basis of laboratory and clinical findings (WCC >12500 × 10^9/L or a temperature of more than 38.5°C) and imaging findings (e.g. air in the gallbladder or gallbladder wall). Antibiotic choice should be guided by local policy and should include coverage against aerobic bowel flora (e.g. *Escherichia coli*, *Klebsiella* spp.), e.g. amoxicillin 1 g IV 6-hourly plus gentanicin 4–6 mg/kg IV once daily. Antibiotics are also recommended for routine use in patients who are elderly or have diabetes or immunodeficiency. Most patients will respond to conservative management, with the gallstone disimpacting and falling back into the gallbladder, thereby allowing the cystic duct to drain. If the gallstone does not disimpact, gangrenous cholecystitis (2–30% of cases), empyema of the gallbladder or gallbladder perforation (10% of cases) may occur.

Surgery

Minimally invasive cholecystectomy is recommended within 7 days for acute cholecystitis to prevent recurrence or other complications. Early surgery appears safe and shortens the total hospital stay. In severe cholecystitis, urgent cholecystectomy or cholecystostomy (percutaneous drainage of the gallbladder) with deferred cholecystectomy is required. Cholecystostomy may also be used in patients who are not candidates for surgery.

Acute acalculous cholecystitis

Acute inflammation of the gallbladder in the absence of gallstones generally occurs in the severely ill patient and accounts for 5–10% of cases of acute cholecystitis. It is associated with greater morbidity and mortality than gallstone cholecystitis. It is most commonly observed in the setting of critically ill patients, often recovering from trauma, burns or major surgery. Acalculous cholecystitis may also occur in elderly patients with coexisting vascular disease, in patients with diabetes, human immunodeficiency virus infection/acquired immunodeficiency syndrome (HIV/AIDS) or patients on long-term total parenteral nutrition (TPN).

Pathophysiology is thought to be due to increased bile viscosity and stasis because of critical illness, fever, dehydration and lack of enteral feeding.

Diagnosis can be difficult as patients usually have other life-threatening illness and may be sedated and ventilated in an intensive care setting. The usual finding on imaging studies is a distended acalculous gallbladder with thickened walls, with or without pericholecystic fluid.

Management consists of urgent cholecystectomy or cholecystostomy with treatment of the underlying illness. Compared with acute calculous cholecystitis, there is a much higher incidence of empyema, gangrene and perforation of the gallbladder and, consequently, an increased mortality rate (up to 50%).

Choledocholithiasis

Pathology and clinical features

Gallstones within the biliary tree almost all originate in the gallbladder, but primary choledocholithiasis (formation of stones within the CBD) can occur. Between 10 and 18% of patients have stones in the CBD at the time of cholecystectomy and the incidence of choledocholithiasis increases with age. Stones may be asymptomatic or cause pain and liver test abnormalities with or without evidence of complications. The common complications are acute cholangitis and acute pancreatitis.

Imaging

Transabdominal ultrasound is less reliable in choledocholithiasis than in gallbladder stones, but is still the preferred initial imaging modality. As well as gallbladder stones, ultrasound can evaluate for CBD stones and CBD dilatation. CBD dilatation is suggestive of CBD stones, but not specific. Sensitivity for CBD stones varies and is poor for stones in the distal duct. ERCP is more accurate and is also therapeutic, but is invasive and associated with complications, such as pancreatitis. Therefore, it is reserved for patients with confirmed CBD stones.

Endoscopic ultrasound, magnetic resonance cholangiopancreatography (MRCP) and intra-operative cholangiography during cholecystectomy are considered the tests of choice for evaluation of possible CBD stones.

Treatment

CBD stones pose a high risk for complications and nearly always warrant treatment. There are various options available, including pre- or postoperative ERCP, open surgery or laparoscopic bile duct exploration. It is not clear yet which one is best.

Cholangitis

Pathology

Cholangitis is defined as an infection of the biliary tree. It most commonly occurs due to biliary obstruction because of choledocholithiasis or a benign or malignant stricture. Infection can also flow in a retrograde direction up the CBD as a result of instrumentation, such as ERCP.

Bacteria are usually Gram-negatives, such as *E. coli*, *Klebsiella*, *Bacteroides* and *Enterobacter* spp., enterococci or Group D streptococci. There is also a subset of Asian patients who develop cholangitis mainly secondary to parasitic infection (recurrent pyogenic cholecystitis).

Clinical features and investigations

Fifty to 70% of patients present with the classic Charcot's triad of jaundice, fever and RUQ pain. Patients may also have features of severe sepsis or septic shock. WCC is raised in the majority of cases. Liver function tests are typically elevated in a cholestatic pattern. One-third of patients have a raised amylase. Blood cultures are positive in 20–30% of cases. If bile fluid is available (e.g. biliary drainage through intervention has occurred), it should also be cultured. Transabdominal ultrasonography is the recommended primary imaging study. Ultrasonography should be followed by ERCP, CT of the biliary tree or MRCP.

Treatment

Resuscitation may be required for patients with severe sepsis or shock. Parenteral antibiotics should be administered once blood cultures have been taken. Antibiotic choice should be guided by local policy but should be effective against anaerobes and Gram-negative organisms, e.g. amoxicillin 1 g IV 6-hourly plus gentamicin 4–6 mg/kg IV once daily. Around 20% of patients fail to respond to antibiotics or have a rapidly deteriorating clinical picture. These patients require urgent biliary decompression, which is achieved through ERCP, percutaneously or via open surgical decompression.

Controversies

- Timing of cholecystectomy.
- Appropriate use of antibiotics in acute cholecystitis.
- The optimal management of choledocholithiasis.

Further reading

Beckingham IJ. ABC of diseases of liver, pancreas, and biliary system: gallstone disease. Br Med J 2001;322:91–4.

British Society of Gastroenterology. Guidelines on the management of common bile duct stones. <http://www.bsg.org.uk/clinical-guidelines/pancreatic/guidelines-on-the-management-of-common-bile-duct-stones-cbds.html>; 2008 [Accessed Dec. 2012].

David GG, Al-Sarira AA, Willmott S, et al. Management of acute gallbladder disease in England. Br J Surg 2008;95:472–6.

Elwood DR. Cholecystitis. Surg Clin N Am 2008;88:1241–52.

Kimura Y, Takada T, Kawarada Y, et al. Definitions, pathophysiology, and epidemiology of acute cholangitis and cholecystitis: Tokyo Guidelines. J Hepato-biliary-pancreat Surg 2007;14:15–26.

NHS Clinical. Knowledge Summaries. Cholecystitis. <http://cks.nice.org.uk/cholecystitis_acute> [Accessed Dec. 2012].

Sanders G, Kingsnorth AN. Gallstones. Br Med J 2007;335:295–9.

Strasberg SM. Acute calculous cholecystitis. N Engl J Med 2008;358:2804–11.

Therapeutic Guidelines (Australia): Therapeutic Guidelines Limited. <http://etg.hcn.net.au>; 2012 [Accessed Dec. 2012].

7.9 Pancreatitis

Kenneth Heng • Eillyne Seow

ESSENTIALS

1 The majority of cases of acute pancreatitis are mild and self-limiting. However, 20% develop severe pancreatitis with a mortality of 20%.

2 When clinical presentation or biochemical tests are equivocal, contrast-enhanced CT is the investigation of choice.

3 Contrast-enhanced CT establishes the diagnosis, excludes alternative diagnoses, anatomically scores severity and detects local complications.

4 At presentation, the focus should be on identification of severe pancreatitis, as these patients require aggressive management in an intensive care setting to reverse organ failure.

Table 7.9.1 Aetiologies of acute pancreatitis

Common
Gallstone (including microlithiasis)
Alcohol
Idiopathic
Dyslipidaemia
Hypercalcaemia (hyperparathyroidism, metastatic bone disease, sarcoidosis)
Sphincter of Oddi dysfunction
Drugs (azathioprine, valproate, pentamidine, didanosine, co-trimoxazole)
Toxins
Post-ERCP
Traumatic
Postoperative

Uncommon
Structural (cancer of the pancreas/periampullary, pancreas divisum)
Vasculitis

Rare
Infective (Coxsackie virus, mumps, HIV, parasitic, ascariasis)
Autoimmune (systemic lupus erythematosus, Sjögren's syndrome)
α1-Antitrypsin deficiency

Acute pancreatitis

Introduction

The twin challenges of acute pancreatitis are to establish the diagnosis and stratify severity. The difficulty in diagnosing pancreatitis lies in its non-specific symptomatology which is shared by a number of other gastrointestinal diseases. Patient outcome depends in part on prompt recognition of severe pancreatitis. These cases require aggressive treatment to reverse organ failure and admission to intensive care or a high-dependency area for ongoing management. The hunt for the aetiology is the next priority, but this may be deferred to the inpatient team.

Aetiology and pathogenesis

The pathogenesis of acute pancreatitis relates to inappropriate activation of trypsinogen to trypsin which, in turn, releases digestive enzymes causing pancreatic injury. In 20% of cases, when pancreatic necrosis occurs, it is coupled with infection due to translocation of gut bacteria. An inflammatory response ensues, resulting in systemic inflammatory response syndrome, multiorgan dysfunction syndrome and, in some cases, death.

The commonest risk factor for recurrent pancreatitis in males is excessive alcohol use and, in females, gallstone disease. In 30% of patients, no obvious aetiology is identified. The other aetiological factors are listed in Table 7.9.1.

Epidemiology

The incidence of pancreatitis is rising, reflecting an increase in alcohol consumption and gallstone disease. The majority of patients have no further attacks. However, despite advances in care, overall mortality remains unaltered at 2–10%.

Clinical features

Gallstone pancreatitis typically presents with a sudden onset of severe, constant epigastric pain radiating to the back. In contrast, pain in pancreatitis from other causes (e.g. alcohol) has a more insidious onset and may be poorly localized. Pain is often accompanied by nausea and vomiting.

Upper abdominal tenderness is usually present but guarding and rebound tenderness are rare. Abdominal signs are often surprisingly few given the severity of the abdominal pain. Abdominal wall ecchymosis around the umbilicus (Cullen's sign), flanks (Grey Turner's sign) and inguinal ligament (Fox's sign) are uncommon findings. They are due to retroperitoneal bleeding from pancreatic necrosis and do not occur till 36–72 hours after the onset of pain. Severe pancreatitis is characterized by tachycardia, hypotension, abdominal distension and shallow respiration from diaphragmatic irritation and associated pleural effusion.

Differential diagnosis

The most important differential diagnoses to exclude are perforated viscus, ischaemic colitis, leaking abdominal aortic aneurysm and myocardial ischaemia.

Clinical investigations

Biochemical tests

Amylase rises in 2–12 hours and normalizes in about a week. In 10% of cases of pancreatitis, amylase is falsely negative due to depleted acinar cell mass. False positives may occur with salivary gland disease, macroamylasaemia, some cancers and decreased renal clearance of amylase in chronic renal impairment.

Lipase rises in 4–8 hours and normalizes in 1–2 weeks. It has superior sensitivity and specificity compared to amylase, as it is only produced in the pancreas. Amylase or lipase levels more than three times the upper limit of normal are diagnostic of acute pancreatitis. Lesser elevations must be interpreted against the timing of the test from symptom onset. The peak amylase and/or lipase level does not correlate with the severity of the disease. Alanine aminotransferase (ALT) $\geq$150 IU/L is 96% specific and 48% sensitive for gallstone pancreatitis.

Full blood examination, urea and electrolyte assays, renal and liver function tests are indicated to provide base-line data, explore differential diagnoses and assist in assessment of severity. Other tests to aid severity scoring include lactate dehydrogenase, alanine aminotransferase, blood gas analysis, calcium and lipid profile. Troponin assay may be indicated if acute coronary syndrome is a differential diagnosis under consideration.

Imaging studies

When clinical signs and biochemical tests are equivocal, a contrast-enhanced computed tomography (CT) scan of the abdomen is the radiological investigation of choice as it can establish the diagnosis, exclude most of the differential diagnoses listed above, stage the disease (see below) and detect complications.

The use of ultrasound is not as helpful as the pancreas is poorly seen in 25–50% of patients. It may, however, show gallstones and/or a dilated common bile duct, giving a clue to its aetiology. Magnetic resonance cholangiopancreatography (MRCP) has strong correlation with contrast-enhanced CT with the advantage of lower risk of nephrotoxicity and greater ability to characterize fluid collections, necrosis, abscess, haemorrhage and pseudocyst formation.

Plain radiography of the chest and abdomen has poor sensitivity for the diagnosis. Chest X-ray may show a pleural effusion or features of acute respiratory distress syndrome and abdominal films may show gallstones, a sentinel bowel loop or peri-pancreatic retroperitoneal gas, the latter signifying infection of the pancreas. Erect abdominal X-rays may identify free intra-abdominal gas in the case of a perforated viscus.

Severity scoring

Severe pancreatitis should be considered at presentation if the following risk factors are present: age >65 years, body mass index >30 kg/m², presence of pleural effusion on chest X-ray, contrast-enhanced CT shows >30% necrosis, APACHE II score >8 or there are symptoms and signs of organ failure (e.g. poor urine output, progressive tachycardia, tachypnoea, hypoxaemia, agitation, confusion, rising haematocrit level).

Biochemical predictors

Severe pancreatitis is identified either using a predictive scoring system or when a patient presents in frank organ failure (e.g. respiratory, renal or cardiovascular). Of the three predictive severity scoring systems in use, only the APACHE II allows scoring at presentation. A score >8 indicates severe pancreatitis with a mortality of 11–18%. Serial APACHE scores in the first 48 hours showing an increasing trend suggests a severe attack. The Ranson and Glasgow scores (Table 7.9.2) can only be completed at 48 hours, which limits their usefulness in the emergency department. Likewise, an elevated C-reactive protein (CRP) >150 mg/dL 24 or 48 hours after presentation also reliably predicts severe pancreatitis.

Radiological predictors

If severe pancreatitis is identified, contrast-enhanced CT can be used to anatomically score the severity using the system described by Balthazar (Table 7.9.3).

Treatment

The treatment for acute pancreatitis is supportive, with emphasis in the emergency department on fluid replacement, prevention of hypoxia and analgesia.

- Supplemental oxygen. Hypoxia may indicate acute respiratory distress syndrome (ARDS) or significant pleural effusions. Mechanical ventilation may be required in patients with respiratory distress. Uncorrected, gut hypoxia promotes translocation of Gram-negative bacteria.
- Fluid resuscitation. Significant third-space losses may occur. Fluid replacement should be titrated to blood pressure and urine output. A worsening haematocrit indicates insufficient replacement. Central venous monitoring should be considered in severe cases.

Table 7.9.2   Biochemical severity scoring systems

Ranson's score (1 point for each positive factor. Score >3 indicates severe pancreatitis)

At presentation	
Age	>55 years
Blood glucose	>10 mmol/L
White cell count	>16 000/mm³
Lactate dehydrogenase	>350 IU/L
Alanine aminotransferase	>250 IU/L
Within 48 hours after presentation	
Haematocrit	>10% decrease
Calcium	<2 mmol/L
Base deficit	>4 mEq/L
Urea	>1.8 mmol/L increase since admission
Fluid sequestration	>6 L
Partial pressure of arterial oxygen	<60 mmHg

Glasgow scoring system for prediction of severity in acute pancreatitis (1 point for each positive factor. Score ≥3 indicates severe pancreatitis)

Partial pressure of arterial oxygen	<60 mmHg
Albumin	<32 g/L
Calcium	<2 mmol/L
White cell count	>15 000/mm³
Aspartate aminotransferase	>200 IU/L
Lactate dehydrogenase	>600 IU/L
Blood glucose	>10 mmol/L
Urea	>16 mmol/L

Table 7.9.3 CT Severity index (score = sum of CT grade and necrosis. Score >6 indicates severe pancreatitis)

	CT grade		Necrosis score
Normal pancreas	0	No necrosis	0
Focal or diffuse enlargement	1	0–30% necosis	2
Intrinsic change, fat stranding	2	30–50% necosis	4
Single, fluid collection	3	>50% necosis	6
Multiple fluid/gas collection	4		

- Analgesia. Opioid analgesia is often required. Morphine, administered intravenously, is the agent of choice and dose should be titrated against response. On occasion, large doses are required for pain control. Patient-controlled analgesia may be appropriate. There are no human studies to support the belief that morphine causes spasm of the sphincter of Oddi.

Other important aspects of treatment include:

- Antibiotics. Prophylactic antibiotics are not indicated in mild pancreatitis. Empirical imipenem has been shown to reduce sepsis in severe pancreatitis with >30% necrosis on contrast-enhanced CT. Antibiotic therapy should be aided by cultures obtained by CT-guided fine needle aspiration.
- Nutritional support. In severe pancreatitis, current evidence supports early nasojejunal tube feeding over total parenteral nutrition (TPN), as it is more physiological, prevents gut mucosal atrophy and eliminates the risk of TPN-associated line sepsis. In mild pancreatitis, a low-fat and low-calorie diet may be started once the pain subsides.
- Surgery. Debridement of infected necrotic pancreatic tissue is required, although current opinion is that it should be delayed for 2 weeks as early surgery is associated with a high mortality.
- Treatment of the cause. In mild gallstone pancreatitis, cholecystectomy and bile duct clearance should occur prior to discharge to prevent a potentially severe and fatal recurrence. In severe gallstone pancreatitis, especially where there is suspicion of cholangitis, current evidence supports endoscopic retrograde cholangiopancreatography with sphincterotomy within the first 24 hours.

Octreotide, aprotinin and glucagon have not been shown to improve outcome.

Disposition

Patients with pancreatitis require admission for treatment and observation of disease progression. Mild pancreatitis can be managed in the general ward, but severe pancreatitis should be managed in intensive care or a high-dependency unit.

Prognosis

The majority of patients with acute pancreatitis experience a mild, self-limiting course with recovery in 5–7 days. Twenty per cent of patients develop severe pancreatitis, with a mortality of 20%. Fifty per cent of deaths occur in the first week from multiorgan dysfunction syndrome, whereas death after 1 week is usually due to infective complications. If organ failure is reversed within 48 hours, the prognosis is good.

Complications

Local complications include pancreatic pseudocyst, abscess, splenic vein thrombosis, duodenal obstruction and progression to chronic pancreatitis. Systemic complications include hypocalcaemia, pleural effusion, ARDS and multiorgan dysfunction syndrome.

Likely developments over the next 5–10 years

New early markers of severe pancreatitis are being developed, such as adipokines and urinary trypsinogen-activating peptide, the level of which correlates with severity. Other markers being investigated include interleukin 6 and 8, polymorphonuclear elastase and phospholipase A2. Mutations in genes for serine protease 1, pancreatic secretary trypsin inhibitor and cystic fibrosis transmembrane conductance regulator

have been identified in patients with recurrent idiopathic pancreatitis. Therapeutic implications are yet to be established.

Chronic pancreatitis

Introduction

Patients with chronic pancreatitis usually present with recurrent abdominal pain radiating to the back. This may be associated with weight loss because of fear of eating due to postprandial exacerbations of pain. There may be symptoms of pancreatic exocrine insufficiency (steatorrhoea) or endocrine insufficiency (diabetes mellitus). Physical examination may reveal a mass in the epigastrium, suggesting a pseudocyst and the patient may assume a characteristic pain-relieving posture of lying on the side with the knees drawn up to the chest.

Aetiology and pathogenesis

The aetiology of chronic pancreatitis is usually metabolic in nature, with excessive alcohol consumption accounting for 60–90% of cases. The primary process is chronic irreversible inflammation, fibrosis and calcification of the pancreas, affecting its exocrine and endocrine functions.

Clinical investigations

In chronic pancreatitis, serum amylase and lipase levels are not as elevated as in acute pancreatitis. Occasionally, enzyme levels may be normal due to atrophy of the gland. Endoscopic retrograde cholangiopancreatography (ERCP) is the gold standard for diagnosis of chronic pancreatitis. Contrast-enhanced CT and MRCP are non-invasive and provide additional information about the pancreatic parenchyma.

Treatment

The key issues in the management of chronic pancreatitis are as follows:

- Continued alcohol intake is associated with increased risk of painful relapses and hastening of pancreatic dysfunction. Alcohol cessation may require a team approach incorporating counsellors and psychiatrists for cognitive therapy and behavioural modification.
- Providing adequate analgesia in chronic pancreatitis is a challenge, with many

patients going on to develop chronic pain syndrome. Opioid dependency is a risk. Analgesia should not be withheld during acute episodes. Early referral to a pain management specialist may attenuate/manage opioid dependence. CT-guided coeliac ganglion blockade provides only temporary relief.

- Malabsorption is treated by a low-fat diet and restoration of pancreatic exocrine function with supplementation of pancreatic enzymes, fat-soluble vitamins and vitamin B12. Diabetes mellitus results from endocrine dysfunction and often requires insulin therapy.
- Relief of mechanical obstruction is achieved by endoscopy or surgical resection or drainage.

Controversies

- The optimal rate, type and the goal of fluid resuscitation in acute pancreatitis.
- The role of adipokines in identification of severe acute pancreatitis.
- The role of haemofiltration in the management of severe acute pancreatitis.
- The role of ultrasound-guided endoscopic drainage of pancreatic fluid collections.

Further reading

AGA Technical. Review. Treatment of pain in chronic pancreatitis. Gastroenterology 1998;115:765–76.

Balthazer EJ. Acute pancreatitis. Assessment of severity with clinical and CT evaluation. Radiology 2002;223:603–13.

Banks P, Freeman M, Practice Parameters Committee. Practice guidelines in acute pancreatitis. Am J Gastroenterol 2006;101:2379–400.

Cahen DL, Gouma DJ, Nio Y, et al. Endoscopic versus surgical drainage of the pancreatic duct in chronic pancreatitis. N Engl J Med 2007;356:676–84.

Dufour MC, Adamson MD. The epidemiology of alcohol-induced pancreatitis. Pancreas 2003;27:286–90.

Neiderau C, Grendell JH. Diagnosis of chronic pancreatitis. Gastroenterology 1985;88:1973.

Papachristou GI, Whitcomb DC. Predictors of severity and necrosis in acute pancreatitis. Gastroenterol Clin N Am 2004;33:871–90.

Pezzilli R, Zerbi A, Di Carlo V, et al. Practical guidelines for acute pancreatitis. Pancreatology 2010;10:523–35.

Ransom JH. Etiological and prognostic factors in human acute pancreatitis: a review. Am J Gastroenterol 1982;77:633–8.

Toouli J, Brooke-Smith M, Bassi C, et al. Working Party Report – Guidelines for the management of acute pancreatitis. J Gastroenterol Hepatol 2002(Suppl 17):S15–39.

UK Working Party on Acute Pancreatitis. UK guidelines for the management of acute pancreatitis. Gut 2005;54(Suppl III):iii1–9.

Whitcomb DC. Acute pancreatitis. N Engl J Med 2006;354:2142–50.

7.10 Acute appendicitis

Ashis Banerjee

ESSENTIALS

1 Appendicitis is the commonest cause of acute abdominal pain requiring surgical treatment.

2 The diagnosis is primarily clinical, but is often difficult to confirm in the absence of a pathognomonic sign or conclusive first-line diagnostic test.

3 Diagnostic delay is the primary cause for morbidity and mortality and is a major reason for litigation related to medical negligence in emergency departments.

4 Specialized imaging techniques enhance diagnostic accuracy and help reduce the negative laparotomy rate for suspected appendicitis.

5 Surgical management is indicated once the diagnosis is confirmed or strongly suspected, although there appears to be an increasingly well-defined role for non-operative management.

Aetiology, pathogenesis and pathology

In the majority of cases, bacterial or viral infection of the colon precedes mucosal ulceration of the appendix and subsequent secondary bacterial invasion by normal colonic flora. In a minority of cases, luminal obstruction is caused by faecoliths, lymphoid follicle hyperplasia, parasites, strictures, adhesions, foreign bodies, tumour (carcinoid or caecal carcinoma) or Crohn's disease. This is followed by increased intraluminal pressure and luminal distension, lymphatic and venous outflow obstruction, arterial inflow occlusion and bacterial overgrowth. Inflammation of the serosa leads to involvement of the parietal peritoneum. Appendiceal perforation may ensue secondary to a high intraluminal pressure.

Clinical features

Appendicitis is a clinical diagnosis, but the clinical presentation may be atypical or equivocal, requiring a period of active observation or recourse to cross-sectional imaging to confirm the suspicion. When evaluating any patient with acute abdominal pain in the emergency

Introduction

Appendicitis remains the commonest cause of acute abdominal pain requiring surgical intervention and is the commonest non-obstetrical surgical emergency in pregnancy. This is in spite of a steady decline in incidence in industrialized countries since the late 1940s, as measured by appendicectomy rates. The peak incidence is in the second and third decades of life. There is a male preponderance (male:female ratio of 1.4:1), with an overall incidence of around 1.9 per 1000 persons per year and an overall lifetime risk of developing appendicitis of 7%. Diagnostic delay is more common in infants and young children, women of reproductive age and the elderly. Early diagnosis is essential to avoid the risk of appendiceal perforation leading to intra-abdominal sepsis, abscess formation and/or generalized peritonitis.

department (ED), one of the focused questions that has to be asked is whether the presentation could be due to appendicitis.

History

The classic presentation of acute appendicitis is with upper midline or periumbilical pain (70%), which represents visceral midgut pain due to appendiceal distension, the afferent fibres being at T10 level. This progresses over a period of 12–24 hours to right lower quadrant pain (50%), which represents somatic pain caused by localized irritation of the parietal peritoneum. The migratory pattern of the pain is the most characteristic symptom of appendicitis.

Pain is associated with nausea, anorexia (often a prominent feature) and vomiting. Low-grade fever – typically 37.5–38.0°C – may be present. Once pain localizes in the right lower quadrant, it becomes persistent, is aggravated by movement, deep inspiration and coughing and tends to progress in severity. Pelvic appendicitis may present with irritative urinary symptoms (frequency of urination and dysuria) or with diarrhoea.

The typical presentation is associated with a retrocaecal or retrocolic position of the appendix. The intraperitoneal position of the appendix depends on the length of the viscus, relationship to the caecum and location of the ascending colon and caecum. Localization of pain may occur in atypical locations, such as the right upper quadrant or right flank with a high retrocaecal appendix (the most common atypical location), or the left lower quadrant with a pelvic appendix or in the presence of situs inversus. Right upper quadrant pain may also be seen in the uncommon event that acute appendicitis complicates pregnancy (on average one per 1000 pregnancies).

Symptoms continuing longer than 72 hours make the diagnosis of appendicitis unlikely unless a mass has developed.

Examination

Examination findings vary according to the stage of evolution. Vital signs may be normal, but a mild tachycardia is usual along with low-grade fever. There may be some facial flushing, fetor oris and a dry, coated tongue.

Typically, there is localized tenderness in the right lower quadrant, classically maximal at McBurney's point (two-thirds of the way from the umbilicus to the anterior superior iliac spine). This is accompanied by reduction in respiratory movement and by involuntary muscle rigidity (guarding). Rigidity may be difficult to elicit in the obese, the elderly, children and in the presence of atypical locations. Attempted demonstration of rebound tenderness is unkind. The same information can be obtained by noting aggravation of pain by deep inspiration or forced expiration (drawing in or blowing out the abdominal wall), with coughing or by percussion of the anterior abdominal wall. Right lower quadrant pain may be provoked by pressure on the left lower quadrant (Rovsing's sign) and there may be accompanying hyperaesthesia of the overlying skin (Sherren's sign).

Unfortunately, the classic constellation of symptoms and signs is seen in only 50–70% of patients with acute appendicitis. Ancillary clinical signs may be of value in arriving at a diagnosis in patients with atypical symptoms, usually related to atypical locations of the tip.

Psoas muscle irritation, caused by a retrocaecal appendix, may be associated with a flexion deformity of the right hip. A positive psoas sign refers to pain with, and resistance to, passive extension of the right hip with the patient in the left lateral position. This has high specificity but low sensitivity. Irritation of the obturator internus muscle, caused by a pelvic appendix, may be associated with a positive obturator sign (pain on passive internal rotation of the flexed right hip). An abdominal mass may be palpable in 10–15% of cases. This represents inflamed omentum and adherent bowel loops in the presence of appendiceal perforation. An appendicectomy scar does not totally exclude the possibility of appendicitis, as recurrent appendicitis in the stump has been reported after both open and laparoscopic appendicectomy.

In most cases, rectal examination in patients with suspected appendicitis is of little value and does not alter management. It may be helpful when the diagnosis is in doubt, particularly in the elderly, when tenderness may be elicited in the right lateral wall of the rectum. Rectal examination may also help diagnose a pelvic abscess in the presence of a ruptured pelvic appendix.

Perforation of the appendix should be suspected in the presence of symptoms of over 24 hours' duration, a temperature higher than 38°C and possibly a white cell count >15 000 cells/mm^3.

Differential diagnosis

Appendicitis can mimic most acute abdominal conditions and should be considered in any

Table 7.10.1 Differential diagnosis
Non-specific abdominal pain
Female genital tract: pelvic inflammatory disease; ruptured tubal gestation; ovarian cyst accident; ovarian follicle rupture
Small intestine: Meckel's diverticulitis; Crohn's disease; ileitis
Colon: caecal carcinoma; caecal diverticulitis; ileocaecal tuberculosis; *Campylobacter* colitis
Renal tract: acute pyelonephritis; ureteric colic
Lymph nodes: mesenteric lymphadenitis
Referred testicular pain

patient with acute symptoms referable to the abdomen. There is a wide range of conditions that may resemble appendicitis (Table 7.10.1). On occasion, the diagnosis of appendicitis may only be confirmed at surgery or laparoscopy; however, there is a 10–20% negative laparotomy rate associated with a preoperative diagnosis of appendicitis. Diagnostic delay can be associated with perforation, progression to abscess formation or to generalized peritonitis. These complications can contribute to wound infection, septicaemia and death.

Clinical investigations

Urinalysis

A urine dipstick examination should be performed in all patients to exclude urinary tract infection, but pyuria and microscopic haematuria can coexist with appendicitis. Qualitative β-hCG testing should be performed in all women of childbearing age in order to exclude pregnancy and the possibility of ectopic gestation.

Blood tests

The white cell count lacks sufficient sensitivity and specificity for the diagnosis of appendicitis. A raised white cell count can also be seen with other causes of an acute surgical abdomen. A raised white cell count is a poor prognostic predictor, lacking correlation with gangrene and perforation. Undue reliance on the white cell count may lead to delays in definitive treatment and a higher perforation rate.

C-reactive protein (CRP) measurement is of no diagnostic value in excluding the diagnosis of appendicitis. It would, however, appear that raised white cell count and CRP add weight to an already highly likely diagnosis of appendicitis and some data suggest that appendicitis is unlikely if both investigations are normal. CRP levels correlate with severity of appendicitis as determined by computed tomography (CT) scanning and could be a useful predictor for appendiceal perforation.

Imaging

Plain abdominal radiography rarely provides helpful information in the work-up of clinical appendicitis and is not indicated, having a low sensitivity and specificity, as well as being frequently misleading. If an X-ray has been inadvertently obtained, the presence of a faecolith in the right lower quadrant may favour a diagnosis of appendicitis.

The normal appendix is visualized in less than 50% of cases at ultrasound scanning, using a 5 or 7.5 MHz transducer with a graded compression technique to displace mobile small bowel loops. If seen, it appears as a hypoechoic tubular structure in continuity with the caecum and has a diameter of <6 mm when compressed with the examining probe. Visualization of a normal appendix excludes appendicitis. Ultrasound signs of acute appendicitis include a non-compressible appendix >6 mm in diameter (measured outer wall to outer wall), >2 mm wall thickness and visualization of an appendicolith. With perforation, a loculated pericaecal fluid collection, a discontinuous wall of the appendix and prominent pericaecal fat are seen. Graded compression ultrasonography may be particularly useful in the presence of atypical presentations. In one study, it had pooled sensitivity and specificity of 88% and 94%, respectively, for the diagnosis of appendicitis in children. It can also potentially identify other pathologies, especially in female patients. Ultrasound is, however, highly operator dependent, relying on skill and experience. Focused bedside ultrasound for evaluation of the appendix is an evolving option, with one study reporting sensitivity of 67%, specificity of 92% and overall accuracy of 80% for the diagnosis of acute appendicitis.

Helical CT is primarily of benefit in equivocal cases. CT signs of appendicitis include distension >6 mm, circumferential thickening of the wall, periappendiceal inflammation (hazy, streaky linear densities), oedema and mass and visualization of an appendicolith. Contrast enhancement can be achieved by the intravenous, oral or rectal routes. Improved diagnostic accuracy with intravenous contrast material

has been reported. Sensitivity and specificity of 98% have been reported. The cost of CT scanning can be offset against the cost savings accruing from reduced rates of hospital admission and of negative laparotomy. Compared to ultrasonography, CT has been reported to have superior accuracy for appendicitis in all reported studies. This must be weighed against radiation exposure, availability and the diagnoses under consideration when selecting the preferred test for an individual patient.

A role has more recently been shown for magnetic resonance imaging (MRI) in the diagnosis of acute appendicitis in the pregnant woman, with one study of 51 patients reporting sensitivity of 100% and specificity of 93.6%. The main MRI sign of acute appendicitis is an enlarged fluid-filled appendix >7 mm in diameter.

Clinical decision tools

Several tools have been described to assist clinical diagnosis. The best known of these is the 10-point Alvarado score for acute appendicitis, also known as the MANTRELS criteria (Table 7.10.2). These criteria were derived from a retrospective study of hospitalized patients with possible acute appendicitis, but have been applied to ED practice. The score was developed as a guide to determine the need for further investigation and to help decide on the need for laparotomy. Diagnostic accuracy may be improved by combining the score with ultrasonography.

Ultimately, improving diagnostic accuracy for appendicitis remains a challenge. A large population-based study concluded that the introduction of CT, ultrasonography and laparoscopy had not led to improved diagnostic accuracy. However, more recent studies have shown that CT scanning has been shown to reduce negative appendicectomy rates.

Treatment

Analgesia, usually small doses of intravenous opioids titrated to the patient's response, should be given as required, even before the diagnosis is confirmed. There is no evidence that the provision of adequate analgesia is associated with delayed diagnosis, as positive abdominal signs related to peritoneal irritation are not eliminated. Intravenous hydration should also be initiated.

The definitive treatment for appendicitis remains appendicectomy, which may be open or laparoscopic. Laparoscopy is being

Table 7.10.2 Alvarado score (MANTRELS criteria)

Criterion	Point(s)
Symptoms	
M migration of pain to RLQ	1
A anorexia	1
N nausea and vomiting	1
Signs	
T tenderness in RLQ	2
R rebound pain	1
E elevated temperature	1
Laboratory findings	
L leucocytosis	2
S shift of WBCs to left	1
Total score (out of)	10
Interpretation	
1–4	Appendicitis unlikely
5–6	Appendicitis possible
7–8	Probable appendicitis
9–10	Surgery indicated

increasingly preferred, as it allows for combined diagnosis and treatment, as well as the recognition and potential treatment of alternative diagnostic conditions. There is an increase in operative time, but a reduction in postoperative analgesia requirements and length of inpatient stay, as well as earlier return to work. Broad-spectrum antimicrobial agents, when given preoperatively or intraoperatively, reduce the incidence of postoperative wound infection and intra-abdominal abscess.

Conservative management (intravenous hydration and broad-spectrum antimicrobial therapy) may be preferred in the presence of an appendix mass (a surgical decision) or in difficult circumstances when surgical help is not readily available, such as remote locations or while at sea. There is an increasing recognition of the potential role of conservative management for uncomplicated appendicitis, typically using antimicrobial therapy with amoxicillin and clavulanic acid, in high-risk patients with significant co-morbidities and increased anaesthetic risk and at extremes of age.

Although a negative laparotomy rate of around 15–20% has been accepted in the past, it must be remembered that a negative laparotomy is associated with a more prolonged stay, higher complication rate and measurable mortality. Reducing this remains a major diagnostic challenge.

Acute appendicitis in pregnancy

Acute appendicitis is the commonest non-obstetric reason for laparotomy in the pregnant woman, occurring in about 1 in 1000 pregnancies. Symptoms of appendicitis are similar to those in the non-pregnant state but, in late pregnancy, the site of tenderness tends to be higher and more lateral. The incidence of perforation is higher. Fetal loss as a result of appendicitis and laparotomy may be as high as 20%.

Likely developments over the next 5–10 years

- Enhanced clinical decision support tools, in combination with selective cross-sectional

imaging, to aid in early definitive diagnosis of appendicitis.
- Portable bedside ultrasound for appendix visualization as part of the emergency physician's repertoire.
- Continued reduction in the negative laparotomy rate to 5% or less.
- Recognition of the role of conservative management of acute appendicitis.

Controversies

- An enhanced role for cross-sectional imaging, including ultrasound, CT and MRI, in confirming the diagnosis in equivocal cases, reducing unnecessary hospital admission and negative laparotomy.
- The role of conservative management of uncomplicated acute appendicitis.
- The role of laparoscopy in diagnosis and treatment.

Further reading

Fox JC, Solley M, Zlidenny A, Anderson C. Bedside ultrasound for appendicitis. Acad Emerg Med 2005;12:76.

Frei SP, Bond WF, Bazuro RK, et al. Is early analgesia use associated with delayed diagnosis of appendicitis? Acad Emerg Med 2005;12:18.

Gupta R, Gernsheimer J, Golden J, et al. Abdominal pain secondary to stump appendicitis in a child. J Emerg Med 2000;18:431–3.

Guttman R, Goldman RR, Koren G. Appendicitis during pregnancy. Can Fam Phys 2004;50:355–7.

Kim HC, Yang DM, Lee CM, et al. Acute appendicitis: relationships between CT-determined severities and serum white blood cell counts and C-reactive protein level. Br J Radiol 2011;84:1115–20.

Mariadason JG, Wang WN, Wallack MK, et al. Negative appendicectomy rate as a quality metric in the management of appendicitis: impact of computed tomography, Alvarado score and the definition of negative appendicetomy. Ann Roy Coll Surg Engl 2012;94:395–401.

Pedrosa I, Levine AD, Eyvazzadeh B, et al. MR imaging evaluation of acute appendicitis in pregnancy. Radiology 2006;238:891–9.

Valdeboncoeur TE, Heister RR, Behling CA, Gass DA. Impact of helical computed tomography on the rate of negative appendicitis. Am J Emerg Med 2006;24:43–7.

van Randen A, Bipat S, Zwinderman AH, et al. Acute appendicitis: meta-analysis of diagnostic performance of CT and graded compression US related to prevalence of disease. Radiology 2008;249:97–108.

Varadhan KK, Neal KR, Lobo DN. Safety and efficacy of antibiotics compared with appendicectomy for treatment of uncomplicated acute appendicitis: meta-analysis of randomized controlled trials. Br Med J 2012;344:14.

7.11 Inflammatory bowel disease

Kim Yates • Louise Finnel

ESSENTIALS

1 The two major forms of inflammatory bowel disease are Crohn's disease and ulcerative colitis. The principal clinical features are diarrhoea and/or abdominal pain.

2 Inflammatory bowel disease is a chronic and relapsing condition. Patients may present to the emergency department with increased disease activity or with complications of the disease process or treatment.

3 Gastrointestinal complications may include dehydration, bleeding, strictures, obstruction, fistulae, sepsis, perforation, neoplasia and toxic megacolon.

4 Acute arthropathy and rashes are the most common extraintestinal manifestations of inflammatory bowel disease.

5 Complications relating to medications may include opportunistic infections in those on corticosteroids, immunomodulators or biological agents.

6 Patients with moderate or severe inflammatory bowel disease require admission to hospital. Most patients are managed initially with medical therapy, such as aminosalicylates and/or corticosteroids, but those with intra-abdominal sepsis, perforation, obstruction or toxic megacolon are likely to require emergency surgery.

Introduction and pathology

Inflammatory bowel disease (IBD) classically refers to Crohn's disease and ulcerative colitis (UC). Both are chronic inflammatory diseases of the gastrointestinal (GI) tract which result from an inappropriate and continuing inflammatory response to commensal microbes and/or environmental factors in a genetically susceptible host. Pathologically, the two major forms of IBD differ. Crohn's disease is a patchy transmural inflammation which can affect any part of the gastrointestinal tract, with ileocolonic disease being most common. It is associated with fistulae, abscesses, strictures and obstruction. In contrast, UC is a continuous, diffuse, colonic mucosal inflammation, often associated with bleeding. Clinical features vary depending on the form and anatomic distribution of the disease. Classification of IBD has changed over the years and newer systems, such as the

Montreal classification, incorporate clinical and endoscopic features that can help select therapy and predict outcome. When assessing patients who present to the emergency department (ED) with known or suspected IBD, assessing disease activity and identifying potentially serious complications of the disease and its treatments are equally important.

Clinical features

History

Bloody diarrhoea is a cardinal symptom of UC and can be associated with colicky abdominal pain, urgency and tenesmus. In Crohn's disease, abdominal pain and anal complaints including fissures, along with diarrhoea without rectal bleeding and weight loss are more common. Abdominal pain in Crohn's disease is commonly right-sided and worse with eating. In UC, pain is less frequent and usually crampy, lower abdominal and relieved by passing a motion. If pain is more severe, other GI complications should be considered.

A search for symptoms and signs of extraintestinal manifestations and past surgical procedures is helpful. Acute arthropathy and rashes are common extraintestinal manifestations of IBD, but thromboembolic, ocular and hepatobiliary complications can be more serious and require specific therapy.

A careful drug history is essential as treatments, such as aminosalicylates, steroids, immunosuppressants (such as methotrexate or azathioprine) and biological agents (such as infliximab), can cause complications. In patients taking immunosuppressants and/or biological agents, symptoms and signs of sepsis and opportunistic infections, such as tuberculosis, should be sought. Patients on biological treatments also have increased risk of hypersensitivity reactions, cancers, such as lymphoma, demyelinating disease and worsening of congestive cardiac failure.

Enquiry about smoking is particularly important in Crohn's disease as smoking increases the risk of relapse.

Examination

Abdominal examination usually reveals a mildly tender abdomen without signs of peritonism. Evidence of dehydration or sepsis should be sought.

The presence of fever, dehydration, orthostatic hypotension, abdominal tenderness, distension and hypoactive bowel sounds suggests fulminant colitis. Abdominal distension raises the question of fulminant colitis, toxic megacolon or obstruction. Toxic megacolon (colonic dilatation with severe colitis) is potentially lethal but uncommon. Rectal examination may show anal fissures, abscesses or fistulae (more common in Crohn's disease).

Severity assessment

Factors to consider when gauging Crohn's disease activity are stool frequency, abdominal pain, general well-being, antidiarrhoeal use, fever, presence of complications, abdominal masses, anaemia and weight loss. Severe UC is defined by Truelove and Witts' criteria as 6 or more bloody stools daily, pulse greater than 90 per minute, fever higher than 37.8°C, anaemia less than 10.5 g/dL and erythrocyte sedimentation rate (ESR) more than 30 mm/h. The Mayo Score (UC symptom score) comprises four factors, namely, stool frequency, amount of rectal bleeding, findings at endoscopy and physician's global assessment. Each feature is scored (0–3) with higher scores indicating more severe disease.

Toxic megacolon (toxic colitis)

Toxic megacolon has the features of non-obstructive colonic distension coupled with evidence of sepsis. Dilatation can be segmental or total. It should be noted that colonic dilatation and sepsis can occur without the presence of the other feature. While originally thought to be only a complication of UC, it is now recognized to occur with other severe colitis including inflammatory, ischaemic, infectious, post-radiation and pseudomembranous colitisies.

Diagnostic criteria for toxic megacolon include:

- radiographic evidence of non-obstructive colonic dilatation (diameter >5.5 cm, caecum >9 cm) and
- any three of fever >38.5°C, tachycardia >120 bpm, leucocytosis >10.5 × 10⁹/L or anaemia and
- any one of dehydration, altered mental state, electrolyte abnormality or hypotension.

Investigation

Blood tests

A full blood count to quantify anaemia and determine the need for transfusion is helpful. Leucocytosis may be present in acute disease, but leucopaenia may be seen in patients on immunosuppressants. ESR and C-reactive protein are frequently used to monitor inflammation. Electrolytes and renal function may be abnormal in dehydration. Iron, folate and vitamin B12 deficiencies and hypoalbuminaemia are common in IBD. Disturbed liver function tests and/or raised amylase/lipase suggest hepatobiliary complications or drug toxicity.

Faecal culture

Faecal cultures should be tested for *Clostridium difficile* toxin as well as standard cultures as *C. difficile* infection has a higher prevalence in patients with IBD and is associated with increased mortality. Cytomegalovirus (CMV) testing should be performed in severe colitis, particularly when patients are on immunosuppressants as CMV colitis is associated with poor outcome. Both of these conditions would require specific therapy.

Imaging studies

On acute presentation, particularly with abdominal pain, abdominal and chest X-rays looking for free gas with perforation, dilated bowel loops and air–fluid levels with obstruction or dilated colon with toxic megacolon (diameter >5.5 cm, caecum >9 cm) may be helpful depending on clinical features (Figs 7.11.1 and 7.11.2). A chest X-ray can be useful in patients on immunosuppressants when considering complications, such as opportunistic infection or malignancy.

Concerns about cumulative diagnostic radiation exposure mean that magnetic resonance

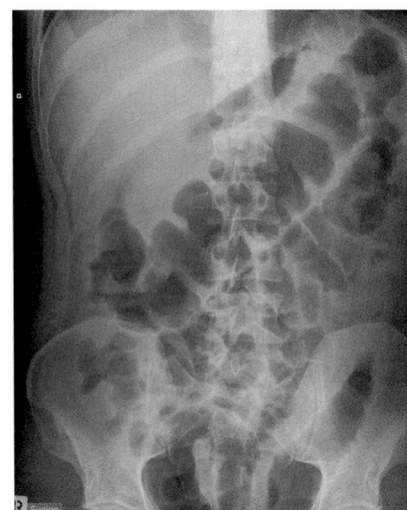

Fig. 7.11.1 Abdominal X-ray in toxic megacolon showing marked oedema.

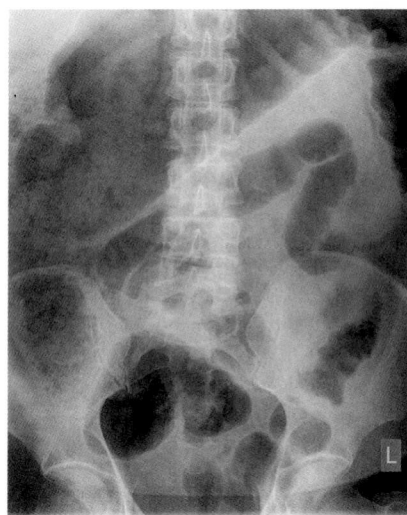

Fig. 7.11.2 Abdominal X-ray in toxic megacolon showing grossly dilated colon.

imaging (MRI) is being used more for diagnosis of disease and complications, particularly in younger patients with Crohn's disease, but availability is an issue. Computed tomography (CT) is more readily available and plays an important role when acute complications, such as obstruction or sepsis, are suspected. Ultrasound can be useful when considering complications of IBD, such as gallstones or kidney stones. Barium studies are used infrequently now.

Endoscopy

Endoscopy is useful for diagnosing IBD, for staging activity and in screening for strictures or cancer. Cautious sigmoidoscopy is safe in the acutely unwell patient, but colonoscopy carries a risk of perforation. The role of wireless video capsule endoscopy is unclear.

Gastrointestinal complications

A life-threatening GI complication of UC is toxic megacolon (toxic colitis), which usually develops in the presence of fulminating disease. Bowel perforation can also occur in patients with fulminant UC, even in the absence of toxic megacolon.

Strictures can cause subacute or acute bowel obstruction, while ulcers present throughout the GI tract have the potential to haemorrhage. Fistulae and abscesses are more common in Crohn's disease, but can occur in up to 20% of patients with UC. Fistulae types include enterovesical (leading to recurrent urinary tract infections and pneumaturia), enteroenteric, enteromesenteric, enterocutaneous, rectovaginal and perianal. Patients with UC and Crohn's disease are also prone to superimposed infectious colitis, such as with *Clostridium difficile*.

Patients with UC have a 10–30-fold increased chance of developing colon cancer, with this risk increasing with extent and duration of disease. Crohn's patients with pancolitis may have the same risk of neoplastic development.

Treatment

General management and disposition

In the ED, detection and treatment of life-threatening conditions, such as septic or hypovolaemic shock, severe anaemia or dehydration, are the priorities. Thereafter, assessment and treatment focuses on disease activity/severity and the presence of complications. Intravenous fluid therapy, correction of electrolytes and/or transfusion may be necessary. For abdominal pain, appropriate analgesia should be provided. Opiates should be used with caution in severe colitis as it has been suggested that toxic megacolon may be precipitated, but tramadol is thought to have less effect on motility. Non-selective non-steroidal anti-inflammatory drugs (NSAIDs) may exacerbate IBD. Selective NSAIDs, such as celicoxib, may not exacerbate IBD but carry other risks. Smokers with Crohn's disease should be given cessation advice as cessation reduces relapse rate.

If toxic megacolon is suspected, nasogastric drainage, intravenous steroids and other medical therapy as discussed below should be commenced and gastroenterology and surgical advice sought. Complications requiring surgery, such as bowel obstruction, intra-abdominal sepsis or perforation, should be ruled out early.

Patients with moderate or severe IBD require admission, usually for a trial of medical therapy. Surgical admission is indicated for perforation, obstruction, intra-abdominal sepsis or toxic megacolon. Treatment for IBD is usually a stepwise approach depending on severity of disease and response to treatment, some of which may need to be initiated in the ED. Patients with mild IBD and no complications can be managed as outpatients, with gastroenterology follow up.

Medical therapy

Vitamin and mineral deficits should be sought and treated, but nutritional therapies, such as probiotics, appear helpful for maintaining remission only in UC.

Aminosalicylates (sulfasalazine, 5ASA/mesalamine) come in topical and oral forms and are most effective in maintaining remission in UC, but may be useful in small-bowel Crohn's disease.

Ciprofloxacin appears more effective than metronidazole in treating perianal Crohn's disease and pouchitis. Infective causes of diarrhoea or colitis will require specific therapy. For *C. difficile* colitis, metronidazole or vancomycin are first-line therapies and, for CMV colitis, antivirals, such as ganciclovir, are indicated.

Corticosteroids induce remission of IBD but are not useful as maintenance therapy. There is no evidence to support particular regimens, but a common approach is oral prednisone 40 mg/day for 1 week then weaned over 8 weeks. Oral prednisone is more effective at inducing remission in mild to moderate UC than aminosalicylates alone and is even more effective when combined with rectal steroids. Rectal steroids are effective in mild distal UC when used with oral aminosalicylates. Budesonide, which has low bioavailability and fewer systemic side effects, is an alternative to prednisone therapy. In the ED, if intravenous steroid is necessary to treat acute severe IBD, hydrocortisone 100 mg every 6 hours can be used until oral therapy is tolerated. In acute severe UC, which can be difficult to distinguish from infective colitis, commence steroids with antibiotic cover until stool microbiology is available.

Thiopurine immunosuppressants, such as azathioprine and 6-mercaptopurine, are used as steroid-sparing agents or in steroid-resistant disease, but allergic reactions, bone marrow suppression, pancreatitis, hepatotoxicity and skin cancers can be problems. Methotrexate is effective in Crohn's disease for induction and maintenance of remission. Cyclosporin may be useful in refractory UC as salvage therapy.

Biological therapies are antitumour necrosis factor (antiTNF) antibodies (e.g. infliximab or adalimumab) and have been shown to be effective for severe, refractory and/or fistulating Crohn's disease. Infliximab appears effective for severe or refractory UC. Antidiarrhoeal agents may be useful for symptom control of mild disease.

Surgical therapy

Indications for surgery in IBD include fulminant colitis, toxic megacolon, perforation, severe GI haemorrhage, intractable IBD, stricture with obstruction, abscesses, fistulae or cancer. In patients with fulminant colitis or toxic mega-colon who do not respond to medical therapy or deteriorate, subtotal colectomy is indicated. Intra-abdominal abscesses, more common in Crohn's disease, can be drained percutaneously using CT or ultrasound guidance but may require laparotomy.

In UC, proctocolectomy is curative; however, subtotal procedures and anastomoses are often performed when disease is limited or when patients wish to avoid a stoma. As Crohn's disease has a high recurrence rate after seg-mental resection, surgery is conservative to preserve bowel length and function.

Prognosis

IBD is characterized by exacerbation and remis-sion. With modern medical and surgical man-agement, overall mortality is only slightly higher than the normal population in the 2 years after diagnosis for both major forms. Severe colitis in UC is potentially life threatening but, overall, Crohn's disease tends to cause greater disabil-ity than UC. IBD with colitis is associated with an increased risk of colonic cancer.

Controversies

- Causes of IBD. Numerous triggers for IBD in the genetically susceptible have been postulated. Pathological interaction of the immune system and gut microbial flora are the basis for the chronic inflammation. Controversial data exist on whether *Mycobacterium paratuberuclosis* or measles infection or high sugar or fat diets increase

prevalence. Although the mechanism is unknown, smoking and appendicectomy appear protective for UC, but are risk factors for Crohn's disease. It is not clear which variables accurately predict clinical relapse in UC.
- Medical therapies. Methotrexate is effective for inducing remission or reducing relapse in Crohn's disease but, owing to toxicity concerns (pneumonitis or hepatotoxicity), is reserved for refractory disease or where azathioprine or 6-mercaptopurine are not tolerated. Salvage therapy with cyclosporin or tacrolimus is limited by the gamut of associated adverse effects (neurotoxicity, gastrointestinal, drug interactions, nephrotoxicity) and long-term failure rate. Other experimental therapies under investigation in UC include alicaforsen, rituximab, probiotics, cytokine inhibitors, golimumab and macrophage inhibitors.
- Biological agents and IBD. There is debate about the use of antiTNF agents including duration of treatment and whether to use them as monotherapy or in combination with immunosuppressants. Use of natalizumab is associated with increased development of progressive multifocal encephalopathy. The long-term safety profile of the antiTNF agents is as yet unknown. Clinical outcomes and quality of life have improved with the advent of the biological agents, but the frequency of surgery required for patients with IBD has only slightly decreased.
- Cancer and IBD. It may be that the same gut microbiota associated with chronic inflammation in IBD can trigger neoplastic transformation, which has major implications for further research. IBD patients with colitis have increased

risk of colorectal cancer and there is debate about the best surveillance strategies, but surveillance guidelines recommend more frequent colonoscopy in higher-risk patients.
- Psychological co-morbidities and support. Up to 60% of IBD patients with relapses suffer anxiety or depression. Antidepressant therapy is common and animal studies suggest a role in reducing inflammation in IBD. Stress may be involved in triggering relapses of IBD by an unknown mechanism. It is unclear whether psychological supports improve the course of IBD, but do improve quality of life.

Further reading

Ahluwalia JP. Immunotherapy in inflammatory bowel disease. Med Clin N Am 2012;96:525–44.

Blonski W, Buchner AM, Lichtenstein GR. Clinical predictors of aggressive/disabling disease: ulcerative colitis and Crohn disease. Gastroenterol Clin N Am 2012;41:443–62.

Cohen R, Stein A. Approach to adults with steroid refractory and steroid-dependent ulcerative colitis. In: UpToDate. Waltham: Wolters Kluwer; 2012 <www.uptodate.com>.

Engel MA, Neurath MF. New pathophysiological insights and modern treatment of IBD. J Gastroenterol 2010;45: 571–83.

Fiocchi C. IBD: advances in pathogenesis, complications, diagnosis, and therapy. Curr Opin Gastroenterol 2012;28:297–300.

Khan KJ, Ullman TA, Ford AC, et al. Antibiotic therapy in inflammatory bowel disease: a systematic review and meta-analysis. Am J Gastroenterol 2011;106:661–73.

Khor B, Gardet A, Xavier RJ. Genetics and pathogenesis of inflammatory bowel disease. Nature 2011;474:307–17.

Larsen S, Bendtzen K, Nielsen OH. Extraintestinal manifestations of inflammatory bowel disease: epidemiology, diagnosis, and management. Ann Med 2010;42:97–114.

Mikocka-Walus AA, Turnbull D, Holtmann G, Andrews JM. An integrated model of care for inflammatory bowel disease sufferers in Australia: development and the effects of its implementation. Inflamm Bowel Dis 2012;18:1573–81.

Mowat C, Cole A, Windsor A, et al. Guidelines for the management of inflammatory bowel disease in adults. Gut 2011;60: 571–607.

Strong SA. Inflammatory bowel disease surgery in the biologic therapy era. Curr Opin Gastroenterol 2012;28:349–53.

Vermeire S, Van Assche G, Rutgeerts P. Classification of inflammatory bowel disease: the old and the new. Curr Opin Gastroenterol 2012;28:321–6.

7.12 Acute liver failure

Abel Wakai • John M Ryan

ESSENTIALS

1 The diagnosis of acute liver failure is based on the presence of increasing coagulopathy, hepatic encephalopathy and deepening jaundice.

2 In developing countries, viral causes predominate, with hepatitis E infection recognized as a common cause in many countries.

3 In developed countries, drug-induced liver injury predominates, often from paracetamol.

4 Diagnosis of ALF must be considered in anyone presenting with the recent onset of hepatic illness associated with prolonged prothrombin time/international normalized ratio (INR).

5 Early diagnosis is important because of the therapeutic option of using antidotes in the presence of a reversible cause.

6 The general principles of care include standard intensive care with additional specific measures aimed at identification and removal or amelioration of the insult that caused hepatic injury. Organ-system support is used to achieve maximum hepatic regeneration, to return to premorbid hepatic function while potential complications are anticipated and prevented.

7 Outcomes have been improved by use of emergency liver transplantation.

8 Public health measures to control patterns of drug use (drug-induced liver injury) and to reduce the incidence of hepatotropic virus infections potentially may significantly reduce the associated morbidity and mortality in future.

Introduction

Acute liver failure (ALF) remains one of the most challenging medical emergencies. It is a rare condition in which rapid deterioration of liver function results in altered mentation and coagulopathy in previously normal individuals. The overall incidence in developed countries is between one and six cases per million people every year. The most prominent causes include viral hepatitis, drug-induced liver injury, autoimmune liver disease and shock or hypoperfusion; many cases ($\approx$20%) have no discernible cause. ALF often affects young persons and carries a high morbidity and mortality. In many countries, it is the most frequent indication for emergency liver transplantation. Prior to the availability of transplantation, mortality of ALF was extremely high, often exceeding

90%; most common causes of death were multiorgan failure, haemorrhage, infection and cerebral oedema. Currently, 1-year survival exceeds 80%. Because of its rarity, ALF has been difficult to study in depth and very few controlled therapy trials have been performed. ALF research has been limited to a handful of large units or to collaborative networks, such as the National Institutes of Health (NIH)-sponsored US Acute Liver Failure Study Group (ALFSG).

Aetiology, pathogenesis and pathology

ALF occurs when the rate of hepatocyte death exceeds the rate of hepatocyte regeneration as a result of various insults that lead

to a combination of apoptosis or necrosis. Apoptosis is associated with nuclear shrinkage but without cell membrane rupture. Therefore, there is no release of intracellular content and no subsequent secondary inflammation. In contrast, necrosis is associated with ATP depletion resulting in a swollen cell that eventually lyses with the release of intracellular content associated with secondary inflammation. Most causes of ALF result in either apoptosis or necrosis; for example, paracetamol toxicity results in apoptosis and ischaemia results in necrosis. The clinical result of the cellular damage is a catastrophic illness that can lead rapidly to coma and death caused by multiorgan failure.

Epidemiology

There is significant worldwide variation in the cause of ALF. It is relatively uncommon in the UK, causing fewer than 500 deaths and being responsible for less than 15% of liver transplantations per annum (less than 100 transplants per year). Meanwhile, ALF affects approximately 2000 people per year in the USA. Although ALF accounts for approximately 7% of all liver transplantations annually in the USA, it accounts for more than two-thirds of transplantations in the Far East.

Drug-induced injury is the second main cause of acute liver failure and predominates in much of the developed world. Paracetamol poisoning is the commonest cause of ALF in the UK and the USA, causing up to 70% of cases in the UK and 51% of cases in the USA. Up to 10% of cases of paracetamol self-poisoning develop severe liver damage, but less than 2% go on to develop ALF, the worst outcomes being in patients with concurrent alcohol use.

Other major causes of ALF in the USA include idiosyncratic drug reactions (13%), secondary to hepatitis B (HBV; 8%) and secondary to hepatitis C (HCV; 4%). Thirteen per cent of ALF cases in the USA are of indeterminate cause. A small number of ALF cases in the USA result from miscellaneous causes, such as Wilson's disease, ischaemia, pregnancy-related, autoimmune disease and Budd–Chiari syndrome.

In the UK, approximately 5% of ALF cases were caused by non-paracetamol drugs, such as antituberculous therapy, anticonvulsants, steroids, non-steroidal anti-inflammatory medications, herbal remedies and recreational drugs (e.g. Ecstasy and cocaine). Less than 0.05% of cases of acute hepatitis A and B lead to ALF, with these viruses contributing less than 5% of all ALF cases. Seronegative (non-A–E) hepatitis, a diagnosis of exclusion, is the commonest presumed viral cause in the UK and other Western countries but contributes less than 10% of all ALF cases. In the UK, unusual viral causes include herpes simplex, Epstein–Barr, cytomegalovirus, and varicella zoster. Small numbers of ALF cases in the UK resulted from miscellaneous causes, such as pregnancy, Wilson's disease, Budd–Chiari syndrome, autoimmune hepatitis, ischaemic hepatitis and malignant infiltration.

While ALF is most commonly drug-induced in the West, in the developing world and Far East, it is most often caused by viral hepatitis. Particularly common causes are exacerbations of chronic HBV, which is endemic in many countries, including Hong Kong, and hepatitis E in India. Flares of chronic HBV may be spontaneous, represent a secondary response to increased levels of replicating wild-type or mutant virus, occur after immunosuppressive and cytotoxic therapy or occur following superinfection with other hepatotropic viruses, such as hepatitis D and HCV.

Prevention

Primary prevention of ALF in the West mainly involves strategies to combat increasing rates of paracetamol-induced ALF including legislation to reduce over-the-counter availability of paracetamol, printing specific warnings about overdose in the packets, use of paracetamol/methionine combination analgesics and promotion of alternative analgesics.

Secondary prevention of ALF involves immunization strategies. Hepatitis A and B vaccination is safe and immunogenic in patients with mild to moderate chronic liver disease (CLD), although vaccination is less effective in those with decompensated liver cirrhosis or after liver transplantation.

Clinical features

History taking should include careful review of possible exposures to viral infection and drugs or other toxins. If severe encephalopathy is present, a collateral history may be all that is available or a history may be unavailable. In this setting, limited information is available, particularly regarding possible toxin/drug ingestions.

Physical examination must include careful assessment and documentation of mental status and a search of stigmata of CLD. Jaundice is often but not invariably seen at presentation. Right upper quadrant tenderness is variably present. Inability to palpate the liver or even to percuss a significant area of dullness over the liver can be indicative of decreased liver volume due to massive hepatocyte loss. Hepatomegaly may be seen early in viral hepatitis or with malignant infiltration, congestive heart failure or acute Budd–Chiari syndrome. History or signs of cirrhosis should be absent as such features suggest underlying CLD, which may have different management implications.

Differential diagnosis

Common causes of ALF are hepatitis viruses or drugs (Table 7.12.1). In Western countries, drug-induced ALF predominates, comprising 19–75% of all cases of ALF. In India, 91–100% of ALF cases are due to viruses, with drug-induced cases responsible for 0–7.4%.

The developed world is particularly subject to rare ALF due to idiosyncratic drug-induced liver injury (DILI), because of the large quantity of drugs ingested. Idiosyncratic drug reactions account for 13% of cases of ALF in the USA and 5% of cases in the UK. Examples of causative drugs include antibiotics (amoxicillin–clavulanic acid, ciprofloxacin, doxycycline, erythromycin, isoniazid, nitrofurantoin, tetracycline, sulphonamides), antivirals (fialuridine), antidepressants (amitriptyline, nortriptyline), oral hypoglycaemic drugs (troglitazone, metformin), anticonvulsants (phenytoin, valproic acid), anaesthetics (halothane, isoflurane), statins (atorvastatin, lovastatin, simvastatin), immunosuppressants (cyclophosphamide, methotrexate, gold), non-steroidal anti-inflammatory drugs (NSAIDs), salicylates (Reye's syndrome), antithyroid drugs (propylthiouracil), antiarrhythmics (amiodarone) disulfiram and flutamide. The presentation

of DILI is more subacute, with lower aminotransferases and higher bilirubin levels. The likelihood of survival in this setting is less than 30% and they more often undergo liver transplantation.

Infectious diseases, such as falciparum malaria, typhoid fever, leptospirosis and dengue fever, may mimic ALF at presentation. They can present with fever, jaundice and features of encephalopathy and should be considered in all patients presenting with ALF, particularly in the tropics or in patients who have recently travelled in the tropics. Baseline routine clinical and laboratory investigations will provide supportive evidence of an infective cause. After reaching a definitive diagnosis, specific therapy for the infectious disease in addition to supportive therapy for ALF reduces mortality.

Clinical investigations

Initial laboratory investigation in the emergency department (ED) is aimed at evaluating both the aetiology and severity of ALF (Table 7.12.2).

Other urgent investigations, mainly aimed at evaluating the aetiology of ALF following hospital admission, include viral hepatitis serologies (anti-HAV IgM, HBSAg, anti-HBc IgM, anti-HEV IgM, anti-HCV IgM), autoimmune markers (antinuclear, antismooth muscle antibodies, immunoglobulin levels) and ceruloplasmin level. Plasma ammonia, preferably arterial, may also be helpful. A liver biopsy, most often done via the transjugular route because of coagulopathy, may be indicated when certain conditions, such as autoimmune hepatitis, metastatic liver disease, lymphoma or herpes simplex hepatitis, are suspected.

Other investigations may be required as clinically indicated. For example, determination of the HIV status for patients who are liver transplantation candidates.

Criteria for diagnosis

The diagnosis of ALF must be considered in anyone presenting with the recent onset of hepatic illness where the prothrombin time/international normalized ratio (INR) has become prolonged. The most widely accepted definition of ALF includes impairment of liver function with evidence of coagulation abnormality (usually an INR ≥1.5) and any degree of mental

Table 7.12.1	Differential diagnosis of ALF
Viruses	Hepatitis A and B viruses (typical viruses causing viral hepatitis) Hepatitis C virus (rare) Hepatitis D virus Hepatitis E virus (often in pregnant women in endemic areas) Cytomegalovirus Haemorrhagic fever viruses Herpes simplex virus Paramyxovirus Epstein–Barr virus
Drugs	Paracetamol hepatotoxicity Idiosyncratic hypersensitivity reactions (e.g. isoniazid, statins, halothane) Illicit drugs (e.g. Ecstasy, cocaine) Alternative medicines (e.g. chaparral and *Teucrium polium*) Traditional Chinese medicine
Toxins	Mushroom poisoning (usually *Amanita phalloides*) *Bacillus cereus* toxin Cyanobacteria toxin Organic solvents (e.g. carbon tetrachloride) Yellow phosphorus
Vasculopathy	Ischaemic hepatitis Hepatic vein thrombosis (Budd–Chiari syndrome) Hepatic veno-occlusive disease Portal vein thrombosis Hepatic arterial thrombosis
Metabolic	Acute fatty liver of pregnancy/HELLP (haemolysis, elevated liver enzymes, low platelets) syndrome α-1 antitrypsin deficiency Fructose intolerance Galactosaemia Lecithin-cholesterol acyltransferase deficiency Reye's syndrome Tyrosinaemia Wilson's disease
Autoimmune	Autoimmune hepatitis
Malignancy	Primary liver malignancy (hepatocellular carcinoma or cholangiocarcinoma) Secondary (e.g. extensive hepatic metastases or infiltration of adenocarcinoma)
Miscellaneous	Adult-onset Still's disease Heat stroke Primary graft non-function (in liver transplant recipients) Indeterminate aetiology (≈20% of ALF cases)

Table 7.12.2	Emergency department investigations for ALF	
Haematology	Full blood count Prothrombin time/INR Blood type and screen
Biochemistry	Liver function tests Urea and electrolytes Arterial blood gas Arterial lactate Arterial ammonia Glucose Calcium Magnesium Phosphate Amylase
Toxicology	Paracetamol level Toxicology screen
Urinalysis	hCG (females)
Imaging studies	Chest radiography Liver ultrasonography
Miscellaneous	Electrocardiogram

Table 7.12.3	Grades of hepatic encephalopathy
Grade 1	Drowsy but coherent, mood change
Grade 2	Drowsy, confused at times, inappropriate behaviour
Grade 3	Very drowsy and stuparose but rousable; alternatively restless, screaming
Grade 4	Comatose, barely rousable

alteration (encephalopathy; Table 7.12.3) in a patient without existing cirrhosis and with an illness of less than 26 weeks' duration. Patients with Wilson's disease, vertically-acquired HBV or autoimmune hepatitis may be included in spite of the possibility of cirrhosis if their disease has only been recognized for less than 26 weeks.

A number of other terms have been used including fulminant hepatic failure and fulminant hepatitis or necrosis. It is intuitively logical that acute liver failure is a better overall term that should encompass all durations up to 26 weeks. Terms used signifying length of illness, such as hyperacute (<7 days), acute (7–21 days) and subacute (>21 days and <26 weeks), are not particularly helpful since they do not have prognostic significance distinct from the cause of the illness.

Treatment

The backbone of management of the ALF patient is good coma care. The most important first step in the treatment of ALF is to identify the cause, since prognosis depends on the cause. Death in ALF is predominantly related to sepsis, multiorgan failure and intracranial hypertension. The circulatory disturbances in ALF, which contribute to the often-associated renal failure, are characterized by a generalized vasodilatation that results in increased cardiac output and reduced systemic vascular resistance and mean arterial pressure.

Emergency liver transplantation is the only proven therapeutic intervention for ALF. While treatments for specific aetiologies are also initiated, emergency management requires intensive care support, because rapid deterioration can occur. Careful attention must be paid to fluid management, haemodynamics and metabolic parameters as well as surveillance for and treatment of infection. Maintenance of nutrition and prompt recognition and resuscitation of gastrointestinal bleeding are crucial as well. Coagulation parameters, complete blood counts, metabolic panels (including glucose) and arterial blood gas should be checked frequently. Liver function tests (LFTs) are generally measured daily to follow the course of the condition, however, changes in aminotransferase levels correlate poorly with prognosis.

General measures

Fundamental to the management of patients with ALF is the provision of good intensive care support. Aggressive monitoring is required to detect respiratory and haemodynamic complications, neurological changes, infections and gastrointestinal haemorrhage. Airway protection and endotracheal intubation may be required because, as patients with ALF become comatose, their ability to protect their airway from aspiration is reduced. Central venous access and invasive and non-invasive arterial blood pressure monitoring are useful for monitoring vascular status. All patients should have a urinary catheter placed to monitor urine output. Volume resuscitation should ideally be with colloids and titrated to a pulmonary wedge pressure of 12–14 mmHg. Intravenous noradrenaline (norepinephrine) may be required for systemic hypotension. Metabolic derangements, such as hypoglycaemia, should be sought and treated aggressively. Hypokalaemia is common and should be managed with intravenous supplements. Intravenous phosphate and magnesium supplements may also be required. Platelets may be required if the count falls below 20 000/mL. H_2-receptor blockers are given for prophylaxis against gastrointestinal bleeding. Nasogastric tube insertion for stomach decompression may be required in comatose patients. Dialysis may be required for deteriorating renal function and worsening acidosis.

Maintaining adequate cerebral perfusion is paramount and the patient should be nursed in a quiet environment with 30° head-up tilt. Intracranial pressure monitoring may be helpful in some patients for directing therapy to prevent brainstem herniation.

Dietary protein withdrawal is commonly recommended to treat acute hepatic encephalopathy, although the traditional use of lactulose for enteral decontamination is now more controversial. Instead, other agents, such as metronidazole and neomycin, have been recommended to treat acute hepatic encephalopathy. Systemic antimicrobial therapy with or without enteral decontamination reduces infection rate in patients with acute liver failure.

Specific measures

N-acetylcysteine (NAC)
Several clinical trials support the use of NAC in ALF. In late-presenting paracetamol overdose, mortality and progression to grade III–IV encephalopathy is reduced in those receiving NAC.

Penicillin G and silibinin
Penicillin G and silibinin (silymarin or milk thistle) are accepted antidotes for mushroom poisoning (usually *Amanita phalloides*), despite no controlled trials proving their efficacy. While some reports have not found penicillin G to be helpful, enough efficacy has been reported to warrant consideration of the drug (given intravenously in doses of 300 000–1 million units/kg/day) in patients with known or suspected mushroom poisoning. Silibinin has generally been reported to be more successful than penicillin G, although penicillin G has been used more frequently. Silibinin/silymarin is not available as a licensed drug in the USA, although it is widely available in Europe and South America. When used for treatment of mushroom poisoning, silymarin has been given in average doses of 30–40 mg/kg/day (either intravenously or orally) for an average duration of 3–4 days.

Drug-induced hepatotoxicity
There are no specific antidotes for idiosyncratic drug reactions; corticosteroids are not indicated unless a drug hypersensitivity reaction is suspected. Current recommendations are: (1) obtain details (including onset of ingestion, amount and timing of last dose) concerning all prescription and non-prescription drugs, herbs and dietary supplement taken over the past year; (2) determine ingredients of non-prescription medications whenever possible; (3) in the setting of ALF due to possible drug hepatotoxicity, discontinue all but essential medications.

Lamivudine and nucleoside analogues
ALF due to reactivation of hepatitis B may occur in the setting of chemotherapy or immunosuppression. The nucleoside analogue, lamivudine (and possibly adefovir), used widely in the treatment of chronic hepatitis B, may be considered in patients with acute hepatitis B, although these dugs have not been subjected to a controlled trial in acute disease. It is currently recommended that nucleoside analogues be given prior to and continued for 6 months after completion of chemotherapy in patients with hepatitis B surface antigen positivity to prevent reactivation/acute flare of disease.

Acyclovir
Although herpes virus infection rarely causes ALF, immunosuppressed patients or pregnant women (usually in the third trimester) are at increased risk. In addition, occurrences of herpes virus ALF have been reported in previously healthy individuals. Meanwhile, other viruses, such as varicella zoster, have occasionally been implicated in causing hepatic failure. Patients with known or suspected herpes virus or varicella zoster as the cause of ALF should be treated with acyclovir.

Corticosteroids
Patients with autoimmune hepatitis may have unrecognized pre-existing chronic disease and yet still be considered as having ALF if their illness is of less than 26 weeks' duration. Such patients represent the most severe form of the disease and would generally fall into the category of patients recommended for corticosteroid therapy (prednisone 40–60 mg/day). Initiation of steroid therapy may constitute a therapeutic trial for some patients, although placement on the transplant list is indicated as, although some patients with ALF due to autoimmune hepatitis respond to steroid therapy, others require transplantation.

Cardiovascular support
In ALF patients with evidence of ischaemic injury, cardiovascular support is the treatment of choice. In such patients, the ability to manage heart failure or other causes of ischaemia (e.g. significant hypovolaemia) will determine outcome.

DIGESTIVE EMERGENCIES

Liver transplantation

Orthotopic liver transplantation (OLT) remains the only definitive therapy for patients who are unable to achieve regeneration of sufficient hepatocyte mass to sustain life. Urgent liver transplantation is indicated in ALF where prognostic indicators suggest a high likelihood of death. Post-transplant survival rates for ALF have been reported to be as high as 80–90%, but accurate long-term outcome data are not yet available.

Patients with ALF secondary to the following causes should be listed for transplantation: mushroom poisoning, Wilson's disease, autoimmune hepatitis and hepatic vein thrombosis (provided underlying malignancy is excluded). In such patients, initial laboratory investigations should include determination of their HIV status, because it has implications for potential liver transplantation. Early liaison with a liver transplantation unit is mandatory and any contraindications to transplantation should be identified with collateral histories through the family, friends and primary care physicians, if necessary. Planning for transfer to a transplant centre should begin in patients with grade I or II encephalopathy (see Table 7.12.3) because they may worsen rapidly. Early transfer is important as the risks involved with patient transport may increase or even preclude transfer once stage III and IV encephalopathy develops.

'Bridging options'

The aim of bridging devices is to provide adequate liver function and maintain the patient well enough until recovery of native liver function occurs or until a graft is found. In one study, only 29% of patients listed for liver transplantation received a liver graft, while 10% of the overall group (one-quarter of patients listed for transplantation) died on the waiting list. Other series have reported death rates of those listed for liver transplantation as high as 40%, despite most organ donor allocation systems prioritizing ALF.

The many and diverse functions of the liver (metabolic, immunological and physiological) make the task of developing bridging devices a major challenge: the effects of the 'toxic liver' itself also require consideration. Bridging devices can be classified into four categories: (1) auxiliary transplant; (2) liver support devices (biological and non-biological); (3) hepatocyte transplantation; (4) innovative/experimental techniques (Table 7.12.4).

Table 7.12.4 'Bridging options' for ALF

Auxiliary transplant	Heterotopic auxiliary liver transplantation (HALT) Auxiliary partial orthoptic liver transplantation (APOLT)
Liver support devices	Bioartifical liver (BAL) devices Demetriou's Hepatassist BAL Amsterdam Medical Centre BAL Extracorporeal liver assist device (MELS) Bioartifical liver support system (BLSS) Non-biological liver devices Molecular Adsorbents Recirculating System (MARS) Prometheus system Plasmapheresis & high volume plasmapheresis
Hepatocyte transplantation	Cryopreserved human hepatocytes via: Intraportal hepatocyte infusions Splenic artery infusion
Innovative/ experimental techniques	Total emergency hepatectomy Portal vein arterialization Auxiliary liver organ formation by implantation of spleen-encapsulated hepatocytes

The current data regarding the efficacy, cost effectiveness and safety of liver support devices, both biological and non-biological (artificial) are conflicting and less promising in ALF. Currently available liver support systems are therefore not recommended outside of clinical trials; their future in the management of ALF remains unclear.

Stem cell transplantation (regenerative medicine)

Liver transplantation is limited by the severely limited supply of human donors.

A regenerative medicine approach employing stem cells has recently been proposed to overcome this problem. Experimentation is underway using infusions of hepatic stem cells that are said to be non-immunogenic, but this is currently highly experimental.

Prognosis

The prognosis of ALF is variable and depends on the cause. Outcomes are much better for patients who have ALF associated with paracetamol, pregnancy or hepatitis A than those who have seronegative hepatitis; non-A, non-B viral hepatitis; idiosyncratic drug reactions or Wilson's disease. Hepatitis B has an intermediate outcome. The age of patients and the rate of disease progression also determine outcome. Generally, patients with slow progression of failure tend to do worse than those with a rapid downhill course to encephalopathy. Other factors associated with a poor prognosis include the presence of a metabolic acidosis and, in cases of paracetamol toxicity, a continuing rise in the prothrombin time at days 3–4, which may rise to 180 seconds.

Given that the only proven beneficial therapeutic intervention in advanced ALF is transplantation, the timing of transplantation and selection of patients is crucial.

Although scoring systems have been proposed, the variety of causes of ALF tends to limit their accuracy. Validating selection criteria is difficult because of poor methodology in several reported series. Furthermore, ALF is rare, therefore, most case series involve small numbers and span long periods of time, during which important supportive medical therapies may have evolved that could affect prognosis.

Two main prognostic scoring systems are currently used: the Clichy and King's College (London) criteria. Both include different demographic, clinical and biochemical variables to identify a group most likely to require transplantation. Other prognostic criteria have been proposed including severity of soluble immune response suppressor (SIRS), alpha-fetoprotein (AFP) levels, ratios of factor VIII and factor V, liver histology, CT scanning of the liver, cytokine levels, serum phosphate levels and adrenal insufficiency. The Model for Endstage Liver Disease (MELD) score, now widely used to predict mortality among patients with chronic liver disease who are under consideration for liver transplantation, has been reported by some studies to have similar or better predictive value than the more established scores.

Likely developments over the next 5–10 years

- Evidence base for NAC in non-paracetamol ALF.
- Mild hypothermia to prevent and treat brain oedema in ALF.
- Optimal biocomponent for liver support devices in ALF.
- Hepatocyte progenitor cells (including fetal liver cells, multipotent hepatic cells and bone marrow derived stem cells) as genuine functional hepatocytes for use in hepatocyte transplantation.
- Auxiliary partial orthoptic liver transplantation as a bridge to transplantation or spontaneous recovery in ALF.

Controversies

- Efficacy of penicillin G and silibinin (silymarin or milk thistle) as antidotes for mushroom poisoning.
- Selection of patients for transplantation.
- Role, selection and efficacy of bridging options for patients awaiting transplantation.

Further reading

Acharya SK, Batra Y, Hazari S, et al. Etiopathogenesis of acute hepatic failure: Eastern versus Western countries. J Gastroenterol Hepatol 2002;17(suppl 3):S268–73.

Bernal W, Auzinger G, Dhawan A, Wendan J. Acute liver failure. Lancet 2010;376:190–201.

Bernal W, Cross TJS, Auzinger G, et al. Outcome after wait-listing for emergency liver transplantation in acute liver failure: a single centre experience. J Hepatol 2009;50:306–13.

Bhatia V, Singhal A, Panda SK, Acharya SKA. 20-year single-center experience with acute liver failure during pregnancy: is the prognosis really worse? Hepatology 2008;48:1577–85.

Broussard CN, Aggarwal A, Lacey SR, et al. Mushroom poisoning–from diarrhea to liver transplantation. Am J Gastroenterol 2001;96:3195.

Brunetto MR, Giarin MM, Oliveri F, et al. Wild-type and e antigen-minus hepatitis B viruses and course of chronic hepatitis. Proc Natl Acad Sci USA 1991;88:4186–90.

Clavien PA. Acute liver failure: where are the challenges? J Hepatol 2007;46:553–4.

Chalasani F, Fontana RJ, Bonkovsky HL, et al. Drug-Induced Liver Injury Network (DILIN). Causes, clinical features, and outcomes from a prospective study of drug-induced liver injury in the United States. Gastroenterology 2008;135:1924–34. e1-e4.

Ellis A, Rhodes A, Jackson N, et al. Acute liver failure (ALF) in a specialist intensive care unit; a 7 year experience. Crit Care 1998;2(Suppl 1):150.

Fukumitsu K, Yagi H, Soto-Gutierrez A. Bioengineering in organ transplantation: targeting the liver. Transplant Proc 2011;43:2137–8.

Ichai P, Samuel D. Etiology and prognosis of fulminant hepatitis in adults. Liver Transpl 2008;14(suppl 2):S67–79.

Jalan R. Acute liver failure: current management and future prospects. J Hepatol 2005;42(Suppl 1):S115–23.

Khan SA, Shah N, Williams R, Jalan R. Acute liver failure: a review. Clin Liver Dis 2006;10:239–58.

Larson AM, Polson J, Fontana RJ, et al. Acetaminophen-induced acute liver failure: results of a United States multicenter, prospective study. Hepatology 2005;42:1364–72.

Lee WM. Acute liver failure. Semin Respir Crit Care Med 2012;33:36–45.

Lee WM. Acute liver failure in the United States. Semin Liver Dis 2003;23:217–26.

Ostapowicz GA, Fontana RJ, Schiodt FV, et al. Results of a prospective study of acute liver failure at 17 tertiary care centers in the United States. Ann Intern Med 2002;137:947–54.

O'Grady J. Modern management of acute liver failure. Clin Liver Dis 2007;11:291–303.

Polson J, William ML. AASLD position paper: the management of acute liver failure. Hepatology 2005;42:1179–97.

Reuben A, Koch DG, Lee WM, Acute Liver Failure Study Group. Drug-induced liver failure: results of a US multicenter, prospective study. Hepatology 2010;52:2065–78.

Rolando N, Grimson A, Wade J, et al. Prospective study comparing prophylactic parenteral antimicrobials, with or without enteral decontamination, in patients with acute liver failure. Hepatology 1993;17:196–201.

Singhal A, Neuberger J. Acute liver failure: bridging to transplant or recovery–are we there yet? J Hepatol 2007;46:557–64.

Stravitz RT, Kramer DJ. Management of acute liver failure. Nat Rev Gastroenterol Hepatol 2009;6:542–53.

Trey C, Davidson CS. The management of fulminant hepatic failure. In: Popper H, Schaffner F, editors. Progress in liver disease. New York: Grune & Stratton, 1970.

Wigg AJ, Gunson BK, Mutimer DJ. Outcomes following liver transplantation for seronegative acute liver failure: experience during 12-year period with more than 100 patients. Liver Transpl 2005;11:27–34.

Weisner R, Edwards E, Freeman R, et al. Model for end-stage liver disease (MELD) and allocation of donor livers. Gastroenterology 2003;124:91–6.

Wesson RN, Cameron AM. Stem cells in acute liver failure. Adv Surg 2011;45:117–30.

Yagi H, Fukumitsu K, Fukuda K, et al. Human-scale whole-organ bioengineering for liver transplantation: a regenerative medicine approach. Cell Transplant 2012. (Epub ahead of print).

DIGESTIVE EMERGENCIES

7

7.13 Rectal bleeding

E Shaun Goh • Francis Lee Chun Yue

ESSENTIALS

1 Rectal bleeding is a common presentation in patients aged over 50 years and can result in shock due to large volume blood loss.

2 Patients aged >50 years with rectal bleeding should have complete investigation of their large bowel, regardless of the presence of anorectal disease.

3 Most cases of lower gastrointestinal haemorrhage are self-limiting and resolve spontaneously.

4 The most common cause of lower gastrointestinal haemorrhage in younger patients (<50 years of age) is anorectal disorders. In elderly patients, diverticular disease is the main cause.

5 Colonoscopy is the investigation of choice, but is unreliable in the unprepared bowel.

6 In patients with significant or massive haemorrhage, an oesophagogastroduodenoscopy (OGD) should be performed to exclude haemorrhage from the upper gastrointestinal tract.

7 CT colonoscopy is increasingly used as a first-line diagnostic modality.

8 Despite improved diagnostic imaging, no source of bleeding will be identified in up to 10–20% of patients.

9 Treatment options consist of colonoscopic, angiographic and surgical techniques.

10 Emergency surgery is necessary in approximately 10% of patients. Morbidity can be reduced by prior haemodynamic stabilization.

Introduction

Rectal bleeding or 'haematochezia' is the passage of blood from the rectum. It may be 'mixed in' with stools or passed separately. Often patients recognize haematochezia as the passage of recognizable blood on or mixed in with bowel movements. In contrast to this is melaena, which is stool with blood that has been altered by the gut flora and digestive enzymes and appears black and is slick and 'tarry'.

Haematochezia is most commonly associated with lower gastrointestinal bleeding (i.e. from beyond the stomach and duodenum; distal to the ligament of Treitz) but clinicians need to keep in mind that brisk upper gastrointestinal bleeding may also present with haematochezia due to rapid transit of blood. In general, rectal bleeding can be subdivided into occult bleeding, mild intermittent bleeding, moderate persistent bleeding and massive active bleeding with haemodynamic instability. It is

important to realize that different patients have different thresholds for symptoms due to blood loss and even repeated episodes of mild intermittent bleeding can present with symptomatic anaemia or haemodynamic instability.

The main priority of care for patients who present with rectal bleeding is the early recognition and management of haemorrhagic shock from massive bleeding, following which is determination of the likely site and aetiology by appropriate investigations and any required interventions.

Occult bleeding is detected as a positive stool test for blood but patients may not have observed haematochezia. Occult bleeding patients can usually be managed as an outpatient unless they exhibit symptoms of anaemia. Mild or intermittent bleeding presents with very short episodes of frank bright red bleeding which ceases spontaeneously and is usually related to defaecation. Moderate bleeding presents with gross haematochezia that may

be persistent but without signs of haemodynamic instability although there may be signs of anaemia. Such patients may require inpatient investigation or observation in a short-stay unit depending on the likely cause and patient risk. The differentiation between mild or moderate bleeding can be difficult in some cases and so it may be prudent to treat as for the latter. Severe or prolonged bleeding or significant re-bleeding within 1 week from initial presentation warrants in-hospital management. Massive lower gastrointestinal haemorrhage is characterized by haemodynamic instability and requiring transfusion of at least 2 units of blood.

Mortality from significant (moderate to severe) acute lower gastrointestinal bleeding is approximately 10–20%. The risk increases with age (particularly in those over 60) and concomitant medical problems relating to haemorrhagic shock (e.g. multiple organ dysfunction, the need for operative management, transfusion requirement of more than 5 units of blood) and stressful conditions, such as recent surgery, sepsis or trauma.

Aetiology

There are many causes of rectal bleeding (Table 7.13.1) and the incidence of causes varies with age. Haemorrhoids are the most common cause for rectal bleeding in patients less than 50 years of age. In a review of the aetiology of lower gastrointestinal bleeding in patients of all ages who presented with significant bleeding and were admitted to hospital or were required to undergo colonoscopy, diverticular disease was the most common aetiology (17–40%), followed by angiodysplasia (2–30%), inflammatory or ischaemic colitis (9–21%) and colonic neoplasia (11–14%). Anorectal conditions, such as haemorrhoids or fissures, made up 4–10% of cases, but were more common in patients under 50 years of age. In up to 25% of patients presenting with rectal bleeding, the source is unidentifiable.

Diverticulosis

'Diverticular disease' or diverticulosis is the result of herniation of colonic mucosa and submucosa through areas of weakness in the

Table 7.13.1   Causes of lower gastrointestinal bleeding
Diverticulosis
Angiodysplasia
Ischaemic colitis
Infective colitis
Malignancy
Haemorrhoids
Other anorectal conditions: anal fissures, anal fistula
Inflammatory bowel disease
Post-polypectomy
HIV/AIDs related
Rectal trauma
Aortoenteric fistula
Radiation-induced colitis
Drug related: NSAIDs, steroids, warfarin
Meckel's diverticulum
Rectal varices
Upper gastrointestinal bleeding

muscle layers of the bowel wall resulting in outpouches. The areas of weakness are usually at the point of entry of nutrient vessels penetrating the circular muscle layer. Usually, they are the result of low dietary fibre intake, slower stool transit time and increased intraluminal pressures. They are present in more than 50% of people over 60 years of age and their incidence increases with age. Diverticula are common in the distal colon and are the source of lower gastrointestinal bleeding in up to 60% of cases in adults. The bleeding is arterial and usually from a single diverticulum. It is acute, painless and can be alarming in its volume. In most patients, the blood loss stops spontaneously, however, it may recur in 10–40% of patients.

Angiodysplasia

Angiodysplastic lesions are acquired submucosal vascular ectasia and account for up to 30% of cases of lower gastrointestinal bleeding in adults. They are the most common vascular anomaly in the gastrointestinal tract and are usually located within the proximal colon. Incidence increases with age but most are asymptomatic. Bleeding is venocapillary and painless but is usually less severe than from

diverticulosis. The main contrast from diverticular bleeding is the high rate of re-bleeding in patients (80%) with self-limiting but untreated bleeding from angiodysplasia.

Rarer vascular anomalies include arteriovenous malformation (3%), haemangioma and syndromes such as hereditary haemorrhagic telangiectasia. These conditions may also affect younger patients.

Colitis

Colitis can be due to parasitic and bacterial infections, such as from *Entamoeba histolytica*, *Salmonella*, *Shigella*, *Escherichia coli* 0157:H7 and *Campylobacter jejuni*. They are characterized by fever, abdominal pain, tenesmus and passage of bloody diarrhoea.

Ischaemic colitis is the result of interruption of mesenteric blood flow causing ischaemia of a segment of colon. Affected areas are typically watershed areas, such as the splenic flexure and the rectosigmoid junction. Patients are usually elderly with cardiovascular or embolic disease. Presentation is usually with abdominal pain out of proportion to clinical findings but may be mild in elderly or immunosuppressed patients. This is followed by haematochezia which is usually minimal and self-limiting in most cases.

Post-radiation colitis is a complication of radiotherapy or radiation exposure. The result is sloughing of mucosa, inflammation and bleeding. Haemorrhagic radiation proctitis is a potential complication of prostate brachytherapy, affecting 4–13% of patients.

Inflammatory bowel disease (see Chapter 7.11)

Small to moderate amounts of rectal bleeding occur in up to 50% of patients with ulcerative colitis and Crohn's disease, usually accompanied by other features, such as weight loss, prolonged diarrhoea, fever and anorectal physical findings. These patients are usually young.

Neoplasia

Neoplasms of the bowel present as painless occult bleeding but may result in mild recurrent bleeding due to erosion or ulceration of mucosa. They have associated symptoms of weight loss, altered bowel habit, abdominal pain or intestinal obstruction. Colon cancer is the predominant cause of rectal bleeding from neoplastic disease and is more common in patients aged older than 50 years of age.

Post-polypectomy bleeding may result in significant blood loss which is often arterial in

nature. This can occur between hours to weeks after polyp removal.

Anorectal disorders (see Chapter 7.14)

Haemorrhoids are the most common cause of distal rectal bleeding. Patients usually complain of the passage of intermittent bright red bleeding associated with defaecation. Often bleeding is dramatic and it is common for patients to report, 'bright red blood all over the toilet bowl' or 'blood dripping into the bowl'. Most episodes are self-limiting and respond well to conservative treatment.

Rectal varices may occur in association with portal hypertension. Other causes of per rectal bleeding from anorectal disease include fissures and fistulae. Clinicians should keep in mind that benign anorectal disease on examination does not exclude the possibility of a more proximal source of bleeding or pathology.

Aortoenteric fistula

This complication occurs as a rare sequela of endovascular abdominal aortic aneurysm repair and is probably due to inflammation and prosthetic leak. There may be a 'herald bleed' prior to catastrophic exsanguinating haemorrhage. High levels of suspicion should be maintained for all patients with gastrointestinal bleeding and previous abdominal aortic aneurysm repair.

Miscellaneous

Rectal ulcers may result from local trauma due to insertion of foreign bodies and aberrant sexual practices. Usually these are self-limiting and do not require further treatment other than symptomatic relief.

Human immunodeficiency virus (HIV) and the acquired immunodeficiency syndrome (AIDS) rarely cause rectal bleeding themselves. Rectal bleeding in such groups is usually related to immunodeficiency and opportunistic infections and AIDS-specific conditions, such as cytomegalovirus colitis, colon ulcers, thrombocytopaenia, Kaposi sarcoma or lymphoma. It is important to note that mortality is high and long-term prognosis is poor in such patients.

Non-steroidal anti-inflammatory drugs (NSAIDs) and the increasing use of antiplatelet agents, such as aspirin or clopidogrel, may result in drug-induced rectal bleeding by complicating existing diseases, such as diverticular disease. The same applies to anticoagulation medications, such as warfarin. NSAIDs themselves are also thought to cause exacerbation of underlying inflammatory bowel disease.

Inherited or acquired bleeding disorders should also be considered as part of the differential diagnosis.

Clinical features

History

Where time and patient condition permit, a detailed history should be taken to assist in determining the likely aetiology and subsequent management. With respect to the actual episode of bleeding, estimation of the volume of blood loss by the patient is almost always unreliable. It is relevant to determine if this is the first or a recurrent episode of bleeding. The nature of bleeding should be noted, whether it is with the passage of hard stools or spontaneously. Symptoms of anaemia should be determined, such as postural giddiness, chest discomfort on exertion or increasing malaise.

The colour of stools is an important aspect of history; as rectal bleeding from the small intestine or the right side of the colon usually manifests as dark red or maroon-coloured stools, while bleeding from the left side of colon is usually brighter red. Anorectal bleeding is bright red. Clinicians should still keep in mind that brisk and massive right colon bleeding may present with bright red blood and that caecum or small intestinal bleeding may present with malaena.

Other important symptoms are the presence of abdominal pain, which may suggest an inflammatory condition, such as inflammatory bowel disease or colitis, as opposed to the absence of pain which is the usual presentation of diverticular disease bleeding or bleeding from angiodysplasia.

A relevant past medical history is important and should include history of cardiovascular conditions, inflammatory bowel disease and previous diagnosis of diverticular disease or angiodysplasia. Other relevant history should include trauma, previous surgery, recent colonoscopy, fever, HIV, liver cirrhosis, coagulopathy and symptoms of colon/rectal cancer (e.g. altered bowel habits, loss of weight, tenesmus, intestinal obstruction or family history). Drug history (NSAIDs, steroids, aspirin, antiplatelet agents, warfarin or chemotherapy) is also relevant.

A history of haematemesis is useful in directing initial investigation to the upper gastrointestinal tract (see Chapter 7.6).

Examination

Initial evaluation should begin with an assessment of haemodynamic stability. Tachypnoea and tachycardia are important early indicators of shock. Orthostatic hypotension suggests a significant blood volume loss, although it can also be caused by drugs and autonomic dysfunction.

A systemic examination should look for anaemia, jaundice, abdominal signs, evidence of chronic liver disease and coagulopathy. Decision as to whether bleeding is from the upper gastrointestinal tract may be assisted with insertion of a nasogastric tube, although this is uncommonly performed in most countries. Positive aspiration of blood indicates that bleeding is likely from the upper gastrointestinal (GI) tract. If needed, a normal temperature saline lavage can be done to determine the presence of blood. Absence of blood in the nasogastric tube should focus determination of bleeding to the lower gastrointestinal tract.

Rectal examination should include an inspection for obvious anorectal disorders. The presence of anorectal inflammation, fistulae and skin tags may suggest the possibility of inflammatory bowel disease. However, the presence of anorectal disorders does not exclude the presence of proximal pathology. A digital rectal examination is strongly indicated in patients presenting with rectal bleeding unless it is unable to be tolerated (e.g. with anal fissures). Digital rectal examination should aim to elicit the presence and colour of blood and clots, colour and consistency of stools and the presence of masses. Should history suggest an anorectal condition and where there are no signs of further proximal lesions, a protoscopy examination may be useful to determine the source of bleeding and whether bleeding is still active.

Clinical investigations

Blood tests

A full blood examination should be performed to determine the haemoglobin (Hb) level and haematocrit (Hct). Typically Hb $<8\,g/dL$ or Hct $<18\%$ or drop by 6% from previous value should prompt consideration for transfusion depending on patient thresholds. Blood should also be sent for type and screen in anticipation of blood-product use. Serum electrolyte analysis is indicated to determine the presence of acute kidney injury or other electrolyte abnormalities. Coagulation profile is also indicated in patients with significant bleeding or in patients with known coagulopathy or who are on medications that cause coagulopathy. Liver function tests should be considered where patients show signs of liver disease, such as jaundice, or in patients with significant bleeding to determine organ injury. In patients with persistent or massive bleeding, a serum lactate should be performed as levels greater than $2.5\,mmol/L$ suggest haemorrhagic shock or ongoing haemorrhage. Other tests will be guided by the clinical presentation and differential diagnosis.

Endoscopy

Sigmoidoscopy

Rigid or flexible sigmoidoscopy enables inspection of the mucosa of the rectum, sigmoid colon and distal descending colon.

Colonoscopy

Colonoscopy is the investigation of choice in stable patients who are bleeding slowly or have already stopped bleeding. Patients with ongoing haemorrhage and persistent shock should undergo emergency surgery and not be considered for colonoscopy. Adequate bowel preparation improves diagnostic accuracy and success of colonsocopic procedures. Bowel preparation itself has not been shown to reactivate or increase bleeding rates.

The origin of bleeding is identifiable on colonoscopy in about 74–82% of patients. It also offers the ability to establish tissue diagnosis by biopsy and perform therapeutic interventions (adrenaline injection, bipolar coagulation or haemoclipping). These have high success rates, particularly in active diverticular bleeding (70–100% success) or post-polypectomy bleeding (95–100% success).

Regarding timing of colonscopy, evidence suggests that urgent colonoscopy (within 8 hours) was more likely to identify a definite source of bleeding compared to delayed colonoscopy (within 48 hours); however there was no significant difference observed in overall patient outcomes.

Oesophagogastroduodenoscopy

Consideration should be made as to whether an oesophagogastroduodenoscope should be done prior or at the same time as the colonoscopy. There is evidence that, in patients with severe haematochezia, 11–15% had upper gastrointestinal lesions, so some authors recommend upper gastrointestinal tract endoscopy as the initial examination in this group.

Imaging

Angiography

Selective mesenteric angiography has for many years been the investigation of choice for localization of bleeding where it may be difficult to perform colonoscopy due to ongoing haemorrhage or following colonoscopy where the bleeding site was not identified. It is performed by an interventional radiologist injecting contrast into the superior mesenteric artery, inferior mesenteric artery and coeliac trunk, in sequential order. A postive study is where there is extravasation of contrast seen during fluoroscopy. Sensitivity varies widely (27–86%), but it is reported to detect bleeding when the rate is more than 0.5 mL/min. Diverticular haemorrhage is the most likely aetiology to be detected by this investigation.

Angiography can also be therapeutic. Selective vasopressin infusion (0.2 units per minute and increased to 0.4 units per minute with active haemorrhage for 6–12 hours) can be administered. The success rate of vasopressin infusion is about 80% with greater success for diverticular bleeding. Complications include myocardial ischaemia, arrhythmia, peripheral ischaemia, aortic and femoral artery thrombosis, mesenteric thrombosis and bowel ischaemia. Transcatheter embolization is another therapeutic option with angiography. Current success rate of this modality is quoted to be greater than 85% in diverticular bleeding but less than 60% in rectal bleeding from other causes.

Computed tomography (CT)

The advent of multidetector row CT (MDCT) has improved the performance of CT as a modality for identifying sites of haemorrhage and identification of lesions. Otherwise known as CT colonoscopy, images obtained by an MDCT are reconstructed to form a three-dimensional image that is easily manipulated to give clearer non-invasive images of lesions of interest. Evidence suggests that MDCT may be superior to endoscopy in identifying site and aetiology of bleeding both in the upper gastrointstinal (sensitivity 100% for site, 90.9% for aetiology in MDCT compared to 72.7% and 54.5%, respectively for endoscopy) and lower gastrointestinal tracts (sensitivity 100% for site, 88.2% for aetiology for MDCT compared to 52.9% and 52.9%,

respectively for endoscopy). Positive indicators of acute haemorrhage include vascular extravasation of contrast, contrast enhancement of bowel wall, thickening of bowel wall, hyperdensity of peri-bowel fat and vascular dilations.

Technetium-labelled red blood cell (^{99m}Tc RBC) scans

The role of nuclear scintigraphic imaging is controversial. It has high sensitivity (up to 85%) and can detect bleeding at a rate as slow as 0.1 mL/min. However, its specificity is low (around 50%) and localization of the bleeding source is often imprecise. Serial scans can be obtained up to 36 hours after injection of the tracer, which may be useful in intermittent bleeding. It is reported to be 10 times more sensitive than mesenteric angiography in detecting ongoing bleeding. Due to its low specificity, nuclear scintigraphy is not used in unstable patients or as a guide for surgical intervention. Its role is more as a screening exam prior to more invasive techniques. A delayed positive result of greater than 2 minutes corresponds to a negative predictive value of 93% for the patient requiring further acute invasive procedures, while an immediate positive result had a positive predictive value of 75%. This suggests a strategy that patients with a positive nuclear scintigraphy require urgent mesenteric angiography or other acute modalities while patient with delayed results can be observed and evaluated later with colonoscopy.

Double-contrast barium enema

Barium studies have no place in the current acute setting as they hamper subsequent diagnostic investigations, including angiography and colonoscopy.

Other imaging modalities

Magnetic resonance imaging (MRI) is a useful modality for rectal cancer and provides good visualization of important local prognostic factors. Endoscopic ultrasound is the modality of choice for small, superficial tumours. Given its current promise of offering high sensitivity, specificity and accuracy, the indications for positron emission tomography (PET) may well expand in the future, but its final role is yet to be confirmed.

Wireless capsule endoscopy (WCE) is the modality of choice for visualization of small bowel bleeding. WCE is indicated where the bleeding source is not identified by the above methods or

after a negative oesophagogastroduodenoscopy and colonoscopy or scintography.

Treatment

Initial management

Detection of haemorrhagic shock and the need for resuscitation is vital. Patients with haemorrhagic shock present with one or more signs of organ failure related to haemorrhage, such as altered consciousness, laboured breathing, continuous chest pain, anuria or oliguria or unstable haemodynamics on initial evaluation. Usually, such patients present with massive haemorrhage, but the development of haemorrhagic shock is dependent on the actual tissue perfusion thresholds of the patient. Critical patients in haemorrhagic shock should be managed in an appropriate area with continuous monitoring of vital signs. The focus is on airway, breathing and circulation with optimization of oxygen delivery. Initial volume replacement (up to 20 mL/kg) may be by administering crystalloids or colloids, but bearing in mind that, in non-responders to fluid challenge, blood products should be given as 'the fluid of choice'. In these patients, early surgical evaluation is advised and immediate reversal of any coagulopathic state (vitamin K, fresh frozen plasma or prothrombin complex).

Further management and disposition

The approach to the patient with rectal bleeding will differ depending on the severity of bleeding. The priorities are haemodynamic stabilization, localization of the bleeding site and the formulation of an interventional plan (Fig. 7.13.1).

Occult bleeding

Haematochezia is usually not observed by the patient or discovered on digital rectal examination. Most patients can be investigated on an outpatient basis unless there are overt symptoms or signs of anaemia. Timing of follow up is dependent on likely aetiology, with signs suggestive of malignancy, such as obvious masses on abdominal examination or on rectal examination, given a higher priority.

Mild intermittent bleeding

Most patients who present with mild intermittent bleeding have anorectal conditions.

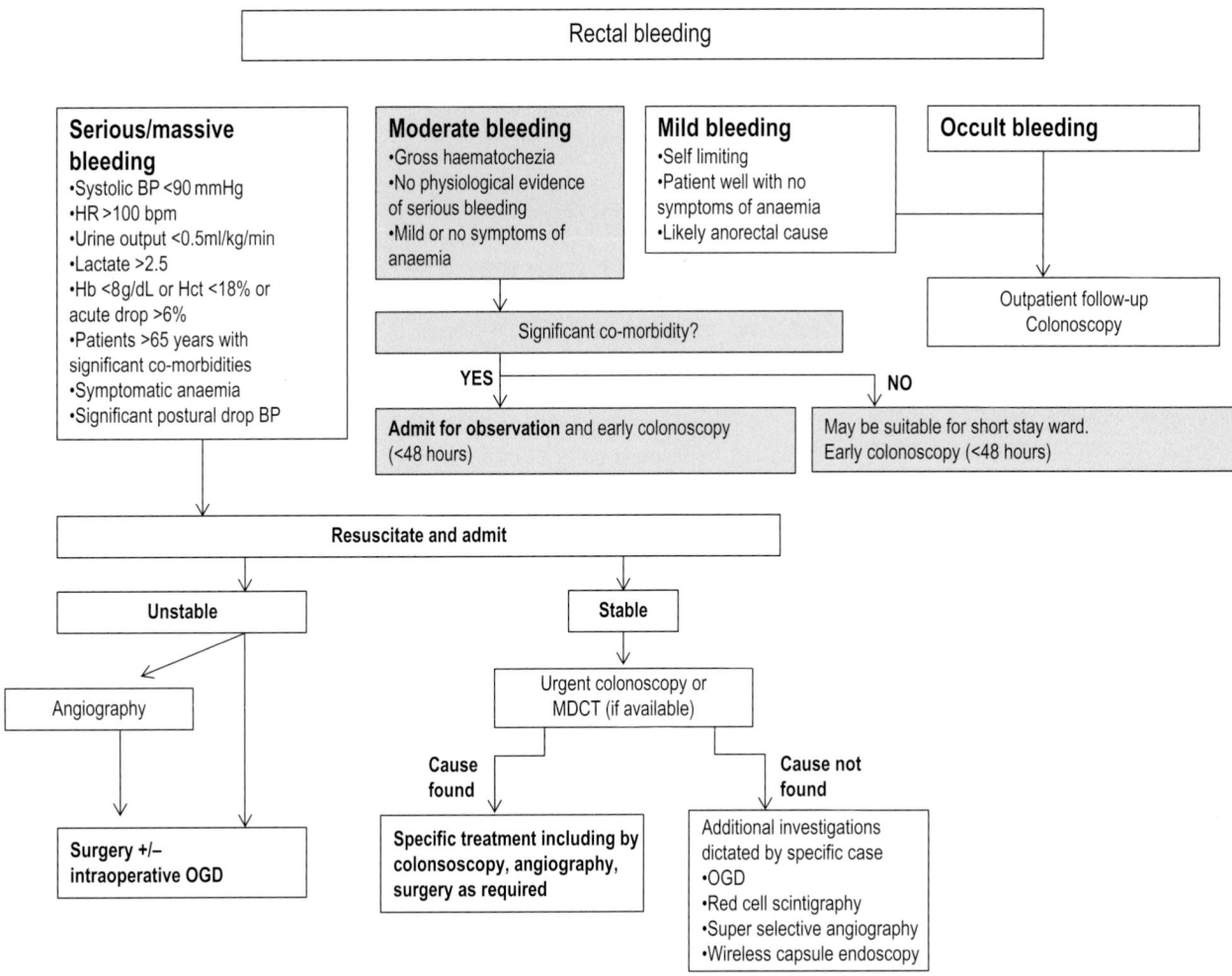

Fig 7.13.1 Management of rectal bleeding.

Proctoscopy and rigid sigmoidoscopy can be performed in the emergency department (ED) at the bedside. Most patients can have further investigations (if necessary) and treatment on an outpatient basis, unless there are overt signs of anaemia then they should be managed as for moderate rectal bleeding. Patients discharged home should have adequate arrangements for outpatient care with either a surgical or a gastroenterology service. For patients more than 50 years of age, an examination of the proximal colon is warranted even if an anorectal condition is found. The extent of further investigation in the younger age group is controversial and dependent on the clinician as well as predisposing factors for malignancy.

Moderate/persistent rectal bleeding

Patients with moderate and persistent bleeding require longer observation, for example in an observational unit or short-stay ward. If such facilities are unavailable or if the patients are of high risk or have significant co-morbid conditions, then they should be managed as an inpatient. These patients would generally require colonoscopy, ideally performed within 48 hours. Treatment should be directed towards the likely aetiology.

Massive rectal bleeding

These patients require resuscitation and inpatient care. Most severe bleeding will cease spontaneously and further investigation can proceed when the bowel has been properly prepared. In some cases, bleeding continues and active management is required on an emergency basis.

Transfusion is indicated in patients with persistent active bleeding refractory to initial resuscitation or in those with haemorrhagic shock.

The cause and site of bleeding should be determined by means of MDCT or early colonoscopy. Mesenteric angiography has a role where MDCT is not available and there is active bleeding or inadequate bowel preparation rendering colonoscopy technically difficult.

Oesophagogastroduodenoscopy should be performed in all cases of massive rectal bleeding prior to colonoscopy or other interventions.

Specific treatment

Treatment should be directed towards the underlying aetiology and is determined by the haemodynamic state of the patient. Colonoscopic control of bleeding is effective in stopping diverticular bleeding and postpolypectomy bleeding. Colonoscopy may also treat rectal bleeding from other causes with variable efficacy. Risks of performing colonoscopy include re-bleeding, failure of procedure and perforation.

Arterial infusion of vasopressin (via interventional radiology) has been shown to reduce splanchnic blood flow by causing vasoconstriction. This allows for plug formation at the bleeding vessel. Vasopressin is effective in bleeding from diverticular disease or other arterial bleeding. It is less effective in cases of venocapillary bleeding, such as in angiodysplasia. Following angiography, initial infusion is at a rate of 0.2 U/min. A repeat angiogram is done after 20 minutes. Bleeding stops in the vast majority of patients ($\approx$90%), but the recurrence rate is reported as high as 50%. In cases of persistent or recurrent bleeding, the infusion can be increased to 0.4–0.6 U/min and angiogram repeated at 6–12 hours. The infusion can then be maintained for 12–48 hours and then tapered over 24 hours. Complications include acute coronary syndrome, arrhythmias or hypertension. Vasopressin is contraindicated in patients with known significant coronary artery disease and peripheral vascular disease.

Transcatheter superselective embolization of angiodysplastic lesions with microcoils, gelatin sponge, polyvinyl alcohol and oxidized cellulose has been reported. Superselective catheterization of the vasa recta has been shown to be successful and safe. Significant complications are intestinal ischaemia and infarction, but this risk is decreased by performing embolization as close to bleeding sites as possible in terminal mural arteries.

Surgey is indicated in patients with persistent haemodynamic instability with active bleeding, persistent recurrent bleeding and haemodynamically unstable patients requiring transfusion of more than 4 units of packed red blood cells in a 24-hour period with active or recurrent bleeding.

Surgery

Subtotal colectomy is the surgical procedure of choice in the management of colonic haemorrhage which is not controlled by other means. It is also indicated in unstable patients where the site of bleeding is unidentifiable or where unstable patients are unable to tolerate prolonged surgery. In these patients, an ileoproctostomy is usually fashioned and the morbidity rate is around 37% and mortality 11–33%. Where possible, efforts should still be made intraoperatively to localize the site of bleeding as a segmental resection can then be performed, which carries less morbidity and postoperative complications.

For 'stable' patients, the bleeding site should be located preoperatively so that segmental bowel resection can be planned. Selective mesenteric angiography followed by intra-arterial vasopressin can be used as a temporizing measure as a bridge towards segmental bowel resection. This approach to surgery has an operative morbidity of 8.6% and mortality 10%, with re-bleeding ranging from 0 to 14%.

Blind segmental bowel resection is now contraindicated due to potential for incorrect bowel segment resection, high re-bleeding rate, need for revisit surgery and higher mortality rates.

Controversies

- The timing of colonoscopy in stable patients presenting with acute bleeding or in unstable patients who have been successfully resuscitated.
- The role of red cell nuclear scintigraphy as a screening test.
- The usefulness of MDCT as a first-line diagnostic tool.

- Timing of outpatient follow up for patients presenting with occult or mild bleeding.
- The extent of investigation in the younger (under 50 years) age group.

Further reading

Adams JB, Margolin DA. Management of diverticular hemorrhage. Clin Colon Rectal Surg 2009;22:181–5.

Browder W, Cerise EJ, Litwin MS. Impact of emergency angiography in massive lower gastrointestinal bleeding. Ann Surg 1986;204:530–6.

Davila RE, Rajan E, Adler DG, et al. Standards of Practice Committee. ASGE Guideline: the role of endoscopy in the patient with lower-GI bleeding. Gastrointest Endosc 2005;62:656–60.

Ernst O, Bulois P, Saint-Drenant S, et al. Helical CT in acute lower gastrointestinal bleeding. Eur Radiol 2003;13:114–7.

Frattaroli FM, Casciani E, Spoletini D, et al. Prospective study comparing multi detector row CT and endoscopy in acute gastrointestinal bleeding. World J Surg 2009;33:2209–17.

Green BT, Rockey DC, Portwood G, et al. Urgent colonoscopy for evaluation and management of acute lower gastrointestinal haemorrhage: a randomized controlled trial. Am J Gastroenterol 2005;100:2395–402.

Jensen DM, Machicado GA, Jutabha R, Kovacs TO. Urgent colonoscopy for the diagnosis and treatment of severe diverticular haemorrhage. N Engl J Med 2000;342:78–82.

Khanna A, Ognibene SJ, Koniaris LG. Embolization as first-line therapy for diverticulosis-related massive lower gastrointestinal bleeding: evidence from a meta-analysis. J Gastrointest Surg 2005;9:343–52.

Laine L, Shah A. Randomized trial of urgent vs elective colonoscopy in patients hospitalized with lower GI bleeding. Am J Gastroenterol 2010;105:2636–41.

Parra-Blanco A, Kaminaga N, Kojima T, et al. Hemoclipping for postpolypectomy and postbiopsy colonic bleeding. Gastrointest Endosc 2000;51:37–41.

Scottish Intercollegiate Guidelines Network (SIGN). Management of acute upper and lower gastrointestinal bleeding. A national clinical guideline. SIGN publication; no. 105. Edinburgh (Scotland): Scottish Intercollegiate Guidelines Network (SIGN); 2008.

Tan BK, Tsang CB, Nyam DC, Ho YH. Management of acute bleeding per rectum. Asian J Surg 2004;27:32–8.

Warner E, Crighton EJ, Moineddin R, et al. Fourteen-year study of hospital admissions for diverticular disease in Ontario. Can J Gastroenterol 2007;21:97–9.

7.14 Perianal conditions

Michael R Augello

ESSENTIALS

1 Anal pain, bleeding and masses are common symptoms in many different types of anorectal pathology. A careful history and anorectal examination is important in making the correct diagnosis.

2 Increasing fibre intake and reducing constipation are effective initial treatments for mild, uncomplicated haemorrhoidal disease and perianal fissures.

3 Anorectal abscesses require incision and drainage. In some cases, this can be done safely in the emergency department, but all supralevator, intersphincteric and ischiorectal abscesses require formal surgical exploration and drainage in theatre.

4 Incision and drainage of cutaneous abscesses is not associated with bacteraemia in immunocompetent, afebrile adults, so routine antibiotic cover is not required.

5 Irreducible haemorrhoids require urgent reduction and surgery.

6 Thrombosed external haemorrhoids presenting early will have a shorter duration of symptoms with incision and excision.

Anorectal abscesses and fistulae

Introduction

Anorectal abscess and fistulae are the acute and chronic phases of the same disease. It is believed to originate from an infection in the anal glands and the various classification patterns seen reflect the direction of spread of the infection. Anorectal abscesses are twice as common in men as in women. Associated factors may include inflammatory bowel disease, infection, trauma, surgery, malignancy, radiation and immunosuppression. Anorectal fistulae arise from a pre-existing abscess or from a history of recurrent abscesses. Fistula formation and recurrence following the first presentation of an anorectal abscess occurs in about 40% of cases. Fistulous tracts may be multiple and be intimately related to the sphincters essential for continence. Treatment of anorectal fistula is complex and the domain of colorectal surgeons. Diagnosis of fistulous disease is suspected on a history of recurrent perianal suppuration and is confirmed by the delineation of fistulous tracks during surgery under anaesthesia.

Clinical features and classification of anorectal abscesses

Clinically, perianal pain is the most common symptom. Swelling and fever may also be present. Examination reveals a tender, erythematous and fluctuant mass.

One commonly used classification system (Fig. 7.14.1) is according to the four potential anorectal spaces they may occupy.

Perianal abscess

Perianal abscess presents as a painful lump around the anal verge, usually lateral and posterior to the anus. It may result from an infected anal gland or, more rarely, is a presentation of Crohn's disease. Systemic symptoms are uncommon. On examination, most will be pointing, with an indurated red area which may be fluctuant. Such abscesses may be suitable for incision and drainage in the emergency department (ED).

Ischiorectal abscess

Ischiorectal abscesses tend to be larger, yet may present with less dramatic cutaneous findings because of the compressibility of ischiorectal fat. Patients may be febrile and systemically unwell. The area of induration is likely to be large and more lateral than a simple perianal abscess. Pointing may not occur until late and initial assessment may seem more like buttock cellulitis.

Supralevator abscess

Supralevator abscesses arise above the levator ani. In reality, it is a pelvic abscess and is often secondary to an intra-abdominal condition, such as diverticular disease or Crohn's disease. Fever is common and it may present as pyrexia of unknown origin. The patient may present with pain on defaecation and altered bowel habit. Inspection of the perineum may be normal, but rectal examination will reveal a firm, spongy, tender mass.

Intersphincteric or submucous abscess

These abscesses may be associated with severe pain and with urinary symptoms. They are within the anal canal, so no external swelling may be visible. They point within the anal canal and may rupture spontaneously.

Treatment

The treatment of all anorectal abscesses is incision and drainage. There is no role for antibiotic treatment alone. Small perianal abscesses can be considered for drainage in the ED. The drained wound should be kept open long enough for the abscess to heal from below and may require placement of a formal drain. Aggressive probing of the cavity should be avoided as it can lead to iatrogenic fistulae. Regular Sitz baths, review and dressing changes should continue until healing is confirmed. Antibiotics are ineffective and are only indicated in patients with valvular or rheumatic heart disease, diabetes, immunosuppression, extensive cellulitis or a prosthetic device.

All other larger and more complicated anorectal abscesses are best treated under general anaesthesia by a surgeon with colorectal expertise to minimize risk of complications. Traditionally, in acute perianal abscesses, the search for a fistulous internal opening followed by fistulotomy has been the standard

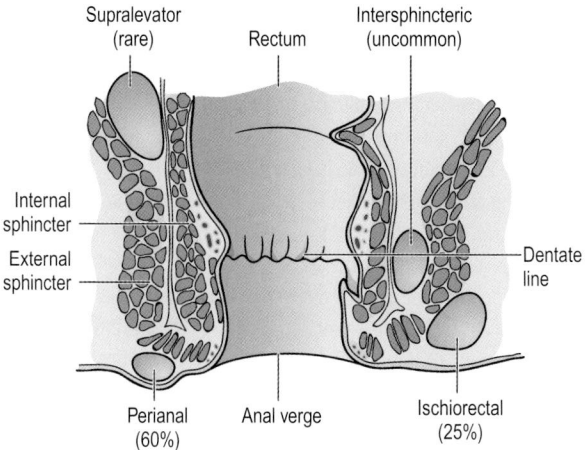

Fig 7.14.1 Anatomic locations of anorectal abscesses. *From John Pfenninger & Grant Fowler: Pfenninger & Fowler's Procedures for Primary Care. Saunders (2011) with permission.*

Table 7.14.1 Grades of internal haemorrhoid and clinical features	
Grade of haemorrhoid	*Clinical features*
Grade 1	Cause painless bleeding. Do not prolapse
Grade 2	Prolapse, usually after straining at stool, but reduce spontaneously
Grade 3	Prolapse and require digital reduction
Grade 4	Prolapsed and irreducible

treatment. Although fistulae are often present, immediate management of associated fistula tracts may result in higher rates of further fistulae, incontinence and unnecessary treatment of fistulae that will resolve spontaneously and not require treatment. Simple drainage is thus advocated for most acute anorectal abscesses.

Pilonidal disease

Introduction

Pilonidal disease is a separate entity to anorectal abscess. It is an acquired recurrent disease of young adults, affecting men twice as often as women. It is uncommon after the fourth decade of life. Its spectrum includes acute abscess, formation of sinus tracts and complex disease with chronic or recurrent abscesses and extensive, branching sinus tracts. Risk factors include hirsutism, obesity, sedentary occupation and local irritation.

The pathological basis of the condition is the migration of loose hair ends into the natal cleft, where they become embedded and cause irritation. A pilonidal sinus or abscess may then form around these loose hairs. Patients usually describe a painful lump in the sacrococcygeal area, with or without seropurulent discharge. Systemic symptoms are uncommon. Examination reveals an abscess in the presacral area about 5 cm cephalad to the anus, with one or more midline draining pits or sinuses. Occasionally hair is seen protruding from a pit.

Treatment

Initial treatment for an acute pilonidal abscess should be incision, preferably off midline, over the area where the abscess is pointing, with drainage and evacuation of pus and hair. This may take place under local or general anaesthesia and, in up to 58% of patients, no further treatment is required. Healing may take up to 10 weeks, so additional surgery should not be considered early. Careful attention to hair control in the natal cleft may have some benefit in preventing recurrence. Shaving, plucking and laser depilation have all been suggested. Failure of initial treatment, as well as delayed recurrence, is not uncommon. More aggressive complex surgical procedures, including various forms of open and closed excision and marsupialization of sinus tracts, is reserved for complex disease that fails more simple procedures, as they produce similar results at greater cost and more loss of working days.

Haemorrhoids

Introduction

Haemorrhoidal tissue is a normal anatomical structure located in the anal canal that plays a role in differentiating between liquids, solids and gas and maintaining anal continence. Haemorrhoids are composed of cushions of submucosal vascular tissue, usually located in the 3, 7 and 11 o'clock positions as viewed through an anoscope with the patient in the lithotomy position. Haemorrhoidal disease occurs when there are symptoms such as

bleeding, prolapse, pain, thrombosis, a mass, discharge or pruritus. Straining, inadequate fibre intake, prolonged sitting on the toilet, constipation, diarrhoea, pregnancy and other conditions with elevated intra-abdominal pressure have been suspected to contribute to the development of the disease.

The dentate line divides haemorrhoidal tissue into internal and external. Internal haemorrhoids are classically painless and are divided into four grades, depending on the degree of any prolapse (Table 7.14.1).

Clinical features and differential diagnosis

Bleeding is the most common symptom and is typically painless and bright red. It is often described as a splash in the pan or streaks on toilet paper. Bleeding between bowel actions or blood mixed with the stool should raise suspicion of other pathologies, such as diverticular disease or neoplasia, and requires further investigation.

Examination involves observing the perineum with the patient straining. Redundant skin tags may be present. Grape-like structures may be seen to bulge around the classic 3, 7 and 11 o'clock positions. Anoscopy may reveal one or more haemorrhoids.

Differential diagnoses to consider include colorectal malignancy, inflammatory bowel disease, anal warts and other anorectal conditions. Some patients with haemorrhoidal symptoms should be evaluated further with colonoscopy to exclude more serious disease. These include patients with any suspicious findings on history or examination, iron-deficiency anaemia, positive faecal occult blood tests, those aged over 40 with a positive family history of neoplasia and those aged over 50 with no recent colonoscopy.

Treatment

Conservative treatment is often successful, especially in lesser-grade disease. Increasing dietary fibre decreases overall haemorrhoidal symptoms by over 50%, especially bleeding. Stool softeners to reduce straining and constipation, as well as Sitz baths, are recommended to assist with symptom control. Topical agents, e.g. 0.2% glyceryl trinitrate paste (Rectogesic), have shown a reduction in overall haemorrhoidal symptoms as well as bleeding.

There are many other popular over-the-counter (OTC) medications available. These include suppositories, creams, ointments and pads that contain various cocktails of local anaesthetics, steroids, vasoconstrictors, antiseptics, keratolytics, protectants (such as mineral oils, cocoa butter) and astringents. There is no evidence to show these agents have any benefit in the prevention or long-term treatment of haemorrhoidal disease. There is also no evidence that spicy food worsens haemorrhoidal symptoms. Haemorrhoidal conditions that require specific treatment including prolapsed irreducible haemorrhoids and thrombosed external haemorrhoids.

Prolapsed irreducible haemorrhoids

Prolapsed irreducible haemorrhoids may become gangrenous and usually cause severe pain. Reduction can sometimes be achieved by the use of adequate analgesia, a foot-up tilted trolley, ice, local anaesthetic and firm slow pressure applied digitally. If successful, the requirement for surgery may change from emergency to urgent elective.

Thrombosed external haemorrhoids

Thrombosed external haemorrhoids present as a painful tender mass in the anus, frequently following an episode of constipation or diarrhoea. Examination reveals a bluish, exquisitely tender skin-covered lump sited lateral to the anus. Pain peaks at 48 hours before gradually easing. If the patient presents with a history of less than 48 hours and severe pain, surgical excision may be considered as it results in earlier pain relief, as well as reduced rates of recurrence at 1 year when compared to incision alone or conservative treatment. Conservative treatment will also ultimately result in resolution of symptoms but averaged 24 days in one study compared to 4 days with surgical excision.

Procedural treatment options

Procedural options for haemorrhoidal disease are reserved for mild disease that has failed conservative procedures, specific situations mentioned above and grade three or four haemorrhoidal disease. Procedural options include rubber band ligation or sclerosant injection (for haemorrhoids above the dentate line), progressing to more invasive surgical procedures including haemorrhoidectomy and stapled haemorrhoidopexy. All surgical techniques may be associated with a significant amount of postoperative pain and bleeding.

Anal fissure

Introduction

Anal fissure is a painful linear ulcer situated in the anal canal. It has a similar incidence in both males and females and is found in the posterior midline in 90% of cases. The anterior midline accounts for almost all other cases. When an anal fissure is not found in the midline, secondary causes, such as Crohn's disease or malignancy, require exclusion. While hard stool is most commonly implicated as the initiating trauma, loose stools may also be associated. Anal spasm and decreased blood flow to the posterior midline anal canal maintains the ulcer. Most acute anal fissures heal with conservative treatment. Some go on to become chronic and develop secondary changes forming a fibrous skin tag, often referred to as a sentinel pile, as well as hypertrophied anal papillae and relative anal stenosis due to scarring.

Clinical features

The history is often strongly suggestive of the condition. Typically, patients describe severe, knifelike, intense anal pain initiated during the passage of stool, described as being 'split open'. The pain may persist for hours, with a tight throbbing quality and is usually accompanied by a small amount of bright red rectal blood, often as a smear on the toilet paper.

Inspection of the perineum may reveal tightening of the corrugator cutis ani, an almost diagnostic sign of anospasm that is usually secondary to a fissure. If a small midline 'sentinel' pile is seen, the diagnosis is confirmed. Gentle retraction of the perianal skin usually allows one to visualize the fissure directly. Rectal examination and anoscopy should be deferred until the acute pain has subsided. Anal

fissure is sometimes complicated by abscess formation in the sentinel pile. This is suggested by a very swollen oedematous tag and requires surgical drainage.

Treatment

In acute fissures, conservative treatment is effective in up to 50% of cases. Warm baths may help relieve sphincter spasm. Stool softeners (such as docusate), bulk-forming laxatives (such as bran) and high-fibre food are the mainstay of medical treatment. Acute relief of pain and spasm can be achieved by the use of local anaesthetic gel.

Avoidance of constipation is probably the single most important non-operative treatment. Recurrence of symptoms after initial success with conservative treatment can occur, but conservative treatment still has a good success rate on recurrent episodes.

Pharmacological agents that reduce internal sphincter tone and improve anodermal blood flow can also be used and have been mainly studied in chronic anal fissures. All agents suffer from relatively poor success rates in the healing of chronic anal fissures. Glyceryl trinitrate (GTN) is more successful than placebo (48.9% vs 35.5%) but headache in 30% caused some patients to abandon treatment. Topical treatments direct to the anus or by distally placed dermal patch have been shown to be equivalent. Calcium channel blockers and injection with botulinum toxin (botox) are also alternative treatments with results slightly better than placebo. Topical calcium channel blocker creams are unavailable in Australia. Botox causes a temporary 'chemical sphincterototomy' that enables healing of a chronic anal fissure, but recurrence may still occur. It is probably no better and no worse than GTN in the latest meta-analysis.

Failure of medical treatment warrants surgical referral. Modern practice achieves long-term cure in over 90%, with the most serious and feared surgical complication of anal incontinence occurring in about 5%. Lateral internal sphincterotomy is safer than controlled anal dilatation.

Pruritus ani

Pruritus ani is a dermatological condition characterized as an unpleasant itchy or burning sensation in the perianal region. Although it may be due to a definable perianal dermatological condition, including psoriasis, eczema and lichen sclerosis, most cases are idiopathic. Fungal, bacterial or parasitic infections, such as pinworm and pediculosis, are rare causes (except in children). Contributing factors may include excessive attempts at hygiene causing local irritation, loose stools, prolapsing haemorrhoids and the frequent use of anorectal creams and ointments which may lead to perianal wetness with maceration of the skin and contact dermatitis. An itch and scratch cycle is then set up which can be very difficult to break resulting in chronic skin changes including lichenification. It is important to note that neoplasms, such as Bowen's disease, lymphoma and Kaposi's sarcoma, may cause pruritus.

Persistent itchiness in the anal region can be a difficult condition to treat. Potential identified causes should be treated appropriately. Idiopathic cases may benefit from reassurance, discontinuation of previously tried anorectal medications and avoidance of irritants, such as bar soap and vigorous scrubbing. Avoiding foods identified as exacerbating symptoms may be tried, as well as air-drying the area after Sitz baths. A short course of topical hydrocortisone or sorbolene cream may provide relief and a break in the itch–scratch cycle.

Proctalgia fugax

Proctalgia fugax is the sudden and unpredictable onset of shearing or knife-like pain in the anus and rectum. It is usually of very short duration and is most common in males. It is thought to be due to dysfunction of the internal anal sphincter. Apart from reassurance, no specific therapy is usually required. Salbutamol inhalation may shorten attacks of severe pain, but the mechanism of action is uncertain.

Injuries to the perianal region

History is paramount and abuse needs to be excluded. Examination should focus on the function of the sphincter and be alert to the possibility of intra-abdominal extension of penetrating injuries. Where there is a history of foreign body insertion, plain films will determine the position of the object and the presence or absence of free intra-abdominal gas.

Other anorectal conditions

Other important local conditions not covered in this chapter but to be considered in the differential diagnosis of most anorectal conditions, include proctitis, rectal prolapse, Fournier's gangrene, faecal impaction, condylomata acuminata (warts associated with human papilloma virus), condylomata lata (flat white lesions associated with secondary syphilis) and carcinoma. A complete anorectal examination reduces the risk of such conditions being missed or misdiagnosed.

Controversies

- If some anorectal abscess can be drained in the ED under local anaesthesia, how do we select the appropriate cases?
- Should thrombosed external haemorrhoids be excised or treated conservatively?
- What is the optimal long-term treatment strategy for pilonidal disease?
- Is botulinum toxin really any more effective than glyceryl trinitrate ointment and topical calcium channel blockers in the treatment of acute anal fissure?

Further reading

Alonso-Coello P, Guyatt GH, Heels-Ansdell D, et al. Laxatives for the treatment of hemorrhoids. Cochrane Database Syst Rev 2005;4:CD004649.

Altomare DF, Rinaldi M, La Tore F, et al. Red hot chili pepper and hemorrhoids: the explosion of a myth: results of a prospective, randomized, placebo-controlled, crossover trial. Dis Colon Rectum 2006;49:1018–23.

Billingham RP, Isler JT, Kimmins MH. The diagnosis and management of common anorectal disorders. Curr Prob Surg 2004;41:586–645.

Clothier PR, Haywood IR. The natural history of the post anal (pilonidal) sinus. Ann Royal Coll Surg Engl 1984;66:201–3.

Greenspon J, Williams SB, Young HA, et al. Thrombosed external hemorrhoids: outcome after conservative or surgical management. Dis Colon Rectum 2004;47:1493–8.

Isenberg G. Anorectal disease. Clin Colon Rectal Surg 2011;24:1–80.

Jensen SL, Harling H. Prognosis after simple incision and drainage for a first episode acute pilonidal abscess. Br J Surg 1988;75:60–1.

Nelson RL, Thomas K, Morgan J, Jones A. Non surgical therapy for anal fissure. Cochrane Database Syst Rev 2012;2:CD003431.

Nelson RL, Chattopadhyay A, Brooks W, et al. Operative procedures for fissure in ano. Cochrane Database Syst Rev 2011;11:CD002199.

Rickard M. Anal abscesses and fistulas. Aust NZ J Surg 2005;75:64–72.

Sklow B. Benign anorectal conditions. Clin Colon Rectal Surg 2007;20:75–137.

Tjandra JJ, Tan Y, Lim JF. Rectogesic® (glyceryltrinitrate 0.2%) ointment relieves symptoms of haemorrhoids associated with high resting anal canal pressures. Colorectal Dis 2007;9:457–63.

DIGESTIVE EMERGENCIES

NEUROLOGY EMERGENCIES

Edited by **Anne-Maree Kelly**

8.1 Headache

Anne-Maree Kelly

ESSENTIALS

1 The pathophysiological basis of headache is traction or inflammation of extracranial structures, the basal dura or the large intracranial arteries and veins or dilatation/distension of cranial vascular structures.

2 Severity of headache is not a reliable indicator of the underlying pathology.

3 History is of paramount importance in the assessment of headache.

4 A normal physical examination does not rule out serious pathology.

5 Sudden, severe headache or chronic, unremitting headache is more likely to have a serious cause and should be investigated accordingly.

6 NSAID and paracetamol are effective treatment for tension headache.

7 As most patients have tried oral medications prior to attending the emergency department, parenterally administered agents are usually indicated for treatment of migraine.

8 Based on current evidence, the most effective agents for treating migraine are phenothiazines and triptans. Pethidine is not indicated because it is less effective than other agents, has a high rebound headache rate and carries the potential for the development of dependence.

9 Carbamazepine is the agent of choice for treatment of trigeminal neuralgia.

Aetiology, pathophysiology and pathology

The structures in the head capable of producing headache are limited. They include:

- extracranial structures, including skin and mucosae, blood vessels, nerves, muscles and fascial planes
- the main arteries at the base of the skull (as arteries branch they progressively lose the ability to produce painful stimuli)
- the great venous sinuses and their branches and
- the basal dura and dural arteries, but to a lesser extent than the other structures.

The bulk of the intracranial contents, including the parenchyma of the brain, the subarachnoid and pia mater and most of the dura mater, are incapable of producing painful stimuli.

The pathological processes that may cause headache are:

- Tension. This usually refers to contraction of muscles of the head and/or neck and is thought to be the major factor in the so-called 'tension headache'.
- Traction. Traction is caused by stretching of intracranial structures due to a mass effect, such as with a space-occupying lesion. Pain caused by this mechanism is characteristically constant, but may vary in severity.

Introduction

Headache is a common ailment that is often due to a combination of physical and psychological factors. The vast majority are benign and self-limiting and are managed by patients in the community. Only a very small proportion of patients experiencing headache attend emergency departments (ED) for treatment. The challenges are to distinguish potentially life-threatening causes from the more benign and to manage effectively the pain of headache.

- Vascular processes. These include dilatation or distension of vascular structures and often results in pain that is throbbing in nature.
- Inflammation. This may involve the dura at the base of the skull or the nerves or soft tissues of the head and neck. This mechanism is responsible for the initial pain of subarachnoid haemorrhage and meningitis and for sinusitis.

The pathophysiological causes of headache are summarized in Table 8.1.1.

Clinical features

In the assessment of a patient with headache, history is of prime importance. Specific information should be sought about the timing of the headache (in terms of both overall duration and speed of onset), the site and quality of the pain, relieving factors, the presence of associated features, such as nausea and vomiting, photophobia and alteration in mental state, medical and occupational history and drug use.

Intensity of the pain is important from the viewpoint of management but is not a reliable indicator of the nature of underlying pathology. This said, sudden, severe headache and chronic, unremitting or progressive headache are more likely to have a serious cause.

Physical examination should include temperature, pulse rate and blood pressure measurements, assessment of conscious state and neck stiffness and a neurological examination, including funduscopy (where indicated). Abnormal physical signs are uncommon, but the presence of neurological findings makes a serious cause probable. In addition, a search should be made for sinus, ear, mouth and neck pathology and muscular or superficial temporal artery tenderness.

Headache patterns

Some headaches have 'classic' clinical features: these are listed in Table 8.1.2. It must be remembered that, as with all diseases, there is a spectrum of presenting features and the absence of the classic features does not rule out a particular diagnosis. Every patient must be assessed on their merits and, if symptoms persist without reasonable explanation, further investigation should be undertaken.

Clinical investigations

For the majority of patients with headache no investigation is required. The investigation of suspected subarachnoid haemorrhage and meningitis is discussed elsewhere in this book. If tumour is suspected, the investigations of choice are magnetic resonance imaging (MRI) or a contrast-enhanced computed tomography (CT) scan. An elevated erythrocyte sedimentation rate (ESR) may be supporting evidence for a diagnosis of temporal arteritis. With respect to sinusitis, facial X-rays are of very limited value.

Tension headache

The pathological basis of tension headaches remains unclear, but increased tension of the neck or cranial muscles is a prominent feature. A family history of headaches is common and there is an association with an injury in childhood or adolescence. The most common precipitants are stress and alteration in sleep patterns.

Table 8.1.1 A pathophysiological classification of headache

	Extracranial	Intracranial
Tension/traction	Muscular headache 'Tension headache'	Intracranial tumour Cerebral abscess Intracranial haematoma
Vascular	Migraine	Severe hypertension
Inflammatory	Temporal arteritis Sinusitis Otitis media Mastoiditis Tooth abscess Neuralgia	Meningitis Subarachnoid haemorrhage

Table 8.1.2 Classic clinical complexes and cause of headache

Preceded by an aura Throbbing unilateral headache, nausea Family history	Migraine
Sudden onset Severe occipital headache; 'like a blow' Worst headache ever	Subarachnoid haemorrhage
Throbbing/constant frontal headache Worse with cough, leaning forward Recent URTI Pain on percussion of sinuses	Sinusitis
Paroxysmal, fleeting pain Distribution of a nerve Trigger manoeuvres cause pain Hyperalgesia of nerve distribution	Neuralgia
Unilateral with superimposed stabbing Claudication on chewing Associated malaise, myalgia Tender artery with reduced pulsation	Temporal arteritis
Persistent, deep-seated headache Increasing duration and intensity Worse in morning Aching in character	Tumour: primary or secondary
Acute, generalized headache Fever, nausea and vomiting Altered level of consciousness Neck stiffness ± rash	Meningitis
Unilateral, aching, related to eye Nausea and vomiting Raised intraocular pressure	Glaucoma
Aching, facial region Worse at night Tooth sensitive to heat, pressure	Dental cause

URTI: upper respiratory tract infection.

Aspirin, non-steroidal anti-inflammatory agents (NSAIDs) and paracetamol (acetaminophen) have all been shown to be effective in the treatment of tension headaches, with success rates between 50 and 70%. Ibruprofen 400 mg or ketoprofen 25–50 mg appear to be the most effective, followed by aspirin 600–1000 mg and paracetamol 1000 mg.

Migraine

Migraine can be a disabling condition for the sufferer. Most migraine headaches are successfully managed by the patient and their general practitioner, but a small number fail to respond or become 'fixed' and sufferers may present for treatment at EDs. As most patients (up to 80% in some studies) have tried oral medications prior to presenting, parenterally administered agents are usually indicated for ED treatment.

Migraine is a clinical diagnosis and, in the ED setting, a diagnosis of exclusion. Other causes of severe headache, such as subarachnoid haemorrhage and meningitis, must be ruled out before this diagnosis is made. Of particular note, the response of a headache to antimigraine therapy should not be used to assume that the cause was migraine. There have been reports that the headaches associated with subarachnoid haemorrhage and meningitis have, on occasion, responded to these agents.

Pathophysiology

The pathophysiology of migraine is complex and not completely understood. It is a chronic neurovascular disorder characterized by dysfunction of the central and peripheral nervous system and intracranial vasculature.

The headache pain of migraine seems to result from the activation of the trigeminovascular system. The triggers for the development of migraine headache are probably chemical and are thought to originate in the brain, the blood vessel walls and the blood itself. These triggers stimulate trigeminovascular axons, causing pain and the release of vasoactive neuropeptides. These neuropeptides act on mast cells, endothelial cells and platelets, resulting in increased extracellular levels of arachidonate metabolites, amines, peptides and ions. These mediators and the resultant tissue injury lead to a prolongation of pain and hyperalgesia.

Serotonin has also been specifically implicated in migraine. By activation of afferents, it causes a retrograde release of substance P. This in turn increases capillary permeability and oedema.

Classification and clinical features

Migraine is defined as an idiopathic recurring headache disorder with attacks that last 4–72 hours. Typical characteristics are unilateral location, pulsating quality, moderate or severe intensity and aggravation by routine physical activity. There is also usually nausea, photophobia and phonophobia.

In some patients, migraine is preceded by an 'aura' of neurological symptoms localizable to the cerebral cortex or brainstem, such as visual disturbance, paraesthesia, diplopia or limb weakness. These develop gradually over 5–20 minutes and last less than 60 minutes. Headache, nausea and/or photophobia usually follow after an interval of less than an hour.

Several variant forms of migraine have been defined, including ophthalmoplegic, abdominal, hemiplegic and retinal migraine, but all are uncommon. In ophthalmoplegic migraine, the headache is associated with paralysis of one or more of the nerves supplying the ocular muscles. Horner's syndrome may also occur. Abdominal migraine manifests as recurrent episodes of abdominal pain for which no other cause is found. Retinal migraine, which is fortunately very rare, involves recurrent attacks of retinal ischaemia which may lead to bilateral optic atrophy. Hemiplegic migraine is a stroke mimic.

Treatment

The complexity of the mechanisms involved in the genesis of migraine suggests that there are a number of ways to interrupt the processes to provide effective relief from symptoms.

A wide variety of pharmacological agents and combinations of agents have been tried for the treatment of migraine, with varying results. Interpreting the evidence is challenging, as the majority of the studies have small sample sizes, compare different agents or combinations of agents, are conducted in settings other than EDs and the outcome measure(s) tested varies widely. For mild to moderate migraine headache in patients who have not taken other medication, aspirin 900 mg combined with metoclopramide 10 mg is effective. Most ED patients, however, have either tried their usual medication or have significant nausea or vomiting making oral therapy inappropriate.

The effectiveness of commonly used agents is summarized in Table 8.1.3. Dosing and administration are summarized in Table 8.1.4. At present, the most effective agents appear to be the phenothiazines (chlorpromazine and prochlorperazine) and the triptans, each of which has achieved >70% efficacy in a number of studies. Note that triptans are contraindicated in patients with a history of ischaemic heart disease, uncontrolled hypertension or with the concomitant use of ergot preparations.

Pethidine (meperidine) is not indicated for the treatment of migraine. Its reported effectiveness is only 56%, it has a high rate of rebound headache and it carries a risk of dependence. The data on dihydroergotamine are difficult to interpret because it is often used in combination with other agents (e.g.

Table 8.1.3 Pooled effectiveness data from ED studies of the treatment of migraine				
Agent	No. of studies	Total patients	Clinical success rate (%)	NNT: clinical success
Chlorpromazine (IV)	6	171	85	1.67
Prochlorperazine (IM or IV)	6	171	71	2.17
Sumatriptan (6 mg SC)	21	3139	71	2.17
Ketorolac (IM or IV)	6	155	66	2.44
Tramadol (IM or IV)	3	191	60	2.86
Metoclopramide (IV)	7	300	58	3.03
Magnesium sulphate (IV)	3	117	41	6.25

Clinical studies in adults, defined 'success' endpoint, minimum of 50 patients studied in aggregate, NNT calculated assuming placebo effectiveness rate of 25%.

Table 8.1.4 Drug dosing and administration

Agent	Drug dosing/administration
Chlorpromazine (IV)	12.5 mg intravenously, repeated every 20 minutes as needed to a maximum dose of 37.5 mg, accompanied by 1 L normal saline over 1 hour to avoid hypotension OR 25 mg in 1 L normal saline over 1 hour, repeated if necessary
Prochlorperazine (IM or IV)	10 mg/12.5 mg (depending on packaging)
Sumatriptan (SC, IN)	6 mg SC, 20 mg IN
Metoclopramide (IV)	10–20 mg
Ketorolac (IM or IV)	30 mg IV, 60 mg IM
Tramadol (IM)	100 mg

metoclopramide); however, it has also been shown to be less effective than chlorpromazine and sumatriptan in acute treatment and to have a high rate of unpleasant side effects. Sodium valproate and haloperidol have also shown moderate effectiveness in small studies, but there are insufficient data to draw a valid conclusion or recommend them as treatment options. Lignocaine (lidocaine) has been shown to be no more effective than placebo. The efficacy of intravenous magnesium sulphate (1 or 2 mg) remains unclear. It was shown in a small placebo-controlled trial to be effective but, in another study, the combination of magnesium with metoclopramide was less effective than metoclopramide and placebo.

Rebound or recurrent headache is common in ED patients treated for migraine (approximately 30%). There is evidence that oral or IV dexamethasone, in addition to standard migraine therapy for selected patients, reduces the proportion of patients who experience early recurrence (so-called rebound headache). A meta-analysis of published papers reports a 26% reduction in the relative risk of headache recurrence within 72 hours. Doses used were 10 mg IV or 8 mg orally.

Trigeminal neuralgia

Trigeminal neuralgia is a debilitating condition in which patients describe 'lightning-'or a 'hot poker-'like pain that is severe and follows the distribution of the trigeminal nerve. Individual episodes of pain last only seconds, but may recur repeatedly within a short period and can be triggered by minor stimuli, such as light touch, eating or drinking, shaving or passing gusts of wind. It is most common in middle or older age.

Aetiology and pathophysiology

Evidence suggests that the pathological basis of trigeminal neuralgia is demyelination of sensory fibres of the trigeminal nerve in the proximal (CNS) portion of the nerve root or, rarely, in the brainstem, most commonly due to compression of the nerve root by an overlying artery or vein.

Trigeminal neuralgia is classified as classic trigeminal neuralgia (no cause identified) and symptomatic trigeminal neuralgia (secondary to another condition). Characteristics associated with symptomatic trigeminal neuralgia are trigeminal sensory deficits and bilateral involvement.

Clinical investigations

In approximately 15% of cases, there is a structural cause for trigeminal neuralgia. For this reason, there is some support for routine neuroimaging (CT, MRI) in these patients. Electrophysiological assessment of trigeminal reflexes can also be helpful in distinguishing classic from symptomatic trigeminal neuralgia. The choice between the two approaches will depend on availability, expertise, cost and patient and treating clinician preference.

Treatment

The mainstay of therapy for trigeminal neuralgia is carbamazepine. The usual starting dose is 200–400 mg/day in divided doses, increased by 200 mg/day until relief up to a maximum of 1200 mg/day. The average dose required is 800 mg/day. Where available, oxcarbazepine 600–1800 mg/day is an effective alternative. For patients who fail first-line therapy, there is some evidence to support the addition of lamotrigine or a change to baclofen. Referral for consideration of surgery is appropriate in patients who are refractory to medical therapy.

Temporal (giant cell) arteritis

Giant cell arteritis is the most common form of vasculitis in patients aged over 50 years. It affects large and middle-sided blood vessels with a predisposition for the cranial arteries arising from the carotid arteries. Loss of vision is the most common severe complication. Involvement of extracranial arteries including the aorta is more frequent than previously assumed. Inflammation markers in blood are usually elevated, but specific laboratory tests for the diagnosis of giant cell arteritis are not available. Imaging using ultrasonography, magnetic resonance imaging and positron emission tomography can be useful to confirm, localize and assess the extent of vascular involvement. Temporal artery biopsy is the gold standard for diagnosis. Glucocorticoids are still the standard therapy (50–100 mg/day). Patients with acute visual changes secondary to giant cell arteritis should receive parenteral corticosteroid therapy and be admitted until their condition stabilizes.

Controversies

- Choice of drug therapy for migraine.
- Role and timing of investigations in atypical migraine. CT or MRI may be indicated acutely to rule out other intracranial pathology.
- The role of corticosteroids in prevention of recurrent/rebound migraine.
- Role and timing of investigations, in particular neuroimaging, for persistent or atypical headache.
- Investigation of trigeminal neuralgia.
- Second-line treatment for trigeminal neuralgia.

Further reading

American Academy for Neurology. AAN summary of evidence-based guideline for clinicians: trigeminal neuralgia. <https://www.aan.com/practice/guideline/uploads/303.pdf> [Accessed Jan. 2013].

Colman I, Friedman BW, Brown MD, et al. Parenteral dexamethasone for acute severe migraine headache: meta-analysis of randomized controlled trials for preventing recurrence. Br Med J 2008;336:1359–61.

Derry CJ, Derry S, Moore RA. Sumatriptan (subcutaneous route of administration) for acute migraine attacks in adults. Cochrane Database Syst Rev 2012;2:CD009665.

Friedman BW, Kapoor A, Friedman MS, et al. The relative efficacy of meperidine for the treatment of acute migraine: a meta-analysis of randomized controlled trials. Ann Emerg Med 2008;52:705–13.

Kelly AM, Holdgate A. Emergency care evidence in practice series, emergency care community of practice: migraine in the emergency department. Melbourne: National Institute of Clinical Studies, 2006. <http://www.nhmrc.gov.au/_files_nhmrc/file/nics/material_resources/Management%20of%20acute%20migraine%20colour.pdf> [Accessed Jan. 2013].

Kelly AM. Specific pain syndromes: headache. In: Mace S, Ducharme J, Murphy M, editors. Pain Management and procedural sedation in the emergency department. New York: McGraw-Hill, 2006.

Kelly AM, Walcynski T, Gunn B. The relative efficacy of phenothiazines for the treatment of acute migraine: a meta-analysis. Headache 2009;49:1324–32.

Sumamo Schellenberg E, Dryden DM, et al. Acute migraine treatment in emergency settings. Comparative effectiveness review No. 84. (Prepared by the University of Alberta Evidence-based Practice Center under Contract No. 290-2007-10021-I.) AHRQ Publication No. 12(13)-EHC142-EF. Rockville, MD: Agency for Healthcare Research and Quality, 2012. <www.effectivehealthcare.gov/reports/final.cfm> [Accessed Jan. 2013].

Yoon YJ, Kim JH, Kim SY, et al. A comparison of efficacy and safety of non-steroidal anti-inflammatory drugs versus acetaminophen in the treatment of episodic tension-type headache: a meta-analysis of randomized placebo-controlled trial studies. Korean J Fam Med 2012;33:262–71.

8.2 Stroke and transient ischaemic attacks

Philip Aplin • Mark Morphett

ESSENTIALS

1 Ischaemic strokes and transient ischaemic attacks (TIAs) are most commonly due to atherosclerotic thromboembolism of the cerebral vasculature or emboli from the heart. Other causes should be considered in younger patients, those presenting with atypical features or when evaluation is negative for the more common aetiologies.

2 Haemorrhagic and ischaemic strokes cannot be reliably differentiated on clinical grounds alone, therefore further imaging, most commonly CT scanning, is required prior to the commencement of antiplatelet, thrombolytic or interventional therapies.

3 The risk of a completed stroke following a TIA is high – up to 15% in the first week. Clinical scoring systems, such as the ABCD^2 score, have been proposed as an assessment tool for a stroke risk following TIA. Patients with TIA identified as low risk for progression to stroke (e.g. ABCD^2 <4) are increasingly managed through integrated rapid TIA assessment clinics in an outpatient setting, with admission reserved for those at higher risk.

4 Differentiating strokes from other acute neurological presentations may be difficult in the emergency department. This issue has implications for the use of high-risk therapies, such as thrombolysis.

5 The early phase of stroke management concentrates on airway and breathing, rapid neurological assessment of conscious level, pupil size and lateralizing signs and blood sugar measurements. Hyperglycaemia may worsen neurological outcome in stroke and so glucose should not be given in likely stroke patients unless a low blood sugar level is objectively demonstrated.

6 Outcomes in stroke patients are improved when they are admitted to a dedicated stroke unit. This involves a multidisciplinary approach to all aspects of stroke management.

7 Treating doctors should be fully aware of the risks/benefits and indications/contraindications of thrombolytic therapy in treating acute strokes. Currently, tPA should be considered for use in selected acute ischaemic strokes when administered within 4.5 hours of symptom onset, but controversies remain.

8 More complex imaging modalities, such as CT perfusion and diffusion/perfusion MRI, continue to be evaluated in acute stroke work-up in an attempt to define better the patient group that will benefit from aggressive vessel opening strategies.

9 In the setting of acute large cerebral vessel occlusion, intra-arterial therapies, such as clot retrieval devices, continue to be evaluated and improved. The place of these interventions in acute stroke therapy is the subject of ongoing research.

Introduction

Cerebrovascular disease is the third highest cause of death in developed countries, after heart disease and cancer. A stroke is an acute neurological injury secondary to cerebrovascular disease, either by infarction (80%) or by haemorrhage (20%). The incidence of stroke is steady and, although mortality is decreasing, it is still a leading cause of long-term disability. Transient ischaemic attacks (TIAs) are defined as transient episodes of neurological dysfunction caused by focal brain, spinal cord or retinal ischaemia, without acute infarction. Causes are similar to those of ischaemic stroke, particularly atherosclerotic thromboembolism related to the cerebral circulation and cardioembolism. Diagnosis of the cause of TIAs with appropriate management is important in order to prevent a potentially devastating stroke.

Pathophysiology

Brain tissue is very sensitive to the effects of oxygen deprivation. Following cerebral vascular occlusion, a series of metabolic consequences may ensue, depending on the extent, duration and vessels involved, which can lead to cell death. Reperfusion of occluded vessels may also occur, either spontaneously or via therapeutic intervention, with the potential for reperfusion injury. An area of threatened but possibly salvageable brain may surround an area of infarction. The identification of this so-called ischaemic penumbra and therapeutic efforts to ameliorate the extent of irreversible neuronal damage, have been the subject of ongoing research efforts.

Large anterior circulation ischaemic strokes can be associated with increasing mass effect and intracranial pressure in the hours to days following onset. Secondary haemorrhage into an infarct may also occur, either spontaneously or related to therapy. Clinical deterioration often follows.

Ischaemic strokes

These are the results of several pathological processes (Table 8.2.1):

- Ischaemic strokes are most commonly due to thromboembolism originating from the cerebral vasculature, the heart or, occasionally, the aorta. Thrombosis usually occurs at the site of an atherosclerotic plaque secondary to a combination of

---

Table 8.2.1 Causes of stroke

Ischaemic stroke

Arterial thromboembolism
　Carotid and vertebral artery atheroma
　Intracranial vessel atheroma
　Small vessel disease – lacunar
　infarction
　Haematological disorders – hypercoagulable
　states
Cardioembolism
　Aortic and mitral valve disease
　Atrial fibrillation
　Mural thrombus
　Atrial myxoma
　Paradoxical emboli
　Hypoperfusion
Severe vascular stenosis or a combination of
these factors
　Hypotension
　Vasoconstriction – drug induced, post-SAH,
　pre-eclampsia
Other vascular disorders
　Arterial dissection
　Gas embolism syndromes
　Moyamoya disease
　Arteritis

Intracerebral haemorrhage

Hypertensive vascular disease
Lipohyalinosis and microaneurysms
Aneurysms
　Saccular
　Mycotic
Arteriovenous malformations
Amyloid angiopathy
Bleeding diathesis
　Anticoagulation
　Thrombolytics
　Thrombocytopenia/disseminated
　intravascular coagulation
　Haemophilia
Secondary haemorrhage into a lesion – tumour
or infarction

---

shear-induced injury of the vessel wall, turbulence and flow obstruction. Vessel wall lesions may also be the site of emboli that dislodge and subsequently occlude more distal parts of the cerebral circulation. Atherosclerotic plaque develops at the sites of vessel bifurcation. Lesions affecting the origin of the internal carotid artery (ICA) are the most important source of thromboembolic events. The more distal intracerebral branches of the ICA, the aorta and the vertebrobasilar system are also significant sites. Acute plaque change is likely to be the precipitant of symptomatic cerebrovascular disease, particularly in patients with carotid stenosis. Hence, the most effective therapies will probably not only target the consequences of acute plaque change, such as thrombosis and embolism, but also aim for plaque stabilization using such agents as antiplatelet drugs, statins and antihypertensive drugs along the lines

---

used in the management of acute coronary syndromes.

- Approximately 20% of cerebrovascular events are due to emboli originating from the heart. Rarely, emboli may arise from the peripheral venous circulation, the embolus being carried to the cerebral circulation via a patent foramen ovale.

- Lipohyalinosis of small arteries is a degenerative process associated with diabetes and hypertension that mainly affects the penetrating vessels that supply areas, such as the subcortical white matter, and is the postulated cause of lacunar infarcts.

- Dissection of the carotid or vertebral arteries may cause TIAs and stroke. This may occur spontaneously or following trauma to the head and neck region, particularly in young people not thought to be at risk of stroke. Distal embolization from the area of vascular injury is the main pathological process involved.

- Haemodynamic reduction in cerebral flow may occur as a result of systemic hypotension or severe carotid stenosis. In these cases, cerebral infarction typically occurs in a vascular watershed area.

- The cerebral vasoconstriction that may occur in association with subarachnoid haemorrhage (SAH), migraine and pre-eclampsia and with drugs, such as sympathomimetics and cocaine, may precipitate stroke.

- Less common vascular disorders, such as arteritis, venous sinus thrombosis, sickle cell disease and moyamoya disease, may be causes of stroke.

- Venous sinus thrombosis may occur spontaneously or in relation to an underlying risk factor, such as an acquired or congenital prothrombotic disorder, dehydration or meningitis. The consequences depend on the extent and localization of the thrombosis. Stroke secondary to venous thrombosis is due to venous stasis, increased hydrostatic pressures and associated haemorrhage.

Haemorrhagic stroke

Haemorrhagic stroke is the result of vessel rupture into the surrounding intracerebral tissue or subarachnoid space. Subarachnoid haemorrhage is the subject of a separate chapter in this book (see Chapter 8.3).

The neurological defect associated with an intracerebral haemorrhage (ICH) is the consequence of direct brain injury, secondary occlusion of nearby vessels, reduced cerebral perfusion caused by associated raised intracranial pressure and cerebral herniation. The causes of ICH include:

- Aneurysmal vessel dilatation. Vascular dilatation occurs at a site of weakness in the arterial wall, resulting in an aneurysm that expands until it ruptures into the subarachnoid space and, in some cases, the brain tissue as well.
- Arteriovenous malformation (AVM). A collection of weakened vessels exists as a result of abnormal development of the arteriovenous connections. AVMs may rupture to cause haemorrhagic stroke or, more rarely, cause cerebral ischaemia from a 'steal' phenomenon.
- Hypertensive vascular disease. Lipohyalinosis, mentioned above as a cause of microatheromatous infarcts, is also responsible for rupture of small penetrating vessels causing haemorrhage in characteristic locations, typically the putamen, thalamus, upper brainstem and cerebellum.
- Amyloid angiopathy. Post-mortem pathological examination has found these changes, particularly in elderly patients with lobar haemorrhages.
- Haemorrhage into an underlying lesion, e.g. tumour or infarction.
- Drug toxicity from sympathomimetics and cocaine.
- Anticoagulation and bleeding diatheses.

Risk factors for TIA/stroke and prevention

This particularly applies to cerebral ischaemic events, both TIAs and strokes. Non-modifiable risk factors for ischaemic stroke include:

- increasing age: the stroke rate more than doubles for each 10 years above age 55.
- gender: stroke is slightly more common in males than females.
- family history.

In terms of primary prevention, hypertension is the most important modifiable risk factor. The benefit of antihypertensive treatment in stroke prevention has been well shown. The other major risk factors for atherosclerosis

and its complications – diabetes, smoking and hypercholesterolaemia – often contribute to increased stroke risk. These should be managed according to standard guidelines.

The most important cardiac risk factor for TIA and stroke is atrial fibrillation (AF), both chronic and paroxysmal. Warfarin is recommended to prevent cardioembolism where the risk:benefit ratio of anticoagulation (target INR 2.0–3.0) favours this. Prediction tools, such as the CHADS$_2$ and CHA$_2$DS$_2$-VASc scores, have been developed to standardize the approach to primary stroke prevention in patients with non-valvular AF. Recently, an oral direct thrombin inhibitor (dabigatran) has been shown to be non-inferior to warfarin for stroke prevention in a large industry sponsored trial (the RE-LY trial). On the basis of this trial, dabigatran has been approved for use as an alternative to warfarin with rapid uptake of this medication in the community. Those with contraindications to warfarin or very low stroke risk should initially receive aspirin.

A carotid bruit or carotid stenosis found in an otherwise asymptomatic patient is associated with an increased stroke risk. However, the role of carotid endarterectomy in these patients is controversial. While early trials suggested some minor benefit, more recent studies have refuted this and it is increasingly clear that intensive

medical therapy in patients with asymptomatic carotid stenosis reduces stroke risk well below that achieved with either endarterectomy or carotid stenting.

Other major cardiac conditions associated with increased TIA/stroke risk include endocarditis, mitral stenosis, prosthetic heart valves, recent myocardial infarction and left ventricular aneurysm. Less common ones include atrial myxoma, a patent foramen ovale and cardiomyopathies.

Secondary prevention involves detection and modification, if possible, of conditions that may have caused a TIA or stroke in order to prevent further events that may result in worse clinical outcomes. As well as the risk factors already mentioned, many other uncommon conditions, such as arterial dissection and prothrombotic states, may cause TIA and stroke. These will be discussed later in the chapter.

Ischaemic stroke syndromes

The symptoms and signs of stroke or TIA correspond to the area of the brain affected by ischaemia or haemorrhage (Table 8.2.2).

In ischaemic brain injury, the history and pattern of physical signs may correspond to a

Table 8.2.2 Location of TIA

Symptom	Arterial territory		
	Carotid	Either	Vertebrobasilar
Dysphasia	+		
Monocular visual loss	+		
Unilateral weakness*		+	
Unilateral sensory disturbance*		+	
Dysarthria**		+	
Homonymous hemianopia		+	
Dysphagia**		+	
Diplopia**			+
Vertigo**			+
Bilateral simultaneous visual loss			+
Bilateral simultaneous weakness			+
Bilateral simultaneous sensory disturbance			+
Crossed sensory/motor loss			+

*Usually regarded as carotid distribution.
**Not necessarily a transient ischaemic attack if an isolated symptom. Reproduced with permission from Hankey GJ. Management of first time transient ischaemic attack. Emerg Med 2001;13:70–81.

characteristic clinical syndrome according to the underlying cause and the vessel occluded. This has a bearing on the direction of further investigation and treatment decisions. Differentiating between anterior and posterior circulation ischaemia/infarction is important in this respect, but is not always possible on clinical grounds alone.

Determining the cause of the event is the next step. Once again, clues, such as a carotid bruit or atrial fibrillation, may be present on clinical evaluation. For accurate delineation of the site of the brain lesion, exclusion of haemorrhage and assessment of the underlying cause, it is usually necessary to undertake imaging studies.

Patterns of clinical features

Anterior circulation ischaemia

The anterior circulation supplies blood to 80% of the brain and consists of the ICA and its branches, principally the ophthalmic, middle cerebral and anterior cerebral arteries. This system supplies the optic nerve, retina, frontoparietal and most of the temporal lobes. Ischaemic injury involving the anterior cerebral circulation commonly has its origins in atherothrombotic disease of the ICA. Atherosclerosis of this artery usually affects the proximal 2 cm, just distal to the division of the common carotid artery. Advanced lesions may be the source of embolism to other parts of the anterior circulation or cause severe stenosis with resultant hypoperfusion distally if there is inadequate collateral supply via the circle of Willis. This is usually manifest by signs and symptoms in the middle cerebral artery (MCA) territory (Table 8.2.3). Less commonly, lesions of the intracranial ICA and MCA may cause similar clinical features.

Embolism to the ophthalmic artery or its branches causes monocular visual symptoms of blurring, loss of vision and field defects. When transient, this is referred to as amaurosis fugax or transient monocular blindness.

The anterior cerebral artery territory is the least commonly affected by ischaemia because of the collateral supply via the anterior communicating artery. If occlusion occurs distally or the collateral supply is inadequate, then ischaemia may occur. This manifests as sensory/motor changes in the leg – more so than in the arm. More subtle changes of personality may occur with frontal lobe lesions, as may disturbances of micturition and conjugate gaze.

Major alterations of consciousness, with Glasgow coma scores <8, imply bilateral hemispheric or brainstem dysfunction. The brainstem may be primarily involved by a brainstem stroke or secondarily affected by an ischaemic or haemorrhagic lesion elsewhere in the brain, owing to a mass effect and/or increased intracranial pressure.

Posterior circulation ischaemia

Ischaemic injury in the posterior circulation involves the vertebrobasilar arteries and their major branches which supply the cerebellum, brainstem, thalamus, medial temporal and occipital lobes. Posterior cerebral artery occlusion is manifested by visual changes of homonymous hemianopia (typically with macular sparing if the MCA supplies this part of the occipital cortex). Cortical blindness, of which the patient may be unaware, occurs with bilateral posterior cerebral artery infarction.

Depending on the area and extent of involvement, brainstem and cerebellar stroke manifest as a combination of: motor and sensory abnormalities, which may be uni- or bilateral; cerebellar features of vertigo, nystagmus and ataxia; and cranial nerve signs, such as diplopia/ophthalmoplegia, facial weakness and dysarthria. Consciousness may also be affected.

Examples of brainstem stroke patterns include (this list is by no means exhaustive):

- ipsilateral cranial nerve with crossed corticospinal motor signs
- lateral medullary syndrome: clinical features include sudden onset of vertigo, nystagmus, ataxia, ipsilateral loss of facial pain and temperature sensation (V) with contralateral loss of pain and temperature sensation of the limbs (anterior spinothalamic), ipsilateral Horner's syndrome and dysarthria and dysphagia (IX and X)

- internuclear ophthalmoplegia manifesting as diplopia and a horizontal gaze palsy due to involvement of the medial longitudinal fasciculus (MLF)
- 'locked-in' syndrome: this is caused by bilateral infarction of a ventral pons, with or without medullary involvement. The patient is conscious due to an intact brainstem reticular formation, but cannot speak and is paralysed. Patients can move their eyes due to sparing of the third and fourth cranial nerves in the midbrain.
- Acute deterioration of conscious state may be the presentation of acute basilar artery occlusion and should be in the differential diagnosis of coma for investigation.

Lacunar infarcts

Lacunar infarcts are associated primarily with hypertension and diabetes. They occur in the small penetrating arteries supplying the internal capsule, thalamus and upper brainstem. Isolated motor or sensory deficits are most commonly seen.

Clinical features

History

This includes the circumstances, time of onset, associated symptoms, such as headache, and any resolution/progression of signs and symptoms. It may be necessary to take a history from a relative or friend, particularly in the presence of dysphasia or reduced conscious state. The history of a stroke is usually of acute onset of a neurological deficit over minutes but, occasionally, there may be a more gradual or stuttering nature to a presentation over a period of hours. A past history of similar events suggestive of a TIA should be carefully sought. The presence of a severe headache with the onset of symptoms may indicate ICH or SAH. However, headache may also occur with ischaemic strokes.

A declining level of consciousness may indicate increasing intracranial pressure due to an ICH or a large anterior circulation infarct – so-called malignant MCA infarction. It may also be caused by pressure on the brainstem by an infratentorial lesion, such as a cerebellar haemorrhage.

The possibility of trauma or drug abuse should be remembered along with the past medical and medication history, particularly anticoagulant/antiplatelet therapy. Risk factors for vascular disease, cardiac embolism, venous

Table 8.2.3 Signs of middle cerebral artery (MCA) occlusion
Homonymous hemianopia
Contralateral hemiplegia affecting face and arm more than leg
Contralateral hemisensory loss
Dysphasias with dominant hemispheric involvement (usually left)
Spatial neglect and dressing apraxia with non-dominant hemispheric involvement

embolism and increased bleeding should be sought.

In young patients with an acute neurological deficit, dissection of the carotid or vertebral artery should be considered. This is often associated with neck pain and headaches/facial pain with or without a history of neck trauma. Trauma if present may be minor, such as a twisting or hyperextension/flexion injury sustained in a motor vehicle accident, playing sports or neck manipulation.

Cardioembolism tends to produce ischaemic injury in different parts of the brain, resulting in non-stereotypical recurrent TIAs, whereas atherothrombotic disease of the cerebral vessels tends to cause recurrent TIAs of a similar nature, particularly in stenosing lesions of the internal carotid or vertebrobasilar arteries.

Examination

Central nervous system This includes assessing the level of consciousness, pupil size and reactivity, extent of neurological deficit, presence of neck stiffness and funduscopy for signs of papilloedema and retinal haemorrhage. Quantifying the neurological deficit using a stroke scale, such as the 42-point National Institute of Health Stroke Scale (NIHSS), is useful in the initial assessment and also for monitoring progress in a more objective way than clinical description alone. Strokes with a NIHSS score >22 are classified as severe.

In the case of TIA, all clinical signs may have resolved. The average TIA lasts less than 15 minutes.

Cardiovascular This includes carotid auscultation and is directed towards findings associated with a cardioembolic source. A carotid bruit in a symptomatic patient is likely to predict a moderate to severe carotid stenosis. Conversely, the absence of a carotid bruit does not exclude significant carotid artery disease as a cause of a TIA or stroke. Major risk factors for cardioembolism that can be identified in the emergency department (ED) include AF, mitral stenosis, prosthetic heart valves, infective endocarditis, recent myocardial infarction, left ventricular aneurysm and cardiomyopathies.

Differential diagnosis (Table 8.2.4)

The acute onset of stroke and TIA is characteristic, however, misdiagnoses (the so-called 'stroke mimics') can occur. The most common stroke mimics are seizures (particularly when there is associated Todd's paresis), hypoglycaemia, systemic infection, brain tumour and toxic metabolic disorders. Others include subdural haematoma, hypertensive encephalopathy, encephalitis, multiple sclerosis, migraine and conversion disorder. This has implications when considering more aggressive stroke interventions, such as thrombolysis.

Complications

CNS complications of stroke include:

- Cerebral oedema and raised intracranial pressure (ICP). This is an uncommon problem in the first 24 hours following ischaemic stroke, but it may occur with large anterior circulation infarcts. It is more commonly seen with ICH, where acutely raised ICP may lead to herniation and brainstem compression in the first few hours.
- Haemorrhagic transformation of ischaemic strokes may occur either spontaneously or associated with treatment.
- Seizures can occur and should be treated in the standard way. Seizure prophylaxis is not generally recommended.
- Non-CNS complications include aspiration pneumonia, hypoventilation, deep venous thrombosis and pulmonary embolism, urinary tract infections and pressure ulcers. In the ED, it is particularly important to be aware of the risk of aspiration.

Clinical investigations

The investigations of TIA and stroke often overlap, but the priorities and implications for management may differ significantly.

General investigations

Standard investigations that may identify contributing factors to stroke/TIA or guide therapy include a complete blood picture, blood glucose, coagulation profile, electrolytes, liver function tests, fasting lipids and, in selected cases, C-reactive protein (CRP). Arterial blood gases should be performed if the adequacy of ventilation is in doubt. An ECG should be performed to identify arrhythmias and signs of pre-existing cardiac disease. Holter monitoring can be considered to identify paroxysmal arrhythmias but has a low yield in unselected patients (i.e. those without any history suggestive of symptomatic arrhythmias or background

Table 8.2.4 Differential diagnosis of stroke
Intracranial space-occupying lesion
Subdural haematoma
Brain tumour
Brain abscess
Postictal neurological deficit – Todd's paresis
Head injury
Encephalitis
Metabolic or drug-induced encephalopathy
Hypoglycaemia, hyponatraemia, etc.
Wernicke–Korsakoff syndrome
Drug toxicity
Hypertensive encephalopathy
Multiple sclerosis
Migraine
Peripheral nerve lesions
Functional

of structural heart disease). A prothrombotic screen may be indicated, particularly in younger patients. Further investigations depend on the nature of the neurological deficit and other risk factors for stroke that are identified on evaluation, but usually involve a combination of brain, vascular and cardiac imaging.

Imaging in TIAs

Prompt diagnosis and management of patients presenting with TIAs and non-disabling strokes has been shown to reduce the risk of subsequent stroke by up to 80%. Risk stratification for patients presenting with TIAs can guide the urgency of investigations required to determine the underlying cause of the TIA – this is discussed more fully below.

Brain imaging A head computed tomography (CT) or magnetic resonance imaging (MRI) scan is indicated in all patients with TIA to exclude lesions that occasionally mimic TIA, such as subdural haematomas and brain tumours. CT and, more particularly MRI, may show areas of infarction which match the symptoms of an ischaemic event that, on clinical grounds, has completely resolved. CT is less sensitive than MRI in detecting posterior territory ischaemic lesions, particularly in the brainstem. In TIAs due to AF or another known cardiac source, brain imaging to exclude ICH is necessary prior to commencing anticoagulation. The exception is in cases of emboli from endocarditis in which anticoagulation is contraindicated owing to the increased risk of secondary ICH.

Imaging vessels *Ultrasound:* if the aetiology of a TIA is likely to be carotid disease, with or without a carotid bruit, then a carotid ultrasound remains the most commonly utilized initial investigation to investigate the presence and degree of a carotid stenosis.

CT angiography (CTA): CTA is increasingly being used to image vessels in cases of TIA – commonly in conjunction with contrast studies examining cerebral perfusion. Advantages include ease of access and avoidance of further delay waiting for second modality imaging. Disadvantages include exposure to contrast dye and ionizing radiation.

Magnetic resonance imaging and magnetic resonance angiography (MRA): this provides non-invasive imaging of the brain and major cerebral vasculature. MRA can show lesions suggestive of a vascular aetiology for TIAs, such as a stenosis due to atheromatous disease and dissection. MRI/MRA is not routine in TIA work-up but may be indicated in more prolonged TIAs, in patients in whom an uncommon cause is suspected or in younger patients.

Angiography: formal angiography may be indicated in selected cases to confirm high-grade carotid stenosis and to confirm/exclude complete carotid occlusions shown on ultrasound. Angiography and MRI/MRA may be performed to investigate for intracranial cerebrovascular disease. The use of formal angiography has declined in recent years, with greater use of both CT angiography and MRA studies as confirmatory tests where atheroma is found on carotid ultrasound.

Cardiac imaging If the clinical evaluation indicates that a cardioembolic source is a likely cause of a TIA, echocardiography is a priority. However, if there is no evidence of cardiac disease on clinical evaluation and the ECG is normal, then the yield of echocardiography is relatively low. A transthoracic echocardiogram (TTE) is the first-line investigation in cardiac imaging. A transoesophageal echocardiogram (TOE) is more sensitive than TTE in detecting potential cardiac sources

of emboli, such as mitral valve vegetations, atrial/mural thrombi and atrial myxoma. TOE should be considered in patients with inconclusive or normal TTE with ongoing clinical concern of a cardioembolic source or patent foramen ovale. This particularly applies to younger patients with unexplained TIAs/non-disabling stroke.

Imaging in stroke

Brain imaging *Computed tomography:* in the setting of completed stroke, the usual first-line investigation is a non-contrast CT scan. The main value of CT is its sensitivity in the detection of ICH and its ready availability. However, CT scans are often normal in the first hours following ischaemic stroke. In only about half of cases will there be changes detected 24 hours after the onset of symptoms.

The early signs of ischaemic stroke include loss of the cortical grey/white matter distinction and hypoattenuation in the affected arterial distribution (e.g. the insular ribbon sign and obscuration of the lenticulostriate territory in MCA infarcts). Occasionally, a hyperdense clot sign will be seen in the region of the MCA. As well as the presence of haemorrhage, the degree of acute ischaemic change, typically change affecting greater than a third of the MCA territory, has been used to exclude patients from thombolytic trials due to possible lack of therapeutic benefit and increased haemorrhage risk. The degree of acute ischaemic change on plain CT can be more reliably quantified by using the ASPECTS score.

A CT scan should be performed as soon as possible following stroke onset. Urgent CT scanning is indicated in patients with a reduced level of consciousness, deteriorating clinical state, symptoms suggestive of ICH, associated seizures, prior to thrombolytic therapy, in younger patients, in patients who are on warfarin and in cases of diagnostic doubt. A CT scan should also be performed to exclude haemorrhage prior to the commencement of antiplatelet therapies. It should, however, be noted that ICH may be subtle and difficult to diagnose, even for radiologists.

CT perfusion/CT angiography: CT perfusion studies are increasingly being used in the setting of acute stroke. Following IV contrast injection, an area of brain is imaged and analysed using computer software with respect to the cerebral blood volume (CBV), cerebral blood flow (CBF) and mean transit time (MTT). Using predetermined cut-offs of these

values, the areas of likely irreversibly infarcted brain (infarct core) and at risk ischaemic brain (ischaemic penumbra) can be demonstrated (E-Fig. 8.2.1). A CT angiogram which includes the carotid vessels is also performed to determine if there is a site of large vessel occlusion. This technology is seen as offering an alternative to diffusion/perfusion MRI and MRA as it is more readily available, generally quicker and less subject to artefact. However, the technique is still in evolution and involves iodinated contrast and radiation exposure.

CT angiography (CTA): CTA is the imaging modality of choice in evaluation of primary ICH to identify the underlying cause, such as an aneurysm or AVM. CTA should be performed in cases of stroke due to suspected arterial dissection and basilar artery thrombosis.

Formal angiography is required occasionally in acute stroke. It will be required if intra-arterial therapy, such as embolectomy, is being considered. This only occurs in specialized centres.

MRI: there are many magnetic resonance modalities available for imaging the brain in acute stroke. Even standard MRI is superior to CT in showing early signs of infarction, with 90% showing changes at 24 hours on T_2-weighted images. Multimodal MRI typically involves additional modes, such as gradient recalled echo (GRE) and fluid-attenuated inversion recovery (FLAIR) sequences for the detection of acute and chronic haemorrhage and diffusion-weighted imaging (DWI) for the detection of early ischaemia or infarction. MR DWI images show areas of reduced water diffusion in the parts of the brain that are ischaemic and likely to be irreversibly injured. This occurs rapidly after vessel occlusion (less than an hour after stroke onset) and manifests as an area of abnormal high signal in the area of core ischaemia. Hence it is much more sensitive in detecting early ischaemia/infarction than standard T_2-weighted MRI modalities or CT. Perfusion-weighted MRI scans (PWI) reveal areas of reduced or delayed cerebral blood flow following MRI contrast injection. This area of the brain is likely to become infarcted if flow is not restored. The DWI and PWI lesions can then be compared. A PWI lesion significantly larger than a DWI lesion is a marker of potentially salvageable brain: the ischaemic penumbra. It is postulated that acute ischaemic stroke patients with this pattern are most likely to benefit from vessel opening strategies, such as thrombolysis. Large areas of diffusion abnormality may also be a marker for increased risk of ICH with thrombolysis. An MRA can be performed at the same time to identify a major vessel occlusion. DWI/PWI imaging is generally considered to be easier to interpret and more reliable than CT perfusion studies. However, MRI may not be as available or feasible. A significant number of patients are unsuitable for MRI and the multimodal imaging takes longer than CT which increases the risk of motion artefact and potential delay to treatment. Radiation and iodinated contrast exposure are absent in MRI.

Recent studies have suggested that MRI is as accurate as CT in diagnosing acute ICH. This is significant as it means that, where facilities are immediately available, CT may be bypassed in acute stroke and MRI can be used both to exclude ICH and to scan for ischaemia/infarction with DWI plus or minus PWI and MRA.

The place of advanced imaging modalities, such as CT perfusion and DWI/PWI MRI, in acute stroke work-up is evolving. For over a decade now it has been hoped that the information provided by these studies will help better select patients who will benefit from aggressive stroke therapies, such as thrombolysis, and extend the current narrow time window for such treatment on the basis of the existence of a significant ischaemic penumbra. They are now a common feature of acute stroke imaging work-up protocols if thrombolysis is being considered. However, at this point, high level evidence of improved clinical outcomes in acute stroke patients based on this approach is lacking. To date, the only published phase III trial (DIAS 2) of thrombolysis 3–9 hours post-onset using penumbral section criteria as shown on advanced imaging CT perfusion or DWI\PWI MRI was negative for the primary outcome of improved neurological outcome. The field of stoke imaging is changing rapidly and ongoing research investigating advanced imaging modalities as a basis for patient selection and mode of treatment is intense.

MRI is indicated in strokes involving the brainstem and posterior fossa where CT has poor accuracy. MRA/MRV is particularly useful in the evaluation of unusual causes of stroke, such as arterial dissection, venous sinus thrombosis and arteritis. Basilar artery thrombosis causes a brainstem stroke with an associated high mortality. If the diagnosis is suspected, urgent specialist consultation should be obtained. If MRA or CTA confirms the diagnosis, aggressive therapies, such as thrombolysis, may improve outcome.

Other investigations

Other investigations may be indicated, particularly in young people, in whom the cause of strokes/TIA may be obscure. These include tests to detect prothrombotic states and uncommon vascular disorders. The list of tests is potentially long and includes a thrombophilia screen, vasculitic and luetic screens, echocardiography and angiography.

Treatment

The treatment of cerebrovascular events must be individualized. It is determined by the nature and site of the neurological lesion and its underlying cause. The benefits and risks of any treatment strategy can then be considered and informed decisions made by the patient or their surrogate. This is particularly the case with the use of more aggressive therapies, such as anticoagulation, thrombolysis and surgery.

Pre-hospital care

The pre-hospital care of the possible stroke patient involves the usual attention to the ABCs of resuscitation and early blood sugar measurement. It is unusual for interventions to be required.

Of potentially greater significance is the development of stroke systems (along the lines of trauma systems) in which the sudden onset of neurological signs and symptoms, identified in the pre-hospital evaluation as being consistent with acute stroke, is used to direct patients to stroke centres with the facilities and expertise to manage them, particularly with regard to the delivery of thrombolytic agents. Closer hospitals without these capabilities may be bypassed.

Pre-hospital evaluation and early hospital triage tools that have been developed for rapid identification of stroke include the Cincinnati Prehospital Stroke Scale or FAST (F – facial movements, A – arm movements, S – speech, and T – test) and the Rosier score. Pre-hospital personnel who identify patients with acute onset of neurological deficits consistent with stroke, using these simple scales, can be potentially directed to stroke centres and in-hospital acute stroke responses can be activated so as to expedite assessment and imaging, particularly if thrombolysis is being considered.

General measures

The ED management of a TIA and stroke requires reassessment of the ABCDs and repeated blood glucose testing. Airway

intervention may be necessary in the setting of a severely depressed level of consciousness, neurological deterioration or signs of raised intracranial pressure and cerebral herniation.

Hypotension is very uncommon in stroke patients, except in the terminal phase of brainstem failure. Hypertension is much more likely to be associated with stroke because of the associated pain, vomiting and raised intracranial pressure and/or pre-existing hypertension, but rarely requires treatment and usually settles spontaneously. It may be a physiological response to maintain cerebral perfusion pressure in the face of cerebral hypoxia and raised intracranial pressure. The use of antihypertensives in this situation may aggravate the neurological deficit. The recently published SCAST trial of candesartan commenced within 30 hours of symptom onset and continued for 7 days in patients with ischaemic (85%) or haemorrhagic (15%) stroke and systolic blood pressure ≥ 140 mmHg showed no benefit in functional outcomes and suggested possible harm. This study excluded patients receiving thrombolysis. Hypertension in the setting of thrombolytic therapy is managed according to local protocols.

Analgesia is appropriate if pain is thought to be contributory and urinary retention should be excluded prior to commencing antihypertensive therapy.

An elevated temperature can occur in stroke and should be controlled. It should also raise the suspicion of other possible causes for the neurological findings or an associated infective focus. Hyperglycaemia should be treated appropriately, however, intensive euglycaemic therapy is not indicated.

TIA

Risk stratification   As already stated, the main aim in therapy in TIAs and minor strokes is to prevent a major subsequent cerebrovascular event. While traditionally patients presenting with TIAs have been hospitalized for work-up, more recently, there has been a move away from this to a more tailored approach where patients are risk stratified into higher risk (inpatient work-up) and lower risk patients who may be suitable for early outpatient follow up, for example in coordinated rapid access 'TIA clinics'.

One popular tool for risk stratification in this population is the ABCD[2] score. The ABCD[2] stroke risk score for TIA has been developed and validated to evaluate the very early risk of a stroke following a TIA. The scoring system is shown in Table 8.2.5. In patients with an $ABCD^2$ score less than 4, there is minimal short-term risk of stroke. With scores of 4–5 and 6–7, the 2-day risk is 4.1%, and 8.1%, respectively. The use of the $ABCD^2$ score is not universally accepted, however, as ongoing validation studies have had mixed results. Other risk stratification strategies, such as the recently published M3T model, use a combination of CT, ECG and carotid ultrasound results to stratify follow-up urgency. Other patient groups are at increased risk of stroke independent of the classical risk stratification systems. These include patients with multiple TIAs within a short period and patients with a probable or proven cardioembolic source.

Antiplatelet therapy Following CT scanning that excludes ICH, aspirin should be commenced at a dose of 300 mg and maintained at 75–150 mg per day in patients with TIAs or minor ischaemic strokes. It has been shown to be effective in preventing further ischaemic events. The ESPRIT trial showed a modest additional benefit from a combination of dipyridamole with aspirin, over aspirin alone. There was no increased risk of bleeding complications but there was a significantly increased rate of withdrawal of patients from the combination arm due to side effects from dipyridamole, principally headache. Clopidogrel may be substituted for aspirin if the patient is intolerant of aspirin or aspirin is contraindicated. There is some evidence that clopidogrel is more effective than aspirin in prevention of vascular events but at greater expense. The combination of aspirin and clopidogrel is not recommended as it does not appear to give any greater therapeutic benefits and there is increased bleeding risk. Anticoagulation with heparin and warfarin has not been shown to be superior to aspirin except in cases of TIA/minor stroke due to cardioembolism (excluding endocarditis).

Anticoagulant therapy Patients with a cardioembolic source of TIA should be considered for full anticoagulation following neurological consultation and normal brain imaging, with the exception of those with endocarditis in whom the risk of haemorrhagic complications is increased.

Surgery Trials have demonstrated a beneficial outcome of urgent surgery for symptomatic carotid stenosis in patients with anterior circulation TIAs and minor stroke with a demonstrated carotid stenosis of between 70 and 99%. The benefit of surgery may extend to lesser grades of stenosis down to 50% in selected patients. The patient's baseline neurological state, co-morbidities and operative mortality and morbidity rate also need to be assessed when considering surgery. The recent CREST trial compared carotid artery stenting (CAS) with endarterectomy (CEA). It revealed slightly superior stroke prevention for CEA in symptomatic patients. In patients with significant co-morbidities, CAS remains an option.

Other medical therapies Risk factors for stroke and TIAs should be identified and treated. Statins should be considered regardless of cholesterol levels. The benefit of lowering LDL cholesterol levels using atorvastatin in preventing further cerebro- and cardiovascular events following an initial episode of cerebral ischaemia was demonstrated in a recent study.

Ischaemic stroke

A more active approach to the acute management of ischaemic stroke is seen as having the potential to improve neurological outcomes. The ED is the place where these important treatment decisions will largely be made. Most patients with a stroke will require hospital admission for further evaluation and treatment, as well as for observation and rehabilitation. Studies of stroke units show that patients benefit from being under the care of physicians with expertise in stroke and a multidisciplinary team that can manage all aspects of their care.

Aspirin In two large trials, aspirin, when administered within 48 hours of the onset of stroke, was found to improve the outcomes of early death or recurrent stroke compared to placebo. A CT or MRI scan should be performed to exclude ICH prior to commencing aspirin. Aspirin should be withheld for at least 24 hours in patients treated with thrombolytics.

Thrombolysis As the most important factor in ischaemic stroke outcome is vessel re-opening, thrombolytic agents are seen as having an important place in the management of acute ischaemic stroke. The evidence on which thrombolysis was originally approved was the NINDs study of 1996. In that study, thrombolysis resulted in improved neurological outcomes in patients receiving tPA compared to placebo, with a 13% absolute increase in the number of patients having good neurological outcomes (numbers needed to treat (NNT) = 8). In the thrombolysis group, there was a significant increase in symptomatic intracerebral haemorrhage rate (6.4% versus 0.6% in the placebo group), of which half were fatal, although there was no overall excess mortality. Factors that may be associated with increased haemorrhage risk include increased age (especially >80 years), increased severity of stroke and early CT changes of a large ischaemic stroke. More recently, three other phase III trials of thrombolysis have been published. The DIAS-2 study was described previously in this chapter. ECASS 3 studied IV tPA versus placebo in

Table 8.2.5	The $ABCD^2$ TIA risk score		
$ABCD^2$	Risk factor		Score
Age	Below 60		0
	Above 60		1
Blood pressure	BP above systolic 140 mmHg, and/or diastolic 90 mmHg on first assessment after TIA		1
Clinical	Unilateral weakness of face, arm, hand or leg		2
	Speech disturbance without weakness		1
Duration	Symptoms lasted >60 mins		2
	Symptoms lasted 10–60 mins		1
	Symptoms lasted <10 mins		0
Diabetes	Presence of diabetes		1

From Johnston SC , Rothwell PM, Nguyen-Huynh MN, et al. Validation and refinement of a score to predict very early stroke risk after transient ischaemic attack. Lancet 2007;369:283-92 with permission.

ischaemic stroke patients 3–4.5 hours from symptom onset. It had a similar design to NINDS but with additional exclusions of patients aged >80, those with severe stroke (NIHSS >25) or acute ischaemic change on plain CT greater than a third of the MCA territory or a history of previous stroke and diabetes. It found a modest but significant improvement in full or very good neurological recovery (Modified Rankin Score [MRS] 0–1), NNT 14. The outcome for full to good neurological recovery (MRS 0–2) was not significantly improved. The risk of a major symptomatic ICH complicating treatment was 5%. The IST-3 trial studied the open label use of IV tPA versus placebo in ischaemic stroke patients from 0 to 6 hours post-onset in whom the treating physician was uncertain if tPA was clearly indicated or not. Over 3000 patients were enrolled over 10 years. The primary outcome of good neurological function at 6 months (Oxford Handicap Score 0–2) was not significantly improved by tPA. There was an excess of early deaths within 7 days in the tPA group but, by 6 months, this was similar in both groups. Symptomatic ICH rate was 7%. The conclusions that can be inferred from these results have been a matter of considerable debate.

Studies of acute stroke patients given tPA outside controlled trials have yielded conflicting results. They suggest that when tPA is used by specialists in well-equipped stroke centres in accordance with strict guidelines, the complication rate for acute stroke patients can be similar to that achieved in trials. The evidence would also strongly suggest that better outcomes are associated with earlier treatment using current treatment guidelines. The percentage of acute ischaemic stroke patients fulfilling the eligibility criteria and receiving thrombolytic treatment is still relatively low. Importantly, protocol violations are associated with an increased risk of poor outcomes, particularly due to haemorrhage. Stroke guidelines in Australia currently recommend the use of tPA if it can be administered in suitable patients up to 4.5 hours post-onset, although every effort should be made to commence treatment as soon as possible.

Patients receiving tPA must be managed in an high dependency type setting. Any deterioration in clinical state, headache or vomiting should instigate cessation of tPA and urgent CT scan. ICH associated with tPA is managed with attention to ABCDs, reversal of thrombolysis

according to local protocols and neurosurgical and ICU involvement as required.

Trials of IV thrombolysis are ongoing with the aims of identifying the best agent, identifying patients most likely to benefit from reperfusion therapy, reducing the risk of symptomatic ICH and extending the time window for treatment. As already discussed, this is particularly through the use of advanced imaging modalities, such as CT perfusion and diffusion/perfusion MRI.

Interventional techniques   Occlusions of the internal carotid and proximal middle cerebral arteries have relatively low rates of recanalization with intravenous tPA. Hence a number of interventional therapies are being investigated either as primary therapy or as a rescue technique post-IV tPA and reperfusion failure. These interventional techniques involve the use of clot retrieval devices and/or intra-arterial thrombolysis and are only available in highly specialized centres. The time window of benefit from interventional therapy may be longer than with IV thrombolysis and may be considered in cases of acute ischaemic stroke due to large vessel occlusion where thrombolysis is contraindicated.

Basilar artery thrombosis has a very poor outcome with conservative management. Case series suggest improved outcomes with interventional techniques, which may be indicated up to 12 hours post-symptom onset.

Anticoagulation   Therapeutic anticoagulation with heparin or clexane is associated with increased risk of haemorrhagic transformation in acute ischaemic stroke. Stroke due to endocarditis has a particularly high risk of this complication. Anticoagulation following acute ischaemic stroke should not be commenced in the ED. In cases of stroke due to cardioembolism, the timing and manner of anticoagulation should be determined by stroke physicians.

Neuroprotection   A range of neuroprotective agents has been trialled in the setting of acute stroke in the hope that modulation of the ischaemic cascade of metabolic changes that follows vascular occlusion may result in improved neurological outcomes. At this stage, however, none of these therapies is recommended for the treatment of acute stroke.

Surgery   As for TIAs, patients with non-disabling stroke should be considered for

investigation with a vascular imaging modality to detect a significant carotid artery stenosis that may be appropriate for urgent surgery. The use of endovascular stents in carotid surgery is also being developed and studied.

Large anterior circulation infarcts have a significant risk of developing cerebral oedema and raised ICP with associated clinical deterioration, particularly manifest by a declining conscious state with or without progression of other signs. These are termed malignant MCA infarcts. Along with standard measures for managing raised ICP, there may be a place for early decompressive craniotomy in selected cases. Intensive care and neurosurgical consultation may be required.

Intracerebral haemorrhage

Primary ICH is most commonly caused by long-standing hypertension-induced small vessel disease. Hypertensive haemorrhage tends to occur in characteristic locations, such as the basal ganglia, thalamus and cerebellum. Berry aneurysms most commonly arise around the circle of Willis, hence ICH due to aneurysmal rupture is often located around this area. Secondary ICH may occur into an underlying lesion, such as a tumour or infarct, and clinical deterioration may result – so-called symptomatic ICH – but this is not always the case.

The clinical presentation of primary ICH is typical of sudden onset of a neurological deficit with associated headache, collapse/transient loss of consciousness, hypertension and vomiting. However, clinical features alone are unable to differentiate ICH from infarction, hence the requirement for brain imaging to confirm the diagnosis. Both CT and MRI (using gradient echo sequences) are equivalent in the detection of ICH.

Treatment

Primary ICH is a medical emergency with a high mortality (between 35 and 50%), with half of these deaths occurring in the first 2 days. There is also a very high risk of dependency. Haematomas can expand rapidly and there is a significant risk of early neurological deterioration and increasing intracranial pressure. General measures as for TIAs and ischaemic stroke should be initiated, in particular attention to airway and ventilatory support. Treatment of raised ICP in a setting of ICH involves a range of modalities similar to those used in head trauma. These include elevation of the head of the bed, analgesia, sedation, an osmotic diuretic, such as mannitol, and hypertonic saline, hyperventilation, drainage of CSF via ventricular catheter and neuromuscular paralysis.

Current consensus guidelines in ICH recommend cautious and controlled lowering of a persistently raised systolic blood pressure >180–200 mmHg or mean arterial pressure (MAP) >130–150 following specialist consultation. Recommended agents include rapidly titratable intravenous drugs, such as sodium nitroprusside, labetolol or glycerine trinitrate at low initial doses, and with continuous haemodynamic monitoring in a critical care setting. The aim is for a 10–15% reduction in blood pressure. The results of the SCAST trial, as mentioned previously, may alter this recommendation; however, the outcome of more aggressive blood pressure reduction in ICH is still being evaluated. The INTERACT trial of intensive BP reduction within 6 hours of symptom onset showed a reduction in haematoma growth. The effect on clinical outcomes is being studied in the INTERACT 2 trial. Treatment should be individualized and take place in consultation with stroke/neurosurgery/intensive care specialists. Sudden falls in blood pressure and hypotension should be avoided as they may aggravate cerebral ischaemia in the setting of raised ICP, which is often associated with ICH.

Use of recombinant Factor VIIa is not recommended. Steroids are also not indicated in ICH. Anticonvulsant prophylaxis is common practice.

Management of ICH associated with anticoagulation or thrombolysis is a matter of urgency and should be done in consultation with a haematologist and a neurosurgeon. Depending on the clinical situation, agents such as protamine sulphate, vitamin K, prothrombin complex concentrate, fresh frozen plasma (FFP) and tranexamic acid may be indicated. Factor VIIa normalizes the INR rapidly, but with a greater potential for thromboembolism. Platelets should be considered if the patient is on antiplatelet therapy.

Surgical management
Surgical management of ICH depends on the location, cause, neurological deficit and overall clinical state. Early neurosurgical consultation should be obtained. High-level evidence for improved outcomes following drainage of supratentorial haematomas by craniotomy is lacking, but the procedure may be indicated

in selected patients, particularly in those with lobar clots within 1 cm of the surface. In patients with deep haemorrhages, craniotomy is generally not recommended.

External ventricular drainage devices (EVDs) may be indicated if hydrocephalus develops.

The presence of a cerebellar haematoma is a particular indication for surgery, with a potential for a good neurological recovery. A variety of other techniques, such as minimally invasive haematoma evacuation, are under investigation.

Controversies

- Thrombolysis is a therapy which may improve neurological outcome in patients with ischaemic stroke when given within 4.5 hours of onset. Problematic issues include the small number of patients who currently present within the time window for treatment; delays in ED assessment and obtaining an expertly reported CT, particularly after hours; identification in the ED of subgroups with higher risk of haemorrhagic complications or lesser treatment benefit; the significant rate of stroke misdiagnosis, with the subsequent potential for unnecessary exposure to a high-risk therapy and the large number of contraindications to thrombolysis. Additionally, protocol violations can increase the risk of a poor outcome.
- Advances in neuroimaging, particularly diffusion/perfusion MRI and perfusion CT/CTA, show promise for improved selection of patients likely to benefit from thrombolytic therapy. The optimal imaging strategy remains unclear.
- The place of interventional therapies in acute ischaemic stroke is the subject of intense research. They have the potential to improve outcome by prolonging the treatment window, increased recanalization rates in large vessel occlusions and reducing haemorrhagic complications. A number of clot retrieval devices are being evaluated as is intra-arterial thrombolysis.
- The place of dabigatran in AF/stroke prevention. Although uptake in the

community has been rapid, more time is needed to see whether industry sponsored trials of efficacy translate into real world benefits.
- The follow-up investigation and management of patients presenting to emergency departments with TIA is moving increasingly to an outpatient model of care. The optimum method of risk stratification and patient selection for this approach has yet to be conclusively determined.
- Treatment of hypertension associated with stroke. Antihypertensive therapy is rarely necessary and recent studies indicate this should not be routinely instituted in the acute phase. Therapy should be considered in patients with persistent very high pressures and intracranial haemorrhage in consultation with treating specialist teams. Ongoing studies are evaluating the value of intensive reduction of high blood pressures in the setting of ICH. Hypertension may require treatment in the setting of thrombolytic therapy in accordance with local protocols.
- Neuroprotective therapies continue to be evaluated but, at this stage, cannot be recommended outside a clinical trial.

Further reading

Barber PA, Demchuk AM, Zhang J, Buchan AM, for the ASPECTS Study Group. The validity and reliability of a novel quantitative CT score in predicting outcome in hyperacute stroke prior to thrombolytic therapy. Lancet 2000;355:1670–4.

Brott TG, Hobson RW, Howard G, et al. for the CREST investigators. Stenting versus endarterectomy for treatment of carotid-artery stenosis. N Engl J Med 2010;363:11–23.

CAST (Chinese Acute Stroke Trial) Collaborative Group. CAST: randomised placebo controlled trial of early aspirin use in 20 000 patients with acute ischaemic stroke. Lancet 1997;349:1641–9.

Connolly SJ, Ezekowitz MD, Yusuf S, et al. Dabigatran versus warfarin in patients with atrial fibrillation. N Engl J Med 2009;361:1139–51.

Hacke W, Furlan AJ, Al-Rawi Y, et al. Intravenous desmoteplase in patients with acute ischaemic stroke selected by MRI perfusion–diffusion weighted imaging or perfusion CT (DIAS-2): a prospective, randomised, double-blind, placebo-controlled study. Lancet Neurol 2009;8:141–50.

Hacke W, Kaste M, Bluhmki E, et al. Thrombolysis with alteplase 3 to 4.5 hours after acute ischemic stroke (ECASS 3). N Engl J Med 2008;359:1317–29.

Johnston SC, Rothwell PM, Nguyen-Huynh MN, et al. Validation and refinement of a score to predict very early stroke risk after transient ischaemic attack. Lancet 2007;369:283–92.

Kidwell CS, Chalela JA, Saver JL, et al. Comparison of MRI and CT for detection of acute intracerebral hemorrhage. J Am Med Assoc 2004;292:1823–34.

National Stroke Foundation. Clinical guidelines for stroke management. Melbourne, 2010.

North American Symptomatic Carotid Endarterectomy Trial Collaborators (NASCET). Beneficial effects of carotid endarterectomy in symptomatic patients with high grade carotid stenosis. N Engl J Med 1991;325:445–53.

Nor AM, Davis J, Sen B, et al. The recognition of stroke in the emergency room (ROSIER) scale: development and validation of a stroke recognition instrument. Lancet Neurol 2005;4:727–34.

Rothwell PM, Giles MF, Chandratheva A, et al. on behalf of the EXPRESS study investigators. Effect of urgent treatment of transient ischaemic attack and minor stroke on early recurrent stroke (EXPRESS study): a prospective population-based sequential comparison. Lancet 2007;370:1432–42.

Sandset EC, Bath PM, Boysen G, et al. The angiotensin-receptor blocker candesartan for treatment of acute stroke (SCAST): a randomised, placebo-controlled, double-blind trial. Lancet 2011;377:741–50.

Sanders LM, Srikanth VK, Jolley DJ, et al. Monash transient ischemic attack triaging treatment. Safety of a transient ischemic attack mechanism-based outpatient model of care. Stroke 2012;43:2936–41.

Spence JD, Pelz D, Veith FJ. Asymptomatic carotid stenosis. Identifying patients at high enough risk to warrant endarterectomy or stenting. Stroke 2011;42:1–3.

The ESPRIT Study Group Aspirin plus dipyridamole versus aspirin alone after cerebral ischaemia of arterial origin (ESPRIT). Lancet 2006;367:1665–73.

The IST 3 Collaborative Group The benefits and harms of intravenous thrombolysis with recombinant tissue plasminogen activator within 6 h of acute ischaemic stroke (the third international stroke trial [IST-3]): a randomised controlled trial. Lancet 2012;379:2352–63.

The National Institute of Neurological Disorders and Stroke rt-PA Stroke Study Group (NINDS). Tissue plasminogen activator for acute ischaemic stroke. N Engl J Med 1995;333:1581–7.

8.3 Subarachnoid haemorrhage

Pamela Rosengarten

ESSENTIALS

1 The diagnosis of subarachnoid haemorrhage (SAH) requires a high index of suspicion.

2 Up to 50% of patients with SAH experience a warning leak – the sentinel haemorrhage – in the hours to days prior to the major bleed.

3 Risk of re-bleeding is maximal in first 2–12 hours and is associated with a poor prognosis and high mortality.

4 Severe sudden headache is the primary clinical feature.

5 Brain CT scan without contrast is the initial investigation of choice.

6 A negative CT scan for SAH should be followed by lumbar puncture and examination of the cerebrospinal fluid.

7 Patients with SAH require urgent neurosurgical referral and management.

8 Early definitive isolation and occlusion of the aneurysm reduces early complications and improves outcome.

9 Endovascular treatment is the treatment of choice in most cases.

Introduction

Patients with headache account for approximately 1% of all emergency department (ED) visits and, of these, 1–4% have a final diagnosis of subarachnoid haemorrhage (SAH). Early accurate diagnosis of aneurysmal SAH is imperative, as early occlusion of the aneurysm has been shown to reduce early complications of re-bleeding and vasospasm and improve outcome.

Epidemiology and pathology

SAH is the presence of extravasated blood within the subarachnoid space. The incidence in Australia is approximately 10 cases per 100 000 patient-years, but is significantly higher (around 20 per 100 000) in Japan and Finland, for reasons that are unclear. Although incidence increases with age, about half of those affected are aged under 55, the condition being most common in the 45–64 age group.

The most common cause of SAH is head trauma which is dealt with elsewhere in this book. Non-traumatic or spontaneous SAH results from rupture of a cerebral aneurysm in approximately 85% of cases, non-aneurysmal perimesencephalic haemorrhage in 10% and the remaining 5% from other rare causes including rupture of mycotic aneurysms, intracranial arterial dissection, arteriovenous malformations, vasculitis, central venous thrombosis, bleeding diatheses, tumours and drugs, such as cocaine, amphetamines and anticoagulants.

Aneurysms

Intracranial aneurysms are not congenital. Rather, they develop during the course of life. An estimate of the frequency for an adult without risk factors is 2.3%, with the proportion increasing with age. Most aneurysms will never rupture, but the risk increases with size. Paradoxically, as the vast majority of aneurysms are small, most aneurysms that rupture are small. An aneurysm of the posterior circulation is more likely to rupture than one of comparable size in the anterior circulation.

Risk factors can be divided into those that are modifiable and those that are not. Modifiable risk factors include cigarette smoking, hypertension, sympathomimetic drug use (e.g. cocaine) and excessive alcohol intake. Non-modifiable factors include history of previous aneurysmal SAH, a family history of first-degree relatives with SAH, inherited connective tissue disorders (particularly polycystic kidney disease and neurofibromatosis), sickle cell disease and α_1-antitrypsin deficiency.

Non-aneurysmal perimesencephalic haemorrhage

This type of SAH is defined by the characteristic distribution of blood in the cisterns around the midbrain in combination with normal angiographic studies. It usually carries a relatively benign prognosis. A small proportion of patients with this distribution of blood may have a ruptured aneurysm of a vertebral or basilar artery.

Clinical features

History

The history is critical to the diagnosis of SAH:

- Headache is the principal presenting symptom, being present in up to 95% of patients with SAH and being the solitary symptom in up to 40% of patients. It is typically severe, of sudden onset, almost instantaneously reaching peak intensity and often being the worst headache ever experienced. Approximately 25% of patients presenting with sudden severe headache will have SAH.
- Up to 50% of patients experience a warning leak (sentinel haemorrhage) in the hours to weeks before the major bleed. This headache may be mild, generalized or localized, of variable duration, resolve spontaneously within minutes to hours or last several days and usually responds to analgesic therapy. It does, however, tend to develop abruptly and differ in quality from other headaches that the patient may have previously experienced. Hence a patient's worst or first headache is suggestive of SAH.
- Upper neck pain or stiffness is common.
- One-third of patients will develop SAH during strenuous exercise, e.g. bending or lifting, whereas in the remaining two-thirds it will occur during sleep or routine daily activities.
- Nausea and vomiting are present in 75% of patients.
- Brief or continuing loss of consciousness occurs in the majority of patients. Severe headache is usually experienced when the patient regains consciousness, although a

Table 8.3.1 Clinical grading schemes for patients with SAH

Grade	Grading scheme of Hunt and Hess	Grading scheme of WFNS	
		GCS	Motor deficit
1	No symptoms or minimal headache, slight nuchal rigidity	15	No
2	Moderate to severe headache, no neurological deficit other than cranial nerve palsy	13–14	No
3	Drowsy, confused, mild focal deficit	13–14	Yes
4	Stupor, moderate to severe hemiparesis, vegetative posturing	7–12	Yes or no
5	Deep coma, decerebration, moribund	3–6	Yes or no

WFNS: World Federation of Neurosurgeons; GCS: Glasgow coma score. Reproduced with permission from Sawin PD, Loftus CM. Diagnosis of spontaneous subarachnoid hemorrhage. Am Fam Phys 1997;55:145–56.

brief episode of excruciating headache may occur prior to losing consciousness.

- Seizures occur in up to 20% of patients and, when associated with a typical headache, are a strong indicator of SAH, even if the patient is neurologically normal when assessed.
- Prodromal symptoms, particularly third cranial nerve with pupillary dilatation and sixth cranial nerve palsies are uncommon, but may suggest the presence and location of a progressively enlarging unruptured aneurysm.
- No clinical feature can reliably identify SAH.

Examination

There is a wide spectrum of clinical presentations, the level of consciousness and clinical signs being dependent on the site and extent of the haemorrhage:

- On ED presentation, two-thirds of patients have impaired level of consciousness – 50% with coma. Consciousness may improve or deteriorate. An acute confusional state can occur which may be mistaken for a psychological problem.
- Signs of meningism, photophobia and neck stiffness, are present in 75% of patients, but may take several hours to develop and may be absent in the deeply unconscious. Absence of neck stiffness does not exclude SAH. Fever may also be present.
- Focal neurological signs are present in up to 25% of patients and are secondary to associated intracranial haemorrhage, cerebral vasospasm, local compression of a cranial nerve by the aneurysm (e.g. oculomotor nerve palsy by posterior communicating aneurysm or bilateral lower limb weakness due to anterior

communicating aneurysm) or raised intracranial pressure (sixth-nerve palsy).
- Ophthalmological examination may reveal unilateral or bilateral subhyaloid haemorrhages or papilloedema.
- Systemic features associated with SAH include severe hypertension, hypoxia and acute ECG changes that may mimic acute myocardial infarction.
- A small proportion of patients present in cardiac arrest. Resuscitation attempts are vital, as half of survivors regain independent function.

Patients are categorized into clinical grades from I to V, according to their conscious state and neurological deficit. Two grading schemes, that of Hunt and Hess and that of the World Federation of Neurosurgeons, which is preferred, are depicted in Table 8.3.1. The higher the score, the worse the prognosis.

Differential diagnosis

Important differential diagnoses include benign thunderclap headache (40%), migraine, cluster headache, headache associated with sexual exertion, vascular headaches of stroke, intracranial haemorrhage, venous thrombosis and arterial dissection, meningitis, encephalitis, acute hydrocephalus, intracranial tumour and intracranial hypotension.

Clinical investigations

Imaging

Computed tomography (CT)
Non-contrast brain CT scan is the initial investigation of choice. In the first 24 hours after

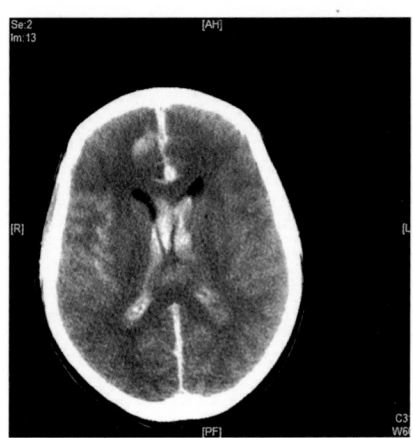

Fig. 8.3.1 Non-contrast head CT scan demonstrating widespread subarachnoid and intraventricular blood.

haemorrhage it can demonstrate the presence of subarachnoid blood in more than 95% of cases (Fig. 8.3.1). The sensitivity, however, decreases with time owing to the rapid clearance of blood, with only 80% of scans positive at 3 days and 50% positive at 1 week. CT will also demonstrate the site and extent of the haemorrhage, indicate the possible location of the aneurysm and demonstrate the presence of hydrocephalus and other pathological changes.

Magnetic resonance imaging
Magnetic resonance imaging (MRI) with FLAIR (fluid attenuated inversion recovery) proton density, diffusion weighted imaging and gradient echo sequences is reliable in demonstrating early SAH and is superior to CT in detecting extravasated blood in the days (up to 40 days) following haemorrhage. Availability and logistical considerations, including longer procedure time, make MRI impractical for use in the initial diagnostic work-up of SAH, but it may be considered in patients who present late.

CT angiography
CT angiography (CTA) is the preferred angiographic technique once SAH has been identified. Compared to catheter angiography, it has a sensitivity of 98% for cerebral aneurysms, is readily available and has a lower complication rate. It should be performed as soon as the diagnosis is made. Where diagnosis has been made by CT, CTA should preferably be performed while the patient is still in the scanner. CTA is usually of sufficient quality to allow planning of endovascular or neurosurgical interventions. It is important to note that small aneurysms <3 mm may not

reliably be detected on CTA and so further investigations may be warranted in CTA-negative SAH.

A CT/CTA approach has been suggested as an alternate diagnostic strategy to CT/LP (lumbar puncture) in the diagnosis of SAH. However, this approach focuses on identifying an aneurysm, rather than the presence of intracranial haemorrhage. The consequence of this strategy may be that the aneurysm detected is an incidental finding, as aneurysms are known to occur in about 2.5% of the normal population. This would then result in unnecessary investigation and treatment of an asymptomatic aneurysm and so is currently not supported.

Cerebral angiography
Cerebral angiography is the gold standard for confirming the presence of an aneurysm, its location and the presence of vasospasm and was previously the preferred angiographic test. It is not, however, without risk. Neurological complications occur in ≈1.8% of cases, with re-rupture of an aneurysm reported in 2–3%. It is also less available than CTA. These factors have seen it become less favoured and used in selected cases only.

Magnetic resonance angiography
MR angiography is currently useful as a screening tool for the diagnosis of intracranial aneurysms in patients at increased risk.

Further imaging when no cause for SAH is found
In patients where SAH is present and no cause is found, then the distribution of extravasated blood on the CT scan should be reviewed. If this conforms to the perimesencephalic distribution of non-aneurysmal haemorrhage, then no further investigations may be warranted. If, however, an aneurysmal pattern of haemorrhage is present, then a second CTA is recommended as occasionally an aneurysm may have gone undetected on the original test.

Lumbar puncture
Lumbar puncture is necessary when there is clinical suspicion of SAH, the CT scan is negative, equivocal or technically inadequate and no mass lesion or signs of raised intracranial pressure are found. In about 3–5% of patients with SAH, the CT scan will be normal. Although it has been suggested that a negative CT scan performed in the first 6 hours following

headache onset is sufficient to exclude a diagnosis of SAH, evidence is inadequate to support this practice and so cannot be recommended to replace a CT/LP strategy.

The diagnosis of SAH, then, is dependent on the finding of red blood cells not due to traumatic tap or red blood cell breakdown products within the CSF. Lumbar puncture should be delayed for at least 6 and preferably 12 hours after symptom onset to allow bilirubin to be formed from cell breakdown in SAH. Detection of bilirubin and xanthochromia is the only reliable method of distinguishing SAH from a traumatic tap. Proceeding to angiographic studies in every patient with bloodstained CSF would be expected to identify an incidental finding of a small unruptured aneurysm in about 2%.

It is important to measure the opening pressure when performing a lumbar puncture, as CSF pressure may be elevated in SAH or in other conditions, such as intracranial venous thrombosis or pseudotumour cerebri, or low in spontaneous intracranial hypotension.

Xanthochromia, the yellow discoloration of CSF caused by the haemoglobin breakdown products oxyhaemoglobin and bilirubin due to lysis of red blood cells, is generally agreed to be the primary criterion for diagnosis of SAH and differentiates between SAH and traumatic tap. It is usually present within 6 hours of SAH and has been demonstrated in all patients with SAH between 12 hours and 2 weeks following the haemorrhage. Xanthochromia is not reliably detected by visual examination of centrifuged CSF. Spectrophotometric analysis of CSF for bilirubin is considered the most sensitive means of detecting xanthochromia.

Controversy exists as to the optimal timing of lumbar puncture. Early lumbar puncture within 12 hours may have negative or equivocal CSF findings, whereas delayed lumbar puncture may result in an increased risk of early re-bleeding as well as having practical implications for the ED. In general, at least 6–12 hours should have elapsed between the onset of headache and lumbar puncture. Although detection of xanthochromia is indicative of SAH, it does not entirely rule out traumatic lumbar puncture and can occur in extremely bloody taps (>12 000 RBC/mL) or where the lumbar puncture has been repeated after an initial traumatic tap.

Other studies of the CSF, such as three tube cell counts, D-dimer assay and detection of erythrophages, have been found to be inconsistent in differentiating SAH from traumatic tap.

General investigations

General investigations to be performed include full blood examination, erythrocyte sedimentation rate, urea, electrolytes including magnesium, blood glucose, coagulation screen, chest X-ray and 12-lead ECG. ECG changes are frequently present and include ST and T-wave changes which may mimic ischaemia, QRS and QT prolongation and arrhythmias. Cardiac biomarkers, including troponin, may also be elevated.

Complications

Early complications

- Re-bleeding: up to 15% within hours of the initial haemorrhage and, overall, 40% of patients re-bleed within the first 4 weeks if there is no intervention. Re-bleeding is associated with 60% mortality and half of the survivors remain disabled.
- Subdural haematoma or large intracerebral haematoma can be life threatening and require immediate drainage. Similarly, a large intracerebral haematoma may be contributing to the poor clinical condition and warrant drainage simultaneously with treatment of the aneurysm.
- Global cerebral ischaemia: irreversible brain damage resulting from haemorrhage at the time of aneurysm rupture. This is probably secondary to a marked rise in intracranial pressure resulting in inadequate cerebral perfusion.
- Cerebral vasospasm: clinically significant vasospasm occurs in approximately 20% of patients with SAH and is a major cause of death and morbidity. It tends to occur between days 3 and 15 after SAH, with a peak incidence at days 6–8. Vasospasm causes ischaemia or infarction and should be suspected in any patient who suffers a deterioration in their neurological status or develops neurological deficits. The best predictor of vasospasm is the amount of blood seen on the initial CT scan.
- Hydrocephalus occurs in approximately 20% of patients with SAH. It can occur within 24 hours of haemorrhage and should be suspected in any patient who suffers a deterioration in mentation or conscious state, particularly if associated with slowed pupillary responses.
- Seizures.
- Fluid and electrolyte disturbances: patients with SAH may develop hyponatraemia

and hypovolaemia secondary to excessive natriuresis (cerebral salt wasting) or, alternatively, may develop a syndrome of inappropriate ADH (SIADH).
- Hyperglycaemia and hyperthermia, both of which are associated with a poor outcome.
- Medical complications include pulmonary oedema, cardiogenic or neurogenic (23%), cardiac arrhythmias (35%), sepsis, venous thromboembolism and respiratory failure.

Late complications

- Late re-bleeding, from a new aneurysm or regrowth of the treated aneurysm, is estimated at ≈1.3% in 4 years for coiling and ≈2–3% in 10 years for surgical clipping.
- Anosmia: up to 30%.
- Epilepsy: 5–7%.
- Cognitive deficits and psychosocial dysfunction are common even in those who make a good recovery; 60% of patients report personality change.

Treatment

The management of SAH requires general supportive measures, particularly airway protection and blood pressure control, as well as specific management of the ruptured aneurysm and the complications of aneurysmal haemorrhage.

General measures

- Stabilization of the unconscious patient, with particular attention to the airway. Endotracheal intubation with oxygenation and ventilation will be required in patients with higher-grade (4–5) SAH.
- Close observation of Glasgow coma scale (GCS) and vital signs.
- In all patients, maintain oxygenation and circulation ensuring adequate (euvolaemic) blood volume.
- Analgesia, using reversible narcotic analgesic agents, sedation and antiemetics as required. Ensure bed rest with minimal stimulation. Avoid aspirin and non-steroidal analgesic agents (NSAIDs).
- Blood pressure control: blood pressure levels are often of the order of 150/90 immediately following SAH and, in most patients, can be adequately controlled by sedation and analgesia. Normotensive levels extending to mild to moderately hypertensive levels, especially in patients with pre-existing hypertension, are

acceptable. Antihypertensive therapy should be reserved for patients with severe (mean arterial pressure >130 mmHg) hypertension or where there is evidence of progressive end-organ dysfunction and short-acting antihypertensive agents (e.g. esmolol or nitroprusside) and intensive haemodynamic monitoring should be employed.
- Fever should be regulated to maintain normothermia which is associated with improved functional outcome.
- Seizures should be treated as they occur. The routine use of long-term prophylactic phenytoin is controversial and has been linked with unfavourable functional and cognitive outcomes.
- Correct electrolyte imbalances. Hyponatraemia of excessive natriuresis must be differentiated from that of SIADH. Hypovolaemia is to be avoided.
- Effective glucose control, importantly avoiding hyper- and hypoglycaemia.
- Venous thromboembolism prophylaxis, initially with compressive devices and later with subcutaneous heparin following treatment of the aneurysm.
- Treatment of hydrocephalus by ventricular drainage may be required.

Specific treatment

Prevention of re-bleeding

Obliteration of the ruptured aneurysm by endovascular coiling or surgical clipping should be performed as early as possible to prevent re-bleeding, remove clot, reduce the incidence of early complications and improve outcomes.

Endovascular occlusion, achieved by placing detachable coils in aneurysms under radiological guidance (coiling), has largely replaced surgical occlusion as the method of choice for prevention of re-bleeding in suitable cases. The method of treatment, however, depends on anatomical considerations, as aneurysms are not equally amenable to this option. In aneurysms that are suitable to treatment by either modality, 4-year outcome has been demonstrated to be better with coiling, although there are higher aneurysm recurrence and re-bleeding rates.

Surgical clipping is now a second-line option for most patients. It is usually done early – within 3 days, and preferably within 24 hours.

Antifibrinolytic agents, including ε-aminocaproic acid, which inhibit clot lysis, reduce the incidence of re-bleeding after initial aneurysmal rupture. Short-term therapy (<72 hours) may be indicated in patients without medical contraindications who have an unavoidable delay in obliteration of the aneurysm and a significant risk of re-bleeding. Although not affecting clinical outcome, their use has been associated with an increase in deep venous thrombosis but not pulmonary embolism.

Prevention of delayed cerebral ischaemia

Cerebral ischaemia is often gradual in onset and involves the territory of more than one cerebral artery. Peak frequency is at 5–14 days after SAH. Nimodipine, a calcium channel antagonist, improves clinical outcome in SAH, with a relative risk reduction of 18% and an absolute risk reduction of 5.1%. The current standard regimen is nimodipine 60 mg orally every 4 hours for 3 weeks. It should be commenced within 48 hours of haemorrhage.

Other treatments including magnesium sulphate, the statins and antiplatelet agents have not been demonstrated to improve clinical outcomes.

There are no definitive treatments for delayed cerebral ischaemia, although improving cerebral perfusion by maintenance of euvolaemia and induced hypertension is recommended where blood pressure and cardiac status permit. In vasospasm unresponsive to medical management, emergency cerebral angiography with intra-arterial vasodilator infusion or transluminal balloon angioplasty may be considered where focal vessel narrowing is demonstrated.

Prognosis

SAH has a 40–60% mortality rate from the initial haemorrhage, with up to one-third of survivors having a significant neurological deficit. The most important prognostic factor is the clinical condition at the time of presentation, with coma and major neurological deficits generally being

associated with a poor prognosis. Survival rates have been reported at 70% for grade I, 60% for grade II, 50% for grade III, 40% for grade IV and 10% for grade V SAH.

It is worth noting, however, that survival without brain damage is possible even after respiratory arrest. Even patients who make a good recovery may suffer cognitive and psychosocial dysfunction.

Aneurysm screening in patients who have survived aneurysmal SAH is advocated, as these patients are at increased risk of new or recurrent aneurysmal bleeds.

Incidental unruptured aneurysms

If an unruptured aneurysm is found incidentally, it raises the dilemma of the risk–benefit rationale between intervention and conservative management. Factors taken into account include age, aneurysm size and location, gender, country, co-morbidity and family history. Such patients should be referred to a neurosurgical service for advice and counselling.

Conclusion

Clinical suspicion of the diagnosis of SAH gained from a history of sudden, severe or atypical headache demands a full investigation, including brain CT scan and, if necessary, lumbar puncture. Once SAH has been diagnosed, urgent neurosurgical referral and management are required.

Controversies

- The timing of lumbar puncture (LP) following a negative CT scan for SAH.
- Non-contrast CT without LP within first 6 hours of headache and CT/CTA as diagnostic strategies for SAH.

- Vascular imaging for patients with a negative CT scan and negative CSF is indicated in those with ambiguous test results, those at high risk for SAH and patients presenting after more than 2 weeks.
- Prophylactic anticonvulsant therapy for patients with SAH.
- Follow up for patients after coiling.

Further reading

Arora S, et al. Evaluating the sensitivity of visual xanthochromia in patients with subarachnoid hemorrhage. J Emerg Med 2010;39:13–16.

Connolly Jr ES, Rabinstein AA, Carhuapoma JR, et al. on behalf of the American Heart Association Stroke Council, Council on Cardiovascular Radiology and Intervention, Council on Cardiovascular Nursing, Council on Cardiovascular Surgery and Anesthesia, and Council on Clinical Cardiology. Guidelines for the management of aneurysmal subarachnoid hemorrhage: a guideline for healthcare professionals from the American Heart Association/American Stroke Association. Stroke 2012;43:1711–37.

Dorhout Mees SM, Rinkel GJE, Vermeulen M, van Gijn J. Calcium antagonists for aneurysmal subarachnoid haemorrhage. Cochrane Database Syst Rev 4:CD000277.

Edlow JA. What are the unintended consequences of changing the diagnostic paradigm for subarachnoid hemorrhage after brain computed computed tomography angiography in place of lumbar puncture? Acad Emerg Med 2010;17:991–5.

Lai L, Morgan MK. Incidence of subarachnoid hameorrhage: an Australian national hospital morbidity database analysis. J Neurosci 2012;19:733–9.

Lysack JT, et al. Asymptomatic unruptured intracranial aneurysms: approach to screening and treatment. Can Fam Phys 2008;54:1535–8.

Mark DG, MD, Hung Y, Offerman SR, et al. for the Kaiser Permanente CREST Network Investigators. Nontraumatic subarachnoid hemorrhage in the setting of negative cranial computed tomography results: external validation of a clinical and imaging prediction rule. Ann Emerg Med ePub; 2012 [Accessed Nov. 2012].

McCormack RF, Hutson AA. Can computed tomography angiography of the brain replace lumbar puncture in the evaluation of acute onset headache after negative non contrast cranial computed tomography scan? Acad Emerg Med 2010;17:444–51.

Naval NS, Stevens RD, Mirski MA. Controversies in the management of subarachnoid haemorrhage. Crit Care Med 2006;34:511–24.

Suarez JI, Tarr RW, Selman WR. Current concepts: aneurysmal subarachnoid haemorrhage. N Engl Med J 2006;354:387–98.

van Gijn J, Kerr RS, Rinkel GJE. Subarachoid haemorrhage. Lancet 2007;369:306–18.

8.4 Altered conscious state

Ruth Hew

ESSENTIALS

1 For clinical purposes, the ability of the individual to respond appropriately to environmental stimuli provides a quantifiable definition of consciousness. The Glasgow coma score is used to quantify conscious state and monitor progress.

2 The causes of altered conscious state can be divided pathophysiologically into structural and metabolic insults.

3 A thorough history and examination is the key to guiding investigation choice and identifying the cause of the primary insult. Management is directed towards resuscitation, specific correction of the primary pathology and minimization of secondary injury.

4 Bedside blood glucose measurement is essential and may be life saving.

Table 8.4.1   The Glasgow coma scale
The GCS is scored between 3 and 15, 3 being the worst and 15 the best. It is composed of three parameters: best eye response, best verbal response, best motor response, as given below
Best eye response (score out of 4) 1 – No eye opening 2 – Eye opening to pain 3 – Eye opening to verbal command 4 – Eyes open spontaneously
Best verbal response (score out of 5) 1 – No verbal response 2 – Incomprehensible sounds 3 – Inappropriate words 4 – Confused 5 – Orientated
Best motor response (score out of 6) 1 – No motor response 2 – Extension to pain 3 – Flexion to pain 4 – Withdrawal from pain 5 – Localizing pain 6 – Obeys commands

Introduction

Consciousness is variously termed lucidness, orientation, awakeness and mentation in the context of patients in the emergency department (ED). None of these terms is a comprehensive definition of consciousness. Neither does the Glasgow coma scale (GCS) (Table 8.4.1), commonly used but developed for head-injured patients in a time when computed tomography (CT) scanning was not yet available, truly measure what we as clinicians mean by conscious state. Ultimately, consciousness is an amalgam of alertness, orientation and clarity of cognition or mentation. Of note, isolated absence or derangement of cognition and mentation (e.g. caused by dementia or psychiatric illness or both) does not result in the clinical entity of altered conscious state. Both these clinical presentations are considered elsewhere. In the same way, the lack of orientation in and of itself does not constitute a clinical alteration in conscious state.

In the clinical context, an alteration in conscious state requires a drop in alertness and 'awakeness'. This drop in alertness may result in a corresponding loss of orientation and/ or a clouding of cognition, thereby altering a patient's response to environmental stimuli or provocation. The reverse, an increase in alertness, could also be considered an alteration in conscious state but, in practice, is most often due to pharmacological agents or a mood elevating psychiatric illness and is beyond the scope of this discussion.

Pathophysiology

The level of consciousness describes the rousability of the individual, whereas the content of consciousness may be assessed in terms of the appropriateness of the individual's response. Broadly speaking, the first is a brainstem function and the second is an attribute of the forebrain.

The physical portions of the brain involved in consciousness consist of the ascending arousal system that begins with monoaminergic cell groups in the brainstem and culminates in extensive diffuse cortical projections throughout the cerebrum. *En route* there is input and modulation from both thalamic and hypothalamic nuclei, as well as basal forebrain cell groups.

The integration of the brainstem and the forebrain is illustrated by individuals who have an isolated pontine injury. They remain awake, but the intact forebrain is unable to interact with the external world, hence the aptly named 'locked-in syndrome'. At the other end of the spectrum are individuals in a persistent vegetative state who, in spite of extensive forebrain impairment, appear awake but totally lack the content of consciousness. These clinical extremes emphasize the important role of the brainstem in modulating motor and sensory systems through its descending pathways and regulating the wakefulness of the forebrain through its ascending pathways.

Differential diagnosis

Given the pathophysiology, the causes of an altered conscious state are myriad and include any cause of insult or injury either directly or indirectly to the brain (Table 8.4.2). Direct injury resulting in structural insults could be traumatic or non-traumatic, e.g. subdural haemorrhage, stroke. Indirect injury could encompass any change in the metabolic and chemical milieu of the brain resulting in a depression of neuronal function, e.g. sepsis, hyper- or hypoglycaemia, drug ingestion.

Structural insults, commonly focal intracranial lesions that exert direct or indirect pressure on the brainstem and the more caudal portions of the ascending arousal system, tend to produce lateralizing neurological signs that can assist in pinpointing the level of the lesion. As there is little space in and around the brainstem, any extrinsic or intrinsic compression will rapidly progress through coma to death, unless the pressure on the brainstem is relieved surgically or pharmacologically.

Metabolic insults, commonly due to systemic pathology that affects primarily the forebrain (although direct depression of the brainstem may also occur), seldom result in lateralizing signs. The appropriate treatment is the correction of the underlying metabolic impairment. Naturally, as in all clinical practice, there are no absolute distinctions. Uncorrected, any of the metabolic causes can eventually cause cerebral oedema and herniation, leading thence to brainstem compression with lateralizing signs, coma and death.

Clinical assessment

In approaching a patient with an altered conscious state, the initial imperatives are to ensure the safety of the airway, the breathing and the circulation and to determine the cause for the alteration with a view to correcting the rapidly reversible causes and offering supportive care while working through the remainder. To this end, assessment and management must proceed concurrently. As in other time critical situations, the primary and secondary survey approach often proves useful, seeking to identify and correct the primary insult while preventing or minimizing secondary injury, such as hypoxia, acidosis and raised intracranial pressure.

Primary survey and resuscitation

An assessment of the airway, breathing and circulation of the patient is urgent to ensure that life-saving measures, such as airway and ventilation support, can be instituted. Initially, supplemental oxygen and non-invasive monitoring should be applied and attention paid to the absolute value and trends in GCS and vital signs. Normotension should be the goal of blood pressure monitoring and this may require inotropic or antihypertensive support.

Early endotracheal intubation may be required if the GCS is less than 8 or ventilatory effort is inadequate. Mechanical ventilation to maintain a pCO_2 of 30–35 mmHg may assist in correcting underlying acidosis and reducing intracranial pressure; however, over-correction may itself be detrimental. Accurate end-tidal CO_2 monitoring correlated to arterial pCO_2 is required. In the setting of trauma, spinal precautions should be maintained until any possibility of trauma is excluded or until clearance of the spine can be obtained.

As hypoglycaemia is an easily identified and corrected cause of altered conscious state, an early bedside glucose determination is vital.

In certain patient populations, pinpoint pupils and a depressed respiratory response may suggest a diagnosis of opiate toxicity and the administration of naloxone as a diagnostic and therapeutic tool. Often this has already been attempted by the pre-hospital services where the practice of intranasal naloxone administration has significantly reduced the risk of needlestick injuries. Although the adverse reactions to naloxone in initial doses is small, the greater risk is in the unmasking of the proconvulsant or proarrhythmic effects of other drugs ingested or injected in combination with opioids. Thus, naloxone should not be given unless clinically indicated. There is also the potential of introducing diagnostic bias as a percentage of non-opioid users also appear to respond clinically to naloxone. The routine use of the 'coma cocktail' of 50% dextrose, naloxone and thiamine intravenously is no longer advocated.

Secondary survey

Following initial assessment and resuscitation, it is important to complete the assessment by obtaining a full history, conducting a full examination and performing any adjunctive investigations. This will assist in identifying the cause of the condition and planning further management.

History

This is often difficult with an obtunded or confused patient and may need to rely heavily on ancillary sources, such as first responders, carers, primary physicians, medical records and patient alert identification.

It is crucial to establish the events leading up to the presentation with specific questioning about prodromal events (e.g. ingestions, IV drug usage, trauma, underlying illness, medications, allergies) and associated seizures and abnormal movements. For example, the presence or absence of a headache and its onset and duration might aid in the clinical diagnosis of a subarachnoid haemorrhage and a history of head injury with loss of consciousness would increase the likelihood of an extra-axial intracranial collection. Patients who are taking anticoagulants also have an increased risk of intracranial haemorrhage with minimal trauma. Patients with a history of hepatic failure may require specific treatment for hepatic encephalopathy.

In the elderly, dementia, itself a progressive illness, may be exacerbated by delirium caused by an acute illness and often, only a careful, corroborated history from care providers and the passage of time will allow the two to be distinguished. Often, the most helpful portion of the history lies in ascertaining the patient's usual pattern of behaviour and the degree and time course of any changes that have occurred. In these patients, it is important to remember that dementia as a cause of altered conscious state is a diagnosis of exclusion.

Examination

A general physical examination, bearing in mind the various differential diagnoses, is very important. In the absence of adequate history, a thorough physical examination may offer the only pointers to initial treatment. Vital signs may suggest sepsis or other causes of shock. A keen sense of smell might detect fetor hepaticus or the sweet breath of ketosis. A bitter almond scent is pathognomonic of cyanide poisoning. Of note, alteration of consciousness can be attributed to alcoholic intoxication only by the process of exclusion. Thus the characteristic odour of alcoholic liquor is indicative but cannot be presumed to be diagnostic. A bedside blood glucose determination is mandatory as deficits are easily correctable.

Neurological examination must be as comprehensive as possible. There are several obstacles to this. Initial resuscitation measures, such as endotracheal intubation, will reduce the ability of the patient to cooperate with the examination and language difficulties will be accentuated as the neurological examination is strongly language orientated. Thus patients who do not share a common language with clinicians and those with dysphasia may be disadvantaged. Also, sensory modalities are difficult to assess in patients with impaired mentation, although these deficits are often paralleled by deficits in the motor system.

The aim of the neurological examination is, primarily, to differentiate structural and non-structural causes; secondly, to identify groups of signs that may indicate specific diagnoses, such as meningitis; and, finally, to pinpoint the location of any structural lesion. Therefore, emphasis needs to be placed on signs of trauma, tone, reflexes, pupillary responses and eye signs, as well as serial calculation of GCS. Circumstances permitting, some or all of the neurological examination should be documented before the patient receives neuromuscular paralysing agents.

Signs of trauma need to be documented and spinal precautions taken as indicated. Palpation of the soft tissues and bones of the skull may detect deformity or bruising and a haemotympanum may herald a fracture of the base of the skull.

Hypotonia is common in acute neurological deficits. Specific examination of anal sphincter tone will uncover spinal cord compromise and is crucial in trauma patients who have a depressed level of consciousness. An upgoing Babinski response is indicative of pyramidal pathology and asymmetry of the peripheral limb reflexes may help to 'side' a lesion. Conversely, heightened tone in the neck muscles (neck stiffness) may indicate meningitis or subarachnoid haemorrhage.

Pupillary responses and eye signs may also be useful to differentiate metabolic and structural insults and, more importantly, to detect incipient uncal herniation. Intact oculocephalic reflexes and preservation of the 'doll's eyes' response indicates an intact medial longitudinal fasciculus and, by default, an intact brainstem, suggesting a metabolic cause for coma. There are four pairs of nuclei governing ocular movements and they are spread between the superior and inferior midbrain and the pons. The pattern of ocular movement dysfunction can be used to pinpoint the site of a brainstem lesion (Table 8.4.3). Likewise, specific testing of the oculovestibular reflex and the cranial nerve examination can be used to locate precisely a brainstem lesion but is of limited use in the emergency setting except as a predictor of herniation (Tables 8.4.3 and 8.4.4).

More generally, skin examination may reveal needle tracks suggestive of drug use, envenomation bite marks or a meningococcal rash. Mucosal changes, such as cyanosis or the cherry-red glow of carbon monoxide poisoning, can be diagnostic. Cardiac monitoring and cardiovascular examination should identify rhythm disturbances, the murmurs of endocarditis and valvular disease or evidence of shock from myocardial ischaemia or infarction. Respiratory patterns may aid in identifying the site of the lesion (see Table 8.4.4). Abdominal examination may detect organomegaly, ascites, bruits or pulsatile masses.

Collections of physical signs, particularly into toxidromes, such as those due to anticholinergic or serotoninergic drugs, should be sought as these are not uncommon causes of alterations in conscious state with or without psychiatric symptoms. Further information on toxidromes can be found in the relevant chapters in this text.

Clinical investigations

Given the breadth of differential diagnoses, these must be guided by the preceding history and examination and their timing dictated by the resuscitation imperatives. The following is an extensive list of possible investigations but there is no suggestion that they should all be performed in every patient with an altered conscious state without due consideration of the patient's context and condition. A comprehensive history and thorough examination are key to the appropriate choice of investigations.

Table 8.4.3 Ocular responses to cold caloric testing of the oculovestibular reflex

Response	Cerebrum	Medial longitudinal fasciculus	Brainstem
Bilateral nystagmus	Intact	Intact	Intact
Bilateral conjugate deviation towards the stimulus	Metabolic dysfunction	Intact	Intact
No response			Structural or metabolic dysfunction
Ipsilateral dysconjugate deviation			Structural dysfunction

Table 8.4.4 Patterns of dysfunction in various parameters determined by the site of the structural or metabolic insult

	Respiratory pattern	Motor response	Pupillary light response	Eye movements
Forebrain	Cheyne–Stokes – waxing & waning	Localizing to pain	Symmetrical, small, reactive Pretectal – symmetrical, large, fixed	
Midbrain	Hyperventilation	Decorticate	Fixed	Upper midbrain CN III palsy Lower midbrain – CN IV deficit – loss of ipsilateral adduction
Pons	Apneusis – halts briefly in full inspiration	Decerebrate	Symmetrical, pinpoint, reactive Uncal – ipsilateral, fixed, dilated	CN VI deficit – loss of ipsilateral abduction
Medulla	Ataxic irregular rate & uneven depth Apnoeic Bilateral ventrolateral medulla lesions			

Haematology

A full blood examination may reveal anaemia, immunocompromise, thrombocytopaenia, inflammation or infection, but is rarely diagnostically specific. In the setting of trauma, a bedside haemoglobin determination can direct immediate blood-product replacement. C-reactive protein (CRP) and erythrocyte sedimentation rate (ESR) are non-specific acute-phase reactants and single determinants are not initially useful, although they may later be followed to monitor resolution of the illness or response to therapy. Coagulation profiles are particularly useful in haematological and liver disease or if patients are taking anticoagulants, such as warfarin, and should lower the threshold for radiological imaging of the brain.

Biochemistry

Serum electrolyte levels aid in the differentiation of the various hypo- and hyper-elemental causes of coma. Electrolyte imbalances may also be secondary to the causative insult and may not need specific correction. In hypotensive patients, a high to normal sodium and low potassium suggests primary or secondary Addisonian crisis.

Cardiac markers, liver, renal and thyroid function tests may confirm focal organ dysfunction. The last may not always be readily available, but hypothyroidism should be considered in the hypothermic patient and hyperthyroidism in the presence of tremor and tachyarrhythmias.

Serum glucose provides confirmation of bedside testing. Serum lactate determinations may reveal a metabolic acidosis and reflect the degree of tissue hypoxia which, again, may be primary or secondary. Creatinine kinase and myoglobinuria are useful to determine the presence and extent of rhabdomyolysis and to predict the likelihood of requiring dialysis. Serum and urine osmolarity may be useful in toxic ingestions, such as ethylene glycol, and in other hyperosmolar states.

Blood gas analysis may give important information regarding acid–base balance, a useful marker of severity of disease and, along with the anion gap and the serum electrolytes, can help distinguish between the various types and causes of acidosis and alkalosis. Knowledge of the partial pressures of oxygen and carbon dioxide is vital to resuscitative efforts.

Microbiology

Sepsis is a major metabolic cause of conscious state alteration and may present with no localizing symptoms or signs, especially in the elderly. In this case, blood cultures – preferably multiple sets obtained before antibiotic therapy – may be the only means of isolating the causative organism. Naturally, system-specific specimens, such as sputum, urine and cerebrospinal fluid, should be collected when clinically indicated. A bedside dipstick of the urine sample can provide valuable information to begin initial treatment. Although as a rule specimens should be obtained prior to therapy, in suspected meningitis or encephalitis, the administration of antibiotics or antiviral agents should not be delayed while a lumbar puncture/CT scan is performed.

Specific laboratory testing

Based on information from the history and examination, specific drug assays and urine screens may be indicated. These may include over-the-counter or prescribed medications, such as paracetamol, lithium or theophylline, or drugs of addiction, such as amphetamine or opiates. Routine urine drug screens are of very limited overall value and no help to emergency management.

Venom detection kits can be used in specific clinical situations and evidence of systemic envenomation can be screened for with other tests, such as coagulation profiles and creatinine kinase.

Imaging

Intracranial imaging is best achieved with a plain CT of the head which, if normal and concern regarding intracranial pathology persists, may be followed by a contrast-enhanced scan or magnetic resonance imaging (MRI). The latter has a higher sensitivity for encephalitis and cerebral vasculitis, although it may not always be easily accessible from the ED. Also, the technical constraints of MRI require a stable patient. Emergency CT angiography has a role in the delineation of cerebral aneurysms and interventional angiography can provide therapeutic options, particularly in a patient who is progressing towards herniation. A normal CT scan does not completely exclude treatable intracranial infection or subarachnoid haemorrhage. Therefore, depending upon the patient's conscious state and the level of clinical suspicion, a lumbar puncture may further assist with diagnosis. However, it must be emphasized that, in suspected intracranial infection, an obtunded patient should be treated empirically with appropriate antiviral agents and antibiotics and the lumbar puncture deferred till the risk of herniation is minimized.

A chest X-ray may reveal primary infection or malignancy. In a patient with an altered conscious state and any suspicion of head trauma, a full cervical spine series is mandatory. Inadequate plain films should be supplemented by CT imaging of the cervical spine, as allowed by resuscitation imperatives while spinal immobilization is maintained. Imaging of the rest of the spine and the pelvis should be guided by clinical assessment.

Other tests

The 12-lead ECG can highlight rate and rhythm disturbances. Specific changes, such as the U wave of hypokalaemia, the J wave of hypothermia and focal infarction and ischaemic patterns, serve to confirm and offer pointers to the cause of the conscious state alteration. It is worth noting that intracranial bleeding, such as subarachnoid haemorrhage, can be associated with an ischaemic-looking ECG. Care is required in cases of depressed level of consciousness with ECG changes, as the use of thrombolysis or anticoagulation based on the ECG in the presence of intracranial bleeding may well be fatal.

Treatment

Management, by necessity, is governed by assessment findings, projected differential diagnoses and the patient's response to initial management. The algorithm in Figure 8.4.1 is aimed at correcting immediate life-threatening pathology and then identifying and treating reversible structural and metabolic causes. Treatment of specific causes is addressed elsewhere in this text.

General measures

The priorities of ED management are the avoidance of hypoxia, hypotension, hyperthermia and hyperglycaemia, the maintenance of normovolaemia and cerebral perfusion and the minimization of any increase in intracranial pressure. It is important to normalize vital parameters and strict monitoring of the same with invasive measures as required.

For monitoring of blood pressure and pCO_2, an arterial line is required in these patients. Strict attention to fluid replacement and the need to monitor end-organ perfusion also dictates the need for a urinary catheter. This can

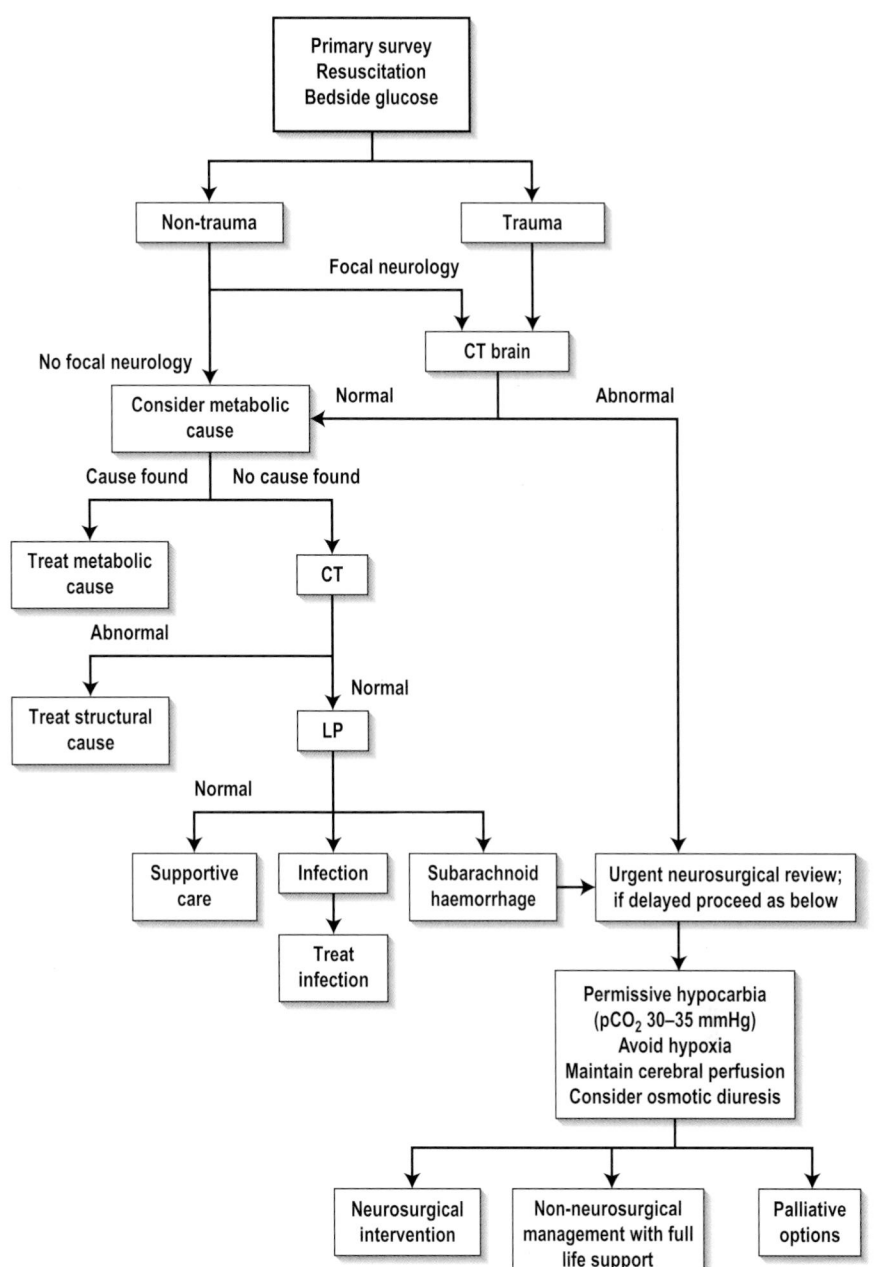

Fig. 8.4.1 Altered conscious state: management algorithm.

also be used to monitor core temperature. The target temperature should be 35°C to avoid hyperthermia.

With regards to drugs required for the management of the airway and ventilation, propofol is a powerful, fast-acting, short-duration sedative that provides potentially neuroprotective effects through decreases in peripheral vascular tension. However, review of multiple small trials and datasets do not suggest any overall

long-term mortality benefits of propofol over the opiate class in the management of sedation and ventilation of the traumatic brain-injured patient. It is important to provide analgesia and sedation as the absence of these will result in physiological stimulation and increase intracranial pressure. Optimization of ventilation is useful to reduce hypoxia and, while neuromuscular paralytic agents may assist in the endeavour, it is important to document as much of the neurological examination as possible prior to paralysing the patient.

Intracranial pressure management

The use of osmotic diuretics may also assist in reducing intracranial pressure but the choice of agent has become more controversial with the introduction of hypertonic saline. There are no class I studies comparing the efficacy of either mannitol (0.5 g/kg) or hypertonic saline (5 mL/kg of 3% saline) with placebo for intracranial pressure reduction, but class II and class III evidence suggests that both may be effective with mannitol potentially being the less effective. Such agents should be used only in consultation with the receiving neurosurgical team due to their potential for additional haemodynamic compromise and secondary neurological embarrassment.

Disposition

Patients with continuing altered consciousness should be admitted to a hospital with the range of services and clinical disciplines to manage the primary diagnosis. This may require stabilization prior to transfer and transport, sometimes over long distances. The exigencies of transfer may also dictate some of the initial management choices. The level of care required will depend on the state of the patient on presentation and their subsequent response to treatment. Patient wishes, premorbid status and prognosis may also temper treatment choices and pathways.

Prognosis

Discussion of prognosis is difficult, as it depends on the cause and patient-specific factors. Effective cerebral resuscitation with optimal oxygenation and minimization of intracerebral hypercarbia and acidosis will promote the best recovery potential while addressing the underlying disease process. Prognosis is naturally dependent on the degree of irreversible cellular damage and the ability to correct the primary insult while minimizing secondary brain injury.

Controversies

- The optimal degree of induced hypercapnoea in the management of the patient with an altered conscious state.
- The role and choice of osmotic diuretics in the management of acute elevations in intracranial pressure.
- The interplay between patient and family wishes, premorbid status, prognosis and medical futility in the decision-making process determining management pathways and dispostion.

Further reading

Adamides AA, Winter CD, Lewis PM, et al. Current controversies in the management of patient with severe traumatic brain injury. Aust NZ J Surg 2006;76:163–74.

Banks CJ, Furyk JS. Hypertonic saline use in the emergency department. Emerg Med Australas 2008;20:294–305.

Casaletto JJ. Is salt, vitamin or endocrinopathy causing this encephalopathy? A review of endocrine and metabolic causes of altered level of consciousness. Emerg Med Clin N Am 2010;28:633–62.

Hoffman JR, Schringer DL, Luo JS. The empiric use of naloxone in patients with altered mental status: a reappraisal. Ann Emerg Med 1991;20:246–52.

Jantzen JAH. Prevention and treatment of intracranial hypertension. Best Pract Res Clin Anaesthesiol 2007;21:517–38.

Kaplan JL, Marsi JA, Calabro JJ, et al. Double-blind randomised study of nalmefene and naloxone in emergency department patients with narcotic overdose. Ann Emerg Med 1999;34:42–50.

Kelly AM, Kerr D, Dietze P, et al. A randomised trial of intranasal versus intramuscular naloxone in prehospital treatment for suspected opioid overdose. Med J Assoc 2005;182:24–7.

Meyer MJ, Megyes J, Meythaler J, et al. Acute management of acquired brain injury part II: An evidence-based review of pharmacological interventions. Brain Injury 2010;24:706–21.

Schreckinger M, Marion DW. Contemporary management of traumatic intracranial hypertension: Is there a role for therapeutic hypothermia? Neurocrit Care 2009;11:427–36.

Sporer KA, Firstone J, Issacs SM. Out-of-hospital treatment of opioid overdose in an urban setting. Acad Emerg Med 1996;3:660–7.

Teasdale G, Jennett B. Assessment of coma and impaired consciousness: a practical scale. Lancet 1974;2:81–4.

White H, Cook D, Venkatesh B. The use of hypertonic saline for treating intracranial hypertension after traumatic brain injury. Anesth Analg 2006;102:1836–46.

8.5 Seizures

Garry J Wilkes

ESSENTIALS

1 Up to 10% of the population will have at least one seizure in their lifetime, but only 1–3% will develop epilepsy.

2 The management of an acute episode is directed at rapid control of seizures, identification of precipitating factors and prevention/correction of complications.

3 Investigation of first seizures should be directed by history and clinical findings. Routine laboratory and radiological investigations are not warranted for uncomplicated first seizures with full recovery.

4 Persistent confusion should not be assumed to be due to a post-ictal state until other causes have been excluded.

5 Benzodiazepines and phenytoin are the principal anticonvulsant agents for acute seizures.

6 Status epilepticus and eclampsia are severe life threats. Management plans for these conditions should be developed in advance.

7 Pseudoseizures are important to distinguish from neurogenic seizures in order to prevent inadvertent harm to patients and allow appropriate psychotherapeutic treatment.

8 Management of drug-related seizures (including those related to alcohol) includes measures to reduce drug absorption and enhance elimination. Specific therapy is available for only a few agents. Phenytoin is usually ineffective in the management of alcohol and drug-related seizures.

9 Severe head injuries are associated with an increased incidence of post-traumatic epilepsy, half of which will be manifest in the first year. Phenytoin is effective as prophylaxis for the first week only.

10 Patients with epilepsy should be encouraged to have ongoing care.

Introduction

The terms 'seizure','convulsion' and 'fit' are often used both interchangeably and incorrectly. A seizure is an episode of abnormal neurological function caused by an abnormal electrical discharge of brain neurons. The seizure is also referred to as an ictus or ictal period. A convulsion is an episode of excessive and abnormal motor activity. Seizures can occur without convulsions and convulsions can be caused by other conditions. The term 'fit' is best avoided in medical terminology, but is a useful term for non-medical personnel.

Epidemiology

Seizures are common. It has been estimated that up to 10% of the population will have at least one seizure in their lifetime and 1–3% of the population will develop epilepsy. A single seizure may be a reaction to an underlying disorder, part of an established epileptic disorder or an isolated event with no associated pathology. The challenge is rapidly to identify and treat life-threatening conditions as well as to identify benign conditions that require no further investigation or treatment.

Diagnosis of epilepsy requires at least two unprovoked seizures more than 24 hours apart. An episode of status epilepticus is considered a single seizure. Simple febrile and neonatal seizures are usually excluded from this definition.

Classification

Epileptic seizures can be classified into partial and generalized. Partial epileptic seizures are further classified into simple partial (preserved consciousness) and complex partial seizures. Either may secondarily become generalized.

Generalized seizures can be divided into convulsive and non-convulsive types. Convulsive seizures are generalized tonic–clonic (grand mal) seizures. Non-convulsive generalized seizures include absence seizures (previously termed petit mal), myoclonic, tonic and atonic seizures. Epilepsy and epileptic syndromes are also classified as focal or generalized. Each disorder can be further classified, according to its relationship to aetiological or predisposing factors, into symptomatic or cryptogenic. The term 'idiopathic' is now discouraged. Seizures can also be classified as provoked (acute symptomatic) or unprovoked (cryptogenic or remote symptomatic).

Different seizure types are associated with differing aetiological and prognostic factors. The details of the classification systems are not as important in emergency medicine as the concept of recognizing the different seizure types and being aware of the accepted terminology when discussing and referring cases.

Management principles

Given the high frequency of this condition in emergency departments (EDs), it is important to have an evidenced-based management strategy formulated in advance. The main management concepts are:

- Altered mental state should be thoroughly assessed and not assumed to be due to a post-ictal state.
- Patients with known epilepsy who have recovered completely from a typical seizure require little further investigation. If they remain obtunded or have atypical features, they must be fully evaluated, e.g. biochemical analysis, computed tomography (CT) scan, etc.
- Patients with epilepsy should be encouraged to seek continuing care.
- Patients at risk of recurrent seizures should be advised about situations of increased personal risk, such as driving, operating power machinery or swimming alone.

Differential diagnosis

Conditions such as syncope may be accompanied by myoclonic activity and are important to distinguish from true seizures. Migraine, transient ischaemic attacks, hyperventilation episodes and vertigo are all important conditions to consider in the differential diagnosis. Pseudoseizures will be discussed below.

First seizures

A generalized convulsion is a dramatic event. Patients and those accompanying them will often be frightened, anxious and concerned, not only for the acute event but for what it may signify. A diagnosis of epilepsy may profoundly influence occupation, social activities, ability to drive a car and long-term health. It is therefore vital the diagnosis is correct and explained fully to the patient and relatives.

Clinical features

The first and most important task is to determine whether a seizure has occurred. As the majority have ceased, the diagnosis is made primarily on history. Patients will not remember seizures other than simple partial seizures and the reports of witnesses may be unreliable or inconsistent. With the exception of partial seizures, generalized seizures are not accompanied by an aura. Most seizures last less than 2 minutes, are associated with impaired consciousness, loss of memory for the event, purposeless movements and a period of post-ictal confusion. Although witnesses may grossly overestimate the duration, prolonged seizures, those occurring in association with a strong emotional event and those with full recall of events should be regarded with suspicion. Similarly, motor activity that is coordinated and not bilateral (such as side-to-side head

movements, pelvic thrusting, directed violence and movement that changes in response to external cues) are less likely to be true seizures.

ED assessment is aimed at identifying associated conditions and treatable causes of seizures. The aetiology of seizures can be classified into five groups on this basis:

- Acute symptomatic: occurring in association with a known central nervous system insult. Causes of this large, important group are listed in Table 8.5.1.
- Remote symptomatic: occurring without provocation in a patient with a previous history (>1 week prior) of central nervous system insult known to be associated with an increased risk of seizures, e.g. encephalopathy, meningitis, head trauma or stroke.
- Progressive encephalopathy: occurring in association with a progressive neurological disease, e.g. neurodegenerative diseases, neurocutaneous syndromes and malignancies not in remission.
- Febrile: patients whose sole provocation is fever. This is almost exclusively confined to children and, as such, is beyond the scope of this book.
- Cryptogenic (previously 'idiopathic'): patients without a precipitating central nervous system insult. This is probably the most common group, however, this classification is by exclusion of the other causes.

A careful history is needed to decide whether this is part of an ongoing process or an isolated event. Patients may not recall previous events, may not recognize their significance or may even avoid reporting previous episodes for fear of being labelled 'epileptic',

with the associated consequences. Particular attention should be paid to any history of unexplained injuries, especially when they occur during blackouts or during sleep. A history of childhood seizures, isolated myoclonic jerks and a positive family history increases the likelihood of epilepsy.

A full physical and neurological examination is mandatory. Evidence of alcohol and drug ingestion and head trauma is particularly important. A comprehensive medication history will include agents known to reduce seizure threshold in susceptible individuals, e.g. tramadol and selective serotonin reuptake inhibitors. A careful mental state examination in seemingly alert patients may reveal evidence of a resolving post-ictal state or underlying encephalopathy. Patients not fully alert should never be assumed simply to be in a post-ictal state until other causes are excluded. Evidence of underlying causes includes fever, nuchal rigidity (meningitis), cardiac murmurs (endocarditis), needle tracks, evidence of chronic liver disease, dysmorphic features and marks such as café-au-lait spots (neurofibromatosis). Complications, such as tongue biting, broken teeth and peripheral injuries, are not uncommon in generalized seizures. Stress fractures can occur, particularly in the elderly. Posterior dislocation of the shoulder is uncommon but significant and easily overlooked.

Clinical investigations

Although it is common practice to order a variety of tests following an uncomplicated seizure, these are rarely of benefit in the fully recovered patient. Elevated neutrophil counts in blood and CSF may be seen as a result of a generalized seizure in the absence of an infectious disorder. Electrolyte abnormalities may cause seizures but are unlikely to be the cause if the patient has recovered. Serum prolactin level 20–60 minutes post-seizure may be helpful if the diagnosis is in doubt. An abnormal neurological examination, features of meningitis, encephalitis or subarachnoid haemorrhage are indications for cranial CT scan and lumbar puncture.

Imaging

There are no clear guidelines to the routine need for or urgency of neuroimaging following a single uncomplicated seizure. Patients with focal neurological signs, those who do not recover to a normal examination and those with a history of head trauma or intracranial pathology should all undergo cranial CT as soon as

Table 8.5.1   Acute symptomatic causes of seizures
Hypoxia
Hypoglycaemia
Head trauma
Meningitis and encephalitis, including HIV disease
Metabolic, including hyponatraemia, hypocalcaemia, hyperthyroidism, uraemia and eclampsia
Drug overdose, including alcohol, tricyclics, theophylline, cocaine, amphetamine and isoniazid
Drug withdrawal, including alcohol, benzodiazepines, narcotics, cocaine and anticonvulsants
Cerebral tumour or stroke

possible. The dilemma arises in patients with complete recovery and no focal signs. The incidence of abnormalities on CT in this group of patients is less than 1%. The decision as to whether to and when to scan patients in this group will be determined largely by local factors. Magnetic resonance imaging (MRI) is more sensitive than CT for infarcts, tumours, inflammatory lesions and vascular lesions but availability may be limited.

Electroencephalography

Electroencephalography (EEG) at the time of a seizure will make a definitive diagnosis. It is not usually performed in the acute setting except when non-convulsive activity is suspected. Typically, an EEG is obtained electively on an outpatient basis, when it may still indicate an underlying focus of activity and may be able to detect specific conditions.

Treatment

Once a diagnosis of first seizure is made and intercurrent conditions are excluded or treated, the patient may be discharged home. It must be stressed to the patient that a diagnosis of epilepsy has not been made but is being considered. When the suspicion is reasonable, the patient should be given the same precautionary advice as epileptic patients with regard to driving and other activities that may place them or others at risk.

The planning of investigation and follow up for patients suspected of having a first seizure is best done in conjunction with a neurology service to ensure appropriate investigations are completed in a timely fashion. Generally, an inter-ictal EEG and contrast CT and/or MRI are completed prior to review.

Status epilepticus

Epidemiology and pathophysiology

Status epilepticus may be defined as 'two or more seizures without full recovery of consciousness between seizures, or recurrent epileptic seizures for more than 30 minutes'.

Status epilepticus accounts for 1–8% of all hospital admissions for epilepsy, 3.5% of admissions to neurological intensive care and 0.13% of all visits to a university hospital ED. It is more common at the extremes of age, with over 50% of all cases occurring in children and a disproportionately high incidence in those

over 60 years of age. Status epilepticus is also more frequent in the mentally handicapped and in those with structural cerebral pathology, especially of the frontal lobes. Four to 16% of adults and 10–25% of children with known epilepsy will have at least one episode of status epilepticus. Notwithstanding, status epilepticus occurs most commonly in patients with no previous history of epilepsy.

Many compensatory physiological changes accompany seizures. As duration increases these mechanisms begin to fail, with an increased risk of permanent damage. Brain damage resulting from prolonged status epilepticus is believed to be caused by excitatory amino acid neurotransmitters, such as glutamate and aspartate, leading to influx of calcium into neuronal cytoplasm and an osmolytic cell destruction. Continuing seizure activity itself contributes to neuronal damage, which is further exacerbated by hypoxia, hypoglycaemia, lactic acidosis and hyperpyrexia. The longer an episode of status epilepticus continues, the more refractory to treatment it becomes and the more likely it is to result in permanent neuronal damage. Mortality increases from 2.7% with seizure duration under 1 hour to 32% with duration beyond this. Generalized convulsive status epilepticus is therefore a medical emergency.

Treatment

Treatment of status epilepticus is along the same lines as the resuscitation of all seriously ill patients. Management is in a resuscitation area with attention to:

- rapid stabilization of airway, breathing and circulation
- termination of seizure activity (clinical and electrical)
- identification and treatment of precipitating and perpetuating factors
- identification and treatment of complications.

Each stage of resuscitation is made more difficult by the presence of active convulsions. Do not prise clenched teeth apart to insert an oral airway: a soft nasal airway will suffice. Oxygen should be given and the patient positioned in the left lateral position to minimize the risk of aspiration. Intravenous access is important for drug treatment and fluid resuscitation, but may be difficult in actively seizing patients. Although status epilepticus cannot be diagnosed until seizures have persisted for 30 minutes, patients still seizing on arrival at

the ED should be treated with anticonvulsants immediately.

The principal pharmacological agents used are benzodiazepines and phenytoin. Opinions vary regarding the optimal benzodiazepine, with little clinical evidence to support any particular one. Lorazepam is preferred by most neurologists because of prolonged central nervous system action (protective effect for 30–120 minutes). Less fat-soluble than diazepam, it typically takes longer to stop seizures (5–10 minutes) and can cause hypotension. Midazolam is popular among emergency physicians for a variety of purposes. Being water soluble, it is non-irritant and can be administered IM with fairly rapid onset of action (between diazepam and lorazepam). It has a short duration of action (another reason for popularity in emergency medicine) and may require further IV doses or ongoing infusion. Diazepam has previously been popular due to its extreme lipid solubility and rapid brain entry. It typically stops seizures in 1–2 minutes. Preparations are, however, irritant, produce complications with IV extravasation and are unsuitable for IM use. Diazepam can be administered rectally if necessary and this technique can be taught to parents with high-risk children. All benzodiazepines share the disadvantages of respiratory depression, hypotension and short duration of clinical effect.

Phenytoin is usually used as a second-line agent in a dose of 15–20 mg/kg at a rate of no more than 50 mg/min. Rapid administration is associated with bradyarrhythmias and hypotension. The common practice of administering 1 g is inadequate for most adults. The effect of phenytoin does not commence until 40% of the dose has been administered; for this reason, it should be commenced at the same time that IV benzodiazepines are given if it is to be used. Most people on anticonvulsants who present in status epilepticus have negligible drug levels and the side effects from a full loading dose on top of a therapeutic level are minimal. The full loading dose should therefore be given even when the patient is known to be on therapy.

The most common causes of failure to control seizures are:

- inadequate antiepileptic drug therapy
- failure to initiate maintenance antiepileptic drug therapy
- hypoxia, hypotension, cardiorespiratory failure, metabolic disturbance, e.g. hypoglycaemia

Table 8.5.2 Doses of drugs used in refractory status epilepticus

Drug	Bolus (IV unless stated otherwise)	Maintenance infusion
Lorazepam	0.05–0.1 mg/kg over 2–5 minutes; not to exceed 4 mg/dose; may repeat every 10–15 min	N/A
Midazolam	0.02–0.1 mg/kg 0.15–0.3 mg/kg IM	0.05–0.4 mg/kg/h
Phenytoin/ fosphenytoin	15–20 mg/kg at up to: Phenytoin max 50 mg/min Fosphenytoin 100–150 mg/min	N/A
Phenobarbitone	10–20 mg/kg at 60–100 mg/min	1–4 mg/kg/day
Thiopentone	5 mg/kg	1–3 mg/kg/h
Pentobarbitone	5 mg/kg at 25 mg/min	0.5–3 mg/kg/h
Propofol	2 mg/kg	5–10 mg/kg/h
Lignocaine	2 mg/kg	3–6 mg/kg/h

- failure to identify an underlying cause
- failure to recognize medical complications, e.g. hyperpyrexia, hypoglycaemia
- misdiagnosis of pseudoseizures.

Causes of failure to regain consciousness following treatment of seizures include the medical consequences of status epilepticus (hypoxia, hypoglycaemia, cerebral oedema, hypotension, hyperpyrexia), sedation from antiepileptic medication, progression of the underlying disease process, non-convulsive status epilepticus and subtle generalized status epilepticus.

When benzodiazepines and phenytoin are ineffective, expert advice should be sought. Drugs that may be used in the control of status epilepticus are summarized in Table 8.5.2. Anaesthetic agents require expert airway control and, in some cases, inotropic support. Management in an intensive care unit is mandatory.

For all patients with status epilepticus, early consultation with intensive care and neurology services is essential in planning definitive management and disposition.

Non-convulsive seizures

Not all seizures are associated with convulsive activity. Convulsive seizures are generally easy to recognize, whereas non-convulsive seizures are more subtle and often require a high index of suspicion. These types of seizure are an important cause of alterations in behaviour and conscious level and may precede or follow convulsive episodes. Seizures can involve any of the sensory modalities, vertiginous episodes, automatism, autonomic dysfunction or psychic disturbances, including *déjà vu* and *jamais vu* experiences. Non-convulsive seizures can easily be confused with migraine, cerebrovascular events or psychiatric conditions. The definitive diagnosis can only be made by EEG during the event.

Non-convulsive seizures may be partial (focal) or generalized. Complex partial seizures and focal seizures account for approximately one-third of all seizures, whereas primary generalized non-convulsive seizures (absence seizures) account for 6%.

Non-convulsive status epilepticus accounts for at least 25% of all cases of status epilepticus and is diagnosed more frequently when actively considered. Absence seizures rarely result in complete unresponsiveness and patients may appear relatively normal to unfamiliar observers. Non-convulsive status epilepticus may precede or follow convulsive seizures and may easily create the perception of a cerebral vascular or psychiatric event. The longest reported episode of absence status is 60 days and that of complex partial status 28 days.

Acute treatment of non-convulsive seizures is the same as for convulsive seizures. An estimated 50% of patients with simple partial seizures have abnormal CT scans. Long-term seizure control uses different agents from those used for convulsive seizures, highlighting the importance of involving a neurological service when planning follow up.

Pseudoseizures

Pseudoseizures or psychogenic seizures are events simulating neurogenic seizures but without the accompanying abnormal neuronal activity. Differentiation from neurogenic seizures may be extremely difficult, even for experienced neurologists. Neurogenic and psychogenic seizures may coexist, making the diagnostic dilemma even more complex. Differentiation will often require video-EEG monitoring, but this facility is not available in the ED and other methods must be used. It is important to recognize pseudoseizures so as to prevent the possible iatrogenic consequences of unnecessary treatment while, at the same time, not withholding treatment from patients with neurogenic seizures.

Pseudoseizures are more common in women, less common after 35 years of age and rare in patients aged over 50. They may be associated with a conversion disorder, malingering, Munchausen syndrome or Munchausen syndrome by proxy.

Pseudoseizures typically last more than 5 minutes, compared to 1–2 minutes for neurogenic seizures. Multiple patterns of seizures tend to occur in individual patients and postictal periods are either very brief or absent. Recall of events during what appears to be a generalized convulsive seizure suggests a psychogenic seizure. Extremity movement out of phase from one side to the other and head turning from side to side typify pseudoseizures. Forward pelvic thrusting occurs in 44% of patients with pseudoseizures and is highly suggestive of the diagnosis.

Several manoeuvres are useful in identifying pseudoseizures. Eye opening and arm drop tests are accompanied by avoidance, eyes turning away from the moving examiner and termination of the event when the mouth and nostrils are occluded are characteristic. Simple verbal suggestion and reassurance are also frequently successful.

The most definitive means of identifying pseudoseizures is by ictal EEG or video-EEG monitoring. Unfortunately, this is of little value in the ED. A fall in SpO_2 on pulse oximetry and a degree of acidaemia on blood gas analysis occur during neurogenic but not pseudoseizures. Serum prolactin levels rise and peak 15–20 minutes after generalized tonic–clonic seizures and then fall with a half-life of 22 minutes. The levels do not consistently rise with partial seizures and remain normal with pseudoseizures.

Patients with pseudoseizures usually demonstrate resistance to anticonvulsant medication and many will therefore present with therapeutic or supratherapeutic levels. Correct diagnosis will prevent unnecessary and potentially harmful treatment. Doubtful cases should be discussed with a neurology service and arrangements made for emergency EEG.

Once the diagnosis is confirmed, it must be presented in an open and non-threatening manner. Patients often have underlying personal and/or family problems that will need to be addressed. Psychotherapy is effective, but seizures often relapse at times of stress.

Alcohol-related seizures

Alcohol contributes to half of seizures presenting to EDs. Acute toxicity and withdrawal are both associated with an increased incidence of seizures. Alcohol intoxication and chronic alcohol abuse are also associated with increased incidences of intercurrent disease, such as trauma, coagulopathy, falls, assaults and other drug intoxication, all of which further increase the likelihood of seizures. The management of seizures presumed to be alcohol related must include a search for associated disease and other causes.

Benzodiazepines are the principal anticonvulsant agent for acute seizures. These agents are also valuable in the treatment of withdrawal. Phenytoin is ineffective in the control of acute alcohol-related seizures or as a preventative for them.

Drug-related seizures

Seizure activity in the setting of acute drug overdose is an ominous sign associated with greatly increased mortality and morbidity. The most commonly reported are in association with cyclic antidepressants, antihistamines, theophylline, isoniazid and illicit drugs, such as cocaine and amphetamines. The diagnosis and management of these are discussed in the section on toxicology.

Some medications are also associated with lowering seizure threshold in susceptible individuals. Tramadol, in particular, has been associated with new-onset seizures at normal therapeutic doses. A complete medication history is therefore essential.

Post-traumatic seizures

Post-traumatic epilepsy develops in 10–15% of serious head injury survivors. More than half will have their first seizure within 1 year. Risk factors are central parietal injury, dural penetration, hemiplegia, missile wounds and intracerebral haematomas. Early treatment with phenytoin for severe head injuries reduces the incidence of seizures in the first week only.

Seizures and pregnancy

Seizures can occur during pregnancy as part of an established epileptic process, as new seizures or induced by pregnancy. The most significant situations are eclampsia and generalized convulsive status epilepticus. At all times, the management is directed at both mother and baby, with the realization that the best treatment for the baby will relate to optimal maternal care.

In previously diagnosed epileptics, there is an increased risk of seizures during pregnancy of 17%. Anticonvulsant levels are influenced by reduced protein binding, increased drug binding and reduced absorption of varying degrees. The final effect on free drug levels is unpredictable and is most variable around the time of delivery.

Isolated simple seizures place both mother and fetus at increased danger of injury, but are otherwise generally well tolerated. Generalized seizures during labour cause transient fetal hypoxia and bradycardia of uncertain significance. Generalized convulsive status epilepticus is life threatening to both mother and fetus at any stage of pregnancy.

All of the anticonvulsants cross the placenta and are potentially teratogenic. The risk of malformation in children is increased from 3.4% in the general population to 3.7% in epileptic mothers. In general, the types of malformation associated are not drug specific, apart from the increased risk of neural tube defects associated with valproate and carbamazepine. Prenatal screening for such defects is advised in patients who become pregnant while taking these agents. The risk from uncontrolled seizures greatly outweighs the risk from

prophylactic medication in patients with good seizure control.

The management of seizures in pregnant patients is along the same lines as for non-pregnant patients. After 20 weeks' gestation, the patient should have a wedge placed under the right hip to prevent supine hypotension and eclampsia must be considered. Investigation will include an assessment of fetal well-being by heart rate, ultrasound and/or tocography, as indicated. Management and disposition should be decided in consultation with neurology and obstetric services.

Eclampsia is the occurrence of seizures in patients with pregnancy-induced toxaemia occurring after the twentieth week of pregnancy. Toxaemia consists of a triad of hypertension, oedema and proteinuria. One in 300 women with pre-eclampsia progresses to eclampsia. Seizures are typically brief, self-terminating, usually preceded by headache and visual disturbances. They tend to occur without warning. Treatment is directed at controlling the seizures and hypertension and expedient delivery of the baby. Magnesium sulphate is effective in seizure control and is associated with a better outcome for both mother and baby than standard anticonvulsant and antihypertensive therapy.

Management of status epilepticus in pregnancy includes consideration of eclampsia, positioning in the left lateral position and assessment and monitoring of fetal well-being. Urgent control of seizures is essential for both mother and baby. Phenobarbital may reduce the incidence of intraventricular haemorrhage in premature infants and should be considered in place of phenytoin in this circumstance. Early involvement of obstetric and neurology services is essential. Pre-eclampsia and eclampsia are addressed specifically in Chapter 19.7.

Future directions

Non-invasive portable modalities allowing definitive precise diagnosis of seizures in the ED will reduce the need for subsequent investigations in the majority of patients who do not have true epilepsy and permit early focused therapy. Advances in pharmacotherapy and neurosurgical techniques will also improve seizure control with minimal side effects, allowing patients to resume normal activities more effectively. Advances in neurobiology understanding of channels, receptors and genetic expression of proteins will allow correction of underlying defects, removing the need for anticonvulsive therapy.

Controversies

- Investigation required for patients with first seizures.
- Place of lumbar puncture in the investigation of first seizures.
- Role of antipyretics in febrile seizures.

Further reading

American College of Emergency Physicians. Clinical policy: critical issues in the evaluation and management of adult patients presenting to the emergency department with seizures. Ann Emerg Med 2004;43:605–25.

Berg AT, Berkovic SF, Brodie MJ, et al. Revised terminology and concepts for organization of seizures and epilepsies: report of the ILAE Commission on Classification and Terminology, 2005–2009. Epilepsia 2010;51:676–85.

Brown AF, Wilkes GJ. Emergency department management of status epilepticus. Emerg Med 1994;6:49–61.

Cavasos JE. Epilepsy and seizures. <http://www.eMedicine.com/article/1184846-overview> [Accessed Nov. 2012].

Dugan EM, Howell JM. Posttraumatic seizures. Emerg Med Clin N Am 1994;12:1081–107.

Gates JR, Ramani V, Whalen S, et al. Ictal characteristics of pseudoseizures. Arch Neurol 1985;42:1183–7.

Hesdorffer DC, Logroscino G, Benn EK, et al. Estimating risk for developing epilepsy: a population-based study in Rochester, Minnestoa. Neurology 2011;76:23–7.

Jagoda A. Nonconvulsive seizures. Emerg Med Clin N Am 1994;12:963–71.

Labate A, Newton MR, et al. Tramadol and new-onset seizures. Med J Aust 2005;182:42–3.

McDonagh TJ, Jelinek GA, Galvin GM. Intramuscular midazolam rapidly terminates seizures in children and adults. Emerg Med 1992;4:77–81.

Riggio S. Psychogenic seizures. Emerg Med Clin N Am 1994;12:1001–12.

Treiman DM. Electroclinical features of status epilepticus. J Clin Neurophysiol 1995;12:343–62.

8.6 Syncope and vertigo

Rosslyn Hing

ESSENTIALS

1 It is important to distinguish between syncope and true vertigo.

2 The most common cause of syncope is neurally-mediated syncope.

3 A detailed history and physical examination are more useful than extensive investigations.

4 It is essential to identify high-risk patients for the serious potential cardiac causes of syncope so that appropriate treatment can be given.

5 A key diagnostic step is to determine whether a central or peripheral cause of vertigo is more likely.

6 Dynamic manoeuvres may be both diagnostic and therapeutic.

Introduction

Syncope and vertigo are relatively common symptoms. They are often described by patients using the term 'dizziness'; however, it is essential to differentiate between the two. Syncope and vertigo both represent a significant diagnostic challenge and it is important to risk stratify patients accurately to distinguish between potentially life-threatening and benign causes.

Syncope

Syncope as a presenting symptom represents about 1–1.5% of all emergency department attendances. It is a symptom, not a diagnosis. It is defined as a loss of consciousness induced by the temporarily insufficient flow of blood to the brain. Patients recover spontaneously, without therapeutic intervention or prolonged confusion.

There is no simple test to distinguish between the benign and the potentially life-threatening causes of syncope, but a careful history, examination and bedside investigations can help determine appropriate disposition.

The causes of syncope are summarized in Table 8.6.1. The most common cause in all age groups is neurally-mediated syncope, also known as neurocardiogenic or vasovagal syncope. Orthostatic hypotension and cardiac causes are the next most common.

Clinical features

Patients with syncope are often completely asymptomatic by the time they arrive at hospital. A thorough history and physical examination is the key to finding the correct cause for the syncope. The history should focus on the patient's recollection of the preceding and subsequent events, including environmental conditions, physical activity, prodromal symptoms and any intercurrent medical problems. Accounts from eyewitnesses or first responders are also vital. Medications that may impair autonomic reflexes need to be scrutinized and a postural blood pressure measurement performed. Physical examination should concentrate on finding signs of structural heart disease, as well as assessing any subsequent injuries.

Neurally-mediated syncope causes a typical prodrome: patients complain of feeling light-headed and faint and often describe a blurring or 'tunnelling' of their vision. This may be accompanied by other vagally-mediated symptoms, such as nausea or sweating. More pronounced vagal symptoms may include an urge to open their bowels. If patients are unable or unwilling to follow their body's natural instincts to lie flat, they may collapse to the ground as they lose consciousness. This reflex brings the head level with the heart, resulting in an improvement in cerebral perfusion and a return to consciousness. During this time, the patient

Table 8.6.1 Aetiology of syncope

Neurally-mediated	Cardiac
Vasovagal/neurocardiogenic Situational: cough, micturition, defaecation Carotid sinus syndrome	Structural valvular disease, such as aortic stenosis Cardiomyopathy Unstable angina Myocardial infarction Bradyarrhythmias, such as sinus node disease, AV block Tachyarrhythmias, such as VT, SVT and *torsades de pointes* Pacemaker/defibrillator dysfunction Pulmonary hypertension Pulmonary embolus Aortic dissection
Orthostatic hypotension	**Neurological**
Dehydration Vasodilatation	Vertebrobasilar transient ischaemic attack Subclavian steal
Medication	**Psychiatric**
Antihypertensives β-Blockers Cardiac glycosides Diuretics Antiarrhythmics Antiparkinsonian drugs Nitrates Alcohol	

Table 8.6.2 Risk stratification for an adverse outcome

High risk	Low risk
Chest pain consistent with IHD History of congestive cardiac failure History of ventricular arrhythmias Pacemaker/defibrillator dysfunction Abnormal ECG (findings such as prolonged QTc interval, conduction abnormalities, acute ischaemia) Exertional syncope/valvular heart disease Age >60 years	Age <45 years Otherwise healthy Normal ECG Normal cardiovascular exam Prodrome (consistent with neurally-mediated syncope or orthostatic hypotension)

IHD: ischaemic heart disease.

may exhibit brief myoclonic movements, which can be mistaken for seizure activity but, in contrast to true epileptic seizures, there are no prolonged post-ictal symptoms. Fatigue is common following syncope.

Orthostatic hypotension occurs when the patient moves from a lying position to a sitting or standing position. If the required autonomic changes fail to compensate adequately, even healthy individuals will experience lightheadedness or blurring of their vision and possibly a loss of consciousness. The most vulnerable people are those with blunted or impaired autonomic reflexes, such as the elderly, those on certain medications (particularly vasodilators, antihypertensive agents and β-blockers) and those who are relatively volume depleted due

to heat, excessive fluid losses or inadequate oral intake.

Cardiac syncope is more likely to present with an absent or brief prodrome. Sudden unexplained loss of consciousness should raise suspicion for a cardiac arrhythmia, particularly in the high-risk patient. Both tachycardia and bradycardia can be responsible. A syncopal event while supine is of particular concern and a predictor for a cardiac cause. Those that occur during exertion should prompt a search for structural heart disease, in particular aortic stenosis.

Risk stratification

Most of the published literature on assessment of patients presenting to emergency

departments (EDs) with syncope has focused on identifying risk factors for mortality or adverse cardiac outcome. These include a number of scores and clinical decision rules. The OESIL score is based on four high-risk factors identified in a multicentre Italian study aimed at predicting mortality at 1 year. These were age over 65 years, a history of cardiovascular disease (which encompasses ischaemic heart disease, congestive cardiac failure, cerebrovascular disease and peripheral vascular disease), an abnormal ECG (including signs of ischaemia, arrhythmias, prolonged QT interval, AV block or bundle branch block) and absence of the typical prodrome. More recently, the San Francisco Syncope Rule (SFSR) has been developed and validated. In this rule, five factors were used to predict serious short-term and longer-term outcomes. These factors are:

❶ history of congestive cardiac failure
❷ haematocrit <30%
❸ abnormal ECG
❹ patient complaining of shortness of breath
❺ systolic blood pressure <90 mmHg at triage.

Based on these factors, patients with syncope can be divided into high- and low-risk groups as shown in Table 8.6.2. Low-risk patients can be safely discharged for outpatient follow up, but controversy over high-risk patients remains. It is likely that there is a significant proportion of patients in the high-risk group who are actually intermediate risk and, given further evaluation in the ED or a short-stay unit, could also be safely discharged; however, it is more difficult to identify this subset.

Other scores/clinical prediction rules have been developed. Available evidence suggests that while most have good sensitivity, specificity is low resulting in recommendations for hospital admission and/or extensive investigations in a significant number of patients who rule out for serious causes. Work continues to refine clinical decision aids of syncope. Recently, a number of authors have published summaries of the various risk stratification rules, most notably:

- Kessler C, et al. The emergency department approach to syncope: evidence-based guidelines and prediction rules. Emerg Med Clin N Am 2010; 28:487–500 and
- Serrano LA, et al. Accuracy and quality of clinical decision rules for syncope in the

emergency department: a systematic review and meta-analysis. Ann Emerg Med 2010; 56:362-73.

The European Society of Cardiology released its guidelines on the diagnosis and management of syncope in 2009.

Differential diagnosis

Seizures are commonly listed as a cause for syncope. Although they do cause a transient loss of consciousness, the pathophysiology is very different. Post-ictal confusion often helps to differentiate the two; however, urinary incontinence may also occur in syncope. True tonic–clonic activity needs to be distinguished from the brief myoclonic jerks occasionally seen in syncope.

Transient ischaemic attacks (TIAs) are often cited as potential causes for syncope, but this is rare. Only vertebrobasilar territory TIAs can affect the reticular activating system of the brain to cause a loss of consciousness; however, TIA should not be named as a cause for the syncope unless associated with other brainstem signs, such as cranial nerve defects or ataxia.

Syncope may also be the presenting symptom of a potentially life-threatening condition such as pulmonary embolus, subarachnoid haemorrhage, gastrointestinal bleed or aortic aneurysm.

Clinical investigations

The only two mandatory investigations are a 12-lead ECG and blood glucose. These should add enough information to the clinical findings to stratify the patient as high or low risk for an adverse outcome. Research has found that a serum troponin taken at least 4 hours after a syncopal event is not a sensitive predictor of an adverse cardiac outcome.

If pulmonary embolus, subarachnoid haemorrhage, gastrointestinal bleed or aortic aneurysm are suspected, appropriate investigations based on clinical suspicion should be initiated.

Treatment

Treatment depends on the presumptive diagnosis. Those with neurally-mediated syncope require explanation and reassurance only. After ensuring that the vital signs have returned to baseline, their blood glucose and ECG are within normal limits and that they

have had something to eat and drink, these patients may be discharged without further investigations.

Patients with orthostatic hypotension often require intravenous fluids and an adequate oral intake to reverse their postural blood pressure changes. Any decision regarding potential changes to chronic medications should ideally include the patient's primary care/treating doctor.

Patients who are deemed high risk for a cardiac cause need continuous cardiac monitoring for at least 24 hours and admission for further evaluation. This may include echocardiography to identify structural heart problems and to quantify an ejection fraction or electrophysiological studies.

Prognosis

Syncope in a patient with underlying heart disease implies a poor prognosis, with data suggesting that a third will die within a year of the episode. Overall, those with syncope on a background of congestive cardiac failure are at the highest risk for an adverse outcome. In the absence of underlying heart disease, syncope is not associated with excess mortality.

Vertigo

Vertigo is defined as the disabling sensation in which the affected individual feels that they or their surroundings are in a state of constant movement. It has a reported 1-year incidence of 1.4%. Like syncope, it is a symptom not a diagnosis and has as many causes. The difficulty is that, whereas many of the causes of vertigo are benign, it may be a symptom of serious neurological conditions, such as vertebrobasilar stroke.

Aetiology

The causes of vertigo may be divided into peripheral and central as shown in Table 8.6.3.

Clinical features

It is vital to establish whether the patient is suffering true vertigo, as opposed to pre-syncope, loss of consciousness or mild unsteadiness. It is also necessary to clarify whether they have a sense of continuous motion (vertigo) or whether they feel 'lightheaded' or 'dizzy'.

If the patient feels they are moving in relation to their surroundings, this is termed subjective vertigo, however, if the patient feels that the surroundings are spinning around them, this is termed objective vertigo.

As previously described, vertigo may be central or peripheral in origin. Peripheral vertigo tends to be more intense and associated with nausea, vomiting, diaphoresis and auditory symptoms, such as tinnitus or hearing loss (although hearing loss can rarely occur with vascular insufficiency in the posterior cerebral circulation, as the auditory apparatus is supplied via the anterior inferior cerebellar artery or the posterior inferior cerebellar artery). There may also be a history of ear trauma, barotrauma, ear infection or generalized illness. The onset of the vertigo tends to be subacute, coming on over minutes to hours. Benign paroxysmal positional vertigo (BPPV) has the classic history of position-induced vertigo lasting only seconds. Central vertigo tends to be less severe and associated with neurological symptoms and signs, such as headache, weakness of the limbs, ataxia, incoordination and dysarthria. These symptoms may be the harbinger of more serious causes, such as cerebellar lesions or demyelinating diseases (Table 8.6.4).

Table 8.6.3 Aetiology of vertigo	
Peripheral	*Central*
Benign paroxysmal positional vertigo (BPPV)	Cerebellar haemorrhage and infarction
Vestibular neuritis	Vertebrobasilar insufficiency
Acute labyrinthitis	Neoplasms
Ménière's disease	Multiple sclerosis
Ototoxicitiy	Wallenberg's syndrome (lateral medullary syndrome)
Eighth-nerve lesions, such as acoustic neuromas	Migrainous vertigo
Cerebellopontine angle tumours	
Post-traumatic vertigo	

Table 8.6.4   Clinical features of vertigo

	Peripheral	Central
Onset	Acute	Gradual
Severity	Severe	Less intense
Duration, pattern	Paroxysmal, intermittent; minutes to days	Constant; usually weeks to months
Positional	Yes	No
Associated nausea	Frequent	Infrequent
Nystagmus	Rotatory – vertical, horizontal	Vertical
Fatigue of symptoms, signs	Yes	No
Hearing loss/tinnitus	May occur	Not usually
CNS symptoms, signs	No	Usually

Physical examination concentrates on any positional factors plus a detailed search for neurological signs, in particular, nystagmus. This is the main objective sign of vertigo. Any spontaneous movement of the eyes needs to be noted, including its direction and persistence. Peripheral vertigo tends to produce unidirectional nystagmus with the slow phase towards the affected side. In addition, patients with vestibular nystagmus are often able to suppress it by fixating on a stationary object.

The 'head impulse' or 'head thrust' test is a simple bedside manoeuvre that can be used to identify the affected labyrinth. With the patient fixating on the examiner's nose, the examiner holds the patient's head and performs a few high acceleration but brief turns to either side. The patient's eyes will automatically move in the opposite direction, in order to maintain visual fixation. The test is positive when this fails to happen and, instead, the patient's eyes are seen to perform a series of catch up movements, or 'saccades' in order to refixate on the examiner's nose. When the 'head impulse' test is positive, the lesion causing the nystagmus is extremely likely to be peripheral. The affected labyrinth is the one in the direction in which the head was moved (see http://www.headimpulse.com/knowledge-center/videos).

Cardiovascular examination should focus on the risk factors for central nervous system thromboembolic events, such as arrhythmias, murmurs and bruits.

Clinical investigations

Most patients who present with vertigo do not need laboratory tests, apart from a blood glucose level. If there is a history of trauma or a space-occupying lesion is suspected, then a computed tomography (CT) or magnetic resonance imaging (MRI) scan of the brain is indicated. An ECG should also be performed to help rule out arrhythmias if differentiation from syncope is problematic.

Dynamic manoeuvres can be both diagnostic and therapeutic. The Dix–Hallpike test can diagnose BPPV. It should not be performed on patients with carotid bruits and patients must be warned that the test may provoke severe symptoms.

Initially, the patient should be seated upright, close enough to the head of the bed so that when they are supine the head will be able to extend back a further 30–45°. To test the right posterior semicircular canal, the head is initially rotated 30–45° to the right. Keeping the head in this position, the patient is quickly brought to the horizontal position with the head placed 30–45° below the level of the bed. A positive test is indicated by rotatory nystagmus towards the affected ear. The test is then repeated on the left side (see http://www.youtube.com/watch?v=cZlXvRlxrRE).

Treatment

Treatment depends on the cause. If BPPV is suspected, the Dix–Hallpike test is performed to identify the affected ear. The Epley

manoeuvre or 'canalith repositioning manoeuvre' aims to move any unwanted particles out of the semicircular canals and thus ease the symptoms for which they are responsible. The steps of this manoeuvre are:

❶ The patient is seated as for the Dix–Hallpike test with the head turned 45° towards the affected ear.
❷ The patient is brought to the horizontal position with the head hyperextended 30–45° below the bed.
❸ The head is gently rotated 45° towards the midline.
❹ The head is then rotated a further 45° towards the unaffected ear.
❺ The patient rolls onto the shoulder of the unaffected side, at the same time rotating the head a further 45°.
❻ The patient is returned to the sitting position and the head returned to the midline (see http://www.youtube.com/watch?v=59ElKztATiw).

These movements may induce nystagmus in the same direction as that seen during the Dix–Hallpike test. Be aware that nystagmus in the opposite direction indicates an unsuccessful test. The manoeuvre may need to be repeated a few times.

Vestibular neuritis is unilateral and thought to be caused by a viral infection or inflammation. Episodes are acute in onset and may be severe, lasting for days, usually associated with nausea and vomiting. The sense of perpetual movement is present even with the eyes closed and is made worse by movement of the head. Symptomatic treatment, with medications, such as antihistamines, antiemetics and benzodiazepines, is often all that is indicated. If nausea and vomiting are severe, intravenous fluid therapy may be needed. There are some reports of trials using steroids for vestibular neuritis, but this treatment remains unproven.

Acute labyrinthitis may be viral or bacterial in origin. If it is viral, the course and treatment are similar to those of vestibular neuritis. Bacterial labyrinthitis may develop from an otitis media. The key feature here is severe vertigo with hearing loss. Patients are febrile and toxic and require admission for intravenous antibiotics.

Ménière's disease has the classic triad of vertigo, sensorineural hearing loss and tinnitus.

Attacks last from minutes to hours and may recur with increasing frequency as the disease progresses. It is caused by dilatation of the endolymphatic system due to excessive production or problems with reabsorption of the endolymph (endolymphatic hydrops). Medical management traditionally involves salt restriction and diuretics, although a 2006 Cochrane review has questioned the efficacy of this.

Vertebrobasilar insufficiency can produce vertigo, often accompanied by unsteadiness and visual changes. Symptoms may be provoked by head position and often include headache. Importantly, however, patients with cerebellar infarction occasionally present with vertigo without other symptoms or signs of neurological impairment. Treatment involves addressing cardiovascular risk factors as well as antiplatelet therapy.

Migrainous vertigo is an increasingly recognized condition that is incompletely understood. In the acute setting, it poses a diagnostic

challenge that will often necessitate exclusion of other central causes for vertigo, such as cerebrovascular disease.

Controversies

- Identifying and determining disposition for syncope patients who do not fall into the high- or low-risk groups.
- Role of a dedicated syncope evaluation unit.
- The use of corticosteroids to treat vestibular neuritis.

Further reading

American College of Emergency Physicians Clinical Policy: critical issues in the evaluation and management of adult patients presenting to the emergency department with syncope. Ann Emerg Med 2007;49:431–44.

Colivicchi F, Ammirati F, Melina D, et al. Development and prospective validation of a risk stratification system for

patients with syncope in the emergency department. Eur Heart J 2003;24:811–9.

Hing R, Harris R. Relative utility of serum troponin and the OESIL score in syncope. Emerg Med Australas 2005;17:31–8.

Jhanjee R, Benditt DG. Syncope. Disease-a-Month 2009;55:532–85.

Kerber A. Vertigo and dizziness in the emergency department. Emerg Med Clin N Am 2009;27:39–50.

Kessler C, Tristano JM, De Lorenzo R. The emergency department approach to syncope: evidence-based guidelines and prediction rules. Emerg Med Clin N Am 2010;28:487–500.

Linzer M, Yang EH, Estes M, et al. Diagnosing syncope Part 1: value of history, physical examination and electrocardiography. Clinical efficacy assessment project of the American College of Physicians. Ann Int Med 1997;126:989–96.

Ouyang H, Quinn J. Diagnosis and evaluation of syncope in the emergency department. Emerg Med Clin N Am 2010;28:471–85.

Quinn JV, Stiell IG, McDermott DA, et al. Derivation of the San Francisco Syncope Rule to predict patients with short-term serious outcomes. Ann Emerg Med 2004;43:224–32.

Quinn JV, Stiell IG, McDermott DA, et al. Prospective validation of the San Francisco Syncope Rule to predict patients with short-term serious outcomes. Ann Emerg Med 2006;47:448–54.

Seemungal BM. A practical approach to vertigo. Pract Neurol 2008;8:211–21.

Serrano LA, Hess EP, Bellolio MF, et al. Accuracy and quality of clinical decision rules for syncope in the emergency department: a systematic review and meta-analysis. Ann Emerg Med 2010;56:362–73.

8.7 Weakness

Tim Green • Eileen M Rogan

ESSENTIALS

1 The differential diagnosis of weakness in the emergency department (ED) is very broad. Careful history taking and examination with targeted investigations will help identify most of the important causes.

2 Causes of weakness must be distinguished as neuromuscular or non-neuromuscular.

3 Most patients presenting to ED with a complaint of weakness have a non-neuromuscular cause underlying their symptoms.

4 Guillain–Barré syndrome is the most common cause of acute onset symmetrical progressive weakness in the developed world. Patients presenting with acute onset symmetrical weakness require early assessment of their airway and ventilation. Early intubation should be considered in high-risk cases. ICU admission is required for any patient with impaired ventilatory function.

5 Patients presenting with a multiple sclerosis relapse should usually be offered pulse steroid therapy in the form of methylprednisolone 1 g IV daily for 3 days (or equivalent oral dosage).

6 Supportive care is the priority in ED management in cases of weakness due to any cause.

7 If a neuromuscular cause is suspected, disposition decisions should be made in consultation with a neurologist.

8 Some patients with weakness will not be definitively diagnosed in the ED and may require referral for further investigations.

Introduction

Weakness is a subjective term that patients use to describe feelings of malaise, fatigue or frailty that they experience as the result of myriad medical and psychological conditions. The Oxford Dictionary defines 'weak' as 'lacking the power to perform physically demanding tasks; having little physical strength or energy'.

For the purpose of this chapter, we will mainly consider the assessment and management of patients presenting with acute onset, generalized, symmetrical or rapidly progressive weakness, primarily in the context of neuromuscular disease. We will not discuss conditions that cause focal or unilateral weakness in any great depth, nor weakness related to non-neuromuscular causes. It should, however, be remembered that the latter group constitutes the majority of patients presenting to the emergency department (ED) complaining of weakness.

Aetiology and pathogenesis

Complaints of weakness are essentially either due to a neuromuscular problem or not. The

Table 8.7.1   Clinical signs that distinguish origin of neuromuscular weakness

Sign	UMN	LMN	NMJ	Myopathy
Atrophy	None	Severe	Mild	Mild
Fasciculation	None	Common	None	None
Deep tendon reflexes	Hyperreflexic	Areflexic/hyporeflexic	Normal/ hyporeflexic	Normal/hyporeflexic
Distribution of weakness	Pyramidal/regional	Distal/segmental	Variable/fatiguable weakness	Proximal > distal
Tone	Spastic	Decreased/flaccid	Decreased/flaccid	Normal/decreased
Plantar response	Upgoing	Downgoing or absent	Downgoing or absent	Downgoing or absent

UMN: upper motor neurons; LMN: lower motor neurons; NMJ: neuro muscular junction

Table 8.7.2   Non-neuromuscular conditions associated with weakness

Condition	Manifestations
Anaemia	Breathlessness, fatigue usually worse if acute onset anaemia
Cardiac failure	Fatigue and weakness are common symptoms of heart failure in elderly patients, especially weakness in females over 50 years
Malignancy	Paraneoplastic syndromes, e.g. generalized wasting
Psychological disorders	Depression/anxiety; psychosis; medication side effects; malingering
Malnutrition	Institutionalized patients; impoverished elderly; anorexia nervosa
Chronic fatigue syndrome	Possibly post-viral syndrome
Rheumatological disorders	Rheumatoid arthritis, systemic lupus erythematosus, fibromyalgia
Medications	Many medications have been associated with weakness but the commonly encountered ones include: glucocorticoids, statins, antiretrovirals, alcohol, colchicine and polypharmacy especially in the elderly
Acute electrolyte derangement, e.g. hypo-, hyperkalaemia, hypo-calcaemia	Acute onset weakness, ± tetany with hypocalcaemia
Sepsis	Acidosis, deranged metabolic state
Dehydration	Lethargy/fatigue
Hypothyroidism	Lethargy, cold intolerance, weight gain, weakness
Chronic disease	Respiratory, renal, hepatic failure

primary goal in ED is to determine if there is actual quantitative loss of muscle strength indicative of a neuromuscular cause or whether weakness is resulting from a non-neuromuscular cause. The latter cases are often the result of multiple system disorders, for example endocrine, cardiac and metabolic factors.

Neuromuscular weakness may reflect deficits anywhere along the neural pathway from cerebral cortex to the myocyte. This pathway includes the pyramidal system as upper motor neurons (UMN) synapse with lower motor neurons (LMN) of the anterior spinal cord. LMN axons then descend through the anterior spinal cord to exit and synapse with myocytes. At the neuromuscular junction, LMNs release the presynaptic neurotransmitter acetylcholine (Ach) into the synaptic cleft and post-synaptic Ach receptors then trigger depolarization of the motor end plate and contraction of the muscle cell. Pathology at any level of this neural pathway will result in weakness. An intact myelin nerve sheath, functioning calcium and sodium channels and the presence of acetylcholinesterase to limit the response are all necessary for normal neuromuscular function.

Specific signs, such as altered deep tendon reflexes (DTRs) and tone, muscle atrophy, fasciculations and distribution of weakness, aid in localizing the site of the neuromuscular pathology (Table 8.7.1).

Non-neuromuscular causes of weakness are myriad and generally reflect a combination of age, general physical and mental health factors and specific systematic disorders that co-exist to result in a general feeling of weakness or malaise (Table 8.7.2).

Pathology

Diverse pathological processes may underlie neuromuscular weakness. Of these, genetic, autoimmune and toxic causes predominate in the ED (Table 8.7.3). Patients with congenital genetic syndromes, such as muscular dystrophies or mitochondrial disorders, are rarely seen in the ED unless they are suffering from acute respiratory decompensation in the context of an acute reversible precipitant, such as pneumonia. Management of these cases will be guided by consideration of the clinical context, the stage of disease and disability and any advance care directives from the patient or their advocates.

In industrialized countries such as Australia, Guillain–Barré syndrome (GBS) is the most common cause of acute onset neuromuscular weakness. GBS variants, multiple sclerosis (MS) and myasthenia gravis (MG) are other autoimmune disorders that precipitate ED presentations, either as *de novo* diagnoses or in the context of acute exacerbations. Toxic triggers, such as organophosphates, tetanus, botulism and envenomations, are relatively rare but can be fatal if not recognized and treated aggressively.

Other pathologies, such as paraneoplastic syndromes (Eaton–Lambert syndrome) and electrolyte disturbances (e.g. hypokalaemic

Table 8.7.3   Key features of conditions associated with the symptom of weakness

Disease	Pathophysiology	Assessment	ED management
Primary neurological			
Guillain–Barré syndrome Most common cause of acute symmetrical weakness	Immune-mediated poly-radiculopathy Post-infective (15–40%), esp. *Campylobacter* or viral infection >50% idiopathic	Suggestive history (e.g. diarrhoea) Symmetrical ascending flaccid weakness; loss of DTRs; early facial palsy common; ± autonomic dysfunction Serial assessment of respiratory function crucial to predict need for intubation/ventilation CSF high protein with normal glucose and cell count	Supportive care; early intubation for respiratory failure Early neurology and ICU consultation Early administration of IVIG ± plasmapheresis beneficial Corticosteroids NOT indicated
Myasthenia gravis Localized variant more common Myasthenic crises/respiratory decompensation are main ED issues (rare)	Immune-mediated Ach receptor dysfunction May be precipitated by thymus disorders	Fluctuating, fatiguable weakness of voluntary muscles especially ocular muscles or proximal limbs. Cranial nerve involvement with ptosis in >25% cases; ± dysphagia, weakness of masticatory muscles; normal sensation; normal reflexes Improves with rest Serial respiratory assessment if severe Ice-pack test if ptosis present	Supportive care Avoid potential precipitants including corticosteroids Anticholinesterase treatment as directed by neurologist
Multiple sclerosis Relapsing/remitting course most common	Immune-mediated scattered neuron demyelination. Affects motor, sensory, visual and cerebellar function Classically ≥2 separate episodes of neurological dysfunction indicating white matter or spinal cord lesions at distinct locations	Acute exacerbations – acute worsening of clinical signs; variable: weakness, hypertonicity, spasticity, clonus, altered pain/temp/vibration and proprioceptive senses Lhermitte's sign Optic neuritis in up to 30% – acute central vision loss, afferent papillary defect, red desaturation LP, MRI, evoked potentials in consultation with neurologist	Pulse methylprednisolone therapy for exacerbations Supportive care for generalized weakness Neurology consultation Long-term disease modification and lifestyle strategies, e.g. vitamin D
Cord compression	Spinal stenosis ± malignancy or infection	Thorough neurological exam Red flags, e.g. fever, malignancy, IVDU warrant MRI	Neurosurgical consultation Decompression, antibiotics, targeted radiotherapy as indicated
Myopathies			
Congenital Dystrophin disorders – DMD/BMD Mitochondrial disorders	X-linked dystrophin gene dysfunction Males affected DMD – more severe; life expectancy early 20s BMD – later onset, less severe	Generalized weakness Usual ED presentation is acute deterioration with respiratory compromise Spirometry/respiratory assessment Mitochondrial disorders – variable episodic weakness and fluctuating consciousness	Supportive care Discussion with patient, advocates, neurologists regarding appropriateness of intensive intervention Consider advance care directives Ventilatory support as appropriate
Acquired Metabolic/electrolyte disorders Hypokalaemic periodic paralysis Endocrine Cushing's Addison's Thyrotoxicosis Toxic Statins, corticosteroids	Variable weakness – may be acute episodic weakness with hypokalaemia ± thyrotoxicosis Drug-induced or endocrine myopathies – history suggestive	Periodic paralysis; may be preceded by vomiting/diarrhoeal illness; may be a family history Check electrolytes especially K+ ECG if K+ deranged Endocrine – assess for other stigmata of endocrinopathy, e.g. Cushingoid, Addisonian	Electrolyte (K+) reconstitution Supportive care Correct endocrine abnormalities Discontinue offending medications
Intoxications			
Botulism *Clostridium botulinum* toxin	Deranged neurotransmission Ingested botulinum toxin prevents Ach release at NMJ	History of ingestion GI symptoms in 50% Descending flaccid paralysis Postural hypotension, diplopia, blurred vision, ptosis, dysphagia, respiratory compromise, progressing to limb weakness Ileus common	Supportive care ICU admission for ventilatory support as needed Specific antiserum in consultation with toxicology/neurology
Tetanus *Clostridium tetani* tetano – spasmin toxin Endemic in developing countries	Impaired inhibitory neurotransmission causing skeletal muscle spasm and rigidity Classically infected deep wounds in non-immunized patients	Suggestive history – recent wound, vulnerable patient, e.g. elderly, non-immune Trismus/dysphagia common early; progressive to painful skeletal muscle spasms; exacerbated by minor stimuli, e.g. touch May be a localized form Clinical diagnosis	Supportive care, ICU for ventilatory support and sedation Tetanus antitoxin Tetanus immunization is protective Antibiotics (penicillin) to treat Clostridial infection

(Continued)

Table 8.7.3 Key features of conditions associated with the symptom of weakness (Continued)

Disease	Pathophysiology	Assessment	ED management
Tick paralysis Tick toxin Ascending flaccid paralysis – mimics GBS	Impaired neurotransmission *Ixodes holocyclus* (Australian paralysis tick) Death from respiratory paralysis	Mostly children in tick endemic area ± tick found on patient; ataxia, weakness, ± extra ocular palsy/dysphagia May progress after tick removal to generalized/respiratory paralysis	Tick removal/observation sufficient in most cases If severe – ventilatory support Antiserum administration as directed by toxicology/neurology
Marine intoxications Ciguatera Puffer fish Blue-ringed octopus	Ciguatera toxin (from reef fish) Tetrodotoxin (puffer fish, blue-ringed octopus) block sodium channels and impairs neurotransmission Tetrodotoxin also acts on CTZ and impairs ventilation	History of tropical fish ingestion; onset of symptoms within a few hours Ciguatera – paraesthesias, electrical sensations in response to hot/cold Tetrodotoxin – progressive flaccid weakness with respiratory compromise	Supportive treatment esp. ventilatory support

periodic paralysis), should be considered if the clinical context is suggestive. Poliomyelitis is an example of an infectious disease that was previously a major cause of acute onset weakness. It has been eradicated in the Western world and is well on the way to eradication in the developing world. Post-polio syndrome is a rare late complication seen in ED.

Differential diagnosis

The differential diagnosis of weakness in the ED is very broad and the definitive diagnosis may not be able to be elucidated during the course of one ED visit. Recognition of neuromuscular disorders that have the potential to deteriorate rapidly and require intensive supportive care with assisted ventilation is the most crucial element of ED diagnosis. In particular, GBS, MS exacerbations, myasthenic crises and intoxications, such as botulism, must be recognized early.

Clinical features

The diagnosis of neuromuscular disease is dependent upon history, examination and specific investigation findings. A starting point for diagnosis should include a thorough history, noting in particular:

- known underlying neuromuscular disorders, such as amyotrophic lateral sclerosis (ALS), muscular dystrophy, MS or MG
- pre-existing medical conditions, such as malignancy suggesting a paraneoplastic syndrome, monoclonal gammopathy associated with chronic inflammatory polymyopathy (CIDP) or HIV infection/

post-transplant immunosuppressive states associated with CIDP, polyradiculopathy or HIV myopathy
- recent infections (diarrhoeal, viral) or major surgery – associated with GBS
- recent exposures/ingestions suggestive of intoxications, for example botulism, organophosphate, ciguatera toxin.

Clinical findings generally reflect the site of the lesion within the motor unit (see Table 8.7.1).

Clinical investigations

Given the broad differential diagnosis possible for weakness, a broad screen of laboratory parameters including full blood count (for anaemia or inflammation), electrolytes and renal function, liver function, thyroid function plus muscle creatine kinase, inflammatory markers (erythrocyte sedimentation rate [ESR] and C reactive protein [CRP]) as indicated, should be measured. ECG should be performed urgently if an electrolyte imbalance is possible. A rheumatoid screen may be suggested by clinical signs. Lumbar puncture may be indicated and can be performed to corroborate the diagnosis of GBS or MS if there are no contraindications. Specific investigations, such as brainstem evoked potentials and magnetic resonance imaging (MRI) scanning for MS should be arranged by specialist neurology services. Chest X-ray or computed tomography (CT) scan may be indicated to exclude thymoma in association with MG.

Treatment and prognosis

The mainstay of treatment for weakness caused by neuromuscular disorders is supportive care with a particular focus on ventilatory support

commenced early rather than later, as emergency intubations are associated with higher complication rates. General supportive measures will also include maintenance of homeostasis with respect to normothermia, euglycaemia, normotension and control of any other autonomic dysregulation, such as paralytic ileus and urinary retention.

Prophylaxis against peptic ulcers and deep vein thrombosis and pressure area care are all crucially important in the mechanically ventilated and sedated patient. This will require ICU admission but treatment is usually commenced in the ED. Early neurological consultation and ICU review is crucial, especially for conditions in which there are effective interventions, such as plasmapheresis or intravenous immunoglobulin (IVIG) administration for GBS. For acute envenomations or intoxications, supportive care is still the priority in combination with antivenoms or antidotes, when indicated.

For non-neuromuscular causes of weakness, the treatment priority is to address the underlying disease state. This will variously include electrolyte reconstitution, rehydration, correction of thyroid function, treatment of systemic diseases and infections, optimization of organ function or psychological assessment as indicated by clinical assessment and investigations. Appropriate referral should follow. In cases where no apparent cause can be found for a complaint of weakness, an expectant approach is warranted.

The prognosis for neuromuscular disease depends on the specific condition.

Criteria for diagnosis

Table 8.7.3 summarizes the key pathophysiology, assessment findings to elucidate and management strategies for the conditions likely to present to the ED with weakness as a predominant feature.

Specific conditions

Guillain–Barré syndrome

Guillain–Barré syndrome is an acute, acquired, inflammatory demyelinating polyradiculoneuropathy (AIDP) caused by autoimmune attack on peripheral nerves/nerve roots. It is the most common cause of acute progressive generalized weakness in the ED. GBS variants exist, such as the Miller–Fisher syndrome with particular ocular muscle involvement, but these are much less common. GBS has an annual incidence in the developed world of about 1–2 cases per 100 000 and mortality of 3–10%. It is more common as people get older.

Pathophysiology

The pathophysiology involves an aberrant autoimmune response associated in about two-thirds of cases with an antecedent respiratory or gastrointestinal tract infection 3 weeks or less before the onset of signs. *Campylobacter jejuni* is the most commonly associated pathogen (up to 40% of cases) and a positive *C. jejuni* IgM titre is associated with a worse prognosis. Cytomegalovirus is the second most common infection associated with GBS. Others include Epstein–Barr virus, *Mycoplasma pneumoniae*, HIV and *Haemophilus influenzae*.

Clinical features

The hallmark of GBS is progressive ascending weakness with loss of DTRs with maximal weakness present within 2–4 weeks after onset. Proximal and distal limb muscles, truncal and respiratory muscles are affected. Cranial nerve involvement is common with facial nerve palsy in up to 70% of cases. Ocular muscle involvement is less common. Sensory symptoms are common but variable with paraesthesias or even severe pain in some patients. Autonomic dysregulation occurs in about two-thirds of patients and can be fatal due to severe fluctuations in blood pressure and cardiac arrhythmias.

The diagnosis of GBS is based on suggestive history (e.g. recent diarrhoeal infection or major surgery), clinical features of an ascending weakness with loss of DTRs and exclusion of other pathologies.

Clinical investigations

Lumbar puncture should be performed and classic CSF findings are of high CSF protein and normal glucose and cell count. Mild CSF pleocytosis is common; however, the presence of CSF leucocytosis should prompt careful consideration of alternative diagnoses, such as lymphoma or HIV.

Complications

Respiratory failure may occur in up to 30% of cases and is the most life-threatening short-term complication of GBS. This is attributed to the high incidence of phrenic nerve involvement.

Treatment

Attention to ventilation is a priority of treatment. Assessment of FVC every 2–4 hours during the acute phase is recommended and FVC of 10–12 mL/kg (<30% of predicted) is generally considered to be an indication for intubation and assisted ventilation. Other suggested criteria for elective intubation and ventilation include significant respiratory distress, fatigue, sweating, tachycardia, active aspiration and $PaCO_2$ >50 mmHg. That said, clinical judgement should guide the decision to intubate as respiratory distress and fatigue often indicate significant respiratory embarrassment prior to $PaCO_2$ or FVC becoming deranged, particularly if the condition is rapidly deteriorating or if the patient has significant co-morbidity, for example, active cardiac ischaemia or heart failure. Swallowing difficulty and inability to lift the head or elbow off the bed are features predicting the need for intubation. Elective intubation is associated with less adverse events than a late emergency intubation so the timing of intervention needs to be carefully considered. About 25% of patients with GBS who cannot mobilize and 30–50% of patients admitted to ICU need mechanical ventilation. Of note, non-invasive ventilation (NIV) is not recommended for GBS and respiratory failure, especially if there is significant bulbar weakness.

Intravenous immunoglobulin (IVIG–usually 2 g/kg over 3–5 days) has largely replaced plasmapheresis in the treatment of GBS after large studies showed them to be equally efficacious. There is also easier access to IVIG in most hospitals.

Prognosis

Most people fully recover but a significant minority (20%) survive with persistent neurological deficits. The most common causes of death are the complications of dysautonomia and respiratory failure.

Multiple sclerosis

Multiple sclerosis (MS) is a chronic demyelinating condition. It is the commonest chronic neurological condition with an estimated prevalence of 40 000 cases in Australia. Incidence is related to latitude with Tasmania having among the highest incidence in the world (1:1000). Sixty per cent of cases occur in women. MS is frequently characterized by exacerbations and remissions. It is usually diagnosed in individuals aged 15–45 years.

Common relapse patterns include ataxia, proximal weakness (more frequently in the lower limbs), urinary symptoms and cranial nerve disorders, such as optic neuritis, diplopia and vertigo. Fatigue is a common symptom in MS and should be distinguished from a focal relapse. Heat sensitivity is a common phenomenon in MS and symptoms are often worse in summer. Exacerbations associated with febrile illness can be minimized with careful antipyretic therapy.

Undiagnosed patients may present to the ED with myriad neurological symptoms, although life-threatening presentations with respiratory compromise are exceedingly rare.

Clinical investigations and diagnosis

The diagnosis is usually made when typical clinical features are supported by the findings of neuroimaging (MRI), CSF examination and evoked potentials. Nearly all MS patients show discrete white matter lesions or homogeneous periventricular lesions on T2-weighted MRI of brain and/or spinal cord. Elevated protein and gammaglobulins (oligoclonal bands) and pleocytosis with mild lymphocytosis are the typical CSF findings. Delays in latencies on visual, somatosensory or brainstem evoked potential testing are diagnostic of demyelination in the visual pathways, posterior columns or auditory pathways, respectively.

Treatment

Relapses usually respond to brief pulse therapy with corticosteroids (methylprednisolone 1g IV daily for 3 days or equivalent oral dosage).

More severe episodes may require high dose corticosteroids and plasmapheresis therapy.

Vitamin D has now been confirmed as an important aetiological factor in MS and a vitamin D level of 150–200 nmol/L obtained by sun exposure and/or vitamin D supplementation is recommended. A range of dietary and lifestyle interventions are also associated with better outcomes in MS. Long-term disease modification therapies are increasingly available and are the remit of the neurologists. It is important to be aware of these therapies, as patients may present with side effects from these increasingly potent immune-modulating drugs.

Disposition

Neurology consultation for directing investigations and management is indicated for all patients with MS exacerbations and hospital admission is often required.

Myasthenia gravis

Myasthenia gravis (MG) is rare but the prevalence is rising in developed countries due to earlier diagnosis and good survival rates. During exacerbations, patients are very likely to attend an ED with localized or, less commonly, generalized weakness. The disease is caused by an idiopathic autoimmune attack of post-synaptic Ach receptors, leading to weakness of the muscle response to stimulus. The weakness tends to be fatiguable and is usually relieved by rest. Most patients experience facial and bulbar muscle weakness so dysphagia and dysarthria are common symptoms. More serious exacerbations are associated with respiratory compromise.

Myasthenic crisis, which occurs in 15–20% of patients (mostly within the first 2 years of diagnosis when the disease has an unpredictable course), refers to generalized weakness with respiratory failure requiring intubation and mechanical ventilation. Respiratory failure rarely presents in isolation. Myasthenic crisis can be precipitated by acute disease progression, intercurrent infections, pregnancy, surgery and by treatment with high-dose glucocorticoids and a long list of other medications that may affect neuromuscular transmission.

Diagnosis

The diagnosis is based on clinical features and demonstration of antibodies to the Ach receptor which are found in about 85% of cases. Clinical suspicion of MG can be supported by a positive bedside ice-pack test in patients with ptosis, where the eyelids are covered with an ice pack for 2 minutes with improvement in the ptosis seen immediately. The Tensilon test is now rarely performed. Electromyography (EMG) may be necessary to differentiate MG from GBS, myopathy or motor neuron disease.

Treatment and disposition

Supportive care is the main priority in ED. Neurological consultation is mandated by suspicion of MG. Treatment for MG should not be commenced until the diagnosis has been confirmed. Many patients take pyridostigmine long term and the dose may be increased in exacerbations. Paradoxically, high-dose pyridostigmine can lead to acute deterioration, so the treatment decisions should always be made in consultation with a neurologist.

Respiratory failure is the main life-threatening issue in acute myasthenic crisis; however, the condition tends to fluctuate so reliable criteria for intubation are difficult to define. Serial measurement of PEF/FVC and $PaCO_2$ are recommended. Intubation is recommended for marginal or deteriorating patients, as elective intubation is associated with fewer complications. Early use of NIV (BiPAP) has been shown to be of benefit in myasthenic crisis in reducing the need for intubation. Plasmapheresis and IVIG (2 g/kg over 3–5 days) have also been shown to be effective in myasthenic crisis. Corticosteroids may exacerbate the condition, so should be avoided unless the patient is mechanically ventilated. In some patients, thymectomy or immunosuppressive strategies are indicated.

Prognosis

The mortality of myasthenic crisis is about 4% overall, with age >50 years and FVC <25 mL/kg predictors of poor outcome and long ICU stay. Most patients with MG have a normal lifespan.

Cord compression/cauda equina syndrome

Patients may present with weakness from acute or chronic conditions that lead to compression of the spinal cord and nerve roots, usually due to a combination of progressive age-related spinal stenosis, infections or malignancy. Progressive spinal stenosis is a common feature of ageing and can occur in isolation or be associated with acute disc herniations. Acute deterioration or sudden onset neurological deficits in the presence of other systemic illness, such as fever, should be 'red flags' that prompt urgent consideration and investigation for sinister pathologies. These include malignancy (e.g. lymphoma or metastatic deposits), infection (e.g. epidural abscess or discitis especially in high-risk groups, such as intravenous drug users (IVDU) or patients who have had recent epidural or spinal anaesthetics) or trauma (e.g. falls in the elderly). Any patient presenting to the ED with lower limb neurological deficits, in particular with signs of bladder or bowel dysfunction, warrants urgent imaging (MRI) to assess for spinal cord compression. Therapeutic interventions including antibiotics, surgical decompression and radiotherapy will be tailored to the individual patient following specialist consultation.

Amyotrophic lateral sclerosis (motor neuron disease)

Motor neuron disease (MND)/amyotrophic lateral sclerosis (ALS) is a rapidly progressive muscle atrophy and weakness caused by degeneration of both upper (UMN) and lower motor neurons (LMN). It causes a variable picture of spasticity, hyperreflexia and muscle weakness with an inexorable decline to respiratory failure and dependence on mechanical ventilation, usually within 2–4 years. UMN or LMN bulbar muscle weakness is invariably present and complicates the condition with aspiration and impaired cough. There is no curative therapy and treatment is therefore supportive. In the ED, ALS patients usually present with acute respiratory compromise as a result an acute precipitant, such as aspiration pneumonia or a choking episode. Management of these patients will be directed at treating the precipitant and increasing respiratory support during the period of acute exacerbation as directed by the patient and any advance care plans they might have in place. NIV should be avoided due to the risks of aspiration and increased work required by already weak respiratory muscles. Medications that reduce respiratory drive, such as opiates, should also be avoided. New diagnoses are rarely made in the ED and, if so, usually present with variable UMN and LMN signs and variable weakness. Neurological consultation is mandated by such presentations.

Eaton–Lambert syndrome

Eaton–Lambert syndrome (ELS) is a rare autoimmune paraneoplastic condition that is usually associated with small cell lung cancer. The major clinical feature is severe limb weakness as a result of autoimmune destruction of voltage-gated calcium channels in the presynaptic membrane at the neuromuscular junction which, in turn, inhibits release of presynaptic Ach vesicles. It often improves with exercise, which distinguishes it from MG. Tendon reflexes are variable but usually reduced. EMG is required to confirm the diagnosis. Management is to treat the underlying malignancy and therefore prognosis depends upon the prognosis of the malignancy. Symptomatic treatments, such as glucocorticoids, are usually ineffective. Supportive care is the goal of ED management.

Myopathies

Congenital muscular dystrophies

The X-linked disorders Duchenne muscular dystrophy and Becker muscular dystrophy are the most common forms of congenital muscular dystrophy. Boys with Duchenne muscular dystrophy are normal at birth but by age ≈5 years exhibit proximal weakness which gradually deteriorates until they are wheelchair-dependent by age 10–12 years. Thereafter, the weakness progresses inexorably and average lifespan is only ≈21 years before death due to respiratory failure. Becker muscular dystrophy has a later onset and slower progression so immobility and respiratory complications may occur in adult life and many patients have a normal life span. ED presentations in both of these conditions are almost always related to respiratory compromise due to disease progression or an acute precipitant, such as pneumonia. The management is supportive and aimed at treating any acute precipitants, as guided by disease stage, patient preference and any advance care directives.

Mitochondrial myopathies, such as those associated with MELAS syndrome, tend to present to ED similarly, with variable weakness and fluctuating conscious state on a known background of mitochondrial disorder. Ventilatory support and the attendant supportive care are the key aspects of treatment. In these cases, a brief period of mechanical ventilation can support the patient through an acute exacerbation and they may return to being relatively independent until the next acute deterioration. Management should be guided by the patient and their neurologist.

Inflammatory myopathies: polymyositis/dermatomyositis

Polymyositis and dermatomyositis are idiopathic inflammatory myopathies that mostly affect women over 30 years of age. Dermatomyositis is associated with a heliotrope rash, erythroderma and other skin changes and is more commonly associated with cancer. Patients present with proximal symmetrical weakness associated with muscle pain and tenderness. Deep tendon reflexes are intact unless weakness is severe. There are no sensory or autonomic deficits. Proximal weakness is demonstrated by asking the patient to stand from a chair while folding their arms or by asking them to lift an object above the head. In severe cases, respiratory function may be affected. Diagnosis is based on clinical findings and elevated ESR and creatine kinase (CK). Management is with immunosuppressive agents, primarily corticosteroids. Differential diagnosis includes HIV myopathy, viral myositis or myositis due to substances, such as alcohol, statins, corticosteroids and AZT. Endocrine myopathies occur rarely.

Acute periodic paralysis

Acute periodic paralyses are an interesting group of rare disorders occasionally seen in the ED. These may be associated with normal, low or elevated serum potassium. Patients are usually well between attacks but some can have residual muscle stiffness. A genetic defect has been linked to these diseases but, in some instances, hypokalaemia may cause acute weakness in healthy individuals.

Acute hypokalaemic periodic paralysis may be primary (i.e. familial) or secondary to excessive renal or gastrointestinal losses or endocrinopathy. Familial periodic paralysis usually occurs in Caucasian males, is autosomal dominant and may last as long as 36 hours. Attacks usually occur at night or in the early morning upon awakening and can be precipitated by a diet high in carbohydrates, rest following exercise or glucose and insulin given intravenously. Supportive care and replenishment of serum potassium are the main management priorities.

Thyrotoxic periodic paralysis associated with hypokalaemia is a condition more common in Asian males. Treatment of the underlying disease and electrolyte disorder are the goals of treatment.

Rhabdomyolysis

Rhabdomyolysis is a disorder with many causes that leads to muscle necrosis and the release of intracellular muscle constituents into the circulation. The characteristic triad in rhabdomyolysis is weakness, muscle pain and dark urine. Causes can be classified as due to trauma or compression, exertional and non-exertional. Non-exertional causes include drugs, toxins, viruses and electrolyte abnormalities. ED management is dependent on the cause and the emphasis is on preservation of renal function.

Intoxications

Botulism

Botulism is an acute paralytic illness caused by a neurotoxin produced by *Clostridium botulinum*. It is characterized by severe descending weakness and gastrointestinal slowing. In adults, the toxin is ingested preformed in foodstuffs whereas, in infants, the disease is usually due to ingestion of foods containing the bacterial spores, such as honey. Botulinum toxin acts at the neuromuscular junction, where it inhibits Ach release from the presynaptic membrane. Early characteristic findings include normal mentation with bulbar weakness manifesting as dysphagia and extraocular palsies with absent papillary light reflex (which distinguishes botulism from myasthenia gravis). Limb weakness is more obvious proximally and deep tendon reflexes are usually intact. Sensation is not affected. Postural hypotension tends to be a feature in adults. Management is supportive with ventilatory support in ICU if necessary. An antitoxin is available.

Tetanus

Tetanus is an acute painful paralytic illness caused by the tetanospasmin toxin of the soil-dwelling organism *Clostridium tetani*. It is characterized by painful severe uncontrolled skeletal muscle spasms. Respiratory muscle involvement leads to hypoxia and death. It remains endemic throughout the world and most of the 1 000 000 cases annually occur in developing countries. In the developed world, tetanus should be considered in the elderly and vulnerable groups like the homeless and poor in particular, where tetanus-prone wounds and lack of immunization are more common. Typically, tetanus is caused by a deep penetrating wound but up to 50%

of patients have only a trivial, if any, wound evident. The onset is highly variable – from days to months. Generalized tetanus is the most common form and causes generalized skeletal muscle spasms, which can be greatly exacerbated by minor stimuli, such as touching or loud noise. Trismus or 'lockjaw' is the classic initial presenting symptom with spasm of the masseter muscle. Other early symptoms include myalgias, cramps, dysphagia and drooling. Violent muscle spasms can cause vertebral and long bone fractures. Death is due to either respiratory failure or autonomic dysfunction. The illness is progressive with an increase in severity over 3–5 days and a gradual reduction after 10 days. Diagnosis is on clinical grounds alone and supportive care with sedation and ventilation, administration of tetanus antitoxin and avoidance of complications are the priorities in treatment. Localized tetanus also occurs with spasms localized near the original wound site and rarely progresses to generalized tetanus. This variant carries a good prognosis with or without treatment.

Envenomations

Several envenomations can present to the ED with weakness as part of the clinical syndrome. These include the *Ixodes holocyclus* paralysis tick, puffer fish and blue-ringed octopus (tetrodotoxin) and reef fish (ciguatera toxin) (see Table 8.7.3). These envenomations are covered in detail elsewhere.

Controversies and future developments

- A number of the causes of weakness discussed in this chapter including GBS, cord compression and MS are misdiagnosed in the ED or diagnosed late and are overrepresented in medicolegal claims arising from the ED. Emergency physicians must maintain a high level of critical thinking to distinguish functional, non-neuromuscular and time-critical neuromuscular emergencies.
- Orthodox neurological opinion stresses the primacy of modern immune modulating therapies for management of relapsing-remitting MS. Recent studies suggest an equally important role for other therapeutic approaches including vitamin D supplementation, avoidance of animal fat, promotion of a whole food diet rich in fish and omega 3 fatty acids and meditation/stress reduction techniques.
- Plasmapheresis and IVIG have both been advocated as definitive therapy for GBS. Recent studies suggest superiority of IVIG.
- Ventilatory support for patients with GBS should be instituted early when indicated, while patients with end-stage muscular dystrophy, MELAS, MND/ALS or MG present difficulties for emergency physicians balancing quality of life, potential reversibility and the patient's expressed advance care directive. Therapeutic decisions must be made with extensive consultation with the treating neurologist, patient and family. NIV may be an effective modality in patients with MG but should be avoided in cases of GBS and MNS/ALS where intubation and mechanical ventilation is preferred.

Further reading

Burton JM, O'Connor PW, Beyene J. Oral versus intravenous treatment for relapses in multiple sclerosis. Cochrane Database Syst Rev 2009;3:CD006921.

Greenberg D, Aminoff M, Simon R. Motor disorders. In: Greenberg D, Aminoff M, Simon R, editors. Clinical neurology (8th ed.). New York: McGraw-Hill, 2012.

Hart IK, Sathasivam S, Sharshar T. Immunosuppressive agents for myasthenia gravis. Cochrane Database Syst Rev 2007;4:CD 005224.

Holmay T, Kampma M, Smolders J. Vitamin D in multiple sclerosis: implications for assessment and treatment. Exp Rev Neurother 2012;12:1101–12.

Hughes RAC, Swan AV, van Doorn PA. Intravenous immunoglobulin for Guillain-Barre syndrome. Cochrane Database Syst Rev 2012;7:CD002063.

Jagannath VA, Fedorowicz Z, Asokan GV, et al. Vitamin D for the management of multiple sclerosis. Cochrane Database Syst Rev 2012;12:CD008422.

Jelinek G. Overcoming multiple sclerosis: an evidence-based guide to recovery. Australia: Allen and Unwin, 2010.

Longo D, Fauci A, Kasper D. Weakness and paralysis. In: Longo D, Fauci A, Kasper D, et al., Harrison's principles of internal medicine (18th ed.). New York: McGraw-Hill, 2012.

Mehndiratta MM, Pandey S, Kuntzer T. Acetylcholinesterase inhibitor treatment for myasthenia gravis. Cochrane Database Syst Rev 2011;2:CD 006986.

Minagar A, Rabinstein A. Neurologic emergencies. Neurol Clin 2012;30:1–404.

Murray L, Daly F, Little M, Cadogan M, editors. Toxicology handbook (2nd ed.). Churchill-Livingstone/Elsevier, 2010.

Ropper A, Samuels M. Motor paralysis. In: Ropper AH, Samuels MA, editors. Adams and Victor's principles of neurology (9th ed.). New York: McGraw-Hill, 2009.

8

NEUROLOGY EMERGENCIES

INFECTIOUS DISEASE EMERGENCIES

Edited by **Peter Cameron**

9.1 Approach to undifferentiated fever in adults

Jonathan Knott

ESSENTIALS

1 Over one-third of patients who have fever for more than 2–3 days with no localizing symptoms and signs are likely to have a bacterial infection; half of these will be in the respiratory or urinary tracts.

2 An unexplained fever in a person over the age of 50 should be regarded as due to a bacterial infection until proved otherwise.

3 An undifferentiated fever in an alcoholic patient, an intravenous drug user or an insulin-dependent diabetic is generally an indication for admission to hospital.

4 Any fever in a traveller returned from a malaria-endemic area should be regarded as due to malaria until proved otherwise.

5 Severe muscle pain, even in the absence of overt fever, may be an early symptom of meningococcaemia, staphylococcal or streptococcal bacteraemia.

6 An unexplained rash in a febrile patient should be regarded as meningococcaemia until proved otherwise.

7 The diagnosis of meningococcaemia should be considered in every patient with an undifferentiated fever.

8 There will always be a small number of febrile patients whose sepsis is not initially recognized because they do not appear toxic and their symptoms are non-specific. It is essential that all patients are encouraged to seek review if they have any clinical deterioration.

Introduction

Fever is a common presenting symptom to the emergency department (ED); about 5% of patients give fever as the reason for their visit. Most patients with fever have symptoms and signs that indicate the site or region of infection. A prospective study of patients aged 16 years or older who presented to an ED with fever ≥37.9°C found that 85% had localizing symptoms and signs that suggested or identified a source of fever and 15% had unexplained fever after the history and examination [1].

Fever with no localizing symptoms or signs at presentation is often seen in the first day or two of the illness. Many patients with such a problem will ultimately prove to have self-limiting viral infections, but others will have non-viral infections requiring treatment. Among this latter group are illnesses that may be serious and even rapidly fatal.

Over one-third of patients who have fever for more than a few days with no localizing symptoms and signs are likely to have a bacterial infection [1,2].

If no cause is found in an adult with fever present for over 3 days, there is a good chance the patient will have a bacterial infection that needs treatment. Over half of these infections are likely to be in the respiratory or urinary tracts [1].

The most important task in the ED for febrile patients without localizing features is not to miss early bacterial meningitis, bacteraemia, such as meningococcaemia and early staphylococcal and streptococcal toxic shock syndromes.

Approach

The management of febrile patients varies according to the severity, duration and tempo of the illness, the type of patient and the epidemiological setting. Although the steps in management of a febrile patient in the ED, listed below, may be set out in a sequential manner, in reality the mental processes involved occur simultaneously by the bedside.

- Step 1: identify the very ill.
- Step 2: find localizing symptoms and signs.
- Step 3: look for 'at-risk' patients.

Step 1: identify the seriously ill patient who requires urgent intervention

The first step in managing febrile patients is to identify those in need of immediate resuscitation, urgent investigations and empirical therapy. The presence of any of the following features justifies immediate intervention: shock, coma/stupor, cyanosis, profound dyspnoea, continuous seizures and severe dehydration.

Step 2: identify those with localized infections or easily diagnosable diseases

Having excluded those who need urgent intervention, the doctor has more time to attempt a diagnosis. The history and physical examination are usually sufficient to localize the source of community-acquired fever in most cases, especially if the illness has been present for several days.

History

A precise history remains the key to diagnosis of a febrile illness. An inability to give a history and to think clearly is a sign of potential sepsis.

Illness

An abrupt onset of fever, particularly when accompanied by chills or rigors and generalized aches, is highly suggestive of an infective illness.

Localizing symptoms, their evolution and relative severity, help to identify the site of infection; localized pain is particularly valuable in this way.

The severity and the course of the illness can be assessed by the patient's ability to work, to be up and about, to eat and sleep and the amount of analgesics taken.

Previous state of health

Underlying diseases predispose patients to infection at certain sites or caused by certain specific organisms. Knowledge of any defects in the immune system is similarly helpful. For example, asplenic patients are more prone to overwhelming pneumococcal septicaemia and renal transplant patients to *Listeria* meningitis.

A past history of infectious diseases, particularly if properly documented, may be useful in excluding infections such as measles and hepatitis.

Predisposing events

Recent operations, accidents and injuries and medications taken may be the direct cause of the illness (e.g. drug fever or rash from co-trimoxazole, ampicillin) or may affect the resistance of the patient, predisposing to certain infections. Concurrent menstruation raises the possibility of toxic shock syndrome.

Epidemiology

Information on occupation, exposure to animals, hobbies, risk factors for blood-borne viruses and travel overseas or to rural areas may suggest certain specific infections, e.g. leptospirosis, acute HIV infection, hepatitis C, malaria, etc.

Contact with similar diseases and known infectious diseases

This information is useful in the diagnosis of problems such as meningococcal infection, viral exanthema, respiratory infection, diarrhoea, and zoonoses.

Examination

Physical examination in the febrile patient serves two purposes: to assess the severity of the illness and to find a site of infection.

Bedside assessment of severity and 'toxicity' based on intuitive judgement is frequently wrong and many patients with severe bacterial infections do not appear obviously ill or toxic.

Physical examination may yield a diagnosis in a febrile patient who has not complained of any localizing symptoms. A checklist of special areas to be examined is useful.

- Eyes: conjunctival haemorrhages are seen in staphylococcal endocarditis and scleral jaundice may be present before cutaneous jaundice is obvious.
- Skin: rashes of any sort, especially petechial rash; cellulitis in the lower legs may present with fever and constitutional symptoms before pain in the leg develops. Evidence of intravenous drug use should be sought at the common injection sites.
- Heart: murmurs and pericardial rubs.
- Lungs: subtle crackles may be heard in pneumonic patients without respiratory symptoms.
- Abdominal organs: tenderness and enlargement without subjective pain may be the only clue to infections in these organs.
- Lymph nodes: especially the posterior cervical glands. Tenderness of the jugulodigastric glands is a good sign of bacterial tonsillitis.
- Sore throat may be absent in the first few hours of streptococcal tonsillitis. Examination of the throat may give the diagnosis. Oedema of the uvula is also a useful sign of bacterial infection in that region.
- Marked muscle tenderness is a frequent sign of sepsis.
- Neck stiffness may be a clue to meningitis in a confused patient who cannot give a history.
- Any area that is covered, e.g. under plasters or bandages, for evidence of sepsis.

There are two caveats when assessing local symptoms and signs:

- localizing features may not be present or obvious early in the course of a focal infection, e.g. the absence of cough in bacterial pneumonia, sore throat in tonsillitis or diarrhoea in gastrointestinal infections in the first 12–36 hours of the illness
- localizing features may occasionally be misleading. For example, diarrhoea, which suggests infection of the gastrointestinal

tract, may be a manifestation of more generalized infection, such as Gram-negative septicaemia, and crepitations at the lung base may indicate a subdiaphragmatic condition rather than a chest infection.

Step 3: look for the 'at-risk' patient

If no diagnosis is forthcoming after the first two steps, the next task is to identify the 'at-risk' patient who may not appear overtly ill but who, nonetheless, requires medical intervention. This applies particularly to those with treatable diseases that can progress rapidly, such as bacterial meningitis, bacteraemia and toxic shock syndromes.

Four sets of pointers are helpful in identifying these 'at-risk' patients: the type of patient (host characteristics), exposure history, the nature of the non-specific symptoms and how rapidly the illness evolves.

Clinical pointers: type of patient

Clinical manifestations of infections are often subtle or non-specific in young children, the elderly and the immunocompromised. The threshold for intervention in these patients should be lowered. The issue of fever in children is not addressed in this chapter.

Elderly patients Elderly patients with infections often do not mount much of a febrile response and fever may be absent in 20–30% of these patients [3].

Infectious diseases in the elderly, as in the very young, often present with non-specific or atypical symptoms and signs and may progress rapidly [4].

In adult patients with unexplained fever, up to one-third may have bacteraemia or focal bacterial infection. This proportion is even higher in those over the age of 50 [1]. In the elderly, a fever >38°C indicates a possible serious infection [5] and is associated with increasing risk of death [6].

The urinary tract is the most frequent site of infection and source of bacteraemia; symptoms of urinary tract infection are frequently absent in the elderly. The respiratory tract is the next most common site of infection; fever and malaise may be the only clues of pneumonia in the elderly. Urinalysis and chest X-ray will identify about half of occult infections [1].

An unexplained fever in a person over the age of 50 should be regarded as being caused by a bacterial infection until proved otherwise and is generally an indication for admission to hospital.

Alcoholic patients Alcoholic patients present with multiple problems, many of which cause fever. Most are caused by infections, the commonest of which is pneumonia. Multiple infections may occur at the same time [7].

Non-infectious causes of fever frequently coexist with infections and conditions such as subarachnoid haemorrhage, alcoholic withdrawal and alcoholic hepatitis and require admission.

The initial history and physical examination in the alcoholic may be unreliable and diagnosis may be difficult.

Alcoholic patients with fever for which no obvious cause is found should be admitted to hospital for investigations and observation.

Injecting drug users The risk of injecting drug users acquiring serious or unusual infections is high through repeated self-injection with non-sterile illicit substances, the use of contaminated needles and syringes and poor attention to skin cleansing prior to injections [8].

Many intravenous drug users presenting with fever have a serious infection. Some have obvious focal infections, such as cellulitis and pneumonia. Others present simply with fever and the presence of bacteraemia and endocarditis must be suspected.

Clinical assessment cannot differentiate trivial from potentially serious conditions in these patients [8]. A history of chills, rigors and sweats strongly suggest the presence of a transient or ongoing bacteraemia. Back pain may be a subtle symptom of endocarditis or vertebral osteomyelitis.

It is difficult to distinguish the patient with endocarditis from other drug users with fever due to another cause. Hospitalization of febrile injecting drug users would be prudent if 24-hour follow up is not possible. Intravenous drug use in the previous 5 days is a predictor of occult major infection and is an indication for admission to hospital [9].

Patients with diabetes mellitus Diabetic patients are more prone to developing certain bacterial infections [1]. A diabetic patient with an unexplained fever is more likely to have an occult bacterial infection than a non-diabetic patient. In general, an insulin-dependent diabetic patient, especially if aged over 50, with

fever and no obvious source of infection, should be investigated and preferably admitted.

Febrile neutropaenic patients Febrile neutropaenic patients (absolute neutrophil count <500/μL or <1000/μL and falling rapidly) must be hospitalized regardless of their clinical appearance. Infections may become fulminant within hours in these patients and the clinical manifestations of their infective illnesses are frequently modified by the underlying disease, therapy received and coexisting problems.

Splenectomized patients Splenectomized patients with fever must be very carefully assessed because of their increased risk of overwhelming bacterial infection. If the fever cannot be readily explained, admission for intravenous antibiotics is usually indicated.

Other immunocompromised patients Fever in transplant patients (renal, hepatic or cardiac) and those with HIV infection is not an absolute indication for admission, but the threshold of intervention should be considerably lowered and they are best assessed by their usual treating doctors.

Patients recently discharged from hospital may have hospital-acquired infections or infections caused by multiresistant organisms. Recent operations or procedures may be a clue to the site of infection.

Clinical pointers: exposure history

Overseas travellers or visitors Returned travellers or overseas visitors may have diseases such as malaria and typhoid fever that need early diagnosis and treatment. Any fever in a traveller returned from a malaria-endemic area should be regarded as due to malaria until proved otherwise.

Influenza in febrile returned travellers is a concern to EDs worldwide. Outbreaks of avian influenza occur periodically in bird populations throughout Asia. Although the virus does not typically infect humans, direct bird-to-human transmission of H5N1 influenza has been documented. The virus is highly pathogenic and the mortality of the disease is high. Travellers acquiring influenza overseas may also introduce this infection. Most cases occur within 2–4 days after exposure, but incubation is as long as 8 days. Suspected influenza infection requires isolation and respiratory precautions. The peak season is generally during the winter months, but can vary, especially in the tropics [10].

Although rare, viral haemorrhagic fever in returned travellers represents a true medical emergency and a serious public health threat. Viral haemorrhagic fevers are caused by several distinct families of virus, including Ebola and Marburg, Lassa fever, the New World arenaviruses (Guanarito, Machupo, Junin, and Sabia) and Rift Valley fever and Crimean Congo haemorrhagic fever viruses. Most exist in Africa, the Middle East or South America. Although some types cause relatively mild illnesses, many can cause severe, life-threatening disease. Viral haemorrhagic fever should be considered in any febrile patient who has returned from an area in which viral haemorrhagic fever was endemic, especially if they have come into contact with blood or other body fluids from a person or animal infected with viral haemorrhagic fever or worked in a laboratory or animal facility handling viral haemorrhagic fever specimens. All these infections have incubation periods of up to 2–3 weeks, so it may be possible to exclude viral haemorrhagic fever on epidemiological grounds alone. Isolation measures should be instituted immediately in these persons [11].

Staff working in emergency departments should be aware of regional outbreaks of unusual pathogens. These are reported by State and National Departments of Health. Returning travellers who are unwell will commonly go directly to an emergency department and this may be a critical point to limit further spread.

Contact with animals A contact history with animals, either at work or at home, is frequently the clue to a zoonosis, particularly if the illness is a perplexing fever of several days' duration. The occurrence of multiple cases at work or at home should also make one suspect these infections early.

Contact with meningococcal and *Haemophilus* meningitis Close contacts of patients with these infections have a high risk of acquiring the same infections. Early symptoms may be subtle and a high index of suspicion must be maintained.

Clinical pointers: non-specific clinical features (Table 9.1.1)
There are several non-specific clinical features whose presence should suggest the possibility

Table 9.1.1 Clinical pointers: non-specific clinical features ('alarm bells')
Severe pain in muscles, neck or back
Impairment of conscious state
Vomiting, especially in association with headache or abdominal pain
Severe headache in the presence of a normal CSF
Unexplained rash
Jaundice
Severe sore throat or dysphagia with a normal looking throat
Repeated rigors

of sepsis. These warrant careful scrutiny even when the patient does not appear toxic. They are by no means specific indicators of serious problems and there will be many false positives. However, ignoring them is frequently the cause of missed or delayed diagnosis of sepsis.

Severe pain in muscles, neck or back Severe muscle pain, even in the absence of overt fever, may be an early symptom of meningococcaemia, staphylococcal or streptococcal bacteraemia. It is also a feature of myositis and necrotizing fasciitis.

Impairment of conscious state A change in conscious state may be the sole presenting manifestation of sepsis, especially in the elderly.

Vomiting Unexplained vomiting, especially in association with headache or abdominal pain, should raise concern. Vomiting without diarrhoea should not be attributed to a gastrointestinal infection. It is a common symptom of CNS infections and occult sepsis.

Severe headache in the presence of a normal CSF This is especially important in a person who seldom gets headaches. Severe headache in a febrile patient with normal CSF should not be diagnosed as a viral infection; many focal infections, e.g. pneumonia and bacterial enteritis, may also present in this manner. CSF may be normal in cerebral abscess and in the prodromal phase of bacterial meningitis.

Unexplained rash An unexplained rash in a febrile patient should be regarded as meningococcaemia until proved otherwise, even in the absence of headache or CSF pleocytosis.

Jaundice Jaundice in the febrile patient is associated with a greatly increased risk of death, admission to ICU and prolonged hospital stay [6]. Jaundice in a febrile patient is unlikely to be due to viral hepatitis, but occurs in serious bacterial infections, such as bacteraemia, cholangitis, pyogenic liver abscess and malaria.

Sore throat or dysphagia Severe sore throat or dysphagia with a normal-looking throat is frequently the presenting symptom of *Haemophilus influenzae* epiglottitis in adults.

Repeated rigors Although repeated rigors may occur in some viral infections, they should generally be regarded as indicators of sepsis, in particular abscesses, bacteraemia, endocarditis, cholangitis and pyelonephritis.

Clinical pointers: evolution of illness (Table 9.1.2)
How rapidly the illness evolves is often an indication of its severity. Previously healthy individuals do not seek medical attention unless they are worried. Notice should be taken of any person seeking help within 24 hours of the onset of illness or a person whose illness appears to have progressed rapidly within 24–48 hours (e.g. from being up and about to being bedridden). Similarly, the patient who presents to the ED on more than one occasion over a 24–48-hour period warrants a careful work-up.

Step 4: a final caveat
A major concern in the management of undifferentiated fever in adults is missing the diagnosis of meningococcal bacteraemia when the patient does not appear ill on presentation.

Table 9.1.2 Clinical pointers: evolution of illness
Those presenting early (<24 hours)
Those presenting with rapidly evolving symptoms
Patients presenting to ED on >1 occasion over a 24–48-hour period

Table 9.1.3 Infections requiring urgent treatment

Disease	Clues
Meningococcaemia	Myalgia, rash. May be none
Falciparum malaria	Travel history, blood film
Bacterial meningitis	Headache, change in conscious state, CSF findings
Post-splenectomy sepsis	Past history, abdominal scar
Toxic shock syndromes	Presence of shock and usually a rash
Infections in the febrile neutropaenic	Past history, blood film
Infective endocarditis	Past history, murmur, petechiae
Necrotizing soft-tissue infections	Pain, tenderness, erythema and swelling in skin/muscle, toxicity
Space-occupying infection of head and neck	Localizing symptoms and signs
Focal intracranial infections	Headache, change in conscious state, neurological signs, CT findings

There are a number of infections that must be treated rapidly to minimize morbidity and mortality (Table 9.1.3). With the exception of meningococcal bacteraemia, there are usually some clues in the history or physical examination.

Meningococcal infection is peculiar in its wide spectrum of severity and variable rate of progression in different individuals. It may be fulminant and cause death within 12 hours or it may assume a chronic form that goes on for weeks.

When the patient presents with fever and a petechial rash, meningococcaemia can easily be suspected if one remembers the golden rule of medicine that 'fever plus a petechial rash is meningococcaemia (or staphylococcal bacteraemia) until proved otherwise'. However, only 40% of meningococcal diseases present with a petechial rash.

It is less well known that the early meningococcaemic rash may be macular, i.e. one that blanches with pressure. This is the basis of another golden rule in infectious disease: early meningococcal rash may resemble a non-specific viral rash.

Rarely, meningococcal disease presents with symptoms and signs of a localized infection other than meningitis, e.g. pneumonia, pericarditis or urethritis. These presentations should not pose any management problems.

The risk of missing the diagnosis increases markedly when the patient with meningococcal disease presents with fever and non-specific symptoms without a rash. Abrupt onset of fever and generalized aches may be due to influenza, but it could be due to meningococcaemia.

It is prudent to single out meningococcal disease and ask oneself: could this patient have meningococcaemia? If in doubt, the safest course is to take cultures, give antibiotics and admit.

Clinical investigations

Most febrile patients seen in the ED justify a fever work-up.

Full blood examination is of limited use. White cell count ($>15 \times 10^9$/L), marked left shift, neutropaenia or thrombocytopaenia are pointers to a possible bacteraemia or occult bacterial infections, but they may also be seen in viral infections [12]. Similarly, non-specific markers of inflammation, such as C-reactive protein and erythrocyte sedimentation rate, have not been shown to be useful in predicting outcomes for febrile patients in the ED [13].

Urinalysis and urine culture should be done in febrile adults over the age of 50 unless the pathology clearly lies in another body system. However, if the history does not suggest urinary sepsis and the dipstick urinalysis is normal, then urine cultures are usually negative [14].

A chest X -ray is usually indicated unless a definite diagnosis has been made, e.g. chicken-pox, tonsillitis.

Blood cultures should be done in anyone suspected of having bacteraemia, endocarditis or meningitis, in compromised patients with a fever, all febrile patients over the age of 50 and, possibly, in anyone with an unexplained high fever. It should be noted that only 5% of blood cultures in this setting will be positive and less than 2% will alter clinical management [15]. In general, a patient considered 'sick enough' to warrant blood cultures should be admitted to hospital or followed up within 24 hours.

Disposition

Patients who have any of the following features are in need of resuscitation, followed by work-up and admission: shock, coma/stupor, cyanosis, profound dyspnoea, continuous seizures and severe dehydration.

With few exceptions, the following groups of febrile adults should be investigated and admitted:

- those over 50 years of age
- patients with diabetes mellitus
- alcoholic patients
- injecting drug users
- immunologically compromised patients
- overseas travellers or visitors
- those with 'alarm bells' as described in Step 3.

In general, there should be close liaison with the admitting unit and the issue of empirical therapy for septic patients should be discussed. For the dangerously ill, e.g. those with septic shock or bacterial meningitis, antibiotics should be commenced almost immediately.

There is an increasing tendency to start antibiotics in the ED as soon as possible to reduce the length of hospital stay. Time to antibiotic therapy is used as a key performance indicator for the ED, e.g. for febrile immunocompromised patients.

Patients who do not require intervention after the basic work-up in the ED are discharged home after a period of observation. Because of the time taken to interview the patient, perform investigations and wait for the results, the patient will usually have been observed for 1–2 hours and progression or lack of progression may be a help in deciding what to do. During observation one must be aware that the apparent improvement of the patient may be the result of pain relief or a fall in temperature due to antipyretics.

Arrangement must be made for the patient to be reviewed by their general practitioner or at the hospital. This is an essential component of the care of a febrile patient seen in an ED.

There is no easy way of detecting occult bacterial sepsis. The infectious process is a dynamic one and the doctor must maintain contact with the patient or family during the 24–72 hours following the initial visit.

Patients with fever >39°C must be seen within 24 hours. Review by a doctor within 6–12 hours may be necessary in those who have had a lumbar puncture and is advisable in those who have had blood cultures taken. A verified phone number should be clearly recorded in the medical history.

All febrile patients discharged from the ED should be encouraged to seek review if there is any adverse change to their condition. A patient re-presenting to the ED has provided an opportunity to ensure that they are being managed appropriately and to rectify any errors.

Fever due to most common viral infections will resolve by about 4 days. Many other infections will be diagnosed when new symptoms or signs appear.

If fever persists beyond 4–5 days without any localizing symptoms or signs, a less common infection or non-infective cause should be suspected and the patient should be thoroughly investigated. In this situation, the threshold of admission to hospital should be low.

The establishment of ED short-stay units allows fast-track treatment and observation, usually for 24–48 hours, for carefully selected febrile patients who are not suitable for immediate discharge home.

Future research directions

- The subject of undifferentiated fever of short duration in the adult has not been well studied. There are few data on the spectrum of diseases producing this clinical problem.

Controversies

- Whether empirical antibiotics should be given to adult patients with undifferentiated fever of short duration in order to minimize the risk of death from unrecognized sepsis or meningitis is a perennial question and there are no algorithms capable of directing management of this problem.
- The safe and ideal course of action is to admit for observation all those patients who are ill enough to warrant a blood culture or a lumbar puncture. The limitation of hospital beds precludes this policy and there will be unnecessary admissions. The introduction of ED short-stay units provides an alternative for selected patients.

References

[1] Mellors JW, Horowitz RI, Harvey MR, et al. A simple index to identify occult bacterial infection in adults with acute unexplained fever. Arch Intern Med 1987;147:666–71.
[2] Gallagher EJ, Brooks F, Gennis P. Identification of serious illness in febrile adults. Am J Emerg Med 1994;12:129–33.
[3] Norman DC, Yoshikawa TT. Fever in the elderly. Infect Dis Clin N Am 1996;10:93–9.
[4] Fontanarosa PB, Kaeberlein FJ, Gerson FW, et al. Difficulty in predicting bacteraemia in elderly emergency patients. Ann Emerg Med 1992;21:842–8.
[5] Marco CA, Schoenfeld CN, Hansen KN, et al. Fever in geriatric emergency patients: clinical features associated with serious illness. Ann Emerg Med 1995;26:18–24.
[6] Tan SL, Knott JC, Street AC, et al. Outcomes of febrile adults presenting to the emergency department. Emerg Med 2002;14:A22.
[7] Wrenn KD, Larson S. The febrile alcoholic in the emergency department. Am J Emerg Med 1991;9:57–60.
[8] Marantz PR, Linzer M, Feiner CJ. Inability to predict diagnosis in febrile intravenous drug abusers. Ann Intern Med 1987;106:823–6.
[9] Samet JH, Shevitz A, Fowle J, et al. Hospitalisation decisions in febrile intravenous drug users. Am J Med 1990;89:53–7.
[10] Beigel JH, Farrar J, Han AM, et al. Avian influenza A (H5N1) infection in humans. N Engl J Med 2005;353:1374–85.
[11] Ufberg JW, Karras DJ. Commentary (viral haemorrhagic fever). Ann Emerg Med 2005;45:324–6.
[12] Wasserman MR, Keller EL. Fever white blood cell count, and culture and sensitivity: their value in the evaluation of the emergency patient. Top Emerg Med 1989;10:81–8.
[13] Van Laar PJ, Cohen J. A prospective study of fever in the accident and emergency department. Clin Microbiol Infect 2003;9:878–80.
[14] Sultana RV, Zalstein S, Cameron PA, et al. Dipstick urinalysis and the accuracy of the clinical diagnosis of urinary tract infection. J Emerg Med 2001;20:13–19.
[15] Kelly A. Clinical impact of blood cultures in the emergency department. J Acad Emerg Med 1998;15:254–6.

Further reading

[1] Talan DA. Infectious disease issues in the emergency department. Clin Infect Dis 1996;23:1–14.

9.2 Meningitis

Andrew Singer

ESSENTIALS

1 Bacterial meningitis can be a rapidly progressive and fatal illness. A high level of suspicion is necessary, as well as rapid diagnosis and treatment.

2 Eighty-five per cent of cases have headache, fever, meningism and mental obtundation, but these are often absent or diminished in very young or old patients, those partially treated with oral antibiotics and those with some form of immunocompromise.

3 Treatment should not be delayed if lumbar puncture cannot be performed within 20 minutes of arrival in the emergency department. Blood cultures should be taken prior to the first dose of antibiotics, if at all possible.

4 The combination of a third-generation cephalosporin and benzylpenicillin will treat most cases of suspected bacterial meningitis and should be given as soon as the diagnosis is suspected (benzyl penicillin is sufficient in the pre-hospital setting).

5 Steroids are potentially of benefit to both adults and children with bacterial meningitis, reducing the incidence of deafness and other neurological complications in *Haemophilus influenzae* and *Streptococcus pneumoniae* infections. They should be given either before or with the first dose of antibiotic.

Introduction

Definition

Meningitis is an inflammation of the leptomeninges, the membranes that line the central nervous system, as well as the cerebrospinal fluid (CSF) in the subarachnoid space. It is usually the result of an infection, but can be due to an inflammatory response to a localized or systemic insult.

Classification

Meningitis is usually classified according to the aetiology or location as bacterial, aseptic (viral, tuberculous, fungal or chemical) or spinal (where the infection specifically affects the spinal meninges).

Aetiology

Bacterial

Bacterial meningitis is a serious cause of morbidity and mortality in all age groups. The causes vary according to age, as shown in Table 9.2.1. *Neisseria meningitidis* serogroups A and C tend to cause endemic cases of meningitis, especially in Aboriginal populations, whereas serogroup B is more commonly associated with epidemics [1]. There has been an increase in the incidence of penicillin-resistant *Streptococcus pneumoniae*, especially in children [2].

Aseptic

Aseptic meningitis may be either due to an immune response to a systemic infection (usually viral) or to a chemical insult.

Viral

Enteroviruses are the most common cause of meningitis, often in clusters of cases. Herpes viruses often cause meningitis as part of a more generalized infection of the brain (meningoencephalitis) or as part of an immune response to a systemic infection. A generalized viraemia may also cause aseptic meningitis, owing to an immune reaction without direct infection.

Fungal

Fungal causes of meningitis, especially that due to *Cryptococcus neoformans*, tend to occur in immunocompromised patients, such as those with HIV/AIDS or those on immunosuppressant medication or cancer chemotherapy. It can occur in immunocompetent individuals as well, particularly the elderly.

Tuberculous

Tuberculous meningitis is rare in industrialized countries, but can occur in all age groups. It

Table 9.2.1	Causes of meningitis	
Viral	*Bacterial*	*Other*
Echovirus 6, 9,11, 30 Coxsackie viruses A9, A16, B1, B5, B6 Enterovirus 71 H Herpes simplex 1 & 2 Cytomegalovirus Varicella zoster Epstein-Barr virus	**Neonates** (<3 months old): Group B streptococcus (*Streptococcus agalactiae*) *Escherichia coli* *Listeria monocytogenes* Coagulase-negative *Staphylococcus aureus* *Pseudomonas aeruginosa* **Children** (<6 years old): *Haemophilus influenzae* type b *Neisseria meningitidis* *Streptococcus pneumoniae* **Adults** *Neisseria meningitidis* (especially in young adults) *Streptococcus pneumoniae* *Listeria monocytogenes* (especially in adults over 50) *Klebsiella pneumoniae* *Staphylococcus aureus* *Escherichia coli* (in the immunocompromised)	*Mycobacterium tuberculosis* *Cryptococcus neoformans* (especially in immunocompromised) Aseptic

tends to follow an insidious course, with a lack of classic signs and symptoms. Diagnosis is often difficult, owing to the low yield from CSF staining and the 4-week time frame required to culture the organism. Suspicion should be high in patients with immunocompromise or chronic illness. It tends to have a high mortality.

Spinal

Spinal meningitis is usually bacterial and due to direct spread from a localized infection in the spine.

Epidemiology

The epidemiology of meningitis is different for groups according to age, as well as immunocompetence:

- Neonates: Table 9.2.1 shows the main causes of bacterial meningitis in neonates. There is an overall incidence of 0.17–0.32 cases per 1000 live births. There is 26% mortality, which is even higher in premature infants [3].
- Children: until the introduction of *Haemophilus influenzae* type b (Hib) immunization in the early 1990s, this organism was the major cause of bacterial meningitis in children under 5 years (until 1990, the incidence of childhood Hib meningitis was 26.3 per 100 000 [152 per 100 000 in Aboriginal children]) [4]. Between 1990 and 1996 there was a 94% reduction in the incidence of Hib disease. *N. meningitidis* and *S. pneumoniae* remain common causes of both meningitis and generalized sepsis [5]. The introduction of immunization programmes for some strains of both of these bacteria will reduce the incidence of meningitis caused by these organisms in the future, although it is important to understand that not all strains are covered by vaccines.
- Adults: *N. meningitidis* and *S. pneumoniae* are common causes in all age groups, with *N. meningitides* predominating in adults under 24 years. *Listeria monocytogenes* is more common in adults over 50 years. The overall incidence in adults is 3.8 per 100 000 population [6]. More unusual organisms occur in patients following neurosurgery or chronic illness, such as alcoholism, hepatic cirrhosis, chronic renal failure and connective tissue disease [7] (GNRs, coagulase-negative *Staphylococcus aureus*,

Mycobacterium tuberculosis, *Klebsiella pneumoniae*).

- Patients with HIV/AIDS: *Cryptococcus neoformans* is relatively common, with an incidence of 5 per million of population or 10% of HIV-infected patients. Tuberculosis, *Listeria*, *Klebsiella* and syphilis are also causes of meningitis in this group, as well as viral causes of meningoencephalitis [8].
- Tuberculous meningitis occurs in around 2% of patients with TB and around 10% of HIV-infected patients with TB. It has a poor prognosis, with 20% mortality.

Pathogenesis

Initially, there is colonization of the infectious agent, commonly in the nasopharynx in the case of the enteroviruses and bacteria, such as meningococcus and Hib. Other infections may spread from already established foci, such as otitis media or sinusitis (e.g. pneumococcus). There is either haematogenous or local spread to the meninges and subarachnoid space, with inflammation of this area and the production of a purulent exudate approximately 2 hours after invasion of the area. The inflammatory response is initiated by bacterial subcapsular components, such as lipoteichoic acid in *S. pneumoniae*, a lipo-oligosaccharide in *H. influenzae* and other Gram-negative endotoxins. These substances stimulate the release of cytokines, such as interleukin-1 and -6, tumour necrosis factor (TNF) and arachidonic acid metabolites, as well as the complement cascade. There is a subsequent increase in neutrophil and platelet activity, with increased permeability of the blood–brain barrier. This response is often worse after the initial destruction of bacteria by antibiotics. If left untreated, fibrosis of the meninges may occur. In viral and aseptic meningitis, there is a more limited inflammatory response, with mild-to-moderate infiltration of lymphocytes. In the more chronic causes, such as fungi or tuberculosis, the exudate is fibrinous, the main cells being a mixture of lymphocytes, monocytes/macrophages and plasma cells. The base of the brain is most commonly affected.

Presentation

History

There are some differences in the history with different causes of meningitis, which may allow an early differential diagnosis to be made.

There are no pathognomonic single symptoms or signs for meningitis, so a high index of suspicion is necessary.

The combination of fever, headache, meningism and mental obtundation is found in approximately 85% of cases of bacterial meningitis [9]. It is also a common pattern in viral or aseptic meningitis, where obtundation is less of a feature. In fungal or tuberculous meningitis, these symptoms are much less common (less than 40% of cases of cryptococcal meningitis). Elderly patients or those who have had recent neurosurgery may present with subtle or mild symptoms and lack a fever [10].

The headache is usually severe and unrelenting. It may be either global or located in a specific area. The main symptoms of meningism are nuchal rigidity (neck stiffness) and photophobia. The nuchal rigidity is something more than merely pain on movement of the neck. It is clinically important when the patient complains of a painful restriction of movement in the sagittal plane (i.e. forwards and backwards only). Up to 35% of cases have associated nausea and vomiting.

As a general rule, the height of the fever is a poor indication of the possible cause, although the fever may often only be mild in tuberculous or fungal meningitis or in bacterial meningitis that has been partially treated by antibiotics. The spectrum of mental obtundation can range from mild confusion, to bizarre behaviour, delirium or coma. The severity of obtundation is a good indication of the severity of the illness.

Focal neurological signs occur in around 10–20% of cases of bacterial meningitis, but are also associated with cerebral mass lesions, such as toxoplasmosis or brain abscess. They are also a feature of tuberculous meningitis. Seizures are relatively uncommon (13–30%), but may occasionally be the only sign of meningitis if the patient has been partially treated with oral antibiotics.

There may also be associated systemic symptoms. Myalgias and arthralgias are often associated with viral causes, but may also be the sole presenting symptom in meningococcal meningitis. HIV/AIDS patients may show stigmata associated with that disease.

The course of the illness may also indicate the cause. Meningococcal or pneumococcal meningitis is often characterized by a rapid, fulminating course, often going from initial symptoms to death over an interval of hours. Viral causes tend to be a slower course over days. Fungal or tuberculous meningitis shows a more chronic course over days to weeks, with milder symptoms.

Risk factors for meningitis include the extremes of age, pre-existing sinusitis or otitis media, recent neurosurgery, CSF shunts, splenectomy, immunological compromise and chronic diseases such as alcoholism, cancer, connective tissue disorders, chronic renal failure and hepatic cirrhosis.

Examination

The physical examination will often reflect symptoms elicited in the history, with fever, physical evidence of meningism, stigmata of AIDS, etc.

As stated above, neck stiffness is only clinically significant when it occurs in the sagittal plane. There will be a restriction of both passive and active movement. Other tests to elicit meningism include Kernig's sign and Brudzinski's sign, although these are only present in 50% of adult cases of bacterial meningitis. Kernig's sign is elicited by attempting to extend the knee of a leg that has been flexed at the hip with the patient lying supine and the other leg flat on the bed. The sign is positive if the knee cannot be fully extended due to spasm in the hamstrings. The test can be falsely positive in patients with shortening of the hamstrings or other problems involving the legs or lumbar spine. In Brudzinski's sign, flexing the head causes the thighs and knees to also flex. It can also be tested in children by the inability to touch the nose with the flexed hips and knees in the sitting position. These are both late signs.

Focal neurological signs should be a cause for concern, as they can indicate a poor prognosis.

Papilloedema is rare and late, as is a bulging fontanelle in infants and should alert one to alternative diagnoses.

A rash, often starting as a macular or petechial rash on the limbs, is seen in sepsis due to *N. meningitidis* and *S. pneumoniae*. A petechial rash is a particularly serious sign and is an indication to start antibiotics immediately. A maculopapular rash is also a feature of viral causes.

Investigations

Lumbar puncture

A CSF sample via a lumbar puncture (LP) is an important source of information for making the diagnosis and determining the likely aetiology and treatment. As the procedure may be time-consuming, treatment should not be delayed if there will be more than a 20-minute delay before the lumbar puncture and there is a reasonable clinical suspicion that a bacterial cause is present. Blood cultures should be taken prior to the administration of antibiotics.

Indications

- Symptoms suggestive of meningitis, especially the combination of fever, headache, neck stiffness and photophobia.
- Any patient with fever and an altered level of consciousness.
- Fever associated with seizures, especially in a neonate, older child or adult.
- Seizures in any patient who has been on oral antibiotics.

Precautions

- Deep coma: a patient with a Glasgow coma score (GCS) of 8 or less should have the lumbar puncture delayed until they are more conscious. A normal brain computed tomography (CT) scan does not exclude the risk of herniation in this group.
- Focal neurological signs: the patient should have CT first, to exclude a space-occupying lesion, which may increase the risk of cerebral herniation following the lumbar puncture.
- Surgery to the lumbar spine.
- Local skin infection around the lumbar spine.

The main features to note during lumbar puncture are the opening pressure and the physical appearance of the CSF. The sample should be sent for Gram staining, culture, sensitivities, polymerase chain reaction (PCR) analysis for bacteria and Herpes simplex virus, a cell count and protein and glucose levels. If fungal meningitis is suspected, an India-ink stain and cryptococcal antigen screen should be requested. If tuberculous meningitis is suspected, multiple 5 mL samples of CSF will be required to increase the likelihood of a positive result. If there has been prior administration of antibiotics, a bacterial antigen screen should also be requested.

Turbid CSF is indicative of a significant number of pus cells and is an indication for immediate administration of antibiotics. The patient should usually rest supine for a few hours after the procedure to prevent a worsening of the headache. This has been known to occur up to 24 hours following the procedure. The evidence for the benefits of enforced rest after lumbar puncture is equivocal.

The pattern of cell counts and glucose and protein levels is shown in Table 9.2.2. This can act as a guide only and the clinician needs to be guided by the complete clinical picture.

A leucocyte count (WCC) of more than 1000/μL with a predominantly neutrophilic pleocytosis is considered positive for bacterial meningitis. Ten per cent of cases, especially early in the course of the illness, may have a

Table 9.2.2 Expected CSF values in meningitis

Parameter	Normal range	Bacterial	Viral	Fungal or TB
Pressure (cm H$_2$0)	5–20	>30	Normal or mildly raised	
Protein (g/L)	0.18–0.45	>1.0–5.0	<1.0	0.1–0.5
Glucose (mmol/L)	2.5–3.5	<2.2	Normal	1.6–2.5
Glucose ratio – CSF/serum	0.6 (0.8 in infants)	<0.4 (allow 2–4 hour equilibration)	0.6	<0.4
White cell count/μL	<3, usually lymphocytes (if the tap is traumatic, allow 1 WBC for every 1000 RBC)	>500 (90% PMN)	<1000, predominantly monocytes (10% are >90% PMN, 30–40% >50% PMN)	100–500
Gram stain	No organisms	60–90% positive	No organisms	

predominance of lymphocytes. As a general rule, bacterial meningitis is characterized by a raised CSF protein and a low CSF glucose level. The ratio of CSF to serum glucose levels is also lowered. The combination of CSF glucose <1.9 mmol/L, CSF to serum glucose ratio <0.23, CSF protein >2.2 g/L and either a total WCC >2000/µL or a neutrophil count of >1180/µL has been shown to have a 99% certainty of diagnosing bacterial meningitis [11]. Aseptic meningitis will often have cell counts near the normal range. This does not exclude infection with less common agents, such as herpes viruses or *L. monocytogenes*.

CT scan

CT scanning of the brain is indicated as a prelude to lumbar puncture in the presence of focal neurological signs, mental obtundation or abnormal posturing. It must be noted though, that a normal CT does not exclude the risk of cerebral herniation in bacterial meningitis [12] and, therefore, those with the above signs should have lumbar puncture delayed until they are conscious and stable.

Microbiology

Apart from microscopy and culture of CSF, there are a number of other methods that may allow the causative organism to be identified.

Skin lesion aspirate

In cases where a petechial rash is present, Gram staining or culture from some of the skin lesions may yield the causative organism. This has a reported sensitivity of 30–70%.

Throat swab

Throat swabs are useful in identifying a bacterial cause spread by nasopharyngeal carriage and should be performed in a case of suspected bacterial meningitis.

Polymerase chain reaction

This potentially allows identification of the causative organism and even the serotype for organisms, such as meningococcus. The test can be performed on CSF or EDTA blood samples and may remain positive for up to 72 hours after the commencement of antibiotics. In CSF, the reported sensitivity is 89% with a specificity of 100% and in blood a sensitivity of 81% with a specificity of 97% [13].

Serology

Tests to detect IgM to specific organisms are available for meningococcus and some viruses.

For meningococcus, the test has a sensitivity and specificity of 97% and 95%, but is only reliable in adults and children over 4 years old and takes 5–7 days after onset of the illness to reach diagnostic levels.

Antigenic studies

Latex agglutination, immunoelectrophoresis or radioimmunoassay techniques can be used to screen for antigens from *S. pneumoniae*, Hib, group B streptococcus (*S. agalactiae*), *Escherichia coli* K1, *N. meningitidis* and *C. neoformans*. The tests can be performed on serum, CSF or urine. Serum or urine samples tend to allow greater sensitivities (around 96–99%) than CSF (82–99%). The test is no more sensitive in untreated cases than either a positive Gram-stain or the presence of CSF pleocytosis [14]. The main purpose of antigenic studies is in allowing rapid identification of the causative organism in cases confirmed by the CSF findings or in cases where partial treatment with antibiotics renders the CSF sterile on culture. In many laboratories, these tests have been superseded by PCR methods.

General investigations

Full blood count (FBC), urea and electrolyte counts (UEC), blood cultures, erythrocyte sedimentation rate (ESR) and a throat swab can assist in building an overall picture.

Blood cultures should be taken prior to parenteral antibiotics, especially in patients where lumbar puncture has been delayed. One study found that blood cultures grew the causative organism in 86% of proven cases of bacterial meningitis and that the combination of blood culture, CSF Gram staining and antigen testing identified the cause in 92% of cases [15].

Differential diagnosis

- Generalized viral infections, with meningism as a component.
- Encephalitis: this is a more generalized viral infection of the brain. Clinically, there may be no difference.
- Brain abscess: this tends to produce focal signs due to local pressure at the site of the abscess.
- Focal cerebral infections, such as those due to *Toxoplasma gondii* in HIV/AIDS patients.
- Subarachnoid haemorrhage: this will often produce identical symptoms of meningism, but generally without any other evidence of infection, such as fever.

- Migraine and other vascular headaches: again, meningism is a similar feature. The patient will often have a known history of the illness.
- Severe pharyngitis with cervical lymphadenopathy causing neck stiffness.

Management

Management depends on the likely causative agents, as well as the severity of the illness.

General

Patients should rest in bed, particularly following a lumbar puncture. A quiet, darkened room will be beneficial to those with headache or photophobia. Simple analgesics may be used to treat the headache, with or without codeine. Opiates may be required in severe headache.

Sedation may be necessary if the patient is very agitated or delirious. Suitable drugs are diazepam 5–10 mg IV or midazolam 2–10 mg IV or IM, with or without the addition of an antipsychotic, such as haloperidol 5–20 mg IV or IM, or chlorpromazine 12.5–50 mg IV or IM.

Seizures should be treated appropriately, initially with a benzodiazepine, then maintenance with phenytoin or phenobarbitone. Meningitis can occasionally be associated with status epilepticus, which should be treated in the standard way.

Patients with raised intracranial pressure may need pressure monitoring and measures to reduce the pressure, such as nursing the patient 30° head up and the administration of hyperosmotic agents, such as mannitol. Hyperventilation is controversial as it may reduce intracerebral pressure at the expense of reduced cerebral perfusion. Obstructive hydrocephalus requires appropriate neurosurgical treatment with CSF shunting.

If septic shock has intervened, it should be treated in the usual way, with IV fluids and inotropes.

Antimicrobials

The choice of antimicrobial agent will be determined by the likely causative organism and is therefore determined primarily by age and immune status. It is important that antibiotic therapy is not delayed by investigations such as lumbar puncture or CT and should be administered as soon as the diagnosis is made. Table 9.2.3 shows the recommended choice of antimicrobial for different situations and

Table 9.2.3   Choice of antimicrobial in meningitis [16]

Organism	First-line drug	Second-line drug	Duration
Pre-hospital	Benzylpenicillin		
Neonates	Ampicillin PLUS cefotaxime PLUS vancomycin		
Organism unknown	Cefotaxime or ceftriaxone PLUS benzylpenicillin		7–10 days
H. influenzae type b	Cefotaxime or ceftriaxone	Ampicillin or chloramphenicol	7–10 days
N. meningitidis	Benzylpenicillin or cefotaxime or ceftriaxone	Ciprofloxacin or chloramphenicol	5–7 days
S. pneumoniae	Benzylpenicillin	Cefotaxime or ceftriaxone or vancomycin	10 days
L. monocytogenes	Benzylpenicillin	Trimethoprim + sulfamethoxazole	3–6 weeks
C. neoformans	Amphotericin PLUS flucytosine	Fluconazole	4–6 weeks
Herpes simplex	Acyclovir		14 days

After eTG complete [internet]. Melbourne: Therapeutic Guidelines Limited; 2013 July with permission.

Table 9.2.4   Antibiotic doses in treating meningitis [17]

Antibiotic	Adult dose	Child dose	Route	Frequency
Cefotaxime	2 g	50 mg/kg	IV	q 6 h
Ceftriaxone	4 g	100 mg/kg	IV	Daily
Benzylpenicillin	2.4 g	60 mg/kg	IV	q 4 h
Ampicillin		50 mg/kg	IV	q 6 h
Trimethoprim + sulphamethoxazole	160 + 800 mg	4 + 20 mg/kg	IV	q 6 h
Chloramphenicol	1 g	25 mg/kg	IV	q 6 h
Acyclovir	10 mg/kg	20 mg/kg in full-term neonates, 10 mg/kg otherwise	IV	q 8 h
Amphotericin B	0.7–1 g/kg	0.7–1 g/kg	IV	Daily
Flucytosine	25 mg/kg	25 mg/kg	IV or PO	q 6 h
Vancomycin	1.5 g	30 mg/kg (if under 12 years old)	IV	q 12 h
Ciprofloxacin	400 mg	10 mg/kg	IV	q 12 h
Moxifloxacin	400 mg	10 mg/kg	IV	q 12 h

After eTG complete [internet]. Melbourne: Therapeutic Guidelines Limited; 2013 July with permission.

organisms. Table 9.2.4 shows the recommended dosage of each. As a general rule, the combination of a third-generation cephalosporin and benzylpenicillin will cover most organisms in all age groups. It is important to note that there is emerging resistance to penicillins in *S. pneumoniae* (currently 7.6% of isolates in Australia). If Gram-positive diplococci are found or *S. pneumoniae* is identified on antigen or PCR testing, vancomycin should be added to the therapy.

Steroids

Steroids have been shown to improve the prognosis of bacterial meningitis in both adults and children. There is a reduction in complications, such as sensorineural deafness and short-term neurological deficits (in high-income countries). The most benefit appears to be derived with infections from *H. influenzae* and *S. pneumoniae*. No clear mortality benefit has been established. Steroids are usually administered as dexamethasone 0.15 mg/kg IV q 6 h (up to 10 mg), started before or with the first dose of antibiotics and continued for 4 days. The main adverse effect is gastrointestinal bleeding, which may be reduced by limiting treatment to 2 days [17].

Disposition

All cases of bacterial meningitis require admission for IV antibiotics, as well as supportive therapy. They often require intensive therapy, especially if septic shock has supervened. Viral meningitis will usually require supportive therapy only, but this may require admission. Mild cases of viral or aseptic meningitis, with a clear diagnosis, can be safely sent home.

Prognosis

Over the last 20 years, the mortality of bacterial meningitis has ranged from 6 to 20% and is higher in the very young or the very old. Meningitis in immunocompromised individuals carries a high mortality of up to 50%. Bacterial meningitis in children can lead to a number of long-term sequelae, such as sensorineural hearing loss, learning difficulties, motor problems, speech delay, hyperactivity, blindness, obstructive hydrocephalus and recurrent seizures. These sequelae are less common in adults.

Prevention

Prophylaxis should be offered in cases of *H. influenzae* type b, or *Meningococcus* infection to:

- the index case
- all household or childcare contacts who have either stayed overnight in the same house or have been in the same room as the index case for any period of 4 hours or more in the preceding 7 days (in Hib, if less than 24 months old or less than 4 years and incompletely immunized against Hib)
- passengers adjacent to the index case on a trip of 8 hours' or longer duration

- any person who has potentially shared saliva (such as eating utensils or drink bottles) with the index case
- healthcare workers who have given mouth-to-mouth resuscitation to an index case
- Appropriate regimens are:
  - for meningococcus:
    - ciprofloxacin 500 mg orally as a single dose – preferred for females on oral contraceptives
    - ceftriaxone 250 mg (125 mg in children <12 years IM in 1% lignocaine – preferred in pregnant women
    - rifampicin 600 mg orally 12-hourly for 2 days (5 mg/kg in neonates <1 month, 10 mg/kg in children).
  - for Hib:
    - rifampicin 600 mg orally daily for 4 days (10 mg/kg in neonates <1 month, 20 mg/kg in children)
    - ceftriaxone 1 g IM daily for 2 days (50 mg/kg in children)
    - if the index case is <24 months old, Hib vaccination should be given as a full course as soon as possible after recovery. Unvaccinated contacts under 5 years of age should be immunized as soon as possible.

Casual, neighbourhood or hospital contacts are not required to receive prophylaxis.

Meningococcal vaccine should be considered in populations where cases are clustered. The vaccine is currently only available for serogroup C.

Controversies

- Whether all patients should have a CT scan before lumbar puncture. In general, it is safe without CT in those with a clear history consistent with meningitis and normal sensorium. Comatose patients should have lumbar puncture delayed until they are conscious.
- The use of steroids. Steroids have been shown to improve hearing and short-term neurological outcome in adults and children in high-income countries, but are known to cause adverse outcomes in patients with generalized sepsis.

References

[1] Munro R, Kociuba K, Jelfs J, et al. Meningococcal disease in urban south western Sydney, 1990–1994. Aust NZ J Med 1996;26:526–32.
[2] Collignon PJ, Bell JM. Drug-resistant *Streptococcus pneumoniae*: the beginning of the end for many antibiotics? Australian Group on Antimicrobial Resistance. Med J Aust 1996;164:64–7.
[3] Francis BM, Gilbert GL. Survey of neonatal meningitis in Australia: 1987–1989. Med J Aust 1992;156:240–3.
[4] Bower C, Payne J, Condon R, et al. Sequelae of *Haemophilus influenzae* type b meningitis in Aboriginal and non-Aboriginal children under 5 years of age. J Paediatr Child Hlth 1994;30:393–7.
[5] Herceg A. The decline of *Haemophilus influenzae* type b disease in Australia. Commun Dis Intell 1997;21:173–6.
[6] Sigurdardottir B, Bjornsson OM, Jonsdottir KE. Acute bacterial meningitis in adults. A 20-year overview. Arch Intern Med 1997;157:425–30.
[7] Segreti J, Harris AA. Acute bacterial meningitis. Infect Dis Clin N Am 1996;10:797–809.
[8] Jones PD, Beaman MH, Brew BJ. Managing HIV. Part 5: Treating secondary outcomes. 5.5 HIV and opportunistic neurological infections. Med J Aust 1996;164:418–21.
[9] Tunkel AR, Scheld WM. Acute bacterial meningitis. Lancet 1995;346:1675–80.
[10] Miller LG, Choi C. Meningitis in older patients: how to diagnose and treat a deadly infection. Geriatrics 1997;52:43–4.
[11] Spanos A, Harrell Jr FE, Durack DT. Differential diagnosis of acute meningitis: an analysis of the predictive value of initial observation. J Am Med Assoc 1989;262:2700–7.
[12] Rennick G, Shann F, de Campo J. Cerebral herniation during bacterial meningitis in children. Br Med Jo 1993;306:953–5.
[13] Communicable Diseases Network Australia, Australian Government Department of Health and Ageing. Guidelines for the early clinical and public health management of Meningococcal Disease in Australia. The 2007 revision of the document is available at: <http://www.health.gov.au/internet/main/publishing.nsf/Content/cda-pubs-other-mening-2007.htm>.
[14] Feuerborn SA, Capps WI, Jones JC. Use of latex agglutination testing in diagnosing pediatric meningitis. J Fam Pract 1992;34:176–9.
[15] Coant PN, Kornberg AE, Duffy LC, et al. Blood culture results as determinants in the organism identification of bacterial meningitis. Pediatr Emerg Care 1992;8:200–5.
[16] Therapeutic Guidelines Limited. Therapeutic Guidelines, Antibiotic, version 14, 2010.
[17] Brouwer MC, McIntyre P, de Gans J, et al. Corticosteroids for acute bacterial meningitis. Cochrane Database Syst Rev 2010;9:CD004405.

INFECTIOUS DISEASE EMERGENCIES

9

9.3 Septic arthritis

Trevor Jackson • Varadarajulu Suresh

ESSENTIALS

1 Delayed or inadequate treatment can lead to irreversible joint damage.

2 Diagnosis is based on clinical features and synovial fluid examination; imaging techniques have a role in difficult cases.

3 *Staphylococcus aureus* and *Neisseria gonorrhoeae* are the most frequent pathogens.

4 Successful treatment hinges on rapid and complete joint drainage and high-dose parenteral antibiotics guided by culture results.

5 Outcomes are good in paediatric and gonococcal subgroups, but the presence of chronic arthritis or polyarticular involvement is associated with up to 15% mortality and 50% chronic joint morbidity.

Introduction

Septic arthritis is defined as bacterial infection of the synovial space. The knee is the most commonly affected joint in adults and the hip joint in the paediatric age group [1].

Aetiology, pathogenesis and pathology

Septic arthritis can be caused by haematological spread or direct invasion. Bacteria are the usual pathogens by haematogenous seeding of the joint. Direct spread from adjacent infection or via trauma are less common. Once inside the joint, bacterial growth and invasion can occur uninhibited. Phagocytic and neutrophil responses to the bacteria lead to proteolytic enzyme release and cytokine production, resulting in synovial abscess formation and cartilage necrosis [2]. Co-morbidity or deficient host defences are risk factors for infection [3] and can be associated with more rapid and severe disease (Table 9.3.1).

The majority of cases are community acquired and occur in children and young adults [4]. Prosthetic joint surgery and invasive management of chronic arthritis are factors in the increased prevalence observed in older age groups.

Epidemiology

The incidence of proven and probable septic arthritis in Western Europe is 4–10 per

Table 9.3.1 Risk factors for septic arthritis

Risk factors	Examples
Direct penetration	Trauma Medical (surgery, arthrocentesis), IV drug use
Joint disease	Chronic arthritis
Host immune deficit	Glucocorticoid or immunosuppressive therapy HIV infection Chronic illness Cancer

100 000 patients per year. This is more in lower socioeconomic groups in both Northern Europe and Australia.

The prevalence is 29 cases per 100 000 of the Aborigine population with a relative risk of 6.6 compared with the white Northern Territory Australian population.

The incidence of septic arthritis is increasing and is linked to an increase in orthopaedic-related infection, an ageing population, more invasive procedures being under taken and an enhanced use of immunosuppressive treatment [5].

Clinical features

History

This will usually reveal the recent onset of a painful, hot and swollen joint, most commonly the hip or knee, although any joint may be affected. Systemic features of fever or rigors should be sought, plus the presence of any risk factors.

Examination

Typical findings include a hot, tender joint with marked limitation of passive or active movement owing to pain. An effusion will be evident in most cases. A polyarticular presentation is more common in gonococcal infection or in the setting of chronic arthritis. In general, fever is low grade and few patients will appear 'toxic' and unwell. The elderly and immunosuppressed may present non-specifically with anorexia, vomiting, lethargy or fever.

Differential diagnosis

Non-septic arthritis or synovitis may be differentiated on clinical features and joint fluid analysis. Fractures will generally be evident on joint radiographs, but detection of osteomyelitis may require more advanced imaging techniques, such as nuclear or computed tomography (CT) scanning. Rheumatic fever and brucellosis are rare causes.

Clinical investigations

Synovial fluid examination and culture

Aspiration should be performed promptly with local anaesthetic and a large-bore needle for cell count, crystals, Gram stain and culture to confirm the diagnosis. Typical findings in septic arthritis and its differential diagnoses are shown in Table 9.3.2 [6].

Most infections are acute and bacterial (Table 9.3.3) [6], although fungal and mycobacterial pathogens have been recognized in chronic infections.

Other laboratory investigations

Blood cultures should always be taken and may be positive in up to 50%. Inflammatory markers (erythrocyte sedimentation rate and C-reactive protein) are elevated, with typically a

Table 9.3.2   Synovial fluid characteristics

Characteristic	Septic arthritis	Non-septic arthritis	Non-inflammatory effusion
Colour	Yellow/green	Yellow	Colourless
Turbidity	Purulent, turbid	Turbid	Clear
Leucocytes/μL	10–100 000	5–10 000	<1000
Predominant cell	PMN*	PMN*	Monocyte

*PMN: polymorphonuclear leucocyte.

Table 9.3.3   Bacterial causes of septic arthritis

Age group	Typical bacteria
Children	Staphylococcus aureus Group A streptococci (B in neonates) Haemophilus influenza
Young adults	Neisseria gonorrhoeae Staphylococcus aureus
Older adults	Staphylococcus aureus Gram-negative species* Group A streptococci

*Pseudomonas spp. and Enterobacteriaceae

neutrophil-predominant leucocytosis. These are non-diagnostic, but aid in monitoring response to therapy.

Imaging studies

Plain radiographs should be performed in all cases: they may reveal effusions or local oedema and help to exclude alternative conditions. Ultrasound is very sensitive in detecting effusions and excellent for facilitating needle aspiration.

Fluoroscopy may also be used. Nuclear medical studies are very sensitive early, but not specific for sepsis. CT and magnetic resonance imaging (MRI) have a small role in difficult joints (e.g. hip and sacroiliac).

Criteria for diagnosis [7]

This depends on positive culture of synovial fluid from an affected joint, a positive Gram stain or blood culture in the context of an inflamed joint suspicious of sepsis, macroscopic pus aspirate and appropriate response to antibiotics.

Management

Joint drainage and empiric parenteral antibiotic therapy must take place without delay. Surgical drainage is usually employed in children, with needle drainage more commonly first line in adults. Newer arthroscopic techniques are increasingly being used [2,8–10]. Repeated drainage procedures will often be necessary to ensure complete resolution of the infection.

Antibiotic therapy is initiated after culture specimens have been obtained, with clinical presentation and Gram stain guiding the choice of agents. All regimens must include an antistaphylococcal agent with Gram-negative cover as indicated by the clinical setting.

Suggested initial empiric regimen [11]

Di(flu)cloxacillin: 2 g (25–50 mg/kg up to 2 g) intravenously, 6-hourly. If Gram-negative bacteria are suspected, add ceftriaxone 2 g (25–50 mg/kg up to 2 g) intravenously daily. If methicillin resistance is suspected, add vancomycin 1 g (25 mg/kg) intravenously 12-hourly.

Definitive therapy will be tailored to later laboratory identification of the organism and its sensitivities.

The duration and route of therapy remain controversial but, in uncomplicated acute cases, parenteral antibiotics will be required for at least 3 days in children and 2 weeks in adults, with a total treatment duration of 3–6 weeks [10,12]. Specific organisms, such as Neisseria spp., will respond more rapidly, whereas chronic infections and co-morbidity will necessitate aggressive and more prolonged therapy.

General care, with initial joint rest, appropriate analgesia and physical therapy, is important. All patients require admission until their joint sepsis is controlled. Thereafter, ongoing therapy may be monitored as an outpatient or via domiciliary hospital services.

Prognosis

This depends upon the organism, patient co-morbidity and the adequacy and rapidity of treatment. Gonococcal and paediatric infections have a generally good response, with low rates of ensuing joint morbidity. Polyarticular sepsis in rheumatoid arthritis has been associated with mortality rates of up to 15% and major morbidity in up to 50% of survivors [2,6,12].

Prevention

Safe sexual practice can reduce gonorrhoeal infections. Strict aseptic technique, good patient selection and prophylactic antibiotics help prevent cases associated with invasive joint procedures. The overall incidence of infection after arthroplasty ranges from 0.5 to 2% [2].

Table 9.3.4   Likely developments in future [14]

Synovial markers to distinguish septic arthritis from other sources of non-traumatic joint pain may become available to the emergency physician

- Synovial fluid lactate assay
- Synovial probe based PCR technique to identify the bacterial pathogen

After Carpenter CR, Schuur JD, Everett WW, Pines JM. Evidence-based diagnostics: adult septic arthritis. Acad Emerg Med 2011;18:781–96.

Controversies

- The total duration of therapy has gradually been reduced, but optimum duration is unclear, as is the balance between parenteral and oral routes [13].
- Consensus has not been reached on the best method of joint drainage. Surgical arthrotomy is usually employed for the hip and in children, but arthroscopic techniques are also available. Most centres still use repeated needle aspiration as first line for most joints.
- Difficulties still exist with the differentiation of septic arthritis from new-onset non-septic arthritis, especially when polyarticular joint fluid analysis and medical imaging are used, but nuclear and CT scanning techniques may have difficulty in distinguishing infective from non-infective inflammation.

References

[1] Visser S, Tupper J. Septic until proven otherwise. Can Fam Phys 55.

[2] Goldenberg DL. Bacterial arthritis. In: Kelley WN, Harris ED, Ruddy S, Sledge CB, editors. Textbook of rheumatology (4th ed.). Philadelphia: WB Saunders, 1993, p. 1449–66.

[3] Goldenberg DL. Septic arthritis. Lancet 1998;351: 197–202.

[4] Sonnen GM, Henry N. Paediatric bone and joint infections. Paediatr Clin N Am 1996;4:933–47.

[5] Matthews CJ, Weston VC, Jones A, et al. Bacterial septic arthritis in adults. Lancet 2010;375: 846–55.

[6] Brooks GF, Pons VG. Septic arthritis. In: Hoeprich PD, Jordan MC, Ronald AR, editors. Infectious diseases (5th ed.). Philadelphia: JB Lippincott, 1994, p. 1382–9.

[7] Ma L, Cranney A, Holroyd-Leduc JM. Acute monoarthritis: what is the cause of my patient's painful swollen joint? Can Med Assoc J 2009;180:1.

[8] Stanitski CL, Harwell JC, Fu FH. Arthroscopy in acute septic knees. Clin Orthop 1989;241:209.

[9] Broy SB, Schmid FR. A comparison of medical drainage (needle aspiration) and surgical drainage (arthrotomy or arthroscopy) in the initial treatment of infected joints. Clin Rheumatol Dis 1986;12:501–22.

[10] Manadan AM, Block JA. Daily needle aspiration versus surgical lavage for the treatment of bacterial septic arthritis in adults. Am J Ther 2004;11:412–5.

[11] Skin, muscle and bone infections. In: Therapeutic guidelines. Antibiotic, 13th ed. <http://www.tg.com.au.qelibresources. health.wa.gov.au/index.php>.

[12] Youssef PP, York JR. Septic arthritis: a second decade of experience. Aust NZ J Med 1994;24:307–11.

[13] Syrogiannopoulos GA, Nelson JD. Duration of antimicrobial therapy for acute suppurative osteoarticular infections. Lancet 1988;1:37–40.

[14] Carpenter CR, Schuur JD, Everett WW, Pines JM. Evidence-based diagnostics: adult septic arthritis. Acad Emerg Med 2011;18:781–96.

9.4 Urinary tract infections

Salomon Zalstein

ESSENTIALS

1 Urinary tract infection (UTI) is the most common bacterial infection.

2 By age 32, 50% of women will report at least one UTI.

3 Sexual activity is the most important risk factor in young women.

4 Most UTIs are caused by *Escherichia coli*, but *Staphylococcus saprophyticus* is responsible for up to 15% of infections in young, sexually active women.

5 There is a genetic predisposition in some women to recurrent UTI.

6 There are specific bacterial virulence factors determining uropathogenic strains of bacteria.

7 Bacteriological diagnosis is based on isolation of 10^5 cfu/mL of urine. Up to half of women presenting with dysuria and frequency will have fewer than this number of bacteria and about half of these do have bacterial UTI.

8 For the majority of outpatients with typical symptoms urine culture is not necessary.

9 In hospitalized patients, urinary catheterization produces infection in 10% of patients per day.

10 In institutionalized elderly patients, non-specific symptoms or decline in function correlate poorly with UTI despite the presence of pyuria and bacteriuria. Non-UTI causes must be sought.

11 Asymptomatic bacteriuria should not be sought or treated except in pregnant women and in patients about to undergo significant urological procedures.

conditions, including asymptomatic bacteriuria, urethritis, cystitis, female urethral syndrome and acute and chronic pyelonephritis. The most common clinical presentations are cystitis and acute pyelonephritis, although the clinical distinction between these diagnoses may not be as straightforward as the terms imply, with up to 50% of patients having unrecognized pyelonephritis [3].

UTI is considered in two main groups: simple (or uncomplicated) and complicated. Simple UTIs occur in an otherwise healthy person with a normal urinary tract, most commonly a young non-pregnant female. A complicated UTI is one associated with anatomical abnormality, urinary obstruction or incomplete bladder emptying due to any cause: instrumentation or catheterization, pregnancy or significant underlying disease, such as immunosuppression or diabetes mellitus.

Significant bacteriuria

Significant bacteriuria most commonly refers to more than 10^5 bacteria/mL of urine, reported as colony forming units per mL (cfu/mL). This usually represents infection as opposed to contamination (see Quantitative culture), although there are significant exceptions to this generalization (see Urethral syndrome).

Asymptomatic bacteriuria

Asymptomatic bacteriuria (ASB) refers to significant bacteriuria in the absence of symptoms of infection.

Introduction

Urinary tract infections are the most common bacterial infections and the major cause of Gram-negative sepsis in hospitalized patients [1,2].

Definitions

Urinary tract infection

The term urinary tract infection (UTI) is non-specific and may refer to a variety of clinical

Epidemiology

UTIs are very common, particularly in women in whom age, degree of sexual activity and the form of contraception used are all factors that affect the incidence and prevalence of infection. While the overall rate of infection is difficult to estimate since UTI is not a reportable disease, in a USA health survey, the self-reported incidence of UTI is 12.1% among women and 3% among men. By age 32, 50% of women will report at least one UTI [4]. In non-pregnant women aged 18–40 years, the rate of infection has been stated to be between 0.5 and 0.7 per person per year, with much higher rates in pregnancy [5].

In males, the prevalence of bacteriuria beyond infancy is 0.1% or less. Between the ages of 21 and 50, infection rates may be as low as 0.6–0.8/1000 [6]. With increasing prostatic disease, the frequency of bacteriuria may rise to 3.5% in healthy men and to more than 15% in hospitalized men by age 70 [7]. Homosexual men are at increased risk of UTI.

In the presence of chronic disease and institutionalization in the elderly, the incidence of bacteriuria may be as high as 50%, although this is most commonly asymptomatic [8].

Aetiology

The aetiology of uncomplicated UTI has remained unchanged for decades, although increased antibiotic resistance in the bacteria responsible has been well documented. In community-acquired UTI, *Escherichia coli* accounts for 75–90% of cases, *Staphylococcus saprophyticus* accounts for 5–15% (especially in young, sexually active women), with enterococci and Gram-negative organisms, such as *Klebsiella* spp. and *Proteus mirabilis*, responsible for 5–10% [9,10]. Which bacteria are isolated is influenced by factors such as whether the infection is initial or recurrent; the presence of obstruction, instrumentation or anatomical abnormalities; and whether the patient is an inpatient or outpatient. In simple acute cystitis, the most common presentation of UTI, a single organism is usually isolated. On the other hand, in complicated UTI, *E. coli* is isolated in 20–50% of cases and non-*E. coli* organisms, such as *Proteus* and *Klebsiella* species, are more commonly seen. In the presence of structural abnormalities, it is more common to isolate multiple organisms and antibiotic resistance is frequently found [10].

Pathogenesis

In healthy individuals, the perineum, vagina, vaginal introitus and urethra and periurethral areas each have their respective flora and are normally colonized by bacteria different from those commonly associated with UTI, that is by non-pathogens. The periurethral area may become colonized by such UTI-causing (uropathogenic) bacteria, which then ascend via the urethra into the bladder and thence may ascend further to the kidney, causing pyelonephritis. The reservoir for these bacteria is the gastrointestinal tract [4]. There are host and bacterial mechanisms involved in determining whether a UTI will occur.

Host mechanisms

Anatomic considerations (men) and prostatic secretions
In males, the length of the urethra, its separation from the anus and the presence of prostatic secretions all contribute to the prevention of colonization and subsequent UTI.

Sexual activity, contraceptive practices, use of diaphragm/spermicides
Sexual activity is the most important risk factor for acute cystitis, with recent or frequent sexual activity increasing that risk. The use of a diaphragm with a spermicide (an inhibitor of normal vaginal flora) promotes vaginal colonization with uropathogenic bacteria and has also been shown to increase the risk of UTI [4].

Secretor/non-secretor status
Blood group antigens are secreted in the body fluids by some women. The urethral and periurethral mucosae in women who do not secrete these antigens (non-secretors) in their body fluids, have a higher affinity for bacterial adhesins (see below) than the mucosae of women who do. These non-secretors are more susceptible to recurrent infections [11].

Entry of bacteria into the bladder
Instrumentation of the bladder (see below) is a well-recognized mechanism by which bacteria are introduced into the bladder. Other factors have been considered but have not been conclusively demonstrated. These include frequency and timing of voiding, hormonal changes and personal hygiene habits [12].

Bladder defence mechanisms
The healthy bladder can normally clear itself of bacteria. There are three factors involved: voiding; urinary bacteriostatic substances, such as organic acids, high urea concentrations and immunoglobulins; and active resistance by the bladder mucosa to bacterial adherence.

Obstruction
This may be extrarenal (congenital anomalies, such as urethral valves, calculi, benign prostatic hypertrophy) or intrarenal (nephrocalcinosis, polycystic kidney disease, analgesic nephropathy). Complete obstruction of the urinary tract predisposes to infection by haematogenous spread. In the absence of such obstruction, haematogenous seeding of bacteria to the kidneys accounts for about 3% of infections. Partial obstruction does not have this effect.

Vesicoureteric reflux
Incompetence of the vesicoureteric valve is a congenital problem that is five times more common in boys than in girls, but tends not to be a significant factor in adults. It allows infected urine to ascend to the kidney and is the most common factor predisposing to chronic pyelonephritic scarring.

Instrumentation
Although any instrumentation of the urinary tract predisposes to infection, catheterization is the most common of these. A single catheterization will result in UTI in 1% of ambulatory patients but, in hospitalized patients, 10% of women and 5% of men will develop a UTI after one catheterization. Once in place, catheters produce infection in up to 10% of patients per day and nearly all catheterized patients will be bacteriuric by 1 month [13]. All chronically catheterized patients are bacteriuric.

Pregnancy
Changes to the urinary tract occur normally during pregnancy as a result of both anatomical alterations and hormonal effects: dilatation of the ureters and renal pelves, decreased peristalsis in the ureters and decreased bladder tone. These changes begin before the end of the second month. The prevalence of bacteriuria rises with age and parity. A large proportion of asymptomatic bacteriuric women develop symptomatic pyelonephritis later in that pregnancy, with significant increases in toxaemia and prematurity (see Asymptomatic bacteriuria).

Diabetes mellitus
The relationship between diabetes mellitus on the one hand and asymptomatic bacteriuria

and UTI on the other has been debated in the past. Current evidence indicates that asymptomatic bacteriuria is more common in diabetic women than non-diabetic women. The evidence in men is less clear cut. Good evidence from prospective studies for increased incidence of symptomatic urinary tract infection in diabetics is lacking. What appears clear is that diabetes is a significant and independent risk factor for pyelonephritis, complicated UTI, urosepsis, hospitalization and other, often rare, complications (such as emphasematous pyelonephritis, papillary necrosis and candidal infections). The precise pathogenetic mechanism is unclear but involves many factors not necessarily related to glycaemic control [14–16].

Ageing
UTI is the most frequent bacterial infection in residents of long-term care facilities. Asymptomatic bacteriuria is highly prevalent in residents of long-term care facilities with up to 30% of men and 50% of women showing such bacteriuria. The likelihood of bacteriuria correlates with the degree of functional impairment. Several factors may be involved: chronic degenerative neurological diseases may impair bladder function as well as bladder and bowel continence, prostatic enlargement in men and oestrogen deficiency in women can both lead to incomplete bladder emptying, the use of devices, such as indwelling catheters or condom drainage, predisposes to bacteriuria [8].

Bacterial factors
A number of studies [17–19] have shown that the strains of *E. coli* (and a number of other Gram-negative bacteria) that cause UTI are not just the most prevalent in the bowel of the patient at the time of the infection, but have specific characteristics, termed virulence factors, that give them certain capabilities: increased intestinal carriage, persistence in the vagina and the ability to ascend and invade the normal urinary tract. Thus, there are clearly uropathogenic strains of these bacteria. In cases of complicated UTI (e.g. those associated with reflux, obstruction or foreign body), these virulence factors are not significantly involved.

Presentation
History
A careful history should be taken in any patient presenting with symptoms of apparent UTI,

looking for risk factors for complicated or recurrent infection (such as previous UTIs and their treatment, the presence of known anatomical abnormalities and investigations or instrumentation, the possibility of pregnancy and history of diabetes mellitus), as well as seeking to identify those patients with urethritis and vaginitis. In men, the most common cause of recurrent lower tract UTI is prostatitis, so evidence of prostatitis, such as chills, dysuria and prostatic tenderness, should be sought.

Lower tract infections (cystitis) typically present with irritative micturition symptoms, such as dysuria and frequency, suprapubic discomfort and, sometimes, macroscopic haematuria. There is usually no fever. Women presenting with dysuria and frequency without vaginal discharge or irritation have a 90% probability of cystitis [20]. The classic symptom complex of loin pain, fever (>38°C), chills and urinary symptoms is usually associated with pyelonephritis. Severe pain should raise the suspicion of a ureteric calculus that, combined with infection, poses a greater risk of sepsis and of permanent injury to the kidney.

Patients with chronic indwelling catheters usually have no lower tract symptoms at all, but may develop loin pain and fever.

In elderly patients, particularly in long-term care facilities, the long-held view that symptoms of increased confusion and reduced mobility in the absence of fever, are due to urinary tract infection has been cast into doubt (see Treatment of specific groups: elderly patients) [8].

Examination
The clinical signs of lower UTI are few and non-specific, however, patients should be examined to exclude other causes for their symptoms, particularly vaginitis in women and prostatitis in men. The presence of renal angle tenderness, associated with fever, chills and dysuria suggests pyelonephritis.

Investigations
The key step in the diagnosis of UTI is examination of the urine, most commonly a midstream specimen (MSU). Catheterization is appropriate in patients with altered mental state or who cannot void because of neurological or urological reasons. Suprapubic aspiration is commonly used in paediatric practice but can be used in adults if other techniques have failed or are unable to be used.

The next step is to look for the presence of pyuria and, subsequently, the specimen may be sent for quantitative culture and antibiotic sensitivity testing. Testing for haematuria, proteinuria and nitrites may be of supportive value but is not diagnostic.

Reagent test strips
In considering the use of reagent strips in the diagnosis of UTI, it should be noted that variations in published sensitivity and specificity exist and are due to: (1) the use of different brands of reagent strips; (2) the use of different 'gold standards' against which comparison is made (e.g. counting chamber or cells/HPF counts, 'cut-off' criterion of the test used); (3) the nature of the study (blinded, unblinded); (4) the reader of the test (lab worker, doctor, nurse); and most importantly, (5) the clinical setting or target population (e.g. symptomatic emergency department patients rather than an asymptomatic population in a clinic or office environment) – in other words, the pre-test probability.

A reagent strip test for leucocyte esterase is now the most common screening test for pyuria (see below). Taken alone, this has a sensitivity of 48–86% and a specificity of 17–93% for detecting pyuria (as defined below). A positive predictive value (in symptomatic individuals) of 50% and a negative predictive value of 92% makes it a valuable test for screening the emergency department population. Most studies indicate that when the combination of leucocyte esterase and nitrite is considered, the sensitivity of the test is 68–88% and a negative test excludes the presence of infection [21]. Recent work by Sultana and others has shown that reagent strips significantly improve the clinician's accuracy in diagnosing UTI in symptomatic emergency department patients [22]. The clinical probability of UTI must be considered when using such screening tests. In the patient with typical urinary tract symptoms, it may provide an adequate screen. It should, however, be used with great caution in the presence of fever of unknown cause in the elderly, the patient with an indwelling catheter or the patient with an impaired mental state, as pyuria and the implied bacteriuria may not be the cause of the problem.

Pyuria
Pyuria, indicates inflammation in the urinary tract and, as an indicator of infection, is second

only to bacteriuria determined by quantitative culture (see below). The 'gold standard' definition of pyuria is based on early work involving the measurement of the rate of excretion of polymorphs in the urine. This work showed that excretion of 400 000 polymorphs per hour was always associated with infection and was also found to be represented by 10 polymorphs per mm^3 in a single (unspun) midstream specimen of urine [23]. Thus, 'significant pyuria' was defined as 10 000 polymorphs per mL of urine. It was subsequently shown that more than 96% of symptomatic patients, defined as having significant bacteriuria, had significant pyuria and conversely less than 1% of asymptomatic people without bacteriuria have this degree of pyuria. Other definitions of pyuria, such as >5 leucocytes/high power field are based on examination of either the urinary sediment or of centrifuged urine and are inherently inaccurate because they cannot be standardized, but are nevertheless often used [24]. 'Sterile' pyuria indicates the presence of significant pyuria without the presence of bacterial growth in standard culture (Table 9.4.1).

Nitrites

This reagent strip-based test is dependent on the bacterial reduction of urinary nitrate to nitrite, a function of coliform bacteria but not of *Enterococcus* spp. nor *S. saprophyticus*. The test has a low sensitivity (45–60%), better specificity (85–98%) but a high false-negative rate (about 45% in many studies). False-negative results are likely if the infecting organism is Gram positive or *Pseudomonas*, if the diet lacks nitrate or if there is diuresis or extreme frequency, as a period of bladder incubation is necessary to form nitrites.

Haematuria

Although a frequent accompaniment of UTI, this finding is non-specific as there are many other causes of haematuria.

Table 9.4.1   Common causes of sterile pyuria
Non-specific urethritis in males
Prostatitis
Renal tract neoplasm
Renal calculi
Catheterization
Renal TB
Previous antibiotic treatment

Proteinuria

Most commonly with UTI protein excretion is less than 2 g/24 h. It is another common but non-specific finding.

Quantitative culture

Urine culture is not essential in the management of the pre-menopausal sexually active female with an uncomplicated UTI as the probability of UTI in these patients is 90% [20]. Culture should always be performed in patients with recurrent infection, possible pyelonephritis, potentially complicated UTI, males, the elderly or in cases where the cause of infection is not clinically evident. In symptomatic patients, a single specimen with a bacterial count in urine of $>10^5$ colony forming units (cfu)/mL has a 95% probability of representing infection [25]. However, it has been shown that 30–50% of women with symptoms of dysuria will have bacterial counts less than 10^5 cfu/mL [26]. Of these, about one-half have bacterial UTI with low numbers of bacteria. The rest may be considered in two groups; one group has urethritis due to *Chlamydia trachomatis* or *Neisseria gonorrhoeae* and the other has negative cultures and may have *Ureaplasma urealyticum* urethritis. In men, counts as low as 10^3 cfu/mL suggest infection [27].

In patients with indwelling urethral or suprapubic catheters, or those who intermittently self-catheterize and have symptoms or signs of UTI, a colony count of $\geq 10^3$ cfu/mL of more than one bacterial species in a single catheter or MSU specimen if the catheter has been removed within the previous 48 hours does indicate UTI [28].

Blood cultures

Blood cultures are normally not taken in afebrile patients with symptoms of cystitis. Current evidence indicates that blood cultures do not alter management and are therefore unnecessary in the majority of cases of uncomplicated pyelonephritis since the infecting organism is able to be isolated from a urine specimen [29,30]. Blood cultures should be taken in the following circumstances:

- recent instrumentation
- known anatomic abnormality
- failure of empiric treatment
- immunosuppression
- significant co-morbidity, such as diabetes mellitus
- major sepsis
- fever of unclear cause.

Imaging

Imaging is not required in cases of uncomplicated cystitis. In pyelonephritis, imaging should be performed if there is:

- pain suggestive of renal colic or obstruction
- failure to defervesce within 72 hours
- rapid relapse on cessation of antibiotic treatment or within 2 weeks
- infection with an unusual organism.

These circumstances have been shown to be associated with stones or renal scarring. CT scanning is the preferred modality as this has greater sensitivity for demonstrating not only stones and obstruction, but rare gas-forming infections, haemorrhage and inflammatory masses.

Management

Ideally, treatment of UTI should rapidly relieve symptoms, prevent short-term complications, such as progression from cystitis to pyelonephritis and subsequent sepsis or long-term sequelae, such as renal scarring, and prevent recurrences by eliminating uropathogenic bacteria from vaginal and perineal reservoirs. Treatment should be cost-effective and have few or no side effects.

There is no evidence that non-specific treatments, such as pushing fluids or attempting to alter urinary pH, improve the outcome of normal antibiotic treatment.

Antibiotic treatment

Serum levels of antibiotics are largely irrelevant in the elimination of bacteriuria. Reduction in urinary bacterial numbers correlates with the sensitivity of the organism to the urinary concentration of the antibiotic. Inhibitory concentrations are usually achieved in the urine after oral doses of the commonly used antibiotics. On the other hand, blood levels are vitally important in the treatment of bacteraemic or septic patients or those with renal parenchymal infections. In considering antibiotic treatment, it is important to recognize the rapidly and constantly evolving antibiotic resistance patterns of common urinary pathogens. In order to ensure effective treatment, while participating in worldwide efforts to mitigate the rapid development of highly resistant forms, clinicians should always refer to the latest available guidelines. Empirically, the choice of antibiotic is based on the clinical presentation and the bacteria likely to be involved (Table 9.4.2).

Table 9.4.2 Choice of treatment depending on bacteria involved (see text)

Condition	Bacteria involved	Suggested treatment [31,32]
Acute simple cystitis	E. coli, E. faecalis, S. saprophyticus, enterococci, Proteus spp., Klebsiella spp., Pseudomonas spp.	1. Trimethoprim 300 mg daily for 3 days¶, **OR** 2. Cephalexin 500 mg 12-hourly for 5 days, **OR** 3. Amoxycillin/clavulanate 500/125 mg 8-hourly for 5 days, **OR** 4. Nitrofurantoin 100 mg 12-hourly for 5 days in women only* Males or patients with recurrent infection should be treated for up to 14 days Norfloxacin 400 mg 12-hourly for 3 days in **resistant infection only** *In men, nitrofurantoin does not achieve reliable concentrations and is therefore not recommended ¶contraindicated in pregnancy
Acute uncomplicated pyelonephritis	E. coli, E. faecalis, S. saprophyticus, enterococci, Proteus spp., Klebsiella spp., Pseudomonas spp.	**Mild infection: oral treatment** 1. Amoxycillin/clavulanate 875/125 mg 12-hourly for 10 days, **OR** 2. Cephalexin 500 mg 6-hourly for 10 days, **OR** 3. Trimethoprim 300 mg/day for 10 days **In cases of proven resistance or Pseudomonas aeruginosa infection:** Norfloxacin 400 mg 12-hourly for 10 days, **OR** Ciprofloxacin 500 mg 12-hourly for 10 days **Severe infection: parenteral treatment (initial empiric treatment)** 1. Gentamycin* 4–6 mg/kg (up to 7 mg/kg for severe sepsis) PLUS amoxy/ampicillin 2 g 6-hourly Use 3rd generation cephalosporin if penicillin hypersensitivity NB: P. aeruginosa and enterococci are not covered by this regimen. Treatment must be continued for at least 14 days in all patients *There are contraindications to aminoglycosides. Clinicians should ensure they are very familiar with these. Dosages indicated here refer to initial dosing only. Subsequent doses must be guided by plasma concentration monitoring
UTI with structural abnormalities (complicated) and inpatients	Increased frequency of Proteus spp., Pseudomonas spp., Klebsiella spp., enterococci, staphylococci	**Treatment should be guided by culture and sensitivity testing. The following are a general indication only [40]** **Mild infection:** Trimethoprim or a fluoroquinolone Amoxy/ampicillin is effective for enterococci and group B strep. Nitrofurantoin may be effective for cystitis due to vancomycin-resistant enterococci **Severe infection:** Aminoglycosides plus piperacillin/tazobactam, ceftazidime or a carbapenem should be considered Treatment may need to be continued (orally) for 4–6 weeks
Catheter-associated	E. coli, Proteus spp., Klebsiella spp., Pseudomonas spp., enterococci, staphylococci	Treat only if symptomatic Change catheter Treat as for 'complicated UTI'
Dysuria with low bacterial numbers (urethral syndrome)	Ureaplasma urealyticum* * NB: may have chlamydial or gonococcal urethritis	Doxycycline in young women
Prophylaxis in patients with recurrent infections		Trimethoprim 150 mg at night, **OR** Cephalexin 250 mg at night

Management of specific groups (Fig. 9.4.1)

Frequency dysuria syndrome: presumed simple cystitis

A non-pregnant, non-diabetic woman first presenting from the community with typical lower urinary symptoms should have vulvovaginitis excluded and an MSU taken and examined or tested by dipstick for pyuria. If pyuria is confirmed, culture of the urine specimen is not necessary and treatment should be commenced empirically.

There is now good evidence that in this group of patients short-course treatment is effective in both treating the infection and eradicating uropathogenic strains of bacteria from reservoirs. Three-day treatment is superior to a single dose in eradicating the reservoirs of uropathogenic organisms, thereby reducing the incidence of recurrence. Longer courses have an increased incidence of side effects but not higher cure rates. The antibiotic of choice for 3-day treatment is trimethoprim [31,32]. The emergence of trimethoprim resistant uropathogens has been

well documented in some communities. The subsequent overuse of fluoroquinolones as first-line agents has resulted in a rapid rate of development of resistance to these agents in parts of Europe and in North America [33,34]. In general, fluoroquinolones should not be used as first-line agents for simple cystitis [31]. Awareness of local antibiotic resistance patterns is thus an important factor in choice of the most appropriate antibiotic.

Amoxycillin/clavulanic acid, nitrofurantoin and cephalexin are suitable for 5-day therapy, but

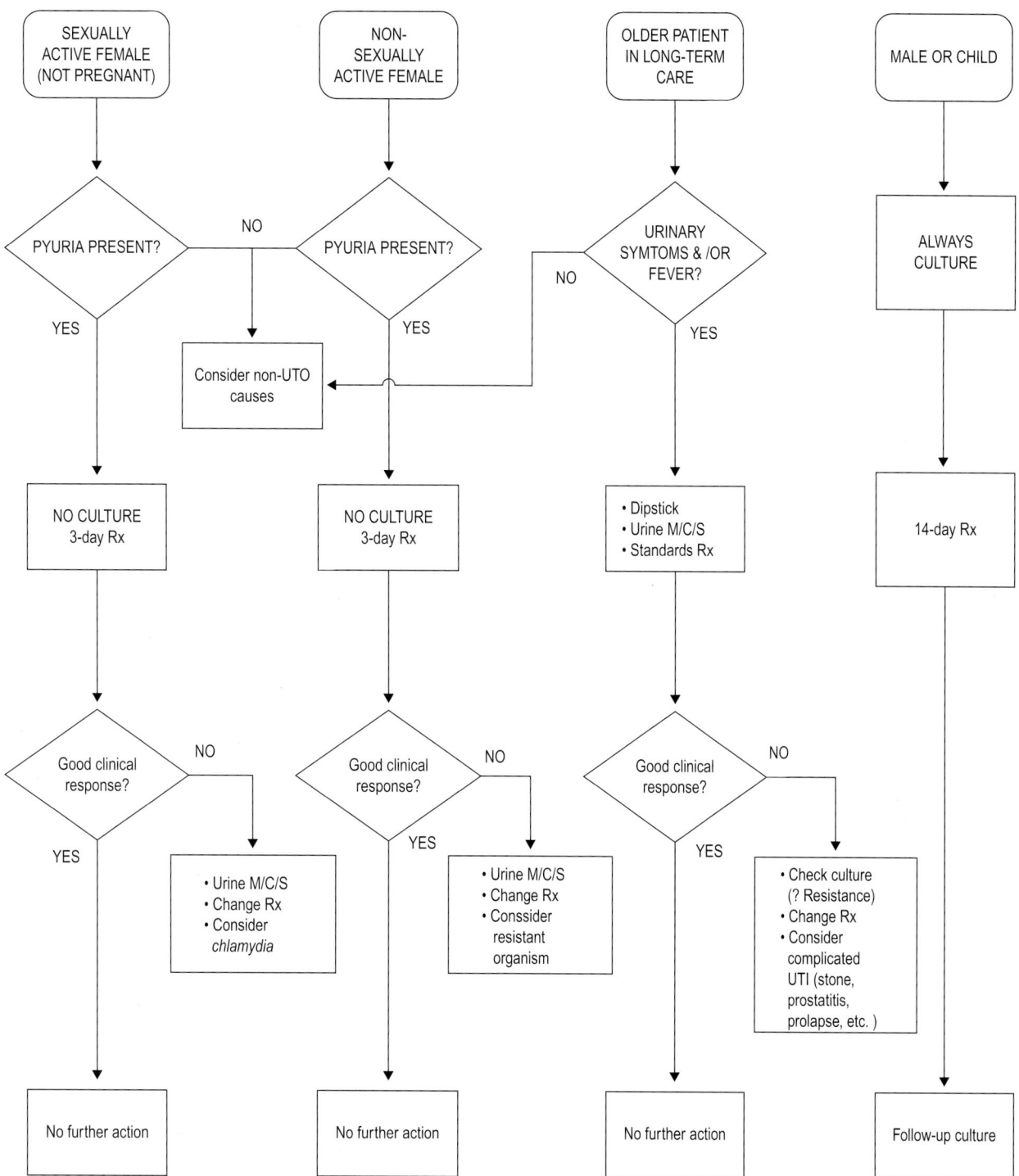

Fig. 9.4.1 Suggested management flow chart for simple cystitis.

amoxycillin alone should not be used as there is a high incidence of resistant *E. coli* in community-acquired UTI. If there is no clinical response, MSU should be sent for culture and, in sexually active women, treatment for *C. trachomatis* commenced (doxycycline 100 mg bd). In non-sexually active women, further treatment is guided by the results of sensitivity testing. Short-course treatment is inappropriate in women who are at risk of upper urinary tract infection (despite lower tract symptoms), which includes those with a history of previous infections due to resistant organisms, with symptoms for more than 1 week or those with diabetes mellitus.

Males with UTI should be investigated for urinary tract abnormality, associated prostatic or epididymal infection, must have urine culture initially and should have at least 14 days of treatment with any of the agents used for treatment of young women with simple cystitis (see Table 9.4.2) [31]. In men over 50 years, there is

447

a high probability of invasion of prostatic tissue and treatment may need to be continued for 4–6 weeks.

Recurrent UTI

Recurrent UTI is defined as a symptomatic UTI which follows resolution of a previous UTI. These may be re-infections (with the same organism or another) or relapses (regrowth of the same organism within 2 weeks of treatment). Re-infections are more common than relapses, but the two may be indistinguishable [35]. It is important to consider the risk factors specific to the age and gender of the patient, e.g. sexual activity and use of spermicides in the young pre-menopausal woman or the higher rate of asymptomatic bacteriuria in the older patient. A careful search for causes and reversible factors (e.g. of complicated UTI due to stone or obstruction, previously undiagnosed diabetes mellitus, prostatitis in males) should be made together with urine culture and sensitivity testing. Treatment is generally as for pyelonephritis, with an appropriate antibiotic guided by the results of sensitivity tests for at least 10–14 days. Female patients may benefit from post-intercourse or maintenance prophylaxis with, e.g. cephalexin 250 mg or trimethoprim 150 mg at night for several months (see Host factors). There has recently been burgeoning interest in the use of cranberry, either as juice or in tablet form, for UTI prophylaxis. Evidence is variable, but a recent Cochrane review of 24 studies concluded that cranberry cannot be recommended for UTI prevention [36].

Acute pyelonephritis

Patients presenting with the typical symptoms of pyelonephritis are at risk of bacteraemia or sepsis syndrome and therefore must rapidly have adequate concentrations of appropriate antibiotics delivered to both the blood and the urine. In order to meet this requirement, particularly in patients who are vomiting, parenteral (intravenous) treatment is usually required initially, but seldom for longer than 24–48 hours, by which time the patient is usually afebrile and not vomiting.

The choice of antibiotics is of necessity empirical at this stage. In cases of mild infection in patients who are not vomiting, 10-day treatment with one of the antimicrobials used for simple cystitis is appropriate, with ciprofloxacin or norfloxacin reserved for resistant organisms or proven Pseudomonas aeruginosa. For severe infections, parenteral ampicillin or amoxycillin (2 g 6-hourly) together with gentamicin

(4–6 mg/kg and up to 7 mg/kg as initial dose for severe sepsis) are appropriate, with a third-generation cephalosporin as an alternative to gentamicin when use of aminoglycosides is contraindicated. In patients with hospital-acquired infections and suspected Gram-negative sepsis or infections with Pseudomonas aeruginosa, broader-spectrum agents, such as ceftazidime, piperacillin/tazobactam, ticarcillin/clavulanic acid and imipenem, perhaps in combination with aminoglycosides, may be required. Parenteral treatment is followed by oral therapy for 2 weeks.

The use of short-stay observation units is now a standard part of the practice of emergency medicine. The safety and efficacy of treatment of pyelonephritis in such units with intravenous antibiotics and fluid administration, followed by oral therapy is widely accepted [37]. 'Hospital in the home (HITH)' programmes are also now commonplace, allowing close supervision of these patients by hospital-based staff and once- or twice-daily intravenous antibiotic administration at home. The efficacy and safety of HITH is well established, but requires careful patient selection to exclude those at risk of complicated infections. Appropriate follow up is essential, although repeat urine cultures are not recommended in asymptomatic patients following simple pyelonephritis [38,39].

Pregnancy

UTI in pregnancy are associated with an increased incidence of premature delivery and low birthweight infants. This has also been demonstrated to occur with asymptomatic bacteriuria, although up to 40% of asymptomatic women develop acute pyelonephritis later in pregnancy. Therefore, screening for bacteriuria and treatment of pregnant women is essential and urine must be sent for culture and antibiotic sensitivity testing. Three-day courses of treatment are not widely recommended, although it may be reasonable to use them with close follow up in an effort to reduce antibiotic usage; however, 10-day treatment courses are the norm. Cephalexin, nitrofurantoin or amoxycillin/clavulanate are appropriate for use in pregnancy, sulphas and trimethoprim being contraindicated [31].

Complicated UTI

As there is a greater range of organisms causing infection in these circumstances and a higher probability of antibiotic resistance, urine culture is essential and initial empiric treatment must cover the broader spectrum of organisms

potentially involved. If possible, antibiotic treatment should be delayed until results of urine culture and antibiotic sensitivities are known and, if empirical therapy is instituted, management should be reviewed as soon as such results are available [40]. Trimethoprim or a quinolone is appropriate for mild infections. More serious infections may need combinations of agents, such as aminoglycosides with amoxycillin or imipenem/cilastatin.

Catheter-associated UTI

Catheter-associated UTI (CA-UTI) are the most common nosocomial infections. In patients with short-term catheters who develop infection, the catheter must be removed or changed and treatment instituted as for complicated UTI. For those with chronic indwelling catheters (such as patients with spinal injuries), bacteriuria is universal and treatment is only indicated in the presence of symptoms such as fever, chills or loin pain. Patients with chronic spinal injuries may present with autonomic dysreflexia syndrome, the symptoms of which include sudden hypertension, muscle spasm and sweating, with or without fever. Antibiotic selection should again be based on culture or empirically as for complicated UTI. The most important strategy for prevention of CA-UTI is minimizing catheter use and duration whenever possible. Preventative strategies based on use of methanemine, cranberry or prophylactic antibiotics at time of catheterization or catheter change are not recommended [28,31].

Elderly patients

As previously stated, asymptomatic bacteriuria and UTI are very common in older patients and more so with increasing functional impairment. Symptomatic infection is a significant cause of morbidity and mortality as this age group also has a higher incidence of bacteraemia associated with pyelonephritis and septic shock commonly follows. Given the high rate of asymptomatic bacteriuria, the diagnosis of UTI in such individuals is difficult. The traditional view that non-specific symptoms, such as increased confusion (without fever), falling or deteriorating mobility are due to UTI has been called into question. Evidence indicates that UTI should only be considered in patients with fever or specific genitourinary symptoms or both. In patients with non-specific symptoms, non-infective causes should be sought and, in the case of fever alone, other potential sources of infection must be considered [8].

Antibiotic treatment of symptomatic UTI in the elderly patient is no different initially to that of younger patients; however, it should be borne in mind that a greater variety of organisms may be cultured in this age group and urine for culture should be obtained at the outset whenever possible.

Asymptomatic bacteriuria

Asymptomatic bacteriuria (ASB) is defined as the presence of significant bacteriuria (as previously defined) in a person without signs or symptoms of UTI. The presence of pyuria *per se* should not be taken to indicate bacteriuria – a quantitative culture is essential for the diagnosis. Current evidence indicates that many patient groups may be harmed, or at least not benefit from antibiotic treatment for asymptomatic bacteriuria. Antibiotics should therefore not be given to:

- pre-menopausal, non-pregnant women
- diabetic women
- older people either living in the community or in institutions
- patients with long-term indwelling catheters.

Conversely, two significant groups receive clear benefit from antibiotic treatment for ASB: pregnant women and patients about to undergo urological procedures in which mucosal bleeding is anticipated (e.g. TURP).

Pregnant women with ASB have a 20–30-fold increased risk of developing pyelonephritis during pregnancy with consequent premature delivery and low birthweight infants. Therefore, pregnant women should be actively screened for ASB in early pregnancy and treated as for uncomplicated cystitis (without nitrofurantoin), with repeat cultures to confirm bacterial clearance. Periodic re-testing is recommended.

Patients who undergo urological procedures with mucosal bleeding (e.g. TURP) have a 60% rate of bacteraemia, with sepsis in 6–10% of these. These patients should be screened for ASB prior to the procedure and antibiotic treatment commenced shortly prior to the procedure and continued until after the procedure or removal of the post-procedure catheter [41].

Disposition

Patients with simple UTI should have follow up to confirm clinical cure. Failure of symptomatic improvement in 48 hours may indicate antibiotic resistance, which requires urine culture to elucidate. Recurrence of symptoms within 1–2 weeks may indicate occult renal infection and necessitates urine culture and at least 7 days' treatment.

Prognosis

In adults with normal urinary tracts, UTI does not cause long-term sequelae. In the presence of urinary-tract abnormalities, infection may be a factor in producing renal damage or altering its rate of onset. Imaging of adults as part of their follow up should detect this group of patients.

Controversies

- The level of bacteriuria representing infection – traditional 10^5 cfu/mL or lower counts, such as 10^2 cfu/mL.
- Best first-line treatment of uncomplicated cystitis in the face of emerging resistance of uropathogens to common antibiotics such as trimethoprim and fluoroquinolones.
- The role of blood cultures as part of the investigation of pyelonephritis. Although traditionally used, they add little to the diagnosis and management.
- Asymptomatic bacteriuria in older, institutionalized patients. Differentiation from symptomatic infection and appropriate management.

References

[1] Bergeron M. Treatment of pyelonephritis in adults. Med Clin North Am 1995;79:619–49.
[2] Kreger BE, Craven DE, Carling PC, McCabe WR. Gram-negative bacteremia. III. Reassessment of etiology, epidemiology and ecology in 612 patients. Am J Med 1980;68:332–43.
[3] Fairley KF, Carson NE, Gutch RC, et al. Site of infection in acute urinary-tract infection in general practice. Lancet 1971;298:615–8.
[4] Foxman B. Epidemiology of urinary tract infections. Transmission and risk factors, incidence, and costs. Infect Dis Clin N Am 2003;17:227–41.
[5] Hooton T, Scholes D, Hughes JP. A prospective study of risk factors for symptomatic urinary tract infection in young women. N Engl J Med 1996;335:468.
[6] Vorland L, Carlson K, Aalen O. An epidemiological survey of urinary tract infections among outpatients in Northern Norway. Scand J Infect Dis 1985;17:277.
[7] Nicolle L, Bjornson J, Harding G, MacDonell J. Bacteriuria in elderly institutionlaized men. N Engl J Med 1983;309:1421–5.
[8] Nicolle LE. Urinary tract infection in geriatric and institutionalized patients. Curr Opin Urol 2002;12:51–5.
[9] Gupta K, Hooton T, Stamm W. Increasing antimicrobial resistance and the managment of uncomplicated community-acquired urinary tract infections. Ann Intern Med 2001;135:41–50.
[10] Ronald A. The etiology of urinary tract infection: traditional and emerging pathogens. Am J Med 2002;113:14S–9S.
[11] Kinane D, Blackwell C, Brettle R, et al. ABO blood group, secretor state and susceptibility to recurrent urinary tract infection in women. Br Med J 1982;285:7–9.
[12] Scholes D, Hooton T, Roberts P, et al. Risk factors for recurrent urinary tract infection in young women. J Infect Dis 2000;182:1177–82.
[13] Turck M, Goffe B, Petersdorf R. The urethral catheter and urinary tract infection. J Urol 1962;88:834–7.
[14] O'Sullivan D, Fitzgerald M, Meyness M, Malins J. Urinary tract infection, a comparative study in the diabetic and general population. Br J Med 1961;1:786.
[15] Ronald A, Ludwig E. Urinary tract infection in adults with diabetes. Int J Antimicrob Agents 2001;17:287–92.
[16] Stapleton A. Urinary tract infections in patients with diabetes. Excerpta Med 2002;113:80S–4S.
[17] Mabeck C, Orskov R, Orskov I. Escherichia coli serotypes and renal involvement in urinary tract infection. Lancet 1971;1:1312–4.
[18] Hagberg L, Hull R, Hull S, et al. Contribution of adhesion to bacterial persistence in the mouse urinary tract. Infect Immun 1983;40:265–72.
[19] Svanborg-Eden C, Hausson S, Jodal Y, et al. Host-parasite interactions in the urinary tract. J Infect Dis 1988;157:421–6.
[20] Bent S, Nallamothu BK, Simel DL, et al. Does this woman have an acute uncomplicated urinary tract infection? J Am Med Assoc 2002;287:2701–10.
[21] Deville WL, Yzermans JC, van Duijn NP, et al. The urine dipstick test useful to rule out infections. A meta-analysis of the accuracy. BMC Urol 2004:4.
[22] Sultana R, Zalstein S, Cameron P, Campbell D. Dipstick urinalysis and the accuracy of the clinical diagnosis of urinary tract infection. J Emerg Med 2001;20:13–19.
[23] Brumfitt W. Urinary cell counts and their value. J Clin Pathol 1965;18:550.
[24] Stamm W. Measurement of pyuria and its relation to bacteriuria. Am J Med 1983;75:53–8.
[25] Kass E. Bacteriuria and the diagnosis of infection of the urinary tract. Arch Intern Med 1957;100:709.
[26] Stamm WE, Counts G, Running K, et al. Diagnosis of coliform infection in acutely dysuric women. N Engl J Med 1982;307:463.
[27] Lipsky B. UTI in men: epidemiology, pathophysiology, diagnosis and treatment. Ann Intern Med 1989;110:138.
[28] Hooton T, Bradley S, Cardenas D, et al. Diagnosis, prevention, and treatment of catheter-associated urinary tract infection in adults: 2009 international clinical practice guidelines from the infectious diseases society of America. Clin Infect Dis 2010;50:625–63.
[29] McMurray B, Wrenn K, Wright S. Usefulness of blood cultures in pyelonephritis. Am J Emerg Med 1997;15:137–40.
[30] Velasco M, Martinez J, Moreno-Martinez A, et al. Blood cultures for women with uncomplicated pyelonephritis: are they necessary? Clin Infect Dis 2003;37:1127–30.
[31] Antibiotic Expert Group. Urinary tract infections eTG Complete [CD-ROM]. Melbourne: Therpeutic Guidlelines Limited, 2012.
[32] Gupta K, Hooton T, Naber KG, et al. Executive summary: international clinical practice guidelines for the treatment of acute uncomplicated cystitis and pyelonephritis in women: a 2010 update by the Infectious Diseases Society of America and the European Society for Microbiology and Infectious Diseases. Clin Infect Dis 2011;52(5):561–4.
[33] Zhanel G, Hisanaga T, Laing N, et al. Antibiotic resistance in *Escherichia coli* outpatient urinary isolates: final results from the North American Urinary Tract Infection Collaborative Alliance (NAUTICA). Int J Antimicrob Agents 2006;27: 468–75.
[34] Naber K, Schito G, Botto H, et al. Surveillance study in Europe and Brazil on clinical aspects and antimicrobial resistance epidemiology in females with cystitis (ARESC): implications for empiric therapy. Eur Urol 2008;54:1164–78.
[35] Franco AV. Recurrent urinary tract infections. Best Pract Res Clin Obstet Gynaecol 2005;19:861–73.
[36] Jepson R, Williams G, Craig J. Cranberries for preventing urinary tract infections. Cochrane Database Syst Rev 2012;10.
[37] Ward G, Jorden R, Severance H. Treatment of pyelonephritis in an observation unit. Ann Emerg Med 1991;20:258–61.
[38] Montalto M, Dunt D. Home and hospital intravenous therapy for two acute infections: an early study. Aust NZ J Med 1997;27:19–23.
[39] Caplan G, Sulaiman N, Mangin D, et al. A meta-analysis of "hospital in the home". Med J Aust 2012;197:512–9.
[40] Nicolle L. Complicated urinary tract infection in adults. Can J Infect Dis Med Microbiol 2005;16:349–60.
[41] Nicolle L, Bradley S, Colgan R, et al. Infectious Diseases Society of America guidelines for the diagnosis and treatment of asymptomatic bacteriuria in adults. Clin Infect Dis 2004;40:643–54.

9.5 Skin and soft-tissue infections

Rabind Charles

ESSENTIALS

1 The time-honoured principles of wound management, together with the judicious evidence-based use of antibiotics remain the basis for preventing and treating skin and soft-tissue infections.

2 All wounds, no matter how trivial, should be assumed to be tetanus prone and treated accordingly.

3 Skin and soft-tissue infections are common and range from mild to life threatening; they occasionally require surgical intervention and usually respond to narrow-spectrum antibiotics.

4 Deep soft-tissue infections have high morbidity and mortality and, unless treated aggressively, can rapidly result in loss of limb or death of the patient.

5 Infections due to unusual organisms, including organisms not usually considered to be pathogenic, frequently cause serious infections in the immunocompromised, patients with diabetes and patients with hepatic disease.

Introduction

Infectious disease is one of the most common reasons for patients to present to the emergency department (ED) and skin and soft-tissue infections (SSTIs) make up an important subset of these. SSTIs are a diverse group of aetiologically and anatomically distinct infections. Bacteria cause the majority of SSTIs encountered in the ED. The pathogenesis of these infections usually involves direct inoculation of bacteria as a result of violation of the skin or its defences, although there may also be spread of infection from a distant source via the haematogenous or lymphatic systems. The severity of infections encountered may range from mild to life threatening. Most recommendations for the diagnosis and treatment of SSTIs are based on tradition or consensus, as there are few randomized clinical trials on the subject. Some of the challenges to the emergency physician include:

- early and accurate diagnosis of the type of infection, based on clinical grounds and limited use of laboratory and radiological investigations
- early identification of potentially high-risk situations when the initial presentation is seemingly innocuous by looking at patient factors (e.g. diabetes, immunosuppression) and local factors (bite wounds, site of infection, e.g. orbital cellulitis)
- role of antibiotics: (1) appropriate choice of pharmacotherapeutic agent where indicated, taking into account the emergence of new infections and changing bacterial resistance patterns; (2) optimal route of delivery, i.e. topical versus oral versus initial intravenous or intramuscular bolus, followed by oral antibiotics versus intravenous therapy; (3) duration of the antibiotic treatment
- need for surgical intervention, e.g. drainage of abscess, early debridement in necrotizing fasciitis
- disposition issues: whether the patient can be discharged with outpatient follow up or will need hospitalization for management.

Aetiology

The majority of SSTIs are caused by aerobic Gram-positive bacteria, commonly *Staphylococcus aureus* and group A streptococcus. Deeper complicated infections, commonly seen in the immunocompromised host, are usually caused by Gram-negative, anaerobic or mixed organisms (Table 9.5.1).

Table 9.5.1   Causes of skin and soft-tissue infections

Risk factor/setting	Expected pathogen
Simple cutaneous infection	*Staphylococcus aureus*. Also *Staph. epidermidis*, *Staph. hominis*, *Streptococcus viridans*
Perianal, genital, buttocks, ungual and cervical areas	*Bacteroides fragilis*, *Escherichia coli*, *Klebsiella* and *Proteus*
Immunocompromised host	*Cryptococcccus neoformans*, *Coccidioides*, *Aspergillus*, *Mycobacterium kansasii*, *M. tuberculosis* and *Yersinia enterocolitica*
Human bite	*Eikenella corrodens*, *Fusobacterium*, *Prevotella*, streptococci
Dog bite	*Pasteuralla multocida*, *Capnocytophaga canimorsus*
Cat bite	*P. multocida*
Injection drug abuse	*S. aureus*, *Clostridium* spp., *E. corrodens*, *S. pyogenes*
Body piercing	*S. aureus*, *S. pyogenes*, *P. aeruginosa*, *C. tetani*
Hot tub/wading pool	*Ps. aeruginosa*
Fresh water injury	*A. hydrophila*
Salt water injury	*V. vulnificus*
Fish tank exposure	*Mycobacterium marinum*

Examination

History

When taking a history, it is important to elicit the following:

- Any event leading to a breach in skin integrity may precipitate an infection, e.g. human, insect or animal bite, 'clenched fist' injury, excoriation, fungal infection or puncture wound. This is important because it will help in determining the likely pathogen and choice of antibiotics, as well as the need to rule out any potential foreign body that may be embedded in the wound.
- The speed with which the infection has progressed serves as a guide as to how aggressive the infection is and the urgency of treatment needed.
- Patient factors that may complicate the treatment of the infection:
  - history of immunosuppression, e.g. diabetes, steroid use, chronic liver disease, alcoholism, malnourishment, HIV, oncology patients on chemotherapy, nephrotic syndrome
  - recent use of antibiotics, i.e. failed treatment
  - history of prosthetic heart valves, mitral valve prolapse with regurgitation, previous history of endocarditis
  - chronic venous stasis or lymphoedema in limbs; surgery that includes lymph node dissection or saphenous vein resection
  - intravenous drug use (IVDU)
- Tetanus status
- Contamination with soil or water, which would suggest unusual pathogens as the cause of the infection.

Physical examination

- Identification of severe sepsis: unstable vital signs, hyperpyrexia, 'toxic'-looking patient.
- Specific features of the infection to help narrow down the diagnosis, e.g. raised erythematous margins in erysipelas; presence of bullae and crepitus or tenderness out of proportion to physical signs, suggestive of necrotizing fasciitis; fetid odour suggesting anaerobic infection or green exudates typical of *Pseudomonas* spp.
- The extent of the infection, e.g. mapping areas of erythema to track progress, fluctuance that indicates fluid and a likely abscess that may need incision and drainage or lymphangitic spread.

- Location of the infection, as involvement of certain critical areas (e.g. head, face, perineum) may require more intensive inpatient management and specialist consultation.
- Complicating factors that might impair successful treatment, e.g. needle tracks in IV drug users, the presence of prosthetic heart valves.

Investigations

SSTIs are usually diagnosed from their clinical presentation. Laboratory and radiological investigations play a secondary and limited role in routine evaluation but may be useful in the ED management of immunocompromised patients or those with signs and symptoms of severe sepsis. In such situations, the following parameters should be considered [1]:

- Full blood examination with differential: presence of marked leucocytosis, leucopaenia or an extreme left shift in the white cell differential; new-onset anaemia or thrombocytopaenia may suggest sepsis syndrome.
- Urea/creatinine: elevated levels suggest intravascular volume depletion or renal failure.
- Creatine kinase: elevated levels may indicate myonecrosis caused by necrotizing fasciitis.
- Blood culture and drug susceptibility tests: the yield from these may be less than 10% and may be compounded by false-positive results [2]. In addition, emergency physicians do not have the luxury of time to await blood culture results before initiating the appropriate antibiotic treatment.
- Other investigations: it is prudent to test for diabetes mellitus in patients presenting with an abscess because of the strong association of the two.

Patients with a chronic, recurrent or unusual infection should have their immune status checked, including serology for HIV. Soft-tissue radiographs may demonstrate a foreign body or gas in deep tissues. Computed tomography (CT) or magnetic resonance imaging (MRI) may be needed to define the depth and extent of the infective process when entertaining the diagnoses of fasciitis or myonecrosis. Ultrasonography in the ED may be a useful adjunct in evaluating soft-tissue infections for the presence of subcutaneous abscesses.

Management

Key points in the management of SSTIs include:

- analgesia
- appropriate use of antibiotics
- appropriate surgical intervention
- tetanus and other prophylaxis
- disposition plans and options.

Analgesia

Oral or parenteral analgesia should be prescribed, as most patients with SSTIs will present with pain. Simple measures, such as immobilization, elevation, heat or moist warm packs, should not be overlooked as they may help to alleviate pain in cellulitis. Abscess pain is best resolved by timely incision and drainage.

It is important to have a high index of suspicion for necrotizing fasciitis in any patient who has cellulitis with an inordinate amount of pain, or exquisite muscle tenderness where there is no history of musculoskeletal trauma.

Antibiotic therapy

Antibiotics are recommended for patients with signs of systemic toxicity, high fever, tachycardia, who are flushed and who look unwell, who are immunocompromised, who have abscesses in high-risk areas (hands, perineal region or face) and where deep necrotizing infection is suspected [2].

It is important for the emergency physician to recognize patients with serious skin and soft-tissue infections and to initiate appropriate care. The choice of antibiotic is often empiric and thus must be guided by the patient's history, where they have been recently institutionalized and knowledge of the typical range of pathogens associated with each type of infection and their resistance patterns. The antibiotic of choice is the one that has proven efficacy against the range of expected pathogens, is associated with minimal toxicity and is cost-effective. Where possible, narrow-spectrum antibiotics should be used in preference to broad-spectrum ones [3]. Published guidance on antibiotic therapy is often deliberately non-prescriptive, reflecting the wide variety between differing patient populations, resistance patterns, methicillin-resistant *Staph. aureus* (MRSA) risk and local governance policies. It is also prudent to remember that SSTI clinical trials often exclude the most severely ill patients and may be powered to demonstrate non-inferiority only. The Infectious

Diseases Society of America recently released guidelines for treating MRSA in SSTIs [4]. Unlike inpatient or chronic care settings, emergency physicians more frequently have to initiate empiric antibiotics based on clinical judgement and prevailing antibiograms, due to absence of culture and susceptibility results.

In the last decade, new agents active against Gram-positive bacteria have emerged and those licensed for treating complicated SSTIs include linezolid, daptomycin and tigecycline.

Surgical intervention

Certain SSTIs are best treated surgically. Effective treatment of abscesses and carbuncles and large furuncles entails incision, drainage of pus and breaking up of loculations, followed by regular dressings. Necrotizing fasciitis requires *early* aggressive surgical debridement together with broad-spectrum antibiotics in order to achieve best morbidity and mortality outcomes [5].

Tetanus and other prophylaxis

All wounds should be considered to be tetanus prone and treated accordingly. The patient's immunization status should be checked and, where appropriate, tetanus toxoid plus tetanus immunoglobulin should be administered. Deep and penetrating wounds and wounds that have significant tissue devitalization or where there is heavy contamination (e.g. soil, dust, manure and wood splinters) are best treated with prophylactic antibiotic cover. The antibiotic of choice is penicillin; patients who are allergic to penicillin should receive cephalexin. If there is a history of severe penicillin allergy, use erythromycin or vancomycin.

Rabies prophylaxis should be considered for all feral and wild animal bites and in geographical areas where there is a high prevalence of rabies.

In cases involving human bites, consideration should also be given to screening for blood-borne pathogens such as hepatitis B virus, hepatitis C virus, HIV and syphilis.

Disposition

SSTIs are among the most frequently encountered conditions in the emergency observation setting. Good candidates for the observation/short-stay unit include patients likely to respond to empirical therapy, with a low likelihood of infection with unusual and/or resistant organisms.

Patients who have systemic toxicity (fever, tachycardia, rigors, altered mentation, severe pain), involvement of vital structures (fingers, hand, face and neck, genitourinary, scrotal and anal regions), those unable to take oral medication, who have failed outpatient therapy or who are immunocompromised (HIV positive, cancer, diabetes mellitus, hepatic or renal failure) are highly likely to require admission. Other prognostic factors include low serum bicarbonate, elevated creatinine, elevated creatine kinase and marked left shift polymorphonuclear neutrophils. The emergency physician must also be alert to scenarios requiring not just inpatient care but also urgent subspecialty consultation, e.g. necrotizing fasciitis.

Superficial skin infections

Clinical presentation

Patients usually present with a complaint of localized pain, redness and swelling. They may have been self-treating or have had previous treatment with oral antibiotics without success. Frequently, an abscess is fluctuant and indurated with surrounding erythema. The patient may also have associated lymphadenitis, regional lymphadenopathy and cellulitis. If the patient is febrile or there is systemic involvement, their immune status needs to be examined.

The possibility of a foreign body associated with an abscess needs to be considered. A careful history needs to be taken to determine whether this is possible and radiography may be necessary. Ultrasound can be useful in identifying the presence of a foreign body. The patient should also be questioned in relation to use of immunosuppressive agents.

Impetigo

This is a localized purulent skin infection, usually caused by group A streptococcus (*Strep. pyogenes*) and is seen more in warm humid climates. Topical therapy with mucipirocin often suffices, but oral antibiotics (first-generation cephalosporin or erythromycin) may be needed in cases with extensive lesions or perioral lesions.

Folliculitis

A superficial infection characterized by reddened papules or pustules of the hair follicles. Most cases are caused by *Staph. aureus*. *Pseudomonas aeruginosa* may be the

cause following swimming pool or hot tub (spa) exposure. Treatment may only require the use of an antibacterial soap or solution. Removal of the hair in limited infections usually results in rapid resolution.

Furuncle and carbuncle

A furuncle arises secondarily to an infected hair follicle, where an abscess forms in the subcutaneous tissue. Furuncles most commonly occur on the back, axilla or lower extremities. *Staphylococcus* species are the most common associated organism. When the infection extends to involve several adjacent follicles, resulting in a coalescent inflammatory mass, the lesion is termed a carbuncle. Small furuncles are best treated with moist heat. Larger furuncles and all carbuncles require incision and drainage. The most common site is the back of the neck and diabetics are particularly prone to this. Systemic antibiotics are usually unnecessary unless there is extensive surrounding cellulitis or fever or if the patient has diabetes or is immunocompromised, in which case di(flu)cloxacillin (500 mg q 6 h oral), cephalexin (500 mg q 6 h) or clindamycin (450 mg q 8 h oral) can be used.

Erysipelas

Erysipelas is a rapidly progressive, erythematous, indurated, painful, sharply demarcated superficial skin infection caused by *Strep. pyogenes* (other causes are non-group A streptococci, *Haemophilus influenzae*, *Staph. aureus* and *Strep. pneumoniae*). The classic description is of a butterfly facial distribution, but recent evidence suggests that erysipelas is commonly found on the lower limbs. There is a clear line of demarcation between involved and uninvolved skin. It is common in young children and the elderly. Systemic symptoms (fever, chills, rigors and diaphoresis) are common and 5% will have bacteraemia. Erysipelas may rapidly progress to cellulitis (i.e. involvement beyond the upper dermis), abscess formation and, occasionally, fasciitis. Treatment consists of the use of antibacterial soap and oral penicillin (di(flu)cloxacillin 500 mg q 6 h oral).

Herpetic whitlow

Herpetic whitlow is a superficial infection with herpes simplex virus and is an occupational hazard of jobs having contact with oral mucosa, e.g. dentistry and anaesthesiology. Incision and drainage is contraindicated and may in fact spread the viral infection.

Cellulitis

Cellulitis is an acute spreading infection of the skin involving the deeper dermis and subcutaneous fat. In patients with a normal immune system who are otherwise healthy, the infection is caused by bacteria that normally colonize skin, principally *Staph. aureus* and group A β-haemolytic streptococci. Predisposing factors include conditions leading to a disrupted cutaneous barrier and/or impaired local host defences, such as trauma and inflammatory dermatoses, e.g. eczema, oedema from venous insufficiency or lymphatic obstruction.

Despite the common occurrence of cellulitis, there is a paucity of published research on issues such as criteria for antibiotics and admission and severity assessment. The presence of an underlying abscess should be considered in patients who 'fail' initial antibiotic therapy: treatment failure may be caused by an undrained abscess rather than inadequate antimicrobial therapy and bedside soft-tissue ultrasonography is a useful tool that is increasingly available in EDs.

Treatment consists of elevation of the affected part and administration of an antistaphylococcal penicillin such as di(flu)cloxacillin (2 g q 6 h IV) or a first-generation cephalosporin, such as cephazolin (2 g q 12 h IV).

Therapy may need to be escalated in special settings, such as diabetes, or particular anatomical areas. Anaerobes or Gram-negative organisms have been identified in 95% of affected diabetic foot ulcers, with *Staph. aureus* found in approximately 33%. Broad-spectrum antibiotic treatment, e.g. metronidazole (400 mg q 12 h orally) plus cephazolin (2 g q 12 h IV), is recommended.

Infections that originate from wounds involving the feet may be due to *Pseudomonas aeruginosa*; this organism is also associated with osteomyelitis of the foot. Antibiotic treatment should consist of an antipseudomonal β-lactam, such as carbenacillin, or a third-generation cephalosporin, such as ceftriaxone, and an aminoglycoside.

Cellulitis is a well-known complication in women who have undergone axillary lymph node dissection and surgery for breast cancer. The major mechanism is thought to be an altered lymphatic and/or venous circulation related to the surgical procedure and to radiation therapy. Empiric antibiotic therapy is targeted at *Staph. aureus* and β-haemolytic streptococci and choices include cephalexin or cefazolin. If the patient has received recent chemotherapy and is neutropaenic, then the antibiotic regimen must be broadened to include coverage for aerobic Gram-negative bacilli, including *Pseudomonas aeruginosa*.

Facial cellulitis, including periorbital and orbital cellulitis is a serious infection occurring in adults and children [6]. The causal organisms include *Staph. aureus*, *H. influenzae* type b and *Staph. pneumoniae*. This type of cellulitis may arise from an infected sinus. Broad-spectrum antibiotic therapy is required, the agent of choice being dicloxacillin 1 g IV 6-hourly. Radiological evaluation, including CT scanning, may be necessary to identify underlying sinusitis.

Abscesses

Pilonidal abscess

Pilonidal abscesses occur in the superior gluteal fold and arise from the disruption of the epithelium, causing the formation of a pit lined with epithelial cells that may become plugged with hair and keratin, leading to an abscess. Treatment involves incision and drainage, usually in the operating theatre, although smaller abscesses can be drained in the ED under local anaesthetic. They are usually associated with mixed organisms, both aerobic and anaerobic.

Hidradenitis suppurativa

This is a chronic suppurative abscess of the upper apocrine sweat glands in the groin and axilla. It is much more common in females, in obesity and in patients who have poor hygiene or who shave the region. Organisms include *Staph. aureus*, *Strep. viridans* and *Proteus* spp. Treatment is incision and drainage, usually in the operating theatre. Definitive treatment may require removal of the apocrine sweat glands from the region.

Bartholin's abscess

This occurs as a result of the obstruction of a Bartholin's duct and is usually composed of mixed vaginal flora. *Neisseria gonorrhoeae* and *Chlamydia trachomatis* may also be involved. Treatment is incision, drainage and marsupialization of the cyst in the operating theatre.

Paronychia

This is a superficial abscess of the lateral aspect of the nail, commonly associated with patients whose hands are frequently wet. Common organisms involved are *Staph. aureus*, *Candida* and anaerobes. Some cases may require incision and drainage, with advice to keep the hands dry.

Perianal abscess

These are thought to originate in the anal crypts and extend into the ischiorectal space. Patients frequently complain of pain on defaecation and sitting. Perianal abscesses may be associated with inflammatory bowel disease and fistula formation. Treatment should be incision and drainage in the operating theatre under general anaesthesia. When the abscess is superficial and 'pointing', drainage in the ED is possible.

Infected sebaceous cyst

Sebaceous cysts become infected when the duct is obstructed. They can occur anywhere on the body, but tend to favour the head and neck region. Treatment is incision and drainage, recurrence is not uncommon.

Treatment

Incision and drainage of cutaneous abscesses is the key to treatment. Some patients require oral antibiotic therapy. Patients who are immunosuppressed or who have diabetes mellitus should be treated with appropriate antibiotic therapy based on a knowledge of the probable pathogen. Patients at risk of developing bacterial endocarditis require prophylactic antibiotics prior to incision and drainage. The treatment of superficial skin abscesses has in recent years been complicated by the emergence of MRSA. Proponents of the practice of 'routine culture' of abscess fluid say that surveillance of antimicrobial susceptibility allows therapeutic adjustment. Detractors point out that for simple abscesses, incision and drainage without antibiotics is usually sufficient and thus if antibiotics are not considered clinically useful it is unlikely that culture results will alter the management.

Deep soft-tissue infections

Necrotizing fasciitis

Necrotizing fasciitis is a rare, rapidly progressing, life-threatening infectious process involving primarily the superficial fascia (i.e. all the tissue between the skin and underlying muscles – the subcutaneous tissue). Patients usually present with the triad of exquisite pain – often out of proportion to initial physical findings – swelling and fever. Early diagnosis is sometimes thwarted by the paucity of cutaneous findings early in the course of the disease. The clinician should have a high index of suspicion based on the clinical presentation as well as the patient's underlying co-morbidities (diabetes, chronic alcoholism, and immunosuppression). Laboratory values may be used in risk scoring, e.g. the Laboratory Risk Indicator for Necrotizing Fasciitis (LRINEC), which has been validated prospectively and has a high sensitivity and positive predictive value of 92% in patients with scores of six points and above. Patients with scores of five points and below are considered at low risk of necrotizing fasciitis [7,8].

Numbness of the involved area is characteristic of advanced necrotizing fasciitis – this is a result of infarction of the cutaneous nerves. Eighty per cent of cases show clear origins for an accompanying skin lesion (insect bite, minor abrasion, furuncle, and IVDU injection site) but, in the remaining 20%, no skin lesion can be found [9,10].

Patients appear extremely toxic with a high fever, tachycardia and malaise. Pathognomonic features include extensive undermining of the skin and subcutaneous tissues, with separation of the tissue planes. The subcutaneous tissues may have a hard, wooden feel. Bullous lesions and skin ecchymoses may also be evident. Crepitation may be clinically evident and gas may be visualized on X-ray in some 80% of patients. The gas is typically layered along fascial planes. CT or MRI may aid in confirming the clinical suspicion.

Bacteria involved in this infection are usually mixed: *Staph. aureus*, haemolytic streptococci, Gram-negative rods and anaerobes. Sometimes only group A streptococci, either alone or in combination with *Staph. aureus*, are found. Aggressive therapy is essential, as mortality approaches 50%. Immediate surgical intervention extensively to open and debride the wound is required, as myonecrosis may be present [11]. Appropriate antimicrobial therapy should be commenced immediately: meropenam (1 g q 8 h IV) plus clindamycin (600 mg q 8 h IV) or lincomycin (600 mg q 8 h IV). Hyperbaric oxygen therapy should be considered.

Fournier's gangrene is a form of necrotizing fasciitis which involves the scrotum, penis or vulva and is usually seen in diabetics. It usually originates from perianal or urinary tract infections (which extend into the periurethral glands)

and can progress explosively. The management is early recognition and surgical debridement and intravenous antibiotics.

Gas gangrene

Gas gangrene is an acute life- and limb-threatening deep-tissue infection, also known as clostridial myonecrosis. Aetiological agents include *Clostridium perfringens*, *Cl. histolyticum*, *Cl. septicum* and *Cl. novyi*. *Cl. perfringens* is the most common cause in traumatic gas gangrene, whereas spontaneous gangrene is principally associated with *Cl. septicum*. This infection is characterized by the rapid development (often within hours) of intense pain in the region of a wound, followed by local swelling and a haemoserous exudate. A characteristic foul smell is also a good indication of the diagnosis. The area becomes tense and may develop a bluish and bronze or dusky discoloration. The presence of gas is typical, although it may be a late finding. It is frequently found on X-ray, where it has a feathered pattern as gas develops within the muscle itself. Aggressive treatment is required as the patient may present in an advanced stage with tachycardia, altered mental status, shock and haemolytic anaemia.

Classically, the gas gangrene occurs in extensive and or deep wounds with predisposing factors, including vascular ischaemia, diabetes and presence of foreign bodies. Gram stain frequently reveals relatively few white blood cells and large numbers of club-shaped Gram-positive rods.

Early surgical intervention is essential, including wide debridement of necrotic muscle and other tissues, administration of high-dose penicillin C (benzylpenicillin 2.4 g q 4 h IV), an aminoglycoside and hyperbaric oxygen therapy. Early hyperbaric oxygen therapy has been demonstrated to result in improved outcome [3,10–13].

One should note that the presence of gas certainly raises the suspicion of a deep-tissue infection, including gas gangrene, but that it may also be present because of previous wound manipulation, self-injection of air, localized gas abscess or other gas-producing organisms, including anaerobes, *E. coli*, streptococci and staphylococci.

Pyomyositis

Pyomyositis is the presence of pus within individual muscle groups and the usual culprit is *Staph. aureus*. A positive blood culture

yield is found in only 5–30% of cases. Typical presenting symptoms included localized pain in a single muscle group, usually in an extremity, and fever. Ultrasonography or CT may be warranted to differentiate the condition from a suspected deep vein thrombosis.

Toxic complications of wound infections

A number of bacteria produce toxins that result in systemic symptoms.

Tetanus

Tetanus, albeit rare in developed countries, still occurs despite the fact that immunization is completely effective in preventing it. All wounds should be treated as tetanus prone. Tetanus may occur with trivial wounds that may not even be apparent. The incubation period is variable, ranging from 3 days to several weeks after inoculation; the disease is more severe at the extremes of age. Difficulty in swallowing and a fever with progression to stiffness and trismus is pathognomonic. Tetanus is also associated with autonomic nervous system dysfunction. Occasionally, localized tetanus may occur with muscle spasm in the area adjacent to the wound. This is sometimes associated with cranial nerve dysfunction. Treatment is largely supportive, often requiring deep sedation, paralysis and ventilation for prolonged periods. Antibiotic therapy with high-dose penicillin should also be given in addition to tetanus immunization and tetanus immunoglobulin (Table 9.5.2).

Toxic shock syndrome

Toxic shock syndrome (TSS) is a life-threatening multisystem disease caused by inflammatory immune responses to toxogenic strains of *Staph. aureus*. TSS has been classically associated with the use of tampons, although 10–40% of cases are non-menstrual related. Onset of menstrual TSS symptoms occurs within 3 days of the menstrual cycle and usually has no preceding clinically apparent infection. Non-menstrual cases occur after childbirth, abortions, in bone and skin infections including postoperative wound infections, burns, mastitis and varicella-related cellulitis. The wound itself may look insignificant. There is a rapid onset of fever, usually >38.9°C, hypotension and an initial diffuse and later desquamating erythematous rash. Multiorgan

Table 9.5.2   Tetanus prophylaxis

Time since vaccination	Type of wound	Tetanus toxoid	Tetanus immunoglobulin
History of 3 or more doses of tetanus toxoid			
<5 years	All wounds	No	No
5–10 years	Clean minor wounds	No	No
	All other wounds	Yes	No
>10 years	All wounds	Yes	No
Uncertain vaccination history or less than 3 doses of tetanus toxoid			
	Clean minor wounds	Yes	No
	All other wounds	Yes	Yes

Reproduced with permission from Antibiotic Expert Group. Melbourne: Therapeutic guidelines Limited, 2013 eTG [14].

involvement may include muscular (myalgia), neurological (headache, and altered sensorium) and gastrointestinal (nausea, and diarrhoea) symptoms. Occasionally, *Staph. aureus* can be cultured locally, although blood cultures are rarely positive. Antibiotics do not affect the course of TSS but may lower the recurrence rate by 59–73% [15]. An antistaphylococcal agent should be given with an aminoglycoside. Patients are frequently haemodynamically compromised, requiring aggressive fluid resuscitation and inotropic support. Debridement of necrotic wounds, if present, and elimination of the source of infections – e.g. removal of the tampon – should be carried out urgently. A similar syndrome can develop due to infection with group A β-haemolytic streptococci. This is known as 'wound' or 'surgical' scarlet fever. Treatment is the same as for TSS.

Special infections

Human bites

Human bite wounds may occur as a result of an accidental injury, deliberate biting or closed fist injuries. The bacteriology reflects the normal oral flora of the biter: streptococci in 50–80% of wounds, staphylococci, *Eikenella corrodens* and anaerobic organisms. Therapy consists of irrigation and topical wound cleansing and prophylactic antibiotics should be initiated as early as possible in all patients, regardless of the appearance of the wound.

Clenched fist injuries over the metacarpophalangeal joint warrant hospitalization for formal washout and intravenous antibiotics. Appropriate antibiotic choices include amoxicillin-clavulanate (875 + 125 mg q 12 h oral), metronidazole (400 mg q 12 h oral) plus either ceftriaxone (1 g daily IV) or cefotaxime (1 g daily IV). In cases of β-lactam allergy, metronidazole plus doxycycline, ciprofloxacin or trimethoprim-sulfamethoxazole may be used.

Animal bites

Most bites are from dogs (80%) or cats, but bites from exotic pets and feral animals also occur. *Pasteurella* and bacteriodes species are the most common bacterial isolates and *Capnocytophaga canimorsus* can cause bacteraemia and fatal sepsis, especially in patients with underlying liver disease or asplenia. Infected bites presenting <12 hours after injury are more likely to be infected with *Pasteurella* spp., whereas those presenting >24 hours post-bite are more likely to be infected with staphylococci or anaerobes. Wounds should be cleansed with sterile normal saline and infected wounds should not be closed. Cat bite wounds have less crush injury and wound trauma than dog bites, but have a higher proportion of osteomyelitis and septic arthritis. The oral agent of choice for both dog and cat bites is amoxicillin–clavulanate, with doxycycline as an alternative. Intravenous options include second-generation cephalosporins, piperacillin–tazobactam and carbapenams. Cellulitis and abscesses usually respond to 5–10 days of therapy. Rabies prophylaxis should be considered for all feral and wild animal bites and in geographical areas where there is a high prevalence of rabies.

Water-related infections

Water-related infections may be caused by unusual organisms. *Vibrio vulnificus*, *V. alginolyticus* and other non-cholera vibrios are found in salt and brackish water and can result in serious and life-threatening infections, especially in patients with hepatic disease. Aggressive infection can progress rapidly over 2–4 hours. It is associated with saltwater exposure or the ingestion of raw shellfish. Infections can mimic gas gangrene, with rapid progression and tissue destruction; septicaemia may occur and can be fatal. If parenteral therapy is required, a third-generation cephalosporin can be combined with an aminoglycoside and/or doxycycline.

Exposure to fresh or brackish water (rivers, mud and caving) can result in infection with the Gram-negative bacillus *Aeromonas hydrophila* [16]. *Aeromonas* infections can result in superficial skin infections, myositis and septicaemia. Treatment consists of administration of cefotaxime 1 g IV 8-hourly or ceftriaxone 1 g IV daily. If oral therapy is possible, consider ciprofloxacin 500 mg orally 12-hourly.

Mycobacterium marinum, *M. ulcerans*, *M. chelonei*, *M. gordanae*. and *M. fortuitum* are found in fish tanks and can result in 'fish fancier's finger'. After 2–6 weeks of incubation, an ulcerating granuloma develops. Treatment options include clarithromycin, trimethoprim–sulfamethoxazole or a combination of ethambutol and rifampicin. Systemic infection is uncommon.

Saltwater fish handlers may develop infections due to *Erysipelothrix rhusiopathiae*; this causes erysipeloid, a type of cellulitis. It also causes infections in people handling fish, poultry, meat and hides. Coral cuts are often infected with *Streptococcus pyogenes*; other marine pathogens may be involved (including *Vibrio* species). Treatment should consist of phenoxymethylpenicillin 500 mg 6-hourly.

Mastitis

Infections of the breast can occur in both sexes and in all ages; however, breast infections are most common in nursing mothers and the prevalence of lactational mastitis in Australia is estimated at 20% [17]. *Staph. aureus* is the most common pathogen in infective mastitis.

Treatment consists of regular emptying of the breast. If breastfeeding needs to be stopped because of the severity of the infection or the risk to the neonate, a pump or manual expression methods should be employed (at least temporarily). If symptoms are not resolving within 12–24 hours of effective milk removal and analgesia, antibiotic treatment should be commenced to prevent abscess formation. Eleven per cent of patients who are not treated appropriately with antibiotics will develop an abscess. Options include di(flu)cloxacillin (500 mg q 6 h oral) or a first-generation cephalosporin, such as cephalexin (500 mg q 6 h oral) or erythromycin (250–500 mg q 6 h oral). Severe infections may require parenteral or more prolonged therapy. Local care to the region is also important, including warm compresses, breast support, analgesia and the application of a moisturizing cream to the nipple and areolar region. Patients who develop an abscess will require percutaneous aspiration or open drainage [18].

Decubitus ulcers

Decubitus ulcers are cutaneous ulcerations caused by prolonged pressure that results in ischaemic necrosis of the skin and underlying soft tissue. They are most commonly found in patients who are bedbound, particularly elderly nursing home patients and patients with sensory deficits, such as paraplegia and quadriplegia. Immobility, compounded by vascular insufficiency and neuropathy, results in ulcer formation and, unless treated aggressively, serious complications can follow [19]. Complications include cellulitis and deep soft-tissue necrosis, osteomyelitis, septic thrombophlebitis, bacteraemia and sepsis. Culture of the ulcer invariably reveals a mixed bacterial flora of both aerobes and anaerobes, which do not distinguish between colonization and tissue infection. The most common organisms found are staphylococci, streptococci, coliforms and a variety of anaerobes. Systemic antibiotics are required for patients with clinical signs of sepsis or osteomyelitis.

Varicose ulcers

Varicose ulcers are cutaneous ulcers caused by oedema and poor tissue drainage as a result of dysfunction of the venous system, including varicose veins. These are more common in the elderly and obese. They may be chronic, and healing is often difficult. Complications include cellulitis and, occasionally, bacteraemia. Culture of the ulcer variably reveals a mixed bacterial flora of both aerobes and anaerobes that cannot distinguish between colonization and tissue infections. The most common organisms found are staphylococci, streptococci, coliforms and a variety of anaerobes.

Treatment consists of debridement of necrotic tissue, pressure area and general nursing care, as well as treatment of infection, if present. Antibiotic treatment is only indicated where there is systemic evidence of infection or where there is a complicating infection, such as osteomyelitis or bacteraemia. Surgical debridement is frequently as important, if not more important, than antibiotic therapy, particularly where the bacterial infection is localized.

Diabetic foot infections

Foot infections are a common complication of diabetes and require both local (foot) treatment and systemic (metabolic) optimization, which is best undertaken by a multidisciplinary team including surgeons, podiatry services and the endocrinologist or physician.

The peripheral neuropathy associated with diabetes results in the loss of protective pain sensation and results in repetitive injuries, followed by the development of ulcers that become infected. Vascular insufficiency and impaired immune function contribute to the increased risk of acute and chronic infection. Infections in foot ulcers are often polymicrobial and both the number of bacterial groups and bacterial density are thought to affect healing [16]. Aerobes include *Staph. aureus*, coagulase-negative staphylococci and streptococci. Enterobacteriaceae and *Corynebacterium* are not uncommon. Anaerobes which have been isolated from up to 48% of patients include *Bacteroides* and *Clostridium* spp. The presence of anaerobes is associated with a high frequency of fever, foul-smelling lesions and the presence of an ulcer. Cultures obtained using curettage following debridement should be used in preference to wound swabs to identify causative organisms and sensitivities.

Local signs and symptoms predominate and include those secondary to infection, vasculopathy and neuropathy. Pain and tenderness are often minimal due to the neuropathy and pulses are frequently reduced or absent. Wound infections must be diagnosed clinically on the basis of local (and occasionally systemic) signs and symptoms of inflammation. Laboratory (including microbiological) investigations are of limited use for diagnosing infection, except in cases of osteomyelitis radiography and/or a bone scan may be warranted to exclude osteomyelitis.

A recent systemic review [20] reported that there is no strong evidence for any particular antimicrobial agent in the prevention of amputation, resolution of infection or ulcer healing. For mild to moderate infections with no evidence of osteomyelitis or septic arthritis, consider amoxicillin–clavulanate (875 + 125 mg q 12 h oral) for at least 5 days. Alternatives include ciprofloxacin 500 mg q 12 h with clindamycin 600 mg q 8 h. For severe limb- or life-threatening infections, intravenous piperacillin–tazobactam 4 + 0.5 g q 8 h or ticarcillin–clavulanate 3 + 0.1 g q 6 h or meropenem 500 mg q 8 h are all acceptable empiric therapy. Prolonged use of appropriate bactericidal antibiotics may be required, especially in the setting of osteomyelitis or septic arthritis.

Surgical-site/postoperative wound infection

Surgical-site infections are the most commonly occurring adverse events in patients who have undergone surgery, accounting for as much as 38% of nosocomial infections in postoperative patients. Surgical-site infections are usually diagnosed by the usual features of inflammation: wound pain, redness, swelling and purulent discharge. These external signs of inflammation may manifest late in morbidly obese patients or those with deep, multilayer wounds. Most bacterial wound infections present with fever only after 48 hours. Earlier symptoms may be seen in *Strep. pyogenes* and clostridial infections.

The mainstay of treatment for surgical site infections is early opening of the incision, coupled with evacuation of any infected material and sending off of wound cultures. This should be done after consultation with the surgeon involved, where possible. There has been a paucity of evidence regarding the use of antibiotics combined with drainage [21], but expert consensus generally advocates the use of empirical antibiotics for patients with temperature >38.5°C and/or pulse rate >100 in the presence of obvious wound infection [5].

Post-traumatic wound infection

The goals of wound care are to avoid infection and to achieve a functional and cosmetically acceptable scar. Adequate wound management requires a thorough history, with particular attention directed at factors adversely affecting healing. Factors, such as the extremes of age, diabetes, chronic renal failure, malnutrition, alcoholism, obesity and patients on immunosuppressive agents, cause an increased risk of infections and impaired wound healing. Wounds located in highly vascular areas, such as the scalp or face, are less likely to become infected than wounds in less vascular areas.

In order to reduce the incidence and severity of infections, wounds need to be thoroughly cleansed and irrigated. Devitalized tissue should be removed, injuries to associated structures need to be excluded and the wound closed appropriately. The method of closure depends on the location of the wound, the level of contamination and whether it is an 'old' wound (over 6 hours old). Wounds that should not be closed because of a high risk of infection, such as heavily contaminated wounds, should be treated by delayed primary closure 3–5 days after initial management. Where primary closure is possible the wound should be closed and a protective non-adherent dressing applied for a minimum of 24–48 hours, with both the wound and the dressing kept dry [22].

The use of prophylactic antibiotics is not recommended except where there is significant bacterial contamination, foreign bodies, the patient is immunosuppressed or the wound is the result of a bite (human or animal) or associated with an open fracture. Most wounds can be treated with amoxicillin–clavulanate (875 + 125 mg q 12h oral) or metronidazole (400 mg q 12h oral) plus di(flu)cloxacillin (500 mg q 6h oral). Broad-spectrum antibiotics should be limited to heavily contaminated and bite wounds and immunosuppressed patients (see Table 9.5.2).

Intravenous drug users

Intravenous drug users frequently develop unusual infections because the needles and the drug paraphernalia used are contaminated. They also have alterations to their skin and flora and frequently have poor nutrition and immune function [23]. Many are hepatitis B, C and HIV positive. Intravenous drug users frequently have mixed organisms, particularly anaerobes, including *Klebsiella*, *Enterobacter*, *Serratia* and *Proteus*. They have mixed Gram-positive and Gram-negative infections. Some develop fungal infections, including candidaemia. Subacute bacterial endocarditis and endocarditis need to be considered in IV drug users. If endocarditis is not suspected, treatment should consist of flucloxacillin 2 g IV 6-hourly and gentamicin 5–7 mg/kg/day as a single daily dose.

Controversies

- The timing and method of closure of contaminated or 'old' (more than 6 hours since injury) wounds.
- The prophylactic use of antibiotics in patients with 'clean' wounds.
- Which antibiotics to use in treating skin and soft-tissue infections: narrow-spectrum, first-generation cephalosporin or broad-spectrum third-generation cephalosporin? Do you use antibiotics to cover Gram-negative, Gram-positive organisms, anaerobes and aerobes?
- Can more patients be treated wholly as outpatients using parenteral therapy or after early discharge once the acute toxic phase is over?
- Management of cutaneous abscesses: are antibiotics necessary after incision and drainage? Are cultures of the abscess fluid needed?

References

[1] Simonart T, Simonart JM, Derdelinckx I, et al. Value of standard laboratory tests for the early recognition of group A beta-hemolytic streptococcal necrotizing fasciitis. Clin Infect Dis 2001;32:E9–12.
[2] Perl B, Gottehrer NP, Raveh D, et al. Cost-effectiveness of blood cultures for adult patients with cellulitis. Clin Infect Dis 1999;29:1483–8.
[3] Antibiotic Expert Group. Therapeutic guidelines: antibiotics. eTG complete [Internet]. Melbourne: Therapeutic Guidelines Limited; 2013. <http://online.tg.org.au.proxy1.athensams.net/ip/> [Accessed Feb. 2013].
[4] Liu C, Bayer A, Cosgrove SE, et al. Clinical Practice Guidelines by the Infectious Diseases Society of America for the Treatment of Methicillin-resistant *Staphylococcus aureus* infection in adults and children. Clin Infect Dis 2011;52:e18–55.
[5] Stevens DL, Bisno AL, Chambers HF, et al. Infectious diseases Society of America. Practice guidelines for the diagnosis and management of skin and soft-tissue infections. Clin Infect Dis 2005;41:1373–406.
[6] Leong WC, Lipman J, Hon H. Severe soft-tissue infections – a diagnostic challenge. The need for early recognition and aggressive therapy. S Afr Med J 1997;87: 648–52, 654.
[7] Wong CH, Khin LW, Heng KS, et al. The LRINEC (Laboratory Risk Indicator for Necrotizing Fasciitis) score: a tool for distinguishing necrotizing fasciitis from other soft tissue infections. Crit Care Med 2004;32: 1535–41.
[8] Hasham S, Matteuci P, Stanley PR, Hart NB. Necrositing fasciitis. Br Med J 2005;330:830–3.
[9] Gabillot-Carre M, Roujeau JC. Acute bacterial skin infections and cellulitis. Curr Opin Infect Dis 2007;20:118–23.
[10] Wong CH, Chang HC, Pasupathy S. Necrotizing fasciitis: clinical presentation, microbiology, and determinants of mortality. J Bone Joint Surg 2003;85A:1454–60.
[11] Bosshardt TL, Henderson VJ, Organ Jr. CH. Necrotizing soft-tissue infections. Arch Surg 1996;131:846–52.
[12] Lille ST, Sato TT, Engrav LH, et al. Necrotizing soft tissue infections: obstacles in diagnosis. J Am Coll Surg 1996;182:7–11.
[13] Ben-Aharon U, Borenstein A, Eisenkraft S, et al. Extensive necrotizing soft tissue infection of the perineum. Isr J Med Sci 1996;32:745–9.
[14] Antibiotic Expert Group. Tetanus prophylaxis. In: eTG complete [Internet]. Melbourne: Therapeutic Guidelines Limited <http://online.tg.org.au.proxy1.athensams.net/ip/>; 2013 [Accessed Feb. 2013].
[15] Nakase JY. Update on emerging infections from the centers for disease control and prevention. Ann Emerg Med 2000;36:268–9.
[16] Weber CA, Wertheimer SJ, Ognjan A. *Aeromonas hydrophila* – its implications in freshwater injuries. J Foot Ankle Surg 1995;34:442–6.
[17] Amir LH, Forster DA, Lumley J, et al. A descriptive study of mastitis in Australian breastfeeding women: incidence and determinants. BMC Publ Hlth 2007;25:62.
[18] File Jr TM, Tan JS. Treatment of skin and soft-tissue infections. Am J Surg 1995;169:27S–33S.
[19] Lertzman BH, Gaspari AA. Drug treatment of skin and soft tissue infections in elderly long-term care residents. Drugs Aging 1996;9:109–21.
[20] Nelson EA, O'Meara S, Golder S, DASIDU Steering Group. Systematic review of antimicrobial treatments for diabetic foot ulcers. Diabet Med 2006;23:348–59.
[21] Huizinga WK, Kritzinger NA, Bhamjee A. The value of adjuvant systemic antibiotic therapy in localised wound infections among hospital patients: a comparative study. J Infect Dis 1986;13:11–16.
[22] Singer AJ, Hollander JE, Quinn JV. Evaluation and management of traumatic lacerations. N Engl J Med 1997;337:1142–8.
[23] Henriksen BM, Albrektsen SB, Simper LB, et al. Soft tissue infections from drug abuse. A clinical and microbiological review of 145 cases. Acta Orthop Scand 1994;65:625–8.

INFECTIOUS DISEASE EMERGENCIES

9.6 Hepatitis

Helen E Stergiou • Biswadev Mitra

ESSENTIALS

1 Acute and chronic viral hepatitis are of global public health importance.

2 Owing to the non-specific symptomatology in the early phases of acute viral hepatitis, definitive diagnosis may be delayed in the emergency setting.

3 Supportive care is fundamental in the management of hepatitis.

4 Prevention of viral hepatitis is possible via the introduction of public health programmes which include appropriate education regarding high-risk practices.

Introduction

Hepatitis is a non-specific clinicopathological term that encompasses all disorders characterized by hepatocellular injury and by histological evidence of a necroinflammatory response [1]. Prolific research has resulted in the identification of specific hepatotrophic viruses. An important distinction is that between acute and chronic viral hepatitis. Acute viral hepatitis refers to a process of self-limited liver injury of less than 6 months' duration [1]. Chronic viral hepatitis is diagnosed on pathological criteria and is characterized by a duration of more than 6 months [1].

Clinical presentations of viral hepatitis

An appropriate clinical pattern of illness and specific laboratory confirmation are necessary for the diagnosis of acute viral hepatitis. Patients with acute viral hepatitis may present quite variably: they may be asymptomatic with only mildly deranged liver function tests (LFTs), they may be symptomatic with or without jaundice or they may present with fulminant disease (severe liver failure which develops within 8 weeks of symptom onset) [2].

Various clinical phases characterize acute viral hepatitis [1–4]. The incubation phase is the time between the original infection and the initial symptoms and is the time of viral replication and laboratory evidence of hepatitis. During the pre-icteric phase non-specific symptoms evolve, such as malaise, fatigue, anorexia, nausea, vomiting, myalgias, arthralgias, abdominal discomfort. If fever is present, it is generally low grade. Cough, coryza, pharyngitis and a distaste for alcohol and tobacco smoke may be evident. Rarely meningoencephalitis may occur.

The icteric phase features a variable degree of jaundice, dark urine (bilirubinuria), pale stools (absence of bile pigment in the stool), pruritus, hepatomegaly and splenomegaly. During the convalescent phase symptoms resolve, as do liver enzyme abnormalities. In patients presenting to the emergency department (ED) during the pre-icteric phase, the diagnosis may be challenging, given their non-specific symptomatology. If the patients present during the icteric phase, focused history taking, examination and the appropriate investigations should result in a definitive diagnosis.

Laboratory investigations

Blood test abnormalities are a prominent aspect of acute viral hepatitis. Serum transaminases are typically elevated at >500 μ/L and often >1000 μ/L [5]. Alanine aminotransferase (ALT) may be characteristically higher than aspartate aminotransferase (AST) [5]. Alkaline phosphatase may be normal or mildly elevated. Serum bilirubin is variably elevated and is usually divided between conjugated and unconjugated fractions. Albumin and the prothrombin time should be normal unless hepatic synthetic function is significantly impaired. Neutropaenia and lymphopaenia may be evident transiently. Severe acute hepatitis may cause hypoglycaemia. Further specific laboratory tests for viral hepatitis will be presented subsequently.

Management

In cases of acute viral hepatitis, the fundamental management is supportive care. Many of these patients can be managed on an outpatient basis. Patients require hospitalization when they have intractable vomiting with inadequate oral intake and when they demonstrate clinical features of liver failure. Bed rest is recommended during the symptomatic phase. A well-balanced diet is beneficial. It is recommended that alcohol be avoided during the acute phase, but there is no definitive evidence that alcohol consumption post-recovery causes either relapses or progression to chronic disease [2]. Given that the liver is involved in the metabolism of a plethora of drugs, all medications must be carefully prescribed to patients with acute hepatitis.

In managing fulminant hepatic failure, it is imperative that potential patients be identified as early as possible. In the emergency setting, intubation and the concomitant critical care are necessary for patients with progressive encephalopathy. Early referral to an appropriate intensive care unit (ICU) is mandatory.

Prevention and immunization

Prevention of viral hepatitis is possible via the introduction of public health programmes, improved sanitation and vaccination programmes. Post-exposure prophylaxis regimens are particularly relevant to healthcare workers.

Hepatitis A virus (HAV)

As the most common cause of viral hepatitis, HAV contributes significantly to the global burden of disease. Multiple genotypes exist and infection with one genotype confers immunity against others [6]. (See Table 9.6.1 for virology.)

Epidemiology

HAV is highly endemic in developing countries and can often be traced to contaminated water or food.

Table 9.6.1	Characteristics of the main hepatitis viruses				
	HAV	*HBV*	*HCV*	*HDV*	*HEV*
Family	Picornavirus	Hepadnavirus	Flavivirus	Incomplete	Calicivirus
Nucleic acid	RNA	DNA	RNA	RNA	RNA
Diameter (nm)	27	42	32	36	34
Incubation period (weeks)	2–6	6–24	2–26	6–9	2–10
Spread					
Faeces	Yes	No	No	No	Yes
Blood	Uncommon	Yes	Yes	Yes	No
Sexual	Uncommon	Yes	Uncommon	Yes	?
Vertical	No	Yes	Uncommon	Yes	No
Chronic infection	No	Yes	Yes	Yes	No
Vaccine	Available	Available	Nil	Nil	Nil

Natural history

Virus is excreted in the stool of the infected person for 1–2 weeks prior to and for 1 week after the onset of symptoms. A non-specific prodrome may be followed by jaundice and tender hepatomegaly. The clinical severity of the illness increases with age, with more than 80% of children being asymptomatic [1]. HAV has been associated with extrahepatic features, such as cutaneous vasculitis, renal failure, pancreatitis, bradycardia and, rarely, convulsions, transverse myelitis and aplastic anaemia [7]. Relapsing hepatitis has been described in 20% of those with HAV infection [2]. Relapses are generally benign and may occur 4–15 weeks after the original illness. Complete recovery is the typical outcome. Fulminant hepatic failure occurs in less than 1% of cases. Chronic infection never ensues.

Laboratory investigations

Serum antibody is present from the onset of HAV disease in both IgM and IgG forms. After approximately 3–12 months, anti-HAV IgM disappears and anti-HAV IgG persists, thereby conferring lifelong immunity against re-infection.

Management

Supportive management is of primary importance. Bed rest is indicated until any jaundice settles. Potentially hepatotoxic medications must be ceased. Alcohol must not be consumed during acute episodes because of the direct nephrotoxic effects.

Prevention and immunization

General measures are imperative – safe water supplies, proper sewage disposal and careful hand washing. HAV vaccines can prevent HAV infection and, importantly, they have excellent safety profiles. Persons who have been exposed to HAV and who have not been previously vaccinated should receive the vaccine within 2 weeks of exposure. Travellers to endemic areas require inactivated hepatitis vaccine, which confers long-term immunity to more than 90% of persons.

Hepatitis B virus (HBV)

Of the viral causes of hepatitis few are of greater global importance than HBV. HBV infection is endemic in certain parts of the world – Southeast Asia, China and sub-Saharan Africa. It is estimated that there are 350 million carriers worldwide [8]. By 2017, it is estimated there will be a two- to threefold increase in the number of hepatitis B-induced liver cancer cases and a marked increase in the number of deaths attributable to hepatitis B under current treatment patterns in Australia [9]. (See Table 9.6.1 for virology.)

Epidemiology

Transmission occurs by percutaneous and mucosal exposure to infected blood products and bodily fluids, hence unprotected sexual contact with infected individuals, the use of contaminated paraphernalia during intravenous drug use and vertical transmission from mother to infant are commonly implicated.

Natural history

Many acute HBV infections are asymptomatic, particularly in younger patients. The non-specific symptoms of the acute episode may be preceded by a serum-sickness syndrome with fevers, urticaria and arthralgias [5].

Approximately 90% of patients completely recover from an acute episode of HBV infection. Fulminant hepatic failure may develop in 1% of patients and has a mortality rate of up to 80%.

Progression to chronic HBV infection occurs in 5–10% of cases, with 90% of these experiencing an asymptomatic carrier state and the remaining 10% proceeding to cirrhosis and hepatocelluar carcinoma. The risk of developing chronic disease is related to the age at which HBV is first contracted – there is a greater than 90% risk of developing chronic HBV in neonates and a less than 5% risk in immunocompetent adults [1,2]. Although chronic HBV infection is generally a lifelong condition, a small percentage of infected individuals will experience complete viral eradication. In chronic HBV infection, the incidence of cirrhosis is about 2–3% per year [10]. Variables associated with progression to cirrhosis are persistence of viral replication, older age, elevation of ALT levels and HBeAg positivity [11].

Laboratory investigations

HBsAg indicates acute hepatitis or a carrier state if it persists beyond 6 months. Anti-HBc IgM indicates acute HBV and high infectivity. Anti-HBc IgG indicates previous infection. HBeAg indicates ongoing viral replication, high infectivity or chronic hepatitis.

Management

Supportive care is the primary aim of management. Household contacts require adequate education. In cases of chronic HBV infection, the aims are to suppress HBV replication and to reduce liver injury. Interferon-alpha (IFN-α) has antiviral, antiproliferative and immunomodulatory effects and is an effective treatment option against HBV. Patients with normal serum ALT levels have a poor response to interferon-alpha because the lack of hepatic dysfunction is suggestive of low immune-mediated hepatic inflammation. The limiting factor in the use of IFN-α is the side-effect profile, which includes an influenza-like illness, gastrointestinal symptoms, psychological sequelae (particularly depression), bone marrow suppression, thyroid dysfunction and possible birth defects [5]. Lamivudine is an oral nucleoside analogue that potently inhibits HBV DNA synthesis. Human monoclonal antibodies may be directed against different epitopes of HBsAg, bind HBV particles and reduce serum viral titres and HBsAg levels. Further research is ongoing.

Prevention and immunization

The pre-exposure administration of HBV vaccine is fundamental to immunoprophylaxis. The vaccine is protective in over 90% of individuals [1]. Current recommendations include all infants at birth and individuals with high exposure risk, such as healthcare personnel, injecting drug users and high-risk sexual workers. Antibody titres may decrease with time, but the protective effects persist. The risk of HBV infection in the occupational setting is related primarily to the degree of contact with blood and to the HBeAg status of the donor. In needle-stick injuries, the risk of developing clinical hepatitis if the blood is both HBsAg- and HBeAg-positive has been estimated to be up to 30%. Post-exposure prophylaxis involves the administration of hepatitis B immunoglobulin in addition to the recombinant vaccine series.

Hepatitis C virus (HCV)

International studies estimate that up to 3% of the world's population is infected with HCV [2,12]. (See Table 9.6.1 for virology.) The identification of six major genotypes of the HCV has important clinical implications in that such genomic sequence variation makes vaccine development extremely difficult.

Epidemiology

Parenteral exposure leads to HCV infection, the use of contaminated needles and syringes being a predominant factor. Sexual and perinatal transmission of HCV is negligible. Transfusion-related HCV transmission has essentially been eradicated via donor screening. Up to 10% of HCV cases do not have an identifiable source of infection.

Natural history

A pre-icteric phase featuring non-specific symptoms develops in 15–20% of patients. When the icteric phase develops it typically lasts for 1–2 weeks. Fulminant hepatic failure rarely results from acute HCV infection.

Following an acute episode, 75–85% of adults and 55% of children will enter a chronic phase [12]. There is a high proportion of subclinical chronic HCV infection, hence patients may not manifest any pathology until incidental blood tests or end-stage liver disease many years after the initial infection. Approximately 20–30% of chronic HCV patients develop cirrhosis, with subsequent hepatocellular carcinoma occurring in up to 20% of the latter group [1,5].

Laboratory investigations

A fluctuating titre of HCV RNA is detectable within days to weeks of the initial HCV infection. The rate at which HCV antibodies develop is variable. Notably, HCV antibodies are neither neutralizing nor protective. It may not be possible to distinguish between acute and chronic HCV infection, given that the same laboratory markers can be present in both conditions. Further specific laboratory tests for viral hepatitis are presented in Table 9.6.2.

Management

Supportive management is fundamental in addressing HCV infection. Relevant education and counselling regarding high-risk behaviours and referrals to appropriate support networks are necessary. Avoidance of alcohol is advisable as some studies indicate that alcohol may promote the progression of HCV infection [13,14]. Standard therapy for HCV infection has consisted of a combination of pegylated interferon-α and ribavirin. However, the combination therapy leads to cure in only abut 50% of cases [15]. Recent advances include the use of HCV protease inhibitors, polymerase inhibitors, NS5A inhibitors and host factor inhibitors, such as cyclophilin antagonists [16,17].

Prevention and immunization

Currently, there is no effective vaccination available against HCV infection, nor is there any specific post-exposure prophylaxis regimen. Vaccination against HAV and HBV is advisable. HCV is not transmitted efficiently

Table 9.6.2 Laboratory tests in viral hepatitis

Test	Interpretation of positive test	Clinical significance
Tests for HAV		
Anti-HAV IgM	Recently acquired HAV	Acute hepatic illness
Anti-HAV IgG	Previous infection/vaccination	Immunity
Tests for HBV		
HBsAg (surface Ag)	Current/chronic infection	Structural viral component
Anti-HBsAg (surface Ab)	Previous infection/vaccination	Immunity
Anti-HBcIgM (core Ab)	Recently acquired HBV	Test for acute HBV
HBeAg	Marker of viral replication	High infectivity
Anti-HBeAg	No viral replication	Low infectivity
HBV DNA	Complete virus present	High infectivity
Tests for HCV		
Anti-HCV	HCV exposure	Variable infectivity
HCV RNA	Virus present	
Tests for HDV		
Anti-HDV IgG/IgM	HDV exposure	Acute or chronic HDV
Delta Ag	HDV present	Acute or chronic HDV
Tests for HEV		
Anti-HEV IgM	Recently acquired HEV	Acute hepatic illness
Anti-HEV IgG	Previous exposure	

Modified from Talley N, Martin C. Clinical Gastroenterology: A Practical Problem-based Approach, 2nd edn. Edinburgh: Churchill Livingstone, 2006 with permission.

through occupational exposures to blood. The average incidence of anti-HCV seroconversion after accidental exposure from an HCV-positive source is <2% [18].

Hepatitis D virus (HDV)

As a defective virus, HDV requires the presence of HBV for virion assembly and for viral replication [1,2]. (See Table 9.6.1 for virology.)

Epidemiology

Only patients with acute or chronic HBV infection are susceptible to infection with HDV. An estimated 5% of HBV carriers are infected with HDV worldwide [1,2,5]. Parenteral exposure is the primary transmission mode. HDV can occur as a co-infection with acute HBV (acquired at the same time) or as a superinfection in chronic HBV carriers.

Natural history

In cases of HDV and HBV co-infection, acute HDV infection generally presents as a benign acute hepatitis with subsequent resolution in up to 80–95% of patients. Chronic HDV/HBV infection may occur in 5–10% of patients [2]. HDV superinfection results in progression to chronic HDV/HBV in 70–80% of cases [5]. Chronic HDV/HBV infection manifests as a chronic healthy carrier state or severe liver disease. HDV superinfection may result in fulminant hepatitis in 2–20% of cases [5]. Chronic HDV infection leads to more severe liver disease than HBV monoinfection and is associated with accelerated fibrosis progression, earlier hepatic decompensation and an increased risk for the development of hepatocellular carcinoma.

Laboratory investigations

HBsAg must be detected to diagnose acute HDV/HBV co-infection. Anti-HDV IgM is transiently present in acute infections. Anti-HDV IgG appears late in acute infections.

Management

There is no specific cure for HDV infection other than suppressing HBV replication. IFN-α treatment has proven antiviral activity against HDV in humans and has been linked to improved long-term outcomes. Studies conducted in the past 2 years on the use of PEG-IFN-α show that a sustained virologic response to therapy, measured in terms of undetectable serum HDV RNA levels, can be achieved in about one-quarter of patients with hepatitis D [19].

Prevention and immunization

Currently, there is no vaccine for preventing HDV infection. HBV immunization has been shown to provide protection against the development of HDV.

Hepatitis E virus (HEV)

See Table 9.6.1 for virology.

Epidemiology

HEV is endemic in developing countries, such as Southeast and Central Asia and the Indian subcontinent. The primary transmission mode is the faecal–oral route, with contaminated drinking water and food supplies being primary sources of infection. Young adults are often predominantly affected.

Natural history

The clinical course is similar to that of acute HAV infection. Full recovery from the acute HEV infection is the norm. There have not been any recorded cases of chronic HEV infection.

Overall mortality from acute HEV infection is about 5%. For reasons which remain unclear, fulminant hepatic failure with a subsequent high mortality rate occurs in 25% of women with HEV infection during the third trimester of pregnancy. Liver transplant recipients may be at a greater risk for HEV infection, which can lead to chronic hepatitis.

Laboratory investigations

Anti-HEV IgM occurs between 1 week and 6 months after the illness onset. Anti-HEV IgG is evident during the convalescent phase or post-exposure.

Management

Supportive management is the key.

Prevention and immunization

Disease control depends on good personal hygiene and improved environmental sanitation. There is no effective vaccine.

Hepatitis G virus (HGV)

Exposure to blood products is a recognized route of acquisition of HGV infection in humans. Chronic viraemia results and reported prevalences of HGV infection range from 1% to 3% in most populations, incidences that are higher than those of either HBV or HCV in these populations [20]. A causal relationship between the prevalence of HGV and hepatitis, however, has not been proven. Although HGV RNA may persist in serum of patients acutely infected with HGV for as long as 16 years, in about 90% of these patients persistence is not accompanied by evidence of hepatocellular injury [21]. Currently, there should be no need to test for HGV in the emergency setting.

Non-hepatotrophic viruses

Several non-ABCDE viruses cause viral hepatitis. The cytomegalovirus (CMV) and Epstein–Barr virus (EBV) commonly contribute to abnormal LFTs and icteric hepatitis may also occasionally be noted. In immunocompromised patients, herpes simplex may lead to a hepatitic picture. Progression to chronic hepatitis has not been demonstrated with any of these viruses.

Non-viral hepatitis

Of the causes of non-viral hepatitis, the following are important in the emergency setting: alcoholic hepatitis, non-alcoholic steatohepatitis (NASH), drug-induced hepatitis and autoimmune hepatitis.

Alcoholic hepatitis

Alcoholic hepatitis is an important clinical syndrome which is variably characterized by anorexia, nausea, jaundice, hepatomegaly and features of portal hypertension, such as ascites and encephalopathy. Cirrhosis and death are possible sequelae if the patients do not cease their alcohol consumption.

Non-alcoholic steatohepatitis

Defects in the processing of fatty acids through the liver may cause steatosis-induced inflammation (steatohepatitis). Ten to 50% of patients with NASH are at risk of developing cirrhosis [14].

Drug-induced hepatitis

Toxic exposure to certain medications, vitamins, herbal remedies and food supplements may result in a drug-induced hepatitis. Drug-induced hepatitis may occur as an expected consequence of a drug's toxicity profile or as an idiosyncratic reaction to a standard dose. Hepatotoxic agents result in variable clinicopathological patterns of liver injury via toxic and immune mechanisms [22]. Commonly, the formation of reactive hepatotoxic metabolites is the primary underlying mechanism [23]. Extensive lists of hepatotoxic drugs can be found in the literature. Acute liver injury may be necroinflammatory (e.g. paracetamol), cholestatic (e.g. chlorpromazine) or of a mixed type. Table 9.6.3 lists drugs which may induce hepatitis and which are encountered in the emergency setting [22,23].

Autoimmune hepatitis

Autoimmune hepatitis is a self-perpetuating hepatocellular inflammation of unknown cause which is associated with hypergammaglobulinaemia and serum antibodies [14]. Fatigue, anorexia and jaundice may progress to liver failure. Corticosteroids are the basis of treatment.

Future directions

- Global emphasis on adequate public health schemes, including vaccination programmes, to control the transmission of viral hepatitis.
- Emphasis on public education regarding high-risk practices.
- Surveillance of the long-term immunity conferred by the hepatitis A and B vaccinations.
- Development of a vaccine for hepatitis C.
- Optimization of the management algorithms for chronic viral hepatitis.

Table 9.6.3 Hepatitis-inducing drugs [13,14]	
Drug	*Pathology*
Allopurinol	Hepatic granulomas
Cloxacillin	Lobular hepatitis
Chlorpromazine	Cholestatic hepatitis
Dantrolene	Cytolytic hepatitis
Erythromycin	Cholestasis with hepatitis
Flucloxacillin	Cholestatic hepatitis
Halothane	Hepatocellular injury
Isoniazid	Cytolytic hepatitis
Non-steroidals	Primarily cholestasis
Paracetamol	Cytolytic hepatitis
Phenothiazines	Cholestatic hepatitis
Phenytoin	Non-caseating granulomas
Sulphonamides	Cytolytic hepatitis

After Thomas D, Astemborski J, Rai R. The natural history of hepatitis C virus infection. Journal of the American Medical Association 2000;284:45; Friedman L, Keeffe E, Schiff E. Handbook of Liver Disease, 2nd edn. Edinburgh: Churchill Livingstone, 2004.

References

[1] Yamada T, Hasler W, Inadomi J, et al. Handbook of gastroenterology, 2nd ed. Baltimore: Lippincott Williams & Wilkins, 2005.

[2] Mandell G, Bennett J, Dolin R. Principles and practice of infectious diseases, 6th ed. Edinburgh: Churchill Livingstone, 2005.

[3] Talley N, Martin C. Clinical gastroenterology: a practical problem-based approach, 2nd ed. Edinburgh: Churchill Livingstone, 2006.

[4] Boon N, Colledge N, Walker B, et al. Davidson's principles and practice of medicine, 20th ed. Edinburgh: Churchill Livingstone, 2006.

[5] Friedman S, McQuaid K, Grendell J. Current diagnosis and treatment in gastroenterology, 2nd ed. McGraw-Hill, 2003.

[6] Lemon S, Jansen RW, Brown EA, et al. Genetic, antigenic and biological differences between strains of hepatitis A virus. Vaccine 1992;10:S40–4.

[7] Schiff E. Atypical clinical manifestations of hepatitis A. Vaccine 1992;10:S18–20.

[8] Kane M, Clements J, Hu D. Disease control priorities in developing countries. In: Jamison D, Mosley W, Measham A, Bobadilla J, editors. Disease control priorities in developing countries. New York: Oxford University Press, 1993, p. 330.

[9] Homewood J, Coory M, Dinh B. Cancer among people living in rural and remote indigenous communities in Queensland: an update 1997–2002. Queensland Health, 2005.

[10] Liaw YF, Tai DI, Chu CM, et al. The development of cirrhosis in patients with chronic type B hepatitis: a prospective study. Hepatology 1988;8:493–6.

[11] McMahon BJ, Holck P, Bulkow L, et al. Serologic and clinical outcomes of 1536 Alaska natives chronically infected with hepatitis B virus. Ann Intern Med 2001;135:759–68.

[12] Lavanchy D. Public health measures in the control of viral hepatitis: a World Health Organization perspective for the next millennium. J Gastroenterol Hepatol 2002;17: S452–9.

[13] Thomas D, Astemborski J, Rai R. The natural history of hepatitis C virus infection. J Am Med Assoc 2000;284:45.

[14] Friedman L Keeffe E, Schiff E. Handbook of liver disease, 2nd ed. Edinburgh: Churchill Livingstone, 2004.

[15] Fried MW, Shiffman ML, Reddy KR, et al. Peginterferon alfa-2a plus ribavirin for chronic hepatitis C virus infection. N Engl J Med 2002;347:975–82.

[16] Gane EJ, Roberts SK, Stedman CA, et al. Oral combination therapy with a nucleoside polymerase inhibitor (RG7128) and danoprevir for chronic hepatitis C genotype 1 infection (INFORM-1): a randomised, double-blind, placebo-controlled, dose-escalation trial. Lancet 2010;376: 1467–75.

[17] Lok AS, Gardiner DF, Lawitz E, et al. Preliminary study of two antiviral agents for hepatitis C genotype 1. N Engl J Med 2012;366:216–24.

[18] Mitsui T, Iwano K, Masuko K. Hepatitis C virus infection in medical personnel after needlestick accident. Hepatology 1992;16:1109–14.

[19] Wedemeyer H, Manns MP. Epidemiology, pathogenesis and management of hepatitis D: update and challenges ahead. Nat Rev Gastroenterol Hepatol 2013;7:31–40.

[20] Yoshibo M, Okamoto H, Mishiro S, et al. Detection of GBV-C virus genome in serum of patients with fulminant hepatitis of unknown origin. Lancet 1995;346:1131–4.

[21] Alter MJ. The cloning and clinical implications of HGV and HGBV-C. N Engl J Med 1996;334:1536–7.

[22] Farrell G. Drug-induced liver injury. New York: Churchill Livingstone, 1994.

[23] Bircher J, Benhamou J-P, McIntyre N, et al. Oxford textbook of clinical hepatology, 2nd ed. Oxford: Oxford University Press, 1999.

9.7 HIV/AIDS

Alan C Street

ESSENTIALS

1 Patients with previously undiagnosed human immunodeficiency virus (HIV) infection may present to the emergency department at any time during the course of infection, from early (acute seroconversion illness) to late (AIDS-defining illness) stages.

2 Patients with previously diagnosed HIV infection may present with complications of antiretroviral therapy or, if therapy has failed or is not taken, with a range of HIV-related clinical syndromes.

3 Globally, heterosexual transmission accounts for most HIV infections but, in Australia, HIV infection remains predominantly a disease of homosexual and bisexual men.

4 Most AIDS-defining illnesses occur when the CD4 T-lymphocyte count is $<0.2 \times 10^9$/L (bacterial pneumonia and tuberculosis are exceptions).

5 Serious non-AIDS events which are not classically associated with HIV infection, such as cardiovascular disease, bone disease, renal disease and cognitive impairment, cause significant morbidity, may occur at higher CD4 cell counts and are possibly related to chronic inflammation.

6 Combination antiretroviral therapy with well-tolerated and potent once-daily regimens dramatically reduces HIV mortality and morbidity, reduces the risk of HIV transmission from the infected individual to his or her partner and may decrease HIV transmission at a population level (treatment as prevention).

7 Close liaison between emergency department staff and the patient's hospital or local doctor is vital for optimal management of HIV-infected patients.

Introduction

HIV medicine is a complex and specialized field and emergency physicians are not the usual primary care providers for people with HIV infection. However, the emergency department (ED) is often the first point of contact for patients presenting with acute HIV-related complications, whether or not they have already been diagnosed with HIV.

Emergency medicine physicians do not need to be HIV experts, but they should develop knowledge and skills in the following areas:

- the natural history and clinical manifestations of HIV infection
- the principles of HIV diagnosis, including the ability to engage patients in discussions about HIV testing and test results
- the principles of early management of patients with common HIV-related disease syndromes
- familiarity with antiretroviral agents in current use, including toxicity and drug interactions.

The first cases of AIDS were recognized in the USA in 1981 and in Australia in 1982. The causative agent, human immunodeficiency virus (HIV), was discovered in 1984 and a diagnostic blood test developed soon thereafter. In 1986, the first effective antiviral drug (AZT, later renamed zidovudine) became available. Since the late 1990s, the use of combination antiretroviral therapy has led to dramatic reductions in HIV-associated morbidity and mortality in resource-rich countries. Antiretroviral use is rapidly increasing in poor countries, but the global HIV situation remains serious; in 2011, the World Health Organization (WHO) estimated that there were 2.5 million new HIV infections, 1.7 million deaths and 34 million people living with HIV, 23.5 million in sub-Saharan Africa and 4.8 million in Asia [1]. A major challenge in the coming years will be to develop an effective HIV vaccine.

Epidemiology

Globally, the great majority of HIV infections arise as a result of heterosexual transmission.

In developed countries, injecting drug use and sex between men account for a greater proportion of HIV infections, although the contribution of specific behaviours to overall transmission varies greatly within and between countries and over time.

In Australia up to December 2011, more than 31 000 people had been diagnosed with HIV infection, of whom an estimated 24 730 are living with HIV. Seventy-nine per cent of people infected with HIV report male-to-male sex, 15% have become infected through heterosexual transmission, 4% of cases have occurred in injecting drug users and 2% in recipients of contaminated blood or blood products. Women account for 9% of HIV-infected people and children for less than 1% [2]. Approximately 1000 new HIV diagnoses have been notified for each of the past few years, mostly among gay men. Compared to some other countries, the prevalence of HIV infection in injecting drug users has remained low, of the order of 1–2%.

Pathogenesis

Once HIV infection becomes established, one billion or more HIV virus particles are produced per day, chiefly in lymph nodes and other lymphoid tissue, accompanied by the daily turnover of up to 1 billion CD4 T lymphocytes. The number of CD4 cells falls secondary to mechanisms such as immune activation and direct infection of CD4 cells, resulting in reduced helper function for cell-mediated and humoral immunity [3].

HIV replication occurs at a relatively constant rate, producing a stable level of HIV in the blood and this can be measured with quantitative HIV RNA detection tests. The HIV viral load is used as a prognostic marker (because it is associated with the rate at which CD4 T lymphocytes are lost) and to monitor the efficacy of antiretroviral therapy.

The peripheral blood CD4 T-lymphocyte count is an accurate indicator of the degree of immunosuppression. The normal count is $0.5–1.5 \times 10^9$/L; susceptibility to opportunistic infection and to most other serious HIV-related complications is greatest when the CD4 cell count is less than 0.2×10^9/L. In untreated patients, the average rate of CD4 cell decline is $0.05–0.1 \times 10^9$/year.

A wide variety of chronic medical conditions not previously associated with HIV infection, such as cardiovascular, bone and kidney disease, mild cognitive impairment and non-HIV related cancers, are more common in HIV-infected patients [4]. Predisposition to these serious non-AIDS events results from a complex interplay between an ageing HIV-infected population, traditional risk factors, side effects of some antiretroviral agents and HIV infection itself. Chronic inflammation induced by HIV infection, which may persist despite effective antiretroviral therapy, is thought to mediate some of the direct HIV effects.

Classification and natural history (Fig. 9.7.1)

HIV infection can be conveniently divided into four stages on the basis of time after infection, CD4 T-lymphocyte count and the presence of complications [5]:

- primary infection: a febrile illness that occurs soon after acquisition of HIV infection (discussed in more detail below)
- early infection: CD4 cell count $>0.5 \times 10^9$/L – generally asymptomatic period
- intermediate infection: CD4 cell count $0.2–0.5 \times 10^9$/L – asymptomatic or less serious complications

- late infection: CD4 cell count $<0.2 \times 10^9$/L – susceptibility to AIDS-defining opportunistic infections and malignancies.

Patients are categorized as having AIDS when they develop a defined opportunistic infection, an HIV-related malignancy, a wasting syndrome or AIDS dementia complex.

Presentation

Patients with underlying HIV infection who present to the ED fall into three distinct groups. First, they may present with a manifestation of previously unrecognized HIV infection. To identify these patients, the physician must know who is potentially at risk of HIV infection (see Epidemiology above) and be aware of the many different ways in which previously undiagnosed HIV infection may present. Prompt consideration of the possibility of HIV infection is important because the differential diagnosis of the presenting problem will broaden to encompass a variety of other conditions, some of which may be life threatening and require a different approach to initial investigation and treatment.

The second group includes those who are already known to be HIV infected. Many of these patients will have been started on anti-retroviral therapy; serious HIV-related infections or malignancies are uncommon in this group, but ED presentations may be related

to complications of therapy or to the chronic medical conditions associated with HIV infection discussed in the section above. A smaller group of patients have developed resistance to or are intolerant of antiretroviral agents or decline to start or remain on treatment; these patients usually present with one of a limited number of classic, HIV-related clinical syndromes, such as fever and cough or shortness of breath, diarrhoea, unexplained fever or neurological symptoms. The initial diagnostic and treatment approach is based on knowledge of the differential diagnosis for each of these syndromes.

Finally, there will be patients whose ED presentation is not related to an HIV complication at all but who have clinically silent, 'incidental' HIV infection. Readily identifiable groups who may be in this category are patients with a sexually transmitted infection and patients with hepatitis B or hepatitis C infection. Otherwise, a brief history, including a sexual history, is required to elicit HIV risk factors. Presentation of these patients to the ED offers an important opportunity to explore HIV risk factors and to discuss the benefits of earlier HIV diagnosis and the desirability of HIV testing.

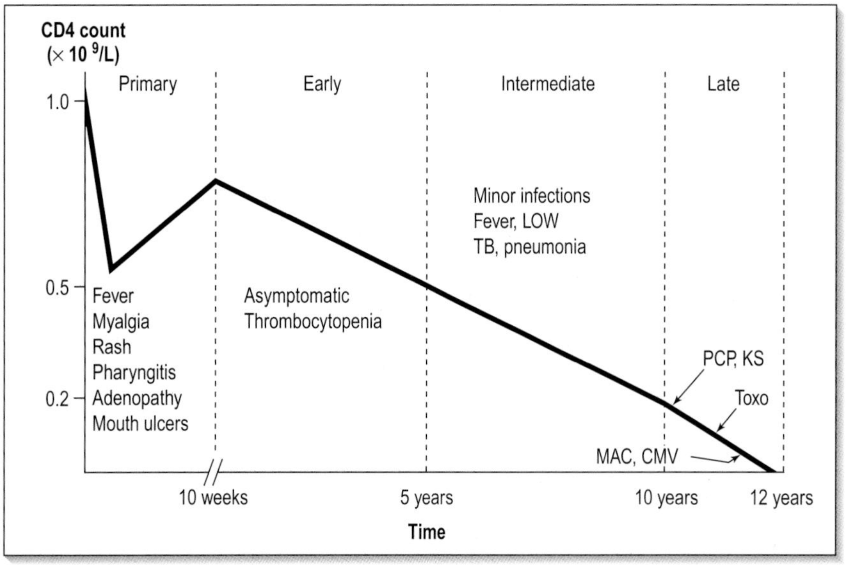

Previously undiagnosed HIV infection [6]

Primary HIV infection (acute seroconversion illness) (Table 9.7.1)

Up to 50% of patients will develop a glandular fever-like illness of varying severity 2–3 weeks after acquiring HIV. The most common features are fever, myalgia, headache, erythematous maculopapular rash, diarrhoea, lymphadenopathy and mouth ulcers. Complications include aseptic meningitis, encephalitis and Guillain–Barré syndrome. The diagnosis is often missed at this stage; patients may be thought to have a 'viral illness', such as infectious mononucleosis or, if a patient develops a complication, more common causes (for example, herpes simplex in a patient with encephalitis) and not HIV are considered.

Early infection (CD4 cell count $>0.5 \times 10^9$/L)

People are generally healthy during this phase. Thrombocytopaenia may occur and so HIV infection should be considered in appropriate patients with idiopathic thrombocytopenia.

Fig. 9.7.1 Natural history of untreated HIV infection. 'Time' represents time after infection. *(Modified with permission from Stewart G (ed.). Managing HIV. Sydney: Australasian Medical Publishing Co, 1997.)*

Table 9.7.1 Manifestations of primary HIV infection

Common (present in >30% of patients)	Less common	Complications
Fever	Diarrhoea	Aseptic meningitis
Rash	Generalized lymphadenopathy	Guillain–Barré syndrome
Myalgia/arthralgia	Painful swallowing	Encephalitis
Headache	Abdominal pain	Interstitial pneumonitis
Pharyngitis	Cough	Rhabdomyolysis
Cervical lymphadenopathy	Photophobia	Haemophagocytic syndrome
Mouth ulcers	Tonsillitis	

Intermediate HIV infection (CD4 cell count 0.2–0.5 × 10⁹/L)

This is a phase when previously undiagnosed HIV-infected patients often present with HIV-related conditions, but the clues may not be recognized as such and the underlying diagnosis can be missed. Manifestations that will alert the astute clinician include:

- minor infections: shingles, severe or very frequent orolabial or genital herpes, oral thrush
- skin conditions: extensive seborrhoeic dermatitis, worsening psoriasis
- constitutional symptoms: fever, weight loss, diarrhoea
- generalized lymphadenopathy
- more serious complications: bacterial pneumonia (especially recurrent), tuberculosis and, rarely, Kaposi's sarcoma or non-Hodgkin's lymphoma.

Late HIV infection (CD4 cell count <0.2 × 10⁹/L)

It is often not appreciated that patients may remain completely well during the early and intermediate stages of HIV infection and only present when they develop a serious HIV-related complication, such as an opportunistic infection; the ED is a common point of initial care for such patients. If the history reveals risk factors for HIV infection, HIV testing can be performed and initial investigations directed at specific HIV-related complications. However, if the patient does not volunteer this information, is not specifically asked about HIV risk factors or does not belong to a 'conventional' HIV risk group, diagnosis of the presenting illness and the underlying HIV infection are often delayed.

The following clinical situations (discussed in more detail in the following section) should prompt consideration of the possibility of underlying HIV infection:

- Diffuse bilateral pulmonary infiltrates (as a manifestation of *Pneumocystis jiroveci* pneumonia, PCP) – this is the commonest serious opportunistic infection in patients with previously undiagnosed HIV infection; it is often misdiagnosed as atypical pneumonia, leading to incorrect initial treatment with a macrolide agent or doxycycline
- Ring-enhancing space-occupying cerebral lesion – in an HIV-uninfected patient, the usual causes are tumour or bacterial brain abscess and brain biopsy is required whereas, in the setting of HIV infection, cerebral toxoplasmosis is the most likely diagnosis and brain biopsy can usually be avoided
- Tuberculosis – although the overlap between those at risk for HIV and tuberculosis is not as great in Australia as in resource-poor countries with a high HIV burden, all patients with tuberculosis should be encouraged to undergo HIV testing after appropriate counselling
- Kaposi's sarcoma – well-developed lesions (purple, oval and nodular) are easy to recognize, but early lesions are often non-descript (brown or pink and flat) and biopsy may be required for diagnosis
- Other presentations – unexplained cytopaenias (anaemia or pancytopenia) and other AIDS-defining conditions, such as non-Hodgkin's lymphoma, cryptococcal meningitis, chronic cryptosporidial diarrhoea or AIDS dementia complex (manifesting as impaired cognition and motor performance) are occasionally the first manifestation of previously unsuspected HIV infection.

Previously diagnosed HIV infection [7]

Patients with known HIV infection are much less likely now than in the past to present with the classic AIDS-related clinical syndromes indicative of advanced immunodeficiency because of the effectiveness of modern anti-retroviral treatment. However, some previously diagnosed patients have failed antiretroviral therapy or have elected not to start or continue treatment and are still susceptible to AIDS-defining conditions. (Otherwise, these presentations involve patients with previously unrecognized HIV infection, as discussed in the above section.) Patients with known HIV infection may also present with complications of antiretroviral therapy, with chronic medical conditions now associated with HIV and of course with a problem not related to HIV at all.

Cough, shortness of breath, fever

Respiratory pathogens are listed in Table 9.7.2. The most important issue to decide is whether the patient has *Pneumocystis jiroveci* pneumonia or not, because this complication is common and potentially serious. Tuberculosis must also be considered because of the need to place the patient in respiratory isolation.

- PCP (occurs in patients with <0.2 × 10⁹ CD4 cells/L): the presentation is subacute or chronic, with a non-productive cough, dyspnoea, fever and chest tightness. Physical examination reveals fever, tachypnoea and reduced chest expansion, but chest auscultation is often normal. PCP is very unlikely in patients taking regular co-trimoxazole because this drug is virtually 100% effective as PCP prophylaxis.

Table 9.7.2 Respiratory complications in HIV-infected patients

Common	Uncommon
Pneumocystis jiroveci pneumonia (PCP)	Tuberculosis
Bacterial pneumonia: pneumococcus *Haemophilus influenzae*	Atypical mycobacteria *Aspergillus* pneumonia
Bronchitis	Other infections: *Rhodococcus equi*, CMV Non-infectious: Pulmonary Kaposi's sarcoma Lymphoma

- Bacterial pneumonia (may occur when the CD4 cell count is >0.2×10^9/L): patients usually present with a short history, a productive cough and sometimes pleuritic chest pain. Physical examination may be normal or reveal signs of consolidation, a pleural rub or pleural effusion.
- Tuberculosis: the clinical features vary according to the degree of immunosuppression. If the CD4 cell count is >0.2×10^9/L, patients usually present with typical symptoms and signs of tuberculosis (chronic cough, haemoptysis, fever and weight loss) but, in late-stage infection, atypical manifestations, such as disseminated disease, are common and diagnosis is more difficult.

Focal neurological signs, convulsions or altered conscious state

These features generally indicate the presence of an intracerebral space-occupying lesion, the most common causes of which are:

- Cerebral toxoplasmosis: this infection occurs when the CD4 cell count is <0.2×10^9/L. The specific focal features depend on the site of the usually multiple lesions and may include hemiparesis, visual field defects, personality change or cerebellar signs.
- Primary intracerebral lymphoma: this complication occurs with advanced HIV infection (CD4 cell count usually <0.05×10^9/L), developed in 2–3% of AIDS patients prior to the development of effective antiretroviral therapy and is closely associated with Epstein–Barr virus (EBV) infection. Clinical presentation is indistinguishable from that of cerebral toxoplasmosis.
- Progressive multifocal leucoencephalopathy: caused by JC virus (a polyoma virus); patients present with cognitive decline or focal signs and seizures are relatively uncommon. Differentiation from cerebral toxoplasmosis and primary cerebral lymphoma requires computed tomography (CT) or magnetic resonance imaging (MRI) (see below).

Diarrhoea, with or without abdominal pain or fever

A wide range of gastrointestinal pathogens cause diarrhoea in HIV-infected patients (Table 9.7.3). Patients should be asked

Table 9.7.3 Gastrointestinal pathogens in HIV-infected patients	
Bacterial	**Protozoal**
Salmonella	Cryptosporidiosis
Campylobacter	Giardiasis
Clostridium difficile	Entamoeba histolytica
Mycobacterium avium complex (MAC)	Microsporidiosis
Viral	**Non-infectious**
CMV	Lactose intolerance
	Gastrointestinal Kaposi's sarcoma
	Lymphoma

about recent travel or antibiotic use. Bloody, small-volume diarrhoea with cramping lower abdominal pain is suggestive of a large bowel pathogen, such as cytomegalovirus, Entamoeba histolytica or Clostridium difficile, whereas profuse watery diarrhoea suggests an infection of the small bowel, such as cryptosporidiosis. However, clinical features are often of limited diagnostic value and the specific diagnosis rests on identification of the pathogen in a faecal or biopsy specimen. Prominent anal pain or tenesmus suggests the possibility of proctitis due to a sexually acquired infection, such as gonorrhoea, Chlamydia (including lymphogranuloma venereum) or herpes.

Fever without localizing features

This is chiefly a problem in those with a CD4 cell count <0.2×10^9/L. The differential diagnosis is extensive, the major causes being:

- disseminated opportunistic infections: disseminated Mycobacterium avium complex (MAC), disseminated tuberculosis, disseminated histoplasmosis (USA and South America), Salmonella bacteraemia, CMV
- focal opportunistic infections with non-focal presentation: PCP, cryptococcal meningitis, tuberculosis
- bacterial infections: sinusitis, bacterial pneumonia, primary bacteraemia (especially in patients with an indwelling long-term intravenous device, or neutropenia)
- non-HIV specific infections: right-sided endocarditis, secondary syphilis
- non-infectious causes: non-Hodgkin's lymphoma, drug fever.

Difficult or painful swallowing

This is usually due to Candida oesophagitis, in which case coexisting oral candidiasis is often present. Other causes include CMV

oesophagitis, herpes simplex oesophagitis and idiopathic aphthous ulceration.

Headache, fever, neck stiffness

Cryptococcal meningitis is the most common cause of this syndrome, although headache may be mild and signs of meningism subtle or absent. Less common causes include tuberculous meningitis, syphilitic meningitis, HIV itself and lymphomatous meningitis.

Complications of antiretroviral therapy

Antiretroviral drugs are discussed in more detail below and drug side effects are outlined in Table 9.7.4. Examples of more serious side effects and treatment complications that may prompt presentation to the ED include:

- pancreatitis – didanosine*
- hepatitis – nevirapine
- drug rash – nevirapine, abacavir, fosamprenavir*, efavirenz
- renal calculi – indinavir*, atazanavir
- lactic acidosis – zidovudine
- renal impairment – tenofovir
- anaemia – zidovudine
- jaundice – atazanavir (unconjugated hyperbilirubinaemia)
- immune reconstitution inflammatory syndrome – patients who commence antiretroviral therapy with a very low CD4 cell count may develop an exacerbation of symptoms and signs of a recently diagnosed opportunistic infection or a previously unrecognized infection may be 'unmasked'; this occurs with mycobacterial infections (notably tuberculosis) and a range of other infections.

Other presentations

- Cutaneous manifestations: Kaposi's sarcoma, infections (e.g. secondary syphilis, zoster, warts, molluscum contagiosum, and crusted scabies), eosinophilic folliculitis, drug rashes
- Abdominal pain: pancreatitis due to antiretroviral therapy, HIV cholangiopathy, intra-abdominal lymphadenopathy secondary to MAC or lymphoma, lactic acidosis and hepatic steatosis associated with antiretroviral therapy

*These agents are no longer in widespread use in Australia.

Table 9.7.4 Side effects of antiretroviral agents*

Agent	Side effect
Nucleoside/nucleotide reverse transcriptase inhibitors (NRTI)	
Zidovudine	Nausea, headache, myalgia, anaemia, neutropenia
Lamivudine (3TC)	Abnormal liver function, neutropenia, pancreatitis (all uncommon)
Emtricitabine (FTC)	Skin pigmentation
Abacavir	Hypersensitivity reaction (challenge contraindicated); associated with HLA-B*5701 (8% of Caucasian populations), perform HLA B locus typing pre-therapy
Tenofovir	Renal tubular dysfunction, renal impairment, reduced bone mineral density
Non-nucleoside reverse transcriptase inhibitors (NNRTI)	
Nevirapine	Rash, hepatitis, fever
Efavirenz	Neuropsychological symptoms (vivid dreams, insomnia, difficulty concentrating, light headedness, sleeping difficulty), rash, abnormal liver function, teratogenic in animals
Etravirine	Rash, abnormal liver function
Rilpivirine	Abnormal liver function, depression and other neuropsychological effects
Protease inhibitors (PI)	
Class effects (variable between individual agents)	Hyperglycaemia, hyperlipidaemia, redistribution of body fat, abnormal liver function, gastrointestinal symptoms
Lopinavir	Diarrhoea, nausea
Atazanavir	Hyperbilirubinaemia, renal calculi
Fosamprenavir	Rash, diarrhoea, nausea
Darunavir	Rash
Tipranavir	Rash, myalgia
Integrase inhibitors	
Raltegravir	Myalgia, abnormal liver function
Entry inhibitors	
Enfuvirtide	Injection site reactions, hypersensitivity
Maraviroc	Gastrointestinal symptoms, myalgia, respiratory infections

*Drugs that are licensed in Australia but are no longer commonly used have been omitted.

- Neuropsychiatric manifestations: depression, mania, cognitive decline
- Visual complaints: CMV retinitis (when CD4 cell count <0.05 × 10^9/L), syphilitic uveitis or chorioretinitis, rarely toxoplasma or cryptococcal chorioretinitis.

Clinically silent HIV infection with risk factors

Sexually transmitted infections

Perianal or rectal sexually transmitted infections (STIs) in men are obvious markers of HIV infection risk and should prompt testing for infection. However, STIs often 'hunt in packs', so any patient diagnosed with gonorrhoea, *Chlamydia*, syphilis, genital warts, genital herpes or another STI should also be investigated for HIV.

Other risk groups

Other patients who present with a problem unrelated to HIV but with whom the desirability of HIV testing should be discussed include those with the following risk factors:

- unprotected male-to-male intercourse
- sharing of injecting equipment

- being from a country with a high HIV prevalence
- being the sexual partner of either an HIV-positive person or a person at risk of HIV.

Investigations

Requesting an HIV test

In Australia, doctors who request an HIV test are obliged to provide patients with information about the medical, psychological and social consequences of a positive or negative HIV test and to provide the result to the patient in person. More detailed information about HIV testing can be found in guidelines issued by Australian authorities [8].

Unfortunately, practical issues mean that the emergency department is usually not an ideal setting for HIV testing. First, discussion about sensitive personal information, such as sexual history (especially if it has to be obtained via an interpreter) is difficult in an open-design, over-crowded and noisy ED. Second, many EDs do not have a mechanism for follow up of patients for provision of test results. For these reasons, a more appropriate arrangement may be to

refer patients who are discharged from the ED to their local doctor or local sexual health clinic for testing, while testing of patients admitted to hospital can be the responsibility of the admitting unit.

Widespread 'opt out' HIV testing of hospital patients is recommended in the USA but has not been adopted in Australia. However, if the 'treatment as prevention' approach is to be effective, increasing rates of testing among groups at risk of HIV will be necessary in order to reduce the number of undiagnosed HIV infections and increase HIV treatment uptake. Rapid point-of-care HIV tests, performed by appropriately trained people (but not patients), are now licensed in Australia and do not require a follow-up visit but whether these tests will have a role in settings such as emergency departments is currently unclear.

Primary HIV infection

- Full blood examination, heterophile antibody test
- HIV antibody/p24 antigen enzyme immunoassay (EIA) test: may be negative initially, in which case it is vital to repeat the test in 2, 4 and 6 weeks. A positive EIA is confirmed with a positive Western blot test
- HIV RNA (viral load) test: not generally recommended for diagnosis of primary HIV infection because false positives may occur (although with a low viral load, whereas true positives usually have a very high viral load).

Previously unrecognized HIV infection (not including primary HIV infection)

The HIV antibody/antigen EIA test will be positive in all patients and other tests are not needed for diagnosis.

Previously diagnosed HIV infection – disease syndromes

Cough, shortness of breath, fever

If the CD4 cell count is >0.2 × 10^9/L, most patients can be managed as if they did not have HIV infection. Investigations required for patients with suspected bacterial pneumonia or tuberculosis include a chest X-ray, full blood examination, sputum examination and blood cultures.

If the CD4 cell count is <0.2 × 10^9/L, investigation is almost always indicated, the extent of which will be guided by the patient's condition and the likely diagnostic possibilities and may include some or all of the following:

- oxygen saturation
- chest X-ray
- blood cultures
- sputum Gram stain, culture and acid-fast bacillus (AFB) smear and culture
- induced sputum for detection (by microscopy or polymerase chain reaction [PCR]) of PCP
- bronchoscopy – usually during inpatient admission.

A high index of suspicion for tuberculosis must be maintained; the diagnosis is generally suggested by one or more suggestive epidemiological, clinical or radiological features.

Focal neurological signs, convulsions or altered conscious state

A brain CT scan (with contrast) should be done in all patients, often as a matter of some urgency, and should always precede a lumbar puncture. MRI will often provide additional important information. The commonest causes of focal lesions are cerebral toxoplasmosis and primary intracerebral lymphoma. A *Toxoplasma gondii* IgG test will have usually been performed in those with previously diagnosed HIV infection: if positive, this indicates prior infection and a predisposition to the development of cerebral toxoplasmosis; if negative, toxoplasmosis is much less likely. Diagnosis of cerebral lymphoma is primarily based on non-response to empiric treatment for cerebral toxoplasmosis; CSF cytology, detection of EBV DNA in CSF by PCR or, occasionally, brain biopsy are required for a specific diagnosis. Progressive multifocal leucoencephalopathy manifests as focal white matter lesions visible on T2-weighted MRI scans.

Diarrhoea, with or without abdominal pain and fever

Faecal examination (preferably two to three fresh specimens collected on different days) for:

- microscopy for ova, cysts and parasites
- Cryptosporidium antigen test or stain, microsporidium stain
- culture for *Salmonella*, *Campylobacter* and *Shigella*
- *Clostridium difficile* culture and toxin, especially if recent antibiotic therapy.

Selected patients with undiagnosed diarrhoea may require colonoscopy or upper GI endoscopy if infections such as CMV, MAC or microsporidiosis are suspected. Swabs for gonorrhoea, *Chlamydia* and herpes should be taken from patients with symptoms of proctitis.

Fever without localizing features

If the CD4 cell count is $>0.2 \times 10^9$/L, serious HIV-related causes are uncommon and so investigation will be guided by clinical features, severity of illness and so on. If the CD4 cell count is $<0.2 \times 10^9$/L, most patients will need investigation, beginning with the following basic work-up:

- blood cultures, including mycobacterial blood cultures if CD4 cell count $<0.05 \times 10^9$/L
- chest X-ray
- serum cryptococcal antigen.

Additional tests for selected patients include faecal examination, sputum examination, abdominal ultrasonography or CT scanning and, occasionally, bone marrow or liver biopsy.

Difficult or painful swallowing

Oesophagoscopy and biopsy are reserved for those who fail an empirical course of antifungal therapy (see below).

Headache, fever, neck stiffness

The serum cryptococcal antigen test is a useful screening test for cryptococcal meningitis because a negative result effectively excludes the diagnosis. A lumbar puncture should only be performed after a CT brain scan and if the CT does not show a space-occupying lesion or evidence of increased intracranial pressure. CSF should be routinely sent for the following:

- protein and glucose
- Gram stain and culture (and AFB smear and culture if tuberculosis is suspected)
- India ink stain and cryptococcal antigen
- cytology
- VDRL or RPR test – only indicated if serum syphilis serology is positive.

Management

Primary HIV infection
- Symptomatic treatment.
- Specific antiretroviral therapy – role not determined.

Specific HIV syndromes

ED physicians should consult doctors experienced in treating HIV-infected patients for advice about the management of specific syndromes and opportunistic infections. The following guidelines focus on initial and empiric therapy and provide examples of treatment options, but detailed information about indications for specific agents, toxicity and so on is omitted. For more comprehensive treatment recommendations, a specialized text should be consulted [9,10].

Cough, fever, shortness of breath

Any person with suspected pulmonary tuberculosis must be placed in respiratory isolation until the diagnosis is excluded. Otherwise, on the basis of the initial diagnostic evaluation, patients can be categorized and management proceed as follows:

- significant infection unlikely: no treatment
- possible PCP: empirical PCP therapy with co-trimoxazole, and corticosteroids if PaO_2 on room air <60 mmHg
- possible bacterial pneumonia:
  - non-severe, outpatient – oral amoxicillin with or without either macrolide (e.g. clarithromycin) or doxycycline
  - non-severe, inpatient – IV penicillin plus either oral macrolide (e.g. roxithromycin) or doxycycline
  - severe – IV ceftriaxone plus IV azithromycin
- possible tuberculosis: admission, and respiratory isolation; treatment with isoniazid, rifampicin, pyrazinamide and ethambutol if diagnosis confirmed; empirical therapy is sometimes necessary depending on clinical circumstances (e.g. suspected coexisting tuberculous meningitis).

Focal neurological signs, convulsions, altered conscious state

Treatment is guided by the results of the brain CT scan. If a space-occupying lesion is found patients are treated empirically for cerebral toxoplasmosis with sulphadiazine and pyrimethamine. The CT scan is repeated after 2–3 weeks and, if no response is evident, a brain biopsy might be considered in selected patients to diagnose cerebral lymphoma. If the CT scan is normal or non-diagnostic, MRI scanning is usually indicated, and supplemented by lumbar puncture.

Diarrhoea, with or without abdominal pain and fever

Any infection identified on initial faecal examinations is treated on its merits. Symptomatic treatment with an antimotility agent, such as loperamide, is contraindicated if bloody diarrhoea and fever are present, but otherwise can be given safely to most patients. Endoscopy is generally reserved for those in whom no specific cause is identified on initial evaluation and whose diarrhoea persists despite antimotility therapy.

Fever without localizing features

Empirical antibacterial therapy (with an anti-pseudomonal agent, such as piperacillin/tazobactam, with or without an aminoglycoside or vancomycin) is indicated for patients with an absolute neutrophil count $<0.5 \times 10^9$/L; otherwise the need for specific treatment is guided by the condition of the patient and the results of the diagnostic work-up. Any long-term IV access device should be removed if infection of the device is confirmed on clinical or microbiological grounds or if diagnostic evaluation reveals no other focus of infection. Treatment for disseminated MAC (with clarithromycin and ethambutol, with or without rifabutin) is generally given only after the organism has been isolated, although occasional patients with debilitating fevers, weight loss and no other diagnosis may be treated empirically.

Difficult or painful swallowing

Empirical antifungal therapy is started with an azole agent, usually oral fluconazole. Patients with resistant *Candida* infections need treatment with an alternative azole agent, such as posaconazole, or a short course of IV amphotericin B. Patients undergo endoscopy if they do not respond to antifungal treatment and the results of histology and cultures determine subsequent treatment.

Headache, fever, neck stiffness

Patients with confirmed cryptococcal meningitis are treated with a combination of IV amphotericin B and oral 5-fluorocytosine for 2 weeks, then remain on suppressive therapy with oral fluconazole. If tuberculous meningitis is suspected empirical therapy should be started immediately, pending the results of CSF cultures.

Specific treatment of other infections

- CMV infections: IV ganciclovir or IV foscarnet
- *Salmonella* infections (non-enteric fever): ciprofloxacin

Antiretrovirals in the management of HIV infection [11]

Combination antiretroviral therapy has transformed the lives of people living with HIV infection, by improving their quality of life and by reducing the incidence of HIV-related complications and deaths by 80% or more. More than 90% of patients starting treatment with one of the current recommended antiretroviral regimens will achieve a non-detectable plasma HIV viral load and a substantial CD4 cell count increase and, in the great majority of patients, these benefits are sustained in the long term. Modern antiretroviral regimens are much more convenient, less toxic and more potent than earlier combination antiretroviral therapy, but antiretroviral therapy is not without its costs: difficulty in maintaining life-long adherence, short- and long-term toxicities of antiretroviral agents and the potential development of antiretroviral resistance.

Effective treatment is also available for patients failing therapy because of drug resistance or intolerance, using antiretroviral agents that belong to the same classes of drugs used for initial therapy or that have novel mechanisms of action. Examples include 'new-generation' protease inhibitors (tipranavir and darunavir) and non-nucleoside reverse transcriptase inhibitors (etravirine), inhibitors of CCR5 (maraviroc), a host chemokine receptor involved in HIV cell entry and the fusion inhibitor enfuvirtide [12].

The emergency physician does not require a detailed knowledge of antiretroviral therapy, but should be aware of the agents in current use, their side effects and the potential for clinically significant drug–drug interactions. More detailed information can be referenced in regularly updated antiretroviral guidelines; examples are those produced by a panel of the US Department of Health and Human Services with an added Australian commentary, accessible at http://www.ashm.org.au/aust-guidelines/ and British HIV treatment guidelines, accessible at http://www.bhiva.org/.

Indications
- Symptomatic HIV infection
- Asymptomatic HIV infection – CD4 cell count $<0.500 \times 10^9$/L
- Asymptomatic HIV infection – CD4 cell count $>0.500 \times 10^9$/L
  - pregnant women with HIV infection [13]
  - patients with chronic hepatitis B that requires treatment
  - patients with HIV-associated nephropathy

- Treatment of the infected individual in a serodiscordant relationship, to prevent transmission to the uninfected partner [14]
- After significant HIV exposure sustained by a healthcare worker (see Chapter 9.10) or following likely or definite exposure to HIV sexually.

Classes of drug[†]
- Nucleoside/nucleotide reverse transcriptase inhibitors (NRTIs): tenofovir, emtricitabine (FTC), abacavir, lamivudine (3TC), zidovudine (ZDV or AZT)
- Non-nucleoside reverse transcriptase inhibitors (NNRTIs): nevirapine, efavirenz, etravirine, rilpivirine
- Protease inhibitors (PIs): atazanavir, lopinavir, fosamprenavir, tipranavir, darunavir (all co-administered with low-dose ritonavir)
- Fusion inhibitors: enfuvirtide
- Entry (chemokine receptor 5 [CCR5]) inhibitors: maraviroc
- Integrase inhibitors: raltegravir

Initial regimens – at least three drugs
- Two NRTIs plus one NNRTI: examples are tenofovir + FTC + efavirenz (Atripla) OR abacavir + 3TC (Kivexa) plus efavirenz OR tenofovir + FTC + rilpivirine (Eviplera)
- Two NRTIs (as listed above) plus one PI (atazanavir) boosted with low-dose ritonavir
- Two NRTIs (as listed above) plus raltegravir.

Side effects [15] (see Table 9.7.4)

If an antiretroviral drug is suspected or known to be the cause of a serious side effect, the patient's treating HIV doctor or a hospital HIV doctor should be consulted. In the interim, or unless advised otherwise by the treating or hospital doctor, all antiretroviral medications, and not just the incriminating drug, should be withheld to reduce the risk of development of resistance on a less than fully suppressive therapy.

Drug–drug interactions

Some commonly used drugs metabolized by or that induce hepatic cytochrome P450 oxidases are contraindicated with certain PIs or NNRTIs; in addition, many other drugs will require dose modification or closer monitoring. Always check before prescribing any new drug to a patient on antiretroviral therapy; a very useful website (from the University of Liverpool, UK) is www.hiv-druginteractions.org.

[†]Drugs that are licensed but are no longer in common use in Australia have been omitted.

Disposition

Patients with newly diagnosed HIV infection should be referred to a specialized HIV clinic or to a doctor with expertise in HIV medicine.

HIV medicine is a complex and rapidly changing field. For this reason, the management of patients with known HIV infection presenting to the ED should always involve consultation with a hospital doctor knowledgeable about HIV infection, such as an infectious diseases physician or immunologist. The patient's usual HIV doctor (a hospital specialist, sexual health physician or general practitioner with a high HIV caseload) can be contacted to obtain important details, such as recent CD4 cell count and current antiretroviral agents, in the event that such information is not otherwise immediately available. In general, patients with a suspected or confirmed serious opportunistic infection will need to be admitted for investigation and management. Patients in the final stages of AIDS (fortunately an uncommon group nowadays in wealthy countries like Australia) or those with less serious complications, can often be managed in the community, in which case liaison with the local doctor, home-care nurses or community-care agencies is vital.

Prognosis

Prior to the widespread use of opportunistic infection prophylaxis and effective antiretroviral therapy, 50% of patients developed AIDS 10 years after becoming HIV infected and 75% of patients after 13 years. Following an AIDS-defining illness, the median survival was 12–24 months. Long-term non-progressors, who have a normal CD4 cell count and no HIV-related complications without antiretroviral therapy after 10 or more years of HIV infection, comprise less than 5% of patient cohorts.

Most AIDS-defining infections, such as PCP, now have low mortality and high 1-year survival rates if the infection is treated appropriately and patients are started promptly on combination antiretroviral therapy, but survival rates following diagnosis of disseminated MAC and CMV end-organ disease are lower because these two opportunistic infections usually occur at a very advanced stage of HIV infection. Combination antiretroviral therapy has reduced the mortality and incidence of opportunistic infections by over 80%.

Data from several large cohort studies indicate that average life expectancy in developed countries for patients on long-term antiretroviral therapy is close to but still lower than that of the HIV-uninfected population [16]. This difference is partly accounted for by an excess of deaths due to chronic conditions not typically associated with HIV infection, such as cardiovascular disease, non-HIV associated malignancy and renal disease (discussed earlier in the chapter); classic HIV complications, such as opportunistic infections or HIV-related malignancies, still occur but do not contribute substantially to this difference.

Prevention

Prevention of HIV transmission

- Public health and educational efforts to encourage the adoption of safer sex practices
- HIV screening of blood, blood products and tissue donors
- Non-sharing and use of clean needles and syringes by injecting drug users
- Observance of standard precautions by workers in healthcare settings
- Use of antiretroviral therapy and avoidance of breastfeeding to prevent transmission from an HIV-infected mother to her baby
- Use of antiretroviral therapy to prevent transmission from an infected individual to an uninfected partner [14]
- Use of antiretroviral prophylaxis after significant occupational exposure (see Chapter 9.10) or sexual exposure to HIV (post-exposure prophylaxis)
- Use of antiretroviral prophylaxis by an uninfected individual before HIV exposure (pre-exposure prophylaxis) [17]
- Male circumcision – shown to reduce the acquisition of HIV infection by 60% in studies in sub-Saharan Africa [18].

Prevention of HIV-related complications [19]

Infection	Preventive measure
Pneumococcal pneumonia	Pneumococcal vaccination
Latent tuberculous infection	Isoniazid
PCP	Co-trimoxazole
Toxoplasmosis	Co-trimoxazole
MAC	Azithromycin or rifabutin

Controversies

- With the availability of more potent, more convenient and better-tolerated antiretroviral drugs, should all patients and not just those below a certain CD4 cell count threshold be treated?
- Will the 'treatment as prevention' approach (broadening treatment indications for people already known to be HIV-infected and increasing testing rates in at-risk groups in order to diagnose and then treat people with unrecognized HIV) lead to a reduction in HIV transmission at the population level?
- What is the role of other prevention measures that are known to be effective, such as pre-exposure prophylaxis and male circumcision?
- What is the relative contribution of HIV infection, antiretroviral therapy and standard risk factors to the risk of developing chronic medical conditions that are responsible for most of the morbidity and mortality in patients on effective antiretroviral therapy, and what is the nature of the association?
- Can an effective HIV vaccine be developed?
- Can HIV ever be eradicated?

References

[1] UNAIDS. Global report: UNAIDS report on the global AIDS epidemic 2012. Geneva: WHO, 2012.

[2] The Kirby Institute. HIV, viral hepatitis and sexually transmissible infections in Australia Annual Surveillance Report 2012. The University of New South Wales, Sydney: The Kirby Institute, 2012.

[3] Cameron PU, Kelly M. HIV immunopathology. In: Hoy J, Lewin S, Post JJ, Street A, editors. HIV management in Australasia: a guide for clinical care. Darlinghurst: Australasian Society for HIV Medicine, 2009, p. 19–37.

[4] Phillips AN, Neaton J, Lundgren J. The role of HIV in serious diseases other than AIDS. AIDS 2008;22:2409–18.

[5] Stewart G, editor. Could it be HIV? Sydney: Australasian Medical Publishing Company Ltd, 1994.

[6] Giles M, Workman C. Clinical manifestations and the natural history of HIV. In: Hoy J, Lewin S, Post JJ, Street A, editors. HIV management in Australasia: a guide for clinical care. Darlinghurst: Australasian Society for HIV Medicine, 2009, p. 125–33.

[7] Post JJ, Kelly C, Clezy M, et al. Key opportunistic infections. In: Hoy J, Lewin S, Post JJ, Street A, editors. HIV management in Australasia: a guide for clinical care. Darlinghurst: Australasian Society for HIV Medicine, 2009, p. 133–66.

[8] National HIV Testing Policy Expert Reference Committee 2011. National HIV testing policy 2011. Commonwealth of Australia, Canberra. <http://testingportal.ashm.org.au/hiv> [Accessed Feb. 2013].

[9] Hoy J, Lewin S, Post JJ, Street A, editors. HIV management in Australia: a guide for clinical care. Darlinghurst: Australasian Society for HIV Medicine, 2009.

[10] Crowe S, Hoy J, Mills J, editors. Medical management of the HIV-infected patient (2nd ed.). Cambridge: Martin Dunitz, 2001.

[11] Pett S, Pierce A. Antiretroviral therapy. In: Hoy J, Lewin S, Post JJ, Street A, editors. HIV management in Australasia: a

guide for clinical care. Darlinghurst: Australasian Society for HIV Medicine, 2009, p. 59–73.

[12] Hirschel B, Perneger T. No patient left behind–better treatments for resistant HIV infection. Lancet 2007;370:3–5.

[13] Panel on Treatment of HIV-Infected Pregnant Women and Prevention of Perinatal Transmission. Recommendations for use of antiretroviral drugs in pregnant HIV-1-infected women for maternal health and interventions to reduce perinatal HIV transmission in the United States (last updated 31 July 2012). <http://aidsinfo.nih.gov/contentfiles/lvguidelines/PerinatalGL.pdf> [Accessed Feb. 2013].

[14] Cohen MS, Chen YQ, McCauley M, et al. Prevention of HIV-1 infection with early antiretroviral therapy. N Engl J Med 2011;365:493–505.

[15] Carr A, Vujovic O. Approaches to the management of antiretroviral therapy toxicity. In: Hoy J, Lewin S, Post JJ, Street A, editors. HIV management in Australasia: a guide for clinical care. Darlinghurst: Australasian Society for HIV Medicine, 2009, p. 103–13.

[16] The ART Cohort Collaboration. Life expectancy of individuals on combination antiretroviral therapy in high-income countries: a collaborative analysis of 14 cohort studies. Lancet 2008;372:293–9.

[17] Grant TM, Lama JR, Anderson PL, et al. Preexposure chemoprophylaxis for HIV prevention in men who have sex with men. N Engl J Med 2010;363:2587–99.

[18] Gray RH, Kigozi G, Serwadda D, et al. Male circumcision for HIV prevention in men in Rakai, Uganda: a randomised trial. Lancet 2007;369:657–66.

[19] Panel on Opportunistic Infections in HIV-Infected Adults and Adolescents. Guidelines for the prevention and treatment of opportunistic infections in HIV-infected adults and adolescents: recommendations from the Centers for Disease Control and Prevention, the National Institutes of Health, and the HIV Medicine Association of the Infectious Diseases Society of America. Available at http://aidsinfo.nih.gov/contentfiles/lvguidelines/adult_oi.pdf. Accessed (25/8/13).

9.8 Sexually transmitted infections

Jane Terris

ESSENTIALS

1 Sexually transmitted infections (STIs) are among the commonest infections worldwide and affect around 340 million new patients per year.

2 STIs account for a significant number of emergency department (ED) visits per year and, despite public health efforts, are increasing each year in Australia.

3 ED staff should be competent to screen, diagnose, treat, notify and improve future sexual health through advice and referral.

4 Emergency physicians should aim to provide effective, confidential, non-judgemental care and this may involve staff challenging their own prejudices around sexual behaviour in order to remain objective.

5 Patients may present at any stage of the STI and with multiple co-existent STIs. Presentation with genital ulcers or with signs of discharge, urethritis or cervicitis are the usual clinical manifestations.

6 STIs may be asymptomatic, missed or undertreated leading to adverse outcomes including chronic infection and infertility.

7 A detailed and specific sexual history should be normalized in the context of the general medical history and should be confidential.

8 The essentials of the sexual history can be summed up by the five Ps: Partners, Practices, Pregnancy, Protection, Past STIs.

9 Empirical treatment may need to be commenced in the ED. Screening test results are rarely available at presentation currently, although point of care testing is becoming more widespread.

10 Syndromic treatment, according to symptoms, is likely to be more successful in males, especially in high prevalence areas. Most cases of vaginal discharge in females are not STI related and many STIs in females are asymptomatic.

Introduction

Sexually transmitted infections (STIs) are among the commonest infections worldwide and continue to be epidemic in all societies. STIs are a major public health problem and are contracted by around 340 million patients per year according to World Health Organization figures [1]. STIs account for a significant number of emergency department (ED) visits per year and notification rates in Australia [2], in common with the UK [3] and the USA [4], currently show a yearly increase. The true incidence of STIs is difficult to ascertain in view of variations in regional reporting and likely under reporting.

EDs should aim to provide effective and confidential care in a sensitive and non-judgemental environment. This may be a challenge for a busy, noisy department with multiple simultaneous care priorities.

The ED management of STIs should include screening, diagnosis, treatment of patients and contacts, notifying confirmed cases to public health authorities and optimizing future sexual health through advice and referral.

Patients will continue to use ED to access general and sexual healthcare needs, therefore, emergency physicians (EPs) must have a sound working knowledge of STI management. This may be the only opportunity to intervene.

Patients may present at any stage of the STI and with multiple coexistent STIs. A detailed and specific sexual history should be normalized within the context of the general medical history.

STIs may be asymptomatic, missed or undertreated, resulting in adverse outcomes including ectopic pregnancy, chronic infection and infertility.

EPs should maintain a high index of suspicion, avoid stereotyping patients and be prepared to treat empirically, especially in males in areas of high prevalence.

Patients should be referred for follow up including HIV and hepatitis screening.

ED patients have high rates of asymptomatic STIs [5] and over half of females presenting with chlamydia or gonorrhoea are discharged without adequate treatment [6]. Conversely, most females presenting with vaginal discharge do not have STIs and are more likely to have candidiasis or bacterial vaginosis. Debates around whether to screen for STIs and HIV in EDs versus specialist clinics continue. The cost of screening, especially if adequate and accessible specialized facilities exist nearby and the potential for increasing antibiotic resistance with empirical treatment must be weighed against the consequences of missed infections and the significant public health, social and economic burden of undiagnosed and untreated STIs. Alternative facilities may not be accessible at the time of presentation. There is, therefore, an important opportunity for the EP to intervene and capture these patients at presentation.

Epidemiology

Sexually transmitted infections are increasing overall in Australia, the UK and the USA, although likely under reporting means that true figures are unknown. There are several well-documented high-risk groups for STIs and some newly emerging patient groups. Those known to be high risk include young people in the 15–24 age group, patients who exchange sex for money or drugs, also known as transactional sex, pregnant women and men who have sex with men (MSM). Recently reported at-risk groups include users of erectile dysfunction medication [7] and widowers. A high index of suspicion should be maintained in view of the fact that STIs can affect any sexually active person and stereotyping should be avoided.

The commonest STI in Australia, the UK and the USA is chlamydia, with an increase in Australia from 103 to 357 cases per 100 000 population between 2001 and 2011 [2]. The next commonest is gonorrhoea with an increase of 53 cases from 31 between 2001 and 2011 [2].

Syphilis is currently increasing overall in Australia, as in the UK [3] and the USA [4] with 659 reported cases in Australia in 2005 to 1285 in 2011 [2]. No cases of chancroid or donovanosis have been reported in Australia for over 10 years [2], although there are still some endemic regions including Papua New Guinea and parts of India and Africa, with reported cases mainly in tropical and subtropical regions.

Prevention

Public health campaigns have been active around STI prevention, although rates of infection continue to increase. It is not clear whether this is linked to increased awareness and reporting. Advice should include discussion around high-risk behaviour and safe sex practices. This should include effective barrier contraception in the form of latex condoms, rather than the less protective non-latex alternatives, the need to abstain from sex until STI treatment is complete and the need for regular STI screening, especially in high-risk groups.

History

Effective communication is especially important within the context of a sexual history and patients are often embarrassed and anxious. Wherever possible a private, clean, comfortable cubicle with a door should be used for taking the sexual history. Attention should be paid to the initial greeting, appropriate body language, eye contact, which varies culturally, and non-verbal cues from the patient. Be prepared that this may take a little longer than the focused history often used in EM. It may be necessary for the EP to reflect on their own personal attitudes to sexual behaviour in order to normalize the sexual history within the overall medical history and make an objective assessment. Communication needs of specific patient groups in ED with regard to language, hearing difficulty and cultural context should be addressed. Resources may include

interpreter services, websites and local support organizations.

Efforts should be made to reinforce the confidential nature of the interview in order to encourage candour. It may help to display local STI clinic posters and literature within the ED. Students and observers will need the consent of the patient to be present and this is not always given due to the sensitive nature of the interview and the need for confidentiality. A detailed and specific history is important to identify those patients at risk for sexually transmitted infections, including HIV, and to ascertain which anatomical sites to focus on for screening. The history may start with open statements and questions, such as telling the patient it is important to ask questions around their sexual behaviour, and progress to closed questions around specifics of the five Ps of the history, below. It may be necessary to explain clearly the need to ask certain questions in order to avoid offence. For example, explaining that asking about the gender of a partner is needed to identify MSM in order to offer rectal, pharyngeal and hepatitis screening tests and that questions around partners are necessary to allow contact tracing and follow up. The history often opens with the presenting local symptoms, including discharge or genital ulcers. Further questions should ask about the characteristics of any discharge, abdominal and pelvic pain, dyspareunia, dysuria, joint and eye symptoms and skin rashes. The history should look for risk factors for STI in general, for specific features of STIs and should also screen for complicated, disseminated or recurrent infection. A previous history of STI, or partner infection and treatment, and the possibility of pregnancy should be explored. It is important to adapt the questioning style within the cultural context as many patients will be unfamiliar and uncomfortable with discussing details of their sexual practices.

The sexual history can be summarized in terms of the five Ps: Partners, Practices, Pregnancy, Protection and Past STIs (Table 9.8.1). The skill of taking a focused sexual history including the points below, in the time available in ED, takes practice.

Partners

Ask how many in the past year and how many in the past 3 months, what gender, current length of relationship, risk factors of partners, for example IV drug use, and other partners outside the relationship.

Table 9.8.1 Essentials of the sexual history

The five Ps of the sexual history	Essential points to cover
Partners	Last 3 months who, how many, where from, risk factors in partners?
Practices	Is sexual contact vaginal, oral, anal and with whom? Are condoms used sometimes, always, never?
Protection	How is risk reduced, e.g. monogamy, condoms?
Pregnancy	Plans around becoming or preventing pregnancy and details of contraception used
Past STIs	In patient and partners – what infections, when and how were they treated, how were they followed up? Screening since?

Practices

Number and genders of recent partners within the past 3 months, whether condoms are used always, sometimes, never and, if not, in which situations condoms are not used, whether sexual acts are vaginal, anal insertive or anal receptive, oral and with whom. A history of recent travel may identify infections in areas where specific pathogens or antibiotic resistance are known.

Pregnancy

Assess for current risk of pregnancy, which may affect treatment options and follow up, whether contraception is used or not and what type, in addition to any pregnancy-related symptoms, including last menstrual period. All females of childbearing age should have a pregnancy test. The need for emergency contraception should be assessed and a cervical cytology history included.

Protection

It is useful to ask what the patient does to protect themselves from STIs and HIV, including monogamy, condoms, safer sexual practices and also to gauge the patient's perception of their own and partners' risks.

Past STIs

Previous STIs may indicate higher risk behaviour and also repeat infection. Ask specifically whether the patient has ever had, and been treated for, gonorrhoea, chlamydia or any other STI, including HIV testing and results, and about hepatitis testing and results.

General principles of examination and screening

Following the full sexual history, a comprehensive STI check should be offered.

A chaperone should be available for all intimate examinations. Examination should be performed in a comfortable private cubicle with a door that closes and, preferably, with screens available for additional privacy. A good light source is essential and swabs and specimen pots should be readily available.

General physical examination including the mouth, pharynx, lymph nodes and skin should then be followed by genital examination, with palpation for inguinal lymph nodes, careful inspection of the genital and perianal areas for discharge, papules, ulcers, warts, lice or nits and signs of local trauma. Examination beneath the foreskin in the male is important and inspection of the urethral meatus for lesions and discharge. The scrotum, testes and epididymis should be examined for lesions and tenderness and the anorectal area examined, including a digital exam and proctoscopy in patients at risk of rectal disease or presenting with anorectal symptoms.

Examination of the vulva, Bartholin's glands, vagina, cervix and perianal area is important in the female and should include bimanual pelvic examination to assess for tenderness and masses. A pregnancy test should be performed on all women of childbearing age.

It is important to confirm with the laboratory which specimen tubes and transport media are needed for which tests and how specimens should be stored, for example gonorrhoea swabs should be kept at room temperature. A ready made testing pack supplied by the laboratory is useful and will generally include swabs with charcoal transport medium for urethral and high vaginal smear and culture, glass slides for high vaginal or urethral smear, wire cottontip swabs with plastic shaft tube for chlamydia, gonorrhoea and herpes NAAT and clotted blood tubes for serological tests.

Specimen collection is a specialist skill upon which the diagnosis rests and advice from laboratory staff prior to collection is invaluable. Swabs should be taken from the appropriate areas as detailed below, for microscopy, culture and sensitivity (M, C and S) and nucleic acid amplification testing NAAT for chlamydia, gonorrhoea, trichomonas and other organisms as indicated. This may include the genital area, anorectal area and pharynx.

Urine should be sent as first void specimen for M, C and S and NAAT testing for specific organisms and a midstream specimen for general M, C and S. Swab or lesion scraping should be sent if ulcers are present. Blood should be taken for syphilis, HIV and hepatitis serology.

Clinical features of specific infections

STIs may be asymptomatic or may present with constitutional or focal symptoms (Table 9.8.2). Focal symptoms are commonly those of urethritis or cervicitis or genital ulcers. Disseminated infection may present with skin rash, joint or eye symptoms. One or more STDs may coexist and, as the clinical features may be indistinguishable, empirical treatment, especially in males in areas of high prevalence, is indicated. Syndromic treatment, according to symptoms, has been shown to be neither sensitive nor specific in females presenting with vaginal discharge because most cases of vaginal discharge are not caused by STIs and many STIs in females are asymptomatic. In areas of high prevalence, a judgement should be taken on each individual case as to whether symptoms are likely to be STI related and whether treatment is indicated prior to results. Around one-third of cases of vaginal discharge presenting to ED remain undiagnosed pathologically [7], which may reflect inadequate specimen sampling or possibly other non-infective physiological causes.

Infections presenting with discharge, urethritis and cervicitis

These symptoms may be caused by chlamydia, gonococcus, *Trichomonas vaginalis*, *Ureaplasma urealyticum* and *Mycoplasma genitalium*. Occasionally, genital herpes may cause discharge, although this is seldom the only symptom. Candida and bacterial vaginosis also

Table 9.8.2 Clinical presentation of STIs and differential diagnosis

Symptoms	Differential diagnosis	
Vaginal discharge	Candida albicans Trichomonas vaginalis Neisseria gonorrhoeae Chlamydia trachomatis Herpes simplex Bacterial vaginosis	
Urethritis or cervicitis	Neisseria gonorrhoeae Chlamydia trachomatis Mycoplasma genitalium Ureaplasma urealyticum Trichomonas vaginalis	
Genital ulcers	Syphilis	Primary chancre, secondary ulcers, tertiary gumma
	Chancroid LGV Donovanosis Herpes virus	

Trichomoniasis

This infection occurs mainly in females and is caused by the protozoan *Trichomonas vaginalis*. The incubation period is up to 1 month. Infection may be asymptomatic or may present with genital irritation and vaginal discharge or urethritis in males. The discharge is rarely frothy and green coloured but, more commonly, clear and offensive. Other symptoms may include dysuria, dyspareunia and pelvic pain. Untreated trichomonas may cause pelvic inflammatory disease. Diagnosis is by visualization of the protozoa if a wet mount is readily available within 20 minutes, but more accurate diagnostic methods include high vaginal or urethral swabs for NAAT. Treatment is with metronidazole 2 g oral single dose or tinidazole 2 g oral if not pregnant. Pelvic inflammatory disease should be treated with combination antibiotics as described previously.

Urethritis or urethral discharge in males

This is usually caused by gonorrhoea or chlamydia, but may also be caused by *Ureaplasma urealyticum*, *Mycoplasma genitalium*, *Trichomonas vaginalis* or the herpesvirus. Diagnosis is made by the clinical history (although this will not indicate the causative organism) plus urethral swab and first void urine specimen for NAAT, culture and cell count. Midstream urine should be sent for general M, C and S as UTI, especially in older males, may be the cause. Treat empirically if STI is likely for gonorrhoea and chlamydia with ceftriaxone 500 mg IM once and azithromycin 1 g oral once.

Candida

Vaginal candidiasis may feature in the differential diagnosis of STIs causing irritation and discharge, but is generally not a sexually transmitted infection. It is caused by the fungus *Candida albicans* in most cases and characterized by an itchy white, curd-like discharge. Swabs for Gram stain or wet mount specimens may confirm the diagnosis by visible yeast and pseudohyphae. Treat with clotrimazole 500 mg single dose vaginal pessary or fluconazole 150 mg oral single dose.

Bacterial vaginosis

Bacterial vaginosis is not caused by any one specific organism and may occur in women who are not sexually active. It is associated with having multiple sexual partners and is a differential diagnosis of STI-related vaginal

present with discharge, although these are not classically sexually transmitted infections.

Chlamydia

Chlamydia is the most common STI in Australia and is increasing yearly in Australia, the UK and the USA. It is caused by the organism *Chalamydia trachomatis* and often coexists with gonorrhoea and other STIs. Chlamydia is often asymptomatic, especially in women [9]. This leads to underdiagnosis and treatment, which may result in long-term complications, including pelvic inflammatory disease and infertility. Screening in sexually active females under 25 and older females with new or multiple sexual partners is advised, although routine screening is not advised in sexually active males [10]. Symptoms, if present, are most commonly a mucopurulent cervical or vaginal discharge, intermenstrual bleeding and dysuria in females, or symptoms of urethritis, proctitis and epididymitis in males including urethral discharge, itching and sterile pyuria. Males may present with Reiter's syndrome.

Diagnosis is made by Gram stain of urethral, vaginal or cervical discharge or first voided urine for NAAT.

Treatment for uncomplicated infection is with azithromycin 1 g oral as a single dose. If pelvic inflammatory disease is likely, ceftriaxone 500 mg IM once and metronidazole 400 mg oral bd for 14 days should be added.

Gonorrhoea

Gonococcal infections are increasing and are the second most common STI in Australia [2],

the UK [3] and the USA [4]. They are caused by the Gram-negative intracellular diplococcus *Neisseria gonorrhoeae* which has an incubation period of 10–14 days. Infection in females is often asymptomatic and may coexist with chlamydia. Untreated gonococcal infection may lead to pelvic inflammatory disease and ectopic pregnancy in females and epididymitis and prostatitis in males. Symptomatic presentation is usually with purulent penile discharge in males and pelvic discomfort and mucopurulent cervicitis in females. Rectal infection is seen in up to 50% of females and in MSM. The latter may also have pharyngeal gonorrhoea which is often asymptomatic. Gonococcus in urban Australia is isolated more commonly in males in pharyngeal and rectal specimens and in genital isolates in both genders in rural areas [11]. Gonococcal infections may disseminate to cause constitutional symptoms of fever and malaise and focal signs of septic arthritis, tenosynovitis and a distinctive skin rash of pustular lesions on an erythematous base on the palms and fingers.

Diagnosis is made by Gram stain of swabs and NAAT testing of swabs and urine. Treatment of uncomplicated infection is with ceftriaxone 500 mg IM with 2 mL 1% lignocaine. Gonococcal antibiotic sensitivities change rapidly, with fluoroquinolone resistance widely documented and some regions, for example the Northern Territory of Australia and Southeast Asia, have penicillin-sensitive strains. Current local advice should always be sought.

discharge. It is characterized by an overgrowth of normal vaginal flora by anaerobic bacteria and may be asymptomatic or present with discharge. Diagnosis is by Gram stain, combined with the characteristic thin, offensive discharge and clue cells on microscopy. Treat with metronidazole 400 mg bd oral for 7 days.

Infections presenting with genital ulcers

Genital ulceration may be caused by the herpes virus, syphilis and, rarely, chancroid, lymphogranuloma venereum (LGV) and lymphogranuloma inguinale (Donovanosis). These infections have higher rates of HIV co-transmission. Genital ulceration may rarely be caused by malignancy and referral should be made for any lesion that does not respond to treatment. There have been recent reports of an increase in vulval cancer in young indigenous Australian females [12].

Herpes simplex

Herpes simplex virus (HSV) infections are common worldwide, although most are asymptomatic. Genital ulceration is more commonly caused by HSV type 2 and occurs in up to one-quarter of patients who are seropositive for the virus. HSV type 1 generally causes oro-labial blisters, but may also cause genital ulceration identical to HSV-2. Subclinical infections may spread by viral shedding during sex. The primary outbreak of genital ulceration is usually accompanied by constitutional symptoms of fever, malaise, headache and painful bilateral regional lymphadenopathy which may precede the ulceration by 1 or 2 days. Prodromal tingling or paresthesia in the affected dermatomes may occur. The lesions are initially vesicular with an itchy, erythematous base and then become ulcerated before forming a scab. They may occur around the vulva, anus, thighs or buttocks in women and on or around the penis, perianal area, thighs and buttocks in males. They are usually very painful and adequate analgesia is important. Females may experience urinary retention due to the pain of voiding and sacral radiculopathy and may require admission for catheterization and intravenous antiviral treatment. The virus is shed for up to 2 weeks after the rash appears and lesions usually heal within 3 weeks. Recurrent episodes are generally less severe. Genital herpes is diagnosed by the characteristic

clinical features and confirmation may be possible from viral swabs of lesion fluid, although treatment should be commenced empirically. Severe or disseminated infection should be treated by high-dose intravenous antivirals with a duration adequate to ensure lesion healing. The patient should be informed that treatment does not cure and there may be recurrent episodes. Future episodes can be attenuated if treatment is commenced at the onset of symptoms. Frequent recurrences (more than six per year) may indicate the need for prophylactic antiviral therapy. Diagnosis is clinical and confirmation is by dry swab of the ulcer base or blister fluid for NAAT. Treatment is with valacyclovir 500 mg bd for 7–10 days for the primary episode or 3 days for recurrent episodes.

Chancroid

Chancroid is a disease mainly seen in Asia, Africa and the Caribbean, with few cases reported in the developed world. There have been no reports in Australia for 10 years to 2012. It is caused by the Gram-negative bacillus *Haemophilus ducreyi* and presents with painful genital ulcers of up to 2 cm diameter. Painful inguinal lymph nodes may go on to suppurate if the infection is untreated. Chancroid may coexist with other genital ulcerating infections including syphilis and herpes simplex. Unlike herpes, chancroid is rarely accompanied by constitutional symptoms and is rarely recurrent. Diagnosis is generally clinical, although lesion swabs for culture and NAAT may confirm the diagnosis. Treatment is with azithromycin 1 g oral once or ceftriaxone 500 mg IM once.

Lymphogranuloma venereum

LGV is caused by *Chlamydia trachomatis* and is endemic in parts of Africa, South America, India, Southeast Asia and the Caribbean, although rarely seen in the developed world. Occasional cases occur in Australia and North America. There are three clinical stages. The initial presentation with a painless ulcer or papule may be missed. The second stage involves painful inguinal lymphadenopathy which is commonly unilateral. The third stage involves strictures, fistulae and scarring around the perianal area. Diagnosis is clinical with exclusion of other causes. Serology is not available everywhere.

Treatment is with doxycycline 100 mg orally twice daily for 21 days or erythromycin 500 mg four times daily for 21 days or azithromycin 1 g oral weekly for 3 weeks.

Donovanosis

This is now a rare infection overall, although there are pockets of increased prevalence in desert areas of central Australia and in rural tropical and subtropical areas including South East India, South Africa, Papua New Guinea and the Caribbean. Despite this, there have been no reported cases for over 10 years in Australia to 2012. It is caused by *Klebsiella granulomatis* and is seen more commonly in males. The incubation period is up to 12 weeks. Red papules in the genital and perianal area evolve into nodules of friable granulation tissue that bleed easily. The initial lesions may resemble chancroid and progress to spread and necrose with loss of genital tissue and depigmentation if untreated. Diagnosis is generally clinical and may be confirmed by lesion swab or scraping for NAAT, although specialized laboratory services may be required for testing. Treat with azithromycin 1 g oral weekly for at least 4 weeks or until fully healed.

Syphilis

Syphilis is currently increasing especially among MSM, with increased reporting worldwide including Australia, the UK and the USA. The causative organism is the spirochaete *Treponema pallidum*. Patients may present with symptoms in any of the three stages of primary, secondary or tertiary infection or may present in the latent phase. Primary syphilis has an incubation period of up to 3 weeks and classically presents with a painless genital ulcer, known as the primary chancre (E-Fig. 9.8.2). This may last for up to 6 weeks and is not accompanied by constitutional symptoms. If untreated, the primary stage may evolve into the secondary stage within 6 weeks, characterized by the distinctive macular pink rash which may resemble pityriasis rosea. It is often present on the flexor surfaces, trunk, palms and soles. The secondary stage is often accompanied by constitutional symptoms of fever, malaise and headache. Tertiary syphilis occurs up to 20 years after the primary infection in around one-third of patients with untreated secondary syphilis. The presentation includes widespread granulomas, known as gummas, or may present with meningitis, dementia, thoracic aneurysm or neuropathy, known as tabes dorsalis. There may be extensive involvement of the cardiovascular and nervous systems.

Diagnosis depends on serological confirmation of treponemal or non-treponemal tests. Treponemal tests remain positive for life.

Table 9.8.3 Treatment guideline summary

Clinical diagnosis and pathogen	Recommended treatment	Alternative choice treatment
Chlamydia (uncomplicated)	Azithromycin 1 g oral once	
Gonorrhoea		
Genital , pharyngeal, rectal	Ceftriaxone 500 mg IM once	If acquired from Top End or Central Australia, amoxicillin 3 g plus probenecid 1 g oral once
Trichomoniasis	Metronidazole 2 g oral once OR Tinidazole (not in pregnancy) 2 g oral once	
Pelvic inflammatory disease	Ceftriaxone 500 mg IM once PLUS Azithromycin 1 g oral once PLUS Metronidazole 400 mg, oral, bd for 14 days PLUS Doxycycline 100 mg oral bd for 14 days	
Bacterial vaginosis	Metronidazole 400 mg oral, bd for 7 days	
Urethritis, dysuria, urethral discharge	Ceftriaxone 500 mg IM once PLUS Azithromycin 1 g oral once OR Doxycycline 100 mg oral bd for 7 days	Erythromycin 500 mg oral qds for 7 days
Chancroid	Azithromycin 1 g oral once OR Ceftriaxone 500 mg IM once	Ciprofloxacin 500 mg oral, bd for 3 days
Lymphogranuloma venereum	Doxycycline (not in pregnancy) 100 mg oral, bd for 21 days	Erythromycin 500 mg oral qid for 21 days OR Azithromycin 1 g oral 1 dose weekly for 3 weeks
Donovanosis	Benzathine penicillin 2.4 million units IM with 2 mL 1% lignocaine once PLUS Azithromycin 1 g oral once weekly for 4 weeks	
Herpes		
Anogenital, primary episode	Valacyclovir 500 mg oral, bd for 7–10 days	
Anogenital, recurrent episode	Valacyclovir 500 mg oral, bd for 3 days	
Severe, disseminated infection	Acyclovir 5–10 mg/kg IV 8-hourly for 5–10 days	
Genital warts		
External genital and perianal	Podophyllin 0.5% lotion topical tds for 3 days, then no treatment for 4 days, repeat 4 cycles or until resolution	
Mucosal warts	Cryotherapy or trichloroacetic acid 80% topical weekly for 2 weeks	Podophyllin resin 25% in benzoin topical for urethral meatus warts once weekly for 2 weeks
Syphilis		
Primary, secondary, early latent, late latent or >2 years' duration	Benzathine penicillin G 2.4 million U IM, with 2 mL 1% lignocaine once Bezathine penicillin G 2.4 million U IM with 2 mL 1% lignocaine weekly for 3 weeks	

Non-treponemal tests respond to treatment. An NAAT for syphilis may be requested from swabs or scrapings from rash or ulcers. Treatment is with benzathine penicillin 2.4 million units IM single dose if under 2 years' duration or three doses at weekly intervals if over 2 years' duration. There is no documented treponemal resistance as yet to penicillin, although treatment failures have occurred occasionally and are thought to be either re-infection or individual variation in decline of the non-treponemal test titres in response to treatment.

Patients should be notified to the regional syphilis register.

Genital warts

Genital warts are caused by the human papillomavirus. Up to three-quarters of sexually active adults are infected, although most infections are subclinical. Multiple warts, which may cluster, are seen over the vulva and penis.

Internal warts may be seen in the rectum and around the cervix. Diagnosis is clinical and the differential diagnosis of molluscum contagiosum, secondary syphilis (condylomata) and carcinoma must be considered. Treatment is with podophllin 0.5% lotion applied twice daily to lesions for 3 days, then no treatment for 4 days, and repeat until lesions resolve. This may take four or more cycles of treatment.

Principles of clinical investigations

Diagnosis is initially clinical and treatment may need to be empirical. Attempts should be made to confirm the diagnosis by laboratory analysis of swabs and urine and it is important to communicate with laboratory staff to discuss collection, transport and testing of specimens and the specific type of swab, transport medium and temperature for each organism. All specimens should be correctly labelled with patient details in leakproof containers. Common tests include dark field microscopy for syphilis, Gram staining for gonorrhoea, chancroid and bacterial vaginosis, Tzanck smear for herpes and Donovanosis, wet mount for trichomoniasis and potassium hydroxide wet mount for candidiasis. NAAT are now seen as the gold standard for confirmation of chlamydia, gonorrhoea and some other STIs. Swabs from the affected areas for M, C and S and swabs and urinalysis for NAAT should be taken. Male swabs should include urethral smear for Gram stain, urethral, throat and rectal swab for culture, urinalysis including NAAT, blood for syphilis, HIV and hepatitis serology.

Female swabs should include lateral vaginal wall smear for Gram stain, vaginal swab for candida and trichomonas, endocervical, urethral, throat and rectal swabs for gonorrhea and urinalysis including pregnancy test, NAAT and culture and sensitivity. Referral for cervical cytology and serology for syphilis, HIV and hepatitis should be made.

If lesions are suggestive, scraping the lesion for syphilis microscopy and specialist swabs for HSV and *Haemophilus ducreyi* may be helpful.

The criteria used for diagnosing urethritis include one or more of: purulent or mucoid urethral discharge showing more than 5 white blood cells (WBC) per high power field, Gram stain of urine sediment showing more than 10 WBC per high power field and positive leucocyte esterase test on early morning first urine. NAAT may identify specific organisms.

Criteria for a diagnosis of cervicitis include purulent endocervical discharge and friable endocervical mucosa which bleeds easily when gently scraped. Direct visualization of organisms in discharge by wet mount, if available, or microscopy, Gram stain and culture of swab material or, if possible NAAT testing of discharge or urine specimens may confirm the diagnosis and add additional diagnoses.

Treatment

See Table 9.8.3 for an example summary guideline.

Treatment is subject to current local guidelines and sensitivities and may vary according to regional strains and sensitivities. Where the infection likely originated is an important part of the history. Always check with local laboratories for current antimicrobial guidelines.

Follow up

Referral to a local STI clinic for follow up and contact tracing and treatment of partners is essential to stop the spread of STIs.

The patient should be advised of the need for partner treatment and of the need to abstain from sex until the infection has been treated adequately. The opportunity for health education around safer sexual practices and STI prevention should be taken. Notifiable diseases include chlamydia, gonorrhoea, syphilis, chancroid, LGV and Donovanosis.

Controversies and future directions

- There are conflicting views over whether the ED is the right place to screen for STIs including HIV, although it should be considered, especially in high prevalence areas. Screening while the patient is in the ED may be the only potential for diagnosis and treatment.
- Debate exists in some regions over whether to treat infections empirically and the potential for increasing antibiotic resistance versus the burden of untreated disease. Syndromic treatment

in areas of low prevalence is likely to be more effective in males as most cases of vaginal discharge in females are not STI related.

- More accurate and easier diagnostic testing, preferably at point of care is needed. Near patient testing is likely to become more accurate and more available in the future.
- Changing antibiotic sensitivities of STIs mandates current local treatment guidelines and close liaison with colleagues in sexual health, infectious disease, microbiology and virology.

References

[1] World Health Organization database. [Accessed Dec. 2012].
[2] Australian Government Department of Health and Ageing. National Notifiable Diseases Surveillance System, Australia. <http://www9.health.gov.au/cda> [Accessed Dec. 2012].
[3] British Association for Sexual Health and HIV (BASHH) Guidelines 2011. <www.bashh.org./guidelines>.
[4] Trends in sexually transmitted diseases in the United States. Centers for Disease Control and Prevention Dec. 2012. <www.cdc.gov/std/stats>.
[5] Mehta S, Hall J, Lyss S, et al. Adult and pediatric emergency department sexually transmitted disease and HIV screening programmatic overview and outcomes. Acad Emerg Med 2007;14:250.
[6] Bachmann L, Pigott D, Desmond R, et al. Prevalence and factors associated with gonorrhoea and chlamydia infection in at risk females presenting to an urban emergency department. Sex Transm Dis 2003;30:335–9.
[7] Smith KP, Christakis NA. Association between widowhood and risk of diagnosis with a sexually transmitted infection in older adults. Am J Publ Hlth 2009;99:2055–62.
[8] Anderson M, Klink K, Cohrssen A. Evaluation of vaginal complaints. J Am Med Assoc 2004;291:1368–79.
[9] Borhart J, Birnbaumer D. Emergency department management of sexually transmitted infections. Emerg Med Clin N Am 2011;29:587–603.
[10] Evans C, Das C, Kinghorn GA. Retrospective study of recurrent Chlamydia infection in men and women: is there a role for targeted screening for those at risk? Int J STD AIDS 2009;3:188–92.
[11] Annual report of the Australian Gonococcal Surveillance Programme 2011. Commun Dis Intell 2012: 36:E166-73.
[12] Condon J, Rumbold A, Thorn J, et al. A cluster of vulval cancer and vulvar intraepithelial neoplasia in young Australian indigenous women. Cancer Causes Control 2009;20:67–74.

Further reading

California STD/HIV Prevention. <www.stdhivtraining.org>.
Hall J, Lyss SB, et al. Adult and paediatric emergency department sexually transmitted disease and HIV screening; programmatic overview and outcomes. Acad Emerg Med 2007;14:250–8.
Northern Territory Government, Department of Health, Australia. Guideline for the management of sexually transmitted infections in the primary care setting, February 2012.
Tapsall JW, Ndowa F, Lewis DA, Unemo M. Meeting the public health challenge of multidrug and extensively drug-resistant Neisseria gonorrhoeae. Expert Rev Anti Infect Ther 2009;7:821–34.

9.9 Antibiotics in the emergency department

John Vinen

ESSENTIALS

1 Patients with infections and infectious diseases commonly present to emergency departments.

2 There are also changing patterns of infectious disease, largely due to immunosuppression from chemotherapy, continuing development of bacterial resistance, HIV-associated infections and new and emerging infections.

3 Many bacteria are becoming increasingly resistant to available antimicrobials, with some resistant to multiple agents including many community-acquired infections.

4 The growing world trade in wildlife, factory farming, increasing air travel and increased population density increases the risk of infectious disease transmission.

5 There are relatively few new antimicrobials to counter these changing patterns of resistance.

6 Antimicrobial prescribing should follow evidence-based guidelines.

7 Some patients with infection can be treated wholly as outpatients using parenteral therapy or after early discharge once the acute toxic phase is over.

8 Early administration of guideline-based antibiotics combined with supportive therapy is the key to a good outcome in patients with serious infections.

9 The increasing incidence of terrorism may result in patients presenting with novel, unusual or clusters of infections caused by biological agents.

Principles of antimicrobial therapy

The first decision to be made regarding antimicrobial therapy is whether the administration of these agents is truly indicated. In many cases, antibiotics are administered without clear indications. This practice is potentially dangerous, as some agents can cause serious toxicity, diagnoses may be masked if appropriate cultures are not taken prior to therapy, serious adverse events can result and microorganism resistance may emerge.

Ideally, antibiotic therapy is determined by isolation of the organism(s) involved and determination of antibiotic susceptibility pattern. As this information is rarely available, it is necessary to make treatment decisions without precise knowledge of infectious source

or microbial species in which case empiric treatment is commenced based on the type of infection (if known) and the likely organisms involved utilizing recognized guidelines.

In specific situations (e.g. suspected meningitis, meningococcal infection, necrotizing fasciitis, sepsis, peritonitis, febrile neutropaenia, and pneumonia), early empiric therapy can be life saving.

The choice of an appropriate antimicrobial agent requires consideration of the following factors.

The microorganism

The identity of the infecting organism(s) needs to be identified or suspected. In the emergency department (ED) setting, almost all antimicrobial decisions will be made without the benefit of cultures, with treatment commencing

based on the most likely to cause infection in a given clinical setting [1]. However, certain 'rapid methods' of microbial identification may be employed. These include Gram-stain preparations (bacterial, some fungal and leucocyte identification) and immunological methods for antigen detection (enzyme-linked immunoabsorbent assay, latex agglutination, polymerase chain reactions).

Microorganism susceptibility

The emergency physician is unlikely to have this information and therapeutic decisions will generally be based on a knowledge of likely susceptibilities [1]. For example, group A streptococci remain susceptible to the penicillins and cephalosporins and virtually all anaerobes (except *Bacteroides* spp.) are susceptible to penicillin G. However, when the identity or susceptibility of the infecting organism is sufficiently in doubt, the patient's clinical condition is atypical, serious or potentially serious or where antimicrobial resistance is suspected, it is good practice to obtain appropriate specimens for culture and susceptibility testing prior to empirical broad-spectrum antimicrobial therapy (Table 9.9.1).

Host factors

An adequate history of drug allergies must be obtained in order to prevent the administration of an antimicrobial that may have serious or fatal consequences. Where this is not possible, avoid administration of penicillin and associated antimicrobials. The age of the patient may have clinically significant effects on drug absorption (e.g. penicillin absorption is increased in the young and the elderly) [2], metabolism (e.g. reduced chloramphenicol metabolism in the neonate) [2] and excretion (e.g. declining renal function with age [3] may reduce the excretion of penicillins, cephalosporins and aminoglycosides). Furthermore, tetracyclines bind and discolour the developing bone and tooth structures in children aged 8 years or less [2]. Pregnant women and nursing mothers may pose certain problems in the selection of appropriate

Table 9.9.1 Antimicrobial agents of choice in selected infections

Microorganism	Diseases	First choice	Second choice
Gram-positive cocci			
Staphylococcus aureus*	Abscesses penicillinase-negative: Osteomyelitis	Benzylpenicillin (penicillin G), phenoxymethyl penicillin (penicillin V)	Cephalosporin (G1), clindamycin
	Bacteraemia penicillinase-positive: Endocarditis	Nafcillin, oxacillin	Cephalosporin (G1) Vancomycin, clindamycin
	Pneumonia methicillin-resistant: Cellulitis	Vancomycin ± rifampicin	Co-trimoxazole + rifampicin Ciprofloxacin + rifampicin
Streptococcus (A, B, C, G and bovis)	Pharyngitis, scarlet fever, otitis media, cellulitis, erysipelas, pneumonia, bacteraemia, endocarditis, meningitis	Benzylpenicillin (penicillin G), phenoxymethylpenicillin (penicillin V), ampicillin	Erythromycin Cephalosporin (G1) Vancomycin
Streptococcus pneumonia*	Pneumonia, arthritis, sinusitis, otitis media, meningitis, endocarditis	Benzylpenicillin (penicillin G), phenoxymethylpenicillin (penicillin V), ampicillin, penicillin G	Erythromycin, cephalosporin (G1–3) Vancomycin + rifampicin Ceftriaxone
Streptococcus viridians*	Bacteraemia, endocarditis	Benzylpenicillin (penicillin G) ± gentamicin	Ceftriaxone, vancomycin ± gentamicin
Enterococcus	Bacteraemia, endocarditis, urinary tract infection	Ampicillin + gentamicin, benzylpenicillin (penicillin G) + gentamicin	Vancomycin + gentamicin, nitrofurantoin Fluoroquinolone, ampicillin + clavulanic acid
Gram-negative cocci			
Moraxella catarrhalis	Otitis, sinusitis, pneumonia	Co-trimoxazole Amoxicillin + clavulanic acid	Cephalosporin (G2,3) Erythromycin, tetracycline
Neisseria gonorrhoeae	Gonorrhoea, disseminated disease	Ceftriaxone, ampicillin + probenecid	Ciprofloxacin, doxycycline spectinomycin
Neisseria meningitides	Meningitis, carrier state	Benzylpenicillin (penicillin G) rifampicin	Cephalosporin (G3), chloramphenicol
Gram-positive bacilli			
Clostridium perfringens*	Gas gangrene Tetanus	Benzylpenicillin (penicillin G)	Clindamycin, metronidazole, cephalosporin
Clostridium tetani	Tetanus	Benzylpenicillin (penicillin G), vancomycin	Doxycycline, clindamycin
Clostridium difficile	Antimicrobial-associated colitis	Metronidazole (oral)	Vancomycin (oral)
Corynebacterium diphtheria	Pharyngitis, tracheitis, pneumonia	Erythromycin	Benzylpenicillin (penicillin G), clindamycin
Listeria monocytogenes	Meningitis, bacteraemia	Ampicillin ± gentamicin	Co-trimoxazole, erythromycin
Gram-negative bacilli			
Brucella	Brucellosis	Doxycycline + gentamicin	Co-trimoxazole + gentamicin/rifampicin
Campylobacter jejuni*	Enteritis	Fluoroquinolone	Erythromycin, azithromycin
Escherichia coli*	Urinary tract infection, bacteraemia	Ampicillin, co-trimoxazole, cephalosporin (G1)	Ampicillin + gentamicin Fluoroquinolone, nitrofurantoin
Enterobacter species	Urinary tract and other infections	Fluoroquinolone imipenem	Gentamicin + broad-spectrum penicillin, co-trimoxazole
Haemophilus influenza*	Otitis, sinusitis, pneumonia	Co-trimoxazole, ampicillin, amoxicillin	Amoxicillin + clavulanic acid, azithromycin, Cefuroxime
	Epiglottitis, meningitis	Cephalosporin (G3)	Chloramphenicol
Klebsiella pneumonia*	Urinary tract infection, pneumonia	Cephalosporin ± gentamicin	Co-trimoxazole, fluoroquinolone
Legionella pneumophila	Legionnaires' disease	Erythromycin ± rifampicin	Ciprofloxacin, azithromycin, co-trimoxazole
Pasteurella multocida	Animal bite infections, abscesses, bacteraemia, meningitis	Benzylpenicillin (penicillin G) Amoxicillin + clavulanic acid	Doxycycline, cephalosporin
Proteus mirabilis*	Urinary tract and other infections	Ampicillin, amoxicillin	Cephalosporin, co-trimoxazole, gentamicin
Proteus (other species)*	Urinary tract and other infections	Cephalosporin (G3), gentamicin	Co-trimoxazole, fluoroquinolone
Pseudomonas aeruginosa*	Urinary tract infection, pneumonia, bacteraemia	Broad-spectrum penicillin ± gentamicin	Ceftazidime ± gentamicin Fluoroquinolone ± gentamicin
Salmonella species*	Typhoid fever, paratyphoid fever, bacteraemia, gastroenteritis	Fluoroquinolone, ceftriaxone	Ampicillin, co-trimoxazole, chloramphenicol
Shigella*	Acute gastroenteritis	Fluoroquinolone	Ampicillin, co-trimoxazole
Vibrio cholera	Cholera	Doxycycline, fluoroquinolone	Co-trimoxazole
Miscellaneous agents			
Chlamydia species	Pneumonia, trachoma, urethritis, cervicitis	Doxycycline	Azithromycin, erythromycin
Mycoplasma pneumonia	Atypical pneumonia	Erythromycin, doxycycline	Azithromycin
Pneumocystis carinii	Pneumonia in impaired host	Co-trimoxazole	Trimethoprim + dapsone, pentamidine
Rickettsia	Typhus fever, Q fever, Rocky Mountain spotted fever	Doxycycline	Chloramphenicol
Treponema pallidum	Syphilis	Benzylpenicillin (penicillin G)	Ceftriaxone, doxycycline

*G1, first-generation cephalosporin; G2, second-generation cephalosporin; G3, third-generation cephalosporin.
All strains should be examined *in vitro* for sensitivity to various antimicrobial agents.

antimicrobial agents, as all of these agents cross the placenta to varying degrees. The administration of antibiotics to pregnant patients must be based on guidelines [4]. Whether or not antibiotic use has an effect on the efficacy of combined oral contraceptive pills (OCPs) has been a matter of controversy. A significant pharmacokinetic interaction between combined OCPs and antibiotics, apart from rifampicin and griseofulvin, has not been proven. It has been suggested that if an interaction does exist, it is likely that it occurs in a small number of predisposed individuals. It is not possible at this time to predict who is at risk for potential interaction [5]. Other host factors that may require consideration include the patient's renal and hepatic function, their genetic (e.g. liver acetylation rate) or metabolic abnormalities (e.g. diabetes mellitus) and the site of the infection [6].

Route of administration

In general, the oral route is chosen for infections that are mild and can be managed on an outpatient basis. In this situation, consideration needs to be given to compliance with treatment, the variability of absorption with food in the stomach and interaction of the agent with concomitant medications [7]. The parenteral route is used for agents that are inefficiently absorbed from the gastrointestinal tract and for the treatment of patients with serious infections in whom high concentrations of antimicrobial agents are required [7]. Intramuscular administration (not in patients on anticoagulants or who are coagulopathic) will provide adequate serum concentrations for most infections and may be appropriate where antimicrobial depots are desirable, e.g. procaine penicillin injections where patient compliance with oral medication is doubtful. Intravenous administration allows large doses of drugs to be given with a minimal amount of discomfort to the patient, e.g. infection prophylaxis in compound fractures, life-threatening infections and shock. For intravenous administration, large veins should be used followed by saline flushing of the veins to help to minimize the incidence of venous irritation and phlebitis.

Supportive care

Supportive care in association with antimicrobial therapy is essential in many infections, fluid resuscitation and vasopressors being essential for a good outcome in sepsis [8].

Adverse drug events involving antibiotics

Antibiotics are one of the top medication classes resulting in ED visits for adverse drug events.

There is a 1:1000 risk that an individual prescribed an antibiotic will require a visit to the ED because of an antibiotic side effect.

Antibiotics are responsible for 19% of ED visits for adverse drug events:

- in children (<18 years), antibiotics are the most common cause of ED visits for adverse drug events
- 79% of ED visits for antibiotic-associated adverse drug events are due to allergic reactions [9].

Antibiotic resistance

Bacteria can be resistant to an antimicrobial agent because the drug fails to reach the target or is inactivated or because the target is altered [10–12]. Bacteria may produce enzymes that inactivate the drug or have cell membranes impermeable to the drug. Having gained entry into the microorganism, the drug must exert a deleterious effect. Natural variation or acquired changes at the target site that prevent drug binding or action can lead to resistance.

Resistance is most commonly acquired by horizontal transfer of resistance determinants from a donor cell, often of another bacterial species, by transformation, transduction or conjugation. Resistance may also be acquired by mutation and passed vertically by selection to daughter cells. Antimicrobial agents can affect the emergence of resistance by exerting strong selective pressures on bacterial populations favouring those organisms capable of resisting them [13].

The increasing emergence of antibiotic resistance is a very serious development that threatens the end of the antibiotic era. Penicillin-resistant strains of pneumococci account for >50% of isolates in some European countries. The worldwide emergence of *Haemophilus* and gonococci that produce β-lactamase is a major therapeutic problem [14]. Methicillin-resistant strains of *Staphylococcus aureus* are widely distributed among hospitals and are increasingly being isolated from community-acquired infections [15]. There are now strains of enterococci (VRE), *Pseudomonas* and enterobacters

that are resistant to all known drugs [16]. Epidemics of multiply drug-resistant strains of *Mycobacterium tuberculosis* have been reported [16].

A more responsible approach to the use of antimicrobial agents is essential to slow the development of multidrug-resistant organisms. Their use should be avoided in viral infections and rational policies for their use in prophylaxis and in established bacterial infections must be developed and followed [1]. The use of narrow-spectrum antimicrobial agents to which the organism is susceptible is encouraged and, in certain circumstances, the use of combinations of agents may prevent the emergence of resistant mutants during therapy.

Prophylactic use of antibiotics

Antimicrobial prophylaxis is the use of antimicrobial agents in order to prevent infection developing. It is indicated in many circumstances, including the prevention of recurrent rheumatic fever, endocarditis, meningitis, tuberculosis and urinary tract and surgical infections [1]. Antimicrobial prophylaxis in the ED is usually indicated to prevent trauma-related infection following contamination of soft tissue, crush injuries, bites, clenched fist injuries and compound fractures. Other risk factors for wound infection include 'old' wounds (>6 hours), penetrating injuries, contaminated wounds, co-morbid illness, shock, colon injury and massive haemorrhage [17].

Antimicrobial prophylaxis should be considered where there is a significant risk of infection, but cannot be relied upon to overcome excessive soiling, damage to tissues, inadequate debridement or poor surgical technique. Adequate wound care, with splinting and elevation of the affected area as indicated, will continue to be important factors in trauma-related infection prophylaxis.

Antimicrobial prophylaxis should be directed against the likely causative organism(s). However, an effective regimen need not necessarily include antimicrobials that are active against every potential pathogen. Regimens that only reduce the total number of organisms may assist host defences and prevent infection [1]. The type, dose, duration and route of administration of antimicrobial therapy will vary according to the nature, site and aetiology of the injury, as well as host factors and should be based on established guidelines. In all cases of open traumatic injury, no matter how trivial, tetanus prophylaxis must be considered.

Penicillins

Chemistry and mechanism of action

The penicillins constitute one of the most important groups of antimicrobial agents and remain the drugs of choice for a large number of infectious diseases. The basic structure of the penicillins consists of a thiazolidine ring connected to a β-lactam ring, and a side chain. The penicillin nucleus is the chief structural requirement for biological activity, whereas the side chain determines many of the antibacterial and pharmacological characteristics of the particular type of penicillin.

Peptidoglycan is an essential component of the bacterial cell wall and provides mechanical stability by virtue of its highly cross-linked latticework structure. Penicillin is thought to acetylate and inhibit a transpeptidase enzyme responsible for the final cross-linking of peptidoglycan layers. Penicillin also binds to penicillin-binding proteins (PBPs), causing further interference with cell wall synthesis and cell morphology. The lysis of bacteria is ultimately dependent on the activity of cell wall autolytic enzymes – autolyses and murein hydrolases. Although the relationship between the inhibition of PBP activity and the activation of autolysins is unclear, the interference with peptidoglycan assembly in the face of ongoing autolysis activity might well lead to cell lysis and death.

Bacterial resistance to penicillins

Microorganisms may be intrinsically resistant to the penicillins because of structural differences in PBPs. Resistance may be acquired by the development of high molecular weight PBPs that have reduced affinity for the antibiotic [12]. Bacterial resistance can also be caused by the inability of the agent to penetrate to its site of action. Unlike Gram-positive bacteria, Gram-negative bacteria have an outer membrane of lipopolysaccharide which functions as an impenetrable barrier to some antibiotics. However, some broader-spectrum penicillins, such as ampicillin and amoxicillin, can diffuse through aqueous channels (porins) of this outer membrane to reach their sites of action.

Bacteria can destroy penicillins enzymatically. Different bacteria elaborate a number of different β-lactamases and individual penicillins vary in their susceptibility to these enzymes. In general, Gram-positive bacteria produce a large amount of β-lactamase, which is secreted extracellularly. Most of these enzymes are penicillinases which disrupt the β-lactam ring and inactivate the drug. In Gram-negative bacteria, β-lactamases are found in relatively small amounts strategically located between the inner and outer bacterial membranes for maximal protection.

Classification of penicillins

Benzylpenicillin (penicillin G) and phenoxymethyl penicillin (penicillin V)

These drugs are the so-called 'natural penicillins'. The antimicrobial spectra of benzyl penicillin (penicillin G) and phenoxymethyl penicillin (penicillin V) are very similar for aerobic Gram-positive microorganisms. Benzyl penicillin is the drug of choice against many Gram-positive cocci (streptococci, penicillin-sensitive staphylococci), Gram-negative cocci (*Neisseria meningitidis* and *N. gonorrhoeae*), Gram-postive bacilli (*Bacillus anthracis*, *Corynebacterium. diphtheriae*), anaerobes (peptostreptococcus, *Actinomyces israelii*, *Clostridium* and some *Bacteroides*), *Pasteurella multocida* and *Treponema pallidum*. Phenoxymethyl penicillin is an acceptable alternative for *Streptococcus pneumoniae*, *Strep. pyogenes* (A) and *Actinomyces israelii*.

The sole virtue of benzylpenicillin compared to phenoxymethyl penicillin is that it is more stable in an acid medium and therefore much better absorbed from the gastrointestinal tract. Benzylpenicillin is administered parenterally but has a half-life of only 30 minutes. Accordingly, repository preparations (penicillin G procaine, penicillin G benzathine) are often used and probenecid may be administered concurrently to block the renal tubular secretion of the drug. Once absorbed, both penicillins are distributed widely throughout the body. Significant amounts appear in the liver, bile, kidney, semen, joint fluid, lymph and intestine. Importantly, penicillin does not readily enter the CSF when the meninges are normal. However, when the meninges are acutely inflamed penicillin penetrates into the CSF more easily. Under normal circumstances, penicillin is eliminated unchanged by the kidney, mainly by tubular secretion.

The penicillinase-resistant penicillins

These drugs remain the agents of choice for most staphylococcal disease. Methicillin is a penicillin resistant to staphylococcal β-lactamase, although the increasing incidence of isolates of methicillin-resistant microorganisms is cause for concern. Methicillin-resistant *Staph. aureus* (MRSA) contain a high molecular weight PBP with a very low affinity for β-lactam antibiotics [12]. From 40 to 60% of strains of *Staph. epidermidis* are also resistant to penicillinase-resistant penicillins by the same mechanism. As bacterial sensitivities are usually not known in the ED, methicillin is rarely administered in this setting.

The isoxazolyl penicillins (oxacillin, cloxacillin, dicloxacillin and flucloxacillin) are congeneric semisynthetic penicillins which are pharmacologically similar. All are relatively stable in an acid medium and are adequately absorbed after oral administration. These penicillins undergo some metabolism but are excreted primarily by the kidney with some biliary excretion. All are remarkably resistant to cleavage by penicillinase and inhibit both penicillin-sensitive and some penicillin-resistant staphylococci. Methicillin-resistant staphylococci are resistant to these penicillins. Isoxazolyl penicillins inhibit streptococci and pneumococci but are virtually inactive against Gram-negative bacilli.

The aminopenicillins

Ampicillin is the prototypical agent in this group. It is stable in acid medium and, although well absorbed orally, is often administered parenterally. Amoxicillin is a close chemical and pharmacological relative of ampicillin. The drug is stable in acid and was designed for oral use. It is more rapidly and completely absorbed from the gastrointestinal tract than is ampicillin. The antimicrobial spectra of these agents are essentially identical, with the important exception that amoxicillin appears to be less effective for shigellosis. Ampicillin is the penicillin of choice for many Gram-negative bacilli (*H. influenzae*, *Escherichia coli*, *Proteus mirabilis*, *Salmonella typhi* and *Salmonella* spp.), some Gram-positive bacilli (*Listeria monocytogenes*) and some Gram-positive cocci (*Enterococcus faecalis*). It also has activity against *Pneumococcus* spp., *Neisseria* spp., *Peptostreptococcus*, *Fusobacterium*, *Clostridium* and *Erysipelothrix*.

Bacterial resistance to these drugs is becoming an increasing problem. Many pneumococcal isolates have varying levels of resistance to ampicillin. *H. influenzae* and the viridans group of streptococci are usually inhibited by very low concentrations of ampicillin. However, strains of *H. influenzae* (type b) that are highly resistant to ampicillin have been recovered from children with meningitis. It is estimated that 30% or more cases of *H. influenzae* meningitis are now caused by ampicillin-resistant strains. Similarly, ampicillin-resistant strains of *H. influenzae* have been increasingly isolated from cases of acute otitis media. An increasing percentage of *N. gonorrhoeae*, *E. coli*, *P. mirabilis*, *Salmonella* and *Shigella* are now resistant to ampicillin and practically all species of *Enterobacter* are now insensitive.

β-Lactamase inhibitors have been introduced to combat many penicillin-resistant microorganisms. These molecules bind to β-lactamases and inactivate them, thereby preventing the destruction of β-lactamase antibiotics. Clavulanic acid binds to the β-lactamases produced by a wide range of Gram-positive and Gram-negative microorganisms. It is well absorbed orally and can also be given parenterally. It has been combined with amoxicillin as an oral preparation (Augmentin) and with ticarcillin (a carboxypenicillin) as a parenteral preparation (Timentin). Augmentin is effective for β-lactamase-producing strains of staphylococci, *H. influenzae*, gonococci and *E. coli*. Sulbactam is another β-lactamase inhibitor which also can be administered orally or parenterally. In combination with ampicillin (Unasyn), good coverage is provided for Gram-positive cocci (including β-lactamase-producing strains of *Staph. aureus*), Gram-negative anaerobes (but not *Pseudomonas*) and anaerobes.

Adverse reactions to penicillin

Hypersensitivity reactions are the major adverse effects of penicillins. Penicillins are capable of acting as haptens to combine with proteins contaminating the solution or with human protein after the penicillin has been administered. Penicilloyl and penicillanic derivatives are the major determinants of penicillin allergy. All acute hypersensitivity reactions to penicillin are mediated by the IgE antibody and range in severity from rash to anaphylaxis. Anaphylactic reactions are uncommon, occurring in only 0.2% of 1000 courses of treatment, with 0.001% out of 100 000 courses resulting

in death [18]. Morbilliform eruptions that develop after penicillin therapy are likely to be mediated by IgM antibodies and the uncommon serum sickness is likely to be mediated by IgG antibodies. All forms of penicillin are best avoided in patients with a history of penicillin allergy.

Otherwise, the penicillins are generally well tolerated. CNS toxicity, in the form of myoclonic seizures, can follow the administration of massive doses of benzylpenicillin (penicillin G), ampicillin or methicillin. Massive doses have also been associated with hypokalaemia. Haematological toxicity – usually neutropaenia – and nephrotoxicity have also been reported. Gastrointestinal disturbances have followed the use of all oral penicillins, but have been most pronounced with ampicillin. Enterocolitis due to the overgrowth of *Cl. difficile* is well documented and abnormalities in liver function have been reported, especially with flucloxacillin [19].

Cephalosporins

The antimicrobial activity of cephalosporins, like that of other β-lactam antibiotics, results at least in part from their ability to interfere with the synthesis of the peptidoglycan component of the bacterial cell wall. However, the exact bactericidal and lytic effects of cephalosporins are not completely understood.

Classification and uses

The first-generation compounds (cephalothin, cefazolin, cefalexin) have a relatively narrow spectrum of activity focused primarily on the Gram-positive cocci, especially penicillin-sensitive streptococci and methicillin-sensitive *Staph. aureus*. These compounds have modest activity against Gram-negative organisms, including *E. coli* and *Klebsiella* spp. Cefaclor has extended Gram-negative activity and is active against *H. influenzae* and *M. catarrhalis*.

The second generation of cephalosporins (cefuroxime, cefamandole) are more stable against Gram-negative β-lactamases. They have variable activity against Gram-positive cocci, but have increased activity against Gram-negative bacteria (*E. coli*, *Proteus*, *Klebsiella*). In spite of relatively increased potency against Gram-negative aerobic and anaerobic bacilli (*Bacteroides fragilis*), the cephamycins (cefoxitin, cefotetan) are included in this generation.

The third-generation cephalosporins (cefotaxime, ceftriaxone, ceftazidime, cefpirome)

have very marked activity against Gram-negative bacteria. Most are useful against *Ps. aeruginosa*, *Serratia* and *Neisseria* species and some Enterobacteriaceae. Some of these compounds have limited activity against Gram-positive cocci, particularly methicillin-sensitive *Staph. aureus*. This generation of cephalosporins is particularly effective in meningitis because of their better penetration into the CSF and higher intrinsic activity. However, as these third-generation drugs are more expensive and have a wide antimicrobial spectrum, their use should be based on established guidelines.

Recently, several compounds have been considered as possibly meriting classification as a fourth generation. Cefepime has activity against Gram-positive cocci and a broad array of Gram-negative bacteria, including *Ps. aeruginosa* and many of the Enterobacteriaceae with inducible chromosomal β-lactamases.

Adverse reactions

Hypersensitivity reactions are the most common side effects of the cephalosporins and all compounds have been implicated. The reactions appear to be identical to those caused by the penicillins. Immediate reactions, such as anaphylaxis, bronchospasm, angio-oedema and urticaria, have been reported. More commonly, a maculopapular rash develops, usually after several days of therapy. Because of the similarity in structure between the penicillins and the cephalosporins, patients allergic to one class of agents may manifest cross-reactivity when a member of the other class is administered. Studies indicate that about 0.5% of patients allergic to penicillin will demonstrate a clinically apparent reaction when a first-generation cephalosporin is administered (0% for second- and third-generation cephalosporins) [20]. Patients with a mild or temporarily distant reaction to penicillin appear to be at low risk of rash or other allergic reactions following the administration of a cephalosporin. However, subjects with a recent history of an immediate reaction to penicillin should not be given a cephalosporin. Other reactions to cephalosporins are uncommon and include diarrhoea, nephrotoxicity, intolerance of alcohol and bleeding disorders.

Penicillin allergy cross-reactivity with cephalosporins is significantly overstated. Cross-reactivity between penicillins and cephalosporins is much less than the 10% commonly cited. Cephalothin, cephalexin, cefadroxil and cefazolin confer an increased risk of allergic reaction among patients with penicillin allergy.

Cefuroxime, cefpodoxime, ceftazidime and ceftriaxone do not increase risk of an allergic reaction.

No cross-reactivity exists between penicillins and third-generation cephalosporins. However, if a patient has known anaphylaxis to penicillin, caution with cephalosporin use is still warranted.

Bacterial resistance

The most prevalent mechanism for resistance to cephalosporins is their destruction by β-lactamase hydrolysis. The cephalosporins have variable susceptibility to β-lactamase, with the later-generation compounds being more resistant to the β-lactamases produced by Gram-negative bacteria. However, third-generation cephalosporins are susceptible to hydrolysis by inducible, chromosomally encoded (type 1) β-lactamases. The induction of type 1 β-lactamases by treatment of infections due to many aerobic Gram-negative bacilli with second- or third-generation cephalosporins may result in resistance to all third-generation cephalosporins.

Macrolides

Erythromycin was originally isolated from soil bacteria and contains a many-membered lactone ring to which are attached one or more deoxy sugars. Clarithromycin, azithromycin and roxithromycin are new semisynthetic derivatives of erythromycin. Clarithromycin differs only by methylation of a hydroxyl group and azithromycin contains a methyl-substituted nitrogen atom in the lactone ring. Roxithromycin is a good alternative to oral erythromycin and has good oral bioavailability, but is more expensive. The macrolides are usually bacteriostatic and inhibit protein synthesis by binding reversibly to 50S ribosomal subunits of sensitive microorganisms. They are thought to inhibit the translocation step wherein a newly synthesized peptidyl tRNA molecule moves from the acceptor site on the ribosome to the peptidyl (donor) site.

Clinical uses

Erythromycin is most effective against aerobic Gram-positive cocci and bacilli. It is active against Strep. pyogenes, Strep. pneumoniae, Cl. perfringens, Cl. diphtheriae, L. monocytogenes and some staphylococci. Useful activity has also been seen with P. multocida, Borrelia spp., B. pertussis, Campylobacter jejuni, Legionella pneumophila, M. pneumoniae, C. trachomatis

and some atypical mycobacteria. It has modest activity in vitro against some Gram-negative organisms, including H. influenzae and N. meningitidis and excellent activity against most strains of N. gonorrhoeae.

Clarithromycin is more potent against erythromycin-sensitive strains of streptococci and staphylococci, but has only modest activity against H. influenzae and N. gonorrhoeae. However, it has good activity against M. catarrhalis, Chlamydia spp., L. pneumophila and Mycoplasma pneumoniae. Azithromycin is generally less active than erythromycin against the Gram-positive organisms and is more active than the other two macrolides against H. influenzae and Campylobacter spp. Azithromycin is very active against M. catarrhalis, P. multocida, Chlamydia spp., M. pneumoniae, L. pneumophila and N. gonorrhoeae.

Adverse reactions

Erythromycin is one of the safest antibiotics and causes serious adverse effects only rarely. Dose-related abdominal cramps, nausea, vomiting, diarrhoea and flatulence occur, but are uncommon in children and young adults. Allergic reactions observed include fever, eosinophilia and skin eruptions. Cholestatic hepatitis, transient hearing loss, polymorphic ventricular tachycardia, superinfection of the gastrointestinal tract and pseudomembranous colitis have been reported. Intravenous use of erythromycin is often associated with thrombophlebitis, but the incidence of this complication can be reduced with appropriate dilution of the dose. Adverse reactions to the other macrolides, at the usual dose, are rare and usually confined to the gastrointestinal tract. For this reason, roxithromycin is often prescribed instead of erythromycin.

Erythromycin and, to a lesser extent, the other macrolides, has been reported to cause clinically significant drug interactions [21]. Erythromycin has been reported to potentiate astemizole, terfenadine, carbamazepine, corticosteroids, digoxin, theophylline, valproate and warfarin, probably by interfering with cytochrome P450-mediated drug metabolism. Care should be used in the concurrent administration of the macrolides with these drugs.

Bacterial resistance

Resistance to erythromycin may be the result of reduced permeability through the cell envelope. This form of resistance is exhibited by the Enterobacteriaceae and Pseudomonas spp. Alteration of ribosomal proteins, especially

the 50S protein, often affects binding of the drug and has led to the emergence of resistant strains of B. subtilis, Strep. pyogenes and Strep. pneumoniae, Campylobacter spp., E. coli, Staph. aureus, Cl. perfringens, Listeria spp. and Legionella spp. Finally, enzymatic degradation of the drug has conferred high-level resistance among strains of Enterobacteriaceae.

Tetracycline

Tetracyclines are generally bacteriostatic and are thought to inhibit bacterial protein synthesis by binding to the 30S bacterial ribosome and preventing access of aminoacyl tRNA to its acceptor site.

Clinical uses

The antimicrobial spectra of all the tetracyclines are almost identical. They possess a wide range of antimicrobial activity against aerobic and anaerobic Gram-positive and Gram-negative bacteria. Clinically, the tetracyclines are useful against Strep. pneumoniae, H. influenzae, Neisseria spp., E. coli, Brucella spp., H. ducreyi, Vibrio cholerae, Campylobacter spp. and some Shigella and Mycobacterium spp. Many pathogenic spirochaetes are susceptible, including Borrelia burgdorferi. They are also effective against some microorganisms that are resistant to cell-wall active antimicrobial agents, such as Rickettsia, Coxiella burnetti, Mycoplasma pneumoniae, Chlamydia spp., Legionella spp. and Plasmodium spp.

Adverse reactions

The tetracyclines all produce gastrointestinal irritation in some individuals, although doxycycline is usually well tolerated. Epigastric discomfort, nausea, vomiting and diarrhoea are commonly reported. Renal and liver toxicity and photosensitivity may occur. Tetracyclines are deposited in the skeleton and teeth during gestation and childhood and can cause abnormalities of bone growth and discoloration of the teeth. It is therefore essential not to administer these agents to pregnant women or children under 8 years of age. Hypersensitivity reactions, including skin reactions, burning of the eyes, pruritus ani, vaginitis, angio-oedema and anaphylaxis, are rarely seen.

Bacterial resistance

Bacteria develop resistance to the tetracyclines mainly by preventing the accumulation of the drug within the cell. This is accomplished by reducing the influx or increasing the ability of the cell to export the antibiotic. Rarely, the tetracyclines are inactivated biologically or inhibited in their ribosomal attachment [22]. Resistance to one tetracycline usually means resistance to all. Clinically, most strains of enterococci are now resistant to tetracycline; group B streptococci are 50% susceptible and only 65% of Staph. aureus remain susceptible. Resistant pneumococci are now found in many geographical areas and many strains of Neisseria spp. are now resistant.

Aminoglycosides

Each aminoglycoside demonstrates concentration-dependent bactericidal activity against susceptible microorganisms. Gentamicin is the most commonly administered aminoglycoside in the ED and is a mixture of three closely related constituents. It binds to a specific area on the interface between the smaller (30S) and the larger (50S) bacterial ribosomal subunits, causing an increase in misreading of messenger RNA and a measurable decrease in protein synthesis. However, these effects do not provide a complete explanation for the rapidly lethal effect of gentamicin on bacteria.

Clinical uses

The antibacterial activity of gentamicin is directed primarily against aerobic and facultative Gram-negative bacilli. It has little activity against anaerobic microorganisms and facultative bacteria under anaerobic conditions and its activity against most Gram-positive bacteria is very limited. Gentamicin is clinically effective against Pseudomonas aeruginosa, Proteus mirabilis, Klebsiella pneumoniae, E. coli, Enterobacter spp. and Serratia spp. It is particularly effective when used in combination with cell-wall active antimicrobial agents, e.g. penicillin, cephalosporin. Interactions between these agents result in synergistic effects on bacterial death and may be useful against enterococci, Strep. pyogenes, some staphylococci, Enterobacteriaceae and Pseudomonas aeruginosa.

Adverse reactions

Like most other aminoglycosides, gentamicin has the potential to cause injury to the renal proximal convoluted tubules, damage to the cochlear and/or vestibular apparatus and neuromuscular blockade. As the drug is eliminated almost entirely by glomerular filtration, gentamicin dosing in renal failure must be undertaken with care and drug-level monitoring is recommended. Gentamicin has little allergenic potential. Anaphylaxis, rash and other hypersensitivity reactions are unusual.

Bacterial resistance

Bacteria defend themselves against the aminoglycosides by a combination of alteration of uptake, synthesis of modifying enzymes and a change of ribosomal binding sites.

In several centers, a significant percentage of clinical isolates are highly resistant to all aminoglycosides. At present, other widespread bacterial resistance to the aminoglycosides remains limited. However, there are reports of resistance emerging among some strains of Ps. aeruginosa, Enterobacteriaceae, E. coli, Serratia spp. and Staph. aureus.

Metronidazole

The toxicity of metronidazole is due to short-lived intermediate compounds or free radicals that produce damage by interaction with DNA and possibly other macromolecules.

Clinical uses

Metronidazole is active against a wide variety of anaerobic protozoal parasites. It is directly trichomonicidal. Sensitive strains of Trichomonas vaginalis are killed by very low concentrations of the drug under anaerobic conditions. The drug also has potent amoebicidal activity against E. histolytica, even in mixed culture, and substantial activity against the trophozoites of Giardia lamblia. Metronidazole manifests antibacterial activity against all anaerobic cocci and both anaerobic Gram-negative bacilli and anaerobic spore-forming Gram-positive bacilli. Bacteroides, Clostridium, Helicobacter, Fusobacterium, Peptococcus and Peptostreptococcus spp. are all susceptible.

Adverse reactions

In general, metronidazole is well tolerated. The most common side effects are headache, nausea, dry mouth and a metallic taste. Vomiting, diarrhoea and abdominal distress are occasionally experienced [23]. Furry tongue, glossitis and stomatitis may occur during therapy and are associated with a sudden intensification of moniliasis. Of clinical importance is metronidazole's well-documented disulfiram-like effect (Antabuse). Some patients experience abdominal distress, vomiting, flushing or headache if they drink alcohol during therapy with this drug.

Bacterial resistance

Fortunately, very few strains of Bacteroides spp. have demonstrated resistance. Some resistant strains of T. vaginalis have been isolated from patients with refractory cases of trichomoniasis, but these patients have usually responded to higher doses of metronidazole and prolonged courses of therapy [24].

Co-trimoxazole

Co-trimoxazole is a combination of sulphamethoxazole, a sulphonamide antibiotic, and trimethoprim, a diaminopyrimidine. The antimicrobial activity of this combination results from actions on two steps of the enzymatic pathway for the synthesis of tetrahydrofolic acid. Sulphamethoxazole inhibits the incorporation of PABA into folic acid and trimethoprim prevents the reduction of dihydrofolate to tetrahydrofolate. The latter is the form of folate essential to bacteria for one-carbon transfer reactions. Mammalian cells utilize preformed folate from the diet and do not synthesize this compound. This combination has been associated with serious sulphonamide-induced side effects. It has been recommended that the combination product be restricted to the few situations where combined use is the treatment of choice [1].

Clinical uses

Trimethoprim is effective in the treatment of most urinary tract infections and should be used alone for this indication. However, co-trimoxazole is active against a wide range of Gram-positive and Gram-negative microorganisms. C. diphtheriae and N. meningitidis are susceptible, as are most strains of Strep. pneumoniae. From 50 to 95% of strains of H. influenzae, Staph. aureus and epidermidis, Strep. pyogenes and viridans, E. coli, Proteus mirabilis, Enterobacter spp., Salmonella, Shigella and Serratia are inhibited. Also sensitive are Klebsiella spp., Brucella abortis, Pasteurella haemolytica and Yersinia spp. Co-trimoxazole has an important place in the treatment and prophylaxis of P. carinii infection and the treatment of L. monocytogenes and Nocardia infection.

Adverse reactions

In routine use, the combination appears to produce little toxicity. About 75% of adverse reactions involve the skin. These reactions are typical of those produced by sulphonamides and include a wide variety of rashes, erythema nodosum, erythema multiforme and Stevens–Johnson syndrome, exfoliative dermatitis and photosensitivity. Severe reactions tend to be more common among the elderly and HIV-infected patients. Gastrointestinal reactions include nausea and vomiting, but rarely diarrhoea. Glossitis and stomatitis are relatively common. Central nervous system reactions (headache, depression and hallucinations) and haematological disorders (anaemias, coagulation disorders and granulocytopaenia) have been reported.

Bacterial resistance

The frequency of development of bacterial resistance to co-trimoxazole is lower than it is to either of the constituent compounds alone. Resistance to sulphamethoxazole is presumed to originate by random mutation and selection or by transfer of resistance by plasmids. Such resistance is usually persistent and irreversible. Resistance to all sulphonamides is now becoming widespread in both community and nosocomial strains of bacteria, including streptococci, staphylococci, Enterobacteriaceae, *Neisseria* spp. and *Pseudomonas* spp. Trimethoprim-resistant microorganisms may arise by mutation, but resistance in Gram-negative bacteria is often associated with the acquisition of a plasmid that codes for an altered dihydrofolate reductase. Increasing incidences of resistance have been found in Enterobacteriaceae, *Ps. aeruginosa*, *Staph. aureus*, *E. coli*, *Salmonella* and *Shigella*.

Quinolones

The 4-quinolones, including nalidixic acid, are a family of compounds that contain a carboxylic acid moiety attached to a basic ring structure. The newer fluoroquinolones also contain a fluorine substituent, e.g. ciprofloxacin, and ofloxacin. Some may also contain a piperazine moiety. Bacterial DNA gyrase is an essential enzyme involved in DNA function. The quinolones inhibit the enzymatic activities of DNA gyrase and promote the cleavage of DNA within the enzyme–DNA complex.

Clinical uses

The early quinolones are most active against aerobic Gram-negative bacilli, particularly Enterobacteriaceae and *Haemophilus* spp. and against Gram-negative cocci, such as *Neisseria* spp. and *M. catarrhalis*. The fluoroquinolones are significantly more potent and have a much broader spectrum of antimicrobial activity. Relative to nalidixic acid, the fluoroquinolones also have additional activity against *Ps. aeruginosa* and some staphylococci. Ciprofloxacin remains the most potent fluoroquinolone against Gram-negative bacteria. Several intracellular bacteria are inhibited by the fluoroquinolones, including *Chlamydia*, *Mycoplasma*, *Legionella*, *Brucella* and some mycobacteria. Recently, a new drug, moxifloxacin, has been released that is useful for sinusitis, community-acquired pneumonia and acute bronchitis.

Adverse reactions

Generally, these drugs are well tolerated. Gastrointestinal symptoms of anorexia, nausea, vomiting, diarrhoea and abdominal discomfort are commonly seen, particularly with the older quinolones. Headache, dizziness, insomnia and alteration in mood are the next most commonly reported symptoms. Allergic and skin reactions, including phototoxicity, may occur. Rarely, arthralgias and joint swelling, leucopaenia, eosinophilia, thrombocytopaenia and haemolysis are reported.

Bacterial resistance

Resistance patterns over time have indicated that resistance increased following the introduction of fluoroquinolones and occurred most often with *Pseudomonas* spp. and staphylococci and in soft-tissue infections and in infections associated with foreign bodies. Possibly reflecting the pressures of extensive use, increasing fluoroquinolone resistance has been reported among strains of *Cl. jejuni* and *E. coli*. Focused quinolone use should be considered to avoid compromising the utility of the fluoroquinolones.

Nitrofurantoin

The mechanism of action is poorly understood, but activity in many cases appears to require enzymatic reduction within the bacterial cell [25]. The reduced derivatives are thought to bind to and damage intracellular proteins, including DNA, and inhibit bacterial respiration, pyruvate metabolism and the synthesis of inducible enzymes.

Clinical uses

Nitrofurantoin is active against over 90% of clinical strains of *E. coli*, *Citrobacter* spp., *Staph. saprophyticus* and *E. faecalis*. However, most species of *Proteus*, *Pseudomonas*, *Serratia*, *Providencia*, *Morganella* and many *Enterobacter* and *Klebsiella* spp. are resistant. Given its spectrum of activity and concentration in the urine, nitrofurantoin is usually administered for the treatment of urinary tract infections or for urinary antisepsis. However, it may have activity against bacteria not usually associated with urinary tract infections, including *Salmonella*, *Shigella*, *Staph. aureus*, *Strep. pneumoniae* and *pyogenes* and *Bacteroides*. Fortunately, bacteria that are susceptible to nitrofurantoin rarely become resistant during therapy.

Adverse reactions

Gastrointestinal upsets, particularly nausea, vomiting and diarrhoea, are the commonest side effects of nitrofurantoin. The frequency of these symptoms may be reduced if the macrocrystalline formulation is administered. Rashes, presumably allergic in nature, have been seen quite commonly. Cholestatic jaundice, acute and chronic hepatitis, pulmonary and haematological reactions and peripheral neuropathies have all been reported.

Colistin link parenteral

Colistin Link Parenteral has activity against Gram-negative bacilli: *Enterobacter aerogenes*, *E. coli*, *Klebsiella pneumoniae* and *Pseudomonas aeruginosa*.

Serious infection due to strains of *Pseudomonas aeruginosa* that exhibit resistance to all common antipseudomonal antimicrobials is an increasingly serious problem.

Pseudomonas aeruginosa is the Gram-negative pathogen that most commonly causes nosocomial pneumonia and is associated with the highest rates of crude and attributable mortality, even among patients who receive appropriate antimicrobial therapy.

Colistin Link Parenteral is eliminated mainly by renal excretion, it should be used with caution when the possibility of impaired renal function exists. The decline in renal function with advanced age should be taken into consideration, it can also cause nephrotoxicity.

Maximum daily dose should not exceed 5 mg/kg/day with normal renal function [26].

Antiviral drugs

Several antiviral drugs are available, although famciclovir, acyclovir and valacyclovir (prodrug of acyclovir that requires a lower dosage frequency) are the most frequently prescribed. Their mechanism of action is similar. Each drug targets virus-infected cells and inhibits viral DNA polymerase. Consequently, viral DNA synthesis and therefore viral replication are inhibited.

Clinical uses

These drugs are primarily used for the management of herpes zoster (within 72 hours of rash onset), treatment and suppression of genital herpes and the management of patients with advanced symptomatic HIV disease. Famciclovir is well absorbed in the gut and has the advantage of three times daily dosage compared to five times daily for acyclovir.

Acyclovir is also used to treat herpex simplex encephalitis (HSE).

HSE needs to be distinguished from herpes simplex meningitis, which is more commonly caused by HSV-2 than by HSV-1 and which often occurs in association with a concurrent herpetic genital infection.

Empiric treatment with acyclovir is essential in patients with suspected HSE pending confirmation of the diagnosis because acyclovir is the drug of choice and is relatively non-toxic and, if commencement of treatment is delayed, the prognosis for untreated HSE is poor.

Adverse reactions

These drugs are generally well tolerated. However, headache, gastrointestinal disturbance, dizziness and fatigue have been reported. Adverse effects are generally mild.

Antiviral agents for influenza

Zanamivir and oseltamivir are related antiviral medications known as neuraminidase inhibitors. These two medications are active against both influenza A and B viruses. They differ in pharmacokinetics, safety profiles, route of administration, approved age groups and recommended dosages.

The two other drugs used to treat influenza, amantadine and rimantadine are related antiviral drugs classified as adamantanes. These medications are active against influenza A viruses but not influenza B viruses. Widespread adamantane resistance among influenza A (H3N2) virus strains has made this class of medications less useful clinically.

Early antiviral treatment can shorten the duration of fever and symptoms and may reduce the risk of complications from influenza (e.g. otitis media in young children, pneumonia, respiratory failure) and death and shorten the duration of hospitalization. Clinical benefit is greatest when antiviral treatment is administered early, especially within 48 hours of influenza illness onset.

Antiretroviral drugs

Emergency physicians are unlikely to initiate these drugs as they form the basis of HIV treatment.

The only exception is prophylaxis following needle stick injury or body fluid exposure where close adherence to the hospital's policy is essential.

However, an appreciation of their uses and side effects is useful. Furthermore, the management of patients with HIV disease can be difficult and advice from an appropriate specialist source is essential.

Standard antiretroviral therapy (ART) consists of the combination of at least three antiretroviral (ARV) drugs to suppress maximally the HIV virus and stop the progression of HIV disease.

Clinical uses

The antiretrovirals are used in the treatment of established HIV infection. This includes patients with HIV-associated illnesses (e.g. CNS disease, malignancies, opportunistic diseases) and asymptomatic patients with low CD4 cell counts and/or high HIV viral loads. The drugs are also of use in the prevention of maternofetal transmission and as post-exposure prophylaxis for significant exposure from a known HIV-infected source.

Three major classes of antiretroviral drugs are available. For initial therapy, two to three drugs are generally used in combination (see Chapter 9.7).

Antifungal agents

Systemic fungal infections are becoming more and more common. Candidiasis and aspergillosis are the most common infections; other systemic fungal infections include histoplasmosis, blastomycosis, coccidioidomycosis.

Severe systemic fungal infection in hospitals are commonly seen in:

❶ neutropaenic patients following chemotherapy and other oncology patients with immune suppression

❷ persons that are immune compromised due to acquired immune deficiency syndrome caused by HIV infection

❸ patients in intensive care (ICU), who are not necessarily neutropaenic, but are compromised due to the presence of long-term intravascular lines or other breaches in their integument, severe systemic illness or burns and prolonged broad-spectrum antibiotic therapy.

Other predisposing factors include:

- APACHE score >10
- renal dysfunction
- haemodialysis
- surgery for acute pancreatitis, splenectomy
- recurrent GIT perforation
- Hickmann catheters.

Systemic fungal infections cause ≈25% of infection-related deaths in leukaemics. Infections due to *Candida* species are the fourth most important cause of nosocomial bloodstream infection.

The mainstay of antifungal therapy for severe systemic mycoses is amphotericin B.

Cryptococcal meningitis

Cryptococcus neoformans is an encapsulated yeast. The most serious infections usually develop in patients with defective cell-mediated immunity including, patients with:

- AIDS
- organ transplantation
- reticuloendothelial malignancy
- corticosteroid treatment
- sarcoidosis.

The incidence of cryptococcosis is increasing and now represents a major life-threatening fungal infection in AIDS patients.

Occupational risk factors for the infection include arborists and those exposed to bird droppings.

The initial site or sites of infection (pulmonary, CNS, and disseminated disease) determine the medical history of patients with symptomatic cryptococcal disease.

Patients with CNS infections, which are usually subacute or chronic in nature, present with headaches, neck pain, confusion, lethargy, malaise, and then, as the untreated infection progresses, focal neurological defects and decreased LOC. Fever, nausea and vomiting are not uncommon.

Treatment

Amphotericin B at 0.7–1 mg/kg/day for 2 weeks, with or without 2 weeks of flucytosine at 100 mg/kg/day in 4 divided doses, followed by fluconazole at 400 mg/day for a minimum of 8–10 weeks.

Initial therapy should be considered successful only after CSF culture is negative for cryptococcal organisms and the patient has had significant clinical improvement.

Initial therapy should be followed with maintenance therapy using fluconazole at 200 mg/day for life.

Amphotericin B

Amphotericin B is useful in treatment of infection with *Blastomyces*, *Coccidioides*, *Histoplasma*, *Paracoccidioides*, *Candida* and *Cryptococcus*, but does have substantial risk of toxicity. It is a 'polyene' and works on fungi by binding to ergosterol in the fungal cell membrane, disrupting the membrane and killing the fungus.

Other antifungal agents include fluconazole, which is mainly used for *C. albicans* infection (and some other susceptible *Candida* spp. but not *C. krusei*, and has variable activity against *C. glabrata*). *C. albicans* may acquire resistance, especially with chronic or recurrent treatment in AIDS patients. Fluconazole may be effective against *Cryptococcus neoformans* meningitis and coccidioidomycosis.

Outpatient parenteral antibiotic therapy

Outpatient parenteral antibiotic therapy (OPAT) has been widely used for the treatment of moderate to serious infections, either as an alternative to hospitalization or following initial hospitalization and early discharge once the patient is over the toxic phase of the infection. A wide range of infections are suitable for OPAT therapy (Table 9.9.2).

Significant savings, both in terms of direct and indirect costs, are possible utilizing OPAT. Appropriate patient selection is essential for safe and effective outpatient parenteral therapy (Tables 9.9.3 and 9.9.4). Patients should be

Table 9.9.2 Conditions that can be treated on an outpatient basis with parenteral antibiotic therapy

AIDS	Soft-tissue infections
Associated infections	Cellulitis Wound infections/abscesses
Cardiac	**Bone and joint infections**
Endocarditis Prosthetic-valve infections	Osteomyelitis Septic arthritis Prosthetic infections Neurological infections Meningitis
Genitourinary	**Other infections**
Pyelonephritis Complicated urinary tract infections Prostatitis Pelvic inflammatory disease	Bacteraemia Mastoiditis
Respiratory	
Pneumonia Lung abscess	

Table 9.9.3 Patient selection process

Condition suitable for outpatient therapy
Patient does not fulfil need to admit criteria (see Table 9.9.5)
OR
Patient meets discharge criteria (see Table 9.9.6) Home environment suitable
Patient/family consent

clinically stable, willing to participate and physically and mentally capable of being treated at home (Table 9.9.4).

Some patients require initial hospitalization (Table 9.9.5), following which they may be suitable for early discharge to continue treatment at home.

Once patients comply with predefined discharge criteria (Table 9.9.6), they may be able to be discharged into an outpatient parenteral therapy programme.

Close patient monitoring is essential, with daily reviews by a nurse either by telephone or face to face while patients are in the programme. Patients should be reviewed at least weekly by a physician.

The benefits of OPAT include a reduction in overall costs of patient care through avoidance or reduction in hospitalization, reduction of the costs associated with the hazards of hospitalization and increased patient satisfaction [27,28].

Table 9.9.4 Patient selection criteria

Able to give consent
Adequate social support at home
The antibiotic(s) chosen is/are appropriate for OPAT use
Patient's condition is stable
Concurrent illness does not require hospital care
Adequate venous access can be maintained Patient is mobile
The infection is amenable to outpatient parenteral therapy
Adequate monitoring by the treating medical team is possible

Table 9.9.5 Criteria for admission to hospital

Confused
Persistent high fever
Systolic blood pressure <100 mmHg
Respiratory rate >30/min
Pulse rate >100/min
Requires specialized nursing care assistance with activities of daily living
Hypoxic on room air (PaO$_2$ <80 mmHg)
Concurrent illness requiring inpatient care
Personal or social reasons
Pneumonic consolidation in more than one lobe

Table 9.9.6 Discharge criteria

Medical
Afebrile
Clinical improvement
No specialized nursing care required
Stable
Bacterial pathogens identified
Response to inpatient therapy
Complications unlikely

Social
Parents interested and motivated
Parents capable
Home environment acceptable
Telephone and transport access

Other issues

The risks associated with bioterrorism need to be taken into account with each and every patient presenting with a febrile illness or signs and symptoms of infection.

Numerous bacterial agents and bacterial toxins have been identified as potential biological agents. Patients presenting in clusters or with unusual or uncommon infections, particularly those that can be used as biological agents, should be quarantined, with staff utilizing post-exposure prophylaxis and strict infection control procedures. It may be necessary to activate the hospital's Mass Casualty Incident Plan when biological agents are suspected [29].

Recent updates from the medical literature

In August 2012, the CDC announced changes to the 2010 sexually transmitted disease guidelines for gonorrhoea treatment. The Gonococcal Isolate Surveillance Project (GISP) described a decline in cefixime susceptibility among urethral *N. gonorrhoeae* isolates in the USA during 2006–2011. Because of cefixime's lower susceptibility, new guidelines were issued that no longer recommend oral cephalosporins for first-line gonococcal infection treatment [30].

Likely developments over the next 5–10 years

The most important challenge regarding infectious disease in the future will be:

- The containment of and management of antimicrobial resistance patterns. In part, these patterns have emerged as a result of poor prescribing habits [31].
- Fewer new antimicrobial drugs are being developed, with the result that with

developing resistance patterns there will be very few effective antibiotics available for use against infection [9].

- The implementation of prescribing guidelines based on scientific evidence will form the basis of all antibiotic prescribing.
- Human behaviour, wildlife trade, factory farming, poor hygiene, global warming and increasing travel will increase the risk of pandemics, evolution and spread of new and old infections [32,33].

Detailed descriptions of the drugs described above are available on the Internet by accessing MIMS Online and Antibiotic Guidelines [1].

References

[1] Therapeutic Guidelines Limited. Therapeutic Guidelines: Antibiotic. Version 2010:14. Therapeutic Guidelines Limited, Melbourne.

[2] Weinstein L, Dalton AC. Host determinants of response to antimicrobial agents. N Engl J Med 1968;279:467.

[3] Moellering RC, Jr. Factors influencing the clinical use of antimicrobial agents in elderly patients. Geriatrics 1978;33:83.

[4] Philipson A. The use of antibiotics in pregnancy. J Antimicrobiol Chemother 1983;12:101.

[5] Black A, Francoeur D, Rowe T. SOCG Clinical Practice Guidelines No. 143, Part 2 2004. Canadian Contraception Consensus.

[6] Moellering Jr. RC. Principles of anti-infective therapy. In: Mandell GL, Bennett JE, Dolin R, editors. Principles and practice of infectious diseases (4th ed.). New York: Churchill Livingstone, 1995, p. 199–212.

[7] Welling PG. Effects of food on drug absorption. Annu Rev Nutrit 1996;16:383–415.

[8] Schlichting D, McCollam JS. Recognising and managing severe sepsis: a common and deadly threat. South Med J 2007;100:594–600.

[9] Cephalosporin-resistant CDC. Neisseria gonorrhoeae Public Health Response Plan. MMWR 2012;61:5.

[10] Davies J. Inactivation of antibiotics and the dissemination of resistance genes. Science 1994;264:375–82.

[11] Nikaido H. Prevention of drug access to bacterial targets: permeability barriers and active efflux. Science 1994;264:382–8.

[12] Spratt BG. Resistance to antibiotics mediated by target alterations. Science 1994;264:388–93.

[13] Kopecko D. Specialized genetic recombination systems in bacteria: their involvement in gene expression and evolution. Proc Mol Subcell Biol 1980;7:135–243.

[14] Elwell LP, Roberts M, Mayer LW, et al. Plasmid-mediated beta-lactamase production in *Neisseria gonorrhoeae*. Antimicrobiol Agents Chemother 1977;11:528–33.

[15] Lyon BR, Skurray R. Antimicrobial resistance of *Staphylococcus aureus*: genetic basis. Microbiol Rev 1987;5:88–134.

[16] Chambers HF, Sande MA. Antimicrobial agents Goodman and Gilman's The pharmacological basis of therapeutics, 9th ed. New York: McGraw-Hill, 1995, 1029–1032.

[17] Stillwell M, Caplan ES. The septic multiple-trauma patient. Infect Dis Clin N Am 1989;3:155.

[18] Kobayashi Y, Takahashi T, Nakae T. Diffusion of beta-lactam antibiotics through liposome membranes containing purified porins. Antimicrobiol Agents Chemother 1982;2:775–80.

[19] Idsoe O, Gothe T, Wilcox RR, et al. Nature and extent of penicillin side reactions with particular reference to fatalities from anaphylactic shock. Bull WHO 1968;38:159.

[20] Pichichero ME. A review of evidence supporting the American Academy of Pediatrics recommendation for prescribing cephalosporin antibiotics for penicillin-allergic patients. Pediatrics 2005;115:1048–57.

[21] Periti P, Mazzei T, Mini E, Novelli A. Pharmacokinetic drug interactions of macrolides. Clin Pharmacokinet 1992;23:106–31.

[22] Spera RV Jr, Farber BF. Multiply-resistant *Enterococcus faecium*. The nosocomial pathogen of the 1990s. J Am Med Assoc 1992; 268:2563–64.

[23] Lau AH, Lam NP, Piscitelli SC, et al. Clinical pharmacokinetics of metronidazole and other nitroimidazole anti-infectives. Clin Pharmacokinet 1992;2:328–64.

[24] Johnson PJ. Metronidazole and drug resistance. Parasitol Today 1993;9:183–6.

[25] McCalla DR, Reuvers A, Kaiser C. Mode of action of nitrofurantoin. J Bacteriol 1970;104:1126–34.

[26] Linden PK, Kusne S, Coley K, et al. Use of parenteral colistin for the treatment of serious infection due to antimicrobial-resistant Pseudomonas aeruginosa. Clin Infect Dis 2003;37:154–60.

[27] Tice AD. Outpatient parenteral antibiotic therapy (OPAT) in the United States: delivery models and indications for use. Can J Infect Dis 2000;11A:45A–8A.

[28] Vinen JD. Intravenous antibiotic treatment outside the hospital: safety and health economic aspects. Rev Contemp Pharmacother 1995; 6:435–44, 525.

[29] <www.bt.cdc.gov/Agent/agentlist.asp> [Accessed Nov. 2007].

[30] Gross EA, Stephens D. Multi-drug resistant bacteria: implications for the emergency physician. Emerg Med Rep 2007;28.

[31] WHO World Health Report. A Safer Future. <www.who. com>; 2007.

[32] Singer JL, Williams M. Imported infections in pediatric travelers. Emerg Med Rep 2007;28.

[33] CDC. 2012 Travellers' Health: Yellow Book <www.n.cdc.gov/travel/contentYellowBook.aspx> [Accessed Nov. 2012].

9.10 Needlestick injuries and related blood and body fluid exposures

Sean Arendse • Muhammad Shuaib Afzal

ESSENTIALS

1 Avoiding blood and other body fluid exposure remains the primary means of preventing occupationally-acquired blood-borne virus infections.

2 The risks of acquiring infection after occupational exposure to blood-borne viruses are: HIV 0.3%, hepatitis B (HBV) 12–30%, hepatitis C (HCV) 1.8%.

3 HBV immunization is an integral part of workplace safety.

4 Effective post-exposure prophylaxis (PEP) is available for both HBV and HIV, but not HCV.

5 Significant emotional distress often complicates needlestick and related occupational injuries.

Introduction

Management of the healthcare worker who sustains an occupational exposure to blood or other potentially infectious body fluids (e.g. semen, vaginal secretions, CSF and fluids containing visible blood) is an important issue for the emergency department (ED) doctor. It is estimated that around 600 000–800 000 needlestick or other percutaneous exposures happen annually in the USA [1]. This figure is a conservative estimate as many needlestick injuries go unreported. HBV, HCV and HIV are the most important occupationally acquired blood-borne pathogens; however, many other organisms, including malaria, syphilis, cytomegalovirus and possibly the prion diseases, such as Creutzfeld–Jakob disease, may also be transmissible via this route.

When evaluating healthcare providers (HCP) at risk for occupational infection with HIV, 'exposure' is defined as contact with potentially infectious blood, tissue or body fluids in a manner that allows for possible transmission of HIV and therefore requires consideration of post-exposure prophylaxis (PEP).

Such potentially infectious contacts are:

- a percutaneous injury (e.g. a needlestick or cut with a sharp object)
- contact of mucous membrane or non-intact skin (e.g. exposed skin that is chapped, abraded, or afflicted with dermatitis).

Body fluids of concern include:

- body fluids implicated in the transmission of HIV: blood, semen, vaginal secretions, other body fluids contaminated with visible blood
- potentially infectious body fluids (undetermined risk for transmitting HIV): cerebrospinal, synovial, pleural, peritoneal, pericardial and amniotic fluids.

Fluids that are not considered infectious unless they contain blood include faeces, nasal secretions, saliva, gastric secretions, sputum, sweat, tears, urine and vomitus.

In addition, any direct contact (i.e. without barrier protection) to concentrated HIV in a research laboratory or production facility is considered an 'exposure' that requires clinical evaluation and consideration of PEP.

Intact skin is an effective barrier against HIV infection and contamination of intact skin with blood or other potentially contaminated fluids is not considered an exposure and does not require PEP.

Most exposures do not result in infection and the risk of infection following significant exposure varies with factors such as:

- the pathogen involved (hepatitis B, hepatitis C or HIV)
- the fluid involved – blood is generally the most infectious body fluid
- the type of exposure – percutaneous or mucous membrane/non-intact skin

- the amount of blood or other infectious body fluid involved in the exposure
- the amount of virus in the patient's blood at the time of exposure.

General issues

Prevention of needlestick injuries

The old adage 'prevention is better than cure' certainly rings true when considering needlestick injuries, as the cost of managing one needlestick injury can range from 376 USD to 2456 USD [2].

The potentially infectious nature of all blood and bodily fluids necessitates the implementation of infection control practices. The universal application of standard precautions should be the minimum level of infection control when treating patients to prevent blood-borne virus transmission. The important elements of standard precautions are:

- the use of gloves when contact with blood, body fluids or secretions is anticipated
- the use of masks and protective eyewear during procedures that have the potential to generate splashes or sprays of blood or bodily fluids
- the use of gowns to protect skin and clothing from soiling by blood and other bodily fluids
- correct handling and disposal of needles and other sharp instruments:
  - disposal of sharps directly from patient immediately into sharps bins
  - locating sharps bins conveniently to reduce the unnecessary transportation of uncapped devices
  - avoiding overfilling sharps containers
  - never re-sheathing or re-capping needles
  - 100% attention when handling sharps.

More than 50 products with features designed to prevent needlestick injuries are currently available and fall broadly into two categories: those providing 'passive' or automatic protection and those with a safety mechanism that the user must activate.

It has been demonstrated that most needlestick injuries are preventable [3] and that use of safety engineered devices reduces needlestick injuries [3,4]. The passive devices are most effective in preventing needlestick injuries [5].

Hospital systems

Hospitals need to have appropriate policies and procedures to deal with occupational exposures to blood and body fluids; these are best implemented through a comprehensive and coordinated occupational exposure programme. Depending on the individual institution, such a programme is usually managed by infection control personnel and also involves staff health, occupational health, laboratory services, the ED and the infectious diseases service.

Staff need to be aware of the appropriate steps to take in the event that they sustain an exposure, such as who to notify, incident reporting requirements and where and how to seek medical evaluation. The programme should develop processes for consent and testing of the source individual (including situations where the individual refuses or is unable to give consent), prompt blood-borne virus testing and communication of results to the exposed person. Clear written guidelines and clinical pathways should be accessible to medical staff involved in managing these exposures (including specific recommendations for exposures involving a blood-borne virus positive source and antiretroviral post-exposure prophylaxis).

Management

The initial management of all needlestick injuries is the same – first aid measures, documentation of the event, determining the status of the source and counselling of exposed worker.

Initial management

Occupational exposure to blood or other potentially infectious body fluids should be considered a medical emergency to ensure timely management. Following exposure, the exposed person should be removed from the area and general first aid measures applied:

- for skin exposures – wash the exposed area well with soap and water; if no water is available, use an alcohol-based antiseptic. Other antiseptics, such as iodophors, chloroxylenol (PCMX) and chlorhexidine (CHG) also inactivate HIV

- for eye exposures – remove contact lenses if present and irrigate eyes with copious amounts of water or saline
- for oral mucous membrane exposures – spit out contaminating material and rinse the mouth with water several times.

Documentation

Clinical information on the source patient for the exposure and the recipient HCP should be documented. This includes risk factors and serological tests for HIV and hepatitis B and C. The nature and time of the exposure should also be described. The exposure should be evaluated and documented on the basis of the definition of exposure given above. All potential exposures to blood or contaminated body fluids as defined above should be promptly evaluated. The following information should be obtained by trained medical personnel:

- name and identification of the source
- time and date of the exposure
- nature of the exposure (i.e. non-intact skin, mucosal, or percutaneous exposure, human bite); type of fluid (i.e. blood, blood-contaminated fluid or other contaminated fluid)
- body location of the exposure and contact time with the contaminated fluid
- infective status of the source (i.e. HIV, HCV, HBsAg), if known, including date of test
- when the source is HIV positive, selection of the post-exposure prophylaxis regimen should consider the comparative risk represented by the exposure and information about the exposure source, including history of and response to antiretroviral therapy based on clinical response, CD4 cell counts, viral load measurements and current disease stage
- for percutaneous injuries, a description of the injury (depth of wound, solid versus hollow needle, sharp use in source patient).

The injured HCP should be questioned about the circumstances of the exposure (activity, time, device type, availability of PPE). The following information should be obtained from the injured person and verified from their medical/occupational health record:

- dates of hepatitis B immunizations
- post-immunization titre, if known
- previous testing (if available) for HIV, HBV and HCV
- tetanus immunization status

- current medications
- current or underlying medical conditions that might influence drug selection (e.g. pregnancy, breastfeeding, renal or hepatic disease).

Determining status of the source

All source cases should be tested for HBsAg, HCV and HIV, unless the source is known to be infectious. If feasible, a system should be devised to allow HIV test results to be obtained as soon as possible (i.e. within 24 hours). The rapid HIV test should be used to make an initial determination of the source patient's HIV status and has the advantage that results are available in less than 60 minutes [6]. All positive tests should be confirmed by Western blot. Negative tests do not require confirmation. Determination of HBsAg status should be obtained as soon as possible, but not later than 7 days. Local and state laws regarding consent and counselling prior to HIV testing should be followed.

Clinicians should also be aware of rare case reports where the source patient tested HIV seronegative and was later found to have primary HIV infection [7]; these rare events do not alter guidelines for routine antibody testing but do highlight the importance of testing for HIV RNA if clinically indicated.

Counselling of exposed worker

Risk assessment is particularly important for the HCP to make educated decisions about PEP since the consequences are huge and the stress is extraordinary. They should also be well informed of the benefits and risks of PEP and of the importance of close follow up. Specifically, the following issues should be discussed with the exposed HCP:

- The HCP should be informed of the risk associated with the specific exposure experienced.
- The efficacy and side effects of PEP should be discussed.
- Risk reduction strategies should be employed to prevent transmission of HIV should the HCP acquire infection. In the event of HIV infection post-exposure, the greatest risk of transmission to other individuals is in the first 6–12 weeks. The exposed HCP should be instructed on condom use or abstinence from sex and refraining from blood, plasma, organ, tissue and semen donation until the 6-month

INFECTIOUS DISEASE EMERGENCIES

serological test is negative. There is no need to modify a healthcare provider's patient-care responsibilities after an exposure.

- Follow up is important to identify HIV infection or adverse effects of the PEP regimen, if administered.
- Specific counselling is warranted for women of childbearing age. The data from an HIV pregnancy registry suggests overall safety of antiretroviral drugs [8]. Temporary discontinuation of breastfeeding following exposure until the 6-month serological test is negative should be considered.

Hepatitis B

Hepatitis B vaccination is recommended for all healthcare workers who are involved in direct patient care or who handle human blood or tissues [9] , and is an important infection control and occupational health strategy. Healthcare workers should be aware of their HBV immunization status and should undergo antibody testing 4–8 weeks after the last dose of the HBV vaccine to ascertain their immune status.

The risk of acquiring HBV from occupational blood/body fluid exposure from a patient positive for hepatitis B surface antigen (HBsAg) is well recognized and related primarily to the degree of contact with blood and the hepatitis B e-anitgen (HBeAg) status of the source. Following contact with a source positive for HBeAg, the risk of clinical hepatitis is 22–31% and serological evidence of HBV infection develops in 37–62% of exposed, non-immune individuals. In contrast, after exposure to HBeAg-negative blood, there is a 1–6% risk of

clinical hepatitis and a 23–37% risk of serological evidence of HBV infection [10]. The average time from exposure to the development of symptoms is 10 weeks (range 4–26 weeks). Routine vaccination against HBV has been recommended for healthcare workers since the early 1980s [11], with a consequent marked reduction in the incidence of infection in this population.

Post-exposure management following an occupational blood/body fluid exposure to HBV requires evaluation of the source's HBsAg status and the HBV vaccination and vaccine response status of the exposed person [12,13]. HB immunoglobulin (HBIG) is indicated for people who are non-immune (either because of no prior vaccination or because of vaccine non-responsiveness) and are exposed to blood or other infectious body fluids from an HBsAg-positive source. HBIG is prepared from human plasma (screened for blood-borne viruses) known to contain a high titre of antibody to HBsAg (antiHBs). The dose of HBIG is 400 IU, given IM. Concomitantly, HBV vaccination should be injected at a separate site and a full course completed. Table 9.10.1 provides more detailed information about specific indications for HBIG and hepatitis B vaccination following occupational exposures. The exposed person does not need to take any special precautions to prevent secondary transmission [14].

There are no apparent risks for adverse effects to developing fetuses when hepatitis B vaccine is administered to pregnant women (CDC, unpublished data, 1990). The vaccine contains non-infectious HBsAg particles which should pose no risk to the fetus. HBV infection during pregnancy might result in severe disease for the mother and chronic infection for the newborn.

Therefore, neither pregnancy nor lactation should be considered a contraindication to vaccination of women. HBIG is also not contraindicated for pregnant or lactating women [15].

Hepatitis C

The risk associated with occupational exposure to hepatitis C following a parenteral injury is estimated to range between 1.8% and 10% [16].

Transmission to healthcare workers has never been documented from skin contamination and rarely from mucous membrane exposure. In contrast to HBV, environmental contamination is not significant [17].

Recommendations for the management of occupational exposures to HCV are aimed at achieving early identification of infection. Recent data suggest that antiviral treatment of acute HCV infection increases rates of HCV clearance [18,19]. If the source HCV antibody test is positive, then polymerase chain reaction (PCR) testing for HCV RNA should be performed. Transmission is much less likely to occur from a source who is PCR negative and the exposed individual can be reassured that the transmission of HCV in this case is negligible. If the source is positive for HCV RNA, a baseline serum from the exposed person is tested for HCV RNA by PCR, anti-HCV antibody testing by enzyme-linked immunosorbent assay (ELISA) and alanine aminotransferase (ALT) with follow-up testing as shown in Table 9.10.2. HCV viraemia can be detected by PCR between 10 days and 6 weeks after infection [20,21].

Currently, there is no proven effective post-exposure prophylaxis for persons exposed

Table 9.10.1 HBV post exposure prophylaxis following occupational exposure			
Vaccination and antibody response status of exposed	Treatment when source		
	HBsAg positive	HBsAg negative	Unknown status
Unvaccinated	HBIG, initiate MB vaccine series	HB vaccine series	Vaccine series, consider HBIG
Vaccinated and known responder*	Reassure	Reassure	Reassure
Vaccinated and known non-responder*	HBIG, initiate HB vaccine series	Reassure, consider revaccine	If high risk source, treat as HBsAg positive
Vaccinated and unknown response*	Test exposed person for anti-HBs If adequate*, reassure If inadequate*, HBIG and course of vaccination	Reassure	Test exposed person for anti-HBs If adequate*, reassure If inadequate*, HBIG and course of vaccination

HBsAg: hepatitis B surface antigen; HBIG: hepatitis B immumoglobulin; anti-HBs: antibody to hepatitis B surface antigen.
From Updated US Public Health Service Guidelines for the Management of Occupational Exposures to HBV, HCV, and HIV and Recommendations for Postexposure Prophylaxis. 29 June 2001; 50:RR-11.

Table 9.10.2   Serology testing for needle stick injury exposed person

		Time			
		At exposure	4–6 weeks	3 months	6 months
Low risk source and negative serology		Anti-HB surface antigen antibody		HIV and HCV antibodies testing may be offered	
High risk source or positive serology	HBV	Anti-HB surface antigen antibody			
	HCV	HCV RNA PCR, Anti HCV antibody by ELISA ALT, AST	HCV RNA PCR ALT, AST	HCV RNA PCR, Anti HCV antibody by ELISA ALT, AST	HCV RNA PCR
	HIV	Anti HIV antibodies	Anti HIV antibodies	Anti HIV antibodies	
Unknown source, serology results not available		Anti HBsAg, Anti HCV, and HIV antibodies		HIV and HCV antibodies	HIV and HCV antibodies

HIV: human immunodeficiency virus, HCV RNA PCR: hepatitis C virus RNA by polymerase chain reaction. ELISA: enzyme linked immunosorbant assay, ALT: alanine amino transferase, AST: aspartate amino transferase, PEP: post exposure prophylaxis.

to HCV blood or contaminated body fluids. Immunoglobulin (Ig) and antiviral agents are not recommended for post-exposure prophylaxis of HCV [22,23]. Post-exposure prophylactic use of interferon has not been demonstrated to reduce the rate of infection and interferon is associated with many side effects [24,25], but early recognition and antiviral treatment of acute HCV infection in healthcare workers vastly increases viral clearance [18].

Currently, no recommendations exist to restrict professional activities of healthcare workers with HCV infection. As recommended for all healthcare workers, those who are HCV-positive should follow strict aseptic technique and standard precautions, including appropriate use of hand washing, protective barriers and care in the use and disposal of needles and other sharp instruments [14].

Human immunodeficiency virus

The average risk of acquiring human immunodeficiency virus (HIV) infection from all types of reported percutaneous exposure to HIV-infected blood is 0.3% [26]. This is increased for exposures considered as high risk involving:

- a deep injury
- visible blood on the device causing the injury
- a device previously placed in the artery or vein of the source patient
- a source with terminal AIDS or who has died as a result of AIDS within 60 days of the exposure and thus is presumed to have a high titre of HIV [27].

These factors are also probably significant for mucous membrane and skin exposures to HIV-infected blood, where the average risk of HIV transmission is approximately 0.09% and <0.09% respectively [28]. Prolonged or extensive skin contact or visibly compromised skin integrity would also suggest a higher risk.

Recommendations for post-exposure prophylaxis with antiretroviral agents have been guided by a better understanding of the pathogenesis of primary HIV infection, which indicates that HIV infection does not become established immediately; this leaves a brief window of opportunity during which post-exposure antiretroviral intervention might modify or prevent viral replication. An early case-control study demonstrated that use of zidovudine decreased the risk of occupational HIV seroconversion by 81% [29], and it is likely (but not proven) that combination antiretroviral therapy provides even greater protection. Animal data also support the use of antiretroviral prophylaxis after exposure to HIV, provided prophylaxis is administered promptly and for an adequate period. Failures of HIV PEP are well documented with both single drug and combination drug regimens [30].

HIV PEP should be initiated promptly, preferably within 2 hours of the exposure, although it may still be effective for up to 72 hours. Given the complexity of choosing and administering HIV PEP, whenever possible, consultation with an infectious diseases consultant or another physician who has experience with antiretroviral agents is recommended, but it should not delay timely initiation of PEP. There is a slight variability in the selection of drugs by different authorities. For the sake of simplicity and ease of understanding, a three-drug regimen is generally recommended

for all high-risk injuries. The preferred PEP regimen is tenofovir + emtricitabine (lamivudine may be used in place of emtricitabine) plus raltegravir. Zidovudine is no longer recommended in the preferred PEP regimen. The recommended duration of PEP is 28 days. A 3–5-day supply of PEP antiretroviral agents (a 'starter pack') should be kept in the ED.

This regimen is now the preferred combination because of its excellent tolerability, proven efficacy, fewer side effects and drug–drug interactions and ease of administration. Studies have shown increased rates of adherence and regimen completion when tenofovir + either emtricitabine or lamivudine have been used as components of the PEP regimen [31–37]. Zidovudine is not a 'must' inclusion in the newer regimens, as it has no clear advantages in efficacy over tenofovir and significant treatment limiting side effects. Efavirenz should not be used in pregnant women or women of childbearing age. Niverapine, abacavir and didanosine should not be used as PEP because of significant side effects.

Most occupational exposures do not result in transmission of HIV and the potential benefits of PEP need to be carefully weighed against the toxicity of the drugs involved. Nearly 50% of healthcare workers taking HIV PEP experience adverse symptoms (e.g. nausea, malaise, headache, diarrhoea and anorexia) and approximately 33% cease taking drugs because of side effects [38,39]. In some other studies, adherence to PEP has been estimated to be around 40–60% [39–41]. The importance of completing the prescribed regimen needs to be stressed and measures taken to minimize side effects.

The emotional effect of an occupational HIV exposure is substantial [42] and often underestimated. The exposed person may need time off work, short-term use of a night-time sedative or even referral for formal psychological or psychiatric counselling. Patients should be advised of measures to prevent secondary transmission (e.g. safer sexual practices) during the follow-up period, especially the first 6–12 weeks.

Maintaining confidentiality for the staff member sustaining exposure is a priority, as it may have lasting implications both personally and professionally.

The circumstances surrounding the exposure should be reviewed as part of the hospital's occupational exposure policy and appropriate preventive and educational measures taken if indicated.

Exposures that occur in the community

Blood or body fluid exposures may be sustained in the community, as well as in healthcare settings; examples include needlestick injuries from improperly discarded needles and syringes or blood splashes to the eye or mouth in the course of an altercation. The exposed person may be a member of the public or of an emergency service, such as a policemen or ambulance officer. These exposures are usually managed in the ED.

Although the principles of management are broadly similar to those for occupational exposures, there are some important differences. First, the source is almost never available for testing. (If the source syringe has been retrieved by the exposed person, this should *not* be tested for blood-borne viruses because such testing is only validated on serum.) Second, needlestick exposures almost always involve old dried blood; this is much less infectious than fresh blood because the viral titre falls with time and dried blood does not pass easily from the lumen of the needle into the exposed person's subcutaneous tissue. Third, these exposures often provoke a considerable degree of distress in the affected person and there may be considerable pressure from the exposed person, a family member or a colleague to 'do something'. Some of these incidents even attract media attention.

In Australia, only 1–2% of injecting drug users are HIV infected, so the risk of HIV transmission from a discarded needlestick injury is negligible: e.g. 1:100 (risk source is HIV positive) times 1:300 (risk of HIV transmission after needlestick) times undefined factor to account for old dried blood (say 1:5) – or approximately 1 in 150 000. Similar calculations show a potentially higher risk of hepatitis B and C transmission but, in reality, documented instances of blood-borne virus infection resulting from these community exposures are extremely rare and people should be reassured about this.

In Australia, antiretroviral prophylaxis is not recommended for these exposures unless there are particularly compelling epidemiological circumstances to indicate a high HIV risk in the source.

People not previously vaccinated against HBV should be given HBIG and the first dose of a hepatitis B vaccination course. Despite the low risk of blood-borne virus transmission, many patients feel more reassured if they are offered baseline and follow-up testing. As with exposures in the hospital setting, the attending doctor needs to provide the affected person with information, support and a sympathetic ear!

Provision of antiretroviral prophylaxis following sexual exposures in the community is a highly specialized field and is outside the scope of this chapter; advice should be sought from a doctor with HIV expertise. Interested readers are referred to guidelines produced by the Australian Department of Health and Ageing, available at http://www.ashm.org.au/pep-guidelines/

References

[1] Report available at <http://www.healthsystem.virginia.edu/pub/epinet/EPINet2011-NeedlestickRpt.pdf>.

[2] O'Malley EM, Scott II RD, Gayle J, et al. Costs of management of occupational exposures to blood and body fluids. Infect Control Hosp Epidemiol 2007;28:774–82.

[3] Cullen BL, Genasi F, Symington I, et al. Potential for reported needlestick injury prevention among healthcare workers through safety device usage and improvement of guideline adherence: expert panel assessment. J Hosp Infect 2006;63:445.

[4] Van der Molen HF, Zwinderman KA, Sluiter JK, et al. Interventions to prevent needle stick injuries among health care workers. Work 2012;41.

[5] Tosini W, Ciotti C, Goyer F, et al. Needlestick injury rates according to different types of safety-engineered devices: results of a French multicenter study. Infect Control Hosp Epidemiol 2010;31:402–7.

[6] Landovitz RJ, Currier JS. Clinical practice. Postexposure prophylaxis for HIV infection. N Engl J Med 2009; 361:1768.

[7] Giulieri S, Schiffer V, Yerly S, et al. The trap: professional exposure to human immunodeficiency virus antibody negative blood with high viral load. Arch Intern Med 2007;167:2524.

[8] Committee, APRS, Antiretroviral Pregnancy Registry International Interim Report for 1 January 1989 through 31 July 2011; 2011.

[9] Australian Immunization Handbook, 8th ed. National Health and Medical Research Council, 2003. <http://www.immunise.health.gov.au>.

[10] Werner BG, Grady GF. Accidental hepatitis-B-surface-antigen-positive inoculations: use of e antigen to estimate infectivity. Ann Intern Med 1982;97:367–9.

[11] CDC. Recommendation of the Immunization Practices Advisory Commitee (ACIP) inactivated hepatitis B virus vaccine. MMWR 1982;31:317–28.

[12] Grady GF, Lee VA, Prince AM, et al. Hepatitis B immune globulin for accidental exposures among medical personnel; final report of a multicenter controlled trial. J Infect Dis 1978;138:625–38.

[13] Seeff LB, Zimmerman HJ, Wrught EC, et al. A randomized, double blind controlled trial of the efficacy of immune serum globulin for the prevention of post-transfusion hepatitis: a veterans administation cooperative study. Gastroenterology 1977;72:111–21.

[14] Updated US Public Health Service guidelines for the management of occupational exposures to HBV, HCV, and HIV and recommendations for postexposure prophylaxis. 29 June 2001;50:RR-11.

[15] HIV/Viral hepatitis – a guide for primary care. Australian society for HIV medicine inc. 2001.

[16] Polish LB, Tong MJ, Co RL. Risk factors for hepatitis C virus infection among health care personnel in a community hospital. Am J Infect Control 1993;21:196–200.

[17] Jaeckel E, Cornberg M, Wedemeyer H, et al. Treatment of acute hepatitis C with interferon alpha-2b. N Engl J Med 2001;345:1452–7.

[18] Gerberding JL. Clinical practice. Occupational exposure to HIV in health care settings. N Engl J Med 2003;348:826.

[19] Zaaijer HL, Cuypers HT, Reesink HW, et al. Reliability of polymerase chain reaction for detection of hepatitis C virus infection. Lancet 1993;341:722–4.

[20] Wang TY, Kuo HT, Chen LC, et al. Use of polymerase chain reaction for early detection and management of hepatitis C virus infection after needlestick injury. Ann Clin Lab Sci 2002;32:137.

[21] Cleveland JL, Cardo DM. Occupational exposures to human immunodeficiency virus, hepatitis B virus, and hepatitis C virus: risk, prevention, and management. Dent Clin N Am 2003;47:681.

[22] Beekmann SE, Henderson DK. Protection of healthcare workers from bloodborne pathogens. Curr Opin Infect Dis 2005;18:331.

[23] Chung H, Kudo M, Kumada T, et al. Risk of HCV transmission after needlestick injury, and the efficacy of short-duration interferon administration to prevent HCV transmission to medical personnel. J Gastroenterol 2003;38:877.

[24] Corey KE, Servoss JC, Casson DR, et al. Pilot study of postexposure prophylaxis for hepatitis C virus in healthcare workers. Infect Control Hosp Epidemiol 2009;30:1000.

[25] CDC. Case-control study of HIV seroconversion in health care workers after percutaneous exposure to HIV-infected blood – France, United Kingdom and United States, Jan. 1988–Aug. 1994. MMWR 1995;44:929–33.

[26] Bell DM. Occupational risk of human immunodeficiency virus infection in health-care workers: an overview. Am J Med 1997;102:9–15.

[27] Gerberding JL. Management of occupational exposure to blood borne viruses. N Engl J Med 1995;332:444–551.

[28] Cardo DM, Culver DH, Ciesielski CA, et al. A case-control study of HIV seroconversion in health care workers after percutaneous exposure. N Engl J Med 1997;337:1485–90.

[29] Jochimsen EM. Failures of zidovudine postexposure prophylaxis. Am J Med 1997;102(suppl 5B):52–5.

[30] Mayer KH, Mimiaga MJ, Cohen D, et al. Tenofovir DF plus lamivudine or emtricitabine for nonoccupational postexposure prophylaxis (nPEP) in a Boston Community Health Center. J Acquir Immune Defic Syndr 2008;47:494–9.

[31] Tosini W, Muller P, Prazuck T, et al. Tolerability of HIV postexposure prophylaxis with tenofovir/emtricitabine and lopinavir/ritonavir tablet formulation. AIDS 2010;24:2375–80.

[32] Mayer K, Mimiaga M, Gelman M, et al. Tenofovir DF/emtricitabine/raltegravir appears safe and well-tolerated for non-occupational post-exposure prophylaxis. Presented

at fifth IAS Conference on HIV Pathogenesis, Treatment, and Prevention. 19–22 July 2009. Cape Town, South Africa. Abstract WEAC104.

[33] Mayer KH, Mimiaga MJ, Gelman M, et al. Raltegravir, tenofovir DF, and emtricitabine for postexposure prophylaxis to prevent the sexual transmission of HIV: safety, tolerability, and adherence. J Acquir Immune Defic Syndr 2012;59:354–9.

[34] Grant RM, Lama JR, Anderson PL, et al. Preexposure chemoprophylaxis for HIV prevention in men who have sex with men. N Engl J Med 2010;363:2587–99.

[35] Baeten J. Antiretroviral pre-exposure prophylaxis for HIV-1 prevention among heterosexual African men and women: the partners PrEP study. HIV-1-infected adults. 6th IAS Conference on HIV Pathogenesis, Treatment and Prevention. 17–20 July 2011. Rome. Abstract MOAX0106.

[36] Thigpen MC, Kebaabetswe PM, Smith DK, et al. Daily oral antiretroviral use for the prevention of HIV infection in heterosexually active young adults in Botswana: results from the TDF2 study. HIV-1-infected adults. Presented at 6th IAS Conference on HIV Pathogenesis, Treatment and Prevention. 17–20 July 2011. Rome. Abstract WELBC01.

[37] Wang SA, Panlilio AL, Doi PA, et al. Experience of healthcare workers taking postexposure prophylaxis after occupational HIV exposure: findings of the HIV postexposure prophylaxis registry. Infect Control Hosp Epidemiol 2000;21:780–5.

[38] Parkin JM, Murphy M, Anderson J, et al. Tolerability and side effects of post-exposure prophylaxis for HIV infection. Lancet 2000;335:722–3.

[39] Day S, Mears A, Bond K, et al. Post-exposure HIV prophylaxis following sexual exposure: a retrospective audit

against recent draft BASHH guidance. Sex Trasm Infect 2006;82:236–7.

[40] Lunding S, Katzenstein TL, Kronborg G, et al. The Danish PEP registry: experience with the use of postexposure prophylaxis (PEP) following sexual exposure to HIV from 1998–2006. Sex Transm Dis 2010;37:49–52.

[41] Armstrong K, Gordon R, Santorella G. Occupational exposures of health care workers (HCWs) to human immunodeficiency virus (HIV): stress reactions and counseling interventions. Social Work Health Care 1995;21:61–80.

[42] Henry K, Campbell S, Jackson B, et al. Long-term follow-up of health care workers with work-site exposure to human immunodeficiency virus. J Am Med Assoc 1990;236:1765.

9.11 Tropical infectious diseases

Sander Manders

ESSENTIALS

1 Tropical diseases are a major cause of morbidity and mortality worldwide.

2 Due to climate change and increasing population mobility (migration and travel), health practitioners in non-tropical areas will increasingly need to diagnose and treat tropical diseases.

3 A significant proportion of northern Australia has a tropical climate and several tropical diseases occur in this area. Vigilant public health surveillance, case tracking and vector control are instrumental in controlling incursions of non-endemic tropical diseases into Australia.

4 Indigenous Australians are disproportionately affected by infections in tropical Australia.

5 Within tropical areas, the aetiological spectrum of common diseases is different from that in temperate areas. This is due to different local prevalences of common pathogens, as well as the existence of specific tropical agents. Knowledge of local protocols is important in choosing appropriate antibiotic cover for the treatment of common diseases in the tropics.

6 In travellers who have returned from the tropics and present to the emergency department, common infections not specific to the tropics should not be forgotten as likely causes. A good history and systematic approach may aid in the correct identification of tropical diseases. Expert consultation may be of great benefit and public health notification is essential.

Introduction

Tropical diseases cause an enormous burden of disease worldwide and many other diseases that are not specific to the tropics disproportionally affect people in developing countries.

Returned travellers or migrants may present to health practitioners with signs and symptoms of tropical diseases. Due to climate change and increasing population mobility (travel and migration), health practitioners in non-tropical areas will increasingly need to diagnose and treat tropical diseases. A high index of suspicion, a systematic approach and expert consultation contribute to the appropriate investigation and management of these cases.

Significant areas of northern Australia have a tropical climate, including the Top End (around Darwin), Far North Queensland (north of Cairns) and the Kimberley (in Western Australia). Several tropical diseases are endemic there, with others occurring only infrequently. Indigenous Australians are disproportionally affected by both tropical and non-tropical disease.

Diseases common to temperate climates also occur in the tropics and it is important to recognize that these may have different aetiologies there. Community-acquired pneumonia in tropical Australia, for instance, is most commonly caused by *S. pneumoniae* but, in severe cases, organisms such as *Burkholderia pseudomallei* and *Acinetobacter baumannii* should also be covered. *Cryptococcus gattii* should be considered in meningitis or subacute pneumonia. In undifferentiated sepsis, melioidosis is an important differential diagnosis. Knowledge of protocols, based on specific local circumstances, is important.

Vigilant public health systems are in place to help prevent spreading disease from endemic areas into non-endemic areas. Many of the diseases discussed in this chapter are notifiable in both Australia and New Zealand. An appropriate public health response may include case surveillance, contact tracing and vector control.

Parasitic tropical diseases

Malaria

Introduction and epidemiology

Malaria is often considered the most important tropical disease worldwide. Half of the world's population is at risk, with over 200 million cases annually. An estimated 655 000 deaths occur each year, of which 90% are in subsaharan Africa [1]. A substantial number of malaria infections occur in South America, Southeast Asia and the Pacific.

In Australia, malaria was only officially considered eradicated in 1981 and there are ongoing concerns regarding the potential re-establishment of the disease due to the widespread presence of appropriate vectors and geographic proximity to endemic areas (particularly Indonesia and Papua New Guinea). An average of 600 cases are notified in Australia each year in travellers and migrants.

Malaria is caused by the protozoan parasite *Plasmodium*, of which six species are currently known to infect humans (Table 9.11.1). They have a complex life cycle and are transmitted by *Anopheles* mosquitoes, which bite from dusk to dawn. Less commonly, malaria can also be transmitted vertically. The parasites enter the blood and spread to the liver, where they replicate and are periodically released back into the bloodstream and then invade red blood cells.

The majority of malaria cases are caused by *P. falciparum*, which is the most severe and lethal form. Groups at particular risk include young children, pregnant women, immunocompromised patients (including those with HIV/AIDS) and travellers (due to a lack of immunity). Conversely, some genetic red blood cell variations, including sickle cell trait, thalassaemia trait, G6PD deficiency [2] and Melanesian ovalocytosis, provide some resistance against malaria.

Prevention

A large number of national and international organizations are involved in malaria prevention. Measures include vector control programmes, indoor residual spraying, insecticide-treated nets and intermittent preventative treatment for pregnant women. Travellers to endemic areas should use appropriate chemoprophylaxis, tailored to the locally occurring *Plasmodium* species and drug resistance patterns and avoid mosquito exposure. Efforts to develop a malaria vaccine are ongoing.

Clinical features

The incubation period is typically 10 days to 4 weeks, but can be longer. Mild cases of acute malaria are characterized by paroxysmal fevers, caused by periodic parasitaemia. Rigors herald 6–10 hours of high fever (>40°C), after which a relatively asymptomatic period follows. The rigors recur after approximately 40 hours ('tertian' fever) with *P. vivax* and *P. ovale* or approximately 64 hours ('quartan fever') with *P. malariae*. In *P. falciparum* malaria, fevers are less predictable and may be continuous. Additionally, there may be flu-like symptoms, diarrhoea, and mild jaundice.

Chronic malaria occurs when low-level parasitaemia persists, causing recurrent attacks and anaemia, hepatosplenomegaly and increased susceptibility to other infections. Secondary complications include massive splenomegaly, malarial nephropathy and Burkitt's lymphoma.

Severe malaria is almost exclusively caused by *P. falciparum*. Important features have been summarized in Table 9.11.2. The WHO has published case definitions for severe malaria [4]. The prognosis is poor, especially in children. Non-falciparum malaria is usually more benign, but death due to splenic rupture can occur.

Table 9.11.1 *Plasmodium* species that cause malaria in humans

Plasmodium *species*	Area	Notes
P. falciparum (≈75%)	Africa, South America, Southeast Asia	Responsible for most severe cases and deaths
P. malariae (≈20%)	Africa, Southeast Asia, Pacific, South America	Quartan malaria
P. ovale curtisi	West Africa, Southeast Asia	Two subspecies of *P. ovale* have recently been described [3]
P. ovale wallikeri	West Africa, Southeast Asia	
P. vivax	USA, South America, Asia, Africa	Relatively benign
P. knowlesi	Southeast Asia (Malaysia)	Can cause severe cases; macaques are reservoir

Table 9.11.2 Features of severe malaria [5]

Feature	Causes	Signs and symptoms
Cerebral malaria	Microvascular obstruction with parasite-containing red blood cells	Drowsiness, confusion, coma Delirium, transient psychosis Seizures Focal neurological signs (rare) Usually absent meningeal signs
Respiratory distress	Direct capillary damage (ARDS) Respiratory compensation of metabolic acidosis Intercurrent chest infection Anaemia	Increased work of breathing Kussmaul breathing pattern
Severe anaemia	Increased RBC clearance (both infected and non-infected RBCs) Hypersplenism and immunological causes Haemolysis Failing bone marrow erythropoiesis	Pallor Fatigue, prostration Failure to thrive Jaundice Haemoglobinuria ('blackwater fever')
Acute renal failure	Pre-renal (dehydration, hypovolaemia) Renal (microvascular obstruction, glomerulonephritis)	Oliguria, anuria
Acidosis	Lactic acidosis	Hyperpnoea (respiratory compensation)
Hypoglycaemia	Abnormal liver function Hyperinsulinaemia from quinine/quinidine administration	Anxiety, diaphoresis Drowsiness, coma Hypothermia
Disseminated intravascular coagulation (DIC)	Inappropriate coagulation cascade activation	Bleeding complications Relatively rare (<10% of severe malaria)

ARDS: acute respiratory distress syndrome; RBC: red blood cell.
After Trampuz A, Jereb M, Muzlovic I, Prabhu RM. Clinical review: severe malaria. Critical Care 2003;7:315–23.

Diagnosis

Clinical findings are of limited utility in diagnosing malaria [6]; microscopic examination of thick and thin blood smears [7] remains essential. A thick smear (drop of blood on a slide) is used to detect the presence of parasites and a thin smear (drop of blood spread thin on a slide) may help to identify the *Plasmodium* species. One negative smear does not exclude malaria and usually three sets are obtained at 12–24 hour intervals. Rapid dipstick immunoassay tests exist, but can be false negative with low or very high levels of parasitaemia. *Plasmodium*-specific polymerase chain reaction (PCR) tests are sensitive and specific but not widely available in endemic areas. Many other laboratory abnormalities, such as thrombocytopaenia and hyperbilirubinaemia, can be seen in malaria, but these are not specific enough to make the diagnosis. Before the diagnosis of cerebral malaria can be made, bacterial meningitis should be ruled out by lumbar puncture.

Treatment

Early treatment reduces morbidity, mortality and malaria transmission. Emerging resistance to antimalarial drugs (chloroquine and sulfadoxine-pyrimethamine) is a recurring problem worldwide. Artemisinin, a compound derived from wormwood, combined with another agent (artemisinin combination therapy) is the best currently available treatment for falciparum malaria [8,9]. It is given orally for uncomplicated cases and intravenously for severe cases. Various regimens are available to treat other *Plasmodium* species. For travellers diagnosed with malaria, different drugs should be used for treatment than were taken for prophylaxis. Initial hospitalization with infectious disease specialist consultation is recommended for all cases.

Schistosomiasis (bilharzia)

This parasitic disease affects more than 200 million people worldwide, with more than 90% of infections occurring in Africa. Its global impact is second only to malaria, with an estimated 200 000 deaths per year and significant chronic morbidity in survivors.

Infected fresh water snails release free-swimming larvae (cercaria) into surface waters, which can penetrate the skin of humans who come into contact with the water. Schistosomula then circulate in the blood and replicate in the portal vessels. Subsequently,

they migrate to blood vessels in other parts of the body and release their eggs, some of which are shed in human faeces and end up back in the surface waters. The eggs hatch in the water and produce miracidia, which enter suitable fresh water snails. After multiplying inside the snail, cercaria are released into the water, awaiting a new human host. The species of *Schistosoma* responsible for human infections are listed in Table 9.11.3; mixed infections occur.

Acute infections are more likely to cause symptoms among non-residents of endemic areas. A pruritic rash in response to cercariae entering the skin (swimmers' itch) can occur within a day, usually subsiding within 10 days. Acute toxaemic schistosomiasis (Katayama fever) is an uncommon but often severe seroconversion illness which may occur 1–3 months after the primary infection. Symptoms include fever, malaise, urticaria, cough, diarrhoea, hepatosplenomegaly and lymphadenopathy. It may last several weeks.

In chronic infection, the parasites migrate to species-specific areas in the host body, where their eggs induce a localized inflammatory response with fibrosis. This causes a high

Table 9.11.3 *Schistosoma* species that infect humans	
S. mansoni	Latin America, Africa, Middle East
S. haematobium	Africa, Middle East, Turkey, India
S. japonicum	East Asia, Pacific
S. intercalatum (≈1%)	Sub-Saharan Africa
S. mekongi (<1%)	Cambodia, Laos (Mekong river basin)

burden of disease [10–12]; common symptoms are listed in Table 9.11.4.

Prevention includes improving sewage management and personal protection, such as rubber boots. Fresh water exposure should be avoided where possible. A vaccine is under development.

The diagnosis is made by a history of fresh water exposure and the demonstration of eggs in the urine or faeces. During Katayama fever, no eggs may yet be seen. Serological tests are available. Abdominal X-rays may show bladder calcification in chronic genitourinary schistosomiasis.

Praziquantel (40–60 mg/kg in two divided doses) is an effective treatment but, due to high rate of re-infection, it may be difficult to achieve a cure in endemic areas. During Katayama fever, prednisone may be given to suppress the acute reaction and a repeat dose of praziquantel is recommended after 1–2 months. Community treatment programmes exist in endemic areas.

Leishmaniasis

Various species of *Leishmania* protozoa occur in South America, Africa, the Middle East and India, but also in southern Europe [13]. They are transmitted by sandflies from human and canine reservoirs. Preventative measures include DEET-containing insect repellents, covering exposed skin and insecticide spraying inside houses. Sandflies are so small they will pass through the mazes of bed nets that have not been treated with insecticide. Insecticide-impregnated dog collars have been shown to be effective.

Leishmania infections can have cutaneous or systemic manifestations, depending on parasite species and host factors; it can remain

Table 9.11.4 Symptoms of chronic schistosomiasis		
S. mansoni S. japonicum S. intercalatum S. mekongi **Hepatosplenic schistosomiasis** (hepatic periportal fibrosis) Hepatomegaly Portal hypertension Splenomegaly Pancytopaenia **Intestinal schistosomiasis** Intermittent bloody diarrhoea Tenesmus Anaemia Hypoalbuminaemia Intussusception	S. haematobium **Genitourinary schistosomiasis** Microscopic haematuria Bladder fibrosis and calcification Ureteric obstruction, hydronephrosis, reflux Squamous cell carcinoma of the bladder	**Neuroschistosomiasis** S. japonicum Meningoencephalitis Focal seizures S. mansoni, S. haematobium Cauda equina syndrome, paraplegia, bladder dysfunction **Pulmonary schistosomiasis** S. haematobium Pulmonary hypertension RV failure, tricuspid incompetence

asymptomatic. HIV co-infection predisposes to severe or recurrent disease. The incubation period is usually 1–2 weeks to 6 months, but there can be a latent period of up to 3 years.

Cutaneous leishmaniasis manifests with skin ulcers, which are usually painless unless a secondary bacterial infection occurs. Most lesions heal spontaneously over a few months, leaving a scar. A mucocutaneous form of the disease causes destruction of the mucous membranes of the nose, mouth, throat and surrounding tissues and can occasionally be fatal.

Visceral leishmaniasis (also known as kala-azar) manifests as fever with rigors, malaise, anorexia, lymphadenopathy and non-tender hepatosplenomegaly. Malnutrition and anaemia occur as the disease becomes chronic. The mortality is very high within 2 years if the disease remains untreated, although milder chronic forms occur.

The diagnosis can be confirmed by microscopy, culture or PCR. Treatment of leishmaniasis varies by clinical manifestation and geographic region; options include amphotericin-B, pentavalent antimony-containing preparations and several other drugs.

Post-kala-azar dermal leishmaniasis (PKDL) can occur several months to years after recovery from visceral leishmaniasis and consists of maculopapular lesions which spread from around the mouth. It typically disappears within a year without treatment, but may require several months of treatment in some regions. PKDL patients can be long-term reservoirs of infection.

Trypanosomiasis

American trypanosomiasis (Chagas' disease)

A major public health concern in Latin and South America, Chagas' disease is caused by the flagellate protozoan *Trypanosoma cruzi*. It is spread to humans and other mammals by the faeces of insects of the Triatominae subfamily ('kissing bugs'). Additionally, it can be spread vertically or by the administration of blood products. Prevention focuses on vector control, including the improvement of housing conditions and the use of insecticides and mosquito nets. Blood products and organ donors in the Americas are screened for *T. cruzi*.

The acute phase of the infection may have no or non-specific flu-like symptoms, but it can be fatal in children. Swelling around the site of inoculation in the face or around the eye (Romaña's sign) is well described. The infection

becomes asymptomatic within approximately 2 months. In the chronic phase, the parasites invade the myocardium and intestinal smooth muscle. The development of cardiomyopathy leads to congestive heart failure and arrhythmias and is fatal in 30%. Dilatation of the oesophagus and colon (10%) and neurological involvement may also occur.

The diagnosis can be made by direct visualization of the parasites in blood smears or serological testing. Benznidazole and nifurtimox are effective treatments if given soon after the infection occurs. Treatment for chronic infections is difficult and side effects are common. Supportive treatment for cardiac and gastrointestinal complications is important.

African trypanosomiasis (sleeping sickness)

This disease of sub-Saharan Africa is caused by *Trypanosoma brucei*, which is spread by bites of the tsetse fly. Several major epidemics have occurred in the last century and vector control programmes have been successful in reducing the number of cases reported.

Approximately 95% of cases are caused by *Trypanosoma brucei gambiense* (West and Central Africa). A chancre may develop at the site of inoculation, followed by an asymptomatic stage which can last months to years. Symptomatic infection then begins with the haemolymphatic stage, characterized by fever, arthralgias and pruritus. Posterior cervical lymphadenopathy (Winterbottom's sign) is common. The neurological stage begins when the trypanosomes invade the central nervous system, causing headaches, personality changes, psychosis and focal motor, extrapyramidal and/or cerebellar signs. The final stages of the

disease are characterized by daytime somnolence, seizures, coma and death.

A second type of the disease is caused by *T. b. rhodesiense* (5%) which occurs in southeastern Africa. Its course is more fulminant, with early multiple organ failure and death.

The diagnosis can be made by direct microscopic observation of the trypanosomes. Several serological screening tests (card agglutination trypanosoma test) exist for Gambian trypanosomiasis. The treatment is complex and depends on parasite subtype, regional drug resistance and the stage of the disease.

Filariasis

This variable disease is caused by a number of helminth species (worms) which occur throughout the (sub)tropics and are spread by mosquitoes and black flies. Lymphatic filariasis is the most common form; the worms develop in the lymphatic system and cause lymphoedema. Elephantiasis is the most extreme manifestation of this disease. Subcutaneous filariasis is caused by different species of helminths, producing a rash and arthritis. *Onchocerca volvulus* inhabits the eyes and is the world's second cause of blindness ('river blindness'). The diagnosis can be made with thick and thin blood smears, obtained on a species-specific time of the day or by PCR. Treatment is with diethyl-carbamazine or ivermectin and albendazole; sequelae often remain chronic.

Gastrointestinal parasites

A variety of gastrointestinal infections are prevalent throughout the tropics (Table 9.11.5); they represent a major cause of morbidity and childhood mortality. Most are transmitted by the faecal–oral route and prevention therefore

Table 9.11.5 Common gastrointestinal pathogens in tropical areas		
Parasites	*Bacteria*	*Viruses*
Protozoa	*Salmonella*	Rotavirus
Giardia lamblia	*Shigella*	Norovirus
Entamoeba histolytica	*Yersinia enterocolitica*	Adenovirus
Cryptosporidium parvum, C. hominis	*Campylobacter jejuni*	Astrovirus
	Eschericia coli (enterotoxigenic)	
Helminths	*Staphylococcus aureus*	
Ascaris lumbricoides (roundworm)	*Clostridium difficile*	
Hookworms	*Clostridium botulinum*	
Ancylostoma duodenale	*Vibrio cholerae*	
Necator americanus		
Trichuris trichuria (whipworm)		
Enterobius vermicularis (threadworm)		
Strongyloides stercoralis (pinworm)		

In Australia, *Strongyloides* is sometimes called 'roundworm'; In American English, 'pinworm' refers to *Enterobius* and 'threadworm' to *Strongyloides*.

includes improving sanitation and access to safe drinking water. The most important feature of management is appropriate oral or intravenous rehydration; specific antimicrobial therapy is secondary.

Protozoa

Giardia lamblia is a protozoan parasite with worldwide distribution, including Australia and New Zealand. It can survive for a long time in freshwater lakes and streams contaminated with animal or human faeces. Mild infections can be asymptomatic but it often causes foul-smelling, loose stools which may become fatty and float on water. It is usually self-limiting (7–10 days) but can become more chronic and contribute to malnutrition. The diagnosis is made by microscopy and treatment is with oral metronidazole (30 mg/kg up to 2 g daily, for 3 days) or tinidazole (50 mg/kg up to 2 g, as a single dose).

Entamoeba histolytica infection is often asymptomatic or causes only mild diarrhoea, but it may lead to severe diarrhoea with mucus, pus and blood in the stools (dysentery). Complications include peritonitis from intestinal perforation and amoebal liver abscesses. Microscopy often needs to be repeated to make the diagnosis. Supportive treatment is important; the specific treatment is oral metronidazole (15 mg/kg up to 600 mg, 8-hourly, for 7–10 days) or tinidazole (50 mg/kg up to 2 g daily, for 3 days).

Table 9.11.6 Clinical features of strongyloidiasis [14,15]

Acute strongyloidiasis
- Diarrhoea
- Hypoproteinaemia
- Hypokalaemia

Chronic uncomplicated strongyloidiasis
- Recurrent diarrhoea
- Epigastric pain
- Cutaneous manifestations
  - Urticaria
  - Transient, migratory, linear erythema (larva currens)
- Respiratory symptoms
  - Cough, haemoptysis
  - Pneumonia, pulmonary abscess

Disseminated strongyloidiasis (hyperinfective syndrome)
- Sepsis (from enteric bacteria spread by migrating larvae)
- Severe diarrhoea
- Paralytic ileus
- Pneumonia, pulmonary haemorrhage

After Adams M, Page W, Speare R. Strongyloidiasis: an issue in Aboriginal communities. Rural and Remote Health 2003; 3 (online); Johnston FH, Morris PS, Spears R, et al. Strongyloidiasis: a review of the evidence for Australian practitioners. Aust J Rural Health 2005;13: 247–54.

Several species of *Cryptosporidium* occur worldwide (including in Australia and New Zealand), causing self-limiting watery diarrhoea. Special microscopic techniques are required to make the diagnosis. Specific treatment is only required in immunocompromised patients (particularly those with AIDS) as it may become severe, even life threatening in this group.

Helminths (worms)

Soil-transmitted helminths infect humans when their eggs are ingested (*Ascaris*, *Trichuris*) or by active penetration of the skin by larvae (hookworms, *Strongyloides*). Most helminthic infections cause chronic abdominal discomfort without significant diarrhoea. Complications include intestinal obstruction (*Ascaris*), chronic diarrhoea (*Trichuris*) and iron deficiency anaemia (hookworms). The eggs and larvae of these species can be distinguished by microscopy. Benzimidazoles (albendazole, mebendazole) as a single dose or short course are effective treatment.

Strongyloides occurs worldwide, but it is hyperendemic in rural and remote indigenous communities in northern Australia with a reported prevalence of up to 60%. Due to a cycle of auto-infection, *Strongyloides* infection can be lifelong if untreated. Clinical features of strongyloidiasis are summarized in Table 9.11.6. Immunocompromised patients, including those given corticosteroids, may develop disseminated strongyloidiasis, which carries a high mortality. The diagnosis can be made by detection of larvae in stool or serology in specialized laboratories. Treatment is with ivermectin (200 μg/kg as a single dose) or albendazole (400 mg daily for 3 days); some authors advocate repeat treatments.

Table 9.11.7 Major viral tropical diseases

Disease & virus*	Areas of common occurrence	Vector
Flaviviruses		
– Yellow fever (YFV)	South America, Africa	Mosquitoes (*Aedes aegypti*)
– Dengue (DENV)	Latin & South America, Africa, South & Southeast Asia	
– West Nile encephalitis (WNV)	Africa, Middle East, Central Asia, North America, Europe, Australia	Mosquitoes (*Culex* spp.)
– Kunjin (KUNV)	Australia, Pacific	
– Japanese encephalitis (JEV)	Southeast and Far East Asia	
– Murray Valley encephalitis (MVEV)	Northern Australia, PNG	
Alphaviruses		
– Ross River fever (RRV)	Australia, PNG, South Pacific	Mosquitoes (*Aedes* spp.)
– Barmah Forest fever (BFV)	Australia	
– Chikungunya (CHIKV)	Africa, South & Southeast Asia	

*Commonly used abbreviation to indicate the causative virus. PNG: Papua New Guinea.

Viral tropical diseases

Many tropical viral infections are arthropod-borne (arboviruses), with flaviviruses being the most important subgroup (Table 9.11.7). Alphaviruses also cause some important infections in tropical and temperate areas.

Yellow fever

In acute yellow fever, a flu-like syndrome develops after 3–6 days' incubation and improves after another 3–4 days. In 15% of cases, a 'toxic phase' then develops, with high fever, liver dysfunction causing jaundice and haemorrhage, and renal impairment. Mortality in this group is approximately 50%; survivors recover without significant sequelae. There is no specific treatment, but an effective vaccine exists. Evidence of vaccination is required by health authorities in many countries for travellers returning from endemic areas.

Dengue

Four distinct serotypes of the dengue virus occur in most tropical areas of the world; most cases occur in Southeast Asia. In Australia, occasional outbreaks occur, mostly in Far North Queensland. Most cases remain asymptomatic. Dengue fever may develop after 3–14 days' incubation; it lasts for 2–7 days. Arthralgias are often severe. The rash resembles that of measles. The most feared complication is dengue haemorrhagic fever (DHF), which may develop if a subsequent infection with another dengue serotype occurs. Features are summarized in Table 9.11.8. Laboratory diagnosis can be made with PCR testing. Supportive management with adequate hydration and analgesia is

Table 9.11.8   WHO case definitions for dengue

Dengue fever (DF)
Acute febrile illness with ≥2 of:
- Headache
- Retro-orbital pain
- Myalgia
- Arthralgia
- Rash
- Haemorrhagic manifestations (not meeting DHF criteria)
- Leukopaenia

AND supportive serology

Dengue haemorrhagic fever (DHF)
ALL of:
- Febrile illness lasting 2–7 days
- Haemorrhagic tendencies
    - Positive tourniquet test
    - Petechiae, ecchymoses or purpura
    - Bleeding from the mucosa, GI tract, injection sites or other
    - Haematemesis or melaena
- Thrombocytopaenia (≤100 000/mm^3)
- Evidence of increased vascular permeability
    - Rise in haematocrit ≥20%
    - Drop in haematocrit ≥20% after rehydration
    - Signs of plasma leakage (pleural effusion, ascites, hypoproteinaemia)

Dengue shock syndrome (DSS)
ALL criteria for DHF
PLUS evidence of circulatory failure:
- Rapid, weak pulse
- Narrow pulse pressure (≤20 mmHg)
- Hypotension
- Cold, clammy skin and restlessness

Table 9.11.9   Important viral haemorrhagic fevers

Virus	Areas of common occurrence	Vector
Arenaviridae		
– Lassavirus	West Africa	Rats
Bunyaviridae		
– Hantaviruses	South & North America, South Asia, Europe	Rodents (rats, mice)
– Crimean–Congo haemorrhagic fever virus	Africa	Ticks (*Hyalomma*)
– Rift Valley fever virus	Africa	Mosquitoes (*Aedes* and *Culex* spp.)
Filoviridae		
– Ebola virus	Central Africa	Bats
– Marburg virus	Equatorial Africa	Bats

important; no specific therapy exists. A vaccine against all four serotypes is in an advanced stage of development [16].

Arboviral encephalitis

Various arboviruses cause encephalitis and, while the vast majority of infections remain asymptomatic, potentially devastating sequelae occur in symptomatic patients. Clinical symptoms do not reliably differentiate between various arboviral causes of encephalitis; a definitive diagnosis can be obtained by serological testing.

In recent years, the West Nile virus (WNV) has been successful in extending its range into temperate areas including North America, Europe and Australia. Kunjin virus is a subtype of WNV endemic to Australia and Papua New Guinea [17]. The Murray Valley encephalitis virus is also endemic to northern Australia and Papua New Guinea and epidemics in the southern states of Australia have been well

described [18]. Japanese encephalitis virus sporadically occurs on the Torres Strait Islands and in the northernmost tip of Queensland.

When symptomatic, these viruses may cause fever with a flu-like syndrome, rash, meningeal signs, convulsions and decreased level of consciousness. Encephalitis, meningitis or a poliomyelitis-like illness with flaccid paralysis have all been described. Disease progression is variable, ranging from full recovery to death. Longterm neuropsychiatric sequelae occur in a large proportion of survivors. Treatment is supportive. A vaccine exists for the Japanese encephalitis virus.

Alphaviruses

Several thousand cases of Ross River virus (RRV) and Barmah Forest virus (BFV) infections occur annually in Australia. They cause flu-like symptoms with arthralgia and a widespread maculopapular rash in 50% of cases. Arthritis, myalgia and fatigue can last for 6 months or

longer. IgM serological tests for RRV or BFV may be false positive in patients with other infections such as malaria and dengue. The closely related chikungunya virus occurs in Africa and Southeast Asia and causes similar symptoms. There is no specific treatment.

Viral haemorrhagic fevers

Several families of viruses can cause fever with haemorrhagic diathesis (Table 9.11.9). They are carried by vectors, but person-to-person spread is mostly responsible for outbreaks. Dengue, yellow fever, and certain other flaviviruses occasionally cause haemorrhagic fever as well.

The clinical presentation is variable, but usually includes a flu-like prodrome with respiratory and sometimes central nervous system symptoms. The disease progresses to multiple organ failure with disseminated intravascular coagulopathy. Case fatality rates are high, up to 90%. Treatment is supportive, with no specific antiviral agents available. Vaccine research is ongoing.

Viral hepatitis

A high incidence of hepatitis A and B (HAV, HBV) occurs in developing countries. HAV is spread via the faecal–oral route, whereas HBV is spread via contaminated blood and other bodily fluids. Vaccinations are recommended for travellers to endemic areas.

The hepatitis C virus (HCV) is a non-arthropod-borne flavivirus. Transmission via non-sterilized medical equipment is a concern in certain countries and recommendations for travellers may include carrying their own needles; no vaccine is available.

Hepatitis E (HEV) causes a self-limiting disease similar to hepatitis A, except during pregnancy when fatal hepatitis is well documented.

Bacterial tropical diseases

Tuberculosis

Introduction

Approximately one-third of the world's human population is infected by *Mycobacterium tuberculosis*, making it a major worldwide public health concern. Tuberculosis is by no means exclusively a tropical disease, but it disproportionally affects people in developing countries. Risk factors include HIV infection and other causes of immune suppression, diabetes, pulmonary disease and malnutrition. It is transmitted via inhalation of droplets produced by a coughing person with tuberculosis. Mortality if untreated is around 50%.

Screening and prevention

For screening purposes, the Mantoux (tuberculin) skin test and interferon-gamma release assays (IGRA) are commonly used. When positive, these tests indicate prior exposure to tuberculosis but do not prove active disease. False negatives and false positives are a concern. The Bacillus Calmette–Guérin (BCG) vaccination offers some protection to people at high risk of contracting tuberculosis. Some controversy remains over the validity of the Mantoux test after BCG vaccination.

Symptoms

Tuberculosis can be asymptomatic, but may produce non-specific symptoms including fever, night sweats, anorexia and cachexia.

The most common presentation is pulmonary tuberculosis, which causes a productive cough, haemoptysis, chest pain and dyspnoea. An exudative pleural effusion may occur. Chronic complications include bronchiectasis and pulmonary fibrosis.

Non-pulmonary tuberculosis can occur in virtually any part of the body, including lymph nodes, bones, meninges, pericardium, abdomen and genitourinary tract. Miliary tuberculosis is an aggressive form of haematogenously disseminated tuberculosis which occurs in infants and immunocompromised patients.

Latent tuberculosis occurs when mycobacteria persist intracellularly; patients are asymptomatic and not infectious. The disease can reactivate later, for example, when the patient becomes immunocompromised.

Diagnosis

Pulmonary tuberculosis may be suggested by chest X-ray appearance (Table 9.11.10). Mycobacteria can be demonstrated on acid-fast (Ziehl–Neelsen) staining of sputum or broncho-alveolar lavage fluid. Culture confirms the diagnosis by identifying the species of mycobacteria and also enables drug susceptibility testing. For non-pulmonary tuberculosis, samples appropriate to the site should be obtained and tested [19].

Management

Within an emergency department or other hospital setting, patients suspected to have infective tuberculosis should be in a negative-pressure room; staff and visitors should

Table 9.11.10 Chest X-ray findings associated with pulmonary tuberculosis
Consolidation
Hilar lymphadenopathy
Ghon focus (calcified nodule that remains after resolution of initial consolidation)
Cavitating lesions
Fibrosis (dominant in upper lobes)
Calcifications
Miliary pattern (small nodules throughout lungs)
Tuberculoma (well-defined tuberculosis mass)

wear appropriate N95 face-masks (aerosol precautions).

Treatment of any form of tuberculosis requires expert consultation. Public health reporting with appropriate contact tracing is essential. A 6-month treatment regimen with four drugs initially ('HRZE', i.e. isoniazid, rifampicin, pyrazinamide, ethambutol) is often used to treat uncomplicated tuberculosis. Emerging multidrug resistance is of increasing concern worldwide [20,21].

Melioidosis

Introduction

The Gram-negative bacterium *Burkholderia pseudomallei* is the cause of melioidosis [22]. It is found throughout Southeast Asia and India and is highly endemic in northeast Thailand, Malaysia, Singapore and northern Australia (with sporadic cases seen further south). The bacteria live in the soil during the dry season but can be found in surface water and mud after heavy rainfall; they may also become airborne. Transmission occurs through the skin (cuts and sores), inhaled airborne dust or droplets and, rarely, through ingestion of contaminated water. Person-to-person transmission is extremely rare.

The most important risk factors are diabetes, renal disease, alcohol excess and chronic lung disease. Indigenous Australians are disproportionally affected. Healthy people can become infected when working in wet, muddy conditions without adequate hand and foot protection.

Symptoms

The most common presentation of melioidosis is pneumonia, which may be severe [23]. It

can also cause multiple abscesses in the skin, prostate, spleen, kidney and liver. Septic arthritis, osteomyelitis and neurological disease also occur. In endemic areas, melioidosis is an important differential diagnostic consideration in community-acquired sepsis. Septic shock develops in approximately 20% and carries a high mortality. Unusual features of melioidosis include the development of sepsis after a long initial period of subclinical infection and its potential for recurrence after apparently appropriate antibiotic treatment.

Diagnosis and management

Melioidosis should be treated empirically when the diagnosis is suspected in endemic areas. Serological tests are of limited utility in populations with high background rates of infection. Cultures of blood, sputum, urine or swabs from an abscess or skin ulcer (in Ashdown's selective medium) can confirm the diagnosis. A chest X-ray should be performed in all suspected cases and a CT-abdomen and pelvis is recommended to seek abscesses in any culture-positive case.

B. pseudomallei is resistant to penicillins, most cephalosporins and aminoglycosides. Although it has some susceptibility to ceftriaxone (2 g IV is recommended initially for adults), to treat melioidosis definitively, meropenem (25 mg/kg up to 1 g, 8-hourly), imipenem (25 mg/kg up to 1 g, 6-hourly) or ceftazidime (50 mg/kg up to 2 g, 6-hourly) needs to be given. Intravenous antibiotic therapy should be continued for at least 14 days and followed by oral therapy (usually with sulfamethoxazole/trimethoprim) for 3–6 months. Abscesses should be drained and septic joints washed out. Expert consultation is recommended.

Leptospirosis

The zoonotic, spirochaete bacteria of the *Leptospira* genus have a worldwide distribution (including Australia and New Zealand), with a higher prevalence in wet and humid tropical areas. Transmission occurs via the urine of infected animals and people with occupational or recreational exposure to animals or their urine are at particular risk.

Leptospira enter the body through damaged skin or mucous membranes, circulate in the blood and then invade kidneys, lungs and liver. The incubation period is 2–20 days. The initial (spiraemic) phase produces non-specific flu-like symptoms with conjunctivitis and occasional jaundice and hepatosplenomegaly. This is followed by a second (immune) phase which may include renal and hepatic failure, aseptic meningitis and pulmonary haemorrhage. Multiorgan failure can lead to death.

The diagnosis is usually made by lepto-spirosis serology (microagglutination test). However, initial serology is often negative, necessitating a convalescent serum sample for diagnosis. Polymerase chain reaction tests are also available. Cultures may only become positive after several weeks of incubation. *Leptospira* are sensitive to a wide variety of antibiotics, including doxycycline (100 mg PO, 12-hourly, for 5–7 days). For more severe disease, intravenous benzylpenicillin (30 mg/kg up to 1.2 g IV, 6-hourly, for 5–7 days) or ceftriaxone (25 mg/kg up to 1 g, daily for 5–7 days) are recommended.

Rickettsia

Rickettsia are a group of pleomorphic, Gram-negative, obligate intracellular bacteria, with various species occurring in different areas throughout the world. They are spread by ticks and several other vectors.

Spotted fever

This group of rickettsial diseases includes Rocky Mountain spotted fever (RMSF), African tick bite fever, Mediterranean spotted fever, Australian tick typhus and others. The disease typically begins with fever, nausea and vomiting, myalgia and headaches. After a few days, a maculopapular rash appears in the majority of cases. RMSF in particular can progress to severe disease with vasculitis involving the lungs, intra-abdominal organs, central nervous system and skin (petechial rash). Treatment with oral or intravenous doxycycline (100 mg, 12-hourly, for 7–10 days) should be commenced when there is sufficient clinical suspicion; confirmation from serological tests should not be awaited.

Typhus

Caused by *Rickettsia* that are spread by lice and fleas; epidemics occur after natural or man-made disasters. Symptoms include a high fever with rigors, cough, myalgias and delirium. After a few days, a centrifugal rash may be seen. Treatment with doxycycline (dosing as above) or azithromycin (500 mg orally on day 1, then 250 mg daily for a further 4 days) may be life saving.

Scrub typhus

This disease is caused by *Orientia* species, a bacterium similar to *Rickettsia*. It is endemic to East and Southeast Asia and northern Australia and is spread by larval stages of mites which occur in dense scrub vegetation. Symptoms include fever with chills, headache, cough, lymphadenopathy and sometimes a rash. An eschar (macule with black scab) often develops when the bite site ulcerates, usually in the groin, on the buttocks or in the axilla. Multiorgan failure can develop and fatal cases within Australia have been described. It is treated with doxycycline or azithromycin (dosing as above).

Enteric fever

Salmonella enterica, serovar Typhi causes a severe, acute febrile illness known as typhoid fever. Paratyphoid fever is a similar but usually less severe disease caused by serovar Paratyphi. Together, these entities are referred to as enteric fever. The causative bacteria occur throughout tropical areas of the world, with the majority of cases occurring in South Asia (India, Pakistan, Bangladesh). They are spread via the faecal–oral route, often via contaminated food or water. Oral and intramuscular vaccines are available, but are not completely effective.

Enteric fever is a systemic illness, different from the 'simple' gastroenteritis caused by non-typhoid *Salmonella* serovars. Initial symptoms include high fever for >2 days with malaise, headache, cough and constipation. After a week, prostration and high fevers with relative bradycardia become prominent. A rash (rose spots) and hepatosplenomegaly can occur. Delirium and profuse diarrhoea often develop in the third week. Most mortality is caused by complications, including intestinal haemorrhage or perforation, septicaemia, encephalitis and secondary abscess formation. Survivors slowly improve over another week or so.

The diagnosis can be made from blood, stool or bone marrow cultures. Management is complicated by increasing rates of antibiotic resistance, with multidrug resistance particularly problematic in Southeast Asia. Fluoroquinolones or third-generation cephalosporins are still largely effective treatments; azithromycin is recommended for Southeast Asia. For infections acquired in areas with less antibiotic resistance, other options may include chloramphenicol, amoxicillin and co-trimoxazole; expert consultation is recommended. Dexamethasone may reduce mortality in septic shock from enteric fever and good supportive management is essential.

Cholera

The flagellated, Gram-negative bacterium *Vibrio cholerae* secretes a toxin which causes profuse, watery diarrhoea [24]. It is transmitted via the faecal–oral route and occurs throughout sub-Saharan Africa, South Asia and South America. Oral vaccines are available.

Cholera causes high-volume watery diarrhoea ('rice water') leading to dehydration with electrolyte loss, metabolic acidosis and hypoglycaemia. Vomiting occurs in the majority of cases. Shock, renal failure and cardiac arrhythmias are the main causes of mortality.

In the event of an outbreak, the diagnosis is often made on clinical grounds alone. *V. cholerae* may be demonstrated on microscopy and cultures in selective media can confirm the diagnosis.

The cornerstone of management is rehydration (oral or intravenous fluids) with electrolyte replacement. In severe cases, antibiotics reduce diarrhoea duration and severity. Doxycycline and azithromycin (20 mg/kg up to 1 g orally as a single dose) are most commonly used; other antibiotics may also be effective, such as ciprofloxacin (25 mg/kg up to 1 g orally, as a single dose).

Approach to the returned traveller

People returning from tropical areas may present to healthcare providers with a variety of symptoms. A systematic approach is important to appropriately investigate and manage these patients. Ordered lists of common presenting symptoms, incubation times and geographical distributions can be found widely on the Internet [25]. Up-to-date information on endemic tropical diseases in the area of the patient's travel should be sought, including any current outbreaks of tropical or non-tropical diseases (such as novel influenza viruses or SARS). It is essential that common non-tropical diseases, such as influenza or meningococcal meningitis, are included in the differential diagnosis.

History

Obtain a detailed previous medical history, including any predisposing factors, such as immune compromise, splenectomy and pregnancy, as well as a list of medications and known adverse drug reactions.

Table 9.11.11 Important tropical diseases by presenting symptom

Fever	Respiratory manifestations	Cutaneous manifestations
Malaria	Tuberculosis	Cutaneous larva migrans
Arboviral infections (dengue)	Melioidosis	(hookworms)
Bacterial diarrhoea	Leptospirosis	Leishmaniasis
Enteric fever	Histoplasmosis	Rickettsia
Rickettsia	Cryptococcosis	Filariasis
Leptospirosis	Pulmonary plague	Trypanosomiasis
Alphaviruses (RRV, BFV)	Tularaemia	Cutaneous myiasis (botfly)
Schistosomiasis	Pulmonary anthrax	
Hepatitis A		
Trypanosomiasis		
Viral haemorrhagic fevers		

The travel history should include:

- exact locations, duration and dates of stay, including any stopovers
- the nature of the accommodation (e.g. air-conditioned hotel or camping), use of bed nets and insect repellents
- vaccination history (routine and travel-related) and adherence to preventative medication (such as antimalarial drugs)
- any behaviour that may have led to disease exposure: known insect or tick bites, contact with sick people, animals, fresh water (including leisure activities), potentially unsafe food or water and sexual or needle exposures.

The history of the presenting complaint should include fever patterns (including rigors) and associated symptoms (e.g. respiratory, cutaneous, gastrointestinal and other symptoms). Ask about appearance and frequency of stools and whether they contained blood or mucus (dysentery).

Examination

The physical examination is often non-specific but can sometimes provide important clues to the diagnosis. Careful examination of the respiratory system, lymph nodes and skin is important (Table 9.11.11). Look for hepatosplenomegaly, jaundice and bleeding.

Investigations

Potential non-tropical causes for the patient's condition should be investigated as usual, e.g. chest X-ray for respiratory infections or a lumbar puncture for meningitis.

If the history and examination have raised suspicion for conditions for which specific tests (such as serology or cultures) are available, these should be sent off. Keep in mind that many of these will take days or longer to come back. Stool samples for culture, ova and parasites may be helpful. Specific tests for *Giardia*, *Cryptosporidium* and *Entamoeba histolytica* can be requested.

Routine blood tests may provide support for certain conditions, but they are rarely diagnostic. There should be a low threshold for obtaining three sets of thick and thin smears for malaria. Malaria rapid antigen detection tests are also very helpful, although relatively low sensitivity of these kits mandates that three blood films are still required to rule out malaria in any traveller with persisting fever who has returned from a malaria-endemic location. Eosinophilia is usually associated with parasitic (helminth) infection, but also with several other infections including HIV, HTLV and tuberculosis. Evidence of haemolysis or coagulopathy may correlate with worse outcome.

Management

Specific treatment may be commenced if available, depending on the likely diagnosis. This may need to be done without the benefit of laboratory confirmation. A low threshold for expert consultation is recommended to help guide investigations and management. Supportive treatment is very important and may include analgesia, fever control measures and the maintenance of adequate hydration and electrolyte replacement.

Patients who are unwell or suspected to have a high-risk condition should be admitted to the hospital. Consideration can be given to discharging low-risk patients, provided that adequate follow up can be arranged, including the results of any outstanding tests. Public health notification of any suspected or proven notifiable diseases is essential.

Acknowledgement

The author wishes to thank Professor Bart Currie, Infectious Diseases Physician at Royal Darwin Hospital and the Menzies School of Health Research, for his helpful suggestions.

The author strongly recommends checking all drug doses and regimens carefully. The latest version of the Australian Therapeutic Guidelines (Antibiotic) or other appropriate local guidelines should be consulted.

References

[1] World Health Organization (WHO). <http://www.who.int/features/factfiles/malaria/en/index.html> and UNICEF <http://www.unicef.org/health/index_malaria.html> [Accessed Feb. 2013].

[2] Hedrick PW. Population genetics of malaria resistance in humans. Heredity 2011;107:283–304.

[3] Sutherland CJ, Tanomsing N, Nolder D, et al. Two nonrecombining sympatric forms of the human malaria parasite *Plasmodium ovale* occur globally. J Infect Dis 2010;201:1544–50.

[4] World Health Organization Guidelines for the treatment of malaria, 2nd ed. Geneva: WHO; 2010.

[5] Trampuz A, Jereb M, Muzlovic I, Prabhu RM. Clinical review: severe malaria. Crit Care 2003;7:315–23.

[6] Taylor SM, Molyneux ME, Simel DL, et al. Does this patient have malaria? J Am Med Assoc 2010;304: 2048–56.

[7] Moody AH, Chiodini PL. Methods for the detection of blood parasites. Clin Lab Haematol 2000;22:189–201.

[8] South East Asian Quinine Artesunate Malaria Trial (SEAQUAMAT) group. Artesunate versus quinine for treatment of severe falciparum malaria: a randomised trial. Lancet 2005;366:717–25.

[9] Dondorp AM, Fanello CI, Hendriksen ICE, et al. Artesunate versus quinine in the treatment of severe falciparum malaria in African children (AQUAMAT): an open-label, randomised trial. Lancet 2010;376:1647–57.

[10] Gryseels B, Polman K, Clerinx J, Kestens L. Human schistosomiasis. Lancet 2006;368:1106–18.

[11] Ross AGP, Bartley PB, Sleigh AC, et al. Schistosomiasis. N Engl J Med 2002;346:1212–20.

[12] MacConnachie Schistosomiasis. J R Coll Physicians Edinb 2012;42:47–50.

[13] Pavli A, Maltezou HC. Leishmaniasis, an emerging infection in travelers. Internatl J Infect Dis 2010;14:e1032–39.

[14] Adams M, Page W, Speare R. Strongyloidiasis: an issue in Aboriginal communities, rural and remote health 2003;3(online). <http://rrh.deakin.edu.au>.

[15] Johnston FH, Morris PS, Spears R, et al. Strongyloidiasis: a review of the evidence for Australian practitioners. Aust J Rural Hlth 2005;13:247–54.

[16] Dengue vaccine roll-out: getting ahead of the game. Bull World Health Org 2011;89:476–7.

[17] Gray TJ, Burrow JN, Markey PG, et al. Case report: West Nile virus (Kunjin subtype) disease in the Northern Territory of Australia – a case of encephalitis and review of all reported cases. Am J Trop Med Hyg 2011;85:952–6.

[18] Knox J, Cowan RU, Doyle JS, et al. Murray Valley encephalitis: a review of clinical features, diagnosis and treatment. Med J Aust 2012;196:5.

[19] National Institute for Health and Clinical Excellence (NICE) clinical guideline 117. Tuberculosis: clinical diagnosis and management of tuberculosis, and measures for its prevention and control, 2011. <www.nice.org.uk/guidance/CG117>.

[20] Ministry of Health. Guidelines for tuberculosis control in New Zealand, 2010; (online) HP 5148. <http://www.moh.govt.nz>.

[21] Lawn SD, Zumla AI. Tuberculosis. Lancet 2011;378: 57–72.

[22] Wiersinga WJ, Currie BJ, Peacock SJ. Melioidosis. N Engl J Med 2012;367:1035–44.

[23] Currie BJ, Ward L, Cheng AC. The epidemiology and clinical spectrum of melioidosis: 540 cases from the 20 year Darwin prospective study. PLoS Neglected Trop Dis 2010;11:e900. <www.plosntds.org>.

[24] Harris JB, LaRocque RC, Qadri F, et al. Cholera. Lancet 2012;379:2466–76.

[25] Centers for Disease Control. <http://wwwnc.cdc.gov/travel/yellowbook/2012/chapter-5-post-travel-evaluation/general-approach-to-the-returned-traveler.htm> [Accessed Feb. 2013].

GENITOURINARY EMERGENCIES

Edited by **George Jelinek**

10.1 Acute kidney injury

Nicholas Adams • Linas Dziukas

ESSENTIALS

1 Acute kidney injury (AKI) is defined as a rapid reduction in the glomerular filtration rate marked by an acute increase in the serum creatinine (SCr) concentration.

2 The early stages of AKI are usually asymptomatic and the diagnosis is based on a decrease in urine output or an elevated SCr. It may take 24 hours or more for an initially normal SCr concentration definitely to increase and up to 48 h to distinguish between early AKI and renal failure.

3 The basic processes causing AKI are: renal hypoperfusion (prerenal causes), damage to glomeruli, tubules, interstitium or blood vessels (renal causes) or obstruction to urine flow (post-renal causes).

4 Prerenal factors are present in about 40% of persons with AKI. They include hypovolaemia, hypotension, oedematous states with a reduced 'effective' circulating volume, renal hypoperfusion and drugs.

5 Bedside correction of hypovolaemia should be based on jugular venous pulse and urine output and their response to intravenous fluid resuscitation.

6 Renal factors are present in about 50% of persons with AKI. Acute tubular necrosis (ATN) is the most common pathological process causing ARF and is classified as ischaemic ATN or ATN due to damage by toxins (e.g. myoglobin) or drugs. No therapeutic intervention has hastened the recovery of renal function in established ATN.

7 Obstruction is present in about 10% of persons with AKI. Hydronephrosis can occur in the absence of obstruction and some persons with obstruction do not have a dilated urinary collecting system.

8 Urine output usually decreases in AKI and the patient may be oliguric (less than 400 mL per day) or anuric (less than 100 mL per day). Only a few conditions cause anuria: complete urinary tract obstruction, vascular lesions, severe ATN or rapidly progressive glomerulonephritis.

9 Intravenous mannitol and sodium bicarbonate to produce an alkaline diuresis as a means of preventing ATN in severe rhabdomyolysis has not been shown to be effective.

Introduction

The basic process in acute kidney injury (AKI) is a rapid (hours to days) reduction in the glomerular filtration rate (GFR) due to renal hypoperfusion, damage to glomeruli, tubules, interstitium or blood vessels, or obstruction to urine flow. The GFR is inversely related to the serum creatinine (SCr) concentration and the diagnosis of AKI is made when there is an acute increase in the SCr concentration, with or without a decrease in the urine output. A simple definition of AKI is an acute and sustained (lasting for 48 hours or more) increase in the SCr of 44 µmol/L if the baseline is less than 221 µmol/L, or an increase in the SCr of more than 20% if the baseline is more than 221 µmol/L. A more comprehensive definition (the RIFLE system) is used to classify persons with acute impairment of renal function (Table 10.1.1) [1].

Table 10.1.1 RIFLE classification of acute renal failure		
Stage	Serum creatinine (SCr) concentration	Urine output
RISK	Increase of 1.5 times the baseline	<0.5 mL/kg/h for 6 h
INJURY	Increase of 2.0 times the baseline	<0.5 mL/kg/h for 12 h
FAILURE	Increase of 3.0 times the baseline or SCr is 355 μmol/L or more when there has been an acute rise of greater than 44 μmol/L for 24 h or anuria for 12 h	<0.3 mL/kg/h
LOSS	Persistent acute renal failure; complete loss of kidney function for longer than 4 weeks	
END-STAGE RENAL DISEASE	End-stage renal disease for longer than 3 months	

Aetiology and pathogenesis

The causes of AKI are grouped according to the source of renal injury: prerenal (hypoperfusion), renal (parenchymal) and post-renal (obstructive). More than one cause can be present simultaneously.

Prerenal acute kidney injury

Prerenal AKI is initially an adaptive response to severe volume depletion and hypotension in structurally intact nephrons. Prerenal AKI that is prolonged or inadequately treated can be followed by parenchymal renal damage (acute tubular necrosis). Prerenal AKI is a potentially reversible cause of acute renal failure (ARF).

Reductions in renal blood flow (RBF) and GFR occur in the setting(s) of hypovolaemia, hypotension, oedematous states with a reduced 'effective' circulating volume (cardiac failure, hepatic cirrhosis, nephrotic syndrome) or impaired renal perfusion (renal artery stenosis, hepatorenal syndrome). Drugs that interfere with renal autoregulation (e.g. prostaglandin inhibitors, angiotensin-converting enzyme [ACE] inhibitors or angiotensin II receptor antagonists) can reduce glomerular perfusion [2]. The physiological responses to volume depletion and hypotension, and the link to prerenal AKI are shown in Figure 10.1.1.

Renal acute kidney injury

Ischaemic, cytotoxic or inflammatory processes may damage the renal parenchyma. The causes of the damage can be grouped according to the major structures that are damaged: vessels, glomeruli, renal tubules or renal interstitial tissue.

Vascular causes involving the larger vessels include acute thrombosis of the renal artery, embolism of the renal arteries, renal artery dissection and renal vein thrombosis. Microvascular causes include vasculitis, malignant hypertension and thrombotic microangiopathy.

The glomeruli are the site of injury in acute glomerulonephritis which can cause proteinuria, haematuria, nephrotic syndrome or nephritic syndrome. A number of different forms of glomerulonephritis have been described, generally diagnosed by the histological changes seen on renal biopsy. The distinction between these forms is not of direct concern for the emergency practitioner.

Acute tubular necrosis (ATN) is the most common pathological process that causes AKI. While the terminology suggests that the main cause is tubular damage, the actual pathophysiology is more complex: impaired autoregulation and marked intrarenal vasoconstriction (the main mechanism for the greatly reduced GFR), tubular damage (with cytoskeleton breakdown), increased tubuloglomerular feedback, endothelial cell injury, fibrin deposition in the microcirculation, release of cytokines, activation of inflammation and activation of the immune system [3].

ATN is often classified as ischaemic ATN or cytotoxic ATN but both processes may be present in some patients. Ischaemic ATN represents an advanced form of prerenal AKI, but the distinction between these two entities is based on histopathological changes and is of little use to the clinician. Important causes of cytotoxic ATN are listed in Table 10.1.2. Nonsteroidal anti-inflammatory drugs (NSAIDs), ACE inhibitors and angiotensin receptor blockers (ARBs) often cause a gradual and asymptomatic decrease in the GFR, but can also cause AKI. NSAIDs do not impair renal function in healthy persons, but can reduce the GFR in the elderly with atherosclerotic cardiovascular disease, in persons with chronic renal failure, when chronic prerenal hypoperfusion is present (e.g. cardiac failure, cirrhosis) or in persons using diuretics and calcium channel blockers [4]. AKI may occur after the administration of intravenous or intra-arterial radiocontrast agents. A number of risk factors have been identified for this, the most important being pre-existing renal impairment, hypovolaemia, a large contrast load and the use of hyperosmolar contrast agents [5]. Drugs that alter angiotensin levels (ACE inhibitors and ARBs) reduce renal perfusion by their antihypertensive effects or by impairing vasoconstriction of the efferent arteriole when renal perfusion is reduced by renal artery stenosis. The nephrotoxicity of haem pigments (myoglobin and haemoglobin) is enhanced by volume depletion, low urine flow rates and possibly low urine pH.

Abnormalities of renal interstitial structure and function are only one feature of ATN, but represent the primary abnormality in acute tubulointerstitial nephritis (ATIN). The damage in ATIN is due to immunological mechanisms, the most important involving cell-mediated immunity. ATIN is usually due to an allergic reaction to a drug, commonly antibiotics (β-lactam antibiotics, sulphonamides, fluoroquinolones), NSAIDs, cyclooxygenase-2 inhibitors, proton pump inhibitors, diuretics, phenytoin, carbamazepine and allopurinol.

Post-renal acute kidney injury

Obstructive uropathy refers to the functional or structural processes in the urinary tract that impede the normal flow of urine and obstructive nephropathy is the renal damage caused by the obstruction. Hydronephrosis and hydroureter refer to dilatation of the renal urinary collecting system and the ureters, respectively. They may occur in the absence of obstruction and, conversely, may be absent in some patients with obstruction.

Casts or crystals within the renal tubular lumen can cause intrarenal obstruction. Extrarenal obstruction can develop in the urethra, bladder, ureter or the pelvi-ureteric junction. Obstructive uropathy in adults is commonly caused by prostate disease or retroperitoneal neoplasm (cancer of the cervix, uterus, bladder, ovary or colon). Metastatic cancer, lymphomas or inflammatory processes in the retroperitoneum (appendicitis, diverticulitis, Crohn's disease) or a neurogenic bladder can also cause obstructive uropathy. Bilateral renal stones are an uncommon cause of obstructive uropathy.

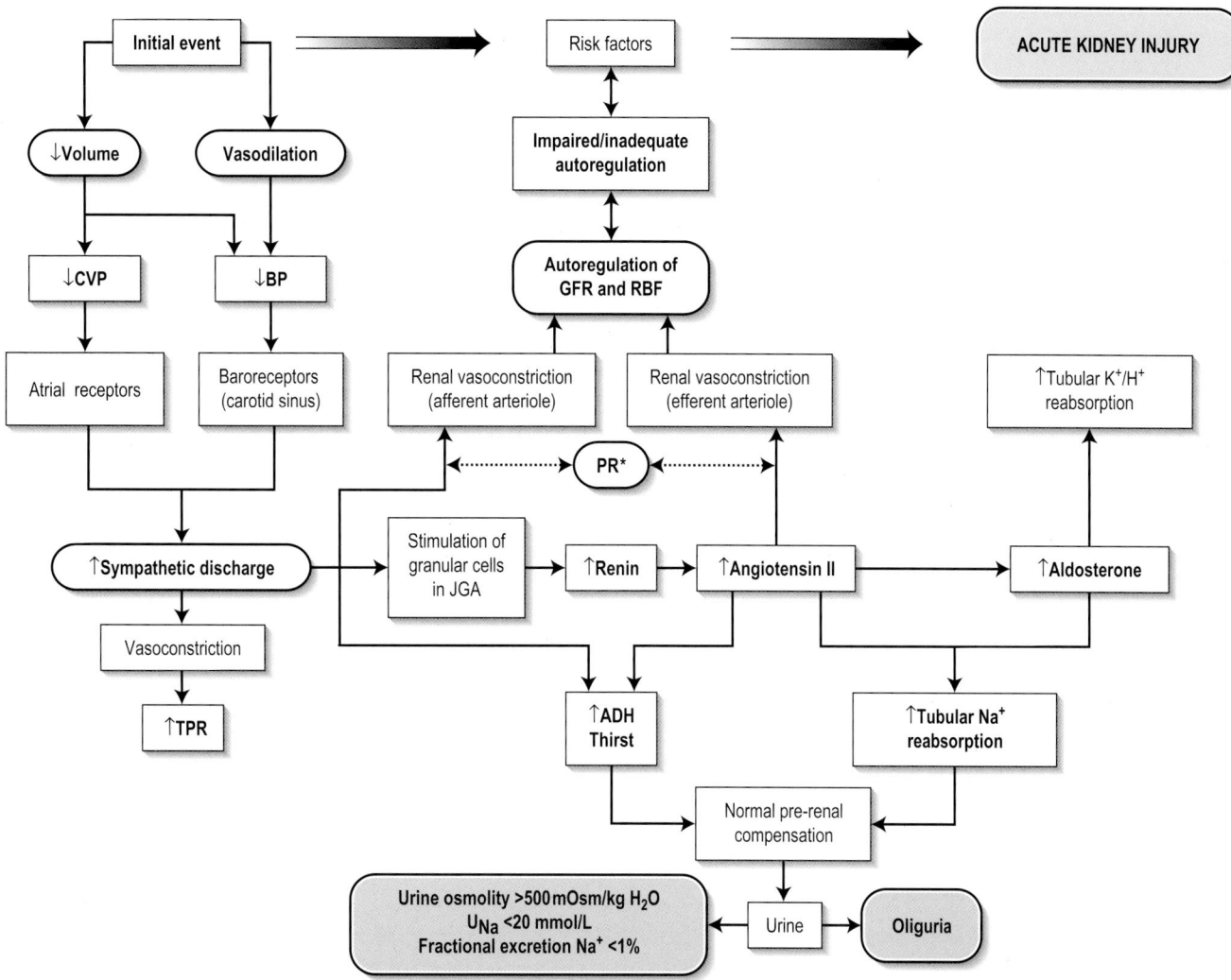

Fig. 10.1.1 Physiological response of the kidney to hypovolaemia or reduced perfusion. The normal response results in a reduced volume of concentrated urine. The presence of risk factors, impaired autoregulation or prolonged hypovolaemia can cause acute kidney injury. ADH: antidiuretic hormone; BP: blood pressure; CVP: central venous pressure; GFR: glomerular filtration rate; JGA: juxtaglomerular apparatus; PR*: renal prostaglandins; RBF: renal blood flow; TPR: total peripheral resistance.

Table 10.1.2   Causes of toxic acute tubular necrosis

Exogenous agents

Radiocontrast
Non-steroidal anti-inflammatory drugs
Antibiotics: aminoglycosides, amphotericin B
Antiviral drugs: acyclovir, foscarnet
Immunosuppressive drugs: ciclosporin
Organic solvents: ethylene glycol
Poisons: snake venom, paraquat, paracetamol
Chemotherapeutic drugs: cisplatin
Herbal remedies
Heavy metals

Endogenous agents

Haem pigments: haemoglobin, myoglobin
Uric acid
Myeloma proteins
Correct intravascular volume depletion
Maintain perfusion pressure
Choice of resuscitation fluid
Diuresis in rhabdomyolysis
Avoid nephrotoxins
Use derived GFR or creatinine clearance when calculating drug doses

Obstructive nephropathy usually develops gradually and can cause chronic renal failure if the obstruction involves the urethra, the bladder or both ureters. Unilateral ureteric obstruction will cause AKI only if it involves a single functioning kidney.

Epidemiology

Studies of the pathogenesis of community-acquired ARF have produced conflicting results. In one study, the major processes were identified as prerenal in 70% of cases, renal in 11% of cases and post-renal in 17% of cases [6]. There are geographical differences in the causes of ATN. In Africa, India, Asia and Latin America, ATN is usually caused by infections (e.g. diarrhoeal illnesses, malaria,

leptospirosis), ingestion of plants or medicinal herbs, envenomation, intravascular haemolysis due to glucose-6-phosphate dehydrogenase deficiency or poisoning.

Prevention

Maintaining intravascular volume and renal perfusion

The rate and volume of intravenous fluid given to hypovolaemic persons depends on the nature of the intravascular depletion, the blood pressure and heart rate, the (estimated) volume of fluid lost, cardiac function and ongoing circulatory losses. The response to treatment is evaluated by simple bedside measurements (heart rate, blood pressure, urine output).

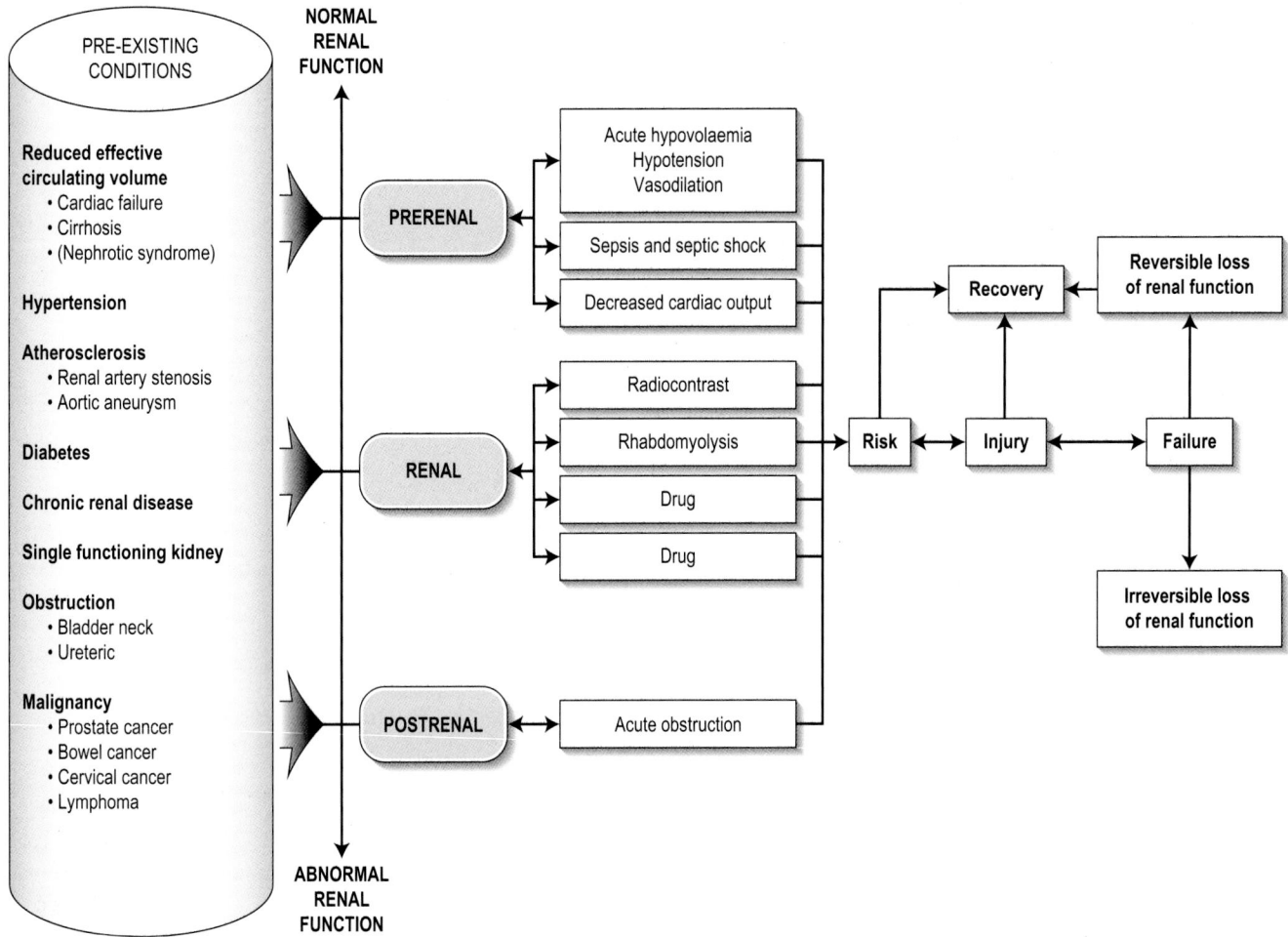

Fig. 10.1.2 The clinical presentation of acute kidney injury depends on the presence of any pre-existing conditions, the precipitating event(s) that caused the acute kidney injury and the severity of the acute kidney injury.

Rhabdomyolysis

Most studies on the prevention of ATN after rhabdomyolysis have been in persons with crush injury after earthquakes, where the incidence of AKI is about 50%. In this situation, fluid resuscitation should, if possible, begin before the crush is relieved. These patients may require massive amounts of fluid because of fluid sequestration in the injured muscles. The goal of intravenous fluid treatment is to produce a urine output of 200–300 mL/h while myoglobinuria (discoloured urine) persists. There is no evidence to support this rate of fluid replacement in persons who have rhabdomyolysis and AKI without crush injury, although a urine output of 100 mL/h would be reasonable while the urine is discoloured. The intravenous administration of mannitol and sodium bicarbonate to produce an alkaline diuresis as a means of preventing ATN in severe rhabdomyolysis has not been shown to be effective [7].

Radiocontrast nephropathy

The incidence of radiocontrast nephropathy can be reduced by saline infusion to produce intravascular volume expansion and by using low osmolar contrast agents. N-acetyl cysteine administration before and after radiocontrast administration does not appear to be effective [5].

Clinical features

The diagnosis of AKI should be considered when there is a decrease in urine output or an elevated SCr concentration. The clinical features depend on the pre-existing conditions that increase the risk of developing AKI, the initiating factor(s) and the effects of AKI (Fig. 10.1.2). The history should include a detailed drug history, enquiry about recent invasive vascular or radiological procedures and any family history of renal disease. This is followed by clinical examination and evaluation

of investigations. A number of key issues then need to be resolved (Table 10.1.3).

Evaluation of prerenal (intravascular volume) status

Imprecise terminology, such as 'dry' or 'dehydrated', should be avoided. 'Dehydration' refers to situations where more water than electrolyte(s) has been lost, shrinking body cells and increasing the serum sodium concentration and osmolality. In other words, 'dehydration' means water depletion. Hypovolaemia is a decrease in the intravascular volume due to loss of blood (haemorrhage, trauma) or loss of sodium and water (e.g. vomiting, diarrhoea, sequestration of fluid in the bowel, etc.).

The (bedside) assessment of the (extracellular) volume status determines the initial resuscitation strategy. This involves evaluation of heart rate and blood pressure, the state of the skin and mucous membranes and the jugular

Table 10.1.3 Evaluation of acute kidney injury
Assess the intravascular volume
Look for renovascular disease
Look for symptoms or signs of obstruction to urine flow
Systematic search for presence of infection or sepsis
Evaluate for pre-existing renal disease or chronic renal failure
Obtain a detailed history of medication or drug use
Consider possibility of glomerulonephritis

venous pulse. The examination also includes auscultation of the lungs (for pulmonary crackles), abdominal examination (for ascites or masses) and examination of the legs (for peripheral oedema).

The 'typical' features of intravascular volume depletion (tachycardia or hypotension or both, in the supine position, or postural hypotension) are not as consistent or reliable as implied by many textbook descriptions. The presence of (supine) tachycardia has low sensitivity as a diagnostic feature of increasing hypovolaemia in healthy persons. An increase in the pulse rate of 30 beats per minute or more between the supine and standing positions is a highly sensitive and specific sign of hypovolaemia after phlebotomy of large volumes (600–1100 mL) of blood, but the sensitivity is much less after phlebotomy of smaller volumes. The inability to stand long enough for vital signs to be measured because of severe dizziness is a sensitive and specific feature of acute large blood loss. A systolic blood pressure of 95 mmHg or less in the supine position has high specificity but low sensitivity for hypovolaemia. Postural hypotension is present in 10% of normovolaemic people younger than 65 years and in up to 30% of normovolaemic people older than 65 years [8].

The textbook descriptions of the signs of saline depletion in adults (dry mucous membranes, shrivelled tongue, sunken eyes, decreased skin turgor, weakness, confusion) are neither specific nor sensitive compared to laboratory tests for hypovolaemia. The presence of a dry axilla argues somewhat for the presence of saline depletion; the absence of tongue furrows and the presence of moist mucous membranes argue against the presence of saline depletion.

The central venous pressure (CVP) is an indicator of the vena caval or right atrial pressure. A vertical distance greater than 3 cm between the top of the jugular venous pulsation (using the external jugular vein or internal jugular vein) and the sternal angle indicates that the CVP is elevated. An elevated venous pressure in persons with pulmonary crackles or peripheral oedema means that the intravascular volume is greater than normal.

The absence of visible venous pulsation in the neck veins when the patient is supine or in a head down position indicates significant intravascular volume depletion. The presence of visible venous pulsations in the neck at or below the level of the sternal angle that is seen only when the patient is supine indicates that the intravascular volume is below normal.

Evaluation of the renovascular state

Acute renal infarction is caused by dissection of the aorta or renal artery, embolism, renal artery thrombosis, renal vein thrombosis or renal artery aneurysm. Acute arterial occlusion is usually symptomatic, with the development of pain (loin, abdominal or back pain), haematuria, proteinuria, nausea and vomiting. Vascular occlusion of a single functioning kidney produces anuria.

Atheromatous disease of the renal arteries is common in persons older than 50 years with widespread atherosclerosis. Persons with stenosis or occlusion of one or both renal arteries can develop an elevation in SCr concentration after starting treatment with ACE or ARB drugs or develop acute on chronic renal failure.

Exclusion of thrombotic microangiopathy (TMA)

TMA is a syndrome of microangiopathic haemolytic anaemia, thrombocytopaenia and varying degrees of organ injury caused by platelet thrombosis in the microcirculation. There are two clinically distinct entities: haemolytic uraemic syndrome (HUS) and thrombotic thrombocytopaenic purpura (TTP). HUS affects young children and causes AKI with absent or minimal neurological abnormalities. TTP occurs in adults and causes severe neurological involvement in most cases and variable degrees of renal damage. Both conditions are rare.

Pre-existing renal disease or chronic renal failure

It can be difficult to distinguish between chronic and acute renal impairment. The following features suggest the presence of chronic renal failure: documented renal impairment in the past, family history of renal disease, polyuria or nocturia, uraemic pigmentation, normochromic and normocytic anaemia or small kidneys on ultrasound or computed tomography (CT) scans. Renal size may be normal or increased in chronic renal failure associated with diabetes, polycystic kidney disease or amyloidosis.

Exclusion of urinary obstruction

The symptoms and signs of urinary tract obstruction depend upon the site, the cause and the rapidity with which it develops. Pain is more common in acute obstruction and is felt in the lower back, flank or suprapubic region, depending on the level of the obstruction. Chronic obstruction is usually painless. Symptoms of prostatic obstruction include frequency, nocturia, hesitancy, post-void dribbling, poor urinary stream and incontinence. Bladder neck obstruction usually results in an enlarged (and palpable) bladder.

Recognition of rhabdomyolysis

Muscle necrosis releases intracellular contents into the circulation. This causes red-brown urine (that tests positive for haem in the absence of visible red cells on microscopy or tests positive for myoglobin with specific tests), pigmented granular casts in the urine, elevated serum creatine kinase (CK) levels that are five times or more above the upper limit of normal and clear serum (serum is reddish in haemolysis). The severity of the rhabdomyolysis ranges from asymptomatic elevations of muscle enzymes in the serum to AKI and life-threatening electrolyte imbalances.

Urine dipstick findings may be normal because myoglobin is renally cleared from the serum more rapidly than CK, thus myoglobinuria may be absent in patients with renal failure or those who present later in the illness. Muscle pain is absent in about 50% of cases and muscle swelling is an uncommon finding. Muscle weakness occurs in those with severe muscle damage. Fluid sequestration in muscles can cause hypovolaemia. Marked muscle swelling can cause a compartment syndrome.

Other blood test abnormalities include hyperkalaemia, AKI with rapid and marked elevation in SCr (e.g. 220 μmol/L per day), hypocalcaemia (which occurs early and is usually asymptomatic), hyperuricaemia, hyperphosphataemia,

Table 10.1.4 Clinical features of acute renal failure
1. Anorexia, fatigue, confusion, drowsiness, nausea and vomiting, and pruritus
2. Signs of salt and water retention in the intravascular and interstitial spaces: an elevated jugular venous pressure, peripheral oedema, pulmonary congestion, acute pulmonary oedema
3. Abnormal plasma electrolyte concentrations, particularly hyperkalaemia
4. Metabolic acidosis
5. Anaemia
6. Uraemic syndrome: ileus, asterixis, psychosis, myoclonus, seizures, pericardial disease (pericarditis, pericardial effusion, tamponade)

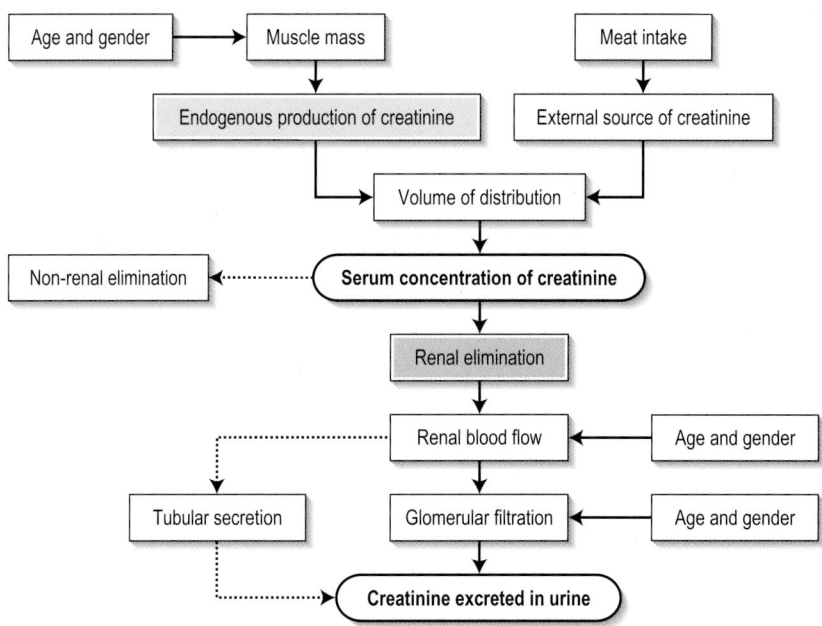

Fig. 10.1.3 Factors that determine the serum creatinine (SCr) concentration.

metabolic acidosis and disseminated intravascular coagulopathy [7].

Acute kidney injury and acute renal failure

The early stages of AKI are usually asymptomatic and the diagnosis is based on an elevated SCr concentration. It may take 24 hours or more for an initially normal SCr concentration to show a definite increase and up to 48 hours after the event(s) that caused the AKI to distinguish between the early stages of AKI (risk and injury) and the development of renal failure.

The urine output usually decreases and the patient may be oliguric (urine output less than 400 mL per day) or anuric (urine output less than 100 mL per day). Persons with AKI and oliguria have more severe kidney impairment than those without oliguria. Only a few conditions cause complete anuria: total obstruction, vascular lesions, severe ATN or rapidly progressive glomerulonephritis. The clinical features caused by ARF are shown in Table 10.1.4.

Differential diagnosis

The diagnosis of AKI requires synthesis of data from the patient's history, physical examination, laboratory studies and urine output. The category of AKI (Risk, Injury or Failure) may be difficult to determine in the emergency department (ED) if the baseline SCr is unknown. The reversibility of the AKI may be inferred if there is a marked increase in urine output after correction of prerenal problems, but a reduction in SCr (due to an increase in GFR) may not be seen for 12–24 hours.

Criteria for diagnosis

Serum biochemistry

The following are measured: serum concentration of electrolytes (sodium, potassium, bicarbonate, chloride, calcium, phosphate), serum urea and SCr concentrations, random blood glucose, liver function tests, coagulation tests and CK concentration.

AKI causes acute elevation in the SCr concentration or serum urea concentrations or both. In prerenal AKI, the low urine flow rate favours urea reabsorption out of proportion to decreases in GFR, resulting in a disproportionate rise of serum urea concentration or blood urea nitrogen (BUN) concentration relative to the SCr concentration. However, serum urea concentrations depend on nitrogen balance, liver function and renal function. Severe liver disease and protein malnutrition reduce urea production, resulting in a low serum urea concentration. Increased dietary protein, gastrointestinal haemorrhage, catabolic states (e.g. infection, trauma) and some medications (corticosteroids) increase urea production and increase serum urea concentration without any change in GFR.

The SCr concentration is the best available guide to the GFR. Acute reductions in GFR produce an increase in the SCr concentration. The changes in SCr concentration lag behind the change in GFR and can be affected by the dilutional effect of intravenous fluid.

Correct interpretation of the SCr concentration extends beyond just knowing the normal values (Fig. 10.1.3). Creatinine is a metabolic product of creatine and phosphocreatine, which are found almost exclusively in skeletal muscle. The SCr concentration is affected by the muscle mass, meat intake, GFR, tubular secretion (which can vary in the same individual and increases as the GFR decreases) and breakdown of creatinine in the bowel (which increases in chronic renal failure). The GFR decreases by 1% per year after 40 years of age, yet the SCr concentration remains unchanged because the decrease in muscle mass with age reduces the production of creatinine. The GFR (corrected for body surface area) is 10% greater in males than females, but men have a higher muscle mass per kilogram of body weight. The SCr concentration in men is thus greater than in women.

The creatinine clearance (CCr) or GFR are estimated indirectly using formulae (Cockcroft–Gault formula or the modification of diet in renal disease (MDRD) study equation) based on the SCr concentration (Fig. 10.1.4) [9]. These equations assume a steady-state SCr concentration and are inaccurate if the GFR is changing rapidly. They will also be less accurate in amputees, very small or very large persons or persons with muscle-wasting diseases.

Knowledge of a patient's baseline SCr concentration is important in assessing the severity and progression of AKI. Small changes

$$CCr = \frac{(140 - age) \times weight}{0.814 \times SCr\,(\mu mol/L)} \quad \text{in males}$$

$$CCr = \frac{(140 - age) \times weight \times 0.85}{0.814 \times SCr\,(\mu mol/L)} \quad \text{in females}$$

Cockcroft–Gault formula

$$\frac{GFR}{(mL/min/1.73\,m^2)} = 186 \times \left[\frac{SCr\,(\mu mol/L)}{88.4}\right]^{-1.154} \times age^{-0.203} \times \underset{(if\ female)}{0.742} \times \underset{(if\ black)}{1.210}$$

MDRD equation

Fig. 10.1.4 Formulae for calculating the creatinine clearance (CCr) or the glomerular filtration rate (GFR) from the serum creatinine concentration (SCr). MDRD: modified diet renal disease.

when the baseline SCr concentration is low are more important than larger changes when the baseline SCr concentration is high. Major decreases in GFR can occur in the normal range of SCr concentration. If the previous SCr concentration is not known, the MDRD equation can estimate the expected (normal) SCr concentration (using a value for the GFR at the lower range of normal).

Hyperkalaemia is a common complication, with the serum K^+ usually rising by 0.5 mmol/L/day in ARF. The serum Ca^{2+} concentration may be normal or reduced in ARF. Both hypocalcaemia and hypercalcaemia may occur at different stages of ARF in rhabdomyolysis. Rhabdomyolysis is characterized by a very high blood CK concentration. Abnormal liver function tests invariably accompany the hepatorenal syndrome associated with hepatic cirrhosis.

Full blood examination

Anaemia develops rapidly in ARF, but its presence or the degree of anaemia does not reliably distinguish between acute and chronic renal failure. Leucocytosis is usually seen if sepsis is the cause of ARF. Eosinophilia is often present in acute interstitial nephritis, polyarteritis nodosa and atheroembolic disease. Anaemia and rouleaux formation suggest a plasma cell dyscrasia. Disseminated intravascular coagulation can complicate ARF due to rhabdomyolysis. A microangiopathic blood film associated with ARF occurs in vasculitis or thrombotic thrombocytopenic purpura.

Serological tests

Tests for the detection of antinuclear antibody (ANA) or antineutrophil cytoplasmic antibody (ANCA) or measurement of complement concentration are indicated in suspected cases of vasculitis or glomerulonephritis.

Urine tests

The results of urine analysis may be normal in AKI. A positive test for leucocytes, nitrates or both is found in urinary tract infections. A positive test for blood, protein or both suggests a renal inflammatory process. The presence of red cell casts on microscopy is diagnostic of glomerulonephritis.

The measurement of the concentration of electrolytes in the urine and the calculation of their fractional excretion is of intellectual interest in understanding the pathophysiological responses of the nephron to different types of AKI. The calculations are cumbersome, the results are inconsistent and the information obtained does not alter the patient's immediate treatment.

Imaging

A chest X-ray is taken to assess the heart size and the presence of cardiac failure, infection, malignancy or other abnormalities. Ultrasound can define renal size and demonstrate calyceal dilation and hydronephrosis, but the findings depend on the expertise of the operator. Obtaining adequate images is difficult in obese patients, in ascites or where there is a large quantity of gas within the bowel. Ultrasound also provides information about bladder size and can detect prostamegaly.

A normal ultrasound examination can occur in the very early stages of obstruction or if ureteric obstruction is due to retroperitoneal fibrosis or to infiltration by tumour. Hydronephrosis not due to obstruction occurs in pregnancy, vesicoureteric reflux or in diabetes insipidus.

Doppler scans are useful for detecting the presence and nature of renal blood flow in thromboembolism or renovascular disease; however, because renal blood flow is reduced in prerenal or intrarenal AKI, test findings are of little use in the diagnosis of AKI. CT scans of the urinary tract evaluate renal size and renal position, renal masses, renal calculi, the collecting system and the bladder. Non-contrast CT is the examination of choice in persons with suspected renal calculi and can be used to assess the urinary tract in persons at risk of radiocontrast AKI. Injection of intravenous contrast is used for CT urography, CT angiography and CT venography, which may be necessary in some circumstances. Radionuclide can be used to assess renal blood flow and tubular function.

Renal biopsy

A renal biopsy provides a tissue diagnosis of the intrarenal cause of AKI and is indicated if the findings will identify a treatable condition. A renal biopsy is also valuable when renal function does not recover after several weeks of ARF and a prognosis is required for long-term management.

Treatment

The basis of emergency management is recognizing that AKI is present, correcting reversible factors, providing haemodynamic support and treating life-threatening complications. This is followed by treatment (if available) of the specific cause of AKI and management of ARF by supportive measures and (if required) renal replacement treatment.

Correction of hypovolaemia

Hypovolaemia not only causes AKI but also worsens all forms of AKI. The clinical diagnosis of hypovolaemia can be difficult if the jugular venous pressure is not easily seen or if there is pre-existing cardiac failure. When there are definite signs of hypovolaemia, the patient is resuscitated with rapid infusion of crystalloid. If hypovolaemia is a possibility, or if the person's urine output has decreased markedly, the patient should have 250–500 mL of crystalloid infused rapidly (fluid challenge) and the response (urine output, vital signs, jugular venous pressure) evaluated. An increase in urine output or an increase in blood pressure following a fluid challenge suggests that hypovolaemia was present.

Invasive measurement of volume status using central venous and pulmonary artery catheters can increase mortality, lengthen hospital stay and increase the cost of care. There is no evidence to justify the routine use of these invasive measures in patients with AKI. The main indications for central venous cannulation in AKI in the ED are difficulties obtaining intravascular access in the limbs or the need to give drugs which can only be given into a large central vein (e.g. noradrenaline).

Haemodynamic support

AKI impairs autoregulation of GFR and renal blood flow throughout all ranges of mean arterial pressure. Renal perfusion in ATN is linearly dependent on mean arterial pressure even in the normal range of blood pressure. Episodes of mild or severe decrease in blood pressure lead to recurrent ischaemic injury. Inotrope/vasopressor drugs (noradrenaline or adrenaline) should be commenced if hypotension persists after correction of hypovolaemia. Dopamine appears to have no clinical advantage compared to other agents and has, in fact, resulted in increased mortality in some studies.

Monitoring and maintaining urine output

Urinary Catheter

Accurate measurement of urine output requires insertion of a urinary catheter, but this is not needed in the less severe forms of AKI if there is frequent spontaneous voiding. A catheter is required initially in persons with oliguria or (apparent) anuria, shock or obstruction to bladder outflow.

Diuretics

Frusemide is used to produce a diuresis in the treatment of AKI due to hypercalcaemia and in the treatment of severe rhabdomyolysis. A trial of high-dose frusemide (80–120 mg intravenously) can be used in persons with AKI who have acute pulmonary oedema if dialysis is not readily available. Persons with less severe forms of AKI (e.g. Risk or Injury) who have a low urine output (less than 0.5 mL/kg/h) that does not increase after correction of hypovolaemia are often given low doses of frusemide (e.g. 20–40 mg intravenously). A subsequent increase in urine output is not necessarily associated with a decrease in the SCr concentration. There is no evidence that the use of diuretics to convert the less severe forms of

AKI from a (presumed) oliguric to a non-oliguric stage affects outcome [11].

Electrolyte abnormalities

Potassium

The serum potassium concentration may be low, normal or high. AKI due to diarrhoea causes hypokalaemia and metabolic acidosis, while AKI due to vomiting or diuretics causes hypokalaemia with metabolic alkalosis. A serum $[K^+]$ less than 3.0 mmol/L is treated with oral or intravenous potassium. Diabetic ketoacidosis (DKA) causes renal loss of K^+, depleting the body of potassium. Persons with AKI due to DKA who have a normal or low serum $[K^+]$ need intravenous potassium during treatment with intravenous fluids and insulin.

Hyperkalaemia is due to an imbalance between potassium intake and renal potassium excretion or follows redistribution of potassium from the intracellular to the extracellular space. Hyperkalaemia in AKI can be asymptomatic, produce electrocardiogram (ECG) changes or cause potentially fatal changes in cardiac rhythm.

The initial ECG changes in hyperkalaemia are shortening of the PR and QT interval, followed by peaked T waves that are most prominent in leads II, III and V2 through V4 (Fig. 10.1.5). Marked ST-T segment elevation (pseudomyocardial infarction pattern) may occur. Bradycardia with sinoatrial (SA) block or atrioventricular block (including complete heart block) can develop and progress to periods of cardiac standstill or asystole. More commonly, the PR interval is prolonged and the QRS complex is widened, with the QRS complex having a left or right bundle branch block configuration (Fig. 10.1.6). At high serum $[K^+]$ (8–9 mmol/L), the sinoatrial (SA) node may stimulate the ventricles without ECG evidence of atrial activity (sinoventricular rhythm). When the serum $[K^+]$ is 10 mmol/L or greater, SA conduction no longer occurs and junctional rhythms are seen. The QRS complex width continues to increase and, eventually, the QRS complexes and the T wave blend, producing a sine wave ECG. At this stage ventricular fibrillation or asystole are imminent [10].

The higher the serum $[K^+]$ concentration, the more likely is the occurrence of ECG changes and life-threatening arrhythmias. However, nearly half of persons with a serum $[K^+]$ greater than 6.8 mmol/L do not have ECG changes of hyperkalaemia. Physicians predict

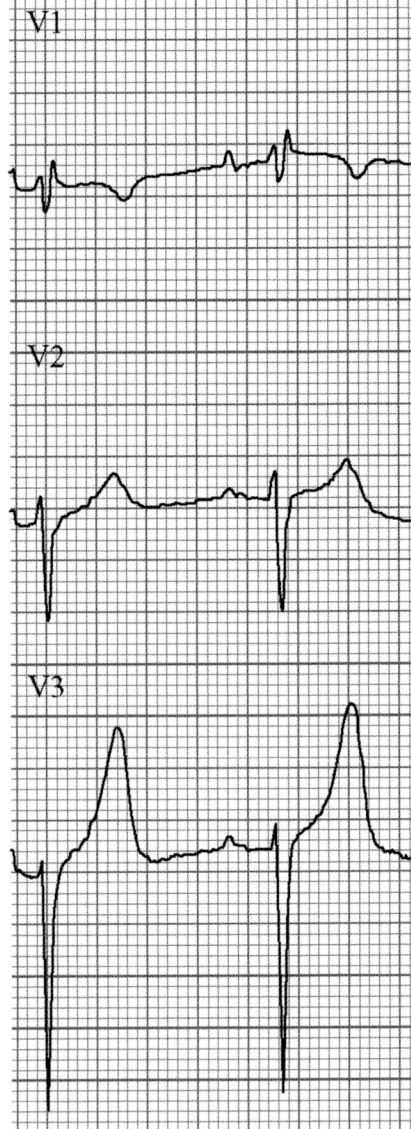

Fig. 10.1.5 The initial electrocardiograph changes in hyperkalaemia. The T waves in leads V3 to V5 are very tall and have a 'peaked' tip. The other findings (which may be unrelated to the hyperkalaemia) are the presence of a right bundle branch block pattern and a slightly prolonged PR interval.

the presence of hyperkalaemia solely on the basis of ECG changes with a sensitivity of less than 50%.

Drugs, such as oral potassium tablets, ACE inhibitors and aldosterone antagonists, should be ceased in AKI. Hyperkalaemia is treated when the serum $[K^+]$ is greater than 6.5 mmol/L (even if there are no ECG changes) or when there are ECG changes of hyperkalaemia. The emergency treatment of hyperkalaemia is covered in Chapter 12.2 Electrolyte disturbances.

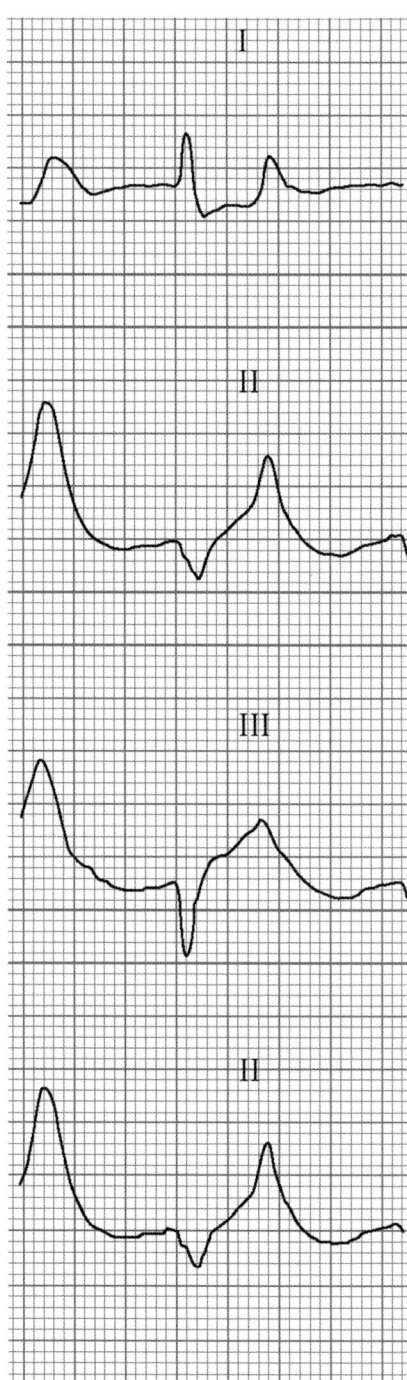

Fig. 10.1.6 Marked electrocardiograph changes in hyperkalaemia. The QRS complexes are widened and have a right bundle branch block type configuration. Tall T waves are seen in the inferolateral leads. P waves are not visible and a junctional rhythm is present.

Sodium

The sodium concentration in AKI may be normal, low (when water excess is present) or high (when water depletion is present). Patients with AKI and symptomatic hyponatraemia should be treated with haemofiltration or dialysis. Hypernatraemia is treated by slow intravenous infusion of hypotonic saline or 5% dextrose.

Calcium, phosphate, uric acid and magnesium

The serum calcium concentration is normal or slightly reduced in the Risk and Injury stages of AKI and is moderately reduced in later stages. Hypocalcaemia does not require therapy unless tetany is present. Hyperphosphataemia is present in nearly all persons with ARF, but does not need treatment in the ED.

Hyperuricaemia is common in AKI, but also occurs in chronic renal failure and in persons without AKI. Episodes of acute gout are very uncommon in AKI and the hyperuricaemia does not need treatment. Hypermagnesaemia is common in AKI, but is usually asymptomatic. Severe symptomatic hypermagnesaemia can occur if magnesium is administered to persons with AKI.

Acid–base abnormalities

Increased loss of bicarbonate-rich intestinal secretions (diarrhoea or an ileal conduit) can cause AKI with a normal anion-gap metabolic acidosis. AKI accompanied by acid loss from the stomach (vomiting or nasogastric suction) or caused by diuretics can result in a hypochloraemic metabolic alkalosis. Persons with the Risk and Injury stages of AKI often have a decrease in the serum bicarbonate concentration. More severe AKI causes a mild-to-moderate metabolic acidosis with an increased anion gap. This acidosis does not usually require specific treatment. Severe acidosis occurs in rhabdomyolysis and in lactic acidosis. The presence of a very severe metabolic acidosis in AKI is an indication for dialysis.

Fluid overload

The management of AKI in patients with peripheral oedema or pulmonary congestion due to cardiac failure is challenging. The clinical diagnosis of hypovolaemia in these patients is difficult and rapid intravenous administration of large volumes of fluid can worsen the pulmonary congestion or heart failure. Hypovolaemia is treated (or excluded) in these cases by assessing the response to small volume (200 mL) fluid challenges.

Patients with acute pulmonary oedema may have a raised SCr, which can be due to chronic renal failure, AKI or acute on chronic renal failure. These patients usually improve following treatment with vasodilators, continuous positive airway pressure (CPAP) ventilation and loop diuretics (40–80 mg frusemide intravenously). Patients with AKI and acute pulmonary oedema who do not respond to these measures need haemofiltration or haemodialysis.

Hypertension

Persons with AKI may have an elevated blood pressure that predated the renal injury or AKI itself may cause hypertension. A markedly elevated blood pressure reading (greater than 180/120 mmHg) in a person with AKI can be treated with glyceryl trinitrate applied as a skin patch (at a dose of 25–50 mg), sublingual nifedipine (5–10 mg) or oral hydralazine (20 mg). Intravenous drugs (glyceryl trinitrate or hydralazine) are used if AKI is associated with a hypertensive emergency, such as acute pulmonary oedema, hypertensive retinopathy or hypertensive encephalopathy.

Specific causes of AKI

Obstruction

Obstruction is relieved by decompression or diversion of the urinary tract. The site of the obstruction determines the technique used: placement of a Foley catheter or insertion of a suprapubic catheter, ureteral catheters (stents) or nephrostomy tubes. Relief of obstruction is often followed by a post-obstructive diuresis. Fluid replacement after relief of obstruction is based on frequent measurements of urine volume and urinary electrolytes.

Other causes

Specific treatments include immunosuppressive agents (glomerulonephritis, vasculitis), plasma exchange (thrombotic microangiopathy), systemic anticoagulation or revascularization (renovascular disease).

Management of ATN

Reduction of damage/accelerating recovery

Despite much experimental laboratory work and numerous clinical trials, no therapeutic intervention has hastened the recovery of renal function in established ATN. Therapeutic trials of dopamine, atrial natriuretic peptide and various growth factors have been ineffective. The use of high-dose loop diuretics to convert oliguric ATN to non-oliguric ATN was based on the observation that patients with non-oliguric ATN had a lower mortality and better renal recovery rates than those with oliguric ATN. The use of high-dose

Table 10.1.5 Indications for renal replacement treatment in acute kidney injury*

Oliguria (urine output <200 mL/12 hours) or anuria (urine output 0–50 mL/12 hours)

Serum urea concentration >35 mmol/L

Serum creatinine concentration >400 µmol/L

Serum potassium concentration >6.5 mmol/L or rapidly rising

Serum sodium concentration <100 mmol/L or >160 mmol/L

Pulmonary oedema not responding to diuretics

Severe (uncompensated) metabolic acidosis with pH <7.1

Uraemic syndrome (asterixis, psychosis, myoclonus, seizures, pericarditis)
Overdose with a toxin that is dialyzable

*Presence of two or more indications in a patient means that renal replacement will be needed.

loop diuretics does not affect the duration of ATN, the need for dialysis or the outcome.

Supportive treatment
This includes monitoring fluid input and fluid output, measuring serum electrolyte values frequently, preventing sepsis by reducing the number of intravenous lines and removing urinary catheters if possible, culturing periodically and using antibiotics when clinically indicated. The fluid intake is restricted to insensible water loss (about 500 mL per day in the absence of fever) plus all measured fluid losses (urine output, gastrointestinal losses, chest tube drainage). Nephrotoxic agents should be avoided and the dosage of renally excreted drugs reduced. Because the increase in SCr lags behind the decrease in GFR, drug doses should be calculated based on a GFR of less than 10 mL/min per 1.73 m^2 rather than on the SCr value.

Renal replacement treatment
Renal replacement treatment (RRT) is required in most patients with oliguric ARF and one-third of patients with nonoliguric ARF. The indications for RRT are summarized in Table 10.1.5.

Prognosis
The prognosis of ARF is largely dependent on the underlying cause and the presence of co-morbidities. Mortality varies from about 40% in those with no co-morbidity to more than 80% in those who have three or more failed organ systems.

References
[1] Bellomo R, Kellum JA, Ronco C. Acute kidney injury. Lancet 2012;380:756–66.
[2] Schetz M, Dasta J, Goldstein S, et al. Drug-induced acute kidney injury. Curr Opin Crit Care 2005;11:555–65.
[3] Gill N, Nally JV, Fatica RA. Renal failure secondary to acute tubular necrosis: epidemiology, diagnosis, and management. Chest 2005;128:2847–63.
[4] Huerta C, Castellsague J, Varas-Lorenzo C, et al. Nonsteroidal anti-inflammatory drugs and the risk of ARF in the general population. Am J Kid Dis 2005;45:531–9.
[5] Tumlin J, Stacul F, Adam A, on behalf of the CIN Consensus Working Panel. Pathophysiology of contrast induced nephropathy. Am J Cardiol 2006;98(suppl):14K–20K.
[6] Ali T, Khan I, Simpson W, et al. Incidence and outcomes in acute kidney injury: a comprehensive population-based study. J Am Soc Nephrol 2007;18:1292–8.
[7] Brown CV, Rhee P, Chan L, et al. Preventing renal failure in patients with rhabdomyolysis: do bicarbonate and mannitol make a difference? J Trauma 2004;56:1191–6.
[8] McGee S., 2nd ed. Evidence based physical diagnosis, vol. 94–96. St Louis: Saunders Elsevier; 2007, 153–73.
[9] Cockcroft DW, Gault MH. Prediction of creatinine clearance from serum creatinine. Nephron 1976;16:31–41.
[10] Dittrich KL, Walls RM. Hyperkalaemia: ECG manifestations and clinical considerations. J Emerg Med 1986;4:449–55.
[11] Ho KM, Sheridan DJ. Meta-analysis of frusemide to prevent or treat acute renal failure. Br Med J 2006;333:420–5.

10.2 The acute scrotum
Gino Toncich

ESSENTIALS

1 Torsion is the most time-critical diagnosis in acute scrotal pain. Early surgery is mandatory if the diagnosis is strongly suspected. No investigation should delay surgery.

2 All males with abdominal pain should have their scrotum and inguinal canals examined.

3 Colour Doppler ultrasound is of limited use in acute torsion and is best used after surgical consultation or in the older patient where torsion is rare.

4 Torsion of a testicular appendage can be diagnosed in early stages by finding a small blue lump in the scrotal sac; however, delayed presentations mimic torsion and surgical exploration is advised.

5 Epididymo-orchitis is rare in adolescence and torsion should be suspected.

6 Masses found on ultrasound should be followed up as traumatic injury can bring attention to an undiscovered tumour.

7 Ultrasound is unreliable in diagnosing testicular rupture.

8 Early surgery in patients with large scrotal haematoma allows diagnosis and treatment of testicular rupture, as well as reducing pain and inpatient admission time.

9 In patients with severe scrotal pain and swelling, particularly in the elderly, diabetic or immunocompromised, necrotizing fasciitis (Fournier's gangrene) should be considered and the patient referred urgently for surgery.

TORSION OF THE SPERMATIC CORD (TESTICLE)

Torsion is a twisting, not of the testicle but of the spermatic cord, which then interferes with the vascularity of the testicle, ultimately leading to infarction.

Aetiology

Torsion is due to a powerful contraction of the cremaster muscles in an abnormally attached testis. A normal testis is anchored posterolaterally to the scrotal sac and is therefore fixed in place. The main abnormality found in patients with torsion is an enlarged tunica vaginalis, which surrounds the whole of the testes and epididymis, preventing the testis from creating any attachment to the scrotal wall. The testis, therefore, floats freely like a clapper inside a bell. The contraction of the cremaster causes the testes and adnexae to rotate, thereby twisting the cord [1].

Pathology

The twisting of the cord causes obstruction of the lymphatic and venous outflows, but allows arterial inflow, leading to venous engorgement. Eventually, the pressure rises and occludes the arterial inflow.

The extent and rapidity of the damage depends on the degree of torsion, that is the number of turns. An incomplete rotation (<360°) may not completely occlude arterial flow, while a complete turn (360°) causes necrosis in 12–24 hours. Two or more turns (>720°) cause necrosis in less than 2 hours because arterial flow is obstructed [1,2].

Clinical presentation

Classically, there is a sudden onset of severe scrotal or abdominal pain. There are no irritative voiding symptoms. Between one-third and one-half of patients have had previous episodes of acute scrotal pain [3,4].

The patient looks pale and may vomit. The testicle is tender and rides high in the scrotum. Other signs include loss of cremasteric reflex, scrotal oedema, testicular swelling and retraction. These clinical signs are unreliable with

sensitivities of 60–91% and specificities of 27–68% [5].

Systemic signs, such as fever, are classically absent. Urinalysis is normal.

Intermittent torsion of the testis

This is a syndrome of recurrent acute scrotal pain, usually lasting less than 2 hours, which resolves spontaneously. Creagh et al. [4] describe a series of 27 patients who underwent elective orchidopexy for these symptoms. Three patients developed acute torsion while on the waiting list; of those coming to operation, one had an atrophic testis and four had evidence of torsion of the appendages of the testis. One patient subsequently had torsion after surgery because absorbable sutures were used [4].

Differential diagnosis of acute testicular pain

Differential diagnoses to consider in acute testicular pain are listed in Table 10.2.1.

Traps in the clinical diagnosis

There are many potential pitfalls in the clinical diagnosis of the acute scrotum:

- Age: the abnormality is present for life, so the torsion could potentially occur at any age. In those under 18 years of age, an acutely painful scrotum should always be considered to be torsion [3]. Most of the literature concerns itself with the under 18-year-old population. Less than 4% of torsions occur in patients over 30 years. It is most common in adolescence (12–18 years) [6]. In teenagers, sexually transmitted disease may confuse the diagnosis. There is an old surgical aphorism: 'Question: When do you diagnose epididymo-orchitis in a teenager? Answer: After you have fixed the torsion.'
- Pain: in 25% of cases there is no sudden onset of pain, nor is it necessarily severe. Some patients with epididymo-orchitis (EDO) have severe pain [1,3].
- Localization: some patients may have no scrotal pain but may have pain referred to the lower abdomen or inguinal area. The author has a case where the pain was referred to the loin with no scrotal symptoms. The scrotum must always be examined in males with any abdominal pain.

Table 10.2.1 Differential diagnosis of acute testicular pain
Epididymo-orchitis
Strangulated hernia
Haematocoele
Hydrocoele
Testicular tumour
Henoch–Schonlein purpura in children
Idiopathic scrotal oedema

- Abnormal position of testis: this is only seen if 360° or greater rotation occurs [3].
- Previous repair: torsion can occur in a testis that has previously been fixed, especially if absorbable sutures have been used [4].
- Dysuria: irritative voiding symptoms rarely occur with torsion and suggest infection [3].
- Fever: temperatures >38.9°C have been noted in up to 15% of torsion patients [1].

Clinical findings remain misleading and none can reliably exclude the diagnosis of torsion [7].

Investigations

Surgical exploration of the scrotum

This is the investigation of choice where the diagnosis of torsion is likely and maximizes the chance of saving the testis.

Delaying the diagnosis has been termed 'castration by neglect' [3,7]. Surgical exploration requires only a skin incision and has no major complications [5,7].

Low rates of torsion diagnosed at operation have led to interest in other tests to predict torsion preoperatively.

Colour Doppler imaging of the testis

It is useful in diagnosing torsion but also in elucidating other scrotal pathology. Comparison of blood flow to the asymptomatic side is crucial. If there is reduced flow to one side then some degree of torsion must be suspected (E-Fig. 10.2.1 and E-Fig. 10.2.2). If the testis has untwisted, hyperaemic flow may be noted. The sensitivity of colour Doppler imaging (CDI) for torsion can be as low as 82%, missing one in five cases, and is affected by:

- lack of sensitivity in low flow states
- inappropriate settings

- inexperience of the operator
- incomplete torsion
- failure to compare low flow to the normal side
- spontaneous untorting, giving an increased flow to the affected side, not reduced or absent flow [2].

Role of investigations in suspected testicular torsion

When the diagnosis of torsion remains probable, then the investigation is surgical exploration of the scrotum; any other investigations that delay theatre are unnecessary. If torsion is unlikely clinically and a surgical opinion concurs, then CDI can be used, provided it is available on an urgent basis [1,3,7]. It is important that there is early communication and discussion with the responsible surgeon to avoid delays between the suspicion of torsion and surgical intervention [1–3].

Treatment

Manual untwisting

This manoeuvre is not universally recommended and should be done only as a temporizing measure or when surgical exploration cannot be performed. The spermatic cord is infiltrated with local anaesthetic and the testis is untwisted. Untwisting is done by turning the left testis anticlockwise (outward) and the right one clockwise, like opening the pages of a book [8].

Surgery

The testes is untwisted and inspected for return of colour and bleeding. An obviously infarcted testis is removed at the initial surgery. A viable testis is sutured into place on the scrotal wall. The tunica should be inverted and also sutured to the scrotal wall. It is vital that the normal side is also explored and fixed to the scrotal wall, as the abnormality is bilateral in most cases. Retorsion following orchidopexy has occurred when absorbable sutures have been used [1,3–6].

Prognosis

Viability depends on the number of twists and the time taken to untwist the testis. There is 100% salvage if the testis is untwisted in less than 4 hours. Up to 24 hours, the rate falls to 50%. There are rare case reports of salvage after 30 hours.

Testicular salvage (return of circulation at surgery) does not mean absence of injury to the testicle. Long-term follow up of salvaged testes shows that 75% have a reduction in volume. Abnormalities are also seen in sperm volume, motility and morphology. These abnormalities are not seen in patients who have had an infarcted testis removed at the initial operation. This suggests some antispermatogenesis effect caused by the damaged testicle [1,3,4].

Torsion of a testicular appendage

Testicular appendages are embryological remnants with no function. They are small (<5 mm) pedunculated structures that may twist on their pedicle. If the appendage can be isolated in the scrotum, a small blue lump may be noted: 'the blue dot sign'. These do not need surgery and can be treated with analgesia. Late presentations may have scrotal or testicular swelling and should be treated as torsion until proved otherwise [1].

Acute epididymo-orchitis (EDO)

Introduction

EDO is a clinical syndrome with pain and swelling of the epididymis (and the testis) of less than 6 weeks' duration. Chronic epididymitis is a long-standing condition of epididymal or testicular pain, usually without swelling [2].

Aetiology

A variety of organisms may be responsible for EDO (Table 10.2.2).

The most likely cause depends on the patient's demographic group. For heterosexual males under 35 years of age, the agent is usually gonococcus or chlamydia. These organisms are also responsible for infection in homosexual males under 35 years (where anal sex is practised), but coliforms and even *Haemophilus* can cause infection. In males older than 35 years, EDO is usually due to obstructive urological disease, so coliforms predominate. EDO may also be part of a systemic disease, for example brucellosis or cryptococcus.

EDO is usually thought to be an ascending infection from the urethra or prostate, but it can be part of a generalized systemic disease. The

Table 10.2.2 Causative agents in EDO
Bacterial: *Neisseria gonorrhoeae*, *Escherichia coli*, *Pseudomonas aeruginosa*, coliforms, *Klebsiella*, *Mycobacterium tuberculosis*
Chlamydial: *C. trachomatis*
Viral: mumps
Drugs: amiodarone epididymitis
Fungal: cryptococcal
Parasitic: filariasis (usually chronic)

infection spreads from epididymis to testicle and, eventually, they may become one large inflammatory mass. Isolated orchitis is rare and usually due to viral causes, spread via the bloodstream [9–11].

Clinical presentation

The exact features depend on the underlying cause and whether both the epididymis and the testicle are involved. The pain may come on suddenly or slowly. There is scrotal swelling and tenderness that is relieved by elevating the testis. The spermatic cord is usually tender and swollen. Associated symptoms of urethritis are common. In younger males (under 35 years), a history of sexually transmitted disease may be elicited. In the older patient, there is often a history of instrumentation, intercurrent urinary tract infection (UTI) or prostatism. Pyuria is common.

Investigations

Urethral swabs

Urethral discharge may not be seen if the patient has just voided, so a urethral swab and smear should be examined for white blood cells (WBC). If there are more than five WBC per high-powered field, then urethritis is likely. The presence of intracellular diplococci confirms the diagnosis of gonorrhoea; their absence suggests chlamydia [9].

Midstream urine

Look for the presence of WBC or Gram-negative organisms.

Differential diagnosis

In the acute non-traumatic setting in those less than 30 years old, the most important differential diagnosis is torsion of the testicle [9]. If the clinical features and midstream urine do not differentiate, then torsion should be considered and surgical opinion obtained. An ultrasound can then be done if surgical opinion agrees. In young men, if CDI is not available and there is no evidence of UTI or urethritis, then surgical exploration may be necessary. Ultrasound can help differentiate other causes of the acute scrotum.

Treatment

Symptomatic treatment consists of bed rest, analgesia and scrotal supports.

If the cause is secondary to a sexually transmitted disease, then appropriate antibiotics should be chosen after urethral swabs have been taken, for instance, a single dose of ceftriaxone (250 mg stat) for gonorrhoea and a 14-day course of doxycycline (100 mg) or roxithromycin (300 mg) for chlamydia. The patient's sexual partners should be investigated and treated. Tests for syphilis or HIV should be performed.

If the infection is secondary to UTIs, then an appropriate antibiotic for 14 days should be used. Refer to antibiotic guidelines that will account for local sensitivities. Antibiotic choice can then be adjusted according to the urine culture results. Investigation for underlying urinary tract obstruction should be undertaken according to clinical features. Symptoms can take many days to settle so, in the absence of systemic illness, no intravenous antibiotics are necessary.

Complications

These include abscess formation, testicular infarction, chronic pain and infertility.

Blunt traumatic injury to the testicle

The mobility of the testicle, cremaster muscle contraction and the tough capsule usually protect the testicle from injury. However, a direct blow that drives the testicle against the symphysis pubis may result in contusion or rupture of the testicle. Typical mechanisms are a direct kick to the groin or handlebar and straddle injuries [12,13].

The types of injury include scrotal-wall haematomas, tunica vaginalis haematoma (haematocoele) or intratesticular (subcapsular) haematoma.

The most serious is testicular rupture, where the tunica splits, allowing blood and seminiferous tubules to extrude into the tunica vaginalis. This occurs in up to 50% of blunt trauma. Complete disruption of the testis may occur [12–14].

Ultrasound examination is not 100% sensitive in detecting testicular rupture, so early surgical exploration is the investigation and treatment of choice. Indications for exploratory surgery include:

- uncertainty in diagnosis after appropriate clinical and radiographic evaluations
- clinical findings consistent with testicular injury
- disruption of the tunica on ultrasound
- absence of blood flow on scrotal ultrasound images with Doppler studies
- clinical haematocoeles that are expanding or of considerable size (e.g. 5 cm or larger) should be explored
- smaller haematocoeles are often explored because it has been shown that such practice allows for more optimal pain control and shorter hospital stays.

It should be noted that 10–15% of testicular tumours present after an episode of trauma and so any abnormalities on ultrasound examination should be followed to resolution if surgery is not performed [15].

Early surgical exploration with evacuation of blood clots in the tunica vaginalis and repair of testicular rupture, if present, results in a shortened hospital stay, a greatly reduced period of disability and a faster return to normal activity compared to patients managed conservatively. Conservative management is complicated by secondary infection of the haematocoele, frank acute necrosis of the testis and delayed atrophy due to pressure effects of haematoma. The orchidectomy rate for early exploration is only 9%, compared to 45% for those managed non-operatively [13].

Necrotising fasciitis of the perineum (Fournier's gangrene)

This is a necrotizing fasciitis caused by a mixture of aerobic and anaerobic bacteria. It usually occurs in frail and elderly men who suffer from diabetes, renal failure or immunocompromise. The initial infection starts in the anterior abdominal wall and spreads to the perineum with scrotal involvement [17].

Features suggestive of this diagnosis are the epidemiological risk factors, severe pain, tense swollen scrotum with possible blisters and crepitus due to gas in the tissues. Often signs of systemic toxicity, not expected in routine EDO, accompany this diagnosis. Diagnosis is often delayed as the diagnosis is mainly clinical [16,17].

The mainstay of treatment is immediate resuscitation with fluids, antibiotics and urgent extensive surgical debridment.

Controversies and future directions

- Some advocate that all patients with scrotal and testicular injury have routine surgical exploration regardless of ultrasound findings.
- It has been argued that all attempts at testicular salvage be abandoned in favour of orchidectomy of the affected side in order to preserve the spermatogenesis of the other side.

References

[1] Lutzker LG, Zuckier LS. Testicular scanning and other applications of radionuclide imaging of the genital tract. Semin Nuclear Med 1990;20:159–88.

[2] Herbener TE. Ultrasound in the assessment of the acute scrotum. J Clin Ultrasound 1996;24:405–21.

[3] Cass AS. Torsion of the testis. Postgrad Med 1990;87:69–74.

[4] Creagh TA, McDermott TE, McLean PA, et al. Intermittent torsion of the testis. Br Med J 1988;297:525–6.

[5] Van Glabeke E, Khairouni A, Larroquet M, et al. Acute scrotal pain in children: results of 543 surgical explorations. Pediatr Surg Internatl 1999;15:353–7.

[6] Rajfer J. Testicular torsion. In: Walsh PC, Retik AB, Darracott VE, Wein AJ, editors. Campbell's urology (7th ed.). London: WB Saunders, 1997, p. 2184–6.

[7] Murphy FL, Fletcher L, Pease P. Early scrotal exploration in all cases is the investigation and intervention of choice in the acute paediatric scrotum. Pediatr Surg 2006;22:413.

[8] Schneider RE. Testicular torsion. In: Tintinalli JE, Ruiz E, Krome RL, editors. Emergency medicine: a comprehensive study guide (4th ed.). New York: McGraw-Hill; 1996.

[9] Berger R. Epididymitis. In: Walsh PC, Retik AB, Darracott VE, Wein AJ, editors. Campbell's urology (7th ed.). London: WB Saunders, 1997, p. 670–3.

[10] Tintanalli JE, Ruiz E, Krome RL. Epididymitis. In: Tintinalli JE, Krome RL, editors. Emergency medicine: a comprehensive study guide (4th ed.). New York: McGraw-Hill; 1996.

[11] Therapeutic Guidelines: Antibiotics, 10th ed. Melbourne: Therapeutic Guidelines Limited; March 2006.

[12] Bertini JE, Corriere JN. The etiology and management of genital injuries. J Trauma 1990;28:1278–81.

[13] Cass AS. Testicular trauma. J Urol 1983;129:299–300.

[14] Kukadia AN, Ercole CJ, Gleich P, et al. Testicular trauma: potential impact on reproductive function. J Urol 1996;156:1643–6.

[15] Cass AS, Luxenberg M. Testicular injuries. Urology 1991;38:528–30.

[16] Hasham S, Matteucci P, Stanley PRW, Hart NB. Necrotising fasciitis. Br Med J 2005;330:830–3.

[17] Evaluation of the Acute Scrotum in Adults. <www.uptodate.com/contients/evaluation-of-the-acute-scrotum-in-adults>

GENITOURINARY EMERGENCIES

10.3 Renal colic

Sean Arendse

ESSENTIALS

1 Renal colic affects 2–5% of the population, with 50% of patients having a recurrence within 5 years.

2 Aproximately 75% of all stones are calcium based.

3 Management usually comprises adequate analgesia and hydration.

4 Computed tomography or intravenous pyelography establishes the diagnosis and evaluates the possibility of obstruction.

5 Most stones (90%) are passed spontaneously within 1 month.

6 Obstruction, infection and intractable pain necessitate admission to hospital.

7 Urology follow up is essential to minimize further episodes.

Introduction

Nephrolithiasis is a common disorder affecting 2–5% of the population at some point in their lives [1]. It occurs most frequently between the ages of 20 and 50 years, with a male:female ratio of approximately 3:1. About 50% of patients only experience a single episode, but the remaining 50% have recurrent episodes within 5 years [2].

Most calculi are believed to originate in the collecting system (renal calyces and pelvis) before passing into the ureter. Supersaturation with stone-forming substances (calcium, phosphate, oxalate, cystine or urate), combined with a decrease in urine volume and lack of chemicals that inhibit stone formation (such as magnesium, citrate and pyrophosphate), result in production of a calculus. In addition to this, infection with urea-splitting organisms that produce an alkaline urinary pH frequently contribute to the growth of 'struvites' or triple phosphate (calcium, magnesium and ammonium phosphate) stones.

Less commonly, mixed stones occur via nucleation with sodium hydrogen, urate, uric acid and hydroxyapatite crystals providing a core to which calcium and oxalate ions adhere (heterogeneous nucleation).

Approximately 75% of all stones are calcium based, consisting of calcium oxalate, calcium phosphate or a mixture of the two. Ten per cent are uric acid based, 1% are cystine based and the remainder are primarily struvite.

Predisposing factors for stone formation include dehydration and low fluid intake, hypertension, prolonged immobilization, strong family history of nephrolithiasis, hyperparathyroidism, peptic ulcer disease (hyperexcretion of calcium), small bowel disease, such as Crohn's disease or ulcerative colitis (hyperoxaluria), and gout (hyperuricaemia). Myeloproliferative disorders, malignancy, glycogen storage disorders, renal tubular acidosis and the use of certain medications (calcium supplements, acetazolamide, vitamins C and D and antacids) may also be conducive to nephrolithiasis [3].

Persistent obstruction of the ureter leads to hydronephrosis of the urinary tract and may precipitate renal failure. Common sites of obstruction are ureteropelvic junction, pelvic brim and vesicoureteric junction.

Pathophysiology of pain

The mechanisms implicated in the production of the pain associated with renal colic are an increase in renal pelvic pressure, ureteric spasm, local inflammatory effects at the level of the calculus and increased peristalsis and pressure proximal to the calculus.

Acute obstruction of the upper urinary tract from a calculus results in increased pressure in the renal pelvis which, in turn, induces the synthesis and secretion of renal prostaglandins, in particular PGE2, which promotes a diuresis by causing dilatation of the afferent arteriole, further elevating the renal pelvic pressure [4,5]. The acute obstruction and renal capsular tension are believed to be the cause of the constant ache in the costovertebral angle.

In experiments utilizing isolated ureteric smooth muscle, prostaglandins have also been shown to increase phasic and tonic contractile activity [6], resulting in ureteric spasm and severe, colicky pain.

Presentation

The pain of renal colic has been described as the worst pain a person can endure. The classic textbook description is of severe, intermittent, flank pain of abrupt onset originating from the area of the costovertebral angle and radiating anteriorly to the lower abdominal and inguinal regions. Testicular or labial pain may be present and may suggest the location of the stone as a low ureteric position. Urinary frequency or urgency often develops as the stone nears the bladder. Nausea and vomiting frequently accompany the pain and about one-third of patients complain of gross haematuria [7].

Examination

Examination usually reveals an agitated, pacing patient unable to find a comfortable position. Pulse rate and blood pressure may be elevated secondary to the pain. Fever is unusual and suggests infection. The abdominal examination may only reveal signs of an early ileus with hypoactive bowel sounds and a distended abdomen, but should not be omitted as it is extremely useful in excluding other intra-abdominal or retroperitoneal causes of the pain (such as pancreatitis, cholecystitis, appendicitis or leaking or rupture of the abdominal aorta).

Investigations

Urinalysis usually shows red blood cells, although the absence of red cells in the urine in the setting of colicky flank loin to groin pain does not rule out nephrolithiasis and between 10 and 30% of patients with documented nephrolithiasis do not have haematuria [8]. Nitrites, leucocytes or microorganisms in the urine suggest either the complication of an infection or a diagnosis of acute pyelonephritis. Urine culture is thus indicated to rule out infection with urea-splitting organisms, such as *Klebsiella* and *Proteus* spp. Electrolyte studies may demonstrate obstruction or suggest an underlying metabolic abnormality, such as hypercalcaemia, hyperuricaemia or hypokalaemia. A slightly elevated white blood cell count may occur with renal colic, but a count greater than 15 000/mm^3 suggests active infection, as does a fever. Renal tract obstruction with concomitant infection is a urological emergency and must be treated immediately and aggressively.

A pregnancy test should be performed in all women of childbearing age, as a positive result needs further investigation to exclude ectopic pregnancy.

Many conditions may have a similar presentation to renal colic and examination and investigations should be directed towards confirming the diagnosis of nephrolithiasis and excluding the other conditions in the differential diagnosis (Table 10.3.1).

Radiological examination

A variety of imaging modalities is used to evaluate renal colic. Their pros and cons are listed in Table 10.3.2.

Most stones (90%) are radiopaque and theoretically should be visible on plain X-ray; if seen, they are irregularly shaped densities on abdominal radiography (KUB). However, a KUB alone is not usually sufficient to make the diagnosis of nephrolithiasis as it has poor

Table 10.3.1 Differential diagnosis of renal colic
Renal carcinoma producing blood clots temporarily occluding the ureter
Ectopic pregnancy
Ovarian torsion
Abdominal aortic aneurysm
Acute intestinal obstruction
Pyelonephritis
Appendicitis
Diverticulitis
Narcotic seekers and Munchausen's syndrome

sensitivity of around 60% [9]. Phlebitis in the pelvic veins and calcified mesenteric lymph nodes may add confusion and many small stones may be obscured by the bony density of the sacrum. Thus, plain X-ray should only be used in conjunction with another imaging modality, such as ultrasound, in the setting of renal colic.

Computed tomography (CT), with or without contrast, is the first-line test in most centres and has become the adopted gold standard with high sensitivity (97%) and specificity (96%) for ureterolithiasis [10]. Nearly all stones are opaque on CT and thus the size of the stone and its position can be accurately measured. Other positive findings include perinephric stranding, dilatation of the kidney (hydronephrosis) or ureter and low density of the kidney, suggesting oedema. Non-contrast CT is equivalent to intravenous urography (IVU) in the diagnosis of obstruction and is more reliable in the detection of ureterolithiasis [11]. It is also useful in the exclusion or confirmation of the other intra-abdominal differential diagnoses, such as appendicitis, abdominal aortic aneurysm or diverticulitis. As no contrast is used, there is not the risk of contrast reaction that is associated with IVU. It is more rapid than IVU and does not depend on the technical expertise required by other imaging modalities, such as ultrasound, but does subject the patient to a larger dose of radiation than IVU.

The intravenous pyelogram had been the standard investigation for the evaluation of renal colic until the widespread adoption of CT. It establishes the diagnosis of calculus disease in 96% of cases and determines the severity of obstruction [12]. Classic findings of acute obstruction include a delay in the appearance of one kidney, a dilated ureter and a dilated renal pelvis [13]. IVU is useful in estimating the size of the stone, in identifying extravasation of dye and in evaluating renal function. Its main disadvantage is the use of ionizing radiation, although less than in CT. In addition, administration of intravenous iodinated contrast media could precipitate a contrast reaction. Compared with CT, it is time-consuming and is not useful in confirming alternative diagnoses.

Table 10.3.2 Pros and cons of imaging modalities in renal colic		
	Pros	**Cons**
CT	High sensitivity (97%) High specificity (96%) Nearly all stones opaque Can accurately measure stone size Can detect obstruction Can diagnose other causes of flank pain Can avoid the use of contrast	Exposes patient to radiation Higher cost
Abdominal radiography (KUD)	Readily available Fast	Low sensitivity Exposes patient to radiation
Intravenous urography	Provides information regarding size and location of stone Measure of renal function	Potential for contrast reaction Exposes patient to radiation More time-consuming than CT Unable to exclude alternative diagnoses
MRI	Useful in pregnant patients Does not use ionizing radiation Does not use contrast	Not readily available Time consuming Accuracy may be less than IVU
Ultrasound	Non-invasive No exposure to ionizing radiation Modality of choice in pregnant patients	Lower sensitivity than IVU Size of stone cannot be accurately measured May not be available 24 hours Requires skilled operator

Ultrasonography is a useful, safe and a non-invasive alternative when renal function is impaired, risk from radiation is high (e.g. pregnancy) or contrast media contraindicated. It can identify the stone, its location and demonstrate proximal obstruction, such as hydroureter or a dilated pelvis, as well as the size and configuration of each kidney but, unfortunately, not size of the stone. Ultrasound has significantly lower sensitivity than IVU and misses more than 30% of stones [14].

Magnetic resonance imaging (MRI) can easily depict a dilated ureter and demonstrate the level of obstruction without using ionizing radiation or contrast, but the accuracy of MRI for stones may be lower than IVU as its spatial resolution is often not high enough to detect small stones. When used in combination with ultrasound, it may have a role in the evaluation of loin pain, especially in the pregnant patient; however, it is expensive, time-consuming and usually not readily available to most emergency departments.

Management

As 90% of stones are passed spontaneously, the most urgent therapeutic step is relief of pain, along with provision of adequate hydration and antiemetics. Opioid analgesics and non-steroidal anti-inflammatory drugs (NSAIDs) remain the mainstay of treatment.

Intravenous narcotics provide rapid analgesia, are titratable to effect and relieve anxiety in most cases. However, prolonged use may cause dependence and tolerance. Side effects are common and include nausea, vomiting, drowsiness, constipation and, with larger doses, precipitation of respiratory depression and hypotension. The data are very variable with regards to the effect of opioids on ureteric tone. Results indicate an increase in ureteric tone or no effect at all [15]. Options include morphine and fentanyl

Codeine, a less potent opioid than morphine, is effective for relieving mild to moderate pain associated with renal colic. Constipation is a significant side effect and limits its long-term use. Another option for analgesia is tramadol, an opioid-like agent, but with fewer side effects. One study showed that 100 mg of tramadol, when used for treating renal colic, was as effective as 50 mg pethidine [16], but more research is needed before adopting tramadol as an alternative to conventional opioids.

NSAIDs appear to be equally effective when compared with opioids [17]. A double-blind study comparing diclofenac and an opioid demonstrated a better effect with diclofenac and fewer side effects, but slower onset of action [18]. There are many NSAIDs available, differing in preparation and route of administration, the major differences between them being the incidence and nature of side effects, predominantly gastric irritation, ulceration and precipitation of renal failure. Ibuprofen has the fewest side effects and the lowest risk of gastrointestinal effects, but the weakest analgesic action. Naproxen and diclofenac provide stronger analgesia and a relatively low incidence of side effects. Oral diclofenac and oral/rectal indomethacin have both been shown to be effective in reducing the number of new renal colic episodes as well as further admission to hospital, but have no effect on spontaneous stone passage rates [19,20]. It has been suggested that one should give both a rapidly acting titratable opioid and a slower acting NSAID, which may result in earlier discharge from the ED [21]. Intravenous preparations of NSAIDs have limited availability in Australian EDs and have been reported to have a faster onset of action but a higher incidence of side effects, with considerably high cost and therefore, if available, should be used with caution. Commonly available alternative options for patients unable to tolerate oral medications include IM ketorolac and PR indomethacin

Buscopan, an antimuscarinic agent used for treating smooth muscle spasm, has been shown to decrease ureteric activity to some degree in 80% of the subjects studied [22]. However, one study comparing its use to an NSAID found that buscopan was less effective [23] and was associated with significant side effects, including dry mouth, photophobia, urgency, urinary retention and constipation, significantly limiting its use in renal colic.

Recently, the use of alpha-blockers in renal colic has been reported, with a number of studies showing that patients treated with alpha-blockers as well as standard therapy achieve stone clearance more often and in less time than controls [24–27].

Intravenous crystalloid should be administered to ensure a urine volume of 100–200 mL/h in those unable to tolerate oral fluids.

The size, shape and site of the stone at initial presentation are factors that determine whether a stone passes spontaneously or

requires removal. Stones less than 5 mm in patients without associated infection or anatomic abnormality pass within 1 month in 90% of cases, stones 4–6 mm pass 50% of the time but only 5% of stones larger than 7 mm pass and hence usually require elective surgical removal [8]. The overall passage rate for ureteral stones is:

- proximal ureteral stones 25%
- midureteral stones 45%
- distal ureteral stones 70%.

Disposition

Most patients with renal colic can be discharged with oral analgesia (codeine, paracetamol and NSAIDs), hydration and a referral for outpatient urology. Rectal administration of indomethacin is particularly effective if tolerated by the patient.

Indications for admission to hospital are listed in Table 10.3.3.

Further intervention is required if obstruction with hydronephrosis is present, the stone is a large stag horn calculus or the patient continues to have pain and no stone is passed within 2–3 days. A percutaneous nephrostomy allows drainage of an obstructed kidney until the blockage can be removed, either by ureteroscopic procedures for low stones or by open surgery for large or infected stones. Extracorporeal shockwave lithotripsy is preferred for single or small (>2 cm) otherwise uncomplicated stones as it has minimal complications and morbidity.

Urology follow up is essential for all patients, for elective removal of stones when complications have not ensued and for the prevention of recurrence. Indications for stone removal include stone diameter >7 mm, stone obstruction associated with infection, single kidneys with obstruction and bilateral obstruction.

Table 10.3.3 Indications for hospital admission in renal colic
Presence of infection
Deteriorating renal function
Persistent pain requiring parenteral narcotics
Stone greater than 5 mm in diameter
Extravasation of dye (uncommon)

Precautions

Renal colic, with its minimal findings on examination, is a commonly used presentation for those seeking narcotics or with Munchausen's syndrome and treating physicians should be aware of this. However, it is essential to give analgesia to those patients suffering from renal colic and it is preferable to give patients analgesia unnecessarily than cause unnecessary suffering. Features suggesting narcotic seeking are discussed in Chapter 21.5.

Conclusion

Renal colic is an acutely distressing medical condition that requires a careful evaluation of symptoms and signs to ensure timely analgesia, recognition of other causes of acute abdominal pain and avoidance of inappropriate narcotic usage.

Controversies and future directions

- Controversies in the management of renal colic relate largely to analgesia. Traditionally, it has been taught that parenteral narcotics provide fast and effective pain relief but, with the advent of injectable NSAIDs, some argue that these should be first line of care.
- The use of alpha blockers in renal colic requires further study.

References

[1] Lingeman J. Calculous disease of the kidney and bladder. Harwood-Nuss A, editor. The clinical practice of emergency medicine. Philadelphia: JB Lippincott; 1991.
[2] Trivedi BK. Nephrolithiasis. Postgrad Med 1996;100:3–78.
[3] Coe FL, Parks JH, Asplin JR. The pathogenesis and treatment of kidney stones. N Engl J Med 1992;327:1141–52.
[4] Holmlund D. The pathophysiology of ureteric colic. Scand J Urol Nephrol 1983;75(suppl):25–7.
[5] Nishikawa K, Morrisin A, Needleman P. Exaggerated prostaglandin biosynthesis and its influence on renal resistance in the isolated hydronephrotic rabbit kidney. J Clin Invest 1977;59:1143–50.
[6] Cole RS, Fry CH, Shuttleworth KED. The action of prostaglandins on isolated human ureteric smooth muscle. Br J Urol 1988;61:19–26.
[7] Smith DR. General urology, 9th ed. Los Altos, California: Lange Medical Publishers; 1978.
[8] Teichman JM. Acute renal colic from ureteral calculus. N Engl J Med 2004;350:684.
[9] Mutgi A, Willliams JW, Nettleman M. Renal colic. The utility of the plain abdominal roentgenogram. Arch Intern Med 1991;151:1589–92.
[10] Kenney PJ. CT evaluation of urinary lithiasis. Radiol Clin N Am 2003;41:979–99.
[11] Sourtzis S, Thibeau JF, Damry N, et al. Radiologic investigation of renal colic: unenhanced helical CT compared with excretory urography. Am J Roentgentol 1999;172:1491–4.
[12] Harrison JH, editor. Campbell's urology, Vol. 1, 4th edn. Philadelphia: WB Saunders; 1987.

[13] Samm BJ, Dmochowski RR. Urologic emergencies. Postgrad Med 1996;100:177–84.
[14] Svedstorm E, Alanen A, Nurmi M. Radiologic diagnosis of renal colic: the role of plain films, excretory urography and sonography. Eur J Radiol 1990;11:180–3.
[15] Lennon GM, Bourke J, Ryan PC, et al. Pharmacological options for the treatment of acute ureteric colic. Br J Urol 1993;71:401–7.
[16] Salehi M, Ghaserni H, Shiery H, et al. Intramuscular tramadol versus intramuscular pethidine for the treatment of acute renal colic. J Endourol 2003;17(suppl 1):A243.
[17] Cordell WH, Larson TA, Lingerman JE, et al. Indomethacin suppositories versus intravenous titrated morphine for treatment of ureteric colic. Ann Emerg Med 1994;23:262–9.
[18] Lundstam SO, Leissner KH, Wahlandar LA, et al. Prostaglandin synthetase inhibition of diclofenac in the treatment of renal colic: comparison with use of a narcotic analgesic. Lancet 1982;1096–7.
[19] Laerum E, Omundsen OE, Gronseth JE, et al. Oral diclofenac in the prophylactic treatment of recurrent renal colic. Eur J Urol 1995;28:108–11.
[20] Grenabo L, Holmlund D. Indomethacin as prophylaxis against recurrent ureteral colic. Scand J Urol Nephrol 1984;18:325–7.
[21] Larkin GL, Peacock WF, Pearl SM, et al. Efficiency of ketorolac tromethamine versus meperidine in ED treatment of acute renal colic. Am J Emerg Med 1999;17:6–10.
[22] Ross JA, Edmond P, Kirkland IS. The action of drugs on the intact human ureter. In: Behaviour of the human ureter in health and disease. Churchill Livingstone, 1972, 118–129, (Chapter 9).
[23] Al-waili NS, Saloom KY. Intravenous tenoxicam to treat acute renal colic: comparison with buscopan. J Pakistan Med Assoc 1998;48:370–2.
[24] De Sio M, Autorino R, Lorenzo GD, et al. Medical expulsive treatment of distal–ureteral stones using tamsulosin. J Endourol 2006;20:12–16.
[25] Hollingsworth JM, Rogers M, et al. Medical therapy to facilitate urinary stone passage: a meta analysis. Lancet 2006;368:1171–9.
[26] Parsons JK, et al. Efficacy of alpha blockers fot the treatment of ureteral stones. J Urol 2007;117:983–7.
[27] Singh A, et al. A systematic review of medical therapy to facilitate passage of ureteric calculi. Ann Emerg Med 2007:50.

11.1 Diabetes mellitus and hypoglycaemia: an overview

Anthony Brown

ESSENTIALS

1 Type I diabetes is characterized by pancreatic beta cell destruction with an absolute insulin deficiency, usually but not exclusively associated with autoimmune damage.

2 Type II diabetes results from a progressive insulin secretory deficiency on the background of insulin resistance.

3 Diabetic ketoacidosis (DKA) and hyperosmolar hyperglycaemic state (HHS) are both life-threatening acute complications of diabetes mellitus.

4 The aim of excellent long-term blood sugar control is an HbA1c (glycated haemoglobin) level of less than 7.5% without frequent disabling hypoglycaemia for the prevention of microvascular disease, and 6.5% in those at increased risk of arterial disease.

5 Oral antidiabetic drug groups include the sulphonylureas, biguanide metformin, alpha-glucosidase inhibitor acarbose, the thiazolidinediones pioglitazone and rosiglitazone, and dipeptidyl peptidase 4 (DDP-4) inhibitors, such as sitagliptin.

6 Optimal blood sugar control aids in reducing the incidence of multisystem diabetic complications.

7 Hypoglycaemic coma requires immediate treatment with intravenous glucose. Intramuscular glucagon 0.5–2.0 mg may be used if liver glycogen stores are adequate and can be given pre-hospital.

DIABETES MELLITUS

Classification system and diagnostic criteria

The classification system and diagnostic criteria for diabetes were revised in 2010 by the American Diabetes Association [1]. The classification of type I and type II diabetes mellitus was retained, with the recommended criteria for the diagnosis of diabetes as a fasting plasma glucose of 7 mmol/L or greater, or a random plasma glucose of over 11 mmol/L associated with polyuria, polydipsia and weight loss. In addition, an HbA1$_C$ (glycated haemoglobin) level of ≥6.5% was added. The oral glucose tolerance test is no longer routinely recommended.

Aetiology

The exact aetiology of diabetes is unclear. Type I diabetes is characterized by pancreatic beta cell destruction with an absolute insulin deficiency usually, but not exclusively, associated with autoimmune damage from a range of antibodies including to islet cells (ICA), glutamic acid decarboxylase (GAD), insulin and tyrosine phosphatases. Genetic and environmental factors are implicated, such as some human leucocyte antigen (HLA) types (most Caucasian patients are HLA-DR3 or DR4 or both), and abnormal immune responses, such as following viral infection. Certain genes are also implicated as co-contributors, particularly sites on chromosomes 6, 7, 11, 14 and 18.

Type II diabetes results from a progressive insulin secretory deficiency on the background of insulin resistance [1]. Genetic factors are implied by strong familial aggregation of cases and environmental factors in the context of genetic susceptibility, including obesity and diet. Thus, the introduction of a high fat and high calorie 'Western' diet rather than traditional crop foods has seen countries such as India record among the fastest growth rate of new diabetes worldwide.

Although type I diabetes occurs most frequently among Caucasians throughout the world, diabetes in Australia is three times more common in the Aboriginal community. Other groups with a high prevalence include Pacific Islanders and Native Americans.

Diabetes secondary to other conditions

Diabetes mellitus may be secondary to conditions that damage the exocrine pancreas including chronic pancreatitis, carcinoma of the pancreas and pancreatectomy, haemochromatosis, cystic fibrosis, pregnancy (gestational) and endocrinopathies, such as Cushing's syndrome, acromegaly, phaeochromocytoma and glucagonoma [2].

Drug-induced diabetic state

Certain drugs can impair glucose tolerance or cause overt diabetes mellitus. These include glucocorticoids, the oral contraceptive pill, thiazide diuretics at higher doses, tacrolimus, sirolimus and ciclosporin, pentamadine (which may also cause hypoglycaemia) and HIV protease inhibitors.

Emergency presentations of a high blood sugar

Diabetic ketoacidosis (DKA) and hyperosmolar hyperglycaemic state (HHS) are both life-threatening acute complications of diabetes mellitus. Although important differences do exist, the pathophysiology and treatment are similar. DKA is usually seen in type I diabetes and HHS in patients with type II, but both complications can occur in type I and type II diabetes. See Chapter 11.2 for the diagnosis and management of DKA and HHS.

General management of diabetes mellitus

Aims of long-term blood sugar control

The aim of optimal long-term blood sugar control is an HbA1c (glycated haemoglobin) level of less than 7.5% without frequent disabling hypoglycaemia for the prevention of microvascular disease, and 6.5% in those at increased risk of arterial disease [3]. This should be represented by a pre-prandial blood glucose level of 4.0–7.0 mmol/L and a post-prandial blood glucose level of less than 9.0 mmol/L.

Insulins

Insulin was first administered to humans in 1922. Animal insulins (bovine, porcine) have been used for many years but, in the 1980s, human insulins became commercially available. Today, with the widespread availability of human insulins, animal insulins are of historical interest only.

Types of insulins

Table 11.1.1 lists the different types of insulins and the important parameters of each type. Mixtures of short- and intermediate-acting insulins are also available: 70/30 (70% NPH/30% regular) and 50/50 (50% NPH/50% regular).

Antidiabetic drugs

Two major groups of oral hypoglycaemic agents used in the management of type II diabetes are the sulphonylureas and the biguanides. The sulphonylurea group of drugs acts by stimulating the pancreatic secretion of insulin, and the biguanide metformin acts by suppressing hepatic glucose production and enhancing the peripheral use of glucose. It is the first choice medication particularly in the overweight patient.

Newer types of oral agents now available for the treatment of diabetes include the alpha-glucosidase inhibitor acarbose, which acts on the gastrointestinal tract to interfere with carbohydrate digestion, but flatulence and diarrhea may be troublesome. The thiazolidinediones, such as pioglitazone and rosiglitazone, act primarily by reducing insulin resistance, thereby enhancing the effect of circulating insulin. Roziglitazone increases the risk of myocardial infarction and cardiovascular deaths and thus should be avoided in ischaemic heart disease [4]. All thiazolidinediones must be avoided in people with moderate or severe heart failure. Finally, the dipeptidyl peptidase 4 (DDP-4) inhibitors, such as sitagliptin, inhibit DDP-4 to prolong the action of the incretin hormones.

Other non-diabetic drugs

Angiotensin-converting enzyme inhibitors delay the onset of diabetic nephropathy even in normotensive patients with diabetes. Statins are important in the strict treatment of dyslipidaemia in diabetic patients.

DIABETIC HYPOGLYCAEMIA

Hypoglycaemia is more common in type I diabetes. The critical plasma level at which hypoglycaemia manifests varies between different individuals, but symptoms are likely below a plasma glucose of 3.5 mmol/L. Precipitants include exercise, a late meal, inadequate carbohydrate intake, errors of insulin dosage and ethanol ingestion.

Hypoglycaemia may also occur in the non-diabetic patient, precipitated by a variety of conditions (Table 11.1.2) [5].

Clinical features

Hypoglycaemia produces neurological and mental dysfunction from tremor, sweating and anxiety to seizures and coma. Less commonly, it can present as hypothermia, depression and psychosis. In some instances, hypoglycaemia is relatively asymptomatic.

Management of hypoglycaemic coma

- The ABC approach is important in the patient with coma.

Table 11.1.1	Pharmacokinetic characteristics of currently available human insulins		
Insulin	*Onset of action*	*Peak of action*	*Duration of action*
Lispro*	5–15 min	1–2 h	4–5 h
Regular	30–60 min	2–4 h	6–8 h
NPH	1–2 h	5–7 h	13–18 h
Lente	1–3 h	4–8 h	13–20 h
Ultralente	2–4 h	8–10 h	18–30 h

*Lispro insulin (Humalog) is the first rapidly acting insulin analogue. It produces a peak blood insulin level 2–3 times higher than regular insulin.

Table 11.1.2   Causes of hypoglycaemia

Table 11.1.2   Causes of hypoglycaemia

Diabetic patients

- Medication change or error, particularly with insulin or oral hypoglycaemic sulphonylurea (very rarely metformin)
- Inadequate dietary intake
- Excessive calorie use, such as exercise

Any patient

- Insulin, sulphonylurea, salicylates, β-blockers, quinine, chloroquine, valproic acid, pentamidine (note ingestion of these may be deliberate or malicious)
- Ethanol
- Liver disease
- Sepsis, other critical illness
- Malnourishment, including anorexia nervosa
- Post-gastrointestinal surgery 'dumping syndrome'
- Adrenal insufficiency
- Hypopituitarism
- Islet cell tumour/extrapancreatic tumour
- Tumour-related, such as mesenchymal, epithelial or endothelial tumours
- Artefact 'Munchausen syndrome'

- Give 50 mL of 50% glucose IV initially after taking a blood sugar level. Further glucose administration is often necessary, such as an infusion of 10% dextrose.
- Alternatively give 0.5–2 mg of glucagon IM when venous access has not been established or has failed. Glucagon is unhelpful in the patient with liver disease and depleted glycogen reserves.

Controversies

- Non-parenteral insulin delivery, such as nasal, oral or intra-pulmonary.
- The combination use and risk–benefit profile of newer antidiabetic drugs, such as the thiazolidinediones and DDP-4 inhibitors.

References

[1] American Diabetes Association. Standards of Medical Care in Diabetes – 2013. Diabetes Care 2013;36(Suppl. 1):S11–66.
[2] McCulloch DK. Classification of diabetes mellitus and genetic diabetic syndromes. <UpToDate.com> [Accessed Jan. 2013].
[3] NICE Clinical Guideline 15. Type 1 diabetes: diagnosis and management of type 1 diabetes in children, young people and adults. July 2004: modified Oct 2011. <http://www.nice.org.uk/CG15> [Accessed Jan. 2013].
[4] Nissen SE, Wolski K. Effect of rosiglitazone on the risk of myocardial infarction and death from cardiovascular causes. N Engl J Med 2007;356:2457–71.
[5] Service J, Cryer PE. Hypoglycaemia in adults: Clinical manifestations, definition, and causes. <UpToDate.com> [Accessed Jan. 2013].

11.2 Diabetic ketoacidosis and hyperosmolar, hyperglycaemic state

Anthony Brown • Richard D Hardern

ESSENTIALS

1 Diabetic ketoacidosis (DKA) consists of the triad of ketonaemia, hyperglycaemia and acidaemia – a high anion-gap metabolic acidosis.

2 DKA is caused by insulin omission or error, intercurrent illness including infection or is a presenting feature of new diabetes.

3 Key management components of DKA include:

- fluids (0.9% normal saline) to replace deficits of sodium of 7–10 mmol/kg and water 100 mL/kg
- soluble insulin infusion at 0.1 unit/kg/h to a maximum of 6 units/h to suppress ketogenesis, reduce blood sugar and help correct the electrolyte abnormalities
- potassium replacement, providing the serum potassium is less than 5.5 mmol/L and there is urine output (anuria is rare in DKA)
- education – all patients on insulin need to know the 'sick day rules', plus be familiar with regular home testing for capillary blood sugar.

4 Meticulous monitoring and documentation of treatment in DKA are essential.

5 Hyperosmolar hyperglycaemic state (HHS) is characterized by hypovolaemia, marked hyperglycaemia (>30 mmol/L) *without* ketonaemia or acidosis and a raised osmolality usually >320 mosmol/kg.

6 Mortality and morbidity of HHS are greater than with DKA, usually related to the older age of patients, co-morbidities and complications, such as stroke.

7 Treatment of HHS is similar to DKA except:

- lower dose insulin infusion rate is used at 0.05 unit/kg/h
- this infusion rate is titrated against the serum osmolarity rather than ketoacids
- 0.9% normal saline is used and *only* changed to half normal (0.45%) saline if the osmolality and glucose are not declining
- low molecular weight heparin (LMWH) thromboprophylaxis is indicated.

Introduction

Diabetic ketoacidosis (DKA) is an acute, potentially life-threatening complication in an insulin-dependent diabetic and in some type II diabetics. It consists of the triad of ketonaemia, hyperglycaemia and acidaemia – a high anion-gap metabolic acidosis. Although DKA is preventable, its prevalence and suboptimal management may highlight shortfalls in the quality of care for patients with diabetes. The mortality rate in developed countries has dropped to <1%.

Hyperosmolar hyperglycaemic state (HHS) is characterized by hypovolaemia, marked hyperglycaemia (>30 mmol/L) *without* ketonaemia or acidosis and a raised osmolality usually >320 mosmol/kg. It comes on more insidiously and has a worse prognosis with an increased mortality of around 15–20% and greater morbidity, in part related to underlying chronic medical disorders.

Epidemiology, aetiology and pathogenesis

An annual incidence of DKA of approximately 1:170 patients with type I diabetes is reported, or 2 episodes per 100 patient years of diabetes, for a prevalence of 4.6–8 episodes per 1000 patients with diabetes [1,2].

DKA may be the presenting feature of diabetes mellitus (3–25% DKA), but is usually seen in patients with autoimmune type I diabetes when there has been an insulin error with inadequate insulin or poor compliance (30% DKA), and/or an intercurrent illness (35% DKA). A variant of type II diabetes is also ketosis prone, 'ketosis-prone (type II) diabetes', usually in the obese with a strong family history. This was originally described in Africans and African-Americans, but is now noted worldwide.

Pathogenesis

DKA arises from an absolute or relative lack of insulin accompanied by an increase in counter-regulatory hormones, such as glucagon, cortisol and growth hormone [1,3]. Insulin absence leads to increased hepatic gluconeogenesis and glycogenolysis, with an incomplete lack of insulin related to greater hyperosmolarity (in HHS). Lack of insulin and excess counter-regulatory hormones increase lipolysis and free fatty acid production as an alternate

energy source. This leads to subsequent ketone body formation produced from acetyl coenzyme A, mainly in hepatic mitochondria, including acetone, beta-hydroxybutyrate and acetoacetate and a reduced ability to prevent ketonaemia.

HHS is the other end of the hyperglycaemia spectrum from DKA, occurring with a relative rather than an absolute deficiency of insulin leading to a greater level of hyperglycaemia, therefore higher hyperosmolarity than is seen in DKA. The degree of dehydration is greater (typically 10–15% body weight), but significant ketosis does not occur. HHS is more insidious in onset than DKA and patients with HHS are typically older with pre-existing type II diabetes. However, HHS is seen in young adults and even teenagers.

Clinical features

Malaise and fatigue on a background of polyuria, polydipsia, weakness and fatigability are common, but gastrointestinal symptoms, such as nausea, vomiting and abdominal pain, may predominate [3]. A lack of history of diabetes does not rule out the diagnosis of DKA, as it may be a first presentation, often presaged by recent, unexplained rapid weight loss.

Laboured, sighing respirations with an increased rate and depth, known as Kussmaul breathing, are characteristic of DKA in association with dehydration causing decreased tissue turgor, a dry mouth and sweet foetor of pear drops (ketotic), which is not always noticed. The conscious level may be reduced, but coma is rare.

Look carefully for signs of an underlying precipitating cause including chest, urine or skin infection, such as boils, as well as meningitis or an acute abdomen, although non-surgical upper abdominal pain is common in DKA. In those with HHS, look out for the complications of acute myocardial infarction, stroke or arterial thrombosis [4,5].

The urine output should be measured regularly, which does not always require urinary catheterization. Likewise, invasive haemodynamic monitoring should not be instituted as a 'routine' for patients with DKA or HHS. It should be reserved for those who fail to respond or in the elderly who are at risk of fluid overload. In addition, venous blood gases are sufficient to monitor progress in DKA, rather than repeated arterial sampling.

Diagnostic criteria

DKA

- Metabolic acidosis with pH <7.3 or serum bicarbonate <15 mmol/L.
- Ketonaemia >3.0 mmol/L, or marked ketonuria >2+ on dipstick (note urinalysis may miss 3-beta hydroxybutyrate early).
- Hyperglycaemia with blood glucose >11 mmol/L.

HHS

Note that there is no precise definition of HHS, but it is characterized by [5]:

- Hyperglycaemia. Serum glucose >30 mmol/L.
- Hyperosmolality. Serum osmolality >320 mOsm/kg. (If unable to measure regularly, use an approximation of the osmolarity = [2 × Na + glucose + urea]).
- Hypovolaemia.
- Minimal ketonaemia (<3.0 mmol/L) with no more than 1+ ketonuria on urinalysis.
- pH >7.30, bicarbonate >15 mmol/L.

Typical deficits per body weight

DKA

- Water 100 mL/kg
- Sodium 7–10 mmol/kg
- Potassium 3–5 mmol/kg.

HHS

- Water 100–220 mL/kg
- Sodium 5–13 mmol/kg
- Potassium 4–6 mmol/kg.

Investigations

Venous blood

Measure capillary blood glucose hourly until near to the normal range, or measure venous urea and electrolytes (U&Es), glucose and pH initially hourly, then 2-hourly once the venous glucose and capillary glucose are in agreement.

A mild leucocytosis is common in DKA, which should not be interpreted as signifying infection. Likewise hyperamylasaemia is common and does not imply pancreatitis.

Urinalysis

DKA is highly likely in the presence of glycos-uria and ketonuria in an unwell patient.

Electrocardiograph (ECG)

Perform an early ECG to look for T-wave changes as a first indicator of hyperkalaemia (tall and peaked) or hypokalaemia (flat or inverted), or a clinically silent myocardial infarction (MI) as a precipitant of HHS or DKA.

Point-of-care testing

Point-of-care testing for blood ketones, such as beta-hydroxybutyrate, is helpful at triage and when monitoring the response to treatment.

Differential diagnosis of DKA

Other causes of high (greater than 16) anion-gap metabolic acidosis include:

- alcoholic or starvation ketoacidosis
- lactic acidosis (multiple causes)
- uraemia
- methanol, ethylene glycol (note ethanol predominantly leads to a lactic acidosis)
- salicylate, iron, isoniazid ingestion.

Other causes of hyperglycaemia include:

- HHS
- drugs, such as corticosteroids, octreotide, thiazide diuretics, ritonavir, diazoxide and atypical antipsychotics (clozapine, olanzapine, risperidone, quetiapine – these may actually precipitate DKA soon after commencement, even in the absence of weight gain) [6]
- critical illness
- endocrine, such as Cushing's, acromegaly, phaeochromocytoma, glucagonoma, VIPoma.

Management

Diabetic ketoacidosis

The treatment of DKA is rigorous and requires careful monitoring of the patient, both clinically and biochemically. Ideally, all observations and results are entered onto a purpose-designed record sheet, such as an integrated care pathway that includes data recording and guidance [7].

Severe DKA

Severe DKA necessitating intensive management includes a venous or arterial pH <7.1,

bicarbonate <5 mmol/L, hypokalaemia on admission (<3.5 mmol/L), Glasgow coma scale (GCS) <12, systolic BP <90 mmHg and SaO$_2$ <92% on room air.

Fluid regimen

Intravenous fluids should be started within 30 min of the patient's arrival in the ED. A shocked patient should receive a fluid bolus on arrival to restore perfusion, although care is needed in patients with co-morbidities, such as the elderly with heart or renal impairment, to avoid fluid overload.

Fluid rate

Give patients who are not shocked 1 L 0.9% normal saline over 1 hour, then at a rate of 500 mL/h for 4 h with added potassium, then 250 mL/h for the next 8 h, again with added potassium [1]. A suggested fluid regimen is shown in Table 11.2.1.

Most intravenous fluid regimens recommend replacing the volume deficit (often 10% of body weight) over 24 h. However, in a patient with significant co-morbidites, it is prudent (although unproven) to aim to correct half the fluid deficit in the first 24 h and the remainder in the next 24 h. Likewise, adopt a slower rate initially in a small, young adult aged 18–25 years with the total volume replaced over 24–48 h to reduce the risk of cerebral oedema (see Table 11.2.1) [1].

Cerebral oedema

The incidence of cerebral oedema is greatest in children under 12 years, possibly related to a lower pH/PaCO$_2$ and a higher potassium and urea at presentation, and smaller increases in serum sodium. The aetiology is unclear but may result from cerebral hypoperfusion followed by reperfusion, with an increased risk associated with early (in first hour) insulin administration (odds ratio OR 12.7) and large volumes of fluid in the first 4 h (OR 6.55) [8].

Choice of fluid

There are no data from randomized controlled trials to support the choice of one crystalloid over another in the treatment of DKA. The risk of hyperchloraemic acidosis from the use of large volumes of normal saline with renal vasoconstriction and slowing of resolution of acidosis is not clinically significant. In addition, colloids are a less physiological replacement for electrolyte losses and are not recommended.

Table 11.2.1 Replacement normal saline fluid regimen in a well 70 kg patient* with DKA, who is not haemodynamically compromised/in shock	
Litre	*Time (hours from starting treatment)*
First at 1000 mL/h	0–1
Second at 500 mL/h + K	1–3
Third at 500 mL/h + K	3–5
Fourth at 250 mL/h + K	5–9
Fifth at 250 mL/h + K	9–13
Reassess cardiovascular status at 12 h and adjust rate accordingly	
Sixth at 166 mL/h + K	13–19

K: potassium; *: in a small (<70 kg), young adult (18–25 years) adopt a slower rate initially, with total volume replacement over 24–48 h.

Addition of 10% dextrose

If serum [glucose] falls to <15 mmol/L, add 10% dextrose at 125 mL/h alongside the 0.9% saline infusion, with continuance of the insulin infusion until the electrolyte and volume losses have been replaced and the ketoacidosis/ketonaemia has been cleared.

Insulin

An intravenous insulin infusion should be started within 60 min of the patient's arrival in the ED.

Insulin infusion regimen

A standard regimen is an infusion of soluble insulin, made up by adding 50 units of soluble insulin to a total of 50 mL with 0.9% saline to produce a solution containing 1 unit/mL. Remember when prescribing insulin always to write 'units' in full rather than as 'u', as the latter is too easily confused with a 0 (zero) and a 10-fold dose increase can be given in error.

Run the infusion at an initial rate of 0.1 units/kg/h (to a maximum of 6 units/h). Adjust the rate to reduce the serum [glucose] by around 3 mmol/L/h, with a rise in the serum bicarbonate of at least 3 mmol/L/h.

When the serum [glucose] is less than 15 mmol/L, halve the insulin infusion rate and then adjust it to maintain the serum [glucose] between 9 and 14 mmol/L [7].

Initial hypokalaemia

Severe hypokalaemia is associated with arrhythmias and sudden death in DKA. Do not start an insulin infusion until the serum [potassium] has been checked to make sure it is not below the lower limit of the reference range, i.e. it should be greater than 3.4 mmol/L. If it is below this, begin the IV fluid with potassium first, prior to commencing the insulin infusion.

Insulin bolus

Although there are few data on the benefits or harm of giving a bolus of insulin before starting an infusion, its short half-life makes this unnecessary. Providing the insulin infusion is prepared and started with minimal delay, there is no justification for a bolus (despite a bolus appearing in many published guidelines).

Intermittent insulin

Switching from an insulin infusion to intermittent insulin is unlikely to occur until the patient is on the medical ward. If ED staff do supervise cessation of an insulin infusion, ensure the first subcutaneous insulin dose is given at least 1 h before the infusion is stopped in association with a meal, providing *all* the following criteria have been met before ceasing the insulin infusion:

- serum [glucose] <11 mmol/L
- pH >7.30
- serum ketones <0.3 mmol/L
- serum bicarbonate >18 mmol/L
- patient is eating and drinking normally, with a normal conscious level.

Potassium replacement

Hyperkalaemia and then hypokalaemia are the most common life-threatening electrolyte problems seen in DKA. Therefore the serum [K] must be monitored closely and treatment planned to treat either condition rapidly, particularly the risk of hypokalaemia. A typical total body deficit of potassium in DKA is 3–5 mmol/kg [1,2].

Hyperkalaemia from intracellular shift from the acidosis and lack of insulin seen in the early phase of DKA may cause life-threatening dysrhythmias. This hyperkalaemia rapidly resolves soon after fluid and insulin commencement.

Conversely, add potassium to intravenous fluids once the serum [K] is below 5.5 mmol/L and the patient is passing urine. However, do not add potassium to the first fluid bolus infused rapidly for volume resuscitation.

Infusion rate

Replacing potassium at 10–20 mmol/h is usually sufficient, with the rate adjusted to the serum [K] measurement, with the aim of maintaining serum [K] in the range 4–5 mmol/L. Use premixed intravenous potassiuim in fluid bags with an intravenous fluid infusor to avoid dosing or infusion rate errors.

Education

Arguably, all episodes of DKA represent a failure of patient education, except for those patients in whom DKA is the first presentation of diabetes mellitus. All patients treated with insulin must understand 'sick day rules' to increase their normal insulin dose by 4 units or more when they have an intercurrent illness, even if they are not eating, as their insulin requirements will rise. Stopping insulin because a person is 'not eating properly' is all too common and an entirely avoidable precipitant of DKA.

Hyperosmolar, hyperglycaemic state

The management of HHS is similar to that of DKA, although patients are older, the water deficit is considerably greater, the sodium and potassium deficits greater and the overall mortality and moribidity higher. Focal or global neurological changes may occur, including an altered conscious level, coma, seizures and stroke (cause or effect).

Give 0.9% normal saline for initial volume resuscitation, with insulin by intravenous infusion and potassium supplementation to maintain serum [K] between 4 and 5 mmol/L, similar to DKA. In addition, the fall in serum osmolality is monitored as a marker of response to treatment.

Severe HHS

Severe HHS necessitating intensive management includes an osmolality >350 mosmol/kg, sodium >160 mmol/L, creatinine >200 μmol/L or urine output <0.5 mL/kg/h, hypokalaemia on admission (<3.5 mmol/L), GCS <12, systolic BP <90 mmHg, SaO_2 <92% on room air and a venous or arterial pH <7.1 (look for other causes, such as a concomitant lactic acidosis).

Management differences in HHS (to DKA)

Insulin infusion

Start fluid replacement first, *before* commencing an insulin infusion at 0.05 units/kg/h to a maximum of 3 units, as a patient with HHS may be more sensitive to insulin, plus the replacement of fluid alone will lead to a fall in serum glucose. Aim for a rate of decline in serum osmolarity of less than 3 mOsm/kg/h and in blood glucose of not more than 5 mmol/L/h.

Reduce the insulin infusion rate when the serum [glucose] drops to 15–18 mmol/L, to maintain serum [glucose] in the range 10–15 mmol/L until the serum osmolarity is less than 315 mOsm/kg. Complete normalization of osmolarity and electrolytes may take up to 72 h.

Fluid choice

Use 0.9% normal saline as the principal fluid to restore circulation volume [5]. An initial rise in serum sodium may occur due to a shift of water intracellularly from a lowering of the blood glucose, which is not an indication to use a more hypotonic solution (normal saline is already relatively hypotonic compared to serum in HHS).

Only change to 0.45% half-normal saline if the serum osmolality *and* blood sugar are not reducing. Avoid a rapid fall in serum sodium, which should not exceed 10 mmol/L per 24 h [5].

Other considerations

- Shock may be partly cardiogenic rather than due to volume depletion. Thus, invasive monitoring, central venous access and the use of vasoactive drugs rather than fluid alone will be required in this circumstance.
- Give LMWH for thromboprophylaxis as there is a higher risk of developing venous thromboembolism including in the 3 months post-hospital discharge [9].

Miscellaneous issues

There are no data to support the use of phosphate or magnesium in the treatment of DKA or HHS, despite there often being hypophosphataemia and hypomagnesaemia.

Heparin thromboprophylaxis is not used routinely in DKA, nor are antibiotics in the absence of a focus of infection or sepsis, even though it is common for the white cell count to be mildly elevated.

Sodium bicarbonate should never be used in DKA if the pH is greater than 7.0 and even below that level its value is unproven. Significant disadvantages of giving IV bicarbonate are a rapid fall in serum [K], worsened intracellular acidosis, reduced tissue oxygen delivery, delay in clearing ketones and a possible association with cerebral oedema.

Controversies

- Choice and rate of intravenous fluid replacement and its impact on the unexpected but devastating development of cerebral oedema (usually seen in children).
- Earlier recognition of ketosis by measuring beta-hydroxybutyrate to reduce the incidence and severity of DKA.
- Titrating insulin use against beta-hydroxybutyrate rather than serum glucose.
- Point-of-care measurement of beta-hydroxybutyrate may become more widespread, although its precise role in the care of patients with DKA is yet to be determined.
- Use of ultrafast-acting insulin analogues subcutaneously in the treatment of DKA in children.

References

[1] Joint British Diabetes Societies Inpatient Care Group. The Management of Diabetic Ketoacidosis in Adults. March 2010. <http://www.diabetes.org.uk/About_us/Our_Views/Care_recommendations/The-Management-of-Diabetic-Ketoacidosis-in-Adults/> [Accessed Mar. 2013].
[2] American Diabetes Association Clinical practice recommendations. Diabetes Care 2004;27(Suppl. 1):S94–102.
[3] Raghavan VA. Diabetic ketoacidosis. eMedicine. Medscape. com, February 2013. <http://emedicine.medscape.com/article/118361-overview> [Accessed Mar. 2013].
[4] Hemphil RR. Hyperosmolar hyperglycemic state. eMedicine. Medscape.com, August 2012. <http://emedicine.medscape.com/article/1914705-overview> [Accessed Mar. 2013].
[5] Joint British Diabetes Societies Inpatient Care Group. The management of the hyperosmolar hyperglycaemic state (HHS) in adults with diabetes. August 2012. <http://www.diabetes.nhs.uk/document.php?o=3778> [Accessed Mar. 2013].
[6] Guenette M, Hahn M, Cohn T, et al. Atypical antipsychotics and diabetic ketoacidosis: a review. Psychopharmacology 2013;226:1–12.
[7] McGeoch SC, Hutcheon SD, Vaughan SM, et al. Development of a national Scottish diabetic ketoacidosis protocol. Pract Diabetes Internatl 2007;24:257–61.
[8] Edge J, Jakes R, Roy Y. The UK case-control study of cerebral oedema complicating diabetic ketoacidosis in children. Diabetologia 2006;49:2002–9.
[9] Keenan C, Murin S, White R. High risk for venous thromboembolism in diabetics with hyperosmolar state: comparison with other acute medical illnesses. J Thromb Haemostas 2007;5:1185–90.

11.3 Thyroid and adrenal emergencies

Andrew Maclean

ESSENTIALS

1 Those thyroid and adrenal emergencies that pose an acute threat to life are thyroid storm, myxoedema coma and acute adrenal insufficiency. Diagnosis of these conditions requires a high index of suspicion and treatment frequently must be initiated on clinical rather than laboratory diagnosis.

2 Common features of thyroid storm are fever, alteration in mental state, cardiovascular complications, such as tachyarrhythmias and cardiac failure, and signs of hyperthyroidism. Treatment is with β-blockers, drugs that block thyroid hormone synthesis and release and corticosteroids.

3 Common clinical signs of myxoedema coma are an alteration in conscious state, hypothermia and features of hypothyroidism. Treatment is with intravenous tri-iodothyronine and corticosteroids.

4 The most important clinical feature of acute adrenal insufficiency is hypotension unresponsive to fluid therapy. Although hyponatraemia and hyperkalaemia are usual in acute adrenal insufficiency, serum electrolytes may be normal. Treatment is with intravenous corticosteroid replacement on suspicion of the diagnosis.

5 General supportive measures and treatment of the precipitating event must parallel the specific treatment regimen in all of these conditions.

Introduction

Four conditions are covered in this chapter: thyrotoxicosis, hypothyroidism, hypoadrenal states and hyperadrenal states. Patients with the first three present relatively infrequently to emergency departments (EDs), but all four conditions are potentially fatal if they go unrecognized and untreated. The most common cause of Cushing's syndrome is exogenous steroid administration. An inability to produce endogenous steroids in times of physiological stress and therefore the potential for adrenal insufficiency occurring with insufficient replacement therapy must be considered in such patients.

THYROTOXICOSIS

Aetiology, genetics, pathogenesis and pathology

Normal secretion of thyroid hormone relies on an intact feedback loop involving the hypothalamus, pituitary gland and thyroid gland. Thyrotropin-releasing hormone (TRH) released from the hypothalamus stimulates thyroid-stimulating hormone (TSH) production in the anterior pituitary, which stimulates thyroid hormone release from thyroid follicular cells. Thyroid hormones suppress TRH and TSH production. Thyroid hormones act at a cellular level, binding with nuclear receptors to enable gene expression and protein synthesis. Thyroid hormone may also have an effect on modulating cellular metabolism.

There are a number of pathological causes of thyrotoxicosis (Table 11.3.1). Graves' disease is an autoimmune condition related to a combination of genetic and environmental factors, including iodine intake, stress and smoking. The thyrotoxicosis of Graves' disease is caused

Table 11.3.1 Causes of thyrotoxicosis

Primary hyperthyroidism	Graves' disease Toxic multinodular goitre Toxic adenoma
Thyroiditis	de Quervain's (subacute) Postpartum Radiation
Central hyperthyroidism	Pituitary adenoma Ectopic thyroid tissue Metastatic thyroid tissue
Drug-induced	Lithium Iodine (including radiographic contrast) Amiodarone Excess thyroid hormone ingestion ('factitious thyrotoxicosis')

Table 11.3.2 Clinical features of thyrotoxicosis

Nervousness, irritability
Heat intolerance and increased sweating
Tremor
Weight loss and alteration in appetite
Palpitations and tachycardia, particularly atrial fibrillation
Widened pulse pressure
Exertional intolerance and dyspnoea
Frequent bowel movements
Fatigue and muscle weakness
Thyroid enlargement (depending on cause)
Pretibial myxoedema (with Graves' disease)
Menstrual disturbance and impaired fertility
Mental changes
Sleep disturbances
Changes in vision, photophobia, eye irritation, diplopia, lid lag or exophthalmos
Dependent lower extremity oedema
Sudden paralysis, with or without hypokalaemia

by autoantibodies, which stimulate the thyroid resulting in excess thyroid hormone production.

Thyroiditis may be acute (rare), subacute or chronic. Inflammation of the thyroid is associated with damage to follicles with release of thyroid hormone. Subacute thyroiditis (de Quervain's, also known as subacute granulomatous) may follow a viral infection and is typically painful, with localized tenderness and neck pain, sometimes with odynophagia.

Multinodular goitre occurs in areas of both iodine deficiency and sufficiency, indicating that a multiplicity of genetic and environmental factors are at play. Fibrosis, hypercellularity and colloid cysts are the main pathological findings.

Epidemiology

Graves' disease accounts for at least 80% of cases of thyrotoxicosis [1]. The prevalence increases in areas with high iodine intake. Graves' disease has a strong female predominance, affecting up to 2% of all women [1,2]. Thyrotoxicosis due to Graves' disease usually occurs in the second to fourth decades of life, whereas the prevalence of a toxic nodular goitre increases with age.

Clinical features

The signs and symptoms of hyperthyroidism are secondary to the effects of excess thyroid hormone in the circulation. The severity of the signs and symptoms is related to the duration of the illness, the magnitude of the hormone excess and the age of the patient. These symptoms and signs are summarized in Table 11.3.2, which illustrates the wide spectrum of possible clinical features.

A comprehensive history and physical examination should be performed, with particular attention to weight, blood pressure, pulse rate and rhythm, looking specifically for cardiac failure, palpation and auscultation of the thyroid to determine thyroid size, nodularity and vascularity, neuromuscular examination and an eye examination for evidence of exophthalmos or ophthalmoplegia.

Clinical investigations and criteria for diagnosis [1–3]

The TSH level is the single best screening test for hyperthyroidism. The recent development of sensitive TSH assays has greatly facilitated the diagnosis of hyperthyroidism. Hyperthyroidism of any cause (except excess TSH production from the anterior pituitary) results in a lower than normal TSH. The reference range is 0.4–5.0 mIU/L depending on the method.

Other laboratory and isotope tests may include:

- Free thyroxine (T4) or free tri-iodothyronine (T3) assay, when there is strong clinical suspicion of hyperthyroidism but the TSH is high or high normal
- Thyroid autoantibodies, including TSH receptor antibody. These are not routine but may be helpful in selected cases
- Radioactive iodine uptake and/or thyroid scan. These tests are helpful in establishing the cause of the hyperthyroidism, but are not part of the ED assessment.

Treatment

Mild hyperthyroidism does not require any treatment in the ED and the patient may simply be referred to an appropriate outpatient clinic. Any features of thyroid storm (see below) mandate admission, as does any significant intercurrent illness. Atrial arrhythmias should be controlled by the use of β-blockers, aiming to achieve a rate of less than 100 beats per minute.

Ensure that all bloods have been collected first if thyroid-blocking drugs are to be commenced in the ED. High doses of thyroid-blocking drugs are often required to gain an initial response, after which the dose can be tapered.

Commence carbimazole 10–45 mg daily or propylthiouracil 200–600 mg daily in two or three divided doses initially, using the larger doses for more severe cases [4]. Ideally, discuss initiation of these agents with the physician who will continue managing the patient after his or her discharge from the ED. Ninety per cent of patients will be controlled within weeks using these drugs [5]. Treatment for 12–18 months will result in a long-term remission in 40–60% of patients with Graves' disease [2].

Thyroid storm

Aetiology

Thyroid storm occurs in about 1% of patients with hyperthyroidism. It usually occurs as an acute deterioration in a patient with poorly controlled or undiagnosed hyperthyroidism, precipitated by factors such as surgery, trauma, infection, radioiodine treatment, use of iodinated contrast, exogenous thyroxine ingestion or any other significant stressor.

The diagnosis is entirely clinical, as there is no test to differentiate a thyroid storm from thyrotoxicosis. The mortality rate if untreated or if the diagnosis is missed is over 90%. Death is usually due to cardiovascular collapse.

Clinical features of a thyroid storm

The symptoms and signs of thyrotoxicosis are present and significantly exaggerated, with the abrupt onset of a combination of the following:

- fever >37.6°C up to 41°C
- cardiovascular complications:
  - tachycardia with pulse rates up to 200–300/min, including rapid atrial fibrillation
  - wide pulse pressure
  - high output cardiac failure
- alteration in mental state, varying from agitation and restlessness to delirium, coma and seizures
- abdominal pain with vomiting and diarrhoea.

Differential diagnosis

The following differential diagnoses of a thyroid storm need to be considered:

- sepsis
- heat stroke
- malignant hyperthermia
- neuroleptic syndrome
- sympathomimetic ingestion
- drug withdrawal (including alcohol)
- phaeochromocytoma crisis.

Treatment

The treatment of thyroid storm is directed to blocking thyroid hormone synthesis and release, the peripheral effects of the thyroid hormones, and corticosteroids.

β-Blockers

β-Blockade is the most important factor in decreasing morbidity and mortality. Many of the peripheral manifestations of hyperthyroidism, in particular the cardiovascular effects, are reduced by the use of propranolol. Propranolol also inhibits the peripheral conversion of T4 to T3 as well as antagonizing the effects of thyroid hormones and the hypersensitivity to catecholamines.

Give intravenous increments of 0.5 mg initially up to 10 mg total with continuous cardiovascular monitoring. Subsequent doses of 40–120 mg 6-hourly orally can be given.

β-Blockers should treat the cardiac failure secondary to the tachyarrhythmia or high cardiac output, but may cause complications in patients with pre-existing heart disease or asthma.

In this situation, use the short-acting β-blocker esmolol, as any adverse effects will be of brief duration. Give a 250–500 μg/kg bolus followed by an infusion starting at 50–100 μg/kg/min titrated to effect. Another option is to use the combination of a β-blocker and digoxin.

Thyroid-blocking drugs

Give propylthiouracil 900–1200 mg loading dose orally or via a nasogastric tube if necessary. This is followed by 200–300 mg 4–6-hourly. Propylthiouracil acts by preventing hormone synthesis by blocking the iodination of tyrosine and also inhibits the peripheral conversion of T4 to T3.

Iodine in large doses inhibits the synthesis and release of thyroid hormones and may be given either orally as Lugol's iodine, 30–60 drops daily in divided doses, or intravenously as sodium iodide 1 g 12-hourly. Lithium carbonate may be used in patients allergic to iodine or be added when there is difficulty with control [4].

Cholestyramine can also be considered, which acts by binding with thyroxine after biliary excretion and hence increasing elimination.

Corticosteroids

Corticosteroids are given to inhibit the peripheral conversion of T4 to T3 and as a relative deficiency may also be present. Hydrocortisone 100 mg IV 6-hourly or dexamethasone 4 mg IV 12-hourly are used.

General supportive measures

Dehydration and electrolyte disturbances need correction. Aggressive treatment of hyperthermia with cooling measures and paracetamol are necessary, but induction of shivering should be avoided. Salicylates are contraindicated as they displace T4 from binding proteins. In addition, it is essential to look for and treat any precipitating cause, which will improve the prognosis.

Prognosis

Mortality rates are high, at 10–75% despite treatment [8].

Apathetic hyperthyroidism

Patients with this condition are generally older, although it has been recorded in all age groups. The clinical picture is of a depressed mental state with cardiac complications, in particular cardiac failure. Weight loss is usually not significant and eye signs are rare. Most of the usual hyperkinetic manifestations of hyperthyroidism are absent. Treatment is as for standard hyperthyroidism.

HYPOTHYROIDISM

Aetiology, genetics, pathogenesis and pathology

Hypothyroidism results from undersecretion of thyroid hormone from the thyroid gland. Causes of primary hypothyroidism include iodine deficiency, chronic autoimmune thyroiditis (Hashimoto's thyroiditis), congenital, surgical removal of the thyroid gland, post-radioactive iodine, thyroid gland ablation and external irradiation. A significant number of cases are idiopathic. Secondary causes of hypothyroidism include pituitary and hypothalamic disease.

Epidemiology

Iodine deficiency is the most common cause worldwide, whereas in areas of iodine sufficiency, autoimmune disease and hypothyoidism secondary to treatment of hyperthyroid disease are more common. The prevalence of hyperthyroidism in adults is around 1.4% in women and <0.1 % in men [6]. Congenital hypothyroidism is rare, occurring in about 1:4000 births.

Clinical features

The symptoms of hypothyroidism are related to the duration and severity of hypothyroidism, the rapidity with which hypothyroidism occurs and the psychological characteristics of the patient. These are summarized in Table 11.3.3.

A complete evaluation, including a comprehensive history, physical examination and appropriate laboratory evaluation should be performed in every patient with a goitre. Patients with chronic thyroiditis have a higher incidence of other associated autoimmune disorders, such as vitiligo, rheumatoid arthritis, Addison's disease, diabetes mellitus and pernicious anaemia.

Clinical investigations and criteria for diagnosis

Laboratory evaluation

Perform a TSH assay as the primary test to establish the diagnosis of hypothyroidism if raised. The reference range is 0.4–5.0 mIU/L depending on the method. Additional tests may include free thyroxine assay and thyroid

Table 11.3.3 Clinical features of hypothyroidism
Dry skin and cold intolerance
Coarse facial features
Enlarged tongue
Coarse brittle hair or loss of hair, loss of outer third of eyebrows
Periorbital oedema
Fatigue
Constipation
Weight gain/obesity
Memory and mental impairment, decreased concentration
Depression, personality changes
Yellow skin (carotenaemia)
Swelling of ankles
Irregular or heavy menses and infertility
Hoarseness
Myalgias
Goitre
Hyperlipidaemia
Delayed relaxation phase of tendon reflexes, ataxia
Sinus bradycardia (atrioventricular block, rare)
Cardiac failure, pericardial effusion (rare)
Hypothermia (uncommon)

autoantibodies. A combination of an elevated TSH and low free thyroxine is diagnostic [3,4,6]. A patient may be hypothyroid with a TSH greater than twice the reference interval, but with a free thyroxine within the normal range. Subnormal thyroxine with a normal TSH can occur in secondary hypothyroidism.

Thyroid autoantibodies are positive in 95% of patients with autoimmune thyroiditis (Hashimoto's thyroiditis). The high titres are of value in making this specific diagnosis.

Other investigations

A thyroid scan and/or an ultrasound are useful if structural thyroid abnormalities are suspected.

Thyroid nodules are not uncommon with chronic thyroiditis and carry a small risk of thyroid cancer.

Treatment

Start thyroxine at 50–100 µg orally daily in adults under 60 years of age without evidence of ischaemic heart disease. Too rapid commencement of full thyroid hormone replacement may cause myocardial ischaemia from increased myocardial oxygen consumption without a corresponding increase in cardiac output. The initial daily replacement dose is therefore 25 µg thyroxine in the elderly and where there is suspicion of heart disease. This dose should remain unchanged for 3–4 weeks to allow a steady state to be reached. It is appropriate to start this in the ED, when a firm diagnosis has been made and appropriate follow up arranged.

The dose of thyroxine is then increased in 25–50 µg increments at not less than 4-weekly intervals, until the optimum dose is reached as determined by clinical response and TSH level. Consider admission for any patient with coexistent unstable angina to monitor cardiac function. Any features of myxoedema coma (see below) also mandate admission.

Myxoedema coma

The clinical syndrome of altered mental state, features of hypothyroidism and hypothermia is referred to as myxoedema coma, or sometimes as myxoedema crisis. There is usually a precipitating event, such as infection, stroke, trauma, myocardial infarction or administration of drugs, particularly phenothiazines, phenytoin, amiodarone, propranolol or lithium, that initiates this terminal decompensation phase of hypothyroidism.

The mortality for myxoedema coma remains up to 50% despite aggressive treatment.

Clinical features
- Altered mental state, usually coma due to cerebral oedema, hypoxia and hypercarbia.
- Seizures may precede coma in 25% of patients.
- Hypothermia with temperature usually less than 32.2°C. Notably, patients do not shiver.
- Hypoventilation resulting in hypoxia and hypercarbia.
- Cardiovascular complications, including hypotension and bradycardia, with heart rate inappropriate for the hypotension.
- Pericardial effusion, rarely with cardiac tamponade.
- Hypoglycaemia (common).
- Hyponatraemia.
- Paralytic ileus, megacolon, and urinary retention.
- Usual clinical features of hypothyroidism (see Table 11.3.3).

Treatment
Treatment should commence on clinical suspicion.

Administration of thyroid hormones

Tri-iodothyronine Intravenous T3 may give a faster clinical response in myxoedema coma, as it is the active form of the hormone, although there is no consensus as to whether T3 or T4 replacement is preferable[7,8]. Give T3 as an initial IV bolus of 25–50 µg followed by 10–20 µg 8-hourly to a maximum of 60 µg per day. Alternatively, commence an infusion with a lower total dose of 20 µg per day, as large initial doses appear unnecessary for recovery and may in fact be harmful. Oral or nasogastric replacement of T3 is not recommended in the initial phase of management because of unreliable gastrointestinal absorption.

Thyroxine The use of T4 is supported as the gradual delivery of T3 through the peripheral conversion of T4 is better tolerated and as the onset of action is more predictable. Give a 400–500 µg IV bolus (300 µg/m^2), followed by 50 µg IV daily until oral therapy is tolerated. Combined approaches are now also described.

Corticosteroids
These are given as there is impaired response to stress and the potential for coexistent adrenal insufficiency. Give hydrocortisone 100 mg IV 6-hourly. If an ACTH stimulation test is being considered, give dexamethasone 4 mg until results are known.

General supportive measures
Requires correction of ventilatory, circulatory, temperature and metabolic abnormalities and includes the use of warm humidified oxygen. Look for and treat any precipitating cause. Finally, avoid sedative drugs and watch out for water overload.

HYPOADRENAL STATES

Aetiology, genetics, pathogenesis and pathology

Glucocorticoids act to produce multiple effects on metabolism, including gluconeogenesis, mobilization of fatty acids and amino acids, inhibiting the effects of insulin and ketogenesis. Glucocorticoids have anti-inflammatory effects related to the inhibition of production and reduction of the effects of cytokines and reduction of cell-mediated immunity. They also maintain the normal response of the vascular system to vasoconstrictors. In addition, glucocorticoids affect the regulation of body water by increasing free water excretion. This occurs by an increase in the glomerular filtration rate as well as inhibition of migration of water into cells. Aldosterone acts primarily to cause the reabsorption of sodium and the excretion of potassium and hydrogen ions.

The adrenals normally respond within minutes by elevating corticosteroid levels in response to any physiological or pathological stress. When glucocorticoid insufficiency is present such stressors may result in hypotension, shock and ultimately death if left untreated.

Primary adrenal insufficiency (Addison's disease)

Primary adrenal insufficiency (Addison's disease) is due to inability of the adrenal cortex to produce adequate levels of adrenal hormones. Hyponatraemia, hyperkalaemia, acidosis and elevated serum creatinine occur mainly due to aldosterone deficiency, whereas hypoglycaemia is related to cortisol deficiency. Hypercalcaemia occurs as a result of reduction in glomerular filtration rate as well as increased proximal tubular reabsorption of calcium. There may also be some increased mobilization of calcium from bone in patients with adrenal insufficiency.

Secondary adrenal insufficiency

Secondary adrenal insufficiency is due to failure of adequate adrenocorticotrophic hormone (ACTH) from the pituitary gland

Table 11.3.4	Causes of adrenal insufficiency
Primary (Addison's)	Autoimmune Surgical removal Infection (TB, viral, fungal) Haemorrhage, including Waterhouse–Friedrichsen syndrome Congenital
Secondary	Exogenous steroid suppression (single most common cause of adrenal insufficiency) Endogenous steroid (from tumour) Pituitary failure (hypopituitarism)

(Table 11.3.4). Hyponatraemia still occurs in secondary adrenal insufficiency, but is due to cortisol deficiency [9,10].

The majority of presentations of acute adrenal insufficiency occur as an exacerbation of a chronic disease process where there is a malfunctioning adrenal system. Acute precipitating factors include sepsis, major trauma, surgery and a myocardial infarct.

Causes of primary or secondary adrenal insufficiency

The cause of 80% of primary adrenal insufficiency is autoimmune. Other causes of acute adrenal gland insufficiency include primary or secondary malignancy, infection, such as tuberculosis, adrenal infarction or haemorrhage (Waterhouse–Friedrichsen syndrome) seen in meningococcaemia or severe sepsis, and drugs. Primary adrenal insufficiency also occurs in up to 20% of patients with AIDS. Up to 60% of patients with sepsis have a low baseline cortisol level, although fewer meet criteria for insufficiency on suppression testing [11,12].

The most common cause of secondary adrenal insufficiency is suppression of the adrenopituitary axis by long-term corticosteroid therapy, although other causes include pituitary failure, such as panhypopituitarism or isolated ACTH production failure.

Clinical features

Suspect adrenocortical failure in any hypotensive patient when no apparent cause is found, particularly anyone who is unresponsive to fluid therapy. Orthostatic postural hypotension is almost always present. Other common features

include abdominal pain, which may be severe, with vomiting.

Less obvious findings are weakness, anorexia, diarrhoea, postural syncope, mucocutaneous pigmentation/vitiligo (only with primary adrenal disease) and a dulled mental state.

Hypercalcaemia and/or hyperkalaemia can be the first sign of adrenal insufficiency in the critically ill patient [10]. The other features of adrenal insufficiency may be masked by coexisting illness, but the possibility of adrenal insufficiency should always be considered.

Differential diagnosis

The diagnosis of adrenal insufficiency in the early stages is difficult as weakness, lethargy and gastrointestinal symptoms are common and non-specific. Consider adrenal insufficiency in any patients presenting with these symptoms once more common causes have been excluded.

Clinical investigations

Laboratory findings

The classical laboratory findings are hyponatraemia (due to sodium depletion and the intracellular movement of sodium), hypochloraemia and hyperkalaemia (due to acidosis and aldosterone deficiency). Mild hypercalcaemia (in 10–20% of cases) and a non-anion-gap metabolic acidosis may be seen. Hypoglycaemia, if present, is usually mild. However, all basic laboratory investigations can be within normal limits, even in the presence of an Addisonian crisis.

Antiadrenal antibodies are positive in 70% of patients with autoimmune adrenalitis.

Criteria for diagnosis

Baseline cortisol and ACTH levels should be taken prior to treatment. The normal reference range for cortisol is 200–650 nmol/L. An ACTH level should be <50 ng/L, although interpretation needs to take into account the time of day when the sample is taken. ACTH should be high in primary adrenal disease and low in pituitary disease.

The Synacthen stimulation test is the definitive investigation and may be required if the initial test results are not diagnostic. It is usually performed as an inpatient, when Synacthen 250 µg is administered intramuscularly and cortisol levels are taken at baseline, 30 minutes and 60 minutes. A baseline or post-Synacthen cortisol level of >550 nmol/L is considered normal.

Treatment

Corticosteroid replacement

Do not delay treatment awaiting confirmatory results if acute adrenal insufficiency is suspected.

Give immediate corticosteroid replacement with either intravenous hydrocortisone or dexamethasone. Dexamethasone is recommended when the diagnosis has not been confirmed by laboratory investigations, as it does not interfere with the cortisol assay. Give 10 mg dexamethasone IV stat followed by 4 mg IV 8-hourly. Alternatively, give hydrocortisone at a dose of 250 mg stat followed by 100 mg IV 6-hourly.

Fluid replacement therapy

Give normal saline 1 L stat, then titrated to response, although the total volume deficit is rarely greater than 10% body weight. Intravenous dextrose should be given at the same time, either separately or as 5% dextrose in normal saline to avoid hypoglycaemia.

General supportive measures

These include treatment of hypoglycaemia and other electrolyte replacement abnormalities, although most will be corrected with saline rehydration alone. Mineralocorticoid replacement is usually not necessary in the acute crisis, if salt and water replacement are adequate.

Once the crisis has been successfully treated, it is important to investigate and manage the cause and to develop a maintenance regimen.

Prognosis

The patient with acute adrenal insufficiency may die if the diagnosis is not made promptly. When the diagnosis is suspected and treatment is early, the outcome is favourable depending on the nature of any precipitating illness.

Response to severe illness

The normal response to severe illness should see cortisol levels rising to at least 500 nmol/L. States of 'relative adrenal insufficiency' are described where glucocorticoid administration diminishes or even eliminates the requirements for vasopressor agents, even though measured cortisol levels are normal or close to normal [11]. There is no concensus on what constitutes 'normal' cortisol levels in severe illness.

Up to 60% of patients with severe sepsis may have some degree of adrenal insufficiency depending upon the threshold cortisol level used [12]. Moreover, it appears that it is the delta cortisol rather than the basal cortisol level that is associated with clinical outcome [13]. Repeat adrenal function testing is indicated in patients with severe illness who remain unstable or who fail to improve with aggressive supportive therapy [14].

The use of hydrocortisone has been recommended in septic shock after an abnormal 250 μg Synacthen stimulation test [15–17]. This should continue for a week if adrenal insufficiency is confirmed.

HYPERADRENAL STATES

Aetiology, pathogenesis and epidemiology

Cushing's disease usually refers to hyperadrenalism due to a pituitary adenoma. Cushing's syndrome occurs as a result of hyperadrenalism from exposure to excess glucocorticoids over a prolonged period. Endogenous causes of Cushing's syndrome are related to primary adrenal disorders, such as adrenal adenoma, carcinoma or hyperplasia, or are secondary to ACTH or CRH stimulation and ectopic ACTH production from bronchogenic carcinoma or carcinoid tumours in particular. However, by far the most common cause of Cushing's syndrome is from the exogenous (iatrogenic) administration of steroids.

The incidence of Cushing's syndrome ranges from 0.7 to 2.4 per million population per year, but the reported prevalence in obese patients with type II diabetes may be between 2 and 5% [18].

Clinical features

The classical clinical features of Cushing's syndrome are increased body weight with central obesity, rounded face, hypertension, fatigue, weakness and proximal myopathy, hirsutism, striae, bruising, decreased libido, amenorrhoea, depression and/or personality changes, osteopaenia or fracture. Proximal weakness or myopathy is useful to differentiate simple obesity (strong limbs) from possible Cushing's syndrome (relative weakness for patient's size).

Clinical investigations and criteria for diagnosis

Laboratory tests

Full blood examination may reveal polycythaemia, neutrophilia and eosinophilia. Electrolytes may show hyperglycaemia, hypokalaemia and metabolic alkalosis.

24-h urinary cortisol level

A measured 24-h urinary cortisol level with a value more than four times the upper normal range is rare except in Cushing's syndrome (normal range 100–300 nmol/24 h).

Overnight dexamathasone suppression test

This is an outpatient screening test for Cushing's syndrome [3]:

- Day 1, 09:00 hours: 5 mL blood taken for baseline cortisol
- Day 1, 23:00 hours: 1 mg dexamethasone taken orally
- Day 2, 5 mL blood for cortisol.

The baseline reference range for cortisol is 200–650 nmol/L. The day 2 cortisol level should drop to lower than 50% of the baseline level, indicating normal suppression and excluding Cushing's syndrome.

Long dexamathasone suppression test

The long dexamathasone suppression test is performed as an inpatient, using increasing doses of dexamethasone to determine at what level suppression occurs, with testing of both cortisol and ACTH levels. Cushing's disease only suppresses at high doses.

Other tests

A chest X-ray is important if bronchogenic carcinoma of the lung is suspected. Magnetic resonance imaging of the adrenals and/or head is used for the identification of tumours.

Treatment

Treatment will depend on the cause. When a pituitary or adrenal adenoma is identified, optimal treatment is removal of the tumour [4,18]. Glucocorticoid replacement is then required for up to 2 years following surgery to allow full recovery of the normal pituitary–adrenal axis.

Pharmacological blockade of adrenal corticosteroid production may be required in some circumstances. Ketaconazole, amino-glutethimide, metapyrone and mitotane may be used for this purpose.

Controversies

- What constitutes 'normal' cortisol levels in severe illness
- Whether T3 or T4 replacement therapy is preferable in myxoedema coma.
- Differentiating simple obesity with hypertension from Cushing's syndrome.

References

[1] Cooper DS. Hyperthyroidism. Lancet 2003;362:459–68.
[2] Pearce EN. Diagnosis and management of thyrotoxicosis. Br Med J 2006;332:1369–72.
[3] Royal College of Pathologists of Australasia On-line Manual. Royal College of Pathologists of Australasia; 2009. <http://rcpamanual.edu.au/> [Accessed Nov. 2012].
[4] Endocrinology Expert Group. Therapeutic Guidelines Endocrinology Version 4. Melbourne: ©Therepeutic Guidelines Limited; 2009.
[5] Cooper DS. Antithyroid drugs. N Engl J Med 2005;352:905–17.
[6] Lindsay RS, Toft AD. Hypothyroidism. Lancet 1997;349:413–7.
[7] Jordan RM. Myxedema coma. Med Clin N Am 1995;79:185–94.
[8] Handy J. Thyroid emergencies Oh's intensive care manual, 6th ed. Butterworth–Heinemann: Elsevier; 2009.
[9] Oelkers W. Adrenal insufficiency. N Engl J Med 1996;335:1206–12.
[10] Nair G, Simmons D. Adrenal insufficiency presenting as hypercalcemia. Hosp Phys 2003:33–5.
[11] de Herder W, van der Lely A. Addisonian crisis and relative adrenal failure. Rev Endocr Metab Disord 2003;4:143–7.
[12] Marik P, Zaloga G. Adrenal insufficiency during septic shock. Crit Care Med 2003;31:141–5.
[13] Lipner Fredman D, Sprung C, et al. Adrenal function in sepsis: the retrospective Corticus cohort study. Crit Care Med 2007;35:1012–8.
[14] Marik P. Adrenal-exhaustion syndrome in patients with liver disease. Intens Care Med 2006;134:275–80.
[15] Cooper MS, Stewart PM. Current concepts: corticosteroid insufficiency in acutely ill patients. N Engl J Med 2003;348:727–34.
[16] Annane D. Glucocorticoids in the treatment of severe sepsis and septic shock. Curr Opin Crit Care 2005;11:449–53.
[17] Luce JM. Physicians should administer low-dose corticosteroid selectively to septic patients until an ongoing trial is completed. Ann Intern Med 2004;141:70.
[18] Newall-Price J, Bertagna X, Grossman AB, et al. Cushing's syndrome. Lancet 2006;367:1605–17.

Further readings

Arlt W. Disorders of the adrenal cortex Longo DL, editor. Harrison's principles of internal medicine (18th ed.). New York: McGraw-Hill; 2012.
Handy J. Thyroid emergencies Oh's intensive care manual, 6th ed. Butterworth–Heinemann: Elsevier; 2009.
Jameson JL, Weetman AP. Disorders of the thyroid gland Longo DL, editor. Harrison's principles of internal medicine (18th ed.). New York: McGraw-Hill; 2012.
Maclean A, Dunn R. Endocrinology The emergency medicine manual, 5th ed. Adelaide: Venom Publishing; 2010.
Venkatesh B, Cohen J. Adrenocortical insufficiency in critical illness Oh's intensive care manual, 6th ed. Butterworth–Heinemann: Elsevier; 2009.

METABOLIC EMERGENCIES

Edited by *Mark Little*

12.1 Acid–base disorders

David McCoubrie • Alan Gault

ESSENTIALS

1 Acid–base homeostasis is one of the most tightly regulated systems within the body. It is maintained by buffering, respiratory and renal mechanisms.

2 Most acid–base disturbances are complex and require a systematic approach to determine underlying processes.

3 High anion-gap metabolic acidosis is significant in emergency medicine and should direct the clinician to determine and treat the aetiology.

4 Acidaemia results in an extracellular shift of potassium that can result in significant hyperkalaemia.

5 Hypoventilation resulting in retention of CO_2 leads to respiratory acidosis.

6 Administration of $NaHCO_3$ is not routine; however, it is indicated in severe hyperkalaemia, sodium channel blockade and other selected poisonings.

7 Lactate levels greater than 4 are associated with raised mortality and should highlight the need for resuscitation and immediate assessment of precipitating pathology.

Introduction

Acid–base disorders are commonly encountered in the emergency department (ED) and their recognition is important for the diagnosis, assessment of severity and monitoring of many disease processes. Although these disorders are usually classified according to the major metabolic abnormality present (acidosis or alkalosis) and its origin (metabolic or respiratory), it is important to realize that acid–base disorders of a mixed type commonly occur and that the recognition and assessment of these are more complex.

CO_2 produces acid when in solution and altering $PaCO_2$ through changes in ventilation can produce or remove acid from the body. The terms respiratory acidosis/alkalosis refer to the pH shifts resulting from alterations in $PaCO_2$ from changes in ventilation. Bicarbonate acts as a base in solution with bicarbonate accumulation resulting in a more alkaline state and its wasting or consumption indicating a more acidic state. The terms metabolic acidosis/alkalosis refer to pH shifts characterized by alterations in bicarbonate levels. By convention, the overall pH abnormality as defined by the blood gas assessment is termed alkalaemia (for pH >7.44) or acidaemia (pH <7.34).

Acid–base homeostasis

Acid–base status is one of the most tightly regulated systems in the body. The term compensation is used to describe the processes by which shifts in plasma pH are attenuated. These mechanisms include buffering, respiratory manipulation of CO_2 and renal handling of bicarbonate. Buffering with plasma proteins, haemoglobin and the carbonic-acid–bicarbonate systems provide the most immediate mechanism. This is followed by respiratory compensation, which occurs within minutes and is achieved by alterations in alveolar ventilation. Renal compensation usually takes hours to days to take effect.

Acidaemia

Systemic acidaemia is defined as the presence of an increased concentration of H^+ ions in the blood. An acidaemia can result from respiratory acidosis, metabolic acidosis or both. The physiological effects of acidaemia are a decrease in the affinity of haemoglobin for oxygen and an increase in serum K^+ of approximately 0.4–0.6 mmol/L for each decrease in pH of 0.1 [1]. Although the presence of acidaemia is often associated with a poor prognosis, the presence of acidaemia *per se* usually has few clinically significant effects. It is the nature and severity of the underlying illness that principally determines outcome. A decrease in measured serum HCO_3^- of up to 5 mmol/L has also been reported as a result of underfilling of vacuum-type specimen tubes [2].

Metabolic acidosis

Metabolic acidosis is defined as an increase in the $[H^+]$ of the blood as a result of increased acid production or bicarbonate wasting from the gastrointestinal (GI) or renal tract. The cause is often multifactorial and can be further classified into 'anion-gap' and 'non-anion-gap' (or hyperchloraemic) metabolic acidosis.

Anion-gap metabolic acidosis (AGMA)

As electroneutrality must exist in all solutions, the anion gap represents the concentration of anions that are not commonly measured. The most commonly used formula for the calculation of the anion gap is:

$$\text{Anion gap} = [Na^+] - ([Cl^-] + [HCO_3^-])$$

The normal value for the anion gap depends on the type of biochemical analyser used and, while the upper limit of normal has been commonly quoted as 14, the mean range with some modern analysers is only 5–12 [3]. In the normal resting state, the serum ionic proteins account for most of the anion gap, with a lesser contribution from other 'unmeasured' anions, such as PO_4^- and SO_4^-. In pathological conditions where there is an increase in the concentration of unmeasured anions, an AGMA results. The anions responsible for the increase in the anion gap depend on the cause of the acidosis. Lactic acid is the predominant anion in hypoxia and shock, PO_4^- and SO_4^- in renal failure, ketoacids in diabetic and alcoholic ketoacidosis, oxalic acid in ethylene glycol poisoning and formic acid in methanol poisoning.

Of the causes of an AGMA, lactic acidosis is the most commonly encountered in the ED and is defined as a serum lactate of >2.5 mmol/L (Table 12.1.1). The presence of lactic acidosis is determined by the balance between lactate production and metabolism. In the seriously ill patient, it is common for increased production and decreased metabolism to be present simultaneously.

Table 12.1.1	Causes of hyperlactataemia
Type A: imbalance between oxygen demand and supply	**Type B: metabolic derangements**
Carbon monoxide poisoning	Beta₂-agonists
Excessive oxygen demand	Cancer
seizure,	Cyanide
hyperpyrexia,	Ethanol
shivering, exercise	Hepatic failure
Shock	Inborn errors of metabolism
Severe anaemia	Ketoacidosis
Severe hypoxia	Metformin
	Sepsis
	Vitamin deficiency (thiamine, biotin)

It is important to realize that, in many conditions, a variety of factors may produce the acidosis and that multiple anions may be involved in the production of an anion-gap acidosis. In a patient with an AGMA, a non-anion-gap metabolic acidosis may also exist (see below).

Non-anion-gap metabolic acidosis

Non-anion-gap metabolic acidosis results from loss of HCO_3^- from the body, rather than increased acid production. To maintain electroneutrality, chloride is usually retained by the renal tubules when HCO_3^- is lost and the hallmark of non-anion-gap acidosis is an elevation of the serum chloride. The causes of non-anion-gap metabolic acidosis are further classified according to the site of HCO_3^- loss. Gastrointestinal losses can occur with lower gastrointestinal tract (GIT) fluid losses that are rich in HCO_3^- or with cholestyramine ingestion due to binding of HCO_3^- in the gut. Renal losses can occur with renal tubular acidosis, carbonic anhydrase inhibitor therapy or adrenocortical insufficiency. Occasionally, direct chloride excess drives the renal bicarbonate loss (again due to electroneutrality) – which can be observed with large volume chloride rich crystalloid administration (chiefly normal saline).

Renal tubular acidosis Renal tubular acidosis (RTA) is a group of conditions where there is an impaired ability to secrete H^+ in the distal convoluted tubule or absorb HCO_3^- in the proximal convoluted tubule. This may result in a chronic metabolic acidosis, with hypokalaemia, nephrocalcinosis, rickets or osteomalacia. There are many subtypes of RTA and many different causes. Most commonly, it is observed in patients with chronic renal impairment but

it may also be drug induced with agents such as ibuprofen, toluene and carbonic anhydrase inhibitors most often implicated.

Treatment of metabolic acidosis

The treatment of acidosis should usually be directed primarily towards correction of the underlying cause. Intravenous HCO_3^- is of use in the presence of acidosis and severe hyperkalaemia, severe sodium channel (e.g. tricyclic antidepressant), salicylate and methanol poisoning. The use of HCO_3^- in patients with diabetic ketoacidosis and lactic acidosis associated with sepsis or severe cardiorespiratory disease does not appear to improve outcome [4–6]. The potential hazards of HCO_3^- therapy include a high solute load, hyperosmolarity, hypokalaemia, decreased ionized serum calcium and worsening of intracellular and cerebrospinal fluid acidosis (which may precipitate hepatic encephalopathy in susceptible patients).

Respiratory acidosis

Respiratory acidosis is defined as an elevation of the arterial partial pressure of carbon dioxide (PCO_2) and is due to alveolar hypoventilation. This can result from central depression in respiratory drive, neuromuscular weakness, mechanical factors, lung parenchymal disorders and ventilation/perfusion mismatch. With significant elevations in CO_2, sweating, tachycardia, confusion and mydriasis occur. When the PCO_2 is greater than 80 mmHg, the level of consciousness is usually depressed, known as CO_2 narcosis.

Treatment

The treatment of respiratory acidosis is directed towards reversal of the causative factors while supporting and promoting ventilation. Indications for and methods of therapy are clinically determined.

Alkalaemia

Alkalaemia is defined as a decrease in $[H^+]$ in the blood. Extreme alkalaemia may cause altered mental status, tetany and seizures. These are predominantly related to a reduction in the concentration of ionized calcium, which is more commonly present in respiratory alkalosis due to anxiety, than from other causes. Alkalaemia in patients with chronic airways disease may exacerbate tissue hypoxia due to

Table 12.1.2   Causes of metabolic alkalosis

Low urine chloride variety (saline-responsive)

Gastric volume loss (vomiting, nasogastric suction, bulimia nervosa)

Diuretics

Licorice

Hypokalaemia

High urine chloride variety (not saline-responsive)

Primary and secondary hyperaldosteronism

Apparent mineralocorticoid excess

Liddle's syndrome

Conn's syndrome (aldosteronoma)

Cushing's disease

Bartter's syndrome

Gitelman's syndrome

Excess bicarbonate administration – antacids, dialysis, milk-alkali syndrome

From Murray L, Daly F, Little M, Cadogan M. Toxicology Handbook, 2nd edn. Churchill Livingstone; 2011.

leftward shift of the oxygen-dissociation curve. Like acidaemia, there are metabolic and respiratory processes by which it occurs.

Metabolic alkalosis

Metabolic alkalosis most commonly results from loss of acid from the GIT, however, renal acid losses or accumulation of bicarbonate from exogenous sources can contribute. Diagnostically and therapeutically, metabolic alkalosis can be divided into two distinct aetiological groups – chloride-responsive and chloride-unresponsive metabolic alkalosis (Table 12.1.2).

Chloride-responsive metabolic alkalosis arises from conditions that result in both chloride and volume loss. Reduction in extracellular volume leads to increased mineralocorticoid activity causing reabsorption of sodium and secretion of hydrogen. This, in turn, causes increased formation of bicarbonate which, ultimately, overwhelms the kidneys' ability further to excrete it. In alkalosis, the urine is usually alkaline with higher concentrations of bicarbonate, there is minimal chloride excreted in order to maintain electroneutrality. Hence a urinary chloride <10 mmol/L is a common finding in these conditions. The commonest causes seen in the emergency department are upper GIT losses as a result of severe and prolonged vomiting and diuretic use.

Chloride-unresponsive metabolic alkalosis is typically due to disease states that either result

in mineralocorticoid excess in the absence of hypovolaemia or chloride wasting, or congenital disorders with defects in the various ionic transport channels within the kidney. As extracellular volume is either normal or increased, urinary chloride is typically >10 mmol/L. These conditions are seen in the emergency department infrequently.

Treatment should be directed primarily towards correction of the underlying cause. In the presence of upper gastrointestinal fluid losses, intravenous fluids with high chloride content (such as 0.9% saline) should be used initially for rehydration and correction of hypokalaemia is also required.

Respiratory alkalosis

Respiratory alkalosis may be acute or chronic, of which the acute form is most commonly encountered in the emergency department.

Respiratory alkalosis may physiologically occur in the general population secondary to exercise, altitude-related hypoxia and stimulation of the medullary respiratory centre by progesterones during pregnancy. Disease states that give rise to respiratory alkalosis are more likely to be seen in the emergency department (Table 12.1.3). Treatment is again directed towards correction of the underlying cause.

Systematic acid–base interpretation

A systematic stepwise approach to acid–base interpretation is beneficial in the evaluation

Table 12.1.3   Causes of respiratory alkalosis

CNS-mediated hyperventilation	Pulmonary
Increased intracranial pressure	Congestive cardiac failure
Cerebrovascular accidents	Mechanical hyperventilation
Psychogenic	Pneumonia
	Pulmonary emboli
Hypoxia-mediated hyperventilation	**Sepsis**
Altitude	**Toxin-induced hyperventilation**
Anaemia	Nicotine
V/Q mismatch	Salicylate
Xanthines	

of disturbances as they are often multiple. What follows is an example of a conventional methodology as outlined by Whittier and Rutecki [7]:

Step 1: what is the pH (primary acid–base disturbance)?

- Acidaemia exists if pH <7.40
- Alkalaemia exists if pH >7.44.

Step 2: determine whether the primary process is respiratory, metabolic or both

- Respiratory acidosis exists if $PaCO_2$ >44 mmHg
- Respiratory alkalosis exists if $PaCO_2$ <40 mmHg
- Metabolic acidosis exists if HCO_3^- <25 mEq/L
- Metabolic alkalosis exists if HCO_3^- >25 mEq/L.

Step 3: calculate the anion gap

$$\text{Anion gap} = [Na^+] - ([Cl^-] + [HCO_3^-])$$

Causes of anion-gap acidosis (mnemonic 'CAT MUDPILES')

C Carbon monoxide, cyanide

A Alcohol, alcoholic ketoacidosis

T Toluene

M Metformin, methanol

U Uraemia

D Diabetic ketoacidosis

P Phenformin, paracetamol, propylene glycol, paraldehyde

I Iron, isoniazid (INH)

L Lactic acidosis (numerous causes)

E Ethylene glycol

S Salicylates, starvation ketoacidosis.

Causes of a low anion gap (<6)

Increased unmeasured cations	Artefactual hyperchloraemia
Hypercalcaemia	Bromism
Hypermagnesaemia	Iodism
Lithium intoxication	Hypertriglyceridaemia
Multiple myeloma and other gammopathies	Propylene glycol
Decreased unmeasured anions	
Dilution	
Hypoalbuminaemia	

Causes of non-anion-gap metabolic acidosis

Abnormal bicarbonate loss or chloride retention	Using the mnemonic 'USED CARP'
Drugs	U Ureterostomy
Acetazolamide (+ others with carbonic anhydrase activity, e.g. topiramate)	S Small bowel fistula
	E Excess chloride
	D Diarrhoea
	C Carbonic anhydrase inhibitors
Acidifying agents (e.g. ammonium chloride)	A Adrenal insufficiency
Cholestyramine	R Renal tubular acidosis
Gastrointestinal bicarbonate loss	P Pancreatic fistula
Diarrhoea	
Pancreatic fistula	
Rapid hydration with normal saline (increased chloride)	
Renal bicarbonate loss	
Renal tubular acidosis	
Ureteroenterostomy	

Causes of respiratory acidosis

Acute	Chronic
Airway obstruction	Lung diseases, e.g. COPD, pulmonary fibrosis
Aspiration	Neuromuscular disorders, e.g. muscular atrophy
Bronchospasm	Obesity
Drug-induced CNS depression	Severe kyphoscoliosis
Hypoventilation of CNS or muscular origin	
Hypoventilation of PNS origin, e.g. GBS, OP poisoning	
Pulmonary disease	

Step 4: check for the degree of compensation

- Metabolic acidaemia: For every 1 mEq/L decrease in HCO_3^-, $PaCO_2$ should decrease by 1.3 mmHg
- Metabolic alkalaemia: For every 1 mEq/L increase in HCO_3^-, $PaCO_2$ should increase by 0.6 mmHg
- Respiratory acidaemia: For every 10 mmHg increase in $PaCO_2$, HCO_3^- should increase by 1 mEq/L (acute) or 4 mEq/L (chronic)
- Respiratory alkalaemia: For every 10 mmHg decrease in $PaCO_2$, HCO_3^- should decrease by 2 mEq/L (acute) or 5 mEq/L (chronic).

Step 5: determine if there is a 1:1 relationship between the anions in the blood (presence of a delta gap)

In an anion-gap metabolic acidosis, this step determines whether there is a non-anion-gap (hyperchloraemic) component as a contributing explanantion of the bicarbonate fall. There should be a 1:1 relationship between the rise in the anion gap over normal and the decrease in the bicarbonate. If the bicarbonate is higher than predicted then a metabolic alkosis is also present. If the bicarbonate is lower than predicted then a non-anion-gap acidosis is also present.

Controversies

- Whether the Stewart approach is advantageous in teaching and characterizing acid–base abnormalities compared to traditional approaches.

References

[1] Natalini G, Seramondi V, Fassini P, et al. Acute respiratory acidosis does not increase plasma potassium in normokalaemic anaesthetized patients. A controlled randomized trial. Eur J Anaesth 2001;18:394–400.

[2] Herr RD, Swanson T. Pseudometabolic acidosis caused by underfill of vacutainer tubes. Ann Emerg Med 1992;21:177–80.

[3] Paulson WD, Roberts WL, Lurie AA, et al. Wide variation in serum anion gap measurements by chemistry analyzers. Am J Clin Pathol 1998;110:735–42.

[4] Cooper DJ. Bicarbonate does not improve haemodynamics in critically ill patients who have lactic acidosis: a prospective controlled clinical study. Ann Intern Med 1990;112:492–8.

[5] Mathieu D, Neviere R, Billard V, et al. Effects of bicarbonate therapy on hemodynamics and tissue oxygenation in patients with lactic acidosis: a prospective, controlled clinical study. Crit Care Med 1991;19:1352–6.

[6] Okuda Y, Adrogue HJ, Field JB, et al. Counterproductive effects of sodium bicarbonate in diabetic ketoacidosis. J Clin Endocrinol Metab 1996;81:314–20.

[7] Whittier WL, Rutecki GW. Primer on clinical acid-base problem solving. Dis Monitor 2004;50:117–62.

12.2 Electrolyte disturbances

John Pasco

ESSENTIALS

1 Sodium disorders are relatively common in hospitalized patients and elderly people.

2 The brain is most at risk from acute hyponatraemia because the osmotically expanded intracellular volume may induce increased intracranial pressure (hyponatraemic encephalopathy).

3 Treatment of hyponatraemia needs to be carefully individualized because of the risk of osmotic myelinolysis.

4 Hypernatraemia has a high in-hospital mortality rate, which often reflects severe associated medical conditions.

5 Although usually benign, hypokalaemia may cause cardiac arrhythmias and rhabdomyolysis. Oral replacement is usually sufficient, except where there is severe myopathy or cardiac arrhythmias.

6 Electrocardiogram changes in the presence of hyperkalaemia require urgent potassium-lowering measures and myocardial protection with calcium.

7 Management of severe hypercalcaemia includes enhancement of renal excretion of calcium, inhibition of osteoclast activity and treatment of the underlying condition.

8 Acute symptomatic hypocalcaemia should be treated with IV calcium.

9 Hypomagnesaemia is difficult to diagnose because its symptoms are non-specific and the serum level often does not reflect the true magnesium status of the patient. It usually exists as a 'deficiency triad' with hypokalaemia and hypocalcaemia.

10 Hypermagnesaemia is often iatrogenic, particularly in elderly patients or patients with renal impairment and/or chronic bowel conditions receiving magnesium therapy.

HYPONATRAEMIA

Introduction

Hyponatraemia, defined as serum sodium concentration of less than 130 mmol/L, is a common condition. The prevalence is estimated at 2.5% in hospitalized patients, of which two-thirds develop the condition while in hospital.

Pathophysiology

Hyponatraemia is almost always associated with extracellular hypotonicity, with an excess of total body water relative to sodium (hypotonic hyponatraemia). The exceptions are:

- Normotonic hyponatraemia (pseudohyponatraemia): an artefactually low sodium measurement seen in hyperlipidaemia and hyperproteinaemia. It is rarely seen now because of the routine use of direction-selective electrodes to measure sodium.
- Hypertonic hyponatraemia: a dilutional lowering of the measured serum sodium concentration in the presence of osmotically active substances, most commonly glucose, but also mannitol, glycerol and sorbitol. In the presence of hyperglycaemia, the true serum sodium can be estimated by adjusting the measured serum sodium upwards by 1 mmol/L for each 3 mmol/L rise in glucose above normal.

Hyponatraemia causes cellular swelling as water moves down an osmotic gradient into the intracellular fluid. Most of the symptomatology of hyponatraemia is produced in the central nervous system (CNS) by the swelling of brain cells within the rigid calvarium, causing raised intracranial pressure (hyponatraemic encephalopathy). As intracranial pressure rises, adaptive responses come into play, returning brain volume towards normal and restoring cellular function.

For this reason, chronic hyponatraemia is generally better tolerated than acute hyponatraemia. Patients can become encephalopathic when hyponatraemia develops rapidly and the adaptive responses have not had time to develop (for example, following rapid ingestion of very large amounts of water, such as in psychogenic polydipsia or post-exercise) or when the adaptive responses fail. Hyponatraemic encepaholopathy carries a high mortality (50%) if left untreated.

Aetiology and classification

Hypotonic hyponatraemia may be classified according to the volume status of the patient (hypovolaemic, euvolaemic or hypervolaemic).

Hypovolaemic hyponatraemia

These patients have deficits in both total body sodium and total body water, but the sodium deficit exceeds the water deficit. Causes include renal and extrarenal fluid losses and are listed in Table 12.2.1. Determination of the urinary sodium concentration can differentiate these two groups. Extrarenal losses

Table 12.2.1 Causes of hypovolaemic hyponatraemia
Renal losses (urinary [Na] 20 mmol/L)
Diuretics
Mineralocorticoid deficiency – Addison's disease
Salt-losing nephropathy
Ketonuria
Osmotic diuresis – glucose, mannitol, urea
Bicarbonaturia with metabolic alkalosis
Extrarenal losses (urinary [Na] <20 mmol/L)
Vomiting – self-induced, gastroenteritis, pyloric obstruction
Diarrhoea
Excessive sweating
Blood loss
Third-space fluid loss – burns, pancreatitis, trauma

are associated with low urinary sodium concentrations (<20 mmol/L) and hyperosmolar urine. The exception is with severe vomiting and metabolic alkalosis, where bicarbonaturia obligates renal sodium loss and urinary sodium is high (>20 mmol/L), despite volume depletion. However, urinary chloride, a better indicator of extracellular fluid (ECF) volume, is low.

Euvolaemic hyponatraemia

Total body water is increased with only minimal change in total body sodium. Volume expansion is mild and usually not clinically detectable. Causes are listed in Table 12.2.2.

Hypervolaemic hyponatraemia

Total body water is increased in excess of total body sodium. Causes include congestive cardiac failure, hepatic cirrhosis with ascites, nephrotic syndrome and chronic renal failure.

Clinical features

In addition to the features of the underlying medical condition and alteration in extracellular volume, clinical manifestations of hyponatraemia *per se* usually develop when serum sodium is less than 130 mmol/L. The severity of symptoms depends partly on the absolute serum sodium concentration and partly on its rate of fall. At sodium concentrations from 125 to 130 mmol/L, the symptoms are principally gastrointestinal whereas, at concentrations below 125 mmol/L, the symptoms are predominantly neuropsychiatric. The principal signs and symptoms of hyponatraemia are listed in Table 12.2.3.

Population groups particularly prone to hyponatraemic encephalopathy have been identified (Table 12.2.4).

Premenopausal women appear at risk of developing hyponatraemic encephalopathy because oestrogen and progesterone are thought to inhibit the brain Na-K-ATPase and increase circulating levels of antidiuretic hormone (ADH).

Psychogenic polydipsia refers to a condition in which kidney function is normal and dilute urine is produced, but free water intake overwhelms the kidney's capabilities and the serum sodium falls. It occurs primarily in patients with schizophrenia or bipolar disorder. These patients develop hyponatraemia with a far lower fluid intake than is usually necessary (over 20 L of water/day in a 60 kg man, in the absence of elevated levels of ADH) and it may arise through a combination of factors: antipsychotics, increased thirst perception, enhanced renal response to ADH and a mild defect in osmoregulation.

Exercise-associated hyponatraemia occurs in endurance athletes and mainly relates to the consumption of excessive fluid, although non-osmotic release of vasopressin and other mechanisms may be implicated.

Hyponatraemia in AIDS is common and associated with a high mortality. It may be secondary to syndrome of inappropriate ADH (SIADH), adrenal insufficiency or volume deficiency with hypotonic fluid replacement.

The use of 'Ecstasy' at 'rave' parties has been associated with acute hyponatraemia. This may be due to a combination of drug effect and drinking large quantities of water in an attempt to prevent dehydration.

Mild chronic 'asymptomatic' hyponatraemia in the elderly contributes to an increased rate of falls, probably due to impairment of attention, posture and gait mechanisms.

Syndrome of inappropriate ADH secretion

This is a diagnosis of exclusion and is characterized by inappropriately concentrated urine in the setting of hypotonicity. It accounts for approximately 50% of all cases of hyponatraemia. These patients have elevated serum ADH levels without an obvious volume or osmotic stimulus. The diagnostic criteria for SIADH secretion are shown in Table 12.2.5 and

Table 12.2.2   Causes of euvolaemic hyponatraemia
Psychogenic polydipsia

Iatrogenic water intoxication
   Absorption of hypotonic irrigation fluids during TURP
   Inappropriate intravenous fluid administration

Postoperative hyponatraemia (elevated ADH levels)

Non-osmotic ADH secretion
   Glucocorticoid deficiency
   Severe hypothyroidism
   Thiazide diuretics

Drugs (ADH analogues, potentiation of ADH release, unknown mechanisms)
   Psychoactive agents: phenothiazines, SSRIs, TCAs, MAOIs, 'ecstasy'
   Oxytocin
   Anticancer agents: cyclophosphamine, vincristine, vinblastine
   NSAIDs
   Carbamazepine
   Chlorpropamide

SIADH
TURP: transurethral resection of prostate; ADH: antidiuretic hormone; SSRI: selective serotonin reuptake inhibitor; TCA: tricyclic antidepressant; MAOI: monoamic oxidase inhibitor; SIAOH: syndrome of inappropriate antidiuretic hormone secretion.

Table 12.2.3   Clinical manifestations of hyponatraemia
Anorexia
Nausea
Vomiting
Lethargy
Muscle cramps
Muscle weakness
Headache
Confusion/agitation
Altered conscious state
Seizures
Coma

Table 12.2.4   Patient groups at risk of hyponatraemia
Postoperative
Menstruating females
Elderly women on thiazide diuretics
Prepubescent children
Psychiatric polydipsic patients
Hypoxaemic patients
AIDS patients
Patients taking 'Ecstasy' (MDMA)
Endurance athletes

Table 12.2.5   Diagnostic criteria for SIADH
Hypotonic hyponatraemia
Urine osmolality >100 mmol/kg (i.e. inappropriately concentrated)
Urine sodium >20 mmol/mL while on a normal salt and water intake
Absence of extracellular volume depletion
Normal thyroid and adrenal function
Normal cardiac, hepatic and renal function
No diuretic use

Table 12.2.6 Conditions associated with SIADH

Neoplasms (ectopic ADH production)
  Bronchogenic carcinoma
  Pancreatic carcinoma
  Lymphoma
  Mesothelioma
  Thymoma
  Carcinoma of the bladder

Pulmonary disease
  Pneumonia
  Tuberculosis
  Aspergillosis
  Cystic fibrosis
  Chronic obstructive airways disease
  Positive-pressure ventilation

CNS disease
  Encephalitis
  Acute psychosis
  Head trauma
  Brain abscess
  Meningitis
  Hydrocephalus
  Brain tumour
  Delirium tremens
  Guillain–Barré syndrome
  Stroke
  Subdural or subarachnoid bleed

HIV infection   *Pneumocystis carinii* pneumonia

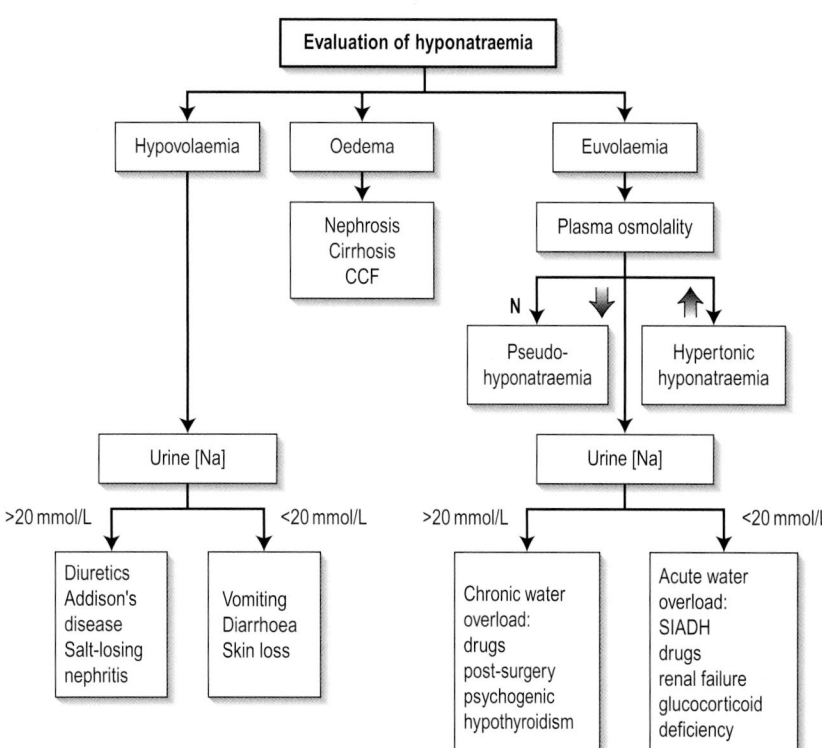

Fig. 12.2.1 Assessment of hyponatraemia. *(Adapted from Walmsley R, Cuerin M. Disorders of fluid and electrolyte balance. Bristol: John Wright & Sons; 1984 with permission.)*

conditions associated with the syndrome are listed in Table 12.2.6.

Clinical investigations

Measurement of serum and urine sodium concentrations and osmolalities, in addition to clinical assessment of volume status, are essential for the assessment of hyponatraemia (Fig. 12.2.1).

Treatment

There is ongoing controversy over the treatment of hyponatraemia because of the risk of osmotic demyelination, which is discussed below.

Treatment should be carefully individualized and depends on the presence of symptoms, the duration of the hyponatraemia and the absolute value of sodium. Ideally, correction of the serum sodium should be of a sufficient pace and magnitude to reverse the manifestations of hypotonicity but not be so rapid and large as to pose a risk of the development of osmotic demyelination. Treatment of the underlying cause is obviously essential and may correct the hyponatraemia. For hypovolaemic hyponatraemia, adequate volume replacement is essential.

Acute symptomatic hyponatraemia (hyponatraemic encephalopathy)

Symptomatic hyponatraemia developing within 48 h is a medical emergency requiring prompt and aggressive treatment. The risks of developing osmotic demyelination are clearly outweighed by those of the encephalopathy. An immediate increase in serum sodium concentration by 8 mEq/L over 4–6 h is recommended. This can be achieved by infusing hypertonic saline (3% NaCl) at a rate of 1–2 mL/kg/h, which should raise the serum sodium by 1–2 mmol/L/h. Where neurological symptoms are severe, hypertonic saline can be infused at 4–6 mL/kg/h. Indications for ceasing rapid correction of hyponatraemia are cessation of life-threatening manifestations, moderation of other symptoms or the achievement of a serum sodium of 125–130 mEq/L. Other measures to reduce intracranial pressure, such as intubation and intermittent positive pressure ventilation (IPPV), may also be required.

Chronic symptomatic hyponatraemia

Hyponatraemia present for more than 48 h, or where the duration is unknown, presents the greatest dilemma. Care must be taken with correction of sodium as these patients are at the greatest risk of developing osmotic demyelination, yet the presence of encephalopathy mandates urgent treatment. Hypertonic saline can be infused so that a correction rate of no more than 1–1.5 mmol/L/h is maintained. Therapy with hypertonic saline should be discontinued when (1) the patient becomes asymptomatic, (2) the serum sodium has risen by 20 mmol/L or (3) the serum sodium reaches 120–125 mmol/L. Thereafter, slower correction with water restriction should follow. The serum sodium should never be acutely elevated to hypernatraemic or normonatraemic levels and should not be elevated by more than 25 mmol/L during the first 48 h of therapy.

Chronic asymptomatic hyponatraemia

In this situation, saline infusion is usually not required and patients can be managed by treating the underlying disorder, discontinuing diuretic therapy or restricting fluids. Fluid restriction is inexpensive and effective but is often limited by patient non-compliance. Other treatment options include pharmacological inhibition of ADH with demeclocycline, which is limited by its neuro- and nephrotoxic side effects, or increasing solute with the use of furosemide or urea.

Osmotic myelinolysis

This is an iatrogenic disorder which develops progressively over 3–5 days following the correction of hyponatraemia. It classically produces symmetrical lesions centred on the midline of the pons and was originally described as 'central pontine myelinolysis'. However, about 10% of cases involve extrapontine lesions. It is reported as occurring in 25% of severely hyponatraemic patients following correction of serum sodium. Clinically, the disorder is initially manifested by dysarthria, mutism, lethargy and affective changes, which may be mistaken for psychiatric illness. Classically, pseudobulbar palsy and spastic quadriparesis are observed. Recovery is usually gradual and incomplete, although both fatalities and complete recovery are reported. Demyelination in the central pons and extrapontine sites can be demonstrated on magnetic resonance imaging (MRI) scan or at autopsy.

It appears that the risk of developing osmotic myelinolysis is associated with severity and chronicity of hyponatraemia. It rarely occurs if the serum sodium is >120 mmol/L or where hyponatraemia has been present for <48 h. Alcoholics, malnourished patients, hypokalaemic patients, burn victims and elderly patients on thiazides seem to be most at risk of developing osmotic demyelination

Both the rate and the magnitude of sodium correction appear important in the development of osmotic myelinolysis. Although there is as yet no agreed rate of correction that is regarded as completely safe, most authorities suggest that the serum sodium concentration should not rise by more than 10–14 mmol/L during any 24-h period.

HYPERNATRAEMIA

Introduction

Hypernatraemia is much less common than hyponatraemia and may be defined as a serum sodium concentration greater than 150 mmol/L.

It is important to recognize hypernatraemia because it is usually associated with severe underlying medical illness. It is a condition of hospitalized patients, elderly and dependent people. The incidence of hypernatraemia in hospitalized patients ranges from 0.3 to 1%, with from 60 to 80% of these developing hypernatraemia after admission. In-hospital mortality is high (40–55%) and may be due to a combination of hypernatraemia and the severity of the underlying disease.

Pathophysiology

Hypernatraemia is a relative deficiency of total body water compared to total body sodium, thus rendering the body fluids hypertonic. The normal compensatory response includes stimulated thirst – the most important response – and renal water conservation through ADH secretion. In the absence of ADH, water intake can match urinary losses because of increased thirst, but where the thirst mechanism is absent or defective, patients become hypernatraemic even in the presence of maximal ADH stimulation. Therefore, hypernatraemia is usually seen where water intake is inadequate, i.e. in patients too young, too old or too sick to drink, with no access to water or with a defective thirst mechanism.

Extracellular hypertonicity causes a shift of water from the intracellular space until there is osmotic equilibrium. The resultant cellular contraction may explain some of the clinical features of hypernatraemia. The brain is especially at risk from shrinkage because of its vascular attachments to the calvarium. Haemorrhage may occur if these vascular attachments tear.

As with hyponatraemia, the rate and magnitude of the rise in sodium determine the severity of the symptoms, which is a reflection of the brain's capacity to adapt to the deranged osmotic conditions.

Aetiology and classification

The clinical causes of hypernatraemia are listed in Table 12.2.7. Population groups at particular risk of developing hypernatraemia are listed in Table 12.2.8.

Hypernatraemia is classified into these categories based on extracellular volume status: hypovolaemic, hypervolaemic and euvolaemic.

Hypovolaemic hypernatraemia

This occurs where there is loss of both total body water and sodium, but with a greater loss of water. Renal causes include osmotic diuresis and diuretic excess. Urinary sodium is usually >20 mmol/L. Extrarenal losses include profuse diarrhoea, sweating, burns and fistulae. Urinary sodium is usually <20 mmol/L.

Euvolaemic hypernatraemia

This is the most common form of hypernatraemia. Patients have pure water losses, with intracellular dehydration as water shifts according to the osmotic gradient. Hypernatraemia in these patients occurs only when there is no accompanying water intake, i.e. restricted access to water or a defect in thirst sensation.

Extrarenal losses are usually seen in skin losses in burns patients and via the respiratory system in respiratory infections and at high altitude. Renal water loss is usually due to diabetes insipidus – a failure of ADH production

Table 12.2.7 Causes of hypernatraemia
Altered perception of thirst
Osmoreceptor damage/destruction
Exogenous: trauma
Endogenous: vasculitis, carcinoma, granuloma
Idiopathic: psychogenic, head injury
Drugs
Normal perception of thirst
Poor intake
Confusion
Coma
Depression
Dysphagia
Odynophagia
Increased water loss and decreased intake
Diuresis
Renal loss
Diabetes insipidus
Chronic renal failure
Diuretic excess
GIT loss: fistulae, diarrhoea
Exogenous increase in salt intake

Table 12.2.8 Groups at particular risk for hypernatraemia
Elderly or disabled, unable to obtain oral fluids independently
Infants
Inpatients receiving:
hypertonic infusions
tube feedings
osmotic diuretics
lactulose
mechanical ventilation
Altered mental status
Uncontrolled diabetes mellitus
Underlying polyuric disorders

or secretion (central diabetes insipidus) or a failure of the collecting duct of the kidney to respond to ADH (nephrogenic diabetes insipidus).

Hypervolaemic hypernatraemia

This is not very common. These patients are typically extracellular volume expanded but intracellular volume depleted. It is seen following resuscitation with sodium bicarbonate, with the use of hypertonic saline solutions, with excess salt intake, in primary hyperaldosteronism and in Cushing's syndrome.

Clinical features

In addition to the features of the underlying medical condition and alteration in extracellular volume, the clinical features of hypernatraemia *per se* are primarily CNS. Early symptoms are anorexia, nausea and vomiting; lethargy, hyperreflexia, confusion, seizures and coma occur later.

Treatment

The speed at which hypernatraemia is corrected should take into account the rate of development and severity of symptoms. Too rapid correction, especially in chronic hypernatraemia, can cause cerebral oedema or isotonic water intoxication. The rate of correction of chronic hypernatraemia should not exceed 0.5–0.7 mmol/L/h.

Treatment is based on clinical assessment of the patient's volume status.

Hypovolaemic hypernatraemia

These patients require restoration of the volume deficit with isotonic saline, colloid or blood in the first instance, to prevent peripheral vascular collapse and treatment of the underlying cause. Following this, the water deficit is corrected with 0.45% saline, 5% dextrose or oral water.

The water deficit is calculated as follows:

$$\text{Water deficit} = \text{total body water} \times (1 - \text{Na2} / \text{Na1})$$

where Na2 = desired sodium, Na1 = actual sodium and total body water is usually 60% of the body weight. The calculated normal daily maintenance fluids should be added to the above volumes.

Euvolaemic hypernatraemia

Calculate the water deficit as above and replace the deficit and ongoing losses with 5% dextrose, 0.45% saline or oral water. To avoid cerebral oedema, particularly in chronic hypernatraemia, 50% of the water deficit should be replaced over the first 6–12 h and the rest given slowly over 1–2 days. Serum sodium estimations should be repeated at regular intervals.

Hypervolaemic hypernatraemia

Removal of sodium is required with the use of diuretics, such as furosemide, and discontinuation of causative agents. Furosemide causes excretion of more water than sodium, so a hypotonic fluid, such as 5% dextrose, may need to be infused. In severe cases or in renal failure, dialysis may be required.

HYPOKALAEMIA

Introduction

Hypokalaemia may be defined as a serum potassium concentration of less than 3.5 mmol/L. It is usually considered to be severe when this is less than 2.4 mmol/L.

Pathophysiology

Hypokalaemia may develop as a consequence of potassium depletion or a shift of potassium into cells. In either case, there is an increase in the ratio of intracellular to extracellular potassium concentrations. This, in turn, produces hyperpolarization across excitable membranes and is responsible for the effects of hypokalaemia on striated muscle and the cardiac conducting system.

Aetiology

The causes of hypokalaemia are listed in Table 12.2.9.

Clinical presentation

Hypokalaemia commonly produces no symptoms in otherwise healthy subjects.

Clinical features may include weakness, constipation, ileus and ventilatory failure. Myopathy may develop, with weakness of

Table 12.2.9   Causes of hypokalaemia
Inadequate dietary intake
Abnormal losses
Gastrointestinal
Vomiting, nasogastric aspiration
Diarrhoea, fistula loss
Villous adenoma of the colon
Laxative abuse
Renal
Mineralocorticoid excess
Conn's syndrome
Bartter syndrome
Ectopic ACTH syndrome
Small cell carcinoma of the lung
Pancreatic carcinoma
Carcinoma of the thymus
Renal tubular acidosis
Magnesium deficiency
Drugs
Diuretics
Corticosteroids
Gentamicin, amphotericin B
Cisplatin
Compartmental shift
Alkalosis Insulin
Na-K-ATPase stimulation
Sympathomimetic agents with β_2 effect
Methylxanthines
Barium poisoning
Hypothermia
Toluene intoxication
Hypokalaemic periodic paralysis

the extremities which characteristically worsens with exercise. If the hypokalaemia is severe and untreated, rhabdomyolysis may occur. Polyuria and polydipsia may result from the effect of hypokalaemia on the distal renal tubule (nephrogenic diabetes insipidus of hypokalaemia). Cardiac effects include ventricular tachycardias and atrial tachycardias, with or without block. Characteristic electrocardiogram (ECG) changes include PR prolongation, T-wave flattening and inversion and prominent U waves

Treatment

Oral replacement is safe for asymptomatic patients and 40–60 mmol of potassium every 1–4 h is usually well tolerated.

Intravenous administration of potassium is recommended when hypokalaemia is associated with cardiac arrhythmias, familial periodic paralysis or severe myopathy. Usual infusion rates are 10–20 mmol/h. Rates greater than 40 mmol/h are not recommended. Potassium is a sclerosant and should, therefore, be given via a large peripheral or central vein. Serum potassium estimations every 1–4 h and continuous cardiac monitoring are mandatory.

HYPERKALAEMIA

Introduction

Hyperkalaemia, defined as a serum potassium concentration greater than 5.5 mmol/L, is less common than hypokalaemia. Moderate (6.1–6.9 mmol/L) and severe (>7 mmol/L) hyperkalaemia can have grave consequences, particularly if acute.

Pathophysiology

Two homeostatic mechanisms are responsible for maintaining potassium balance. The renal system maintains external potassium balance by excreting 90–95% of the average daily potassium load (100 mmol/day); the gut excretes the remainder. This is a relatively slow process: only half the administered load of potassium will have been excreted in the urine after 3–6 h. The extrarenal system involves hormonal and acid–base mechanisms that rapidly translocate potassium intracellularly. This system is critical in the management of acute hyperkalaemia.

Aetiology

The causes of hyperkalaemia are listed in Table 12.2.10.

Table 12.2.10   Causes of hyperkalaemia

Pseudohyperkalaemia
   Delay in separating red cells
   Specimen haemolysis during or after
     venesection
   Severe leucocytosis/thrombocytosis
Excessive intake
   Exogenous: IV or oral KCl, massive blood
     transfusion
   Endogenous: tissue damage
   Burns
   Trauma
   Rhabdomyolysis
   Tumour lysis
Decrease in renal excretion
   Drugs
     Spironolactone, triamterene, amiloride
     Indomethacin
     Captopril, enalapril
   Renal failure
   Addison's disease
   Hyporeninaemic hypoaldosteronism
Compartmental shift
   Acidosis
   Insulin deficiency
   Digoxin overdose
   Succinylcholine
   Fluoride poisoning
   Hyperkalaemic periodic paralysis

Clinical features

The clinical features of hyperkalaemia are often non-specific. Diagnosis depends on clinical suspicion, measurement of potassium concentration in the plasma and the characteristic changes on the ECG.

Generalized muscle weakness, flaccid paralysis and paraesthesia of the hands and feet are common, but there is poor correlation between the degree of muscle weakness and serum potassium concentration.

The ECG changes (Table 12.2.11) are characteristic, but are an insensitive method of evaluating hyperkalaemia.

Serum biochemistry in almost all patients with hyperkalaemia shows some degree of renal impairment and metabolic acidosis. In dialysis patients, hyperkalaemia may develop without concomitant metabolic acidosis.

Treatment

Pseudohyperkalaemia is common and, if hyperkalaemia is an unexpected finding, the serum potassium should be remeasured.

Hyperkalaemia with ECG changes requires urgent management. The priorities are as follows:

❶ Antagonize potassium cardiac toxicity:
  - IV calcium chloride 10%, 5–10 mL or
  - IV calcium gluconate 10%, 15–30 mL. The effects of calcium should be evident within minutes and last for 30–60 min. A calcium infusion may be required. Calcium antagonizes the myocardial membrane excitability induced by hyperkalaemia. It does not lower serum potassium levels

❷ Shift potassium into cells:
  - IV soluble insulin, 20 U with dextrose 50 g or
  - salbutamol nebulized (10–20 mg) or IV (0.5 mg diluted in 100 mL over 10–15 min) or
  - IV sodium bicarbonate, 50–200 mmol

❸ Enhance potassium excretion:
  - oral and/or rectal resonium A 50 g. This is a cation exchange resin; as the resin passes through the gastrointestinal tract, Na and K are exchanged and the cationically modified resin is then excreted in the faeces
  - furosemide diuresis
  - haemodialysis. This is usually reserved for cases of acute renal failure or end-stage renal disease. It is the most effective treatment for acutely lowering serum potassium, but there is usually a time delay in instituting dialysis and the temporizing measures outlined above must be employed in the interim.

The use of insulin and glucose is well supported in the literature. A response is usually seen within 20–30 min, with lowering of plasma potassium by up to 1 mmol/L and reversal of ECG changes. Transient hypoglycaemia may be observed within 15 min of insulin administration. In some patients, particularly those with end-stage renal failure, late hypoglycaemia may develop. For this reason, a 10% dextrose infusion at 50 L/h is recommended and the blood glucose should be monitored closely. The exact mechanism by which insulin translocates potassium is not known; it is thought to be stimulation of Na-K-ATPase independent of cAMP.

β_2-Agonists significantly lower plasma potassium when given intravenously or via a nebulizer. Potassium levels are reduced by up to 1.00 mmol/L within 30 min following 10–20 mg of nebulized salbutamol. The effect is sustained for up to 2 h. Adverse effects of salbutamol administration include tachyarrhythmias and precipitation of angina in patients with coronary artery disease. Patients on non-selective β-blockers may not respond. Some patients with end-stage renal disease are also resistant to this therapy. The reason for this is unknown. Greater decreases in potassium have been observed when

Table 12.2.11   ECG changes of hyperkalaemia

Plasma potassium (mmol/L)	ECG characteristics
6–7	Tall peaked T waves (>5 mm)
7–8	QRS widening, small-amplitude P waves
8–9	Fusion of QRS complex with T wave producing sine wave
>9	AV dissociation, ventricular tachycardia, ventricular fibrillation

salbutamol treatment is combined with insulin and glucose. The additive effect is thought to be due to stimulation of Na-K-ATPase via different pathways. Transient hyperglycaemia may occur with combined therapy, but delayed hypoglycaemia does not occur.

HYPOCALCAEMIA

Introduction

A reduction in serum calcium concentration manifests principally as abnormal neuromuscular function.

Pathophysiology

Calcium is involved in smooth and skeletal muscle contraction and relaxation, platelet aggregation, neurotransmission, hepatic and adipose glycogenolysis, thermogenesis and neutrophil function. In addition, most endocrine and exocrine gland function is calcium dependent.

Aetiology

Hypocalcaemia occurs when calcium is lost from the extracellular fluid at a rate greater than can be replaced by the intestine or bone. The major cause of severe hypocalcaemia is hypoparathyroidism, as a result of surgery for thyroid disease, autoimmune destruction or from developmental abnormalities of the parathyroid glands. Other causes are listed in Table 12.2.12.

Table 12.2.12 Causes of hypocalcaemia
Factitious EDTA contamination
Hypoalbuminaemia

Decreased PTH activity
  Hypoparathyroidism
  Pseudohypoparathyroidism
  Hypomagnesaemia

Decreased vitamin D activity
Acute pancreatitis

Hyperphosphataemia
  Renal failure
  Phosphate supplements

'Hungry bone' syndrome

Drugs
  Mithramycin
  Diuretics: furosemide, ethacrynic acid

Clinical features

Patients with acute hypocalcaemia are more likely to be symptomatic than those with chronic hypocalcaemia. Symptomatic hypocalcaemia is characterized by abnormal neuromuscular excitability and neurological sensations. Early signs are perioral numbness and paraesthesia of distal extremities. Hyperreflexia, muscle cramps and carpopedal spasm follow. Chvostek's sign (ipsilateral contraction of the facial muscles elicited by tapping the facial nerve just anterior to the ear) and Trousseau's sign (carpopedal spasm with inflation of a blood pressure cuff for 3–5 min) are signs of neuromuscular irritability. If muscle contractions become uncontrollable, tetany results and this can prove fatal if laryngospasm occurs. Seizures may occur when there is CNS instability. Cardiovascular manifestations include hypotension, bradycardia, impaired cardiac contractility and arrhythmias. ECG evidence of hypocalcaemia includes prolonged QT interval and possibly ST prolongation and T-wave abnormalities.

Treatment

Acute symptomatic hypocalcaemia

In the emergency situation where seizures, tetany, life-threatening hypotension or arrhythmias are present, IV calcium is the treatment of choice. Infusion of 15 mg/kg of elemental calcium over 4–6 h increases the total serum calcium by 0.5–0.75 mmol/L.

Administration of 10–20 mL of 10% calcium gluconate (89 mg elemental calcium per 10 mL) IV over 5–10 min is recommended. This should be followed by a continuous infusion because the effects of a single IV dose last only about 2 h. The infusion rate should be adjusted according to serial calcium measurements obtained every 2–4 h. Over-rapid infusion may cause facial flushing, headache and arrhythmias.

Calcium chloride 10% may also be used. This contains more calcium per ampoule (272 mg in 10 mL), resulting in a more rapid rise in serum calcium, but is more irritant to veins and can cause thrombophlebitis with extravasation.

Where hypcalcaemia and metabolic acidosis are present (usually in sepsis or renal failure), correction of the acidosis with bicarbonate may result in a rapid fall in ionized calcium as the

number of calcium-binding sites is increased. Therefore, hypocalcaemia must be corrected before the acidosis. Bicarbonate or phosphate should not be infused with calcium because of possible precipitation of calcium salts.

Cardiac monitoring is recommended during rapid calcium administration, especially if the patient is taking digoxin, when calcium administration may precipitate digitalis toxicity.

If coexisting magnesium deficiency is suspected, or when symptoms do not improve after calcium administration, $MgSO_4$ 1–5 mmol IV over 15 min may be given.

Chronic asymptomatic hypocalcaemia

These patients are usually managed with oral calcium supplements taken between meals. Calcitriol, the active hormonal form of vitamin D, 0.5–1.5 mg daily, can also be given.

HYPERCALCAEMIA

Introduction

The normal total serum calcium concentration is 2.15–2.55 mmol/L. Hypercalcaemia is a relatively common condition with a frequency estimated at 1:1000–1:10 000. Although there are many causes, the most frequent are malignancy and hyperparathyroidism, with the former the most likely to cause hypercalcaemia requiring urgent attention.

Pathophysiology

Total serum calcium is made up of protein-bound calcium (40%, mostly albumin and not filterable by the kidneys), ion-bound complexes (13%, bound to anions such as bicarbonate, lactate, citrate and phosphate) and the unbound, ionized fraction (47%). The ionized fraction is the biologically active component of calcium and is closely regulated by parathyroid hormone (PTH). Total serum calcium is affected by albumin and does not necessarily reflect the level of plasma ionized calcium. Normal ionized calcium levels are 1.14–1.30 mmol/L. Protein binding, in turn, is influenced by extracellular fluid pH and alterations in serum albumin. Acidaemia decreases protein binding and increases the level of ionized calcium. To correct for pH: ionized calcium rises 0.05 mmol/L for each 0.1 decrease in pH.

To correct for serum albumin:

$$\text{Corrected } [Ca^+] = \text{measured } [Ca^+] + (40 - \text{albumin g/L}) \times 0.02 \text{ mmol/L}$$

Corrected calcium is used for all treatment decisions except where direct measurement of ionized calcium using an ion-specific electrode is available.

Three pathophysiological mechanisms may produce hypercalcaemia:

- Accelerated osteoclastic bone resorption. This is the most common cause of severe hypercalcaemia. Osteoclasts are activated by PTH and various humoral tumour products, the most common being parathyroid hormone-related protein (PTHRP).
- Increased gastrointestinal absorption (rarely important).
- Decreased renal excretion of calcium. PTH and PTHRP stimulate renal tubular reabsorption of calcium. Hypercalcaemia *per se* causes polyuria by interfering with renal mechanisms for reabsorption of water and sodium. If there is inadequate fluid intake to compensate, extracellular volume depletion occurs, reducing glomerular filtration and exacerbating the hypercalcaemia.

Aetiology

The majority of cases of hypercalcaemia requiring urgent treatment are due to malignancy or, less commonly, primary hyperparathyroidism (parathyroid crisis). Malignant hypercalcaemia is most commonly seen with the solid tumours: lung and breast cancer, squamous cell carcinoma of the head and neck and cholangiocarcinoma and the haematological malignancies, multiple myeloma and lymphoma. Other causes of hypercalcaemia are uncommon (Table 12.2.13).

Clinical features

Hypercalcaemia causes disturbances of the gastrointestinal, cardiovascular, renal and central nervous systems.

Gastrointestinal manifestations include anorexia, nausea, vomiting and constipation. Cardiovascular manifestations include hypertension and a shortened QT interval on the ECG. Renal manifestations include polyuria,

Table 12.2.13   Causes of hypercalcaemia

Factitious
  Haemoconcentration
  Postprandial

Malignancy
Primary hyperparathyroidism

Drugs
  Thiazides
  Vitamin D
  Lithium
  Vitamin A

Hormonal
  Thyrotoxicosis
  Acromegaly
  Hypoadrenalism
  Phaeochromocytoma

Granulomas
  Tuberculosis
  Sarcoidosis

Renal failure
Milk alkali syndrome
Immobilization

polydipsia and nephrocalcinosis (rare). CNS symptoms include psychotic behaviour, seizures, apathy, cognitive difficulties, obtundation and coma. Renal elimination of digoxin is also impaired.

Moderately elevated total serum calcium (3.00–3.50 mmol/L) is usually associated with symptoms. Markedly elevated total serum calcium (>3.5 mmol/L) mandates urgent treatment regardless of symptoms.

Treatment

Irrespective of the cause, the management of hypercalcaemic crisis is the same. There are three primary treatment goals:

❶ hydration of the patient ± enhancement of renal excretion of calcium
❷ inhibition of accelerated bone resorption
❸ treatment of the underlying problem.

Hydration and diuresis

Hydration expands intravascular volume, dilutes calcium and increases calcium clearance. Infusion rates of 200–300 mL/h of 0.9% saline, depending on the degree of hypovolaemia and the ability of the patient to tolerate fluid, may be required and, once adequate rehydration has been achieved, the infusion rate can be adjusted to maintain a urine output of 100–150 mL/h.

This treatment, although effective, results in a relatively modest reduction in serum calcium and patients with severe hypercalcaemia usually require additional treatment with bisphosphonates.

The use of frusemide to enhance the excretion of calcium once the patient is adequately hydrated has fallen out of favour and should only be used to treate fluid overload.

Enhancement of renal excretion

Haemodialysis is the treatment of choice to decrease rapidly serum calcium in patients with heart failure or renal insufficiency

Inhibition of bone resorption

Pharmacological inhibition of osteoclastic bone resorption is the most effective treatment for hypercalcaemia, particularly hypercalcaemia of malignancy. Bisphosphonates, analogues of pyrophosphate, are the principal agents used. They inhibit osteoclast function and hydroxyapatite crystal dissolution. Unfortunately, normalization of calcium levels may take 3–6 days, which is too slow in critically ill patients.

Disodium pamidronate is currently one of the bisphosphonates of choice. The dose is 60 mg IV (in 500 mL 0.9% saline over 4 h) if serum calcium is <3.5 mmol/L, and 80 mg IV if serum calcium is >3.5 mmol/L. Calcium levels normalize in up to 80% of patients within 7 days and this effect can persist for up to a month. Common adverse reactions include a mild transient elevation in temperature, local infusion site reactions, mild gastrointestinal symptoms and mild hypophosphataemia, hypokalaemia and hypomagnesaemia.

An alternative treatment to pamidronate is zoledronic acid 4 mg/100 mL (N saline or 5% dextrose) IV over 15 minutes. It is more potent and effective than pamidronate.

Glucocorticoids, after rehydration, are the treatment of choice in selected patient populations where there is inappropriately high production of 1.25-dihydroxyvitamin D as the mechanism for causing hypercalcaemia. Such conditions include vitamin D toxicity, sarcoidosis, other granulomatous diseases and haematological malignancies, such as multiple myeloma and lymphoma. The usual dose is 200–300 mg hydrocortisone IV for 3–5 days. However, the maximal calcium-lowering effect does not occur for several days and glucocorticoids should only be regarded as adjunctive therapy in hypercalcaemic crises.

Treat the underlying disorder

The definitive treatment for hypercalcaemia is to treat the underlying disease: surgery for hyperparathyroidism and tumour-specific therapy for hypercalcaemia of malignancy.

HYPOMAGNESAEMIA

Introduction

The diagnosis of magnesium deficiency is difficult and often overlooked largely because the symptoms are non-specific and do not usually appear until the patient is severely deficient.

Serum magnesium concentration (normal range: 0.76–0.96 mmol/L) is not a sensitive indicator of magnesium deficiency as it may not truly reflect total body stores. However, it is commonly used in the absence of other reliable methods to estimate the 'true' magnesium status. A low serum magnesium concentration is usually present in symptomatic magnesium deficiency, but it is important to remember that it may be normal in the presence of significant intracellular depletion.

Pathophysiology

Magnesium plays a critical role in metabolism: as an enzyme co-factor, in the maintenance of cell membranes and in electrolyte balance. It is the fourth most common cation in the body and is predominantly an intracellular ion with the majority found in bone (>50%) and soft tissue. Only 0.3% of total body magnesium is located extracellularly, of which 33% is protein bound, 12% is complexed to anions, such as citrate, bicarbonate and phosphate, and 55% is found in the free ionized form.

Hypokalaemia is present in 40–60% of cases of magnesium deficiency, due to renal wasting of potassium. The hypokalaemia is resistant to potassium replacement alone, as a result of a combination of factors, including impaired cellular cation pump activity and increased cellular permeability to potassium.

Hypocalcaemia is usually present at serum magnesium concentrations below 0.49 mmol/L. This may be due to impaired PTH synthesis or secretion or to PTH resistance as a result of magnesium deficiency.

Aetiology

From an emergency medicine perspective, hypomagnesaemia is most frequently encountered in the context of acute and chronic diarrhoea, acute pancreatitis, diuretic use, in alcoholics and in diabetic ketoacidosis, secondary to glycosuria and osmotic diuresis. Table 12.2.14 details causes of magnesium deficiency.

Hypomagnesaemia has been found in 30% of alcoholics admitted to hospital and results from a combination of the direct effect of alcohol on the renal tubule, which increases magnesium excretion, and associated malnutrition, diarrhoea and metabolic acidosis.

Table 12.2.14 Causes of magnesium deficiency

Gastrointestinal losses

Acute and chronic diarrhoea
Acute pancreatitis
Severe malnutrition
Intestinal fistulae
Extensive bowel resection
Prolonged nasogastric suction

Renal losses

Osmotic diuresis – diabetes, urea, mannitol
Hypercalcaemia and hypercalciuria
Volume expanded states
Chronic parenteral fluid therapy

Drugs

ACE inhibitors
Alcohol
Aminoglycosides
Amphotericin B
Cisplatin
Ciclosporin

Diuretics – thiazide or loop

Other

Phosphate depletion

From Weisinger JR, Bellorin-Font E. Magnesium and phosphorus-electrolyte quintet. Lancet 1998; 352:391–6 with permission.

Clinical features

The clinical manifestations of severe magnesium deficiency include metabolic, neurological and cardiac effects (Table 12.2.15).

The presenting symptoms are non-specific and can be attributed to associated metabolic abnormalities, such as hypocalcaemia, hypokalaemia and metabolic alkalosis. In particular, patients may present with symptoms of hypocalcaemia: neuromuscular hyperexcitability, carpopedal spasm and positive Chvostek's and Trousseau's signs.

Early ECG changes of magnesium deficiency include prolongation of the PR and QT intervals, with progressive QRS widening and U-wave appearance as severity progresses. Changes in cardiac automaticity and conduction, atrial and ventricular arrhythmias, including torsades des pointes, can occur. Administration of a magnesium bolus can abolish torsades des pointes, even in the presence of normal serum magnesium levels. Magnesium is a co-factor in the Na-K-ATPase system and so magnesium deficiency enhances myocardial sensitivity to digitalis and may precipitate digitalis toxicity. Digitalis-toxic arrhythmias, in turn, can be terminated with intravenous magnesium.

Treatment

Oral replacement is the preferred option in asymptomatic patients, although this route takes longer.

Table 12.2.15 Clinical manifestations of severe magnesium deficiency

Cardiac effects	Metabolic effects	Neurological effects
Atrial fibrillation	Hypokalaemia	Grand mal seizures
Atrial flutter	Hypocalcaemia	Focal seizures
Supraventricular tachycardia	Hyponatraemia	Paraesthesias
Ventricular tachycardia	Hypophosphataemia	Dizziness
Torsades des pointes	Metabolic alkalosis	Vertigo
Coronary artery spasm	Hyperglycaemia	Ataxia
Hypertension	Hyperlipidaemia	Nystagmus
ECG changes		Tremor
Atherosclerosis		Myopathy
		Dysphagia
		Oesophageal spasm
		Delirium, personality changes
		Depression
		Coma

From Fawcett WJ, Haxby EJ, Male DA. Magnesium: physiology and pharmacology. Br J Anaesth 1999; 83:302–20 with permission.

Table 12.2.16 Magnesium doses (in mmol magnesium)

Emergency – IV route
  8–16 mmol *statim*
  40 mmol over next 5 h
Severely ill – IM route
  48 mmol on day 1
  17–25 mmol on days 2–5
Asymptomatic – oral route
  15 mmol/day

Symptomatic moderate-to-severe magnesium deficiency should be treated with parenteral magnesium salts. The patient should be closely monitored and therapy discontinued if deep tendon reflexes disappear or serum magnesium exceeds 2.5 mmol/L. Suggested dosing regimens are outlined in Table 12.2.16.

HYPERMAGNESAEMIA

Hypermagnesaemia (serum magnesium above 0.95 mmol/L) is rare and usually iatrogenic.

The elderly and patients with renal impairment or chronic bowel disorders are particularly at risk, especially when IV magnesium or magnesium-containing cathartics or antacids are used.

Clinical manifestations include mental obtundation progressing to coma, cardiac arrhythmias, loss of deep tendon reflexes, refractory hypotension and respiratory arrest, nausea and vomiting, muscle paralysis and flushing.

Magnesium administration should be immediately discontinued. Further management is largely supportive. Maintain urine output at greater than 60 mL/h with fluid administration to enhance renal excretion. Furosemide (40–80 mg IV) may also be given once the patient is adequately hydrated. Haemodialysis may be of benefit in severe cases, particularly if there is impaired renal function.

Controversies

- The safest and most effective ways of correcting hyponatraemia remain controversial because of the risk of inducing osmotic myelinolysis.
- The usefulness of bicarbonate for the acute therapy of hyperkalaemia has been questioned. A number of studies have shown that bicarbonate fails to lower potassium levels sufficiently in the acute, life-threatening situation to justify its use as first-line treatment. It is still recommended, however, when hyperkalaemia is associated with severe metabolic acidosis (pH <7.20).

Further reading

Almod CS, Shin AY, Fortescure EB, et al. Hyponatremia among runners in the Boston Marathon. N Engl J Med 2005;352:1550–6.
Androgue HJ, Madias NE. Hyponatremia. N Engl J Med (Baltimore) 2000;342:1581–9.
Bilezikian J. Management of acute hypercalcemia. N Engl J Med 1992;326:196–1203.
Box SA, Prescott LF, Freestone S. Hyponatraemia at a rave. Postgrad Med J 1997;73:53–4.
Bushinskey D, Monk R. Calcium-electrolyte quintet. Lancet 1998;352:306–11.
Decaux G. Is asymptomatic hyponatraemia really asymptomatic? Am J Med 2006;119:S79–82.
Fawcett WJ, Haxby EJ, Male DA. Magnesium: physiology and pharmacology. Br J Anaesth 1999;83:302–20.
Halperin M, Kamel K. Potassium-electrolyte quintet. Lancet 1998;352:135–40.
Mandel A. Hypokalemia and hyperkalemia. Med Clin N Am 1997;81:611–39.
Noakes TD, Sharwood K, Speedy D, et al. Three independent biological mechanisms cause exercise-associated hyponatraemia: evidence from 2,135 weighed competitive athletic performances. Proc Natl Acad Sci USA 2005;102:18550–5.
Sterns RH, Cappuccio JD, Silver SM, et al. Neurologic sequelae after treatment of severe hyponatremia: a multicenter perspective. J Am Soc Nephrol 1994;4:1522–30.
Yeong-Hau HL, Shapiro JI. Hyponatremia: clinical diagnosis and management. Am J Med 2007;120:653–8.

HAEMATOLOGY EMERGENCIES

Edited by *Mark Little*

SECTION

13

13.1 Anaemia

Lindsay Murray

ESSENTIALS

1 Anaemia is a condition in which the absolute number of red cells in the circulation is abnormally low.

2 Anaemia is not a diagnosis: it is a finding, which should prompt the search for an underlying cause.

3 The anaemic patient is doing at least one of three things: not producing enough red cells, destroying them too quickly or bleeding.

4 Bleeding is the most common cause of severe anaemia encountered in the emergency department.

Introduction

Anaemia is a condition in which the absolute number of red cells in the circulation is abnormally low. The diagnosis is usually made on the basis of the full blood count (FBC). This, together with the blood film, offers qualitative as well as quantitative data on the blood components and a set of normal values is shown in Table 13.1.1.

The average lifespan of a normal red blood cell in the circulation is from 100 to 120 days. Aged red cells are removed by the reticuloendothelial system but, under normal conditions, are replaced by the marrow such that a dynamic equilibrium is maintained. Anaemia develops when red cell loss exceeds red cell production. It follows that the anaemic patient is doing at least one of three things: not producing enough red cells, destroying them too quickly or bleeding.

The overriding functional importance of the red cell resides in its ability to transport oxygen, bound to the haemoglobin molecule, from the lungs to the tissues. Functionally, anaemia may be regarded as an impairment in the supply of oxygen to the tissues and the adverse effects of anaemia, from whatever cause, are a consequence of the resultant tissue hypoxia. Anaemia is not a diagnosis: rather, it is a clinical or a laboratory finding that should prompt the search for an underlying cause (Table 13.1.2).

ANAEMIA SECONDARY TO HAEMORRHAGE

Aetiology

By far the most common cause of severe anaemia encountered in the emergency department (ED) is haemorrhage. Therefore, the assessment of the anaemic patient is often chiefly concerned with the search for a site of blood loss. The most common causes of haemorrhage are outlined in Table 13.1.3. However, the emergency physician must remain alert to the possibility that the patient is not bleeding but manifesting a rarer pathological condition.

Clinical features

While it may be obvious on history and examination that a patient is bleeding, occasionally, the source of blood loss is occult and the extent of loss underestimated.

In the context of trauma, the history often gives clear pointers to both sites and extent of blood loss. Consideration of the mechanism of injury may allow anticipation of occult pelvic, intraperitoneal or retroperitoneal bleeding. Intracranial bleeding is never an explanation for hypovolaemic shock in an adult. In the context of non-trauma, it is essential to obtain an obstetric and gynaecological history in women of childbearing age. The remainder of the formal history may supply information essential in determining the aetiology of anaemia. The past medical history may point to a known haematological abnormality or to a chronic disease process. A drug and allergy history is always relevant. Many drugs cause marrow suppression, haemolytic anaemia and bleeding. The family history points to hereditary disease; the social history may alert the clinician to an unusual occupational exposure in the patient's

Table 13.1.1 Full blood count: normal parameters

Haemoglobin (Hb)

Males	135–180 g/L
Females	115–165 g/L

Red blood cell count

Males	4500–6500 × 10⁹/L
Females	3900–5600 × 10⁹/L

Males	4500–6500×10^9/L
Females	3900–5600×10^9/L

Haematocrit

Males	42–54%
Females	37–47%

Other values

MCH	27–32 pg
MCHC	32–36 g/dL
MCV	76–98 fL
Reticulocytes	0.2–2%
White blood cells	4–11×10^9/L
Neutrophils	1.8–8×10^9/L
Eosinophils	0–0.6×10^9/L
Basophils	0–0.2×10^9/L
Lymphocytes	1–5×10^9/L
Monocytes	0–0.8×10^9/L
Platelets	150–400×10^9/L

MCH: Hb divided by RBC; MCHC: Hb divided by HCT; MCV: HCT divided by RBC. Most automated counting machines now give the red cell distribution width (RDW), a measure of degree of variation of cell size.

Table 13.1.2 Causes of anaemia

Haemorrhage

Traumatic
Non-traumatic
  Acute
  Chronic
Megaloblastic anaemia
Vitamin B12 deficiency
Folate deficiency
Aplastic anaemia
Pure red cell aplasia
Myelodysplastic syndromes
Invasive marrow diseases
Chronic renal failure

Decreased RBC survival (haemolytic anaemia)

Congenital
Spherocytosis
Elliptocytosis
Glucose-6-phosphate-dehydrogenase deficiency
Pyruvate kinase deficiency
Haemoglobinopathies: sickle cell diseases
Acquired autoimmune haemolytic anaemia, warm
Acquired autoimmune haemolytic anaemia, cold
Microangiopathic haemolytic anaemias
RBC mechanical trauma
Infections
Paroxysmal nocturnal haemoglobinuria

RBC: red blood cell.

Table 13.1.3 Common causes of haemorrhage in the emergency department

Trauma

Blunt trauma to mediastinum
Pulmonary contusions/haemopneumothorax
Intraperitoneal injury
Retroperitoneal injury
Pelvic disruption
Long bone injury
Open wounds: inadequate first aid

Non-trauma

Gastrointestinal haemorrhage
  Oesophageal varices
  Peptic ulcer
  Gastritis/Mallory–Weiss
  Colonic/rectal bleeding
Obstetric/gynaecological bleeding
  Ruptured ectopic pregnancy
  Menorrhagia
  Threatened miscarriage
  Antepartum haemorrhage
  Postpartum haemorrhage
Other
  Epistaxis
  Postoperative
  Secondary to bleeding diathesis

past or, more likely, to recreational activities liable to exacerbate an ongoing disease process. The systems review is particularly relevant to the consultation with middle-aged or elderly male patients, who must be asked about symptoms of altered bowel habit and weight loss.

The symptomatology of anaemia proceeds from vague complaints of tiredness, lethargy and impaired performance through to more sharply defined entities, such as shortness of breath on exertion, giddiness, restlessness, apprehension, confusion and collapse. Co-morbid conditions may be exacerbated (the dyspnoea of chronic obstructive airway disease) and occult pathologies unmasked (exertional angina in ischaemic heart disease).

Anaemia of insidious onset is generally better tolerated than that of rapid onset because of cardiovascular and other compensatory mechanisms. Acute loss of 40% of the blood volume may result in collapse whereas, in certain developing countries, it is not rare for patients with haemoglobin concentrations 10% of normal to be ambulant. Trauma superimposed on an already established anaemia can lead to rapid decompensation.

The cardinal sign of anaemia is pallor. This can be seen in the skin, the lips, the mucous membranes and the conjunctival reflections. Yet, not all anaemic patients are pallid and not all patients with a pale complexion are anaemic. Patients who have suffered an acute haemorrhage may show evidence of hypovolaemia: tachycardia, hypotension, cold peripheries and sluggish capillary refill. The detection of postural hypotension is an important pointer towards occult blood loss.

Conversely, patients with anaemia of insidious onset are not hypovolaemic and may manifest high-output cardiac failure as a physiological response to hypoxia.

Other features of the physical examination may provide clues to the aetiology of anaemia. The glossitis, angular stomatitis, koilonychia and oesophageal web of iron-deficiency anaemia are uncommon findings. Bone tenderness, lymphadenopathy, hepatomegaly and splenomegaly may point to an underlying haematological abnormality. The rectal and gynaecological examinations can sometimes be diagnostic.

Clinical investigations

The full blood count often reveals an anaemia that has not been clinically suspected and that must be interpreted in the light of the history and examination. If the anaemia is mild it may be a chance finding with little relevance to the patient's presenting complaint, but such a finding should never be ignored. At the very least a follow-up blood count should be arranged.

Anaemic patients have a low red cell count, a low haematocrit and a low haemoglobin, but some caveats need to be borne in mind:

- patients who are bleeding acutely may initially have a normal FBC
- normal or high haematocrits may reflect haemoconcentration
- mixed pictures can be difficult to interpret, e.g. that of a polycythaemic patient who is bleeding.

Red cell morphology, particularly the mean corpuscular volume (MCV), can help elucidate the cause of anaemia. The finding of a pancytopaenia suggests a problem in haematopoiesis, rather than haemolysis or blood loss. In women of childbearing age, assay of blood or urine β-HCG is important.

Treatment

The principles of management of haemorrhage are as follows:

- maintain the circulation
- identify the site of bleeding
- control the bleeding
- identify the underlying pathological process
- arrange for definitive treatment
- restore the blood volume.

The indications for red cell transfusion are discussed in Chapter 13.5. The faster the onset of the anaemia, the greater the need for urgent replacement. Patients who are tolerating their anaemia may require no more than an appropriate diet with or without the addition of haematinics. Elderly patients with severe bleeding often need red cells urgently. Excessive administration of colloid and/or crystalloid precipitates left ventricular failure and it can then be difficult to administer red cells.

Chronic haemorrhage

The finding of a hypochromic microcytic anaemia on blood film is usually indicative of iron deficiency and, in the absence of an overt history of bleeding, should prompt the search for occult blood loss. Iron deficiency anaemia may be due to malnutrition, but inadequate dietary intake of iron is not usually the sole cause of anaemia in developed countries: much more commonly it is the result of chronic blood loss from the gastrointestinal (GI) tract, the uterus or the renal tract. More unusual causes are haemoptysis and recurrent epistaxes.

Patients present with insidious and rather vague symptoms. They may be unaware that they are bleeding and will probably show none of the trophic skin, nail and mucosal changes of iron deficiency. The automated cell count, in addition to showing a hypochromic, microcytic picture, may also show a raised red cell distribution width, which reflects anisocytosis on the blood film.

Iron studies may confirm the diagnosis of iron deficiency without pointing to the underlying cause. Serum iron and ferritin are low and total iron-binding capacity is high.

Disposition

If the source of blood loss is obvious, for example heavy menstrual bleeding, then appropriate referral may be all that is indicated. If the source is not obvious, particularly in older patients, then sequential investigation of the GI tract and the renal tract may be indicated. Decisions to admit or discharge these patients depend on the red cell reserves, the patient's cardiorespiratory status, home circumstances and the likelihood of compliance with follow up.

The anaemia itself can be corrected with oral iron supplements: 200 mg of ferrous sulphate three times daily is an appropriate regimen,

although single daily doses are often more acceptable to the patient and have fewer GI side effects.

ANAEMIA SECONDARY TO DECREASED RED CELL PRODUCTION

Megaloblastic anaemia

The finding of a raised MCV is common in the presence or absence of anaemia. Alcohol abuse is a frequent underlying cause and other causes are listed in Table 13.1.4. MCVs greater than 115 fL are usually due to megaloblastic anaemia which, in turn, is usually due to either vitamin B12 or folate deficiency. Vitamin B12 and folate are essential to DNA synthesis in all cells. Deficiencies manifest principally in red cell production because of the sheer number of red cells that are produced. B12 deficiency is usually the result of a malabsorption syndrome, whereas folate deficiency is of dietary origin. Tetrahydrofolate is a co-factor in DNA synthesis and, in turn, the formation of tetrahydrofolate from its methylated precursor is B12-dependent. Unabated cytoplasmic production of RNA in the context of impaired DNA synthesis appears to produce the enlarged nucleus and abundant cytoplasm of the megaloblast. These cells, when released to the periphery, have poor function and poor survival.

B12 deficiency is an autoimmune disorder in which autoantibodies to gastric parietal cells and the B12 transport factor (intrinsic factor) interfere with B12 absorption in the terminal ileum. Patients have achlorhydria, mucosal atrophy (a painful smooth tongue) and, sometimes, evidence of other autoimmune disorders, such as vitiligo, thyroid disease and Addison's disease. This is so-called 'pernicious anaemia'.

A rare, but important, manifestation of this disease is 'subacute combined degeneration of the spinal cord'. Demyelination of the posterior and lateral columns of the spinal cord manifests as a peripheral neuropathy and an abnormal gait. The central nervous system abnormalities worsen and become irreversible in the absence of B12 supplementation. Treatment of B12 deficient patients with folate alone may accelerate the onset of this condition.

Undiagnosed untreated pernicious anaemia is not a common finding in the ED, but the laboratory finding of anaemia and

Table 13.1.4   Some causes of a raised mass cell volume
Alcohol
Drugs
Hypothyroidism
Liver disease
Megaloblastic anaemias (B12 and folate deficiency)
Myelodysplasia
Pregnancy
Reticulocytosis

megaloblastosis should prompt haematological consultation. The investigative work-up, which includes B12 and red cell folate levels, autoantibodies to parietal cells and intrinsic factor, a marrow aspirate, and Schilling's test of B12 absorption, may well necessitate hospital admission.

The work-up for folate deficiency is similar to that for B12. Occasionally, patients require investigation for a malabsorption syndrome (tropical sprue, coeliac disease), which includes jejunal biopsy. Folate deficiency is common in pregnancy because of the large folate requirements of the growing fetus. It can be difficult to diagnose because of the maternal physiological expansion of plasma volume and also of red cell mass, but diagnosis and treatment with oral folate supplements are important because of the risk of associated neural tube defects.

Both B12 and folate deficiency are usually manifestations of chronic disease processes. Rarely, an acute megaloblastic anaemia and pancytopaenia can develop over the course of days and nitrous oxide therapy has been identified as a principal cause of this condition.

Anaemia of chronic disorders

Patients with chronic infective, malignant or connective tissue disorders can develop a mild-to-moderate normochromic normocytic anaemia. Evidence of bleeding or haemolysis is absent and there is no response to haematinic therapy. The pathophysiology of this anaemia is complex and probably involves both decreased red cell production and survival. Possible underlying mechanisms include reticuloendothelial overactivity in chronic inflammation and defects in iron metabolism mediated by a variety of acute-phase reactants and cytokines, such as interleukin-1, tumour necrosis factor and interferon γ, which impair renal erythropoietin production and function.

Anaemia of chronic disorders (ACD) is generally not so severe as to warrant emergency therapy. The importance of ACD in the ED lies in its recognition as a pointer towards an underlying chronic process. Difficulties can arise in distinguishing ACD from iron deficiency and the two conditions may coexist – in rheumatoid arthritis, for example. Iron studies generally elucidate the nature of the anaemia. In iron deficiency, iron and ferritin are low and total iron binding is high, whereas in ACD iron and total iron binding are low and ferritin is normal or high.

Other causes of decreased red cell production

Bone marrow failure is rarely encountered in emergency medicine practice. The physician must be alert to the unusual, insidious or sinister presentation and be particularly attuned to the triad of decreased tissue oxygenation, immunocompromise and a bleeding diathesis that may herald a pancytopaenia. An FBC may dictate the need for haematological consultation, hospital admission and further investigation.

Among the entities to be considered are the aplastic anaemias, characterized by a pancytopaenia secondary to failure of pluripotent myeloid stem cells. Half of cases are idiopathic, but important aetiologies are infections (e.g. non-A, non-B hepatitis), inherited diseases (e.g. Fanconi's anaemia), irradiation, therapeutic or otherwise and, most important in the emergency setting, drugs. Drugs that have been implicated in the development of aplastic anaemia include, in addition to antimetabolites and alkylating agents, chloramphenicol, chlorpromazine and streptomycin.

Characteristic of patients with a primary marrow failure is the absence of splenomegaly and the absence of a reticulocyte response. There is a correlation between prognosis and the severity of the pancytopaenia. Platelet counts less than 20×10^9/L and neutrophil counts less than 500/mL equate to severe disease. Depending on the severity of the accompanying anaemia, patients may require red cell

Table 13.1.5 Classification of the myelodysplastic syndromes

Refractory anaemia
Refractory anaemia with ringed sideroblasts
Refractory anaemia with excess of blasts
Chronic myelomonocytic leukaemia

and sometimes platelet transfusion in the ED, as well as broad-spectrum antibiotic cover. It is imperative to stop all medications that might be causing the marrow failure. Other forms of marrow failure include pure red cell aplasia, where marrow red cell precursors are absent or diminished. This can be a complication of haemolytic states in which a viral insult leads to an aplastic crisis (see haemolytic anaemias).

The myelodysplastic syndromes are a group of disorders primarily affecting the elderly. In these states there is no reduction in marrow cellularity but the mature red cells, granulocytes and platelets generated from an abnormal clone of stem cells are disordered and dysfunctional. There is peripheral pancytopaenia. These disorders are classified according to observed cellular morphology (Table 13.1.5). These conditions were once termed 'preleukaemia' and one-third of patients progress to acute myeloid leukaemia.

Two more causes of failure of erythropoiesis might be mentioned. One is due to invasion of the marrow and disruption of its architecture by extraneous tissue, the commonest cause being metastatic cancer. Finally, but not at all uncommon, is the anaemia of chronic renal failure, where deficient erythropoiesis is attributed to decreased production of erythropoietin. Most patients with chronic renal failure on dialysis treatment tolerate a moderate degree of anaemia, but occasionally require either transfusion or treatment with erythropoietin. Emergency physicians should recognize anaemia as a predictable entity in patients with chronic renal failure, usually not requiring any action.

ANAEMIA SECONDARY TO DECREASED RED CELL SURVIVAL: THE HAEMOLYTIC ANAEMIAS

Patients whose main problem is haemolysis are encountered rarely in the ED. The most

fulminant haemolytic emergency one could envisage is that following transfusion of ABO-incompatible blood (discussed in Chapter 13.5), a vanishingly rare event where proper procedures are followed. Haemolysis and haemolytic anaemia are occasionally encountered in decompensating patients with multisystem problems. Rarely, first presentations of unusual haematological conditions occur.

Some of the haemolytic anaemias are hereditary conditions in which the inherited disorder is an abnormality intrinsic to the red cell, its membrane, its metabolic pathways or the structure of the haemoglobin contained in the cells. Such red cells are liable to be dysfunctional and to have increased fragility and a shortened lifespan. Lysis in the circulation may lead to clinical jaundice as bilirubin is formed from the breakdown of haemoglobin. Lysis in the reticuloendothelial system generally does not cause jaundice but may produce splenomegaly. The anaemia tends to be normochromic normocytic; sometimes a mildly raised MCV is due to an appropriate reticulocyte response from a normally functioning marrow. Serum bilirubin may be raised even in the absence of jaundice. Urinary urobilinogen and faecal stercobilinogen are detectable and serum haptoglobin is depleted. The antiglobulin (Coombs') test is important in the elucidation of some haemolytic anaemias. In this test, red cells coated *in vivo* (direct test) or *in vitro* (indirect test) with IgG antibodies are washed to remove unbound antibodies, then incubated with an antihuman globulin reagent. The resultant agglutination is a positive test.

Any chronic haemolytic process may be complicated by an 'aplastic crisis'. This is usually a transient marrow suppression brought on by a viral infection which can result in a severe and life-threatening anaemia. Red cell transfusion in these circumstances may be life saving.

Hereditary spherocytosis

A deficiency of the red cell wall protein, spectrin, leads to loss of deformability and increased red cell fragility. These cells are destroyed prematurely in the spleen. The condition may present at any age, with anaemia, intermittent jaundice and cholelithiasis. Patients are Coombs' negative and show normal red cell osmotic fragility. Splenectomy radically improves general health. Hereditary elliptocytosis is a similar disease, with usually a milder course.

Glucose-6-phosphate dehydrogenase deficiency

Glucose-6-phosphate dehydrogenase (G6PD) generates reduced glutathione, which protects the red cell from oxidant stress. G6PD deficiency is an X-linked disorder present in heterozygous males and homozygous females. The disorder is commonly seen in West Africa, southern Europe, the Middle East and Southeast Asia. Oxidant stress leads to severe haemolytic anaemia. Precipitants include fava beans, antimalarial and analgesic drugs and infections. The enzyme deficiency can be demonstrated by direct assay and treatment is supportive.

Sickle cell anaemia

Whereas in the thalassaemias there is a deficiency in a given globin chain within the haemoglobin (Hb) molecule, in the haemoglobinopathies a given globin chain is present but structurally abnormal. HbS differs from normal HbA by one amino acid residue: valine replaces glutamic acid at the sixth amino acid from the N-terminus of the β-globin chain. Red cells containing HbS tend to 'sickle' at states of low oxygen tension. The deformed sickle-shaped red cell has increased rigidity, which causes it to lodge in the microcirculation and sequester in the reticuloendothelial system – the cause of a haemolytic anaemia.

Sickle cell disease is encountered in Afro-Caribbean people. The higher incidence in tropical areas is attributed to the survival value of the β-S gene against falciparum malaria. Heterozygous individuals have 'sickle trait' and are usually asymptomatic. Homozygous (HbSS) individuals manifest the disease in varying degrees. The haemolytic anaemia is usually in the range of 60–100 g/L and can be well tolerated because HbS offloads oxygen to the tissues more efficiently than HbA.

A patient with sickle cell disease may occasionally develop a rapidly worsening anaemia. This may be due to:

- a production defect – reduced marrow erythropoiesis may be secondary to folate deficiency or to a parvovirus infection; this is an aplastic crisis
- a survival defect – increased haemolysis is usually secondary to infection
- splenic sequestration.

In any of these circumstances, transfusion may be life saving. However, these events are unusual and more commonly encountered is the vaso-occlusive crisis. A stressor – for example infection, dehydration, or cold – causes sickle cells to lodge in the microcirculation. Bone marrow infarction is one well-recognized complication of the phenomenon, but virtually any body system can be affected. Common presenting complaints include acute spinal pain, abdominal pain (the mesenteric occlusion of 'girdle sequestration'), chest pain (pulmonary vascular occlusion), joint pain, fever (secondary to tissue necrosis), neurological involvement (transient ischaemic attacks, strokes, seizures, obtundation, coma), respiratory embarrassment and hypoxia, priapism, 'hand–foot syndrome' (dactylitis of infancy), haematuria (nephrotic syndrome, papillary necrosis), skin ulcers of the lower limbs, retinopathies, glaucoma and gallstones.

Most patients presenting with a vaso-occlusive crisis know they have the disease but, otherwise, the differential diagnosis is difficult. Sickle cells may be seen on the blood film and can also be induced by deoxygenating the sample. Hb electrophoresis can establish the type of Hb present. Other investigations are dictated by the presentation and may include blood cultures, urinalysis and culture, chest X-ray, arterial blood gases and electrocardiograph.

Pain relief should commence early. A morphine infusion may be required for patients with severe ongoing pain. Other supportive measures are dictated by the presentation. Intravenous fluids are particularly important for patients with renal involvement. Aim to establish a urine output in excess of 100 mL/h in adults. Antibiotic cover may be required in the case of febrile patients with lung involvement. It may be impossible to differentiate between pulmonary vaso-occlusion and pneumonia. Many patients with sickle cell disease are effectively splenectomized owing to chronic splenic sequestration with infarction and are prone to infection from encapsulated bacteria. The choice of antibiotic depends on the clinical presentation. Indications for exchange transfusion are shown in Table 13.1.6. The efficacy of exchange transfusion in painful crises remains unproven.

Haemoglobin S-C disease

Sickle trait or Hb S-C disease occurs in up to 10% in the black population. The clinical presentation resembles that of sickle cell disease but is usually less severe.

Table 13.1.6 Indications for exchange transfusion in sickle cell crisis
Neurological presentations: TIAs, stroke, seizures
Lung involvement (PaO$_2$ < 65 mmHg with FiO$_2$ 60%)
Sequestration syndromes
Priapism
TIA: transient ischaemic attack.

Haemoglobin C disease

In HbC, lysine replaces glutamic acid in the sixth position from the N terminus of the β-chain. Red cells containing HbC tend to be abnormally rigid, but the cells do not sickle. Homozygotes manifest a normocytic anaemia but there is no specific treatment and transfusion is seldom required.

Thalassaemias

There is a high incidence of β-thalassaemia trait among people of Mediterranean origin although, in fact, the region of high frequency extends in a broad band east to Southeast Asia.

Thalassaemias are disorders of haemoglobin synthesis. In the haemoglobin molecule, four haem molecules are attached to four long polypeptide globin chains. Four globin chain types (each with their own minor variations in amino acid order) are designated α, β, γ and δ. Haemoglobin A comprises two α and two β chains; 97% of adult haemoglobin is HbA. In thalassaemia, there is diminished or absent production of either the α chain (α-thalassaemia) or the β chain (β-thalassaemia). Most patients are heterozygous and have a mild asymptomatic anaemia, although the red cells are small. In fact, the finding of a marked microcytosis in conjunction with a mild anaemia suggests the diagnosis.

There are four genes on paired chromosomes 16 coding for α-globin and two genes on paired chromosomes 11 coding for β-globin. α-Thalassaemias are associated with patterns of gene deletion as follows: (−/−) is Hb-Barts hydrops syndrome, incompatible with life and (α/-) is HbH disease.

Patients who are heterozygous for β-thalassaemia have β-thalassaemia minor or thalassaemia trait. They are usually symptomless. Homozygous patients have β major.

Diagnosis of the major clinical syndromes is usually possible through consideration of the presenting features in conjunction with an FBC, blood film and Hb electrophoresis.

HbH disease patients present with moderate haemolytic anaemia and splenomegaly. The HbH molecule is detectable on electrophoresis and comprises unstable β tetramers. α Trait occurs with deletion of one or two genes. Hb, MCV and mean corpuscular haemoglobin (MCH) are low, but the patient is often asymptomatic.

β major becomes apparent in the first 6 months of life with the decline of fetal Hb. There is a severe haemolytic anaemia, ineffective erythropoiesis, hepatosplenomegaly and failure to thrive. With improved care, many of these patients survive to adulthood and may possibly present to the ED, where transfusion could be life saving. Patients with β trait may be encountered in the ED relatively frequently. They are generally asymptomatic, with a mild hypochromic microcytic anaemia. It is important not to work-up these patients continually for iron deficiency and not to subject them to inappropriate haematinic therapy.

Acquired haemolytic anaemias

Many of the acquired haemolytic anaemias are autoimmune in nature, a manifestation of a type II (cytotoxic) hypersensitivity reaction. Here, normal red cells are attacked by aberrant autoantibodies targeting antigens on the red cell membrane. These reactions may occur more readily at 37°C (warm autoimmune haemolytic anaemia, or AIHA), or at 4°C (cold AIHA). Warm AIHA is more common. Red cells are coated with IgG, complement or both. The cells are destroyed in the reticuloendothelial system. Fifty per cent of cases are idiopathic, but other recognized causes include lymphoproliferative disorders, neoplasms, connective tissue disorders, infections and drugs (notably methyldopa and penicillin). Patients have haemolytic anaemia, splenomegaly and a positive Coombs' test. In the ED setting, it is important to stop any potentially offending drugs and search for the underlying disease. The idiopathic group may respond to steroids, other immunosuppressive or cytotoxic drugs or splenectomy.

In cold AIHA, IgM attaches to the I red cell antigen in the cooler peripheries. Primary cold antibody AIHA is known as cold haemagglutinin

Table 13.1.7 Causes of microangiopathic haemolytic anaemia
Disseminated intravascular coagulation
Haemolytic uraemic syndrome
HELLP
Malignancy
Malignant hypertension
Snake envenoming
Thrombotic thrombocytopaenic purpura
Vasculitis

disease. Other causes include lymphoproliferative disorders, infections such as mycoplasma, and paroxysmal cold haemoglobinuria. Patients sometimes manifest Reynaud's disease and other manifestations of circulatory obstruction. Symptoms worsen in winter. Red cell lysis leads to haemoglobinuria.

Microangiopathic haemolytic anaemia

In this important group of conditions, intravascular haemolysis occurs in conjunction with a disorder of microcirculation. Important causes are shown in Table 13.1.7.

Haemolytic uraemic syndrome and thrombotic thrombocytopaenic purpura

These are probably manifestations of the same pathological entity, with haemolytic uraemic syndrome occurring in children and thrombotic thrombocytopaenic purpura most commonly in the fourth decade, especially in women. The primary lesion is likely to be in the vascular endothelium. Fibrin and platelet microthrombi are laid down in arterioles and capillaries, possibly as an autoimmune reaction. The clotting system is not activated. Haemolytic anaemia, thrombocytopaenia and acute renal failure are sometimes accompanied by fever and neurological deficits.

In adults, the presentation is usually one of a neurological disturbance (headache, confusion, obtundation, seizures or focal signs). The blood film reveals anaemia, thrombocytopaenia, reticulocytosis and schistocytes. Coombs' test is negative.

Patients require hospital admission. Adults with this condition may require aggressive therapy with prednisone, antiplatelet therapy, further immunosuppressive therapy and plasma exchange transfusions.

HELLP syndrome

HELLP stands for haemolysis, elevated liver enzymes and a low platelet count and is seen in pregnant women in the context of pre-eclampsia. Treatment is as for pre-eclampsia, early delivery of the baby being of paramount importance.

Disseminated intravascular coagulation

The introduction of procoagulants into the circulation resulting in the overwhelming of anticoagulant control systems may occur as a consequence of a substantial number of pathophysiological insults, obstetric, infective, malignant and traumatic. Disseminated intravascular coagulation has an intimate association with shock, from any cause. The widespread production of thrombin leads to deposition of microthrombi, bleeding secondary to thrombocytopaenia and a consumption coagulopathy, and red cell damage within abnormal vasculature leading to a haemolytic anaemia.

Recognition of this condition prompts intensive care admission and aggressive therapy. Principles of treatment include definitive management of the underlying cause and, from the haematological point of view, replacement therapy that may involve transfusion of red cells, platelets, fresh frozen plasma (FFP) and cryoprecipitate. There may be a role for heparin and other anticoagulant treatments if specific tissue and organ survival is threatened by thrombus.

Paroxysmal noctural haemoglobinuria

This entity is unusual in that an intrinsic red cell defect is seen in the context of an acquired haemolytic anaemia. A somatic stem cell mutation results in a clonal disorder. A family of membrane proteins (CD55, CD59 and C8 binding protein) is deficient and renders cells prone to complement-mediated lysis. Because the same proteins are deficient in white cells and platelets, in addition to being anaemic, patients

Table 13.1.8   Infections associated with haemolysis

| Babesiosis |
| Bartonella |
| Clostridia |
| Cytomegalovirus |
| Coxsackie virus |
| Epstein–Barr virus |
| Haemophilus |
| Herpes simplex |
| HIV |
| Malaria, especially *Plasmodium falciparum* (Blackwater fever) |
| Measles |
| Mycoplasma |
| Varicella |

Table 13.1.9   Drugs and toxins associated with haemolysis

| Antimalarials |
| Arsine (arsenic hydride) |
| Bites: bees, wasps, spiders, snakes |
| Copper |
| Dapsone |
| Lead (plumbism) |
| Local anaesthetics: lidocaine, benzocaine |
| Nitrates, nitrites |
| Sulphonamides |

sometimes seen in association with a number of infectious diseases, notably malaria. Other infections that have been implicated are listed in Table 13.1.8. Certain drugs and toxins are associated with haemolytic anaemia (Table 13.1.9). The haemolytic anaemia that is commonly seen in patients with severe burns is attributed to direct damage to the red cells by heat.

Further reading

Bain BJ. Morphology in the diagnosis of red cell disorders. Hematology 2005;10S:178–81.

Bayless PA. Selected red cell disorders. Emerg Med Clin N Am 1993;11:481–93.

Carbrow MB, Wilkins JC. Haematologic emergencies. Management of transfusion reactions and crises in sickle cell disease. Postgrad Med 1993;93:183–90.

Evans TC, Jehle D. The red blood cell distribution width. J Emerg Med 1991;9(suppl 1):71–4.

Gaillard HM, Hamilton GC. Hemoglobin/hematocrit and other erythrocyte parameters. Emerg Med Clin N Am 1986;4: 15–40.

Glassberg J. Evidence-based management of sickle cell disease in the emergency department. Emerg Med Pract 2011;13:1–20.

Shander A, Javidroozi M, Ashton ME. Drug-induced anaemia and other red cell disorders: a guide in the age of polypharmacy. Curr Clin Pharmacol 2011;6:295–303.

Stuber SP. Clinical practice. Vitamin B12 deficiency. N Engl J Med 2013;368:149–60.

Thomas C, Thomas L. Anemia of chronic disease: pathophysiology and laboratory diagnosis. Lab Hematol 2005;11:14–23.

are prone to infections and haemostatic abnormalities. They may go on to develop aplastic anaemia or leukaemia. Treatment is supportive. Marrow transplant can be curative.

Other causes of haemolysis

Haemolysis may be due to mechanical trauma, as in 'March haemoglobinuria'. Artificial heart valves can potentially traumatize red cells. Historically, ball-and-cage type valves have been most prone to cause haemolysis, whereas disc valves are more thrombogenic. Improvements in design have made cardiac haemolytic anaemia very rare. Haemolysis is

13.2 Neutropaenia

Mark Little

ESSENTIALS

1 The risk of infection increases significantly as the absolute neutrophil count drops below 1.0×10^9/L.

2 Life-threatening neutropaenia is most likely to be due to impaired haematopoiesis.

3 A detailed medication history is vital to the 'work-up' of neutropaenia.

4 Fever in the presence of severe neutropaenia constitutes a true emergency that mandates rapid assessment and aggressive management to prevent progression to overwhelming sepsis.

5 Strategies of early empiric broad-spectrum antibiotic administration have significantly reduced the overall mortality of febrile neutropaenia.

Introduction

Neutropaenia is defined as a decrease in the number of circulating neutrophils. The neutrophil count varies with age, sex and racial grouping. The severity of neutropaenia is usually graded as follows:

- mild: neutrophil count 1.0–1.5×10^9/L
- moderate: neutrophil count 0.5–1.0×10^9/L
- severe: neutrophil count $<0.5 \times 10^9$/L

The risk of infection rises as the neutrophil count falls and becomes significant once the neutrophil count drops below 1.0×10^9/L. Recent Australian guidelines have defined

Table 13.2.1   Features of systemic compromise

Systolic BP ≤90 mmHg or ≥30 mmHg below patients usual BP or inotropic support
Room air arterial pO_2 ≤60 mmHg ot SpO_2 <90% or need for mechanical ventilation
Confusion or altered mental state
Disseminated intravascular coagulation or abnormal PT/aPTT
Cardiac failure or arrhythmia, renal failure, liver failure or any major organ failure (only if new or deteriorating and not AF or CHF)
From Tam CS, OReilly M, Andersen D, et al. Use of empiric antimicrobial therapy in neutropenic fever. Int Med J 2011; 41:90-101.

Table 13.2.2   Important causes of neutropaenia

Decreased production
Aplastic anaemia
Leukaemias
Lymphomas
Metastatic cancer
Drug-induced agranulocytosis
Megaloblastic anaemias
Vitamin B12 deficiency
Folate deficiency
CD8 and large granular lymphocytosis
Myelodysplasic syndromes

Decreased survival
Idiopathic immune related
Systemic lupus erythematosus
Felty syndrome
Drugs

Redistribution
Sequestration (hypersplenism)
Increased utilization (overwhelming sepsis)
Viraemia

febrile neutropaenia as a patient with a temperature above 38.3°C (or above 38°C on two occasions) with a neutrophil count less than 0.5×10^9/L or with less than 1.0×10^9/L and likely to fall to less than 0.5×10^9/L. These patients need to be examined for signs of systemic compromise (Table 13.2.1).

Neutropaenic patients are at greater risk of overwhelming infection if the onset of the neutropaenia is acute rather than chronic and, in the case of patients receiving cancer chemotherapy, if the absolute neutrophil count is in the process of falling rather than rising.

Signs or symptoms of infection in the presence of severe neutropaenia, especially with features of systemic compromise, constitute a true emergency that mandates rapid assessment and aggressive management to prevent progression to overwhelming sepsis. In the emergency department (ED) setting, this is most commonly encountered when a patient presents with fever in the context of chemotherapy for cancer.

Pathophysiology and aetiology

Polymorphonuclear neutrophils are formed in marrow from the myelogenous cell series. Pluripotent haematopoietic stem cells are committed to a particular cell lineage through the formation of colony forming units, which further differentiate to form given white cell precursors. The mature neutrophil has a multilobed nucleus and granules in the cytoplasm. The cells are termed 'neutrophilic' because of the lilac colour of the granules caused by the uptake of both acidic and basic dyes.

The neutrophils leave the marrow and enter the circulation, where they have a lifespan of only 6–10h before entering the tissues. Here they migrate by chemotaxis to sites of infection and injury and then phagocytose and destroy foreign material. In health, about half of the available mature neutrophils are in the circulation. 'Marginal' cells are adherent to vascular endothelium or in the tissues and are not measured by the full blood count. Some individuals have fixed increased marginal neutrophil pools and decreased circulating pools; they are said to have benign idiopathic neutropaenia.

For a previously normal individual to become neutropaenic there must be decreased production of neutrophils in the marrow, decreased survival of mature neutrophils or a redistribution of neutrophils from the circulating pool. The important causes are shown in Table 13.2.2.

It is a defect in neutrophil production that is most likely to prove life threatening. Consumption of neutrophils in the periphery, as occurs early in infectious processes, is likely to be rapidly compensated for by a functioning marrow. Fortunately, most of the primary diseases of haematopoiesis are rare and, in practice, many of the acquired neutropaenias are drug induced. Processes interfering with haematopoiesis, often involving autoimmune mechanisms, may affect neutrophils both in the marrow and in the periphery. Some drugs cause neutropaenia universally but many more reactions are idiosyncratic, be they dose-related or independent of dose. Some commonly implicated drugs are listed in Table 13.2.3.

Cancer chemotherapy drugs are now recognized as the commonest cause of neutropaenia.

Clinical features

Neutropaenia is frequently anticipated based on the clinical presentation, such as fever developing in the context of cancer chemotherapy, by far the most common scenario in which severe neutropaenia is seen in the ED. Alternatively, it may be identified in the course of investigation for a likely infective illness or it might be an incidental finding during investigation for an unrelated condition.

Chronic neutropaenia may be asymptomatic unless secondary or recurrent infections develop. Acute severe neutropaenia may present with fever, sore throat and mucosal ulceration or inflammation. Symptoms or signs of an associated disease process may also be present, such as pallor from anaemia or bleeding from thrombocytopaenia, as might occur in conditions causing pancytopaenia.

The history of the mode of onset and duration of the illness is important. Systems enquiry may reveal cough, headache and photophobia, a diarrhoeal illness or urinary symptoms. The past history may reveal a known haematological illness or previous evidence of immunosuppression, such as frequent and recurrent infections. A detailed drug history is vital. Most neutropaenic drug reactions occur within the first 3 months of taking a drug.

In the ED, vital signs, including pulse, blood pressure, temperature, respiratory rate and pulse oximetry, should be performed at initial assessment and monitored regularly until disposition. Attention should be paid to identifying early signs of severe sepsis and the progression to septic shock.

Physical examination may reveal necrotizing mucosal lesions, pallor, petechial rashes, lymphadenopathy, bone tenderness, abnormal tonsillar or respiratory findings, spleno- or other organomegaly. Careful examination of the skin of the back, the lower limbs and the perineum for evidence of infection is important. The presence of indwelling venous access devices should be noted and insertion sites inspected for evidence of inflammation or infection.

Clinical investigations

Investigation in the ED is first aimed at confirming and quantifying the severity of neutropaenia, identifying the cause and then at

Table 13.2.3   Drugs commonly associated with neutropaenia
Antibiotics: chloramphenicol, sulphonamides, isoniazid, rifampicin, β-lactams, carbenicillin
Antidysrhythmic agents: quinidine, procainamide
Antiepileptics: phenytoin, carbamazepine
Antihypertensives: thiazides, ethacrynic acid, captopril, methyldopa, hydralazine
Antithyroid agents
Chemotherapeutic agents: especially methotrexate, cytosine arabinoside, 5-azacytidine, azathioprine, doxorubicin, daunorubicin, hydroxyurea, alkylating agents
Connective tissue disorder agents: phenylbutazone, penicillamine, gold
H_2-receptor antagonists
Phenothiazines, especially chlorpromazine
Miscellaneous: imipramine, allopurinol, clozapine, ticlopidine, tolbutamide

identifying the focus and severity of infection. An urgent full blood count and blood film should be ordered in any patient who is suspected of suffering febrile neutropaenia. A coagulation profile and biochemistry, including electrolytes and creatinine, serum lactate, glucose and liver function tests may be indicated once severe neutropaenia is confirmed. Anaemic patients may require a group-and-hold or cross-match.

Microbiological cultures aimed at isolating a causative organism should be taken but antibiotics should not be unreasonably delayed in the presence of fever and confirmed significant neutropaenia. Blood cultures should be taken at the time of cannulation and, if possible, prior to the instigation of antibiotic therapy. Throat swab, swabs of skin lesions and indwelling venous access device sites, urinalysis and urine culture may be indicated depending on the clinical picture. Patients with apparent central nervous system infections might require a lumbar puncture, but this should be postponed or even cancelled in the presence of an uncorrected coagulopathy, signs of raised intracranial pressure, focal neurological signs or haemodynamic instability. Antibiotics, if clinically indicated, should be commenced prior to lumbar puncture.

Treatment

Management of the patient with confirmed febrile neutropaenia in the ED involves early recognition and treatment of bacterial infection and institution of supportive care to prevent progression to overwhelming sepsis and shock. Evolving or established haemodynamic instability requires immediate, aggressive resuscitation.

Empiric broad-spectrum antibiotic therapy should be started in the ED after drawing blood for culture in any patient with fever and suspected or confirmed significant neutropaenia. This strategy has played a pivotal role in reducing mortality rates in febrile neutropaenia. Australian consensus-based clinical recommendations for the management of neutropaenic fever in adults were recently published. They reinforce the need for the administration of early antibiotics. In general, antibiotics should provide good cover for both Gram-positive and Gram-negative organisms. With increased use of indwelling venous access devices for cancer chemotherapy, there has been an increase in the incidence of sepsis due to Gram-positive organisms, such as coagulase-negative staphylococci, *S. aureus* and methicillin-resistant *Staph. aureus* (MRSA). Although occurring infrequently, bacteraemia due to *Pseudomonas aeruginosa* is associated with a high morbidity and mortality and therefore should also be covered.

Recent evidence has suggested that antibiotic monotherapy is as efficacious as combined therapy. Therefore, for clinically stable patients, Australian consensus guidelines recommend a beta lactam monotherapy (such as pipperacillin–tazobactam 4.5 g 6-hourly or cefepime 2 g 8-hourly or ceftazidime 2 g 8-hourly). These antibiotics should be administered within 1 hour of presentation and after at least one set of blood cultures.

For patients with systemic compromise, the Australian consensus guidlelines recommend the above beta lactam antibiotics plus gentimicin (5–7 mg/kg daily) given within 30 minutes of presentation and after at least one set of blood cultures. If the clinicians believed the shocked patient was colonized with Gram-positive organisms (e.g. MRSA or has clinical evidence of a catheter-related infection in a unit with a high incidence of MRSA), then vancomycin (1.5 g 12-hourly if normal renal function) should be added. Empiric antifungal therapy is not generally required unless there is persistent fever in high-risk patients beyond 96 hour of antibacterial therapy.

Disposition

The presence of significant neutropaenia with fever generally mandates admission to hospital. Patients with severe acute neutropaenia without an established aetiology will also generally require admission regardless of the presence or absence of fever. Both the haematological abnormality and the likely presence of infection require investigation. Sometimes the aetiology of the neutropaenia will be evident; on other occasions marrow aspiration and biopsy will be required.

There is emerging evidence that a subset of febrile neutropaenic patients can be identified who are at low risk of life-threatening complications and in whom duration of hospitalization and intensity of treatment may be safely reduced. Strategies that involve outpatient treatment of low-risk patients with oral antibiotics have also been evaluated. Such regimens are reliant upon accurate prediction of risk, as well as the availability of structured programmes and resources and are not yet in widespread use.

Prognosis

The prognosis of the neutropaenic patient is largely dependent upon the underlying aetiology of the condition. Febrile neutropaenia has in the past been associated with a significant mortality rate which varies depending on the organism causing the infection. Improvements in therapy, such as rapid treatment with empiric broad-spectrum antibiotics, have significantly reduced mortality rates from this condition. Overall mortality rates for patients with febrile neutropaenia have reduced from more than 20% to less than 4% in recent data sets.

Controversies

- The prophylactic use of granulocyte colony-stimulating factors, such as filgrastim and pegfilgrastim, to reduce the incidence of febrile neutropaenia during cancer chemotherapy.
- The indications for and efficacy of granulocyte transfusions in the management of febrile neutropaenia.
- The development and validation of clinical decision rules to stratify risk patients with febrile neutropaenia and the use of these to determine suitability for oral antibiotic and/or outpatient therapy.

Further reading

Bishton M, Chopra R. The role of granulocyte transfusions in neutropenic patients. Br J Haematol 2004;127:501–8.

Chisholm JC, Dommett R. The evolution towards ambulatory and day-case management of febrile neutropenia. Br J Haematol 2006;135:3–16.

Dale DC. Neutropenia and neutrophilia In: Lichtman MA, editor. Williams haematology (7th ed.). New York: McGraw-Hill; 2006.

Glasmacher A, von Lilienfeld-Toal M, Schulte S, et al. An evidence-based evaluation of important aspects of empirical antibiotic therapy in febrile neutropenic patients. Clin Microbiol Infect 2005;11(suppl 5):17–23.

Lingaratnam S, Slavin MA, Koczwara B, et al. Introduction to the Australian consensus guidelines for the management of neutropenic fever in adult cancer patients, 2010/2011. Int Med J 2011;41:75–81.

Palmblad J, Papadaki HA, Eliopoulos G. Acute and chronic neutropenias. What's new? J Intern Med 2001;250:476–91.

Picazo JJ. Management of the febrile neutropenic patient: a consensus conference. Clin Infect Dis 2004;39:S1–S6.

Severe sepsis: empirical therapy (no obvious source of infection): febrile neutropenic patients. In: eTG. Therapeutic Guidelines Limited; 2007.

Tam CS, OReilly M, Andersen D, et al. Use of empiric antimicrobial therapy in neutropenic fever. Int Med J 2011;41:90–101.

Viscoli C, Varnier O, Machetti M. Infections in patients with febrile neutropenia: epidemiology, microbiology, and risk stratification. Clin Infect Dis 2005;40:S240–5.

Waladkhani AR. Pegfilgrastim 2004: a recent advance in the prophylaxis of chemotherapy-induced neutropenia. Eur J Cancer Care 2004;13:371–9.

13.3 Thrombocytopaenia

Mark Little

ESSENTIALS

1 A low platelet count detected on automated blood count should always be confirmed by examination of the blood film prior to further investigation or treatment.

2 The cause of isolated thrombocytopaenia can often be determined by a careful history and physical examination in addition to assessment of the full blood count and blood film.

3 Platelet transfusion is unnecessary in the management of the thrombocytopaenic patient unless the platelet count is extremely low or there is ongoing bleeding.

4 In the absence of other clotting disorders or abnormal platelet function, bleeding in the thrombocytopaenic patient is often amenable to local measures of haemostasis.

Introduction

Thrombocytopaenia is defined as a reduction in the number of circulating platelets, the normal circulating platelet count being $150–400 \times 10^9$/L. It is the most common cause of abnormal bleeding. Like anaemia, thrombocytopaenia itself is not a diagnosis, but rather a manifestation of another underlying disease process.

In the emergency department setting, thrombocytopaenia may present as an incidental finding on a routine blood count or may be diagnosed in the context of abnormal bleeding. In most cases, the underlying aetiology can be determined by a careful history and physical examination combined with interpretation of the blood count.

Aetiology

The clinically important causes of thrombocytopaenia are outlined in Table 13.3.1. Diagnoses are classified by pathological process. It should be noted that more than one pathological process may be present. The causes can be divided into three different groups: pseudo-thrombocytopaenia, increased destruction of platelets or reduced production of platelets.

Pseudothrombocytopaenia

Pseudothrombocytopaenia results from an underestimation of the platelet count as measured by an automated particle counter. The most common mechanism is platelet clumping. Clumping is most often due to the anticoagulant EDTA, but may also result from autoantibodies, such as cold agglutinins. The presence of giant platelets and platelet satellitism may also yield falsely low automated platelet counts.

Pseudothrombocytopaenia should be suspected when the automated platelet count is low in the absence of symptoms or signs of abnormal bleeding or disorders associated with thrombocytopaenia. It is best excluded by examination of the blood film by an experienced observer. Any case of thrombocytopaenia found on an automated blood count should be confirmed by examination of the peripheral smear prior to further investigation or treatment.

Thrombocytopaenia due to increased platelet destruction

Immune-related thrombocytopaenia

Immune thrombocytopaenia

Immune thrombocytopaenia (ITP) is defined as an isolated thrombocytopaenia (low platelet count with an otherwise normal complete blood count and peripheral blood smear) in a patient with no clinically apparent associated conditions that can cause thrombocytopaenia.

Table 13.3.1   Causes of thrombocytopaenia

Pseudothrombocytopaenia
Platelet clumping
Collection into anticoagulant (EDTA)
Platelet agglutinins
Giant platelets

Increased platelet destruction
Immune
  Primary
    Idiopathic thrombocytopaenic purpura (ITP)
  Secondary
    Autoimmune thrombocytopaenia associated with other disorders
      Graves' disease, Hashimoto's thyroiditis, systemic lupus erythematosus
    HIV-related thrombocytopaenia
    Drug-induced thrombocytopaenia
      Heparin, gold salts, quinine/quinidine, sulphonamides, rifampicin, H2-blockers, indomethacin, carbamazepine, valproic acid, ticlopidine, clopidogrel, monoclonal antibodies (infliximab, efalizumab, rituximab)
  Post-transfusion purpura
Non-immune
  Thrombotic thrombocytopaenic purpura – haemolytic uraemic syndrome
  Pregnancy
  Gestational benign thrombocytopaenia
  Pre-eclampsia/HELLP
  Disseminated intravascular coagulation

Decreased platelet production
Congenital
  TAR (thrombocytopaenia with absent radius), Wiskott–Aldrich syndrome, Fanconi anaemia
Acquired
  Viral infection
  Epstein–Barr virus, rubella, dengue fever
  Marrow aplasia
  Malignant bone marrow infiltrates
  Chemotherapeutic agents
  Radiation therapy
Abnormal distribution and dilution
  Splenic sequestration (hypersplenism)
  Splenic enlargement
  Hypothermia
  Massive blood transfusion

It is a common cause of low platelet count and abnormal bleeding in both children and adults. ITP is thought to be caused by the development of autoantibodies to platelet membrane antigens.

Treatment is aimed at modulating the immune response and reducing the rate of platelet destruction and is indicated in all patients who have counts less than 20×10^9/L and those with counts less than 50×10^9/L accompanied by significant mucous membrane bleeding. First-phase treatment includes parenteral glucocorticoids (e.g. prednisolone 1 mg/kg/day for 4–6 weeks in tapered doses) and intravenous IgG. Splenectomy is usually reserved for patients who do not respond to medical therapy and have ongoing bleeding symptoms. Platelet transfusions may cause temporary increases in platelet count and may be used in cases of life-threatening haemorrhage but are otherwise not usually indicated.

In addition to the primary idiopathic form, immune thrombocytopaenia may also accompany autoimmune disorders, such as Graves' disease and systemic lupus erythematosus. It is the main mechanism of the thrombocytopaenia related to HIV infection.

Drug-related thrombocytopaenia

A large number of drugs have been reported to cause immune-related thrombocytopaenia. By far the most commonly implicated are quinine, quinidine and heparin. Heparin is associated with a syndrome of thrombosis due to diffuse platelet activation accompanied by a consumptive thrombocytopaenia. Some platelet inhibitors, particularly ticlopidine and, less commonly, clopidogrel, are associated with severe thrombocytopaenia and other signs and symptoms of thrombotic thrombocytopaenic purpura. Recently developed monoclonal antibodies, such as infliximab (antitumour necrosis factor-α antibody), efalizumab (anti-CD11α antibody) and rituximab (anti-CD20 antibody) are also associated with an acute, severe, but usually self-limited thrombocytopaenia.

In most cases of drug-related thrombocytopenia, recovery occurs rapidly after withdrawal of the offending agent. The exception is patients with gold sensitivity who may remain thrombocytopaenic for months due to the slow clearance of this drug.

Post-transfusion purpura

Post-transfusion purpura is clinically distinct from thrombocytopaenia due to dilution of platelets following massive transfusion. It is an acute, severe thrombocytopaenia occurring about 1 week after blood transfusion and is associated with a high titre of platelet-specific alloantibodies. It is most commonly reported in multiparous women following their first blood transfusion. The mechanism for alloantibody formation is unclear. Spontaneous recovery occurs within weeks, although fatalities from severe haemorrhage have been reported.

Non-immune platelet destruction

Thrombotic thrombocytopaenic purpura

Thrombotic thrombocytopaenic purpura (TTP) is considered to be the adult form of the haemolytic uraemic syndrome (HUS). Essentially a thrombotic microangiopathy, the classic pentad of clinical findings is: (1) fever, (2) thrombocytopaenia, (3) microangiopathic haemolytic anaemia, (4) neurological abnormalities and (5) renal involvement.

TTP can occur sporadically as an idiopathic disorder or may be associated with pregnancy, epidemics of verotoxin-producing *Escherichia coli* and *Shigella dysenteriae*, malignancy, chemotherapy, marrow transplantation and drug-dependent antibodies. Treatment with plasma exchange has dramatically influenced the outcome of TTP. Mortality has fallen from more than 90% prior to introduction of plasma exchange to less than 20% with this treatment.

Thrombocytopaenia in pregnancy

Gestational thrombocytopaenia develops during an otherwise normal pregnancy and is clinically distinct from autoimmune thrombocytopaenias such as ITP. It is thought to be due to decreased platelet survival consequent to activation of the coagulation system. Thrombocytopaenia is usually mild and there is no corresponding thrombocytopaenia in the infant. The platelet count returns to normal after delivery, although thrombocytopaenia may recur in subsequent pregnancies.

Autoimmune thrombocytopaenias, on the other hand, are often associated with more severe reductions in the platelet count. Antiplatelet antibodies are capable of crossing the placenta and may result in significant thrombocytopaenia in the fetus and newborn. This can lead to complications, such as intracranial haemorrhage, during the delivery. Treatment of the mother with autoimmune thrombocytopaenia is similar in principle to the treatment of non-pregnant cases.

In the context of pregnancy, thrombocytopaenia may also be seen as part of the HELLP (haemolysis, elevated liver enzymes, low platelets) and pre-eclampsia syndromes. The two syndromes are thought to be related. Common to both is a process of microvascular endothelial damage and intravascular platelet activation. This leads to release of thromboxane A and serotonin, which provoke vasospasm, platelet aggregation and further endothelial damage. In both syndromes, the process is terminated by delivery.

Disseminated intravascular coagulation

Thrombocytopaenia is one manifestation of the syndrome of disseminated intravascular coagulation (DIC). DIC is an acquired syndrome of diffuse intravascular coagulation up to the level of fibrin formation, accompanied by secondary fibrinolysis or inhibited fibrinolysis. It occurs in the course of severe systemic diseases or may be provoked by toxins, such as snake venoms.

Thrombocytopaenia due to impaired platelet production

Congenital disorders of impaired platelet production usually present in childhood and will not be discussed.

Of the acquired disorders of impaired platelet production, the most commonly seen in the emergency setting is the incidental finding of reduced platelet count in patients suffering viral illness. Causative viruses include Epstein–Barr virus, rubella and dengue fever. Thrombocytopaenia in these cases is reversible and requires no specific therapy other than monitoring of the platelet count to ensure normalization.

Disorders of bone marrow dysfunction, such as malignant infiltration and bone marrow suppression, cause thrombocytopaenia accompanied by reductions in numbers of other blood components. Examination of the full blood count (FBC) and blood film usually distinguishes these from other causes of isolated thrombocytopaenia. Further investigation is best referred to a haematologist.

Massive blood transfusion and thrombocytopenia

Massive blood transfusion is defined as the transfusion of a volume equivalent to the patient's normal blood volume within a 24-h period. Thrombocytopaenia results from dilution of the patient's remaining platelets and, where whole blood is used, decreased survival of platelets in stored blood. It is possibly the most important factor contributing to the haemostatic abnormality seen in massively transfused patients. Platelet transfusion should be reserved for cases where the platelet count falls below 50×10^9/L.

Hypersplenism

Hypersplenism refers to the thrombocytopaenia due to pooling in patients with splenic enlargement. It is the primary cause of thrombocytopaenia in hepatic cirrhosis, portal venous hypertension and congestive splenomegaly. In these cases, thrombocytopaenia is rarely severe and not usually of clinical importance.

Transient thrombocytopaenia has been described in patients suffering severe hypothermia and is due to splenic sequestration. Platelet counts usually return to normal within days of rewarming.

Clinical features

Thrombocytopaenia may be an incidental finding on the FBC or may be diagnosed in the context of abnormal bleeding. There are distinct differences in the patterns of abnormal bleeding associated with disorders of platelet deficiency and disorders of impaired coagulation.

Spontaneous bleeding related to thrombocytopaenia typically manifests as cutaneous petechiae and/or purpura, most commonly in dependent areas, such as the legs and buttocks. Other spontaneous manifestations include multiple small retinal haemorrhages, epistaxis, gingival and gastrointestinal bleeding. Bleeding following trauma or surgery in thrombocytopaenic patients is often immediate and may respond to local methods of haemostasis. In contradistinction to this, the bleeding associated with coagulation disorders is most commonly in the form of large haematomas or haemarthroses that occur spontaneously or develop hours to days following trauma.

In addition to the haemorrhagic manifestations of platelet insufficiency, patients with thrombocytopaenia may present with the clinical features of the underlying causative disorder. Splenic enlargement may be present in cases where thrombocytopaenia is due to hypersplenism but is not a feature of immune-related thrombocytopaenia.

The level of platelets associated with clinically significant abnormal bleeding is not precisely defined. It varies depending on the platelets' functional integrity and with the presence or absence of other risk factors, such as coagulation disorder, trauma, and surgery. There is evidence that platelet counts above 5×10^9/L are sufficient to prevent bleeding when the platelets are functionally normal and there are no other risk factors. Severe haemorrhage is uncommon at platelet counts above 20×10^9/L and, in the setting of surgery, the risk of abnormal haemorrhage is reduced at counts above 50×10^9/L.

Clinical investigation

The FBC and examination of the blood film are diagnostic of thrombocytopaenia. The pattern of deficiency should be considered. Isolated thrombocytopaenia refers to a low platelet count in the presence of an otherwise normal FBC and blood film. In these cases, FBC combined with a careful clinical history and examination is often sufficient to lead to a final diagnosis. Coexistent anaemia and/or leucopaenia suggest bone marrow dysfunction as the primary aetiological process.

Other useful investigations may include coagulation studies and D-dimer (DIC, pre-eclampsia), electrolytes, urea and creatinine (TTP), liver function tests (HELLP, and liver disease) and thyroid function tests (autoimmune thyroid disorders). Platelet antibody titres are indicated in the work-up of pregnancy-related thrombocytopaenia and bone marrow aspirate may be indicated in investigation of thrombocytopaenia due to bone marrow dysfunction, but neither of these tests is useful in the emergency department setting.

Treatment

Treatment for specific causes of thrombocytopaenia has already been discussed. Bleeding in the face of low platelet count may be responsive to local methods of haemostasis if the remaining platelets are functionally normal and there is no other disorder of coagulation present. Individual case reports provide some support for the use of recombinant Factor VIIa as an enhancer of haemostasis in the treatment of bleeding in the context of severe thrombocytopaenia, although evidence from randomized clinical trials is lacking. Platelet transfusion may be helpful in cases of severe haemorrhage and is sometimes used prophylactically to prevent bleeding in patients with very low platelet counts

Platelet transfusion is primarily indicated in patients in whom thrombocytopaenia is due to impaired platelet production and who are bleeding or have very low counts. The threshold for prophylactic transfusion in these patients is controversial. It is indicated when the platelet count is below 5×10^9/L, but is probably not indicated above this level unless other risk factors for bleeding are present.

Platelet transfusion is rarely indicated in immune-related thrombocytopaenias as the transfused platelets are rapidly destroyed. Transfusion of platelets may aggravate TTP. In DIC, platelet transfusion has not been proven to be effective but may be indicated in bleeding patients. There is little evidence to support the suggestion that blood component therapy aggravates DIC. In cases of massive blood transfusion, platelets are not routinely indicated unless there is ongoing bleeding and the platelet count is below 50×10^9/L.

Raising the platelet count to $20–50 \times 10^9$/L is sufficient to prevent serious bleeding. In patients undergoing surgery or other invasive procedures, counts up to $60–100 \times 10^9$/L may be required. A useful rule of thumb is that in a 70-kg adult, transfusion of one unit of platelets will increase the platelet count by 11×10^9/L.

At present, platelet preparations for transfusion are stored in liquid at 22°C. Problems include the continued risk of febrile non-haemolytic reactions, transmission of infectious agents and graft-versus-host disease. Alternatives to conventional liquid storage include frozen storage, cold liquid storage, photochemical treatment and lyophilized platelets. None of these methods is currently widely available. Several platelet substitutes have been developed but remain untested in the clinical setting. Some examples are red cells with surface-bound fibrinogen, fibrinogen-coated albumin microcapsules and liposome-based haemostatic agents.

Disposition

Disposition will depend on the presence and extent of abnormal bleeding, the degree of thrombocytopaenia and the underlying aetiology. In general, patients who present with abnormal bleeding and a low platelet count should be admitted for further evaluation and treatment. In the absence of bleeding, patients who have isolated thrombocytopaenia with counts above 20×10^9/L may be investigated on an outpatient basis.

Controversies

- The platelet count at which prophylactic platelet transfusion is indicated.
- The development and clinical testing of alternative methods of platelet preparation and platelet substitutes.
- The role of recombinant Factor VIIa in the treatment of bleeding in the context of severe thrombocytopaenia.

Further reading

Aster RH, Bougie DW. Drug-induced immune thrombocytopenia. N Engl J Med 2007;357:580–7.

Erkurt MA, Kaya E, Berber I, et al. Thrombocytopenia in adults: review article. J Haematol 2012;1:44–53.

George JN. Thrombocytopenia: pseudothrombocytopenia, hypersplenism, and thrombocytopenia associated with massive transfusion. In: Beutler E, Beutler E, Williams WJ, editors. Williams hematology (5th ed.). New York: McGraw-Hill, 1995, p. 1355–60.

George JN, El-Harake M, Aster RH. Thrombocytopenia due to enhanced platelet destruction by immunological mechanisms. In: Beutler E, Beutler E, Williams WJ, editors. Williams hematology (5th ed.). New York: McGraw-Hill, 1995, p. 1315–54.

Goodnough LT, Lublin DM, Zhang L, et al. Transfusion medicine service policies for recombinant factor VIIa administration. Transfusion 2004;44:1325–31.

Lee DH, Blajchman MA. Novel treatment modalities: new platelet preparations and substitutes. Br J Haematol 2001;114: 496–505.

Levi M, de Jonge E, van der Poll T. Novel approaches to the management of disseminated intravascular coagulation. Crit Care Med 2000;28(9 suppl):S20–4.

Myers B. Diagnosis and management of maternal thrombocytopenia in pregnancy. Brit J Haematol 2012;158:3–15.

Neunert C, Lim W, Crowther M, et al. Amercian Society of Haematology. The American Society of Haematology 2011 evidence based practice guidelines for immune thrombocytopenia. Blood 2011;117:4190–207.

Padden MO. HELLP syndrome: recognition and perinatal management. Am Fam Phys 1999;60:829–36.

Schwartz KA. Gestational thrombocytopenia and immune thrombocytopenias in pregnancy. Hematol Oncol Clin N Am 2000;14:1101–16.

Ten Cate H. Pathophysiology of disseminated intravascular coagulation in sepsis. Crit Care Med 2000;28(9 suppl):S9–11.

13.4 Haemophilia

Sean Arendse

ESSENTIALS

1 Haemophilia is a disorder which should be managed by the emergency physician in consultation with their nearest haemophilia centre.

2 Patients should carry their treatment regimen cards with them. If not, they should be encouraged to do so.

Introduction

Haemophilia is a group of congenital disorders of blood coagulation that arise as a result of a deficiency of clotting factor proteins, which are essential to the normal intrinsic coagulation pathway. The classic form, haemophilia A, is attributable to deficiency of Factor VIII, while haemophilia B (also known as Christmas disease) is attributable to deficiency of Factor IX. Both these diseases have a classic X-linked pattern of inheritance and thus affect males, although female carriers may also have mild deficiency of the appropriate coagulation factor.

Haemophilia A is the commoner disease (80%), with an incidence of 1 in 8000–10 000 live male births, compared to an incidence of 1 in 25 000–30 000 for haemophilia B (20%).

Pathophysiology

The normal clotting system is activated in the presence of vascular injury to produce: (1) vascular spasm, (2) platelet plug formation, (3) coagulation: factor activation and the production of fibrin. Normal coagulation of blood is dependent on the generation of adequate thrombin via the clotting cascade. Deficiency of Factor VIII or IX reduces the amplification of the clotting cascade thus causing haemophilia. The severity of the bleeding disorder is inversely related to the level of functional factor present and is categorized into mild, moderate and severe disease:

- Mild disease (6–30% of normal factor level) – manifests with persistent bleeding after surgery, dental extractions and trauma. Spontaneous bleeds do not occur in this group of patients.
- Moderate disease (1–5% of normal factor level) – manifests with bleeding into joints and muscles after minor trauma and excessive bleeding after surgery and dental extractions.
- Severe disease (<1% of normal factor level) – manifests with spontaneous joint and muscle bleeding and excessive bleeding following minor trauma, surgery or dental extractions.

Clinical features

Haemophilia A and B are clinically indistinguishable and symptoms vary according to the severity of the inherited disorder. Mild disease may not present until adulthood, whereas moderate to severe disease usually presents in infancy or early childhood.

Bleeding in haemophilia tends to occur spontaneously or following minor trauma and is typically delayed and persistent. This is because, although initial platelet 'plugging' function is normal, the subsequent coagulation 'cascade' response is abnormal. This delay is usually hours, and occasionally days. Once bleeding occurs it may persist for days or even weeks. Patients who are severely affected may present with bleeding episodes on a weekly basis.

The most common manifestations of haemophilia are:

- bleeding into joints (knees, elbows, ankles, shoulders, hips, wrists in descending order of frequency)
- bleeding into soft tissues and muscles (the iliopsoas muscle around the hip, calf, forearm, upper arm, Achilles tendon, buttocks)
- bleeding in the mouth from a cut, bitten tongue or loss of a tooth
- haematuria
- superficial bruising
- haemarthroses – the bleeding is from synovial membrane appendicular structure, with inflammation of the synovium, and leads to degenerative arthritis, joint destruction and loss of joint mobility and function
- bleeding into tissue planes – tense flexor haematomas in limbs can cause compartment syndromes and haemorrhage into muscles may lead to atrophy and contracture
- bleeding into the neck (may cause airway compromise)
- central nervous system bleeding
- retroperitoneal bleeding.

Patients may also present with a complication of therapy. Most haemophiliac patients treated before 1985 have been exposed to pathogenic viruses, of which the most important are hepatitis C, hepatitis B and HIV. Of those who received plasma prior to the mid-1980s, 90% are hepatitis B positive, 85–100% are hepatitis C positive and 60–90% are HIV positive.

Clinical investigations

Investigations are tailored to the individual presentation. A full blood count, blood film and coagulation profiles are useful in the evaluation of first presentations, or major bleed, but unlikely to be helpful in patients with an established diagnosis. It is important to note that in an acute presentation, investigation and awaiting their results should not delay treatment with factor. The most important role for us in the emergency department is to administer factor as soon as is possible, blood results are not used to guide our use of factor in this group of patients. Generally, we always administer factor if we have any suspicion of a bleeding, regardless of how small we may think that bleed is.

Plain radiography of affected joints and computed tomography (CT) scanning of the head, chest, abdomen and pelvis may be essential to establish the presence or absence of bleeding complications.

The prothrombin time measures primarily Factors II, VII, V and X, thus patients with both haemophilia A and B have a normal prothrombin time and a normal thrombin clotting time. The partial thromboplastin time measures activation of all factors other than Factor VIII and is prolonged in haemophilia (although it can be normal if factor activity exceeds 30%). Specific factor assays are required to distinguish between haemophilias A and B.

Treatment

Treatment of haemophilia has evolved dramatically in the past 40 years with the discovery in the 1960s that coagulation Factor VIII was concentrated in cryoprecipitate. More recently, highly purified concentrates of Factor VIII and Factor IX have been developed.

Products currently available for the treatment of haemophilia include:

❶ 'Recombinate' (recombinant Factor VIII)
❷ 'BeneFix' (recombinant Factor IX)
❸ 'Biostate' (plasma-derived Factor VIII, includes von Willebrand factor)
❹ 'Monofix' (plasma-derived Factor IX)
❺ DDAVP (desmopressin).

Treatment of acute bleeding episodes primarily involves administration of factor replacement therapy. Complications of bleeding may require specific intervention. Adjunctive therapies include pain relief, rest and immobilization. Specific treatment is influenced by:

- the type of haemophilia
- the severity of haemophilia
- the severity of the bleed.

Haemophilia patients presenting with suspected bleeds should be triaged as ATS 3 and receive prompt assessment by a senior doctor. For muscle and joint bleeds 'RICES' should be initiated on arrival to limit bleeding and reduce pain:

- R = rest (in position of comfort)
- I = ice (cold pack to reduce bleeding and pain)
- C = gentle compression bandage
- E = elevation
- S = splint (severe/recurrent bleeds).

Options for adequate analgesia include:

- paracetamol and/or codeine
- inhaled nitrous oxide
- tramadol
- IV morphine
- may require patient controlled analgesia (PCA)/opioid infusion.

In the context of pain relief, aspirin (or other platelet-modifying drugs) should be avoided and non-steroidal anti-inflammatory drugs (NSAIDs) used with caution. Intramuscular injections should never be administered. In major bleeds, there may be a requirement for red cell transfusion. Developing limb compartment syndromes may require surgical decompression and intracranial bleeds may require neurosurgical intervention. In all of these cases, factor replacement must commence as quickly as possible. Management of complex presentations requires a multidisciplinary approach and early consultation with the relevant state haemophilia centre, especially if the presentation is a major bleed or the patient has inhibitors.

Intravenous cannulation is best performed by a skilled practitioner to help ensure vein preservation. Invasive procedures, such as arterial puncture and lumbar puncture, must only be performed after clotting factor replacement.

Some patients with Factor VIII levels higher than 10% may be successfully treated with 1-amino-8-D-arginine vasopressin (desmopressin, DDAVP), which acts by releasing von Willebrand factor stored in the lining of the blood vessels. Von Willebrand factor is a protein that transports Factor VIII in the bloodstream and, as such, plays an important role in blood clotting. Desmopressin appears to mobilize available Factor VIII stores and may raise Factor VIII activity by a factor of three. If the patient has previously had a documented good response to desmopressin, this can be used as first-line therapy for minor bleeding, such as haemarthroses.

Desmopressin can be administered intravenously, subcutaneously or by nasal spray. The intravenous dose is 0.3 μg/kg in 100 mL saline over no less than 45 min. A response should be evident within the first hour. More rapid administration can be associated with blood pressure changes. Side effects, including facial flushing and headache, are usually well tolerated. Tachyphylaxis tends to develop after three or four doses. The antidiuretic properties of desmopressin (which can last up to 24 h after a dose) can produce fluid retention and hyponatraemia (leading to seizures) and the serum sodium levels should be measured before giving further doses. Desmopressin is useful in treating mild and very rarely moderate haemophilia A. It is not of value in severe haemophilia A or with any type of haemophilia B. In serious bleeds or major surgery, desmopressin alone will not control bleeding. In such a case, most patients should also receive Factor VIII concentrate, recombinant Factor VIII replacement and recombinant Factor IX replacement.

Most haemophiliac patients are usually well known to their state haemophilia centres, who often hold specialized treatment protocols for difficult or complex patients. Patients should have their treatment regimen cards with them. If not they should be encouraged to do so.

One unit of Factor VIII concentrate provides the amount of Factor VIII activity in 1 mL of normal plasma. Given that a 70-kg adult has a plasma volume of 3500 mL, we can expect that an infusion of 3500 units of Factor VIII will produce 100% Factor VIII activity in a haemophiliac with negligible activity prior to treatment. The half-life of Factor VIII is approximately 12 h. Accordingly, a further dose of 1750 units in 12 hours' time will again restore 100% activity.

It is not always necessary to provide 100% Factor VIII activity in order to ensure haemostasis: levels of 30–50% may be sufficient in the context of haemarthrosis or dental extraction. Larger infusions should be reserved for life-threatening situations.

Treatment of bleeding

Minor bleed (e.g. spontaneous haemarthrosis or muscle bleed):

- Recombinate 20 units/kg single dose only
- BeneFIX 40 units/kg single dose only
- DDAVP (0.3 μg/kg in patients proven to be responsive).

Moderate bleed (e.g. epistaxsis, traumatic haemarthrosis, excluding hip):

- Recombinate 30 units/kg for first dose then 20 units/kg at 12 and 24 h
- BeneFIX 60 units/kg for first dose then 30 units/kg at 24 h
- DDAVP.

Major bleed (e.g. intracerebral, hip, neck, throat, psoas muscle):

- Recombinate 45 units/kg stat and urgent haematology consultation
- BeneFIX 90 units/kg stat and urgent haematology consultation.

Many patients can administer Factor VIII concentrate at home 'on demand'. Indeed, the availability of Factor VIII and the ease of administration have revolutionized the care of haemophiliac patients in the community. However, the following are indications for hospital admission:

- suspected intracranial haemorrhage
- a large bleed
- ongoing bleed
- suspected bleeding into the head, neck or throat
- need for ongoing therapy, especially infusions

- suspected compartment syndrome (especially of forearm and calf)
- bleeding into hip or inguinal area, suspected iliopsoas haemorrhage
- undiagnosed abdominal pain
- persistent haematuria
- ongoing analgesia requirements
- inadequate social circumstances.

Antifibrinolytic agents, such as tranexamic acid (cyclokapron) and aminocaproic acid (amicar), have been used as adjunctive therapy in episodes of gastrointestinal and mucosal bleeding, for example, following dental extraction. Fibrin tissue adhesives containing fibrinogen, thrombin and Factor XIII have also been successfully placed in tooth sockets and similar surgical sites.

Tranexamic acid and aminocaproic acid are useful in treating both haemophilia A and B. These drugs help to hold a clot in place once it has formed. They act by stopping the activity of plasmin, which dissolves blood clots. They do not actually help to form a clot which means they cannot be used instead of desmopressin or Factor VIII or IX concentrate, but can be used to hold a clot in place on mucous membranes, including in the oral cavity, nasal cavity, intestinal and uterine walls. Tranexamic acid and aminocaproic acid are associated with minor side effects including nausea, lethargy, vertigo, diarrhoea and abdominal pain.

Oral/dental bleeds

First-line therapy should be topical tranexamic acid mouthwash (5%). Patients hold 10 mL of the solution in the mouth near the site of bleeding (without gargling) for 2 min repeated 5 times a day for a week.

Haematuria

Factor replacement and antifibrinolytic therapy is not usually recommended in these cases due to the risk of clot retention and renal tract obstruction.

Head injury

Haemophiliac patients with even apparently minor head trauma need hospital assessment and CT head scanning. Beware of subtle signs of a developing subdural haematoma. If an intracranial bleed is suspected, replacement therapy should be initiated prior to radiological investigation.

Compartment syndrome

Compartment syndromes are relatively common in patients with hereditary and acquired bleeding disorders. As compartment syndrome is a clinincal diagnosis, measuring compartment pressure is generally not needed to make the diagnosis.

Four of the classic signs of compartment syndrome, pallor, pulselessness, paraesthesia and paralysis are all (very) late signs.

Pain is the earliest sign and has the following characteristics:

- pain out of proportion to the expected
- associated with hard/tense compartment on clinical examination
- severe pain on gentle passive stretch of that compartment (e.g. plantar flexion of ankle/toes thus stretching anterior compartment)
- unremitting/increasing pain with increasing requirement of pain medications.

The treatment for this condition is urgent fasciotomy.

Patients who present to the emergency department with bleeding disorders and suspected compartment syndrome should have the usual management for these conditions plus immediate referral to the orthopaedic unit and haematology unit.

Surgical decision making and indications for fasciotomy are the same as for patients without bleeding disorders and factor replacement dosage and frequency for these patients is the same as for any major surgery.

Antibodies to Factor VIII

Some patients develop antibodies to Factor VIII, known as 'inhibitors'. Treatment has to be modified according to the titre of inhibitor present (measured by the Bethesda inhibitor assay). Patients are classified as 'high responders' if their baseline inhibitor titre exceeds 10 Bethesda units (BU) or if the titre rises above 10 BU on exposure to Factor VIII. Different management strategies are employed according to the severity of the bleed. These include increasing the dose of Factor VIII or alternative therapies, such as activated prothrombin complex, porcine Factor VIII or recombinant Factor VIIa.

Most patients who develop inhibitors do so early in life and are known to have severe hereditary haemophilia, but inhibitors can also arise in previously normal individuals to produce an acquired haemophilia. The incidence of this phenomenon is from 0.2 to 1/1 000 000/year. Patients tend to be elderly and some have autoimmune disease, but there is also an association with pregnancy as well as with some drugs, notably penicillin. Patients haemorrhage into muscle and soft tissues and may present with haematemesis or with unusual postoperative bleeding. In the laboratory, the patient's blood shows a prolonged APPT that is not corrected by 'mixing', that is, by the addition of normal plasma. Factor VIII levels are low. Management is directed towards control of the bleeding episode, replacement therapy and the prevention of further reactions using a variety of immunosuppressive remedies.

Disposition

- Patients with 'minor' bleeds and no other complicating issues may be discharged after treatment in the emergency department but management should ideally be discussed first with the treating haemophilia unit and early review arranged.
- Patients with 'moderate' bleeds may need admission, preferably at the state treatment centre. These cases must be discussed with the treating unit before discharge from the emergency department.
- All patients with 'major' bleeds *must* be admitted and management discussed on an urgent basis with the treating haemophilia unit, prior to transferring care.

von Willebrand disease

Factor VIII has an intimate association with von Willebrand factor (vWF). This is an adhesive glycoprotein, secreted by endothelium and megakaryocytes, which is required for the normal instigation of platelet plug formation and for stabilization and transport of Factor VIII within the circulation. Thus von Willebrand disease (vWD) is a result of dysfunction, reduction or a complete lack of the vWF and is often associated with low Factor VIII activity. It is the most common inherited bleeding disorder, affecting 0.1–1% of the population and affects males and females equally.

Three types of von Willebrand disease are recognized:

- type I (common): reduced levels of vWF – clinically associated with mild bleeding
- type II (uncommon): abnormally functioning vWF – clinically associated with a variable bleeding pattern
- type III (rare): a near absence of vWF – clinical presentation is similar to that of moderate-to-severe haemophilia.

Common symptoms of vWD are:

- frequent nose bleeds
- easy bruising
- bleeding from gums following tooth extractions
- menorrhagia
- gastrointestinal bleeding.

Treatment

If the patient has previously had a documented good response to DDAVP, this can be used as first line in type I vWD. It is occasionally also effective in type II vWD, but never effective in type III vWD. The dose is the same as used in haemophilia (0.3 µg/kg). Antifibrinolytic agents, such as tranexamic acid, are often helpful for mucosal bleeding, epistaxis and menorrhagia. 'Biostate' (plasma derived Factor VIII, includes von Willebrand factor) may be required in type I vWD if bleeding is severe or unresponsive to DDAVP and it can also be used to treat bleeding in patients with type II and type III vWD.

Useful contacts

Websites

Australian Haemophilia Centre Directors' Organisation: www.ahcdo.org.au
Haemophilia Foundation Australia: www.haemophilia.org.au
Canadian Hemophilia Society: www.hemophilia.ca
Hemophilia Federation of America: www.hemophiliafed.org
Haemophilia Foundation Australia: www.haemophilia.org.au
Haemophilia Foundation of New Zealand: www.haemophilia.org.nz
Haemophilia Society (UK): www.haemophilia.org.uk
World Federation of Hemophilia: www.wfh.org

Contact numbers for advice/referrals

ACT
Canberra
The Canberra Hospital
Haemophilia Centre
Ward 14 A Yamba Drive Garran ACT 2605
Telephone 02 6244 2188/2286
Emergency 02 6244 2222
Fax 02 6244 2271

NSW
Newcastle
Mater Misericordiae Hospital
Haemophilia Centre
Edith Street Waratah NSW 2298
Telephone 02 4921 1240
Emergency 02 4921 1211
Fax 02 4960 2136

Sydney
Royal Prince Alfred Hospital
Haemophilia Centre
Page Building, Level 9 Missenden Road
Camperdown NSW 2050
Telephone 02 9515 7013
Emergency 02 9515 6111
Fax 02 9515 8946

The Children's Hospital
Cnr Hawkesbury Rd & Hainsworth St
Westmead NSW 2145
Telephone 02 9845 0000 and page haematologist on call
Emergency 02 9845 0000 and page haematologist on call
Fax 02 9845 3082

NT
Darwin
Royal Darwin Hospital
Rocklands Drive, Tiwi NT 0812
Telephone 08 8920 6176
Emergency 08 8922 8888
Fax 08 8920 6183

QLD
Brisbane
Royal Brisbane & Women's Hospital
Queensland Haemophilia Centre
Level 4, West Block, Butterfield Street,
Herston QLD 4029
Telephone 07 3636 5727/8760
Emergency 07 3636 8111
Fax 07 3636 4221

Royal Children's Hospital
Haemophilia Centre
Banksia Ward, Level 3 Woolworths Building,
Herston Road, Herston QLD 4029
Telephone 07 3636 9030
Emergency 07 3636 7472
Fax 07 3636 1552

SA
Adelaide
Royal Adelaide Hospital

Haematology Day Centre
Level 7 East Wing, North Terrace,
Adelaide 5000
Telephone 08 8222 4308/5632
Emergency 08 8222 4000
Fax 08 8222 4358

Women's and Children's Hospital
McGuinness – McDermott Foundation
Children's Clinic
72 King William Road, North Adelaide
SA 5006
Telephone 08 8161 7411
Emergency 08 8161 7000
Fax 08 8161 6567

TAS
Hobart
Royal Hobart Hospital
Paediatric Ambulatory Care Unit
Liverpool Street, Hobart TAS 7000
Telephone 03 6222 8045
Emergency 03 6222 8308
Fax 03 6222 8900

VIC
Melbourne
The Alfred
Ronald Sawers Haemophilia Centre
Commercial Road, Melbourne Vic 3004
Telephone 03 9076 2178
Emergency 03 9076 2000
Fax 03 9076 3021

Royal Children's Hospital
The Henry Ekert Haemophilia Treatment Centre
Flemington Road Parkville Vic 3052
Telephone 03 9345 5099
Emergency 03 9345 5522
Fax 03 9345 5099

WA
Perth
Royal Perth Hospital
Haemophilia Centre
Kirkman House, 10 Murray Street, Perth
WA 6000
Telephone 08 9224 2937/2897
Emergency 08 9224 2244
Fax 08 9224 8475

Princess Margaret Hospital for Children
Oncology & Haematology Ward 3B
Roberts Road, Subiaco WA 6008
Telephone 08 9340 8682/8234
Emergency 08 9340 8222
Fax 08 9341 9842

Fremantle

Fremantle Hospital

Alma Street, Fremantle WA 6160

Telephone 08 9431 2210/2886

Emergency 08 9431 3333

Fax 08 9431 2881

Further reading

Bell BA, Birch K, Glazer S. Experience with recombinant factor VIIA in an infant with haemophilia with inhibitors to FVIII:C undergoing emergency central line placement. A case report. Am J Pediatr Hematol Oncol 1993;15:77–9.

Bush MT, Roy N. Hemophilia emergencies. J Emerg Nurs 1995;21:531–8.

De Behnke DJ, Angelos MG. Intracranial hemorrhage and hemophilia: case report and management guidelines. J Emerg Med 1990;8:423–7.

Pfaff JA, Geninatti M. Hemophilia. Emerg Med Clin N Am 1993;11:337–63.

Warrier I, Ewenstein BM, Koerper MA, et al. Factor IX inhibitors and anaphylaxis in hemophilia B. J Pediatr Hematol Oncol 1997;19:23–7.

13.5 Blood and blood products

Sean Arendse • Biswadev Mitra

ESSENTIALS

1 The decision to transfuse packed red cells should ultimately be based on the knowledge that the patient's oxygen carrying capacity has dropped to an unacceptably low level.

2 The administration of blood products carries substantial risk. The emergency physician should always ensure that potential benefits outweigh potential risks and communicate these risks and benefits in order to obtain informed consent where possible.

3 Rigorous risk management of administrative and clinical processes minimize the risk of serious adverse reaction from transfusion of blood products.

Introduction

Blood is living tissue composed of blood cells suspended in plasma; it transports nutrients and oxygen and facilitates temperature control. An average 70-kg male has a blood volume of about 5 L. The cellular elements comprise red blood cells, white blood cells and platelets and make up about 45% of the volume of whole blood. Plasma, which is 92% water, makes up the remaining 55%.

Early attempts at blood transfusion were thwarted by adverse reactions. In 1900, Karl Landsteiner demonstrated the ABO blood group system and explained many of the observed severe incompatibility reactions (Table 13.5.1). He won the Nobel prize for medicine in 1930 and went on to discover the Rhesus factor in 1940. The next major advance in transfusion medicine occurred with the development of long-term anticoagulants, such as sodium citrate, which allowed extended preservation of blood. Development of refrigeration procedures allowed storage of anticoagulated blood. The addition of a citrate–glucose solution extended the viability of collected blood to several days. The ability to preserve blood for longer than a few hours paved the way for the establishment of the first blood bank in a Leningrad hospital in 1932.

Transfusion of blood and blood products is now routine and vital to the practice of emergency medicine. As with any prescribed treatment, these products are associated with potential hazards as well as advantages. The hazards are more likely to be encountered with blood products used during emergencies. The blood products available in most Australian emergency departments (EDs) are packed red blood cells, platelets, fresh frozen plasma (FFP), cryoprecipitate, activated Factor VII, prothrombin complex concentrates and other factor concentrates.

In the Australian urban hospital setting, 50% of packed red cells are used for the treatment of anaemia, 22% pre- or perioperatively and 13% for abnormal, excessive or continued bleeding. Medical oncology uses 78% of all platelets. Forty-one per cent of all FFP is used to correct coagulopathy associated with surgery, 27% to correct coagulopathy in bleeding, 16% to reverse haemostatic disorders in patients having massive blood transfusion, 11.5% for reversal of warfarin effect and the remaining 4.5% for a number of miscellaneous conditions, including liver disease and disseminated intravascular coagulation (DIC).

In the ED setting, blood products are most often administered to patients with acute rather than chronic blood loss. In trauma centres, severely injured patients are the major consumers of blood products while, in non-trauma centres, patients with gastrointestinal haemorrhage account for the majority of transfusions. In these settings of acute blood loss, transfusion may be required rapidly and in large quantities. However, as short stay units are developed, non-time critical transfusions of blood products for other medical indications are increasingly the responsibility of ED staff.

Packed red blood cells

Packed red blood cells are produced from whole blood collections by removing most of the plasma by centrifugation and then resuspending the red cells in citrate-based anticoagulant-preservative solution to prolong storage time. Each unit of packed cells contains approximately 200 mL of red cells. Transfusion of one unit can be expected to raise the haematocrit by 3% and the haemoglobin by 10 g/L provided there is no ongoing blood loss.

Packed red cells are the blood product most commonly prescribed in the ED, the usual indication being the replacement of acute blood loss. Transfusion of packed red cells is

Table 13.5.1	The ABO group system	
ABO blood group	Antigens on red cells	Antibody in serum
O	None	Anti-A, anti-B
A	A	Anti-B
B	B	Anti-A
AB	A, B	None

Table 13.5.2 Potential indications for red cell transfusion

Haemorrhage
Dilutional anaemia following severe burns
Iron-deficiency anaemia
Megaloblastic anaemia
Anaemia of chronic disorders
Chronic renal failure
Failure of erythropoiesis
Sickle cell disease
Septic shock
Disseminated intravascular coagulopathy

Table 13.5.3 Guidelines for transfusion of blood components

Indications	Considerations
Red blood cells	
Hb	
<70 g/L	Lower thresholds may be acceptable in patients without symptoms and/or where specific therapy is available
70–100 g/L	Likely to be appropriate during surgery associated with major blood loss or if there are signs or symptoms of impaired oxygen transport
>80 g/L	May be appropriate to control anaemia-related symptoms in a patient on a chronic transfusion regimen or during marrow suppressive therapy
>100 g/L	Not likely to be appropriate unless there are specific indications
Platelets	
Bone marrow failure	At a platelet count of $<10 \times 10^9$/L in the absence of risk factors and $<20 \times 10^9$ in the presence of risk factors (e.g. fever, antibiotics, evidence of systemic haemostatic failure)
Surgery/invasive procedure	To maintain platelet count at $>50 \times 10^9$/L. For surgical procedures with high risk of bleeding (e.g. ocular or neurosurgery), it may be appropriate to maintain at 100×10^9/L
Platelet function disorders	May be appropriate in inherited or acquired disorders, depending on clinical features and setting. In this situation, platelet count is not a reliable indicator
Bleeding	May be appropriate in any patient in whom thrombocytopaenia is considered a major contributory factor
Massive haemorrhage/transfusion	Use should be confined to patients with thrombocytopaenia and/or functional abnormalities who have significant bleeding from this cause. May be appropriate when the platelet count is $<50 \times 10^9$/L ($<100 \times 10^9$/L in the presence of diffuse microvascular bleeding)
Fresh frozen plasma	
Single factor deficiencies	Use specific factors if available
Warfarin effect	In the presence of life-threatening bleeding. Use in addition to vitamin-K-dependent concentrates
Acute DIC	Indicated where there is bleeding and abnormal coagulation. Not indicated for chronic DIC
TTP	Accepted treatment
Coagulation inhibitor deficiencies	May be appropriate in patients undergoing high-risk procedures
Following massive transfusion or cardiac bypass	Use specific factors if available. May be appropriate in the presence of bleeding and abnormal coagulation
Liver disease	May be appropriate in the presence of bleeding and abnormal coagulation
Cryoprecipitate	
Fibrinogen deficiency	May be appropriate where there is clinical bleeding, an invasive procedure, trauma or DIC

TTP: idiopathic thrombocytopaenia purpura; DIC: disseminated intravascular coagulation. Adapted from the National Health and Medical Research Council and Australasian Society Clinical Practice Guidelines on appropriate use of blood components. http://www.nhmrc.gov.au/publications/synopses/-files/cp82.pdf.

indicated where the patient's oxygen-carrying capacity is so impaired that control of bleeding alone, if indeed it can be readily achieved, is regarded as insufficient to prevent tissue hypoxia. In patients with primary haematological conditions, failure of erythropoiesis or a haemolysis, the indication for transfusion is usually the same as for haemorrhage: a severe reduction in oxygen-carrying capacity. In patients with associated complex multisystem failure, such as DIC or septic shock, red cell transfusion may be life saving by improving the oxygen debt in tissues (Table 13.5.2).

The indication of transfusion in haemorrhagic shock has been traditionally defined as persistent haemodynamic instability post-3 L of crystalloids. However, a further two patient factors must be considered. First is the concept of hypotensive resuscitation, which states that prior to definitive cessation of bleeding, relative hypotension may stabilize clots and reduce further bleeding. The clinican must therefore alter their thresholds of haemodynamic instability. Patient factors must be borne in mind, including the cardiovascular co-morbidities and the presence of head injuries. Secondly, both high volume crystalloid and blood transfusion have been associated with adverse outcomes, suggesting limitations of both, instead focusing resuscitation on the management of coagulopathy and early surgical management of haemorrhage.

Transfusion is not indicated when alternative haematinic therapy is deemed safe and appropriate. A moderately anaemic patient who is asymptomatic and not bleeding, with some reserve oxygen-carrying capacity, does not require blood transfusion. A haemoglobin of 7 g/dL is sometimes taken as the failsafe point in the decision whether to transfuse, although of course the patient's unique circumstances need to be taken into account: treat the patient, not the number. It should be also considered that, in an acutely bleeding patient, the initial haemoglobin result, measured at a time of volume contraction, may be an inaccurate representation of circulating oxygen carrying capacity. The National Health and Medical Research Council together with the Australasian Society of Blood Transfusion have published transfusion guidelines for red blood cells and other products (Table 13.5.3).

Prior to any blood product transfusion, informed consent should be sought, obtained and documented, except in emergent cases where the delays may result in substantial adverse effects. The following sections discuss the risks of red cell transfusion.

Effect of storage on red blood cells

Although it makes intuitive sense that blood loss should be replaced by blood products, there is evidence that the immediate observed benefit is from volume replacement rather than improved oxygen carriage. Red blood cells may not be fully functional until 2–6 h after transfusion because storage affects the oxygen-carrying capacity of blood. This is probably due to decreased intracellular 2,3-diphosphoglycerate (2,3-DPG), loss of red cell viability, decreased red cell deformability, relative acidosis and potassium leakage.

Storage reduces 2,3-DPG levels, leading to a leftward shift of the oxyhaemoglobin dissociation curve and increased affinity of oxygen binding. The transfused red cell does regenerate 2,3-DPG to normal levels but this can take 6–24 h post transfusion. With increasing age of stored red cells, levels of 2,3-DPG progressively fall such that by 5–6 weeks the level is 10% of normal. It is still uncertain whether this abnormality is physiologically important, even in critically ill patients. In addition, hypocalcaemia, cell lysis, release of free haemoglobin, changes in nitric oxide levels, alterations in pH and increases in lipids, complement and cytokines are other effects of red cell storage. These changes are accompanied by increased membrane fragility, which can compromise microcirculatory flow and lead to increased red cell–endothelial cell interaction and inflammatory cytokine release. Such changes could explain recent findings associating age of red blood cells with adverse outcomes and may be particularly disadvantageous to critically ill patients with a higher mortality risk.

When red cells are transfused, some of the cells are removed from the circulation within a few hours, with the rest surviving normally; as the storage time increases to 42 days, more cells are removed immediately after transfusion. This loss of viability is highly dependent upon the anticoagulant-preservative solution used.

Potassium gradually leaks out of stored red cells and this raises the plasma potassium by approximately 1 mEq/L per day. Citrate toxicity results when the citrate in the transfused blood begins to bind calcium in the patient's body, resulting in hypocalcaemia. Clinically significant hypocalcaemia does not usually occur unless the rate of transfusion exceeds 1 unit every 5 minutes or so. Citrate metabolism is primarily hepatic – so hepatic disease or dysfunction can cause this effect to be more pronounced.

Choice of red cell product

The choice of red cell product is determined by time and safety considerations. O-negative red cells, the universal donor group, are readily available in most major hospitals. Supplies of O-negative blood are limited and the product should be used with care. The transfusion of O-negative blood is generally reserved for transfusion immediately during patient reception and the initial stages of resuscitation, switching to cross-matched blood as soon as available. It is preferable that blood be collected prior to transfusion so as to characterize the recipient's blood group serology. Premenopausal female patients should be given group O Rhesus negative, Kell negative blood in an emergency situation in order to avoid sensitization and possibility of haemolytic disease of newborn in subsequent pregnancies. Male patients, however, can be transfused either Rhesus positive or negative blood. The incidence of adverse reaction using this type of blood is approximately 3%. By contrast, the provision of group-specific blood requires matching a blood sample to the major (ABO) and Rhesus D compatibility groups only. Group-specific blood can be available for transfusion within 35 min depending on the logistic support and staffing levels within the haematology laboratory. It has an incidence of adverse reaction similar to O-negative blood. As O-negative blood is usually in short supply, it is preferable where possible to infuse group-specific blood. A more comprehensive cross-match where there are no atypical antibodies identified in the initial screening can take 30 min or more and the incidence of adverse transfusion reaction is reduced to 0.01%.

Precautions when cross-matching and transfusing blood

Although most patients do not require transfusion in the ED, it is often appropriate to 'group and hold' or cross-match the patient while in the department. Many hospitals have written protocols detailing the anticipated requirements for a given surgical procedure. Documentation should be meticulous. It should be mandated that the person drawing the blood for cross-matching should also fill in and sign the laboratory request form. Most severe incompatibility reactions to blood transfusion result not from exposure to unusual antigens but from administrative errors. Any systematic change in documentation protocols, for example, the adoption of an electronic record, needs to be accompanied by obsessive risk management strategies.

The checking of the compatibility details of blood to be transfused must be meticulous. Blood products should not be left lying around workbenches. Universal precautions must be observed by staff setting up transfusions. Rapid or large transfusions should be via a blood warmer. Blood is transfused intravenously through sterile giving sets containing 170 μm filters. Alternative routes (arterial, intraperitoneal or intraosseous) are only used in exceptional circumstances. Lines for transfusion should be dedicated lines; drugs and other additives should be administered at separate sites. Normal saline is compatible with all blood components.

Pulse, blood pressure and temperature are measured at regular intervals and particular attention is paid to the patient during the first 25 min of the transfusion. The transfusion is started slowly. The rate at which it continues depends on clinical urgency. As a general rule, the faster the anaemia has developed the more rapidly it needs to be corrected. Rapid infusion techniques may be indicated in patients who appear to be exsanguinating, but over-rapid infusion may precipitate cardiac failure in the elderly. Hypothermia may be a problem if a blood warmer is not used.

Adverse reactions to transfusion

The principal adverse reactions to blood transfusion are listed in Table 13.5.4. Serious adverse reactions are relatively rare (Table 13.5.5), although some are more likely to occur when blood is administered urgently.

Immunological transfusion reactions

Immunological transfusion reactions may be immediate or delayed in onset.

Immediate

Febrile non-haemolytic reactions The most common transfusion reaction is a febrile, non-haemolytic transfusion reaction (FNHTR), which is defined as an increase in temperature of 1°C or more over baseline during a transfusion. It manifests as fever and occasionally shortness of breath 1–6 h after transfusion. FNHTRs are benign, but their presentation is very similar to acute haemolytic transfusion reaction and infection, which have a higher rate of mortality and morbidity, mandating early clinical review to exclude more serious complications.

Acute haemolytic reactions Acute haemolytic transfusion reactions (ATHRs) result from the rapid destruction of donor red cells by preformed recipient antibodies and are a

Table 13.5.4 Adverse effects of blood transfusion

Immunological transfusion reactions	Transmission of infection
Immediate	Bacterial
Febrile non-haemolytic reactions	Brucella
Acute haemolytic transfusion reactions	Pseudomonas
Allergic reactions and anaphylaxis	Salmonella
Transfusion-related acute lung injury	Treponema pallidum
Delayed	Parasites
Delayed haemolytic transfusion reactions	Babesia
Alloimmunization	Plasmodium
Transfusion-associated graft versus host disease	Toxoplasma
Hypothermia	Trypanosoma
Dilutional coagulopathy	Viruses
Volume overload	Cytomegalovirus
	Hepatitis B and delta agent
	Hepatitis A
	Hepatitis C
	Other hepatitis 'non-A, non-B'
	HIV-1 and HIV-2
	HTLV-1 and HTLV-2
	Parvovirus

HIV: human immunodeficiency virus; HTLV: human T-cell lymphotropic virus.

Table 13.5.5 Incidence of adverse transfusion reactions (per unit packed red cells transfused)

Adverse transfusion reaction	Incidence	Mortality
Bacterial sepsis	1 in 40 000–500 000	1 in 4–8 million
Acute haemolytic reaction	1 in 12 000–38 000	1 in 600 000–1.5 million
Delayed haemolytic reaction	1 in 1000–12 000	1 in 2.5 million
Anaphylaxis	1 in 20 000–50 000	
Transfusion-related acute lung injury	1 in 5000–100 000	1 in 5 million
Fluid overload	1 in 100–700	
Transfusion-associated graft versus host disease	Rare	90% fatality

Adapted from Australian Red Cross website: http://www.transfusion.com.au/adverse_events (Accessed April 2013).

medical emergency. They are usually due to ABO incompatibility and most often the result of clerical or procedural errors. ABO and Rhesus compatibility between donors and recipients is presented in Table 13.5.6. Some acquired alloantibodies, such as anti-Rh or anti-Jka, are occasionally implicated, but AHTRs more typically occur when a group O recipient is transfused with non-group O red cells. This may lead to DIC, shock and acute tubular necrosis precipitating acute renal failure. These reactions usually manifest with fever and rigors, lumbar pain, crushing chest pain, tachycardia, hypotension and haemoglobinaemia with subsequent haemoglobinuria. The symptoms usually develop within the first 30 min of transfusion.

Anaphylactoid transfusion reactions Anaphylactoid reactions usually begin within 1–45 min of the start of transfusion of blood products but less severe reactions can be delayed up to 2–3 h. Generally, a shorter time between commencement of the transfusion and onset of symptoms is associated with a more severe reaction. These reactions are manifested by rapid onset of shock, hypotension, angio-oedema and respiratory distress. They are almost always due to the presence of class-specific IgG, anti-IgA antibodies in patients who are IgA deficient. Selective IgA deficiency is not uncommon, occurring in about 1 in 300–500 people. The incidence of anaphylactic transfusion reactions can be reduced by the use of washed products (e.g. washed red cells) and by premedicating the patient with antipyretics and antihistamines.

Treatment of an anaphylactoid transfusion reaction consists of immediate cessation of transfusion and standard treatment of anaphylaxis including, oxygen fluids and adrenaline (see Chapter 28.7).

Transfusion-related acute lung injury Transfusion-related acute lung injury (TRALI) is a syndrome characterized by acute respiratory distress following transfusion. All plasma-containing blood products have been implicated including rare reports involving IVIG and cryoprecipitate. It is a rare complication of allogeneic blood transfusion but the incidence has not been well established due to difficulty in defining the syndrome and variable reporting mechanisms worldwide. Symptoms of TRALI typically develop during, or within 6 hours of a transfusion. Patients present with the rapid onset of dyspnoea and tachypnoea. There may be associated fever, cyanosis and hypotension. Clinical exam reveals respiratory distress and pulmonary crackles may be present with no signs of congestive heart failure or volume overload. Chest X-ray (CXR) shows evidence of bilateral pulmonary oedema unassociated with heart failure (non-cardiogenic pulmonary oedema), with bilateral patchy infiltrates, which may rapidly progress to complete 'white out' indistinguishable from acute respiratory distress syndrome. The central venous pressure

Table 13.5.6 ABO and Rhesus compatibility between donors and recipients

Donors		O +	A +	B +	AB +	O –	A –	B –	AB –
Recipients									
	O +	C				C			
	A +	C	C			C	C		
	B +	C		C		C		C	
	AB +	C	C	C	C	C	C	C	C
	O –					C			
	A –					C	C		
	B –					C		C	
	AB –					C	C	C	C

C: compatible.

Table 13.5.7 Risks of transfusion transmitted infection (per unit tested blood transfused)

Infection	Residual risk
CMV	1 in 127 000
Hepatitis B	Approximately 1 in 660 000
Syphilis	Considerably less than 1 in a million
Hepatitis C	<1 in 10 million
HIV	<1 in 10 million
HTLV I and II	<1 in 10 million
Variant CJD	Possible and cannot be excluded

CMV: cytomegalovirus; HIV: human immunodeficiency virus; HTLV: human T-cell lymphotropic virus; CJD: Creutzfeldt–Jakob disease.
Adapted from Australian Red Cross website: http://www.transfusion.com.au/adverse_events (Accessed April 2013).

is normal, which helps distinguish the condition from transfusion-associated circulatory overload. Treatment is supportive. There is no role for diuretics or corticosteroids The blood bank needs to be notified as reporting of TRALI allows better understanding of the true incidence of this reaction, in addition to its clinical course and associated mortality

Delayed

Delayed haemolytic transfusion reaction These reactions occur in patients who have developed antibodies from previous transfusions or pregnancy but, at the time of pretransfusion testing, the antibody in question is too weak to be detected by standard procedures. Subsequent transfusion with red cells having the corresponding antigen results in an anamnestic antibody response and haemolysis of transfused red cells. These delayed reactions are seen generally within 2–10 days after transfusion. Haemolysis is usually extravascular, gradual and less severe than with acute reactions, but rapid haemolysis can occur. A falling haematocrit, slight fever, mild increase in serum unconjugated bilirubin and spherocytosis on the blood smear may be noted.

Treatment of a delayed haemolytic transfusion reaction is usually not required unless anaemia is severe enough to require treatment. However, future transfusions containing the implicated red cell antigen need to be avoided. Alternatives to transfusion should be explored whenever possible.

Red cell alloimmunization When antibodies are formed against foreign antigens from one's own species, the process is termed alloimmunization and the antibodies are called alloantibodies (as opposed to forming autoantibodies to one's own antigens or forming xenoantibodies to antigens from a foreign species). Transfused (non-leucocyte depleted) red cells and platelets contain leucocytes to which antibodies can be made. This may cause patients to become resistant to subsequent platelet transfusions. Approximately 50% of patients undergoing multiple blood transfusions become alloimmunized and are refractory to further platelet transfusions. Refractory patients require platelets matched to their specific platelet/human leucocyte antigen (HLA) type. Patients receiving leucocyte reduced blood products are at a much lower risk for refractoriness to platelet transfusion than are recipients of non-leucocyte reduced blood products. Although debate exists about its merits, for selected high-risk patients with transfusion-dependent diseases (e.g. sickle cell anaemia, thalassaemia, etc.), some transfusion services phenotype patients and provide phenotypically matched donor RBC, even to those patients without alloantibodies (i.e. to prevent the formation of antibodies). There is general agreement that this is useful for Rhesus and Kell blood group antigens in these groups of patients, but debate exists about its merits for more extensive phenotyping.

Transfusion-associated graft-versus-host disease (TA-GVHD) Transfusion-associated graft-versus-host disease results from transfusion of viable T lymphocytes which proliferate and damage the recipient's tissue, particularly skin, gastrointestinal tract, liver, spleen and bone marrow. This is a rare and almost always fatal complication of transfusion. Clinical manifestations typically develop 10–14 days following transfusion and consist of fever, erythematous skin rash, pancytopaenia, diarrhoea and abnormal liver function. High-risk patients for this complication include bone marrow transplant recipients, patients receiving granulocyte transfusions, transfusions from a biologically related donor (directed donation), the fetus (intrauterine transfusion), exchange transfusion, patients with Hodgkin lymphoma and patients with congenital cellular immune deficiency.

The investigation begins with the confirmation of the presence of GVHD. This is a pathological diagnosis requiring a skin or intestinal biopsy. Currently, the only method of preventing TA-GVHD is to gamma irradiate cellular components at risk of causing TA-GVHD or destined for at-risk recipients. Current techniques to leucoreduce cellular blood components are not adequate to prevent TA-GVHD

Transmission of infection

In Australia, blood is tested for ABO and Rh (D) blood groups, red cell antibodies and the following infections:

- human immunodeficiency virus 1 and 2
- hepatitis B and C
- human T-cell lymphotropic virus I and II
- syphilis.

In terms of viral safety, Australia has one of the safest blood supplies in the world (Table 13.5.7).

Hypothermia

Red blood cells are stored at 4°C. Rapid infusion of large volumes of stored blood can contribute to hypothermia. Blood warmers should be used during massive blood transfusion.

In addition, other intravenous fluids should be warmed and other measures instituted to maintain patient body temperature (see Chapter 28.2).

Dilutional coagulopathies

Clinically significant depletion of coagulation proteins and platelets is a complication of massive transfusion, secondary to dilution and the consumptive coagulopathy of trauma. Stored red cells are deficient in platelets and clotting factors and transfusion of large amounts can complicate bleeding when not accompanied by assessment and correction of coagulation disturbances. Coagulation parameters including the prothrobin time (PT), activated partial thromboplastin time (APTT), platelet count and fibrinogen level should be monitored and corrected if deficiencies occur in the presence of abnormal bleeding. In actively bleeding patients, however, these parameters may not provide an accurate estimate of clot strength and results are often delayed by 30–60 minutes. Thromboelastography has the advantage of providing real-time assessment of clot strength and should be utilized where available.

Volume overload

This complication occurs when excessive volume of fluid is administered. Pulmonary oedema is a particular risk in the elderly, in infants and in patients with chronic severe anaemia where the red cell mass is decreased but the blood volume is normal. Abdominal compartment syndrome may result in bowel ischaemia and should be watched for.

Management of transfusion reactions

The first action to be taken in the management of any suspected transfusion reaction is to stop the transfusion immediately and assess the patient. The bag containing the transfused cells, along with all attached labels, should not be discarded so as to allow repeat typing and cross-matching of this unit by the blood bank. Management then proceeds as follows:

- maintain the patient's airway, blood pressure and heart rate
- from a different limb to the one transfused, obtain a sample for a direct antiglobulin test, plasma-free haemoglobin and repeat

blood group and cross-match. Save a urine sample for haemoglobin testing
- culture the patient's blood
- commence broad-spectrum antibiotics to cover Gram-positive skin organisms and Gram-negative organisms.

The laboratory which tested and issued the blood should be alerted immediately and a search for any clerical error instituted. Every hospital has a protocol for evaluating transfusion reactions, which should be rigorously followed. The haematology unit should notify the local blood bank, who have a haematologist on-call at all times and are responsible for the recall of any other implicated components from the same donor in the case of suspected infection or transfusion-related acute lung injury. If there is any suggestion (e.g. clerical mistake, hypotension, pink plasma or urine) that an AHTR is possible, oxygen should be applied to the patient and fluid resuscitation with saline to maintain a urine output of 2–3 mL/kg/h, in an attempt to prevent acute oliguric renal failure. A vasopressor, such as adrenaline, may be required. If massive intravascular haemolysis has already occurred, hyperkalaemia is likely and cardiac monitoring and acute haemodialysis may be required.

Platelets

Platelets are one of the main cellular components of blood and are central to haemostasis. Platelet products commonly available for transfusion are obtained by apheresis from a single donor or from donated blood using buff-coat or platelet-rich plasma techniques. Modifications to reduce the risk of viral transmission and prevent graft-versus-host disease include leucocyte reduction, irradiation, plasma depletion and the use of platelet additive solutions.

Platelets are transfused to prevent or treat haemorrhage in patients with thrombocytopaenia or defects in platelet function. Specific indications for platelet transfusion are shown in Table 13.5.3. Use of platelets is not generally considered appropriate in the treatment of immune-mediated platelet destruction, thrombotic thrombocytopaenic purpura, haemolytic uraemic syndrome or drug-induced or cardiac bypass thrombocytopaenia without haemorrhage.

In general, one platelet unit will raise the platelet count about $5–10 \times 10^9/L$ in an average adult. Depending on the method of

manufacture, the volume of each unit of platelets varies from 100 to 160 mL, with a storage life of about 5 days at 20–24°C.

Compatibility testing is not necessary in routine platelet transfusion, although platelet components should preferably be ABO and Rh type compatible with the recipient. ABO-incompatible platelets may be used if ABO compatible platelets are not available. The usual dose in an adult patient is 4 units, which is equivalent to 1 unit of apheresis platelets or 1 unit of pooled platelets.

Fresh frozen plasma

FFP is prepared from anticoagulated blood by separating the plasma from the blood cells through centrifugation of whole blood or apheresis. It is stored frozen until used. It contains all coagulation factors including small amounts of Factor V and approximately 200 units of Factor VIII. Fresh frozen plasma can be stored at below −25°C for up to 12 months. Indications for use of FFP are shown in Table 13.5.3.

The appropriate dose depends on the clinical indication, patient size and results of laboratory tests. A general guide is 10–15 mL/kg per dose but, in some situations, dosages greater than this may be required (e.g. dilutional coagulopathy in the context of massive transfusion). On average 1 mL of FFP/kg patient weight will raise most coagulation factors by 1%, therefore a dose of 10–15 mL/kg would be expected to increase levels by 10–15%. Compatibility testing is not required, however, ABO compatible plasma should be used wherever possible. Group AB plasma can be used for all patients in an emergency.

Cryoprecipitate

Cryoprecipitate is prepared by thawing FFP to between 1 and 6°C and recovering the precipitable protein fraction. It contains most of the Factor VIII, fibrinogen, Factor XIII, von Willebrand factor and fibronectin from the FFP. It may be stored for up to 12 months at −25°C or below. Once thawed it must be used immediately or stored at 2–6°C for up to 24 h. Cryoprecipitate is indicated in fibrinogen deficiency with clinical bleeding or prior to an invasive procedure and in DIC. Cryoprecipitate is transfused to keep fibrinogen levels above 1.0 g/L in the acutely bleeding patient. Compatibility tests before transfusion are not necessary. It is preferable to use an ABO group compatible with the recipient's red cells, however, ABO incompatible can be used with caution. Up to 4 units/10 kg body weight may be required to raise the fibrinogen concentration by approximately 0.5 g/L in the absence of continued haemorrhage.

The use of cryoprecipitate is not generally considered appropriate in the treatment of haemophilia, von Willebrand's disease or deficiencies of Factor XIII or fibronectin, unless alternative therapies are unavailable.

Refusal of blood and blood product transfusion

Patients with certain religious beliefs may refuse blood and blood product transfusion, e.g. Jehovah's witnesses. Healthy volunteers can tolerate Hb levels of 50 g/L without evidence of end-organ hypoxia. However, it is estimated that the median Hb concentration associated with mortality is about 25 g/L. The patient's wishes must be rigorously protected and blood products avoided. Several strategies may be used to manage the anaemia. Sedation should be instituted to minimize metabolic demand. A ventilation cycle of 2 hours of 90% FiO_2, followed by 2 hours of 90% SpO_2 and then 20 hours of 95% SpO_2 may be employed to maximize oxygen delivery while minimizing shunt from absorption atelectasis and to promote erythropoiesis. Recombinant erythropoietin (36 000 units daily), folic acid (5 mg daily), vitamin B12 (1 mg daily) and iron infusions are options to maximize haematopoiesis. In female patients, where applicable, menses should be inhibited with progesterone. Blood testing should be rationalized and performed using paediatric-sized samples.

A few case studies on the use of synthetic haemoglobin have been published. HBOC-201 is the commonest product used and is a modified lactated Ringer's solution containing 130 g/L of polymerized Hb of bovine origin. It is compatible with all blood types, stable for 3 years when stored at 2–30°C and stable for 2 years when stored at 40°C. When fully saturated, HBOC-201 has the same oxygen-carrying capacity as whole blood with the same Hb concentration. The partial pressure of oxygen at which HBOC-201 is 50% saturated (40 mmHg) is higher than that for cellular Hb (27 mmHg), which facilitates oxygen delivery to tissues. The half-life of HBOC-201 is approximately 20 hours. Polymerization of the Hb reduces its glomerular diffusion and nephrotoxicity. The use of synthetic haemoglobin remains experimental at this stage and outcomes of further trials currently underway aim to determine the efficacy and safety profile of such products.

Controversies

- While the changes observed during red cell storage affect overall red cell viability and function, there are no randomized controlled studies examining the effect of storage duration on recipient morbidity and mortality.
- Acute coagulopathy has been observed in up to 40% of cases of massive acute haemorrhage, associated with tissue injury and shock. Best practice guidelines for use of platelets, cryoprecipitate or FFP in the shocked patient are determined primarily from observational studies and expert opinion. Prospective randomized controlled trials are required to determine optimal management strategies in the acutely haemorrhaging and coagulopathic patient.
- The potential for prions, thought to be the infective molecules in the variant form of Creutzfeldt–Jakob disease, to be transmitted by blood transfusion has become a subject for intense scrutiny for transfusion medicine.

Further reading

Beckwith H, Manson L, McFarlane C, Reed MJ. A review of blood product usage in a large emergency department over a one-year period. Emerg Med J 2010;27:439–42.

Clinical Practice Guidelines on the Use of Blood Components (red blood cells, platelets, fresh frozen plasma, cryoprecipitate). National Health and Medical Research Council and Australasian Society of Blood Transfusion Clinical. <http://www.nhmrc.gov.au/_files_nhmrc/publications/attachments/cp78_cp_blood_components.pdf>; 2002 [Accessed Apr. 2003].

Council of Europe. Guide to the preparation, use and quality assurance of blood components. Recommendation R (95) 15, 11th ed. Strasbourg: Council of Europe Publishing 2005;1–266.

Dabrowski GP, Steinberg SM, Ferrara JJ, et al. A critical assessment of endpoints of shock resuscitation. Surg Clin N Am 2000;80:825–44.

Koch CG, Li L, Sessler DI, et al. Duration of red-cell storage and complications after cardiac surgery. N Engl J Med 2008;358:1229–39.

McKinley BA, Valdivia A, Moore FA. Goal orientated shock resuscitation for major torso trauma. Curr Opin Crit Care 2003;9:292–9.

Neal D, Hoffman MK, Cuschieri J, et al. Crystalloid to packed red blood cell transfusion ratio in the massively transfused patient: when a little goes a long way. J Trauma Acute Care Surg 2012;72:892–8.

Popovsky MA, Chaplin Jr HC, et al. Transfusion-related acute lung injury: a neglected, serious complication of hemotherapy. Transfusion 1992;32:589–92.

Reiss RF. Hemostatic defects in massive transfusion: rapid diagnosis and management. Am J Crit Care 2000;9:158–65.

Walsh TS, McArdle F, McLellan SA, et al. Does the storage time of transfused red blood cells influence regional or global indexes of tissue oxygenation in anaemic critically ill patients? Crit Care Med 2004;32:364–71.

Weiskopf RB. Emergency transfusion for acute severe anemia: a calculated risk. Anesth Analg 2010;111:1088–92.

RHEUMATOLOGY AND MUSCULOSKELETAL EMERGENCIES

Edited by *Anthony Brown*

SECTION **14**

14.1 Rheumatological emergencies

Michael J Gingold • Adam B Bystrzycki • Flavia M Cicuttini

ESSENTIALS

1 Rheumatological emergencies relate to either the disease, extra-articular manifestations or toxicity from treatment.

2 Understanding the inflammatory basis of the conditions helps early emergency diagnosis.

3 Infection must be considered and promptly treated in patients on antirheumatic and immunosuppressive medication, including those on biological therapies.

Introduction

Rheumatological conditions are common and encompass inflammatory or connective tissue diseases and mechanical/musculoskeletal conditions. Life-threatening emergencies are rare and relate to either the underlying condition or its treatment. The challenge is in making the distinction between the two, as treatment is frequently diametrically opposed; for example, the difference between administering further immunosuppression and giving antibiotics.

The most common rheumatological emergency seen in the emergency department (ED) is acute monoarthritis (see Chapter 14.2). This chapter discusses the important general emergencies associated with rheumatological conditions. Many of these are multisystem diseases and emergencies relate to either a primary joint problem, an extra-articular manifestation or sometimes to the drugs used in management.

Many of these conditions are autoimmune, thus immunosuppression is usually central to their management making infection a frequent complication. More targeted, so-called biological therapies, which inhibit proinflammatory cytokines as well as B- and T-cell activity have been developed. They carry their own set of potential complications, again including infection.

RHEUMATOID ARTHRITIS

Rheumatoid arthritis (RA) affects 1–2% of the population across most ethnic subgroups and is two to three times more common in females than males. RA is a systemic inflammatory condition of unknown aetiology characterized by widespread synovitis resulting in joint erosions and destruction. It may also produce extra-articular manifestations including vasculitis and visceral involvement.

Management typically involves symptom relief with non-steroidal anti-inflammatory drugs (NSAIDs) and/or corticosteroids and early initiation of conventional disease modifying antirheumatic drugs (DMARDs). These include methotrexate, leflunomide, sulphasalazine and hydroxychloroquine and, if these agents fail to control disease progression, biological agents are commenced. The latter act by inhibiting tumour necrosis factor-α (TNF-α) (infliximab, etanercept, adalimumab, golimumab, certolizumab pegol), interleukin-6 (IL-6) (tocilizumab), T-cell co-stimulation (abatacept) or by depleting B cells (rituximab). See Chapter 14.3 for further details on the clinical features of RA, its diagnosis, investigation and management.

ARTICULAR MANIFESTATIONS OF RHEUMATOID ARTHRITIS

Acute monoarthritis

A patient with established RA may present with an acutely painful, hot, swollen joint that may be due to the underlying condition or, alternatively it may be due to a septic arthritis. Patients with RA are two to three times more susceptible than matched controls [1]. The risk is approximately twofold higher again in RA patients on TNF-α inhibitors compared to RA patients on conventional DMARDs [2]. Thus, the possibility of septic arthritis must be considered in a patient with RA who has acute

Table 14.1.1 Symptoms and signs of cervical myelopathy
Symptoms
Pain
Weakness
Peripheral paraesthesia
Gait disturbance
Sphincter dysfunction
Changes in consciousness
Respiratory dysfunction
Signs
Spasticity
Weakness
Hyperreflexia of deep tendon reflexes
Extensor plantar response
Gait ataxia
Respiratory irregularity

monoarthritis out of keeping with their disease activity. See Chapter 14.2 for an approach to acute monoarthritis.

Cervical spine involvement

Cervical spine involvement in RA is common with a prevalence of up to 61%. It is more likely in those with long-standing, erosive disease and disease of greater severity and activity [3]. Cervical spine involvement is associated with increased mortality [4] and may manifest as atlanto-axial subluxation (most commonly anterior movement on the axis) or subluxation of lower cervical vertebrae. Either of these can result in cervical myelopathy.

Cervical spine subluxation is often asymptomatic – up to 44% in one study [3]. The most common symptom is neck pain that may radiate towards the occiput. Other suggestive symptoms include sensory loss in hands or feet, paraesthesia or weakness in the distribution of cervical nerve roots and slowly progressive spastic quadriparesis.

Important 'red flags' suggesting cervical myelopathy are listed in Table 14.1.1.

Imaging

Plain X-rays of the cervical spine (lateral view) may demonstrate an increase in separation between the odontoid and arch of C1. Prior to taking flexion–extension films, perform plain 'peg' X-rays through the open mouth to exclude odontoid fracture or severe atlanto-axial subluxation. Computed tomography (CT) can provide additional useful information, although if there is concern regarding myelopathy, magnetic resonance imaging (MRI) is more sensitive.

Management

The main implication of RA of the cervical spine in the ED is when endotracheal intubation is required. Excessive manipulation (neck flexion with head extension) of the rheumatoid cervical spine in preparation for intubation can result in significant morbidity and even mortality from atlanto-axial and subaxial subluxation.

Whenever possible, a patient with RA who is scheduled to undergo surgery should have imaging of his or her cervical spine prior to endotracheal intubation. Anaesthetic consultation is recommended.

Patients with subluxation and signs of spinal cord compression represent a neurosurgical emergency and prompt referral is essential.

EXTRA-ARTICULAR MANIFESTATIONS OF RHEUMATOID ARTHRITIS

Rheumatoid vasculitis

Vasculitis in RA can occur in both small- and medium-sized vessels. Patients typically have long-standing, aggressive joint disease. This presentation, although important, is becoming less frequent.

Clinical features

Rheumatoid vasculitis presentations are varied and non-specific. Patients frequently have constitutional symptoms and fatigue. The most common manifestation is cutaneous vasculitis with deep skin ulcers on the lower limbs [5], digital ischaemia and gangrene (medium vessels) or palpable purpura (small vessels). Mononeuritis multiplex is another frequent presentation resulting from vasculitic infarction of the vasa nervorum, which typically has an acute onset.

Medium vessel rheumatoid vasculitis may cause organ infarction and necrosis. Rheumatoid vasculitis can mimic polyarteritis nodosa (PAN) with involvement of the renal arteries and, less commonly, the mesenteric circulation. Pericarditis may accompany rheumatoid vasculitis, but coronary vasculitis is rare. Ocular manifestations include episcleritis and peripheral ulcerative keratitis. Central nervous system (CNS) involvement is rare.

Investigations

Rheumatoid factor titre is typically elevated in rheumatoid vasculitis, although this is a non-specific finding. Rheumatoid vasculitis in the absence of rheumatoid factor is rare. Erythrocyte sedimentation rate (ESR) and C-reactive protein (CRP) are also elevated. Check a full blood count, urea and electrolytes and a midstream urine specimen for active urinary sediment including abnormal red cells or casts, as well as infection.

Further investigations are directed at the relevant organ system involved usually after specialist consultation:

- skin biopsy
- nerve conduction studies/electromyography (EMG)
- sural nerve biopsy
- kidney biopsy.

Angiography findings are non-specific and not always diagnostic.

Diagnosis

Suspect rheumatoid vasculitis in patients with a long-standing history of seropositive RA who presents with constitutional symptoms and one of the above features, such as a typical rash, digital gangrene, red eye, neurological complaint or an active urinary sediment.

Management

Systemic rheumatoid vasculitis has a poor prognosis without immune-suppressive therapy. Urgent rheumatology consultation is required as treatment usually consists of high-dose corticosteroids as well as cyclophosphamide, often necessitating hospital admission.

Other extra-articular manifestations of RA

Pulmonary disease

Pulmonary manifestations include pleural-based disease, such as pleurisy or pleural effusions, or parenchymal disease, such as interstitial lung disease (the most common manifestation), organizing pneumonia and rheumatoid nodules. Caplan's syndrome occurs when RA is associated with pneumoconiosis. Important differential diagnoses include infection due to immune suppression, treatment-related toxicity, such as methotrexate-induced pneumonitis, and other medical co-morbidities including chronic obstructive pulmonary disease.

Pleural disease often resolves without treatment, although an NSAID may be used symptomatically. Parenchymal disease documented on chest X-ray or high-resolution CT requires specialist treatment.

Cardiac disease

Pericarditis occurs in 30% of RA patients based on echocardiography, but less than 10% have clinical features. It generally presents when there is active joint and other extra-articular disease and management consists of NSAIDs or prednisolone.

Myocarditis is a rare manifestation of RA. It may be granulomatous and, depending on its location, can produce valvular (especially mitral) incompetence or conduction defects.

Sjögren's syndrome

Sjögren's syndrome may present in a primary form as a systemic disease, but can also occur secondary to RA and other connective tissue disorders. The classic symptoms are dry gritty eyes, dry mouth or both. Treatment is usually symptomatic in patients with no other features.

Felty's syndrome

Felty's syndrome is characterized by seropositive RA, splenomegaly and neutropaenia. There may be other cytopaenias, as well as leg ulcers, and infection is a risk.

Renal disease

Renal involvement with RA is rare and includes vasculitis and glomerulonephritis. Secondary amyloidosis can occur in patients with long-standing active disease. However, many medications used in RA are nephrotoxic, in particular NSAIDs and ciclosporin.

Neurological disease

Vasculitis may produce mononeuritis multiplex, otherwise central nervous system involvement is rare.

Ischaemic heart disease in RA and other connective tissue diseases

Patients with RA and other connective tissue diseases, such as systemic lupus erythematosus (SLE), have an increased risk of ischaemic heart disease (IHD) [6]. This occurs independently of traditional risk factors, such as smoking, dyslipidaemia, hypertension, etc. and is more common in those with extra-articular disease [7]. The higher incidence of IHD appears related to disease factors, such

as widespread inflammation, but medications, such as NSAIDs (including selective COX-2 inhibitors) and corticosteroids, may play a role.

Thus there should be a heightened awareness when ruling out ischaemic chest pain in the RA patient. Cardiac investigations are no different to those undertaken for non-RA patients and a patient with a history suggestive of acute coronary syndrome (ACS) but negative serial cardiac biomarkers and electrocardiograms must proceed to provocative testing. Management of ACS in RA is no different (see Chapter 5.2).

SYSTEMIC LUPUS ERYTHEMATOSUS

Systemic lupus erythematosus is a multisystem, autoimmune disease. It is the prototype disease of immune complex deposition resulting in tissue damage across a wide range of organ systems and one of the most common autoimmune conditions in women of childbearing age.

Clinical features

Common presenting features of SLE include general constitutional symptoms, such as fatigue, malaise and weight loss. There is a variety of skin manifestations in SLE which are lupus-specific (malar rash, discoid lupus, subacute cutaneous lupus erythematosus) or non-specific (panniculitis, alopecia, oral ulceration). Arthralgias or an acute non-erosive arthritis are the most common presenting symptoms of SLE.

Another common manifestation is serositis causing pleurisy, pericarditis or peritonitis. SLE also causes renal and CNS disease (see below) and, rarely, can involve the lung parenchyma (pneumonitis, pulmonary hypertension) and heart (myocarditis, endocarditis). Myositis may also occur.

Investigations

A full blood examination often reveals cytopaenias which are a common feature of SLE. Biochemistry may indicate renal impairment. ESR and CRP may be raised.

Clotting abnormalities can include a prolonged activated partial thromboplastin time due to the lupus anticoagulant (LA), one of the antiphospholipid antibodies along with

anticardiolipin antibody (aCL) and others. Paradoxically, there is an associated predisposition to both venous and arterial blood clots when these are positive.

Serological abnormalities

The antinuclear antibody (ANA) is present in 95% of patients with SLE, but may also occur in other connective tissue and inflammatory diseases, as well as at low levels in healthy adults. The anti-Smith (Sm) and anti-dsDNA (double-stranded DNA) antibodies are more specific but less sensitive for SLE. Anti-Sm is obtained as part of a panel of antibody tests for extractable nuclear antigens (anti-ENA). Serological abnormalities also include decreased levels of complement components C3 and C4.

Other tests are directed towards the organ system involved, for example, midstream urine specimen looking for proteinuria or glomerular haematuria (>70% dysmorphic red blood cells or red-cell casts) and chest X-ray in the patient with serositis.

Assessing SLE disease activity

It is important to determine SLE disease activity in the ED. Useful symptoms of activity include mouth ulcers, alopecia and constitutional symptoms, as well as organ-specific symptoms, such as arthralgia or pleuritic chest pain.

Investigations used to assess disease activity include complement levels (low in active SLE), CRP and ESR (elevated), as well as anti-dsDNA titre. These are not diagnostic and many people with quiescent SLE may also have hypocomplementaemia or elevated anti-dsDNA titres.

A midstream urine for urinary sediment is an essential marker of renal involvement.

Management

Management of SLE is directed by the organ system involved and includes topical therapies for cutaneous lupus and NSAIDs for arthralgias and mild serositis. Most patients with SLE will be on an antimalarial, such as hydroxychloroquine, helpful for skin and musculoskeletal manifestations as well as organ involvement. Many patients will also be on corticosteroids. Those with major organ involvement will also be taking other immuno-suppressants, such as methotrexate, cyclo-phosphamide or azathioprine. Mycophenolate mofetil is frequently now used as an alternative to cyclophosphamide for lupus nephritis.

Lupus nephritis

Early diagnosis of lupus nephritis is essential to prompt management and prevent progression of renal damage. Patients may be asymptomatic or present with nocturia, haematuria or proteinuria. Other presentations include hypertension, rapidly progressive glomerulonephritis and the nephrotic syndrome.

Urinalysis is the most useful investigation in detecting lupus nephritis and proteinuria is the most common abnormality detected. The fresh urine specimen should be sent for phase contrast microscopy in order to detect the presence of dysmorphic erythrocytes (>70% indicates glomerular disease) or cellular casts.

Urinalysis can expedite the investigation and further management of this potentially organ-threatening condition. Prompt referral to a rheumatologist or renal physician for consideration of renal biopsy and further management is indicated.

Neuropsychiatric SLE

There is a myriad of neuropsychiatric manifestations of neuropsychiatric SLE. Neurological presentations include:

- stroke (due to vasculitis, emboli, atherosclerosis or antiphospholipid antibodies)
- seizure
- migraine
- aseptic meningitis.

Psychiatric presentations include:

- headache and mood disturbance, including anxiety
- cognitive dysfunction 'lupus fog'
- dementia
- psychosis.

These presentations are non-specific and have a broad differential diagnosis or can be subtle and progress. Unfortunately, there is no specific diagnostic test which helps differentiate SLE from other potential aetiologies. Thus, the diagnosis is made from a range of clinical features and tests. The role of the emergency department is first to exclude the more common non-SLE presentations, such as meningitis or intracranial haemorrhage.

Investigations

Imaging studies are needed as well as tests for SLE activity (see above). CT brain scan may detect changes of acute infarction, but is also useful in excluding other non-SLE causes, such as haemorrhage or tumour. MRI is more sensitive in detecting white matter abnormalities, although they are frequently non-specific.

Cerebrospinal fluid (CSF) analysis is essential to exclude infection, but may be normal in SLE. Changes, such as elevated protein, low glucose or even a positive ANA, are non-specific and do not always reflect active SLE. The electroencephalogram is occasionally useful in cases of unexplained altered conscious level with suspected non-convulsive status epilepticus.

TEMPORAL (GIANT CELL) ARTERITIS AND OTHER VASCULITIDES

Temporal (giant cell) arteritis

Giant cell arteritis (GCA) is the most frequent vasculitis and almost exclusively affects Caucasians. It is a large and medium vessel vasculitis of unknown aetiology, which predominantly affects the cranial branches of arteries originating from the aortic arch and, commonly though not exclusively, the temporal artery.

Polymyalgia rheumatica (PMR) is a syndrome of inflammatory pain and stiffness in the shoulder and pelvic girdles that occurs alone or frequently in association with GCA.

Epidemiology

GCA and PMR rarely ever occur before the age of 50 years [8], with a mean age at diagnosis of approximately 72 years. The incidence of GCA is roughly 1 in 500 of people over the age of 50 years, although the incidence and prevalence of PMR are less well studied.

Clinical features

The most common symptom of GCA is new headache, usually localizing to the temporal region, although it can be more diffuse. The area is often tender and worsened by brushing the hair. Most patients complain of constitutional symptoms, such as malaise, fatigue, anorexia and weight loss. Jaw claudication (pain after a period of chewing) is the most specific symptom for GCA, although not sensitive, as it is present in only 34% [8]. On examination, the temporal arteries may be thickened, 'ropey' and tender with a reduced or absent pulse.

The most serious complication of GCA is anterior ischaemic optic neuropathy (AION) resulting in sudden painless loss of vision which can be bilateral, particularly if untreated. Less commonly, other branches of the aorta may be involved resulting in hemiparesis, arm claudication, aortic dissection or myocardial infarction.

Polymyalgia rheumatica

PMR usually affects the neck, shoulder and pelvic girdles resulting in stiffness and inflammatory pain, worse in the morning and after rest. The pain is often poorly localized and muscle atrophy may occur late in the disease. There may also be synovitis affecting the shoulders, knees, wrists and hands.

The relationship between onset of symptoms of GCA and PMR is highly variable. PMR symptoms may occur before, after or with GCA symptoms. At some point, 5–15% of patients with PMR will have a diagnosis of GCA and about 50% of patients with GCA have symptoms of PMR.

Differential diagnosis of GCA and PMR

GCA can mimic any of the other vasculitides. Non-arteritic anterior ischaemic optic neuropathy can also mimic GCA. The differential diagnosis of PMR includes late-onset RA, polmyositis and other myopathies, fibromyalgia, malignancy and hypothyroidism.

Investigations

The classic non-specific laboratory finding in GCA and/or PMR is a markedly elevated ESR (often >100 mm/h). CRP is also usually elevated and a full blood count often shows a mild normochromic normocytic anaemia.

A temporal artery biopsy confirms the diagnosis of GCA and is particularly useful when the diagnosis is doubtful or the presentation atypical. However, as there is a false negative rate of 10–30%, a negative biopsy does not exclude GCA.

Criteria for diagnosis

The ACR classification criteria for GCA are helpful in differentiating GCA from other forms of vasculitis [9]. They include age at onset >50 years, a new headache, temporal artery tenderness or decreased pulsation and an ESR >50. An abnormal artery biopsy showing vasculitis with mononuclear infiltrate or granulomatous inflammation with multinucleated giant cells also confirms the diagnosis.

Although various classification criteria for PMR have been published, having excluded other diagnoses (except GCA), the presence of all three of the following clinical and laboratory criteria defines the diagnosis [10]:

- age ≥50 at onset of symptoms
- bilateral aching and stiffness for over 30 minutes after waking, in two of the following three areas; neck and torso, shoulder girdle, hips/pelvic girdle
- ESR >40.

In practice, rapid response to prednisolone ≤20 mg daily is also used as an additional criterion with 50–70% improvement within 72 hours.

Management

Corticosteroids are essential for GCA and should not be withheld to perform a biopsy. The initial dose for GCA is unclear, but prednisone 1 mg/kg/day is used especially for ischaemic complications. However, lower doses, such as prednisone 40–60 mg, are recommended for uncomplicated disease [10].

The dose of prednisone for PMR uncomplicated by GCA is lower at 10–20 mg/day; 15 mg is generally agreed as an appropriate standard dose [11]. Most GCA patients do not require hospital admission, provided a temporal artery biopsy can be organized within a few days. However, patients with visual loss at diagnosis require urgent treatment often with pulsed parenteral corticosteroids and inpatient admission. Patients with GCA should also be commenced on aspirin.

Approach to the other systemic vasculitides

The systemic vasculitides are a group of disorders characterized by an inflammatory infiltrate in the walls of blood vessels resulting in damage to the vessel wall. The clinical manifestations depend upon the size of vessel and location in the vascular tree and may result

Table 14.1.2 Classification of systemic vasculitis according to vessel size	
Vessel size	**Vasculitis**
Large	Takayasu's arteritis Temporal (giant cell) arteritis
Medium	Polyarteritis nodosa Kawasaki's disease
Small	Wegener's granulomatosis (ANCA +) Microscopic polyangiitis (ANCA +) Churg–Strauss syndrome (ANCA + / −) Henoch–Schönlein purpura Cryoglobulinaemic vasculitis Leucocytoclastic cutaneous vasculitis

in systemic or organ-specific manifestations. Table 14.1.2 classifies vasculitic syndromes according to vessel size (there is much overlap).

Clinical features

An underlying vasculitis should be considered in patients who present with one or more of the following:

- unexplained systemic illness – fatigue, fevers, night sweats, malaise
- unexplained ischaemia of an organ or limb
- rash with palpable purpura
- chronic inflammatory sinusitis and chronic discharge or bleeding from the nose or ears
- mononeuritis multiplex
- pulmonary infiltrates
- microscopic haematuria, especially if dysmorphic glomerular erythrocytes
- any of the above in the setting of atopy and peripheral blood eosinophilia.

Investigations and diagnosis

Baseline investigations should include full blood count (FBC), urea and electrolytes (U&E), liver function tests (LFTs) and clotting studies as well as CRP and ESR. Blood cultures should be taken if the patient is systemically unwell.

A panel of autoimmune serological tests is carried out including ANA, ENA, rheumatoid factor, dsDNA, anticyclic citrullinated peptides (anti-CCP), complement levels (C3, C4), antineutrophil cytoplasmic antibodies (ANCA) and cryoglobulins. PAN is associated with hepatitis B and cryoglobulinaemic vasculitis with hepatitis C infection.

Collection of a midstream urine specimen to look for glomerular haematuria is mandatory when vasculitis is suspected. Imaging is

indicated, such as chest X-ray, CT scan of the chest or sinuses or other areas depending on the suspected organ involved. The definitive diagnosis of vasculitis requires biopsy of affected tissue or angiography.

Differential diagnosis of systemic vasculitis

Other conditions which may mimic systemic vasculitis include:

- infections, such as infective endocarditis, meningococcaemia, gonococcaemia
- disorders of haemostasis and thrombosis, such as thrombotic thrombocytopaenic purpura (TTP), antiphospholipid syndrome
- malignancy, such as lymphoma, myxoma
- sarcoidosis.

Management of systemic vasculitis

Treatment is usually with high-dose corticosteroids and, depending on the condition, additional immunosuppression, such as cyclophosphamide. Urgent specialist referral is essential.

ANKYLOSING SPONDYLITIS

Ankylosing spondylitis (AS) is an inflammatory arthritis of the axial skeleton which can result in progressive spinal fusion. It affects <1% of the general population and its prevalence is linked to the prevalence of HLA-B27.

The hallmark pathological feature of AS is new bone formation and spinal fusion which, combined with the increased prevalence of low bone mineral density in these patients, makes spinal injury a particular risk. Also a range of features including reduced mobility and muscle atrophy lead to a higher falls risk.

Spinal fractures are up to four times more common in AS patients than in the general population and the risk of spinal cord injury is even higher. Fractures can occur at any point in the spine and do not have the classical appearance of wedge or endplate compression. In advanced fusion, the spine may fracture in a similar way to a long bone and not respect traditional spinal anatomical boundaries. There is also a higher rate of atlanto-axial subluxation, with similar precautions required as in those with RA. Furthermore, patients with advanced fusion may also develop cauda equina syndrome in the absence of a fracture.

Fractures in AS can be missed by plain X-ray and the onset of new spinal pain or a change in spinal pain necessitiates further imaging with either CT or MRI.

RHEUMATOLOGICAL THERAPY EMERGENCIES

The medications used in rheumatology include NSAIDs, corticosteroids, DMARDs and biological DMARDs. These medications are all associated with adverse effects which occasionally result in serious morbidity.

Non-steroidal anti-inflammatory drugs

NSAIDs are commonly used for relief of arthralgia in both inflammatory and non-inflammatory conditions. They are of equal efficacy, although those with shorter half-lives appear to have less gastrointestinal toxicity [12]. NSAIDs should be used in the lowest possible dose for the shortest duration and combinations of NSAIDs (except aspirin) should be avoided [12].

The most common adverse effects of NSAIDs include peptic ulcer disease and acute renal failure, both related to inhibition of prostaglandin synthesis. Gastrointestinal (GI) toxicity is more common in the elderly, those on anticoagulants and with high doses or prolonged duration of NSAIDs. Prescribe a proton pump inhibitor when there is concern about GI toxicity. The COX-2 selective inhibitors, such as celecoxib, have a reduced incidence of peptic ulcer disease, but a similar incidence of other adverse effects including hypertension, peripheral oedema and cardiac failure. There is an increased risk of cardiovascular deaths with prolonged courses.

Corticosteroids

Corticosteroids are the mainstay of treatment for most inflammatory rheumatological conditions. At high doses, they provide rapid control of inflammatory disease and are often required for long-term management at low doses. Long-term use is associated with numerous adverse effects, such as diabetes, hypertension and osteoporosis. In addition, psychosis and mood disorders related to corticosteroid use, as well as peptic ulcer disease, may present as an emergency.

Table 14.1.3   Adverse effects of disease modifying antirheumatic drugs (DMARDs)

DMARD	Adverse effects
Methotrexate	Nausea and other GI upset, mouth ulcers, abnormal liver function (transaminases), bone marrow suppression, rash, alopecia, pneumonitis Increased bone marrow toxicity in renal impairment – withhold in acute renal failure Teratogenic
Leflunomide	Abnormal liver function (transaminases), diarrhoea, rash, alopecia, hypertension, peripheral neuropathy Teratogenic
Hydroxychloroquine	Nausea, rash, dizziness ('cinchonism'), retinal toxicity at higher doses (all uncommon)
Sulphasalazine	GI upset, uncommonly abnormal liver function and bone marrow suppression, rashes (rarely, Stevens–Johnson syndrome)
Ciclosporin	Renal impairment, hypertension, electrolyte disturbance, hyperuricaemia and gout, gingival hyperplasia, hirsutism
Cyclophosphamide	Bone marrow suppression especially neutropaenia, GI upset, bladder toxicity, including haemorrhagic cystitis (acute) and bladder cancer (chronic), opportunistic infections Teratogenic
Azathioprine	GI upset, rash, systemic symptoms, abnormal liver function, bone marrow suppression, skin cancers, infections

GI: gastrointestinal.

Although there is concern about infection among patients on DMARDs, prednisolone contributes considerably (possibly more) to the immune-suppressed patient's overall infection risk.

Immunosuppressants/ disease modifying antirheumatic drugs

This heterogeneous group of medications is used to prevent joint destruction in the inflammatory arthritides and as steroid-sparing therapy in many connective tissue diseases. They include methotrexate, leflunomide, hydroxychloroquine, sulphasalazine, ciclosporin, azathioprine and cyclophosphamide. Each drug has its own range of adverse effects, but common adverse effects include cytopaenias, rashes including Stevens–Johnson syndrome, abnormal liver function tests, GI toxicity and heightened susceptibility to infections (Table 14.1.3).

Biological disease modifying antirheumatic drugs

The so-called 'biological' DMARDs are a newer and expanding collection of therapies directed against molecules and cells that mediate joint destruction and help drive the inflammatory process. These therapies are being increasingly used for those who fail conventional DMARD therapy for RA and TNF inhibitors are also used for treatment-resistant psoriatic arthritis and ankylosing spondylitis, as well as other non-rheumatological conditions.

Adverse effects associated with biological DMARDs include an increased risk of infections, particularly soft-tissue and joint infections, as well as reactivation of tuberculosis. Other opportunistic infections appear more common, such as listeriosis. Patients may also develop local injection site reactions and infusion-related reactions, which can be delayed. Less common adverse effects include a form of drug-induced lupus and demyelination.

Presentations of treatment-related emergencies

Infections

As treatment of rheumatological conditions is directed at immunosuppression, infections are a common and expected adverse effect of therapy. Although studies have shown RA patients to have a *de novo* increased risk of infection, biological DMARDs further increase this risk. Although most of the larger studies have focused on TNF inhibitors, which have been available the longest, there is an increased risk of serious infections compared to the general RA population. This risk may be highest in the first 6 months of therapy [13].

Patients on biological therapy who develop an infection are advised temporarily to cease their treatment and to commence antibiotics. If in doubt, they should be admitted to hospital to receive parenteral antibiotics. There is also an increased risk of reactivation of tuberculosis and infections such as *Listeria* and *Salmonella* [13]. Rigorous tuberculosis screening prior to commencement of anti-TNF therapy should now be universal.

Special mention must be made of the biological agent tocilizumab directed against interleukin-6. Tocilizumab causes marked suppression of acute phase reactants, particularly CRP and, even in the presence of active infection, a patient on this may have a normal CRP. Thus if there is a clinical suspicion of infection, appropriate antibiotic therapy must be instituted regardless.

Bone marrow suppression

Anaemia, leucopaenia and thrombocytopaenia all may occur in patients taking DMARDs, such as methotrexate, cyclophosphamide, sulphasalazine and azathioprine, with neutropaenic sepsis a particular danger.

Cytopaenia in a patient taking methotrexate is uncommon but those at increased risk include the elderly and those with renal impairment, related to the drug's mechanism of action as an inhibitor of dihydrofolate reductase. Management includes temporary cessation of treatment and administration of folinic acid, the active form of folic acid which does not require to be converted by dihydrofolate reductase.

The most common adverse effect of cyclophosphamide is myelosuppression, particularly leucopaenia. The white cell nadir occurs at 2 weeks post-infusion following intravenous therapy. Patients on oral therapy may experience a gradual decrease in white cell count, which is typically less predictable than on intravenous therapy.

Bone marrow suppression may also occur as a side effect of azathioprine treatment, especially if given in combination with allopurinol which inhibits its metabolism, thus potentiating bone marrow toxicity. Cytopaenias are also more common in patients with deficient thiopurine methyltransferase enzyme. Sulphasalazine therapy is uncommonly complicated by bone marrow suppression.

DMARD-related pneumonitis

Methotrexate and leflunomide may both result in lung toxicity. The incidence of methotrexate-induced lung toxicity is difficult to assess but uncommon, with those patients at higher risk who have prolonged duration of methotrexate treatment, pre-existing rheumatoid involvement of the lungs and pleura, increased extra-articular manifestations, diabetes mellitus, previous DMARD use and a low serum albumin [14]. Age and smoking also appear to be important. The most frequent is a hypersensitivity pneumonitis, but other forms of lung injury may occur both acute and chronic, with rapid progress to respiratory failure in more acute situations. Clinical features are non-specific and include constitutional symptoms, cough and progressive dyspnoea. Subacute presentations are more common.

Imaging reveals interstitial opacities and patchy consolidation. High-resolution CT scanning typically shows a ground-glass appearance. The main differential diagnosis is of a respiratory infection which may be due to typical pathogens or opportunistic infections, such as *Pneumocystis jirovecii.*

Management is supportive with empiric antibiotic therapy in case of infection. Corticosteroids are also used. Patients may become seriously ill and require intensive care, but mortality is still low (1%).

Leflunomide may also cause lung injury, typically in the first few months of therapy and usually when given in combination with methotrexate.

Allopurinol hypersensitivity syndrome

Minor hypersensitivity reactions to allopurinol occur in about 2% of patients and usually consist of a mild rash. Rarely, a severe hypersensitivity syndrome may present in an unwell patient with fever, rash including toxic epidermal necrolysis, erythema multiforme or a diffuse macropapular or exfoliative dermatitis, abnormalities of liver function, peripheral blood eosinophilia and acute renal failure due to interstitial nephritis. It is more common in those with renal impairment who do not have an appropriate dose reduction. This presentation has a mortality rate of 25%. Treatment is supportive.

References

[1] Margaretten ME, Kohlwes J, Moore D, et al. Does this adult patient have septic arthritis?. J Am Med Assoc 2007;297:1478–88.

[2] Galloway JB, Hyrich KL, Mercer LK, et al. Risk of septic arthritis in patients with rheumatoid arthritis and the effect of anti-TNF therapy: results from the British Society for Rheumatology Biologics Register. Ann Rheum Dis 2011;70:1810–4.

[3] Neva MH, Hakkinen A, Makinen H, et al. High prevalence of asymptomatic cervical spine subluxation in patients with rheumatoid arthritis waiting for orthopaedic surgery. Ann Rheum Dis 2006;65:884–8.

[4] Riise T, Jacobsen BK, Gran JT. High mortality in patients with rheumatoid arthritis and atlantoaxial subluxation. J Rheumatol 2001;28:2425–9.

[5] Genta MS, Genta RM, Gabay C. Systemic rheumatoid vasculitis: a review. Semin Arthrit Rheum 2006;36:88–98.

[6] Turesson C, Jarenros A, Jacobsson L. Increased incidence of cardiovascular disease in patients with rheumatoid arthritis: results from a community based study. Ann Rheum Dis 2004;63:952–5.

[7] Turesson C, Jarenros A, Jacobsson L. Severe extra-articular disease manifestations are associated with an increased risk of first ever cardiovascular events in patients with rheumatoid arthritis. Ann Rheum Dis 2007;66:70–5.

[8] Smetana GW, Shmerling RH. Does this patient have temporal arteritis? J Am Med Assoc 2002;287:92–101.

[9] Hunder GG, Bloch DA, Michel BA, et al. The American College of Rheumatololgy 1990 criteria for the classification of giant cell arteritis. Arthrit Rheum 1990;33:1122–8.

[10] Salvarani C, Cantini F, Hunder GG. Polymyalgia rheumatica and giant cell arteritis. Lancet 2008;372:234–45.

[11] Dasgupta B, Borg FA, Hassan N, et al. BSR and BHPR guidelines for the management of polymyalgia rheumatic. Rheumatology 2010;49:186–90.

[12] Therapeutic Guidelines: Rheumatology, Version 2. Melbourne: Therapeutics Guidelines Ltd; 2010.

[13] Galloway JB, Hyrich KL, Mercer LK, et al. Anti-TNF therapy is associated with an increased risk of serious infections in patients with rheumatoid arthritis especially in the first 6 months of treatment: updated results from the British Society for Rheumatology Biologics Register with special emphasis on risks in the elderly. Rheumatology 2011;50:124–31.

[14] Alarcon GS, Kremer JM, Macaluso M, et al. Risk factors for methotrexate-induced lung injury in patients with rheumatoid arthritis: a multicentre, case control study. Ann Intern Med 1997;127:356–64.

Further reading

D'Cruz DP. Clinical review: systemic lupus erythematosus. Br Med J 2006;332:890–94.

Hochberg M, et al. Rheumatology, 3rd ed. Edinburgh: Mosby; 2003.

Savage COS, et al. ABC of arterial and vascular disease: vasculitis. Br Med J 2000;20:1325–8.

Therapeutic Guidelines: Rheumatology, Version 2. Melbourne: Therapeutics Guidelines Ltd; 2010.

UpToDate. <http://www.utdol.com/utd/content/search.do> [Accessed Nov. 2012].

14.2 Monoarthritis

Michael J Gingold • Adam B Bystrzycki • Flavia M Cicuttini

ESSENTIALS

1 Presenting features alone, including absence of fever, do not reliably exclude a septic arthritis.

2 Synovial aspirate in appropriate pathology transport media may be diagnostic performed prior to antibiotics in septic arthritis.

3 Acute monoarthritis affecting a prosthetic joint or the hip should *not* be aspirated in the emergency department. It requires urgent orthopaedic assessment.

Table 14.2.1 Common presentations with acute monoarthritis to an emergency department

Gout
Reactive arthritis such as post-viral, Reiter's syndrome
Acute exacerbation of pre-existing inflammatory arthritis
Rheumatoid arthritis
Septic arthritis

Note: Orthopaedic-related joint problems, such as trauma and/or haemarthrosis, plus osteoarthritis (OA) were not included in this series [4].

SEPTIC ARTHRITIS

The assessment of a patient with acute monoarthritis is focused on excluding a septic arthritis. Septic arthritis can cause rapid joint destruction and mortality has been reported as high as up to 15% [1].

Pathogenesis and pathology

Non-gonococcal bacterial arthritis occurs when bacteria enter the synovial lining of a joint via the haematogenous route, local spread from nearby soft-tissue infections or following penetrating trauma or injury to a joint.

When the bacteria reach the synovium, they trigger an inflammatory response and bacteria and inflammatory cells enter the synovial fluid in the joint space, causing swelling and destruction of articular cartilage. These destructive changes may extend to subchondral bone and produce irreversible damage within days. The commonest causative organisms are staphylococci and streptococci.

Epidemiology and risk factors

The prevalence of septic arthritis ranges between 4 and 10:100,000 patients per year and appears to be rising. It is also almost seven times more common in indigenous Australians [2].

Risk factors for septic arthritis include inflammatory arthritis (especially rheumatoid arthritis), diabetes mellitus and systemic factors, such as age greater than 80 years, as well as local factors, such as recent joint surgery, joint prosthesis and overlying skin infection. These individual risk factors increase the risk of septic arthritis by two- to threefold [3]. Skin infection overlying a prosthetic joint increases the risk of infection by 15-fold [3].

Clinical features

Septic arthritis presents with joint pain and swelling in over 80% of cases, which may or may not be associated with systemic symptoms, such as sweats and rigors [3]. The hip and knee joints are the most commonly involved joints.

The patient may be febrile and the affected joint is usually swollen, warm, erythematous and tender. Classically, there is reduced ability to actively move the joint and marked pain on passive movement. Unfortunately, the symptoms and signs are not sensitive and a patient with septic arthritis may present with only certain of these features. Thus, septic arthritis cannot be excluded with confidence on the history and examination alone.

Differential diagnosis

The differential diagnosis of acute monoarthritis is shown in Table 14.2.1. Ask the patient about a history of previous rheumatological disease, such as rheumatoid arthritis, gout or other inflammatory arthritis, as well as risk factors for infection, such as immunosuppression, including diabetes and steroids. Recent trauma or history of a bleeding diathesis or anticoagulation are also relevant. Finally, ask the patient about any recent sexually transmitted infection, including gonococcal infection or non-specific urethritis, or any systemic features including uveitis and/or gastrointestinal infection, which may point towards a reactive arthritis.

Clinical investigations

Blood tests

Send blood for a full blood count, which may reveal an elevated peripheral white blood cell count, as well as C-reactive protein (CRP) and erythrocyte sedimentation rate (ESR). ESR and CRP are non-specific and not sensitive for septic arthritis, but may help in the differential diagnosis. Blood cultures are taken in the presence of fever. Finally, a serum urate may be elevated, but can be normal in acute gout.

Imaging

X-ray may be normal in septic arthritis, as it takes at least one week for destructive changes to appear on plain X-ray. Magnetic resonance imaging when available, while non-specific, is frequently helpful to determine if the pathology is in the joint or juxta-articular bone.

Joint aspiration

The single most important investigation is synovial fluid aspiration and analysis. Send the aspirate in a sterile container for Gram stain and culture, as well as for polarizing light microscopy to look for the presence of urate (strongly negative birefringent) crystals or calcium pyrophosphate crystals (weakly positive birefringent crystals). Using blood culture bottles does not appear to increase the yield of a positive culture.

Place some of the aspirate in an EDTA tube for a white cell count to be performed. The likelihood of septic arthritis increases from 2.9% with a synovial white cell count above 25,000/μL up to 28% with a synovial white cell count of greater than 100,000/μL. Synovial glucose and protein levels are unhelpful.

Criteria for diagnosis of septic arthritis

There is no 'gold standard' test for the diagnosis of septic arthritis. Synovial fluid Gram stain has a sensitivity of up to 50% only, while culture has a sensitivity up to 85% [3]. However, combined with an appropriate clinical presentation, the presence of microorganisms in synovial fluid on Gram stain and/or a positive synovial fluid culture with high synovial white cell count are diagnostic.

Treatment

Treatment of septic arthritis requires parenteral antibiotics and urgent referral to orthopaedics for surgical drainage with admission to hospital. Commence empirical antibiotic therapy with dicloxacillin or flucloxacillin 2 g IV 6-hourly or cephalothin 2 g IV 6-hourly (or cephazolin) if patient is allergic to penicillin to cover against *Staphylococcus*, until guided by microbiology results.

The patient with suspected hip sepsis or sepsis affecting a prosthetic joint must be referred to orthopaedics urgently without attempting joint aspiration.

GOUT

Gout is an intra-articular inflammatory response to monosodium urate crystal deposition usually related to hyperuricaemia. It is more common in males than females, but is extremely rare in the premenopausal female.

Aetiology and pathogenesis

Uric acid is derived from purine metabolism. Hyperuricaemia is the strongest predictor for gout and relates to either overproduction or underexcretion of uric acid. Hyperuricaemia may also cause radiolucent renal calculi.

Overproduction of uric acid is due to dietary factors, such as beer, fructose-containing soft drinks, shellfish and other purine-rich foods, or endogenous factors associated with high cell turnover, such as a haematological malignancy. Reduced excretion is related to chronic kidney disease, hypovolaemia, acidosis and medications, such as diuretics, ciclosporin, pyrazinamide, ethambutol and low-dose aspirin. There is frequently a family history of gout.

Epidemiology

The peak incidence of acute gout occurs in men between the ages of 30 and 60 years and in women between 55 and 70 years. The presentation of gout in younger patients should prompt a search for a secondary cause (including lifestyle factors). Gout is more common in Maori and Polynesian populations.

Clinical features

The classic presentation is of acute onset of a hot, swollen and painful first metatarsophalangeal joint (75% of cases) known as podagra. Other commonly affected joints include joints in the foot, the ankle, knee and small joints of the hand.

Common triggers of an acute attack are binges of alcohol or purine-rich foods, dehydration, severe illness such as sepsis, trauma and surgery. Sudden cessation or the introduction (especially in an acute attack) of hypouricaemic agents, such as allopurinol or probenecid, may also precipitate gouty arthritis, as can the introduction or a dose change of a diuretic.

Untreated, the symptoms will abate over the course of several days to 2 weeks. Occasionally, the patient may appear systemically unwell during an acute attack with malaise and systemic inflammatory response features. Examination reveals a tender, warm and erythematous joint with severely restricted range of movement. The patient may also be febrile. Presentations of acute gout may also be polyarticular (see Chapter 14.3).

Recurrent untreated acute gout and hyperuricaemia results in chronic tophaceous gout, where the patient is no longer pain-free between attacks. Examination reveals tophus formation on the ears, around the elbows and in the fingers with marked joint deformity.

Investigations and diagnosis

Synovial fluid aspiration

Synovial fluid aspirate to identify monosodium urate crystals is diagnostic of acute gout. The crystals may be phagocytosed (intracellular) and the synovial fluid will have a high white cell count. Send fluid for Gram stain and culture to rule out septic arthritis, which may rarely coexist with gout. Podagra with a typical clinical scenario has a sensitivity of 96% and specificity of 95% for acute gout, so aspiration is not indicated [5].

Blood tests

Hyperuricaemia on blood testing is not diagnostic of gout as, although up to 5% of adults may have a raised serum uric acid at some point, only one-fifth (1% overall) will ever have an attack of gout. Conversely, in about one-third of patients with gout, the serum uric acid level is normal during an acute attack. Other blood tests, such as FBE, ESR and CRP are sent and may be abnormally elevated. Check the renal function with serum urea and creatinine both to identify a potential aetiology and help guide treatment, such as avoidance or reduced doses of non-steroidal anti-inflammatory drugs (NSAIDs) or colchicine.

Imaging

Plain X-ray is performed to exclude injury, but should be normal in the acute attack other than soft-tissue swelling. Punched-out periarticular erosions are seen in chronic gouty arthritis which, when associated with calcium deposition, deforming arthritis and soft-tissue swelling, are characteristic of chronic tophaceous gout.

Management

The aim is to treat acute pain and then prevent chronic relapse with hypouricaemic drugs. Colchicine is losing favour due to the frequency of its side effects and potential for serious toxicity. Educate all patients to correct lifestyle factors where appropriate.

Acute attack

Non-steroidal anti-inflammatory drugs

After excluding infection, give either an NSAID, corticosteroid and/or colchicine in the absence of contraindications. Give diclofenac 50 mg tds orally followed by 25 mg tds orally or naproxen 500 mg followed by 250 mg tds orally until symptoms subside. A selective COX-2 inhibitor, such as celecoxib 100 mg bd orally, is preferred in patients with a history of peptic ulcer disease, although there is a similar risk of renal dysfunction in the elderly or with pre-existing renal disease.

Corticosteroids

Patients with gout refractory to the above treatment or in whom other treatment is contraindicated may be given corticosteroids, such as prednisolone 25–50 mg daily for 3 days, then weaned over 1–2 weeks [6,7]. An alternative approach is intra-articular corticosteroid for monoarticular gout provided sepsis has been excluded.

Colchicine

When NSAIDs and prednisone are contraindicated, colchicine may be used. Doses of 0.5 mg 6- or 8-hourly orally have equivalent efficacy and a lower rate of gastrointestinal toxicity compared to higher doses [8]. Higher doses, such as colchicine 1.0 mg followed by 0.5 mg up to four times daily, with a maximum cumulative dose of 6–8 mg per acute attack are no longer recommended, due to increased toxicity with nausea, vomiting, diarrhoea and the risk of renal impairment. All colchicine doses should thus be less with renal impairment, as these patients are at risk of severe neuromyopathy and/or who are on statins, as this combination may increase the risk of myopathy and rhabdomyolysis.

Recurrent attacks

Urate lowering therapy

A second attack of gout usually requires urate lowering therapy, although this is not usually commenced in the emergency setting, as treatment should be delayed until the acute flare up has settled. Allopurinol, a xanthine oxidase inhibitor, prevents the production of uric acid from xanthine. It is introduced at a low dose once the acute attack has settled and gradually titrated up to a maximum of 300 mg daily [9]. Typically, the patient will remain on a low-dose NSAID (or prednisolone/low-dose colchicine) as prophylaxis against precipitating further acute attacks.

Febuxostat is a new orally administered selective xanthine oxidase inhibitor for gout that may be used to reduce urate levels, particularly in patients with poor kidney function or intolerant of allopurinol, such as due to a hypersensitivity reaction.

An alternative uricosuric agent to allopurinol is probenecid, which should be avoided in renal impairment.

ACUTE PSEUDOGOUT

Acute pseudogout causes an acute monoarthritis and is one of the several potential presentations of calcium pyrophosphate dihydrate (CPPD) deposition disease. It is more common in females and patients over 65 years old.

Aetiology and pathogenesis

Calcium pyrophosphate disease is characterized by deposition of CPPD crystals in cartilage causing chondrocalcinosis. When released, there may be uptake in other synovial structures and an inflammatory response producing acute synovitis, tenosynovitis or bursitis.

Advanced age is the strongest risk factor. Other associations are a family history, metabolic diseases such as haemochromatosis, Wilson's disease, hyperparathyroidism, hypophosphataemia or hypomagnesaemia and mechanical factors, such as previous injury or osteoarthritis (OA).

Clinical features

CPPD deposition disease presents in a variety of ways. The two most common are acute pseudogout and chronic pyrophosphate arthropathy, which may mimic OA. Other presentations include tenosynovitis, bursitis or as an incidental radiographic finding of chondrocalcinosis. CPPD deposition disease may also mimic rheumatoid arthritis or ankylosing spondylitis, as well as the neuropathic joint.

Acute pseudogout typically presents in older patients and the knee is the most commonly affected joint. Other common sites include the wrist, shoulder, elbow and ankle. Occasionally, there may be an oligoarticular presentation. Presentation is with a hot, red and swollen joint. There may be systemic inflammatory response features and the patient may be febrile. Triggers include trauma, surgery or illness, but most cases are spontaneous.

Investigations and clinical diagnosis

Joint aspiration

Diagnosis of pseudogout depends on the demonstration of CPPD crystals in synovial fluid, which is frequently blood stained. Polarizing light microscopy demonstrates weakly positive birefringent rhomboid-shaped crystals.

Laboratory studies and imaging

Younger patients presenting with polyarticular chondrocalcinosis should be screened for an underlying metabolic cause, checking serum calcium, magnesium, phosphate, alkaline phosphatase, parathyroid hormone, thyroid function and iron studies.

Plain X-rays of the joint may reveal chondrocalcinosis seen in fibrocartilage, such as the knee menisci, triangular cartilage of the wrist and pubic symphysis. Other characteristic findings are of marked degenerative change in joints that are not usually affected by OA.

Management

Symptoms of acute pseudogout frequently improve once the joint has been aspirated. Intra-articular injection of corticosteroid is also appropriate for acute monoarthritis, once infection has been excluded. In addition, rest and splintage for 48–72 h is beneficial.

Give oral analgesics and NSAIDs similar to acute gout, particularly for polyarticular pseudogout as performing multiple joint injections is impractical and painful.

Take care using NSAIDs in the elderly and use the smallest doses to avoid renal impairment and precipitating heart failure.

HAEMARTHROSIS

Haemarthrosis is bleeding into a joint which may be traumatic and related to intra-articular injury or non-traumatic related to an underlying bleeding diathesis.

Aetiology

The causes of haemarthrosis are listed in Table 14.2.2.

Clinical features

A haemarthrosis causes a painful swollen joint with a reduced range of movement. The joint is often warm. Ask about a history of trauma and, if minimal or absent, consider a bleeding disorder, such as haemophilia or anticoagulant

Table 14.2.2 Causes of haemarthrosis
Traumatic
• Fracture
• Ligamentous (e.g. anterior cruciate or peripheral meniscal tear in the knee)
Non-traumatic
• Bleeding diathesis, e.g. haemophilia, von Willebrand's disease
• Anticoagulation
• Neuropathic joint
• Acute pseudogout
• Septic arthritis
• Pigmented villonodular synovitis
• Vascular abnormalities, such arteriovenous malformation, haemangioma

use. Also ask about troublesome bleeding during a previous operation or following dental instrumentation and about a family history.

Investigations

Perform plain radiography to exclude a fracture. Consider a computed tomography scan if there is a high index of clinical suspicion but normal plain imaging. Send a full blood count and a coagulation screen if there is no history of significant trauma.

Haemarthrosis is diagnosed on aspiration of synovial fluid. An intra-articular fracture is indicated by observing fat globules floating on the surface of the blood.

Management

Management includes rest, immobilization, ice and compression as well as analgesia. Aspiration frequently provides pain relief if performed within 24 h of onset. NSAIDs should be avoided in patients with a bleeding diathesis.

Haemophilia or other bleeding diathesis

Haemarthrosis due to haemophilia or other disorders of clotting factor deficiency requires *immediate* factor replacement therapy to a level of 40–50% of normal. This should be performed

as soon as possible after the presentation, in consultation with a haematology specialist.

Often the patient will be able to advise on their normal treatment (and usually knows what factor they are deficient in, their usual basal level and how much replacement is necessary in an acute bleed).

Vitamin K and administration of fresh frozen plasma may be required in patients with elevated INR related to warfarin toxicity.

SPONDYLOARTHRITIS

Monoarthritis is occasionally a presentation of a spondyloarthritis, such as reactive arthritis, psoriatic arthritis or inflammatory bowel disease-associated arthritis.

Clinical features suggesting a reactive arthritis include a recent history of infective diarrhoea, uveitis or sexually transmitted infection, such as urethritis. The patient may appear ill and be febrile with a tachycardia. The patient should be asked about a history of psoriasis or inflammatory bowel disease in the past.

Check for sites of enthesitis with inflammation at a tendon insertion points, such as the Achilles tendon or plantar fascia around the heel, or dactylitis causing 'sausage-shaped' digits.

GUIDELINE APPROACH TO THE MANAGEMENT OF ACUTE MONOARTHRITIS

The British Society for Rheumatology, in conjunction with other medical associations, published guidelines in 2006 regarding an approach to the hot swollen joint. No changes were recommended on review in 2012 [10]. These guidelines are summarized below:

❶ The hot, swollen and tender joint should be considered as septic arthritis until proven otherwise. This may occur in the absence of fever.

❷ Synovial fluid must be obtained and sent for appropriate investigations prior to commencement of antibiotics. In situations of high clinical suspicion, a negative Gram stain or culture does not exclude septic arthritis.

❸ Other investigations should include blood cultures, CRP, ESR and full blood count.

❹ X-ray of the affected joint should be performed as a baseline.

❺ Septic joints require aspiration to dryness in addition to parenteral antibiotics.

❻ Prosthetic joints and suspected hip sepsis require an urgent orthopaedic opinion.

❼ The presentation of a hot and swollen first metatarso-phalangeal joint is almost always gout, and is diagnosed clinically.

References

[1] Gupta MN, Sturrock RD, Field M, et al. Prospective comparative study of patients with culture proven and high suspicion of adult onset septic arthritis. Ann Rheum Dis 2003;62:327–31.

[2] Matthews CJ, Weston VC, Jones A, et al. Bacterial septic arthritis in adults. Lancet 2010;375:846–55.

[3] Margaretten ME, Kohlwes J, Moore D, et al. Does this adult patient have septic arthritis?. J Am Med Assoc 2007;297:1478–88.

[4] Sharma M, Leirisalo-Repo M. Arthritis patient as an emergency case at a university hospital. Scand J Rheumatol 1997;26:30–6.

[5] Zhang W, Doherty M, Pascual E, et al. EULAR evidence based recommendations for gout. Part 1: diagnosis. Ann Rheum Dis 2006;65:1301–11.

[6] Cronstein BN, Terkeltaub R. The inflammatory process of gout and its treatment. Arthrit Resp Ther 2006;8(suppl 1):S3.

[7] Therapeutic Guidelines: Rheumatology, Version 2. Melbourne: Therapeutics Guidelines Ltd; 2010.

[8] Morris I, Varughese G, Mattingly P, et al. Colchicine in acute gout. Br Med J 2003;327:1275–6.

[9] Zhang W, Doherty M, Bardin T, et al. EULAR evidence based recommendations for gout. Part 1: management. Ann Rheum Dis 2006;65:1312–24.

[10] Coakley G, Mathews C, Field M, et al. BSR and BHPR, BOA, RCGP and BSAC guidelines for management of the hot swollen joint in adults. Rheumatology 2006;45:1039–41. Revision 2012 available at < http://www.rheumatology.org.uk/ > [Accessed Feb. 2013].

Further reading

Antibiotic Guidelines, Version 14. Melbourne: Therapeutic Guidelines Ltd; 2010.

Matthews CJ, Weston VC, Jones A, et al. Bacterial septic arthritis in adults. Lancet 2010;375:846–55.

Rider TG, Jordan KM. The modern management of gout. Rheumatology (Oxford) 2010;49:5–14.

14.3 Polyarthritis

Shom Bhattacharjee • Adam B Bystrzycki • Flavia M Cicuttini

ESSENTIALS

1 Polyarthritis is a common adult rheumatological presentation with a wide differential diagnosis.

2 Recording articular and extra-articular involvement facilitates decision making, particularly with regards to patient admission.

3 Joint aspiration is useful for both diagnosis and excluding a septic arthritis. Other valuable tests include full blood examination, erythrocyte sedimentation rate and plain radiography.

4 Emergency management is with anti-inflammatory medication that may include systemic or intra-articular corticosteroids.

5 Early rheumatological consultation and/or admission is essential, particularly in the presence of extra-articular or systemic inflammatory response features.

6 Otherwise organize multidisciplinary follow up on discharge from the emergency department.

Table 14.3.1   Differential diagnosis of polyarthritis syndromes

Inflammatory
Rheumatoid arthritis
Inflammatory osteoarthritis
Systemic connective tissue disease, including SLE, vasculitis, Behçet's disease, relapsing polychondritis
Seronegative spondyloarthropathies, commonly psoriatic arthropathy
Gout
Pseudogout (calcium pyrophosphate arthropathy)
Drug induced, including lupus syndromes
Infectious arthritis – bacterial including mycobacteria, endocarditis, protozoal, viral
Reactive or post-infectious arthritis including rheumatic fever

Non-inflammatory
Neoplastic/paraneoplastic disease, including hypertrophic pulmonary osteoarthropathy
Sarcoidosis
Endocrine disease, such as haemochromatosis, acromegaly
Haematological disease, such as haemophilia, leukaemia

Introduction

Polyarthritis is a frequent rheumatological presentation to the emergency department in adults. This chapter focuses on the initial assessment, management and most appropriate follow up of the more common conditions encountered. These include rheumatoid arthritis (RA), seronegative spondyloarthritis including psoriatic arthritis, reactive arthritis with reference to arthritides occurring in association with enteric and urogenital infections, and infectious arthritis including viral arthritis and rheumatic fever. Management principles include establishing the diagnosis, treating the acute problem and arranging appropriate follow up.

ACUTE POLYARTHRITIS

Polyarthritis syndromes may be difficult to diagnose accurately due to the wide range of differential diagnoses, as seen in Table 14.3.1 [1]. Important principles are to rule out infection, quantify underlying inflammation and document extra-articular involvement.

Clinical features and diagnosis

History
Take a focused history to include the following [2,3].

Mode of onset
- Acute (less than 6 weeks): gonococcal, viral including human immunodeficiency virus (HIV), reactive arthritis, rheumatic fever.
- Chronic: RA, psoriatic arthropathy, systemic lupus erythematosus (SLE), scleroderma, dermatomyositis, other autoimmune diseases.

Distribution
- Symmetric or asymmetric: large or small joint involvement.

Course
- Progressive, intermittent or migratory.

Constitutional symptoms
- Fever, night sweats, fatigue, significant weight loss >10%.

Rheumatological systems review
- Symptoms including early morning stiffness, Raynaud's phenomenon, sclerodactyly, sicca syndrome, uveitis, scleritis, oral, nasal, digital or genital ulcers, rash, alopecia, urethritis, cervicitis, chronic bowel symptoms and serositis with pleuritis or pericarditis.

Extra-articular organ involvement
- Cough, dyspnoea, hypertension, haematuria, symptomatic peripheral neuropathy.

Other history
History of recent sore throat, febrile illness, new sexual contact, features of a sexually transmitted disease, diarrhoea, rash or uveitis.

Past medical history of gout, rheumatic fever, inflammatory bowel disease (IBD), malignancy and juvenile polyarthritis.

Family history of gout, psoriasis, IBD, uveitis or chronic back pain suggesting ankylosing spondylitis (AS) and other seronegative arthritis.

Examination

Perform a detailed physical examination [4] and document:

- vital signs
- painful joints and soft-tissue swelling and their distribution
- cutaneous stigmata of underlying diseases, such as nail changes (psoriatic), rash and subcutaneous nodules, oral, genital or digital ulceration
- features of organ involvement, such as a pleural or pericardial rub, cardiac murmur or pulmonary crackles
- lumbosacral spine and pelvis including sacroiliac joints.

Investigations

Laboratory studies

Send blood for full blood count (FBC), urea, electrolytes and liver function tests (ELFTs) and inflammatory markers including erythrocyte sedimentation rate (ESR) and C-reactive protein (CRP) [1,2].

Send serum antibody or antigen tests as indicated by the history for infectious exposure, such as hepatitis B serology, streptococcal antigen test (ASO titre) and an autoantibody panel including antinuclear antibody (ANA), rheumatoid factor (RF) and antibodies against citrullinated peptides (ACPA) usually ordered as anticyclic citrullinated peptide (anti-CCP). Antibody tests in particular should be interpreted with caution and in the context of each individual patient, due to their varying sensitivity and specificity [5].

Joint aspiration

Joint aspiration and analysis of synovial fluid are essential to diagnose septic arthritis and crystal arthropathy (see Chapter 14.2).

Imaging studies

Imaging studies, such as plain X-rays, may demonstrate diagnostic features in erosive arthropathy, but these do not occur for some time after the acute onset.

RHEUMATOID ARTHRITIS

Rheumatoid arthritis (RA) is a chronic systemic inflammatory disorder of unknown aetiology

Table 14.3.2   Classification criteria for RA
A. Joint involvement 1 large joint – 0 pts 2–10 large joints – 1 pt 1–3 small joints (with or without involvement of large joints) – 2 pts 4–10 small joints (with or without involvement of large joints) – 3 pts >10 joints (at least 1 small joint) – 5 pts
B. Serology (at least 1 test result is needed for classification) Negative RF and negative ACPA – 0 pts Low-positive (<3 × ULN) RF or low-positive ACPA – 2 pts High-positive (≥3 × ULN) RF or high-positive ACPA – 3 pts
C. Acute-phase reactants (at least 1 test result is needed for classification) Normal CRP and normal ESR – 0 pts Abnormal CRP or abnormal ESR – 1 pt
D. Duration of symptoms <6 weeks – 0 pts ≥6 weeks – 1 pt
Add score of categories A–D: a score of >6/10 classifies a patient as having definite RA
ACPA: antibodies against citrullinated peptides; ULN: upper limit normal; RF: rheumatoid factor; RA: rheumatoid arthritis. Adapted from [7]

characterized by symmetric synovitis, erosive polyarthritis and numerous extra-articular manifestations. It occurs in up to 2% of the general population and is two to three times more common in women [6]. The onset is often indolent and may lack the characteristic symmetrical joint involvement. Uncommonly, it presents as an acute monoarthritis.

Diagnosis

The diagnosis in adults is guided by the American College of Rheumatology/European League Against Rheumatism critera. These criteria were revised in 2010 [7] to identify features predictive of erosive disease earlier in the illness, compared with the 1987 criteria which defined the disease by its later stage features. Constitutional features, such as malaise and fatigue, are common.

'Definite RA' is based on the confirmed presence of:

- synovitis in at least one joint
- absence of an alternative diagnosis that better explains the synovitis
- a total score of 6 or greater (of a possible 10) from individual scores in four domains: number and site of involved joints (score range 0–5); serologic abnormality (score range 0–3); elevated acute-phase response (score range 0–1) and symptom duration (2 levels; range 0–1) (Table 14.3.2).

Morning stiffness, symmetric involvement and radiographic erosions are no longer included.

Clinical features

Characteristic presentations in RA include the following [8–10].

Cervical spine

Cervical arthritis is common and may result in critical spinal problems from degeneration of the transverse ligament of the C1 vertebra that produces C1–2 instability in up to 5% of patients and can result in cervical cord compression or vertebral artery insufficiency. In addition, decreased motion and myelopathy may result from longstanding joint involvement.

Upper limb

The wrist, metacarpophalangeal and proximal interphalangeal joints are typically affected, with sparing of the distal interphalangeal joints. Swan-necking and boutonnière deformities are common, together with ulnar deviation at the metacarpophalangeal joints. Fixed flexion deformities may result in entrapment neuropathies, in particular, carpal tunnel syndrome with median nerve involvement. Tenosynovitis may lead to tendon rupture, particularly of the extensor pollicis longus, or degenerative changes in the long extensors of the middle, ring and the little fingers with rupture of these tendons.

Lower limb

The hip and knee are frequently involved. Metatarsophalangeal joint subluxation may occur. Talonavicular joint inflammation causes pronation and eversion deformity, with overlying muscle spasm. A Baker's cyst due to posterior herniation of the joint capsule of the knee joint may occur and require differentiation from a deep vein thrombosis by Doppler ultrasound. Entrapment of the posterior tibial nerve causes burning paraesthesiae on the sole of the foot.

Extra-articular manifestations

The extra-articular manifestations of RA are protean and may involve any organ system due to local inflammation causing functional or neurological deficits, rheumatoid vasculitis or distant inflammation (see Chapter 14.1). Patients may also present with the side effects of the treatment, including sepsis related to immunosuppression. Sepsis with encapsulated organisms is of particular concern in patients with Felty's syndrome of RA with splenomegaly and neutropaenia [11].

Investigations

Laboratory studies

Send blood for FBC and ELFTs and non-specific markers of inflammation, such as ESR, and CRP, with assays for serum rheumatoid factor and anti-CCP [12]. Anti-CCP is as sensitive but more specific than rheumatoid factor for RA and is more frequently positive early in the disease process. It is also thought to identify individuals at higher risk of erosive disease [13]. Send blood cultures as well as midstream urine for suspected sepsis.

Joint aspiration

Joint aspiration is essential to exclude coexistent or primary sepsis in any sudden hot, swollen joint.

Imaging

Initial plain imaging of affected joints at first presentation does not usually demonstrate erosive changes, but is useful in patients with longstanding disease. However, always request X-rays of the cervical spine in any patient with cervical or neurological features to look for an atlanto-dens interval of greater than 2.5 mm, which is diagnostic of instability [14]. Include a chest X-ray if there is a fever and/or any respiratory features. Request an ultrasound examination to differentiate deep vein thrombosis from a Baker's cyst.

Emergency management

Emergency therapy aims to relieve acute pain and reduce joint inflammation. Longer-term goals include restoration and maintenance of joint function and the prevention of periarticular bony and cartilage destruction. Important principles include medication, education, rest and exercise, with the input of a multidisciplinary allied health team incorporating occupational therapy and physiotherapy.

Medication falls broadly under the categories of non-steroidal anti-inflammatory drugs (NSAIDs) and disease-modifying antirheumatic drug (DMARD) therapy. Readers are referred to Chapter 14.1 for a brief overview of these medications and common adverse effects, as well as the references at the end of this chapter [15–18].

Other long-term measures include orthopaedic and orthotic intervention. Surgery involving joint fusion, synovectomy, total joint arthroplasty and reconstruction may be required.

Early consultation with a rheumatologist is essential, particularly for patients with acute or first presentations. Exclusion of infection even for mild or moderate features is imperative and to control symptoms with simple analgesics with discharge for specialist follow up. Admit patients if there is evidence of multisystem involvement, severe symptoms requiring nursing or allied health management or if they are unable to tolerate oral therapy.

Prognosis

The spontaneous remission rate in RA is less than 10% [19,20]. High titres of anti-CCP or rheumatoid factor, which are present in up to 75% of patients with rheumatoid arthritis, the presence of nodules and human leucocyte antigen (HLA)-DR4 haplotype are markers of severity. A patient's life expectancy is shortened by 10–15 years by accelerated cardiovascular disease, infection, pulmonary and renal disease and gastrointestinal bleeding.

SERONEGATIVE ARTHRITIS

The seronegative spondyloarthritis disorders are characterized by inflammation of the axial spine with sacroiliitis and spondylitis in particular, enthesitis, which is inflammation at the attachments of tendons and ligaments to bones, dactylitis, asymmetric polyarthritis often of the lower limb, eye inflammation and varied mucocutaneous features [21]. They are labelled 'seronegative' as the serum rheumatoid factor is negative.

Epidemiology

The term 'seronegative spondyloarthritis' covers conditions such as ankylosing spondylitis (AS), reactive arthritis occurring in the setting of viral or bacterial infection, psoriatic arthritis and arthritis associated with inflammatory bowel disease (IBD). It is further differentiated into *axial* and *peripheral* spondyloarthritis.

The prevalence of the seronegative spondyloarthritis disorders varies widely and may parallel the prevalence of the HLA-B27 gene.

However, the exact role of HLA-B27 in the pathogenesis of these disorders has not been clearly defined. The proportion of HLA-B27 positive individuals who develop symptomatic arthropathy varies widely from 16% in patients with AS to 70% of patients with spondylitis in the setting of IBD [22]. HLA-B27 positive individuals may be less efficient at the intracellular removal of certain inciting bacteria, although this is controversial [23].

The Assessment of SpondyloArthritis international Society (ASAS) recently advanced classification criteria for axial and peripheral spondyloarthritis (Fig. 14.3.1). These criteria have better sensitivity and comparable specificity to previous criteria and are well validated [24].

PSORIATIC ARTHRITIS

Psoriatic arthritis is a heterogeneous disease distinct from other inflammatory arthritides. It occurs in 10% of patients with psoriasis, but may affect up to 40% of hospitalized psoriasis patients with widespread skin involvement [25]. It occurs between the ages of 30 and 60 years, with an equal prevalence in males and females. It is thought to be inherited in a polygenic pattern significantly influenced by environmental factors, including trauma and infectious agents. Multiple studies have confirmed the important role of class I HLA, particularly B13, B16 and B27 and certain C-subclasses [26,27]. The arthropathy pattern may be pauci-articular, but more than five peripheral joints are usually involved.

In patients with ≥3 months back pain (with/without peripheral manifestations) and age at onset ≤45 years:

| Sacroiliitis on imaging plus ≥1 SpA feature | OR | HLA-B27 plus ≥2 other SpA features |

SpA features:
- Inflammatory back pain (IBP)
- Arthritis
- Enthesitis (heel)
- Uveitis
- Dactylitis
- Psoriasis
- Crohn's/ulcerative colitis
- Good response to NSAIDs
- Family history for SpA
- HLA-B27
- Elevated CRP

In patients with peripheral manifestations ONLY:

Arthritis* or enthesitis or dactylitis plus

≥1 SpA feature:
- Uveitis
- Psoriasis
- Crohn's/ulcerative colitis
- Preceding infection
- HLA-B27
- Sacroiliitis on imaging

OR

≥2 other SpA features
- Arthritis
- Enthesitis
- Dactylitis
- IBP ever
- Family history for SpA

Fig. 14.3.1 Combined use of the Assessment of SpondyloArthritis international Society (ASAS) criteria for axial spondyloarthritis and the ASAS criteria for peripheral SpA in the entire SpA population. *Peripheral arthritis: usually predominantly lower limb author asymmetric arthritis combined sesitivity 79.5% and combined specificity 83.3% n = 975. (From Rudwaleit M, et al. Ann Rheum Dis 2011;70:25–31 with permission.)

Clinical features and diagnosis

The diagnosis of psoriatic arthritis is essentially clinical, requiring the demonstration of coexisting synovitis and psoriasis. A set of simple clinical diagnostic criteria, the ClASsification criteria for Psoriatic ARthritis (abbreviated to the CASPAR criteria) were proposed by a large international study group in 2006 [28].

CASPAR diagnostic criteria for psoriatic arthritis

Established inflammatory joint disease and at least three points from the following features:

- current psoriasis (2 points)
- history of psoriasis (in the absence of current psoriasis) (1 point)
- family history of psoriasis (in the absence of current or past history) (1 point)
- dactylitis (1 point)
- juxta-articular new bone formation (1 point)
- rheumatoid factor negativity (1 point)
- nail dystrophy (1 point).

Five clinical subtypes are recognized, including asymmetric oligoarthritis, symmetric small joint polyarthritis, predominant distal interphalangeal joint involvement, psoriatic spondyloarthropathy and arthritis mutilans [29]. Major extra-articular organ manifestations, such as aortic insufficiency and pulmonary fibrosis, occur rarely. However, up to 30% of patients have mild inflammation at the eye, most commonly conjunctivitis.

Asymmetric oligoarthritis

This occurs in 30–50% of patients [30]. It presents as an oligoarthritis involving a single large joint, in association with a 'sausage-shaped' or dactylitic digit or toe. Dactylitis occurs due to a combination of arthritis and tenosynovitis. Distal interphalangeal joint involvement is typical, almost invariably associated with psoriatic nail changes of pitting, ridging and onycholysis. Enthesitis occurs most frequently with this form of the disease and commonly manifests as plantar fasciitis or epicondylitis at the elbow.

Symmetric small joint polyarthritis

This occurs in 30% of patients, in a pattern strongly resembling RA, but with more frequent distal interphalangeal joint involvement [30].

Psoriatic spondyloarthritis

This occurs in 5% of patients [30]. It is often asymptomatic, but may present with inflammatory low back pain due to sacroiliitis in up to 30% of cases.

Arthritis mutilans

'Arthritis mutilans' is a rare (<5% of patients), but well-characterized feature of psoriatic arthritis with severely deforming arthritis including telescoping of the fingers or toes from osteolysis of the metacarpal or metatarsal bones and phalanges [30].

Dermatological features

Dermatological features include typical erythematous, scaling plaques on the extensor surfaces of the elbows and knees, scalp and ears and nail changes. The nail changes include pitting with usually greater than 20 pits, ridging with transverse depressions and onycholysis with separation of the nail from the underlying nail bed [25]. Nodules and vasculitic features such as digital ulcers are not seen.

Psoriatic arthritis can be difficult to distinguish from the other seronegative spondyloarthritides in the absence of dermatological features or a positive family history.

Investigations

ESR and CRP are raised, but the rheumatoid factor and autoantibody screen are negative. Plain X-rays of affected joints may reveal typical radiographic features including soft-tissue swelling, bone proliferation at the base of digital phalanges coupled with resorption of the distal tufts (the 'pencil-in-cup' deformity) and fluffy periostitis [31]. Chest radiographs are useful as a baseline when clinical examination suggests cardiac or pulmonary involvement.

Emergency management

Emergency treatment involves the relief of pain and reduction of joint inflammation, with appropriate specialist follow up. Education, rest and exercise and referral to a multidisciplinary allied health team are the mainstay of ongoing management. Admit patients if their symptoms are severe enough to preclude oral therapy or safe discharge pending outpatient specialist follow up.

NSAIDs are useful for acute symptomatic relief and intra- or peri-articular corticosteroids may be used for short-term relief of painful arthritis or enthesitis. Long-term therapy with disease modifying agents, such as sulphasalazine or methotrexate, is instituted at specialist review [32]. Oral corticosteroids are usually avoided as their cessation often exacerbates the psoriasis. Therapy with tumour necrosis factor-α antagonists, such as infliximab, etanercept and adalimumab, has been approved for rheumatologists under strict access criteria for severe disease resistant to other DMARD therapy.

Emergency management of skin disease includes topical treatments, such as emollients and keratolytic agents [33]. Phototherapy and photo-chemotherapy may be instituted on early dermatological consultation.

Prognosis

Psoriatic arthritis generally runs a more benign course than RA but, nonetheless, patients suffer from considerable morbidity. Adverse prognostic factors include onset before 20 years of age, erosive disease and extensive skin involvement [30].

REACTIVE ARTHRITIS

Reactive arthritis is an aseptic peripheral arthritis following certain infections, which include bacterial infections of the urogenital tract usually by *Chlamydia trachomatis*, or of the gastrointestinal tract with organisms, such as *Shigella*, *Salmonella* and *Campylobacter*. It may also follow viral infections, such as HIV, although in the case of HIV, co-infection with sexually transmitted organisms rather than the virus itself is thought to be the cause [34]. The seroconversion illness of HIV has its own constellation of articular symptoms and is considered to be a separate entity.

Epidemiology

The prevalence of reactive arthritis is difficult to define owing to diagnostic uncertainty particularly in the setting of asymptomatic sexually transmitted infection. The male preponderance is up to 9:1 following sexually transmitted infection, but males and females are equally affected following gastrointestinal tract infection [35]. The peak incidence is around age 35 years and up to 75% of patients are HLA-B27

positive [35]. An important exception is with the reactive peripheral arthritis that occurs in 20% of patients with idiopathic IBD, a condition that may mimic gastrointestinal tract infection, but where patients are usually HLA-B27 negative.

Clinical features and diagnosis

The diagnosis of reactive arthritis is clinical. It typically manifests within a month of gastrointestinal or genitourinary infection, although the latter is frequently asymptomatic [36]. Musculoskeletal manifestations include myalgias and asymmetric polyarthritis affecting the knees, ankles and small joints of the feet in particular, although peripheral upper limb involvement is seen. Affected joints demonstrate marked inflammatory features with erythema, swelling, warmth and exquisite pain on active or passive movement. Fever and malaise are common.

Arthritis and extra-articular manifestations

Symptomatic spondylitis and sacroiliitis cause low back and buttock pain and occur frequently. Dactylitis and enthesitis are characteristic features of this disease with heel pain from plantar fasciitis or Achilles tendonitis [36].

Extra-articular features associated with reactive arthritis include keratoderma blennorrhagica, the scattered, thickened, hyperkeratotic skin lesions with pustules and crusts seen in Reiter's syndrome and circinate balanitis. Keratoderma blennorhagica on the soles or palms may coalesce to form plaques virtually indistinguishable from those of psoriasis [37]. Circinate balanitis causes shallow meatal ulcers that are moist in uncircumcised men or hyperkeratotic and plaque-like in circumcised men [37]. An inflammatory aortitis occurs in 1% of patients and may result in aortic valvular incompetence and/or heart block

The peripheral arthritis associated with IBD is migratory and occurs in a similar distribution. Common features include large joint effusions, particularly involving the knee, and sacroiliitis or spondylitis [38]. Unlike peripheral arthritis following genitourinary infection, the spondylitis of IBD-associated arthritis does not tend to settle with treatment of the bowel inflammation. Cutaneous features associated with this form of arthritis occur mainly on the lower limbs and include erythema nodosum and pyoderma gangrenosum [38].

Investigations

Laboratory

An active inflammatory response is seen in the acute phase with a neutrophil leucocytosis and thrombocytosis and raised ESR and CRP. The presence of a mild normochromic, normocytic anaemia suggests chronic disease. Send blood for HLA-B27.

Document the preceding gastrointestinal or genitourinary organism by stool culture or cervical/urethral swabs [39]. Rheumatoid factor and ANA are negative.

Joint aspiration

Joint aspiration may be necessary to exclude intra-articular sepsis (see Chapter 14.2). The synovial fluid may be turbid, viscous and with a neutrophil leucocytosis up to 50000/mm³, but Gram stain and bacterial culture are negative and, unlike true septic arthritis, the synovial glucose level is not significantly reduced compared to serum levels [39]. Macrophages with intracytoplasmic vacuoles containing ingested neutrophils are occasionally seen.

Imaging

X-ray changes are unusual with acute arthritis, but are seen after several months. As with psoriatic arthritis, a common finding is a 'fluffy' periosteal reaction, particularly at the calcaneus, and evidence of sacroiliitis or spondylitis with bridging syndesmophytes in long-standing disease.

Emergency management

Exclude infection by synovial aspiration and culture with a markedly inflamed joint and consult early with a rheumatologist, particularly in a patient with a first presentation. Admit patients with suspected septic arthritis until it is excluded or if they are unable to tolerate simple oral therapies. Request a cardiology opinion for major cardiac involvement with valvular disease or a conduction abnormality and a gastroenterology opinion when IBD is suspected, although the role of treatment and the effect on the arthropathy is unclear.

Otherwise provide symptom relief with NSAIDs as the mainstay of treatment. Corticosteroids may be given after rheumatological consultation, either systemic or topically for the skin manifestations. Disease modifying therapy with sulphasalazine is initiated at specialist follow up if NSAID therapy fails to control symptoms. Multidisciplinary physical therapy is essential on an outpatient basis.

Give antibiotics, such as doxycycline 100 mg orally bd for 7 days or azithromycin 1 g orally once for documented urethritis or cervicitis, and remember partner contact tracing and treatment. An infectious diseases opinion is useful in these cases [39].

Prognosis

Signs and symptoms usually remit within 6 months. However, up to 50% of patients suffer from recurrent arthritis and up to 30% develop chronic arthritis [40]. Post-dysenteric cases have a better prognosis than post-chlamydial cases. Poor prognostic signs include early onset under the age of 16 years, hip involvement and the presence of dactylitis.

POLYARTICULAR CRYSTAL ARTHRITIS

Crystal-induced arthritis disorders result from the deposition of crystal in joint spaces, such as in gout or pseudogout. Both diseases cause debilitating joint inflammation resulting from the lysis of neutrophil polymorphs that have ingested monosodium urate in the case of gout, or calcium pyrophosphate crystals in pseudogout. Although usually monoarticular, polyarticular involvement can occur in up to 5% of cases. See Chapter 14.2 for a detailed discussion of these diseases.

INFECTIOUS POLYARTHRITIS

Septic bacterial arthritis is most often monoarticular, although it can present with polyarticular involvement. Infectious polyarthritis may also occur as aseptic manifestation of certain viral infections and following streptococcal infection in acute rheumatic fever (ARF).

Viral arthritis

Arthralgia affecting several joints is common in many viral infections, but few cause frank polyarthritis. In general, these are self-limiting and managed symptomatically. Viruses involved include alphaviruses, such as the Ross River virus (RRV), parvovirus B19 and hepatitis A, B and C viruses.

Alphaviruses

Alphaviruses are a mosquito-borne genus of the *Togaviridae* family. They are responsible for epidemics of febrile polyarthritis, including Ross River, Barmah Forest and Sindbis viruses (SINV) in Australia; West Nile virus which has recently been documented in the USA; Chikungunya virus in East Africa, South and Southeast Asia; O'nyong-nyong virus in East Africa and the Mayaro virus in South America [41].

Ross River virus

RRV is endemic to Australia, New Zealand and South Pacific islands and is the most common arboviral disease in Australia. RRV is transmitted by the *Ochlerotatus* (formerly *Aedes*) *vigilex* mosquito via a marsupial reservoir [42]. Epidemics of acute febrile polyarthritis are most common between January and May, but can occur after periods of heavy rains.

Clinical features and diagnosis

A detailed travel history is essential. There is usually low grade fever and other constitutional symptoms. A rash varying in distribution, character and duration occurs up to 2 weeks before, during or after the other features. Polyarticular symptoms are present in most patients with a symmetric arthritis or arthralgia primarily affecting the wrist, knee, ankle and small joints of the extremities. Cervical lymphadenopathy occurs frequently and paraesthesiae and tenderness of the palms and soles in a small percentage of cases [43].

The diagnosis is predominantly clinical, particularly in endemic areas in the event of a local outbreak, and confirmed by serology.

Investigations

Serology testing distinguishes RRV from other causes of febrile polyarthritis, such as Barmah Forest virus. A significant rise in IgM antibody titre to RRV indicates acute infection or the virus itself may be isolated from the serum of acutely unwell patients. Radiographs are unremarkable and unnecessary as the disease is largely self-limiting [44].

Emergency management

Patients with RRV require symptomatic treatment with simple analgesics or NSAIDs. Occasionally, a brief course of low-dose prednisolone may be used. RRV is a notifiable disease [42]. Refer to a rheumatologist if symptoms are severe or refractory to simple treatment measures.

Conventional personal preventative measures, such as protective clothing, effective mosquito repellent and avoidance of mosquito-prone areas should be recommended, as no vaccine currently exists.

Prognosis

RRV is usually self-limiting, but prolonged symptoms may occur and there may be relapses of decreasing intensity, separated by remissions for up to a year or more.

Parvovirus B19

Human parvovirus B19 infection is caused by a small, single-stranded DNA virus that has a predilection for erythroid precursor cells and is transmitted by respiratory secretions. It causes the self-limiting illness *erythema infectiosum* known as 'slapped cheek disease' or 'fifth disease' in children. In adults, however, parvovirus B19 manifests with severe 'flu-like symptoms and as many as 75% develop joint symptoms. It may be responsible for up to 12% of adult patients presenting with acute polyarthritis, most notably in those who have frequent exposure to children [45].

Clinical features and diagnosis

The characteristic 'slapped cheek' rash is usually absent in adults. An acute polyarthritis improves over 2 weeks, with symmetric involvement of peripheral small joints, including the hands (proximal interphalangeal and metacarpophalangeal joints in particular), wrists, knees and ankle joints. Morning stiffness is prominent. These features are similar to those seen in patients with RA, with up to 50% of affected patients found to meet the (now superceded) 1987 ACR diagnostic criteria for RA [46].

Uncommon but important extra-articular features of parvovirus B19 infection include [47]:

- development of an aplastic crisis in patients with chronic haemolytic anaemia
- bone marrow suppression in immunocompromised patients
- *hydrops fetalis* in women infected during pregnancy
- Henoch–Schönlein purpura
- thrombotic thrombocytopaenic purpura
- Wegener's granulomatosis or polyarteritis nodosa (rare).

Investigations

Send a FBC, particularly given the potential for an aplastic crisis and bone marrow suppression. Non-specific markers of inflammation are likely to be elevated. Specific serological diagnosis is made by a high IgM antibody titre specific to the virus and by isolation of the viral DNA by polymerase chain reaction (PCR). IgG antibodies to parvovirus B19 indicate past infection and are common in the adult population [48].

Transient, moderate elevations of rheumatoid factor, anti-DNA, antilymphocyte or anticardiolipin antibodies sometimes occur [48]. Radiographs of the affected joints are normal.

Emergency management

Rest and NSAIDs are the mainstay of emergency treatment, except in pregnant women when NSAIDs are contraindicated in the third trimester [49]. A short course of prednisolone may be required. Significant extra-articular manifestations may require admission and consultation with the appropriate specialist. Blood transfusion or intravenous immunoglobulin infusions may be necessary.

Prognosis

Joint symptoms are self-limited in the majority of adult patients, but up to 10% may have prolonged relapsing and remitting symptoms lasting up to 9 years [50].

Hepatitis A, B and C viruses

The hepatitis viruses A, B and C all cause viral polyarthritis. Hepatitis B virus (HBV) is responsible for 20–25%, and hepatitis A (HAV) up to 14% of causes in patients with viral polyarthritis [51]. The polyarthritis of HAV tends to occur during the infectious phase and is self-limiting. The polyarthritis of HBV occurs in early infection during a period of significant viraemia and is thought to be due to immune complexes.

Clinical features and diagnosis

HBV polyarthritis is acute and severe and manifests in a symmetric, migratory or additive fashion, most commonly involving the hand and knee joints [52]. Other large axial joints may be involved and significant early morning stiffness is often present. The arthritis may precede the development of jaundice and persist for several weeks after jaundice has developed.

Hepatitis C virus (HCV) polyarthritis is rapidly progressive and symmetrical, involving the hands, wrists, shoulders, knees and hips [53]. Carpal tunnel syndrome and tenosynovitis may occur. It is unusual for polyarthritis to be the first manifestation of the underlying disease in either HBV or HCV. Nonetheless, ask about exposure risk factors for these viruses, such as intravenous drug abuse, unprotected sexual intercourse, past blood transfusions, tattoos, as well as about previous jaundice.

Both hepatitis B and hepatitis C disease are associated with a number of important extra-articular, extra-hepatic manifestations which include:

- HBV: polyarteritis nodosa, systemic necrotizing vasculitis, membranous glomerulonephritis [54]
- HCV: mixed cryoglobulinaemia causing palpable purpura, arthritis and serum cryoglobulinaemia with cutaneous phenomena, such as Raynaud's syndrome and digital ulcers, membranous glomerulonephritis and lymphoma [53,55].

Laboratory investigations and imaging

Send blood for ELFTs for raised transaminases with elevated bilirubin, hepatitis B surface antigen, antihepatitis B surface antigen IgM to indicate acute infection and/or viral DNA quantification by PCR. Check also for anti-HCV IgM and for viral DNA quantification by PCR.

Also check FBC and for ESR, CRP, cryoglobulins and rheumatoid factor in the presence of a rash, ulcers or other vasculitic phenomena.

Radiographs are normal other than showing soft-tissue swelling.

Emergency management

Commence symptomatic treatment with NSAIDs and refer refractory HBV- or HCV-associated polyarthritis to a rheumatology specialist and/or combined hepatology clinic. Disease modifying agents, such as prednisolone and sulphasalazine, may be used cautiously with careful monitoring of the liver function tests and for increasing viraemia [56].

Prognosis

This varies depending on the underlying disease and on the presence of vasculitic phenomena. The polyarthritis of HBV is usually limited to the pre-icteric phase, but patients with chronic active hepatitis or chronic HBV viraemia may have recurrent arthritis.

RHEUMATIC FEVER

Acute rheumatic fever (ARF) refers to the constellation of non-infectious symptoms occurring after a pharyngeal infection with group A streptococci (GAS). Evidence suggests that it may also occur in high-risk populations following skin infections with GAS [57].

Epidemiology

ARF is characterized by inflammation of connective tissue including the joints, subcutaneous tissue, heart and blood vessels. Its prevalence has declined over time in developed countries, but it remains a major public health problem in indigenous populations in the more socially isolated parts of Australasia and in developing countries. In fact, the highest documented rates in the world occur in the Aboriginal Australian population and Torres Strait Islander populations of New Zealand and the Pacific Islands [58].

ARF is primarily a disease of children aged 5–14 years. The annual incidence may reach 350:100 000 in Aboriginal children [59]. However, the polyarthritis of ARF is most common in adolescents and young adults.

Diagnosis and clinical features

The diagnosis of ARF worldwide is made using the 1944 Jones, or more recent World Health Organization major and minor criteria. However, these criteria appear too restrictive for diagnosing ARF in Australian indigenous populations. Therefore, new criteria for use in high- and low-risk populations in Australia have been proposed (Table 14.3.3) [60].

The polyarthritis of ARF is usually the earliest symptom of the disease and is classically described as migratory, affecting several joints in quick succession for a short time, commencing with the large joints of the lower limb then the large joints of the upper limb [61]. Affected joints are painful but objective signs of inflammation, such as erythema and swelling, are not prominent.

Fever and constitutional symptoms are common. Other important extra-articular major criteria (with polyarthritis) of the disease include the following [61]:

- carditis: symptomatic pericarditis with pain and/or congestive cardiac failure

Table 14.3.3	2005 Australian guideline for the diagnosis of acute rheumatic fever	
	High-risk groups	All other groups
Initial episode of ARF	Two major or one major and two minor manifestations plus evidence of a preceding GAS infection	Two major or one major and two minor manifestations plus evidence of a preceding GAS infection
Recurrent attack of ARF in a patient with known past ARF or RHD	Two major or one major and two minor or three minor manifestations plus evidence of a preceding GAS infection	Two major or one major and two minor or three minor manifestations plus evidence of a preceding GAS infection
Major manifestations	• Carditis, including subclinical evidence of rheumatic valve disease on echocardiogram • Polyarthritis or aseptic monoarthritis or polyarthralgia • Chorea • *Erythema marginatum* • Subcutaneous nodules	• Carditis, excluding subclinical evidence of rheumatic valve disease on echocardiogram • Polyarthritis • Chorea • *Erythema marginatum* • Subcutaneous nodules

ARF: acute rheumatic fever; GAS: group A streptococci; RHD: rheumatic heart disease.

with breathlessness, new murmurs, cardiomegaly, electrocardiographic evidence of heart block

- Sydenham's chorea (St Vitus' dance): choreiform movements particularly of the face and upper limbs, emotional lability, rarely transient psychosis
- subcutaneous Aschoff nodules: firm, painless, mobile nodules near bony prominences on the extensor surfaces of wrists, elbows and knees
- rash (*erythema marginatum*): occurs in around 5% of ARF. This consists of blanching ring-like pink macules with a serpiginous edge and central clear portion occurring on the trunk and inner surfaces of the arms and legs, which are not itchy and can come and go for months. They may be slightly raised, but spare the face. The rash may change from hour to hour and may seem to appear, disappear or move rapidly in front of you. It is exacerbated by heat and fades when the patient is cool.

Laboratory investigations and imaging

Measure antistreptolysin O and antideoxyribonuclease B (anti-DNase B) titres [61]. As these titres can take 6 weeks after infection to peak, interpretation in the acute phase should be cautious and serial tests should be performed. Note that antistreptococcal antibody titres are useful in low-risk populations, but are difficult to interpret in high-risk populations due to pre-existing high background titres [62].

Send a throat swab, although this is positive in less than 10% of high-risk populations. Other important tests include:

- ESR and CRP, which are almost invariably elevated
- FBC, which may demonstrate a leucocytosis and, less commonly, a normochromic, normocytic anaemia
- ECG to document the P-R interval
- chest X-ray to look for cardiomegaly or symptomatic cardiac failure.

Synovial fluid aspirate is usually inflammatory with an elevated white cell count and sterile on microscopy and culture. Radiographs of affected joints generally demonstrate soft-tissue swelling only.

Emergency management

This depends on establishing the diagnosis and treating the manifestations. Patients are markedly symptomatic and often require admission for initial observation and management. Request rheumatology and infectious disease opinions and a neurology opinion if chorea is troublesome. The presence of heart block or, more importantly, frank cardiac failure or acute valvular regurgitation mandate cardiology admission.

The polyarthritis of rheumatic fever is exquisitely responsive to NSAID therapy, particularly aspirin, so much so that failure of NSAID therapy rapidly to relieve symptoms should prompt consideration of an alternative diagnosis [63]. Give high-dose aspirin at 80–100 mg/kg/day in 4–5 divided doses in adults, usually for 1–2 weeks [64].

Commence antibiotic therapy with phenoxymethylpenicillin 10 mg/kg up to 500 mg orally 12-hourly for 10 days to eradicate streptococcal pharyngitis, after obtaining appropriate diagnostic investigations as detailed above. Commence prophylaxis following resolution of the acute episode in high-risk indigenous communities.

Ongoing rheumatology and infectious diseases specialist follow up is recommended. Note that penicillin reduces the frequency and severity of post-streptococcal rheumatic fever, but has little effect on the course of the immune-complex mediated post-streptococcal glomerulonephritis (PSGN).

Prognosis

Recurrence of ARF commonly occurs within 2 years of the initial attack, despite prophylactic therapy. Most affected connective tissues do not sustain long-lasting damage, with the exception of the heart, which is prone to additive subclinical damage resulting in rheumatic heart disease [65].

Controversies

- DMARD therapy in the various causes of acute polyarthritis.
- The exact role of HLA-B27 in the pathogenesis of the spondyloarthritis disorders.
- Pathogenic mechanisms leading to reactive arthropathy.

References

[1] Klinkhoff A. Rheumatology: 5. Diagnosis and management of inflammatory polyarthritis. Can Med Assoc J 2000;162:1833–8.
[2] Pinals RS. Polyarthritis and fever. N Engl J Med 1994;330:769.
[3] Richie A, Francis M. Diagnostic approach to polyarticular joint pain. Am Fam Phys 2003;68:1075–88.
[4] Talley NJ, O'Connor S. The rheumatological system. In: Talley NJ, O'Connor S, editor. Clinical examination: a systematic guide to physical diagnosis, 5th ed. 2005. Sydney: Churchill Livingstone.
[5] Woolf SH, Kamerow DB. Testing for uncommon conditions. The heroic search for positive test results. Arch Intern Med 1990;150:2451–8.
[6] Rindfleisch JA, Muller D. Diagnosis and management of rheumatoid arthritis. Am Fam Phys 2005;72:1037–47.
[7] Aletaha D, Neogi T, Silman AJ, et al. Rheumatoid arthritis classification criteria: an American College of Rheumatology/ European League Against Rheumatism collaborative initiative. Arthritis Rheum 2010;62:2569–81.
[8] Rindfleisch JA, Muller D. Diagnosis and management of rheumatoid arthritis. Am Fam Phys 2005;72:1037–47.

[9] Scott DL. Rheumatoid arthritis: acute presentations and urgent complications. Br J Hosp Med 2006;67:235–9.

[10] Tutuncu Z, Kavanaugh A. Rheumatic disease in the elderly: rheumatoid arthritis. Rheum Dis Clin N Am 2007;33:57–70.

[11] Balint GP, Balint PV. Felty's syndrome. Best Pract Res Clin Rheumatol 2004;18:631–45.

[12] Westwood OM, Nelson PN, Hay FC. Rheumatoid factors: what's new? Rheumatology 2006;45:379–85.

[13] Bose N, Calabrese LH. Q: should I order an anti-CCP antibody test to diagnose rheumatoid arthritis? Cleve Clin J Med 2012;79:249–52.

[14] Macarthur A, Kleiman S. Rheumatoid cervical joint disease–a challenge to the anaesthetist. Can J Anaesth 1993;40:154–9.

[15] Emery P. Treatment of rheumatoid arthritis. Br Med J 2006;332:152–5.

[16] O'Dell JR. Therapeutic strategies for rheumatoid arthritis. N Engl J Med 2004;350:2591–602.

[17] Strand V, Hochberg MC. The risk of cardiovascular thrombotic events with selective cyclooxygenase 2 inhibitors. Arthritis Rheum 2002;47:349–55.

[18] Olsen NJ, Stein CM. New drugs for rheumatoid arthritis. N Engl J Med 2004;350:2167–79.

[19] Alarcon GS. Predictive factors in rheumatoid arthritis. Am J Med 1997;103:19S–24S.

[20] Wagner U, Kaltenhauser S, Sauer H, et al. HLA markers and prediction of clinical course and outcome in rheumatoid arthritis. Arthritis Rheum 1997;40:341–51.

[21] Nash P, Mease PJ, Braun J, van der Heijde D. Seronegative spondyloarthropathies: to lump or split? Ann Rheum Dis 2005;64(Suppl 2):ii9–13.

[22] Braun J, Bollow M, Remlinger G, et al. Prevalence of spondylarthropathies in HLA-B27 positive and negative blood donors. Arthritis Rheum 1998;41:58–67.

[23] Young JL, Smith L, Matyszak MK. HLA-B27 Expression does not modulate intracellular Chlamydia trachomatis infection of cell lines. Infect Immun 2001;69:6670–5.

[24] Rudwaleit M, van der Heijde D, Landewé R, et al. The Assessment of SpondyloArthritis International Society classification criteria for peripheral spondyloarthritis and for spondyloarthritis in general. Ann Rheum Dis 2011;70:25–31.

[25] Myers WA, Gottlieb AB, Mease P. Psoriasis and psoriatic arthritis: clinical features and disease mechanisms. Clin Dermatol 2006;24:438–47.

[26] Eastmond CJ. Psoriatic arthritis. Genetics and HLA antigens. Baillières Clin Rheumatol 1994;8:263–76.

[27] Espinoza LR, van Solingen R, Cuellar ML, et al. Insights into the pathogenesis of psoriasis and psoriatic arthritis. Am J Med Sci 1998;316:271–6.

[28] Taylor W, Gladman D, Helliwell P. Classification criteria for psoriatic arthritis: development of new criteria from a large international study. Arthritis Rheum 2006;54:2665–73.

[29] Cuellar ML, Silveira LH, Espinoza LR. Recent developments in psoriatic arthritis. Curr Opin Rheumatol 1994;6:378–84.

[30] Mease P, Goff BS. Diagnosis and treatment of psoriatic arthropathy. J Am Acad Dermatol 2005;52:1–19.

[31] Ory PA, Gladman DD, Mease PJ. Psoriatic arthritis and imaging. Ann Rheum Dis 2005;2(64 suppl):ii55–7.

[32] Mease P. Management of psoriatic arthritis: the therapeutic interface between rheumatology and dermatology. Curr Rheumatol Rep 2006;8:348–54.

[33] Menter A, Griffiths CE. Current and future management of psoriasis. Lancet 2007;370:272–84.

[34] Hamdulay SS, Glynne SJ, Keat A. When is arthritis reactive? Postgrad Med J 2006;82:446–53.

[35] Toivanen A, Toivanen P. Reactive arthritis. Best practice and research. Clin Rheumatol 2004;18:689–703.

[36] Amor B. Reiter's syndrome. Diagnosis and clinical features. Rheum Dis Clin N Am 1998;24:677–95.

[37] Angulo J, Espinoza LR. The spectrum of skin, mucosa and other extra-articular manifestations. Baillières Clin Rheumatol 1998;12:649–64.

[38] Holden W, Orchard T, Wordsworth P. Enteropathic arthritis. Rheum Dis Clin N Am 2003;29:513–30. viii.

[39] Petersel DL, Sigal LH. Reactive arthritis. Infect Dis Clin N Am 2005;19:863–83.

[40] Colmegna I, Espinoza LR. Recent advances in reactive arthritis. Curr Rheumatol Rep 2005;7:201–7.

[41] Suhrbier A, La Linn M. Clinical and pathologic aspects of arthritis due to Ross River virus and other alphaviruses. Curr Opin Rheumatol 2004;16:374–9.

[42] Ross River virus infection factsheet. Australian Government Department of Health and Ageing, May 2004. <http://www.health.gov.au/> [Accessed Aug. 2008].

[43] Mylonas AD, Brown AM, Carthew TL, et al. Natural history of Ross River virus-induced epidemic polyarthritis. Med J Aust 2002;177:356–60.

[44] Cheong IR. Ross River virus: are we wasting money doing tests? Med J Aust 2003;178:143.

[45] Servey JT, Reamy BV, Hodge J. Clinical presentations of parvovirus B19 infection. Am Fam Phys 2007;75:373–6.

[46] Naides SJ, Scharosch LL, Foto F, et al. Rheumatologic manifestations of human parvovirus B19 infection in adults. Initial 2-year clinical experience. Arthritis Rheum 1990;31:1297–309.

[47] Calabrese LH, Naides SJ. Viral arthritis. Infect Dis Clin N Am 2005;19:963–80. x.

[48] Moore TL. Parvovirus-associated arthritis. Curr Opin Rheumatol 2000;12:289–94.

[49] Jacqz-Aigrain E, Koren G. Effects of drugs on the fetus. Semin Fetal Neonatal Med 2005;10:139–47.

[50] Broliden K, Tolfvenstam T, Norbeck O. Clinical aspects of parvovirus B19 infection. J Intern Med 2006;260:285–304.

[51] Franssila R, Hedman K. Infection and musculoskeletal conditions: viral causes of arthritis. Best Pract Res Clin Rheumatol 2006;20:1139–57.

[52] Chi ZC, Ma SZ. Rheumatologic manifestations of hepatic diseases. Hepatobil Pancreat Dis Internatl 2003;2:32–7.

[53] Sanzone AM, Bégué RE. Hepatitis C and arthritis: an update. Infect Dis Clin N Am 2006;20:877–89. vii.

[54] Farrell GC, Teoh NC. Management of chronic hepatitis B virus infection: a new era of disease control. Internatl Med J 2006;36:100–13.

[55] Hoofnagle JH. Course and outcome of hepatitis C. Hepatology 2002;36(5 Suppl 1):S21–9.

[56] Ramos-Casals M, Trejo O, García-Carrasco M. Therapeutic management of extrahepatic manifestations in patients with chronic hepatitis C virus infection. Rheumatology (Oxford) 2003;42:818–28.

[57] McDonald M, Currie B, Carapetis J. Acute rheumatic fever: a chink in the chain that links the heart to the throat? Lancet Infect Dis 2004;4:240–5.

[58] Carapetis JR, et al. The global burden of group A streptococcal diseases. Lancet Infect Dis 2005;5:685–94.

[59] Australian Institute of Health and Welfare. Rheumatic heart disease in Australia – all but forgotten except in Aboriginal and Torres Strait Islander peoples. Canberra: AIHW; 2004.

[60] National Heart Foundation of Australia (RF/RHD guideline development working group) and the Cardiac Society of Australia and New Zealand. Diagnosis and management of acute rheumatic fever and rheumatic heart disease in Australia – an evidence based review. National Heart Foundation of Australia; 2006; 6–24. <http://www.heartfoundation.org.au/Professional_Information/Clinical_Practice/ARF_RHD.html> [Accessed Aug. 2008].

[61] Carapetis JR, McDonald M, Wilson NJ. Acute rheumatic fever. Lancet 2005;366:155–68.

[62] Nimmo GR, Tinniswood RD, Nuttall N, et al. Group A streptococcal infection in an Aboriginal community. Med J Aust 1992;156:537–40.

[63] Cilliers AM. Rheumatic fever and its management. Br Med J 2006;333:1153–6.

[64] Thatai D, Turi DG. Current guidelines for the treatment of acute rheumatic fever. Drugs 1999;57:545–55.

[65] Figueroa FE, Fernández MS, Valdés P. Prospective comparison of clinical and echocardiographic diagnosis of rheumatic carditis: long term follow-up of patients with subclinical disease. Heart 2001;85:407–10.

14.4 Musculoskeletal and soft-tissue emergencies

Anthony Tzannes • Anthony Brown

ESSENTIALS

1 The mechanism of injury and biomechanics predict the soft-tissue damage caused.

2 Soft-tissue injuries may be as debilitating and painful and take longer to heal than fractures in the same area.

3 The so-called 'minor injury' can be associated with significant and prolonged morbidity that could be permanent if managed incorrectly. Adopting a careful, consistent approach which considers potential pitfalls is important to patient outcome.

4 Exclude potentially serious causes of back pain by assessing for 'red flags' in every patient presenting with this complaint.

COMMON CAUSES OF SOFT-TISSUE INJURIES

All injuries have a soft-tissue component. The simplest way of dividing the causes of soft-tissue injuries is into 'acute' (specific event that exceeds tissue tolerance) and 'chronic' (repetitive minor damage in excess of ability to heal). Both types may be further subdivided by the tissue affected (bone, tendon, muscle, etc.).

Acute soft-tissue trauma can also be subdivided by the mechanism:

- Penetrating:
  - puncture vs incised
  - solid object vs fluid stream (high pressure hose, etc.).
- Blunt:
  - crush injury ± laceration
  - shear/degloving (open or closed).

Many of the types of trauma above are covered in other chapters.

General evaluation of a soft-tissue injury

Assessment

History
Obtain a history of:

- the nature of the injury: when, where and how it was sustained with specific attention to the forces involved, especially any potential crush or shear injury with devitalized tissue
- the possibility of a foreign body, wound contamination and/or damage to deeper structures
- patient function pre and post the injury
- pain associated with the injury, including time course, nature and aggravating factors
- co-morbidities and drug therapy
- allergies and tetanus immunization status.

Examination
This should potentially be delayed until after an X-ray if a radiopaque foreign body (metal or glass) is suspected, after giving analgesia.

The extent of any nerve damage should be determined *before* using local anaesthetic, although tendon damage may be best elucidated after adequate analgesia is obtained, so the wound can be adequately explored.

PUNCTURE INJURY

Management

Refer immediately to the appropriate surgical team all high-pressure gun injuries, such as from grease, paint or oil where the skin has been broken, even if no damage is apparent initially. They require extensive wound debridement and tissue plane cleaning, however innocuous they may seem.

Otherwise, clean the wound with antiseptic and evaluate the need for tetanus prophylaxis and antibiotics. A puncture wound to the sole of the foot will require exploration if it has occurred through the sole of footwear, or potentially has a foreign body. Otherwise, if there was direct skin penetration, this can be managed with a 30 min soak in an iodine/alcohol solution.

Prophylactic antibiotics are controversial as they do not adequately lower the risk of infection to offset the difficulty in managing likely resistant bacteria if infection then occurs. If prophylaxis is chosen, give amoxicillin/clavulanate 875/125 mg bd for 5 days. As these wounds are at high risk of infection, instruct the patient to return if increasing pain, redness or swelling occurs.

ACUTE MECHANICAL OVERLOAD INJURIES

These include fractures, ligament sprains, muscle strains or tears and tendon ruptures. Many are covered in Section 4 Orthopaedic Emergencies.

See Table 14.4.1 for a classification system for ligamentous sprains.

Management

General principles

The initial management principles are the same for both ligament sprains and muscular strains. This includes rest, ice, compression and elevation (RICE) with analgesia, usually a combination of paracetamol 1 g orally qid, plus a non-steroidal anti-inflammatory drug (NSAID), such as ibuprofen 400 mg orally tds (in the absence of NSAID-sensitive asthma, peptic ulcer disease and renal impairment).

Ligament sprain

Ligament sprains that are grade I or II (see Table 14.4.1) are managed with a protective brace or strapping and reduction in, but not cessation of, physical activity. Consider

Table 14.4.1 Classification of ligament sprains/muscle strains

Grade	Features
I	Small number of fibres injured, pain on loading, but no laxity or loss of strength
II	Significant number of fibres injured, with laxity and/or weakness and pain on loading
III	Complete tear with gross laxity and no strength

immobilizing grade III sprains with a splint or plaster of Paris (POP) cast and/or operative repair if there is gross instability and warn the patient that they can take up to 3 months or longer to heal. This is of particular relevance to the manual labourer and high-level athlete. Proprioception retraining at physiotherapy is important in ankle injuries to prevent recurrence, especially with grade II or III injuries.

Muscle strain

Muscle strains require initial RICE to minimize bruising and haematoma formation followed by a graded return to activity. Physiotherapy may aid in return of function and prevent re-injury, although research is limited by high rates of programme non-compliance in completed studies.

Assess the functional limitations imposed by these injuries, particularly in patients who live alone and/or who are elderly and infirm, as loss of independence is likely. A complete muscle tear, especially in an active individual, may benefit from operative repair following referral to an orthopaedic specialist. Consider the need for community services, respite care or admission in those who are initially unable to care for themselves.

Tendon rupture

Evaluation

Acute rupture of the supraspinatus tendon, long head of biceps and Achilles tendon are the most common serious tendon injuries that present to an emergency department (ED). Injury may be secondary to an acute event or chronic overload that is often asymptomatic until a tear occurs, and the extent of the rupture may be partial or complete.

Management

Request an ultrasound to confirm the diagnosis. Magnetic resonance imaging (MRI) is equally or more sensitive and specific depending on which tendons are being imaged, although is much less readily available.

Treatment is aimed at the earliest return to normal function, with the least likelihood of recurrence. Refer a complete tear, particularly in active people, for orthopaedic surgery repair. Manage partial tears conservatively, but they too may have a better outcome if repaired surgically, depending on local hospital practice and surgical availability.

PRETIBIAL LACERATION

These are most common in elderly patients, often from trivial trauma that tears a flap of skin, particularly if taking steroids. Ask about general mobility and safety issues at home.

Management

Clean the wound, remove blood clots, trim obviously necrotic tissue and unfurl the rolled edges of the wound to determine actual skin loss. Refer the patient immediately for consideration of early skin grafting if there is significant skin loss or marked skin retraction preventing alignment of the skin edges.

Otherwise, lay the flap back over the wound and hold in place with adhesive skin-closure strips (Steristrips). Then cover the wound with a non-adhesive dressing, and apply a firm crêpe bandage and instruct the patient to keep the leg elevated whenever possible. Determine the need for tetanus immunization or booster.

Arrange follow up in 5 days for review and a dressing change, or earlier if blood or serum has seeped through the wound dressing, known as 'strike-through', which increases the risk of secondary infection.

Expect the wound edges to heal by granulation tissue, with new epidermal tissue laid down at the rate of approximately 1 mm per week. If healing has not started to occur by the time of review, then skin grafting may be necessary and appropriate referral made. Otherwise, arrange follow up with the GP, with community nurse input as necessary.

DEGLOVING INJURY

Evaluation

Degloving injuries are caused by either a shearing or traction force on the skin, causing it to be torn from its underlying capillary blood supply. When the skin actually peels off it leaves an obvious exposed open injury, or the skin may remain intact causing a closed injury.

A closed degloving injury is much harder to diagnose. It may only cause the skin to feel less tethered than prior to injury but with poor capillary return with the failure to blanch on pressure and, most importantly, altered cutaneous sensation. This is most accurately assessed by 2-point discrimination. If 2-point discrimination is normal, a significant degloving injury has not occurred. Pain may or may not be prominent and/or may relate to an underlying bony injury.

Management

Arrange specialist assessment and admission for all degloving injuries by the appropriate surgical team, usually plastic and/or orthopaedic surgery. Keep any degloved skin, as it may be used as a skin graft.

Do *not* be tempted simply to replace the skin into its original position and hold it there with sutures or adhesive skin-closure strips (Steristrips), as this is inadequate. Degloving injuries are also a high-risk wound for tetanus.

CHRONIC OVERUSE (OVERLOAD) INJURIES

Chronic overuse injuries develop wherever tissue microtrauma occurs at a rate that exceeds the body's natural ability to heal. Few require emergency treatment, but general knowledge of these conditions is valuable to advise patients on cause and management.

Classification

Bony overuse injuries follow a continuum from pain on activity only, through local tenderness to pain at rest, with loss of function. Many will have led to a stress fracture by the time of presentation to an ED.

Other overuse injuries are classified by the tissue type and extent of injury and are often best diagnosed by the timing of the pain in relation to physical activity. They are further classified by the presence or absence of inflammation. See Table 14.4.2 for a classification of chronic overuse syndromes.

Table 14.4.2 Classification of chronic overuse syndromes

Grade	Symptom
I	Pain after activity
II	Pain early on and after activity; activity not limited
III	Pain throughout activity, which is limited
IV	Pain at rest

Management

Most chronic overuse injuries are managed with a decrease in activity and NSAIDs. Arrange referral to a physiotherapist or specialty physician, such as sports or performing arts physician, as appropriate. Tendon-related injuries may benefit from steroid injection, which should only be performed by doctors trained in the technique (orthopaedic surgeons, rheumatologists, sports physicians or some ED doctors).

Specific chronic overuse injuries that require more extensive management are summarized in Table 14.4.3.

NON-ARTHRITIC JOINT AND SOFT-TISSUE DISORDERS

General management of non-arthritic joint and soft-tissue disorders

Joint pain, swelling and tenderness mimicking arthritis may be due to inflammation of periarticular structures. Most patients can be treated with NSAIDs, such as ibuprofen 200–400 mg orally tds or naproxen 250 mg orally tds and/or with paracetamol in combination with codeine, usually as paracetamol 500 mg plus codeine 8 mg.

Underlying or secondary true arthritis may also be present and complicate the presentation. Joint aspiration is indicated to rule out a septic arthritis and, when this is suspected, follow local guidelines as to who performs it. Refer the patient back to their GP or outpatients unless mobility is so significantly affected that they require admission.

Do not perform steroid injection in the emergency department, as complications, such as septic arthritis and joint destruction do occur.

This is best left to the specialist who undertakes long-term care. Some of the more common presentations include the following.

Torticollis ('wry neck')

Diagnosis

Torticollis is abnormal unilateral neck muscle spasm, resulting in the head being held in a bent or twisted position. The aim of the history and examination is to exclude a serious underlying cause such as local sepsis, from a quinsy or submandibular abscess, recent trauma, cervical disc prolapse, acute drug dystonia or even a carotid artery dissection.

Management

Benign 'wry neck' most commonly occurs on waking after sleeping in an awkward position or follows unaccustomed activity or minor trauma. Arrange for cervical imaging if there is a history of possible bony trauma or cervical pathology. Give benztropine 1–2 mg IV when drug-induced dystonia is suspected.

Once serious causes have been excluded, use NSAIDs or paracetamol in combination with codeine 8 mg. Recommend gentle manipulation or muscle energy techniques to slowly work loose the muscles in spasm. Discharge the patient back to their GP with analgesia and ongoing exercises/stretches to maintain neck alignment.

Frozen shoulder (adhesive capsulitis)

Diagnosis

Frozen shoulder (adhesive capsulitis) has a natural history lasting 1–5 years, with an average duration of 2.5 years. It begins with an acutely painful period of 3–9 months with a progressively decreasing range of motion at the glenohumeral joint, 'freezing phase', over 4–12 months starting soon after the pain. Pain tends to be worse at night or when lying flat. The decreased range of motion usually resolves in the 'thawing' phase, but this may take from 1 to 4 years.

A frozen shoulder may occur spontaneously, but more commonly follows local trauma (which can be trivial), immobilization, a cerebrovascular accident or shingles. There is an increased risk in diabetic patients where the condition may present bilaterally, in smokers, with hyperlipidaemia and in those on treatment

with protease inhibitors. It is more common in females with a peak incidence age of 55 years and in the non-dominant arm.

On examination, the most sensitive sign is loss of external rotation at the glenohumeral joint. Test for this by first immobilizing the scapula by placing a hand over the top of the shoulder to exclude scapulothoracic movement.

Management

Treatment includes high-dose intra-articular steroid injection that reduces early pain but without effect on the range of motion and physical disruption of the joint capsule, for instance by arthroscopic capsule release. There is no evidence that NSAIDs or physiotherapy alone have an effect on outcome, with physiotherapy in the painful and freezing phases specifically found to increase pain with no effect on range of movement.

Rotator cuff tear (usually rupture of supraspinatus)

Diagnosis

Sudden traction on the arm may tear the muscles that make up the 'rotator cuff' which include supraspinatus, infraspinatus, subscapularis and teres minor. Although the onset of pain may be insidious, a traumatic incident may complete a tear, causing sudden severe pain and reduced shoulder function.

The vast majority (95%) of tears occur in patients over 40 years with a component of chronic tendon damage. Any movement of the shoulder may be markedly painful after an acute injury, limiting assessment. Where able, evaluate active and passive ranges of motion, with limitation of abduction (supraspinatus) most commonly found. The combination of weakness of supraspinatus (tested with downwards pressure on the abducted, 30° forward flexed arm) and impingement in both internal (shoulder 90° flexion) and external (shoulder 90° abduction) rotation is highly sensitive (95%) for a rotator cuff tear.

Radiography

Shoulder X-ray may show a decrease in the space between the head of the humerus and the acromion in a large chronic tear. Ultrasound is best at characterizing the extent of a full thickness rotator cuff tear and/or a biceps tendon dislocation, but is less sensitive for a partial-thickness tear. MRI is highly sensitive and specific for delineating the degree, location and

Table 14.4.3   Stress fractures which require active specialist management

Injury	Associated with	Symptoms	X-ray	Other imaging	Management
Pars interarticularis	Gymnasts, ballet dancers, fast bowlers	Unilateral low back pain, worse on extension	Pars # often seen	CT or MRI definitive. XR + Bone scan alternative option	Avoiding hyper extension for 6/52, consider brace for 6-12/52. Core stability retraining once healed
Femoral neck	Athletes/military increased activity	Vague thigh/groin pain with loading	Often normal	Bone scan or MRI, CT less sensitive	if <50% of bone fractured, decrease activity, if >50% ORIF
Femoral shaft	Dancers	Vague thigh/knee pain with loading	# Usually visible	CT or bone scan	Lateral cortex – ORIF, medialcortex (much rarer) non-weightbearing 6/52
Anterior cortex of midtibia	Distance runners, ballet dancers	Progressive anterior leg pain with activity	Anterior # line, thickened cortex	Bone scan? Non-union vs recent injury	Decrease activity, intermedulary nail if progresses
Talus	Repeated falls/jumping from height	Foot/ankle pain worse with weightbearing	Usually normal	Bone scan, CT or MRI	6/52 Non-weightbearing in POP
Navicular	Increased running/marching	Vague midfoot pain with point tenderness over navicular	May show #	Bone scan, CT or MRI	6-8/52 Non-weightbearing, ORIF if fails to heal
Base 2nd metatarsal	Ballet dancers	Forefoot pain on exercise	# Usually visible	Bone scan, CT or MRI but usually not needed	Non-weightbearing on crutches for 4-6/52
Base 5th metatarsal	Ballet dancers	Midfoot pain with activity	# Usually visible	Bone scan, CT or MRI but usually not needed	Non-weightbearing with POP for 6/52 or direct ORIF as often fail to heal
Sesamoid bone of hallux	Increased running/marching	Forefoot pain, tender/swelling over ball of foot	Often hard to interpret	Bone scan or MRI	6/52 Non-weightbearing with crutches then orthotics to correct biomechanics

CT = computed tomography; MRI = magnetic resonance imaging; ORIF = open reduction internal fixation; 6/52 = 6 weeks.

characteristics of rotator cuff pathology, when available.

Management

Refer a young patient with an acute full thickness tear to the orthopaedic specialist for consideration of early operative repair, as it becomes technically more difficult after 2–3 weeks due to tissue retraction. Otherwise, conservative management consists of analgesia, an immobilizing sling and referral to the physiotherapy department for a physical therapy rehabilitation programme.

Supraspinatus tendonitis

Diagnosis and management

Supraspinatus tendonitis is one of the causes of the 'painful arc' occurring between 60° and 120° of shoulder abduction. Perform a shoulder X-ray, which may reveal calcification in the supraspinatus tendon and/or 'hooking' of the acromion, decreasing the subacromial space and predisposing to this condition. Ultrasound is used for both diagnosis and to facilitate aspiration and local steroid injection.

Give an anti-inflammatory analgesic and consider referral to the orthopaedic (especially if there is a hooked acromion) or rheumatology clinic for aspiration and local steroid injection or via ultrasound by an interventional radiologist.

Subacromial bursitis

Diagnosis and management

Subacromial bursitis may follow rupture of calcific material into the subacromial bursa that again causes a 'painful arc' on attempted shoulder abduction or constant severe pain in the shoulder. Manage as for supraspinatus tendonitis above.

Tennis and golfer's elbow

Diagnosis and management

Tennis elbow (incorrectly termed lateral epicondylitis) causes pain over the lateral epicondyle of the humerus from chronic angiofibroblastic tendinosis. There is disorganized tissue and neovascularization but minimal actual inflammation of the extensor origin of the forearm muscles involved in repetitive movements, such as using a screwdriver or playing tennis. Advise the patient to avoid the activity causing the pain and to rest the arm.

Give an anti-inflammatory analgesic and refer for physiotherapy. Eccentric and isometric exercises are most effective in treating and preventing recurrence. A tension strap can also be used to control symptoms, particularly when a patient presents within the first 6 weeks. Local steroid injection often reduces short-term pain and improves movement in the first 6 weeks, but has a worse longer-term outcome.

Golfer's elbow (medial epicondylitis) is a similar condition affecting the medial epicondyle and the flexor origin. Management is the same.

Olecranon bursitis

Diagnosis and management

Painful swelling of the olecranon bursa is due to local trauma, gout or infection, usually with *Staphylococcus aureus*. Aspiration under sterile conditions is indicated in the presence of severe pain and/or systemic features of sepsis, with microscopy for both crystals and bacteria and culture if there is adequate fluid to allow drainage. Imaging is indicated when a foreign body is suspected.

Refer the patient for drainage of the bursa under anaesthesia if significant bacterial infection or a foreign body is confirmed, or if a septic arthritis is suspected due to markedly reduced movement at the elbow (see Chapter 14.2). Otherwise, give an antistaphylococcal antibiotic, such as di- or flucloxacillin 500 mg orally qid for 7–10 days for overlying cellulitis and/or a non-steroidal anti-inflammatory analgesic and refer back to the GP.

Prepatellar bursitis (housemaid's knee)

Diagnosis and management
This is a prepatellar bursitis secondary to friction or, occasionally, infection. Treat by giving an anti-inflammatory analgesic, avoiding further trauma and, if necessary, by aspiration and steroid injection by an orthopaedic or rheumatology specialist, or by arrangement with the patient's GP. When local infection is suspected, start an antistaphylococcal antibiotic, such as di- or flucloxacillin 500 mg orally qid for 7–10 days and, again, refer back to the GP.

Refer the patient to the orthopaedic specialist for intravenous antibiotics and/or local drainage if systemic infection is suspected.

De Quervain's stenosing tenosynovitis

Diagnosis and management
This causes tenderness over the radial styloid, a palpable nodule from thickening of the fibrous sheaths of the abductor pollicis longus and extensor pollicis brevis tendons and pain on moving the thumb. Treat by resting the thumb in a splint and by using an anti-inflammatory analgesic.

Refer to a rheumatology specialist for consideration of local steroid injection, although it may require surgical release of the tendon sheaths if local steroid injection fails.

Plantar fasciitis

Diagnosis and management
Plantar fasciitis presents as a painful midfoot, especially in the sole or arch, that is worse on first weight bearing and improves after 10–15 min of walking, recurring again during load bearing for an extended period. It is one of the most common causes of recurrent foot pain and may be one manifestation of the spondyloarthropathy seen in Reiter's syndrome, ankylosing spondylitis and psoriatic arthritis (see Chapter 14.3). On examination, there is tenderness of the plantar fascia, especially at the calcaneal attachment.

X-ray may reveal a bony spur extending along the plantar fascia, but this has no bearing on the initial management. Symptomatic relief may be obtained by a soft heel pad. Longer-term management and prevention is best achieved by a properly fitted orthotic splint.

Carpal tunnel syndrome

Diagnosis and management
This is a compressive neuropathy of the median nerve at the wrist, most commonly affecting middle-aged females. Secondary causes include rheumatoid arthritis, diabetes, post-trauma, such as a Colles' fracture, pregnancy and, rarely, myxoedema, acromegaly and amyloidosis. Most cases though are idiopathic or related to minor repetitive trauma.

Patients complain of pain and burning paraesthesiae in the distribution of the median nerve in the hand, primarily the thumb, index, middle and lateral aspect of the ring finger. It is typically worse at night or following repetitive strain, especially with higher loads or vibrating tools.

Perform Phalen's test by reproducing paraesthesiae in the distribution of the median nerve following 60 s of wrist hyperflexion, or look for Tinel's sign eliciting median nerve paraesthesiae by tapping on the volar aspect of the wrist over the median nerve. Test for reduced sensation over the palmar aspect of the affected digits and weakness of thumb abduction, associated with thenar muscle wasting in chronic cases.

Treat with an anti-inflammatory analgesic and immobilize the wrist in a volar splint in the neutral position, particularly at night. Refer resistant cases to an orthopaedic specialist for consideration of carpal tunnel decompression.

BACK PAIN

This is a common problem that usually simply requires analgesia and patient education.

Assessment is targeted at determining whether concerning features, 'red flags', are present which mandate further investigation. Back pain may be subdivided into four major categories:

- direct major spinal trauma
- indirect mechanical back trauma (non-specific low back pain)
- back pain with radiculopathy
- back pain with focal 'hard' neurology, or a specific serious cause suspected.

Direct major thoracic and lumbosacral spine trauma is covered in Chapter 3.3.

Back pain 'red flags'
Every patient presenting to the ED with acute low back pain must be assessed for the presence of 'red flag' symptoms or signs suggesting a potentially serious underlying cause. These 'red flags' include unexplained weight loss, unexplained fever, immunosuppression, history of cancer, intravenous drug use (IVDU), duration greater than 6 weeks, focal neurological deficit/progressive or disabling symptoms, particularly pain at night, prolonged use of glucocorticoids, osteoporosis (note chronic alcoholism leads to osteopaenia) and age over 70 years.

Although the majority will still just end up having a diagnosis of musculoskeletal pain, laboratory testing with a full blood count (FBC), C-reactive protein (CRP) and erythrocyte sedimentation rate (ESR), plus imaging with CT or MRI is indicated. See Table 14.4.4 for the differential diagnosis and investigation of the possible underlying disorders from malignancy, spinal cord compression to discitis and epidural abscess.

Indirect mechanical back trauma (non-specific low back pain)

Clinical features

History
Bending, lifting, straining, coughing or sneezing may precipitate acute, severe low back pain, causing intense muscle spasm or even complete immobility. It is common for patients to have apparently minor back discomfort on one day, then wake with severe spasm the next.

Examination
This is focused on excluding any focal 'hard' neurology or radiculopathy. Giving adequate

Table 14.4.4 Differential diagnosis and investigation of serious disorders causing back pain

Suspected diagnosis	Symptoms/findings	Investigations

Infection
  osteomyelitis
  discitis
  epidural abscess
	Fever
	IVDU
	Immunosuppression
	Recent infection or instrumentation
		FBC/CRP/ESR
		ESR most sensitive
		MRI best imaging

Cancer
  primary
  secondary
	Previous cancer
	Unexplained weight loss
	Age >50 (65 years some series)
	Failure to improve after 4 weeks
		X-ray
		+MRI if neurology

Fracture	Osteoporosis Pain still significant at rest Steroid use	X-ray
Spinal cord compression (includes cauda equina)	Urinary retention Incontinence Saddle anaesthesia Sensory and/or motor level	MRI
Ankylosing spondylitis	Age <30 years Pain worse at night Morning stiffness Improves with exercise	ESR/CRP HLA-B27 Pelvis X-ray

FBC: full blood count; CRP: C-reactive protein; ESR: erythrocyte sedimentation rate; IVDU: intravenous drug user; MRI: magnetic resonance imaging.

analgesia so that pain does not limit strength is an important part of the assessment. See Chapter 3.3 for a description of the myotomes, dermatomes and nerve roots in the leg.

Hard neurology is characterized by the loss of sensation, reflexes or true weakness. A radiculopathy is characterized by pain or subjective altered sensation following a dermatome. These should both be absent. Imaging is not usually indicated unless symptoms are continuous for greater than 6 weeks and/or are not previously investigated.

Management

The mainstay of management is to limit normal activities with some directed range of movement exercises and stretches. The ED management consists of excluding more serious causes, then education and reassurance while ensuring adequate analgesia to allow movement. Combinations, such as paracetamol 1 g qid, ibuprofen 400 mg tds ± addition of oral opioids, are usually effective. The addition of diazepam 2–5 mg PO tds for patients with a particularly spasmodic and/or anxiety component is also effective.

Patients who are able to mobilize with this management may be discharged to the care of their GP for ongoing follow up and education concerning posture and lifting. Patients who fail initial management will require admission, either to an ED short-stay ward for nursing care and regular analgesia prior to physiotherapy review, or to an inpatient ward according to hospital policy, most commonly under orthopaedics or general medicine.

Back pain with radiculopathy

Clinical features

These patients have a similar presentation to those with non-specific low back pain, but also have neuropathic pain following one or more lower leg dermatomes. Examination may reveal subjectively altered sensation but with intact sharp/dull (or hot/cold), 2-point discrimination and proprioception. Straight leg raising may exacerbate radicular symptoms. Strength and reflexes are also intact, with no reported incontinence or urinary retention.

Imaging is again not indicated unless symptoms are progressing with increasing numbers of dermatomes or there are continuous symptoms for greater than 6 weeks.

Management

Management is the same as for non-specific back pain, with the addition of more specific neuropathic pain analgesia, such as tramadol (trial in ED first as may cause vomiting) 150–200 mg SR bd if effective, added to either amitriptyline 25 mg nocte or pregabalin (a GABA analogue that reduces the release of neurotransmitters by interfering with the calcium channels in nerve terminals) 75 mg bd.

Back pain with focal 'hard' neurology, or a specific serious cause suspected

This small group of patients with hard neurology consisting of true weakness, loss of sensation and/or reflexes requires further investigation and specialist referral (usually neurosurgery or orthopaedics). The timing of this investigation will depend on the acuity and extent of the symptoms or signs. Acute onset or ongoing progression mandate emergent investigation and referral for treatment. Subacute or chronic symptoms (especially if from a single nerve root) may be investigated and managed on a less urgent basis in discussion with the specialist team, particularly if they are unlikely to be reversible.

Other patients with 'red flag' symptoms or signs must also be investigated urgently (see Table 14.4.4). They may have any of the following conditions.

Spinal infection

Clinical features

Spinal infections include epidural abscess, discitis and vertebral osteomyelitis. Risk factors are recent instrumentation (prolonged epidural catheter > surgery > brief, such as obstetric epidural catheter), immunosuppression, alcoholism, diabetes, IVDU, contiguous infection or distal infection with bacteraemia. The classic progression of symptoms is from back pain to radiculopathy, to weakness, to paralysis with progression from radiculopathy to paralysis sometimes occurring over hours. Fever is absent in over one-third of cases.

Investigations

A normal WCC, ESR and CRP virtually exclude the diagnosis, with ESR being the most (110 out 117 confirmed cases in one study) and

WCC the least sensitive. Blood cultures should be taken, although CT-guided or surgical specimens are more likely to culture the causative microbe. MRI is the imaging modality of choice to confirm or exclude the diagnosis.

Management

Progressive neurology requires urgent operative intervention with the decision on which antibiotic(s) prior to surgery discussed with the treating team. Patients without neurology may be treated conservatively. Empirical antibiotic therapy is targeted at skin flora including methicillin-resistant *Staphylococcus aureus* (MRSA) and dental flora, unless spread from a focal infection, such as from *Escherichia coli* or *Strepotococcus pneumoniae* is suspected.

Spinal cancer

Clinical features

Acute symptoms are most likely in the setting of previous cancer, particularly those that metastasize to bone (lung, breast, prostate, renal, thyroid and melanoma). Unexplained weight loss, age >50 years and symptoms failing to improve after 1 month are risk factors. Examination should thus include skin (melanoma), breasts, chest, abdomen and prostate to look for a primary tumour.

Investigations

Plain X-ray may be adequate to find a bony lesion, but more information with high sensitivity is obtained from CT scanning. An MRI is indicated if there is any focal neurology.

Management

If cancer is found or highly suspicious, admit to hospital. Spinal cord compression may respond to radiotherapy and a pathological fracture may require stabilization. Otherwise, management is with analgesia and investigation aimed at determining the primary tumour, which will dictate definitive treatment.

Fracture (vertebral compression)

Clinical features

Suspect this with significant pain at rest, long-term steroid use or known osteoporosis even with minor trauma. Examination is aimed at excluding focal neurological complications.

Investigations

Plain X-ray is the initial investigation. CT is indicated if there is greater than 50% vertebral height loss or retropulsion of fragments into spinal canal noted.

Management

Analgesia is as per non-specific back pain. It is extremely rare for these injuries to be unstable or require immobilization or surgical stabilization, although admission for analgesia and bedrest may be necessary.

Spinal cord compression or cauda equina syndrome

Clinical features

Spinal cord compression or cauda equina syndrome (lesion at or below the first lumbar vertebra) may be due to tumour, infection or central disc prolapse. Urinary retention is the most sensitive sign of cauda equina syndrome, which is seen in ≈90% of cases. A history of incontinence and perineal or perianal 'saddle area' anaesthesia or bilateral leg weakness may also occur. The neurology findings will correspond to a specific level in the case of spinal cord compression, but may be inconsistent and patchy in cauda equina syndrome.

Investigation

Urgent MRI is the investigation of choice, with CT of some value, particularly if bony injury is suspected or if MRI is unavailable. Imaging should not delay urgent transfer to definitive treatment under the care of a spinal surgeon.

Management

Urgent surgery. Corticosteroids are not supported unless due to a steroid-responsive tumour.

Ankylosing spondylitis

Clinical features

Ankylosing spondylitis is a chronic inflammatory enthesopathy affecting the axial skeleton. It usually occurs in males (5:1) below the age of 30 years, causing pain that improves with exercise and worsens with rest, sometimes resulting in waking in the second half of the night due to discomfort. Examination may be unremarkable or show a general decreased range of spinal motion in more advanced cases.

Investigations

The ESR and CRP are usually raised. HLA-B27 is sensitive for the disease and is present in around 95% of Caucasian and Chinese patients. Pelvic X-ray often shows sacroiliitis.

Management

Commence NSAIDs at a maximum dose and refer to rheumatology outpatients follow up. Regular physiotherapy including hydrotherapy is essential.

Controversies

- Indications for surgical versus conservative management for soft tissue or chronic overuse injuries, particularly in elite athletes/young manual workers to reduce the time to return to elite or work activity.
- Timing of a rotator cuff repair.
- Who should perform joint aspiration and/or intra-articular/intralesional steroid injections and its safety.
- Sensitivity of inflammatory markers to exclude spinal infection and which imaging is required.

Further reading

Bassett RW, Cofield RH. Acute tears of the rotator cuff: the timing of surgical repair. Clin Orthop Relat Res 1983;175:18–24.

Bone School. <http://www.boneschool.com.au> [Accessed Nov. 2012].

Booth C. High pressure paint gun injuries. Br Med J 1977;2:1333–5.

Brukner P, Khan K. Clinical review of sports medicine, 3rd ed. Sydney: McGraw-Hill; 2010.

Chou R, Qaseem A, Snow V, et al. Diagnosis and treatment of low back pain: a joint clinical practice guideline from the American College of Physicians and the American Pain Society. Ann Intern Med 2007;147:478–91.

Petersen SA, Murphy TP. The timing of rotator cuff repair for the restoration of function. J Shoulder Elbow Surg 2011;20:62–8.

UpToDate. Online version 19.5. <http://www.uptodate.com> [Accessed Nov. 2012].

DERMATOLOGY EMERGENCIES

Edited by **Anthony Brown**

15.1 Emergency dermatology   598

15.1 Emergency dermatology

Rebecca Dunn • George Varigos • Vanessa Morgan

ESSENTIALS

1 Emergency dermatology presentations may be divided into potentially life-theatening dermatoses, other bullous and vesicular conditions, petechial and purpuric rashes, pruritic (itchy) conditions, exzema and psoriasis, and other.

2 The potentially life-threatening include toxic epidermal necrolysis and Stevens-Johnson syndrome, Sweet's syndrome, drug rash with eosinophilia (DRESS), and erythroderma.

3 Petechial or purpuric rashes can have non-palpable purpura and be thrombocytopaenic with or without splenomegaly, or non-thrombocytopaenic; or they may have palpable purpura usually relating to a vasculitis.

Table 15.1.2	Definitions of patterns in skin disorders
Annular	Ring-like or part of a circle
Linear	Line-like
Arcuate	Arch-like
Grouped	Local collection of similar lesions
Unilateral	One side
Symmetrical	Both sides

Introduction

The pattern and form of acute dermatological conditions that present to the emergency department (ED) are confusing in that the clinical features, such as vasodilatation, exfoliation, blistering or necrosis, are the common endpoint of many different inflammatory processes in the skin.

The pathological process involves cytokines or chemokines and their effects create the visible response(s). The important clinical differences seen in these acute reactions should be recognized by the trained observer (Tables 15.1.1 and 15.1.2). This chapter aims to provide a clinical pathway from taking an appropriate history to having knowledge of the distinguishing clinical features of the likely differential diagnoses. The emergency presentations discussed are limited to specific dermatological conditions that may be seen in an ED as a true urgency.

It is important to use other resources with this chapter, such as a dermatology atlas or specialized texts, to provide greater detail on the conditions mentioned. The presentation of skin and soft-tissue infections (Chapter 9.5) and anaphylaxis (Chapter 2.8) are covered elsewhere.

Table 15.1.1	Definition of macroscopic skin pathological lesions
Papule	Circumscribed firm raised elevation, less than 0.5 cm in diameter
Nodule	A solid or firm mass more than 0.5 cm in the skin which can be observed as an elevation or can be palpated
Purpura	Discoloration of skin or mucous membranes due to extravasation of red blood cells
Pustule	A visible accumulation of fluid, usually yellow, in the form of a vesicle or papule containing the fluid It may be centred around a pore, such as a hair follicle or sweat glands, and sometimes appears in normal skin, not uncommonly palmar/plantar
Vesicle	A visible accumulation of fluid in a papule of <5 mm The fluid is clear, serous-like and is located within or beneath the epidermis
Blister or bulla	Large fluid-containing lesion of more than 5 mm
Plaque	An area or sheet of skin elevated and with a distinct edge, of any shape and usually wider than 1 cm

With permission from Rook AJ, Burton JL, Champion RH, Ebling FJG. Diagnosis of skin disease. In: Bolognia J, Jorizzo J, Rapini R (eds). Textbook of Dermatology. Oxford: Blackwell Scientific; 1992.

POTENTIALLY LIFE-THREATENING DERMATOSES

Toxic epidermal necrolysis and Stevens–Johnson syndrome

Toxic epidermal necrolysis (TEN) and Stevens–Johnson syndrome (SJS) are acute severe reactions characterized by extensive necrosis and detachment of the epidermis defined by mucosal ulceration at two or more sites usually with cutaneous blisters. Confusion exists between these two diagnoses and erythema multiforme (EM). EM was previously considered a variant of SJS/TEN, but it is now commonly accepted that they are clinically distinct disorders with different causes and prognosis. Most consider EM minor and major to be related to infections and SJS/TEN as variants (mild and severe) or a separate disorder, usually due to drugs. However, this distinction is not important in the emergency setting, but rather it is the recognition of a potentially serious dermatosis that is important.

The difference between TEN and SJS is defined by the extent of skin involvement. TEN affects more than 30% of the body surface area, whereas SJS affects 10% or less (Fig. 15.1.1). 'TEN/SJS

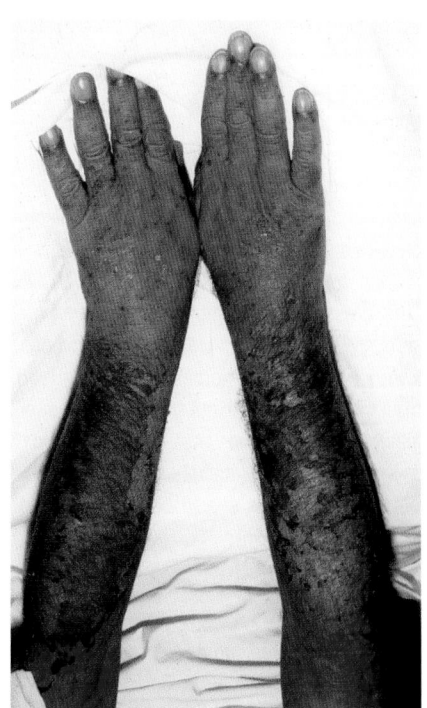

Fig. 15.1.1 Toxic epidermal necrolysis.

overlap' refers to patients where there is between 10 and 30% body surface area involvement. The extent of necrolysis must be carefully evaluated since it is a major prognostic factor. Patients with HIV, collagen vascular disease and malignancy are at increased risk of TEN.

Clinical features

Clinical features of SJS/TEN include a prodrome with upper respiratory tract- (URTI) like symptoms, fever, malaise, vomiting and diarrhoea. Skin pain may herald the development of SJS/TEN and should not be dismissed. Symmetrical erythematous macules, mainly localized on the trunk and proximal limbs, evolve progressively to dusky erythema and confluent flaccid blisters leading to epidermal detachment.

The key to making the diagnosis is recognizing mucosal involvement, which may include conjunctival, oral mucosal, genital and sometimes perianal erosions, as well as an often severe haemorrhagic cheilitis. Gastrointestinal and respiratory mucosa can also be involved. Nikolsky sign is positive, that is dislodgement of the epidermis by lateral finger pressure in the vicinity of a lesion causes an erosion, or pressure on a bulla leads to lateral extension of the blister.

TEN is almost always due to drug ingestion which may, in rare instances, include illicit drug ingestion. Therefore, ask about prescribed and over-the-counter drugs, such as non-steroidal anti-inflammatory drugs (NSAIDs), sulphonamides, allopurinol, nevirapine and anticonvulsants, such as sodium valproate and lamotrigine, as well as illicit drug use.

Investigations

Request a full blood count (FBC), urea and electrolytes (U&E), liver function tests (LFT) and a blood glucose. These may also be used to calculate the prognostic SCORTEN (see below). Other tests to consider include antinuclear antibody (ANA), extractable nuclear antigens (ENA), double stranded DNA (dsDNA), C-reactive protein (CRP), erythrocyte sedimentation rate (ESR), anti-skin antibodies, HIV and mycoplasma serology. Skin swabs for viral polymerase chain reaction (PCR) and bacterial culture should be taken and chest X-ray (CXR), urine and blood cultures as indicated.

Biopsies are taken from the edge of a blister for histology and a perilesional site for immuno-fluorescence. Clearly state on the request slip that the differential diagnosis is of toxic epidermal necrolysis. Epidermal (keratinocyte) necrosis is the histological hallmark of this condition.

Management

Cease the triggering drug or agent immediately and involve the intensive care unit and/or the burns unit. Rapid institution of resuscitation measures is associated with a more favourable prognosis. Arrange assessment and treatment by the ophthalmology and ear, nose and throat teams for ocular and oral/pharyngeal involvement, respectively.

TEN may continue to evolve and extend over days, unlike a burn, where the initial insult occurs at a defined time. The SCORTEN severity scoring system for TEN (Table 15.1.3) is similar in concept to the Ranson's score for pancreatitis. Calculate the SCORTEN severity score within 24 h of admission and again on day 3 to aid the prediction of possible death (Table 15.1.4).

Table 15.1.3 SCORTEN severity score for toxic epidermal necrolysis (TEN)

- Age >40 years
- Heart rate >120/min
- Presence of cancer or haematological malignancy
- Epidermal detachment involving body surface area >10% on day 1
- Blood urea nitrogen >10 mmol/L (28 mg/dL)
- Glucose >14 mmol/L (252 mg/dL)
- Bicarbonate <20 mEq/L

(One point is given for each variable.)

Table 15.1.4 SCORTEN mortality prediction*

Score	Mortality (%)
0–1	3.2
2	12.1
3	35.3
4	58.3
5 or greater	90.0

*Guegan S, Bastuji-Garin S, PoszepczynskaGuigne E, et al. Performance of the SCORTEN during the first five days of hospitalization to predict the prognosis of epidermal necrolysis. J Invest Dermatol 2006;126:272–6.

Erythema multiforme

While not life threatening, EM is part of the differential of a potentially life-threatening reaction, such as SJS/TEN. EM is an acute usually mild, self-limited cutaneous and/or mucocutaneous syndrome that presents with the rapid onset of lesions within a few days, favouring acral sites. These are often mildly pruritic or painful papular or urticarial lesions, as well as the classical 'target' lesions, but with only one mucous membrane involved (EM major) or none (EM minor). Typically, the oral mucosa is involved showing a few, discrete, mildly symptomatic erosions. Rarely, the eye, nasal, urethral or anal mucosa may be involved. A mild prodrome may precede development of the rash.

Most cases of EM are due to infection, most commonly Herpes simplex virus (HSV) or *Mycoplasma*. Drugs are now considered to be an uncommon cause (Fig. 15.1.2).

Investigations

Send a baseline FBC, U&E, LFT and CRP, as well as a skin biopsy if the diagnosis is uncertain, swabs and/or serology for HSV. Request a CXR and mycoplasma serology if there are respiratory symptoms.

Management

Usually, only symptomatic treatment is required with topical steroids, antihistamines, antiseptic mouthwashes and local anaesthetic preparations for oral involvement. For severe cases, treat erythema multiforme with a systemic steroid, such as predinosolone (0.5–1 mg/kg/day). In recurrent EM due to HSV, oral antivirals are effective.

Sweet's syndrome

Sweet's syndrome (acute febrile neutrophilic dermatosis) may resemble severe EM in the acute oedematous phase, presenting with fever, arthralgia, neutrophilia and sterile, non-infective but painful pustules, plaques or nodules over the head, trunk and arms. It may recur and can be associated with inflammatory bowel disease, rheumatoid arthritis or other connective tissue diseases, haematological malignancy, such as myeloid leukaemia, pregnancy or infection, such as streptococcal or *Yersinia* (Fig. 15.1.3).

Sweet's syndrome is highly responsive to systemic steroids, however, any underlying association must be sought and excluded by appropriate investigations.

Drug rash with eosinophilia (DRESS)

DRESS is a severe skin reaction with systemic manifestations that carries significant morbidity and a mortality rate of 10%.

It usually occurs during the first prolonged course of a responsible associated drug, typically within 2–6 weeks of starting. It has been reported with the aromatic antiepileptics (phenytoin, carbamazepine, phenobarbital), lamotrigine, sulphonamides (including sulphamethoxazole and trimethoprim combinations and dapsone), minocycline, allopurinol, terbinafine, abacavir and nevirapine. Up to 70% cross-reactivity occurs between different aromatic anticonvulsants which should therefore be avoided if someone has previously had a major reaction to an aromatic antiepileptic.

Fever and rash are the most common symptoms. Cutaneous involvement is often polymorphic usually starting as a maculopapular rash which may later become oedematous, exfoliative or erythrodermic and/or include non-follicular pustules. Often, rash involving the face indicates a more serious drug reaction and facial oedema and lymphadenopathy are frequent hallmarks of this syndrome.

Prominent eosinophilia is a characteristic feature that occurs in 60–70% of cases. Potentially serious internal organ involvement, such as hepatitis, nephritis, pneumonitis, myocarditis, thyroiditis, encephalitis and haemophagocytic lymphohistiocytosis (HLH) syndrome, can occur. Fever, skin rash and organ involvement may fluctuate and persist for weeks or months after drug withdrawal, with the delayed onset of sequelae reported.

Investigations

Diagnosis can be difficult because of the polymorphic rash and variable organ involvement. A skin biopsy should be taken for histopathology and, although not diagnositic, histological features of a drug reaction will assist in making the diagnosis. Also request a basline FBC, U&E and LFT. Immunoglobulins and viral serology (Epstein–Barr virus (EBV), cytomegalovirus (CMV), human herpesvirus 6 or 7 (HHV6, HHV7) should be sent, as transient hypogammaglobulinaemia and viral reactivation may be associated with fluctuations in symptoms. Other investigations should be as directed for systemic involvement.

Management

This usually includes admission to hospital and ceasing the suspected drug. Corticosteroids are first line of therapy despite no consensus on dose or regimen. Fluctuation in symptoms and

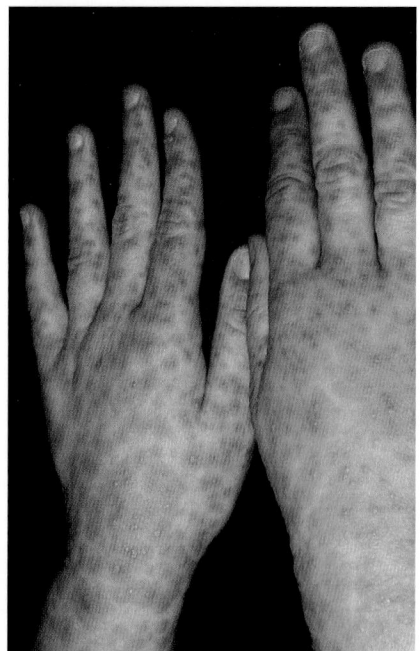

Fig. 15.1.2 Erythema multiforme.

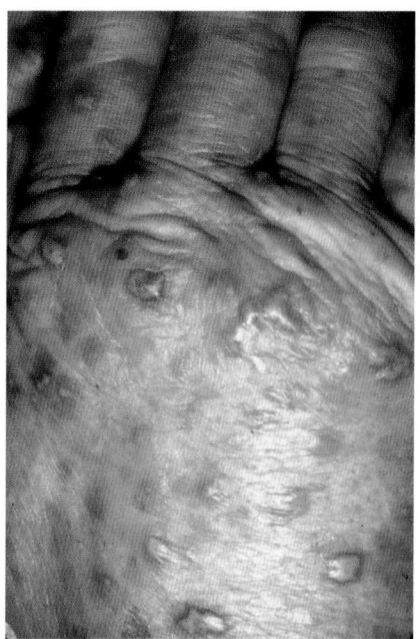

Fig. 15.1.3 Sweet syndrome.

DERMATOLOGY EMERGENCIES

relapse can occur when the dosage is tapered. As a result, steroid therapy sometimes has to be maintained for several weeks, even months and a steroid-sparing agent may be required. Antivirals and intravenous immunoglobulin (IVIG) are emerging as potentially useful therapies for this condition. In milder cases, topical high-potency corticosteroids may be helpful for skin manifestations.

Erythroderma

The causes of erythroderma include eczema (40%), psoriasis (22%), drugs (15%), lymphoma (Sezary syndrome) (10%) and idiopathic (8%). Seek a history of previous skin disease, recent medications or recent changes to skin management, assess hydration and cardiac status, check for oedema, respiratory infection and a deep vein thrombosis (DVT).

Complications of erythroderma

These include:

- high output cardiac failure
- dehydration, which may result in renal failure
- protein loss with oedema that contributes to the fluid loss and renal failure
- hypothermia/temperature dysregulation
- thrombophlebitis/DVT
- infection, both cutaneous and respiratory, with pneumonia a major cause of death
- side effects of treatment.

Investigations

Send an FBC with film and differential, U&E, LFTs and blood cultures if the temperature is greater than 38°C, or if the patient appears unwell with rigors, even if the temperature is normal, as the patient may have become poikilothermic but is still septic.

Send skin swabs for microscopy and culture and request a chest X-ray. Arrange biopsy of the skin if the cause of the erythroderma is uncertain.

Management

Arrange to admit the patient. Treatment is general and supportive and includes:

- attention to temperature control, avoiding hypothermia
- IV fluid replacement with careful charting of the fluid balance, monitoring urine output in particular

- referral to dietitian for high protein diet in the first 24 h
- chest physiotherapy
- DVT prophylaxis.

Specific treatment includes:

- bath oil daily in bath or shower
- 50% white soft paraffin, 50% liquid paraffin all-over strictly every 6 h
- antibiotics for proven infection.

Supervision should be under the direction of the dermatology team. Intensive care may be necessary.

OTHER BULLOUS AND VESICULAR CONDITIONS

There are many causes of blistering skin rashes that range from common and harmless (but still distressing) to the uncommon and potentially life threatening, such as TEN and SJS described above. See Table 15.1.5 for the differential diagnosis of a vesicobullous rash.

Always ask about recent drug ingestion and also about drug allergy in the event that a bacterial skin infection is diagnosed and antibiotics are required.

Pemphigus vulgaris

Pemphigus vulgaris is characterized by flaccid bullae and erosions, together with oral ulceration. The bullae often breakdown readily to form erosions as the split is epidermal. The Nikolsky sign is positive with dislodgement of the epidermis by lateral finger pressure in the vicinity of a lesion, causing an erosion or

pressure on a bulla leading to lateral extension of the blister. Vegetating lesions, particularly in flexures, such as the axillae or on the scalp, may occur as 'pemphigus vegetans'.

Investigations

Send blood for FBC, U&E, LFTs and glucose as a baseline and for thiopurine methyl-transferase (TPMT) levels, reduction of which increases the risk of toxicity if adjuvant immunosuppression with azathioprine is required.

Send a serum autoantibody profile for anti-skin antibodies directed against a 130-kDa glycoprotein designated desmoglein 3 and located in desmosomes. Arrange biopsy of lesional skin for histology and perilesional skin, which should be sent fresh and not in formalin, for direct immunofluorescence. An alternative medium is Michel's if fresh transport is not possible.

Management

Start high-dose prednisolone initially at a dose of 1 mg/kg/day to achieve remission (prior to the introduction of systemic steroids this disease was uniformly fatal). Admit the patient under the care of a dermatologist for consideration of other therapies, such as immunosuppression with azathioprine, mycophenolate mofetil, rituximab or cyclophosphamide. Plasmapheresis, intravenous gamma-globulin and rituximab may have an additive drug-sparing effect.

Bullous pemphigoid

The usual presentation is an elderly patient with tense skin bullae that may occur on an urticarial base, particularly in the axillae, medial thigh, groin, forearm and abdomen. Itch is a common accompaniment (Fig. 15.1.4).

Table 15.1.5   Causes of a vesicular or bullous skin rash

Most common	Less common	Rare
Viral: • herpes zoster • herpes simplex Impetigo Scabies Insect bites and papular urticaria Bullous eczema and pompholyx Drugs: • sulphonamides • penicillin • barbiturates	Erythema multiforme major ('target lesions' rash, plus one mucous membrane involved) or erythema multiforme minor (1–2 cm 'target lesions' only): • mycoplasma pneumonia • herpes simplex • drugs such as sulphur, penicillins • idiopathic (50%) SJS and TEN with epidermal detachment and mucosal erosions: • drugs such as anticonvulsants, sulphonamides, NSAIDs and penicillins Staphylococcal scalded-skin syndrome (children) Dermatitis herpetiformis (gluten sensitivity) Pemphigus and pemphigoid	Porphyria cutanea tarda Epidermolysis bullosa

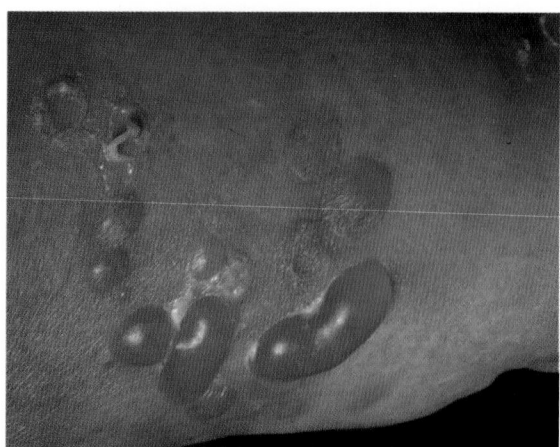

Fig. 15.1.4 Bullous pemphigoid.

Investigations

Send for FBC, electrolytes, LFTs and glucose level as a baseline, plus serum for indirect immunofluorescence for autoantibodies to Bullous pemphigoid antigens 1 or 2, components of the hemidesmosome. Also send a TPMT level, as adjuvant immunosuppression with azathioprine may be required. Arrange biopsy of an urticated or bullous lesion for histology and perilesional skin for direct immunofluorescence. If this is not possible, blister fluid may be sent for indirect immunofluorescence.

Management

Start prednisolone at a moderate dose, such as 0.5–0.75 mg/kg daily. A tetracycline antibiotic, such as doxycycline 100 mg daily and nicotinamide 500 micrograms orally tds, may be used for their anti-inflammatory properties as adjuvant therapy. Admit patients for supportive care if blistering is widespread.

In more severe disease, steroid-sparing agents, such as azathioprine, methotrexate or mycophenolate mofetil, may be required. Superpotent topical steroids are also effective and may be used as monotherapy for localized disease.

PETECHIAL AND PURPURIC RASHES

Petechiae, bruising and ecchymoses

Consider and exclude potentially life-threatening causes, such as thrombocytopaenia and vasculitis, platelet abnormalities such as those associated with thrombasthenia or uraemia, or over-anticoagulation (see Table 15.1.6 for causes of a petechial or purpuric rash). Take a full drug history, including anticoagulant medications, and ask about systemic symptoms including fever, bleeding tendency, travel history, alcohol abuse and known HIV disease.

'Senile purpura' are usually due to sun damage and ageing with subsequent loss of dermal support for blood vessels which then bleed into the skin. Sometimes they can be dramatic but are always benign and resolve. When simple trauma is considered, remember non-accidental injury in all cases where the history is suspicious, 'hollow' or changes over time.

Cutaneous vasculitis

There are many potential causes of cutaneous vasculitis, such as viral and bacterial infection, autoimmune and connective tissue diseases including systemic lupus erythematosus and rheumatoid arthritis, systemic vasculitis, such as Wegener's granulomatosis, polyarteritis nodosa and other causes that include inflammatory bowel diseases. Rarely, malignant tumours and leukaemia may present with vasculitis.

However, 50% of all cases of cutaneous small vessel vasculitis remain of undetermined aetiology or 'idiopathic' after extensive investigation and are presumed to be of post-infectious origin. Cutaneous vasculitis is clinically best diagnosed when lesions are palpable and on the lower limbs, although they may spread to the buttocks and arms (Fig. 15.1.5). Sharp edges with stellate or irregular shapes indicate full thickness ischaemia and are seen in septic embolic lesions or meningococcal infection and in thrombotic occlusion states, such as calciphilaxis in, for instance, chronic renal failure.

Table 15.1.6 Causes of petechiae or purpura						
	Non-palpable purpura					**Palpable purpura (vasculitis)**
Non-thrombocytopaenic	**Thrombocytopaenic disorders**					
	with splenomegaly		*without splenomegaly*			
	Normal marrow	*Abnormal marrow*	*Normal marrow*	*Abnormal marrow*		

Cutaneous disorders:
• trauma, sun
• steroids, old age
Systemic disorders:
• uraemia
• von Willebrand's disease
• scurvy, amyloid
	Liver disease with portal hypertension
	Myeloproliferative disorders
	Lymphoproliferative disorders
	Hypersplenism
		Leukaemia
		Lymphoma
		Myeloid metaplasia
			Immune: idiopathic thrombocytopaenic purpura, drugs, infections including HIV
			Non-immune: vasculitis, sepsis, disseminated intravascular coagulation, haemolytic-uraemic syndrome, thrombotic thrombocytopaenic purpura
				Cytotoxics
				Aplasia, fibrosis or infiltration
				Alcohol, thiazides
						Polyarteritis nodosa (PAN)
						Leucocytoclastic (allergic)
						Henoch–Schönlein purpura
						Infective:
						• meningococcaemia
						• gonococcaemia
						• other infections:
						  • staphylococcus
						  • rickettsia (Rocky Mountain spotted fever)
						  • enteroviruses
						Embolic

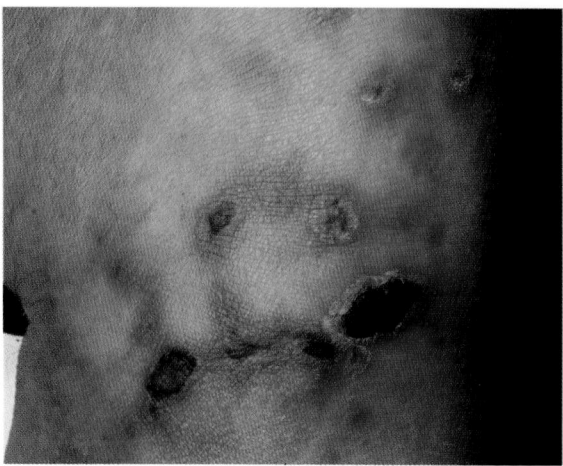

Fig. 15.1.5 Palpable purpura due to vasculitis.

Pyoderma gangrenosum

Pyoderma gangrenosum is frequently a differential diagnosis of cutaneous vasculitis. It may begin as a discrete painful haemorrhagic pustule or grouped lesions that rapidly ulcerate, usually on the lower leg, causing larger lesions with neutrophilic inflammation with abscesses and necrosis, but not vasculitis on biopsy. It may be associated with inflammatory bowel disease, rheumatoid arthritis, blood dyscrasias, Behçet's syndrome and malignancy, such as myeloma and leukaemia (Fig. 15.1.6).

Investigations for vasculitis

Send blood for a vasculitis screen including FBC, ESR, CRP, U&E, LFTs, hepatitis B and C

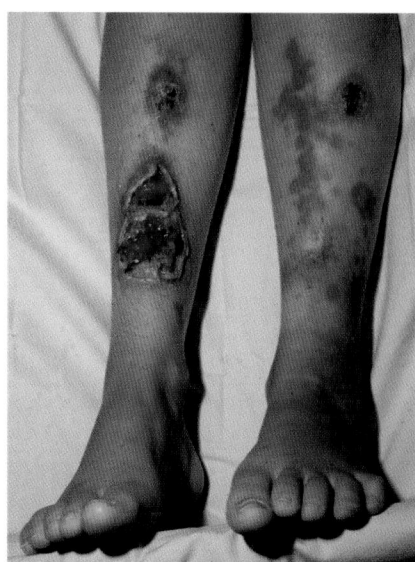

Fig. 15.1.6 Pyoderma gangrenosum.

serology, ANA, rheumatoid factor, antinuclear cytoplasmic antibodies (ANCA), antistreptolysin O (ASO) titre, cryoglobulin screen, anticardiolipin and antiphospholipid screen, serum protein electrophoresis and C3 and C4 complement levels.

Send two sets of blood cultures prior to any antibiotic therapy, such as ceftriaxone 2 g IV, if meningococcal infection is possible. Send a fresh urine specimen for phase contrast microscopy, looking specifically for glomerular red cells and casts indicating renal involvement (over 70% dysmorphic red cells or the presence of red cell casts indicate glomerular disease).

Arrange biopsy, although this is usually performed after admission or dermatology referral to clinic. Send a fresh specimen for both immunofluorescence (Henoch–Schönlein purpura suspected) and culture (infection suspected), as well as a specimen in formalin for histology.

Management

Potential triggers (see above) should be sought and treated appropriately. General measures include rest and elevation of the legs, supportive stockings and topical steroids. If systemic treatment is required, NSAIDs may be trialled before prednisolone. Antibiotics, steroids and cytotoxic immunosuppression are indicated based on the aetiology and severity of the disease, in consultation with a dermatologist.

PRURITIC (ITCHY) DERMATOSES

Itch can be localized or generalized and may present with or without rash. While not an urgent problem, itch must be recognized as being distressing to the patient. The causes are many and varied and the prevalence of chronic itch (like chronic pain) increases with age. See Table 15.1.7 for causes of pruritus with or without skin disease.

Urticaria

Urticaria may occur alone and be acute, relapsing or chronic (Fig. 15.1.7). It may also be a warning of impending anaphylaxis that necessitates immediate assessment for upper airway swelling, wheeze and/or hypotension (see Anaphylaxis, Chapter 2.8).

The causes of urticaria are heterogeneous and include immunological such as IgE-related, immune-complex or autoimmune; or non-immunological including physical such as cold, heat, sweating, exercise, pressure, sunlight,

Table 15.1.7 Causes of pruritus with, and without, skin disease	
With skin disease	*Without skin disease*
Drugs Scabies, pediculosis, insect bites, parasites (roundworm) Eczema Contact dermatitis Urticaria Lichen planus Pityriasis rosea ('Herald' patch) Dermatitis herpetiformis (gluten sensitivity)	Hepatobiliary – jaundice, including primary biliary cirrhosis Chronic renal failure Haematological: • lymphoma • polycythaemia rubra vera Endocrine: • myxoedema • thyrotoxicosis Carcinoma: • lung • stomach Drugs

water and vibration; drug-related such as NSAIDs and radiocontrast media, or food and food additives. Or they they may be related to an underlying systemic condition such as infection including bacterial, viral, parasitic and fungal, systemic lupus erytematosus (SLE) or other vasculitis, malignancy including lymphoma, or urticaria pigmentosa (mastocytosis).

However, in many acute cases, no clear cause is found, 'idiopathic' and, in chronic urticaria, defined as lasting more than 6 weeks, frequently there is no known aetiology, although autoimmune causes are eventually found in 30–40%.

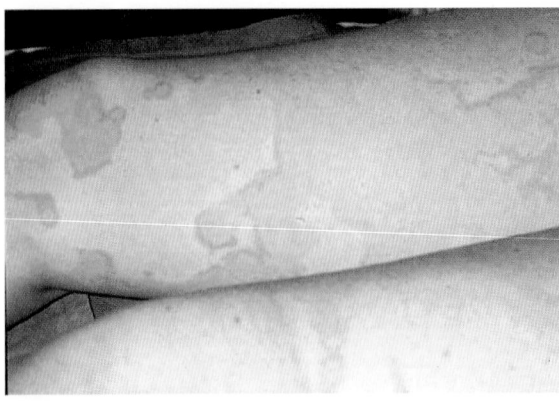

Fig. 15.1.7 Urticaria.

Scabies

Scabies must be excluded in the elderly patient with pruritus, particularly nursing home residents, and adolescents or young adults. This requires careful examination of web spaces, flexural wrist and the instep of the foot for scabies burrows and the penis and scrotum for nodules.

Crusted 'Norwegian' scabies is predisposed to by glucocorticoid therapy, organ transplant and HIV infection and in the elderly. It is usually not particularly itchy, but an affected patient who is infested with countless mites is often the source of large-scale outbreaks in nursing homes and hospitals (Fig. 15.1.8).

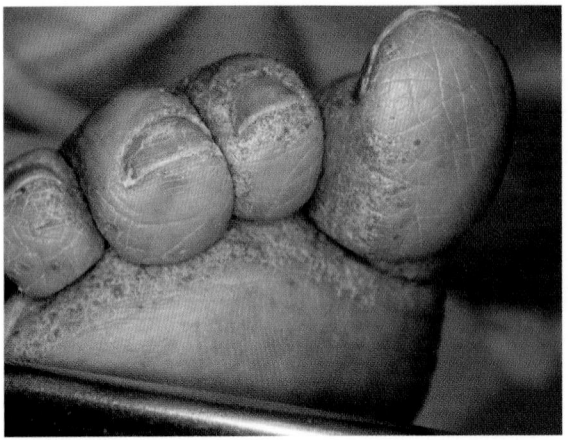

Fig. 15.1.8 Crusted 'Norwegian' scabies.

Tinea

Tinea incognito refers to tinea corporis which has been suppressed and modified in appearance due to the inappropriate use of topical steroids. The topical steroid suppresses the erythema and allows for excessive growth of the causative fungus.

Investigations for pruritus

Send blood for the following:

- FBC for eosinophilia (a non-specific finding seen in atopy, scabies and parasitic infections) and to look for iron deficiency anaemia
- iron studies and ferritin level if there is a hypochromic, microcytic blood picture
- glucose level to screen for diabetes
- urea, electrolytes and creatinine to exclude renal failure
- liver function tests to exclude hepatic impairment with jaundice, including from primary biliary cirrhosis

- serum protein electrophoresis to look for a monoclonal gammopathy, particularly in patients over 70 years
- thyroid stimulating hormone to exclude hypothyroidism or hyperthyroidism
- coeliac serology, such as IgA tissue transglutaminase (IgA tTG) antibodies.

Take skin scrapes from any suspicious areas for fungal culture and microscopy. In suspected scabies, send material to look for scabies mites, eggs or faeces on microscopy.

Management

General measures include avoiding triggers, in particular overheating, and rehydrating the skin with an emollient, such as aqueous cream combined with an anti-itch preparation (0.5% menthol). Prescribe an antihistamine for short-term use, particularly if sleep is impaired, such as promethazine 10 mg 8-hourly or chlorpheniramine 4 mg 6-hourly, with a clear warning to avoid alcohol and not to drive or operate machinery.

Attempt to identify a cause in every case. Resist giving prednisolone for an itchy dermatosis when no cause has been identified. Arrange appropriate investigations and refer the patient for dermatological follow up to avoid missing a treatable but otherwise chronic condition, such as dermatitis herpetiformis from gluten sensitivity.

ECZEMA AND PSORIASIS

Eczema

Atopic eczema is a common skin complaint often affecting the flexures (Fig. 15.1.9). It may present as an emergency in a number of ways. See Table 15.1.8 for an overview of aetiology, clinical features and management principles.

Eczema is one of the most common causes of erythroderma. See earlier for management principles, which should always involve a dermatologist and may require intensive care unit admission.

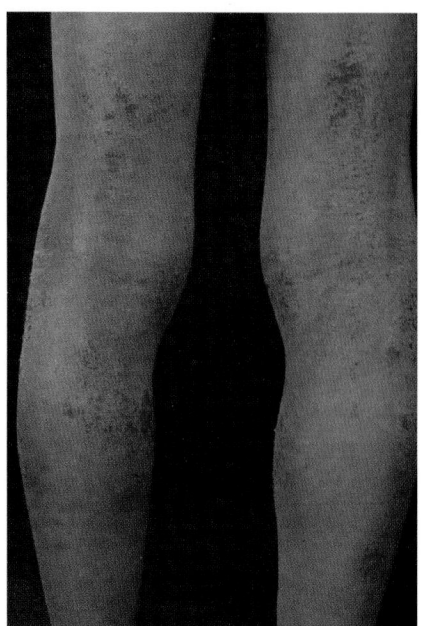

Fig. 15.1.9 Atopic flexural eczema.

Discoid eczema

Discoid eczema presents as discrete coin-like or 'nummular' erythematous plaques that may develop significant exudate and crusting. 'Satellite' lesions are common and skin involvement is often progressive, as one area of involvement 'drives' other areas of skin to become eczematous.

Investigation

Take swabs to exclude staphylococcal super-infection.

Management

Prescribe a potent topical steroid, such as mometasone 0.1% or betamethasone 0.1% cream or ointment. Advise the patient that more than 1 week of daily or twice daily application may be required and that lesions will tend to recur at the same site. Relapses should be treated in the same manner. Topical coal tar preparations may be used as a steroid alternative, such as 5–10% coal tar in either white soft paraffin or aqueous cream. Preparations are also available as a shampoo.

Allergic contact dermatitis

Allergy to plants typically presents in a 'streaky' or linear pattern. A severe facial flare of eczema may suggest an airborne allergen as a trigger. The use of hair dyes following a 'henna tattoo' (which may have been applied months or years before) can result in severe scalp and facial dermatitis, as henna used on hair is adulterated with paraphenylene diamine. The patient becomes sensitized to this compound, which is found in most hair dyes.

Some allergens are activated by the ultraviolet (UV) in sunlight to become symptomatic. This occurs in phytophotodermatitis (often a streaky or linear dermatitis on exposed areas that may be blistered or hyperpigmented) which is seen after contact with photosensitising compounds found naturally in some plants, fruit and vegetables. Nickel sensitivity is a common cause of reactions to jewellery, particularly costume jewellery and, occasionally, to the clasp of a bra. These causes may or may not be obvious to the patient, so a careful focused history is essential.

Irritant contact dermatitis

The hands are commonly involved and may become secondarily infected. Patients may be severely incapacitated if both hands are affected and may need admission. Patients commonly have an atopic background, especially atopic eczema. Ask the patient how many times they wash their hands each day, as irritant contact dermatitis may be one of the first signs of an obsessive–compulsive disorder.

Psoriasis

Psoriasis may present acutely in the following patterns:

- Erythroderma: an unstable state that may be caused by systemic or external factors, including treatment. Clinically, it is indistinguishable from the other causes of erythroderma, as there is total body redness with no typical features of psoriasis. At presentation, hypothermia and sepsis and high output cardiac failure must be recognized.

- Pustular psoriasis: triggered by systemic or external factors, including pregnancy, topical treatments, medication and oral steroids. Examination reveals yellow sterile pustules on plaques, diffuse generalized (Fig. 15.1.10) or localized red areas beginning around the paronychium of the digits or pulp. Arthritis may be present and consider Reiter's syndrome if there is a history of gastrointestinal or genitourinary symptoms. Hypocalcaemia may develop if the pustular psoriasis is generalized.

- Immune activated psoriasis flares: caused by bacterial or viral infective foci in respiratory, bowel, gallbladder or urinary bladder sites. Typically, there are new guttate lesions or flares in old psoriatic plaques. Often there have been similarly

Table 15.1.8 Atopic eczema: acute attacks and complications					
	Infective eczema	**Erythroderma**		**Acute eczema**	
	Eczema herpeticum	*Impetiginized eczema*	*Unstable eczema*	*Psychological*	*Contact*
Cause	Infection with herpes simplex, Varicella, which can rapidly disseminate over the skin	Staphylococcal	Due to many factors systemic or external	Stressors	Allergen?
Examination	Grouped locally or generally Pinhead-sized papules or vesicles Clear or closed pustules Excoriated sharply defined circular erosions	Discharge and weeping Yellow and crusted blisters or erosions	Total body redness Scale or weeping. Pruritus Hypothermia. Fever, sepsis	Severe Red Pruritus Disturbed sleep	Sharp edges Localized
Management	Antivirals if severe, early and eyes at risk	Oral antibiotics. Antiseptic (triclosan) soaks and wet dressings	Admission Oral steroids Ciclosporin	Admission topicals Oral steroids Paraffin, etc.	Oral steroids Admission

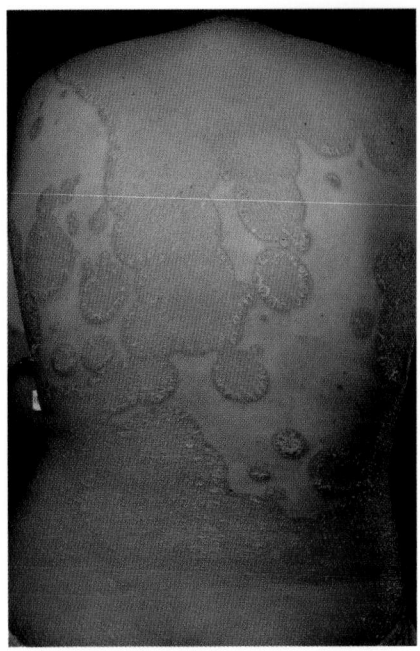

Fig. 15.1.10 Generalized psoriasis.

triggered attacks in the past. Streptococcal pharyngitis is a common precipitant.

- Flare or rebound psoriasis: following cessation or poor compliance with therapy or after treatment with oral steroids.
- Palmar plantar psoriasis: may be pustular or may show a keratoderma (thickened skin) which can be difficult to distinguish from eczema, or even inflammatory tinea pedis. Patients are debilitated and unable to walk or care for themselves and therefore may require admission.

Investigations for acute psoriasis
Send blood for FBC, U&E and LFTs, including a serum calcium (which may be low with pustular psoriasis). Send other investigations for systemic complications such as infection, including a skin swab and/or blood cultures, as well as monitoring for the side effects of therapy. A skin biopsy is usually performed in the ward or dermatology clinic if the diagnosis is in doubt.

Management
Treatments include UV therapy, methotrexate, ciclosporin, acitretin or antitumour necrosis factor (TNF) therapy, such as etanercept or infliximab. These all require a dermatology consultation and careful review of past treatment. Admission is required if the patient has extensive areas involved, is systemically unwell or unable to manage at home.

Older treatments, such as Ingram's or Goerkerman's regimens, used the combination of dithranol or coal tar respectively, and UV phototherapy. They can be particularly effective, have low toxicity and may therefore be considered as one option for patients. Rotating therapies in psoriasis may be beneficial and a past treatment failure does not necessarily indicate that treatment will always be ineffective.

OTHER DERMATOSES

Skin cancer
Patients may present to an ED with lesions they, or a concerned family member or partner, are worried about. Important differential diagnoses not to miss include melanoma and non-melanoma skin cancer, including squamous cell and basal cell carcinoma. Refer the patient for prompt assessment by a dermatologist if the lesion looks suspicious, which will usually require a biopsy.

Eczema herpeticum
Eczema herpeticum is widespread herpes simplex infection complicating a pre-existing skin disease, most often atopic eczema. Consider this in any patient with an acute flare of eczema, particularly if the skin is painful. It presents as an acute eruption of monomorphic vesicles and/or erosions often with purulent exudate and crusting, not necessarily with herpetiform grouping.

A preceding herpetic cold sore may or may not have been present. Some episodes present as a severe systemic illness with high fever, malaise and a widespread generalized eruption. However, there may be no systemic disturbance and the eruption may be quite localized, often to areas of pre-existing eczema.

Ocular HSV infection should be suspected if there is periorbital involvement or if ocular symptoms are present, such as eyelid oedema, tearing, photophobia, chemosis or preauricular lymphadenopathy, whether the eruption involves the face or not. An urgent ophthalmology opinion should be sought for complications, such as corneal ulceration, scarring and blindness.

Investigations
Viral swabs for PCR should be taken of vesicle fluid or the base of an erosion to confirm the diagnosis of HSV. Bacterial superinfection is common, so send a swab for bacterial M, C&S as well.

Management
Antiviral therapy is essential, such as acyclovir 400 mg 5 times daily for 7 days or valaciclovir 1 g bd for 7 days. Antiviral prophylaxis may be required for recurrent attacks. If secondary bacterial infection is suspected, start an antistaphylococcal antibiotic, such as cephalexin 500 mg qid for 5 days. Optimizing the management of eczema is also important.

Herpes zoster
The first manifestation of herpes zoster (HZV) is usually pain, which may be severe and accompanied by fever, headache, malaise and regional lymphadenopathy. Closely grouped red papules evolve to classical vesicles and then often pustules, in a dermatomal distribution. Rarely, the eruption may be multidermatomal or bilateral, particularly if the patient is immunosuppressed.

Diagnosis can be a challenge unless the dermatomal distribution of the eruption is appreciated. Vesicles on the side of the nose indicate involvement of the nasociliary branch of the ophthalmic division of the trigeminal nerve, which also innervates the cornea. Nasal herpetic infection (Hutchinson's sign) may precede or accompany ophthalmic involvement, which necessitates urgent ophthalmologic referral. Vesicles within the external auditory meatus associated with deep ear pain and lower motor neuron facial nerve palsy is the classic triad of Ramsay Hunt syndrome. Early diagnosis and treatment with oral prednisolone and antivirals is indicated.

Investigations
Take swabs for bacteriology and viral polymerase chain reaction for HZV to confirm the diagnosis.

Management
Prompt treatment with antiviral medication, such as acyclovir 800 mg orally five times a day or famciclovir 250 mg orally tds, when seen within 72 h of vesicle eruption, may prevent post-herpetic neuralgia.

Controversies

- The treatment of TEN is controversial with IVIG, prednisolone and ciclosporin at one time or another being advocated and then discredited. Currently, evidence suggests that IVIG improves survival. Qualifying criteria for IVIG therapy for TEN or SJS/TEN overlap and include: (1) diagnosis by a dermatologist; (2) body surface area of 10% or more: (3) evidence of rapid evolution. IVIG should be initiated as quickly as possible, preferably within 24 h of diagnosis. As it does not always limit the progression of TEN, further investigation is required. Several studies have concluded corticosteroids did not stop the progression of the disease and were even associated with increased mortality and adverse effects, particularly sepsis.
- The use of immunomodifying agents and immunosuppressants, with their potential for toxicity, opportunistic infections, unusual side effects or severe rebound of cutaneous disease following cessation or poor compliance.
- The take up of teledermatology makes it easier to obtain a second opinion in isolated areas or to triage patients better for dermatological review. Studies have now shown that teledermatology can provide rapid and accurate diagnosis and treatment advice for dermatological presentations to ED. Research is in progress to improve telemedicine services.

Further reading

Bolognia JL, Jorizzo JL, Schaffer JV. Dermatology, 3rd ed. London: Mosby; 2012.
Burns T, Breathnach S, Cox N, et al. Rook's textbook of dermatology, 8th ed. Oxford: Blackwell; 2010.
Goldsmith L, Katz S, Gilchrest B, et al. Fitzpatrick's color atlas & synopsis of clinical dermatology, 8th ed. New York: McGraw-Hill; 2012.
Muir J, et al. Incorporating teledermatology into emergency medicine. Emerg Med Australas 2011;23:562–8.
Smith S, Dennington PM, Cooper A. The use of intravenous immunoglobulin for treatment of dermatological conditions in Australia: a review. Aust J Dermatol 2010;51:227–37.
Wallett A, Sidhu S. Management pathway of skin conditions presenting to an Australian tertiary hospital emergency department. Aust J Dermatol 2012;53:307–10.
Zuberbier T, Asero R, Bindslev-Jensen C, et al. EAACI/GA2LEN/EDF/WAO guideline: definition, classification and diagnosis of urticaria. Allergy 2009;64:1417–26.

SECTION 16 OCULAR EMERGENCIES

Edited by **Peter Cameron**

16.1 Ocular emergencies

David V Kaufman • James K Galbraith • Mark J Walland

ESSENTIALS

1 Always assess and record visual acuity.

2 Chloramphenicol eyedrops are not a universal panacea.

3 Never provide local anaesthetic drops for the patient to take away.

Injuries

1 Gentle examination with magnification is essential.

2 X-ray/computed tomography where bony or penetration injury is suspected.

3 Copious free irrigation for all corneal acid or alkali burns with subsequent removal of any particulate matter.

Inflammation

1 Bacterial keratitis requires intensive, specific, topical antibiotic therapy.

2 Acute primary angle closure produces a rock-hard, inflamed eye with a fixed, mid-dilated pupil and a steamy cornea.

Loss of vision

1 Test the pupils for a relative afferent pupillary defect, which is an objective sign.

2 Central retinal artery occlusion requires immediate referral to an ophthalmologist.

3 Elderly patients with acute visual failure have giant cell arteritis until proven otherwise and need oral steroid cover until the diagnosis is excluded.

4 Recent onset of distorted vision requires ophthalmic review within 1–2 days to exclude exudative age-related macular degeneration.

5 New onset of floaters, particularly in association with flashes, requires early ophthalmic review to exclude retinal detachment.

6 Local ocular pathology does not cause a visual field defect respecting a vertical midline.

Introduction

Acute ocular presentations are common. A seemingly trivial trauma may mask a more serious underlying injury. Similarly, a relatively transient episode of visual loss with no abnormality found on examination may indicate potentially life-threatening cerebrovascular disease. Therefore, all eye presentations in an emergency department (ED) should be carefully evaluated with the necessary equipment.

Basic sight testing equipment should include a Snellen 6-metre chart and a black occlusive paddle with multiple pinhole perforations. A slit-lamp biomicroscope is needed for examination of the anterior segment and the removal of foreign bodies. A portable slit lamp for examining reclining patients can be a valuable asset in the emergency department. An intraocular pressure-measuring device, such as a Tono-pen or iCare tonometer which is portable, accurate and easily used, is desirable.

Emergency eye trolley setup

Examining equipment
- Torch
- Magnifying loupe
- Desmarres lid retractors/lid speculum
- Sterile dressing packs
- Normal saline for irrigation
- Fluorescein strips (sterile)
- Topical anaesthetic (e.g. tetracaine 1%).

Treating
- Mydriatics (dilating): tropicamide 1%, homatropine 2%
- Miotic (constricting): pilocarpine 2%
- Antibiotic ointment (e.g. chloramphenicol)

- Pressure control: acetazolamide 250 mg tablets; ampoules 500 mg (Diamox)
- Eye pads, plastic shields, skin adhesive tape
- Cotton-tipped applicators (sterile)
- 25 G, 23 G disposable hypodermic needles (foreign body removal).

OCULAR TRAUMA

History

The incidence of injuries varies with the environment and protective measures taken. The major injuries result from blunt trauma or penetrating injuries to the globe, with or without the retention of a foreign body. Mechanical interference with eye movement may result from orbital injury, either haematoma or interference with muscle function. Similarly, neurotrauma may disturb the visual pathways or ocular motor nerves.

It is necessary to elicit a history of the patient's prior visual status, including the wearing of glasses or contact lenses and ocular medication.

Examination

Visual acuity

After an eye toilet to remove any debris from the eyelids, vision is tested by a distance Snellen chart, if necessary using a pinhole device as a rough focussing aid. Vision less than 6/60 Snellen may be graded by the patient's ability to count fingers (CF) at a measured distance, discern hand movements (HM) or to project the direction of a light (PL) from various angles. The eye not being tested must be completely shielded by an opaque occluder.

It is essential to assess early whether the patient has sustained a relatively minor superficial injury or a severe injury, which may be either blunt or penetrating. Reassurance and extreme gentleness in examining the eye will allow a more definite assessment to be made in the ED. Fresh local anaesthetic drops—preferably single use Minims – may be instilled to ease discomfort. With penetrating trauma, any external pressure on the eye may result in ocular structures being squeezed out of the wound, drastically worsening the prognosis. Desmarres retractors (Fig. 16.1.1) can be useful to open the lids yet avoid globe pressure. To open lids that are adherent due to blood or

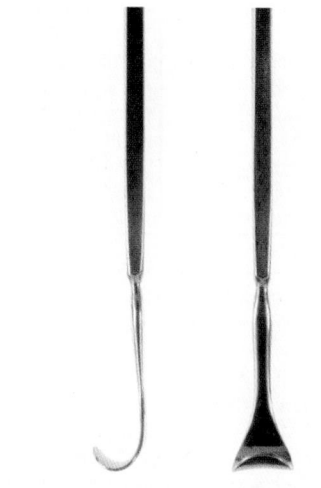

Fig. 16.1.1 Desmarres retractors for opening eyelids.

discharge, gently bathe with sterile saline. Wipe the eyelid skin dry and apply gentle distractive pressure to skin below the brow and below the lower lid, i.e. over bony orbital rim to open the lids.

Investigation

All patients in whom a penetrating injury is suspected require X-ray or computed tomography (CT) scanning to exclude a radiopaque intraocular foreign body (IOFB). If there is any possibility of metallic IOFB, magnetic resonance imaging (MRI) scans are contraindicated. When an adequate examination cannot be made, or where occult perforation is suspected, examination under anaesthesia is mandatory.

Management of specific injuries

Superficial injury

Corneal abrasion

The corneal epithelium is easily dislodged by a glancing blow from fingers, twigs, stones or a paper edge. The trauma produces an acute sensation of a foreign body, with light sensitivity and excessive tearing.

After fluorescein staining, the size of the epithelial defect is recorded. Antibiotic ointment (chloramphenicol) is instilled and an eye pad applied if local anaesthetic was used. The condition heals spontaneously within 24–48 h. Large abrasions produce reflex ciliary spasm, which may require short-acting mydriatics, such as homatropine 2%, in addition to oral

analgesia to relieve the pain. *Under no circumstances can a patient ever be discharged with local anaesthetic drops for their own use.*

Corneal foreign body

Small ferrous particles rapidly oxidize when adherent to the corneal epithelium, producing a surrounding rust ring within hours. The rusted particle requires removal under adequate topical anaesthesia using a slit-lamp microscope. An adherent rust ring may be loosened by the application of antibiotic ointment and padding for 24 h, after which it is easily shelled out with the edge of a fine hypodermic needle. Mechanical dental burrs can be difficult to sterilize and may cause large areas of epithelial removal and delay return to work. Wooden splinters are particularly dangerous as they may easily penetrate the eye and cause violent suppuration. In all suspected foreign body injuries, the upper and lower lids should be everted and examined with suitable lighting and magnification. The conjunctival fornices may be swept gently with a moist cotton bud under topical anaesthesia.

Technique for upper eyelid eversion: the patient must look down at all times; grasp the upper lid lashes and draw the lid down, then with a cotton bud in the other hand, depress the lid 11 mm above the central lid margin (i.e. above the tarsal plate) and counter-rotate the grasped lashes and lid around this cotton-bud fulcrum. The lashes may be held against the superior orbital margin with a finger and the cotton bud removed. When the examination is complete, release the lid and allow the patient finally to look up and the lid will revert to the normal position.

Conjunctival laceration

Unless large, it is rare that these require suturing. It is, however, vital to ensure that this superficial laceration does not hide a deeper penetration of the globe. After instillation of local anaesthetic, the conjunctiva may be gently moved aside with a cotton bud to examine the bed of the laceration.

Penetrating injury

A careful history is important in assessing penetrating injury, including prior visual status and the use of contact lenses or spectacles. Occupational trauma may be due to high-speed penetrating metal fragments. Agricultural trauma often involves heavily contaminated implements. Australian seatbelt legislation has markedly reduced the incidence of penetrating eye injuries in road trauma, but eye problems still occur from violent head and facial trauma, in addition to the neurological complications of head injury [1,2].

Examination of the eye involves the instillation of sterile topical anaesthetic drops, followed by a gentle eye toilet removing debris, clot and glass from the face and lids. The lids should be opened without pressure (Fig. 16.1.2). The penetration may be evidenced by an obvious laceration or presence of prolapsed tissue with collapse of the globe. Conjunctival oedema (chemosis) and low intraocular pressure (IOP) may indicate an occult perforation or bursting injury.

When a penetrating injury is either suspected or established, the patient must be transferred without delay to a centre where appropriate surgical facilities are available. During transport, the eye should be covered with a sterile pad and a plastic cone. Vomiting should be prevented with antiemetics and the fasted patient given intravenous fluids as necessary. Extruded tissue or projectiles should not be removed: intraocular contents will surely follow. Removal can only be undertaken in the controlled environment of an operating theatre. Prognosis depends on the extent of globe disruption.

Blunt injury

Concussion of the globe may cause tearing of the iris root, resulting in blood in the anterior chamber (hyphaema). A hyphaema greater than one-third of the anterior chamber usually indicates some damage to the drainage angle and may also be associated with concussive lens damage. Uninterrupted absorption of the hyphaema is essential and is aided by sedation and an admission to hospital. Traditional treatment is to pad the affected eye and to nurse the patient semirecumbent to encourage sedimentation of the blood in the anterior chamber to clear as much of the angle as possible. A hyphaema may cause considerable pain due to raised IOP. To lower the pressure, oral or intravenous acetazolamide 500 mg initially is required. Atropine drops to 'splint' the ocular interior are logical but theoretically risk a re-bleed with the initial dilating effect.

Pain is relieved by paracetamol or narcotics, with antiemetics if necessary. Aspirin in any form should be avoided as it increases the risk of secondary haemorrhage. The patient should remain in bed until the blood has completely

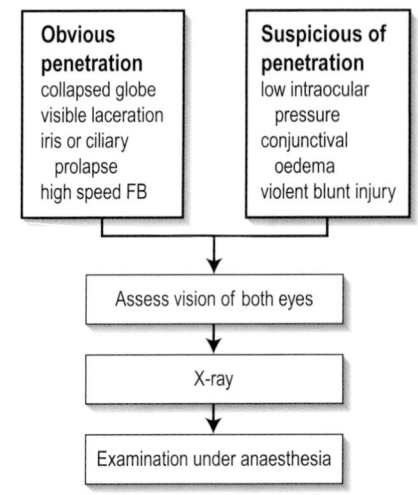

Fig. 16.1.2 Emergency department diagnosis of penetrating injury. FB: foreign body.

cleared from the anterior chamber. Bleeding recurs in up to 10% of patients, usually due to early mobilization in those with extensive iris damage. Total hyphaema has a poor prognosis because of secondary glaucoma, field loss and corneal opacification. When angle damage occurs, long-term follow up after hyphaema is required to determine whether the IOP is raised. The fundus requires careful examination after the hyphaema has cleared completely, to exclude a traumatic retinal tear, which may be heralded by sudden onset of flashes and floaters.

Smaller hyphaemas may be managed on an outpatient basis, perhaps with rest at home and the use of atropine drops and can be considered only if daily IOP monitoring is not required.

Chemical burns

The first principle of management at the location where the injury was sustained is copious irrigation of the eyes for at least 10 min with running water. Chemical trauma requires priority assessment on arrival at an emergency centre and immediate irrigation if this has not been done or was inadequate.

Alcohol and solvent burns occur from splashes while painting and cleaning. Although the epithelium is frequently burnt, it regenerates rapidly. The condition is very painful initially, but heals with topical antibiotic and patching for 48 h.

Alkali and acid burns are potentially more serious because of the ability of the burning agent to alter the pH in the anterior chamber of

the eye and inflict chemical damage on the iris and lens. Caustic soda, lime and plaster, commonly used in industry, may inflict painful, deep and destructive ocular burns. Splashes of acids, such as sulphuric and hydrochloric, if concentrated, will cause equally destructive injury.

Assessment of the ocular burn should be done using topical anaesthetic drops and fluorescein staining to determine the area of surface injury. The eyelids should be everted and the fornices carefully examined and swept gently with a cotton bud to ensure there is no particulate caustic agent remaining.

Chemical burns where the epithelium is intact or minimally disturbed can usually wait 24 h before review by an ophthalmologist. Burns involving more than one-third of the epithelium and the corneal edge, with any clouding of the cornea, are potentially more serious as subsequent melting of the cornea by collagenase action may ensue. These burns should all be further irrigated in the ED with a buffered sterile solution, such as lactated Ringer's (Hartmann's). The irrigation should continue until the tears are neutral to litmus testing.

More serious caustic injuries have shown a significant improvement in outcome with the introduction of 10% citrate and ascorbate drops, commencing 2-hourly for 48 h and reducing over the week, in combination with 1 g oral ascorbic acid daily. This regimen has an inhibitory effect on corneal melting. Topical antibiotic (e.g. chloramphenicol) is used; topical steroid is used under ophthalmic supervision.

Flash burns

Exposure of the eyes to prolonged or severe ultraviolet radiation results in widespread punctate epithelial loss from the corneal surface. This is most frequently seen in welders who have not used sufficient eye protection while working or workers who have been inadvertently adjacent to welding. Patients complain of moderate to severe ocular discomfort with excessive watering and foreign body sensation. This usually occurs some hours after exposure to the inciting ocular radiation.

Ocular examination shows widespread punctate fluorescein staining, usually with no ulceration and no evidence of foreign body present. It is usual to elicit a history of exposure to welding. Other instances in which excessive ultraviolet radiation may be encountered are in alpine snowfields and tanning beds.

Treatment is supportive with oral analgesia and explanation of the cause and likely time course. The symptoms generally settle within 24–48 h as the epithelium recovers. While local anaesthetics give short-term relief, it is not appropriate to use these as a treatment.

ACUTE INFLAMMATORY CONDITIONS

Acute primary angle-closure (glaucoma)

Acute primary angle-closure (APAC) is characterized by an acute impairment of the outflow of aqueous from the anterior chamber in an anatomically predisposed (crowded) eye. This results in a rapid and severe elevation in IOP. Usual IOP lies between 10 and 21 mmHg but, in cases of APAC, can rise to >60 mmHg. This is manifested as severe pain, blurring of vision and redness. The pain may be severe enough to cause nausea and vomiting and may be poorly localized to the eye. Visual disturbance can be preceded by halos around lights and, in established cases, is due to corneal oedema. Relative hypoxia of the pupillary sphincter due to elevated pressure results in a pupil unresponsive to light stimulation. The pupil is classically fixed and mid-dilated. The associated inflammation induces congestion of conjunctival and episcleral vessels. The term 'acute angle-closure glaucoma' is no longer regarded as appropriate, as there may be no optic nerve head cupping or visual field loss – the features that define glaucoma – at the acute presentation.

Treatment of APAC is aimed at lowering the IOP and allowing the flow of aqueous from the posterior to the anterior chamber. Acetazolamide 500 mg IV and/or topical apraclonidine or brimonidine may be effective in acutely lowering the pressure and thereby reducing pain. If ineffective, subsequent constriction of the pupil with 2% pilocarpine, a parasympathomimetic, may alleviate the forward bowing of the iris, relieve the pupil block and re-establish aqueous flow and angle drainage. One drop is initially instilled every 5 min for 15 min and then half-hourly. If the pressure is very high, however, the ischaemia induced will render the pupillary sphincter unresponsive to the pilocarpine. In these cases, it may be necessary to move to early laser treatment.

A peripheral iridotomy (PI) is performed using the yttrium:aluminium:garnet (YAG) laser to allow aqueous permanently to bypass the

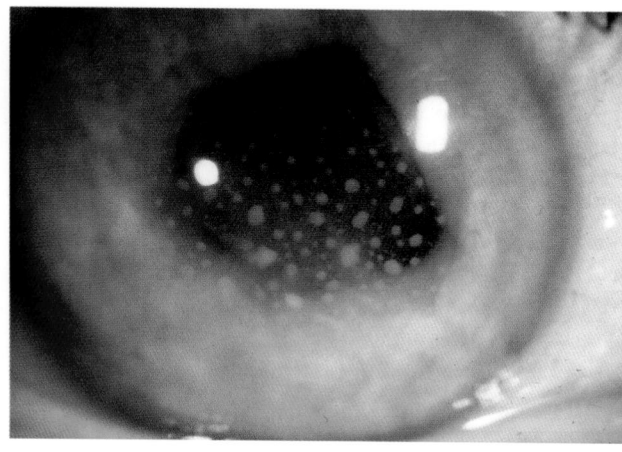

Fig. 16.1.3 Anterior uveitis with keratic precipitates (KP) and adhesions between the iris and anterior lens surface (posterior synechiae).

pupil and remove the risk of further episodes of APAC. This may be done acutely or electively. The anatomical predisposition to APAC is usually bilateral and a PI is also performed in the other eye as an elective procedure. Until this is done, miotics are instilled (G. pilocarpine 2% qid) in the unaffected eye to avoid the risk of APAC.

Early YAG laser PI in the affected eye may be hampered by corneal oedema. Argon laser peripheral iridoplasty may be used in the acute phase for resistant attacks or where corneal oedema precludes YAG laser PI [3,4].

Acute iritis

Acute iritis (AI) is an inflammatory response in the ciliary body and the iris. As part of this response there is an increase in vascular dilatation and permeability, with release of inflammatory mediators and cells that can damage intraocular structures.

Acute iritis is usually an idiopathic condition with no systemic cause or association. Less commonly, associated conditions may include HLA-B27-related disease, sarcoidosis, inflammatory bowel disease, including ulcerative colitis and Crohn's disease, connective tissue disorders, such as ankylosing spondylitis and ocular infection, including herpetic disease or toxoplasmosis. A complete history will often give clues to these associations.

Acute iritis is generally unilateral, although bilateral involvement is seen. It is characterized by pain, redness and visual disturbance. The pain is constant and exacerbated by light owing to movement of the inflamed iris. Dilatation

of the conjunctival and episcleral vessels is apparent, particularly in the vessels adjacent to the corneal limbus, often referred to as limbal flush. Visual acuity can be reduced by varying degrees depending on the severity of inflammation. The pupil is constricted due to irritation.

Examination of the anterior segment with the slit lamp will reveal evidence of increased vascular permeability, seen as fibrin clumps, flare and inflammatory cells in the aqueous released from the vessels. In some cases, small collections of neutrophils can be seen aggregating on the posterior surface of the cornea as keratic precipitates (KP) (Fig. 16.1.3). In cases of severe inflammation, cells can accumulate in the inferior anterior chamber and a sediment level can be seen as a hypopyon. The IOP may be raised.

Treatment of AI is directed towards resolution of the inflammatory response and limiting the ocular effects of this response. The mainstay of treatment is intensive, topical steroid eye drops (prednisolone acetate 1%, up to hourly in severe cases). In severe cases, orbital steroid injections or oral steroids may be necessary. Mydriatic eye drops (G. homatropine 2% qid) are used to break any lens–iris adhesions and to limit the extent of permanent adhesions. In 'splinting' the iris, these drops also provide pain relief by limiting pupil movement.

As the degree of inflammation decreases on slit-lamp examination, the topical treatment is decreased in frequency. The long-term use of topical steroid drops is not without risk and can be associated with the development of glaucoma, cataract and concurrent ocular surface infection, such as herpes simplex keratitis.

Acute infectious keratitis

The surface of the eye is protected by several mechanisms from penetration by infectious agents, both bacterial and viral. The flow of tears over the surface washes debris away and contains antibodies and lysozymes. The smooth surface of the corneal epithelium hinders the adherence of infectious agents and the rapid repair of any defect in the epithelium limits the likelihood of penetration by such agents. If these defences are impaired in any way, there is the possibility of penetration into the corneal stroma and active infection may occur.

Bacterial keratitis is characterized by a focus of infection with an associated inflammatory response. Patients complain of pain, redness, watering and a decrease in visual acuity. Fluorescein staining shows an area of ulceration over the infection, which appears as an opacity or area of whiteness within the cornea. Marked conjunctival and episcleral injection results in a unilateral red eye. Evidence of intraocular inflammation is usually present, with cells and flare being seen in the anterior chamber on slit-lamp examination. In severe cases, a collection of inflammatory cells can be seen in the inferior part of the anterior chamber as sediment, called a hypopyon.

The most important aspect of management is to identify the infectious agent and to commence appropriate antibiotic treatment. A specimen is taken via a scraping for microbiological assessment, including Gram staining and culture. Under topical anaesthetic, using a preservative-free single-use dispenser of benoxinate or tetracaine, a sterile 23 G needle is used to gather a small specimen. This is transferred directly to glass slides and also plated on to HB and chocolate agar plates for culture. Fungal cultures may be indicated. Antibiotic therapy is not delayed until the results are available, but is commenced on a broad-spectrum basis, such as the intensive use of a fluoroquinolone eye drop (e.g. G. ciprofloxacin) on an hourly basis. Daily monitoring with slit-lamp examination is mandatory and severe infections require hospital admission. This regimen can be modified when culture and sensitivity results are available.

Herpes simplex keratitis usually presents initially as an infection of the epithelial cell layer, although with recurrent episodes, stromal involvement may be seen. It is most often a unilateral infection. As with other herpetic infections, it is not possible to eradicate the

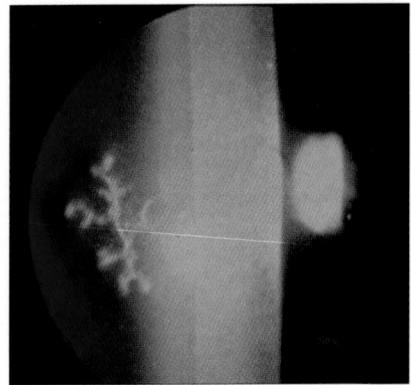

Fig. 16.1.4 Herpetic dendrite.

virus, but limitation of inflammatory-mediated damage is important. Patients complain of foreign body sensation, redness, watering and a variable decrease in visual acuity. On examination, the areas of infected epithelium can be seen as a branching irregularity or *dendrite* on the surface of the eye (Fig. 16.1.4). Multiple dendrites may be scattered over the surface, particularly in immunocompromised patients. These are best seen when the cornea is stained with fluorescein and viewed by the slit lamp

Treatment is directed to clearing the virus from the cornea to promote epithelial healing and limit stromal involvement and damaging corneal inflammation. A single pass with a sterile cotton bud rolled across the ulcer will deplete the viral load; an antiviral ointment (acyclovir) is then instilled five times daily until there is resolution of the epithelial lesions and then ceased as long-term usage may be toxic to the unaffected corneal epithelium. Steroid eye drops are contraindicated except under the strict supervision of an ophthalmologist.

Adenoviral conjunctivitis

This highly contagious conjunctival infection is the commonest cause of viral conjunctivitis.

Initial presentation is usually with a short history of discomfort or aching, watery discharge, redness, crusting of the eyelid margins and ocular foreign body sensation. While ultimately often bilateral, it may be unilateral on initial presentation. There is often a history of either recent upper respiratory tract infection or contact with someone with a current episode of adenoviral infection.

Examination shows a follicular pattern of conjunctivitis, particularly in the subtarsal conjunctiva. In severe cases, subconjunctival

haemorrhage and pseudomembrane formation can occur. The bulbar conjunctiva is often inflamed and a watery discharge is noted. There is often crusting of the lid margin and eyelashes. Uncommonly, the cornea can be involved with focal subepithelial infiltrates noted with minimal overlying epithelial disturbance. This is an immune response and can affect the visual acuity if in the visual axis. There is no evidence of intraocular inflammation and preauricular lymphadenopathy is often noted. The appearances may be asymmetrical.

It is an acute, self-limiting disease (2–3 weeks) for which no specific treatment is required. There is no evidence that topical antibiotics or antiviral agents affect the course of the infection. Lid hygiene and cold compresses may be helpful for symptomatic relief. Topical steroid eyedrops are only given under strict ophthalmic supervision for corneal infiltrates if vision is affected. It is also important to stress the contagious nature of this condition and to encourage hand washing and the use of one's own towel, pillow and face washer.

ACUTE VISUAL FAILURE

Introduction

Acute visual failure is any acute loss of visual acuity, visual field or colour vision. Most of the sinister causes of acute visual failure are painless (Table 16.1.1) and the absence of apparent distress may result in the patient being triaged in error to a non-acute review. Effective emergency management depends upon rapid recognition of those conditions for which acute therapy is available (Table 16.1.2). Some conditions have no effective therapy or are more appropriately managed on an outpatient basis.

Clinical assessment

History
Particular attention should be paid to the rapidity of onset, degree and location in space of visual loss, previous episodes and associated symptoms. One should distinguish history between acute onset and acute *discovery* of visual loss, as a patient may discover decreased vision from, for example, cataract, by inadvertently covering one eye for the first time.

Table 16.1.1 Symptoms significant for cause in acute visual failure

Symptom	Condition
Floaters (if recent onset)	Posterior vitreous detachment Vitreous haemorrhage Retinal detachment
Flashes (especially temporal)	Retinal detachment Migraine aura
Shadow (billowing curtain/ cloud)	Retinal detachment Vitreous haemorrhage
Distortion	Exudative macula disease
Amaurosis fugax	Retinal artery occlusion Anterior ischaemic optic neuropathy
Pain on eye movement	Optic neuritis
Visual field loss	
Horizontal hemifield	Anterior ischaemic optic neuropathy Branch retinal vein occlusion Branch retinal artery occlusion
Vertical hemifield (bilateral)	Retrochiasmal CVA/ compression
Whole-field (unilateral)	Vitreous haemorrhage Central retinal artery occlusion Anterior ischaemic optic neuropathy Central retinal vein occlusion Retinal detachment
Bilateral total loss of vision	Bilateral occipital infarction Toxic (methanol/quinine)

Table 16.1.2 Acute visual failure for which acute therapy is available

Condition	Therapy
Central (or branch) retinal artery occlusion	Acetazolamide CO_2 rebreathing Pulsed ocular compression Anterior chamber paracentesis
Anterior ischaemic optic neuropathy	Steroids
Exudative age-related macula degeneration	Anti-VEGF injections Laser
Retinal detachment	Surgery

Examination

Testing of the visual acuity and visual field will clarify uni- or binocular involvement.

Examination of the pupils is mandatory before pharmacological dilatation. *Test for a relative afferent pupillary defect (RAPD), one of the few objective signs.* When required, pupils will dilate in 10–15 min with tropicamide 1.0% drops, which last 1–2 h. Pupils should not be dilated if the patient requires monitoring for a head injury.

Bilateral vision loss

Bilateral visual field loss usually implicates a retrochiasmal and, therefore, non-ocular cause. This visual field defect will, however, respect a vertical midline. In contrast, the retinal nerve fibre layer and retinal vascular elements within the eye are distributed around a horizontal midline and may thus involve a superior or inferior (i.e. horizontal) hemifield. *Localized ocular pathology does not cause a visual field defect respecting a vertical midline.*

Bilateral acute, complete, visual failure is uncommon. Bilateral occipital infarction may present with bilateral blindness, but pupil responses would be expected to be intact. Rapidly progressive bilateral sequential visual loss from temporal arteritis is occasionally encountered. Other prechiasmal causes of bilateral, simultaneous, ocular involvement include toxic causes, such as poisoning with either quinine or methanol, where the patient presents with bilateral blindness and fixed, widely dilated pupils. Visual recovery in these cases is variable and the efficacy of a range of therapeutic interventions is controversial [5–7].

Central retinal artery occlusion (CRAO)

The history is typically of sudden, painless loss of vision in the affected eye over seconds. This may have been preceded by episodes of transient loss of vision (amaurosis fugax) in the previous days or weeks. Mean age of presentation is in the 70s. Men are more frequently affected and the patient may be a 'vasculopath'. Carotid disease is frequently implicated, with an embolus often being the cause of the obstruction, but its absence does not preclude the diagnosis, as the obstruction may lie behind the lamina cribrosa. Erythrocyte sedimentation rate (ESR) and C-reactive protein (CRP) should be tested when an embolus is not seen: temporal arteritis causes 5% of cases of CRAO.

The visual acuity is drastically reduced, often to the level of light perception, with an RAPD present on the affected side. Fundus examination shows creamy-white retinal oedema (cloudy swelling) with a central red fovea – the 'cherry-red spot' – caused by the absence of oedema in the thinner retina at the fovea. The arterioles may be attenuated, with segmentation ('cattle-trucking') of the blood column. An embolus may be seen at any point along the retinal arterioles, from the disc to the periphery.

Acute treatment proceeds on the assumption that the cause is embolic. The principles of therapy are, therefore, to vasodilate the retinal arterial circulation in order to promote dislodgement of the embolus from a proximal position and encourage its movement downstream to a less strategic site. All the measures currently used are directed to lowering the IOP, thereby relieving the compressive effect on the intraocular vasculature. Intravenous or oral acetazolamide 500 mg will lower IOP within 15–30 min; pulsed ocular compression ('ocular massage') involves cyclical sustained compression of the globe for 10–15 s before sudden release of this compression, continuing for 5–10 min. The release of pressure may result in a momentary marked increase in the perfusion pressure gradient and dislodge an embolus. The use of carbogen gas (95% oxygen/5% carbon dioxide) is now largely historical, but carbon dioxide rebreathing may be tried for its central vasodilatory effect. Definitive reduction of IOP is achieved with anterior chamber paracentesis by the removal of aqueous from the eye, but this is a procedure that cannot realistically be undertaken by the inexperienced and consultation by an ophthalmologist is needed. Timely intra-arterial fibrinolytic therapy is often beyond the logistical capabilities of many institutions and trials have so far shown a discouraging level of co-morbidity from the treatment [8–11]. The place of hyperbaric therapy is uncertain at this time [12]. Visual outcomes are generally poor in CRAO, but occasional successes justify aggressive intervention if the patient presents within 12 h. Non-acute management must include investigations to define the embolic source.

Central (branch) retinal vein occlusion

Central or branch retinal vein occlusion may present as a painless blurring of vision that is not sudden. Patients are usually in the older age group, often with systemic hypertension, diabetes mellitus and glaucoma. Visual acuity varies with severity, as does the presence of an RAPD. The characteristic fundus appearance is of extensive intraretinal haemorrhage with a variable number of cotton wool spots ('margherita pizza'). There may be disc oedema, with venous tortuosity and a generally congested appearance. If an insufficiently wide fundus view is obtained and this diagnosis missed, the patient may be subjected to unnecessary investigations to determine the cause of presumed 'papilloedema'.

There is no emergency management specific to the vein occlusion that will positively influence the visual outcome – systemic hypertension and raised IOP rarely require acute control – and the patient should therefore be referred to the next ophthalmic outpatient clinic.

Anterior ischaemic optic neuropathy

Arteritic anterior ischaemic optic neuropathy (AION) is the feared visual loss of giant cell (temporal) arteritis (GCA). The patient is commonly mid-70s or older and more often female. Presentation is with profound vision loss in one eye. This may have been preceded by brief premonitory visual obscurations or double vision, to which the patient may not have ascribed significance. Systematic questioning may reveal specific features, such as jaw claudication, headache, scalp tenderness, anorexia, malaise, weight loss or night sweats, and there may be a history of polymyalgia rheumatica in up to 50% of cases. Giant cell arteritis is a systemic illness with the potential for devastating visual loss, as well as long-term life-threatening non-ophthalmic complications.

Vision may be reduced at presentation to the level of perception of light only. An RAPD

will be present. Total field loss in the affected eye is usual. The optic disc is almost invariably oedematous, but the fundus may be otherwise normal. Evidence of decreased acuity, colour vision deficits and disc oedema should also be sought in the other eye. Palpation of the temporal arteries will often be abnormal, with the pulses perhaps absent or the arteries thickened and tender.

Clinical suspicion requires blood to be drawn for ESR and CRP. Treatment should then be started on an urgent basis and must not be delayed or deferred until after temporal artery biopsy. The biopsy will remain positive for at least several days despite steroids. Elevation of both ESR and CRP is highly specific for a diagnosis of GCA, but does not avoid the need for biopsy [13]. Urgent referral to an ophthalmologist is required.

Prednisolone 1 mg/kg daily is an accepted dose, although recent experience has suggested that 'pulse' methylprednisolone 500 mg IV daily or twice daily over 1–2 h is safe and more efficacious in suppressing the inflammation and this has become standard therapy in a number of centres. This is generally used for 3 days and oral prednisolone is then substituted [14–16]. Treatment will be prolonged (at least 6 months) and should be undertaken in cooperation with a physician. Attention must be directed to the avoidance of steroid complications in this aged patient group.

Non-arteritic AION is classically seen in males in the late 50s and 60s who have a history of cardiac or vascular disease, hypertension, diabetes or smoking. The visual presentation may be similar to that seen with GCA – although the visual acuity and field loss may not be as profound (may be a hemifield loss) and the specific systemic symptoms are absent – so that management must be as for arteritic AION until GCA is excluded.

Retinal detachment

Retinal detachment is usually a result of retinal hole formation, with seepage of fluid into the subretinal space and lifting of the retina. This may occur as a result of trauma, but is more often seen in an older age group as a result of vitreous traction in spontaneous posterior vitreous detachment (PVD) and is predisposed to by high myopia (short-sightedness). Exudative retinal detachment is less common and is associated with underlying pathology.

Posterior vitreous detachment (PVD)

Shrinkage and detachment of the vitreous is common in the older population and produces a new onset of floaters – wispy spots, threads or 'spider webs' in the vision. As part of this process, vitreous traction on the retina may produce flashes of light (photopsia) seen particularly in the temporal periphery of vision in that eye. These flashes can usually be distinguished from the visual aura of migraine. While PVD is usually not serious in its own right, early elective ophthalmic review is required as it is not possible to exclude related changes predisposing to retinal detachment without dilated examination of the retinal periphery.

Retinal detachment

With a history of flashes and floaters, the presence of pigmented cells ('tobacco dust') in the anterior vitreous should alert one to the possibility of a retinal hole and subsequent retinal detachment. A detached retina shows a visual field defect, which will be described as a shadow or curtain, corresponding to the area of detachment, i.e. inferior field defect equals superior retinal detachment. Vision loss is painless. There may be an RAPD, depending on the amount of retina involved. Treatment will usually require surgery. If the visual acuity is normal, the macula is likely to be still attached and referral to an ophthalmologist specializing in vitreo-retinal surgery is urgent.

Vitreous haemorrhage

The common causes are proliferative diabetic retinopathy, chronic branch retinal vein occlusion, posterior vitreous detachment or trauma. Patients with an acute vitreous haemorrhage may have symptoms varying from a few floaters causing blurred vision to a total loss of vision to a level of light perception, depending on the density of the haemorrhage. Any loss of vision is painless. The red reflex may be poor and the view of the retina may be similarly impaired. Media opacities do not affect pupil light reflexes, so *there should be no RAPD, unless the underlying retina is damaged or detached.*

The patient should be referred for early ophthalmic assessment – urgent if an RAPD is present – which may include B scan ultrasonography to exclude retinal detachment if the retinal view is inadequate. Anticoagulants should be avoided where possible.

Age-related macular degeneration

In 10–20% of cases of age-related macular degeneration (AMD), an exudative-type disease is seen and, in its most sinister form, this will involve subretinal neovascularization (SRNV). These patients may present with painless distortion of vision, particularly 'metamorphopsia' – a complaint that objects that they know to be straight appear curved. Visual acuity is reduced, depending on the stage of the disease; an RAPD is rarely seen owing to the relatively small area of retina involved, which manifests as a central scotoma on field testing. Macular drusen (yellow spots), retinal thickening and haemorrhage may be seen, with at least drusen usually also seen in the fellow eye.

Acute symptoms must not be dismissed. With appropriate treatment, central vision may be preserved in a proportion of these patients. Rapid ophthalmic review is therefore appropriate. Recent advances in treatment with antivascular endothelial growth factor (VEGF) agents, such as ranibizumab (Lucentis) or bevacizumab (Avastin), have revolutionized the prognosis and sight can often now be preserved [17,18].

Optic neuritis

Optic neuritis classically presents in young females and may be the first presentation of a demyelinating illness. Visual symptoms are not usually sudden and presentation is thus seldom acute. The vision declines gradually over days, perhaps to the level of 6/36–6/60, with loss of colour vision being prominent. The common visual field defect is a central scotoma, but many variations are possible and an RAPD should always be present. If disc oedema is not seen, the diagnosis may be retrobulbar neuritis. There may be pain on medial or superior eye movement.

Good spontaneous recovery has made the value of treating optic neuritis controversial: the results of the Optic Neuritis Treatment Trial [19] would suggest that there is no place for oral prednisolone alone in management. The benefit of 'pulse' intravenous methylprednisolone seems restricted to shortening the acute episode, without influencing the possibility of progression to multiple sclerosis or the final visual outcome [20]. However, there is usually no role for acute intervention and referral within a day or two to a neurologist is satisfactory.

Controversies

- What are the roles of hyperbaric oxygen and intra-arterial fibrinolytic therapy in central retinal artery occlusion?
- Does padding speed the recovery of corneal abrasions?
- Are anti-VEGF injections for exudative age-related macula degeneration required for the rest of the patient's life?

References

[1] McCarty CA, Fu CLH, Taylor HR. Epidemiology of ocular trauma in Australia. Ophthalmology 1999;106:1847–52.
[2] Colby K. Management of open globe injuries. Internatl Ophthalmol Clin 1999;39:59–9.
[3] Lai JSM, Tham CCY, Chua JK, et al. Laser peripheral iridoplasty as initial treatment of acute attack of primary angle-closure: a long-term follow-up study. J Glaucoma 2002;11:484–7.
[4] Lam DSC, Lai JSM, Tham CCY, et al. Argon laser peripheral iridoplasty versus conventional systemic medical therapy as first line treatment of acute angle closure: a prospective, randomised controlled trial. Ophthalmology 2002;109:1591–6.
[5] Canning CR, Hague S. Ocular quinine toxicity. Br J Ophthalmol 1988;72:23–6.
[6] Bacon P, Spalton DJ, Smith SE. Blindness from quinine toxicity. Br J Ophthalmol 1988;72:219–24.
[7] Stelmach MZ, O'Day J. Partly reversible visual failure with methanol toxicity. Aust NZ J Ophthalmol 1992;20:57–64.
[8] Beatty S, Au Eong KG. Local intra-arterial fibrinolysis for acute occlusion of the central retinal artery: a meta-analysis of the published data. Br J Ophthalmol 2000;84:914–6.
[9] Chen CS, Lee AW, Campbell B, et al. Efficacy of intravenous tissue-type plasminogen activator in central retinal artery occlusion: report from a randomized, controlled trial. Stroke 2011;42:2229–34.
[10] Feltgen N, Neubauer A, Jurklies B, et al. Multicenter study of the European assessment group for lysis in the eye (EAGLE) for the treatment of central retinal artery occlusion: design issues and implications. EAGLE Study report no. 1. Graefe's Arch Clin Exp Ophthalmol 2006;244:950–6.
[11] <http://clinicaltrials.gov/show/NCT00637468> [Accessed Nov. 2012].
[12] Beirna I, Reissman P, Scharf J, et al. Hyperbaric oxygenation combined with nifedipine treatment for recent-onset retinal arterial occlusion. Eur J Ophthalmol 1993;3:89–94.
[13] Hayreh SS, Podhajsky PA, Raman R, et al. Giant cell arteritis: validity and reliability of various diagnostic criteria. Am J Ophthalmol 1997;123:285–96.
[14] Hayreh SS. Anterior ischaemic optic neuropathy. Differentiation of arteritic from non-arteritic type and its management. Eye 1990;4:25–41.
[15] Liu GT, Glaser JS, Schatz NJ, et al. Visual morbidity in giant cell arteritis. Clinical characteristics and prognosis for vision. Ophthalmology 1994;101:1779–85.
[16] Cornblath WT, Eggenberger ER. Progressive visual loss from giant cell arteritis despite high-dose intravenous methylprednisolone. Ophthalmology 1997;104:854–8.
[17] Rosenfeld PJ, Brown DM, Heier JS, et al. Ranibizumab for neovascular age-related macular degeneration. N Engl J Med 2006;355:1419–31.
[18] Brown DM, Kaiser PK, Michels M, et al. Ranibizumab versus verteporfin for neovascular age-related macular degeneration. N Engl J Med 2006;355:1432–44.
[19] Beck RW, Cleary PA, Anderson MA, et al. A randomized controlled trial of corticosteroids in the treatment of acute optic neuritis. N Engl J Med 1992;326:581–8.
[20] Kapoor R, Miller DH, Jones SJ, et al. Effects of intravenous methylprednisolone on outcome in MRI based prognostic subgroups in acute optic neuritis. Neurology 1998;50:230–7.

Further reading

Kanski J. Clinical ophthalmology, a systematic approach. 7th ed. Oxford: Butterworth-Heinemann Ltd; 2011.
Riordan-Eva P. Vaughan and Asbury's general ophthalmology, 18th ed. New York: McGraw-Hill Medical; 2011.
The Wills Eye Manual: office and emergency room diagnosis and treatment of eye disease, 6th ed. Philadelphia: Lippincott Williams and Wilkins; 2012.

17.1 Dental emergencies

Sashi Kumar

ESSENTIALS

1 An avulsed tooth reimplanted within 30 min has a 90% survival rate.

2 Dental caries is the most common cause of dental emergency attendance.

3 Dental caries requires analgesia in the emergency department and referral to a dentist for definitive care. Antibiotics are not required unless complicated by abscess.

Anatomy

The tooth consists of the crown, which is exposed, and the root, which lies within the socket covered by the gum and serves to anchor the tooth. The gingival pulp carries the neurovascular structures via the root canal and is covered by dentine which, in turn, is covered by enamel, the hardest substance in the body (Fig. 17.1.1).

The deciduous teeth are 20 in number and erupt between the ages of 6 months and 2 years. The permanent dentition begins to erupt at around age 6 and, in the adult, consists of 32 teeth.

Dental caries

The most common cause of toothache or odontalgia is caries. Dental caries-related emergencies account for up to 52% of first contact with a dentist for children below the age of 3 years [1]. Dental caries is the cause of emergency visits to a dentist in 73% of paediatric patients [2]. Pain associated with dental caries is of a dull, throbbing nature, localized to a specific area and aggravated by changes in temperature in the oral cavity (hypersensitivity to hot and cold food or fluids).

Examination reveals tenderness of the offending tooth when tapped with a tongue depressor or a mirror. Management includes symptomatic pain relief using analgesics, such as paracetamol with or without codeine, non-steroidal anti-inflammatory drugs (NSAIDs) and urgent referral to the dentist.

Periodontal emergencies

Pain is the most common cause of self-referral to the emergency department for dental problems. The common conditions causing dental pain are acute apical periodontitis and reversible and irreversible pulpitis resulting from dental caries [3]. Symptoms include painful swollen gums with or without halitosis. On occasions, frank pus or bleeding from the gums may be the presenting symptom. At all stages, varying degrees of pain associated with inflammation are invariably present [4].

Infected gums could be an early clinical sign of undiagnosed diabetes, HIV, graft-versus-host disease in radiation therapy for head and neck malignancy and bone marrow transplantation.

Management includes diagnosis of the periodontal disease and the offending tooth. Symptomatic pain relief can be achieved with analgesics, NSAIDs and warm saline rinses. Routine antibiotic therapy is not required unless there is evidence of gross infection locally, regional lymphadenopathy or fever. In all cases, urgent review by the dentist is mandatory.

Acute necrotizing ulcerative gingivitis (ANUG) is a severe form of gingivitis which could be related to stress and needs antibiotic cover and urgent referral to the dentist.

Alveolar osteitis (dry socket)

Dry socket occurs between 2 and 5 days following dental extraction. The dull throbbing pain is due to the collection of necrotic clot and debris in the socket. The condition is diagnosed on the history and examination, which confirms the acutely tender extraction site.

Treatment consists of irrigation of the extraction site to remove the necrotic material and packing the socket with sterile gauze soaked in local anaesthetic, such as cophenylcaine, followed by urgent dental review [5].

Postdental extraction bleeding

Bleeding from the socket post-extraction within 48 h is due to reactionary haemorrhage due to opening up of the small divided blood vessels. Bleeding after 5 days is secondary haemorrhage due to infection that destroys the organizing blood clot.

General causes, such as hypertension and warfarin therapy, need to be addressed to control the bleeding.

Management is essentially reassurance, careful suction to clear the debris and clot in the socket, followed by packing with gauze soaked in lignocaine with adrenaline or cophenylcaine and pressure.

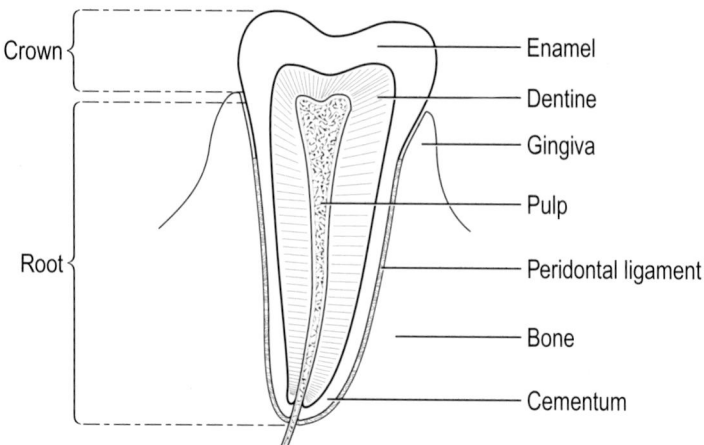

Fig. 17.1.1 The anatomy of the tooth. *(From an original drawing by Ian Miller RN.)*

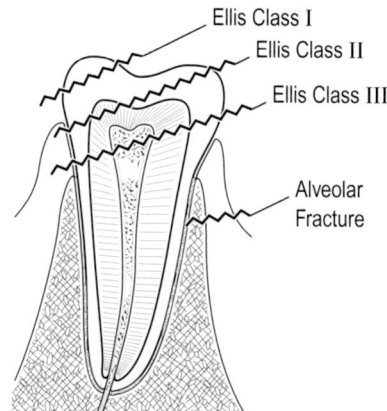

Fig. 17.1.2 Ellis classification. *(From an original drawing by Ian Miller RN.)*

Dilute aminocaproic acid (IV Amicar) 5 mL in 10 mL of normal saline to rinse the mouth. Use Amicar or tranexamic acid-soaked gauze to bite on, applying direct pressure for about 30 min and repeat as required to control the bleeding. Occasionally, the gingival flaps may need to be sutured under local anaesthetic.

Traumatic dental emergencies

Tooth avulsion is probably the most serious tooth injury. An avulsed tooth, if reimplanted in the socket within 30 min, has a 90% survival rate [6]. The mechanism of injury in such cases is usually either accidental sports-related facial injuries or assault.

Management

If the patient makes telephone contact with the emergency department, the patient is advised to locate the tooth because, even if the crown is broken, the root may be intact. The tooth should not be handled by the root to avoid damage to the periodontal ligament fibres; it is washed in running cold water and replaced in the socket. If this is not possible, place the tooth in the cheek or under the tongue and proceed immediately to the dentist. Do not scrub the tooth [7,8].

The best transportation medium for an avulsed tooth is saliva. Cold milk or iced salt water are suitable alternatives.

If the patient arrives in the emergency department with the tooth, clean it by holding it by the crown in cold running water; any foreign debris should be removed with forceps. The tooth should not be allowed to dry. Following irrigation, the tooth should be placed in the

socket as near the original position as possible and the patient referred to a dentist for stabilization with an archbar or orthodontic bands.

If the reimplanted tooth remains mobile after 2 weeks, it should be extracted. The complications of reimplantation are ankylosis and loss of viability.

The 2010 Dental Trauma Guide by the Danish Dental Association supported by the International Association of Dental Traumatology provides an interactive drop down menu on how to deal with every possible dental trauma [9].

Dentoalveolar trauma in children

Concussion and subluxation

Concussion is an injury to the tooth without displacement or mobility. Subluxation is when the tooth is mobile but not displaced.

Management

Periapical X-rays as baseline, soft diet for a week and local dentist follow up.

Intrusive luxation

Most common injury to upper primary incisors after a fall.

Management

If the crown is visible leave the tooth to re-erupt. If the whole tooth is intruded, extraction is required as it might affect the permanent dentition underneath.

Extrusive and lateral subluxation

If there is excessive mobility or displacement, extraction is recommended.

Avulsion

Avulsed primary teeth should not be replanted. Unless there is extensive soft-tissue damage, antibiotics are not required.

Dental fractures

The incidence of fractured teeth is reported to be 5 and 4.4 per 100 adults per year for all teeth and posterior teeth, respectively [10]. Based on the above statistics, it can be deduced that the likelihood of experiencing a fractured frontal/anterior tooth is about 1 in 20 in a given year in adults and 1 in 23 for posterior teeth.

Traumatic injuries to the teeth have been classified as follows [11]:

Class I: simple fracture of the enamel of the crown.
Class II: extensive fracture of the crown involving dentine.
Class III: extensive fracture of the crown involving dentine and dental pulp.
Class IV: extensive involvement and exposure of the entire pulp.
Class V: totally avulsed or luxated teeth.
Class VI: fracture of the root with or without loss of crown structure.
Class VII: displacement of tooth without fracture of crown or root.
Class VIII: fracture of the crown in its entirety (Fig. 17.1.2).

Management

Emergency management includes reassurance, adequate analgesia, replacement of an avulsed tooth in the socket and immediate referral to a dentist for further evaluation and appropriate management.

Specific treatment depends on the type of fracture [12]:

- Class I: treated by smoothing the enamel margins and applying topical fluoride to the fracture site.
- Class II A: calcium hydroxide dressing is applied as a bandage to provide a stable form of temporary restoration, which will be replaced by a more aesthetic restoration as soon as the vitality of the pulp is assured.
- Class III: if seen within 6 h of the accident, calcium hydroxide direct pulp capping. If more than 6 h but less than 24 h, pulpotomy. If more than 24 h since the accident, total pulpectomy.
- Class IV: conventional filling for permanent teeth and total pulpectomy for a primary tooth.
- Class V: managed as for an avulsed tooth.
- Class VI: if the pulp is necrotic, pulpectomy and root canal therapy.
- Class VII: if the tooth is intruded it should be extracted. If driven through the labial plate of bone, extraction and, if not, it should be left alone to re-erupt. If the tooth is extruded, slowly move it back to its original position using finger pressure. Primary teeth, if mobile after 2 weeks after the injury, should be extracted. Parents should be warned about possible damage to the developing permanent tooth.
- Class VIII: in a permanent tooth, pulpotomy or pulpectomy. Primary teeth with this amount of destruction should be extracted.
- When a tooth is missing following facial trauma, a thorough intraoral examination is followed by appropriate radiographs to avoid missing an intruded tooth. When full intrusion of a tooth is suspected, a facial computed tomography (CT) scan may aid definite diagnosis [13].

Temporomandibular dislocation

Temporomandibular dislocation can result from congenital weakness of ligaments, iatrogenic causes (traumatic extractions, prolonged dental procedures and direct laryngoscopy), trauma, drugs, epilepsy and even simple yawning. The dislocation may be unilateral but is more commonly bilateral. The condyle is most frequently dislocated anterior to the articular eminence.

The patient presents with an open bite and malocclusion. If unilateral, the mandible deviates to the unaffected side. The patient

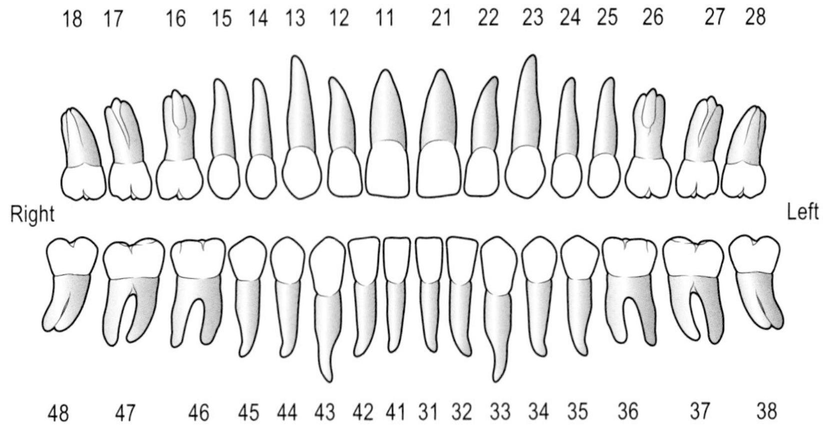

Fig. 17.1.3 Dental nomenclature. *(From the FDI World Dental Federation Two-Digit Notation. ISO 3950:2009: Dentistry – Designation system for teeth and areas of the oral cavity.)*

complains of severe pain in the ear and is unable to open or close the mouth fully. Management includes diagnosis and reduction. The patient is seated, with posterior head support, and the muscle spasm is overcome by using intravenous benzodiazepines, such as midazolam, and narcotic analgesia, such as fentanyl.

The mandible is held by the clinician by both hands, with the gloved thumbs intraorally just lateral to the lower molars. The mandibular condyle is then manipulated in a downward and backward direction below the articular eminence. In bilateral dislocation, it may be easier to reduce one side at a time using a lateral rocking motion.

Following the procedure, a post-reduction radiograph is taken to confirm enlocation. The patient is discharged with a supportive bandage to the mandible and a soft diet advised for the next few days. Follow up by the maxillofacial surgeon is essential, as temporomandibular dysfunction due to damage to the fibrous cartilage can lead to ongoing symptoms or recurrent dislocations.

Dental infection and abscess (odontogenic infection)

Dentofacial infections usually arise from necrotic pulps, periodontal pockets or pericoronitis.

The symptoms are pain and swelling of the adjacent gingival tissue with facial swelling and fever.

Examination reveals erythema and tender swelling of the gingiva and, in severe cases, frank pus with halitosis. The offending tooth is tender on percussion.

Gingival probing, X-rays and orthopontomogram (OPG) confirm the diagnosis.

Management
Periapical abscess requires root canal (endodontic) treatment and extraction in severe cases.

Periodontal abscess requires scaling and root planing (periodontal) treatment and extraction in severe cases.

Complications include spread of infection into the submental, submandibular, parapharyngeal spaces of the neck and Ludwig's angina (cellulitis of the floor of the mouth), which requires intravenous antibiotic therapy and drainage if a collection is diagnosed on the CT scan.

Dental nomenclature

The international numbering system of teeth should be strictly adhered to in any form of communication. The mouth is divided into four quadrants. The right maxillary as 1, left maxillary as 2, left mandibular as 3 and the right mandibular as 4 (Fig. 17.1.3).

There are five primary teeth and eight permanent teeth in each quadrant.

Controversies

- Dental services are generally not part of acute health service funding, therefore, low-income patients may have to wait for medical complications of poor dental hygiene before being able to access appropriate care.

- Oil of cloves originated from India and was traditionally used topically for relief of dental pain, such as dry socket prior to the availability of safe approved topical anaesthetic agents. However, it is highly toxic to human cells even at relatively low concentrations.
- 0.03% (v/v) and even small amounts can be life threatening if ingested.

References

[1] Sheller B, Williams BJ, Lombardi SSM. Diagnosis and treatment of dental caries related emergencies in a children's hospital. Am Acad Pediatr Dent 1997;19:470–5.

[2] Wilson S, Smith GA, Preisch J, Casamassimo PS. Non traumatic dental emergencies in a pediatric emergency department. Clin Pediatr 1997;36:333–7.

[3] Matthews RW, Peak JD, Skully C. The efficacy of management of acute dental pain. Br Dent J 1994;176:413–6.

[4] Ahl DR, Hidgeman JL, Snyder JD. Periodontal emergencies. Dent Clin N Am 1986;30:459–72.

[5] Laskin DM, Steinberg B. Diagnosis and treatment of common dental emergencies. Med Dent 1984;77:41–52.

[6] Gaedeve Norris MK. Emergency treatment for tooth avulsion. Nursing Springhouse International edn. 1992;92:33–35.

[7] Scheer B. Emergency treatment of avulsed incisor teeth. Br Med J 1990;301:4.

[8] Rice RT, Bulford OG Jr. Clinical notebook. Emergency treatment of injured teeth. J Emerg Nurs 1988;14:32–3.

[9] <www.dentaltraumaguide.org>.

[10] Bader JD, Martin JA, Shugars DA. Preliminary estimates of the incidence and consequences of tooth fracture. J Am Dent Assoc 1995;126:1650–4.

[11] Ellis RG, Davey KW. The classification and treatment of injuries to the teeth of children, 5th ed. Chicago: Yearbook Medical Publishers; 1970.

[12] Braham RL, Roberts MW, Morris ME. Management of dental trauma in children and adolescents. J Trauma 1977;17:857–65.

[13] Tung-Chain T, Yu-Ray C, Chien-Tzung C, Chia-Jung L. Full intrusion of a tooth after facial trauma. J Trauma 1977;2:357–9.

18.1 Ears, nose and throat emergencies

Sashi Kumar

ESSENTIALS

1 Removal of foreign bodies from the ear requires good lighting, a cooperative or fully restrained patient and a patient/gentle approach by the clinician.

2 Haematoma of the auricle requires urgent release by aseptic incision and immediate application of a firm mastoid bandage.

3 It is important to exclude septal haematoma in patients with a fractured nose. In general, X-rays are not warranted.

4 Patients presenting with odynophagia but no dysphagia following ingestion of a fish bone and negative physical examination and radiology, can be safely discharged for review within 48 h.

5 Sudden sensory neural hearing loss constitutes an ENT emergency, which requires urgent ENT consultation and audiometry.

THE EAR

Introduction

Emergency presentations for ear, nose and throat (ENT) problems are common and all emergency physicians need to be familiar with the basic skills required for assessment and management of these problems.

Foreign body

Foreign bodies in the ear are most common in children under the age of 5 and in mentally handicapped adults. Animate objects, such as insects in the ear, can affect all ages, especially adults who enjoy the outdoors, particularly at dusk.

Accidental foreign bodies, such as the end of a cotton bud or a matchstick, occur in people

obsessed with cleaning their ears with such objects.

Management

Two simple rules in managing foreign bodies in the ear are:

- Do not attempt to remove a foreign body that is not there! (Identify the foreign body prior to attempts at removal.)
- Unless the object is alive, there is no emergency to remove it if it can be done safely at a later time under better conditions.

Removal of a live foreign body

This is a true ENT emergency. The insect should be killed as a matter of urgency, as considerable damage is being done to the sensitive skin of the bony meatus and the tympanic membrane by the flapping wings and

appendages of the desperate insect trying to escape.

The movement of the insect also causes intense pain and tinnitus, thereby creating further anxiety and distress.

Any liquid used to kill the insect should be carefully chosen so as to avoid damage to the sensitive skin and tympanic membrane: strong corrosive agents, knockdown spray or alcohol should be avoided. The common agents of choice are lignocaine 2%, olive oil, water for injection or normal saline.

One of the preferred methods is to instil some water for injection from a 10 mL plastic ampoule and leave an examination light on the pinna. The insect swims up to surface towards the light and can be helped to safety by holding the tip of the ampoule [1].

Removal of a foreign body in a child or a mentally handicapped adult may be done in one of two ways. The patient is either cooperative and unrestrained or fully restrained. It is vital not to attempt any procedure with partial restraint, as any movement of the patient during the attempt could cause trauma to the ear canal and the tympanic membrane.

There are two techniques used to remove a foreign body. The dry method is by using a Jobson Horne probe for solid objects, such as beads, or alligator forceps for an insect or a cotton bud. The wet method is by syringing the ear canal with tepid water. The water should be close to body temperature to avoid a caloric effect, which produces nystagmus and vertigo.

The key to success is good lighting, preferably through a head lamp, a cooperative or fully restrained patient and a patient, gentle approach by the clinician, who knows when to stop if unsuccessful.

Impacted cerumen

Impacted hard cerumen or wax causes pain and hearing loss.

Sudden onset of hearing loss after a swim is classical of impacted ceruman as the wax swells up when in contact with water.

A 3–5-day course of Waxsol or Cerumol ear drops 3–5 drops three times a day followed by syringing of the ear canal with warm water should clear up the ear canal.

Trauma

Trauma to the ear canal requires the ear to be kept dry for about a week with antibiotic ear drops for 4–5 days in severe cases to avoid progressing into otitis externa.

Penetrating trauma can cause perforation of the eardrum and, occasionally, disruption of the ossicular chain. Dislocation of the footplate of the stapes following such an injury can cause permanent sensorineural hearing loss. Referral to an ENT specialist is essential in all cases of traumatic perforation with suspected ossicular chain disruption.

Blunt trauma

Boxing and other contact sports can lead to blunt trauma to the pinna. Accumulation of blood under the perichondrium, if not treated properly, may progress to cartilage necrosis and the end result is a 'cauliflower ear'.

A slap on the ear can also produce a ruptured tympanic membrane with or without ossicular chain disruption.

Assessment

Assessment of the injury includes a clinical assessment of the hearing loss. A ruptured eardrum without ossicular chain disruption does not usually cause a significant hearing loss. Any evidence of nystagmus or tinnitus suggests damage to the inner ear.

Management

A simple traumatic perforation of the eardrum is managed by simple analgesics and keeping the ear dry. On no account should any drops or water be allowed into the ear, as this may precipitate otitis media.

If ossicular chain disruption or inner ear trauma is suspected, an urgent ENT opinion is required to assess the need for urgent tympanotomy and repair.

Haematoma of the pinna requires urgent release of the accumulated blood by aseptic incision and drainage and the immediate application of a firm mastoid bandage, to prevent reaccumulation, and this should be left in place for up to a week. The patient should be placed on broad-spectrum antibiotics to prevent infection.

Infection

Otitis externa

Infection of the external ear is common and affects between 3 and 10% of the patient population [2]. It can be localized (furuncle) or diffuse. The symptoms are pain, itching and tenderness to palpation, followed by aural fullness, hearing loss and discharge. The common pathogens responsible are *Pseudomonas aeruginosa*, *Proteus* spp. and *Staphylococcus aureus*[3].

The diagnosis is usually self-evident, but the diagnostic signs of otitis externa are tragal tenderness or pain on pulling the pinna. This is a disease of the cartilaginous ear canal, with swelling and discharge causing occlusion of the meatus. It may be extremely painful to pass the ear speculum and often the tympanic membrane is not able to be visualized.

Management

The most important step in the treatment is thorough and atraumatic cleansing of the ear canal [4]. Tolerance and cooperation between the patient and the clinician is vital. Pope Otowick (Xomed) is very useful in the management of this condition. This is a semirigid foam wick that, when inserted into the ear canal, swells, absorbing moisture to increase the size of the ear canal. Topical otic drops, such as Sofradex (Roussel), are used three to four times a day and the patient is reviewed on a daily basis to change the wick and continue the ear toilet. Occasionally, oral antibiotics, such as ciprofloxacin or flucloxacillin, may be required [5], particularly if there is evidence of cellulitis. The patient is advised to keep the ear clear of any water. Strong analgesics are usually required.

Fungal otitis externa (otomycosis) tends to be not that painful and is treated with ear toilet as described and topical antifungal ear drops, such as Loco corten vioform.

Otitis media

Acute otitis media is a common infection and is due to blocking of the eustachian tube

(eustachian catarrh) and negative pressure in the middle ear cavity. Although viral in origin, secondary bacterial infection often supervenes. The most frequently isolated pathogens are *Streptococcus pneumoniae*, *Haemophilus influenzae* and *Moraxella catarrhalis* [6]. The symptoms are earache, fullness, hearing loss and fever, with ear discharge if the drum has perforated. The development of discharge usually marks an improvement in the pain and fever.

The clinical findings vary from a retracted dull eardrum to a congested bulging drum or a white eardrum with pus behind and a perforated tympanic membrane with discharge in the ear canal. A perforated eardrum without much pain is usually a sign of chronic otitis media.

Management

Treatment is almost always empiric and amoxicillin is a good first-line therapy. Cephalosporins and trimethoprim/sulpha are also used with considerable success. The newer macrolides, such as azithromycin and clarithromycin, are rational alternatives [6].

In otitis media with a perforated eardrum, the mainstay of treatment should be toilet by dry mopping followed by antibiotic drops, such as Sofradex. The ear should be kept dry and regular follow up arranged until the perforation has healed.

Labyrinthitis

Acute labyrinthitis usually has cochlear symptoms, such as hearing loss and tinnitus, which should be referred for audiometry and urgent ENT evaluation. If the symptoms are limited to vertigo and nystagmus, it is more likely to be due to acute vestibular neuronitis.

Management

The management of labyrinthitis includes bed rest, antiemetics, e.g. prochlorperazine, benzodiazepine, e.g. diazepam, and admission if severely debilitating. In the presence of hearing loss, a course of oral steroids or intratympanic dexamethasone may be started after discussions with the ENT surgeon.

Otitis media with effusion (glue ear)

This is most common in children in developed countries. The symptoms are fullness and hearing loss and, occasionally, pain. Management includes the diagnosis based on history and examination, which reveals a dull, retracted drum or fluid behind the drum without redness.

The most reliable sign of a glue ear is an immobile eardrum on Valsalva manoeuvre or pneumatic otoscopy. Repeated attacks of glue ear are an indication for the insertion of tympanostomy tubes.

Mastoiditis

Acute mastoiditis is a complication of acute or chronic otitis media. It is a rare condition in the developed world, although still quite prevalent in the developing world and the Aboriginal population of Australia. Otitis externa with a painful and tender postauricular lymph node is usually mistaken for acute mastoiditis due to the postauricular tenderness. Extension of infection can cause meningitis or temporal lobe abscess, with life-threatening complications if untreated.

Examination reveals infection in the middle ear cavity by way of an injected drum or a perforated drum with discharge. The cardinal sign of acute mastoiditis is tenderness at the base of the mastoid on digital pressure. The diagnosis is confirmed by computed tomography (CT) scan.

Management

Admission, intravenous antibiotics and surgical intervention, such as mastoidectomy, to remove the infected mastoid air cells and drain any abscess collection.

THE NOSE

Foreign body

A foreign body in the nose is common in preschool children and adults with mental retardation. The most common types of foreign body are beads, buttons and pieces of paper.

The diagnostic sign of a neglected nasal foreign body is a unilateral foul-smelling nasal discharge. The patient or the parent usually provides the history as to the type of foreign body and for how long present.

Management

The removal of the foreign body follows the same rules as for a foreign body in the ear. An additional method is to blow forcefully through the patient's mouth while occluding the unaffected nostril. This could be done by the parent with instruction.

The suggested method of removal is to pass the ring end of a Jobson–Horne probe

above and behind the foreign body and to roll it along the floor of the nose. The patient should be cooperative and unrestrained, or fully restrained. At the first sign of trauma or bleeding, removal should be organized under general anaesthesia as soon as practically possible.

Trauma

Fractured nose

This is a common presentation in the emergency department. The history is often quite clear and the findings include pain and tenderness over the nasal bones with or without crepitus and swelling at the bridge of the nose with or without epistaxis.

Careful examination will usually rule out CSF rhinorrhoea due to cribriform plate fracture and any external deformity. Active bleeding from the nostril should be controlled by direct pressure by pinching the nostril; if it does not settle it may require nasal packing.

Radiographs are not indicated for nasal bone fracture as this is a clinical diagnosis. It is often difficult to visualize the fracture line on the X-rays and radiographs do not help in the management. If associated facial fractures are suspected, X-ray facial views or CT scan should be taken.

Management
Acute intervention is required in the following circumstances:

- Continuing epistaxis should be managed along the lines described later.
- Obvious external deformity of the nose needs cosmetic correction, either by immediate reduction under local anaesthetic or by referral to an ENT surgeon for review and reduction in 7–10 days' time. A formal rhinoplasty may be required in severe cases. The acute management of a fractured nose is reassurance, analgesia and ice packs, followed by a review by the general practitioner or an ENT surgeon in 7–10 days. The patient is advised to avoid any form of contact sport for a week.
- CSF rhinorrhoea requires a CT scan and neurosurgical referral.
- A septal haematoma, which is clinically apparent as a widened and bulging septum, can become infected, causing a septal abscess that could result in the collapse of the septum causing a saddle nose. The diagnosis is made by visualizing the boggy

swelling on one or both sides of the septum and management requires admission, drainage under local or general anaesthesia, followed by nasal packing.

Sinusitis

Approximately 90% of upper respiratory infections have associated sinus cavity disease [7]. Viral rhinosinusitis is the most common cause and is associated with the common cold. Approximately 0.5–2% of these cases progress to bacterial sinusitis.

Clinical features

Symptoms of viral sinusitis are rhinorrhoea, nasal obstruction and sneezing and facial pressure with or without headache. With bacterial superinfection, a purulent or coloured nasal discharge and fever of 38°C or higher develop. Significant facial pain and maxillary toothache with no obvious dental cause also occurs. The common organisms involved are *Streptococcus pneumoniae* and *H. influenzae*. Patients with allergic sinusitis typically have sneezing and itching, with watery eyes, as a leading symptom.

Radiographs of the sinus are not very helpful unless they demonstrate a distinct air–fluid level, as this increases with the likelihood of bacterial sinusitis. CT can indicate the presence of sinus abnormalities and evidence of infection. A raised white cell count is neither sensitive nor specific in the diagnosis of bacterial sinusitis.

Management of viral rhinosinusitis is symptomatic and it is generally self-limiting. Bacterial sinusitis must be treated with antibiotics: amoxicillin, augmentin or keflex could be used as first-line drugs. Although of unproven value, an oral decongestant or antihistamine is commonly used. Complications of sinus disease include meningitis, orbital extension and brain abscess. Diagnosis is by CT scan and treatment is intravenous antibiotics with surgical intervention by an otolaryngologist.

Epistaxis

Nose bleeding is the most common ENT emergency: a Scottish study reported an incidence of 30/100 000 people [8] in which the cause could only be found in 15% [9]. The common identified causes are trauma, blood dyscrasias, anticoagulation therapy and, occasionally,

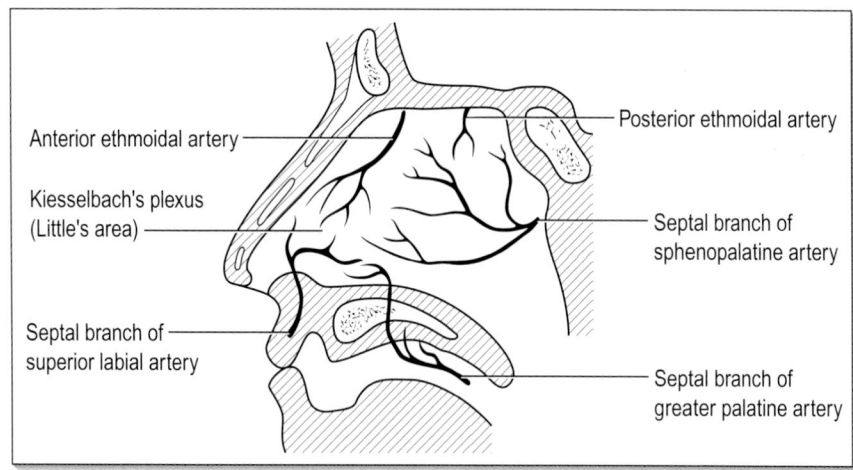

Fig. 18.1.1 Arterial supply to the nasal septum. *(From an original drawing by Ian Miller RN.)*

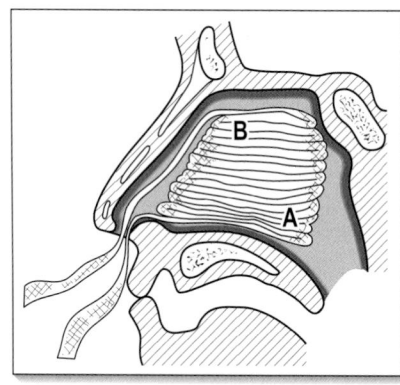

Fig. 18.1.2 Insertion of anterior nasal pack (begin at A and finish at B). *(From an original drawing by Ian Miller RN.)*

hereditary haemorrhagic telangiectasia [10]. Although hypertension has been traditionally labelled as a cause of epistaxis, studies have shown that blood pressure in these patients is no higher than in the control population [11,12].

The history is vital and all patients should be asked where the blood appeared first – anteriorly in the nose or in the back of the throat. Anterior epistaxis can usually be controlled in the emergency department and the patient safely discharged home without a nasal pack after cautery.

Management

The control of epistaxis due to a general cause, such as uncontrolled warfarin therapy or a bleeding disorder, is to reverse the cause. Local measures can still be used to stem the flow.

Idiopathic epistaxis, or that due to a local cause such as trauma, can be dealt with using local measures. The most common cause of anterior epistaxis is bleeding from Kiesselbach's plexus in the Little's area of the septum [13] (Fig. 18.1.1), which can easily be controlled by simple measures in the emergency department. Careful examination of a seated patient applying direct pressure to the bleeding vessel by pinching the anterior nares with the thumb and forefinger for up to 10 min will usually slow or cease the bleeding. At this point, it is essential to remove all the blood clots from the nasal cavity and the postnasal space using suction.

Following this, the application of cotton pledgets soaked in 5 or 10% cocaine or lignocaine with adrenaline or cophenylcaine (phenylephrine and lignocaine) will provide analgesia and vasoconstriction to the septum and the anterior part of the lateral wall.

Examination may reveal the bleeding vessel on the septum, which can be cauterized under direct vision using silver nitrate sticks. Following this, the patient is observed for a short time and can be discharged from the emergency department. The patient is advised not to pick, rub or blow the nose for 10 days and is advised to keep the cauterized area moist by applying chloromycetin eye ointment or Vaseline twice a day.

If the bleeding cannot be controlled by the above measures, or the bleeding point is posteriorly placed, the nasal cavity should be packed. There are several ways to pack the nose, the most traditional being to use ribbon gauze to fill the entire nasal cavity in layers (Fig. 18.1.2). A Foley urinary catheter can be used to control the posterior bleed, but it can be better controlled with a specifically designed epistaxis catheter, such as a Brighton's epistaxis catheter, which has a double balloon for anterior and posterior tamponade. A Merocel nasal pack (Xomed) can be used as a nasal tampon for anterior bleeds. Posterior bleeds require a Rapid Rhino which has inflatable anterior and posterior balloons with hydrocolloid fabric on the outside surface, that promotes clotting when soaked in sterile water for a few minutes prior to insertion to activate the ingredient. Almost all patients with nasal packing need admission and observation. When the above measures are unsuccessful, further invasive procedures, such as postnasal packing, examination under anaesthesia and septal surgery or arterial ligation may be required under general anaesthesia.

Summary
Patients with anterior nasal bleeds can usually be managed by chemical cautery with silver nitrate and then be discharged. Posterior bleeding or failure to control by simple measures may require nasal packing and admission for further invasive procedures.

THE THROAT

Foreign body

Coins are a common oesophageal foreign body in children. In adults, the foreign body is usually a fish, chicken or meat bone and, occasionally, objects such as partial dentures, safety pins, etc.

The common lodgement sites include the cricopharynx, the oesophagus at the level of the aortic arch and the gastro-oesophageal junction. Fish bones can lodge in the tonsil, the posterior third of the tongue or the vallecula prior to entering the oesophagus.

Management

Careful examination of the oropharynx initially, especially if the patient localizes the foreign body above the level of the hyoid and to one side. If the foreign body is found it should be removed under direct vision.

A foreign body at or below the cricopharynx requires general anaesthesia and endoscopy.

Lateral X-ray of the neck for soft tissues is useful in identifying and localizing radiopaque foreign bodies, such as coins and bones, including large fish bones.

Patients presenting with odynophagia but no dysphagia following the ingestion of a fish bone and a negative physical examination, can be discharged safely for review in 48 h. Symptoms of increasing odynophagia, fever, haematemesis or dysphagia warrant admission for endoscopy. Patients with a confirmed foreign body should be admitted for endoscopy and removal.

ENT surgeons use a rigid scope for visualizing and removal of foreign bodies at the cricopharynx and the proximal one-third of the oesophagus and gastroenterologists use a flexible scope for distal oesophageal foreign bodies which can be removed or more commonly pushed distally into the stomach.

A food bolus not containing bone causing obstruction should have a trial of IV glucagon 1 mg, IV buscopan 20–40 mg and sips of a fizzy drink before arranging for an endoscopy, as one of these may dislodge the obstruction, thereby avoiding an urgent endoscopy. Recurrent food bolus obstructions require an endoscopy to rule out stricture or malignancy.

Button batteries

A button battery lodged in the oesophagus can cause liquefaction necrosis and perforation so urgent endoscopy and removal is recommended [14].

If the battery is lodged past the oesophagus in the stomach most, if not all, will pass in the next 48–72 h and the patient can be safely discharged following reassurance [15].

Inhaled foreign body

History of choking, coughing or gagging while eating.

Immediate treatment is firm back blows to dislodge the foreign body. Examination may reveal unilateral wheeze. Inspiratory and expiratory chest X-ray may reveal the foreign body or air trapping distal to it.

Urgent referral for a bronchoscopy and removal of the object, especially if the foreign body is organic material, such as nuts, which can cause excessive tissue reaction and pneumonitis if there is excessive delay.

Infection

Tonsillitis

Patients with acute tonsillitis present to the general practitioner and, occasionally, to the emergency department. The emergency department patients usually have severe symptoms or are not responding to oral antibiotics. They are often dehydrated, toxic, with a high temperature and unable to take adequate oral fluids. Treatment includes intravenous penicillin in high doses (e.g. 2 g 4-hourly), intravenous fluids, one off dose of 8 mg of intravenous dexamethasone and adequate analgesia.

Infectious mononucleosis (glandular fever)

The symptoms are similar to severe tonsillitis with odynophagia, fever and a hot potato voice. The tonsils are quite swollen but have a smooth diffuse swelling with not much exudate on the fossa. The cervical lymph nodes are enlarged and tender and there may also be axillary and inguinal lymphadenopathy with or without hepatosplenomegaly.

The diagnosis is made by abnormal lymphocytes in the blood film and monospot test.

Treatment is symptomatic. Amoxicillin should not be used as it produces a rash.

Quinsy

Peritonsillar abscess or quinsy is a condition which occurs mostly in young adults in which the infection in the tonsil has breached the capsule and caused cellulitis in the adjacent soft palate (peritonsillitis) and, eventually, a collection of pus (quinsy).

Examination reveals a congested tonsil being pushed medially and downwards by a diffuse swelling of the soft palate. The opposite tonsil may look injected. There are often unilateral or bilateral enlarged and tender jugulodigastric lymph nodes in the neck. The patient is usually febrile, toxic and dehydrated. There is marked trismus due to masseteric spasm and referred otalgia.

Management includes admission to hospital for intravenous fluids, penicillin or cephalosporin and adequate analgesia. Aspiration of the pus using a large-bore needle or incision and drainage of the quinsy can be done in the emergency department under local anaesthesia in a conscious patient sitting up. Sometimes this needs general anaesthesia. Intubation of such patients should be performed by a skilled anaesthetist preferably by awake fibreoptic technique and every effort must be made to avoid rupturing the abscess to avoid aspiration of pus.

A second attack of quinsy usually requires tonsillectomy.

Retropharyngeal abscess

This is predominantly a disease of young children, as the retropharyngeal lymph nodes atrophy after the age of 5. In older patients, it could be secondary to trauma or lodgement of a foreign body, such as a fish bone. Diagnosis is made on symptoms of fever, swelling of the neck due to cervical lymphadenopathy and, especially in young children, stridor. Clinical suspicion leads to imaging procedures, such as CT, which is diagnostic.

Management includes admission to hospital, intravenous antibiotics and urgent ENT consultation. Treatment is incision and drainage of the abscess under general anaesthesia.

Epiglottitis

Childhood epiglottitis is rare these days due to a highly successive immunization programme against *Haemophilus influenzae*. Adults with epiglottitis are still occasionally seen in emergency departments. The classical symptoms are acutely painful throat, drooling, odynophagia and increased pain to speech with enlarged tender bilateral cervical lymph nodes.

A quick bedside test is to ask the patient to poke his or her tongue out and wiggle it from side to side as this will increase the pain substantially.

Management is mainly intravenous antibiotics and analgesia. If the patient is showing signs of imminent upper airway obstruction, an attempt should be made to intubate by the most skilled emergency doctor available with the surgical airway kit readily available in case of failure.

All other patients should be taken to the operating theatre for a gaseous induction by a skilled anaesthetist with an ENT surgeon standing by for immediate surgical airway if unable to intubate.

Post-tonsillectomy bleed

Haemorrhage from the tonsillar fossa that occurs 24 h after tonsillectomy is termed 'secondary haemorrhage'. This differs from primary, which happens during surgery, and reactionary haemorrhage, which occurs within 24 h of surgery while the patient is still in the hospital. The cause of secondary haemorrhage is usually infection and this occurs classically 10 days postoperatively. This incidence is about 1% and is usually not very severe. The management is intravenous antibiotics, usually penicillin. The patient should be admitted and bloods taken for estimation of haemoglobin and cross-matching. Application of a swab soaked in 1 in 1000 adrenaline (epinephrine) to the tonsillar fossa after removal of the clot may help to stop the bleeding. Rarely, the patient may need to have a general anaesthetic to cauterize/ligate the bleeder [16].

Controversies

- Timing of nasal fracture reduction. This may be performed either immediately or after 7–10 days.
- The method used for control of epistaxis. There is no clear advantage in using one method over another.

References

[1] Kumar S. An interesting method of removal of live foreign body from the ear. Emerg Med 1998;10:278.

[2] Bojrab DI, Bruderly T, Razzak YA. Otitis externa. Otolaryngol Clin N Am 1996;29:761–82.

[3] Briggs RJ. Otitis externa: presentation and management. Aust Fam Phys 1995;24:1859–64.

[4] Ali Raza S, Denholm SW, Wong JCH. An audit of the management of acute otitis externa in an ENT casualty clinic. J Laryngol Otol 1995;109:130–3.

[5] Mirza N. Otitis externa – management in the primary care office. Postgrad Med 1996;99:153–8.

[6] Block SL. Causative pathogens, antibiotic resistance and therapeutic considerations in acute otitis media. Paediatr Infect Dis J 1997;16:449–56.

[7] Bukata R. Sinusitis, a ubiquitous, yet enigmatic disease. Emerg Med Acute Care Essays 1997;21:1–4.

[8] Kotecha B, Fowler S, Harkness P, et al. Management of epistaxis: a national survey. Ann Roy Coll Surg Engl 1996;78:444–6.

[9] Small M, Maran AGD. Epistaxis and arterial ligation. J Laryngol Otol 1984;98:281–4.

[10] Juselius H. Epistaxis. J Laryngol Otol 1974;88:317–27.

[11] Shaheen OH. Studies of nasal vasculature and problems of arterial ligation for epistaxis. Ann Roy Coll Surg Engl 1970;47:30–44.

[12] Weiss NS. The relation of high blood pressure to headache and epistaxis and selected other symptoms. N Engl J Med 1972;287:631–3.

[13] Darry KW, Barlow F, Deleyiannis WB, Pinczower EF. Effectiveness of surgical management of epistaxis at a tertiary care center. Laryngoscope 1997;107:21–4.

[14] Gordon AC, Gough MH. Oesophageal perforation after button battery ingestion. Ann Roy Coll Surg Engl 1993;75:362–4.

[15] Kumar S. Management of foreign bodies in the ear, nose and throat. Emerg Med 2004;16:17–20.

[16] Evans JNG, editor. Scott Brown's otolaryngology, 5th ed. London: Butterworth; 1987:96.

19.1 Emergency delivery and complications

Stephen Priestley

ESSENTIALS

1 Perform a rapid assessment of a pregnant patient arriving in labour at the emergency department to decide the most appropriate site for management.

2 Emergency department staff must be prepared to provide newborn resuscitation following an emergency delivery. Preparedness for newborn resuscitation requires preparation of a suitable, warmed area, special equipment and trained personnel and a structured approach to assessment and intervention.

3 Equipment, drugs and protocols must be placed within emergency departments so that unexpected deliveries can be managed safely.

4 Be prepared to manage sudden complications of delivery, such as shoulder dystocia, breech delivery or postpartum haemorrhage.

5 Establish and maintain lines of communication with regional obstetric services so that decisions regarding management of labour and transfer of mothers and babies are optimum.

Introduction

Occasionally, a doctor working in an emergency department (ED) is faced with caring for a patient in labour and is required to manage a spontaneous vaginal delivery. This situation is generally accompanied by much anxiety on the part of the ED medical and nursing staff, but it is important that a calm, systematic approach is taken to minimize the risk of an adverse fetal or maternal outcome.

This chapter describes the management of a normal delivery in the ED and provides a brief outline of the recognition and management of abnormal deliveries and selected peripartum complications.

Setting

There are a number of settings when childbirth may need to occur in an ED. Pregnant patients at different gestational ages may present to the ED in varying stages of labour. Immediate management will depend on the availability of obstetric services, the gestational age and on both the stage of labour and its anticipated speed of progression.

Safe transfer to a delivery suite when there is adequate time is always preferable to delivery in the ED. If there is no delivery suite available, or a patient arrives with full cervical dilatation and the fetal presenting part is on the perineal verge and there is no time for transfer to an appropriate facility, then arrangements need to be made rapidly to perform the delivery in the ED. In these situations, the emergency physician should prepare for two patients, both potentially needing care.

Precipitate labour

Patients who have precipitate labour – an extremely rapid labour lasting less than 3 hours from onset of contractions to delivery, more common in the multiparous – may have to stop in the ED even when *en route* to the delivery suite, or another hospital, because of the rapidity of the labour.

Concealed or unrecognized pregnancy

The diagnosis of a concealed or unrecognized pregnancy may also be made in the ED. Concealed pregnancies occur most commonly in teenage girls who do not tell anyone that they are pregnant and receive no antenatal care. Unrecognized pregnancy occurs most commonly in obese females who may present to the ED complaining of abdominal pain or a vaginal discharge and are found to be pregnant and/or in labour. Women with intellectual impairment or mental illness are another group who may present with an unrecognized pregnancy.

'Born before arrival'

The term 'precipitous birth' or 'born before arrival' (BBA) is commonly associated with precipitate labour and refers to women who deliver their baby prior to arrival at a hospital, usually without the assistance of a trained person. On arrival in the ED, both the mother and baby require assessment and may need resuscitation and completion of the third stage of labour. The term precipitous birth is also commonly used to describe deliveries that occur in the emergency department or areas outside of a labour and delivery suite.

The incidence of BBA is low but depends on the population studied. In Australia, the incidence of precipitate labour is approximately 1–2% in spontaneous non-augmented labours.

History

Assessment of the patient in labour in the ED includes obtaining information regarding gestational age, antenatal care, progression of the pregnancy, past obstetric and a medical history. Always enquire if the patient has a copy of her antenatal care record with her. Take a careful history regarding the onset and timing of contractions and the presence and nature of fetal movements, in addition to a history of vaginal bleeding or discharge, which may represent the rupture of membranes.

Delivery in a hospital where there is no delivery suite should include immediate contact by telephone with the nearest or most appropriate obstetric unit to obtain advice and to organize transfer of the mother and newborn.

Gestational age

The gestational age may be determined from the last normal menstrual period (LNMP) if this is known. Naegle's rule is the most common method of pregnancy dating. The estimated date of delivery (EDD) is calculated by counting back three months from the last menstrual period and adding seven days. As an example, if the last menstrual period is December 20, then the EDD will be September 27. This method assumes the patient has a 28-day menstrual cycle with fertilization occurring on day 14. Inaccuracy occurs because many women do not have regular 28-day cycles, or do not conceive on day 14 and many others are not certain of the date of their last period.

Antenatal ultrasound

Antenatal ultrasound is useful in gauging the estimated date of confinement (EDC) where dates are uncertain, remembering that scans performed later in the pregnancy are less accurate in dating the gestational age of the baby than those performed early. Additionally, a rough estimation of the gestational age of the baby can be made by abdominal examination; between 20 and 35 weeks there is correlation between gestational age and the height of the uterine fundus measured in centimetres from the pubic symphysis.

Past obstetric history

The past obstetric history should include the duration and description of previous labours, the types of deliveries and the size of previous babies, in addition to a history of a previous caesarean section, the use of forceps or vacuum extraction, a neonatal death and history of abnormal presentation, shoulder dystocia, prolonged delivery of the placenta or a postpartum haemorrhage.

Maternal medical conditions

Maternal conditions, such as cardiac and respiratory disease, diabetes, bleeding diathesis, hepatitis B and herpes simplex, should be documented. Record all drugs whether prescribed, over-the-counter or illicit that the patient is taking. The presence of any bleeding or other complications during the pregnancy should also be noted. Obtain the results of antenatal investigations, including a full blood count, blood group, hepatitis-B status, HIV and syphilis serology.

Examination

General examination

A general physical and obstetric examination to confirm the progression of labour, the number of babies and the presence or absence of any complications related to the pregnancy and labour is made. In hospitals where there is a delivery suite, a member of that unit (usually a midwife) is called to attend the ED either to assist with immediate transfer to the delivery suite if possible, or with the assessment and conduct of the labour within the ED. Occasionally, a member of the ED staff will hold a midwife certificate and this staff member should be tasked to assist with labour and delivery.

The general examination includes particular emphasis on vital signs and the abdominal and pelvic examination. Examine the breast, nipples, heart and chest and perform a urinalysis looking for evidence of infection, glucose or proteinuria, which may be associated with pre-eclampsia (see Chapter 19.7).

Abdominal examination

Perform an abdominal examination to ascertain the height of the fundus, the lie and presentation of the fetus and to make an assessment of the engagement of the presenting part. The presence of scars and extrauterine masses should be noted. Assess the frequency, regularity, duration and intensity of uterine contractions.

Fetal heart rate

Count the fetal heart for 1 minute using an ordinary stethoscope, Pinard or a Doppler stethoscope, which should normally be between 110 and 160 beats/min. Count the fetal heart for at least 30 seconds following a contraction. If bradycardia is detected, give the mother oxygen and position her in the left lateral position to ensure that uterine blood flow and fetal oxygenation is optimized.

If post-contraction bradycardias persist despite these measures give an intravenous fluid bolus and seek specialist obstetric advice. Note any vaginal bleeding or discharge and record the amount, remembering haemorrhage may also be concealed. Assess the colour and character of any amniotic fluid, looking for evidence of meconium staining.

Vaginal examination

Perform an aseptic vaginal examination with the patient in the dorsal lithotomy position to assess the effacement, consistency and dilatation of the cervix, the nature and position of the presenting part (i.e. vertex or breech) and to exclude a cord prolapse. If unsure of the nature of the presenting part, a portable ultrasound can aid in diagnosis.

The exception to performing a vaginal examination is the gravid patient with active vaginal bleeding who should be evaluated with an ultrasound to exclude placenta praevia, *before* performing any pelvic examination.

If the membranes are intact, there is no indication to rupture them if the labour is progressing satisfactorily, as there is an increased risk of cord prolapse when the presenting part is not engaged in the pelvis. After the vaginal examination, apply a sterile perineal pad and allow the mother to assume whichever position gives her the most comfort, while avoiding a totally supine position as this has the potential for inferior vena cava (IVC) compression by the gravid uterus.

Transferring the patient

After this assessment, the decision whether to transfer the patient to a delivery suite either within the hospital, or at a distant hospital, must be made. Cervical dilatation greater than 6 cm in a multiparous patient and 7–8 cm in the primiparous makes transfer to a distant hospital a hazardous process, because of the risk of rapid progression to full cervical dilatation and imminent delivery of the baby.

The availability and type of transport and personnel and the distance to be travelled must be carefully considered. Consult with the obstetric unit regarding the safety of transfer and make arrangements for reception of the patient.

Management

Preparation for delivery

Ongoing assessment of maternal temperature, blood pressure, heart rate and contractions should be performed and recorded. Fetal heart rate should be counted every 15–30 minutes up to full cervical dilatation and every 5 minutes thereafter. The fetal heart rate is best measured with a Doppler device, commencing towards the end of a contraction and continuing for at least 30 seconds after the contraction has finished.

Unless there is a clear indication for an intravenous line, such as a history of postpartum haemorrhage or antepartum haemorrhage, bleeding tendency, evidence of pre-eclampsia or history of a previous caesarean section, then placement for the normal delivery is unnecessary. Perform simple venepuncture for a haemoglobin and blood group and put some blood aside for cross-matching.

Table 19.1.1 Equipment and drugs required for emergency delivery	
Equipment	*Drugs*
Three clamps – straight or curved (e.g. Pean)	Adrenaline 1:10 000
Episiotomy scissors	Oxytocin 10 units
Scissors	Ergometrine 250 µg
Suture repair set	Vitamin K 1 mg
Absorbable suture material	Lignocaine 1%
Sterile drapes	Naloxone 400 µg/1 mL
Huck towels	Glucose 10%
Sterile gloves	
Soap solution	
Sterile bowls	

Neonatal resuscitation equipment including appropriately-sized suction catheters, oropharyngeal airways, masks, self-inflating bag (approximately 240 mL), endotracheal tubes, stylets, laryngoscopes, end-tidal CO_2 detector device, neonatal oxygen saturation probe

Umbilical vein catheters, overhead warmer, clock with timer in seconds, warmed towels, and feeding tubes for gastric decompression

Equipment and drugs

Obtain a delivery pack, sterile surgical instruments and oxytocic drugs and place close by (Table 19.1.1). Resuscitation equipment and drugs should be available. Assemble personnel with clear task delegation, remembering that reassurance and emotional support for the mother and the mother's partner is crucial during the entire labour. A specific member of staff may be delegated to provide this.

If a midwife or doctor experienced in delivery is available then they should assume control of the procedure and continue the assessment of the progression of labour and conduct the delivery of both the baby and the placenta. A doctor or nurse with some experience in neonatal or paediatric resuscitation should perform a rapid assessment of the newborn immediately after the delivery of the baby, to ascertain the need for resuscitation.

Conduct of labour

Labour is divided into three stages: the first stage is from the onset of regular contractions to full (10 cm) dilatation of the cervix. The second stage is from full dilatation of the cervix to delivery of the baby and the third stage is from the birth of the baby until delivery of the placenta. A full description of the detailed management of the three stages of labour is beyond the scope of this chapter, but a brief summary of the management of a normal vertex delivery is described.

First stage

Examine the patient abdominally and vaginally as necessary to follow the progress of the labour. As mentioned earlier, perform measurement and recording of maternal vital signs and fetal heart rate. Gently wash the perineum with a non-irritating soap solution, such as 0.1% chlorhexidine, particularly when operative vaginal delivery by forceps or vacuum extraction is anticipated. Shaving, urinary catheterization or enema administration are not required.

The average duration of the first stage of labour in primiparous patients is 14 hours and, in subsequent pregnancies, is 6–8 hours.

Analgesia

Analgesics are helpful for the patient with significant discomfort and are not injurious to the fetus. The timing and dose of analgesia must be decided with due regard to the stage and rate of progression of labour, in addition to the mother's wishes and birth plan.

Inhaled nitrous oxide is simply delivered, acts quickly, is rapidly eliminated and does not affect the fetus. It is usually provided initially in a dose of 50% N_2O mixed with 50% oxygen but the N_2O dose can be increased to 70% maximum by delivery systems available in many emergency departments.

Opiate analgesia is also commonly used, though is generally not recommended within 4 hours of predicted delivery, meaning that it is unlikely to be used in a precipitous delivery in the emergency department. Morphine is preferred to pethidine as the active metabolite of IM pethidine has a longer half-life in the newborn, compared to IM morphine. Major opiate side effects include maternal drowsiness, nausea and vomiting. While there is no clear evidence of major adverse effects at birth, the newborn may have respiratory depression and drowsiness which may interfere with breastfeeding [1].

Second stage

Spontaneous delivery of the fetus presenting by vertex is divided into three phases: delivery of the head, delivery of the shoulders and delivery of the body and legs. The second stage of labour begins when the cervix is fully dilated and delivery will occur when the presenting part reaches the pelvic floor.

The normal duration of this stage in the absence of regional anaesthesia ranges from 20 to 60 minutes in the primiparous, down to 10–30 minutes in the multiparous patient. Prolongation of the second stage is defined as 2 hours or more in the primiparous patient and 1 hour or more in the multiparous patient. Preparations for delivery including cleansing are made as described earlier. Drape the patient in such a manner that there is a clear view of the perineum.

Maternal position

Either a dorsal lithotomy or lateral Sims' position may be used for delivery. The dorsal lithotomy position is recommended for inexperienced operators, as it is easier to visualize and manually control the delivery process, or perform an episiotomy. In the dorsal lithotomy position, the mother should be tilted over to the left side using a pillow or soft wedge, to avoid compression of the inferior vena cava by the gravid uterus and possible maternal hypotension and fetal hypoxia.

Episiotomy

When the presenting part distends the perineum, delivery is imminent. Consider an episiotomy at this time, but this should not be routine. Episiotomy refers to a surgical incision of the female perineum performed by the accoucheur at the time of parturition. The primary reason to perform an episiotomy is to prevent a larger spontaneous, irregular laceration of the perineum, particularly one that extends into the rectum. It is performed with scissors when the perineum is stretched and distended, just prior to crowning of the fetal head, following infiltration of a posterior area of the peritoneum with 5–10 mL of 1% lignocaine (lidocaine) between contractions.

Commonly, a mediolateral perineal incision is made beginning at the posterior fourchette and extended towards the ischiorectal fossa. A midline episiotomy is no longer recommended due to an increased risk of tears extending through to the rectum. The patient should be encouraged to bear down during contractions and to rest in between.

Delivery of the head

Delivery of the head must be controlled by the accoucheur so that the head extends slowly after crowning and does not 'pop out' of the vagina. Placing the palm of one hand over the head to control its extension most easily achieves this. At this point, the patient should cease actively pushing and may need to be instructed to pant or breathe through her nose, in order to overcome a desire to push. The accoucheur's second hand covered with a sterile gauze pad or towel may be used gently to lift the baby's chin, which can be felt in the space between the anus and the coccyx.

As the occiput descends under the symphysis pubis, extension of the head occurs and progressively the forehead, nose, mouth and finally chin emerge. Suctioning of the nasopharynx and oropharynx prior to birth of the shoulders and trunk should not be done routinely even in the presence of meconium-stained liquor [2,3].

In 25–30% of patients, the umbilical cord is looped around the neck (nuchal cord), which should be checked for. Usually, it is only loosely looped and can be drawn over the head. If this is unsuccessful, another method is to bring the cord caudally over the shoulders and deliver the baby through the cord and then unwind it after delivery. When these manoeuvres are unsuccessful, delivery of the baby without reduction of the cord may be possible (somersault manoeuvre). If none of the techniques seem feasible and the cord is too tight to be reduced, the cord is divided by placing two clamps on the cord 2–3 cm apart and cutting the cord in between them. Release of additional loops is now straightforward by unwinding the clamped ends around the neck.

The baby's head, having been delivered face down in the most common occipito-anterior position, is allowed to 'restitute' (or correct) to one or the other lateral position.

Restitution and delivery of the shoulders

Once the head has restituted, the shoulders will lie in an antero-posterior plane within the pelvis and delivery of the shoulders is now effected taking great care not to allow the perineum to tear. Usually, the anterior shoulder slips under the symphysis pubis with the next contraction by exerting gentle downward and backward traction on the head to facilitate this. Do not use excessive force as this may result in a brachial plexus injury.

On delivery of the anterior shoulder, lifting the baby up will deliver the posterior shoulder followed by the body and lower limbs. Grasp the baby firmly with one hand, securing the infant behind the neck and the other encircling both ankles and place on the mother's abdomen. The baby is slippery as a result of being covered with vernix and should never be held with one hand alone. Dry the baby and wrap in a warm blanket to minimize heat loss and record the time of birth.

Clamping the cord

There is no need to cut the cord immediately if the baby is breathing spontaneously and is close to term. There is benefit in delaying cord clamping in preterm and possibly term infants, as more blood is transferred from the placenta to the infant when clamping is delayed [4]. Perform an assessment of the baby with Apgar scoring to determine the need for resuscitation.

If the baby is preterm or requires resuscitation, quickly clamp the cord following delivery and transfer the baby for further assessment and resuscitation to a resuscitation trolley that has a radiant heat source. Apply an umbilical clamp 1–2 cm from the baby's abdomen to cut the umbilical cord and trim the cord approximately 0.5 cm above the plastic clamp.

Apgar score

If circumstances permit, the Apgar score should be calculated. This score allows easy communication of a baby's status between providers and indicates a basic prognosis for the newborn. It is obtained at 1 minute and 5 minutes after birth, with a score from 0 to 10.

The following acronym approach can be used to remember the five categories, with each scored on a scale from 0 to 2:

A: **A**ppearance (0: pale or blue; 1: pink body, blue extremities; 2: pink body and extremities)
P: **P**ulse (0: absent; 1: less than 100 beats/min; 2: more than 100 beats/min)
G: **G**rimace (0: absent; 1: grimace or notable facial movement; 2: cough, sneezes, or pulls away)
A: **A**ctivity (0: absent; 1: some flexion of extremities; 2: active and spontaneous movements of limbs)
R: **R**espiration (0: absent; 1: slow and irregular; 2: good breathing with crying).

The Apgar score can be calculated after the delivery and resuscitation is complete [5].

Use of oxytocics
Following the birth of the baby, palpate the woman's abdomen to exclude the possibility of a second fetus when an antenatal ultrasound result is unavailable and administer an oxytocic agent if none is present. The most common is oxytocin at a dose of 10 units given intramuscularly, or 5 units intravenously as a slow bolus. An alternative is ergometrine in a dose of 250 μg intramuscularly, or slowly intravenously but, as this agent is associated with nausea, vomiting and hypertension, it is unsuitable for use in pre-eclampsia, eclampsia or hypertension.

Third stage
After administration of the oxytocic agent, look for signs of separation of the placenta from the uterine wall. Three classic signs of placental separation are: (1) lengthening of the umbilical cord; (2) a gush of blood from the vagina signifying separation of the placenta from the uterine wall; and (3) change in the shape of the uterine fundus from discoid to globular, with elevation of the fundal height.

Following separation, and once the uterus is firmly contracted, apply traction on the cord in a backward and downward direction with one hand, while the other is placed suprapubically to support the uterus. Cease traction if the cord feels as though it is tearing.

Placental inspection
As the placenta appears at the introitus, traction is then applied in an upward direction and the placenta is grasped and gently rotated to ensure that the membranes are delivered without tearing. Inspect the placenta and membranes to look for any missing segments or cotyledons, or evidence of a missing succenturiate 'accessory' lobe, which may prevent the uterus from contracting properly if they remain within the uterus.

Uterine tone
Rub over the uterus to facilitate contraction and expulsion of clots. A common cause of postpartum haemorrhage is incomplete uterine contraction as a result of clots or tissue remaining within the cavity, which may be expelled by massaging the fundus or by manual removal under anaesthesia. Further oxytocics may be necessary.

Bleeding may also occur from other sites, so always perform a careful examination of the cervix, vagina, episiotomy wound and perineum following delivery. Full examination of the cervix for ongoing bleeding will require anaesthesia. The episiotomy wound and any other lacerations may be repaired with a synthetic absorbable suture.

Observations
Observations taken following the birth of the baby should include:

- maternal – temperature, pulse, blood pressure, uterine tone, lochia and fundal height
- examination of placenta and membranes – assessment of their condition and structure, cord vessels and completeness
- maternal emotional/psychological condition in response to labour and birth
- successful bladder emptying.

Newborn care
Keep the baby warm and dry and record the baby's vital signs, Apgar scores and weight. If vitamin K is available, administer it to the baby as a deep intramuscular 1 mg injection.

Disposition
Disposition of mother and baby to an obstetric unit either within the hospital or at a distant hospital should then be made once both are stable. The important information that should be provided includes the time of birth, drugs given to either mother or baby and the Apgar scores of the baby. Include the results of any blood tests and a copy of the observations. If either mother or baby is unstable, then early consultation with the appropriate referral service is mandatory regarding the optimum timing and nature of the transfer.

Complications of delivery

Breech delivery
Breech presentation occurs in 3–4% of all deliveries, reducing in incidence with advancing gestation. It is associated with a morbidity rate three to four times greater than that of a normal cephalic delivery. Breech presentation is more common with prematurity, as the final natural rotation in the pelvis may not have occurred, and is associated with a greater incidence of fetal distress and umbilical cord prolapse. The most feared complication is head entrapment, which can lead to fetal asphyxiation and death.

In the normal cephalic presentation, the head maximally dilates the birth canal, allowing the rest of the body to descend unobstructed. However, with a breech presentation, the head emerges last and can become entrapped by incomplete cervical dilatation [6,7]. Delivery of a breech presentation is often performed by caesarian section when available [7,8].

Circumstances, such as precipitous delivery, lack of prenatal care, prematurity and the mother's preference for vaginal delivery, can place an emergency medicine physician in the situation of managing a breech delivery. The following is relevant to the emergency department when vaginal delivery is imminent without obstetric backup or if the physician is concerned about fetal demise.

Management of breech delivery
Immediate obstetric expertise should be requested urgently, while preparations are made for neonatal resuscitation. It is critical for the emergency physician to avoid manipulating the fetus, but rather to allow the delivery to occur spontaneously as far as possible.

Perform an episiotomy as the fetal anus is climbing the perineum. Allow maternal effort to deliver the baby spontaneously to the umbilicus, delivering the legs with knee flexion. Do not apply traction to the fetus, as this may cause fetal head extension which leads to entrapment of the head and greatly increases the risk of asphyxiation [9]. A loop of umbilical cord may be pulled down and allowed to hang. The mother is encouraged to bear down until the trunk becomes visible up to the scapula.

Then rotate the trunk until the anterior shoulder delivers. Subsequent rotation of the trunk in the opposite direction results in delivery of the posterior shoulder.

Once the shoulders are delivered an assistant should provide downward pressure in the suprapubic area to keep the fetal head flexed while the accoucheur delivers the head either with the application of forceps, or by placing the left hand into the vagina and pressing on the maxilla to cause further neck flexion while the other hand grasps a shoulder and applies firm traction in the line of the baby's hips, taking care not to extend the head. The combined neck flexion, traction on the fetus toward the hip/pelvis and the suprapubic pressure on the mother/uterus allows for delivery of the head of a breech infant (Mauriceau Smellie Veit manoeuvre).

Shoulder dystocia

Shoulder dystocia occurs when the anterior shoulder of the baby cannot be delivered under the pubic symphysis. It is one of the more frightening complications of vaginal delivery and, while some at-risk patients may be identified, it is frequently unexpected. Estimates of the incidence is between 0.2 and 3.0% depending on the exact definition used [9]. Important steps in management are recognizing the at-risk patient, calling for assistance early and understanding the manoeuvres to deliver the fetus. At-risk patients may have a large baby, gestational diabetes or have had a previous shoulder dystocia. Notably, the most relevant risk factor for an emergency physician performing emergency delivery is in fact a precipitous delivery – which is frequently the antecedent to the mother delivering in the emergency department in the first place [9]. However, in many cases, there are no predisposing factors.

Recognizing shoulder dystocia

As it is not possible to predict which deliveries will be complicated by shoulder dystocia, the emergency physician must be prepared for it. Following delivery of the fetal head, the anterior shoulder does not deliver spontaneously, or with gentle traction by the accoucheur. Instead, the anterior shoulder becomes caught immediately above the symphysis. The first sign of shoulder dystocia is retraction of the fetal chin into the perineum, following the delivery of the head.

Delivery in less than 5 minutes is essential to prevent asphyxia as a consequence of compression of the umbilical cord, compression of the carotid vessels and potential premature separation of the placenta.

Morbidity with shoulder dystocia

Fetal mortality and morbidity rates are significant. There is a linear decline in cord arterial pH with increasing time to delivery. Although the incidence of devastating hypoxic–ischaemic encephalopathy as a consequence of asphyxia is low, it can be minimized when the head-to-body delivery time is less than 5 minutes [10]. Brachial plexus injuries result from lateral traction on the fetal head during delivery. Erb's palsy is caused by damage to the C5 and C6 nerve roots, with paralysis of the deltoid and short muscles of the shoulder and of brachialis and biceps which flex and supinate the elbow. The arm hangs limply by the side with the forearm pronated and the palm facing backwards ('waiter's tip position'). Around 90% of these lesions recover fully or almost fully. Fractures of the clavicle and humerus can occur which heal with conservative treatment without permanent sequelae.

Maternal consequences of shoulder dystocia include postpartum haemorrhage, uterine rupture and third and fourth degree vaginal lacerations [11].

Treatment of shoulder dystocia

McRobert's manoeuvre involves placing the mother's hips in hyperflexion against the abdomen, while being slightly abducted and externally rotated in an effort to widen the pelvic diameter. This should be the initial manoeuvre performed as it is successful in reducing up to 40% of cases [11].

The addition of downward suprapubic pressure applied just proximal to the symphysis by an assistant – either continuously or in a rocking motion – may also be successful and is commonly used in association with McRobert's manoeuvre. Suprapubic pressure adducts the shoulders and disimpacts the baby from the pubic symphysis into an oblique position. These two manoeuvres result in successful shoulder delivery in over 50% of episodes.

Additional manoeuvres include the Wood's corkscrew and the Rubin II manoeuvres, which seek to rotate the shoulder girdle into a different orientation and free the anterior shoulder from under the symphysis pubis. Both these rotational manoeuvres require the physician's hands to be placed into the vagina and a large episiotomy.

Further alternatives include placing the mother 'on all fours' in a hands and knees position, which can facilitate spontaneous delivery. Zavanelli's manoeuvre involves replacing the head in the birth canal and proceeding to immediate emergency caesarian section.

Postpartum haemorrhage

Primary postpartum haemorrhage (PPH) is defined as excessive bleeding in the first 24 hours after birth, which is diagnosed clinically as excessive bleeding making the patient symptomatic with lightheadedness, vertigo and syncope. Or it results in signs of maternal hypovolaemia with hypotension, tachycardia and oliguria [12]. Blood loss is frequently underestimated, with usual losses at vaginal delivery being under 500 mL.

Other definitions of PPH include blood loss in excess of 500 mL after vaginal birth, or >1000 mL after caesarean section. Severe PPH is blood loss greater than or equal to 1000 mL while a critical or major PPH is blood loss of greater than 2500 mL.

The common causes of PPH are referred to as the '**four Ts**', which in order of decreasing frequency include:

- Tone (70 %):
  - atonic uterus
- Trauma (20%):
  - laceration of the cervix, vagina and perineum
  - extension lacerations at CS
  - uterine rupture or inversion
  - non-genital tract (e.g. subcapsular liver rupture)
- Tissue (10%):
  - retained products, placenta (cotyledon or succenturiate lobe), membranes or clots, abnormal placenta
- Thrombin (<1%):
  - coagulation abnormalities (See Table 19.1.2).

Management of PPH

Prevention is essential by identifying the at-risk patient and the aggressive use of oxytocin, along with active management of the third stage of labour. These measures reduce the incidence of PPH by 40%. The initial response to PPH requires a multidisciplinary team approach to restore the woman's haemodynamic state while simultaneously identifying and treating the cause of bleeding.

Resuscitate with intravenous fluids and cross-match blood, carefully estimating the

Table 19.1.2 Risk factors for PPH

Risk factors	Aetiology
Antenatal	
Increased maternal age – more than 35 years	Tone
Asian ethnicity	Tone/trauma
Obesity – body mass index (BMI) of more than 35	Tone
Grand multiparity – uncertain as mixed findings	Tone/tissue
Existing uterine abnormalities (e.g. anatomical anomalies, fibroids)	Tone
Maternal blood disorders:	Thrombin
Von Willebrand's disease	
idiopathic thrombocytopaenic purpura	
thrombocytopaenia caused by pre-eclampsia/gestational hypertension	
disseminated intravascular coagulation (DIC)	
History of previous PPH or retained placenta	Tone/tissue
Anaemia of less than 9g/dL at onset of labour	No reserve
Antepartum haemorrhage associated with:	Tissue/tone/
suspected or proven placental abruption	thrombin
known placenta praevia	
Overdistension of the uterus:	Tone
multiple pregnancy	
polyhydramnios	
macrosomia – greater than 4kg	
Intrauterine fetal death	Thrombin
Intrapartum	
Precipitate labour	Trauma/tone
Prolonged labour – first, second or third stage	Tone/tissue
Chorioamnionitis, pyrexia in labour (e.g. prolonged membrane rupture)	Tone/thrombin
Amniotic fluid embolism/DIC	Thrombin
Uterine inversion	Trauma/tone
Genital tract trauma (e.g. episiotomy, ruptured uterus)	Trauma
Postnatal	
Retained products (e.g. placenta, cotyledons or succenturiate lobe, membranes or clots)	Tissue
Amniotic fluid embolism/DIC	Thrombin
Drug-induced hypotonia (e.g. anaesthetic, magnesium sulphate)	Tone
Bladder distension preventing uterine contraction (e.g. obstructed IDC, unable to void)	Tone

Adapted from Queensland Maternity and Neonatal Clinical Guideline: PPH, with permission from the Queensland Maternity and Neonatal Clinical Guidelines Program.

amount of blood loss including blood-soaked linen and dressings. O negative may be required followed by cross-matched blood. Fresh frozen plasma (FFP), platelets and cryoprecipitate may all be indicated in severe postpartum haemorrhage, with initiation of the department's Massive Transfusion Protocol. Currently, there is no evidence or consensus to guide the optimal ratio of blood component replacement in obstetric haemorrhage, although most use similar ratios as for trauma (1:1:1 for RBC:FFP:platelets) [12]. Consultation with a haematologist is important and the use of tranexamic acid or recombinant activated Factor VII considered.

Before massaging the fundus, ensure that the placenta has been delivered and is complete. An adherent or incomplete placenta in the setting of postpartum haemorrhage may necessitate transfer to the operating suite for operative removal. If the placenta is delivered and complete, check that the third stage oxytocic has been given and massage the uterine fundus to promote contraction. Expel any uterine blood clots and ensure the bladder is empty.

Ensure a careful inspection of the vagina, cervix and perineum is made to confirm or exclude genital trauma as a cause of ongoing bleeding. Clamp obvious arterial vessels and repair lacerations. Transfer to an operating suite may be necessary to allow a full inspection of the vagina, cervix and uterus and effective repair. Suspect uterine rupture in a patient with severe abdominal pain.

Uterine atony

If uterine atony is causal, give oxytocin 5 units IV followed by an infusion of 20–40 units oxytocin in 1 L of 0.9% saline. Use an initial rate of 250 mL/h with the rate slowed as uterine contraction occurs. Other drugs used for uterine atony include misoprostol 800–1000 μg per rectum (PR) and/or ergometrine 250 μg by the intravenous or intramuscular route. Persisting uterine atony necessitates immediate transfer to theatre to identify and remove retained products; bimanual uterine compression may be employed as a temporizing measure.

Second line drugs, such as PGF$_2$-α 250 μg IM or intramyometrially may be used up to a maximum of 2 mg, which is successful in 60–85% cases of refractory uterine atony. Side effects include nausea, vomiting, diarrhoea, pyrexia, hypertension and bronchoconstriction. Its use is therefore contraindicated in women with asthma and hypertension.

Coagulopathy

Coagulopathies must be considered and blood sent for full blood count, clotting studies, including serum fibrinogen, and baseline electrolytes and renal and liver function tests. If a coagulation or platelet defect is present correct with either FFP or platelets.

Other surgical causes

Continuing severe postpartum haemorrhage and haemodynamic instability after management of all of reversible causes requires urgent theatre with possible laparotomy. Causes include uterine rupture or inversion and persistent atony; or causes such as subcapsular liver rupture or amniotic fluid embolism. Surgical procedures for intractable bleeding include placement of B-Lynch compression suture to the uterus, bilateral uterine artery ligation and hysterectomy [12].

NEONATAL RESUSCITATION

Approximately 10% of infants require some assistance to begin breathing at birth, although less than 1% require extensive resuscitation. Of those requiring some assistance, the majority simply require basic manoeuvres, such as stimulation, airway positioning and transient mask ventilation. Few require intubation and ventilation, with the need for chest compressions and medications uncommon [13].

The need for resuscitation may be completely unexpected and so prior preparation to manage a newborn requiring resuscitation is essential. This includes suitable equipment and training and an appropriate location to conduct resuscitation. Early contact is made with the neonatal or paediatric team to plan for transfer or retrieval.

Neonates in need of resuscitation

The need for resuscitation in the newborn is more likely in circumstances such as preterm birth, absent or minimal antenatal care, maternal illness, complicated or prolonged delivery, antepartum haemorrhage, multiple births, previous neonatal death and a precipitate birth.

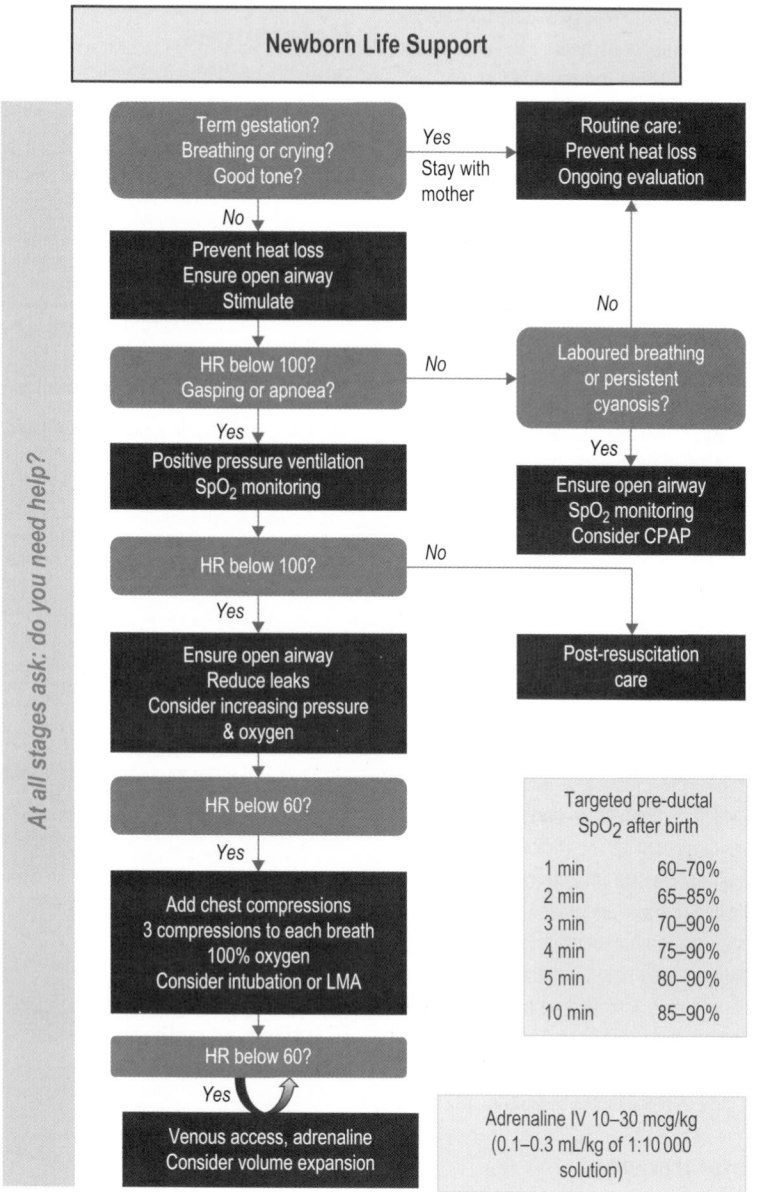

Fig. 19.1.1 Neonatal resuscitation flowchart. *(Reproduced with permission from the Australian Resuscitation Council.)*

This suggests that all emergency department deliveries should be treated as possibly high risk, with appropriate preparations made to provide neonatal resuscitation.

Assessment and resuscitation of the newborn

The initial assessment should focus on tone, breathing and heart rate while subsequent assessment during resuscitation is based on the infant's heart rate, breathing, tone and oxygenation. The Australian Resuscitation Council Neonatal Resuscitation Flowchart illustrates the assessment and resuscitation of a newborn baby (Fig. 19.1.1).

Infants who are born at term, have had low or no risk factors for needing resuscitation, are breathing or crying and have good tone should be dried and kept warm. These actions can be provided on the mother's chest and do not require separation of mother and baby. Poor tone and minimal response should be managed with brisk but gentle drying with a soft towel to stimulate the infant to breathe.

Positive-pressure ventilation

If the infant remains apnoeic or breathing is inadequate, positive-pressure ventilation is started using a self-inflating bag, T-piece device or a flow-inflating bag via a face mask or even

endotracheal tube. Persistent apnoea, particularly associated with hypotonia and a heart rate <100/min is an ominous sign. The main measure of effectiveness of ventilation is prompt sustained improvement in heart rate. This can be determined by listening to the heart with a stethoscope or initially by feeling for pulsations at the base of the umbilical cord. It should be consistently above 100/min within 1 minute of birth in a non-compromised infant. Rates <100/min are managed with ventilation, while a rate <60/min requires both positive pressure ventilation and chest compressions.

Chest compressions

The preferred technique for chest compression is an 'encircling technique' with two thumbs on the lower third of the sternum, with the fingers surrounding the thorax to support the back. A chest compression should be performed each half second with a half second pause after each third compression to deliver a breath, resulting in a 3:1 ratio with a total of 90 compressions and 30 breaths per minute [13].

Oxygenation

Oxygenation is assessed using pulse oximetry, noting that the healthy term newborn takes up to 10 minutes to achieve oxygen saturations of 85–90%. While insufficient oxygenation can impair organ function or cause permanent injury, there is increasing evidence that even brief exposure to excessive oxygenation is harmful to the newborn during and after resuscitation. Emergency physicians should recognize this aspect of a newborn's normal respiratory physiology and not provide high dose oxygen in an attempt to attain unnecessarily high oxygen saturations. A guide to expected oxygenation saturations in the first 10 minutes after birth is listed on the Australian Resuscitation Council Neonatal Resuscitation Flowchart (see Fig. 19.1.1).

Air should be given initially for ventilation of the term infant while pulse oximetry is commenced. Supplemental oxygen delivered by a blender with air is used when the infant's oxygen saturations do not reach the lower end of the target saturations despite effective ventilation. Increased concentrations of oxygen should be used if the infant's heart rate fails to increase or oxygenation as measured by oximetry remains lower than expected.

Attempting to increase the oxygen saturation over 90% in a newborn is potentially harmful. In all cases, the first priority is to ensure adequate inflation of the lungs followed by increasing the concentration of inspired oxygen only if needed [13].

Adrenaline

Adrenaline is recommended if the heart rate remains <60 beats/min after 1 minute of effective ventilation and chest compressions. The recommended intravenous adrenaline dose is 10–30 µg/kg (0.1–0.3 mL/kg of a 1:10 000 adrenaline solution) followed by a small saline flush. This dose is repeated if the heart rate remains below 60 beats/min despite effective ventilation and cardiac compressions. Higher doses of adrenaline are not recommended.

The preferred route of administration of adrenaline is via the umbilical vein. Other routes include an intraosseous catheter or peripheral vein catheter, although these are more technically challenging in the newborn. Adrenaline can also be administered via the endotracheal tube, although there is little evidence to support this route [8]. If the endotracheal route is used, a dose of 50–100 µg/kg (0.5–1 mL/kg of a 1:10 000 solution) is recommended.

Intravenous fluids

Consider intravenous fluids when there is suspected blood loss and/or the infant appears shocked (pale, with poor perfusion and a weak pulse) and has not responded adequately to the other resuscitative measures outlined above. Normal saline is used initially in a dose of 10 mL/kg, but blood may be required early in the setting of blood loss. In the absence of a history of blood loss, give a single dose of fluids to an infant who fails to respond adequately to chest compressions, adrenaline and ventilation; repeated doses are not indicated.

Naloxone

Naloxone is not used routinely as part of the initial resuscitation of newborns with respiratory depression in the delivery room. It may be considered in continuing respiratory depression following restoration of heart rate and colour by standard resuscitation methods as outlined above. The current recommended naloxone dose is 0.1 mg/kg intravenously or intramuscularly, though evidence to support this recommendation is lacking [8].

Meconium-stained liquor

Meconium-stained liquor (light green tinge) is relatively common, occurring in up to 10% of births. Notwithstanding this, meconium aspiration is a rare event and has usually occurred *in utero* before delivery. Suctioning the infant's mouth and pharynx before the delivery of the shoulders makes no difference to the outcome of babies with meconium-stained liquor and is not recommended. Similarly, routine endotracheal suctioning of babies with meconium-stained liquor who are vigorous (breathing or crying, good muscle tone) is discouraged, as it does not alter their outcome and may cause harm.

In the non-vigorous baby with depressed vital signs, there is no clear evidence to support or refute the practice of endotracheal suctioning which is frequently performed. It must not delay other critical resuscitative measures and, if tracheal suction is performed, it must be accomplished before spontaneous or assisted respirations are commenced to minimize delay in establishing breathing. Endotracheal suctioning of meconium is achieved via an endotracheal tube which is then removed. There is no need to repeat this intervention and efforts should be then directed to establishing respiration [3].

Neonatal transfer

Neonates requiring resuscitation following emergency delivery will need to be referred to a regional or tertiary neonatal unit for ongoing care. Transfer of these babies requires careful communication and coordination between the two centres, with transport usually undertaken by a specialized neonatal transport team.

References

[1] Queensland Maternity and Neonatal Clinical Guideline: Normal Birth. Queensland Maternity and Neonatal Clinical Guidelines Program April 2012. <http://www.health.qld.gov.au/qcg/documents/g_normbirth.pdf> [Accessed Feb. 2013].

[2] National Institute for Health and Clinical Excellence. Intrapartum care: care of healthy women and their babies during childbirth CG55. London: National Institute for Health and Clinical Excellence; 2007.

[3] Advanced Life Support Group. Advanced paediatric life support: the practical approach, 5th ed. (Australia and New Zealand). Melbourne: Blackwell Publishing Ltd; 2012.

[4] Rabe H, Reynolds G, Diaz-Rossello J. Early versus delayed umbilical cord clamping in preterm infants. Cochrane Database Syst Rev 2004;4:CD003248.

[5] Casey B, McIntire D, Leveno K. The continuing value of the Apgar score for the assessment of newborn infants. N Engl J Med 2001;344:467–71.

[6] Tintinalli J, Stapczynski J, Cline D, et al. Tintinalli's emergency medicine, 7th ed. New York: McGraw-Hill; 2011.

[7] Hearne A, Driggers R. The Johns Hopkins manual of gynecology and obstetrics, 2nd ed. Baltimore (MD): Johns Hopkins University Press; 2002.

[8] Hofmeyr GJ, Hannah M, Lawrie TA. Planned caesarean section for term breech delivery. Cochrane Database Syst Rev 2003;2:CD000166.

[9] Silver DW, Sabatino F. Precipitous and difficult deliveries. Emerg Med Clin N Am 2012;30:961–75.

[10] Leung T, Stuart O, Sahota D. Head-to-body delivery interval and risk of foetal acidosis and hypoxic ischaemic encephalopathy in should dystocia: a retrospective review. Br J Obstet Gynaecol 2011;118:474–9.

[11] Gottlieb A, Galan H. Shoulder dystocia: an update. Obstet Gynecol Clin N Am 2007;26:501–31.

[12] Queensland Maternity and Neonatal Clinical Guideline: Postpartum Haemorrhage. Queensland Maternity and Neonatal Clinical Guidelines Program November 2012. <http://www.health.qld.gov.au/qcg/documents/g_pph.pdf> [Accessed Jan. 2013].

[13] Neonatal Guidelines. 2010 Australian Resuscitation Council. Guidelines 13.1–13.10 <http://www.resus.org.au/> [Accessed Feb. 2013].

Further reading

Advanced Life Support Group. Advanced paediatric life support: the practical approach, 5th ed. (Australia and New Zealand). Melbourne: Blackwell Publishing Ltd; 2012.

Beischer N, Mackay E, Colditz P, editors. Obstetrics and the newborn: an illustrated textbook (3rd ed.). Philadelphia: WB Saunders; 1997.

DeCherney AH, Nathan L, Goodwin TM, et al. Current diagnosis and treatment: obstetric and gynecology, 11th ed. New Jersey, Lange: McGraw Hill; 2013.

Perlman JM, Wylie J, Kattwinkel J, et al. Part 11: Neonatal resuscitation: 2010. International Consensus on Cardiopulmonary Resuscitation and Emergency Cardiovascular Care Science with Treatment Recommendations. Circulation 2010;122:S516–38.

Sommerkamp SK, Wittels K, editors. Ob/Gyn emergencies. Emerg Med Clin N Am 2012; 30:837–1028.

19.2 Ectopic pregnancy and bleeding in early pregnancy

Sheila Bryan

ESSENTIALS

1 Approximately 25% of all clinically diagnosed pregnancies are associated with bleeding in the first 12 weeks, of which approximately 50% of cases will be due to a failed pregnancy.

2 Ectopic pregnancy occurs at a rate of around 11:1000 diagnosed pregnancies.

3 The management of ectopic pregnancy and failed pregnancy may be surgical, medical or conservative.

Introduction

Bleeding in early pregnancy is a common problem affecting approximately 25% of all clinically diagnosed pregnancies and, of these, approximately 50% will have bleeding due to a failed pregnancy [1]. Other causes of bleeding include ectopic pregnancy and molar pregnancy; however, *most* bleeding is incidental or physiological and has no bearing on the outcome of the pregnancy.

Terminology

The terminolgy used to describe early pregnancy bleeding conditions is defined below:

Miscarriage

A miscarriage is defined as pregnancy loss occurring before 20 completed weeks' gestation or a fetus less than 400 g weight, if the gestation is unknown.

Threatened miscarriage

A threatened miscarriage is any vaginal bleeding other than spotting before 20 weeks' gestation.

Inevitable miscarriage

Inevitable miscarriage is a miscarriage that is imminent or in the process of happening.

Complete miscarriage

A complete miscarriage is when all products of conception have been expelled.

Failed pregnancy

A failed pregnancy is defined on ultrasound criteria. These include the finding of a crown rump length (CRL) greater than 6–10 mm with no cardiac activity or a gestational sac equal to or greater than 20–25 mm with no fetal pole (previously referred to as an anembryonic pregnancy or a blighted ovum).

A failed pregnancy may then remain in the uterus (previously termed a missed abortion) or may progress to either an incomplete or complete miscarriage, as defined by the presence or absence of pregnancy-related tissue in the uterus.

Pregnancy of unknown location

A pregnancy of unknown location refers to the situation where the beta subunit of human chorionic gonadotrophin (β-hCG) is elevated, but no pregnancy can be identified on ultrasound.

Ectopic pregnancy

An ectopic pregnancy is a pregnancy that is implanted outside of the normal uterine cavity. The most common location for an ectopic pregnancy is in the fallopian tube. Other sites include cervix (≈1%), ovary (1–3%), interstitial (1–3%), abdomen (1%) and, rarely, in a uterine scar.

The natural history of an ectopic pregnancy may be one of resorption, spontaneous miscarriage (vaginal or tubal) or it may continue to grow and disrupt the surrounding structures (rupture).

History

History should include the date of the last normal menstrual period (LNMP) and a complete obstetric and gynaecological history including the use of assisted reproductive technology (ART).

Risk factors for ectopic pregnancy include a past history of tubal damage, a previous ectopic pregnancy, pelvic infection, tubal surgery, assisted reproductive technology, increased age, smoking and progesterone-only contraception. Also intrauterine contraceptive devices (IUD) not only decrease the chance of intrauterine pregnancies, but increase the likelihood of an ectopic pregnancy [2].

When estimating the amount of vaginal bleeding, it is useful to quantify the blood loss compared to the woman's normal menstrual loss. Heavy bleeding and the passage of clots are more common with failed intrauterine pregnancy, as ectopic pregnancy is rarely associated with heavy bleeding.

However, the history of passage of fetal products should not be used as the basis for diagnosis of a miscarriage. Blood clots or a decidual cast may be misinterpreted as the products of conception. In addition, the correct identification of the products of conception does not exclude the possibility of a live twin or of a coexistent ectopic pregnancy (known as a heterotopic pregnancy).

Examination

Determination of the patient's haemodynamic status and the rate of ongoing bleeding are a priority. Hypotension, tachycardia and signs of peritoneal irritation suggest a ruptured ectopic pregnancy or bleeding from a corpus luteal cyst.

Bimanual examination can localize tenderness and identify adnexal masses and can also give an estimate of the size of the uterus. However, bimanual examination lacks sensitivity and specificity in identification of a small, unruptured ectopic pregnancy [3] and gives no information about the viability of the pregnancy. Speculum examination allows visualization of the vaginal walls and the cervix and allows identification of the source of bleeding.

A complete physical examination should be performed, including assessment of the woman's mental state, as pregnancy loss may have a profound psychological impact on some women.

Investigations

Biochemistry

Beta subunit of human chorionic gonadotrophin

The beta subunit of human chorionic gonadotrophin (β-hCG) is produced by the outer layer of cells of the gestational sac (the syncytiotrophoblast) and may be detected as early as 9 days after fertilization [4]. The β-hCG level increases by approximately 1.66 times every 48 hours, then plateaus, before falling at around 12 weeks to a lower level.

At any stage of the pregnancy there is always a large range of normal values and a single value cannot be used to determine the location or viability of the pregnancy. There is also potentially significant laboratory-to-laboratory variation and, as such, serial hormone levels may only be compared if they are from the same laboratory.

The half-life of β-hCG is approximately 48 hours, which results in the β-hCG level remaining elevated for a number of weeks post-miscarriage or termination. Therefore, a positive pregnancy test or a single β-hCG level is unreliable to confirm ongoing pregnancy and cannot be used to identify retained products of conception. High levels of β-hCG may be associated with multiple or molar pregnancies.

Urine pregnancy test

Urine pregnancy tests are sensitive to a β-hCG level of 25–60 IU/L. Thus false negatives may rarely occur in the setting of early pregnancy or dilute urine.

Haematology

A full blood count and cross-match should be arranged for haemodynamically unstable patients. Blood group and Rhesus factor should be determined on all patients.

Ultrasound

Ultrasound should be performed in every patient to identify the anatomical location of the pregnancy and to assess fetal viability. The introduction of emergency department (ED) ultrasound provides a cost-effective method for the assessment of a patient presenting with bleeding in early pregnancy [5].

Transvaginal ultrasound

A gestational sac can be identified as early as 31 days' gestation using transvaginal ultrasound. A yolk sac can be identified within the gestational sac at 5–6 weeks when the β-hCG is around 1500 IU/L (except in the case of anembryonic pregnancy). Embryonic cardiac activity should be identified by approximately 39 days' (5.5 weeks') gestation, at which stage the crown rump length of the embryo is approximately 5 mm [6].

Transabominal ultrasound

The findings on transabominal ultrasound are similar approximately 1 week later. Previously a β-hCG of approximately 1500 IU was called the discriminatory zone, meaning that if no pregnancy was identified in the uterus at this level, then an ectopic pregnany could be diagnosed. However, ultrasound is still valuable even when the β-hCG level is less then 1000 IU/L, as direct or indirect signs of an ectopic pregnancy can often be found at levels lower than 1500 IU [7].

The two most common errors in the interpretation of early pregnancy ultrasound include the misidentification of a pseudo-sac or an endometrial cyst as an early gestational sac. A pseudo-sac is a small collection of fluid seen in the uterine cavity, often in association with an ectopic pregnancy. Secondly, assuming that an ultrasound finding of a uterus with no signs of pregnancy is a complete miscarriage, rather than correctly identifying the situation as that of a pregnancy of unknown location. One study of 152 women with a history and examination supporting a complete miscarriage had a 6% rate of ectopic pregnancy.

Heterotopic pregnancy

Identification of an interuterine pregnancy does *not* exclude a coexistent ectopic (heterotopic) pregnancy. The incidence of heterotopic pregnancy in the general population is around 1:3889 but, in patients who have undergone assisted reproductive technology (ART), the incidence is as high as 1:100–1:500 [8]. Thus, in the patient with risk factors and clinical features of an ectopic pregnancy, finding an intrauterine gestation cannot rule out a coexistent ectopic.

Management

Rh(D) immunoglobulin

All patients should have their blood group and Rhesus (Rh) factor determined. As little as 0.1 mL of Rh(D) positive fetal blood will cause maternal Rh iso-immunization. A dose of 250 IU Rh(D) immunoglobulin is given as soon as possible in early pregnancy bleeding with a singleton pregnancy to an Rh-negative woman, certainly within 72 hours of onset of the bleeding. This dose prevents immunization from a feto-maternal haemorrhage of up to 2.5 mL of fetal cells. Further doses may be required in repeat or prolonged bleeding [9].

A dose of 625 IU Rh(D) is recommended in multiple pregnancies or with a gestation of greater than 13 weeks. The Kleihauer test is used in later pregnancy to quantify the amount of fetal cells in the maternal circulation, but is unreliable in early pregnancy.

Note that international guidelines on the use of Rh(D) immunoglobulin differ, such that in the UK no anti-D Ig is required for spontaneous miscarriage before 12 weeks gestation, provided there is no instrumentation of the uterus.

ECTOPIC PREGNANCY

Haemodynamically unstable patient

A haemodynamically unstable patient with suspected ectopic pregnancy should be resuscitated and referred for surgical intervention. A ruptured corpus luteal cyst may rarely cause similar haemodynamic compromise and is also diagnosed at laparoscopy.

Haemodynamically stable patient

The management options for a haemodynamically stable patient with an ectopic pregnancy found on ultrasound include observation, medical treatment or surgical intervention.

Factors to be considered in reaching a management decision include the location of the ectopic pregnancy, the β-hCG level, the size of the ectopic pregnancy, the presence of fetal cardiac activity and patient factors.

Selection criteria for conservative or medical management depend upon the gynaecological team, but may include stable patients with a low β-hCG (<1000 IU/L) which is falling, non-tubal ectopic pregnancy or a small tubal ectopic pregnancy (<3 cm) with no cardiac activity and a β-hCG level less than 5000 IU/L [10].

MISCARRIAGE

Haemodynamically unstable patient

Any patient with heavy vaginal bleeding, hypotension and bradycardia should have an immediate speculum examination as, occasionally, the products of conception cause dilatation of the cervix, which leads to cervical shock, a form of neurocardiogenic shock. Removal of the clot and products of conception from the cervix usually results in cessation of bleeding and reversal of the shock.

Haemodynamic compromise may also be secondary to significant blood loss related to the miscarriage. Fluid resuscitation should be instituted simultaneously with attempts to control the bleeding by removal of blood clot and the products of conception from the cervix and vagina. Uterine contraction may be induced by administering ergometrine 200 micrograms IM if removal of clot and tissue fail to control the bleeding. Emergency surgical evacuation of the uterus is then required.

Haemodynamically stable patient

A haemodynamically stable patient has traditionally been treated by surgical evacuation of uterine contents following the diagnosis of a miscarriage. There have been a number of systematic reviews comparing conservative management with surgical or medical managment (such as prostaglandin E1) [11,12]. Currently, there is insufficient evidence to support the superiority of any one of these three treatment options. Although studies have assessed the time to achieve complete miscarriage and the frequency of complications, they suffer from different inclusion criteria and duration of conservative management.

The success of conservative treatment is variable, but 78.6% of women in one study had an empty uterus at 8 weeks [13]. Conservative management is usually associated with slightly longer duration of bleeding and pain and possibly the need for transfusion. The incidence of infection was similar or higher in the surgical group. Complications of surgery, such as cervical trauma, uterine perforation and intrauterine adhesions, were uncommon.

Currently, the view is that the woman's preference should be the major consideration in recommending a treatment option and the haemodynamically stable patient may be discharged for ongoing care by the gynaecology team [11]. Discharge advice should include explicit indications of when to return, such as heavy bleeding or signs of infection, and advice regarding pelvic rest and a clear follow-up plan.

Prognosis

Approximately 50% of patients with bleeding in early pregnancy will proceed to term. Only 60% of women with an ectopic pregnancy will conceive again naturally, and will have a recurrent ectopic rate of 25–30% in subsequent pregnancies.

Disposition

Patients with a threatened miscarriage and an ultrasound confirming a live intrauterine gestation have an 85–90% chance of the pregnancy progressing to term. Poor prognostic indicators include advanced maternal age, ultrasound findings of an enlarged yolk sac and fetal bradycardia after 7 weeks' gestation. Patients should be advised to avoid sexual intercourse and not to use tampons until after the bleeding has settled. There is no evidence to support improved pregnancy outcomes from recommending bed rest [14]. Referral for counselling or psychological support may be indicated in some women.

Investigation for an underlying cause is generally not indicated until after a third consecutive miscarriage. These include anatomical uterine abnormalities, thrombophilic disorders such as antiphospholipid syndrome and Factor V Leiden, chromosomal abnormalities, immune disorders, hormonal disorders, infection and environmental and lifestyle factors.

Patients with a non-viable intrauterine pregnancy or an ectopic pregnancy are referred to a gynaecology service for ongoing management.

Controversies

- Role of emergency physician ultrasound within the ED.
- Indications for anti-D immunoglobulin.
- Management of patients with pregnancy of unknown location.
- Best practice for emptying the uterus following a failed pregnancy.
- Best practice for managing an ectopic pregnancy.

References

[1] Beischer NA, MacKay EV, Colditz PB. Obstetrics and the newborn, 3rd ed. Philadelphia: WB Saunders; 1999.

[2] Tay JI, Moore J, Walker JJ. Ectopic pregnancy. Br Med J 2000;320:916–9.

[3] Dart R, Kaplan B, Varakis K. Predictive value of history and physical examination in patients with suspected ectopic pregnancy. Ann Emerg Med 1999;33:283–90.

[4] Guyton AC, Hall JE. Textbook of medical physiology, 11th ed. Pennsylvania: WB Saunders; 2005.

[5] Durston W, Carl M, Guerra W, et al. Ultrasound availability in the evaluation of ectopic pregnancy in the ED: comparison of quality and cost effectiveness with different approaches. Am J Emerg Med 2000;18:408–17.

[6] Cacciatore B, Titinen A, Stenman U-H, et al. Normal early pregnancy: serum hCG levels and vaginal ultrasonography findings. Br J Obstet Gynaecol 1990;97:899–903.

[7] Dart RG, Kaplan B, Cox C. Transvaginal ultrasound in patients with low beta-human chorionic gonadotrophin values: how often is the study diagnostic. Ann Emerg Med 1997;30:135–40.

[8] Society for Assisted Reproductive Technology (SART)/ The American Fertility Society. In vitro fertilization embryo transfer (IVF-ET) in the United States. 1990 results from the IVF-ET registry of the Medical Research International and Society for Assisted Reproductive Technology (SART)/The American Fertility Society. Fertil Steril 1992;57:15–24.

[9] NHMRC. Guidelines on the prophylactic use of Rh D immunoglobulin (Anti-D) in obstetrics. NHMRC 2003. <http://www.nhmrc.gov.au/guidelines/publications/wh33> [Accessed Feb. 2013].

[10] Hajenius PJ, Mol F, Mol BWJ, et al. Interventions for tubal ectopic pregnancy. Cochrane Database Syst Rev 2007:CD000324.

[11] Nanda K, Lopez LM, Grimes DA, et al. Expectant care versus surgical treatment for miscarriage. Cochrane Database Syst Rev 2012;3:CD003518.

[12] Neilson JP, Gyte GM, Hickey M, et al. Medical treatments for incomplete miscarriage (less than 24 weeks). Cochrane Database Syst Rev 2010;1:CD007223.

[13] Shelly JM, Healy D, Grover S. A randomised trial of surgical, medical and expectant management of first trimester spontaneous miscarriage. Aust NZ J Obstet Gynaecol 2005;45:122–7.

[14] Aleman A, Althabe F, Belizan J, et al. Bed rest during pregnancy for preventing miscarriage 2005. Cochrane Database Syst Rev 2005;2:CD003576.

19.3 Bleeding after the first trimester of pregnancy

Jenny Dowd • Sheila Bryan

ESSENTIALS

1 Up to 4% of pregnant women will have significant bleeding after 20 weeks' gestation.

2 Resuscitation of the mother followed by ultrasound localization of the placenta are the priorities of management for patients with heavy vaginal bleeding after 20 weeks' gestation.

3 Secondary postpartum haemorrhage is commonly caused by endometritis or retained products of conception.

Introduction

Vaginal bleeding after the first trimester may be due to a number of causes. The most common is classified as 'incidental', where the bleeding is not directly related to pregnancy.

Antepartum haemorrhage

Bleeding that occurs after 20 weeks' gestation is classified as an antepartum haemorrhage (APH). Obstetric causes of bleeding include placenta praevia, accidental haemorrhage or placental abruption and vasa praevia. Various amounts of blood loss from 60 to 200 mL have been used as a definition threshold for an APH but, in practice, any bleeding beyond minor spotting should be assessed.

Postpartum haemorrhage

Primary post-partum haemorrhage (PPH) is defined as heavy (>500 mL) vaginal bleeding within 24 hours of delivery and is discussed in Chapter 19.1.

Secondary postpartum haemorrhage

Secondary PPH is most commonly due to infection and/or retained tissue and may cause significant bleeding up to 6 weeks' postpartum.

ANTEPARTUM HAEMORRHAGE

Differential diagnosis

Incidental causes

These include bleeding from the lower genital tract, most commonly from physiological cervical erosion or ectropion, where the bleeding may be either spontaneous or post-traumatic, such as post-coital. Other causes that need to be excluded include bleeding from cervical polyps, cervical malignancy and cervical or vaginal infection.

Bleeding from haemorrhoids or vulval varices may also be mistakenly reported as vaginal bleeding.

Placenta praevia

Placenta praevia occurs when the placenta is situated in the lower part of the uterus and therefore is in front of the presenting part of the fetus. It occurs in 0.5% of pregnancies [1]. Bleeding in this situation is usually painless, unless associated with labour contractions and often presents with several small, 'warning' bleeds.

Accidental haemorrhage (marginal bleed or placental abruption)

This is bleeding from a normally situated placenta. It may come from the edge of the placenta, known as a marginal bleed, or from behind the placenta associated with placental separation (placental abruption). Vaginal bleeding may not always be present with a placental abruption, but it is usually associated with pain. A placental abruption that causes significant detachment of the placenta may cause fetal compromise and fetal death in up to 30% of cases [2].

The retroplacental clot consists of maternal blood with up to 2–4 L being concealed behind the placenta without vaginal loss. A placental abruption may follow relatively minor blunt trauma, such as a fall onto the abdomen, or a shearing force, such as that applied in a motor vehicle deceleration crash. Placental abruption may also occur spontaneously associated with hypertension, inherited disorders of coagulation or with cocaine use [3].

Vasa praevia

This is the presence of fetal vessels running in the amniotic membranes distant from the placental mass and across the cervical os, such as with a succinturate lobe of placenta or a villamentous insertion of the cord, so that an earlier ultrasound may have described a fundal placenta. These vessels occasionally rupture, often in association with rupture of the amniotic membranes.

When this happens, the bleeding is from the fetus, which may quickly lead to fetal compromise. The first indication of this may be fetal bradycardia or other abnormalities of the fetal heart rate seen on cardiotocographic (CTG) tracing.

Physiological

Vaginal blood mixed with mucus is called a 'show' and is due to the mucus plug or operculum within the endocervical canal dislodging as the cervix begins to dilate. This usually occurs at the time of, or within a few days of, the onset of labour and is not significant unless the pregnancy is preterm or associated with rupture of the membranes. As a general guide, when a woman needs to wear a pad to soak up blood, she should be assessed as having an APH.

History

The history should specifically include details of recent abdominal trauma or drug use suggesting a diagnosis of placental abruption. A history of recent coitus is commonly identified in bleeding from a cervical ectropion. The history should also include details regarding the presence and quality of fetal movements.

Constant pain over the uterus or sometimes in the lower back from separation of a posteriorly situated placenta is suggestive of a placental abruption. Intermittent pains in the lower abdomen or back may represent uterine contractions. Women may describe this as 'period pains' or tightenings and may notice a general hardening over the whole uterus in association with the pain. Painless bleeding is suggestive of either an incidental cause or of placenta praevia.

An increase in pelvic pressure associated with a mucous vaginal fluid loss and spotting or mild bleeding suggests cervical incompetence. This usually presents between 14 and 22 weeks' gestation. Prior cervical damage secondary to either a cone biopsy or a cervical tear is a risk factor for cervical incompetence.

Examination

Assess the mother as a priority. A relatively low blood pressure with a systolic of 90 mmHg and a resting tachycardia of up to 100 bpm is normal in pregnancy.

Examination after 30 weeks' gestation should be performed with the right hip elevated by a pillow to give a 15° tilt of the pelvis to the left. This avoids the problem of vena caval compression (supine hypotension syndrome) from pressure of the gravid uterus reducing inferior vena caval venous return.

Speculum or digital vaginal examination

Speculum or digital vaginal examination should *never* be performed until the site of the placenta is determined by ultrasound, to avoid disrupting a low-lying placenta and precipitating torrential haemorrhage.

Once an ultrasound scan has excluded a low-lying placenta, an experienced operator may proceed to a speculum examination to look for liquor within the vagina in suspected rupture of the membranes, or to assess the cervix to localize the site of bleeding and to look for cervical dilatation.

A sterile speculum examination is indicated, again by an experienced operator, if preterm pre-labour rupture of the membranes is possible, to decrease the risk of introducing infection. Digital vaginal examination should be performed to assess the cervix for dilatation if labour is suspected.

Ideally, a CTG should be applied to assess the status of the fetus beyond 24 weeks' gestation. Auscultation of the fetal heart for several minutes should be attempted if this is not available. The baseline rate and variations related to contractions are important. The normal range of the fetal heart rate is 120–160 bpm, but a healthy term or post-term fetus may have a heart rate of between 100 and 120 bpm. Decelerations of the fetal heart rate may indicate fetal distress.

Investigations

Laboratory blood tests

Blood should be taken for baseline haemoglobin and platelet count, coagulation screen, Kleihauer test, blood group, Rhesus factor, Rhesus antibodies and a cross-match.

A pre-eclampsia screen should be ordered if the patient is hypertensive, including liver function tests and uric acid as well as the platelet count.

Ultrasound

Ultrasound is used to assess fetal gestation, presentation, liquor volume and placental position. Many 'low-lying' placentas at 18 weeks are no longer classified as placenta praevia by 30–32 weeks, owing to the differential growth of the lower uterine segment as pregnancy progresses. A placental edge at least 2 cm away from the cervical os at term is considered safe to allow a planned vaginal delivery.

As only 50% of placental abruptions will be seen on ultrasound, it is unreliable for excluding this problem with the diagnosis usually made on clinical grounds alone. Transvaginal ultrasound with an empty bladder is best to visualize the cervix to look for shortening or 'beaking' of the amniotic sac into the internal os which are signs of early cervical incompetence.

Management

Incidental causes of bleeding usually require no specific therapy apart from explanation and reassurance. Cervical polyps are rarely removed during pregnancy due to the risk of heavy bleeding.

Minor amounts of bleeding due to placenta praevia distant from term are managed by close observation, usually initially as an inpatient or later as an outpatient.

Small placental abruptions may also be managed conservatively with serial ultrasound scans to monitor fetal growth and regular CTG assessments. Delivery is usually advised round 37 weeks to pre-empt a massive placental abruption developing. Sometimes, a small retroplacental clot will cause weakening of the amniotic membranes and subsequent rupture of the amniotic sac 1–2 weeks after the initial bleed.

Massive antepartum haemorrhage, often with fetal demise when associated with placental separation, requires urgent delivery, possibly by caesarean section. Hypovolaemia and coagulopathies are treated as per usual guidelines.

Prognosis

A decision needs to be made in a hospital where there are no obstetric or neonatal facilities about when to transfer a patient to an obstetric unit. Corticosteroids should be administered to the mother if the fetus is between 23 and 34 weeks and delivery can be delayed for 24 hours. Two intramuscular doses of betamethasone or dexamethasone given over 24 hours decrease the baby's risk of developing respiratory distress syndrome, necrotizing enterocolitis and intraventricular haemorrhages [4].

There are new national guidelines for the infusion of magnesium sulphate in pregnancies less than 30 weeks' gestation where delivery within 24 hours is expected. This significantly decreases the rate of subsequent cerebral palsy in such infants [5]. Discussion about dose and timing should be with the obstetric staff receiving the woman if transfer is being planned.

The current survival rate of a baby admitted to a neonatal intensive care unit (NICU) is 40%, 50%, 60% and 70% at 24, 25, 26 and 27 weeks, respectively [4].

Disposition

Discharge home may be appropriate if the diagnosis of a benign physiological cause for bleeding can be made with certainty.

SECONDARY POSTPARTUM HAEMORRHAGE

Introduction

Secondary PPH is defined as excessive or prolonged bleeding from 24 hours to 6 weeks' postpartum. Normal lochia is moderately heavy, red vaginal loss for some days that settles to light bleeding or spotting by 2–4 weeks. Some women have a persistent brownish vaginal discharge for up to 8 weeks [6].

Differential diagnosis

Common causes of secondary PPH

Common causes of secondary PPH include retained products of conception and endometritis. The bleeding is usually prolonged, moderate blood loss or a recurrence of blood loss after an initial decline.

Less common causes of secondary PPH

Less common causes include trophoblastic disease, uterine arterio-venous malformation (AVM) and any of the incidental causes outlined in the previous section. Reactivation of bleeding from an episiotomy or vaginal laceration may also be responsible. Annoying spotting may occur for several weeks in women using progestogen-only contraception, especially when concurrently breastfeeding, in the setting of an oestrogen-deficient endometrium.

History

Distinguishing endometritis from retained products may be difficult clinically and the two conditions often coexist. Endometritis may follow any type of delivery, but is more common in women with a history of prolonged rupture of the membranes and multiple vaginal examinations during labour.

Examination

Abdominal examination may show subinvolution of the uterus with retained tissue, while offensive lochia, uterine tenderness and systemic signs of infection support the diagnosis of endometritis.

An AVM presents with heavy vaginal bleeding and, occasionally, haemodynamic compromise.

Investigations

Full blood examination and two paired sets of blood cultures are indicated if the woman is clinically septic. Send cervical swabs for microscopy and culture and *Chlamydia trachomatis* detection to help guide the management of endometritis.

Ultrasound is necessary to quantify the amount of retained products of conception and to confirm a diagnosis of an AVM.

Treatment

Empirical treatment with amoxicillin/clavulanic acid 875 mg/125 mg bd PO for 5–7 days as an outpatient is appropriate if endometritis is suspected but the woman is systemically well. Erythromycin may be substituted in penicillin-sensitive patients. Admit those who are systemically unwell for intravenous antibiotics.

Perform an ultrasound examination if bleeding persists to look for retained products of conception. Patients with small amounts of retained products may be treated conservatively. Uterine curettage in the postpartum period is associated with the risks of uterine perforation or Asherman syndrome due to intrauterine adhesions and/or fibrosis.

Controversies

- Suppression of labour in patients with APH.
- Timing of delivery in patients with mild APH due to placental abruption.
- The timing and interpretation of ultrasound investigation in patients with secondary PPH.

References

[1] Cotton D, Ead J, Paul R, et al. The conservative aggressive management of placenta praevia. Am J Obstet Gynecol 1980;17:687–9.

[2] Saftlas A, Olsen D, Atras H, et al. National trends in the incidence of abruptio placenta. Obstet Gynecol 1991;78:1081–6.

[3] Paterson M. The aetiology and outcome of abruptio placentae in Sweden. Obstet Gynecol 1986;67:523–8.

[4] Koh THHG. Simplified way of counselling parents about outcomes of extremely premature babies. Lancet 1996;348:963.

[5] Doyle L, Crwother C, Middleton P, et al. Antenatal magnesium sulfate and neurologic outcome in preterm infants: a systematic review. Obstet Gynecol 2009;113:1327–33.

[6] Bonnar J. Massive obstetric haemorrhage. Best Pract Res Clin Obstet Gynaecol 2000;14:1–18.

19.4 Abnormal vaginal bleeding in the non-pregnant patient

Sheila Bryan • Anthony Brown

ESSENTIALS

1 Start the assessment of any patient with vaginal bleeding by excluding pregnancy.

2 Locate the anatomical site of bleeding and assess the severity.

3 Consider coagulopathy as a cause of heavy uterine bleeding in all patients, especially adolescents.

Introduction

Vaginal bleeding may be divided into two major categories, bleeding which occurs in a pregnant patient and bleeding in the non-pregnant patient. Therefore, the first step in a patient presenting with vaginal bleeding is to exclude pregnancy. See Chapter 19.2 if the woman is pregnant.

This chapter deals exclusively with bleeding in non-pregnant women. Bleeding may be from the external genitalia, vaginal walls, cervix or uterus. The pathological basis for bleeding from the vulva, vagina and cervix includes infection, trauma, atrophy or malignancy. Uterine bleeding may be physiological or pathological.

Physiological uterine bleeding

Physiological uterine bleeding is associated with ovulatory menstrual cycles, which occur at regular intervals every 21–35 days, and last for 3–7 days. The average volume of blood loss is 30–40 mL with >80 mL being defined as menorrhagia.

The menstrual cycle is controlled by the hypothalamic–pituitary–ovarian (HPO) axis. During the first 14 days, oestrogen is produced by the developing follicle, leading to proliferation of the endometrium, which reaches a thickness of 3–5 mm. Oestrogen acts on the pituitary gland to cause the release of follicle stimulating hormone (FSH) and luteinizing hormone (LH) which result in ovulation. The corpus luteum then releases progesterone in excess of oestrogen.

Progesterone causes stabilization of the endometrium during the secretory phase of the menstrual cycle. In the absence of fertilization, there is involution of the corpus luteum and a fall in oestrogen and progesterone levels. This results in vasoconstriction within the endometrium, which consequently becomes ischaemic and is shed as normal menstrual bleeding.

Pathological uterine bleeding

Pathological causes include infection, structural abnormalities, such as polyps, fibroids, arteriovenous malformations (AVM) or malignancy, drugs, hyperprolactinaemia, coagulopathy and thyroid endocrinopathy. Terms associated with abnormal uterine bleeding are inconsistently defined, but may be broadly considered as abnormal uterine bleeding with ovulatory menstrual cycles and abnormal uterine bleeding with anovulatory menstrual cycles.

Abnormal uterine bleeding with ovulatory menstrual cycles

The most common cause of abnormal uterine bleeding is menorrhagia occurring in ovulatory menstrual cycles. This presents as regular heavy bleeding and may result in anaemia. In these women, the menstrual blood has been shown to have increased fibrinolytic activity and/or increased prostaglandins.

Abnormal uterine bleeding with anovulatory menstrual cycles

Abnormal uterine bleeding or metrorrhagia due to anovulatory menstrual cycles, sometimes referred to as dysfunctional uterine bleeding (DUB), presents as irregular bleeding of variable volume. In anovulatory menstrual cycles and other high oestrogen states, there is a relative lack of progesterone to oppose the oestrogenic stimulation of the endometrium. This results in excessive proliferation and occasionally hyperplasia/metaplasia of the endometrium. The endometrium also becomes 'unstable' and prone to erratic sloughing.

Clinically, this presents as irregular, often heavy, menstrual bleeding. Anovulatory cycles are due to immaturity or disturbance of the normal HPO axis. This is seen at the extremes of reproductive ages in the first decade after menarche and in premenopausal women, as well as in polycystic ovary syndrome (PCOS) and during times of either physical or emotional stress.

CAUSES OF ABNORMAL VAGINAL BLEEDING

It is essential initially to review all the possible causes of vaginal bleeding which may be considered by pathophysiology and/or pathological location (Table 19.4.1).

History

A careful menstrual history helps determine the cause of the vaginal bleeding. A history of vaginal trauma may indicate vulval or vaginal wall bleeding. The vaginal trauma may be associated with either consensual or non-consensual intercourse or a vaginal foreign body. Exposure *in utero* to diethyl stilboestrol (DES) should raise suspicion of vaginal malignancy.

The patient's estimate of the amount of vaginal bleeding is often inaccurate and has limited use in diagnosis, other than the presence of clots, which is abnormal and suggests heavy bleeding [1]. Ask about additional information including known gynaecological cancer, a known bleeding disorder or a family history of a bleeding diathesis and exogenous sex steroid use.

Postcoital or intermenstrual bleeding

Postcoital or intermenstrual bleeding may be symptomatic of cervical or uterine pathology. Common causes include ectropion or polyps on the cervix, infection or malignancy causing bleeding from the vagina, cervix or uterus.

Postmenopausal bleeding

Postmenopausal bleeding is related to vaginal or uterine conditions, which include infection,

Table 19.4.1 Differential diagnosis of abnormal vaginal bleeding

- Ovulatory bleeding *'menorrhagia'*
  Anovulatory bleeding: sometimes known as dysfunctional uterine bleeding (DUB)

- Uterine and ovarian pathology:
    uterine fibroids (pelvic pain, dysmenorrhoea)
    endometriosis; adenomyosis (dysmenorrhoea, dyspareunia, pelvic pain, infertility)
    pelvic inflammatory disease and pelvic infection (fever, vaginal discharge, pelvic pain, intermenstrual and postcoital bleeding)
    endometrial polyps (intermenstrual bleeding)
    endometrial hyperplasia; endometrial carcinoma (pelvic pain, abnormal bleeding, postcoital bleeding)
    polycystic ovary syndrome (irregular bleeding, infertility and hirsutism)
- Systemic disease:
    coagulation disorder; bleeding diathesis such as von Willebrand's disease
    liver or renal disease
    hypothyroidism (fatigue, constipation, coarse features, alopecia)
- Iatrogenic cause:
    anticoagulation
    intrauterine device
    chemotherapy
    sex steroids

atrophy, trauma or malignancy. Risk factors for uterine malignancy include obesity, age >40 years, nulliparity, tamoxifen use, infertility and chronic anovulatory cycles.

Anovulatory bleeding

A diagnosis of anovulatory bleeding is classically made from the history of irregular menses with periods of amenorrhoea followed by heavy bleeding, in the absence of features suggesting a structural or a histological uterine abnormality [2]. A menstrual cycle of less than 21 days or more than 35 days, even if regular, is usually anovulatory.

Physical examination

First determine the haemodynamic stability of the patient. Physiological menorrhagia alone is rarely a cause of shock and other diagnoses, such as cervical malignancy or endometrial AVM, should be considered. Also look for evidence of anaemia, petechiae suggesting a bleeding tendency and thyroid endocrinopathy.

Abdominal and pelvic examination

Palpate the abdomen to assess for uterine enlargement. Inspect the vulva for local causes of bleeding, including trauma and infection. Vaginal speculum examination should include assessment of the vaginal walls and the cervix, ideally, with a clear plastic speculum for ease of view. Speculum examination will also allow an assessment of the site and amount of bleeding. Bimanual examination is indicated to assess for local tenderness, uterine size and/or masses and adnexal masses or cervical motion tenderness.

Investigations

These are based around laboratory tests and ultrasound scanning.

Laboratory investigations

- *Serum or urinary β-hCG pregnancy test.* Perform this immediately on all women of childbearing age, even in the face of assurances from the patient that pregnancy could not be possible. Urine pregnancy tests are highly sensitive, detecting β-hCG levels as low as 25 IU/L.
- *Full blood count.* Perform this in all patients to identify anaemia. Add iron studies if the blood count shows a hypochromic, microcytic picture.
- *Thyroid function tests.* These are only indicated in women with menorrhagia and anovulatory bleeding or with clear evidence of thyroid endocrinopathy (see Chapter 11.3). Do *not* send routinely.
- *Coagulation profile.* Perform on all adolescents and any women with unusually heavy uterine bleeding.

Radiology

- Ultrasound is requested to assess the pelvic organs. Particular attention is paid to the myometrium looking for fibroids or adenomyosis, the endometrial thickness and the endometrial cavity for polyps or retained products of conception (positive β-hCG).
- Ultrasound may also identify an AVM, which may be congenital or acquired either postpartum or, more commonly, post-instrumentation of the uterus.

Management

Management may be considered as general supportive measures and then specific treatment.

General supportive measures

Resuscitation should proceed in the usual manner with initial therapy determined by the degree of haemodynamic instability or severity of anaemia.

Specific treatment for structural lesions

Vaginal wall bleeding

Vaginal wall bleeding secondary to trauma generally settles spontaneously. Examination under anaesthesia (EUA) is indicated for vaginal trauma if the laceration extends beyond the mucosa or if examination is too uncomfortable for the woman.

Cervical bleeding

Cervical bleeding rarely requires immediate therapy. However, cervical bleeding from malignancy may occasionally be difficult to control as lesions tend to be friable. Attempt cautery with silver nitrate and, if this fails to control the bleeding, consider placing a vaginal pack. Refer the patient immediately to the gynaecology team.

Specific treatment for vaginal and endometrial infection

Vaginal and endometrial infections are dealt with as outlined in Chapter 19.5. Arrange for the partner(s) to have contact tracing and simultaneous antibiotic treatment as necessary.

Specific treatment for menorrhagia associated with ovulatory cycles

Progestins

Oral progestins, such as norethisterone 5 mg bd or tds or medroxyprogesterone acetate 10 mg one to three times a day, on days 1 to 21 of a 28-day cycle reduce blood loss by up to 87%, although adherence can be poor due to nausea, lethargy, headache, bloating with fluid retention and acne [3].

Tranexamic acid

Tranexamic acid is a plasminogen activator inhibitor that promotes local haemostasis. The usual dose is 1 g tds for 3–4 days. Side effects include nausea and leg cramps, but it is generally well tolerated. Although long-term studies have not shown an increase in thromboembolic events, active thromboembolic disease is a contraindication to use [4]. It reduces blood loss by around 47%.

Non-sterioidal anti-inflammatory drugs

Non-steroidal anti-inflammatory drugs (NSAIDs) block prostaglandin PGE_2, a vasodilator found in excess in patients with menorrhagia [5]. The efficacy of NSAIDs is less than other therapies with only a 29% reduction in blood loss. However, they are well tolerated and are particularly helpful if there is associated dysmenorrhoea.

Usual doses are mefenamic acid 500 mg tds, naproxen 250 mg tds or ibuprofen 400 mg tds.

Combined oral contraceptive

As a longer-term therapy, the combined oral contraceptive pill reduces the mean menstrual blood loss by about 43% using a pill containing 35 μg of ethinyloestradiol. Contraindications include the desire for fertility and all contraindications to oestrogens.

Specific treatment for heavy anovulatory uterine bleeding

Acute irregular heavy bleeding is most commonly secondary to anovulatory bleeding. There are many different treatment regimens and emergency department (ED) physicians should select a range of agents with which to become familiar [1–3,6]. The underlying pathology is a relative lack of progesterone and so treatment should include progestin therapy to stabilize the endometrium. This may be combined with tranexamic acid and/or an NSAID, which decreases the amount of blood loss. If anovulatory cycles are expected to continue, then progestin therapy may need to be long term.

Progestin therapy

Medroxyprogesterone acetate 20 mg orally every 8 hours for one week then reducing to 20 mg daily for 3 weeks [7]. Side effects include bloating, headache, acne and breast tenderness.

Tranexamic acid and NSAIDs

These can be added to progestin therapy for heavy anovulatory bleeding.

Combined oral contraceptive pill

The combined oral contraceptive pill (COCP) may be used to decrease blood loss in ovulatory cycles and to regulate and decrease blood loss in anovulatory cycles. It also provides contraception. Start a monophasic COCP that includes at least 30 μg of ethinyloestradiol and a progestin.

Consider histological assessment of the endometrium in patients over 35 years of age, prior to commencing hormone therapy.

Other treatments not usually commenced in the ED

Surgical procedures

Dilatation and curettage is a method of endometrial sampling and *not* a long-term treatment for menorrhagia or irregular menstrual cycles. The procedure is often combined with hysteroscopy, which allows visual assessment of the uterine cavity and biopsy if indicated.

Other drug treatments

Other treatments that are not usually commenced in the ED include the levonorgestrel-releasing intrauterine system, such as Mirena, or long-acting progestogens, such as medroxyprogesterone acetate (Depo-Provera), which may prove successful if oral agents fail.

Gonadotrophin-releasing hormone (GnRH) analogues should only be commenced by a gynaecologist when other medical and surgical treatments are contraindicated or prior to proposed surgery.

Disposition

Admit patients with haemodynamic instability or profound anaemia. Consult the gynaecology team if a significant underlying cause for the abnormal bleeding is likely. However, most patients may be discharged and followed up in an outpatient clinic.

Controversies

- Precise regimen for progestins in the management of anovulatory bleeding.
- Indications for endometrial sampling, especially in postmenopausal women.
- Role of surgical versus medical therapy in the long-term management of menorrhagia.

References

[1] National Health Service. Menorrhagia (heavy menstrual bleeding). Clinical knowledge summaries, Oct 2010. <http://www.cks.nhs.uk/menorrhagia/management/scenario_diagnosis_and_assessment/view_full_scenario> [Accessed Feb. 2013].
[2] National Institute for Health and Clinical Excellence. Heavy menstrual bleeding. NICE Clinical Guideline 44, Jan 2007. <http://www.nice.org.uk/nicemedia/pdf/CG44FullGuideline.pdf> [Accessed Feb. 2013].
[3] Cirilli A, Cipot SJ. Emergency evaluation and management of vaginal bleeding in the nonpregnant patient. Emerg Med Clin N Am 2012;30:91–106.
[4] Sundstrom A. The risk of VTE associated with use of tranexamic acid. Br J Obstet Gynaecol 2009;116:91–7.
[5] Duckitt K., Collins S. Menorrhagia. Clinical evidence (online), 18 Sept. 2008. BMJ Publications. <http://www.ncbi.nlm.nih.gov/pmc/articles/PMC2907973/> [Accessed Feb. 2013].
[6] Hicky M, Higham JM, Fraser I. Progestogens with or without oestrogen for irregular uterine bleeding associated with anovulation. Cochrane Database Syst Rev 2012:9.
[7] Menorrhagia. Therapeutic Guidelines: eTG complete. Nov. 2012. <www.tg.org.au/> [Accessed Feb. 2013].

19.5 Pelvic inflammatory disease

Sheila Bryan

ESSENTIALS

1 Pelvic inflammatory disease (PID) is infection and/or inflammation of the upper genital tract.

2 The clinical features cover a spectrum of presentations which depend on the extent of infection and/or inflammation, the anatomical structures involved and the specific microorganisms.

3 *Chlamydia trachomatis* is the most common pathogen identified in sexually transmitted PID. Other pathogens include *Neisseria gonorrhoeae* and mixed anaerobes.

4 The sequelae of PID include ectopic pregnancy, infertility and chronic pelvic pain.

5 Screening high-risk patients for sexually transmitted infections reduces the incidence of PID.

Introduction

Pelvic inflammatory disease (PID) refers to a clinical syndrome resulting from infection or inflammation involving the usually sterile upper genital tract in women. The term PID is generally reserved for infection initiated by sexually transmitted organisms rather than for pelvic infections secondary to a medical procedure, pregnancy or other primary abdominal infections which have a similar clinical presentation.

Most cases of PID are caused by ascent of microorganisms from the vagina and endocervix into the upper genital tract [1]. The passage of organisms through the cervix is facilitated by disruption of the cervical barrier, e.g. by a sexually transmitted infection (STI), such as *Chlamydia trachomatis* and *Neisseria gonorrhoeae*, or by a surgical procedure.

Early identification and treatment are important to reduce the serious sequelae of PID, which include ectopic pregnancy, chronic pelvic pain and infertility.

Epidemiology

The true incidence of PID is indeterminable as there are no standardized clinical criteria for diagnosis, plus the fact that asymptomatic or subclinical disease and under-diagnosis occur.

Up to 300 000 women are treated as outpatients and 10 000 are admitted to Australian hospitals each year with a diagnosis of PID.

The highest reported incidence is between ages 20 and 29 years. The rate of hospitalization is up to nine times higher in the indigenous population.

Risk factors

Risk factors for PID include STIs and procedures or conditions that involve disruption of the normal cervical barrier. Chlamydial infection is the most common cause of sexually transmitted PID in Australia. The presence of an intrauterine contraceptive device (IUCD) increases the risk of PID in the first 3 weeks following insertion [2]. There is also an increased risk of PID during or shortly after the menses [3].

Presentation

No symptom or sign is pathognomic of PID and the diagnosis of PID includes a spectrum of clinical conditions determined partly by the anatomical location of the infection and by the pathogen involved. The diagnosis encompasses endometritis, salpingitis, tubo-ovarian abscess (TOA) and/or pelvic peritonitis.

The assessment of a patient with suspected PID must involve the exclusion of other possible diagnoses, such as ectopic pregnany, endometriosis, ruptured ovarian cyst, appendicitis and urinary tract infection. However, in view of the significant sequelae of untreated PID, the current recommendation is to consider treatment for PID in an at-risk woman with adnexal tenderness, if no other cause for the local signs can be found [4].

History

The history should assess recognized risk factors for STIs, such as young age at first sexual intercourse, younger age, high frequency of sexual intercourse, multiple sexual partners and non-barrier methods of contraception. History should also enquire about non-sexually transmitted causes, such as recent uterine instrumentation, including operative termination of pregnancy.

Abdominal pain of less than 3 weeks' duration is the most sensitive symptom of PID, which is usually suprapubic and diffuse, but may lateralize. However, significant lateralization suggests an alternate diagnosis or a tubo-ovarian abcess. Other symptoms may include a new or changed vaginal discharge, dyspareunia, postcoital and/or intermenstrual bleeding.

Examination

Adnexal tenderness on bimanual examination is the most sensitive examination finding and is present in 95% of cases, but only has a specificity of just 3.8% [4]. Other examination findings with high sensitivity include lower abdominal tenderness, cervical motion tenderness or uterine tenderness. However, as isolated findings, all lack sensitivity.

The presence of fever is associated with a more severe infection, but the absence of fever does not exclude the diagnosis.

Fitz–Hugh–Curtis syndrome (perihepatitis)

Fitz–Hugh–Curtis syndrome (FHCS) is a perihepatitis with focal peritonitis resulting from the transcoelomic spread of inflammatory peritoneal fluid to the subphrenic and subdiaphragmatic spaces.

FHCS is usually an incidental finding in patients with PID but, occasionally, right upper quadrant (RUQ) pain is the presenting symptom and the diagnosis is considered when upper abdominal ultrasound rules out biliary tract disease [5].

Investigations

Haematology

There are no specific laboratory tests to diagnose PID. The white cell count, erythrocyte sedimentation rate and C-reactive protein are all raised as non-specific markers of inflammation, but lack sensitivity and specificity for the diagnosis.

Biochemistry

Check a beta subunit of human chorionic gonadotrophin (β-HCG) level on all women of childbearing age. Although PID is uncommon in pregnancy, especially after the first trimester, the diagnosis of PID when pregnant has significant implications.

Pelvic pain secondary to a complication of pregnancy, such as an ectopic pregnancy, is an important differential diagnosis.

Microbiology

Collect and send endocervical swabs for microscopy and culture and polymerase chain reaction (PCR) for *N. gonorrhoeae* and *C. trachomatis*. A positive result retrospectively supports the diagnosis of PID, defines antibiotic sensitivities and identifies the need to treat a sexual partner [6]. However, a negative result does not exclude the diagnosis.

The presence of either mucopus or white blood cells (WBCs) in the vaginal discharge is a sensitive marker for PID. The diagnosis of PID is thus unlikely if the cervical discharge appears normal and there are no WBCs in a wet slide preparation [7]. All patients who are diagnosed with acute PID should be considered for a full sexual health evaluation including hepatitis B, syphylis and HIV serology, plus partner contact tracing [8].

Ultrasound

Ultrasound, particularly transvaginal, is valuable in the assessment of suspected PID to identify complications, such as tubo-ovarian abscess, and to exclude other causes of pelvic pain. However, ultrasound features, such as free fluid in the pouch of Douglas, lack sensitivity in the diagnosis of mild to moderate PID.

Laparoscopy

Laparoscopy is no longer considered to be a gold standard to diagnose PID as, although it has a specificity approaching 100%, the sensitivity is as low as 50–80%. The main indications for laparoscopy incude acute pain of uncertain origin and the diagnosis of chronic pelvic pain.

Differential diagnosis

Important differential diagnoses include ectopic pregnancy, endometriosis, complications of ovarian cysts and tumours, appendicitis, diverticulitis and urinary tract infection.

Management

Patients with mild to moderate PID may be treated as outpatients. There is no evidence of improved outcomes between inpatient and outpatient treatment with respect to fertility, chronic pelvic pain or recurrence of PID [9].

Indications for inpatient treatment include severe PID, inability to tolerate oral antibiotics, failed oral therapy and/or compliance issues, pregnancy and when a surgical emergency cannot be excluded.

Antibiotic therapy

Sexually acquired PID
- *Mild-to-moderate infection:* ceftriaxone 500 mg IM or IV as a single dose and azithromycin 1 g orally as a single dose, plus metronidazole 400 mg orally 12-hourly for 14 days, plus either azithromycin 1 g orally as a single dose 1 week later or doxycycline* 100 mg orally bd for 14 days [10].
- *Severe infection:* ceftriaxone 1 IV daily, plus azithromycin 500 mg IV daily, plus metronidazole 500 mg IV 12-hourly.
- Treat sexual partners in all proven cases of *N. gonorrhoeae* and *C. trachomatis*.

Non-sexually acquired PID
- *Mild-to-moderate infection:* amoxicillin plus clavulanate 875/125 mg orally bd for 14 days, plus azithromycin 1 g orally as a single dose, plus either azithromycin 1 g orally as a single dose 1 week later or doxycycline* 100 mg orally bd for 14 days.

---

*Substitute roxithromycin 300 mg orally once daily for 14 days if the patient is pregnant or breast feeding or when doxycycline is contraindicated (category B1).

- *Severe infection:* amoxicillin or ampicillin 2 g IV 6-hourly, plus gentamicin 4–6 mg/kg IV (then either 1 or 2 days further doses of gentamicin based on renal function), plus metronidazole 500 mg IV bd.

Disposition

Patients discharged on oral medication should be reviewed within 24–48 hours to assess the response to therapy. All patients with sexually acquired PID should be counselled regarding safe sex practices and other sexual health issues, such as hepatitis B and human papilloma virus vaccination.

Prognosis

Women with PID are at increased risk of ectopic pregnancy, chronic pelvic pain and infertility.

Controversies

- Clinical criteria for initiation of treatment in PID.
- Role of ultrasound in the primary diagnosis of PID.
- Indications for laparoscopy in PID.

References

[1] Cunningham FG, Hauth JC, Gilstrap LC. The bacterial pathogenesis of acute pelvic inflammatory disease. Obstet Gynecol 1978;52:161–4.
[2] Farley TM, Rosenberg MJ, Rowe PJ. Intrauterine devices and pelvic inflammatory disease: an international perspective. Lancet 1992;339:785–8.
[3] Nowicki S, Tassell AH, Nowiki B. Susceptibility to gonoccoccal infection during the menstrual cycle. J Am Med Assoc 2000;283:1291–2.
[4] Peipert JF, Ness RB, Blume J, et al. Clinical predictors of endometritis in women with symptoms and signs of pelvic inflammatory disease. Am J Obstet Gynecol 2001;184:856–63.
[5] Lopez-Zeno JA, Keith LG. Berger. The Fitz–Hugh–Curtis syndrome revisited. Changing perspectives after half a century. J Reprod Med 1985;30:567–82.
[6] Livengood CH, Chacko MR. Clinical features and diagnosis of pelvic inflammatory disease. UpToDate Sept 2012. <www.uptodate.com> [Accessed Feb. 2013].
[7] Peipert JF, Boardman J, Hogan JW. Laboratory evaluation of acute upper genital tract infection. Obstet Gynecol 1996;87:730–6.
[8] Centers for Disease Control and Prevention. Sexually Transmitted Diseases Treatment Guidelines 2010. Pelvic inflammatory disease. <http://www.cdc.gov/std/treatment/2010/pid.htm> [Accessed Feb. 2013].
[9] Ness R, Soper D, Holley R, et al. Effectiveness of inpatient and outpatient treatment strategies for women with pelvic inflammatory disease: results from the pelvic inflammatory disease evaluation and clinical health (PEACH) randomized trial. Am J Obstet Gynecol 2002;186:929–37.
[10] Pelvic inflammatory disease. Therapeutic Guidelines: eTG complete. Nov 2012. <www.tg.org.au/> [Accessed Feb. 2013].

OBSTETRICS AND GYNAECOLOGY EMERGENCIES

19

19.6 Pelvic pain

Michael Cadogan • Anusch Yazdani • James Taylor

ESSENTIALS

1 First consider the possibility of pregnancy in *all* patients of reproductive age with abdominal or pelvic pain, under the well iterated tenets:
- 'all female patients are pregnant until proven otherwise'
- 'all pregnant patients have an ectopic pregnancy until proven otherwise'.

2 Give effective analgesia with the regular administration of non-steroidal anti-inflammatory drugs.

3 A negative pelvic examination should not preclude gynaecological referral, even in the absence of other findings.

4 'Psychogenic pain' is a diagnosis of exclusion.

Introduction

Pelvic and lower abdominal pain in female patients is a complex and challenging complaint. It is the second most common gynaecological symptom after vaginal bleeding. The large differential diagnosis for female pelvic pain makes a definitive diagnosis in the emergency department (ED) difficult. A systematic approach is essential.

The emergency physician should aim to stabilize the haemodynamically unstable patient, identify those conditions that require early surgical intervention and to expedite the investigation and further management of females with pelvic pain, giving adequate analgesia.

Classification

Pelvic pain may be acute, acute-on-chronic or chronic pain. Conditions causing pelvic pain can be life threatening or inconsequential, gynaecological or non-gynaecological and/or non-organic. These presentations are often complex and require ongoing care and management often by multiple specialties.

Presentation

This chapter outlines the initial presentation and management of the most common gynaecological conditions associated with acute and chronic pelvic pain.

History

Parietal pelvic pain may be well localized and occurs secondary to peritoneal irritation, such as in appendicitis and Mittelschmerz. More generalized and diffuse abdominal pain is associated with intraperitoneal blood or pus resulting from the rupture of an ectopic pregnancy or tubo-ovarian abscess.

Pain of sudden onset is associated with ovarian cyst rupture or adnexal torsion. Gradually worsening pain is suggestive of a long-term process, such as endometriosis or chronic pelvic inflammatory disease (PID). Pain with sexual intercourse (dyspareunia) may be associated with any pelvic process, including adnexal pathology and endometriosis.

Sexual and menstrual history

The patient's sexual and menstrual history will help define potential pregnancy-related problems or sexually transmitted diseases (STD) and determine whether chronic pain is cyclic or acyclic. This should include time of last intercourse, contraception, number of partners, possibility of physical or sexual abuse, menarche, menopause, last normal menstrual period (LNMP), previous STD, gravida, parity, tubal surgery and previous ectopic pregnancy.

Radiation of the pain

The pain may radiate and provide a clue to the underlying origin, such as pain referred via the hypogastric nerve plexus to the lower abdomen from the uterine fundus, adnexae and bladder dome. The S2–4 sacral nerve roots transmit pain from the lower uterine segment, cervix, bladder trigone and rectum to the lower back, buttocks, perineum and legs. Ask about associated urological, gastrointestinal and musculoskeletal symptoms.

Psychosocial impact

Finally, consider psychosocial factors particularly in the evaluation of chronic pain. The symptoms of fatigue, loss of energy and depressed mood are commonly associated with chronic pelvic pain, thus a screen for anxiety, depressive and somatoform disorders is essential.

Enquire about marital distress, the partner's understanding and response to the pain and the family's response to how the patient is handling the pain.

Examination

As in all intimate examinations, it is important to provide early analgesia and establish rapport with the patient who may be reticent, frightened or embarrassed. Note the temperature, pulse, blood pressure and respiratory rate to indicate life-threatening haemorrhage, such as an ectopic pregnancy, or overwhelming sepsis associated with tubo-ovarian abscess.

Abdominal examination

Commence the abdominal examination with inspection for distension associated with obstruction, ascites or abdominal masses. Palpation and percussion delineate areas of generalized or localized tenderness and may replicate the patient's pain. Check for hernias, inguinal nodes and other non-gynaecological causes for the patient's symptoms at the same time (Table 19.6.1).

Pelvic examination

A pelvic examination is essential. Only perform this in the presence of a chaperone, after providing careful explanation of the procedure and gaining verbal consent. The pelvic examination includes:

- visual examination of the vulva and urethral meatus to identify varicosities, infection or abnormal lesions

Table 19.6.1   Causes of acute pelvic pain

Gynaecological	Non-gynaecological		
	Intestinal	Urological	Other
Complication of pregnancy: ectopic, miscarriage	Appendicitis	Cystitis	Hernia
Complication of ovarian and adnexal cysts and masses	Diverticulitis	Acute urinary retention	Pelvic vein thrombophlebitis
Pelvic inflammatory disease	Inflammatory bowel disease	Urolithiasis	
Adnexal torsion	Gastroenteritis	Pyelonephritis	
Leiomyoma complication	Bowel obstruction Constipation		

- speculum examination to visualize the cervix, cervical os and the vaginal vault. Note any vaginal discharge and take endocervical and vaginal swabs. However, performing a PAP smear is *not* encouraged and, if done, this should only be by an experienced operator when follow up of the result can be guaranteed
- bimanual (vagino–abdominal) examination to examine the cervix, uterus and adnexae.

The uterus is normally mobile, but conditions, such as endometriosis or adhesions, may cause fixation. An enlarged uterus is associated with pregnancy, fibroids or adenomyosis. The uterine axis is dependent on a number of other local pelvic factors, such as the content of the bladder or bowel. A retroverted uterus can be normal, but a fixed retroverted uterus is classically associated with pouch of Douglas pathology, such as endometriosis.

Uterine tenderness occurs with any cause of pelvic peritonism, but also conditions such as adenomyosis or fibroid degeneration. An open cervical os may be associated with the passage of intrauterine pathology, such as a failed pregnancy or clots. Cervical excitation pain on moving the cervix is non-specific and associated with conditions producing pelvic peritonism, such as blood or other irritants in the peritoneal cavity, including PID (see Chapter 19.5). Palpable adnexal masses are associated with more gross pathology, such as ovarian cyst including endometriomata ('chocolate cyst'), again associated with adnexal tenderness.

A normal pelvic examination does not exclude pelvic pathology, but provides valuable information and helps in the selection of further definitive investigations, such as ultrasound scan (USS) and laparoscopy.

Rectal examination

A rectal examination completes the pelvic examination, taking note of stool consistency, faecal occult blood and the presence of a mass lesion. A rectovaginal examination allows palpation of the posterior cul-de-sac for ovarian masses, the posterior wall of the uterus and the uterosacral ligaments for nodularity and tenderness in association with endometriosis. This should only be performed once, preferably by the doctor with ongoing clinical care.

Laboratory investigations

Laboratory studies depend on the history and physical examination and are tailored to the individual patient. They include the following tests.

Blood tests

Beta human chorionic gonadotrophin

Screening for pregnancy is essential in a patient of reproductive age and a serum (or urine) pregnancy test is performed. The beta subunit of human chorionic gonadotrophin (β-hCG) is produced by the outer layer of cells of the gestational sac (the syncytiotrophoblast) and may be detected as early as 9 days after fertilization (see Chapter 19.2). False-positive and even false-negative serum and urine tests do occur, but are extremely rare.

Full blood count, erythrocyte sedimentation rate (ESR) and C-reactive protein

A full blood count may show anaemia and a leucocytosis may indicate underlying infection

or inflammation. An elevated ESR or C-reactive protein are non-specific markers of acute inflammation and are included in the clinical diagnosis of PID in some centres.

Tumour markers

Tumour markers have a limited role in the evaluation of pelvic pain in the ED. Markers such as the CA 125 may be sent in the evaluation of an adnexal mass or when endometriosis is suspected. Serial levels improve the sensitivity and specificity of such markers, usually on an outpatient basis.

Urinalysis

Urinary β-hCG is rapid, inexpensive and accurate. Perform this in all sexually active patients. The presence of leucocytes in the urine may indicate infection with a sensitivity of around 70–75%, but may also be associated with inflammation of adjacent pelvic organs. The presence of red cells may indicate urolithiasis.

Send the urine for microscopy, culture and sensitivity if urinary tract pathology is suspected. The urine should also be sent for chlamydial polymerase chain reaction (PCR) in suspected PID (see Chapter 19.5).

Microbiological swabs

Take endocervical swabs for chlamydia, gonorrhoea and ureaplasma during the speculum examination. Specific viral and bacterial swabs vulval swabs should only be taken in the presence of a vulval lesion, such as suspected Herpes simplex infection.

Imaging

Ultrasound scan (USS)

Ultrasound should be considered a non- or minimally invasive extension of the physical examination in females. It is the single most useful ED test in diagnosing acute gynaecological presentations.

Ultrasound may determine the uterine size, presence of fibroids and the thickness and characteristics of the endometrium and myometrium. It can delineate adnexal pathology, such as ovarian cysts, endometriomata, hydro/pyosalpinx, tubo-ovarian abscess and tumours.

USS is more accurate at predicting abnormal pelvic pathology, as confirmed by laparoscopy, than pelvic examination alone. However, when using laparoscopy as the gold standard, studies still find that half of the patients with either a normal pelvic examination or USS have abnormal laparoscopic findings.

Computed tomography scan

A computed tomography (CT) scan is helpful to define a pelvic mass, such as malignancy or complex abscess formation. A CT scan may also help identify a urinary calculus, a Spigelian hernia and appendicitis. The radiation risk should be considered, particularly if a repeat scan is needed.

Magnetic resonance imaging

Magnetic resonance imaging (MRI) most appropriately defines adenomyosis, congenital reproductive abnormalities and endometriotic lesions, but has a limited role in an emergent ED assessment.

DIFFERENTIAL DIAGNOSIS

Patients attending the ED present with:

- acute pelvic pain
- acute-on-chronic pelvic pain
- chronic pelvic pain

Acute pelvic pain

Table 19.6.1 lists conditions that present to the ED with acute pelvic pain. The causes may be considered under the following.

Pregnancy-related

Pregnancy is tested for in all women of reproductive age and, if diagnosed, an ectopic pregnancy must then be excluded (see Chapter 19.2).

Pelvic inflammatory disease

See Chapter 19.5 on the evaluation of pelvic inflammatory disease (PID).

Adnexal mass or cyst

Ovarian mass or cyst

- 'Functional' ovarian cysts are either follicular cysts that develop during the first 14 days of the menstrual cycle prior to ovulation or corpus luteum cysts that develop during the last 14 days following ovulation. 'Functional' cysts are usually asymptomatic unless a complication occurs. As these cysts are related to normal ovarian activity, an ovarian cyst in the postmenopausal woman should never be considered 'functional'.

- Neoplastic masses may be benign or malignant. Features that increase the risk of malignancy include being postmenopausal, the presence of ascites and increasing size or complexity.
- Infective masses usually arise as part of a tubo-ovarian mass in association with PID.
- Endometriomata are deposits of endometriosis in association with the ovary, forming a collection of altered blood and cellular debris, hence the term 'chocolate cyst'.

Non-ovarian adnexal mass or cyst

- Para-ovarian and paratubal cysts are related to either the ovary or, more commonly, the fallopian tube.
- A hydrosalpinx arises in the blocked fallopian tube.

Any of these structures may present acutely due to rupture, haemorrhage or torsion.

Rupture of an ovarian cyst   Follicular cyst expansion and/or rupture at ovulation is accompanied by ovarian bleeding and peritoneal irritation during the mid-cycle known as Mittelschmerz. Rupture of a corpus luteum cyst usually occurs between days 20 and 26 of the menstrual cycle and is associated with intraperitoneal bleeding. This bleeding may be catastrophic depending on the size of the torn ovarian blood vessel.

A USS helps differentiate a ruptured ectopic pregnancy from a bleeding corpus luteum cyst, although they may coexist.

Intra-ovarian haemorrhage   Haemorrhage may occur into a functional cyst or tumour. The sudden onset of sharp unilateral pain with increasing intensity results from ovarian capsule distension. There may be localized or generalized peritonism dependent on the degree of peritoneal irritation and haemorrhage extravasation. Pelvic examination may reveal a focal expanding adnexal mass, which is confirmed by USS.

Haemorrhagic ovarian cysts may be managed conservatively. Indications for intervention include haemodynamic instability, failure to obtain adequate analgesia and failure of symptom resolution.

Torsion of adnexae   The adnexae include the ovary and fallopian tube. Torsion occurs when these structures twist on their supportive appendages causing compromise of their

vascular supply. This most commonly occurs in the third decade of life and accounts for 3–5% of emergency gynaecological surgery.

Over 90% of cases of adnexal torsion are associated with cystic tumours or simple cysts of the ovary. Torsion of the fallopian tube is less common and is associated with a hydrosalpinx, tubal ligation and pelvic adhesions. Both adnexal torsion and torsion of the fallopian tube include an enlarging adnexal mass, secondary to venous obstruction and secondary oedema.

Pain character   Pain associated with adnexal torsion is commonly sudden in onset, sharp, unilateral and increasingly severe on a background of a dull pelvic ache. Classically, it radiates from the pelvis to the flank, 'reverse renal colic', and is associated with nausea, vomiting, low-grade pyrexia and urinary symptoms secondary to bladder irritation. Late cases can present with ovarian necrosis, frank peritonitis and shock.

Pelvic examination   Pelvic examination reveals cervical motion tenderness, adnexal tenderness and a discrete adnexal mass in the majority. USS defines an adnexal mass and Doppler studies are of assistance in the differential diagnosis. Definitive diagnosis and treatment may require laparoscopy or laparotomy.

Ovarian infection   This may rarely occur as a primary event with mumps or tuberculosis, but most commonly occurs in the setting of PID with the formation of a tubo-ovarian abscess (see Chapter 19.5).

Acute-on-chronic and chronic pelvic pain

Chronic pelvic pain is defined as pain lasting more than 6 months, localized to the anatomic pelvis causing functional disability requiring medical or surgical treatment. It affects millions of women worldwide and accounts for 10% of gynaecology outpatient attendances.

The commonest diagnoses associated with chronic pelvic pain are endometriosis and pelvic adhesions. However, up to 60% of patients have no visible pathology at laparoscopy and 25% remain without a definitive diagnosis.

Patients usually present to the ED with an acute exacerbation of their chronic condition (acute-on-chronic pelvic pain), an unrelated acute cause of pelvic pain or are simply unable to cope with their debilitating condition.

Table 19.6.2	Causes of cyclic and acyclic pelvic pain
Cyclic	**Acyclic**
Mittelschmerz	Chronic PID
Endometriosis*	Pelvic adhesions
Adenomyosis	Uterine prolapse
Cervical stenosis*	Chronic urethritis
Intrauterine device	Diverticulitis
Leiomyoma (fibroid)	Irritable bowel syndrome
Primary and secondary dysmenorrhoea	Levator syndrome of the perirectal area
Pelvic congestion*	Detrusor instability
	Interstitial cystitis
	Abdominal hernia
	Abdominal wall myofascial pain
	Abuse syndromes: physical and sexual
	Depression

*May become 'acyclic'. PID, pelvic inflammatory disease.

Cyclic pelvic pain

Cyclic pelvic pain occurs in 30–50% of women of reproductive age and interferes with normal daily activities in up to 12% of cases. It is usually related to ovulation or menstruation. Many conditions that cause cyclic pain may ultimately develop acyclic pain, such as endometriosis (Table 19.6.2).

Mittelschmerz

Mittelschmerz is defined as a transient mid-cycle pain occurring at or after ovulation. Increasing ovarian capsular pressure is associated with poorly localized pain, which becomes localized following follicular rupture and the release of fluid and/or blood causing peritoneal irritation.

There are usually minimal findings on physical examination, but a thorough evaluation is essential to rule out other pelvic pathology. A slightly enlarged ovary may be palpated on the affected side.

Mittelschmerz is a clinical diagnosis, but USS may reveal the presence of a recently ruptured follicle. Provide regular non-steroidal anti-inflammatory drugs (NSAIDs) and reassurance; although the pain on presentation may be severe, it usually resolves spontaneously.

Endometriosis

Endometriosis is defined as the presence of ectopic endometrial glands and stroma outside the uterine cavity. Initially, the pain may be cyclic and associated with menses but, as the disease progresses, for instance with the development of pelvic adhesions, the pain often becomes continuous and acyclic.

Endometriosis affects women of reproductive age and is the second most common cause of cyclic pain in this age group. Over 70% of sufferers are nulliparous and up to 60% of patients investigated for infertility are found to have endometriosis.

Pain character Typically, the pain commences a few days prior to the menses and extends variably into or beyond this period. Persistent, unilateral mid-cycle pain is suggestive of an endometrioma. Patients commonly present with dysmenorrhoea (75%), dyspareunia (20%), tenesmus or following the finding of an adnexal mass (endometrioma).

Examination Physical examination is normal in the majority of women with endometriosis. Retrocervical (uterosacral ligament and pouch of Douglas disease) and/or rectovaginal nodularity is characteristic of severe endometriosis, but is not always palpable.

USS may reveal endometriomata or focal endometriotic lesions. The definitive diagnosis is made on histology at laparoscopy. Excision is both diagnostic and therapeutic.

Adenomyosis

Adenomyosis is a benign condition characterized by the ingrowth of endometrial glands and stroma into the myometrium. The majority (>80%) of cases involve multiparous women in the fourth and fifth decade of life. Patients usually present with menorrhagia and dysmenorrhoea.

Pelvic examination reveals a symmetrically enlarged, slightly tender uterus with a diffusely boggy consistency. Rarely, a large mass (adenomyoma) may be palpated.

USS may reveal generalized uterine enlargement with indistinct myo-endometrial margins. An MRI will more clearly demonstrate the pathology, but is rarely indicated or available in the ED.

Hysteroscopy and uterine biopsy may demonstrate adenomyosis, but the definitive diagnosis is usually made at hysterectomy.

Leiomyomata (fibroids)

Leiomyomata or fibroids are benign tumours of myometrial origin. They are the most common pelvic tumour and occur in 25% of Caucasian women and 50% of Negro women. Their aetiology is unknown but they enlarge in pregnancy and recede in the climacteric.

Symptoms relate to the space-occupying effect of the lesion, but they may lead to chronic pelvic pain with or without bleeding. Acute pain occurs with torsion or degeneration; torsion usually involves pedunculated subserosal lesions. Degeneration is associated with pregnancy and results from the rapidly expanding lesion restricting its own blood supply.

Examination Fibroids may be palpated on bimanual pelvic examination and are usually painless unless associated with acute degeneration, when uterine tenderness, pyrexia and leucocytosis occur.

Treatment of chronic leiomyomata is conservative unless associated with anaemia. The patient with acute torsion or degeneration of a fibroid requires opiate analgesia and urgent gynaecological review for definitive management.

Primary or secondary dysmenorrhoea

Primary dysmenorrhoea This is painful menstruation in the absence of pelvic pathology and is a diagnosis of exclusion. Primary dysmenorrhoea is associated with the release of prostaglandins, principally PGF2α from the endometrium during menstruation. This causes uterine contractions, arteriolar vasoconstriction and uterine ischaemia, with the most intense pain occurring as the menstrual flow is subsiding. Primary dysmenorrhoea usually coincides with the onset of ovulatory cycles 4–12 months after menarche and affects up to 10% of young nulliparous women.

Primary dysmenorrhoea is associated with spasmodic, crampy lower abdominal pain radiating to the lower back and upper thighs and lasts 24–48 hours. Associated symptoms include headache, nausea and vomiting. Symptoms may be alleviated by the regular administration of NSAIDs or by suppressing ovulation with the oral contraceptive pill.

Secondary dysmenorrhoea This is painful menstruation associated with pelvic pathology, such as cervical stenosis, adenomyosis, leiomyomata, pelvic congestion syndrome and the intrauterine contraceptive device. It usually affects women later in life and symptoms often start earlier in the menstrual cycle and can precede menstruation.

Acyclic pelvic pain

Chronic pelvic inflammatory disease (PID)
See Chapter 19.5.

Pelvic adhesions
Adhesions occur when anatomical structures are abnormally bound to one another by bands of fibrous tissue. They are believed to account for pain suffered by up to 33% of patients with chronic pelvic pain, although their exact role is uncertain. They are associated with PID, endometriosis, abdominal surgery, perforated appendix and inflammatory bowel disease.

Adhesions contain their own nerve fibres and the pain perceived by patients is thought to originate within the fibrous tissue when it is under tension. The pain is often consistent in location and aggravated by sudden movements, intercourse or physical activity. Laparoscopy is the gold standard for diagnosis and treatment.

Pelvic congestion syndrome
Pelvic congestion syndrome is characterized by dilatation, congestion and venous stasis of the pelvic veins. This syndrome is associated with multiparity, polycystic ovarian syndrome (PCOS), tubal ligation and lower limb varicosities. Patients commonly present with a chronic, dull ache localized to the pelvis and lower back with exacerbations of sharp stabbing pain. Other symptoms include dyspareunia (75%), dysfunctional uterine bleeding (54%) and mucoid vaginal discharge (47%).

Deep abdominal palpation, particularly over the adnexae, reproduces the pain. On external examination, superficial vulval varices are seen and speculum examination may reveal a bluish tinge to the engorged cervix.

Ultrasound may demonstrate uterine enlargement and venous incompetence. Pelvic venography can establish the size of varicosities and the site of incompetence.

Psychological
There is an association between chronic pelvic pain and somatization disorders. In addition, many women with chronic pelvic pain have suffered physical, sexual and emotional abuse and psychiatric disease is often related.

Conclusion
Female pelvic pain presents a complex and challenging problem in the ED. A systematic evaluation may find a diagnosis in acute pelvic pain, but chronic conditions require review and follow up by a specialist unit.

The resuscitation of the acutely unwell patient, exclusion of pregnancy-related problems, provision of adequate analgesia, prompt initiation of appropriate investigations and specialist referral for ongoing evaluation are fundamental to the management of gynaecological pelvic pain.

Controversies
- Accuracy of emergency physician focused pelvic ultrasound scan to evaluate pelvic pain.
- Diagnosis and management of acute-on-chronic and chronic pelvic pain syndromes.

Further reading
Berchuk A, Boente MP, Bast RB. The use of tumour markers in the management of patients with gynaecological carcinomas. Clin Obstet Gynaecol 1992;35:45–54.

Carter JE. A systematic history for the patient with pelvic pain. J Soc Laparoendosc Surg 1993;3:245–52.

Howard FM. The role of laparoscopy as a diagnostic tool in chronic pelvic pain. Best Pract Res Clin Obstet Gynaecol 2000;14:467–94.

Howard FM, Perry CP, Carter JE, editors. Pelvic pain: diagnosis and management. New York: Lippincott; 2000.

Muse KN. Cyclic pelvic pain. Obstet Gynecol Clin N Am 1990;17:427.

Scialli AR, Barbieri RL, Glasser MH, et al. Chronic pelvic pain: An integrated approach. Medical Education Collaborative. Association of Professors of Gynaecology and Obstetrics 2000:3–9.

Sturgeon C. Practice guidelines for tumor marker use in the clinic. Clin Chem 2002;48:1151–9.

19.7 Pre-eclampsia and eclampsia

Marian Lee

ESSENTIALS

1 Pre-eclampsia is a multiorgan condition with non-specific symptoms at presentation that may go on to have a fulminant course.

2 Definition has been broadened by the Society of Obstetric Medicine of Australia and New Zealand (SOMANZ) to include evidence of end-organ dysfunction besides proteinuria, although worldwide this is not universally accepted.

3 Knowledge of the underlying pathophysiology is incomplete.

4 Eclampsia is a complication of pre-eclampsia but not a natural progression of the condition (<1% in Australasia).

5 Haemolysis, Elevated Liver enzymes and Low Platelet count (HELLP) syndrome is a life-threatening complication of pre-eclampsia.

6 Delivery is the definitive treatment for pre-eclampsia. Other treatments are supportive only, which aim to mitigate the adverse effects of pre-eclampsia on maternal and perinatal morbidity and mortality.

7 Magnesium sulphate is the first-line drug treatment for eclampsia.

8 There is no one antihypertensive medication superior to another in the treatment of hypertension in pre-eclampsia.

Introduction

Pre-eclampsia is part of the spectrum of hypertensive disorders of pregnancy. It has the most devastating consequence for the mother and fetus compared to chronic/pre-existing hypertension and gestational hypertension.

Incidence

Worldwide, pre-eclampsia is estimated to affect over one million women annually with 780 perinatal deaths globally per day (about one-quarter of cases) [1]. In Australia, mild pre-eclampsia affects 5–10% of pregnancies and severe pre-eclampsia affects 1–2% of pregnancies [2].

Pre-eclampsia is the cause of 15% of direct maternal mortality and 10% of perinatal mortality [2]. Timely diagnosis and management of pre-eclampsia are critical to maternal and fetal outcomes. Emergency physicians must be familiar with the non-specific presentation of this multiorgan disease, as they are frequently involved in the acute management of these patients.

Definition of pre-eclampsia

Pre-eclampsia is traditionally defined by hypertension arising beyond 20 weeks' gestation together with proteinuria. Hypertension is defined as a systolic blood pressure (sBP) of ≥140 mmHg and/or a diastolic blood pressure (dBP) of ≥90 mmHg.

The Society of Obstetric Medicine of Australia and New Zealand (SOMANZ) has broadened this definition [3]. While SOMANZ recognizes the traditional definition as essential for research purposes, it proposes the clinical definition extends beyond proteinuria to emphasize that pre-eclampsia is a multiorgan disease.

Hence, pre-eclampsia is recognized when hypertension is associated with evidence of dysfunction of maternal end-organs and/or the fetus. This definition of pre-eclampsia is not universally accepted, but neither is there worldwide consensus on the classification of hypertensive disorders of pregnancy [4,5]. None of the classification systems have been proven to be more reliable in identifying pre-eclampsia than another [4].

Table 19.7.1 illustrates the classification used by SOMANZ for hypertensive disorders of pregnancy [3].

Pathophysiology

The pathophysiology of pre-eclampsia remains incompletely understood [4–6]. However, it is accepted that the placenta is responsible and that the condition is systemic affecting multiple organs, but how this occurs is unclear.

Normal pregnancy

In the normal pregnancy, trophoblasts invade the myometrium to get to the spiral arteries, which are remodelled into low resistance and high capacity vessels, to assist the increasing demands of the growing placenta.

Pre-eclamptic pregnancy

In contrast, trophoblastic invasion of the myometrium is not as successful in the pre-eclamptic pregnancy. The spiral arteries are not remodelled and remain as highly resistive vessels, thus the placenta is poorly vascularized. Reduction of angiogenic factors released by the placenta is also contributory.

Multiorgan involvement

The multiorgan involvement of pre-eclampsia may be explained by maternal endothelial inflammation due to the presence of placental debris, which may account for the widespread vascular reactivity in the maternal circulation and the consequent systemic involvement. The fetus is also involved through suboptimal perfusion of the placenta.

Immunological intolerance

Immunological intolerance of fetal tissues in the maternal circulation is thought to account for some of the risk factors for pre-eclampsia. Thus reduced exposure to paternal tissue prior to conception may increase the risk of pre-eclampsia, hence the predisposing factors of nulliparity, inter-pregnancy interval of greater than 10 years, new partner and artificial donor insemination.

Table 19.7.1   Classification of hypertensive disorders of pregnancy

Hypertensive disorder of pregnancy	Features
Chronic hypertension	Hypertension that predates the pregnancy or onset prior to 20 weeks' gestation
Gestational hypertension	Onset of hypertension after 20 weeks' gestation without any maternal or fetal features of pre-eclampsia, followed by return of blood pressure to normal within 3 months' postpartum
Pre-eclampsia/eclampsia	Onset of hypertension after 20 weeks' gestation together with features of end-organ dysfunction. Hypertension resolves within 6 weeks' postpartum
Pre-eclampsia superimposed on chronic hypertension	Development of end-organ dysfunction after 20 weeks' gestation in women with chronic hypertension

Table 19.7.2   Risk factors for pre-eclampsia

Maternal general	Age over 40 years – note that the previous predisposing factor of <16 years is no longer current [4]
Obstetric history	Previous pre-eclampsia Previous gestational hypertension Multiple pregnancies Nulliparity or interpregnancy interval greater than 10 years Artificial insemination with donor sperm
Pre-existing conditions	Chronic hypertension Diabetes mellitus Congenital heart conditions: coarctation of the aorta, transposition of great vessels, pulmonary atresia with VSD and pulmonary stenosis Chronic renal disease Thrombophilia, such as antiphospholipid syndrome Increased body mass index Migraine
Fetal factors	Gestational trophoblastic disease Hydrops fetalis Triploidy

VSD: ventricular septal defect.

Table 19.7.3   End-organ dysfunction in pre-eclampsia

Renal	Oliguria Urine dipstick showing greater than 1+ protein Elevated serum creatinine
Neurological	Seizure (known as eclampsia) Headache Visual disturbance Hyperreflexia
Hepatic	Right upper quadrant pain Epigastric pain Elevation of transaminases to at least 2 × normal
Haematological	Haemolytic anaemia Thrombocytopaenia Disseminated intravascular coagulation (DIC)
Pulmonary	Pulmonary oedema
Fetal/placental	Fetal growth restriction Fetal death in utero Placental abruption Premature labour Premature delivery

Gestational hypertension

Gestational hypertension and pre-eclampsia are separate entities. The total circulatory volume is reduced in pre-eclampsia due to disruption of sodium and water homeostasis whereas, in gestational hypertension, the circulating volume is unaffected. Additionally, placental and renal pathology is not present in gestational hypertension.

Risk factors

The risk factors for pre-eclampsia may be divided into general maternal, obstetric, pre-existing conditions and fetal factors (Table 19.7.2).

Clinical features

Two critical features of pre-eclampsia are that it is a progressive multiorgan disease that can become fulminant and that it frequently presents with non-specific symptoms [3–6]. Hence an active search for organ dysfunction in a pregnant patient with hypertension beyond 20 weeks' gestation is essential.

Table 19.7.3 is a summary of clinical and investigative features of end-organ dysfunction that form part of the symptomatology.

Pre-eclampsia presentations

Pre-eclampsia superimposed on chronic hypertension

In a patient with chronic hypertension, worsening of hypertension control, the onset of proteinuria and end-organ dysfunction are evidence of superimposed pre-eclampsia.

Eclampsia

Eclampsia is pre-eclampsia complicated by a generalized tonic–clonic seizure, but it is not a natural progression of pre-eclampsia [6]. In Australia, one in 200–300 pre-eclamptic pregnancies is complicated by eclampsia [2]. It may occur any time after 20 weeks' gestation with 35% of seizures occurring prepartum, 9% intrapartum and up to 28% postpartum, usually within 24 hours [5].

Unfortunately, no factor(s) reliably predicts eclampsia, which has an immediate risk of intracranial haemorrhage. Headache, visual disturbance, including cortical blindness and epigastric pain in the preceding week, may be important [5]. One-third of eclamptic patients do not have hypertension preceding the seizure, thus eclampsia may be the first presenting feature of underlying pre-eclampsia. Other causes of seizure must also be considered.

HELLP syndrome

This syndrome is the combination of haemolysis, elevated liver enzymes and low platelets (HELLP). It is a laboratory diagnosis with presenting symptoms indistinguishable from those of pre-eclampsia. It occurs in 5–20% of pre-eclampsia, particularly with severe disease [6]. Up to 70% of cases are in the postpartum period [5].

The underlying pathology is a microangiopathic haemolysis with consumptive thrombocytopaenia. Hepatocellular necrosis accounts for the elevated transaminases. Placental abruption, disseminated intravascular coagulation and acute renal failure may result or, less commonly, acute pulmonary oedema, subcapsular liver haematoma and eclampsia.

Table 19.7.4 Features of severe pre-eclampsia

Onset	Less than 32 weeks' gestation
Magnitude of hypertension	sBP ≥170 mmHg or dBP ≥110 mmHg
Renal	Dipstick protein ≥3+ on 2 occasions over 3 hours apart Oliguria <500 mL/day
Neurological	Severe headache Persistent visual symptoms
Hepatic	Severe epigastric or RUQ pain
Haematological	Thrombocytopaenia <100 × 10⁹/L
Pulmonary	Pulmonary oedema
Fetal	Intrauterine growth restriction

SBP: systolic blood pressure; dBP: diastolic blood pressure; RUQ: right upper quadrant.

Table 19.7.5 Investigations and their interpretation in pre-eclampsia

Urinalysis	Proteinuria – dipstick protein of >1+ necessitates follow up with a spot urinary protein:creatinine ratio Abnormal is >30 mg/mmol
Full blood count	Haemolytic anaemia Thrombocytopaenia <100 × 10⁹/L may indicate DIC <50 × 10⁹/L may indicate need for platelet transfusion Haemolytic anaemia with thrombocytopaenia may indicate HELLP syndrome check LFTs
Electrolytes and creatinine	Elevated creatinine
Liver function tests	Transaminases >70 IU/L consistent with hepatic parenchymal damage Raised bilirubin from haemolysis
Lactate dehydrogenase	Raised in haemolysis
Abnormal coagulation profile Fibrinogen level	Evidence of DIC (↓ fibrinogen,↑ FDPs) DIC likely in placental abruption, and hepatic subcapsular haematoma
Group and hold	For RBC and platelet transfusion
Fetal assessment	Ultrasound for oligohydramnios or fetal growth restriction CTG for fetal distress

DIC: disseminated intravascular coagulation; HELLP: haemolysis, elevated liver enzymes and low platelets; LFTs: liver function tests; IU/L: international units per litre; FDPs: fibrinogen degradation products; RBC: red blood cells; CTG: cardiotocograph.

Risk stratification of pre-eclampsia

Risk stratification is essential in the emergency department (ED) approach. Table 19.7.4 shows the features suggestive of severe disease [5].

Investigations

The aim of the investigations is to determine the involvement of organ systems (Table 19.7.5).

Significant proteinuria is defined as ≥0.3 g/day. A 24-hour collection is not always possible and of little use to decisions made in the ED.

SOMANZ recognizes significant proteinuria and hence renal involvement as a spot urine protein:creatinine ratio of >30 mg/mmol. A urine dipstick of greater than 1+ protein mandates following up with this test. A negative spot urinary ratio is a reasonable 'rule out' test for detecting proteinuria of ≥0.3 g/day in hypertensive pregnancy, but does not equate to a 24-hour collection of urinary protein [7].

Management

Delivery of the fetus and placenta is the only definitive treatment. All other measures are symptomatic and have no impact on the progression or the severity of the disease. The timing of delivery is recognized as a fine balance of maternal and fetal factors and the decision to proceed is a multidisciplinary one.

Hypertension

Stabilizing the hypertension is essential to mitigate against the adverse effects on end-organs, in particular to prevent intracerebral haemorrhage [3]. Urgent treatment using parenteral medications is indicated for sBP ≥170 mmHg and/or a dBP ≥110 mmHg (Table 19.7.6).

Target ranges

The target ranges are an sBP of 140–160 mmHg and a dBP of 90–100 mmHg, which are important in reducing the likelihood of a second seizure in the eclamptic patient [3]. Concurrent fetal monitoring is essential.

Oral antihypertensives may be used for hypertension falling outside the severe range, such as labetalol 100–400 mg tds or nifedipine slow release 20–60 mg bd. Methyldopa 250 mg has a slow onset over 24 hours and may cause sedation. Prazosin may cause precipitous orthostatic hypotension with the first dose.

Choice of antihypertensive

As no antihypertensive has been found superior to another, no single drug can be recommended [8]. Hydralazine is commonly used, with efficacy falling between that of nifedipine and labetalol, but it is more likely to cause maternal hypotension, thus a bolus of 250 mL normal saline is recommended.

Although nifedipine is one of the drugs used for the urgent treatment of hypertension, it is not available in parenteral form and the capsular form is no longer available in Australia. Although effective, its onset of action in tablet form is 30–45 minutes.

Infusions may be given for severe or intractable hypertension, such as hydralazine or labetalol. Nitroprusside and glyceryl trinitrite are rarely used in pre-eclampsia.

Some antihypertensives are *not* recommended in pregnancy, such as ACE inhibitors (ACEIs) and angiotensin receptor blockers (ARBs) due to teratogenicity in the first trimester and fetal renal failure and oligohydramnios. Likewise, a diuretic is not recommended

Table 19.7.6   Antihypertensive drugs plus side effects in pre-eclampsia

Drug	Dose	Practice points	Adverse effects
Labetalol	20–50 mg IV	Onset: 5 min Duration: 45 min – 6 h May repeat at 15–30 min	Bronchospasm in asthmatics Heart block
Hydralazine	5–10 mg IV	Onset: 15 min Duration: 2–6 h May repeat in 30 min	Rapid fall in blood pressure Palpitations Fluid bolus first
Diazoxide	15–45 mg IV Maximum: 300 mg	Onset: 5 min Duration: 3–5 h May repeat in 5 min	Flushing, Hyperglycaemia Tachy- or bradycardia Sodium and water retention
Nifedipine	10–20 mg PO	Onset: 30–45 min May repeat after 45 min	Tachycardia Not used in aortic stenosis

Table 19.7.7   Acute management of eclampsia

Acute treatment	Magnesium 4 g IV over 10–15 min Magnesium infusion at 1–2 g/h continued for 24 h *after* the last seizure Diazepam up to 10 mg IV or clonazepam 1–2 mg IV may be used when magnesium is not immediately available
Second seizure	Repeat magnesium 2–4 g IV over 10 min Continue infusion
Monitoring	Cardiorespiratory monitoring Urine output Deep tendon reflexes Fetal monitoring Serum Mg level in renal impairment
Hypertension treatment	Urgent reduction of hypertension to range of <160/<100 mmHg to prevent intracranial haemorrhage and further seizures
Delivery of fetus	Urgent indication for delivery

in pre-eclampsia as the maternal circulatory volume is already reduced. Additionally, β-blockers and calcium channel antagonists other than labetalol and nifedipine are not used in pregnancy.

Eclampsia

Acute treatment

The acute treatment of eclampsia includes standard resuscitation with monitoring and concurrent treatment of the seizure to reduce the risk of intracranial haemorrhage [1,3,4,6].

Magnesium sulphate

Magnesium sulphate (MgSO$_4$) is the first-line drug that reduces the recurrence of eclampsia by 50% [9]. It is superior to both intravenous diazepam [10] or phenytoin [11] in the acute treatment of eclampsia. See Table 19.7.7 for the acute management of eclampsia.

Magnesium acts by slowing neuromuscular conduction and raising the threshold for subsequent seizures. The intravenous form is excreted renally, thus the serum level is important in patients with renal impairment, with the adverse effects of hypermagnesaemia including respiratory depression, bradycardia and sedation. It may cause local tissue necrosis if extravasation occurs. Monitoring for toxicity with serum levels monitoring is recommended for patients with renal impairment.

Bolus doses and duration of infusion

There is no consensus on bolus doses and duration of infusion with magnesium use. No regimen has been shown to be more effective than another [12]. Prophylactic use of magnesium is not routine practice in developed countries. However, in developing countries where maternal and perinatal morbidity and mortality are higher, local practice will determine when prophylaxis is indicated. Indicators may include worsening of hypertension, proteinuria, headache, epigastric pain and/or the onset of hyperreflexia with clonus. Alternatively, it may be given in severe pre-eclampsia during labour, birth and immediately postpartum.

Table 19.7.7 acute management is outlined in accordance with the recommendation from SOMANZ. Local practice may vary. Note that urgent reduction of the hypertension forms part of the acute management.

Delivery of the fetus

Delivery is the definitive treatment for pre-eclampsia. The timing is based on balancing the maternal risks and benefits with those of the fetus. The decision is necessarily multidisciplinary, but severe and/or uncontrollable hypertension and/or worsening of end-organ dysfunction are indications for immediate delivery.

The impact of fetal maturity on perinatal morbidity and mortality is relevant.

Delivery is indicated when the gestation is under 24 weeks or at term. Under 34 weeks, expectant treatment is only indicated in a specialized obstetric unit [3]. After 34 weeks, expectant treatment must be balanced against developing fulminant pre-eclampsia, with the risk in 25–30% of placental abruption, HELLP or pulmonary oedema within 24–48 hours [3].

Intravenous fluid

The use of intravenous fluid in pre-eclampsia is challenging as, although the intravascular volume is reduced, no maternal or fetal benefit above maintenance has been demonstrated. Conversely, there is a risk of pulmonary oedema and the worsening of peripheral oedema, due to the increased vascular permeability and lowered serum albumin. Aim for a urine output of no more than 1 mL/kg/h.

In the event of oliguria, a 250 mL bolus of fluid may lead to improvement, but ongoing management in an intensive care unit (ICU) is needed.

Prevention of pre-eclampsia

Until the pathophysiology is clear, prevention of pre-eclampsia is unlikely to be successful. Pre-eclampsia tends to recur in subsequent pregnancies, with risks of recurrence for pre-eclampsia (7–10%) and gestational hypertension (4–11%) in subsequent pregnancies [6]. Those at greatest risk are patients with severe pre-eclampsia. Additionally, there is an increased lifetime risk of cardiovascular disease, diabetes and hyperlipidaemia.

Currently, low-dose aspirin (75–100 mg) is recommended for pregnancies with a high risk of pre-eclampsia. Calcium supplementation is only recommended for patients with a low calcium diet [3].

References

[1] Preeclampsia Research Laboratories (PEARLS). <www.preeclampsia.org.au/index.php> [Accessed Feb. 2013].

[2] The Royal Women's Hospital, Victoria. Pre-eclampsia. <www.thewomens.org.au/Preeclampsia> [Accessed Feb. 2013].

[3] Lowe SA, Brown MA, Dekker G, et al. Society of Obstetric Medicine of Australia and New Zealand (SOMANZ). Guidelines for the management of hypertensive disorders of pregnancy 2008. <www.somanz.org/pdfs/somanz_guidelines_2008.pdf> [Accessed Feb. 2013].

[4] Vest AR, Cho LS. Hypertension in pregnancy. Cardiol Clin 2012;30:407–23.

[5] Steegers EA, von Dadelszen P, Duvekot JJ, et al. Pre-eclampsia. Lancet 2010;376:631–44.

[6] Deak TM, Moskovitz JB. Hypertension and pregnancy. Emerg Med Clin N Am 2012;30:903–17.

[7] Côté AM, Brown MA, Lam E, et al. Diagnostic accuracy of urinary spot protein:creatinine ratio for proteinuria in hypertensive pregnant women: systematic review. Br Med J 2008. http://dx.doi.org/10.1136/bmj.39532.543947.BE.

[8] Duley L, Henderson-Smart DJ, Meher S. Drugs for treatment of very high blood pressure during pregnancy. Cochrane Database Syst Rev 2006;3:CD001449.

[9] Duley L, Gülmezoglu AM, Henderson-Smart DJ, Chou D. Magnesium sulphate and other anticonvulsants for women with pre-eclampsia. Cochrane Database Syst Rev 2010;11:CD000025.

[10] Duley L, Henderson-Smart DJ, Walker GJA, Chou D. Magnesium sulphate versus diazepam for eclampsia. Cochrane Database Syst Rev 2010;12:CD000127.

[11] Duley L, Henderson-Smart DJ, Chou D. Magnesium sulphate versus phenytoin for eclampsia. Cochrane Database Syst Rev 2010;10:CD000128.

[12] Duley L, Matar HE, Almerie MQ, Hall DR. Alternative magnesium sulphate regimens for women with pre-eclampsia and eclampsia. Cochrane Database Syst Rev 2010;8:CD007388.

OBSTETRICS AND GYNAECOLOGY EMERGENCIES

20 PSYCHIATRIC EMERGENCIES

Edited by **George Jelinek**

20.1 Mental state assessment

George Jelinek • Sylvia Andrew-Starkey

ESSENTIALS

1 Prevalence of mental health disorders appears to be increasing in Western society.

2 Regardless of diagnosis and presentation, three brief risk assessments must be performed within the first few minutes of an individual's arrival in the emergency department (ED). These are:
- suicide risk assessment
- violence risk assessment
- absconding risk assessment.

3 The role of organic illness presenting as a behavioural disorder should not be forgotten.

4 Substance use/misuse resulting in presentations to EDs also appears to be increasing in the general population.

Epidemiology

Mental health disorders are one of the three leading causes of total burden of disease and injury in Australia, alongside cancer and cardiovascular disease [1–3]. In middle age, it is the leading cause of non-fatal disease burden in the Australian population. There is no doubt that mental health disorders have a high prevalence, are disabling and are high cost in both human and socioeconomic terms [1,2].

In terms of disability, it has been estimated that having moderate to severe depression is the equivalent of having congestive cardiac failure [3], chronic severe asthma or chronic hepatitis B [2]. Severe post-traumatic stress syndrome was comparable to the disability from paraplegia and severe schizophrenia was comparable to quadriplegia, in terms of disability [2]. Over the 10 years to 2007, emergency department (ED) presentations rose 8% in the USA, whereas mental health presentations for the same time period rose 38%, contributing significantly to ED overcrowding [4]. This trend has been mirrored in Australia.

Contributing to this may be:

- lack of private health insurance
- lack of social supports
- lack of alternatives to care
- 24-hour accessibility of the ED [4].

The Australian Institute of Health and Welfare report into Mental Health Services in 2012 estimated that there were nearly a quarter of a million occasions of service to Australian EDs in 2009/10 where the primary problem was thought to be due to a mental health disorder, with an average annual increase of 3.6% between 2005–06 and 2009–10 [1]. A little over 3% of Australian public hospital ED presentations are for mental health related problems, correlating well with other studies and US figures, which estimate 2–6% of emergency medicine presentations are primarily due to mental health disorders [4–7].

Two-thirds of these people are between the ages of 15 and 44 years (compared to 42% for the general population presenting to a suburban ED); 29% have anxiety and neurotic disorders, 21% mental and behavioural disorders due to psychoactive substance abuse, 19% mood disorders and 17% schizophrenia or delusional disorders [4].

This is a significant underestimate of the prevalence of mental health disease in the ED as many patients remain undiagnosed and many have active medical conditions and a mental health diagnosis may be secondary [6].

It is estimated that 17.7% of adult Australians admitted to hospital report a mental health issue in the previous 12 months. An estimated 0.4–0.7% of the adult population suffer from a psychotic episode in any 1 year [2]. Mental health issues are highly prevalent and relevant.

Introduction to the mental state examination

The mainstreaming of mental health patients into general EDs has brought problems and anxieties for staff. Staff often feel a lack of confidence because they are dealing with a population of patients unfamiliar to them. They can also feel inadequate due to poor assessment skills [7,8].

Recent Australian studies have shown ED clinicians are most concerned about knowledge gaps in risk assessment, particularly related to self-harm, violence and aggression, and distinguishing psychiatric from physical illness [9]. ED clinicians routinely report the need for more education on mental health related presentations [10]. A high proportion of mental health patients have drug and alcohol intoxication. This confounds the evaluation and treatment, lengthens the stay of these patients within the ED and delays their disposition.

Mental health patients can be assigned lower triage categories and longer waits to be seen by staff than mainstream patients and there is more variation in triage categorization for mental health patients [11]. They have a higher chance of leaving before assessment has begun or is complete and the overall increase in length of assessment time has the potential to increase violence in the ED [7,8].

With this in mind, there has been much work over the last 10 years on the assessment of mental health patients in a general ED.

Bias and discrimination

It is important for health professionals assessing the mentally ill to be aware of their own potential biases. An interviewer's past history and personal beliefs can influence a mental state assessment and the interviewer should be aware of this. These beliefs may stem from past personal or professional experience (Table 20.1.1).

ABC of the MSE

A mental state examination (MSE) is analogous to the management of severe trauma. There is an initial risk assessment looking for immediately life-threatening risks to the patient or staff. The triage nurse and the treating doctor should then obtain a brief collateral history from the emergency services or carers and initial management is based on this assessment. Regardless of threat, all assessments should balance the safety of both patient and staff with privacy and dignity [7].

Assessment should be based on [12]:

- appearance and affect
- behaviour
- conversation
- drug and/or alcohol intoxication.

If the situation is relatively controlled, the formal mental health assessment should then take place. Further information is gathered from the community. A provisional assessment and management plan is developed in conjunction with the mental health team and appropriate disposition is arranged (Fig. 20.1.1).

Triage

The Mental Health Triage Scale (Table 20.1.2) has been developed and modified to be included into the Australian Triage Scale (ATS) [7,13,14]. It is very broad and asks the triage nurse to make four assessments: risk of suicide/self-harm, risk of aggression/harm to others, risk of absconding and whether the patient is intoxicated. From this, the triage nurse determines the ATS and urgency of initial treatment. It is also helpful to determine if the patient is known to a mental health service.

Many centres have developed a triage risk assessment proforma. For ease of use, many of these have included 'tick box' areas. A compilation of multiple assessment tools used throughout Australia is shown in Tables 20.1.3–20.1.5 [2,5,12–15].

It is recommended that any patient who scores 'high risk' in any one area or 'medium

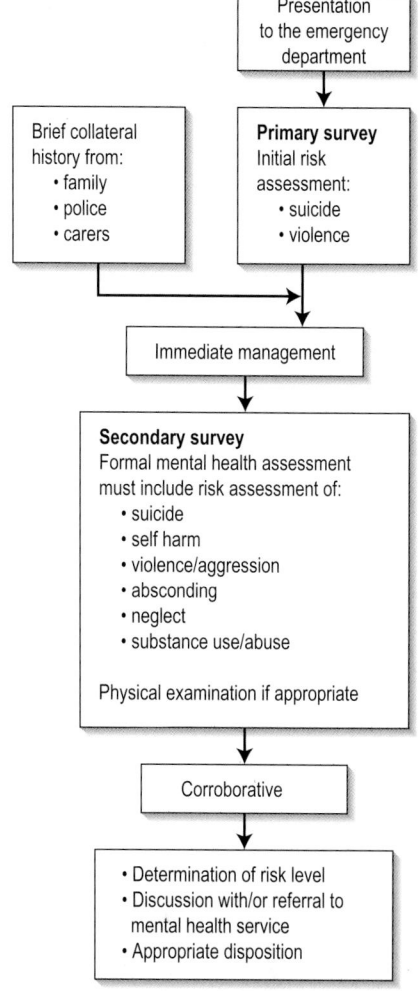

Fig. 20.1.1 The mental health assessment process.

risk' in two areas is treated as a 'high-risk' patient. Ensuing management of 'high-risk' patients depends on: local protocols, levels and presence of security, police intervention, restraint and sedation guidelines and guidelines for the urgent assessment by ED and/or by mental health services.

Table 20.1.1 Factors which may influence an objective MSE
• Religious beliefs
• Race/ethnicity/cultural beliefs and practices
• Political opinion
• Philosophical beliefs
• Sexual preference or orientation (provided not criminal)
• Promiscuity or immorality
• Intellectual disability
• Intoxication

Table 20.1.2	The mental health triage scale
ATS 2	Patient is violent, aggressive or suicidal, or is a danger to self or others Requires police escort/restraint
ATS 3	Very distressed or acutely psychotic Likely to become aggressive May be a danger to self or others
ATS 4	Long-standing or semi-urgent mental health problem and/or has supporting agency/escort present
ATS 5	Patient has a long-standing non-acute mental health disorder but has no support agency Many require referral to an appropriate community resource

Table 20.1.3 Brief screening suicide risk template

Mental state	☑ Active disease ☑ Depression ☑ Psychosis ☑ Hopelessness/despair/guilt/ shame ☑ Anger/agitation ☑ Impulsivity
Suicide attempts/thoughts	☑ Continual/specific thoughts ☑ Formulated plan ☑ Intent ☑ Past history of attempt with high lethality ☑ Means ☑ Suicide note ☑ Risk of being found ☑ Organizing personal affairs
Substance abuse	☑ Current misuse
Supports	☑ Lack of or hostile relationships
Loss	☑ Recent major loss (even perceived): significant relationship, job, housing, financial difficulties, independence ☑ Recent/new diagnosis of major illness or chronic illness

Patients then stratified into high, medium or low risk

Table 20.1.4 Aggression risk tool

☑ Alert on chart
☑ Previous history of violence/threatening behaviour: verbal or physical
☑ Aggressive behaviour/thoughts
☑ Homicidal ideation
☑ Use of weapons previously
☑ Access to weapons
☑ Intoxicated
☑ Middle-aged male

Patients then stratified into high, medium or low risk

Aims of mental health assessment

The aims of the formal mental health assessment are to determine the following:

- Does the patient have a mental illness?
- Is there a question of safety for the patient or for others?
- Does the patient have insight into the illness?
- Will the patient comply with suggested treatment?
- Can the patient be managed in the community or is hospitalization required?

Table 20.1.5 Risk of absconding

Mode of arrival
☑ Police
☑ Handcuffed
☑ Family/carer coercion
☑ Voluntary
☑ Past history of absconding behaviour
☑ Alert on chart
☑ Verbalizing intent to leave
☑ Lack of insight into illness
☑ Poor/non-compliance with medication

Patients then stratified into high, medium or low risk

Only if all of the above are answered, can management and appropriate disposition be considered.

The formal psychiatric interview

Introduction

The environment in which the mental state assessment is conducted is important. Behaviourally disturbed people tolerate noise poorly and have short concentration spans. The interview room should be quiet, private, make the patient feel safe and the interviewer should avoid all interruptions. These prerequisites are increasingly difficult to attain in current access-blocked environments.

The interviewer should sit at the same level as the patient and impart empathy. The voice should be quiet and calming. The interviewer should use non-judgemental language and open-ended questions [13,16]. It is important that the interviewer also feels safe and secure. If any risk is felt, the interviewer should have security or police present in the room or just outside. Depending on state legislation and hospital policy, the interviewer may request to have the patient searched. The interviewer should also note the nearest duress alarm and may choose to wear a personal alarm. The interviewer should sit within easy access of an exit and should never be boxed into a corner. If an interviewer begins to feel uncomfortable, there is always the option of leaving and returning to complete the assessment at a later stage. All threats, attempts and gestures suggestive of violence should be treated seriously.

First part of the interview: direct questioning

Basic demographic information

The formal interview has become less diagnosis focused and more problem based.

Table 20.1.6 Demographic information required

Age/date of birth
Address
Accommodation history
Other persons in household
Occupation
Occupational history
Social resources: • family, friends, partners • social history
Past medical history
Previous hospital admissions
Previous mental health admissions: • length of stay • type of treatment: medication/ECT • medications on discharge • follow-up arrangements
Forensic history: • trouble with police • jail terms/convictions
Alcohol
Drug use
Tobacco use

Management is centred around the alleviation of symptoms and return to function. Thus, the psychiatric interview has become somewhat less structured.

It is wise to establish rapport with the patient by personal introduction and explaining the purpose of the interview. The interviewer can begin by asking a series of non-threatening questions, such as demographics. This information is often required as many mental health services rely on an appropriate post code to determine follow-up management.

These questions assist by building a profile of lifestyle, relationships and thought processes. Likelihood of success or failure of particular treatment modalities may be assisted by knowledge of previous hospital admissions, both general hospital and mental health (Table 20.1.6).

The process of obtaining a mental health assessment is different to that of a general medical assessment. In a general medical history, a series of questions is asked and the response is written. In a mental health assessment, responses are also interpreted. The interviewer is asked to form an opinion as to how thoughts are processed, based on observations.

The interviewer is asked to interpret the patient's thought patterns by what, and how, the patient tells the interviewer.

Presenting complaint

The patient is asked to recall the sequence of events prior to presentation to the ED. The interviewer should explore the circumstances of the behaviour, reasons for it, degree of planning or impulsivity and its context. Were drugs and alcohol involved? Was there a recent precipitating event? It is often useful to get the patient to recall the previous 48–72 hours leading up to the event.

This usually leads to questioning regarding current difficulties. The interviewer should explore the nature of current problems. They may be financial or legal problems, isolation, bereavement, impending or actual loss, or diagnosis of major illness. Have there been any recent changes and who are their usual support people? An exploration of significant relationships is important along with the depth and duration of these relationships. It is useful to explore the patient's usual coping methods when under stress.

Mood and affect

There should be formal questioning regarding the patient's mood (internal feelings) and whether it is in keeping with affect (external expression). The mood may be incongruent with affect, swing wildly between extremes (labile) or be inappropriate.

Usually mood is assessed by asking about the patient's ability to cope with activities of daily living, such as eating, weight loss or gain, sleep disturbance (early morning wakening or trouble getting to sleep) and general hygiene. The patient's ability to concentrate may also diminish with increasing mood disturbance, reflected by the ability to perform normal work duties.

This may lead to direct questioning regarding mood and thoughts of suicide. It is important to be direct in asking the patient about suicide and whether there is a formulated plan. A well thought out plan with clear means of carrying out threats is of great concern.

Delusions and hallucinations

Delusions and hallucinations are often personal and the patient may not want to disclose intimate thoughts and beliefs to the interviewer. Hallucinations may be auditory, visual, tactile, olfactory, somatic or gustatory. The

context in which they occur should be explored. Hypnagogic (occurring just before sleep) and hypnopompic (occurring on wakening) hallucinations are more benign than others. Common themes for all types of hallucinations include suicide, persecution, religion, control, reference, grandeur or somatization.

Insight and judgement

Insight is the degree of understanding of what is happening and why. This may be:

- denial of illness
- awareness of being sick and needing help but denying it at the same time
- awareness of being sick but blaming it on external factors
- awareness that illness is due to something unknown within the patient
- intellectual insight: admission that the patient is ill and that symptoms are due to irrational feelings, but inability to apply this to the future
- true insight: being aware of motives and feelings and being aware of what can lead to changes in behaviour.

It is important to determine the patient's level of insight. This determines appropriate treatment and management, level of supervision required and the likelihood of compliance with treatment.

Second part of interview: observation

Key elements

The second part of the MSE can be more difficult to conceptualize. It relies on the interviewer actively observing the patient's behaviour and conversation and interpreting thoughts. A summary is given in Table 20.1.7.

This part of the interview can be difficult to remember and different services have developed a multitude of acronyms for remembering the various elements of the remaining mental health assessment. Listed below are two.

ABC of Mental Health Assessment [12]:

- Appearance
- Affect
- Behaviour
- Conversation and mood.

GFCMA – 'Got Four Clients on Monday Afternoon' [13]:

Table 20.1.7 Overview of mental state examination
General description: • appearance • behaviour • attitudes
Mood and affect: • mood • affect • appropriateness
Motivation/energy
Appetite
Sleep
Speech: • perception
Thought process: • form • content
Cognition: • consciousness • orientation • memory • intelligence
Insight and judgement
Impulse control

- General appearance
- Form of thought
- Content of thought
- Mood and affect
- Attitude.

Appearance, attitude and behaviour

This determines the patient's ability to self-care. Table 20.1.8 lists features that may require particular attention. Attitude is important as it may indicate whether a patient is compliant with management and treatment. Abnormal posturing or repetitive behaviours should be noted. These may indicate increasing thought disturbance. With increasing aggression and agitation, there may be motor restlessness, pacing and hand wringing. Tension may escalate rapidly and steps should be taken early to diffuse the situation.

The interviewer should note the rate, volume and rhythmicity of speech. This can range from completely mute, through monosyllabic answers, to rapid, loud speech indicative of pressure of speech. The tone, inflection, content and structure of speech should be noted. The interviewer should determine if the speech is fluent, if the thoughts behind it are logical and whether it flows appropriately for the situation.

Table 20.1.8 Appearance, attitude and behaviour
General: • clothes   • application   • appropriate for climate?
Cleanliness: • general grooming (hair, nails)   • tattoos, track marks on arms
Eye contact: • avoids direct gaze   • decreases with increasing anxiety
Facial expression: • variation in facial expression, voice, use of hands and body movements
Reaction to interviewer: • aggressive, submissive, cooperative, guarded, evasive, passive or hostile
Motor: • restless   • repetitive behaviour, e.g. rocking, hand wringing   • tremor   • posturing   • tics   • tardive dyskinesia
Speech: • rate, volume and rhythm   • mute   • poverty of speech (slow, monosyllabic responses)   • pressure of speech (extremely rapid, loud speech)   • normal inflection or flat and monotonous

Table 20.1.9 Thought disorders	
Circumstantiality	Delays in reaching goals by long-winded explanations, but eventually gets there
Distractible speech	Changes topic according to what is happening around the patient
Loosening of associations	Logical thought progression does not occur and ideas shift from one subject to another with little or no association between them
Flight of ideas	Fragmented, rapid thoughts that the patient cannot express fully as they are occurring at such a rapid rate
Tangentiality	Responses that superficially appear appropriate, but which are completely irrelevant or oblique
Clanging	Speech where words are chosen because they rhyme and do not make sense
Neologisms	Creation of new words with no meaning except to the patient
Thought blocking	Interruption to thought process where thoughts are absent for a few seconds and are unable to be retrieved

Thought disorder

This is speech that does not reach its goal, is not fluent and is interrupted often with many pauses or changes in direction. A list with explanations is given in Table 20.1.9.

Thought content

There are often recurrent themes in the speech of an acutely disturbed patient. These may revolve around suicide, persecution, control, reference, religion or somaticism (the extremes of which are nihilistic delusions – the belief that part of the self does not exist, is dead or decaying) or they may be grandiose in nature.

Perception

A patient may be actively hallucinating despite denying this on questioning. It is important to note if the patient's eyes suddenly switch direction for no apparent reason or they appear to be listening to a voice. These movements are often quite subtle and easily missed if observation is not active.

Cognitive assessment and physical examination

A formal examination of cognitive function and a thorough physical examination complete the full psychiatric assessment. The interviewer should ensure that the patient does not have an acute confusional state secondary to a physical condition that may account for a behavioural problem.

A number of tools are available to assess cognitive functioning. These comprise assessments in orientation, concentration, memory, language, abstraction and judgement. An assessment of a patient's cognitive functioning and intelligence may assist in deciding the best way to deal with problems.

Approximately 20% of mental health patients have a concurrent active medical disorder requiring treatment and possibly contributing to the acute behavioural disturbance [6]. Investigations depend on physical findings but may include creatine kinase, urine drug screen, electroencephalogram, computed tomography and lumbar puncture. Only after this can an emergency medicine practitioner plan the most appropriate management.

Conclusion

Although time consuming, a good mental health assessment is vital for the appropriate management and disposition of what is an increasingly large group of patients in the ED. If able to formulate an opinion on the risk assessments regarding suicide, violence and flight risk and the aims of the MSE, the emergency clinician will be able to present to mental health services a comprehensive picture of the patient.

The mental health professional is then able to administer mental health first aid [2], the principles of which are:

- assess the risk of suicide/harm to others
- listen non-judgementally
- give reassurance and information
- encourage getting professional help
- encourage self-help strategies.

Controversies

- Whereas most general hospitals have integrated the assessment of mental health patients within the ED, there is now a growing trend towards the development of stand-alone psychiatric emergency centres – a separate area attached to the ED where mental health patients are assessed after initial triage. This is staffed by dedicated mental health professionals and has the potential to deskill emergency medicine personnel, both nursing and medical. It is uncertain whether this model or mainstreaming is more effective in the management of mental health patients.
- Despite an overall improvement in assessments, mainstreaming of mental health patients has exposed them to the increasing levels of access block within general hospitals and increasing overcrowding in EDs. This has resulted in mental health patients spending prolonged periods of time in the ED while waiting for inpatient beds to become available. This has the potential

for increased violence, unnecessary use of sedation and increased morbidity and mortality of mental health patients while placing other patients, their carers and staff members at unnecessary risk.

References

[1] The Australian Institute of Health and Welfare. Mental health provided in emergency departments (updated Aug 2012). Canberra: Australian Institute of Health and Welfare; 2012. <http://mhsa.aihw.gov.au/services/emergency-departments/> [Accessed Mar. 2013].

[2] Kitchener B, Jorm A. Mental health first aid manual. Melbourne: Orygen Research Centre; 2002.

[3] Clinical Practice Guidelines Team for Depression, Royal Australian and New Zealand College of Psychiatrists Australian and New Zealand clinical practices. Practice guidelines for the treatment of depression. Aust NZ J Psychiatr 2004;38:389–407.

[4] Larkin GL, Classen CA, et al. Trends in US Emergency Departments. Visits for mental health conditions, 1992–2001. Psychiatr Serv 2005;56:671–7.

[5] Crowe M, Carlyle D. Deconstructing risk assessment and management in mental health nursing. J Adv Nurs 2003;43:19–27.

[6] ACEP Clinical Policies Subcommittee. Clinical policy: critical issues in the diagnosis and management of the adult psychiatric patient in the emergency department. Ann Emerg Med 2006;47:79–99.

[7] Smart D, Pollard C, Walpole B. Mental health triage in emergency medicine. Aust NZ J Psychiatr 1999;33:57–66.

[8] Happell B, Summers M, Pinikahana J. Measuring the effectiveness of the national Mental Health Triage Scale in an emergency department. Internatl J Mental Hlth Nurs 2003;12:288–92.

[9] Jelinek GA, Weiland T, Mackinlay C, et al. Knowledge and confidence of Australian emergency department clinicians in managing patients with mental health-related presentations: findings from a national qualitative study. Internatl J Emerg Med 2012;6:2.

[10] Weiland T, Mackinlay C, Hill N, et al. Optimal management of mental health patients in Australian emergency departments: barriers and solutions. Emerg Med Australas 2011;24:667–88.

[11] Gerdtz MF, Hill N, Weiland TJ, et al. Perspectives of emergency department staff on the triage of mental health related presentations: implications for education, policy and practice. Emerg Med Australas 2012;24:492–500.

[12] McSherry B. Risk July 2004 Assessment by mental health professionals and the prevention of future violent behaviour. Australian Government: Australian Institute of Criminology.

[13] NSW Department of Health. Framework for suicide risk assessment and management. Emergency Department Online. <www.health.nsw.gov.au>; 2004.

[14] Department of Health and Ageing. Emergency triage education kit. Australian Government; 2007; 37–48.

[15] Department of Human Services, Victorian Emergency Department. Mental health triage tool. <www.health.vic.gov.au/emergency/mhtriagetool.pdf> [Accessed Mar. 2013].

[16] Meyers J, Stein S. The psychiatric interview in the emergency department. Emerg Med Clin N Am 2000;18:173–83.

20.2 Distinguishing medical from psychiatric causes of mental disorder presentations

David Spain

ESSENTIALS

1 Morbidity and health costs are reduced by correct distinction of medical from psychiatric causes of mental disorder in presentations to emergency departments.

2 The question of whether any medical condition exists in addition to the psychiatric complaints should be asked. This will identify most medical causes of mental disorder.

3 Missed medical diagnosis is most commonly associated with failure to undertake an adequate medical history, mental state examination and physical examination.

4 Substance-related disorders are most easily identified on direct or collateral history.

5 The presence of delirium or other significant cognitive defects makes an organic or substance-related illness almost certain.

6 The diagnosis of delirium may require repeated assessments over time.

Introduction

Emergency physicians often assess patients who have suspected mental disorder. The critical question posed is: what is the cause of this? Causes are many but broadly include psychiatric, medical, intoxication and behavioural. Identifying the likely cause and careful consideration of the capability of local facilities usually leads to correct disposition, reducing medical costs and morbidity [1]. In practice, emergency physicians need a simple classification defining the principal diagnosis of the presenting mental disorder consistent with the Diagnostic and Statistical Manual of Mental Disorders, 4th edition (DSM-IV) terminology. This allows us to communicate with psychiatric colleagues and should assist diagnostic, management and disposition accuracy. Table 20.2.1 is such a suggested classification.

This patient group is diverse and many factors increase the difficulty of assessment including poor cooperation, intoxication, violence and minimal information referrals. Additionally, many presentations are subtle, can mimic other conditions and may not have absolute or clear distinguishing criteria. The historical approach of 'medical clearance' aims to screen for emergent medical causes that are unsuitable for psychiatric care. Medical issues are traditionally called organic. That terminology persists but is increasingly challenged by a postulated medical basis for some psychiatric disorders. Medical clearance has been used for over 30 years, but there is still no accepted universal agreement of what that means or should entail. Overall, the process should be considered an imperfect risk reduction strategy.

Table 20.2.1   A simple classification of principal diagnosis of mental disorder for emergency physicians

DSM-IV terminology	Broad traditional clinical grouping	Likely principal management and disposition
Axis 1		
Clinical disorder due to a general medical disorder	Organic	Medical
Delirium, dementia and amnestic and other cognitive disorders	Organic	Medical
Substance-related disorder – intoxication or withdrawal disorder	Organic	Medical
Substance-related disorder – substance induced persistent disorder	Organic	Psychiatric
Clinical disorder (not identified to above or axis II principal diagnosis)	Psychiatric	Psychiatric

Table 20.2.2   Triage safety questions [8]

Is the patient a danger to him- or herself?
Is the patient at risk of leaving before assessment?
Is the patient a danger to others?
Is the area safe? Does the patient need to be searched?

Pollard C. Psychiatry reference book – nursing staff. Hobart: Department of Emergency Medicine Royal Hobart Hospital; 1994 with permission.

General approach

Patients with abnormal behaviour labelled as psychiatric after routine medical and psychiatric assessment frequently have a final diagnosis of a medical cause or precipitant for the mental disorder. The incidence of missed medical diagnosis ranges between 8 and 46% [1–3]. One study of first psychiatric presentations found a higher rate of medical diagnosis of 63% [4]. Deciding whether a particular presentation of mental disorder is medical or psychiatric is often difficult, as there are very few absolutes that distinguish medical from psychiatric illness. Careful collection and weighting of appropriate information commonly only leads to a differential diagnosis.

Some diagnoses and dispositions can be determined quickly after a medical and psychiatric history, with the addition of a mental state and full physical examination. This may sometimes take place without expensive diagnostic procedures. Other presentations are difficult and require extensive and intensive evaluation, repeat evaluation, observation in hospital and significant investigations before the diagnosis is clear.

Medical clearance in emergency departments (EDs) can be inaccurate due to the presence of intoxicating substances or patient factors that limit necessary assessments. A non-judgemental approach with prudent intervention based on known or likely risks, close monitoring in a safe environment and repeated reassessment of physical and mental state over time are often necessary to obtain an accurate diagnosis and optimal outcome.

Studies on medical clearance by ED staff, primary-care physicians and psychiatrists have repeatedly shown a poor ability to discover medical conditions. This failure is commonly due to one or more of the following factors: inadequate history; failure to seek alternative information from relatives, carers and old records; poor attention to physical examination, including vital signs; absence of a reasonable mental state examination; uncritical acceptance of medical clearance by receiving psychiatric staff; and failure to re-evaluate over time [5]. One study noted that medical conditions were most easily identified in the ED by the triage nurse or medical officer asking whether any medical conditions existed in addition to the patient's psychiatric complaints [6].

Evaluation requires a thorough approach and a commitment of time and effort. Special skills are required for medical clearance and psychiatric interview. A coordinated and focused medical and psychiatric assessment has the highest yield of correct diagnoses [1]. Proformas or clinical pathways may improve compliance and documentation of important details, but have not been clearly demonstrated to improve patient outcomes [7].

National Emergency Access Targets (NEAT) in Australia will change the management of mental disorder clients. The approaches will vary dependent on institutional capabilities and local agreements. Universal medical clearance for every patient presenting will be unlikely, with many known psychiatric patients being triaged directly for psychiatric assessment. Additionally, medical processing when required will need to occur concurrently with psychiatric assessments, thus replacing traditional sequential processing where medical assessment and often investigation precedes psychiatric involvement. High yield presentations for organic disease will be directed to Medical Assessment Units when available to allow investigations, observation and reassessment over a reasonable period of time.

Triage

Triage is vital, as many patients presenting with apparent psychiatric problems have medical conditions. Correct identification at the point of entry by nursing staff facilitates correct management and reduces morbidity and mortality. Many patients with psychiatric illness are also a significant risk to themselves or others and require urgent intervention. Questions regarding safety should always be raised (Table 20.2.2) [8].

Nursing staff should use a triage checklist to identify likely organic presentations (Table 20.2.3). These are indications for urgent medical assessment. If these are absent and a psychiatric diagnosis is likely, then an appropriate urgency rating by Australasian Triage Scale for psychiatric presentations should be applied. This triage categorization for psychiatric presentations has been developed and verified and allows reasonable waiting time standards for urgency to be applied in Triage Category 2–5 (Table 20.2.4) [9]. A Triage Category 1 when there is severe behavioural disturbance with immediate threat of serious violence has been sensibly added to that scale by the Australasian College for Emergency Medicine.

Triage should consider patient privacy issues if the history obtained is to be accurate. Collateral information from the carers with the patient should always be diligently obtained, carefully considered and documented. This information should allow the patient to be placed in an appropriate and safe environment where continuing visual and nursing observations can occur while further assessment occurs. An emerging trend is to use nursing

PSYCHIATRIC EMERGENCIES

Table 20.2.3 High-yield indicators of organic illness
First presentation of mental disorder or distinctly different mental disorder in patient with known psychiatric illness

Delirium
  Abrupt onset change in mental state
    Hours to days
    Fluctuates
  Change in cognition
    Disorientation
    Memory deficit
    Language disturbance
  Disturbance of consciousness
    Fluctuating or decreased
    Poor attention
  Perceptual disturbance
    Hallucinations (especially visual)
    Illusions
    Misinterpretations

Drug or alcohol use
  Recreational/illicit
  Overdose
  Prescribed or over-the-counter

Recent or new medical problems
Neurological signs or symptoms
Abnormal vital signs

Table 20.2.4 Guidelines for Australasian Triage Scale coding for psychiatric presentations [9]
Emergency: Category 2
Patient is violent, aggressive or suicidal or is a danger to self or others or requires police escort
Urgent: Category 3
Very distressed or acutely psychotic, likely to become aggressive, may be a danger to self or others. Experiencing a situation crisis
Semi-urgent: Category 4
Long-standing or semi-urgent mental health disorder and/or has a supporting agency/escort present (e.g. community psychiatric nurse*)
Non-urgent: Category 5
Long-standing or non-acute mental disorder or problem, but the patient has no supportive agency or escort. Many require a referral to an appropriate community resource

*It is considered advantageous to 'up triage' mental health patients with carers present because carers' assistance facilitates more rapid assessment.
Smart D, Pollard C, Walpole B. Mental Health triage in emergency medicine. Aust NZ J Psychiatr 1999;33:57–66 with permission.

triage immediately to refer likely psychiatric presentations to mental health clinicians without formal medical clearance. This method identifies clients who have presented with an aggravated or past similar psychiatric condition, who have normal vital signs, without recent medical concerns and who are not under the influence of drugs or alcohol. This streaming will become more widespread with National Emergency Access Targets and appears effective and efficient for both patient and clinicians. These triage referral systems require a medical safety net if referral was inappropriate. They have been operating now for some years without obvious increase in adverse outcomes. They are yet to be validated by scientific studies.

The interview environment

A climate of trust is very important, as many details of the psychiatric interview are quite sensitive. The psychiatric interview should take place in as quiet and private an environment as possible. The choice of the interview site may be limited in emergencies to ensure safety for both patient and staff.

History

A careful traditional medical history is the most common identifier of medical illness as a cause of a mental disorder presentation. Substance-related disorders are also most easily identified on history. A careful drug history, including prescribed, recreational and over-the-counter medications, should always be included. A slow onset and a previous psychiatric history are more commonly associated with psychiatric illness. Conversely, rapid onset, no premorbid decline and no past psychiatric history favour a medical cause. Poor recall of recent events may indicate delirium.

Family history is often a key indicator of psychiatric or medical cause. For example, a newly depressed 30-year-old man with a family history of Huntington's disease or porphyria is more likely to have a physical cause. Conversely, an 18-year-old man with a hypomanic presentation and a strong family history of bipolar disorder is more likely to have a psychiatric cause. Suicidal and homicidal risk should be assessed routinely to ensure safety. Escalating immediate risk can often be recognized by combining patient perceived lethality and inquiry about any transition from thoughts, to actual plans and finally to actions. For patients with previous psychiatric illness, the system review is a useful screen for organic illness.

HIV is an increasingly important area as HIV-related illness becomes the new great mimic of modern psychiatry and medicine. Practices likely to have put the patient at risk should be explored. These may have been in the distant past. Known positive HIV status always warrants assessment for an organic cause of any new behavioural disturbance. Clinically, these problems often initially present with symptoms of mild anxiety or depression. Many treatable medical causes are only evident after significant investigations.

Delirium, a highly specific but not absolute indicator of medical or substance-induced disorders, should always be sought. By definition, this requires a history of recent onset and of fluctuation over the course of the day. Classically, there will be subtle changes in level of consciousness or the sleep–wake cycle. Patients may not be able to attend sufficiently to give this history if delirious. The psychiatric history, including life profile, may give evidence of the presence or absence of premorbid decline. An abrupt onset of abnormal behaviour with no premorbid decline is more suggestive of an organic cause.

Collateral history

Collateral history is important as the patient is not always capable of or willing to give full information. This history often crystallizes a diagnosis that would otherwise be uncertain or completely missed. Previous discharge summaries may provide relevant information regarding alcohol and drug use, previous behaviour and diagnosis. The family should be asked to bring in all medications, including over-the-counter items. Family, friends and caregivers may give more rapid access to collateral history than waiting for past admission details. Family and friends may be the only source for obtaining a history of a patient's fluctuating mental status suggesting delirium, even when the patient appears quite lucid in the ED.

Examination

Lack of attention to important details of the examination is a frequently identified cause of missed medical illness. Areas that commonly yield positive findings, but which are frequently omitted, are the neurological examination, a search for general or specific appearances of endocrine disease, the toxidromes, examination for signs of malignancy, drugs or alcohol abuse and vital sign examination. Poor cooperation can prevent detailed examination and should be documented so that future consulting clinicians are aware of a deficient entry examination.

Vital signs

Abnormal vital signs are frequently the only abnormality found on examination of patients with serious underlying medical disease. They must always be acknowledged and explained. Pulse oximetry should be included rapidly to exclude hypoxia. A bedside blood sugar level should be routine for patients with abnormal behaviour.

Mental state examination

This is an account of objective findings of mental state signs made at the time of interview. It is the psychiatric equivalent of the medical examination and specifically details the current status. Observations made by other staff in the department, such as hallucinations, may be very significant and can be included with the source identified. Careful consideration of the mental status frequently clearly distinguishes medical from psychiatric illness and guides further investigation and management. For example, the presence of delirium or other significant cognitive defects make an organic illness almost certain. Disorientation is highly suggestive of delirium. Delirium can be very subtle. Sometimes, owing to the fluctuating nature, the patient may appear normal on a single interview. Other less obvious features, such as lability of mood, variability of motor activity or lapses in patient concentration making the interview more difficult, can be the only clues and can be easily overlooked. The importance of formulation using collateral history

and repeated mental state examination is stressed. Documentation is important so that mental status changes with time during repeat assessment can be appreciated.

Examination tools

Cognitive defects may be rapidly and reliably identified in the ED during mental status examination by the use of Folstein's Mini Mental State Examination (MMSE) [10]. A score of less than 20 suggests an organic aetiology. A fall of two or more points on serial MMSE is highly suggestive of delirium. Elderly patients with delirium or cognitive defects are frequently not recognized by emergency physicians. These patients are at high risk of morbidity and mortality [11]. Simple assessment methods, such as the confusion assessment method (CAM), are rapid, reliable methods of identifying delirium in older patients, suitable for ED use [12]. Use of such simple methods should be encouraged to reduce inappropriate disposition. The tests above are suitable screening tools for EDs but are not intended to replace formal neuropsychological assessment. Proformas of medical history, mental state examination and physical examination may improve thoroughness of assessment and documentation.

Investigations

Investigations should always be guided by clinical findings and must be tailored to each individual presentation. A combined Massachusetts Emergency Physician and Psychiatry Task Force in 2009 identified criteria for low medical risk. Patients must meet all criteria. The criteria were adults aged 15–55, no acute medical complaints, no new psychiatric or physical symptoms, no evidence of substance abuse pattern, normal vital signs, normal gait and speech with normal memory and concentration. Patients with low medical risk were not recommended for any routine testing in the ED as they are of very low yield.

First presentations and suspicion of a medical cause that needs to be confirmed or excluded are the major indications for emergency investigations. Baseline blood tests, such as full blood profile, blood sugar level, electrolytes, liver function tests, calcium and thyroid function tests, may at times detect clinically unsuspected problems. Examination and culture of urine and cerebrospinal fluid should

be undertaken if occult infection is considered a possible cause. A urine drug screen may on occasion be the only way to confirm clinical suspicions of drug-related illness. Time delays for results, low specificity from cross-reactivity and uncertainty caused by drugs with long half-lives limit their usefulness. Newer drug-screening stat tests at the bedside may improve their usefulness in the ED. Mandatory brain computed tomography (CT) is not indicated, but the threshold for imaging in first presentations of altered mental state without obvious cause should be low. HIV and syphilis testing should be done on all patients with significant risk profile. Herpes encephalitis may not produce imaging changes but should be considered when fever, delirium or cognitive changes are present with sudden alterations in behaviour. Newer imaging modalities, such as magnetic resonance imaging, magnetic resonance spectroscopy, positron emission tomography and single-photon emission CT, continue as research tools but may have a role in the future. Electroencephalogram examination is rarely a current ED test for psychiatric patients.

Diagnostic formulation

Emergency physicians should suspect organic disease until proved otherwise. In particular, reversible medical causes of abnormal mental state should be sought. Proformas improve documentation and summation. Consideration of the factors in Table 20.2.5 may help to determine doubtful cases. There are few absolutes that distinguish organic from psychiatric patients. Use of the five-axis DSM-IV system improves the ability to look at the patient's presentation in the context of total functioning. It also allows emergency physicians to communicate with psychiatric peers in the recognized language.

Some patients require periods of observation, re-examination and further investigations before a definitive answer is obtained. Intoxicated patients frequently are not assessable till sober. NEAT will pressure hospitals to look for safe disposition sites for this often difficult patient group. Interim care and disposition varies depending on presentation, prior history and facilities available. A common expectation of emergency physicians for patients referred to psychiatrists is to document that the patient is 'medically cleared'. The assessment is known to be imprecise and difficult [1–4,7]. Better documentation is to state that the ED

Table 20.2.5 Factors influencing the likelihood of medical or psychiatric illness as the principal diagnosis

Organic	Psychiatric
Abnormal vital signs	Family history of psychiatry disorder
Age >40 with first psychosis	Past psychiatric illness
Delirium	Fully orientated
Conscious level fluctuates	Clear sensorium
Inability to attend	
Memory impaired	
Impaired cognitive abilities	Intact cognition
Neurological signs, e.g. dysarthria	
Abnormal physical signs	
Abrupt onset	Slow onset
Dramatic change in general status (hours to days)	Premorbid slow deterioration in employment/family/socially
Recent medical problem	Recent significant life event
Medication, drugs/alcohol/withdrawal	Non-compliance psychiatric medication
Marked new personality changes	
Visual, tactile or olfactory hallucinations more common Agitation/irritability HIV/AIDS Failed psychiatric treatment	Auditory hallucinations more common especially: Voices arguing Voices commentary Two voices discussing Audible thoughts
Disorganized delusions	Structured delusions
Movement disorders	Somatic passivity experiences
Perseveration	
Confabulation	
Illusions or misinterpretations	
Circumstantiality	
Concretism	Thought withdrawal, insertion or broadcasting
FH degenerative brain disease	
FH heritable metabolic	

FH: family history.

assessment has revealed no evidence of an emergent medical problem that would preclude admission to psychiatric care.

Conclusion

A thorough medical history, psychiatric history, collateral history, physical examination, mental state examination and judicious specific investigation will identify most patients likely to have an underlying physical cause for a mental disorder presentation. Omission of any of these steps may lead to missed medical diagnosis and incorrect disposition.

Controversies and future directions

- Where and when assessment of mental disorder ideally occurs is somewhat controversial. Urgent assessment in the traditional hospital-based general ED with strict medical clearance is ideal and safest for rapid and new onset illness. Patient volume and time demands with resource restraints are forcing alternative models for entry to care. Many EDs are triaging patients in crisis as likely medical, emergent psychiatric or non-emergent psychiatric. Depending on local service availability, early streaming based on this triage allows many psychiatric clients (some emergent and most non-emergent) to be directed away from the ED to appropriate community mental health services. Additionally, community-based psychiatric services are increasingly managing acute episodes of behaviour disorder in the community without the need for hospitalization or emergency department involvement. Hard outcome studies are yet to be undertaken on these new models.

- Driven by new access targets, there is some pressure for early referral to an acute care psychiatric team after triage, rather than all mental disorder patients receiving medical clearance by a doctor. Many believe that this has produced significant benefits to patients, with shorter waiting times and better psychiatric assessments by psychiatric trained nurses and psychologists when compared to junior medical staff. Experience to date indicates they need ready access to safety net medical systems and consultant psychiatric supervision to operate effectively and safely.

- Providing adequate resources and a safe physical environment for assessment, management and disposition of the rapidly escalating number of patients with substance-related disorder is a major ED challenge. Assessments during intoxication are typically unhelpful. Intoxication may last hours to days and require medical therapy. NEAT targets will likely force new care pathways for this patient group. Some health services are exploring memorandums of understanding with local police services to care for selected high-risk clients until sober.

References

[1] Hoffman RS. Diagnostic errors in the evaluation of behavioural disorders. J Am Med Assoc 1982;248:964–7.

[2] Koranyi EK. Morbidity and rate of undiagnosed physical illnesses in a psychiatric clinic population. Arch Gen Psychiatr 1979;36:414–9.

[3] Hall RC, Popkin MK, Devaul RA, et al. Physical illness presenting as psychiatric disease. Arch Gen Psychiatr 1978;35:1315–20.

[4] Henneman PL, Mendoza R, Lewis RJ. Prospective evaluation of emergency department medical clearance. Ann Emerg Med 1994;24:672–7.

[5] Tintinalli JE, Peacock FW, Wright MA. Emergency medical evaluation of psychiatric patients. Ann Emerg Med 1994;23:859–62.

[6] Olshaker JS, Browne B, Jerrard DA, et al. Medical clearance and screening of psychiatric patients in the emergency department. Acad Emerg Med 1997;4:124–8.

[7] Zun LS, Downey L. Prospective medical clearance of psychiatric patients. Primary Psychiatr 2008;15:60–6.

[8] Pollard C. Psychiatry reference book – nursing staff. Hobart: Department of Emergency Medicine Royal Hobart Hospital; 1994.

[9] Smart D, Pollard C, Walpole B. Mental health triage in emergency medicine. Aust NZ J Psychiatr 1999;33:57–66.

[10] Folstein MF, Folstein SE, McHugh PR. 'Mini Mental State': a practical method for grading the cognitive state of patients for the clinician. J Psychiatr Res 1975;12:189–98.

[11] Trzepacz P, McIntyre Charles SC, et al. Practice guideline for the treatment of patients with delirium. Am J Psychiatr 1999;156:1–20.

[12] Inouye SK, van Dyck CH, Alessi CA, et al. Clarifying confusion. The confusion assessment method. A new method for detection of delirium. Ann Intern Med 1990;113:941–8.

20.3 Deliberate self-harm/suicide

Jennie Hutton • Grant Phillips • Peter Bosanac

ESSENTIALS

1 Deliberate self-harm is a frequent presentation to emergency departments and is a symptom of diverse underlying problems, be they biological, social or psychological.

2 Patients with deliberate self-harm form a heterogeneous group, most of whom do not have ongoing suicidal behaviour.

3 Assessment of suicide risk following deliberate self-harm is to inform treatment, to identify risks amenable to intervention and protective factors. It involves assessment of background demographic, psychiatric, medical and psychosocial factors.

4 There is no 'gold standard' for suicide risk assessment and level of risk can change quickly.

5 The most consistent factors predicting fatal and non-fatal repetition following deliberate self-harm are psychiatric illness, personality disorder, substance abuse, multiple previous and types of attempts, hopelessness, social disconnectedness and intoxication.

6 Management requires coordinated care with emergency, mental health and primary care clinicians, as well as carers.

7 A planned strategy to deal with these patients should address triage, restraint and observation, medical and suicide risk assessment, treatment and disposition.

8 The legal framework for the location in which individuals practice should be known and considered.

Introduction

Suicide is a deliberate act of intentional self-inflicted death. It is the most extreme manifestation of deliberate self-harm, where the spectrum also comprises suicidal ideation, plans and intent. Although suicide is uncommon, 10% of people who commit suicide are seen in an emergency department (ED) in the month prior to death, with a substantial proportion not having psychosocial assessment, thus providing an opportunity for intervention [1,2]. The major ED impact, however, is in the identification and assessment of large numbers of patients potentially at risk of suicide, with initial management of co-morbidities and modifiable risk factors.

Deliberate self-harm (DSH) is a maladaptive response to internal distress and may not have suicidal intent; it may, however, indicate a risk for suicide. Deliberate self-harm is a common ED presentation (approximately 0.4% of all ED visits [3]) and the goals of management include treatment of the physical health sequelae, assessment of risk of non-fatal or fatal repetition and diagnosing and commencing treatment of potentially reversible psychosocial causes.

Epidemiology

In Australia, there were approximately 2300 deaths per year from suicide in 2010, with age-standardized rates of approximately 16.4 per 100 000 in males and 4.8 in females (Table 20.3.1) [4]. Suicide accounts for 1.6% of deaths in Australia. Suicide remains the leading cause of death among Australians between 15 and 34 years of age. Despite some decreases in suicide rate over the past decade, suicide remains a major external cause of death, accounting for more deaths than road traffic crashes [5].

Across OECD (Organisation for Economic Cooperation and Development) countries, suicide rates were lowest in Greece, Mexico, Italy, the UK and Spain at less than 7 deaths per 100 000. They were highest in Hungary, Japan, Korea, Finland and Belgium at more than 19 deaths per 100 000 [6]. WHO estimates the low and middle income countries account for 84% of global suicides with India and China accounting for 49%. In these countries, rural young women are at an increased risk of suicide [7].

The trends involving completed suicide vary internationally, as well as subnationally, in addition to variance over time. Figure 20.3.1 shows this change over 62 years for New Zealand.

Table 20.3.1 Suicide summary statistics, Australia, 2001–2010 [6]										
Year of registration										
Rate of suicide deaths (age standardized)	2001	2002	2003	2004	2005	2006	2007	2008	2009	2010
Male	20.3	18.8	17.8	16.8	16.5	15.8	16.3	17.2	16.0	16.4
Females	5.3	5.0	4.7	4.3	4.3	4.7	4.9	4.7	4.8	4.8
Persons	12.7	11.8	11.1	10.4	10.3	10.1	10.5	10.8	10.3	10.5
Rate ratio M:F	3.8	3.7	3.8	3.9	3.9	3.4	3.3	3.7	3.4	3.4
Suicide as % of total deaths	1.9	1.7	1.7	1.6	1.6	1.6	1.6	1.6	1.6	1.6
Suicide as percentage of all deaths from external causes	31.2	29.7	28.6	26.3	26.2	26.2	27.1	26.3	25.3	26.5

OECD Factbook 2009. [Internet homepage] [cited 2012, Nov 4]. <http://www.oecd-ilibrary.org/economics/oecdfactbook-2009/suicide-rates_factbook-2009-graph162-en>

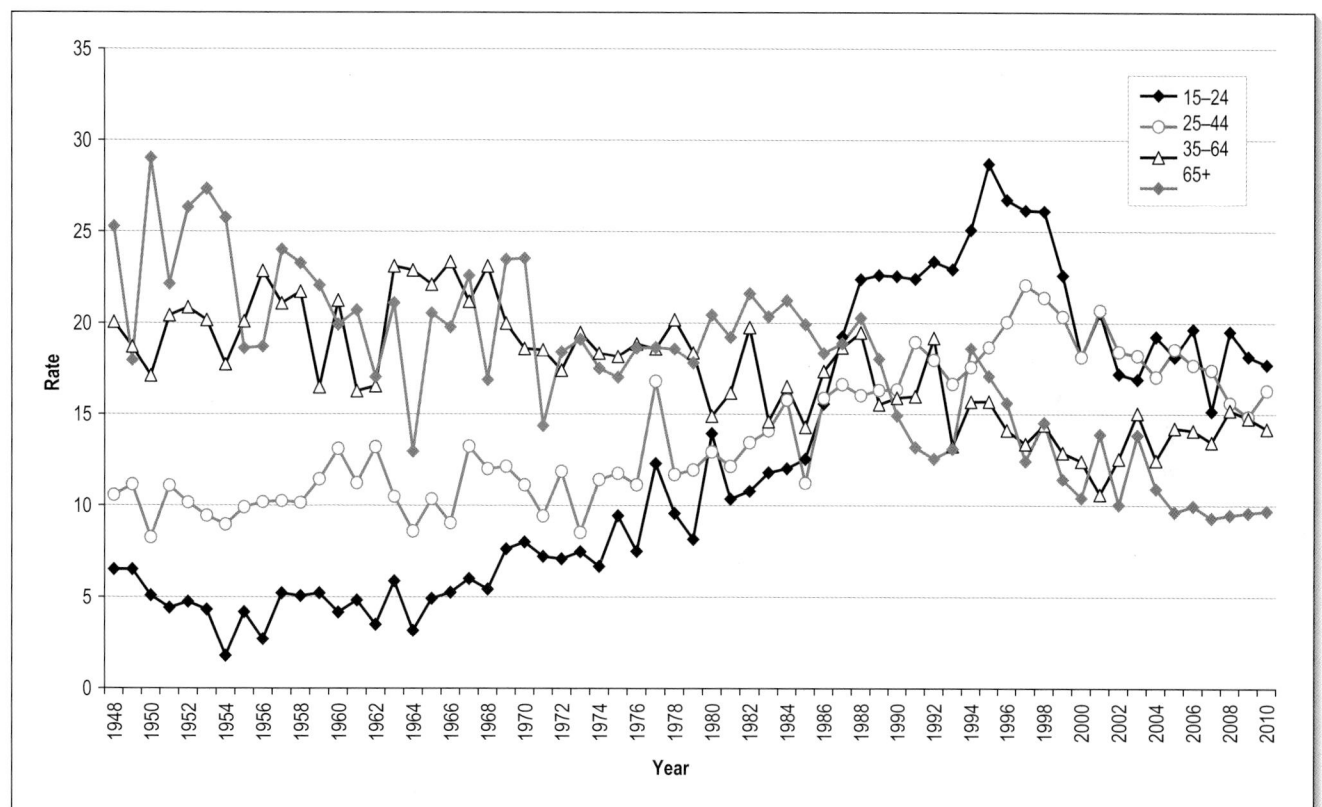

Fig. 20.3.1 New Zealand suicide age-specific death rates, by life-stage age group, 1948–2010 as an example of changing rates over time in a developed country.
Notes: The rates in this figure are age-specific rates, measuring the frequency of suicides per 100 000 population relative to particular population age groups. *(With permission from Ministry of Health, New Zealand Government. New Zealand Mortality Collection.)*

Some inconsistencies across reporting systems should also be considered when interpreting suicide rates.

Hospital presentations for DSH are at least 10 times higher than suicide rates [4]. In the 2007 Australian National Survey of Mental Health, 0.3% of males and 0.5% of females reported they had made a suicide attempt in the previous 12 months. Most of these are not reported or are reported as accidents. Hence, unrecognized DSH is at least as frequent as that recognized. The same survey reported 1.9% of males and 2.7% of females experienced suicidal ideation within 12 months [8]. This rate may be as high as 25% in certain populations and age groups [9,10].

Risk of suicide

An episode of DSH is one historical risk factor predictive of future suicide attempts. Approximately 1–2% of patients commit suicide during the year following an attempt and in approximately 40% of suicides there is a history of a previous self-harm. A systematic review of fatal and non-fatal repetition of self-harm reported a suicide rate of 2% at 1 year and 7% after 9 years [11]. In a prospective Finnish 14-year follow-up study and a UK 18-year follow-up study, the rate of suicide after an episode of DSH was 6.7% [12,13]. A 10-year follow-up study in New Zealand documented a suicide rate of 4.6% in patients admitted for DSH [14]. An emergency centre-based retrospective cohort study in New Zealand demonstrated an 18% re-presentation and a 1.1% suicide rate at 1-year follow up [15]. Hospitalization and aftercare decrease short-term risk of suicide, but have little impact on long-term risk of suicide. However, this may be due to undertreatment of psychiatric illness [16–18].

Exposure to suicide in adolescents tends not to cause an increased risk of suicide among friends, but may cause an increased incidence of depression anxiety and post-traumatic stress disorder [19].

Repeated episodes of DSH

DSH usually invokes help from friends, family and the medical profession so that the patient's social situation and psychological well-being tends to improve [20]. This effect is prominent in younger patients, but may not occur in patients aged over 60 years [21]. The risk of repetition is 12–16% in the following year, with 10% of these occurring in the first week [11]. This is more likely in females who are unemployed, have cluster B (e.g. borderline, narcissistic and histrionic) personality traits or have substance-abuse problems. A younger age at first attempt, presence of long-standing affective disorders, drug/alcohol misuse disorders and anxiety all correlate with repeated attempts. Some patients have chronic suicidal ideation and multiple repetitions of DSH. They often suffer from personality disorders, psychotic disorders, chronic medical conditions, alcohol or drug use, a history of childhood sexual abuse [22,23] and violent behaviour. They use DSH as a means of fighting off anxiety, hopelessness, loneliness or boredom, or for inter-personal secondary gains with regard to family, friends or healthcarers. These patients are at increased risk of eventual suicide. Reversible potentiating factors should be addressed where possible.

Patients with DSH who leave the ED prior to a psychosocial assessment may have a higher risk for repeat DSH, probably associated with lack of specialist follow up and treatment of reversible factors [18,24].

Increased mortality

A suicide attempt is associated with a severe risk of premature death with the increased mortality rate not entirely due to suicide [25]. There is a higher than expected rate of accidents, homicides and death from other medical conditions. This may indicate social disadvantage, disengagement with the health system, underlying chronic illnesses or lifestyle factors.

Patient characteristics

Demographic factors

Age

Suicide and DSH are rare in children under 12 years of age. Australian data suggest similar rates of suicide from the age of 20–50, with a peak at 40–44 years in males (27.7 per 100 000) and 45–49 years in females (7.6 per 100 000) [4]. There is another peak in the elderly, with suicide rates increasing with age from 65 years. This bimodal distribution is also evident from USA and New Zealand data, with males aged over 80 years having the highest age-specific rates of suicide.

The incidence of DSH increases throughout puberty, reaching a peak at 15–24 years of age and decreasing thereafter. The ratio of rates of DSH to suicide decreases markedly with age. DSH is uncommon in the elderly, who have a high ratio of successful to unsuccessful attempts [26].

Gender

In Australia, the overall rate ratio of M:F suicide is 3.4 in 2010 compared with 2.7 in New Zealand and 3.2 in the UK in the same year [27,28]. The rate for male DSH has been increasing in Western countries recently with the male to female ratio approximately 1:2. Females choose methods that are less likely to be fatal and may be more likely to present to hospital following DSH.

Employment

Unemployment increases the risk of DSH by 10–15 times, with the risk increasing with duration of unemployment. This may not be a cause or effect, but may be due to some underlying factor, such as psychiatric illness, personality disorder or substance abuse. There is a more pronounced increased in the risk factors of unemployment rate and lower socioeconomic status for young men in Australia [29].

Social and cultural factors

Suicide rates are higher in those who live alone or are in a lower social group, especially in urban areas characterized by social deprivation and overcrowding. Being single, separated, divorced or widowed increases the risk of suicide two- to threefold in the high-income countries [7]. In these countries, being partnered reinforced by children decreases the risk of suicidal behavior. In India and China, there is a reduced risk of suicide versus other causes of death in women widowed, divorced or separated compared with married women and men [7].

Recent data in Australian Aboriginal people report substantially higher suicide rates that commence at a lower age than in the non-Aboriginal population [4]. Suicide has become more common in recent years; in 2010 the percentage of deaths by suicide among Aboriginal and Torres Strait Islander people was 4.2% compared with non-indigenous Australians 1.6% (does not include states of Victoria, Tasmania and Australian Capital Territory data). It is of concern that the age-specific suicide rate for Aboriginal males aged 25–29 was 90.8 deaths per 100 000 in a combined 10-year period 2001–2010 [4]. A higher suicide rate is seen in indigenous groups of other developed countries, for example, in New Zealand, the age standardized rate was 16 per 100 000 in 2010 compared with a rate of 10.4 in the non-Maori population [28].

Suicide rates of migrants initially reflect rates in the country of origin and converge toward the Australian rate over time. Rural areas in Australia and New Zealand and remote areas in the UK have a higher rate than urban areas [4,28,30]. Incarceration is a risk factor for suicide; in any form of custody, the suicide rate is three times that of the general population [31].

Some social groups, such as doctors, dentists, musicians, lawyers and law-enforcement officers, are more prone to suicide [32]. Most adults (75%) with DSH have relationship problems with their partners and teenagers with their parents. A major argument or separation often precedes the act on a background of ongoing social difficulties or substance use.

Medical factors

There is an increased risk of suicidal ideation in people with chronic ill health, terminal illness or chronic pain and epilepsy. The majority of such patients have sought medical advice in the 6 months before suicide. Most patients with DSH have good health.

Psychiatric factors

There is a pre-existing psychiatric disorder in 90–100% of cases of suicide, with depression accounting for 66–80%, but this rate may be based on retrospective psychological autopsy and therefore be open to dispute. The lifetime rate of suicide among psychiatric inpatients is 3–12 times higher than in the general population and involves a greater proportion of more violent methods, such as jumping from buildings, hanging or jumping in front of vehicles. One-third of these episodes occur after self-discharge from hospital, with another third occurring during approved leave. The high-risk time is the first week of admission and during the first 3 months after discharge [33].

Psychiatric disorders are present in up to 60% of patients who commit DSH, but may be transient and secondary to acute psychosocial difficulties. Da Cruz et al. examined the cases of 286 individuals who died within 12 months of mental health contact in North West England; 43% of the sample attended the ED on at least one occasion and 12% of the sample attended an ED on more than three occasions and could be considered 'frequent attenders'. Most frequent attenders had a history of self-harm (94%), 68% had a history of alcohol abuse, 63% were unemployed at the time of deaths and 49% had a history of drug abuse [34].

Affective disorders

The psychiatric diagnosis that carries the greatest risk of suicide is mood disorder, particularly major depressive disorder if associated with borderline personality disorder, anxiety or agitation [35]. Fifteen per cent of these high-risk patients commit suicide over a lifetime. Depression correlates well with the occurrence of suicidal desire and ideation, but may not be as strong a predictor of planning and preparation (intense thoughts, plans and capability) and, therefore, suicide completion [36]. Hopelessness is the most important factor associated with suicide completion and may be of greater importance than suicidal ideation or depression itself [36]. Depressed patients should, therefore, have their attitudes towards the future carefully assessed.

Substance abuse

Individuals with alcohol use disorders have an overall approximately 7% lifetime risk of dying by suicide, with women being at greater risk than men. Fifteen per cent of alcohol-dependent persons eventually commit suicide. The majority of these are also depressed. The risk is higher if associated with social isolation, poor physical health, unemployment and previous suicidal behaviour. The increased risk may be more pronounced in males aged below 35 years [37]. Young males dependent on heroin have 20 times the risk of the general population. Chronic alcohol dependence is uncommon in DSH, but alcohol intoxication is involved in 50–90% of suicide attempts. Wyder found that 65% of people presenting with deliberate self-harm in Australia were substance affected at the time [38]. Acute alcohol ingestion is found in approximately 35% of people who die by suicide and between 15 and 60% of people who die by suicide have been found on psychological autopsy to have lifetime alcohol-use disorders [39].

Schizophrenia

Up to 10% of people with schizophrenia die by suicide. Young adult males are at high risk, especially if there is associated depression with feelings of hopelessness, previous DSH or suicide attempts, unemployment or social isolation.

Personality disorders

Patients with cluster B personality disorders are at high risk of DSH and suicide, especially if associated with labile mood, impulsivity, alienation from peers and associated substance abuse. This may be due to precipitation of undesirable life events, predisposition to psychiatric and substance-abuse disorders and social isolation. Adjustment disorders are associated with 25% of adolescent suicide [23].

Frequent attenders

Frequent attenders to EDs (defined as greater than three presentations in a year) are also at high risk. This group has seven times the risk of the general population and rates of suicide similar to clinical psychiatric populations. This risk is particularly pronounced in patients who present with panic attacks, especially if associated with depressive symptoms.

Aetiology

No specific psychological or personality structure is associated with suicide and patients who commit suicide or DSH do so for many unrelated reasons. The precipitant may be a personal crisis or life change amplified by poor social support, substance abuse or psychiatric disorder. Intoxication may decrease inhibitions enough to allow an act to proceed. A study by Wyder interviewed 112 people following a deliberate self-harm attempt. She found that 51% had considered deliberate self-harm for 10 minutes or less, but of those who had been affected by alcohol that number jumped to 93% [40].

The most frequent methods of suicide in Australia are hanging, strangulation and suffocation, these modes being used in 56% of all suicide deaths in 2010 in Australia. Poisoning by drugs was used in 12% of suicide deaths in 2010, followed by poisoning by other methods including alcohol and motor vehicle exhaust (10%). Firearms accounted for 7% of suicide deaths in Australia in 2010, a rate which has declined from 20% a decade prior, possibly due to firearm restriction legislation [5]. Proportions due to each method vary according to region, residence, age and sex [1,41]. In the USA, firearms accounted for 57% of male and 32% of female suicide deaths. In trauma centres in the USA, stab wounds are a far more common method of deliberate self-harm than gunshot wounds and people (more often men) at the extremes of age are more likely to use firearms with fatal consequences [3]. In many developing countries, organophosphate or antimalarial poisoning and charcoal burning are more common methods of suicide [42]. One-third of patients with DSH express a wish to die, but most do so to communicate distress. DSH may serve many functions for the person. At its most simple, it serves an integrative function calming the person at a time of great distress. It may also be a way of mobilizing assistance for someone who is feeling overwhelmed by circumstances. Many patients threaten suicide or magnify being at risk of suicide to increase the likelihood of admission to hospital. These patients are more likely to be substance dependent, have personality diatheses (for example, marked borderline, antisocial or dependent traits or disorder) or homelessness and be unpartnered and in legal difficulty. However, these instances of goal directed behaviour should not be discounted and the behaviour should be taken seriously. A presentation to an ED is a declaration that the person is in a self-defined crisis for which they are using maladaptive coping measures.

Most cases of medically serious DSH are due to self-poisoning, with 90% associated with alcohol intoxication. The most common drugs are non-prescription analgesics and psychotropic drugs. Many overdoses are related to alcohol or illicit substance intoxication and may be accidental rather than deliberate, although this distinction is often difficult to ascertain. Self-injury may involve cutting of the skin in various sites about the body but may also involve self-inflicted cigarette burns, excoriation of the skin or hitting themselves or other objects. More violent forms of self-injury are less common and suggest serious suicidal intent. Bizarre self-mutilation may occur in psychotic patients who may not necessarily have an intention to die but are acting in accordance with delusional beliefs or in response to command hallucinations.

Assessment

A person who expresses suicidal ideation or engages in DSH is sending a distress signal that emergency physicians must acknowledge. Suicidality should also be assessed in patients with symptoms or signs of depression, unusual behavioural changes, substance abuse, psychiatric disorders, complainants of sexual violence [27] and those who present with injuries of questionable or inconsistent mechanism, such as self-inflicted lacerations and gunshot wounds or motor vehicle accidents involving one victim. Many would argue that assessment of suicidality should be a routine part of any ED assessment. A retrospective study by Da Cruz et al. found that 40% of persons who died by suicide had presented to the ED at least once during the year prior to their death [34]. Assessment in the emergency department ideally will contain elements that provide the person with the opportunity to discuss psychosocial aspects of their life. Within this discussion, it may be that suicidal ideation or thoughts of deliberate self-harm may be elicited. This may allow early referral to psychosocial supports thereby providing the person with holistic care to help address their needs.

Assessment requires a systematic, multidisciplinary approach involving prior staff education, appropriate triage, observation and restraint procedures (in the setting of imminent risk and the absence of less restrictive options) and a planned strategy for assessment followed by treatment and disposition. The priorities are to define the physical sequelae of the act, risk of further DSH behaviour, psychiatric

diagnoses and acute psychosocial stressors. These aspects are those that can then be targeted for short-term interventions.

Triage

In a patient who has attempted DSH, initial management involves resuscitation, treatment of immediate life threats and preventing complications. The patient should be triaged according to the physical problem as well as current suicidality, agitation and aggressiveness and mental state. The mental health triage scale can be used for this purpose [43]. A triage score of 2 or 3 should be applied if patients are violent, actively suicidal, psychotic, distressed or at risk of leaving before full assessment can occur. Constant observation is required at this point and nursing staff, security or police may be needed. In Australia, a number of different triage scales can be used. There is some evidence that a mental health triage scale improves outcomes; however, the accuracy of the assessment can be limited by a number of environmental, staff and patient factors [44].

Medical assessment

The patient's safety in the ED should be optimized by limiting availability of drugs, removing sharp implements, removing car keys, ropes, belts or sheets and securing nearby windows. Other concurrent and concealed methods of self-harm should be sought. This may be facilitated by changing into hospital gowns, whereby the patient is more easily identified if they abscond. In addition, other means to increase visibility, such as security cameras, high visibility cubicles or assigning a special nurse, should be considered. Assessment of the patient may be difficult, either due to a general medical cause or being unsettled from the precipitant of the act, or from not wanting to be in hospital or allow medical intervention. This may necessitate the therapeutic utilization of anxiolytic medication; the use of physical restraint may be considered if at high risk or unable to be fully assessed and wanting to self-discharge. This may be done under a duty of care to the patient or the local mental health act may be utilized in extreme situations. Emotional support of patient, friends and relatives is required during and after this phase, with clear explanation of the rationale and the procedures. Distinguishing medical from psychiatric causes of mental disorder presentations is discussed elsewhere in this book (see Chapter 20.2).

Suicide risk assessment

Initially, an assessment needs to be done in the ED so as to determine patient disposition, but a more comprehensive psychiatric assessment may need to wait until substance or anxiolytic medication effects wear off. Other sources of information need to be accessed since patient history can be unreliable or incomplete. Friends, family, local doctor, ambulance officers, helping agencies already involved and previous presentations documented in the medical record can all add useful information in order to advise an assessment. A therapeutic relationship should be formed and the clinician should be non-judgemental, non-threatening and clearly willing to help. A positive attitude has been shown to improve outcomes with this group of patients [45]. People presenting in crisis are hypersensitive to any negative transference. This may intensify the patient's already low self-esteem, increasing future suicide potential and making a therapeutic relationship difficult to establish [46]. When managing a patient who may be suicidal, the suicidal ideation should be discussed openly. Expressions of self-harm carry individual meaning for each person. It is important, in a therapeutic relationship, to explore the meaning that this carries for the person and alternatives.

Risk factors may be divided into two main categories, namely static and dynamic. Static factors have been historically identified by Durkheim [47] who showed some, less socially integrated groups within society to be at greater risk of suicide than others. These static factors are enduring and in context of a person's developmental history and social circumstances. Hence, being male, unemployed, single, poorly educated, from a lower socioeconomic group, with a history of mental disturbance and substance-use disorders would all place someone in a higher risk group.

Dynamic factors are the more fluid day-to-day factors that intensify the risk posed by the static factors. Flewett [48] divides these factors into internal and external factors. The internal factors include current feelings of abandonment, desperation, hopelessness, co-morbid depression, current drug use or physical illness. External factors are those of increased social dislocation, including homelessness, bereavement, intoxication, adverse life event, such as the recent loss of a job or relationship.

Table 20.3.2 Factors associated with suicide [1]

Variable	High risk	Low risk
Static factors		
Gender	Male	Female
Marital status	Separated, divorced, widowed	Married
Employment	Unemployed or retired	Employed
Medical factors	Chronic illness, chronic pain, epilepsy	Good health
Psychiatric factors	Depression, bipolar, schizophrenia, panic disorder, previous psychiatric inpatient, substance abuse	No psychiatric history
Social background	Unresponsive family, socially isolated or chaotic, indigenous background, refugee from conflict areas, past history of trauma, developmental trauma	Supportive family, socially stable and integrated
Dynamic factors		
Suicidal ideation	Transient, intense suicidal ideation, plan and intent, intoxication and impulsivity with impaired judgement	Infrequent, transient
Attempts	Multiple	First attempt
Lethality	Violent, lethal and available method	Low lethality, poor availability
Planning	Planned, active preparation, extensive premeditation	No realistic plan, telling others prior to act
Rescue	Act performed in isolation, event timed to avoid intervention, precautions taken to avoid discovery	Rescue inevitable, obtained help afterwards
Final acts	Wills, insurance, giving away property	
Coping skills	Unwilling to seek help, feels unable to cope with present difficulties	Can easily turn to others for help, can plan to overcome present difficulties, willing to become involved in aftercare
Current ideation	Admitting act was intended to cause death, no remorse, continued wish to die, hopelessness or helplessness	Primary wish to change, pleased to recover, suicidal ideation resolved by act, optimism
Precipitant	Similar circumstances can recur, acute precipitant not resolved	Stressful but transient life event, acute precipitant addressed

Salter A, Pielage P. Emergency departments have a role in the prevention of suicide. Emergency Medicine 2000; 12: 198–203 with permission.

The role of dynamic risk is highlighted by Rosenman [49] when he states:

for conditions with multiple risk factors... each factor adds a little to the risk, but only when it interacts with other factors. No single predictor or combination of predictors is present in every individual, and membership of the high risk group changes from moment to moment. Half a bottle of whiskey may create a high suicide risk within an hour.

Assessment of suicide risk involves assessing background demographic, psychiatric, medical and social factors, these are the static factors that underlie any presentation and will determine the chronic suicidal risk that the person presents. Dynamic risk factors as well as the current circumstances and risk of suicidal behaviour itself are outlined in Table 20.3.2. There are epidemiological differences between people who attempt suicide and those who complete suicide. Although the groups are different, there is an important overlap. The more an individual's characteristics resemble the profile of a suicide completer, the higher the risk of future suicide or suicide attempts. Despite this, in long-term follow-up studies very few of these factors have been shown to be good independent predictors of suicide following DSH. The most consistent factors are psychiatric illness, personality disorder, substance abuse, multiple previous attempts and current suicidal ideation and hopelessness. Guidelines are available to assist in suicide-risk stratification and describe characteristics associated with suicide-risk levels and the appropriate further assessment and disposition for each group [50].

Use of scales

Many screening tools have been devised to identify high-risk groups within those presenting with DSH. PATHOS [51], the Suicidal Intent Scale [52], the Sad Persons Scale [53] and other scoring systems have been devised to complement medical assessment of suicide risk. However, many of these scales use outdated risk factors and patient populations unrepresentative of EDs. Scales need to be sensitive, but this misclassifies a large number of individuals as potentially at risk of suicide. These deficiencies need to be considered when applying suicide risk scales in the ED and these scales should not be used as an absolute assessment of suicide risk or of the need for psychiatric admission [54,55]. In addition to validated questionnaire assessment, there are a number of validated interview assessment tools, such as the Suicide Attempt Self-Injury Interview [56]. Problems clinicians report in using these tools is that of the time taken to administer them. In any event, these tools have been shown to be as accurate as a mental health clinician's global assessment [9].

The problems associated with suicide-risk assessment are summarized in Table 20.3.3.

Definitive treatment and disposition

Following necessary medical treatment and suicide-risk stratification, disposition may involve involuntary or voluntary admission to a psychiatric or medical ward, short-term observation or discharge with appropriate follow up. Restraint and involuntary admission may be necessary for the high-risk patient who wishes to self-discharge. Approximately 30% of DSH patients are admitted for psychiatric inpatient care, but the factors involved in the decision for psychiatric hospitalization following DSH involve a complex evaluation of risk, potential for treatment and social supports [57].

Patients who are intoxicated with alcohol can be both behaviourally disinhibited and

Table 20.3.3 Problems in assessing suicide risk

Suicide is rare, even in high-risk groups, so it cannot be predicted without a high rate of false-negative or false-positive errors
Suicidality presents in heterogeneous ways that may not be recognized
Suicidality is transient and affected by intoxication, stress and being in hospital
The patient may be reluctant, oppositional or manipulative
The patient may present in an atypical fashion, especially the elderly with physical complaints
Suicide risk factors identify high-risk subgroups but not individuals
The demographic factors associated with suicide have changed recently, thus changing the make-up of risk groups
Risk factors are based on studies of long-term follow up and, therefore, long-term risk
Subtle changes in mental status and behaviour may be missed if not assessed by the usual doctor
Unexplained improvement in psychological status may be the result of increased motivation to die
Patients may deny their true intentions due to embarrassment, fear of being stopped in carrying out their own wishes, fear of being institutionalized or fear of the confidentiality of the interview
Patients may say life is not worth living or that they feel they would be better off dead, but not necessarily have an increased risk of suicide, unless they have made suicidal plans or attempts, or if they have pervasive hopelessness
Correlation between medical danger and suicidal intent is low unless the patient can accurately assess the probable outcome of their attempts if treatment had not been received

emotionally labile and, as discussed, are at higher risk of intentional self-injury. Short-term observation allows intoxication to resolve so that more comprehensive and longitudinal psychiatric assessment can take place. A short-term stay in hospital can also help resolution of many acute areas of conflict and make psychiatric evaluation more accurate. ED short-stay wards or psychiatric assessment and planning units are appropriate for these admissions, especially if a multidisciplinary team is available to review the patient and institute management and follow up.

Important elements of management involve addressing the modifiable elements of the precipitating problem, treatment of psychiatric illness and environmental interventions, such as family counselling, encouraging a support network and developing coping and problem-solving skills [58]. Adaptive solutions to the current crisis should be reinforced utilizing short-term solutions. Factors that should be addressed while patients are in hospital include referral to services to help address the dynamic risk issues, such as problems with relationships, employment, finances, housing, legal problems, social isolation, bereavement, alcohol and drug abuse and dependence. In this regard, social workers or mental health nurses are invaluable [59]. For greatest effect, these should be available after hours and on weekends since the majority of DSH presentations are after hours [60]. For repeat attenders who are often socially isolated, hospitalization should not be a substitute for social services, substance-abuse treatment and legal assistance, although admission may be necessary while appropriate supports are put in place [61].

Dispositional decisions need to be taken, weighing up the relative and potential iatrogenic harm generated by hospitalization and the now common legal mandate for treatment in a least restrictive environment. Discharge will be with referral to community agencies with responsibility for supporting the person in the community and, according to risk assessment, may include community mental health teams, GPs, non-government support agencies, etc. The aim of disposition is to minimize risk factors while empowering the person to develop more positive and capable coping styles for future crises.

Pharmacotherapy has been shown to be useful in addressing the debilitating symptoms of a major depressive disorder and, along with psychotherapy, can help the person regain their previous level of functioning. Once risk and disposition have been addressed, the pharmacotherapeutic management and ongoing assessment can be by the local medical officer, who can refer as necessary to mental health specialists. Pharmacotherapy involves the treatment of the underlying psychiatric disorder. Antidepressants decrease the risk of attempting suicide, although the lethality of suicide attempts is increased if tricyclic antidepressants are taken in overdose. Selective serotonin reuptake inhibitors and other newer classes of antidepressants (including SNRIs, NassA, NRI, etc.) may have a more selective effect in decreasing suicidal behaviour and are less toxic in overdose than tricyclic antidepressants – the latter are no longer prescribed as first-line antidepressant medications by psychiatrists. These factors make the newer class of drugs an attractive choice for depressed patients who are suicidal.

Prevention

Comprehensive strategies for prevention of suicide have been or are being developed in Finland, Norway, Sweden, Australia and New Zealand [62]. Suicide prevention focuses on psychiatric, social and medical aspects and usually involves public education, media restrictions on reporting of suicide, school-based programmes with teacher education, training of doctors in detection and treatment of depression and other psychiatric disorders, alcohol and drug abuse information, enhanced access to the mental health system and supportive counselling after episodes of DSH. Decreasing the availability of lethal methods may involve legislative changes, such as more stringent gun control, restricting access to well-known jumping sites or changes to availability or packaging of tablets [63]. Overall, studies into the effectiveness of suicide-prevention strategies have shown inconsistent reductions in suicide rates following interventions [64]. Approaches to reduce DSH repetition have also shown disappointing results [65]. Improved recognition and treatment of mental illness, improved social services and drug and alcohol-support services may be of greater benefit than specific suicide-prevention strategies.

Ethical considerations

In assessing and managing patients with deliberate self-harm and suicidality, the patient's desire for autonomy and self-determinism (e.g. declining recommended or reasonable treatment options, follow up or support) must be considered in terms of their mental state, static and imminent dynamic risk factors, protective factors and available support (e.g. social, family, carer, accommodation, financial, etc.) These considerations must also be balanced with the patient's capacity to provide informed consent and their human rights and dignity, against that of the paternalism of clinicians initiating immediate treatment or restricting immediate care to the emergency department or other inpatient setting (e.g. psychiatric inpatient unit).

Often, in circumstances of imminent risk to self, the patient's requests or demands for confidentiality may not be absolute, in so far as it is often necessary to obtain collateral history from others (e.g. general practitioners, psychiatrists, family, carers, etc.) and communicate with others about the immediate assessment and management of risk. Other aspects of confidentiality include local governance around accessing electronic mental health databases or clinical records that record service contact data about patients.

The framework of care in which the above issues and dilemmas are considered is also informed by relevant local mental health, medical treatment and human rights legislation. Emergency department clinicians should familiarize themselves with the relevant local legislation and the processes of invigilation.

The disposition of emergency department patients who have presented with deliberate self-harm or a suicide attempt must also be considered through the prism of the health service's key performance indices. For example, such key performance indices may cover response times for triage and target times for disposition from the department. Accordingly, the patient's disposition must also be considered in terms of balancing non-maleficence with utilitarianism (the 'greater goods' of accessibility, responsiveness and quality of healthcare for a community) in the context of these indices.

Conclusion

Assessment of suicide risk is an important skill in emergency medicine, since many patients present to EDs with suicidal thinking or behaviour. Although the risk of suicide for an individual patient is difficult to predict, emergency physicians can provide a system for assessment and identification of risk groups. Acute interventions can attempt to prevent short-term completion of suicide or repetition of DSH, since emergency physicians are predominantly involved in the care of these patients, often using short-stay wards. It is during this period

in the emergency department that linkage to ongoing support services can be effected. A team approach involving psychiatry and social work is necessary in most cases, with many problems resolved by a short-term hospital admission, brief crisis intervention and intensive short-term follow up.

Controversies

- The legal position is clear in not assisting suicide, meaning we have a duty of care for people who are suicidal.
- Dispositional decisions need to be taken, weighing up the relative and potential iatrogenic harm generated by hospitalization and the now common legal mandate for treatment in the least restrictive environment.
- Consideration must be given to the issue of competency when taking into consideration patients' preferences for disposition.
- Clinical trials of ED assessment and brief intervention strategies, including short-stay admissions, need to occur since more patients are managed entirely in EDs.
- Currently available guidelines and triage scales need to be validated and refined.

References

[1] Salter A, Pielage P. Emergency departments have a role in the prevention of suicide. Emerg Med 2000;12:198–203.
[2] Gairin I, House A, Owens D. Attendance at the accident and emergency department in the year before suicide: retrospective study. Br J Psychiatr 2003;183:28–33.
[3] Ting S, Sullivan A, Boudreaux E, Miller I, Camargo C. Trends in US emergency department visits for attempted suicide and self-inflicted injury, 1993–2008. Gen Hosp Psychiatr 2012;34:557–65.
[4] Australian Bureau of Statistics. 3309.0 Suicides, Australia, 2010 [Internet homepage] [updated 2012, July 24; cited 2012, Nov 4]. <http://abs.gov.au/AUSSTATS/abs@.nsf/mf/3309.0/>
[5] Australian Bureau of Statistics. 3303.0 Causes of Death, Australia, 2010 [Internet homepage] [updated 2010, Mar 20; cited 2012, Nov 4]. <http://www.abs.gov.au/ausstats/abs@.nsf/mf/3303>
[6] OECD Factbook 2009. [Internet homepage] [cited 2012, Nov 4]. <http://www.oecd-ilibrary.org/economics/oecd-factbook-2009/suicide-rates_factbook-2009-graph162-en>
[7] WHO The global burden of disease: 2004 update. Geneva: World Health Organization; 2008. [Internet homepage]; cited 2012, Nov 4]. <www.who.int/evidence/bod>
[8] National Survey of Mental Health and Wellbeing: Summary of Results, 2007. [Internet homepage] [updated 2008, October; cited 2012, Nov 8]. <http://www.abs.gov.au/ausstats/abs@.nsf/mf/4326.011>.
[9] Repper J. A review of the literature on the prevention of suicide through interventions in Accident and Emergency Departments. J Clin Nurs 1999;8:3–12.
[10] Bertolote JM, Fleischmann A, De Leo D, et al. Suicide attempts, plans, and ideation in culturally diverse sites: the WHO SUPRE-MISS community survey. Psychol Med 2005;35:1457–65.

[11] Owens D, Horrocks J, House A. Fatal and non-fatal repetition of self-harm. Br J Psychiatr 2002;181:193–9.
[12] Suokas J, Suominen K, Isometsa E, et al. Long-term risk factors for suicide mortality after attempted suicide – findings of a 14-year follow-up study. Acta Psychiatr Scand 2001;104:117–21.
[13] De Moore GM, Robertson AR. Suicide in the 18 years after deliberate self harm. Br J Psychiatr 1996;169:489–94.
[14] Gibb SJ, Beautrais AL, Fergusson DM. Mortality and further suicidal behaviour after an index suicide attempt: a 10-year study. Aust NZ J Psychiatr 2005;39:95–100.
[15] Howson M, Yates K, Hatcher S. Re-presentation and suicide rates in emergency department patients who self-harm. Emerg Med Australas 2008;20:322–7.
[16] Kurz A, Moller HJ. Attempted suicide: efficacy of treatment programs. Psychiatr Clin Neurosci 1995;49:S99–S103.
[17] McNeil DE, Binder RL. The impact of hospitalization on clinical assessments of suicide risk. Psychiatr Serv 1997;48:204–8.
[18] Kapur N, Cooper J, Hiroeh U. Emergency department management and outcome for self-poisoning: a cohort study. Gen Hosp Psychiatr 2004;26:36–41.
[19] Brent DA, Moritz G, Bridge J. Long-term impact of exposure to suicide: a three-year controlled follow-up. J Am Acad Child Adolesc Psychiatry 1996;35:646–53.
[20] Sarfati Y, Bouchaud B, Hardy-Bayle M-C. Cathartic effect of suicide attempts not limited to depression: a short-term prospective study after deliberate self-poisoning. Crisis 2003;24:73–8.
[21] Matsuishi K, Kitamura N, Sato M, et al. Change of suicidal ideation induced by suicide attempt. Psychiatr Clin Neurosci 2005;59:599–604.
[22] Soderberg S, Kullgren G, Salander Renberg E. Childhood sexual abuse predicts poor outcome seven years after parasuicide. Soc Psychiatr Psychiatr Epidemiol 2004;39:916–20.
[23] Vajda J, Steinbeck K. Factors associated with repeat suicide attempts among adolescents. Aust NZ J Psychiatr 2000;34:437–45.
[24] Hickey L, Hawton K, Fagg J, et al. Deliberate self-harm patients who leave the accident and emergency department without a psychiatric assessment: a neglected population at risk of suicide. J Psychosom Res 2001;50:87–93.
[25] Ostamo A, Lonnqvist J. Excess mortality of suicide attempters. Soc Psychiatr Psychiatr Epidemiol 2001;36:29–35.
[26] Hawton K, Harris L. Deliberate self-harm in people aged 60 years and over: characteristics and outcome of a 20-year cohort. Internatl J Geriatr Psychiatr 2006;21:572–81.
[27] Office of National Statistics, United Kingdom 2012. Statistical Bulletin. Suicide rate in the UK 2006–2010.[Internet Homepage][Updated Jan 2012; cited 2012, Nov 4] <http://www.ons.gov.uk/ons/rel/subnational-health4/suicides-in-the-united-kingdom/2010/stb-statistical-bulletin.html>
[28] New Zealand Ministry of Health, New Zealand 2010. [Internet Homepage] Updated August 2012, Cited 2012, Nov 2]. <http://www.health.govt.nz/publication/suicide-facts-deaths-and-intentional-self-harm-hospitalisations-2010>
[29] Taylor R, Page A, Morrel S, et al. Mental health and socio-economic variations in Australian suicide. Soc Sci Med 2005;61:1551–60.
[30] Gunnell D, Wheeler B, Chang S, et al. Changes in the geography of suicide in young men: England and Wales 1981–2005. J Epidemiol Commun Hlth 2012;6:536–43.
[31] Fazel S, Grann M, Kling B, Hawton K. Prison suicide in 12 countries: an ecological study of 861 suicides during 2003–2007. Soc Psychiatr Psychiatr Epidemiol 2011;46:191–5.
[32] Kaplan HI, Sadock BJ, Grebb JA. Kaplan and Sadock's synopsis of psychiatry, 7th ed. Baltimore: Williams & Wilkins, 1994, p. 803–9.
[33] Shah AK, Ganesvaran T. Inpatient suicides in an Australian mental hospital. Aust NZ J Psychiatr 1997;31:291–8.
[34] Da Cruz D, Pearson P, Saini P, et al. Emergency department contact prior to suicide in mental health patients. Emerg Med J 2011;28:467–71.
[35] Gilbody S, House A, Owens D. The early repetition of deliberate self harm. J R Coll Physicians Lond 1997;31:171–2.
[36] Hawton K. Assessment of suicide risk. Br J Psychiatr 1987;150:145–53.
[37] Cooper J, Kapur N, Webb R, et al. Suicide after deliberate self-harm: a 4-year cohort study. Am J Psychiatr 2005;162:297–303.
[38] Wyder M, De Leo D. Behind impulsive suicide attempts: indications from a community study. J Affect Disord 2007;104:167–73.

[39] Schneider B. Substance use disorders and risk for completed suicide. Arch Suicide Res 2009;13:46–51.

[40] Wyder M. Understanding deliberate self harm: an enquiry into attempted suicide. Sydney: University of Western Sydney; 2004.

[41] Dudley MJ, Kelk NJ, Florio TM. Suicide among young Australians, 1964–1993: an interstate comparison of metropolitan and rural trends. Med J Aust 1998;169:77–80.

[42] Eddleston M. Patterns and problems of deliberate self-poisoning in the developing world. Q J Med 2000;93:715–31.

[43] Smart D, Pollard C, Walpole B. Mental health triage in emergency medicine. Aust NZ J Psychiatr 1999;33:57–66.

[44] Gerdtz M, Weiland T, Jelinek G, et al. Perspectives of emergency department staff on the triage of mental health-related presentations: implications for education, policy and practice. Emerg Med Australas 2012;24:492–500.

[45] Anderson M. Nurses attitudes towards suicidal behavior – a comparative study of community mental health nurses and nurses working in accident and emergency departments. J Adv Nurs 1997;25:1283–91.

[46] Rund DA, Hutzler JC. Behavioral disorders: emergency assessment and stabilization. In: Tintinalli JE, Kelen GD, Stapczynski JS, (eds). Emergency medicine: a comprehensive study guide (6th ed.). New York: American College of Emergency Physicians, McGraw-Hill, 2004, p. 1812–6.

[47] Durkheim E. Suicide: a study in sociology. New York: Free Press; 1951.

[48] Flewett T. Clinical risk management, an introductory text for mental health clinicians. Sydney: Elsevier; 2010.

[49] Rosenman S. Preventing suicide: what will work and what will not. Med J Aust 1998;69:100–2.

[50] Australasian College for Emergency Medicine and the Royal Australian and New Zealand College of Psychiatrists Guidelines for the management of deliberate self harm in young people. Victoria: ACEM and RANZCP; 2000.

[51] Kingsbury S. PATHOS: a screening instrument for adolescent overdose: a research note. J Child Psychol Psychiatr Allied Discip 1996;37:609–11.

[52] Beck AT, Schuyler D, Herman J. Development of suicidal intent scales. In: Beck AT, Resruk HLP, Lettieri DJ, (eds). The prediction of suicide. Maryland: Charles Press; 1974.

[53] Hockberger RS, Rothstein RJ. Assessment of suicide potential by nonpsychiatrists using the SAD PERSONS score. J Emerg Med 1988;6:99–107.

[54] Cochrane-Brink KA, Lofchy JS, Sakinofsky I. Clinical rating scales in suicide risk assessment. Gen Hosp Psychiatr 2000;22:445–51.

[55] Harris L, Hawton K. Suicidal intent in deliberate self-harm and the risk of suicide: the predictive power of the Suicide Intent Scale. J Affect Disord 2005;86:225–33.

[56] Kerr PI, Muehlenkamp JJ, Turner JM. Non-suicidal self-injury: a review of current research for family medicine

and primary care physicians. J Am Board Fam Med 2010;23:240–59.

[57] Carter GL, Safranko I, Lewin TJ, et al. Psychiatric hospitalisation after deliberate self-poisoning. Suicide Life-Threaten Behav 2006;36:213–22.

[58] Brent DA. The aftercare of adolescents with deliberate self harm. J Child Psychol Psychiat Allied Discip 1997;383:277–86.

[59] Brakoulis V, Ryan C, Byth K. Patients seen with deliberate self-harm seen by a consultation – liaison service. Austral Psychiatr 2006;14:192–7.

[60] Bergen H, Hawton K. Variations in time of hospital presentation for deliberate self-harm and their implications for clinical services. J Affect Disord 2007;98:227–37.

[61] Lambert MT, Bonner J. Characteristics and six-month outcome of patients who use suicide threats to seek hospital admission. Psychiatr Serv 1996;47:871–3.

[62] Taylor SJ, Kingdom D, Jenkins R. How are nations trying to prevent suicide? An analysis of national suicide prevention strategies. Acta Psychiatr Scand 1997;95:457–63.

[63] Cantor CH, Baume PJM. Access to methods of suicide: what impact? Aust NZ J Psychiatr 1998;2:8–14.

[64] Gunnell D, Frankel S. Prevention of suicide: aspirations and evidence. Br Med J 1994;308:1227–33.

[65] Burns J, Dudley M, Hazel P. Clinical management of deliberate self-harm in young people: the need for evidence-based approaches to reduce repetition. Aust NZ J Psychiatr 2005;39:121–8.

20.4 Depression

Simon Byrne

ESSENTIALS

1 Clinical depression is common, affecting 2–5% of the population at any time.

2 Depressive symptoms can be accurately assessed through a systematic interview.

3 The diagnosis of depressive syndrome depends on the severity, pervasiveness and persistence of the symptoms.

4 Management decisions include inpatient admission and referral to appropriate community outpatient services.

Introduction

The need to determine the presence and severity of a depressive syndrome is a very frequent task in the emergency department (ED). Assessment of depression is necessary in relation to a variety of patient presentations. The classic ED situation is the overdose or other attempted suicide or self-harm, where the assessment of depression forms part of further evaluation after the patient has been medically stabilized.

It is also becoming more common for patients to present to the ED complaining of depression (often on the advice of family, friends or crisis help lines) without having

harmed themselves. Patients with a variety of medical conditions, especially conditions which are chronic or disabling, also often develop a depressive syndrome that can form a major part of the reason behind an ED attendance. Some patients who present to EDs with personal crisis or self-harm may have been identified as suffering from a personality disorder but, nevertheless, need assessment for co-morbid depression. The evaluation of depressive symptoms is also an important aspect of the assessment of patients seen in the ED with alcohol and drug abuse problems.

In these assessments, it is very important to have a clear concept of the syndrome of 'clinical depression'. This syndrome is called

'depressive episode' in The International Classification of Disease – 10th edition [1] (ICD-10) and 'major depression' in the Diagnostic and Statistical Manual of Mental Disorders – 4th edition (DSM-IV) [2]. The importance of diagnosing a depressive episode lies principally in determining the presence of a clinical syndrome which is in need of treatment, is likely to respond to treatment and is likely to persist without treatment. The clear delineation of a depressive episode is also an essential basis for differential diagnosis from other medical and psychiatric conditions and for distinguishing between the clinical syndrome of depression and the day-to-day fluctuations of mood and states of dejection, pessimism, frustration and disappointment which are the lot of all human beings.

The diagnosis of a depressive episode depends on the pervasive presence of enduring mood change, marked loss of interest in usual activities or marked loss of energy and drive, as well as a number of other associated symptoms. The list of symptoms contributing to the depressive episode syndrome in ICD-10 is shown in Table 20.4.1. The DSM-IV syndrome of major depression has the same list of symptoms, with the exception of 'loss of confidence

Table 20.4.1 Symptoms contributing to the diagnosis of a depressive episode in ICD-10 [1]
1. Depressed mood, most of the day, nearly every day, largely uninfluenced by circumstances
2. Markedly diminished interest or pleasure in all, or almost all, activities, most of the day, nearly all day
3. Loss of energy or fatigue, nearly every day
4. Loss of confidence or self-esteem
5. Unreasonable feelings of self-reproach, or excessive or inappropriate guilt, nearly every day
6. Recurrent thoughts of death or suicide or any suicidal behaviour
7. Diminished ability to think or concentrate or indecisiveness, nearly every day
8. Psychomotor agitation or retardation, nearly every day
9. Insomnia or hypersomnia, nearly every day
10. Change in appetite (decrease or increase with corresponding weight change)

or self-esteem'. An adequate number of these symptoms must be present for at least 2 weeks before the diagnosis of depressive episode can be made. The pervasiveness of the symptoms is defined principally by the specifications that they must be present 'most of the day' and for 'nearly every day.'

ICD-10 further classifies depressive episodes into mild, moderate and severe, according to the total number of symptoms present (mild = 4/10 symptoms, moderate = 6/10 symptoms and severe = 8/10 symptoms). However, it is important to note that, even in mild or moderate depression, the patient must have at least two of the first three symptoms; that is the patient must have two of depressed mood, loss of interest or loss of energy, most of the day, nearly every day, for at least 2 weeks. The diagnosis of severe depressive episode requires the presence of all three of the first three symptoms.

The diagnosis of a depressive episode does not in any way depend on the presence or absence of a precipitating life event or situation. The ICD-10 also has a category of brief depressive reaction (one of the 'adjustment disorders'), which forms part of the differential diagnosis of a depressive episode. This syndrome is defined by the presence of a precipitating life event and depressive symptoms. However, if the depressive symptoms are of sufficient number, pervasiveness and duration as to qualify for the description of a depressive episode, then this diagnosis should be made regardless of the presence of a precipitant. The notion that 'this patient's depression is understandable given the circumstances' should never detract from a proper evaluation of the severity and duration of the symptoms.

Epidemiology

Clinical depression, defined as 'major depression' or an ICD-10 'depressive episode', is a very common condition. Extensive epidemiological community surveys in many populations around the world have established that the 6-month prevalence rate of major depression is in the range of 2–5% in any population [3]. The epidemiological research has also shown that only a minority of persons with current depressive syndromes are receiving active treatment [3].

The age onset of the first depressive episode is typically in the third decade, but can be at any age. The male to female ratio is 1:2. A person who has had one episode of clinical depression has an 80% chance of recurrence and patients with recurrent depression have an average of four episodes in their lifetime [4].

Incomplete recovery is common. Studies of hospitalized patients have shown that, while at least 50% of patients recover from an index episode within 6 months, 30% remain symptomatic for more than a year and 12% for more than 5 years [5].

There is some evidence for an increase in the prevalence of major depression and a younger age of onset, over the last 40 years [6].

Aetiology

The aetiology of depression is complex, involving both genetic and environmental factors. Important environmental factors include childhood experiences of adversity or neglect and stresses in adult life. The effect of genetic factors may be mediated in part through inherited predispositions to excessive worry and anxiety [3].

Precipitating life events, especially those involving loss, are known to play a part in triggering individual episodes of depression [7]. This effect is greatest for the first episode of depression. Second and subsequent episodes are more likely to occur without identifiable precipitating events [8], suggesting that the first episode has a neurobiological priming effect [9].

Neurobiological changes in depression are also complex. Based in part on the supposed mechanism of action of antidepressant medication, early work focused on evidence of depletion of amine neurotransmitters in the central nervous system [10]. More recent research has suggested depression may involve alterations in neural cell populations, especially in the hippocampus [11].

Prevention

Depression is a major public health problem. The World Health Organization has determined that, in 1990, depression was the fourth leading cause of disease burden in the world and that by 2020 it would be the second leading cause of disease burden [12]. Public health measures have included campaigns to raise awareness of depression both in the general public and in healthcare providers. ED staff can play a very significant role in case identification and in ensuring referral for effective treatment.

Clinical features

The syndrome described as a 'depressive episode' (or 'major depression') is defined principally by its symptoms and, to a lesser extent, signs. As the severity of the depressive episode is also dependent on specific characteristics of the individual symptoms and signs (as well as the total number of symptoms), it is also important to understand the varieties of their manifestations.

Symptoms

It is useful to start the history with an exploration of the problem that has brought the person to the ED. This problem may be an overdose or other attempted suicide or self-harm, a personal or relationship crisis, a period of alcohol or other drug abuse, an exacerbation of a chronic medical condition or chronic pain or some other complaint. It is also important during the clinical assessment to begin to form some picture of who the patient is, including whether he or she lives alone or with others, the nature and quality of his or her personal relationships and his or her daily occupation, interests and activities. These inquiries assist in building rapport through demonstrating an interest in the patient, but also elicit information that is necessary for understanding the patient's symptoms in context.

At some point, the patient can be told that the interviewer would now like to explore the symptoms of depression in more detail. It may be helpful to group the symptoms of the depressive episode (see Table 20.4.1) into various domains of the patient's experience. The first group ('depressed mood', 'markedly diminished interest' and 'loss of energy') refers to the pervasive mood state and the quality of the patient's spirits or enthusiasm for life. The second group ('loss of self-esteem', 'unreasonable self-reproach or guilt' and 'recurrent thoughts of death or suicide') refers to the cognitive contents of the patient's thoughts. The third group ('diminished concentration' and 'psychomotor agitation or retardation') refers to the degree of agitation or lethargy associated with the patient's thought processes and physical activity. The final group ('insomnia or hypersomnia' and 'change in appetite') refers to physiological changes.

Both the pervasiveness and duration of these symptoms should be assessed. The syndrome is, by definition, one in which the symptoms have become persistent and inescapable, not the occasional or sporadic experience of these symptoms which nearly everybody endures sometimes. Duration is important because the syndrome must be present for at least 2 weeks before the diagnosis can be made, although often the patient may have been unwell much longer than this.

The timing of onset of a depressive episode can be difficult to establish because the onset is often very gradual and insidious (although it can be relatively rapid). The patient may have experienced previous episodes which become confused with the present one and patients often confuse long-term feelings of low self-esteem with the current episode. Hence, the question 'How long have you been feeling like this?' is often unproductive. It is more useful to ask the patient to describe the presence and pervasiveness of each of the symptoms 'during the last 2 or 3 weeks or so' and, in particular, to try to identify some recent time at which there has been a change in the clinical state or function of the patient.

The pervasiveness and duration criteria taken together imply a diminished ability to carry out normal activities and meet responsibilities. Although many depressed patients push themselves to keep going, careful enquiry reveals that this has become more arduous. Difficulty in attending to tasks may range from diminished effectiveness at work, child care or study to, eventually, neglect of self-care and nutrition. Thus, impairment in function is another indicator of the severity of the episode.

'Depressed mood, most of the day, nearly every day' is perhaps the most difficult of the symptoms to characterize. 'Mood' refers to a person's underlying emotional state, the emotional baseline that permeates each day. It is useful to ask not only 'Do you feel depressed?' but also 'What is that like for you?' Some patients describe feeling much more unhappy than usual or sad all the time or unexpectedly tearful; others report feeling more irritable with others or more inclined to worry. The severity of the mood change may be shown in a loss of mood reactivity, which can be elicited by asking 'Can you cheer yourself up, take your mind off your worries?' and 'Do you find that the things which normally make you happy don't seem to cheer you up as much as usual?'

'Markedly diminished interest or pleasure in all, or almost all, activities, most of the day, nearly every day' is somewhat easier to assess, especially if the interviewer takes the time to build up a picture of the patient's usual day. With careful inquiry, a nuanced picture can be built up of the extent of the patient's withdrawal from his or her usual activities. Included within this criterion is a lack of pleasure or interest in sexual activity which, in more severe cases, can be experienced as a profound loss of sexual feelings.

'Loss of energy or fatigue, nearly every day' is an important symptom which is sometimes overlooked. The emphasis should be on the loss of energy, that is, whether the patient is aware of having much less energy or drive than usual. In severe cases, the patient may describe feeling the body is heavy or thoughts sluggish, at which point this symptom overlaps with 'psychomotor retardation'. Loss of energy is an important symptom in differential diagnosis, which may point to such conditions as anaemia, hypothyroidism, diabetes or other undiagnosed medical conditions.

The cognitive symptoms of depression ('loss of self-esteem', 'unreasonable self-reproach or guilt' and 'recurrent thoughts of death or suicide') can to some extent be observed in listening to the patient's spontaneous comments and, as such, form a part of the mental state examination. However, patients who are more introspective have some awareness of a change in thought processes and are able to describe the ways in which their thoughts have become more gloomy than usual. This insight is lost when depression becomes more severe and the patient tends to regard the self-reproach or thoughts of suicide as entirely justified.

In assessing 'loss of confidence or self-esteem', the emphasis should be on the loss or change in the person's self-concept. It can be helpful to approach the issue with suggestive questions, such as 'Tell me about a time when you felt better about yourself', 'Did you used to feel more confident at work?' or 'Was there a time when you felt more adequate as a parent?'

'Unreasonable feelings of self-reproach or excessive or inappropriate guilt, nearly every day' is probably one of the most consistently reliable symptoms pointing to a diagnosis of depressive episode. Sometimes, a very conscientious person may habitually find fault with him- or herself without being clinically depressed. However, a person who is not depressed will usually be able to consider other points of view, to debate the sense of culpability internally and to consider whether the sense of guilt may be 'excessive', 'inappropriate' or 'unreasonable'. This capacity to rationalize about thought processes becomes progressively more impaired as the patient becomes more severely depressed, until the patient's guilt appears unquestionable.

In psychotic forms of depression, the sense of guilt may take on bizarre dimensions in which the patient can feel responsible for all the evil in the world or for distant events. A not uncommon experience is for the patient to see a report on the television of a calamity, such as an earthquake, and to feel responsible for the event.

'Recurrent thoughts of death or suicide' can arise in a depressive episode in a variety of ways. Not uncommonly, the thoughts may simply come into the patient's mind; the patient reports having thoughts of being dead, wanting to be dead or thoughts of suicide that are uncharacteristic, unbidden and unwanted, without any intention to act on these thoughts. Sometimes the suicidal thoughts are directly linked to excessive or delusional guilt, in which the patient feels his or her death to be necessary and inevitable; here the risk of suicidal action is very high.

In other cases, the suicidal thoughts are a logical consequence of a sense of hopelessness, a lack of faith in the future. This last type of suicidal ideation is less specific for the diagnosis of depressive episode, as it may also reflect an apparently realistic appraisal of life circumstances, an attitude of philosophical pessimism or poor coping skills in a person with impaired personality function. These distinctions are important because the suicidal ideation, which is a part of a depressive episode, may be expected to resolve with treatment of the depression, whereas the other forms may not.

'Diminished ability to think or concentrate or indecisiveness, nearly every day' is a relatively straightforward symptom to assess and is useful as an indicator of the severity of the depressive episode. It can be assessed by asking about ability to focus on work or a recreational activity, such as watching television or reading a book. Some patients report that their mind is easily distracted or restlessly inattentive. Many report the intrusion of negative ruminations (concerning lack of worth, sense of failure or guilt, thoughts of suicide or other worries) which go round and round in their minds. Progressive impairment in the capacity to concentrate will demonstrate increasing severity of depression; a severely depressed patient may not even be able to focus on one newspaper story and take in the contents.

'Psychomotor agitation or retardation, nearly every day' refers to abnormalities of movement, facial expression, speech and thought processes which are directly assessed in the mental state examination and are discussed more fully below. However, this can also to some extent be assessed through the history from the family. 'Psychomotor agitation' includes restless, fidgety behaviour, inability to sit still or attend to a task and anxious, repetitive speech or even perseveration. 'Psychomotor retardation' includes lack of spontaneous bodily movement, lack of facial expression, lack of verbal communication and slowness of response. Retardation is the more common and the patient or family may report progressive withdrawal and decrease in activity to the point where the patient sits for long hours apparently doing nothing. The presence of significant psychomotor agitation or retardation is usually indicative of a severe depressive episode.

Changes in sleep pattern ('insomnia or hypersomnia, nearly every day') are very common in depression, even in mild episodes. It is worth enquiring in detail about the specific changes in sleep pattern, as these relate to the severity of the depressive episode. Initial insomnia or delay in the onset of sleep is not specifically associated with depression, as it can be strongly associated with anxiety or primary insomnia. Middle insomnia (waking after 2 or 3 hours of sleep) and early morning waking are more specific to depression. The extent of difficulty the patient has in going back to sleep and the mood and thought content when awake during the night are also relevant.

Change in appetite may involve an increase or decrease with corresponding weight change. Severe loss of appetite with marked loss of weight, in the absence of medical illness or deliberate dieting, is associated with severe depression.

Signs

The most important signs are:

- signs of psychomotor agitation or retardation
- the affective state of the patient
- the thought content
- the degree of insight.

The patient with psychomotor agitation demonstrates, in milder forms, fidgety or repetitive behaviours, such as hand wringing or sighing. This can progress to an inability to sit still and, eventually, continuous pacing. The patient may say little while looking very apprehensive and preoccupied or may importune all the staff with repetitive, anxious questions, apparently seeking reassurance which is never achieved. In severe cases, speech becomes perseverative.

By contrast, the psychomotor-retarded patient maintains a relative immobility, lying in bed or sitting in a chair for long periods, with infrequent changes in posture. The face may be relatively expressionless, look sad or show an anxious dread. Both the facial expression and the body language show diminished reactivity during interview. There is little spontaneous speech and, if responses to questions can be elicited, the responses lack richness, depth or elaboration. Slowness of thought processes is shown especially by a marked increase (sometimes as long as several minutes) in the time taken to supply an answer to a question. In severe cases, the patient may be mute.

The affective state of the depressed patient during the interview is most often sad, but sometimes anxious or even hostile. As the depression becomes more severe, the patient tends to show a diminished range of affects and has an impaired affective reactivity (for example, the patient does not smile in response to social cues).

During the interview it is important to observe the themes evident in the patient's spontaneous conversation. Themes of despair, failure, guilt and death are typical of a depressive episode. The degree of insight may be a marker of the severity of the depressive episode.

Variants

Melancholic (somatic) depression

Some severe depressive episodes can be distinguished which have severe mood symptoms, marked changes in physiological function and significant psychomotor agitation or retardation.

This form of the depressive syndrome is designated 'major depression with melancholia' in DSM-IV and 'depressive episode with somatic syndrome' in ICD-10. The ICD-10 criteria for the 'somatic syndrome' are shown in Table 20.4.2. At least four of the eight symptoms must be present to make the diagnosis. Most 'depressive episodes with somatic syndrome' are also likely to meet the criteria for 'severe depressive episode'.

The clinical significance of making the diagnosis of melancholic depression is that this form of depression is likely to require intensive biological treatment.

Table 20.4.2 ICD-10 criteria for the 'somatic syndrome' (melancholia) [1]
1. Marked loss of interest in activities that are normally pleasurable
2. Lack of emotional reactions to events or activities that normally produce an emotional response
3. Waking in the morning 2 hours or more before the usual time
4. Depression worse in the morning
5. Objective evidence of marked psychomotor retardation or agitation
6. Marked loss of appetite
7. Marked loss of libido

Most of the symptoms contributing to the diagnosis of the 'somatic syndrome' are more severe and more specific forms of the symptoms of a 'depressive episode.' It is not just any sleep disturbance, but marked early morning waking which is important. Similarly, it is not just a change in appetite, but a significant (more than 5% of body weight) loss of weight which is important. The presence and severity of the psychomotor agitation or retardation is the most important sign, since these phenomena can be objectively and systematically observed and rated [13].

Psychotic depression

This is discussed in Chapter 20.5. The patient with a psychotic depression will usually meet the criteria for a severe depressive episode, often with the 'somatic syndrome.'

Mild and moderate depressive episodes

In clinical practice, it is usually not difficult to recognize a 'severe' depressive episode.

Greater uncertainty may be associated with making the diagnosis of 'mild' or 'moderate' depressive episode, especially in patients who have a long-term history of poor self-esteem or are temperamentally inclined to worrying, moodiness or irritability. Some research evidence [14] suggests that these temperamental factors can affect the presentation of the depressive syndrome. Thus, a person who is a habitual worrier who develops a depressive episode is likely to worry more and perhaps to withdraw from social contact or abuse alcohol or anxiolytic drugs. A person who tends to be moody or irritable is likely to become more so in a depressive episode and may appear demanding, complaining and unreasonable.

Nevertheless, the essential and salient characteristic of even a mild or moderate depressive episode is that the patient has a persistent mood change for at least 2 weeks. The interviewer should focus on the symptoms of depressed mood, loss of interest and loss of energy because it is the enduring presence of these symptoms which makes the diagnosis clear. Of the additional symptoms contributing to the diagnosis of depressive episode, probably the most common are difficulty with sleep and diminished ability to think and concentrate.

A patient with persistent depressed mood and impaired concentration almost certainly has some functional impairment. A useful approach to this question is to ask the patient about normal daily activities and then assess the extent to which these activities are disrupted by the symptoms. Can the patient do household chores? Does this require unusual effort? Can the patient go to work? Is the patient functional at work? Are even simple leisure activities like watching television disrupted by the patient's mood state? It is this evidence of change in function that permits the identification of a mild or moderate depressive episode, regardless of pre-existing temperamental vulnerabilities.

Depression in the elderly

The symptoms of depression in older people are generally very similar to those in younger age groups and should be assessed in a similar way [15]. Symptoms, such as loss of energy, insomnia or change in appetite, may also be influenced by co-morbid medical illness, but a persistent mood change or loss of interest should prompt consideration of a depressive episode. Older people may tend to minimize their feelings of depression and, in these cases, a collateral history of loss of interest in usual activities may be found. Not uncommonly older people are seen in the ED following an overdose that may appear medically trivial. These patients should always be carefully assessed for the presence of a depressive syndrome.

'Pseudo-dementia' is a term used to describe patients with a depressive syndrome who present with an apparent change in cognitive function. The patient with depressive pseudo-dementia is likely to have a relatively recent and relatively abrupt change in concentration and memory. In contrast to the patient with dementia, the patient with pseudo-dementia usually shows a great awareness of having memory difficulties and will tend to demonstrate the impairment to the interviewer with considerable anxiety. In addition, the patient with depressive pseudo-dementia manifests other symptoms of a depressive episode.

Differential diagnosis

The differential diagnosis of the depressive syndrome is important because there are several other clinical disorders involving depressed mood or other symptoms of depression which have a different prognosis and treatment.

Brief depressive reaction

A brief depressive reaction (also called 'adjustment disorder with depressed mood' in DSM-IV) can be diagnosed when a person experiences some depressive symptoms without meeting the full criteria for a depressive episode, following stressful life events. Typically, the person describes a depressed mood which is not persistent, that is there are good days and bad days and the depressed mood can be relieved by distraction or pleasant activities. Common stressful life events include relationship crises or other interpersonal conflicts.

This is often the diagnosis in patients who are seen in the ED following overdose, although care should be taken to inquire about symptoms of a depressive episode. Treatment involves brief psychotherapy aimed at helping the person achieve some resolution of the personal crisis. If the hospital has a crisis counselling service, the patient can be referred to that service for brief therapy. Alternatively, the patient can be referred to their GP or other community counselling service. Social work staff in the ED often have good knowledge of local crisis counselling services.

Grief

The symptoms of acute grief can be mood disturbance, guilt, impaired concentration, sleep and appetite disturbance, impaired function in daily activities and preoccupation with memories of the deceased [16]. There is a considerable overlap with the symptoms of a depressive episode. However, it is customary to respect the feelings of the bereaved and to recognize that it is usually beneficial for the person to be supported through the natural process of grief, preferably by family, friends or other familiar persons, such as the family GP.

However, if the symptoms become more severe or more prolonged (such as beyond 6 months), it is appropriate to consider the diagnosis of a depressive episode. Symptoms suggestive of the development of a depressive episode include persistent and progressive lowering of self-esteem, persistent thoughts of death and suicide, markedly impaired concentration and psychomotor retardation.

Bipolar depression

ICD-10 specifies that in a person who has a history of bipolar disorder, a diagnosis of 'depressive episode' should not be made even if the patient meets the criteria for a depressive episode. Instead, the diagnosis of 'bipolar affective episode, current episode mild, moderate or severe depression' should be made. The

PSYCHIATRIC EMERGENCIES

Table 20.4.3   Signs contributing to the diagnosis of a manic episode in ICD-10 [1]
1. Increased activity or physical restlessness
2. Increased talkativeness ('pressure of speech')
3. Flight of ideas or subjective experience of thoughts racing
4. Loss of normal inhibitions, resulting in behaviour that is inappropriate to the circumstances
5. Decreased need for sleep
6. Inflated self-esteem or grandiosity
7. Distractibility or constantly changing activity or plans
8. Behaviour that is foolhardy or reckless
9. Marked sexual energy or sexual indiscretions

Table 20.4.4   Medical conditions associated with depressive syndrome
Hypothyroidism
Hypercalcaemia
Pernicious anaemia
Pancreatic cancer
Lung cancer
Stroke
Alzheimer's dementia
Vascular dementia
Parkinson's disease
Huntington's disease
AIDS
Central nervous system tumour
Multiple sclerosis
Neurosyphilis
Brucellosis

distinction is important because of the treatment and prognosis. In particular, antidepressant medication should be used very cautiously in the person with bipolar disorder because of the risk of provoking a switch to mania.

The symptoms of a bipolar depressive episode are in themselves not different from the symptoms of any other episode of depression. The distinction therefore rests on a previous history of treatment for bipolar disorder or a history of a manic episode that may not have been treated.

A manic episode, as defined in ICD-10 [1], involves an elevated or irritable mood sustained for at least a week and at least three (or at least four if the mood is only irritable) of the signs shown in Table 20.4.3. Mania is discussed in more detail in Chapter 20.5.

The depressed patient seen in ED who is suspected of having a bipolar disorder should usually be referred to a psychiatrist for assessment and treatment. Bipolar disorder is a lifelong condition, with a high rate of recurrent episodes, which requires specialized pharmacological and psychological management.

Organic mood disorder
Many medical conditions (Table 20.4.4) are especially associated with a typical depressive syndrome. Because the medical condition is considered likely to have a pathophysiological significance in the development of the depressive syndrome, these conditions are termed 'organic mood disorders.'

Occasionally, the depressive syndrome may be the first presentation of a previously undiagnosed medical illness. Clinical or laboratory evidence of hypothyroidism was found in 5% of patients with a depressive syndrome in one series [17]. Hypercalcaemia due to unsuspected hyperparathyroidism very occasionally presents with depressed mood, lethargy or cognitive change as the presenting symptoms [18]. The first presentation of pancreatic cancer with a depressive syndrome is well recognized [19]. A depressive syndrome may be the first presentation of Huntington's disease, before the onset of the movement disorder and the diagnosis will only be suggested by the family history [20]. Some patients with HIV infection have been found to present with a mood disorder before manifesting other symptoms of AIDS [21]. Because many medical conditions associated with depressive symptoms involve central nervous system disease, any neurological signs should prompt investigation for, for example, unsuspected cerebral tumour.

However, more commonly the depressive syndrome presents in a patient with an already recognized medical illness. In these cases, it is important to evaluate carefully the severity and persistence of the depressive symptoms and not dismiss them as an understandable reaction to the illness. Symptoms, such as loss of energy, sleep disturbance and anorexia, may be difficult to evaluate as they may be related to other pathophysiological change, but the patient with persistent depressed mood, loss of pleasure in activities, marked loss of self-esteem and feelings of guilt or hopelessness is likely to be experiencing a depressive episode. If such a depressive episode is diagnosed and treated, the patient will experience relief of suffering and a greater ability to deal effectively with other medical problems.

Many drugs have been associated with depressive symptoms, often based on only a few case reports [22]. Medications with a particularly strong association with depression include interferon, isotretinoin, methyldopa, benzodiazepines, digitalis, β-blockers, oral contraceptives and corticosteroids. A useful approach is to consider drugs which have recently been introduced in relation to the time course of the depressive symptoms.

Mood disorder due to psychoactive substance use
Chronic alcohol misuse is frequently associated with depressed mood, low self-esteem and feelings of guilt and hopelessness. Severe sleep disturbance can also be precipitated by rebound wakefulness as blood alcohol levels fall during the night. The person who regularly abuses alcohol is also likely to experience fatigue, impaired concentration, appetite disturbance and loss of sex drive. These symptoms may mimic those due to a depressive episode, such that it is not possible to make a differential diagnosis of a depressive episode while the patient continues to drink, nor is it likely that the depressive symptoms will remit without abstinence. Patients with alcohol-induced mood disorders should be encouraged to attend alcohol detoxification and rehabilitation programmes. There is some evidence that antidepressant medication may help to reduce both depressive symptoms and alcohol consumption [23].

Amphetamine withdrawal is often associated with a markedly depressed mood which usually improves within a few days if the patient remains abstinent.

The abuse of alcohol and other drugs is sometimes an attempt to self-medicate for a pre-existing depressive syndrome. This history should be especially sought in the patient whose abuse of alcohol or other drugs is of recent onset or follows important life change, such as bereavement or divorce. Even if a pre-existing depressive syndrome is identified, however, the patient should be informed that abstinence is necessary for recovery.

Depressive stupor, catatonia and hysterical stupor

Sometimes a patient with profound psycho-motor retardation presents with 'depressive stupor', that is the patient is mute but alert and lacking spontaneous bodily movement. This presentation can give rise to a diagnostic uncertainty in the ED. Neurological conditions, such as pontine haemorrhage causing a 'locked-in syndrome', may have to be considered. Collateral history, if available, generally reveals that the patient with depressive stupor has a preceding history of the gradual onset of a depressive syndrome. Occasionally, the condition of depressive stupor may be confused with the catatonic form of schizophrenia. However, in catatonia the patient is likely to display 'waxy flexibility' (maintenance of an uncomfortable posture, such as an arm held up for a prolonged period against gravity), echopraxia (imitation of movements) and bizarre posturing and grimacing. These specific motor abnormalities are not usually associated with depressive stupor. Furthermore, the catatonic form of schizophrenia is now quite rare, especially as a first presentation. A final differential diagnosis of depressive stupor is hysterical stupor: in this condition, the collateral history shows that the patient was well preceding the abrupt onset of apparent paralysis and mutism. There will usually be a history of a markedly stressful event.

Dysthymia

Dysthymia refers to a chronic form of depression in which the patient experiences symptoms, such as lack of enjoyment in life and a gloomy or pessimistic outlook, without meeting the full criteria for a depressive episode. The depressed outlook tends to become interwoven with the personality of the patient, who tends to be sombre, self-critical and lacking in confidence and motivation. Dysthymia often has onset in early adult life and can persist for many years. The disorder has been well characterized [24] and found to be relatively common (about 3% of the general population) in epidemiological studies [25].

Sometimes, patients with a dysthymic disorder develop further symptoms indicating a superimposed depressive episode, which can be termed a 'double depression'.

Patients with dysthymia may present to EDs as a consequence of suicidal ideation or behaviour. The condition should be regarded as serious because of its chronicity. The patient should be referred to a psychiatrist or mental health service as the treatment can be difficult [26].

Anxiety

Anxiety disorders include panic disorder (recurrent panic attacks), generalized anxiety disorder (persistent worrying associated with muscular tension and autonomic symptoms), obsessive–compulsive disorder and phobic disorders, such as agoraphobia or social phobia. Any of the symptoms of each of these anxiety disorders may occur as part of the symptoms of a depressive episode if a person with a pre-morbid anxious temperament becomes depressed. However, primary anxiety disorders are also common. In these cases, the patient gives a history of typical anxiety symptoms usually extending over many months or even years. Many patients with primary anxiety disorder go on also to develop a depressive syndrome.

Because of both the overlap in symptoms and the frequent co-morbidity, it may be difficult to distinguish primary anxiety disorders from primary depressive disorders in the emergency setting. Probably the most important symptoms are persistent depressed mood and suicidal ideation, which may require inpatient treatment. Patients who do not have persistent depressed mood and suicidal ideation, but who have a mixture of other depressive symptoms and anxiety symptoms, can be safely directed to their GP or to an outpatient mental health service for further evaluation.

Personality disorder

The concept of personality disorder refers to enduring patterns of behaviour, including especially interpersonal behaviours, which are well outside the usually sanctioned range of behaviours in a particular culture and which are associated with substantial subjective distress or conflict with others. The diagnosis of personality disorder should only be made if the behaviour patterns are persistent, relatively inflexible and have been present since a young age, often beginning in childhood or adolescence.

Although a variety of specific personality disorders have been described, the two most common forms in the ED are antisocial personality disorder and borderline personality disorder.

Persons with antisocial personality have a long-term history of disregard for social rules, usually resulting in a chequered employment history, broken relationships and often violent or criminal behaviour. As a result of personal crisis precipitated by these behaviours, persons with antisocial personality not infrequently present to ED with acute brief depressive reactions, helplessness and suicidal ideation or behaviour. Assessment should be especially directed at clarifying if a superimposed persistent depressive episode is present and the severity of this episode.

Inpatient psychiatric treatment is problematic because the patient often has difficulty adhering to ward rules and expectations. If the depressive symptoms are not severe and seem to be reactive to recent stressors, it is preferable to try to engage the patient in a realistic discussion of the current problems and, if possible, make a referral to crisis counselling. In some cases, however, when the depressive symptoms are more severe and the risk of suicidal behaviour is high, it may be necessary to arrange inpatient admission.

The person with borderline personality disorder displays persistent severely immature interpersonal behaviour, as well as considerable impulsivity and recklessness. The interpersonal behaviours include a strong tendency to see others in 'all good' or 'all bad' terms and to blame others for the patient's own feelings and behaviours. Reckless and impulsive behaviours include abrupt breaches in relationships, alcohol and other drug abuse and self-damaging acts, such as cutting. Persons with borderline personality often describe chronic feelings of emptiness and loneliness, often associated with suicidal ideation. These features are sometimes misdiagnosed as depression when they may actually represent the patient's usual way of feeling rather than a discrete depressive episode. Because borderline personality disorder is a long-term condition, intervention with the patient who presents in the ED in crisis should, if possible, be directed towards facilitating or enhancing the patient's engagement with outpatient treatment services.

As many as 50% of patients with borderline personality may also meet the criteria for a depressive episode at any one time [27]. Although a diagnosis of borderline personality may have been made on the basis of the longitudinal history, it is therefore also important to try to assess the severity, persistence and duration of current depressive symptoms. If the patient is already engaged with an outpatient mental health clinician, it is useful to liaise with the therapist regarding recent symptoms and function.

Assessment

The assessment of the patient for depression should cover:

- the current social circumstances of the patient
- recent stressors or precipitating events
- thorough evaluation of the symptoms of the syndrome of clinical depression and their severity
- consideration of previous depressive or manic episodes
- mental state examination
- risk assessment
- consideration of possible medical illness as cause of symptoms
- detailed evaluation of alcohol and other drug use
- identification of treatment services already available to patient.

It is generally a good idea to start the interview with some basic social information. Does the patient live alone? How is he or she occupied or employed? Is there a supportive relationship or other family? This information assists in understanding the context of the symptoms and helps with treatment planning.

Exploration of precipitating events is important partly because these worries are likely to be occupying the mind of the patient and discussion of these issues helps to build rapport in the interview.

Identification of the presence and severity of the depressive symptoms is the most important part of the assessment. Unfortunately, it is often not done systematically and the 'diagnosis' of depression is made only on the basis of a patient's statement about 'being depressed' and one or two other symptoms, such as sleep and appetite disturbance. Systematic evaluation requires detailed exploration of the symptoms described above. Particular attention should be paid to the persistence, pervasiveness and duration of the symptoms. If this systematic approach is taken it is possible to determine:

- if the syndrome of clinical depression is present or not
- the severity of the syndrome.

The proper diagnosis of a depressive syndrome and the assessment of the severity of the syndrome are of major importance in treatment planning.

There may be insufficient time in an emergency interview to explore fully the previous psychiatric history. However, it is useful to ask if the patient has been depressed before, whether or not any previous episodes were treated and what was the response to previous treatment. It is also important to identify any previous episodes of mania in case the depressive episode may be a presentation of bipolar disorder.

Mental state examination focuses on the signs described above. Persistently sad affect and noticeable psychomotor agitation or retardation are indicators of more severe depression. Similarly, if the patient's conversation is very preoccupied with themes of failure, despair, guilt or death, the depression is likely to be more severe. Inquiry about these matters should be extended to look for delusional beliefs. Useful questions may include 'Do you feel responsible for bad things happening?', 'Do you feel there is something drastically wrong with you?' or 'Do you believe you deserve punishment?' Understanding the patient's level of insight into his or her condition is also important to treatment planning, particularly if involuntary treatment should become necessary due to the risk of suicide.

Risk assessment is multifaceted. If the patient has attempted suicide through overdose or other means, inquiry should be made about the circumstances of this attempt, the patient's understanding of the lethality of the attempt and whether or not the patient sought help afterwards or made an effort to conceal the attempt. The patient's current thoughts about suicide and his or her attitude to suicide are also relevant. Many patients admit to having thoughts of suicide but indicate that they would be deterred from suicidal action by, for example, having responsibility for dependent children. The disappearance of these 'protective factors' from a patient's considerations is an indicator of worsening risk. Patients with psychotic depression may be at higher risk because they lack such 'emotional' constraints on suicidal behaviour. Other factors associated with increased suicide risk include lack of supportive relationships, living alone, being unemployed and current alcohol abuse.

A primary medical condition causing depressive symptoms is likely to be suggested by other symptoms and signs or be pre-existing. There are no mandatory investigations for the assessment of a depressive episode, although checking thyroid biochemistry is sensible.

Inquiry should be made about alcohol and other drug-use patterns and, especially, recent changes in pattern use. A person with long-standing alcohol or other drug abuse is likely to have a substance-induced mood disorder and needs to address this as the major focus of treatment. A recent marked increase in alcohol or other drug use may indicate an attempt to self-medicate for a depressive syndrome.

It is always useful to ask the patient if she or he is currently seeing a psychiatrist, psychologist or other mental health therapist or has a good relationship with a trusted GP. These existing healthcare professionals can often be the natural starting point in planning treatment interventions.

Treatment

Treatment for a depressive episode involves the prescription of specific antidepressant medication or a specific course of psychotherapy or both.

Medications

Commonly used first-line antidepressant medications are shown in Table 20.4.5. Because no one of these medications has been shown consistently to have superior efficacy, choice of medication is based on the acceptability of the side-effect profile and previous treatment response.

The selective serotonin re-uptake inhibitors (SSRIs) are usually well tolerated and are a good first choice. Some patients experience agitation, nausea or gastrointestinal hypermotility when they start SSRI medications. These symptoms usually settle in a week or two. The most troublesome long-term side effect of SSRIs is sexual dysfunction (especially delayed ejaculation or anorgasmia). These side effects sometimes require a change of medication. The side effects of venlafaxine are similar to SSRIs, with the addition of excessive sweating and itch at high doses.

Mirtazapine has useful sedating properties and can be very helpful in a patient with marked insomnia or agitation. Because it stimulates appetite, its use is limited in patients

Table 20.4.5 Commonly used antidepressant medications

Drug	Class	Usual daily oral dose range (mg)	Half life (hours)
Fluoxetine	SSRI	20–60	24–144
Citalopram	SSRI	20–40	23–45
Escitalopram	SSRI	10–20	27–32
Fluvoxamine	SSRI	100–300	9–28
Paroxetine	SSRI	10–40	3–65
Sertraline	SSRI	50–200	22–36
Venlafaxine	SNRI	75–225	3–7
Moclobemide	RIMA	450–600	1–3
Mirtazapine	–	30–60	20–40
Reboxitene	–	8–10	12–13

SSRI: selective serotonin re-uptake inhibitor; SNRI: serotonin and noradrenaline re-uptake inhibitor; RIMA: reversible monoamine oxidase inhibitor.

with a weight problem. Mirtazapine, reboxitine and moclobemide are useful alternatives for patients who experience sexual dysfunction with SSRIs or venlafaxine.

Tricyclic antidepressants (e.g. imipramine, amitriptyline and dothiepin) and irreversible monoamine oxidase inhibitors (MAOIs; phenelzine and tranylcypromine) continue to be prescribed for some patients, but they tend not to be first-line drugs. The use of tricyclics has decreased because of side effects (especially anticholinergic) and because of their cardiac toxicity in overdose. Irreversible MAOIs are generally inconvenient to take because of the need for dietary restrictions.

Psychotherapy

The psychotherapies commonly used for depression include supportive psychotherapy, cognitive behavioural therapy (CBT) and interpersonal psychotherapy (IPT). Most psychiatrists and clinical psychologists have appropriate training and skills to offer one or more of these therapies. Many GPs and other health professionals, such as social workers, nurses and occupational therapists, have also often received training in these therapies.

Supportive psychotherapy is the least well defined of the psychotherapeutic treatments. The core of the treatment is a supportive relationship, education about the nature of depression and practical advice. CBT is a structured psychotherapy, usually involving 10–20 sessions. The behavioural techniques include reversing social isolation, scheduling relaxing or pleasurable activities and working with family members to provide incentives for helpful behaviours. The main part of the therapy involves 'cognitive restructuring', a systematic exploration of the patient's unhelpful thought patterns, followed by collaborative work to help the patient substitute more positive responses [28].

IPT is also a structured psychotherapy, typically of about 16 sessions. The therapy focuses on helping the patient to make changes in his or her interpersonal relationships which may be contributing to the depressive syndrome [29].

Evidence

All currently available antidepressants have been shown to achieve better symptom reduction than placebo, with no one antidepressant consistently demonstrating superior efficacy [30]. In drug trials, up to 40% of patients in the placebo arm show improvement, which may include the non-specific effects of supportive interventions, as well as spontaneous remissions [31]. As the natural history of depression in a community sample (which includes relatively minor, untreated cases) shows a median episode duration of 12 weeks, spontaneous remission appears to be not uncommon [32]. Patients with psychotic depression respond better to the combination of an antidepressant and an antipsychotic medication than to an antidepressant medication alone [33].

Both CBT and IPT have been shown to be effective in achieving symptom reduction compared to pill placebo control [34,35]. CBT and IPT have been shown to be as effective as medication for mild-to-moderate depression [35]. For a severe depressive episode, psychotherapy alone is not as effective as medication alone or a medication–psychotherapy combination [36].

There are no systematic data regarding supportive psychotherapy (as it is not a standardized treatment) but substantial clinical experience attests to its efficacy.

Mild-to-moderate depressive episodes

As long as the suicide risk is containable, the great majority of these patients can be treated as outpatients. The most important part of treatment planning in the ED is therefore to identify an appropriate referral pathway. If the patient is already in contact with a mental health professional or has a trusted GP, it is preferable to refer the patient back to these persons and, if possible, make phone contact with that doctor or therapist with advice regarding the emergency presentation. If the patient does not have their own doctor or mental health professional, it is appropriate to refer the patient to an outpatient mental health service.

Patients with mild-to-moderate depressive episodes can improve with either medication or psychotherapy and can be advised to discuss these treatment options with the follow-up doctor. It is not essential to start the antidepressant medication in the ED; it is probably more appropriate to leave this to the follow-up doctor who can monitor for efficacy and side effects.

Some patients may only have mild-to-moderate symptoms but, nevertheless, be at significant suicidal risk, associated with recent suicidal behaviour and persistent suicidal ideation. The risk is increased if the patient lives alone. Such patients require admission to a psychiatry ward, where the options for medication and psychotherapy can be further explored.

Severe depressive episodes

Most patients with severe depressive episodes will be admitted because of significant suicide risk or substantial functional impairment. The evidence suggests that these patients require treatment with antidepressant medication and are often initially too symptomatic to engage in psychotherapy. Classical indications for electroconvulsive therapy are psychotic depression and severe retarded depression (especially if the patient has inadequate oral intake).

Controversies and future directions

- Population-based studies indicate that clinical depression is very common, possibly increasing in prevalence and significantly undertreated.
- A major challenge for all health services is to improve the rate of case identification.
- Equally important will be the further development of effective referral pathways to appropriate treatment.

References

[1] World Health Organization The ICD-10 classification of mental and behavioural disorders. Geneva: WHO; 1993.

[2] American Psychiatric Association. Diagnostic and statistical manual of mental disorders, 4th ed. Washington DC: American Psychiatric Association; 1994.

[3] Joyce P. Epidemiology of mood disorders. In: Gelder M, Lopez-Ibor J, Andreasen N, editors. New Oxford textbook of psychiatry. Oxford: Oxford University Press, 2000, 695–701.

[4] Judd J. The clinical course of unipolar major depressive disorders. Arch Gen Psychiatr 1997;54:989–91.

[5] Katz M, Secunda S, Hirschfeld R, et al. NIMH clinical research branch collaborative program on the psychobiology of depression. Arch Gen Psychiatr 1979;36:765–71.

[6] Cross National Collaborative Group. The changing rate of major depression. Cross national comparisons. J Am Med Assoc 1992;268:3098–105.

[7] Tennant C. Life events, stress and depression: a review of recent findings. Aust NZ J Psychiatr 2002;36:173–82.

[8] Frank E, Anderson B, Reynolds C. Life events and research diagnostic criteria endogenous subtype. Arch Gen Psychiatr 1994;51:519–24.

[9] Kendler K, Thornton L, Gardner C. Stressful life events and previous episodes in the etiology of major depression in women: an evaluation of the 'kindling' hypothesis. Am J Psychiatr 2000;157:1243–51.

[10] Schildkraut J. The catecholamine hypothesis of affective disorders: a review of supporting evidence. Am J Psychiatr 1965;122:509–22.

[11] Jacobs B, Praag H, Gage F. Adult brain neurogenesis and psychiatry: a novel theory of depression. Mol Psychiatr 2000;5:262–9.

[12] Murray C, Lopez A. The global burden of disease and global health statistics. Boston: Harvard University Press; 1996.

[13] Parker G, Hadzi-Pavlovic D. Melancholia: a disorder of movement and mood. Cambridge: Cambridge University Press; 1996.

[14] Parker G, Hadzi-Pavlovic D, Roussos J, et al. Non-melancholic depression: the contribution of personality, anxiety and life-events to subclassification. Psychol Med 1998;28:1209–19.

[15] Musetti L, Perugi G, Soriani A, et al. Depression before and after age 65: a re-examination. Br J Psychiatr 1989;155:330–6.

[16] Lindemann E. The symptomatology and management of acute grief. Am J Psychiatr 1944;101:141.

[17] Gold M, Pottash A, Extein I. Hypothyroidism and depression. J Am Med Assoc 1981;245:1919–22.

[18] Watson L. Clinical aspects of hyperparathyroidism. Proc Roy Soc Med 1968;61:1123.

[19] Joffe R, Rubinow D, Denicoff K, et al. Depression and carcinoma of the pancreas. Gen Hosp Psychiatr 1986;8:241–5.

[20] Folstein S, Abbott M, Chase G, et al. The association of affective disorder with Huntington's disease in a case series and in families. Psychol Med 1983;13:537–42.

[21] Atkinson J, Grant I, Kennedy C, et al. Prevalence of psychiatric disorders among men infected with human immunodeficiency virus. Arch Gen Psychiatr 1988;45:859–64.

[22] Hales R, Yudofsky S. The American psychiatric publishing textbook of clinical psychiatry, 4th ed. Washington: American Psychiatric Publishing, 2003, 462–3.

[23] Cornelius J, Salloun I, Ehler J, et al. Fluoxetine reduced depressive symptoms and alcohol consumption in patients with co-morbid major depression and alcohol dependence. Arch Gen Psychiatr 1997;54:700–5.

[24] Akiskal H, Cassano G, editors. Dysthymia and the spectrum of chronic depressions. New York: Guildford Press; 1997.

[25] Waintraub L, Guelfi J. Nosological validity of dysthymia. Part 1, historical, epidemiological and clinical data. Eur Psychiatr 1998;13:173–80.

[26] Haykal R, Akiskal H. The long-term outcome of dysthymia in private practice. Clinical features, temperament and the art of management. J Clin Psychiatr 1999;60:508–18.

[27] Gunderson J. Borderline personality disorder: a clinical guide. Washington: American Psychiatric Publishing; 2001.

[28] Seligman M. Learned optimism. New York: Random House; 1991.

[29] Weissman M, Markowitz J, Klerman G. Comprehensive guide to interpersonal psychotherapy. New York: Basic Books; 2000.

[30] Nemeroff C, Schatzberg A. Pharmacological treatment of unipolar depression. In: Nathan P, Gorman J, editors. A guide to treatments that work. New York: Oxford University Press, 1998, p. 212–5.

[31] Paykel E, Scott J. Treatment of mood disorders. In: Gelder M, Lopez-Ibor J, Andreasen N, editors. New Oxford textbook of psychiatry. Oxford: Oxford University Press, 2000, p. 724–6.

[32] Eaton W, Anthony J, Gallo G, et al. Natural history of diagnostic interview schedule/DSM-IV major depression: the Baltimore epidemiologic catchment area follow-up. Arch Gen Psychiatr 1997;54:993–9.

[33] Schatzberg A, Rothschild A. Psychotic (delusional) major depression: should it be included as a distinct syndrome in DSM-IV? Am J Psychiatr 1992;149:733–45.

[34] Dobson K. A meta-analysis of the efficacy of cognitive therapy for depression. J Consult Clin Psychol 1988;57:414–9.

[35] Elkin I, Shea M, Watkins J, et al. National Institute of Mental Health treatment of depression collaborative treatment programme. Arch Gen Psychiatr 1992;46:971–82.

[36] Thase M, Greenhouse J, Frank E, et al. Treatment of major depression with psychotherapy or psychotherapy pharmacotherapy combinations. Arch Gen Psychiatr 1997;54:1009–15.

20.5 Psychosis

Simon Byrne

ESSENTIALS

1 In the age of community mental health treatment, emergency departments have become major sites for the assessment of patients with psychosis.

2 It is important to distinguish psychiatric causes of psychosis from psychosis due to medical conditions or to drug abuse.

3 Attention must be given to the proper management of the patient with psychosis in the emergency department environment.

4 Disposition decisions, including community referral or hospitalization, depend on the collection of information about treatment history, community supports and risk assessment, as well as assessment of the mental state of the patient.

Table 20.5.2   Pragmatic classification of patients with psychotic symptoms

1. Psychotic symptoms due to general medical condition
   1.1. Delirium
   1.2. Dementia
   1.3. Psychosis in clear consciousness without cognitive impairment
   1.4. Psychosis caused by medications
2. Acute and chronic schizophrenia
3. Mania with psychosis
4. Depression with psychosis
5. Substance-induced psychosis
6. Psychotic-like reactive states

Introduction

Psychotic illness is a frequent cause of presentation to the emergency department (ED), accounting for 0.5–1.0% of all visits and 10–20% of all mental health presentations [1,2]. Because these patients are usually severely mentally unwell, they also account for a significant share of the workload of EDs.

The tasks of the ED staff in relation to patients with psychotic illness are complex and varied. Initially, there is usually a need for containment and stabilization of an aroused and frightened patient with impaired reality testing. The patient is often in the hospital unwillingly and frequently following a major crisis in the community or at home. There is often a need to manage behavioural disturbance, potentially involving risk of harm to the patient, staff or others, while the patient remains in the ED for often lengthy periods of assessment and for the implementation of disposition plans. It is also important to exclude medical causes for the psychotic symptoms and to consider the presence of co-morbid medical conditions. In determining disposition, consideration must be given to the need for voluntary or involuntary admission or, alternatively, referral to an array of community-based treatment services. Finally, it is often useful to involve families and other carers in both the assessment phase and in treatment planning. These tasks are summarized in Table 20.5.1.

Table 20.5.1   Tasks of the ED in relation to the patient with psychosis

1. Stabilization of the aroused or frightened patient
2. Management of behavioural disturbance in the ED
3. Exclusion of medical causes for the psychiatric presentation
4. Assessing the presence of co-morbid medical illness
5. Determining the need for voluntary or involuntary admission
6. Arranging referral to community services
7. Liaison with family and other carers

ED, emergency department.

Classification

Traditionally, psychotic illnesses were classified into 'functional' (i.e. non-organic) psychoses and 'organic' psychoses. Developments in psychiatric nosology have expanded this classification and the ICD-10 Classification of Mental and Behavioural Disorders [3] now contains at least 16 different diagnoses, many with several subtypes, which could be used to describe patients with psychotic symptoms.

In emergency practice, however, the differentiation of the specific psychiatric syndrome is not always possible. The pragmatic classification shown in Table 20.5.2 is based on:

- excluding medical causes for the psychotic presentation

- considering the role of alcohol and other drugs of abuse
- making a provisional psychiatric diagnosis as a guide to initial management and
- considering the possibility that the symptoms may be related primarily to psychological stress.

A description of each of these categories is given in the section on clinical features.

Epidemiology and prognosis

The two principal 'non-organic' conditions which involve psychotic presentations are schizophrenia and bipolar affective disorder.

The prevalence of schizophrenia is 0.2–0.5% of the population. It is not a rare disorder. The male:female ratio is 1:1. Onset can be at any age, but mostly before the age of 30 [4].

Schizophrenia is usually a chronic condition, but with a variable course. In the long term, about 20% of cases have a good recovery, 20% have recurrent episodes with good recovery between episodes, 40% have recurrent episodes with incomplete remission and 20% have a severe chronic course [5]. The 20-year suicide rate may be as high as 14–22% [5].

The prevalence of bipolar disorder (which by definition means that the patient has had at least one manic episode) is about 1.0% of the population. The male:female ratio is 1:1. The onset is often in late adolescence and 95% of cases have onset before the age of 26 [6].

A patient who has had one episode of mania has about an 80% chance of a recurrence within 5 years. Although there is usually a good recovery between episodes, there is a very high rate of recurrence, with an average of one episode of mania or depression every 2 years, although the frequency of episodes in the individual case varies greatly [7]. The 22-year suicide rate is 13% [7].

Aetiology and prevention

The aetiology of schizophrenia and bipolar disorder is not well understood, despite intensive research. Both disorders involve genetic and environmental factors. A person who has one parent with schizophrenia has about a 10% chance of developing the disorder; this is similar for bipolar disorder. There is insufficient knowledge about the aetiology of either disorder to suggest effective strategies for primary prevention.

There is considerable scope for secondary prevention, which is early diagnosis and prompt treatment, especially in relation to recurrent episodes. Strategies include education of patients and families, the identification of early warning signs of relapse and the use of maintenance and prophylactic medication [8]. ED staff can make a major contribution to this preventative work by emphasizing the importance of continuing treatment and facilitating engagement with generalist and specialist mental health services.

Clinical features

Psychotic symptoms due to a general medical condition

Delirium

Delirious patients often manifest psychotic symptoms. Visual illusions (misperception of real objects, such as mistaking an innocuous object for a malevolent figure or animal) and delusions of persecution (such as the patient believing he is being poisoned by the doctors and nurses) are particularly common. Other symptoms include auditory hallucinations, affective lability, apparent formal thought disorder and grandiose or religious delusions.

The pathognomonic features of delirium are disorientation (especially for time and place) and a fluctuating conscious state. Not uncommonly, the patient plucks at the air or the bedclothes in apparent response to visual illusions or hallucinations. The abnormalities of mental state can fluctuate widely over the course of a day from relative lucidity to marked disturbance.

The delirious patient usually has a history or symptoms of a medical disorder and manifests abnormalities of vital signs or other abnormalities on physical examination or laboratory investigation.

The differentiation of medical and psychiatric causes of altered mental state is discussed in detail in Chapter 20.2.

Dementia

Psychotic symptoms in dementia can include auditory and visual hallucinations, delusions (often persecutory) and delusional misidentification (e.g. the delusion that a person closely related to the patient has been replaced by a double). These psychotic symptoms are common in dementias of all types, including Alzheimer's and vascular dementias. A mean prevalence of 44% has been found across several cross-sectional samples [9]. The diagnosis of dementia depends on the presence of multiple cognitive deficits and will usually be evident from other features of the history and presentation. A change in the mental state of a patient with dementia should prompt consideration of superimposed delirium.

Psychosis in clear consciousness without cognitive impairment

Occasionally, patients present with psychotic symptoms of organic cause, without features of delirium or dementia. The variety of medical conditions associated with psychotic presentations is shown in Table 20.5.3. Although these disorders are relatively rare as the cause of psychiatric presentation, they should be especially considered in relation to a patient with new-onset psychosis over the age of 40 (i.e. older than the usual age of onset of the much more common schizophrenia and bipolar disorder).

In emergency practice, the psychoses associated with epilepsy are probably those most likely to be associated with uncertainty in management. These psychoses are of two types. Some patients with established epilepsy develop chronic inter-ictal psychosis, that is, a psychosis without specific temporal relationship to seizure activity. The clinical picture is often like schizophrenia and the disorder should be treated in its own right with antipsychotic medication [10]. The second presentation is of a post-ictal psychosis, usually following a cluster of seizures and sometimes with a lucid interval of 1 or 2 days. The patient can present with both schizophrenia-like and mood symptoms. The mental state spontaneously returns to

Table 20.5.3 Medical causes of psychotic presentations
Epilepsy
Hypo- or hyperthyroidism
Huntington's disease
Wilson's disease
Porphyria
B12 deficiency
Cerebral neoplasm
Stroke
Viral encephalitis
Neurosyphilis
AIDS

normal within a few days, as in the more common post-ictal delirium [11].

Psychoses caused by prescribed medications

A long list of medications, many based on sporadic case reports, can sometimes be associated with psychotic symptoms [12]. The two most common are corticosteroids and dopamine agonists.

Steroid psychosis usually presents a manic-like picture and can show florid psychosis. It is most often associated with doses greater than 40 mg equivalents of prednisolone per day [13].

Dopamine agonists used in the treatment of Parkinson's disease like levodopa and bromocriptine are associated with auditory and visual hallucinations, persecutory delusions and hypomania. The psychotic symptoms are dose-related but dose reductions may be associated with severe exacerbation of Parkinsonian symptoms [14].

Acute and chronic schizophrenia

The symptoms of schizophrenia include the 'positive' symptoms of acute psychosis and the 'negative' symptoms, such as apathy and social withdrawal.

Positive symptoms involve delusions, hallucinations and formal thought disorder. The content of delusions may include beliefs that the patient is an important person (grandiose), that the patient has special communication with deities or spirits (religiose) or that there is something awry with the patient's body or the world (hypochondriacal and nihilistic). The most common delusions are beliefs that other persons or the TV or radio are making special reference to the person (delusions of reference) and beliefs that certain persons or agencies are engaged in conspiracies to harm the patient (delusions of persecution).

Hallucinations are usually auditory but can be in any sensory modality. The specific types of auditory hallucinations first described by Schneider [15], although not specific to schizophrenia, are strongly supportive of the diagnosis. These include a voice making a running commentary on the patient's actions, two or more voices discussing or arguing about the patient and a voice repeating the patient's thoughts aloud.

Sometimes the most obvious positive symptom of psychosis is formal thought disorder. This usually takes the form of loosening of associations (lack of logical connection between statements) and tangential (off the point) replies to questions. The effect of these symptoms is to make it difficult or impossible to take a sequential history. In more severe cases, the language itself becomes incoherent as grammatical conventions are abandoned and invented words ('neologisms') are used. In the emergency setting, the less severe forms of formal thought disorder may also be shown by highly anxious, delirious or intoxicated patients.

The negative symptoms include blunting of affect (lack of emotional response), apathy (loss of volition), poverty of speech (severely diminished verbal communication) and autistic withdrawal from social interaction. These symptoms can be difficult to distinguish in the acute setting from the effects of co-morbid depression or from the bradykinesia caused by antipsychotic medications.

In emergency practice, the three most common types of presentation of schizophrenia are the first psychotic episode, acute psychotic relapse of an established illness and a social crisis in a patient with chronic schizophrenia. It is useful to distinguish these types of presentation because of the management implications.

The patient with a first episode of psychosis is typically a young adult who has been brought to the ED by family or police often following months of concern about deterioration in the patient's mental state or behaviour. Sometimes there will have been an acute episode of bizarre, suicidal or aggressive behaviour. Exclusion of medical causes of psychosis is important in the first episode, especially in the older patient. It may be difficult to be certain whether the syndrome is one of mania (see below) or schizophrenia, but this distinction is not crucial in

emergency assessment. More important is the fact that the patient is likely to be frightened and confused, as is also the family. The patient may require involuntary hospitalization.

The acute relapse of an established illness can also involve considerable distress to the patient and family. In these cases, it is useful to look for changes in medication, problems in compliance, changes in the treatment system, such as absence of the treating doctor, alcohol and other drug abuse and recent stressful events. It may be possible to avoid hospitalization.

Patients with chronic schizophrenia are now treated most frequently through community mental health services. They may present with an exacerbation of the psychosis for the reasons outlined above. However, the presentation is often related to social problems, such as conflict with family or difficulties with accommodation or finances. In these cases, it can be very useful to communicate with the community mental health services to clarify the patient's baseline level of function and current problems. Some patients with chronic illness are effectively homeless and have poor engagement with community services, irregular medication use and ongoing drug abuse. Although it is difficult in a busy ED, these patients ideally need some work towards establishment of continuity of care and long-term treatment plans.

The term 'schizo-affective disorder' has been used to describe an illness in which patients show typical symptoms of schizophrenia as well as having definite manic or depressive episodes. In practice, in the ED, such patients can be assessed and managed in a similar way to patients with schizophrenia.

Mania with psychotic symptoms

The manic syndrome is one form of presentation of bipolar disorder, the others being a depressive episode and mixed affective psychosis.

The typical manic syndrome is very distinctive. The patient presents with euphoric or irritable affect, pressure of speech (rapid, continuous speech which is difficult to interrupt), distractibility and disinhibited or over-familiar behaviour. If delusions are present, they are grandiose (that the patient has an important mission) or persecutory (e.g. that other persons are engaged in a conspiracy to prevent the patient fulfilling his or her destiny). Collateral history will usually show that the patient has been well until the last few days when the patient has become overactive and disorganized with a markedly decreased need for sleep.

In mixed affective psychosis, the patient often shows typically manic arousal and irritability, but may have a depressive theme evident in the content of speech. Depressive psychosis is discussed below.

Sometimes a delirious patient with affective lability, irritability, disinhibition and distractibility may be misdiagnosed as manic. The diagnosis should be considered in the older patient without previous history of bipolar disorder. The distinction can be made on the basis of the impairment of cognitive function (disorientation, fluctuating conscious state and memory impairment) in delirium and clinical or laboratory evidence of medical illness.

It may be difficult to distinguish acute mania from acute schizophrenia in the emergency setting, especially in first episode cases. Being certain of the diagnosis is not crucial, as the short-term management is similar (see below).

Major depression with psychotic features

Patients who exhibit psychotic features during a depressive syndrome are severely depressed. The content of delusions and hallucinations relates to the patient's feelings of worthlessness or guilt and may include the conviction that the patient should die. Because the patient is unable to evaluate these beliefs rationally, the risk of suicidal actions is high and these patients should be closely supervised.

The patient with a depressive psychosis will show the other typical features of a depressive syndrome. Most often, the mental state assessment will show a patient who lacks spontaneity and is withdrawn and sad. Occasionally, however, the patient may be agitated and irritable.

The differential diagnosis and management of depressive syndromes are discussed in Chapter 20.4.

Substance-induced psychosis

Drugs of abuse are associated with psychotic presentations in several ways: psychosis as a manifestation of acute intoxication, psychosis during withdrawal reactions, chronic psychosis following prolonged use and the exacerbation of pre-existing psychotic illness due to drug abuse. Drugs of abuse which may contribute to psychosis are listed in Table 20.5.4.

The psychosis associated with intoxication may include auditory and visual hallucinations and persecutory or grandiose delusions. The patient is usually agitated, highly anxious and incoherent and often shows autonomic signs,

Table 20.5.4 Drugs of abuse associated with psychosis
Amphetamine and methamphetamine
Methylenedioxymethamphetamine (MMDA, ecstasy)
Cocaine
Phencyclidine
Ketamine
LSD
Cannabis
Alcohol
Benzodiazepines

such as dilated pupils. Some drugs, such as phencyclidine, are particularly associated with disinhibited rage. Management is focused on ensuring safety and maintaining vital functions in the expectation that the psychosis will clear when the intoxication resolves.

Alcohol and benzodiazepines can lead to psychotic symptoms (most commonly visual hallucinations) in the context of withdrawal delirium. The psychotic symptoms resolve through management of the withdrawal with benzodiazepines.

Amphetamine (and amphetamine derivatives), phencyclidine and lysergic acid diethylamide (LSD) have all been associated with chronic psychosis which can persist for weeks or months after cessation of drug use [16–18]. Whether or not the patients who develop these chronic psychoses may have been predisposed to psychotic illness is controversial but, nevertheless, the psychosis should not be regarded purely as an intoxication effect but treated in its own right. Amphetamine dugs are most frequently associated with this chronic psychosis, usually following prolonged heavy amphetamine abuse. The clinical picture can be quite distinctive, including beliefs that the patient is being watched or followed or that thoughts may be monitored with an implanted device. 'Running commentary' auditory hallucinations may occur as well as tactile hallucinations, which may lead the patient to excoriate the skin in pursuit of a supposed infestation with insects.

The role of cannabis as a cause of chronic schizophrenia-like psychosis is uncertain, although cannabis frequently exacerbates psychotic symptoms in patients with an existing illness [19].

Alcoholic hallucinosis is a relatively uncommon condition found in some patients with long-term alcohol abuse histories. The patient experiences auditory hallucinations of a derogatory or 'running commentary' type in clear consciousness, without being in a withdrawal state. This disorder may persist for weeks or months and the symptoms may respond to antipsychotic medications.

Because alcohol and drug abuse can exacerbate psychosis in patients with an established schizophrenic or bipolar disorder, inquiry should be made into their use with every patient.

Psychotic-like reactive states

Patients with histories of severe personality disorder, post-traumatic stress disorder and dissociative disorder sometimes present with quasi-psychotic states [20,21]. These episodes usually follow acute stress, such as a relationship or other social crisis, or events which trigger recall of traumatic experiences. The patient is usually extremely anxious and may have impaired verbal communication, further complicating assessment. Psychotic-like experiences can include intense subjective experiences of a derogatory internal monologue, which can seem like auditory hallucinations or intense fears of being harmed which mimic persecutory delusions. Some patients' recall of traumatic experiences is so persistent and vivid that it seems as if it is actually happening again.

When such patients are seen in emergency settings, they often need containment and assessment in a similar manner to patients with true psychoses. Benzodiazepines and sedative antipsychotic medications (see below) are often useful in reducing the high level of arousal.

Assessment

Objectives and sources of information

The assessment of the psychotic patient in ED has several objectives. The basic questions are:

- Is the altered mental state primarily due to a medical condition?
- To what extent are drugs or alcohol contributory?
- Can a primary psychiatric diagnosis be made?
- Can the patient be treated at home or is hospitalization necessary?
- Should the patient be detained under the mental health act?

These questions cannot be answered by considering only the clinical state of the patient. Decisions about risk assessment and disposition depend on a careful consideration of the social circumstances of the patient, recent events that have led to the emergency presentation and past and current engagement with community mental health treatment services. Diagnostic clarification is often greatly assisted by previous treatment records, which can usually be fairly quickly accessed.

Information should be sought from family and community mental health teams about recent function, symptoms, dangerous behaviours and alcohol and other drug use. The police who sometimes bring patients with psychosis to ED can often give important information about the circumstances that led to the presentation.

The assessment process is not a single one-off review of the patient's mental state, nor is it a linear process in which the various objectives of assessment can be serially addressed. It tends rather to be a back and forth process as multiple lines of inquiry are simultaneously pursued and the clinical data re-evaluated in the light of new information.

At the end of the assessment process, it should be possible to record a summary of the various parameters of assessment as outlined in Table 20.5.5, which can then form the basis for management planning.

Initial stabilization of the patient

In order that conditions can be created for an adequate assessment, there is an immediate need to stabilize the patient. The acutely

Table 20.5.5 The psychotic patient – brief assessment schedule
1. Circumstances of referral
2. Presenting problem
3. Social circumstances
4. Previous treatment
5. Current mental health services
6. Current medication
7. Alcohol and other drug use
8. Mental state examination
9. Medical assessment and investigations
10. Provisional diagnosis
11. Risk assessment
12. Treatment and disposition plan

psychotic patient has distorted understanding and may be an unwilling participant in the process. It is preferable to try to engage the patient in a calm manner with straightforward and clear explanation of the need for assessment. The patient's own concerns and perceptions of the problem are worth listening to without initially trying to seek answers to specific questions. This attention is reassuring to the patient and provides an opportunity for observation of the mental state, even if the patient's account lacks coherence.

Patients who are aroused and agitated, intoxicated or have persecutory delusions may pose a risk of violent or aggressive behaviour. In these cases, it is important to monitor safety by having security staff present, by not assessing the patient in a confined space and by remaining out of striking distance and not turning one's back on the patient. Sometimes the patient may have to be sedated before much assessment can be made. Sedating the aroused patient is discussed in Chapter 20.6.

Moderate use of benzodiazepines need not significantly complicate the mental state assessment, although these drugs may exacerbate delirium. High doses of benzodiazepines (especially diazepam which has active metabolites with long half-lives) can produce a prolonged delirium, which will delay the assessment process.

Mental state assessment

Especially in the aroused patient, it is often difficult to carry out a formal mental state examination. Nevertheless, it is possible to collect a lot of information by simple observation. The general appearance can give clues to the patient's level of self-care. The rate and mode of speech can suggest the presence of formal thought disorder. Hostile or euphoric affects may suggest a manic syndrome or intoxication. Patients may spontaneously reveal delusional ideas or auditory hallucinations or may admit to these on specific questioning. Orientation to time and place and recent events should always be assessed because of the strong association of disorientation with delirium. Although detailed cognitive assessment is usually not possible, an attempt should be made to assess short-term memory function and attention and concentration.

As with all aspects of assessment, the assessment of mental state should not be based on a single evaluation but on serial assessments by medical staff and the observations of the nursing staff throughout the time the patient is in the ED.

Risk assessment

It is important to inquire directly about suicidal and homicidal ideation and to record the patient's statements. However, risk assessment depends on an objective evaluation of the whole situation. A patient with persistent persecutory beliefs may be at significant risk of behaving aggressively towards perceived persecutors, even though he or she may deny hostile intent. Conversely, a patient's expression of suicidal ideation may reflect long-standing frustration and dissatisfaction (which may be alleviated by receiving help) rather than intent to act in a suicidal manner. The degree to which the patient can exercise judgement is also important. A floridly psychotic or grossly disorganized patient is at greater risk than a patient with chronic symptoms who presents with a social crisis. The home situation and the views of family should also be considered and taken very seriously. Inquiry should be also made into the provision of care for dependent children.

Decisions about hospital admission and involuntary detention usually focus appropriately on danger to self and others. Uncertainty may sometimes arise regarding the use of mental health act detention powers in relation to manic (and some schizophrenic) patients who clearly deny any intent to harm themselves or others, but who are clearly in need of treatment, lack insight and are very unlikely to receive treatment unless compulsorily detained. Most jurisdictions, however, make some provision in their mental health legislation for such patients to be detained in the interests of their health or to prevent other 'harms', such as harm to reputation. The decision to detain involves balancing the patient's right to autonomy against the probable risks of not receiving treatment. In general, such a patient has only been brought to ED because family, friends or other carers have been concerned about the behaviour or mental state of the patient and it is therefore wise to consult with these concerned others if there is doubt about the decision to detain.

Medical evaluation and investigation

Medical evaluation has three goals: excluding delirium (or dementia), considering other organic causes of psychosis and assessing for the presence of co-morbid medical illness.

The practice of 'medical clearance' prior to psychiatric evaluation may detract from a comprehensive evaluation of the patient. A more satisfactory process is to compile an adequate history of the presenting illness, assess the mental state, review the medications and alcohol and other drug use, consider previous medical history, check vital signs and carry out as comprehensive a physical examination as possible, with particular attention to signs of injury, poisoning or intoxication [22]. In services where both emergency physicians and psychiatrists are available, direct discussion about cases of uncertain diagnosis is useful.

Medical causes for an altered mental state will usually be suggested by the history, mental state assessment, abnormal vital signs and physical examination. As noted above, particular consideration should be given to medical causes in a first presentation of psychosis, especially in an older patient.

Investigations should be driven by history and examination findings, such as neurological signs or signs of infection. Nevertheless, because of the difficulties in compiling comprehensive medical histories, it is often appropriate to do a number of 'screening' investigations as indicators of unsuspected medical illness. The range of suggested tests varies, but usually includes urea and electrolytes, full blood count, liver function tests, random blood sugar, blood alcohol level, thyroid function tests and B12 and folate levels [23].

The availability of computed tomography (CT) scanning in more centres has facilitated the use of neuroimaging as an aid to diagnosis. This investigation is likely to be indicated in patients where stroke, neoplasm, haemorrhage or central nervous system infection may be suspected. It is also appropriate to consider a CT scan of the brain in first episode psychosis cases to assess further the possibility of neurological disease presenting with only psychotic or affective symptoms. However, the yield of positive results with this investigation is low [24], especially in the younger patient [25], and neuroimaging is therefore generally not required as an emergency investigation if the patient is otherwise medically well.

It is well established that patients with chronic psychotic illness tend to have poorer physical health than the general population [26]. Common conditions include obesity, late onset diabetes, hypertension, arteriosclerotic disorders, smoking-related disorders and alcohol and other drug-related disorders. The prevalence of these problems can be related to lifestyle factors, the side effects of medication and difficulties in making effective use of primary medical care. It is worth considering the possible presence of these common conditions as they sometimes need acute treatment or contribute to an exacerbation of the mental state.

Treatment

Management in the ED

Once medical causes have been excluded, the primary psychiatric diagnosis is likely to fall into one of the following groups:

- drug-induced psychosis
- acute schizophrenia
- mania
- chronic schizophrenia
- psychosis-like reactive state
- depressive psychosis.

Patients with psychotic illness often stay in the ED for prolonged periods. Sometimes this is due to delays in the assessment process, but it is also significantly a result of access block, that is the lack of ready availability of beds in psychiatric wards. In some hospitals, these circumstances have resulted in the establishment of specific psychiatric 'holding beds', within or closely related to the ED, where patients may be observed and treated for up to 48 hours while further management and disposition plans are being made [27,28]. The availability of such specialized psychiatric observation units is likely to reduce the need for reliance on sedative medications to manage behavioural disturbance. The patient can move around more freely, preferably with access to an outside secure area and specialized mental health staff can provide assessment, supervision, explanation and reality orientation.

In the more conventional ED setting, behavioural management is more difficult as a balance must be achieved between imposing restrictions on the patient and maintaining the safety of all patients and staff. Psychotic patients should be in areas which can be easily observed and often one-to-one supervision will be necessary, preferably with trained mental health nurses. If possible, this should be in a quiet area without too much coming and going. Engagement of the patient in reality-based conversation (explanation of what is happening, attention to personal concerns) is often useful. It may be possible to enlist the help of family members in providing reassurance and comfort.

The use of specific medications will depend in part on the diagnostic picture. Patients with drug-induced psychosis are usually quite aroused and require significant levels of sedation. Benzodiazepines, such as midazolam and diazepam, are usually preferred as they are less likely to lead to medical complications (especially arrhythmias) in a person who has already taken other drugs and has a high sympathetic drive. The period of sedation may become prolonged for several hours (or even days if high doses of diazepam are used). The mental state needs to be reassessed for the presence of persistent psychosis when the sedation abates.

Patients with acute schizophrenia, mania or persistent psychosis following drug use all have similar management in the short term. These patients tend to be aroused and agitated and to have considerable difficulty in coping with the restrictions and the stimulation of the ED environment. If the patient will take oral medications, sedative antipsychotics (such as olanzapine) or benzodiazepines (such as lorazepam) can be used. These are better prescribed as regular doses (e.g. olanzapine 5 mg tds or 7.5 mg qid or lorazepam 1 mg qid or 2 mg qid) than on a pro re nata (PRN) basis to ensure consistency in dosing. Repeated divided doses to maintain a more constant level of sedation are preferable to infrequent large doses. Estimates of the probable appropriate dose can be made on the basis of the size of the patient and degree of arousal and then titrated upward or downward on the basis of response in the first 24 hours.

If the patient refuses oral medication, lorazepam (if available) or clonazepam can be used intramuscularly or intravenously. Olanzapine can also be used effectively intramuscularly. Patients who are likely to stay in the ED for more than 24 hours can be given zuclopenthixol acetate 50–150 mg IM (dose dependent on the size of the patient). This is a medium-acting depot antipsychotic preparation which will last for 3–4 days. However, the onset of action is delayed for 6–8 hours, and this medication should be avoided in neurolept-naïve patients because of the risk of prolonged dystonia.

The patient who presents with acute schizophrenia who is not aroused may benefit from explanation and only small doses of medication, such as olanzapine 5 mg at night. Similarly, the patient with chronic schizophrenia should be maintained on usual medications, possibly with the addition of a PRN benzodiazepine if very anxious.

Patients with psychotic depression can be quite agitated, but also may be quiet and withdrawn. They should be considered at high risk of suicidal behaviour and need close supervision. Their mental anguish may be helped in the short term with the use of benzodiazepines or sedative antipsychotics (olanzapine or quetiapine). Regular doses are better than PRN, although smaller doses are needed than in the treatment of the acutely schizophrenic or manic patient. It is not essential to commence an antidepressant medication during the time the patient is in the ED.

The patient with severe personality disorder or a history of severe trauma who presents with a psychosis-like reactive state often requires similar treatment to a patient with acute schizophrenia. The patient may require containment in a place of safety and will benefit from explanation and reassurance. Benzodiazepines and sedative antipsychotics can be very useful in lowering arousal.

Admission to inpatient care

The decision to admit the patient for inpatient psychiatric care depends on the acuity of the presentation, the supports available at home, the degree of risk and the availability of community mental health services.

Patients with an acute episode of schizophrenia, especially a first episode, often require admission because they are often very disorganized, lack insight and are likely to be non-compliant with medication and may be at risk of suicide or aggressive behaviour. However, the increasing availability of mobile crisis teams (community mental health teams with the capacity for rapid and intensive follow up in the home) has made it more possible to treat even these acutely unwell patients at home. This is usually preferred by the patient and sometimes by the family, especially where the patient is an adolescent or young adult still living with their family. In these cases, careful assessment of potential risks to the patient or others and frank discussion of these issues with the family is advisable.

The acutely manic patient who has been brought to the ED almost certainly requires admission. Once established, the manic syndrome is likely to persist for several weeks if untreated. In some cases, especially those involving recurrence of a previous bipolar disorder, the patient presents relatively early in the relapse and with sufficient insight to accept advice about increasing or changing medications. If such a patient is discharged to outpatient care, specific arrangements should be made with the family and the community mental health services for monitoring and follow up.

The patient with an acute psychotic depression almost always requires admission because of the high risk of suicidal behaviour.

On the other hand, patients with chronic schizophrenia who present with a mild exacerbation of symptoms or family or social crisis should generally be managed in the community if possible. These are chronic conditions analogous to diabetes or asthma and quality of life can be enhanced if the patient can be helped to engage with community treatment services, achieve stability of accommodation and daytime activity and learn to self-manage the condition [29].

For patients with reactive psychoses in the context of personality disorder or trauma history, the individual circumstances vary widely and the decision to admit depends on careful assessment of the risk factors. Every effort should be made to return the patient as quickly as possible to reality-based perceptions of the world and to restore a sense of autonomy and personal responsibility. It is sometimes not possible to achieve this during the course of an ED stay and a brief crisis admission to a psychiatric unit may be necessary.

Criteria for involuntary treatment

When inpatient admission is considered desirable but refused by the patient, consideration should be given to the use of mental health act powers for referral and detention. Contemporary mental health legislation requires the person considering this option (which may be a doctor or other authorized mental health practitioner) to review options for less restrictive treatment before making this decision.

Mental health acts generally stipulate that persons can only be referred under the act if they suffer from a 'mental disorder' and are also at some 'risk'. Risks involving danger to self through suicidal intent or behaviour and danger to others as a result of aggression or persecutory delusions are usually straightforward grounds for referral and detention. The decision may be more difficult in relation to the mildly manic patient or the schizophrenic patient with partial insight. The need for detention involves weighing up the potential consequences of not receiving treatment, the

possibility of access to community services and the availability of family or other social supports.

Where mental health specialists are not readily available to the ED, ED doctors may appropriately refer a patient under the mental health act so that assessment by a psychiatrist can take place at another location. Especially in cases where the need for involuntary treatment is uncertain, it is good practice for the ED doctor to make this referral to ensure that the decision to detain or release can be made by a psychiatrist, who is in a clearer position to take medico-legal responsibility.

Community referral

The range of potential community treatment options is now wide. Patients may receive outpatient treatment through GPs, private psychiatrists and psychologists, community mental health clinics, public and private drug and alcohol services, relationship counselling agencies and various other specialized services (e.g. non-government community support services, services for indigenous persons and services for victims of trauma). In planning outpatient care, a good approach is to determine initially what service providers may be already involved in helping the patient and the strength of the patient's relationship with those services. Direct communication between the ED staff and the community service providers is very desirable, especially if the patient is a new referral to those services.

Some of the more effective psychiatric emergency services work in close liaison with mobile crisis teams or acute care teams, who actively and intensively follow up discharged patients in their own homes or in crisis accommodation [28,30].

Controversies and future directions

- As a result of the contemporary mental health community focus, EDs will continue to have a major role in the assessment and stabilization of patients with psychosis.
- Should this assessment occur within traditional EDs or should EDs facilitate

the development of co-located psychiatric emergency services?
- The models of care which will achieve the best integration of emergency mental health assessments with community services require better definition.

References

[1] Gregory LL, Claassen CA, Edmond JA, et al. Trends in US emergency department visits for mental health conditions, 1992 to 2001. Psychiatr Serv 2005;56:671–7.
[2] Kalucy R, Thomas L, King D. Changing demand for mental health services in the emergency department of a public hospital. Aust NZ J Psychiatr 2005;39:74–80.
[3] World Health Organization. The ICD-10 classification of mental and behavioural disorders. Geneva: WHO; 1993.
[4] Jablensky A. Epidemiology of schizophrenia. In: Gelder MG, Lopez-Ibor JJ, Andreasen NC, editors. New Oxford textbook of psychiatry. London: New Oxford Press; 2000.
[5] Jablensky A. Course and outcome of schizophrenia and their prediction. In: Gelder MG, Lopez-Ibor JJ, Andreasen NC, editors. New Oxford textbook of psychiatry. London: New Oxford Press; 2000.
[6] Joyce PR. Epidemiology of mood disorders. In: Gelder MG, Lopez-Ibor JJ, Andreasen NC, editors. New Oxford textbook of psychiatry. London: New Oxford Press; 2000.
[7] Angst J. Course and prognosis of mood disorders. In: Gelder MG, Lopez-Ibor JJ, Andreasen NC, editors. New Oxford textbook of psychiatry. London: New Oxford Press; 2000.
[8] McGorry PD. The concept of recovery and secondary prevention in psychiatric disorders. Aust NZ J Psychiatr 1992;26:3–17.
[9] Douglas S, Ballard C. Psychotic symptoms in dementia. In: Hassett A, Ames D, Chiu E, editors. Psychosis in the elderly. London: Taylor Francis; 2005.
[10] Bredkjoer SR, Mortensen PB, Parnas J. Epilepsy and non-organic non-affective psychosis: national epidemiologic study. Br J Psychiatr 1998;172:235–8.
[11] Logsdail SJ, Toone BK. Post-ictal psychoses. Br J Psychiatr 1988;152:246–52.
[12] Hales RH, Yudofsky SC. Textbook of clinical psychiatry, 4th ed. Washington: American Psychiatric Publishing, 2003, p. 462–3.
[13] Boston Collaborative Drug Surveillance Program. Acute adverse reactions to prednisolone in relation to dosage. Clin Pharmacol Ther 1972;13:694–8.
[14] Young BK, Camicioli R, Ganzini L. Neuropsychiatric adverse effects of antiparkinsonian drugs: characteristics, evaluation and treatment. Drugs Aging 1997;10:367–83.
[15] Mellor CS. First rank symptoms of schizophrenia. Br J Psychiatr 1970;117:15–23.
[16] Flaum M, Schultz SK. When does amphetamine-induced psychosis become schizophrenia? Am J Psychiatr 1996;153:812–5.
[17] Javitt DC, Zukin SR. Recent advances in the phencyclidine model of schizophrenia. Am J Psychiatr 1991;148:1301–8.
[18] Abraham HD, Aldridge AM, Gogia P. The psychopharmacology of hallucinogens. Neuropsychopharmocology 1996;14:285–98.
[19] Hall W. Cannabis and psychosis. Drug Alcohol Rev 1998;17:433–4.
[20] Chopra HD, Beatson JA. Psychotic symptoms in borderline personality disorder. Am J Psychiatr 1986;143:1605–7.
[21] Butler RW, Mueser KT, Sprock J, et al. Positive symptoms of psychosis in post-traumatic stress disorder. Biol Psychiatr 1996;39:839–44.
[22] Olshaker JS, Brown B, Jerrard DA, et al. Medical clearance and screening of psychiatric patients in the emergency department. Acad Emerg Med 1997;4:124–8.
[23] Thienhaus OH. Physical evaluation and laboratory tests Hillard JP, editor. Manual of clinical emergency psychiatry. Washington: American Psychiatric Press; 1990.

[24] Rock DJ, Wynn Owen P. An investigation of criteria used to indicate cranial CT in males with schizophrenia. Acta Neuropsychiatr 2003;15:284–9.
[25] Adams M, Kutcher S, Antonio E, et al. Diagnostic utility of endocrine and neuroimaging screening tests in first-onset adolescent psychosis. J Am Acad Child Adolesc Psychiatr 1996;35:67–73.
[26] Phelan M, Stradius L, Morrison S. Physical health of people with severe mental illness. Br Med J 2001;322:443–4.

[27] Allen MM. Level 1 psychiatric emergency services: the tools of the crisis sector. Psychiatr Clin N Am 1999;22:713–33.
[28] Frank R, Fawcett L, Emmerson B. Development of Australia's first psychiatric emergency centre. Austral Psychiatr 2005;13:266–72.
[29] Bennett C, Fumall J, Fossey E, et al. Assessing and responding to the needs of people with schizophrenia and related disorders. In: Meadow G, Singh B, editors. Mental

health in Australia: collaborative community practice. Melbourne: Oxford University Press, 2001, p. 283–312.
[30] Breslow RE. Structure and function of psychiatric emergency services. In: Allen MH, editor. Emergency psychiatry review of psychiatry, Vol 21. Washington: American Psychiatric Press, 2002, p. 1–34.

20.6 Pharmacological management of the aroused patient

Mark Monaghan • Simon Byrne

ESSENTIALS

1 Benzodiazepines and antipsychotics, often used most effectively in combination, are the first-line drugs for sedation of the aroused patient.

2 As much information as possible should be collected before the patient is sedated.

3 The risks involved in giving sedative drugs need to be considered, particularly at higher doses.

4 Dose adjustments are necessary in the older or medically compromised patient.

Introduction

Aroused patients who present to the emergency department (ED) of their own accord can generally be best assisted by verbal reassurance and prompt mental health evaluation. Reducing the waiting time and arriving quickly at an action plan will provide the best response to the patient's anxiety and agitation.

For highly aroused patients who have been brought to the hospital reluctantly, the immediate need is to gain control of the situation to permit further evaluation, while ensuring the safety of the patient, staff and the public.

Where possible, it is desirable to collect some information about the patient before sedation. The patient should be approached in a calm manner in a safe, observed area of the ED, with security staff in the background if necessary. The patient should be asked about his or her understanding of the problems and listened to attentively, even if the account is incoherent. This attention will be reassuring to the patient and helps in building rapport. During this process observations can be made about the mental state. If possible, vital signs should be recorded and a brief physical examination

carried out, with particular attention to signs of injury, intoxication or overdose.

In the hostile or frightened uncooperative patient, it will often be necessary to proceed to rapid tranquilization. This is a familiar procedure to the emergency physician and the practice can be enhanced by attention to the basic principles of care, an awareness of the risks and knowledge of the characteristics of the available drugs.

Pharmacological management should always be tailored to the particular patient. The medically compromised patient will be at greater risk of the complications of sedation. In elderly patients, decreased and delayed metabolism and elimination can result in prolonged therapeutic and adverse effects. Dose adjustments and agents with shorter half-lives and more favourable side-effect profiles must be considered for these patients.

General principles of rapid tranquillization

The general principles of care are:

❶ Use sedative benzodiazepines and/or antipsychotics as the first-line agents.

❷ Should the situation allow, oral dosing is the least distressing approach for patients and staff.

❸ Treating physicians should use agents with which they are familiar. In particular, they should be aware of maximal safe dosing and expected adverse effects.

❹ The endpoint should be a calm cooperative patient. Sedation to the point of loss of airway protection is dangerous.

❺ The patient should be nursed in a quiet, calm and gently lit environment if possible.

❻ Sedated patients should be monitored with basic observations; a 12-lead ECG should be performed on any patient being administered repeat doses of antipsychotics.

❼ Supportive care, such as hydration, indwelling catheterization, pressure care and deep vein thrombosis prophylaxis, are essential for patients requiring ongoing sedation. This is particularly relevant in overcrowded EDs and if patients are detained in the ED for prolonged periods.

❽ Maintenance of patient dignity by using single rooms and limiting visual exposure of the patient to the public is often forgotten but should be a basic standard of care.

Risks of rapid tranquillization

There are inherent risks in attempting to gain control of the aroused patient, including risks of injury to the staff and patient. If physical restraint is necessary to administer parenteral medication, adequate staff, trained in restraint procedures should be on hand. Sometimes mechanical (padded strap) restraint may be necessary in the early stages or to limit the dose of medication if the patient is developing toxic effects. Mechanical restraint should not be maintained in the absence of chemical sedation due to the risks of physical injury and rhabdomyolysis, as well as for ethical reasons.

The risks of adverse events from medication administration are well recognized.

Over-sedation and resultant respiratory depression and pulmonary aspiration are relatively common and for the most part avoidable with proper care.

Sudden cardiac death, particularly with agents that prolong the QT interval and precipitate torsade des pointes and ventricular tachycardia (VT), is a rare but catastrophic complication of rapid tranquilization [1,2]. This risk is heightened in the aroused patient with increased circulating catecholamines and in patients with pre-existing heart disease or conduction disturbance. Antipsychotics combined with other medications that prolong the QT interval pose an increased risk. The agents most associated with risk of sudden death are thioridazine and clozapine. Droperidol and haloperidol are associated with QT prolongation but rarely with the risk of torsade des pointes. Quetiapine and chlorpromazine are associated with QT prolongation but this is probably less clinically significant than with the above agents. The atypical agent olanzapine appears to be relatively safe from this perspective.

Hypotension can occur with administration of any agent with alpha blockade effects, but is especially associated with chlorpromazine (particularly when given intravenously). Dystonic reactions are seen with all antipsychotics, most frequently with the butyrophenones, such as haloperidol, and less commonly with atypical agents, such as olanzapine. Neurolept malignant syndrome is a risk with any antipsychotic agent, even following a single dose.

Anticholinergic effects, such as delirium and urinary retention, are risks with virtually all antipsychotics and are generally seen at high doses. Delirium is also caused by high doses of benzodiazepines, particularly diazepam, which accumulates with recurrent dosing. All antipsychotics have the potential to lower the seizure threshold.

Elderly patients are at significantly greater risk of drug accumulation and adverse effects. They are also at far greater risk of delirium, particularly with the combination of possible underlying cognitive impairment and environment change. Age-related reductions in hepatic metabolism and renal function make

it reasonable to assume that all agents will have prolonged elimination half-lives in these patients. Even small doses of benzodiazepines can produce significant and prolonged respiratory depression in the elderly. Standard doses of antipsychotics, such as haloperidol, may result in prolonged extrapyramidal effects that impair mobility for days to weeks post-administration.

Specific agents

Benzodiazepines

Midazolam This water-soluble benzodiazepine has major benefits over diazepam in that it produces fewer site reactions and can be given intramuscularly. It has a rapid effect by intramuscular or intravenous injection (2–5 minutes), with a half-life of 1–3 hours. The active metabolite has a similar half-life. The elimination half-life is significantly prolonged in the elderly. The major adverse effect is respiratory depression. It is available in ampoules (5 mg/mL, 15/3 mL, 5 mg/5 mL and 50 mg/10 mL).

Diazepam Diazepam can be used orally or intravenously. It is not recommended for intramuscular use due to unpredictable absorption. Diazepam demonstrates biphasic elimination with rapid redistribution of 1–3 hours, followed by a prolonged terminal elimination phase of up to 20 hours. Hepatic metabolism produces active metabolites and excretion is renal. Elimination is significantly prolonged in the elderly. Major adverse effects are respiratory depression and accumulation causing delirium. It is available in ampoules (10 mg/2 mL), tablets (2 mg and 5 mg) and elixir (10 mg/10 mL).

Clonazepam Clonazepam can be used by oral, intravenous or intramuscular routes. Clonazepam has a prolonged elimination half-life (20–50 hours) with hepatic metabolism and renal excretion. The major adverse effects are excessive sedation and risk of accumulation. It is available in ampoules (1 mg/mL), tablets (0.5 mg and 2 mg) and oral liquid (2.5 mg/mL).

Lorazepam In Australia, lorazepam is only used orally as the parenteral preparation is not available. However, in other countries, it is widely used intramuscularly in the sedation of psychotically aroused patients. It is well absorbed orally, with an elimination half-life of 12–15 hours. The hepatic metabolites are non-active. The major adverse effect is excessive

sedation, but it is less likely to accumulate than diazepam or clonazepam. It is available in tablets (1 mg and 2.5 mg).

Antipsychotics

Droperidol Droperidol can be administered intramuscularly or intravenously. Clinical effects are seen within 3–10 minutes, maximum at 30 minutes and the elimination half-life is approximately 2 hours. It is significantly more sedating than haloperidol, which makes it an attractive choice for the aroused patient. It is also a potent antiemetic. The black box labelling of droperidol is highly controversial as there appears to be little evidence that there is greater cardiovascular risk with this agent than with haloperidol. QT prolongation is seen with greater frequency at higher dose, but deterioration to torsade de pointes is rare. The risk is greater when combined with agents that prolong the QT interval or in patients with pre-existent QT prolongation. As with haloperidol, there is risk of dystonic reactions and neurolept malignant syndrome. (Ampoules 2.5 mg/mL.)

Haloperidol Haloperidol can be given by oral, intramuscular or intravenous routes. Peak plasma levels occur 20 minutes after intramuscular injection and 2–6 hours post-oral dose. Mean elimination half-life is 20 hours, but this includes initial rapid elimination followed by a prolonged elimination over days. Hepatic metabolites are renally excreted. Major adverse effects are extrapyramidal effects that may persist for days (particularly in the elderly), prolongation of QT interval with risk of torsade and neurolept malignant syndrome. It is available in tablets (0.5 mg, 1.5 mg and 5 mg), liquid (2 mg/mL) and ampoules (5 mg/mL).

Olanzapine Olanzapine is licensed for oral, sublingual (SL) and intramuscular use. There are also common reports in the literature of intravenous use. It is an atypical antipsychotic that is well absorbed orally with peak plasma levels 2–5 hours post-oral dose and 30 minutes post-intramuscular injection. It has a half-life of approximately 33 hours and is hepatically metabolized to inactive metabolites that are renally and faecally excreted. There is also now a long-acting preparation with a half-life of 30 days. Major adverse effects include excessive sedation, mild anticholinergic effects and neurolept malignant syndrome (NMS). Extrapyramidal side effects, including dystonias, are rare. Cardiotoxicity is also rare. It is available in tablets (2.5 mg, 5 mg, 7.5 mg and 10 mg), dissolvable tablets, wafers (5 mg and 10 mg) and ampoules (10 mg).

Risperidone Risperidone is for oral and sublingual use. It is an atypical antipsychotic that is well absorbed orally with a peak effect in 1–2 hours. It is hepatically metabolized to an active metabolite that is renally excreted. The half-life of the parent compound is 3 hours in extensive metabolizers and 17 hours in poor metabolizers; the active metabolite elimination half-life is 24 hours. Risperidone's adverse effect profile is benefited by the absence of anticholinergic effects, but includes postural hypotension with initial dosing, extrapyramidal effects and NMS. Extrapyramidal reactions, including dystonias, are less frequent with risperidone than with haloperidol. There has been an increased mortality associated with risperidone and elderly patients on frusemide, so caution should be taken to ensure adequate hydration in these patients. It is available in tablets and sublingual 'quicklets' (0.5 mg, 1 mg, 2 mg, 3 mg and 4 mg) and solution (1 mg/mL).

Chlorpromazine Chlorpromazine is for oral, intramuscular or intravenous use. It has variable and incomplete absorption and a large first-pass metabolism, with peak plasma levels 1–4 hours after oral and 30 minutes after intramuscular administration. Metabolism is hepatic with many metabolites that are renally excreted. Elimination is complicated with early (2–3 hours), intermediate (15 hours) and late (60 days) elimination phases. Major adverse effects are postural hypotension, strong anticholinergic effects, excessive sedation and the risk of NMS. Extrapyramidal effects are relatively uncommon. It is available in tablets (10 mg, 25 mg and 100 mg), syrup (25 mg/mL) and ampoules (50 mg/2 mL).

Zuclopenthixol acetate ('Acuphase')
This is given intramuscularly. Zuclopenthixol acetate is a medium-acting depot preparation of a typical thioxanthene antipsychotic. Maximal plasma levels are achieved 24–36 hours post-intramuscular injection, declining to 30% of maximum levels by day 3. It is hepatically metabolized to inactive metabolites and faecally excreted. Zuclopenthixol acetate should be avoided in neurolept-naïve patients and those with organic brain disorders, cardiac disease and lowered seizure threshold. This is because any adverse effects, including

NMS, will be prolonged because of the slow absorption and elimination. The usual dose is 50–100 mg.

Dexmedetomidine and clonidine
These central alpha-agonists have a significant sedative effect. Dexmedetomidine is used as an infusion, primarily in the ICU setting. Clonidine has a recognized role in opiate and, to a lesser extent, alcohol withdrawal. It may be administered by the oral, SC, IM or IV route. It has a rapid onset of action when given parenterally and a half-life of greater than 12 hours. There is the potential for both these agents to have an increasing role in the emergency department for the management of hyperaroused patients. Both have a risk of bradycardia and hypotension and should be avoided in patients with pre-existent cardiac conduction abnormalities and used with caution in patients on rate lowering agents.

A rapid tranquillization algorithm

There are a variety of published algorithms for rapid tranquillization [3–15]. The following is a reasonable approach in terms of effectiveness, risk of adverse effects and availability. This algorithm applies to the management of a previously well adult patient. It must be remembered that, in general, the risk of adverse events is increased the greater the doses used. Elderly patients as a general rule should have lower initial doses and smaller daily doses.

First-line treatment
Try to develop rapport with the patient and use oral medication if possible. Oral agents of choice include:

- benzodiazepines: diazepam 10 mg, clonazepam 2 mg or lorazepam 2.5 mg (elderly: lorazepam 0.5–1 mg)

and/or:

- antipsychotic: olanzapine 5–10 mg oral/SL (elderly: olanzapine 2.5 mg oral/SL or risperidone 0.25–0.5 mg oral/SL).

Second-line treatment
If oral therapy is not achievable or is not effective, parenteral medications must be given. Agents of choice include:

- benzodiazepines: midazolam 2.5–5 mg IV/IM repeated as required to a maximum of around 100 mg (elderly or compromised

patients may develop respiratory depression with as little as 1 mg midazolam, so 0.5–1 mg is a safer initial dose, with maximal dose many times lower than 100 mg)

and/or:

- antipsychotic: olanzapine 10 mg IM, which can be repeated up to a maximal daily dose of 30 mg (elderly patients can be given olanzapine in doses of 2.5 mg IM, but may be better managed with sublingual olanzapine 2.5 mg or sublingual risperidone 0.5 mg)

or:

- droperidol 2.5–5 mg IM/IV, up to max of 25 mg/24 h. Risks include dystonic reactions, QT prolongation, anticholinergic delirium and NMS, with QT prolongation risk greater with increasing dose or if combined with QT prolonging agents. Doses less than 10 mg seem to be relatively safe from this perspective [15]. It would seem sound clinical advice to obtain a 12-lead ECG in any patients treated with droperidol or haloperidol, particularly if doses exceed 10 mg.

There is evidence of more rapid onset of sedation and less adverse events when a combination of midazolam and antipsychotics is used rather than midazolam alone [12].

Third-line treatment
If the maximal doses of the above agents have been reached with the first- or second-line drugs without adequate effect, it is necessary to try other options. Sometimes also the first- or second-line drugs may have to be avoided because of previous adverse effects. The maximum doses described here are based on the likelihood of very limited greater benefit (and the probability of greater adverse effects) of exceeding these doses.

Third-line agents include:

- diazepam 2.5–5 mg IV, up to a maximum of around 100–150 mg. (Risks include accumulation, delirium and respiratory depression; should not be given intramuscularly)
- clonazepam 1–2 mg IM/IV up to a maximum of 8 mg per day. Clonazepam can also be given as an infusion at a rate of 4–6 mg/24 h; the rate of the infusion can be varied according to the arousal level of the patient. (Risks include accumulation, delirium and respiratory depression)

- haloperidol 2.5–5 mg IM/IV, up to a maximum of around 30–50 mg/24 h. Risks similar to droperidol
- chlorpromazine can also be given as an intravenous infusion, with an initial rate of 6.25–12.5 mg/h to gain initial control and then reduced to a maximum of around 200 mg/24 h. (Risks include anticholinergic effects, hypotension, delirium, accumulation, QT prolongation and NMS.)

Aroused patients with amphetamine intoxication should be managed with benzodiazepines and supportive care, sometimes requiring large doses for initial control. Both intravenous midazolam and oral/intravenous diazepam are reasonable first choices. Severe intoxication with hyperthermia and rigidity requires paralysis and intubation. In patients who present with paranoid psychosis associated with amphetamine abuse, addition of an antipsychotic, such as olanzapine (oral or intramuscular), is appropriate.

Maintenance therapy

Following initial rapid tranquillization, the patient will remain sedated for several hours, during which collateral history may be obtained. When the patient awakes, a further psychiatric assessment should be made, especially with a view to deciding whether the patient needs to be admitted to a psychiatric unit.

If the patient does need to remain in hospital, consideration must be given to further appropriate medication. A general approach is to use lorazepam (1 or 2 mg three times a day) or sedative antipsychotics (olanzapine 5 or 10 mg three times a day). It is better to prescribe regular medication (rather than 'PRN') to ensure consistency of dosing. The appropriateness of the prescribed medication and the side effects should be reviewed at least daily.

If the patient remains uncooperative, intravenous benzodiazepines or intramuscular olanzapine can be used on an as needed basis. If adequate facilities are available for monitoring respiratory function, the use of an infusion of clonazepam or chlorpromazine can help to achieve control. Alternatively, some patients who are likely to remain in the ED for more than 24 hours may benefit from a one-off dose of zuclopenthixol acetate.

Controversies and future directions

- The role of butyrophenones versus atypical antipsychotics is controversial from a drug safety perspective.
- There is debate about the appropriateness of prolonged restraint and sedation of patients 'stranded' in emergency departments.
- The role of the central alpha-2 agonists in the management of hyperaroused patients in the emergency department is yet to be determined.

References

[1] Abdelmawla N, Mitchell AJ. Sudden cardiac death and antipsychotics. Part 1: risk factors and mechanisms. Adv Psychiatr Treat 2006;12:35–44.

[2] Abdelmawla N, Mitchell AJ. Sudden cardiac death and antipsychotics. Part 2: monitoring and prevention. Adv Psychiatr Treat 2006;12:100–9.

[3] McAllister-Williams RH, Ferrier IN. Rapid tranquillisation: time for a reappraisal of options for parenteral therapy. Br J Psychiatr 2002;180:485–9.

[4] MacPherson R, Dix R, Morgan S. A growing evidence base for management guidelines. Adv Psychiatr Treat 2005;11:404–15.

[5] Battaglia J, Moss S, Rush J, et al. Haloperidol, lorazepam or both for psychotic agitation? A multicentre, double-blind, emergency department study. Am J Emerg Med 1997;15:4335–40.

[6] Atakan Z, Davies T. ABC of mental health: mental health emergencies. Br Med J 1997;314:1740–2.

[7] Pilowski LS, Ring H, Shine PJ, et al. Rapid tranquillisation: a survey of emergency prescribing in a general psychiatric hospital. Br J Psychiat 1992;160:831–5.

[8] Alexander J, Tharyan P, Adams C, et al. Rapid tranquillisation of violent or agitated patients in a psychiatric emergency setting: pragmatic randomized trial of intramuscular lorazepam versus haloperidol plus promethazine. Br J Psychiat 2004;185:63–9.

[9] TREC Collaborative Group. Rapid tranquillisation for agitated patients in emergency psychiatric rooms: a randomized trial of midazolam versus haloperidol plus promethazine. Br Med J 2003;327:708–13.

[10] Currier GW. Atypical antipsychotic medications in the psychiatric emergency service. J Clin Psychiatr 2000;61(Suppl. 14):21–6.

[11] Department of Pharmacy. Clinical management of agitation in the older patient. Fremantle Hosp Hlth Serv Drug Bull 2006;30:2.

[12] Chan EW, Taylor DM, Knott JC, et al. Intravenous droperidol or olanzapine as an adjunct to midazolam for the acutely agitated patient: a multicenter, randomized, double-blind, placebo-controlled clinical trial. Ann Emerg Med 2013;61:72–81.

[13] Shale JH, Shale CM, Mastin WD. A review of the safety and efficacy of droperidol for the rapid sedation of severely agitated and violent patients. J Clin Psychiatr 2003;64:500–5.

[14] Wilson MP, Pepper D, Currier GW, et al. The psychopharmacology of agitation: consensus statement of the american association for emergency psychiatry project BETA psychopharmacology workgroup. West J Emerg Med 2012;13:26–34.

[15] Isbister GK, Calver LA, Page CB, et al. Randomized controlled trial of intramuscular droperidol versus midazolam for violence and acute behavioral disturbance: the DORM study. Ann Emerg Med 2010;56:392–401.

SECTION

21

CHALLENGING SITUATIONS

Edited by **George Jelinek**

21.1 Death and dying

William Lukin • Bryan G Walpole

ESSENTIALS

1 Death and management of the dying process is core business for emergency medicine.

2 Death in the emergency department can either be sudden and unexpected or the natural and expected evolution of a disease process.

3 Emergency physicians have a responsibility to understand the principles of a good death and to manage departmental deaths in alignment with these principles.

4 Communication skills for discussing death and dying are part of the skill set of an emergency physician.

5 How a death is managed in the emergency department has a profound impact on the grieving process of the next of kin. Emergency physicians should understand and be able to manage their role in establishing a normal grieving process for bereaved families.

6 Organ donation services should be offered unless there are clinical contraindications.

7 Local statutory obligations for coronial reporting must be well understood and observed.

8 Emotional health of emergency medicine practitioners should be monitored and external assistance sought when appropriate.

Introduction

For most people, the normal expectations are that they will live a full life, that parents will pre-decease their children and that the dying person will be able to deal with any unfinished business and die surrounded by loved ones, as portrayed in the media. There is an expectation that death will be natural, peaceful and, for the majority, pain free. In marked contrast to such expectations is the unexpected death of a loved one at an emergency department (ED) where sudden unexpected and violent death is not uncommon.

Death and dying patients are an inevitable part of emergency medicine practice.

In 2011/12, 1956 people died in emergency departments in Australia and a further 5477 were pronounced dead on arrival [1]. These deaths can be either be sudden and unexpected or the natural evolution of a dying process. Sudden unexpected death from trauma or rapid overwhelming disease processes is somewhat unique to emergency medicine and management of patients and families in this situation is something with which all emergency physicians must be familiar. The management of the patient dying from a life-limiting illness in the emergency department needs a different skillset to unexpected death but is just as important. For some, facing a surviving family or counselling a dying patient may symbolize failure in the battle against disease; however, it is a privilege and, done correctly, can be an extremely fulfilling part of emergency medicine practice. In emergency medicine, one does not have the benefit of a long-standing doctor–patient relationship. The support and mutual understanding that are the cornerstones of family practice are missing and so rapport must be forged in the heat of the moment. Families need space and time to come to grips with death, but both are limited in the ED. Access block and overcrowding should not preclude sensitive, empathetic grief management.

To follow the strain and pace of a difficult resuscitation with the grace and emotional energy required to care for a family requires

Box 21.1.1   Principles of a good death (adapted from Smith [2])

To know when death is coming and to understand what can be expected

To be able to retain control

To be afforded dignity and privacy

To have control over pain and symptom relief

To have choice and control over where death occurs

To have access to necessary information and expertise

To have access to required spiritual or emotional support

To have access to hospice care in any location

To have control over who is present and who shares the end

To be able to issue advance directives that are respected

To have time to say goodbye and control over timing

To be able to leave when it is time to go and not have life prolonged pointlessly

Adapted from Smith R. A good death. British Medical Journal Jan 2000 Vol 320 pp129–130 with permission.

considerable effort. Emergency physicians also have a duty of care to the survivors who deserve compassion as much as the recently deceased.

Similarly, management of the patient dying from a life-limiting illness can be a complex and challenging task. Patients and their families in this setting attend emergency departments for many reasons including fear, unrelieved symptomatology and the inability to access appropriate services. This is not always a failure of the system; sometimes an emergency department is the only place that can deliver the care they require. ED clinicians should have sufficient knowledge of local processes to enable advocacy roles for these patients with special needs and foster partnerships with local care providers to facilitate transition into other services.

The 12 principles of a good death were outlined in an editorial in 2000 (Box 21.1.1) [2]. These apply equally to unexpected and expected deaths. Death in an emergency department of necessity violates some or all of these principles. Emergency physicians should apply these to practice as best they can within the constraints of a busy, crowded emergency department.

Quality management of grief states can prevent significant morbidity, as pathological or unresolved grief can lead to later problems with physical and mental health.

The death process

Diagnosing dying

Death does not occur at a finite moment. Cardiac death, cerebral death, brainstem death and cellular death form a continuum over minutes or hours. Considerable effort has gone into diagnosing death. Legal definitions for diagnosing brain death, cardiac death and the staff involved are outlined in the relevant transplantation and organ donation acts in various jurisdictions. This has been done largely to facilitate organ transplantation.

There is a paucity of research in the area of diagnosis of the dying process and the part emergency physicians can play in this. Diagnosing dying is a skill best exemplified by specialists in palliative care. It can be hard to estimate and comes with experience. Making this diagnosis can enable the emergency physician to engage patients on a dying trajectory and allow them to take control and plan for the time they have remaining (see Chapter 21.6).

Managing the dying process

When the point of dying is reached, the practitioner needs to be acutely aware of the needs of the dying person. While physical needs, such as analgesia, are relatively easily met, other domains can easily be ignored.

For patients whose death is inevitable or not unexpected, a protocol, such as the Liverpool care of the dying pathway, can be instituted in the emergency department [3]. This tool focuses team care on the needs of the dying patient and avoids unnecessary interventions. The intent is to provide hospice level care in other clinical settings. At this point, the principles of a good death can act as an aspirational target as clinicians attempt to rationalize the care provided to patients.

A large family may need significant space, which can interfere with the routine work of the ED so a private room should be available. Then all can pay special attention to physical comfort, symptom management, privacy and the confidentiality of the patient and family.

Death

Families should be encouraged to be present during resuscitation efforts. A senior support person should be available for the family if at all possible during this time. If the outcome is hopeless, family members can be encouraged to be involved in decision making around abandoning resuscitation. After death, families should be encouraged to view, touch and talk to the deceased. It is well recognized that this improves the grieving process. They will remember these moments for the rest of their lives. Having participated in the resuscitation and in the decision to stop can be helpful

Initiation of the grieving process

Quality management of grief states can prevent significant morbidity, as pathological or unresolved grief can lead to later problems with physical and mental health. Emergency physicians have a duty of care to the survivors to play their part in the initiation of family grief.

Grief is not like an illness, to be fought and cured as so often is the case in Western medicine. Generalizations can be made about human behavioural tendencies and time lines can be drawn for predicted recovery, but each person's grieving process is unique. Some people never get better and nobody survives grief unchanged.

All relatives need time to receive the clear message of death, which they may need to be given again and again. Some need to make meaning of the event and the clinical art of managing perceptions is paramount. For the families of the deceased, this time will be recalled with unrivalled clarity. It is a great privilege to be part of those memories and it carries the responsibility to manage the family in keeping with best practice principles for the initiation of grieving.

Breaking bad news

The interview with the family of the recently deceased can be more difficult than the resuscitation. Handled with sensitivity, however, it can be a positive start to successful grieving and recovery.

The room in which such information is given should be private and comfortable and contain a telephone. Tea, coffee, iced water and simple food should be readily available. If refreshments arrive soon after the news has been broken, this can help diffuse tension. The offering of food is a time-honoured expression of warmth and comfort and facilitates communication and the grieving process.

The emergency physician should greet the family by name, confirm the relationship of each with the patient and shake hands or touch them gently. All parties should be seated and a helpful way to start is to ask the family members what they know. They may have been present at the scene, where CPR was under way, or have come to hospital independently with no preconceived ideas. A simple unambiguous summary of events should be given. This often needs to be repeated and the family members given time to ask questions.

It is important to use the word 'dead' or 'died'; euphemisms such as 'passed away', 'she's gone' and 'departed this life' are unclear messages that can mislead. The grieving process cannot start until there is acknowledgement of death. A truthful explanation can be comforting. There is no curriculum for teaching this type of interaction. Junior staff should be able to be present when a more senior staff member is conducting these discussions to facilitate role modelling. Over time, junior staff should be encouraged to facilitate these discussions in the presence of more senior mentors.

Tranquillizers

Requests for tranquillizers can come from survivors or a third party, who may ask that the bereaved be given sedation. It is now recognized that the use of anxiolytic medication is contraindicated in early grieving. This must be carefully explained to families when it is requested. It may be part of the management of morbid grief weeks or months later but has no place in early management. Anxiety, sadness and insomnia can be a natural part of early grief.

Reactions

There is a range of responses to the information that a close relative has died. The mode of death can be a guide. Homicide can lead to great distress, along with suicide and unintended injury. Some common reactions are:

- Disbelief: some will immediately deny the event, claiming that it must be somebody else or that they are dreaming. Reinforcement is required.
- Numbness: some sit mute, appearing not to take in the information. They need time to absorb it.
- Expressive: a sudden flood of tears or loud cries with upsetting or disturbing noises should be allowed to run its course. Such acknowledgement can be a positive response.
- Guilt: particularly with homicide and suicide, such news is often followed by 'if only' or 'why couldn't I have?' Here, gentle repeated reassurance and discussion can be important. These people are at risk of pathological grief reactions and can be helped by seeing the body and talking to it.
- Displacement activity: an immediate call to inform relatives, organize the funeral and discuss family matters is a poor prognostic sign. These people are often seen as mature, rational and born organizers, but they are at risk of pathological grief reactions months later. They will need careful follow up to see that they grieve eventually.

Offers of follow up can be made at this time. If the family members have unresolved questions they need a contact in the emergency department to arrange further meetings if required.

Viewing the body

Relatives and their invited friends should be encouraged to view the body. By seeing the body, by feeling and touching, the grieving process, separation and rebuilding can start. People should be encouraged to speak, touch, kiss, stroke, caress, even to argue, negotiate and cajole in private for as long as they wish. This facilitates natural grieving. The presence of a bereavement or viewing room can make this process much easier as, particularly with children, visiting can go on for several hours. A hospital morgue may be used, some have a purpose-built facility and appropriate staff support. Relatives should be informed of the necessity for police involvement if the matter has been referred to the coroner.

Cultural issues

Various ethnic and religious groups have differing practices for the handling and disposal of bodies. Emergency physicians should be able to manage different family requests in a sensitive manner while bearing in mind local statutory obligations.

For Australians of Aboriginal or Torres Strait Island descent, cultural practices and beliefs vary from region to region and families will guide practitioners. In larger hospitals, Aboriginal liaison services can help.

Death certificates

Doctors managing deaths in the ED must understand and have a sound knowledge of reporting requirements for the coroner's court (see Chapter 25.2 The coroner). Any death suspected to be not entirely from natural causes or where the cause is unknown requires reporting. Local regulations stipulate the circumstances under which a death certificate may be issued and by whom. For instance, in some states, it is not necessary for the issuer to have seen the person while alive. Coroner's courts are proactive in assisting medical practitioners to complete certificates where possible.

Organ donation

A thorough knowledge of local definitions is crucial for the emergency physician to participate in efforts to improve organ transplantation rates (see Chapter 21.7). Relatives can ask later why donation was not suggested and some really appreciate the opportunity to contribute to the welfare of others. All Australian states have access to professional transplant coordinators to facilitate the process once permission has been obtained.

Bereavement counselling

Most hospitals have qualified practitioners to support the recently bereaved. Referral should be arranged prior to departure if counsellors have not already made contact. Ministers of religion are trained in grief counselling and are usually available after hours. People can feel unprepared to ask for them and it is not necessary for the deceased to have had any religious affiliation to make use of such counsellors. The general practitioner is also a useful resource and should always be informed promptly of the death of a practice patient. Social workers are expert in grief counselling and many funeral companies and coroner's offices now provide counselling services.

Subsequent issues

Permission to leave

Recently bereaved people are sometimes confused, frightened, stunned and at a loss as to what to do next. When forensic issues (identification and statements) and viewing have been completed, they can be given the dead person's possessions and politely given permission to leave the hospital. 'There is nothing more you can do' or 'Can I phone someone or get a taxi to take you home?' may be usefully offered.

Information about contacting a funeral office to arrange for collection of the death certificate and the body and to discuss burial rites should be in an explanatory leaflet, readily available.

Professional issues

One of the important aspects of looking after survivors is caring for the carers, who are often overlooked. Patient death has been reported to lead to physical and emotional symptoms in emergency medicine practitioners [4]. There is no evidence that psychological debriefing prevents or ameliorates post-traumatic stress disorder and it may cause harm to some. Often, after an unsuccessful resuscitation, professionals need to talk about the events within the team environment. This should be done to foster reflective practice around teamwork in crisis situations. It is uncertain whether this improves psychological outcome. There is, however, a distinct propensity for those who spend their lives among misery to become cynical and full of black humour. The cultural norms of emergency medicine can become so integrated into personal values that the physician does not even recognize their presence. We should regularly assess our own emotional fatigue and, if there is a significant divergence between our personal values and career activities, we may be motivated to seek support from a trusted source. This area awaits further research.

Controversies and future directions

- The role of protocols, such as the Liverpool care of the dying pathway, in emergency medicine is currently unclear and is controversial in some health systems where it has been implemented.

The challenge for emergency physicians is to improve the care of the dying in our busy emergency departments.

- Increasingly, attention will be paid to ensuring the well-being of staff who are constantly exposed to death and dying in the course of their duties.

References

[1] Australian Institute of Health and Welfare: Australian hospital statistics 2011–12: emergency department care <http://www.aihw.gov.au/WorkArea/DownloadAsset.aspx?id=10737423039>.
[2] Smith R. A good death. Br Med J 2000;320:129–30.
[3] Marie Curie Palliative Care Institute. Liverpool care pathway for the dying patient. <http://www.liv.ac.uk/mcpcil/liverpool-care-pathway> [Accessed Jan. 2013].
[4] Strote J, Schroeder E, et al. Academic emergency physicians' experiences with patient death. Acad Emerg Med 2011;18:255–60.

Further reading

Carey G, Sorensen R, editors. The penguin book of death. Melbourne: Penguin Books, Melbourne University Press; 1997.
Shears R. Emergency physicians' role in end-of-life care. Emerg Med Clin N Am 1999;17:2.

21.2 Sexual assault

Ian Knox • Roslyn Crampton

ESSENTIALS

1 Sexual assault is defined as an act of a sexual nature carried out against a person's will.

2 There is widespread under reporting of this criminal offence.

3 The complex medical, legal and psychological sequelae mandate a team-based approach for victims involving doctors, police and counsellors in a collaborative effort.

4 Management by a sympathetic non-judgemental physician helps the victim to regain control.

5 The medical evaluation is specifically directed at the issues of injury assessment and management, infection risk and emergency contraception.

6 The forensic aspects of the examination require vigilant examination and documentation by the physician to assist the court in legal proceedings.

Introduction

Sexual assault is defined as an act of a sexual nature carried out against a person's will. Following sexual assault, a patient presenting should first be evaluated for acute traumatic physical injuries and drug or alcohol intoxication. The victim should be offered prophylaxis for sexually transmitted infection (STI) and pregnancy as appropriate. If required to collect forensic evidence to assist in any police investigation, consent is obtained for recording the victim's account of the assault, the findings on physical examination and for the collection of forensic material. Follow-up medical care and psychological support should be arranged prior to safe discharge.

Definitions

Every jurisdiction in Australia has its own legislation and definitions used to describe all types of sexual offences. Sexual assault has a number of elements. It is an act of a sexual nature that is carried out against the will of the victim. Consent is the crucial issue. The victim does not give consent, is intimidated to consent, or is legally incapable of giving consent because of youth or incapacity. It includes attempts to force the victim into sexual activity and includes rape (intentional penile penetration of the vagina, including the vulva), attempted rape, aggravated sexual assault (assault with a weapon or infliction of injury), indecent assault (oral or anal intercourse), penetration by objects and forced sexual activity that did not result in penetration. Penetration is not an essential element to sexual assault.

The absence of physical resistance by the victim is not regarded as consent. Consent by intimidation or coercive conduct without physical threat is also a criminal act. Consent requires free agreement and a person may be incapable of consenting because of the influence of drugs or alcohol.

Sexual assault by a carer upon a child is termed sexual abuse. This is sexual activity in which consent is not at issue and involves the child in sexual activity that is either beyond the child's understanding or contrary to accepted community standards. There are legal definitions regarding age, generally in the order of 15–17 years depending on the jurisdiction. Sexual violence involving a disabled person may also be either abuse or assault depending on the nature of the act or the circumstances of the victim.

Epidemiology

Global statistics indicate at least one in five women experiences rape or attempted rape during her lifetime [1]. Crime statistics are limited; it is estimated, for example, in the Australian Bureau of Statistics Personal Safety Survey 2005 that only 19% women who were sexually assaulted reported the incident to police [2]. Victims hesitate to report because of humiliation, fear of retribution, fear they will not be believed, self-blame and lack of understanding of the criminal justice system.

In this survey, based on sampling the Australian population of women, 5.8% (443 800)

experienced violence in the previous 12 months, including 1.3% experiencing sexual assault. Males experienced sexual assault less frequently at 0.6%. For females, only 22% were assaulted by a stranger, 21% by a previous partner, 39% by a family member or friend and 32% by another known person. Stranger assaults were more common in males (33%). An estimated 17% of women had experienced sexual assault since the age of 15 versus 4.8% of men.

Sexual assault is more common in vulnerable populations. Individuals in psychiatric facilities may be targeted and their report may not be believed as may occur with intellectually or physically disabled persons with diminished ability to detect or escape from such danger. Homeless women with serious mental illness have a very high lifetime risk for this violent victimization. Young adult male prisoners are also at risk [3].

Barriers to care

The ABS study [4] found that once an incident of sexual assault has been reported to the police, one in four cases result in the perpetrator being charged, but the conviction rate is low with less than 50% of defendants found guilty. The study showed 12.5% of women also did not report the assault to the police because of shame and embarrassment. Emergency physicians and nurses need to be aware of these attitudes that the victim and they themselves may have when approaching the sexual assault victim. A non-judgemental, accepting stance by care providers is essential. The victim has enough self-doubt without healthcare providers adding to that. It is not the health professional's role to make a judgement as to whether the rape occurred; the courts will decide this. False allegations of rape are made, but given the perceived penalties associated with reporting a rape, such a person is likely to be disturbed and in need of help in any event.

The role of the doctor in attending to victims of sexual assault who have consented to forensic examination and evidence collection is not the usual model of a therapeutic relationship. There is a dual obligation, as it is recognized that they have both a therapeutic role and a duty to the court to provide completely objective expertise in collecting evidence and interpreting the findings on examination to a court of law, where the impartiality of experts is key to their duty.

Consent

Victims who experience sexual assault may have experienced a loss of control and feel in danger. For the person to regain control, every step of the process must be explained and consent gained. Consent must be obtained for the forensic examination and evidence collection and for the release of the information to the police. Consent must be informed, specific and freely given. The consent must be witnessed. The capacity of the victim to give consent has to be carefully assessed. The mental competence to understand the information can be impaired, for example, by drugs or alcohol and mental state should be first tested. Certain patients are bound by formal legal requirements, which vary in each jurisdiction, for consent or responsibility for medical treatment. These include intellectually disabled persons, psychiatric patients under involuntary admission and children under custody orders or under the care of the state.

The evidence collected under this consent must be accurately labelled and secured.

Chain of evidence

Once a forensic specimen has been collected from its origin, all aspects of its existence must be recorded. All persons coming into custody of the specimen must be identified and the details of all transfers of custody and maintained security of the material must be recorded. A forensic register must be maintained for all items in a dedicated and secure storage facility.

Medical evaluation of the victim

The medical, forensic and psychological needs of a complainant depend on the nature and timing of the assault. The immediate medical needs are paramount. Medical care for victims of sexual assault includes consideration of physical injury, toxicological issues and the risks of acquiring an infection or pregnancy.

Evaluation of acute traumatic injuries is the first priority. The literature typically describes about half the victims having some sort of physical injury [5], although less than 5% of victims require admission to hospital for treatment. An analysis of over 1000 cases in the USA [6] revealed that physical examination showed evidence of general body trauma in

64% of victims. Genital trauma was noted in 52%, while 20% had no injuries documented. An Australian study confirmed non-genital injuries in 46% of women and genital injury in only 22% [7]. These findings indicate that many sexual assault victims may not have either general or genital trauma on examination and this absence does not mean that an assault did not occur.

Potentially life-threatening injuries may include attempted strangulation, blunt traumatic injury to the head or face and torso and penetrating injuries, which may be occult. These should be fully evaluated prior to referring for forensic processes.

A study from Florida found that one in 1500 sexual assaults resulted in the death of the victim, with asphyxiation being the most common cause of death. While there has been no comparable Australian study, the Australian Institute of Criminology reports that there were 288 homicides committed in Australia in 2003 and a sexual assault was the precipitating factor in nine [8].

Non-fatal strangulation is an important risk factor for homicide of women [9]. Of 300 survivors of strangulation reported from the San Diego City attorney's office [10], 150 had no visible markings. Examination findings, where present, can include ligature abrasions, finger tip bruising from the assailant's grasp and curvilinear abrasions caused by finger nail markings, occurring singly or in sets, caused by the victim's struggle to pry the grasp from her neck. Subconjunctival haemorrhage and petechial haemorrhages in the skin may be identified.

Strangulation is a form of asphyxia characterized by closure of the blood vessels or air passages of the neck as a result of external pressure usually by hands (throttling) or ligature strangulation (garrotting). External injury may appear trivial but is a marker of potentially significant sequelae that can develop in surviving victims, both acute and delayed.

Compression of the airway can lead to laryngeal injuries including fractures, soft-tissue swelling and mucosal oedema with potential development of airway compromise. Significant gulping of air together with vomiting and an episode of loss of consciousness may precipitate aspiration. Hypoxic cerebral damage depends on the duration of hypoxia and most victims either die or survive without obvious brain damage, but post-hypoxic encephalopathy has been reported. Carotid artery intimal

dissection with subsequent thrombus formation has also been reported. This may present as a delayed focal deficit from subsequent stroke up to 2 weeks after the incident [11]. Attempted strangulation warrants a high index of suspicion to rule out injuries and a period of observation may be required.

Penetration with foreign bodies can cause overt or occult pelvic injury. Further investigation or operative intervention may be necessary.

Forensic history, examination and evidence collection

The forensic examination is carried out for the purpose of obtaining evidence of the rape or assault that could be used in a prosecution. The aim is to record the victim's report of the assault and collect and record evidence related to this report and collect DNA. Specific consent should be sought before this examination is undertaken, as therapeutic benefit is not intended. Specific consent must be additionally obtained to turn over the specimens to the police. Police services produce kits that give a comprehensive guide to the history and examination including body charts required for various aspects of the prosecution. Emergency departments should have access to a multidisciplinary team with a clinician trained in such collection.

Physical examination recorded for the forensic record must include every wound detected on meticulous forensic examination. Injury could have been inflicted by the assailant or in the victim's attempted defence or escape; in the interpretation of the injury, even minor wounds that may not require treatment take on key forensic significance. Physical examination requires a sympathetic but professional and methodical approach of every body surface as with the collection of relevant forensic samples. Every injury must be carefully recorded on a body chart. Height and weight is required for interpretation of toxicological results.

Standard nomenclature including lacerations, abrasions and bruises should be used in wound description. Correct anatomical sites must be recorded and labelled in genital examination. Evidence collection kits provided in each jurisdiction contain anatomical body charts for recording all body areas, which must be assessed for evidence of injury including the ears, mouth and throat.

A wound is a disruption in the continuity of tissues produced by physical injury. Description of the physical characteristics of a wound includes the site, size, shape and depth of the wound as well as the appearance of the wound edges and adjacent tissue, the contents of the wound and whether there is evidence of healing.

An abrasion is a superficial injury of the skin caused by pressure and movement applied simultaneously. Abrasions can be of importance in the forensic context, as they may identify direction, as with friction abrasions, or patterns of the causative object as with imprint abrasions or they may contain embedded trace materials.

A bruise is an area of haemorrhage within or beneath the skin due to blunt trauma. This is also known as a haematoma, contusion or haemorrhage. The discoloration is caused by blood leaking from damaged blood vessels. The age of a bruise cannot be determined by its colour as this can undergo considerable variation. It takes more than 18 hours to develop any yellow discoloration [12]. Bruises may not occur at the site of the trauma and their size does not always correlate with the applied force; they may be altered by coincident conditions, such as anticoagulant therapy.

A laceration is a ragged or irregular tear in the skin, subcutaneous tissue or organs resulting from blunt force. Lacerations can be distinguished by irregular or crushed margins, bands of intact tissue forming bridges across the wound and intact structures, such as tendons, within the wound. The term laceration is often misused to describe an incised wound. An incised wound is an injury produced by sharp-edged objects. The edges of incised wounds are sharply defined and blood loss may be extensive as the vessels are divided rather than crushed. The correct classification of injuries can assist in determining the mechanism of injury or the object or weapon that caused the injury.

Patterns of injury may be observed. Blows to the head, face and neck may cause bruising, lacerations and fractures and include hyphaemas, dental trauma and tympanic membrane perforation. Fingertip bruising and imprint bruising may be evident. Defensive responses may show warding off injuries to the hands, for example, incised wounds to the palm or bruising on extensor surfaces of the arms. Fingertip bruising can be present on the medial thighs. Bite marks may be seen on breast or buttocks. Abrasions from contact with unshaven skin may be detected. Postmenopausal women are significantly more likely to need surgical management and repair of genital injuries than are younger women [13].

Examination of the genitalia includes inner thighs, buttocks and anus. Common locations for genital injuries include tears or abrasions of the posterior fourchette (where the two labia meet posteriorly), abrasion or bruising of the labia minora and fossa navicularis (directly anterior to the fourchette) and bruising or tears of the hymen. After relevant forensic specimens have been collected, it may be necessary to use a Foley catheter to tease out any folds in hymenal tissue to facilitate the inspection of hymenal injury. An examination of the vagina and cervix can then be completed using a speculum, any evidence of injury recorded and any bleeding or discharge recorded with the source identified. Perianal injury may need a moistened swab to tease out folds for inspection and proctoscopy may be required for inspection as appropriate.

Despite the relatively low frequency of obvious injury, the documentation of such injuries increases the chance of successful prosecution [14]. Photography must have the specific consent of the victim and is best performed by an experienced practitioner and the secure storage of images must be ensured.

Collection of forensic specimens

The perpetrator may have left evidence on the victim. Sampling from sites of contact between the victim and assailant is the basis of evidence collection. Specimens collected are guided by the circumstances. Standardized evidence collection kits used in each jurisdiction contain both forms of swabs and slides appropriate to obtain trace evidence of saliva, semen, blood and skin-to-skin contact. Samples should be sampled, allowed to dry, sealed and packaged with all contents carefully labelled and the chain of evidence maintained. Slides should be made where the presence of semen is suspected.

Any sample collected from the victim that contains cellular material from the victim's assailant can be used for DNA testing. This includes spermatozoa, semen if it contains cells or blood or tissue from under fingernails, which should be clipped. DNA evidence left on or in the body of a victim, particularly in moist areas, degrades quickly over 2–10 days. The forensic assessment should thus be made as soon as possible. Underpants and panty liners

worn during or after the assault may be contaminated with forensic material and should be retained. As DNA degrades quickly if moist, with the overgrowth of organisms, underclothes should be stored in paper not plastic bags.

Proof of sexual contact is established by the detection of spermatozoa or semen either on or within the victim or on the victim's clothes. The likelihood of detecting spermatozoa or semen from the vagina is generally very low by 72 hours. However, under some circumstances, spermatozoa may persist for days longer and can be obtained from the endocervical os or cervix. The detection of sperm or semen from the rectum or mouth is possible but very dependent on the actions of the victim after the assault, which should be recorded. The presence of DNA in deposited saliva may give a positive result for up to 2 days. Skin swabs for epithelial cells are generally unhelpful after 12 hours.

Care must be taken when the victim undresses for the examination. Hair or clothes fibres from the offender or other traces from the crime scene may have adhered to the body or clothes of the victim. The victim should undress standing over a drop sheet, which should then be included in a bag into which clothes are placed. This becomes part of the physical evidence.

The most accurate laboratory method currently available to identify the assailant is DNA testing. The chance of incorrectly identifying an alleged assailant as the source of DNA material is very small. However, the risk of contamination of the evidence samples with that of DNA belonging to other individuals is significant and has resulted in wrongful incarceration [15]. Accordingly, forensic collection and analysis techniques are under increasing scrutiny by the legal system and sources of contamination must be excluded. All measures to minimize DNA cross-contamination in the clinical setting, including the consistent use of gloves, gowns, mask and drapes and in the techniques of collection must be taken and recorded.

Toxicological issues

Drugs may be administered to the victim in order to facilitate sexual assault. The commonest drug is alcohol, but large numbers of drugs, including flunitrazepam and gamma hydroxybutyrate (GHB), have been implicated and the victim may be unaware or have no memory of events surrounding the assault. Self-reported alcohol consumption immediately prior to

assaults is very common, including up to 77% of those reporting drug-facilitated sexual assault [16] and this study revealed levels in 37% of those reporting with an average blood alcohol concentration of 0.11% at the time of examination. This is likely to have had a significant impact on conscious state and the ability to consent at the time of assault and may impair the victim's subsequent recall of events. The victim is at additional risk, particularly where there is a combination with prescription or recreational drugs. Covert administration of drugs in the setting of sexual assault appears uncommon in this Australian study. The interpretation of drug levels and their possible effects is difficult. In general, urine is the preferred specimen, although blood samples should be collected within 24 hours of the assault and these must be refrigerated prior to laboratory analysis.

Medical aftercare

The risk of genital infection after sexual assault

The risk of sexually transmitted infections (STIs) following rape is reported to be 4–56%, with infection reflecting those organisms that are locally prevalent. One study showed that with baseline testing, 43% of victims had evidence of pre-existing infection [17]. The finding of pre-existing infection is not admissible in court under Australian law. Most experts discourage testing for STIs in the emergency department unless symptomatic.

Baseline screening [18] for the following infections is recommended in follow up:

- HIV: HIV antibody
- Hepatitis B: hepatitis B surface antigen, HbsAg, core antibody, anti-HBc and surface antibody, anti-HBs
- syphilis: rapid plasma reagin (RPR) and *Treponema pallidum* haemagglutination assay (TPHA)
- chlamydia: polymerase chain reaction (PCR) endocervical swab, first void urine
- gonorrhoea: endocervical swab, PCR and microscopy culture and sensitivity
- trichomonas: high vaginal swab, microscopy culture and sensitivity.

While the risk of acquiring an infection is difficult to define, antibiotic prophylaxis is not generally recommended for the victim unless the person committing the assault is known to be suffering from an STI, is at high risk for having an STI or it is thought unlikely to return for follow up. Poor follow-up rates are the norm and all patients should be offered prophylaxis in the emergency department if urgent follow up cannot be ensured. Intramuscular ceftriaxone 250 mg together with 1 g azithromycin orally plus either metronidazole 2 g or tinidazole 2 g as a single dose is the suggested antibiotic regimen [19].

Given the low prevalence of syphilis in the general community, it is reasonable not to give benzathine penicillin routinely but to have syphilis serology performed at 3 months, depending on the circumstances and whether follow up can be assured. Chlamydia trichomatis is the most common notifiable sexually transmitted infection in Australia. If the victim has a pre-existent infection and receives treatment with azithromycin without follow up or contact tracing there is a risk of re-infection and increased risk of serious morbidity, including infertility.

Hepatitis B virus can be transmitted by sexual intercourse but the risk of transmission is undefined. By comparison, the risk of infection following a percutaneous needle stick from an HBAg-positive individual to an HBAb-negative recipient is 5–43% [20]. Prophylaxis with hepatitis B vaccine 1 mL IM is indicated. HBV vaccination and hepatitis B immune globulin (HBIG) (400 IU IM) should be available where the assailant is either known to be HBV positive or the woman is considered to be particularly at risk of infection. Hepatitis B vaccination without HBIG is highly effective in preventing HBV infection in sexual contacts of persons who have chronic HBV infection. Persons exposed to an assailant with acute HBV infection additionally require HBIG which prevents 75% of such infections [21]. Unless victims have a reliable vaccination history and serological conversion, the full hepatitis B course should be initiated, even when the completion of the vaccine series cannot be ensured [22]. Hepatitis C is not efficiently transmitted sexually.

It is likely that the victim will be concerned about HIV or will become concerned at a later date. The offer of HIV testing should be made accompanied by the usual full explanation and written consent needs to be obtained if the test is done. HIV seroconversion has occurred in persons whose only known risk factor was sexual assault, although the frequency of this occurrence is thought to be low [22]. In consensual sex, the risk for HIV transmission from vaginal intercourse is 0.1–0.2% and for receptive anal intercourse 0.5–3.0%. The risk of transmission from oral intercourse is much lower. Specific circumstances of an assault that might increase risk for HIV transmission include the site of penetration, site of exposure to ejaculate and the presence of mucosal trauma, genital lesions or another STI.

Other factors that should be considered in the recommendation for post-exposure prophylaxis (PEP) include multiple assailants, the likelihood of an assailant having HIV given the local epidemiology for HIV and whether the assailant is from a high-risk group including men who have sex with men or use drugs by injection.

HIV PEP should be offered as soon as possible after the assault up to 72 hours post-exposure. PEP appears to be well tolerated. Local protocols for the initial 3–5-day medication supply, collection of baseline testing and prompt referral for specialist consultation must be in place. National guidelines [23] recommend the use of two and three antiretroviral drug regimens according to the calculated risk of HIV exposure, increased to a three-drug regimen using stavudine 40 mg twice daily when calculated exposure risk exceeds 1 in 1000. The full 28-day course must be undertaken with both regimens.

Tetanus prophylaxis must be considered as part of the management of any injuries in the usual way.

Pregnancy prophylaxis

The risk of pregnancy following a single unprotected episode of coitus has proven difficult to define. However, a large prospective study from North America rated the risk of pregnancy from rape as 5% [24]. Emergency contraception is readily available in Australian pharmacies and it is the responsibility of the medical practitioner to ensure the patient knows of the availability and has immediate access to the medication.

The progestagen levonorgestrel is used alone for emergency contraception in a dose of 1.5 mg and can be given up to 5 days from the time of unprotected intercourse. If this single dose is given within 72 hours, the proportion of pregnancies prevented was 85% in the WHO multicentre study [25]. The earlier it is given, the more effective it is.

The literature demonstrates that there is poor compliance with follow-up instructions in this setting. Arrangements for follow-up testing for pregnancy, sexually transmitted diseases, HIV and hepatitis B vaccination should be supplied as written instructions as victims may subsequently remember little of their interview.

Crisis intervention

Acute reactions to rape range from emotional numbing to shame, self-blame and severe emotional distress. The predominant reaction is a devastating sense of loss [26] based on the fear for survival and the gross invasion of bodily boundaries which removes the victim's control over that which she finds most personal to her. Longitudinal data [27] suggest sexual assault survivors are at increased lifetime risk of post-traumatic stress disorder (30%) and major depression (30%). The input of sexual assault counsellors in evaluating the patient's immediate and ongoing emotional and safety needs must be in place prior to discharge. The role of various psychological therapies in decreasing long-term sequelae is not yet clear.

It has been found that the greater support the doctor provides the victim, the better the outcome [28]. However, this study found doctors were the least supportive health professionals in this setting.

Children

Child sexual assault is ideally managed by a team with specific paediatric expertise. The circumstances regarding children who are the victims of sexual assault differ from those relating to adults. First, the child is likely to have been the victim of chronic abuse rather than an attack by a stranger. Second, almost always the offender will be a man known to the child, often in a position of authority and trust. This introduces the issue of protecting the child from further molestation. The injury pattern is highly variable. Chronic sexual abuse tends to develop as a pattern of behavior between the victim and the offender beginning with touching and possibly leading to penetrative intercourse. This escalation of activity may evolve over a lengthy period and physical trauma may not be a feature. If the child has been the victim of a stranger assault, the risk of physical injury is greater than for an adult victim [29].

Conclusion

A patient presenting for care after sexual assault should first be evaluated for acute traumatic injury and any intoxication issues.

The victim should be assessed in order to offer appropriate post-exposure prophylaxis to pregnancy and sexually transmitted diseases including gonorrhoea, chlamydia, trichomoniasis, hepatitis B and HIV, plus routine tetanus prophylaxis. Specific informed consent must be obtained prior to forensic evaluation. The involvement of a multidisciplinary team with an experienced forensic examiner and sexual assault counsellor is of value. Discharge must not occur until the immediate safety of the victim is ensured. Follow up for medical issues and ongoing psychological support should be arranged prior to discharge. Maintaining a sympathetic non-judgemental approach by the physician improves the victim's outcome.

Controversies and future directions

- The incidence of sexual assault has previously been under recognized in the disabled, mental health inpatients, military and police recruits in academies and a range of other institutional and educational settings.
- One of the most challenging areas is the endemic problem of violence, including sexual violence inflicted on indigenous women. Some groups of Aboriginal girls and women report that half of them have been the victims of incest or

sexual assault. Crime statistics recorded in 2008 found that the indigenous victimization rate for sexual assaults in NSW was nearly 3.5 times the rate for the non-indigenous population [30].
- It is now recognized that every precaution must be taken to reduce possible cross-contamination of DNA during collection and storage of forensic specimens.

References

[1] International Medical Advisory Panel. Statement of gender based violence. London: International Planned Parenthood Federation; 2000.
[2] Australian Bureau of Statistics. Personal safety survey Australia. ABS Catalogue 4906.0 Commonwealth of Australia; 2005.
[3] Heilpern D. Fear or favour: sexual assault of young prisoners. Southern Cross University Press; 1992.
[4] Australian Bureau of Statistics. Sexual assault in Australia: a statistical overview. ABS Catalogue 4523.0 Commonwealth of Australia; 2004.
[5] Rambow B, Adkinson C, Frost TH, et al. Female sexual assault: medical and legal implications. Ann Emerg Med 1992;21:727–31.
[6] Riggs N, Houry D, Long G, et al. Analysis of 1076 cases of sexual assault. Ann Emerg Med 2000;35:358–62.
[7] Palmer C. Genital injuries in women reporting sexual assault. Sexual Hlth 2004;1:55–9.
[8] Australian Institute of Criminology. Homicide in Australia 2003–2004. National Homicide Monitoring Program. Research and Public Policy Series No. 66.
[9] Glass N, et al. Non fatal strangulation is an important risk factor for homicide of women. J Emerg Med 2008;35:329–35.
[10] Hawley D, Mc Clane E, Strack G. A review of 300 attempted strangulation cases part III. J Emerg Med 21: 315.
[11] Malek AM, et al. Patient presentation angiographic features and treatment of strangulation induced bilateral dissection of the internal carotid artery. J Neurosurg 2000;92:481–7.
[12] Langlois NE, Gresham GA. The aging of bruises a review and study of the colour changes with time. Forens Sci Internatl 1991;50:227–38.
[13] Ramin SM, Satin AJ, Stone IC, et al. Sexual assault in postmenopausal women. Obstet Gynecol 1992;80:860–4.
[14] Linden JA, Care of the adult patient after sexual assault. N Engl J Med 2011;365(9):834–41.
[15] Vincent FHR. Inquiry into the circumstances that lead to the conviction of Mr F.A.J. Victorian Government Printer; 2010.
[16] Hurley M, Parker H, Wells DL. The epidemiology of drug facilitated sexual assault. J Clin Forens Med 2006;13:181–5.
[17] Hampton HL. Care of the woman who has been raped. N Engl J Med 1995;332:234–7.
[18] Mein J, Palmer C, Shand MC, et al. Management of acute adult sexual assault. Med J Aust 2003;178:226–30.
[19] Workowski KA, Berman S. Sexually transmitted disease treatment guidelines, 2010. Centers for Disease Control and Prevention. Morbid Mortal Wkly Rep 2010; 59:91.
[20] Gerberding JL, Henderson DK. Management of occupational exposures to blood-borne pathogens: Hepatitis B virus, hepatitis C virus, and human immunodeficiency virus. Clin Infect Dis 1992;14:1179–85.
[21] Centers for Disease Control and Prevention. Post-exposure prophylaxis Hepatitis B. Recommendations and reports. Morbid Mortal Wkly Rep 1997;47:101–4.
[22] Centers for Disease Control. Post-exposure prophylaxis Hepatitis B. Recommendations and reports. Morbid Mortal Wkly Rep 2010; 59:80–8.
[23] Australian Government Department of Health and Aging. National Guidelines for post exposure prophylaxis after non occupational exposure to HIV. Copyright Commonwealth of Australia; 2006.
[24] Holmes MM, Resnick HS, Kilpatrick DG, et al. Rape-related pregnancy: estimates and descriptive characteristics from a national sample of women. Am J Obstet Gynecol 1996;175:320–5.
[25] Von Hertzen H, Piaggio G, Pregoudov A, et al. Low dose mifeprostone and two regimes of levonorgestrel for emergency contraception: a WHO multicentre randomised trial. Lancet 2002;360:1803–10.
[26] Rose DS. Worse than death: psychodynamics of rape victims and the need for psychotherapy. Am J Psychiatr 1986;143 817–4.
[27] Linden JA. Care of the adult patient after sexual assault. N Engl J Med 2011;365:834–41.
[28] Popiel DA, Susskind EC. The impact of the rape: social support as the moderator of stress. Am J Commun Psychol 1985;13:645–76.
[29] Cartwright PS, the Sexual Assault Study Group. Factors that correlate with injury sustained by survivors of sexual assault. Obstet Gynecol 1987;70:44–6.
[30] Australian Bureau of Statistics. Recorded Crime: Victims. Catalogue No 4510.0, 22. Commonwealth of Australia; 2008.

21.3 Family violence

Sandra L Neate • Lyndal Bugeja • Carolyn Walsh

ESSENTIALS

1 Family violence encompasses physical, sexual and psychological violence.

2 All forms of family violence are inter-related in a complex way. Victims of violence may suffer many forms of abuse over their lives.

3 Between 30 and 50% of women and approximately 15% of men experience family violence over their lifetime.

4 Family violence occurs across all socioeconomic, religious and cultural groups.

5 There is a range of barriers to disclosure and reporting to authorities.

6 Effectively responding to family violence requires a multidisciplinary and coordinated approach, involving health practitioners, social services and justice agencies.

Definition

Family violence involves all types of violence within intimate or family relationships. It includes physical and sexual abuse, threats and intimidation, psychological, emotional and social abuse and financial deprivation and can occur across the lifespan [1].

Physical violence is defined as intentionally inflicted harm using bodily force or a weapon. It encompasses sexual violence, such as non-consensual or coercive sexual activity using physical force, sexual harassment, stalking, forced or deceptive sexual exploitation, threats or intimidation [2] and non-personal violence, such as intentional property damage. Psychological abuse, which frequently precedes physical abuse, may take the form of threats, verbal harassment, ridicule or behaviours designed to intimidate, humiliate, control and isolate the victim.

Family violence most often occurs within current or former intimate relationships and is described as a gendered phenomenon, as it is largely perpetrated by men against women [3]. However, while women account for the larger proportion of victims, males can also be affected [4] and this form of violence may also feature in same sex relationships [5]. Family violence may involve any family member related by blood or law. Children may be directly victimized or suffer harmful consequences as a result of hearing or witnessing violence [6].

The subjective experience and definition of family violence are strongly influenced by cultural beliefs and previous life experiences and the individual's perceptions of their experience may vary greatly.

Family violence is also referred to as domestic violence or intimate partner violence. The more inclusive term of family violence accounts for violence within a range of intimate and family relationships.

Incidence

The prevalence of family violence varies according to definition (whether sexual and emotional abuse are included), timing of the abuse (current, during adult life or cumulative life time prevalence) and whether the violence is actual or threatened. Australian prevalence surveys indicate that approximately 30% of women and 15% of men report a lifetime history of (actual, personal) family violence, with around 20% of women and 8% of men disclosing a history of family violence during adult life [7,8]. US studies report a higher cumulative lifetime prevalence of approximately 50%, but include actual and threatened, personal and non-personal violence [9].

The 2005 Australian Personal Safety Survey reported that 15% of Australian women had experienced physical or sexual violence by a previous partner and 2.1% by a current partner since the age of 15. In contrast, 4.9% and 0.9% of Australian men had experienced violence by a previous or current partner, respectively [10]. The Australian component of the International Survey of Violence against Women survey reported that 34% of women had experienced physical and/or sexual violence since the age of 16 [3]. The 2005 Personal Safety Survey also reported that 61% of women who had experienced violence had children in their care at the time of the violence and 31% of these children had witnessed the violence. Of women who had experienced violence, 59% had been pregnant during that relationship, 36% reported violence during pregnancy and 17% reported the first instance of violence occurring during pregnancy [10].

Overall, women have a four times higher risk of experiencing family violence than men and those who have been victims of child abuse have six times the risk of experiencing adult family violence. Men and women report a similar incidence of approximately 7% of childhood abuse alone [8].

Approximately 2% of women presenting to emergency departments (EDs) have experienced physical violence within the 24 hours preceding the presentation [7,8]. The incidence is approximately 10% if psychological abuse is included [9].

Vulnerable groups

Certain groups within the population may be more vulnerable to the effects of family violence. Among these are indigenous communities, culturally and linguistically diverse communities (CALD), people with disabilities and the elderly.

Indigenous communities

Members of indigenous communities may be exposed to heightened levels of family violence. In 2010, 14% of Australian homicide victims were identified as Aboriginal or Torres Strait Islander and the majority of these victims (68%) died in a family homicide incident, most commonly involving an intimate partner [11]. One New Zealand general practice survey found a life-time incidence of partner violence of 75% for Maori women [12].

CALD communities

CALD communities experience additional complexities with respect to family violence. While it is important to avoid generalizations and stereotypes, cultural values and beliefs can have implications for the way in which the individual experiences and responds to violence. CALD victims may encounter greater difficulty obtaining assistance and support from mainstream service providers for reasons including: discrimination and marginalization; lack of awareness of legal rights and protections; concerns of bringing dishonour to the family; fear of authority figures; and communication barriers.

Disability

Women with disabilities can be disproportionally affected by family violence. Victims with cognitive and physical disabilities experience greater difficulty in accessing mainstream services due to: communication barriers; lack of appropriate transport and accommodation; reliance on the perpetrator of violence; and limited recognition of their victimization status.

Elderly

The elderly are at risk of abuse from people on whom they depend. Physical or cognitive impairments add to their vulnerability. Older persons can become socially isolated due to a decline in social contacts and supports, increasing the risk that abuse will go undetected.

Risk factor identification

The identification of risk and contributory factors for family violence within intimate relationships has allowed for improved understanding of the nature, form and degree of danger to victims, as well as the conditions under which incidents of family violence are more likely to occur.

While the growing evidence base about risk factors has informed the development of a variety of tools and measures designed to improve and detect those at risk, the presence of these factors is not an infallible predictor of violence. For example, some victims with multiple risk factors will not experience escalating or severe violence, while fatal family violence can occur in the absence of clearly defined risk and contributory factors.

Despite this caveat, knowledge and recognition of these factors is an important step toward improved identification and intervention

in violent behaviour. To this end, risk factors are generally classified at the level of the individual, relationship and social environment [13].

Individual level risk factors have been identified for both victims and perpetrators of violence. Individual characteristics associated with men having an increased risk of perpetrating violence are alcohol abuse, drug use, low education standards, unemployment and being a former rather than current partner [12]. Alcohol abuse is the most identifiable risk factor and the risk is proportional to the degree of abuse, although it is not necessarily causal. Pregnancy and new birth have been associated with both emerging and escalating violence [14]. There is some association between perpetrator mental health and violence, particularly conditions such as depression and psychosis [15].

At the level of the relationship, a history of abusive and violent behaviour is one of the strongest predictors of further violence [16]. Separation or the announcement of an intention to end an intimate relationship is associated with an increased risk of violence. Separated or divorced women are four times more likely to be abused than women who have never married, are married or are widowed [17]. Men who are abused are commonly assaulted by the women whom they abuse [18].

Social environment factors affecting family violence include gender inequality supported by societal norms and economic or social policies that create or sustain inequalities [13].

Outcomes

Family violence affects health outcomes in a multitude of physical and psychological ways. Most presentations to health professionals by victims of violence are a complex mix of indirectly related physical and psychological problems and are not trauma related [9].

Physical injury and illness

Physical injuries resulting from family violence may have patterns similar to other forms of non-accidental injury, such as a history inconsistent with the injury, injuries of varying temporal stages or unreasonable delay in presentation. Non-accidental injuries are often in central compared with peripheral areas of the body. Injuries to defensive areas of the body or to the back, legs, buttocks, back of the head and soles of the feet reflect attempts at self-protection. Injuries inflicted on females

are likely to be contusions, abrasions, lacerations, fractures and dislocations [19]. Women are more likely to be choked, beaten or sexually abused. Men have a greater risk of having objects thrown at them or weapons used against them. Although family violence-related injuries may follow certain patterns, injury pattern is of low positive predictive value in the identification of family violence [19].

Abuse before, during and after pregnancy represents a threat to the well-being of the mother and baby. Approximately 40% of women who are physically abused are forced into non-consensual sex at some stage. This results in high rates of sexually transmitted disease, unintended and adolescent pregnancy and termination of pregnancy. There is also an established complex link between family violence and preterm labour, low-birthweight babies and postnatal depression [20].

Prevention of access to or interference with general healthcare or antenatal care may occur with up to 17% of abused women reporting partner interference with accessing healthcare [21].

In Australia, homicide among intimate partners and other family members forms a substantial proportion of annual homicide incidents. Between 1989 and 2002, 38% of homicide victims were murdered by a family member [22]. Approximately 25% of USA female homicides are family violence related. Many homicide victims had presented to an ED in the 2 years preceding their death. Documentation of violence and intervention were rare [23].

Psychological impact

Family violence is an independent risk factor for mental illness. Women who have experienced family violence have an approximately 11-fold increase of dissociative disorders, 6-fold increase in somatization disorders, 5 times higher incidence of anxiety and are three times more likely to suffer depression, phobias and drug dependence [17,18]. Exposure to family violence has also been shown to be associated with the onset of post-traumatic stress disorder. Abused women have twice the rates of hazardous alcohol consumption and dependence [17]. Abuse occurring both in childhood and adulthood causes a further significant increase in the incidence of mental illness. The experience of psychological abuse, especially ridicule and humiliation, are particularly responsible for causing low self-esteem.

Impact on children

The impact of family violence on children includes potential victimization, witnessing violence, separations from family, foster care, risks of future mental illness and an increased potential to perpetrate violence in the future [6].

Children living in a home where violence is perpetrated against a parent are 15 times more likely to be a victim of abuse or neglect themselves [20]. Family violence is a risk factor for becoming a perpetrator of homicide in the pre-teenage group [24].

The outcome of the experience of violence is directly proportional to the duration and frequency of violent episodes. Overall, approximately one-third of the population risk for all mental illness is attributable to family violence [25].

Social

Control by the perpetrator who fears disclosure by the victim can lead to social isolation, prevention from paid employment or contact with medical practitioners.

Financial dependence and the responsibility of children increase isolation, loss of choices and difficulties of separation from the perpetrator. Poverty is prevalent and multifactorial. Separation from or incarceration of the perpetrator may lead to further loss of income.

Homelessness may be relative, where there is no sense of safety or security in the home, or absolute, where there is need for interim or emergency accommodation or families may be living on the streets. Children or elderly people living in violent circumstances may be institutionalized by authorities or carers.

Outcomes for male victims differ from female victims in several significant ways. Male victims typically express fewer feelings of fear and terror and less frequently feel trapped and controlled. Men are also generally less constrained by financial dependence. As fear, control, dependence and isolation contribute greatly to the psychological outcomes of family violence, women still suffer approximately 95% of the serious physical and psychological consequences of family violence [18].

Economic cost

The costs of family violence are vast. Costs include pain, suffering and premature mortality costs, health costs (victim, perpetrator and children), production-related costs (lost productivity), consumption-related costs (property replacement), second-generation costs (child-care, child protection), administrative (legal and forensic) and transfer costs (income support, lost taxes). The total annual cost of family violence in Australia in 2002–03 was AUD $8.1 billion. The lifetime cost per victim was AUD $224 470 [26]. The National Council to Reduce Violence Against Women and their Children has more recently projected that family violence will cost Australia $9.9 billion in the years 2021–22, if appropriate action is not taken [27]. International studies estimate costs in the billions of dollars annually [28].

Barriers to detection and reporting of family violence

Detection rates of family violence in EDs are low. Only 10% of those who present with acute family violence-related injuries or issues will be asked by the attending nurse or physician or volunteer information about the violence issue. Documentation of violence in the medical record is rare [9]. Barriers to detection may include system factors, such as inadequate privacy, health-practitioner's lack of time and education, health-practitioner's attitudes and cultural, social and gender issues.

Crime statistics in Australia show a general increase in reporting of family violence. Rates of women reporting physical and sexual assault to the police rose from 19% and 15% in 1996, respectively to 36% and 19%, respectively in 2005 [10,29].

A range of barriers can inhibit victims' disclosure, including feelings of fear and shame, concerns about not being believed or about further victimization, anxiety about possible medical or legal processes, as well as familial, cultural or religious pressures. In some cases, individuals do not recognize themselves as victims of violence or may not have yet considered seeking assistance in respect to their violent partner.

Indigenous women in Australia report violence rarely. Historical interactions with police, such as forcible removal of children and high rates of Aboriginal death in custody, contribute to indigenous women fearing for the safety of themselves and their families when police or social services are involved [20] and the lack of accessible and culturally appropriate legal processes create further barriers to reporting. The elderly may be prevented from reporting by fear of further abuse, neglect or the threat of institutionalization [20].

Screening

The high prevalence of family violence, low positive predictive values of demographic factors and clinical presentations, low detection rates and high incidence of subsequent physical and psychological illness have supported the argument for universal screening. Opportunistic screening may increase detection rates of family violence. Detection rates without screening are in the order of 0.4%. Rates of detection rise to approximately 14% with the use of simple direct questioning [30]. The use of a single screening question may be as effective as asking several questions. Screening questions should be simple and direct such as 'Do you feel safe at home?' or 'Are you afraid of your partner?' Explanation that these questions are routine may improve patient comfort.

Screening may indicate to the victim that channels of communication are open and that help will be available. It educates women about violence, its nature and prevalence. Screening may also be important in detection of perpetrators. Approximately 40% of family violence perpetrators have sought medical attention in the preceding 6 months with half having attended an ED [31].

Most women find screening an acceptable practice, however, up to two-thirds of medical practitioners and 50% of nurses are not in favour of performing screening. Reported barriers include a lack of education on how to ask questions about abuse, language barriers, a personal or family history of abuse and time constraints [32]. In the USA, the legal implications of mandatory reporting add to reluctance to screen.

Screening may improve detection rates and referral rates to external agencies. However, currently, no evidence exists that screening leads to improved health outcomes for victims [33].

Management

The management of family violence is complex. Leaving a violent relationship is no guarantee of safety and may precipitate increased levels of violence. Leaving a violent relationship is a process and not an event and requires support through all phases. Help may best be offered by validating the disclosure, expressing concern, listening, providing support, ensuring safety and offering a bridge to services.

Understanding

Interviews with survivors of family violence provide a framework for understanding the stages through which a victim must work before leaving a violent relationship [34]. The pre-contemplative phase is where the victim is not consciously aware of or is in denial about the abuse. A contemplation phase follows where the abuse is acknowledged, but the victim is unable to decide to leave. A preparation stage follows where steps are taken in preparation to leave and take action. The action phase involves leaving the relationship but is typically characterized by episodes of return to the relationship. A maintenance phase occurs when a period of 6 months without return to the relationship has occurred.

Listening and understanding where the victim is in terms of progress through these phases assists in assessing readiness for change and guides intervention. The aim is to validate the person's experience, emphasize that they did not deserve or cause the abuse and empower the making of independent decisions that lead to improvements in safety and well-being.

Referral

There are multiple agencies to assist victims of family violence. Community services include hotlines for emergency advice through to counselling services, emergency shelters, police and legal services.

Safety

Safety is paramount and emergency accommodation or hospital admission may be required to ensure immediate safety. Safety is an ongoing issue as the greatest risk of injury occurs while leaving the relationship. Seventy per cent of family violence homicides occur as the woman is leaving or has left the home [35]. Continued contact with the perpetrator due to custody arrangements make the risk of abuse a continuing one.

Reporting

Most Australian states and territories have not implemented mandatory reporting of family violence for adults. The exception is the Northern Territory, where mandatory reporting provisions were introduced in 2009. In contrast to adult victims of family violence, all Australian states and territories have some description of mandatory reporting of suspected cases of child abuse and neglect. Variations exist regarding which professionals are legally required to report, however, these generally include doctors, nurses and midwives. Most jurisdictions protect the identity of persons making a notification whether mandated or not.

Documentation

Documentation in the medical record may provide vital evidence and should be objective and accurate. Direct quotes and descriptions of behaviours and appearances increase objectivity. Body maps and photographs assist documentation of physical injury. Sexual assault examinations ideally should be performed by specially trained staff to ensure legal admissibility of evidence.

The management of family violence requires a coordinated response from all practitioners and service providers involved from when the victim first discloses the violence. This includes the health system, social services and the police and judicial system if the victim chooses to pursue this course of action. At all times, the victim's wishes must be paramount and the service providers should do their utmost to support these wishes.

Conclusion

Family violence is a pervasive social problem that does not discriminate across age, cultural background, religion or socioeconomic status. The implications of family violence are substantial, including physical injury, mental illness, economic and social costs and fatal outcomes. Despite the commonness of family violence, it frequently remains undetected and unreported. Identification of risk factors for violence and interventions aimed at increased identification and referral can be considered in the ED environment. When violence is disclosed, the expression of concern and a willingness to listen, risk assessment, safety planning, support and stage-appropriate referral are the mainstays of management.

Controversies and future directions

- While there has been considerable research on screening for family violence in emergency departments, further research regarding the outcomes after screening interventions is required to ensure efficacy and safety of screening.
- Mandatory reporting of violence among adults remains controversial.

- Management strategies should not be aimed at encouraging the woman immediately to leave the violent relationship. Risk assessment, safety planning, support and stage-appropriate referral are the mainstays of management.

References

[1] Council of Australian Governments. The national plan to reduce violence against women and children 2010–2022. Canberra; 2010.

[2] Mitchell L. Domestic violence in Australia – an overview of the issues. Canberra: Department of Parliamentary Services; 2011.

[3] Mouzos J, Makkai T. Women's experience of male violence; findings from the Australian component of the International Violence Against Women Survey (IVAWS). In: Australian Institute of Criminology, (ed.). Research and Public Policy Series 56. Canberra; 2004.

[4] Reid RJ, Bonomi AE, Rivara FP, et al. Intimate partner violence among men: prevalence, chronicity and health effects. Am J Prevent Med 2008;34:478–85.

[5] Duke A, Davidson M. Same-sex intimate partner violence: lesbian, gay and bisexual affirmative outreach and advocacy. J Aggress Maltreat Trauma 2009;18:795–816.

[6] Australian Domestic and Family Violence Clearinghouse. The impact of domestic violence on children: a literature review. Sydney: Australian Domestic and Family Violence Clearinghouse; 2011.

[7] Bates L, Redman S, Brown W, et al. Domestic violence experienced by women attending an accident and emergency department. Aust J Publ Hlth 1995;19:293–9.

[8] Roberts GL, O'Toole BI, Raphael B, et al. Prevalence study of domestic violence victims in an emergency department. Ann Emerg Med 1996;27:741–53.

[9] Abbott J, Johnson R, Koziol-McLain J, et al. Domestic violence against women. Incidence and prevalence in an emergency department population. J Am Med Assoc 1995;273:1763–7.

[10] Australian Bureau of Statistics. Personal Safety Survey, Australia, 2005 reissue. Canberra: Australian Bureau of Statistics; 2006.

[11] Virueda M, Payne J. Homicide in Australia: 2007–08 National Homicide Monitoring Program annual report. Canberra: Australian Institute of Criminology; 2010.

[12] Koziol-McLain J, Webster D, McFarlane J, et al. Risk factors for femicide-suicide in abusive relationships: results from a multisite case control study. Violence Victims 2006;21:3–21.

[13] World Health Organization. Multi-country study on women's health and domestic violence against women: initial results of prevalence, health outcomes and women's responses. Geneva: World Health Organization; 2010.

[14] Gartland D, Hemphill SA, Hegarty K, et al. Intimate partner violence during pregnancy and the first year postpartum in an Australian pregnancy cohort study. Matern Child Hlth J 2011;15:570–8.

[15] Shorey RC, Febres J, Brasfield H, et al. The prevalence of mental health problems in men arrested for domestic violence. J Fam Violence 2012;27:741–8.

[16] Riggs DS, Caulfield MB, Street AE. Risk for domestic violence: Factors associated with perpetration and victimization. J Clin Psychol 2000;58:1289–316.

[17] Roberts GL, Williams GM, Lawrence JM, et al. How does domestic violence affect women's mental health? Women Hlth 1998;28:117–29.

[18] Frank JB, Rodowski MF. Review of psychological issues in victims of domestic violence seen in emergency settings. Emerg Med Clin N Am 1999;17:657–77, vii.

[19] Muelleman RL, Lenaghan PA, Pakieser RA. Battered women: injury locations and types. Ann Emerg Med 1996;28:486–92.

[20] Astbury J, Atkinson J, Duke JE, et al. The impact of domestic violence on individuals. Med J Aust 2000;173:427–31.

[21] McCloskey LA, Williams CM, Lichter E, et al. Abused women disclose partner interference with health care: an unrecognized form of battering. J Gen Intern Med 2007;22:1067–72.

CHALLENGING SITUATIONS

707

[22] Mouzos J, Rushforth C. Family homicide in Australia, no.255, Trends and Issues in Crime and Criminal Justice. Canberra: Australian Institute of Criminology; 2003.

[23] Wadman MC, Muelleman RL. Domestic violence homicides: ED use before victimization. Am J Emerg Med 1999;17:689–91.

[24] Shumaker DM, Prinz RJ. Children who murder: a review. Clin Child Fam Psychol Rev 2000;3:97–115.

[25] Roberts GL, Lawrence JM, Williams GM, et al. The impact of domestic violence on women's mental health. Aust NZ J Publ Hlth 1998;22:796–801.

[26] Access Economics. The cost of domestic violence to the Australian economy. Canberra: Access Economics Pty Ltd; 2004.

[27] National Council to Reduce Violence Against Women and their Children 2009. The cost of violence against women and their children. Department of Families, Housing, Community Services and Indigenous Affairs, Canberra; 2009.

[28] Laing L. Economic costs of domestic violence: Australian Domestic and Family Violence Clearing House. University of New South Wales; 2002.

[29] Australian Bureau of Statistics. Women's Safety Australia 1996. Canberra; 1996.

[30] Morrison LJ, Allan R, Grunfeld A. Improving the emergency department detection rate of domestic violence using direct questioning. J Emerg Med 2000;19:117–24.

[31] Coben JH, Friedman DI. Health care use by perpetrators of domestic violence. J Emerg Med 2002;22:313–7.

[32] Yonaka L, Yoder MK, Darrow JB, et al. Barriers to screening for domestic violence in the emergency department. J Contin Educ Nurs 2007;38:37–45.

[33] Ramsay J, Richardson J, Carter YH, et al. Should health professionals screen women for domestic violence? Systematic review. Br Med J 2002;325:314.

[34] Gerbert B, Caspers N, Bronstone A, et al. A qualitative analysis of how physicians with expertise in domestic violence approach the identification of victims. Ann Intern Med 1999;131:578–84.

[35] Haywood YC, Haile-Mariam T. Violence against women. Emerg Med Clin N Am 1999;17:603–15, vi.

21.4 Alcohol-related illness

Venita Munir, Ioana Vlad

ESSENTIALS

1 Acute alcohol intoxication and withdrawal are responsible for many emergency department attendances and carry significant morbidity and mortality.

2 Chronic gastrointestinal and hepatic disease, coagulopathy and secondary bleeding complications, confusional states, mental illness, central nervous system disease with neuropathy and immunosuppression are common in alcohol-dependent persons, with complications that increase the morbidity and mortality further.

3 Wernicke's encephalopathy is an uncommon but serious illness related to vitamin B1 deficiency. It requires high-dose parenteral thiamine 500 mg IV tds.

4 Many serious illnesses mimic alcohol intoxication or are masked by it. Maintain a high index of suspicion in the intoxicated patient with an altered conscious state.

5 Emergency physicians are uniquely placed to screen for high-risk drinking and to offer brief advice or intervention to this group to reduce the burden of recurrent alcohol abuse.

Introduction

Alcohol-related illness is common across the world and has a high prevalence in emergency department (ED) presentations. Alcohol misuse not only places the individual at risk of acute intoxication and injury but also poses significant long-term health issues.

Acute alcohol intoxication causes much morbidity and mortality from all forms of violence from motor vehicle and other accidents, interpersonal to self-harm. Chronic alcohol use contributes to many hospitalizations and deaths due to alcohol-related medical conditions and brain injury, resulting in both physical and psychosocial impairment.

Many acutely intoxicated patients presenting with an altered conscious state have significant co-morbidities masked by alcohol, which must be considered on each presentation.

Emergency physicians should not only recognize and treat alcohol-related emergencies, but also intervene in patients at high risk from their alcohol intake who present with other conditions. Early opportunistic screening using recognized alcohol screening tools and standardized brief interventions reduce 'at-risk' drinking and the morbidity and mortality from alcohol-related illness.

Epidemiology

Australia ranks 30th of 180 countries for alcohol consumption per capita. Australian alcohol consumption per capita is estimated at 9.8 L of pure ethanol per person per annum [1]. The percentage of Australian drinkers who report consuming more than the National Health and Medical Research Council (NHMRC) recommended levels for preventing chronic harm is decreasing (10% in 2008 vs 44% in 2001); however, 35% of Australian drinkers still consume more than the recommended amount for preventing short-term harm [2]. Alcohol misuse, morbidity and mortality among indigenous Australians is appreciably higher than the non-indigenous; certain populations, such as in central Northern Territory and north Western Australia, experienced double the national alcohol-attributable death rate in 2004 [3]. Death rates attributable to alcohol are higher in rural than metropolitan areas. Deaths from acute alcohol-related causes are most common in younger people aged 15–29 years, but chronic alcohol-related deaths mostly occur in those over 45 years [1].

Alcohol use is implicated in more frequent attendance at EDs [4] with presentations most commonly due to acute intoxication and injuries sustained by violence or motor vehicle trauma. Alcohol consumption is an important reason for repeat ED attendance and is the most common reason for repeat use of an ambulance to attend EDs [5]. In one study, a core group of alcohol-related attendees accounted for 4.3% of ED presentations, but 28% of ambulance transports to ED, 70% of those transports being for episodes of acute intoxication [5].

Six per cent of young persons attending city hospital EDs are for alcohol-related reasons, with injury significantly more likely among alcohol users than illicit drug users [6]. Among young people attending the ED, nearly 38% may be drinking harmfully, 18% may have consumed alcohol in the previous 6 hours and 15%

consider their attendance to be alcohol-related [7]. Up to 45% of injured patients attending ED may have consumed alcohol within the past 24 hours and almost 30% in the last 6 hours [8].

The natural history of alcohol dependence is to remit and relapse, with a relentless progression to early death. Risk factors for alcoholism are a family history of alcohol dependence or total abstention, parental divorce, youngest child, other substance misuse, availability of alcohol and extremes of income.

Pharmacology

Pharmacokinetics

Alcohol is passively absorbed from the entire gastrointestinal tract (GIT), with about 25% from the stomach. Absorption is rapid within 60–120 minutes of intake and may be slowed by food. Alcohol is distributed throughout body water; females and obese people with lower body water-to-fat ratio reach higher blood alcohol concentrations (BAC) sooner than lean counterparts. Hepatic oxidative metabolism occurs via alcohol dehydrogenase. Alcohol-tolerant people also utilize the hepatic microsomal ethanol oxidizing system, which is upregulated with increasing drinking. First-order elimination kinetics becomes saturated as the BAC increases, changing to zero-order kinetics and slower sobering at higher BAC.

Pharmacodynamics

Alcohol is thought to act on γ-aminobutyric acid A (GABA$_A$) inhibitory neuroreceptors in the brain causing central nervous system (CNS) depression. The characteristic euphoria is thought related to the release of endogenous opioids (endorphins). Rapidly rising BAC causes quicker and more pronounced behavioural changes than the same level achieved over hours. A steady state of absorption to metabolism and excretion can be achieved at about one standard drink per hour. A standard drink is defined as containing 10 g or 12.5 mL of pure alcohol. Behavioural intoxication depends on factors such as habituation, food co-ingestion, body habitus and the concentration of alcohol in the drink.

Measurement of blood alcohol concentration

The blood alcohol concentration may be estimated using a portable breathalyser that estimates BAC after measuring alcohol concentration of alveolar air. This is a useful non-invasive screening tool but relies on a cooperative and awake patient being able to exhale adequately for the reading. There is an approximate difference of 15–20% between breath alcohol readings and serum BAC. Readings are influenced by temperature, hyper- or hypoventilation prior to exhalation, haematocrit level, other substances, such as ketones, and machine error. Directly measured serum blood alcohol concentration is more reliable. The Australian legal limit for driving is 0.05%; in New Zealand it is 0.04%, while in the USA and UK it is 0.08%.

Chronic alcohol-related illness

Gastrointestinal

Chronic alcohol use results in disease of the gastrointestinal tract (GIT), liver and pancreas. Morbidity most frequently arises from GIT bleeding, liver disease and pancreatopathy.

Gastrointestinal bleeding

The most common causes of alcohol-related GIT haemorrhage are peptic ulcer disease (PUD) and the consequences of portal hypertension, such as oesophagogastric varices or subepithelial gastropathy. Mallory–Weiss tears, oesophagitis and alcoholic gastropathy are less frequent causes of alcohol-related GIT haemorrhage. Heavy alcohol use may be a risk factor for development of PUD, although the exact pathogenesis is poorly understood and the role of alcohol may be additive to the effects of *Helicobacter pylori*, non-steroidal anti-inflammatory drugs (NSAIDs) and tobacco [9].

Variceal bleeding in portal hypertension results from raised portal blood flow and portal vascular resistance due to hepatic fibrosis. Fifty per cent of cirrhotic patients develop varices and, once present, variceal bleeding occurs in 10–30% per annum. Variceal bleeding may be catastrophic with a 30% mortality for a first bleed. The 5-year survival was estimated at 26% in one patient series of variceal bleeding, of which 80% were alcohol dependent [10].

While Mallory–Weiss tears are less common, up to 44% are associated with alcohol use and may have significant morbidity due to blood loss [11]. Alcohol-induced vomiting against a closed glottis can also result in oesophageal rupture (Boerhaave's syndrome).

Management of GIT bleeding Close attention to airway, breathing and circulation is the first priority. Aggressive initial fluid resuscitation is necessary in shock with an initial crystalloid bolus of 500–1000 mL, followed by transfusion of blood products if required. Vitamin K 10 mg IV is indicated in patients with known or suspected liver cell failure. Replacement of clotting factors with factor concentrate or fresh frozen plasma and platelets will also be required if the patient requires massive transfusion or has abnormal coagulation secondary to chronic liver disease or to major haemorrhage [12].

An intravenous proton pump inhibitor, such as omeprazole 80 mg stat, followed by an infusion at 8 mg/h is often initiated for bleeding from presumed PUD, oesophagitis, gastritis or duodenitis. This decreases hospital length of stay and the need for endoscopic therapy but does not reduce transfusion requirement, re-bleeding, the need for surgery or death at 30 days [13].

Variceal bleeding After the initial resuscitation and replacement of clotting factors if needed, acute variceal bleeding should be managed with a bolus of octreotide or terlipressin, followed by an infusion, while urgent upper gastrointestinal endoscopy is arranged. Terlipressin is a synthetic analogue of vasopressin, that reduces splanchnic blood flow and portal pressure. It is the only agent that has been shown to improve mortality (34% relative risk reduction) in the setting of acute variceal bleeding [14]. Octreotide is a synthetic somatostatin analogue that reduces splanchnic blood flow. Endoscopy is diagnostic for the site of bleeding, as well as being both therapeutic and prognostic. Therapy is usually by banding ligation, sclerotherapy or tissue adhesive. Sclerotherapy with the injection of varices with sclerosant with octreotide is more effective than sclerotherapy alone at controlling bleeding but may not improve longer-term mortality. Gastroesophageal balloon tamponade with Sengstaken–Blakemore or Minnesota tube can provide temporary haemostasis when sclerotherapy is not available or is unsuccessful. It controls bleeding in up to 80% of cases, but it does not affect long-term mortality and it is associated with a high rate of complications, especially if it is performed by individuals who are not familiar with its use [15].

Early variceal surgery by oesophageal transection or selective portocaval shunt or interventional radiology, such as transjugular intrahepatic portosystemic shunting (TIPSS), may enhance short- and long-term survival, but both techniques are complicated by the risk of encephalopathy. TIPSS is preferred if liver transplantation is being considered. When the acute episode of variceal bleeding is over, oral propranolol and isosorbide mononitrate are used as maintenance therapy for portal hypertension.

Alcoholic liver disease

Alcoholic liver disease (ALD) comprises a spectrum of disorders from alcoholic fatty liver (steatosis), inflammation (hepatitis) to progressive fibrosis (cirrhosis) and hepatoma. These occur from chronic insult to the liver due to oxidative stress, damage from free radicals and the immunogenicity of alcohol metabolites. Many factors are involved in the aetiology of ALD, including genetic predisposition, gender, ethnicity, nutrition, obesity and co-existent chronic viral hepatitis, non-alcoholic fatty liver and other liver diseases, such as autoimmune.

The duration and amount of alcohol consumed play important roles; drinking at levels above the NHMRC recommendations (more than two standard drinks a day, both in men and women) is a defined risk for the development of alcohol-related injuries, ALD and eventual cirrhosis. NHMRC also recommend drinking less than 4 standard drinks per occasion to reduce the short-term adverse effects of alcohol use, in particular alcohol-related injuries. Alcohol dependence does not inevitably lead to cirrhosis, as only 10–20% of heavy drinkers progress [16]. Alcoholic fatty liver is a common finding among alcohol-dependent patients but is not a frequent cause for presentation to an ED.

Alcoholic hepatitis and cirrhosis Alcoholic hepatitis may present as acute anorexia, nausea, vomiting, right upper quadrant pain and jaundice. Treatment is supportive and abstinence from alcohol is essential (see Chapter 9.6).

Cirrhosis typically presents late, with subtle malaise, anorexia, weight loss, weakness and fatigue, with a combination of liver cell failure and the development of portal hypertension. Acute decompensation results in symptomatic ascites, jaundice, pruritus, spontaneous bacterial peritonitis (SBP), hepatic encephalopathy, variceal bleeding and coagulopathy.

Ascites Ascites due to hypoalbuminaemia, secondary hyperaldosteronism and portal hypertension is usually recurrent. Sudden exacerbations may be caused by SBP, the development of portal vein thrombosis, a hepatoma or medication non-compliance. Symptoms include abdominal discomfort, girth increase and anorexia. Fever, chills and abdominal pain occur with SBP or, conversely, signs of sepsis are minimal but there is sudden worsening of jaundice or encephalopathy.

The long-term treatment of ascites includes sodium restriction and diuretics, especially spironolactone and/or furosemide. Problematic ascites may require fluid restriction, recurrent abdominal paracentesis and albumin transfusion. It is important to exclude SBP by paracentesis and polymorphonuclear (PMN) cell count, with greater than 250 PMN cells/mm² being diagnostic. The treatment of SBP includes intravenous broad-spectrum antibiotics, such as ceftriaxone 1 g IV daily or timentin 3.1 g 6-hourly daily, followed by oral antibiotic prophylaxis with trimethoprim 160 mg and sulphamethoxazole 800 mg tablets once daily.

Coagulopathy and encephalopathy

Coagulopathy results from the failure of hepatic synthesis of coagulation factors, thus administration of vitamin K 10 mg IV and factor concentrate or fresh-frozen plasma is required in the bleeding cirrhotic patient. GIT bleeding may also precipitate hepatic encephalopathy, with confusion and characteristic asterixis. This potentially reversible decrease in neuropsychiatric function must be distinguished from other causes of an altered conscious level in the cirrhotic patient.

Hepatic encephalopathy is associated with an increased nitrogenous GIT load (such as from a gastrointestinal bleed), dehydration, sepsis, certain drugs, hyponatraemia or hypokalaemia, worsening liver function and increasing jaundice. The treatment includes supportive care, GIT cleansing with lactulose (oral and enema) and oral non-absorbable antibiotics, such as neomycin to reduce bacterial counts, although their efficacy is unclear [16].

Thrombocytopaenia Thrombocytopaenia is a common finding in alcoholic liver disease and several factors contribute. The aetiology is multifactorial: direct toxicity of the alcohol on the bone marrow, portal hypertension and platelet sequestration in the enlarged spleen, decreased thrombopoietin (TPO) synthesis in the liver, with subsequent reduction in the proliferation and differentiation of megakaryocytes and platelet formation.

Alcoholic pancreatopathy

Alcoholic pancreatopathy is used to describe a group of pancreatic diseases caused by chronic heavy alcohol intake. It includes acute alcoholic pancreatitis, recurrent abdominal pain or GIT symptoms induced by alcohol, high serum levels of pancreatic enzymes or an abnormal pancreatic ultrasound. Recurrent bouts of acute alcoholic pancreatitis precede the development of pancreatic pseudocysts, chronic pancreatitis and pancreatic malignancies.

Alcohol is the most common aetiology of chronic pancreatitis (70–80%), although as few as 10% of heavy drinkers will develop it. Like cirrhosis, its aetiology is multifactorial; other risk factors include tobacco smoking and hyperlipidaemia, which should be addressed if early signs of pancreatopathy are recognized. Acute and chronic alcoholic pancreatitis are managed conservatively, with abstinence from alcohol, intravenous fluids, parenteral analgesia and antibiotics if pancreatic necrosis or an abscess are suspected (see Chapter 7.9).

Chronic pancreatitis can be debilitating with recurrent cycles of pain and admissions to hospital. Progressive pancreatic calcification, failure of exocrine and endocrine function and chronic pain can all be mitigated if alcohol is avoided. Recurrent pancreatic insults and chronic pancreatitis increase the risk of pancreatic carcinoma by up to 16 times.

Mental health and mental state issues

Depression and suicidal intent

Alcohol is a recognized risk factor for suicide. Mood expression and self-harm intent are often underestimated in the ED intoxicated patient. A Scandinavian study showed that 62% of 1207 'parasuicides' who presented to an ED involved alcohol use, with even higher rates in young males. Psychiatric referral was less likely if alcohol was involved yet, after 5.6 years, 3.3% had completed suicide. This represented a 51-fold increased risk compared to the general population, with the risk of completed suicide being greatest in the first year [17].

Alcoholic hallucinosis

Alcohol misuse causes psychotic symptoms by several mechanisms, including direct intoxication, alcohol withdrawal, delirium tremens (DTs), Wernicke's encephalopathy, Korsakoff psychosis and alcoholic dementia. Alcohol dependence doubles the risk of psychotic symptoms.

Alcoholic hallucinosis is a schizophrenia-like syndrome that differs from the other causes in that it occurs at a younger age, in a setting of clear consciousness and not related to acute withdrawal. There are no associated physical symptoms of autonomic dysfunction as in the DTs and its duration is longer with predominantly auditory hallucinations as opposed to visual. Its chronicity and derogatory auditory hallucinations are similar to schizophrenia, but thought disorder is not a feature.

Alcohol withdrawal states

The alcohol withdrawal syndrome follows prior alcohol dependence. Its clinical importance lies in the potential severity of the symptoms and signs, the need to consider alternative or concomitant pathology and the likelihood of seizures occurring. The principal symptoms are tremor, agitation, nausea and vomiting, sweating, anxiety and autonomic nervous system overactivity with tachycardia, tachypnoea and fever. Sleep disturbance, hallucinations and generalized tonic–clonic seizures generally begin within 10 hours of reduced alcohol intake, with a peak intensity by day 2. The withdrawal syndrome may occur in an individual who usually drinks an 'eye opener' or 'hair of the dog' but is prevented from doing so.

Alcohol withdrawal scales A number of scales measure alcohol withdrawal. One simple one is to rate symptoms as mild (tremulousness), moderate (agitation) and severe (confusion). Most EDs use an alcohol withdrawal scale (AWS) to measure symptoms and predict likelihood of seizure and direct preventative management. The most commonly used AWS is the Clinical Institute withdrawal assessment – alcohol, revised scale (CIWA-R). This scale measures 10 items and was primarily developed for planned detoxification or for use on general medical and psychiatric wards [18]. Surprisingly, blood pressure and pulse, although often abnormal, are not included in the scale. A modified version that includes seizures in the AWS is also used [19]. Patients with high scores have an increased risk of seizure if they remain untreated. The higher the score, the greater the relative risk. However, some patients experience complicated withdrawal despite initial low scores.

Pharmacological therapy Benzodiazepine (BZD) therapy reduces signs and symptoms of alcohol withdrawal and prevents complications [20]. All BZDs appear to have similar efficacy. Longer-acting agents, such as diazepam used with symptom-triggered dosing (as opposed to regular), decrease the total of drugs given and both shorten and smooth the clinical course. Early treatment is preferred to waiting for advanced withdrawal.

Published data on ideal doses are lacking. High-dose oral diazepam 20 mg 1- to 2-hourly may be needed for symptom control and up to 160 mg per day may be required to allow for BZD tolerance, which is common in alcohol-dependent patients. Under-dosing for fear of over-sedation is common.

Antipsychotics such as droperidol, haloperidol or olanzapine are commonly used to manage the agitation and other behavioural disturbances induced by severe alcohol withdrawal. However, they lower the seizure threshold and can cause anticholinergic syndrome if given in excessive doses. They can also cause prolongation of the QT interval and increase the risk of torsade de pointes in the alcoholic patients who are often hypokalaemic, hypocalcaemic and hypomagnesaemic. Carbemazepine is used in Europe and appears as effective as fixed-dose BZDs. β-Blockers decrease tremulousness but may worsen delirium and are not anticonvulsant. Clonidine improves symptoms of withdrawal but is not anticonvulsant. Vigabatrin has shown promise in reducing sedation, BZD use and the total withdrawal treatment time. Ethanol, of course, would 'treat' the symptoms of withdrawal.

Alcohol withdrawal seizures Around 3–5% of those with severe alcohol use disorder experience withdrawal seizures within 48 hours of stopping drinking and 15% will have a seizure in their lifetime. Previous withdrawal seizure is the strongest predictor of recurrent seizure. Most alcohol withdrawal seizures are short lived and self-terminating. Localizing signs or prolonged seizure should prompt a search for alternate pathology. Intravenous BZD, such as midazolam 0.1–0.2 mg/kg, is given for prolonged seizure. Phenytoin is not recommended for alcohol withdrawal seizures, unless there is coexistent epileptic disorder.

Delirium tremens DTs is characterized by confusion, altered conscious state and autonomic hyperactivity. The incidence of DTs has been reduced by effective early management of withdrawal and excluding intercurrent illness. DTs occur in less than 1% during any single withdrawal episode. The diagnosis is important, as the mortality approaches 15% if untreated. As symptoms usually manifest within 48 hours, DTs may be encountered in EDs experiencing access block or in short-stay observation units.

Risk factors for DTs: five risk factors are associated with the development of the DTs [21]. These include current infection, tachycardia greater than 120 beats/min, signs of alcohol withdrawal accompanied by BAC of more than 0.1%, seizure history and history of delirious episodes. DTs are rare in the absence of these factors. The treatment includes management in an intensive care with regular intravenous BZD, such as midazolam 0.1–0.2 mg/kg, and a search for underlying conditions, such as sepsis.

Wernicke's encephalopathy

The classical features of Wernicke's encephalopathy are ataxia, confusion and ophthalmoplegia, usually lateral rectus palsy. It is caused by thiamine deficiency, but severe deficiency may be present without these signs. In alcohol-dependent persons, oral thiamine absorption is poor. Malabsorption, reduced storage and impaired utilization of thiamine increase the risk of Wernicke's encephalopathy.

Post-mortem studies suggest that thiamine deficiency sufficient to cause irreversible brain damage remains undiagnosed ante-mortem in 80–90% of alcohol-dependent persons. Wernicke's encephalopathy should be considered in all patients in coma, as replacement of depleted brain thiamine is necessary. The mortality approaches 20% if left untreated.

Treatment of Wernicke's encephalopathy High-dose oral thiamine may be ineffective, thus parenteral therapy with thiamine 500 mg IV tds is recommended for at least 5 days. The risk of anaphylaxis is low with the current drug formulations [22,23]. The recommended prophylactic thiamine dosage has been increased to 200 mg parenterally tds.

Other alcohol-related neurological problems

Alcohol is a neurotoxin and chronic heavy use causes CNS damage, peripheral neuropathy, myopathy and movement disorders such as tremor, Parkinsonism, dyskinesias, cerebellar ataxia and asterixis.

Peripheral neuropathy

Peripheral neuropathy is common in alcohol misuse and has multiple aetiologies, including direct toxic effect of ethanol and malnutrition with thiamine deficiency. The prevalence among chronic drinkers is unclear but is estimated at between 9 and 50%. Other contributing factors are increased age, total lifetime dose of alcohol, nutritional status (malnutrition and thiamine deficiency) and family history of alcohol misuse. Alcoholic peripheral neuropathy is most commonly sensory in the lower limbs.

Alcoholic autonomic neuropathy

Alcoholic autonomic neuropathy is uncommon. It is often asymptomatic or causes erectile dysfunction in males, postural hypotension and/or diarrhoea. It is related to different pathological processes than sensory peripheral neuropathy.

Ataxia

Ataxia is a common presenting symptom and sign and may be due to peripheral neuropathy affecting proprioception, cerebellar degeneration or a combination of both. Cerebellar ataxia is possibly an extension of the insult from thiamine deficiency as in Wernicke's encephalopathy. Whereas in Wernicke's encephalopathy the ataxia may be reversible by thiamine administration, full recovery is rare and permanent damage occurs affecting the superior cerebellar vermis.

Blackouts

Neuronal failure resulting in blackouts and amnesia is a direct toxic result of alcohol on the CNS. This is especially common in binge drinkers. Orthostatic hypotension from autonomic failure is differentiated on the clear relationship to posture.

Respiratory illness in alcohol-dependent persons

Chronic obstructive airways disease

Chronic obstructive airways disease (COAD) is common among alcohol-dependent persons, mostly due to the high prevalence of concurrent tobacco smoking (see Chapter 6.5).

Pneumonia

Alcohol dependence increases the risk of community-acquired pneumonia due to immunosuppression, as well as general lifestyle factors, such as hygiene and smoking. Typical organisms include *Streptococcus pneumoniae* and *Haemophilus influenzae*. There is also a higher frequency of cavitating disease, empyema and unusual pathogens. Anaerobic and Gram-negative organisms are frequent colonizers of the oropharynx and GIT and aspiration pneumonia is common. Opportunistic disease, such as tuberculosis, *Pneumocystis carinii* pneumonia, now known as *Pneumocystis jiroveci*, and *Legionella* are also more frequent in alcohol-dependent persons.

Metabolic problems with alcohol use

Alcohol use and metabolic acidosis

Alcoholic ketoacidosis There is contention about the existence and frequency of alcoholic ketoacidosis. This refers to high anion-gap metabolic acidosis associated with the acute cessation of alcohol on a background of chronic alcohol abuse and relative starvation. Clinical features include nausea, vomiting, abdominal pain, tachycardia, tachypnoea and hypotension, all of which may occur in other alcohol-related emergency presentations.

Chronic alcohol intake can lead to depleted carbohydrate and protein stores in the body due to relative starvation. Reduced hepatic gluconeogenesis from substrates, such as lactic acid, glycerol and amino acids, can cause hypoglycaemia. In dehydrated states, the combination of hypotension and hypoglycaemia results in reduced insulin production and raised catecholamines, cortisol, glucagon and growth hormone. These hormones promote utilization of fatty acids for energy, resulting in ketogenesis.

Alcoholic ketoacidosis has been described as 'a common reason for investigation and admission of alcohol-dependent patients', although research data appear limited. There may be an increased frequency of sudden death among patients who present in this fashion [24].

Diabetic ketoacidosis Acute alcohol intoxication can precipitate ketoacidosis in known insulin-dependent diabetics.

Acute alcohol ingestion can cause a state of acute insulin resistance. Alcohol-induced post-prandial hyperinsulinaemia occurs without significant decrease in blood glucose levels, consistent with impaired insulin sensitivity. Relative starvation may result in hypoglycaemia and reduced insulin release. Alcohol-induced insulin resistance is important in these patients to recover from hypoglycaemia. Conversely, there is a reduced risk of type II diabetes mellitus in moderate drinkers (18–48 g per day) compared to light or heavy drinkers.

Other metabolic acidosis Metabolic acidosis is rare in alcohol intoxication alone. One study of 60 ED patients with BAC greater than 0.1% described seven patients with a raised serum lactate, all of whom had alternative reasons for this, such as seizure, hypoxia and sepsis [25]. The treatment of an alcohol-dependent patient with metabolic acidosis is symptomatic with intravenous crystalloid fluid resuscitation and rehydration, thiamine 200 mg IV, 5% or 10% dextrose for hypoglycaemia, electrolyte replacement (see below) and a search for and treatment of another underlying cause, such as sepsis.

Electrolyte disturbance

There are no direct correlations between acute or chronic use of alcohol with specific electrolyte disorders, although certain deficiencies are characteristic, such as hypokalaemia, hyponatraemia, hypomagnesaemia, hypophosphataemia and hypocalcaemia. The causes include poor intake, malabsorption, excessive losses from vomiting, diarrhoea and fluid diuresis, reduced renal tubular reabsorption and dilutional changes due to polydipsia.

Electrolyte imbalances result in disturbance of other endocrine systems. Thus, hypomagnesaemia suppresses parathyroid hormone release, resulting in hypocalcaemia. Electrolyte disturbances are also related to alcohol-induced illness, such as pancreatitis or pneumonia.

Cardiovascular

Coronary heart disease

There is a reduced mortality from coronary heart disease in diabetic moderate drinkers (approximately 28 g per day). However, alcohol use in diabetes increases the risk of retinopathy, peripheral neuropathy and foot ulcers. Coronary protective effects of alcohol are due to influences on increased high-density lipoprotein (HDL) cholesterol, platelet function and fibrinogen.

Hypertension

Acute alcohol intake is a vasodilator, whereas drinking alcohol over the longer term causes systolic hypertension and increased aortic stiffness. An assessment by the World Health Organization Global Burden of Disease 2000 Comparative Risk Analysis attributed 16% of all hypertensive disease to alcohol intake. These findings may be confounded by other lifestyle factors and there are many contrasting effects of alcohol at various intakes, depending on gender and body mass index (BMI). Thus, raising HDL cholesterol is cardioprotective, but developing central obesity 'beer gut' is not. Overall, any benefits of moderate alcohol consumption on coronary disease are likely to be outweighed by harmful effects.

Cardiac arrhythmias

Heavy alcohol use is associated with an increased risk of sudden cardiac death, most commonly due to ventricular arrhythmias. Atrial arrhythmias including atrial fibrillation occur commonly after heavy binge drinking, 'holiday heart', in both acute and chronic drinkers. They are not necessarily associated with cardiomyopathy. The risk of a cardiac arrhythmia is increased by electrolyte abnormalities, such as hypokalaemia, hypomagnesaemia and hypocalcaemia.

The treatment of arrhythmias is as recommended by the current Advanced Cardiovascular Life Support guidelines.

Cardiomyopathy

Concentric left ventricular hypertrophy is common in chronic alcohol users. Dilated cardiomyopathy may ensue with progressive dilatation and fibrosis, leading to congestive cardiac failure. This myotoxic process has a worse prognosis than idiopathic dilated cardiomyopathy, particularly if drinking continues. Myocyte function can improve with total abstention.

Aggressive anti-failure therapy should be implemented with dietary measures, such as reduced sodium intake, an angiotensin converting-enzyme inhibitor and other pharmacotherapy, even if total abstention cannot be achieved.

The so-called 'wet beri-beri' cardiomyopathy is caused by severe thiamine deficiency that leads to myocardial dysfunction and peripheral vasodilation. Thiamine absorption is impaired by alcohol and long-term use of frusemide depletes the body of water-soluble vitamins, including thiamine. Changes in myocardial function occur within 1 hour of starting parenteral thiamine therapy and are back to normal within 1 week of treatment [26].

Malignancy

Alcohol has been causally linked to many types of neoplasia, most commonly those of the GIT. Oropharyngeal and other head and neck cancers have a direct link to alcohol. Drinking more than 1.5 bottles of wine daily elevates the risk of oesophageal cancer 100 times. Hepatocellular carcinoma (HCC) is usually preceded by alcoholic cirrhosis in the Western world, although other causes include hepatitis B and C viruses. Progression of cirrhosis to HCC is more rapid if drinking continues. Chronic alcohol consumption is also related to laryngeal, breast, pancreatic and colorectal carcinomas.

Important illnesses to be excluded that mimic alcohol intoxication

It is hard to know when to look for another cause for altered conscious state in the habitual drinker or intoxicated person, as many alternative conditions must be considered that mimic apparent alcohol intoxication (Table 21.4.1). The mean length of altered conscious state in an ED for intoxication alone has been reported at 3.2 hours with a wide standard deviation of 3.6 hours, with the likelihood of another pathology being present increasing rapidly after 4 hours. Close observation looking for trends in autonomic responses and neurological signs and detailed examination looking for other pathology are more appropriate than waiting for, or intervening after, a certain period of time.

Metabolic disturbance

There is little evidence that hypoglycaemia occurs in adults with simple alcohol intoxication alone; with one large study of ED patients screened for alcohol use and serum blood glucose finding no linear relation between blood alcohol and glucose levels. The incidence of hypoglycaemia is not increased in alcohol-related ED attendances compared to sober patients. Intravenous glucose administration has not been shown to be useful in changing rates of alcohol elimination or decreasing periods of intoxication. However, it is essential in each patient with an altered mental state to measure the blood glucose and treat if it is low. Chronic alcoholics have limited hepatic glycogen stores due to malnutrition, so administering glucagon is not effective as it cannot initiate gluconeogenesis. In the intoxicated or alcohol-dependent patient, an alternative cause for hypoglycaemia should still be sought.

Hyponatraemia may occur with sepsis and general debility. Diabetic ketoacidosis or hyperglycaemic, hyperosmolar non-ketotic syndrome should also be excluded (see Chapter 11.2).

Head injury

Head injuries are not only more common in intoxicated and alcohol-dependent patients, they are easily missed due to a presumption that intoxication is the main cause of the altered conscious state. Head injuries may be complicated by coexisting coagulopathy and thrombocytopaenia from liver disease, cerebral atrophy and underlying metabolic problems. A computed tomography (CT) brain scan is essential to rule out intracranial pathology, particularly cerebral contusion, extradural haematoma, subdural haematoma and base of skull fracture.

Close neurological observation in a monitored resuscitation area is necessary in the intoxicated person with an altered conscious level and a possible head injury. Worsening confusion, deteriorating level of consciousness or focal neurology necessitate an urgent

Table 21.4.1 Illnesses not to be missed in the presumed intoxicated person	
Metabolic and encephalopathic	Hypoglycaemia
	Hyperglycaemia
	Wernicke's encephalopathy (thiamine deficiency)
	Hyponatraemia
	Liver failure
	Renal failure
Head injury	Skull fracture
	Cerebral contusion
	Subdural and extradural haematoma
Other intracranial pathology	Infection
	Cerebrovascular accident
	Seizure and post-ictal state
	Space-occupying lesion
Toxicological including CNS depressant Illicit drugs	Opioids, GHB
	Ecstasy and related drugs, e.g. ketamine, amphetamines and cocaine
Prescription medications	BZD, antidepressants and anticonvulsants
Other alcohols	Methanol, ethylene glycol and isopropyl alcohol
Other sepsis	CNS, UTI, pneumonia and aspiration

CNS: central nervous system; GHB: γ-hydroxybutyrate; BZD: benzodiazepine; UTI: urinary tract infection.

CT brain scan, which may be challenging in a poorly compliant patient. Intravenous sedation or even endotracheal intubation may be necessary to obtain a CT scan safely.

Other intracranial pathology

Altered conscious state: differential diagnosis

A patient with any significant intracranial pathology may present with an altered conscious state mimicking alcohol intoxication. The chronic alcohol-dependent patient may present with an unusual cerebral infection, such as cryptococcal meningitis, cerebral abscess or herpes encephalitis. Also a cerebrovascular accident, either embolic or haemorrhagic, is more likely in the habitual drinker, due to co-morbid vascular disease and smoking, hypertension and coagulopathy.

An altered conscious state may be due to a seizure from alcohol excess or withdrawal, status epilepticus or a post-ictal state. Cerebral neoplasia, particularly metastases, may present late in this population. Again a CT scan is usually indicated in the alcohol-dependent patient following a seizure, particularly if there is persisting or deteriorating confusion or focal neurology. A lumbar puncture may be needed to exclude meningitis or a subarachnoid haemorrhage if there is clinical suspicion, even if the CT brain scan was normal.

Other toxicological states in the alcohol-dependent patient

Multiple drug ingestion

Multiple drug ingestion, whether prescription or illicit, is common in regular drinkers for recreational reasons, due to dependence, to 'come down' from other drug effects, in accidental overdose or in deliberate self-harm. The most common and important ingested drugs to consider include BZDs, opiates, paracetamol, often as over-the-counter analgesics, antidepressants including tricyclics and selective serotonin reuptake inhibitors, γ-hydroxybutyrate, ecstasy and other sympathomimetics, such as cocaine and ketamine.

Other alcohols

Other alcohols, such as methanol, ethylene glycol and isopropyl alcohol, although rare, should be considered in the significantly intoxicated, self-harm patient. 'Methylated spirits'

bought over the counter in Australia only contains 95% ethanol v/w with no methanol at all and, in New Zealand, the methanol content has been reduced to 2% or less, due to deaths attributed to chronic misuse and methanol poisoning there.

Serum drug levels

The only clinically useful screening serum drug levels are paracetamol and ethanol. Other drug levels take hours to days to perform (institution dependent); thus they are not of use at the time and should only be requested if there are specific indications. The only safe antidotes to consider are naloxone, thiamine and glucose. Flumazenil is not recommended due to the risk of inducing seizures and then not being able to manage them effectively.

Other sepsis

Sepsis must be considered in any person with an altered conscious state potentially masked by alcohol intoxication and a directed septic work-up carried out.

Treatment of alcohol-related illness

Alcohol intoxication

Intoxication starts with a feeling of well-being and an increasing sense of relaxation, followed by impairment of judgement and incoordination. At BAC of 0.1%, dysarthria, ataxia and disinhibition are common. At BAC of 0.2%, confusion occurs and new memories are not formed. At BAC of 0.25%, cortical depression is seen with the onset of stupor. At BAC of 0.4%, most are unconscious and at risk of respiratory depression and death. The mean BAC found in fatal alcohol intoxication is 0.45%.

'Pathological intoxication'

Some people have idiosyncratic responses to alcohol, the so-called 'pathological intoxication', which is more common among certain ethnic groups. A clear indicator of alcohol tolerance and neuroadaptation is the recording of high BAC in a person functioning at an otherwise reasonable level, for example the patient capable of normal conversation and gait with a BAC 0.3%. This may follow a continuous prolonged drinking binge.

Treatment of the acutely intoxicated person

The treatment of an acutely intoxicated person is supportive, protecting the at-risk airway and placing in the semi-prone position to reduce the risk of gastric aspiration. Gastric emptying procedures are not recommended under any circumstances. Intravenous fluids in simple alcohol intoxication do not increase the elimination or decrease the BAC. Likewise, IV 5% dextrose administration has not been shown to be useful in changing the rates of alcohol elimination or decreasing periods of intoxication.

There remains no antidote to alcohol intoxication. As alcohol affects endogenous opiate GABA receptors, both naloxone and flumazenil have been tried with no effect. Flumazenil use in the alcohol-intoxicated patient is dangerous as it renders benzodiazepines ineffective in the treatment of seizures for about 45 minutes after its use. It can also precipitate seizures if the patient is a chronic benzodiazepine user. Various substances have been tried in animals, but none so far is safe and/or effective. There has been interest in pyridoxine and, more recently, its analogue metadoxine in hastening alcohol metabolism and reversing both the biochemical and the clinical symptoms of intoxication, but studies are small [27].

'Hangover'

It was estimated in the UK in 2003 that £2 billion in lost work value was due to post-alcohol-related headache and malaise 'hangover', which may be a greater economic problem than habitual intoxication. Paradoxically, light or binge drinkers' hangovers cause the most lost work time as the hangover is more common and the sufferer is more commonly in regular employment than the heavy drinker.

Diagnosis and management

A hangover is distinguished from the alcohol withdrawal syndrome as it follows a defined single episode of intoxication. Symptoms include headache, feeling generally unwell, diarrhoea, anorexia, nausea, tremulousness and fatigue. The presence of two or more of these symptoms following alcohol intake has been used to define a hangover [27]. Acetaldehyde, the dehydrogenated metabolite of alcohol, has been implicated. Alcohol alters cytokine production and thromboxane B2 is increased, an effect blocked by prostaglandin inhibitors. This may explain why prostaglandin inhibitors, such as NSAIDs, including aspirin, may have some limited prophylactic effect on hangover development.

Hangover is not solely dose related. Hangovers are worse with dehydration, no food intake, decreased sleep, increased physical activity while intoxicated and poor general physical condition. Congener byproducts of some alcohols including aldehydes, esters, histamine, phenols, tannins, iron, lead and cobalt are found, especially in darker liquors, which are associated with an increased severity and incidence of hangover. Clear liquors, such as gin, vodka and rum, may lead to fewer hangovers. The evidence for hangover treatment and prevention is minimal [28,29].

The habitual alcohol-dependent emergency attender

Most EDs, particularly in metropolitan areas, have a group of recurrent ED attenders who keep presenting with alcohol intoxication and chronic alcohol-rela ted disease. Such people are usually male, aged 30–40 years and often have no fixed place of abode. They usually are well known to neighbouring EDs, community services and police. They tend to attend in cycles and an absence of attendance may indicate a prison term, a medical illness and/or hospital admission, an attempt at sobriety, use of an adjacent ED or sudden death. Over a year they may accumulate multiple investigations, especially CT scans of the head. This group has an increased mortality over time from assault and other trauma, as well as alcohol-related illness associated with neglect.

The ED as a temporary refuge

The ED provides a temporary refuge in an otherwise chaotic lifestyle and an opportunity for a health assessment and intervention. It is important to realize that providing care for this group of people is core business for every ED, despite any frustrations felt. Interventions to alter lifestyle and prevent recurrent attendances are successful. ED initiated case management involving community linkages and assistance with accommodation improves health outcomes but may increase ED utilization. Serial inebriate programmes may target this group, often commencing with socialization skills, such as personal hygiene and nutrition management [30]. Acceptance to such programmes is often precipitated by the threat of

imprisonment. Such programmes have been demonstrated to be cost-effective.

Assessment of alcohol misuse

Alcohol screening tools

Emergency physicians witness daily the effects of lifestyle abuse on ED presentations and thus may find many opportunities to intervene opportunistically to affect the long-term health of the patient, as well as treating the immediate presentation. This is particularly valuable for patients with irregular contact with other medical services, such as the itinerant and the homeless [31].

Screening for chronic alcohol abuse or dependence

Any screening tool to be of value must have adequate sensitivity and specificity for detecting the illness involved and there should be an effective, cost-effective intervention available. Many screening tools for chronic alcohol abuse or dependence have been developed for primary care, with the best known being the CAGE questionnaire [32]. This poses four questions on behaviour and a positive answer to two or more indicates probable chronic alcohol abuse (Table 21.4.2).

Paddington alcohol test

An effective and quick alternative in the time-pressured setting of an ED is the Paddington alcohol test (PAT), which includes 'routine' focused selective screening combined with education, audit and feedback [32]. PAT has reduced screening time to 1 minute, simply

---

Table 21.4.2 CAGE screening questionnaire for alcohol abuse

C = 'Have you ever felt you should **C**ut down on your drinking?'

A = 'Have people **A**nnoyed you by criticizing your drinking?'

G = 'Have you ever felt bad or **G**uilty about your drinking?'

E = 'Have you ever had a drink as an **E**ye-opener first thing in the morning to steady your nerves or help get rid of a hangover?'

'Yes' to two or more indicates probable chronic alcohol abuse or dependence

---

quantifying the amount of alcohol consumed, how often and whether in the opinion of the patient the reason for ED attendance is due to alcohol.

Opportunistic screening and brief intervention

Brief intervention usually consisting of counselling lasting 10–15 minutes and a pamphlet on safe levels of regular alcohol consumption reduce the frequency of dangerous drinking by 30% and recurrent ED attendances by as much as 50%, after ED-initiated PAT screening and trained alcohol health worker follow up [33].

Focused PAT screening of high-risk patients (Table 21.4.3) followed by brief advice and referral for trained alcohol health worker brief intervention appear the most time- and cost-effective methods of reducing alcohol-related harm and ED attendances [34]. Brief advice consists of informing the patient during the ED 'teachable moment' that they have a drinking problem [35]. This advice increases compliance to attend brief intervention later by 20%. Using PAT to screen all ED attendances as opposed to only those presentations considered at 'high risk' may increase the incidental pick-up of at-risk drinkers but may also decrease the enthusiasm of ED staff to provide screening because of the time required and the many negative screens [36]. Although it has been demonstrated that ED doctors and nurses with empathy and volition can be trained to provide ED-based brief intervention on the spot, the long-term benefit of this type of brief intervention is uncertain.

Table 21.4.3 The top 10 ED presenting conditions associated with alcohol use [33]

Falls	Unwell
Collapse	Non-specific gastrointestinal problems
Head injury	Psychiatric-behavioural
Assault	Cardiac
Accident	Repeat attender

To be used with the Paddington alcohol test (PAT).
Crawford MJ, Patton R, Touquet R, et al. Screening and referral for brief intervention of alcohol misusing patients in an emergency department: a pragmatic randomised controlled trial. Lancet 2004;364:1334–9 with permission.

Pharmacotherapy for alcohol use disorder

Acamprosate

Acamprosate acts on GABA receptors in the CNS to reduce the craving for alcohol after detoxification. It is safe and well tolerated, suitable for use in treatment of alcohol-use disorder aimed at maintaining abstinence. The usual dose is 666 mg (two 333 mg tablets) orally three times daily. Mild gastrointestinal side effects may occur and therapeutic levels take 5–7 days to become established.

Naltrexone

Naltrexone is a partial opioid agonist that is useful in reducing the effects of endogenous opioids. It has had success in opioid addiction treatment, as well as in alcohol-use disorder. The usual dose is 50 mg orally daily.

These agents may be used safely in combination, although this has not been shown to have superior effect. Pharmacotherapy produces better results when used in combination with cognitive behavioural therapy and motivational sessions.

Likely developments over the next 5–10 years

- ED-initiated screening and intervention for alcohol-use disorder are likely to become more widespread in EDs in coming years.
- ED-initiated case management of the chronic recurrent alcohol-affected ED attender ('inebriate programmes') is also likely to gain favour.
- Novel pharmacological agents may appear to assist treatment of alcohol intoxication, withdrawal and hangover.

Controversies

- The true prevalence and incidence of alcoholic ketoacidosis is uncertain.
- Use of high-dose parenteral thiamine to prevent Wernicke's encephalopathy is somewhat controversial.

- There is a question about who to target for brief intervention by emergency clinicians; high-risk attendances or unselected patients.

References

[1] Australia: the healthiest country by 2020. Technical Report No 3: Preventing alcohol-related harm in Australia: a window of opportunity (including addendum for October 2008 to June 2009). Australian Government Preventative Taskforce. <http://www.health.gov.au/internet/preventativehealth/publishing.nsf/Content/09C94C0F1B9799F5CA2574DD0081E770/$File/alcohol-jul09.pdf>; 2009 [Accessed Apr. 2013].

[2] National Health and Medical Research Council Australian Guidelines to Reduce Health Risks from Drinking Alcohol. Published February 2009. <http://www.nhmrc.gov.au/_files_nhmrc/publications/attachments/ds10-alcohol.pdf> [Accessed Apr. 2013].

[3] Chikritzhs T, Pascal R, Gray D, et al. Trends in alcohol-attributable deaths among indigenous Australians, 1998–2004 National Alcohol Indicators, Bulletin 11. Perth: National Drug Research Institute; 2007.

[4] Reynaud M, Schwan R, Loiseaux-Meunier MN, et al. Patients admitted to emergency services for drunkenness: moderate alcohol users or harmful drinkers? Am J Psychiatr 2001;158:96–9.

[5] Brokaw J, Olson L, Fullerton L, et al. Repeated ambulance use by patients with acute alcohol intoxication, seizure disorder, and respiratory illness. Am J Emerg Med 1998;16:141–4.

[6] Hulse GK, Robertson SI, Tait RJ. Adolescent emergency department presentations with alcohol or other drug related problems in Perth, Western Australia. Addiction 2001;96:1059–67.

[7] Thom B, Herring R, Judd A. Identifying alcohol-related harm in young drinkers: the role of accident and emergency departments. Alcohol 1999;34:910–5.

[8] Roche AM, Watt K, Mclure R. Injury and alcohol: a hospital emergency department study. Drug Alcohol Rev 2001;20:155–66.

[9] Rosenstock S, Jorgensen T, Bonnevie O. Risk factors for peptic ulcer disease: a population based prospective cohort study comprising 2416 Danish adults. Gut 2003;52:186–93.

[10] Pinto HC, Abrantes A, Esteves AV. Long-term prognosis of patients with cirrhosis of the liver and upper gastrointestinal bleeding. Am J Gastroenterol 1989;84:1239–43.

[11] Kortas DY, Haas LS, Simpson WG, et al. Mallory-Weiss tear: predisposing factors and predictors of a complicated course. Am J Gastroenterol 2001;96:2863–5.

[12] National Health and Medical Research Council/Australasian Society of Blood Transfusion Clinical Practice Guidelines for the Use of Blood Components. Module 1 – Critical Bleeding/Massive Transfusion (released 31 March 2011) <http://www.nba.gov.au/guidelines/module1/cbmt.pdf> [Accessed Apr. 2013].

[13] Lau JY, Leung WK, Wu JC, et al. Omeprazole before endoscopy in patients with gastrointestinal bleeding. New England J. Med. 2007;356:1631–40.

[14] Ioannou GN, Doust J, Rockey DC. Terlipressin for acute esophageal variceal hemorrhage. Cochrane Database of Syst. Rev. 2003, Issue 1.

[15] Roberts: Clinical procedures in emergency medicine, 5th edn. Chapter 41: Balloon tamponade of gastroesophageal varices: 754–759.

[16] Gramenzi A, Caputo F, Biselli M, et al. Review article: alcoholic liver disease – pathophysiological aspects and risk factors. Aliment Pharmacol Ther 2006;24:1151–61.

[17] Suokas J, Lonnqvist J. Suicide attempts in which alcohol is involved: a special group in general hospital emergency rooms. Acta Psychiatr Scand 1995;91:36–40.

[18] Sullivan JT, Sykora K, Schneiderman J, et al. Assessment of alcohol withdrawal: the revised clinical institute withdrawal assessment for alcohol scale (CIWA-Ar). Br J Addiction 1989;84:1353–7.

[19] Williams D, Lewis J, McBride A. A comparison of rating scales for the alcohol withdrawal syndrome. Alcohol Alcoholism 2001;36:104–8.

[20] Mayo-Smith MF. Pharmacological management of alcohol withdrawal: a meta-analysis and evidence based guidelines. J Am Med Assoc 1997;278:144–51.

[21] Palmstierna T. Model for predicting alcohol withdrawal delirium. Psychiatr Serv 2001;52:820–3.

[22] Galvin R, Brathen G, Ivashynka. EFNS guidelines for diagnosis, therapy and prevention of Wernicke encephalopathy. Eur J Neurol 2010;17:1408–18.

[23] Sechi GP, Serra A. Wernicke's encephalopathy: new clinical settings and recent advances in diagnosis and management. Lancet Neurol 2007;6:442–55.

[24] McGuire LC, Cruickshank AM, Munro PT. Alcoholic ketoacidosis. Emerg Med J 2006;23:417–20.

[25] MacDonald L, Kruse JA, Levy DB. Lactic acidosis and acute ethanol intoxication. Am J Emerg Med 1994;12:32–5.

[26] Constant J. The alcoholic cardiomyopathies – genuine and pseudo. Cardiology 1999;91:92–100.

[27] Shpilenya LS, Muzychenko AP, Gasbarrini G. Metadoxine in acute alcohol intoxication: a double-blind, randomized, placebo-controlled study. Alcohol Clin Exp Res 2002;26:340–6.

[28] Weise JG, Shiplak MG, Browner WS. The hangover. Ann Intern Med 2000;132:897–902.

[29] Pittler MH, Verster JC, Ernst E. Interventions for preventing or treating alcohol hangover: systematic review of randomised controlled trials. Br Med J 2005;331:1515–8.

[30] Phillips GA, Brophy DS, Chenhall AJ, et al. The effect of multidisciplinary case management on selected outcomes for frequent attenders at an emergency department. Med J Aust 2006;184:602–6.

[31] Greane J. Serial inebriate programmes: what to do about homeless alcoholics in the emergency department. Ann Emerg Med 2007;49:701–3.

[32] Nilssen O, Ries RK, Rivara FP. The CAGE questionnaire and the Short Michigan Alcohol Screening Test in trauma patients: comparison of their correlations with biological alcohol markers. J Trauma 1994;36:784–8.

[33] Crawford MJ, Patton R, Touquet R, et al. Screening and referral for brief intervention of alcohol misusing patients in an emergency department: a pragmatic randomised controlled trial. Lancet 2004;364:1334–9.

[34] Touquet R, Brown A. Alcohol misuse: positive response. Alcohol health work for every acute hospital saves money and reduces repeat attendances. Emerg Med Australas 2006;18:103–7.

[35] Williams S, Brown A, Patton R, et al. The half-life of the 'teachable moment' for alcohol misusing patients in the emergency department. Drug Alcohol Depend 2005;77:205–8.

[36] Weiland TJ, Dent AW, Phillips GA, et al. Emergency clinician-delivered screening and intervention for high-risk alcohol use: a qualitative analysis. Emerg Med Australas 2008;20:121–8.

21.5 The challenging patient

Sandra L Neate • Georgina A Phillips

ESSENTIALS

1 Many patients characterized as 'challenging' share common characteristics, including complex and chronic medical disease, mental illness, marginalization, poverty, high levels of drug and alcohol use and lack of social supports, safety and security.

2 An understanding of the issues that contribute to the challenging nature of some patients may assist the practitioner in developing a management approach characterized by sound knowledge, clear and achievable goals and compassion.

3 Management strategies may help to alleviate the dissatisfaction and frustration frequently experienced by the clinician.

4 Allied health and psychiatric services in the emergency department facilitate multidisciplinary and holistic care for the patient with complex needs.

5 Safety and security for all patients and staff must be assured.

Introduction

The emergency department (ED) may be the only easily accessible healthcare for patients with multiple and challenging needs. For those impaired due to chronic illness, drugs and alcohol, mental illness or social circumstances, the ED is an environment where services are available 24 hours a day or during crisis. The challenges posed by complex patients are compounded by system factors, such as decreased after hours' services, ED overcrowding and access block. Some patients require urgent management for reasons other than medical issues, for example, a behaviourally disturbed patient who causes disruption and threatens violence within the ED, a VIP who may distract the attention of staff or someone who poses a security risk. The management of a complex patient in a difficult environment represents a common challenge for emergency physicians. All emergency staff may find dealing with challenging patients tiring and frustrating and experience feelings of dissatisfaction. Several types of patients are described and discussed, with the aim of understanding the circumstances that contribute to these presentations and assisting the practitioner to develop an approach to management.

THE HOMELESS PATIENT

ESSENTIALS

1 Multidisciplinary management of the homeless person is required.

2 Discharge planning is difficult and short-stay admission is frequently required.

Definition and epidemiology

Definitions of homelessness vary. A homeless person is often considered to be someone living on the streets without shelter. A broader definition includes any person without a conventional home who lacks most of the economic and social supports that a home normally affords. These persons are often cut off from the support of relatives and friends, have few independent resources and often no immediate means and, in some cases, little prospect of self-support.

The most widely accepted definition in Australia, and the one used by government and other specialist agencies to gather data, describes three kinds of homelessness:

- Primary homelessness, such as sleeping rough or living in an improvised dwelling.
- Secondary homelessness including staying with friends or relatives and with no other usual address, people in specialist homelessness services.
- Tertiary homelessness including people living in boarding houses or caravan parks with no secure lease and no private facilities, both short and long term [1].

Concepts of homelessness vary with culture. People from Aboriginal and Torres Straight Islander cultures may experience homelessness when separated from their spiritual home despite adequate shelter and, conversely, may feel a spiritual connection to the land on which they live independent of the presence of shelter. Three broad categories of indigenous homelessness are identified in Australia: those living in public places, those at risk of losing their house and those who are spiritually homeless [2].

Estimates of prevalence of homelessness are difficult due to variations in definition and methodologies of identification. Every night in Australia, around 105 000 people are homeless [3]. More than 160 000 Australians experience homelessness each year, one-third of them children, while resources allocated in response to homelessness are grossly inadequate. Homelessness is more prevalent in women and is closely related to the experience of domestic violence and inequity in general. Homelessness among children, families and older people is increasing. The Australian indigenous population comprises 2–3% of the Australian population but accounts for 18% of those accessing homeless services primarily as a result of domestic and family violence, overcrowded dwellings and evictions [4]. Ex-prisoners, war veterans, the mentally and physically ill, people leaving healthcare facilities and protective services, youths and people in rural communities experience increased incidence of homelessness.

Clinical features

Homeless patients presenting to the ED exhibit high rates of complex physical and mental illness and substance dependence. Due to poverty and social isolation, access to healthcare is impeded with a subsequent cycle of deterioration in health. Lack of housing stability, social supports and points of reference within the local community lead to a high rate of utilization and re-presentation to the ED despite the development of outreach programmes or case management strategies [5]. Homeless patients may present to the ED up to 10 times more frequently than the rest of the population [6].

Re-presentation rates within 28 days of discharge are high and may account for up to 48% of all re-presentation episodes and 23% of all patients who re-present to the ED [6]. Certain features, such as sociodemographics (age <65 years, receiving government pension), service utilization history (case management and discharge at own risk) and clinical features (primary psychiatric presentation, complex medical history and high numbers of prescribed medications), are highly predictive of re-presentation [6,7]. Presentations by homeless people are often of low acuity. Triage categories are non-urgent in up to 91% of attendances [6].

Presentations with infectious diseases (e.g. TB and HIV), penetrating trauma, depression, schizophrenia and ethanol and drug abuse are common. Deliberate self-harm presentations are more frequent and are followed by a higher rate of re-presentation with recurrent self-harm and approximately double the rate of death from successful completion of suicide than in the domiciled population [8]. Homeless patients presenting with deliberate self-harm are more likely to be a recent victim or perpetrator of violence or have a criminal record or a personality disorder, thus highlighting the complex links between these variables.

Management

The management of the homeless patient requires a multidisciplinary approach and an understanding of the social and financial constraints the patient faces. Allied health services may be able to provide background information or links to established community services, assist with discharge planning or assist with emergency accommodation or other social services. Discharge planning may be especially difficult and short-stay admission for management of simple conditions normally treatable at home or admission to low acuity facilities may

assist with improvements in health and other social parameters. A compassionate approach to the homeless patient, where patients were assigned a volunteer who offered food and conversation, was found to decrease significantly rates of re-presentation, dispelling the myth that increasing patient satisfaction encourages homeless patients to re-attend [9].

THE PRISONER

ESSENTIALS

1 The prison population is disadvantaged and vulnerable.

2 Prisoners' health needs differ from the general public.

3 Presentations are often injury related and are generally of high acuity.

4 Security events are uncommon.

Definition and epidemiology

In all states and territories except Queensland, prisoners are defined as persons greater than 18 years remanded or sentenced to adult custody (age 17 in Queensland) [10]. The patient brought to the ED by police from the community under arrest differs from the patient who is residing in prison. Both types of patients may pose security issues, but their health needs and demographics differ.

The prisoner poses several challenges when seen in the ED (Table 21.5.1).

Table 21.5.1 Challenges involving the prisoner in the ED

Security issues	Patient care issues
Perceived threat to safety of staff and other patients	Clinical management of complex illness
Potential for violent incidents	Medical, psychiatric and addiction co-morbidities
Presence of non-hospital security staff	Maintenance of confidentiality
Weapons in the ED	Discharge planning

The prison population in general, has low educational achievements, poor records of employment, high reliance on social welfare, poor nutrition and more complex physical and mental health needs when compared with the general population and, from a health perspective, represents a cohort of patients distinct from the wider community [11].

Prisoners have a high rate of pre-existing mental and physical illness, substance use and dependence and high rates of hospitalization. Twenty-five per cent of prisoners report having been hospitalized in the preceding year [11]. Prisoners have a high rate of risk-taking behaviours that increase the risk of poor health, such as tattooing and heavy alcohol and substance use, and display behaviours with addictive or compulsive orientations and low impulse control. These factors contribute to the illnesses experienced, modes of presentation and the responses to health staff and treatments offered.

Clinical features

The mean age of prisoners presenting to the ED is approximately 30 years, however, as with the general community, the prison population is ageing rapidly [12]. Presentations are most commonly injury related, with approximately one-third self-inflicted injury, one-third accidental and one-third as a result of assault or unclear mechanisms. Prisoner injuries seen in the ED are overall more severe when compared with those in the general male population, with a higher frequency of fractures, blunt head injuries, greater rates of hospital admission and death [13].

Mental health issues are common among prisoners and incarceration is more common in those with mental illness. Risk factors for incarceration for those with mental illness include prior incarcerations, substance-related diagnoses, homelessness, schizophrenia, bipolar or other psychotic disorder diagnoses and male gender [14]. Risk of suicide is high among prisoners with factors specifically related to incarceration, such as isolation, punitive sanctions, severely restricted living conditions and acquisition of new charges or imposition of an unexpected sentence, elevating risks substantially [15].

Substance withdrawal is implicated in approximately 9% of presentations and 6% of admissions [16]. Due to the increased risk of overdose following periods of abstinence, recently released inmates who use opiates are at particularly high risk of overdose and overdose deaths are eight times more likely in the 2 weeks following release than in a comparable non-incarcerated group of men [17].

Prisoners have a high rate of admission to hospital (range 36–49%), which may be due to higher acuity of illness, with approximately 80% of prisoners triaged as category 3 or above, and the practical and logistical difficulties in managing unwell people in custody. Prisoners have a decreased length of stay in the ED compared with the non-prisoner population [16].

Violence and security issues

Episodes of violence are uncommon. The rate of security incidents may be lower than for the non-prisoner population [16]. Perceived threat and the accompanying stress caused to staff are yet to be quantified.

The presence of weapons provides the potential for serious injury to the patient if escape is attempted or to staff if the patient removes a weapon from security staff. Fatalities have been documented [16].

Management

The urgency with which a prisoner is assessed depends on a combination of medical issues and security considerations; prioritization, in order to expedite managment and decrease length of stay in the ED, is reasonable.

Prisoners may perceive the ED as a threatening, embarrassing environment that lacks privacy, where they can be seen by members of the public to be under guard and restrained. Most express feelings of distress when removed from their familiar environment. Prisoners are unable to have the normal reassurance and support of family while in hospital. The presence of guards during medical assessment raises confidentiality concerns for the patient. These concerns need to be weighed against security issues. Guidance from custodial staff as to whether it is safe for them leave the cubicle or remove restraints may be helpful. If the clinician feels insecure, custodial staff should remain within the room. The history obtained in the presence of guards may be inaccurate. Patients may be fearful of disclosing the mechanism of injuries due to fears of reprisal or prison guards in attendance overhearing the circumstances of injury.

In many Australian states, psychiatric services are not resourced or mandated to care for prisoners and mental health acts do not cover those incarcerated under separate forensic laws. This may render the ED care of the mentally unwell prisoner even more difficult, as psychiatric illness may be undiagnosed or undertreated and access to normal mental health clinicians to aid in assessment and treatment may not be available.

Opportunities for follow up of medical conditions are limited. There may be little possibility for observation of the person's condition upon return to detention. Outpatient follow up is time and resource intensive and logistically difficult for the prison staff. There is therefore often a need for more extensive investigation while in the ED. A low threshold for ruling out potential illnesses and for admission to hospital is generally required.

If the patient is returning to prison, clear written discharge instructions should be formally communicated and discharge medication with dispensing instructions provided. Liaison with the prison nurse or forensic medical officer should establish whether their facilities and staffing can provide the expected management.

THE BEHAVIOURALLY DISTURBED AND VIOLENT PATIENT

ESSENTIALS

1 Complex co-morbidities of organic illness, psychosocial issues and substance misuse can manifest as acute behavioural disturbance.

2 Understanding legal and ethical considerations can inform rapid decisions and humane treatment in behavioural emergencies.

3 A safe environment and team approach can maximize containment of disturbed and violent behaviour, while respecting the privacy and dignity of patients.

4 A strategic approach to understanding and managing violence in the ED may minimize the harmful effects of violence to staff, patients and carers.

Aetiology and epidemiology

A behavioural emergency can be defined as an unarmed threat by a patient or others characterized by agitation, aggression, violence and irrational or altered behaviour. Violent and unarmed threats involving patients in the ED have been described with an incidence of between 0.3% [18] and 2% [19]. Accurate information on the incidence and subsequent management of acute behavioural disturbance is limited by the lack of clarity around what constitutes a behavioural emergency and significant differences in treatment response both within and between EDs. Heavy recreational drug use and alcohol binge drinking in the community have contributed to the public perception that behavioural disturbance requiring urgent medical care has increased. It has also been argued that psychiatric deinstitutionalization and limited community supports have led to an influx of unstable, mentally ill patients to the ED.

Approximately half of the patients presenting with acute behavioural disturbance have an acute flare of a primary mental illness, while 40–50% are intoxicated with drugs or alcohol [18]. A smaller number have an organic illness, including dementia, manifesting as a behavioural emergency [20]. A combination of psychiatric illness and substance intoxication commonly occurs. Most patients are male (approximately 65%) and under the age of 40 [18,21], and around 20% are brought to the ED in police custody [18,22]. The majority of unarmed threats occur in the late afternoon, evening and overnight, with a weekly peak on a Saturday [18]. Between 58 and 80% of these require some form of chemical or physical restraint as part of management [18,19,21].

Prevention

There are no validated tools or clinically useful predictive factors for violence and acute behavioural disturbance in the ED; however, experienced clinicians are able to recognize environmental and individual factors that can lead to unstable and dangerous behaviour. Crowded, noisy and brightly lit departments are the antithesis of the calm and stable surrounds that promote controlled behaviour and de-escalate aggression. Fear, confusion and inadequate communication can trigger anger and aggressive behaviour in both patients and carers, while long waiting times and negative waiting room environmental factors have been suggested as contributors to violence in the ED.

In order to prevent anger or illness from escalating to a behavioural emergency, recognition of verbal and non-verbal cues is required, as well as an ability to utilize environmental and clinical resources to ensure a calm, controlled situation. EDs are now incorporating separate rooms or areas that are quiet, private and secure, as sites for the assessment and containment of behavioural disturbance. This model has become the recommended standard in Australia for assessing and containing aggressive and agitated patients both at a national [23] and state level [24]. Physical separation from the main ED and removal of stimulation may be enough to reverse the trend to increased aggression. Respectful and clear communication with lowered voice level, eye contact and non-threatening body language may establish a rapport that enhances a therapeutic bond between clinician and patient. Explanation of treatment decisions and the reasons for them may alleviate confusion, while bargaining and rewarding compliance can diffuse tension. Allowing a semblance of autonomy and control to the patient, while setting clear behavioural limits, is recommended.

A 'security response' is utilized in the ED to contain behaviour when disturbance and aggression can be anticipated [25]. This is aided by prior police and ambulance notification of the imminent arrival of a patient with a behavioural emergency. A team comprising hospital security service, nursing and medical staff can in itself be a disincentive for increased aggression, when confronting an aroused patient. In the event of violence, the team response carried out in a separate area of the ED can quickly control behaviour safely and thus prevent further episodes or prolongation of aggression.

Clinical features

Clinical assessment comprises three components: diagnostic, evaluation of risk and assessment of arousal (Table 21.5.2).

Signs of acute intoxication or withdrawal may follow recognized patterns or drug toxidromes, while psychiatric instability may manifest with features of psychosis. Differentiating between organic illness, delirium and substance intoxication or psychosis can

Table 21.5.2 Aims of clinical assessment in acute behavioural assessment	
Diagnosis	What is the aetiology of the behaviour: psychiatric, substance related, organic, personality?
Risk assessment	Can the patient's autonomy be over-ridden? Can I keep them in the ED against their will?
Arousal assessment	Does the patient require containment or sedation and how rapidly?

be extremely difficult in the initial assessment and may only be clarified after immediate management and behaviour containment. A breath alcohol determination is useful and intravenous puncture sites may suggest substance misuse. In an agitated and aroused patient, the act of taking a blood pressure or putting a stethoscope on the chest may be recognized as a familiar and non-threatening action and thus be better tolerated than attempting to get a detailed history or expecting a rational response to verbal requests.

The role of investigations in the behaviourally disturbed patient is controversial. Routine laboratory blood testing is of low yield and diagnostic evaluation should be directed by history and examination. Urine drug screens have no role in the acute assessment or management. Cognitive abilities should guide the readiness for psychiatric assessment, rather than the suspected presence of drugs or alcohol. A positive breath alcohol should not preclude mental health assessment in the patient who is alert and orientated [26].

Risk assessments are often made rapidly and intuitively in the highly agitated and aggressive patient. The decision to contain and restrain an aroused patient with extreme behaviour is primarily based around the perceived threat of harm to self or others. If patient competence cannot be assessed, then the assumption of risk of harm and the doctor's duty of care override patient autonomy. Clinical features that are suggestive of high risk include threats or actual self-harm, suicidal behaviour or ideation, threats or actual violence to others, altered conscious state due to illness, injury or substance intoxication and incompetence. Risk assessments and restraint can only be made within an acute framework (i.e. pertaining to hours rather than weeks or months), as this is the length of time a person can humanely be contained within an

ED setting. Patients with longer-term high-risk behaviours are not suitable for physical or chemical restraint in the ED and may be managed more appropriately in a mental health or forensic setting.

Assessment of arousal requires utilization of collaborative and clinical tools and informs decisions about urgency and methods of restraint. Information about behaviour immediately prior to ED presentation can be gathered from police and ambulance officers. Physical struggle and violence requiring restraint during transport to the ED is an indication of the need for ongoing restraint. Physical intimidation, threats or acts of violence to self, people or property, attempts to escape, uncontrollable verbal abuse and aggressive acts, such as spitting, all indicate extreme arousal and the need for immediate containment and restraint. Signs that a patient is increasingly aroused and that violence may be imminent, include physical agitation and restlessness, pacing, sweating, loss of rational thinking, increased voice tone, swearing or foul language, eye widening and pupil dilation. Early recognition of these prodromal features may prevent the escalation of aggression and ensure the safety of both staff and patient.

Legal and ethical considerations

Sedation and restraint for behaviour containment represent significant deprivations of personal liberty. Australasian law strongly upholds the fundamental principle of individual autonomy and mental health legislation mandates a 'least restrictive' approach to involuntary care. Emergency physicians must also respect patient autonomy and be mindful of employing the least restrictive practices when making decisions to restrain aroused and aggressive patients (see Chapter 25.1).

The ability to detain and treat people without their consent is lawfully recognized in emergency situations, committal under legislation (e.g. mental health acts), suicide prevention, to protect others from harm, self-defence, 'necessity' or 'in best interests' and for incompetent patients [27]. Thus, ED staff are comprehensively protected under the law if they act in good faith and with integrity when managing acute behavioural disturbance. Doctors are also legally required to maintain confidentiality, to take reasonable care, not to take advantage of a patient and to meet professional standards. Containment and restraint often take place in highly visible sites within the ED, where the patient is exposed to the scrutiny of other staff, patients and visitors, which can undermine personal privacy and confidentiality. Similarly, abusive and aggressive patients may provoke anger and frustration in ED staff. Competent patients are responsible for their actions and are expected to behave within a reasonable and legal framework. Damage to property and assault to person are crimes which are subject to prosecution if they occur in an ED and towards ED staff. There are occupational health and safety requirements that mandate a safe working environment and can inform structural changes and clinical practices in the management of violence in the ED.

Medical ethics and the law complement each other when recognizing personal autonomy and human rights. A compassionate approach that respects the human dignity of all patients and recognizes the medical duty to provide care is likely to result in both a lawful and an ethical framework for managing patients with behavioural emergencies.

Management

Once the decision to contain and restrain a patient with behavioural disturbance has been made and preventative, de-escalation measures have been unsuccessful, it is worth determining the desired endpoint of management. Containment methods differ significantly according to the desired outcome, which may range from a calmed, awake patient through to one who is fully tranquillized and physically restrained. In an ED setting, containing and restraining a patient is not therapeutic and should be viewed as a transient departure from the normal physician–patient collaboration.

Containing a highly aroused and aggressive patient requires a team of trained staff: a minimum of six people comprising hospital security staff and orderlies, with medical and nursing staff to assist with team leadership, documentation, drug administration and subsequent monitoring [28]. Smaller hospitals may need to utilize police in their initial team response, but this is not recommended, given the differing training and aims of hospital- and police-based restraint practices. Police should be involved when a weapon is present or the violent person is not a patient receiving treatment. The importance of prior planning, regular aggression management training and good communication cannot be overemphasized.

Chemical restraint

The pharmacological management of the acutely aroused patient is discussed in detail elsewhere (see Chapter 20.6), but the principles should be emphasized. The least traumatic measures are advocated, depending on the desired endpoint of chemical restraint and the risks to staff and patient in administration.

Oral benzodiazepines are preferred where possible and may allow patients a small sense of control if they are able to choose this option ahead of parenteral sedation. Choice between intramuscular or intravenous administration of sedation depends on perceived risks to staff, ease of obtaining intravenous access, need for blood tests or other intravenous therapy and desired rapidity of sedative effect. Where rapid tranquillization is desired, the intravenous route of administration is required, as the onset of action is within the first 5 minutes rather than the approximate 15–20 minutes of intramuscular drugs [29,30]. Commonly used drugs for rapid tranquillization include benzodiazepines (diazepam and midazolam), neuroleptics (droperidol and haloperidol) and newer antipsychotics (olanzapine). A combination of intravenous midazolam with droperidol or olanzapine has been shown to be more effective than midazolam alone with respect to time to adequate sedation and need for re-sedation [31]. Intravenous midazolam alone may cause more adverse events relating to airway obstruction and oversedation and is more likely to require re-sedation within an hour. High dose parenteral midazolam is not supported due to concerns about effect and safety [32].

Other drugs used for less urgent or longer-term sedation include benzodiazepines administered intramuscularly or orally, intramuscular neuroleptics and other antipsychotics, including olanzapine. Combinations of these drugs are often used, although unpredictable intramuscular absorption and an additive sedative effect can result in oversedation. Careful monitoring in a high acuity area of the ED is required when parenteral chemical restraint is used.

Physical restraint

Physical restraint can initially proceed on the floor and move to a trolley as soon as practical. A five-point hold is recommended, involving securing the head, upper and lower limbs in firm grasps. Personal protective gear of gown, safety goggles and gloves should be worn by all involved and an oxygen mask or loosely applied towel over the face can be used if the patient is spitting. While it is paramount not to inflict harm on the patient, the safety of staff is also a priority and may justify the use of moderate physical force. Using staff physically to restrain a patient is a temporary measure only and should be followed by more definitive restraint in the form of sedating drugs, physical shackles or both.

Physical restraint with shackles provokes emotional distaste in many clinicians, but it can be used safely and humanely in an ED setting. There have been reported deaths in restrained, agitated patients, described largely in the USA where 'hobble' restraints including prone positioning with hands and feet secured together behind the back are used [33]. Where supine positioning is used, physical shackles have been shown to be safe [34], although caution should be employed with restraints around the upper chest and neck area. Soft-edged, strong, fabric shackles securing the wrists and ankles of a supine patient to the trolley are recommended. Concomitant chemical sedation is advised with appropriate monitoring. Prolonged shackling is inhumane and carries risks of musculoskeletal injury, respiratory compromise and psychological trauma. All Australian states have laws that mandate careful and close observation of physically restrained patients, as well as regular review of the need for such ongoing, extreme restraint.

While few EDs have appropriate resources, it may be possible to contain patients with behavioural disturbance in a less restrictive manner by using seclusion rooms. Such areas must be visible to ED staff, be easily accessible to a security response team and have no dangerous furniture or fittings with which patients could potentially harm themselves or others.

Patient perspective

Emergency clinicians rarely consider patient preferences when faced with the need urgently to control aggressive or threatening behaviour and there is limited evidence to inform this issue. The majority of patients prefer chemical restraint rather than physical for interventions and seclusion is preferred over physical shackles. Benzodiazepines are the preferred drug for chemical sedation rather than neuroleptics [35].

Disposition

Behaviourally disturbed patients commonly spend many hours in the ED, both for accurate assessment and for diagnostic purposes. Increasingly, the lack of access to general medical, psychiatric and detoxification inpatient beds means that timely transfer for definitive care is delayed. The result is prolonged, inhumane containment of behaviourally disturbed patients, which is likely to lead to worse therapeutic outcomes. For this reason, ED doctors must be strong advocates on behalf of their patients, as well as maintaining vigilant clinical review of physical and mental state and the need for ongoing restraint. Patients who are transferred to inpatient wards for ongoing care must be alert, have stable vital signs, not require further monitoring and be declared safe for transfer by the most senior available ED clinician. Respiratory depression and death have occurred in patients transferred to psychiatric wards after receiving chemical sedation from the ED; therefore, the time, nature and route of drug administration must be taken into account when considering safety for transfer.

The decision to admit a patient depends on the result of clinical and investigative findings, ongoing mental health and risk assessment and the progress of the patient over time. It is appropriate to keep behaviourally disturbed patients under ED observation for up to 24 hours in order to clarify the aetiology of the altered behaviour and determine a safe disposition. Patients with aggression and arousal due to substance intoxication often wake up several hours later with normal behaviour and no recollection of their earlier violent behaviour. This presents a preventative health opportunity to counsel, educate and refer the patient for ongoing drug and alcohol review. Patients should be informed that their substance misuse resulted in dangerous behaviour both for themselves and others, but many will already be socially marginalized and vulnerable as a result of homelessness, substance addiction and psychosocial stressors. A multidisciplinary care-coordination approach optimizes a safe discharge for these patients.

Normal clinical and investigative findings, the absence of substance intoxication and exclusion of acute mental illness mean that the patients do not require further ED care. Such patients may still present a behavioural challenge and, if ongoing risk to self or others exists, then they should be discharged to the care of the police. Collaborative decision making with mental health clinicians is often required in such situations, as these patients often suffer antisocial or other personality disorders that are difficult to manage in both forensic and health settings. For those discharged to the community, mental health and social work follow up is recommended.

At all stages in the assessment, containment, restraint and disposition of patients with acute behavioural disturbance, clear documentation is mandatory. The importance of recording management events and the reasons behind containment or discharge decisions protects staff from clinical and legal criticism, as well as aiding care in potential future ED presentations.

Violence

The impact of violence is under-recognized in Australasian EDs, although it has been increasingly documented [36]. Aggression and violence most often stem from acutely disturbed patients, although violence in the ED can also come from visitors and carers, as well as hospital staff. Internationally recognized as a growing problem, ED violence is also generally poorly documented and under-reported, with limited formal hospital support for those exposed and rare conviction for the perpetrators [37,38]. While conventional definitions of violence centre around the act of intent to cause physical or psychological harm, in an ED setting, aggression and violence are commonly a manifestation of underlying illness or substance intoxication. The absence of a malicious intent to cause harm may be a reason why violence has been under-recognized in the hospital environment and has led to an alternative workplace definition: any episode in which staff experience either implicit or explicit challenges to their personal safety, health or sense of well-being [39].

Other reasons for under-reporting of ED violence stem from hospital systems which act as barriers by burdening staff with excessive and time-consuming paperwork, confusing policies, inadequate confidentiality and lack of peer support. While most episodes of violence in the ED do not result in serious physical injury, staff who experience violence may be traumatized, which can lead to feelings of stress and anger.

The cumulative effect of violence may result in clinician 'burnout' and staff attrition.

Three core components comprise a strategic approach to managing violence in the ED: environment (appropriateness, safety); staff (education, training, teamwork); and systems (reporting, follow up, peer support). Prevention and early intervention within a safety and patient-care framework is emphasized.

Generally, a comfortable environment with clear visibility that facilitates good communication will have a greater effect on behaviour modification than increasing fortification of waiting rooms, triage and clinical areas in the ED. Violence minimization is assisted by security cameras and televisions at triage so potential aggressors can see that they are being monitored, the visible proximity of security staff, high visibility within the clinical workspace, restricted access areas, minimizing access to potential weapons, widely dispersed and simple-to-use duress alarm devices. Weapon searches and metal detectors are rarely used in Australasian EDs and the introduction of such measures may compromise the welcoming and therapeutic atmosphere that should characterize an ED. Introducing armed security personnel into EDs increases risk to staff and patients and is not recommended [24]. Staff training and support is paramount in managing ED violence. Interdisciplinary programmes that involve role-play and real scenario discussions can enhance cooperation between all ED staff, while clarifying roles and responsibilities during actual security responses. Peer education sessions can serve to change culture towards a preventative and proactive approach, based on good communication skills and sound knowledge about behavioural emergencies. Hospital security staff are experts in the containment of aggressive and violent patients within a healthcare framework and can lead team-based prevention and safety training for ED staff.

In general, ED doctors are required to take a leadership role when managing a violent episode, although collaboration with experienced nursing colleagues improves care. Awareness of personal factors that may affect the escalation of violence and the subsequent outcomes is therefore essential. Anger, fear and personal insult can lead to interactions with aroused patients that may escalate aggression rather than diffuse tension. The role of peer support and follow up in such situations is vital.

Similarly, issues of gender, language and culture are often under-recognized as factors influencing the escalation and management of a behavioural emergency. Male staff may experience higher levels of physical violence than women. Self-awareness and consideration of these issues can optimize management of the violent episode, as well as minimize the potential negative outcomes for staff and others.

The final component of the structured approach to ED violence management is ensuring adequate documentation and follow-up systems, which include debriefing and support. Reporting should be incorporated into the standard documentation of any security incident within the ED, rather than the onus of staff who have been victims of violence. As the issue of workplace violence is one of occupational health and safety, follow up of violent incidents should fall within this framework, thus depersonalizing the impact of aggression and owning violence as an organizational responsibility rather than one belonging to the individual.

THE FREQUENT ATTENDER

ESSENTIALS

1 Frequent attenders to the ED have increased morbidity and mortality.

2 Assumptions about inappropriate use of the ED have been shown to be false.

3 ED-based multidisciplinary care coordination can lead to improved psychosocial status for frequent attenders.

Definition and epidemiology

Patients who present to hospital EDs more than three times a year can be defined as 'frequent attenders' [40] and represent a particularly vulnerable population [41]. Both internationally and within Australasia, the frequent attender population has consistent characteristics that include poverty, homelessness, chronic and complex medical illness, psychiatric illness and drug and alcohol abuse [42–44]. Frequent

attenders also suffer a high mortality, with an increased risk of death from violent causes, such as suicide and substance misuse [45]. They are known to use health services in a frequent, chaotic and episodic way, often attend multiple EDs and are difficult to engage in any long-term care. Importantly, availability and engagement with primary healthcare providers does not alter ED use by frequent attenders [46].

While representing a small number of people, frequent attenders can be responsible for up to 8% or more of annual ED attendances [47]. Demographic details vary according to how the frequent attender population is defined and analysed in the literature, although they are consistently more likely to be male, older and socially isolated [5,41]. A range of 27–55% have chronic and complex medical illness as the key reason underlying their frequent ED use, while the remainder suffer primarily psychiatric, social or drug- and alcohol-related illness [5,48]. Commonly, heavy ED users display a combination of all of these co-morbidities. Patterns of attendance generally fall into two categories, with those suffering primarily psychosocial illness or substance abuse sustaining consistently frequent ED use over many years, while those with primarily chronic medical illness showing peak ED attendance over 1–2 years [48]. Recent research from New Zealand demonstrates the natural attrition of frequent ED attenders over time [49]; however, the principal finding in studies around the world is the high mortality of this population.

Clinical features

There is great variability in the clinical presentation of frequent attenders. Acute exacerbations of underlying chronic medical illness are common as are traumatic injuries or injuries and illness sustained through violence or substance misuse, including acute substance intoxication. Infections in the respiratory, gastrointestinal and dermatological systems are frequent. Deterioration in mental state or self-harm and suicide attempts are also common reasons for ED attendance [47]. Compared with the whole population, frequent attenders are more likely to present out of hours [50], have more serious and urgent illness and more often require inpatient services [41]. Frequent attenders are more likely to discharge themselves from the ED prior to completing their ED

care or self-discharge before assessment after the initial triage process [47].

There is a pervasive assumption that frequent attenders present to the ED excessively and unnecessarily and are therefore suitable for diversion to general practitioners. Evidence suggests that this belief is false and that the majority of patients presenting frequently for ED care do so appropriately and are unsuitable for diversion to primary-care providers [47]. Patients may be adversely affected if their symptoms are belittled and attendance classified as 'inappropriate' [51].

Management

Understanding the vulnerability of frequent attenders and their complex co-morbidities while adopting a humane approach is fundamental. Medical care follows standard procedures. Access to past history and information from all healthcare and community services involved in the care of the frequent attender provides an essential context enabling timely, focused and relevant care, without unnecessary duplication of services and investigations. The development and wide dissemination of individualized acute care plans can assist in streamlining assessment and management when frequent attenders re-present to the ED after hours. Utilization of ED-based multidisciplinary services for care coordination has been shown to be of benefit when caring for the frequent attender [5].

Attempts to reduce perceived unnecessary ED attendance have met with varying results. Neither education of patients nor management care plans has reduced the frequency of ED attendance. The most successful international diversion strategies have adopted multidisciplinary approaches, including social worker support [52,53]. ED-based multidisciplinary case management has been shown to increase ED utilization but also to lead to improvement in psychosocial factors, such as housing status and engagement with primary- and community-care providers [5]. ED use may need to increase for frequent attenders if psychosocial improvements are desired.

Frequent attenders are a complex, unwell and chaotic population. Diversion away from the ED has no proven patient benefit, therefore, it may be that the ED is the best site of care for such vulnerable patients and can have a role in improving overall well-being.

THE PATIENT WITH DRUG-SEEKING BEHAVIOUR

ESSENTIALS

1 Drug addiction can be viewed as a chronic, organic disease.

2 Drug-seeking behaviour is problematic for the patient and the clinician.

3 Physicians managing these patients may experience dissatisfaction, frustration and feelings of manipulation.

Definition and aetiology

Drug abuse is defined as a maladaptive pattern of drug use indicated by continued use despite knowledge of having a social, occupational, psychological or physical problem that is caused or exacerbated by the use [54]. Addiction is defined as a primary, chronic neurobiological disease that develops as a result of genetic, psychosocial and environmental factors and manifests as use of a substance to the extent that the user is periodically or chronically intoxicated, exhibits compulsive use, has great difficulty in voluntarily ceasing or modifying substance use and exhibits determination to obtain psychoactive substances by almost any means. Typically, tolerance is prominent and a withdrawal syndrome frequently occurs when substance use is interrupted [54]. Drug-seeking behaviour can be defined as behaviour aimed at obtaining controlled substance prescriptions for reasons of dependence, abuse or illicit use in a manner that is problematic to the prescriber [55]. Patients may have a range of underlying disorders, such as psychiatric illness, substance misuse, chronic pain and complex medical conditions, which have resulted in drug dependence and institutionalized behaviour on many levels.

The concept of addiction as a disease is useful in modifying the clinician's approach to patients with addiction issues. The illness model has countered the widely held view of addiction as a wilful behaviour with moral implications. Likening addiction to other chronic illnesses, such as hypertension and diabetes, helps to understand the chronicity of the problem and the vulnerability to relapse. The rehabilitation of patients with substance-abuse problems has, however, been handled largely by non-physicians who work closely with their patients. The ongoing nature of the treatment and the relationship required to effect treatment makes intervention in the ED challenging.

Clinical features

Identification of the patient seeking drugs may be difficult. Features raising suspicion of drug seeking include previous suspicions of drug seeking documented in the medical record, inconsistent history or examination findings, requests for specific narcotic or other drugs of dependence, unwillingness to try simple analgesia, higher than expected analgesia requirements and demanding or aggressive behaviour. Other features that may raise suspicion include complaints of lost or stolen prescriptions or medications, letters from remote medical practices supporting the provision of medications and presentations that are possible to feign, such as migraine or ureteric calculus.

Presenting problems of those diagnosed as drug seeking include acute and chronic pain, primary psychiatric disorder or drug and alcohol dependence or specific request for medication. Patients exhibit a high rate of previous attendances with drug-seeking behaviour and, commonly, have a past history of mental illness, drug dependence and self-harm [56].

The possibility of missing organic illness is considerable in patients suspected of drug seeking, as nearly 20% require hospital admission and 17% self-discharge against medical advice. Missed, too, is the opportunity to acknowledge drug dependence and refer appropriately. Of drug-seeking patients seen in the ED, only 11% have a documented discussion around this issue in the medical record and only 23% are referred to addiction, psychiatric or chronic pain services [56].

Management

There is considerable individual variation in the management of patients who are drug seeking. Clinicians often find these interactions frustrating and unsatisfying and may feel abused or manipulated. The development of a general approach may assist (Table 21.5.3).

Limit setting requires confidence, experience and familiarity with local laws that limit the

Table 21.5.3 General approach to the drug-seeking patient

Attempt to develop rapport with the patient
Ensure that new organic pathology does not exist
Determine that genuine pain has been adequately treated
Once the physician has some degree of certainty that problematic drug-seeking behaviour exists, set clear limits regarding medications requested
Consider the possibility of open discussion with the patient regarding the behaviour
Consider referral to appropriate services for ongoing care
Develop management protocols for particular patients if frequent attendance or threatening behaviours develop

prescribing of controlled drugs. A departmental policy regarding the drugs available within the ED available for dispensing after hours and which may be prescribed on an outpatient basis can give guidance. Approaches vary, but a factual and dispassionate explanation about the inability to prescribe controlled substances due to departmental policy or legal requirements may be of assistance.

The physician needs to determine the appropriateness and utility of an open discussion surrounding the perceived problem behaviour. If open discussion is possible, referral for assistance may be more successful. Opportunities for interdisciplinary discussion of particular patients and an approach to their management with the development of an easily accessible electronically available protocol may assist those in front-line management.

THE VERY IMPORTANT PERSON (VIP)

ESSENTIALS

1 Management of the VIP should be based on the maintenance of standard clinical procedures.

2 Management may be aided by the establishment of a plan resembling a disaster plan aimed at coordination of clinical and administrative issues.

3 Specific issues include security, confidentiality and management of the media.

Definition

A VIP in the ED can be defined as anyone whose presence in the ED may, by virtue of the fame or public position, disrupt normal ED functioning [57]. The VIP may be a person of worldwide repute or may also be someone of local fame or importance, such as a prominent staff member. A 'VIP syndrome' can occur where the treating staff become so overwhelmed by the person's presence that they cease to operate in their normal way and the patient's care is compromised. Disaster plans are formulated in hospitals to deal with situations that overwhelm normal ED operations. In a similar manner, the formulation of a plan to deal with VIPs to ensure optimal management of the patient may help prevent poor outcomes. Ideally, clinical and administrative issues should be individually managed by senior clinical staff.

Management

Medical issues

The key goals of management should be the maintenance of standard clinical procedures. The clinician should perform a standard clinical evaluation without omitting questioning, examinations or procedures that would normally occur due to other considerations, such as embarrassment. Consultation with inpatient specialists should proceed as appropriate and the frequency and timing should reflect standard practice. Deviation from normal procedures, whether in assessment, referral or disposition, invites errors and lack of clarity in management decisions. Healthcare providers function most efficiently when performing their normal roles and nursing staff, junior medical staff and allied health should be involved as appropriate.

Access to the ED should be restricted after the arrival of the patient. Heads of state may be accompanied by their own teams of physicians. The treating clinician should liaise and consult with these physicians when immediate concerns, such as resuscitation, have been addressed.

EDs are accustomed to managing multiple complex patients at once. However, the presence of a VIP may consume the attention of many staff. The senior medical and nursing clinicians need to ensure that adequate staff are assigned to the management of other patients in the ED and that other patients do not suffer adverse outcomes due to the presence of the VIP.

Different issues arise when treating medical colleagues or their families, other staff members or friends and relatives who are 'relative' VIPs. While aiming to expedite the management and ensure the comfort of someone who is known to the treating clinician, as with the VIP, the safest pathway for the patients is not to deviate from standard medical care. In general, a conservative clinical approach to the VIP is recommended, with a lower than normal threshold for observation or admission.

Administrative issues

The essential administrative issues are security for the VIP and the hospital staff, protection of privacy and confidentiality, containment of the press, timely release of appropriate information and a coordinated response to the VIP's needs. If the patient is of national importance, the response may resemble a disaster response and require the appointment of a central coordinator to manage the initial crisis, security control and media liaison [57].

Liaison with hospital security is essential to minimize entry of unnecessary people to the ED and to ensure the safety of the VIP. Assistance from clinical staff may be required to identify those required to enter the ED. Internal security may need to liaise and cooperate with external security teams. The VIP's security team must not impede medical management.

Confidentiality should be respected and consent to release information should be obtained as with any other patient. Release of information to the media should occur in a graded and accurate manner. Disclosure should occur on two levels: the first is the acknowledgement that the VIP is present and seeking medical attention and the second level involves the graded release of medical information [57]. One senior clinician should be appointed to convey this information. Ideally, a centre for the media should be set up on a site remote from the ED.

While the presence of a VIP in the ED may not overwhelm services in the same way as disaster, a similar approach with a pre-formulated plan of management may assist with the management of these rare and unexpected events and assist in attaining positive outcomes for the VIP and all other patients in the ED.

Controversies and future directions

- The development of acute behavioural centres similar to trauma centres may assist in streamlining the management of acute behavioural disturbance.
- Given the significant deprivations of rights and liberty that are applied when containing those with behavioural disturbance, there is a need to learn more from patients about their experiences.
- The perception of inappropriate ED use by frequent attenders remains controversial, while some healthcare workers and health policy makers continue to assume that frequent attenders can and should be diverted to primary-care providers.
- Understanding of drug dependence as a chronic, organic brain disease may reduce stigma and lead to the development of better medical models of treatment that can enhance the behavioural and social therapies currently practised.

References

[1] Chamberlain C, MacKenzie D. Understanding contemporary homelessness: issues of definition and meaning. Aust J Social Iss 1992;27:274–97.

[2] Pinkney S, Ewing S. The costs and pathways of homelessness: developing policy-relevant economic analyses for the Australian homelessness service system. Melbourne: Institute for Social Research Swinburne University of Technology; 2006: 243.

[3] Commonwealth of Australia. The road home: a national approach to reducing homelessness. In: Department of Families H, Community Services and Indigenous Affairs; 2008.

[4] Australian Bureau of Statistics. Health and Welfare of Australia's Aboriginal and Torres Straight Islander peoples, 2008, ABS cat. no. 4704.0. Canberra: Commonwealth of Australia; 2008.

[5] Phillips GA, Brophy DS, Weiland TJ, et al. The effect of multidisciplinary case management on selected outcomes for frequent attenders at an emergency department. Med J Aust 2006;184:602–6.

[6] Moore G, Gerdtz M, Manias E, et al. Socio-demographic and clinical characteristics of re-presentation to an Australian inner-city emergency department: implications for service delivery. BMC Public Health 2007;7:320.

[7] Moore G, Hepworth G, Weiland T, et al. Prospective validation of a predictive model that identifies homeless people at risk of re-presentation to the emergency department. Austral Emerg Nurs J 2012;15:2–13.

[8] Haw C, Hawton K, Casey D. Deliberate self-harm patients of no fixed abode: a study of characteristics and subsequent deaths in patients presenting to a general hospital. Soc Psychiatr Psychiatr Epidemiol 2006;41:918–25.

[9] Redelmeier DA, Molin JP, Tibshirani RJ. A randomised trial of compassionate care for the homeless in an emergency department. Lancet 1995;345:1131–4.

[10] Australian Bureau of Statistics. Prisoners in Australia, 2010. Canberra; 2010.

[11] Department of Justice. Victoria prisoner health study. Melbourne; 2003.

[12] Williams BA, Goodwin JS, Baillargeon J, et al. Addressing the aging crisis in U.S. criminal justice health care. J Am Geriatr Soc 2012;60:1150–6.

[13] Kuzak N, O'Connor M, Pickett W, et al. Impact of a prison triage system on injuries seen in emergency departments. Can J Emerg Med 2001;3:199–204.

[14] Hawthorne WB, Folsom DP, Sommerfeld DH, et al. Incarceration among adults who are in the public mental health system: rates, risk factors, and short-term outcomes. Psychiatr Serv 2012;63:26–32.

[15] Patterson RF, Hughes K. Review of completed suicides in the California Department of Corrections and Rehabilitation, 1999 to 2004. Psychiatr Serv 2008;59:676–82.

[16] Augello M. Patients in custody: why do they present to an emergency department? Australasian College for Emergency Medicine (Victorian Faculty) Scientific Meeting. Melbourne; 2004.

[17] Wakeman SE, Bowman SE, McKenzie M, et al. Preventing death among the recently incarcerated: an argument for naloxone prescription before release. J Addict Dis 2009;28:124–9.

[18] Knott JC, Bennett D, Rawet J, et al. Epidemiology of unarmed threats in the emergency department. Emerg Med Australas 2005;17:351–8.

[19] Phillips G. Senate Select Committee on Mental Health (written and oral submissions). Melbourne: Hansard; 2005.

[20] Cannon ME, Sprivulis P, McCarthy J. Restraint practices in Australasian emergency departments. Aust NZ J Psychiatr 2001;35:464–7.

[21] Brookes J, Dunn R. The incidence, severity and nature of violent incidents in the emergency department. Emerg Med (Fremantle) 1997;9:5–9.

[22] Emergency Medicine Research Unit Royal Melbourne Hospital. Mental health presentations to the emergency department. Melbourne: Department of Human Services, Victorian State Government; 2006.

[23] Australian Federal Government. Senate Select Committee on Mental Health: recommendations; 2006.

[24] Parliament of Victoria DaCPC. Inquiry into Violence and Security Arrangments in Victorian Hospitals, recommendations. December 2011.

[25] Downes MA, Healy P, Page CB, et al. Structured team approach to the agitated patient in the emergency department. Emerg Med Australas 2009;21:196–202.

[26] Lukens TW, Wolf SJ, Edlow JA, et al. Clinical policy: critical issues in the diagnosis and management of the adult psychiatric patient in the emergency department. Ann Emerg Med 2006;47:79–99.

[27] Wallace M. Health care and the law, 3rd ed. Sydney: Lawbook Co; 2001.

[28] Brayley J, Lange R, Baggoley C, et al. The violence management team. An approach to aggressive behaviour in a general hospital. Med J Aust 1994;161:254–8.

[29] Knott J, Taylor D, Castle D. Randomised clinical trial comparing intravenous midazolam and droperidol for sedation of the acutely agitated patient in the emergency department. Ann Emerg Med 2006;47:61–7.

[30] Nobay F, Simon BC, Levitt MA, et al. A prospective, double-blind, randomized trial of midazolam versus haloperidol versus lorazepam in the chemical restraint of violent and severely agitated patients. Acad Emerg Med 2004;11:744–9.

[31] Chan EW, Taylor DM, Knott JC, et al. Intravenous droperidol or olanzapine as an adjunct to midazolam for the acutely agitated patient: a multicenter, randomized, double-blind, placebo-controlled clinical trial. Ann Emerg Med 2013;61:72–81.

[32] Spain D, Crilly J, Whyte I, et al. Safety and effectiveness of high-dose midazolam for severe behavioural disturbance in an emergency department with suspected psychostimulant-affected patients. Emerg Med Australas 2008;20:112–20.

[33] Stratton SJ, Rogers C, Brickett K, et al. Factors associated with sudden death of individuals requiring restraint for excited delirium. Am J Emerg Med 2001;19:187–91.

[34] Zun LS. A prospective study of the complication rate of use of patient restraint in the emergency department. J Emerg Med 2003;24:119–24.

[35] Sheline Y, Nelson T. Patient choice: deciding between psychotropic medication and physical restraints in an emergency. Bull Am Acad Psychiatr Law 1993;21:321–9.

[36] Jones J, Lyneham J. Violence: part of the job for Australian nurses? Aust J Adv Nurs 2000;18:27–32.

[37] Jenkins MG, Rocke LG, McNicholl BP, et al. Violence and verbal abuse against staff in accident and emergency departments: a survey of consultants in the UK and the Republic of Ireland. J Accid Emerg Med 1998;15:262–5.

[38] Wyatt JP, Watt M. Violence towards junior doctors in accident and emergency departments. J Accid Emerg Med 1995;12:40–2.

[39] Gerdtz M, Maude P, Santamaria N, et al. Occupational violence in nursing: an analysis of the phenomenon of code grey/black events in four Victorian hospitals. Published report. Melbourne: Policy and Strategic Project Division, Victorian Department of Human Services; 2005.

[40] Hunt KA, Weber EJ, Showstack JA, et al. Characteristics of frequent users of emergency departments. Ann Emerg Med 2006;48:1–8.

[41] Jelinek GA, Jiwa M, Gibson NP, et al. Frequent attenders at emergency departments: a linked-data population study of adult patients. Med J Aust 2008;189:552–6.

[42] Byrne M, Murphy AW, Plunkett PK, et al. Frequent attenders to an emergency department: a study of primary health care use, medical profile, and psychosocial characteristics. Ann Emerg Med 2003;41:309–18.

[43] Helliwell PE, Hider PN, Ardagh MW. Frequent attenders at Christchurch Hospital's emergency department. NZ Med J 2001;114:160–1.

[44] Mandelberg JH, Kuhn RE, Kohn MA. Epidemiologic analysis of an urban, public emergency department's frequent users. Acad Emerg Med 2000;7 637–6.

[45] Hansagi H, Allebeck P, Edhag O, et al. Frequency of emergency department attendances as a predictor of mortality: nine-year follow-up of a population-based cohort. J Publ Hlth Med 1990;12:39–44.

[46] Lucas RH, Sanford SM. An analysis of frequent users of emergency care at an urban university hospital. Ann Emerg Med 1998;32:563–8.

[47] Dent AW, Phillips GA, Chenhall AJ, et al. The heaviest repeat users of an inner city emergency department are not general practice patients. Emerg Med (Fremantle) 2003;15:322–9.

[48] Kne T, Young R, Spillane L. Frequent ED users: patterns of use over time. Am J Emerg Med 1998;16:648–52.

[49] Peddie S, Richardson S, Salt L, et al. Frequent attenders at emergency departments: research regarding the utility of management plans fails to take into account the natural attrition of attendance. NZ Med J 2011;124:61–6.

[50] Moore L, Deehan A, Seed P, et al. Characteristics of frequent attenders in an emergency department: analysis of 1-year attendance data. Emerg Med J 2009;26:263–7.

[51] Olsson M, Hansagi H. Repeated use of the emergency department: qualitative study of the patient's perspective. Emerg Med J 2001;18:430–4.

[52] Okin RL, Boccellari A, Azocar F, et al. The effects of clinical case management on hospital service use among ED frequent users. Am J Emerg Med 2000;18:603–8.

[53] Pope D, Fernandes CM, Bouthillette F, et al. Frequent users of the emergency department: a program to improve care and reduce visits. Can Med Assoc J 2000;162:1017–20.

[54] World Health Organization. Lexicon of alcohol and drug terms.

[55] Weaver M, Schnoll S. Addiction issues in prescribing opioids in chronic non malignant pain. J Addiction Med 2007;1:2–10.

[56] McNabb C, Foot C, Ting J, et al. Profiling patients suspected of drug seeking in an adult emergency department. Emerg Med Australas 2006;18:131–7.

[57] Smith MS, Shesser RF. The emergency care of the VIP patient. N Engl J Med 1988;319:1421–3.

21.6 End of life decision making and palliative care

William Lukin • Sandra L Neate • Ben White

ESSENTIALS

1 An emergency department attendance represents an opportunity to set goals for care during the attendance and beyond.

2 End of life discussions and advance care planning assist early decision making about treatment goals and end of life care.

3 Knowledge of the law assists decision making at the end of life.

4 Not all dying patients require the skill set of a palliative care specialist but every dying patient will benefit from a palliative approach.

5 Palliative care does not preclude active treatment where the intent is understood by patient and family.

6 Failure to diagnose dying can compromise patient care.

7 The emergency department should foster close relationships with local specialist palliative care providers to improve and ensure timely access for patients and families and so that emergency staff have access to the knowledge and skills provided.

Definitions

Definitions are given in Table 21.6.1.

General legal principles in end of life decision making

Patients have the right to decide whether to accept or refuse medical treatment. This right is underpinned by Western liberal concepts of self-determination and individual autonomy [3] (see Chapter 25.5). Although the state has an interest in preserving the life and health of citizens, this interest is subject to an individual's right to self-determination.

Therefore, a patient's informed consent must be obtained before treatment commences. To perform a medical procedure against the wishes of a patient can amount to trespass and battery in common law and can also contravene guardianship and medical treatment legislation [4]. A legitimate refusal of treatment must be respected, even if it is contrary to medical opinion. Where a person lacks capacity and so cannot give consent, he or she may have an advance directive or consent should be obtained from a legally authorized decision maker, such as a substitute decision maker or parent if the patient is a child.

There are exceptions to the need for consent to treat. One is cases of emergency where both the common law and various legislation (including guardianship legislation) permit the provision of life-saving or other urgent treatment. Another exception is where mental health legislation authorizes treatment [5].

A patient generally has no legally enforceable right to demand a particular treatment. Medical practitioners are not obliged to offer treatment that is not in a patient's best interests, such as treatments that are futile and where the burdens exceed the benefits of treatment. In Australia, an exception exists under Queensland's guardianship legislation for adults who lack decision-making capacity as then consent *is required* to withhold life-sustaining treatment [6].

Introduction

Improved socioeconomic conditions and advances in medicine, including improved management of chronic disease, have resulted in extended life expectancy. Prior to death, many people now experience a period of progressive deterioration in health and loss of independence due to complex multisystem disease and possible cognitive impairment. It is estimated that up to 40 000 adult deaths occur in Australia annually in the setting of a medical decision to withhold, limit or withdraw treatment [1]. End of life decision making, such as decisions not to provide, to limit or to discontinue life-sustaining treatments and the decision to transition care to a palliative approach are now a common part of the practice of emergency medicine.

End of life discussions and decision making can be challenging due to the complexity of balancing family wishes with the best interests of the patient and dealing with families in times of great stress. End of life decisions require an understanding of the law and the ethical positions of peak medical bodies and are greatly assisted by patients and their families having considered, discussed and documented their wishes. These discussions and decisions may be communicated informally or formally in advance care plans and directives supported by common law and legislation.

Palliative care is the provision of care to those facing life-limiting or life-threatening illness and focuses on the needs of the patient as a whole across various domains, not just the physical. In addition, it looks at the family as a unit also requiring care. For patients for whom the palliative approach should be adopted, palliative care skills enable the emergency physician to engage patients on a dying trajectory and allow them to take control of this process and plan for the time they have remaining, be it hours, days or months. This enables planning for the non-physical aspects of the dying process and reduces time lost to futile medical endeavours.

The most important aims of end of life discussions and palliative care are the identification of what the patient sees as an acceptable outcome from any proposed treatment, to make early and wise decisions about the appropriateness of treatment and to improve communication with patients and families to enable the provision of patient-centred care [2].

Table 21.6.1   Definitions of terms

Term	Definition
Advance care planning (ACP)	A process that allows competent individuals to express their views regarding future healthcare decisions if the capacity to express those views is lost
Advance directive (AD)	A statement that allows competent individuals to state in advance how they wish to be treated if they lack decision-making capacity in the future. Making an AD can be part of ACP. Different terms are used for ADs in different jurisdictions
Futile treatment	The definition of futile treatment is contested, but treatment may be considered futile when it is no longer providing a benefit to a patient or the burdens of providing the treatment outweigh the benefits
Good medical practice	Practice that is consistent with currently recognized medical standards, practices and procedures and currently recognized ethical standards of the medical profession
Life-limiting illness	An illness where it is expected that death will be a direct consequence of the specified illness
Life-sustaining treatment	Medical treatment that supplants or maintains the operation of vital bodily functions that are temporarily or permanently incapable of independent operation. This includes assisted ventilation, artificial nutrition and hydration and cardiopulmonary resuscitation but excludes measures of palliative care
Palliative care	An approach that improves the quality of life for patients and their families facing life-threatening illness, through the prevention and relief of suffering by means of early identification and rigorous assessment and treatment of pain and other problems, physical, psychosocial and spiritual
Substitute (surrogate) decision maker ('person responsible' in some jurisdictions)	The person legally responsible for making decisions about healthcare, including its limitations, on behalf of an adult patient who lacks decision-making capacity. State guardianship or medical treatment legislation determines a patient's substitute decision maker
Enduring guardian, attorney or agent (depending on jurisdiction)	A substitute decision maker who is given authority by a patient to make healthcare decisions on behalf of that patient if capacity is lost

While the vast majority of disagreements about end of life care are resolved informally, recourse may also be had to the courts and, for adults who lack capacity, to guardianship tribunals and the statutory office of public advocate or guardian.

Expected legal knowledge of medical practitioners

Despite attempts to harmonize the law that regulates end of life decision making, it varies across Australian states and territories [7] and the rest of the world. Medical practitioners play significant legal roles at the end of life including: assessing a patient's capacity to understand and make decisions for themselves; determining the scope of any consent or refusal and whether it applies to current circumstances; and understanding the operation of guardianship laws to find a patient's substitute decision maker when the individual is not competent.

Medical practitioners have knowledge gaps regarding their legal roles and obligations [8,9]. The importance of the doctor's role in ensuring the legality of all decisions and medical treatments and the apparent gap in current knowledge of practitioners suggests that regular systematic legal training for the medical profession would be ideal.

Advance care planning and advance directives

Advance care planning (ACP) is planning and expressing wishes for future health and personal care for a time in the future when the individual cannot make or communicate decisions. ACP provides a means for people to ensure their wishes and preferences are known. Most doctors, nurses and members of the community support ACP but rates of formal planning are low despite evidence that ACP leads to improvement in end of life care, patient and family satisfaction and reduction of anxiety and depression in surviving relatives [10].

Advance directives (ADs) are generally a form of written advance care plan made by a competent person recognized by common law or legislation depending on the jurisdiction. An AD can be written at any time of life and may relate to periods of temporary or permanent incapacity. Content may vary from an expression of personal values and wishes to specific medical directions by a person with a life-limiting illness.

ADs are recognized in many parts of the world, including all Australian jurisdictions and six Australian states and territories now have specific legislation relating to ADs. All jurisdictions, except the Northern Territory, also have legislative provisions that allow patients to appoint a substitute decision maker, called an enduring guardian, enduring attorney or agent depending on the jurisdiction. The guardianship legislation of all states and territories allows for the appointment of a guardian, but this only occurs where less formal mechanisms are inadequate [6].

A National Framework for Advance Care Directives authored by the Clinical, Technical and Ethical Principal Committee of the Australian Health Minister's Advisory Council aims to provide a practical and ethical basis to the development of a national framework for advanced directives [7].

Limitation or withdrawal of treatment

Emergency medicine practitioners may be confronted with circumstances where the patient and family have not considered the desired outcomes of their ongoing treatment or that death may be a possible outcome of their current condition. Up to 35% of deaths in EDs involve patients in the terminal phases of existing chronic illness who attend the ED for conditions that represent the natural evolution of the illness [11]. The ED has become a place where terminally ill patients frequently die and where decisions regarding limitation or withdrawal of care are now often made.

While doctors generally must not cause or hasten a patient's death, there are circumstances where limiting or withdrawing treatment is lawful. These include when a competent adult refuses treatment, when another person (such as a substitute decision maker or parent) has lawfully refused treatment on behalf of the patient and when the treatment is not in the patient's best interests, either because it is considered futile or the burdens are not justified by the potential benefits [4].

The Australian Medical Association states that if a medical practitioner acts in accordance with good medical practice, the following forms of management at the end of life do not constitute euthanasia or physician assisted suicide: not initiating life-prolonging measures; not continuing life-prolonging measures and the administration of treatment or other action intended to relieve symptoms which may have a secondary consequence of hastening death [12].

Despite growing community interest in ADs and an increasing burden of chronic disease, the majority of patients presenting to EDs have not discussed their end of life wishes with family or expressed their wishes in an AD [13]. In these situations, discussions should focus on the desired outcomes of treatment and the delivery of treatments consistent with those desires and which offer some comfort and assistance to the patient.

Resuscitation and not for resuscitation (NFR) orders

When first described in the 1960s, cardiopulmonary resuscitation (CPR) involved simple resuscitative measures to reverse physiological instability. Although CPR can 'stay' death on occasion, it is frequently applied in circumstances that will not result in a return to previous health and is applied in patients who are, in reality, dying [14]. American healthcare culture has been described as one of medical optimism, characterized by an unwillingness to give up hope for a miracle, which has led to patients choosing distressing and burdensome treatment options which eventually end in death, whether or not these treatments had been instituted [15]. Unrealistic expectations of outcomes from CPR are common [16].

The combination of knowledge deficits, unrealistic expectations of outcomes and medical optimism have left patients and doctors with a sense that there is a presumed consent to CPR unless otherwise indicated [14]. NFR orders have developed in response to CPR being universally applied and such presumed consent to CPR. The absence of an NFR order has become considered an order to perform CPR unless otherwise instructed [14]. CPR is no longer seen as a medical intervention with specific indications but one of many patient choices.

The American Heart Association defines the goals of resuscitation as to preserve life, restore health, relieve suffering, limit disability and respect the individual's decisions, rights and privacy [17]. Decisions to commence, continue or to terminate resuscitation are based on the difficult balance between the benefits, risks and cost these interventions place on patient, family members and the healthcare system [18]. Ethical reasons for withholding attempted resuscitation include respecting the patient's autonomy and choices, weighing maleficence against beneficence (avoiding treatment that may cause more harm than benefit), trying to provide good 'quality of death' and the consideration of resources [19].

Some peak medical bodies provide ethical guidance on these issues [17,18,20,21]. The General Medical Council (UK) advises that: 'in cases where you assess that such treatment is unlikely to be clinically appropriate, you may conclude that CPR should not be attempted' [22]. The Medical Board of Australia recognizes that: 'doctors have a vital role in assisting the community to deal with the reality of death and its consequences' and good medical practice involves both 'understanding the limits of medicine in prolonging life and recognizing when efforts to prolong life may not benefit the patient'. The Medical Board also states that there is no duty to prolong life at all cost but a duty exists to know when not to initiate and when to cease attempts at prolonging life [23].

The ability to 'refuse' an NFR order perpetuates the paradigm that CPR is solely a patient choice and that all deaths can potentially be prevented. The performance of CPR, under the guidance of the bodies such as the GMC and the Medical Board of Australia, is a medical decision that the patient can refuse, but on which the patient cannot insist (although the situation under Queensland's guardianship legislation discussed above should be noted).

Palliative care

The World Health Organization defines palliative care as an approach that improves the quality of life of patients and their families who are living with a life-limiting illness through the prevention and relief of suffering by means of early identification and impeccable assessment and treatment of pain and other problems, physical, psychosocial and spiritual [24].

Palliative care is an emerging area in emergency medicine with international evidence suggesting that the care of the patient who is imminently dying is not done well in emergency departments. In addition, the care of the patient who is on a dying trajectory who presents to the emergency department needs further research. Palliative care focuses on the needs of the patient as a whole across various domains, not just the physical. In addition, it looks at the family as a unit also requiring care. Emergency physicians should adhere to the principles of a good death for all of the patients who die in emergency departments [25]. For patients for whom the palliative approach should be adopted, skills in palliative care enable the emergency physician to engage patients on a dying trajectory and support them in taking control of this process and putting in place a plan for end of life. This allows for choice of place of death outside of the acute setting, which requires appropriate social and clinical supports. The discussions surrounding such planning include the non-physical aspects of the dying process and may reduce time lost to futile medical endeavours that are likely to ensue in the acute setting.

Specialist palliative care versus a palliative approach

Not all dying patients need the skill set of a specialist palliative care provider. However, all patients living with a life-limiting disease and those dying in the emergency department can benefit from a palliative approach to care. This approach focuses on quality of life remaining for those with life-limiting disease. This approach can be adopted by all clinicians who deal with dying patients. The complexity (in respect to palliation) of a patient fluctuates as the patient approaches end of life. For patients whose needs are complex, timely referral to specialist palliative care providers may be helpful.

Palliative care skills for the emergency physician

Communication skills in the palliative domains (physical, spiritual and psychosocial)

Appropriate discussion around these domains enables patients to regain some control of the dying process and improves the experience for patients and families. While there is often not time for in-depth exploration of all these themes in a patient encounter, simple acknowledgement of their existence by the clinician can help shape the priorities for the presentation. Conversations that begin in the ED can be a stimulus for further discussions with treating teams and also encourage and prompt families to have these discussions. While traditionally viewed as difficult, such discussions are generally welcomed by patients and families. To walk away from a dying patient without this engagement is a failure of care and a loss of opportunity for the patient.

Impeccable assessment skills

The needs of these patients for comprehensive evaluation are the same as any other patient coming into the ED. To deal with physical symptoms appropriately, a diagnosis is required and appropriate investigations may be undertaken if there is likely to be a benefit. For example, delirium in an older person may be relatively simply resolved through appropriate investigation and treatment of the underlying cause and should not be ignored or generically treated with sedation.

Pain relief and symptom control

Uncontrolled pain or other distressing symptoms may prevent engagement in appropriate end of life discussions and planning. It is imperative that these needs be met promptly in the ED. Where these needs are complex, early referral to specialist palliative care providers may assist. No patient should have uncontrolled pain in an ED and processes should address this with pain score assessments, protocol-driven analgesia and fostering a culture where patients and families can speak up and voice concern. For patients under the active care of palliative providers who are on opioid analgesics other than morphine, understanding the relative potency of these opioids is critical to providing appropriate titration of medication in the ED.

Diagnosing dying

The concept of diagnosing dying implies recognition of the fact that the patient will not recover from a given illness. The need for this emphasis stems from our place in a society that denies death and an acute care system that can see death as the enemy. Failure to diagnose the dying process can result in over-investigation, inappropriate treatment and instillation of false hope and shortens the time dying patients have to plan for what is to come. A simple question often posed by palliative care providers is 'Would you be surprised if your patient were to die in the next 12 months?' For emergency clinicians it could be posed as 'Would you be surprised if this patient

died during this admission?' If the answer is 'no' to the 'surprise question', then there is an opportunity to engage patients and families in discussions about the goals of this admission. Referral to palliative care providers from the ED can shorten length of stay in hospital and increase the likelihood that goals of care around end of life care are established. This reduces the burden on the medical emergency response teams within the hospital.

The dying pathway

For patients whose death is imminent (hours), it may not be appropriate to transfer them out of the emergency department. In this case, compassionate, understanding care is necessary, perhaps involving the use of a clinical pathway, such as the Liverpool care pathway [26], that enables hospice level care to be delivered in other care settings, such as a short-stay unit. The use of continuously delivered medication via syringe driver may be appropriate in this setting to control pain and other symptoms.

The role of the medical practitioner in end of life care

The Australian Medical Association states that good quality end of life care should ensure that the patient is treated with respect, dignity and compassion and is free from unnecessary suffering; should be treated in their environment of choice; that goals for end of life care, privacy and confidentiality are respected; that the physical, psychological, emotional, religious and spiritual needs of the patient, their family and carers are supported; patients and family members are encouraged, where appropriate, to participate in managing their treatment; and that counselling and other support are provided throughout the patient's condition and beyond the patient's death [12].

The provision of high quality end of life care requires early discussions and planning with the patient and family so that all concerned with the patient's care are clear about the goals of treatment. Silvester identifies three opportunities to ensure that patient-centred care is delivered at the end of life [27]. First, a competent person may consider and express their wishes via advance care planning. Second, when a person is no longer competent, healthcare professionals should determine whether advance directives exist and have discussions with substitute decision makers about what outcome the patient would have wished. Third, the delivery of care at the end of life should provide a 'good

death': avoiding suffering and the prolongation of dying, achieving a sense of control, relieving burdens placed on the family and strengthening relationships with loved ones.

Controversies and future directions

- Close partnering between emergency providers and palliative care providers will provide timely intervention in the emergency departments so that opportunities to establish goals of care are not lost.
- Short-stay units should be able to provide hospice level care to the dying with support as required from specialist palliative care services or the use of care of the dying pathways.
- End of life and palliative care may become subspecialty areas for emergency physicians.
- Short-stay units may incorporate palliative care beds for the care of those imminently dying in whom transfer may be impractical.

Acknowledgements

Thanks to Dr Carol Douglas, Director Palliative Care Royal Brisbane and Women's Hospital, for her suggestions.

References

[1] White B, Willmott L, Trowse P, et al. The legal role of medical professionals in decisions to withhold or withdraw life-sustaining treatment: Part 1 (New South Wales). J Law Med 2011;18:498–522.
[2] Cartwright CM, Parker MH. Advance care planning and end of life decision-making. Aust Fam Phys 2004;33:815–9.
[3] Willmott L, White B, Mathews B. Law, autonomy and advance directives. J Law Med 2010;18:366–89.
[4] Skene L. Law and medical practice–rights, duties, claims and defences, 3rd ed. Australia; 2008.
[5] Ryan CJ, Callaghan S. Legal and ethical aspects of refusing medical treatment after a suicide attempt: the Wooltorton case in the Australian context. Med J Aust 2010;193:239–42.
[6] White B, McDonald L, Willmott L. Health law in Australia. Sydney: Thomson Reuters; 2010.
[7] Australian Health Minister's Advisory Council. A National Framework for Advance Care Directives; 2011.
[8] Willmott L, White B, Parker M, et al. The legal role of medical professionals in decisions to withhold or withdraw life-sustaining treatment: Part 2 (Queensland). J Law Med 2011;18:523–44.
[9] Willmott L, White B, Parker M, et al. The legal role of medical professionals in decisions to withhold or withdraw life-sustaining treatment: Part 3 (Victoria). J Law Med 2011;18:773–97.
[10] Detering KM, Hancock AD, Reade MC, et al. The impact of advance care planning on end of life care in elderly patients: randomised controlled trial. Br Med J 2010;340:c1345.
[11] Tardy B, Venet C, Zeni F, et al. Death of terminally ill patients on a stretcher in the emergency department: a French speciality? Intensive Care Med 2002;28:1625–8.
[12] Australian Medical Association. The role of the medical practitioner in end of life care; 2007.

[13] Le Conte P, Riochet D, Batard E, et al. Death in emergency departments: a multicenter cross-sectional survey with analysis of withholding and withdrawing life support. Intens Care Med 2010;36:765–72.

[14] Bishop JP, Brothers KB, Perry JE, et al. Reviving the conversation around CPR/DNR. Am J Bioeth 2010;10:61–7.

[15] Scripko PD, Greer DM. Practical considerations for reviving the CPR/DNR conversation. Am J Bioeth 2010;10:74–5.

[16] Kaldjian LC, Erekson ZD, Haberle TH, et al. Code status discussions and goals of care among hospitalised adults. J Med Ethics 2009;35:338–42.

[17] Morrison LJ, Kierzek G, Diekema DS, et al. Part 3: ethics: 2010 American Heart Association Guidelines

for Cardiopulmonary Resuscitation and Emergency Cardiovascular Care. Circulation 2010;122:S665–75.

[18] Lippert FK, Raffay V, Georgiou M, et al. European Resuscitation Council Guidelines for Resuscitation 2010: Section 10. The ethics of resuscitation and end-of-life decisions. Resuscitation 2010

[19] Fritz Z, Fuld J. Ethical issues surrounding do not attempt resuscitation orders: decisions, discussions and deleterious effects. J Med Ethics 2010;36:593–7.

[20] American College of Emergency Physicians. Ethical issues at the end of life. Ann Emerg Med 2008; 52:592–3.

[21] American College of Emergency Physicians. Ethical issues of resuscitation. Ann Emerg Med 2008; 52:593.

[22] General Medical Council end of life care: When to consider making a Do Not Attempt CPR (DNACPR) decision. London: General Medical Council; 2010.

[23] Medical Board of Australia. Good medical practice: a code of conduct for doctors in Australia. Australia.

[24] World Health Organization. Cancer. Palliative care; 2012.

[25] Ellershaw J, Dewar S, Murphy D. Achieving a good death for all. Br Med J 2010;341:c4861.

[26] The Marie Curie Palliative Care Institute. Liverpool care pathway for the dying patient; 2012.

[27] Silvester W, Detering K. Advance care planning and end-of-life care. Med J Aust. 2011;195(8):435–6.

21.7 Organ and tissue donation

Sandra L Neate • David Pilcher

ESSENTIALS

1 Significant numbers of missed potential organ and tissue donors have been identified in emergency departments and intensive care units.

2 Clinical triggers have been introduced in Australian emergency departments to assist with early identification of potential donors.

3 Knowledge of pathways to donation and the skills required to commence donation discussions may decrease the numbers of missed potential donors and improve the numbers of organ and tissue donors.

Introduction

Transplantation has become the therapy of choice for patients with end-stage organ failure. However, worldwide, there are insufficient organs available to meet demand for those on transplantation waiting lists. In Australia in 2012, there were 1600 people awaiting organ transplantation. In 2011, there were 337 deceased organ donors in Australia and 1001 transplant recipients [1]. Between 2008 and 2011, 474 patients were admitted to Australian and New Zealand intensive care units (ICUs) primarily to assess suitability for organ donation and, of these, almost two-thirds came directly from the emergency department (ED) [2].

In Australia, there is a relatively small pool of potential donors [3], as less than 2% of patients who die in hospital are eligible to donate their organs. However, there is potential to increase the number of organ donors. Despite high rates of community support for donation, consent rates to donation by families of donor-eligible patients remain a major limiting factor to donation [4]. In Australia, fewer than 60% of families consent to donation. Another factor limiting donation rates is missing opportunities for donation. Missed opportunities include situations where life-sustaining therapies are withdrawn in patients with imminent or potential brain death, particularly in the ED; patients who may be suitable for donation for whom donation is never raised due to clinician unwillingness to discuss donation with family; resource pressures; and a perception by clinicians that the patient may not be medically suitable for donation [5,6].

Although donation of solid organs is a rare opportunity, eye and tissue (e.g. skin, bone, heart valves and connective tissues) donation can occur up to 24 hours after death regardless of where death occurred and may apply to a larger population of patients, especially those in the ED.

Emergency practitioners play an important role in the donation process. Donors identified in the ED, although small in number, have a greater rate of proceeding to successful donation than those referred from other in-patient critical care settings [7]. Emergency clinicians are ideally placed to exhibit positive attitudes toward donation, support donation, identify potential donors and assist families to make informed decisions about donation.

Donation pathways

The initial critical step in making organ donation a reality is to recognize the potential donor. These are usually ventilated patients in the ED or ICU who are expected to die either through brain death or following cessation of the circulation. The majority of donations in Australia and worldwide occur following brain death. The donation of heart, lungs, liver, pancreas, bowel and kidneys from one brain dead donor can lead to up to eight organ transplants. For a minority of patients, donation may be possible when death is diagnosed after cessation of the circulation. This is known as donation after cardiac (or circulatory) death (DCD) or non-heart beating donation and may lead to the donation of kidneys, lungs or liver but rarely other organs. Kidneys are the only organs donated commonly from living donors, although lobar liver and lung donation has occasionally been performed.

Donation after brain death (DBD)

Criteria to diagnose brain death vary slightly in different countries [8,9] but essentially depend on the loss of capacity for consciousness and the ability to breathe. If certain preconditions are met (e.g. no effects of sedating drugs and a diagnosis consistent with producing severe brain injury), brain death may be diagnosed clinically by demonstrating loss of all brainstem reflexes. Making a clinical diagnosis of brain death cannot be done until a period of observation has elapsed (minimum 4 hours in Australia). Thus, brain death is rarely diagnosed in the ED, but patients who might become brain

731

dead are commonly identified here. When clinical testing is not possible, imaging tests (e.g. cerebral angiograms, nuclear medicine scans and computed tomography (CT) angiogram) may be performed.

Donation after cardiac death

Although donation after brain death has remained the most common route for organ donation throughout the world, the 2000s saw renewed interest in achieving donation from patients in whom death was diagnosed after cessation of circulation. Unlike brain dead donation, the practices and processes for DCD vary widely across countries and reflect differing social, medical and legal environments. Patients considered for DCD in Spain and France are those who present following cardiac arrest (with or without failed attempts at resuscitation) – so-called 'uncontrolled DCD'. In contrast, in Australia, the UK and the USA, DCD is usually performed in patients who undergo elective withdrawal of cardiorespiratory support in ICU after determining that a person will not recover – so-called 'controlled DCD' [10]. DCD has been increasingly implemented across Australia and has led to an increase in overall donor numbers and organs transplanted without a reduction in brain dead donors. The widespread implementation of DCD across Australia may help reduce the shortfall of organs for transplantation [11].

Introducing uncontrolled DCD to emergency departments

The recognition that patients who died following cardiac arrest might still be suitable donors has led to the creation of 'rapid response teams' or 'mobile donor units' to facilitate organ donation when such patients are identified either within the ED or prior to admission to hospital. These have resulted in successful donations in Spain, France, Japan and the USA. However, some programmes started in the USA have closed down due to a failure to identify more than a handful of patients [12]. In addition, concerns over the use of vascular cannulation techniques for organ perfusion which are similar to extra-corporeal membrane oxygenation – cardiopulmonary resuscitation (ECMO–CPR), lack of consistency over an appropriate observation period ('hands-off' time) prior to instituting organ preservation therapy (varying from 2 minutes in some US states to 20 minutes in Italy) and the large

resources required for small numbers of suitable patients [13], are likely to limit uptake of these techniques outside a few specialized centres worldwide.

Initiatives to improve organ donation rates

There is wide variation in rates of organ donation throughout the world with Spain's 30+ donors per million population often highlighted as a target for others. Many factors influence these numbers, including the number of road traffic fatalities, attitudes towards ongoing treatment of patients who are going to die but in whom wishes about donation are not known, access to intensive care beds (lower in the UK than in Spain and Australia), end of life practices in general and public support for organ donation among others. However, countries that have successfully increased donation rates have concerted approaches towards identification of potential donors, support for clinicians involved in donation, pubic promotion about the benefits of organ donation and transplantation, clear legislation, infrastructure and funding.

In the late 1980s and early 1990s, Spain established a system of transplant donor coordinators (predominantly doctors supported by specialized nurses) in all major hospitals. It was only with the implementation of this system (a decade after Spain's presumed consent laws) that the major increase in Spain's donation rates occurred. The USA has a long history of federal legislation which supported the creation of the united network for organ sharing (UNOS) which coordinates 11 different organ procurement organizations (OPOs) [14].

For many years, Australia's donation rate lagged a long way behind that of similar developed countries. In the late 2000s, building on experiences from abroad, federal funding of over $150 million led to the formation of the Australian Organ and Tissue Donation and Transplantation Authority and thus a coordinated national approach to increasing organ donation. This has led to a progressive increase in donor numbers to 15 per million population in 2011, from below 10 per million in 2000 [15]. One of the key strategies has been to focus on identification of the potential donor. Recognizing that nearly half of the unrecognized potential brain dead donors died in the

ED [3], clinical triggers have been adopted in the ED and ICU.

Clinical triggers for identification of potential donors

Clinical triggers have been developed worldwide and aim to minimize the number of missed potential donors, particularly those in whom life-sustaining therapies are withdrawn in the ED and ICU who would be likely to progress to brain death if supportive treatment was continued [3].

In the UK, the National Institute for Health and Clinical Excellence has published guidelines for the identification of potential DBD and DCD donors [16]. In the USA, the use of clinical triggers that utilize clinical signs suggestive of irrecoverable brain injury or where withdrawal of life-sustaining therapies is being considered, assist the identification and (often mandatory) referral of patients to OPOs.

In Australia, the GIVE clinical trigger was introduced in 2010. The trigger aims to identify patients with a Glasgow coma scale (GCS) equal to or less than 5 (G) from an irrecoverable brain injury who are intubated (I), ventilated (V) and in whom withdrawal of life-sustaining measures and end of life care (E) is being discussed. It is important to note that there are no medical exclusions to activation of the trigger. Following identification of a potential donor and discussions with families regarding consideration of their family member's wishes, admission to the ICU can be undertaken to continue the assessment of the potential for organ and tissue donation (OTD).

With the increasing availability of DCD, it is worth remembering that missed opportunities may also occur in patients who do not fit the clinical triggers exactly as implemented in Australia or elsewhere. Although the majority of potential DCD patients are those with a low GCS due to neurological injuries, patients about to undergo withdrawal of cardiorespiratory support following terminal heart or lung disease may still be liver or kidney donors. Education and training in donor recognition, referral pathways and in OTD is vital to ensure patients such as these can be given the opportunity to be organ donors. This is known to increase rates of successful donation and the comfort and competence of practitioners and is supported by the public within Australia [17,18].

Emergency clinicians attitudes to, knowledge and perceptions of OTD

An Australian survey of ED clinicians showed high levels of general support for OTD, a willingness to donate their own organs and tissues after death and to consent to OTD of family members [19]. In general, ED clinicians agree that facilitation of OTD is a vital part of emergency medicine [20] but that barriers exist to facilitation, such as time, resource pressures and access block [21]. Resources in EDs may pose a barrier to the facilitation of OTD. Most EDs operate at full capacity with time pressures limiting time available for complex discussions with families and continued support of the potential donor if ICU facilities are not immediately available. Hospital overcrowding compounds the problem. Imposed performance indicators requiring a definitive destination for patients within 4 hours may also compound perceived and real barriers [21].

Cultural and religious barriers to facilitation of OTD exist both with respect to the clinician's comfort in discussing and facilitating OTD [19] and to family acceptance of and consent to donation. Despite common perceptions, most religions, including all major religions, support OTD and transplantation as acts of generosity and merit because they benefit others [22]. Early consultation with religious elders may assist if families express concerns.

Attitudes of healthcare providers to OTD are known to affect the outcome of donation-related conversations, with this effect extending even to the perceived level of care and concern displayed by treating physicians, independent of any discussions around donation [4,23].

The acceptance of brain death as a valid determination of death is essential for clinician support of OTD. While acceptance of brain death is high among emergency clinicians, some knowledge deficits about brain death exist [24]. While it is uncommon for emergency clinicians to need to explain brain death and very rare to have to assist in determination of brain death, understanding brain death assists both the clinician and family.

OTD discussions in the ED

Discussions with families about OTD in the ED may arise infrequently for the individual practitioner, but knowledge of donation pathways and expertise in communication ensures accurate information is imparted to families to enable informed decision making when the occasion arises. With growing public education about OTD, families may raise OTD or discussions may be required following activation of clinical triggers in end of life discussions. Depending on pathways within hospitals, specialists in donation discussions may be available to talk with families, but this may not be the case in many environments.

Enhanced knowledge and experience with OTD-related tasks increase comfort and competence in organ donation discussions [18]. Specific training in donation conversations and related communication skills and behaviours increase the clinician's comfort in speaking with patients' families about donation and answering donation-related questions and consent to both organ donation [25] and tissue donation following death [26].

As with all aspects of end of life communication, normalization of the discussion of OTD assists both the clinician and the family in feeling comfortable about such discussions. The offer of OTD as a routine part of end of life care, when appropriate, can assist families and clinicians in this respect. Failing to offer donation to families may result in families feeling they were unable to fulfil their loved one's wishes in the future. The offer of OTD may also offer the possibility for converting an otherwise negative discussion and circumstance into a discussion with a potentially positive outcome for the family.

An understanding of the common factors influencing decisions regarding OTD may assist practitioners in delivering factual information that can address concerns and support the family's right to make a choice that is based on complete information [27]. Families cannot make informed choices when the information they receive is incomplete and this information may include the potential benefits of OTD to others. Reasons that families support donation in principle and consent to donation include altruism; the positive impact that donation will make on others' lives; pre-existing knowledge of their loved one's wishes; and the solace which may be derived from organ donation. Reasons given for not supporting donation and non-consent to donation include fear of disfigurement; the belief the body must be buried whole; fear of medical neglect of potential donors; religious concerns; and not knowing the family member's wishes [4,28,29].

The aim of ED discussions regarding organ donation is not to obtain formal consent to donation, as this is would be premature in the ED setting. The aim is to offer donation as one of the possibilities that may be considered at the end of life, in a patient who may have the potential to become an organ donor. Following the identification of a potential donor and the discussion of the possibility of donation in the end of life setting with the family, early involvement of intensive care specialists and then donation agency staff to continue donation discussions should occur.

Eye and tissue donation

The donation of tissues, such as eye and corneal tissue, musculoskeletal tissues including bone, tendons and menisci, cardiac tissue including heart valves and pericardium and skin tissues, can both enhance and save lives, for example by restoring vision, improving mobility, replacing diseased heart valves and as skin grafts in burns victims [30].

Tissue donation can occur following death, independent of the donation of solid organs and the place of death. Unlike solid organ donation, the patient does not need to be managed in an ICU setting prior to donation. Patients who die in the ED commonly have fewer exclusions to the donation of eyes and tissues (e.g. sepsis, massive blood product transfusion). However, the current rates of tissue donation are paradoxically low given that the pool of potential tissue-eligible donors is much larger than the potential solid organ donor pool.

Community awareness of eye and tissue donation may be less than that of solid organ donation. Because many families have limited knowledge about tissue donation, the knowledge and communication skills of the clinician may affect the next of kin's perceptions of donation and thus affect the likelihood of consent to donation [31]. The knowledge and communication skills that affect organ donation discussions also affect the discussion regarding eye and tissue donation [25]. Quality of communication skills and the level of comfort of the requester are known to affect outcome of these discussions just as they do for organ donation [26].

In some jurisdictions in the USA, reporting of hospital deaths to OPOs is mandated in law. The family of every deceased patient who may be considered a potential eye and tissue donor will be approached by phone by an OPO. In Australia, consideration of the potential for eye and tissue donation rests, in general, with the treating clinician and the discussion with families regarding potential tissue donation should ideally be part of routine end of life care. Eye donation can frequently occur on the hospital premises. Tissue retrieval often needs to occur in a controlled environment within 24 hours of death, so identification of potential donors, discussion with families and notification of eye and tissue donation agencies must occur in a timely fashion.

Controversies and future directions

- With the increasing frequency of DCD, clinical triggers for the identification of potential donors may need to be extended to include all those in whom withdrawal of life-sustaining therapies is being considered.
- Although the number of donors from patients presenting to EDs in cardiac arrest is low, this is an ongoing area of research and interest.
- Rates of eye and tissue donation could be increased by identification of potential tissue donors in the ED.

Acknowledgements

Thanks to Stefan Poniatowski, Head, Donor Tissue Bank of Victoria, for advice regarding eye and tissue donation.

References

[1] Organ and Tissue Authority. Performance Report 2011: Australian Government Organ and Tissue Authority; 2011
[2] ANZICS Centre for Outcome and Resource Evaluation. ANZICS Adult Patient Database. Carlton, Victoria.
[3] Opdam HI, Silvester W. Potential for organ donation in Victoria: an audit of hospital deaths. Med J Aust 2006;185:250–4.
[4] Siminoff LA, Gordon N, Hewlett J, Arnold RM. Factors influencing families' consent for donation of solid organs for transplantation. J Am Med Assoc 2001;286:71–7.
[5] Aubrey P, Arber S, Tyler M. The organ donor crisis: the missed organ donor potential from the accident and emergency departments. Transplant Proc 2008;40:1008–11.
[6] Riker RR, White BW. Organ and tissue donation from the emergency department. J Emerg Med 1991;9:405–10.
[7] Michael GE, O'Connor RE. The importance of emergency medicine in organ donation: successful donation is more likely when potential donors are referred from the emergency department. Acad Emerg Med 2009;16:850–8.
[8] Australian and New Zew Zealand Intensive Care Society. The ANZICS Statement on Death and Organ Donation. 3.1 edn. Melbourne; 2010.
[9] Gardiner D, Shemie S, Manara A, Opdam H. International perspective on the diagnosis of death. Br J Anaesth 2012;108(Suppl 1):i14–28.
[10] Manara AR, Murphy PG, O'Callaghan G. Donation after circulatory death. Br J Anaesth 2012;108(Suppl 1):i108–21.
[11] Coulson TG, Pilcher DV, Graham SM, et al. Single-centre experience of donation after cardiac death. Med J Aust 2012;197:166–9.
[12] Green J. Organ donation in the emergency department. A missed opportunity? Ann Emerg Med 2012:59.
[13] Blackstock M, McKeown DW, Ray DC. Controlled organ donation after cardiac death: potential donors in the emergency department. Transplantation 2010;89:1149–53.
[14] Rudge C, Matesanz R, Delmonico FL, Chapman J. International practices of organ donation. Br J Anaesth 2012;108(Suppl 1):i48–55.
[15] Australia and New Zealand Dialysis and Transplant Registry. Australia and New Zealand Organ Donation Registry 2012 Report; 2012.
[16] National Institute for Health and Clinical Excellence. CG 135 Organ donation: identification and referral of potential organ donors; 2012.
[17] Riker RR, White BW. The effect of physician education on the rates of donation request and tissue donation. Transplantation 1995;59:880–4.
[18] Neate S, Marck CH, Weiland TJ, et al. Australian emergency clinicians' perceptions and use of the GIVE clinical trigger for identification of potential organ and tissue donors. Emerg Med Australas 2012;24:501–9.
[19] Marck CH, Weiland TJ, Neate SL, et al. Personal attitudes and beliefs regarding organ and tissue donation: a cross-sectional survey of Australian emergency department clinicians. Prog Transplant 2012;22:317–22.
[20] Jelinek GA, Marck CH, Weiland TJ, et al. Organ and tissue donation-related attitudes, education and practices of emergency department clinicians in Australia. Emerg Med Australas 2012;24:244–50.
[21] Marck CH, Jelinek GA, Neate SL, et al. Resource barriers to the facilitation of organ and tissue donation reported by Australian emergency clinicians. Australian health review: Australian Hospital Association; 2012.
[22] Organ and Tissue Authority. Religion and donation. Canberra; 2012.
[23] Siminoff LA, Arnold RM, Hewlett J. The process of organ donation and its effect on consent. Clin Transplant 2001;15:39–47.
[24] Marck CH, Weiland TJ, Neate SL, et al. Australian emergency doctors' and nurses' acceptance and knowledge regarding brain death: a national survey. Clin Transplant 2012;26:E254–60.
[25] Siminoff LA, Marshall HM, Dumenci L, et al. Communicating effectively about donation: an educational intervention to increase consent to donation. Prog Transplant 2009;19:35–43.
[26] Siminoff LA, Traino HM, Gordon N. Determinants of family consent to tissue donation. J Trauma 2010;69:956–63.
[27] Mulvania P, Wise C. Dual advocacy: a value-positive approach to obtaining consent for organ donation. Philadelphia: Gift of Life Institute training material; 2012.
[28] Irving MJ, Tong A, Jan S, et al. Community attitudes to deceased organ donation: a focus group study. Transplantation 2012;93:1064–9.
[29] Siminoff L, Mercer MB, Graham G, Burant C. The reasons families donate organs for transplantation: implications for policy and practice. J Trauma 2007;62:969–78.
[30] Siminoff LA, Traino HM, Gordon NH. An exploratory study of relational, persuasive, and nonverbal communication in requests for tissue donation. J Hlth Commun 2011;16:955–75.
[31] Dorflinger L, Auerbach SM, Siminoff LA. The interpersonal process in tissue donation requests with "undecided" next of kin. Prog Transplant 2012;22:427–35.

PAIN RELIEF

Edited by **Anthony Brown**

22.1 General pain management

Daniel M Fatovich

ESSENTIALS

1 Acute pain is the most common presenting complaint to an emergency department.

2 Pain is a complex, multidimensional, subjective phenomenon.

3 Patient self-reporting is the most reliable indicator of the presence and intensity of pain.

4 Patients with pain should receive timely, effective and appropriate analgesia, titrated according to response.

5 There is a wide range of pharmacological and non-pharmacological techniques available for the treatment of acute pain. Effective pain relief should always be achievable.

6 Titration of intravenous opioids remains the standard of care for acute severe pain.

Introduction

Pain is defined by the International Association for the Study of Pain as: 'An unpleasant sensory and emotional experience associated with actual or potential tissue damage or described in terms of such damage' [1]. Acute pain is defined as: 'Pain of recent onset and probable limited duration. It usually has an identifiable temporal and causal relationship to injury or disease' [2]. However, once a patient presents for medical care, severe acute pain has ceased to serve a useful purpose. Whereas in some conditions the nature and progression of the pain may be helpful in making the diagnosis of the underlying pathology, too great a reliance has been placed upon this feature, thereby allowing the patient to suffer needlessly for prolonged periods [2,3].

When severe pain is inadequately relieved it produces pathophysiological and abnormal psychological reactions that often lead to complications. This is important as acute pain is the most common presenting complaint to an emergency department (ED) [4] and its management forms part of the daily practice of emergency medicine. It should be considered poor patient care not to treat pain while attempting to arrive at a diagnosis. There can be no greater gift to one's neighbour than to practise, teach and discover more effective methods to relieve pain and suffering [2,3]. Unfortunately, the management of acute pain is often not a specific component of medical training.

Physiology

Pain is one of the most complex aspects of an already intricate nervous system [2]. A number of theories have been developed to explain the physiology of pain, but none is proven or complete.

'Gate Control Theory'

In 1965, the Melzack–Wall 'Gate Control Theory' emphasized mechanisms in the central nervous system that control the perception of a noxious stimulus and thus integrated afferent, upstream processes with downstream modulation from the brain [5]. However, this theory did not incorporate long-term changes in the central nervous system to the noxious input and to other external factors that impinge upon the individual [5].

Nociceptor function

Most pain originates when specific nerve endings (nociceptors) are stimulated, producing nerve impulses that are transmitted to the brain. Nociception is the detection of tissue damage by specialized transducers [5]. It is now recognized that nociceptor function is altered by the 'inflammatory soup' that characterizes a region of tissue injury [5]. The final pain experience is subject to a complex series of facilitatory and inhibitory events that precede pain awareness, such as past experience, anxiety or expectation [6].

There are two types of nociceptors [7]:

❶ Mechanoreceptors, which are present mainly in the skin (also muscle, joints, viscera, meninges) and respond rapidly to pinprick or heat via Aδ, myelinated afferent neurons.

❷ Polymodal, which are widely distributed throughout most tissues and are the nerve endings of unmyelinated C-type afferent neurons. These respond to tissue damage caused by mechanical, thermal or chemical insults and are responsible for the slow onset, prolonged, poorly localized, aching pain following an injury.

Once transduced into electrical stimuli, conduction of neuronal action potentials is dependent on voltage-gated sodium channels [2]. A number of chemicals are involved in the transmission of pain to the ascending pathways in the spinothalamic tract. These include substance P and calcitonin gene-related peptide, but many others have been identified [2,8,9]. Opioid receptors are present in the dorsal horn and it is thought that encephalins (endogenous opioid peptides) are neurotransmitters in the inhibitory interneurons [7].

Phospholipids released from damaged cell membranes trigger a cascade of reactions, culminating in the production of prostaglandins that sensitize nociceptors to other inflammatory mediators, such as histamine, serotonin and bradykinin [7].

The threshold for the perception of a painful stimulus is similar in everyone and may be lowered by certain chemicals, such as the mediators of inflammation. The discrete cognitive processes and pathways involved in the interpretation of painful stimuli remain a mystery. The cognitive and emotional reactions to a given painful stimulus are variable among individuals and may be affected by culture, personality, past experiences and underlying emotional state [2,5,10]. In addition, intense and ongoing stimuli further increase the excitability of dorsal horn neurons, leading to central sensitization [2]. With increased excitability of central nociceptive neurons, the threshold for activation is reduced and pain can occur in response to low intensity, previously non-painful stimuli known as allodynia [2]. Pain is a complex, multidimensional, subjective phenomenon [10].

Assessment of pain and pain scales

There is no truly objective measurement of pain. Doctors use a variety of methods for determining how much pain a patient feels. These include the nature of the illness or injury, the patient's appearance and behaviour and physiological concomitants. None of these is reliable.

Pain scales have been developed because there are no accurate physiological or clinical signs to measure pain objectively. Three scales have become popular tools to quantify pain intensity [11,12]: the visual analogue scale (VAS), the numeric rating scale and the verbal rating scale.

Visual analogue scale

The VAS usually consists of a 100-mm line with one end indicating 'no pain' and the other end indicating the 'worst pain imaginable'. The patient simply indicates a point on the line that best indicates the amount of pain experienced. The minimum clinically significant change in patient pain severity measured with a 100-mm visual analogue scale is 13 mm [13]. Studies of pain experience that report less than a 13 mm change in pain severity, although statistically significant, may have no clinical importance [13].

Numeric rating scale

The patient is asked in the numeric rating scale to choose a number from a range (usually 0–10) that best describes the amount of pain experienced, with zero being 'no pain' and 10 being the 'worst pain imaginable'. This has been used for cardiac ischaemia pain and is also useful in illiterate patients.

Verbal rating scale

The verbal rating scale simply asks a patient to choose a phrase that best describes the pain, usually 'mild', 'moderate' or 'severe'.

The use of pain scales has been restricted predominantly to research, where experimental pain is not associated with the strong emotional component of acute pain. In the clinical setting, anxiety, sleep disruption and illness burden are present [9]. It is difficult to use a unidimensional pain scale to measure a multidimensional process. Using pain intensity alone will often fail to capture the many other qualities of pain and the overall pain experience. The best illustration of this problem is that the same pain stimulus can be applied to two different people with dramatically different pain scores and analgesic requirements [14]. At best, the use of pain scales is an indirect reflection of 'real' pain, with patient self-reporting still being the most reliable indicator of the existence and intensity of pain [15].

Nevertheless, pain scales are simple and easy to use. They are now routine in many EDs, often being a standard part of the triage process, which leads to substantially faster provision of initial analgesia [4] (see Vazirani J, Knott JC in Further reading).

General principles

Patients in pain should receive timely, effective and appropriate analgesia, titrated according to response [2]. Therefore, essentially there is no role for the intramuscular route for parenteral analgesia, which simply delays the onset of analgesia. The following points should be stressed:

- The correct analgesic dose is 'enough', that is, whatever amount is needed to achieve appropriate pain relief.
- A patient's analgesic requirements should be reviewed frequently. Do not wait for pain to return to its previous level before re-dosing with analgesia. Larger early doses and more frequent doses of analgesia are associated with lower total doses and shorter duration of analgesic use. Some patients have been misled into believing that pain medicine is dangerous, so it is important to explain the safety and efficacy of this approach.
- EDs should have specific policies relating to pain and analgesia.
- Senior clinicians should lead by example.

Specific agents

Opioids

The term 'opioid' refers to all naturally occurring and synthetic drugs producing morphine-like effects. Morphine is the standard opioid agonist against which others are judged [16]. These drugs are the most powerful agents available in the treatment of acute pain. A number of specific opioid receptors have been identified.

Opioid receptor effects

Opioids are responsible for a variety of effects, including analgesia, euphoria, respiratory depression and miosis (μ receptor); cough suppression and sedation (κ); dysphoria and hallucinations (σ); nausea and vomiting, and pruritus (δ) [7]. Opioids act on injured tissue to reduce inflammation in the dorsal horn to impede transmission of nociception and supraspinally to activate inhibitory pathways that descend to the spinal segment [9].

Unfortunately, many doctors use opioids inappropriately as there are particular concerns regarding the risks of respiratory depression and inducing iatrogenic addiction. Less than 1% of patients who receive opioids for pain develop respiratory depression [17]. Tolerance to this side effect develops simultaneously with tolerance to the analgesic effect. If the opioid dose is increased so that at least half the pain is relieved, the chance of respiratory depression is small. Further, naloxone will reverse the effects of opioids. In relation to fears of addiction, large studies have shown that inducing this following opioid analgesia use is exceedingly rare [18].

Use of intravenous opioids

From a clinical practice point of view, many patients who require intravenous opioid will also require admission to hospital, as there will be ongoing opioid requirements that can only be administered in hospital. There have been occasions where patients have received opioid analgesia that has relieved their pain and they have then been discharged without a final diagnosis. This is an unacceptable practice. A patient may present with abdominal pain with vomiting and, for instance, a provisional diagnosis of gastroenteritis is made. After opioid analgesia is given the patient may feel better and be discharged. A diagnosis, such as appendicitis or bowel obstruction, has not been excluded.

It is therefore necessary for patients to have an appropriate diagnostic evaluation to confirm a benign cause and to reassess the patient after the opioid effects have waned. For patients in whom the final diagnosis is certain, such as in anterior shoulder dislocation, discharge is appropriate after a suitable period of observation until the patient is deemed clinically fit for discharge. This is a different scenario from that described previously, as it is a single system problem in which there is no doubt about the diagnosis. In summary, pain that is considered severe enough to warrant intravenous opioid analgesia requires a high index of suspicion for significant pathology.

Side effects

All potent opioid analgesics have the potential to depress the level of consciousness, protective reflexes and vital functions. It is mandatory that these are closely monitored during and after administration [7]. Specific side effects include:

- respiratory depression: rare <1%
- nausea and vomiting: nausea occurs in approximately 40% and vomiting in 15% [7]

- hypotension: opioids may provoke histamine release
- constipation
- spasm of the sphincter of Oddi, therefore patients with biliary colic may initially experience more pain. There is no good evidence to suggest that pethidine has any clinically significant advantage at equianalgesic doses over other opioids for biliary or renal colic [16]
- miosis.

Routes of administration

Opioids may be administered by many routes, including oral, subcutaneous, intramuscular, intravenous, epidural, nebulized, intrapleural, intranasal, intra-articular and transdermal. All may have a role in a specific clinical situation [4]. There is a good rationale for the use of the intravenous route in moderate-to-severe pain [4] and titration of intravenous opioids remains the standard of care for acute severe pain.

Opioid analgesics

Morphine The standard intravenous morphine dose is 0.1–0.2 mg/kg or more with a duration of action of 2–3 h. This should be initiated as a loading dose of opioid to provide rapid initial pain relief aiming for an optimal balance between effective pain relief and minimal side effects. This means tailoring the approach to each individual patient. Thus, a young fit healthy man with renal colic may require an initial bolus of 0.1 mg/kg morphine, followed by further increments of 0.05 mg/kg. Conversely, a frail elderly patient may only tolerate 1.0–2.5 mg morphine total to begin with. There may also be considerable inter-individual variation in response to analgesia. Procedural pain may require higher-dose opioid analgesia, which has been found to be well tolerated and safe [19]. Appropriate monitoring and resuscitation equipment should be available to maximize safety.

Rapid pain relief and titration to effect are obvious advantages. Intramuscular administration results in unreliable and variable absorption and older routine practices, such as prescribing '5–10 mg morphine IM', take no account of an individual's requirements [7].

Pethidine Pethidine should be used with caution in patients with renal failure, as there is increased risk of central nervous system toxicity due to the toxic metabolite, norpethidine. Norpethidine causes tremor, twitching, agitation

and convulsions [16]. Also pethidine is contraindicated in patients receiving monoamine oxidase (MAO) inhibitors, as they interfere with pethidine metabolism, increasing the likelihood of toxicity [20]. Finally, pethidine may trigger the serotonin syndrome if used concomitantly with selective serotonin reuptake inhibitors (SSRIs).

Pethidine has approximately one-eighth the potency of morphine and causes the same degree of bronchospasm and increased biliary pressure as morphine [2]. Its use has now declined and it should continue to be discouraged in favour of other opioids [2].

Fentanyl Allergic reactions are extremely rare with opioids. Fentanyl does not release histamine, making it ideal for treating patients with reactive airways disease. There are advantages in using fentanyl for brief procedures in the ED because of its short half-life. The intravenous dose of fentanyl is 1–2 µg/kg or more with a duration of action of 30–60 min. High doses of fentanyl may produce muscular rigidity, which may be so severe as to make ventilation difficult, but which responds to naloxone or muscle relaxants. Intranasal fentanyl is an effective analgesic in the ED and in the pre-hospital setting [2].

Oral opioids

Oral opioids tend to be underused in the ED, but are effective for all levels of pain and are associated with improved patient satisfaction. Their side effect profile may be better than paracetamol/codeine combinations. Oxycodone (immediate release) reaches peak levels at 45 min to 1 h but the dose should be reduced and dosing interval increased in the elderly and in those with hepatic or renal dysfunction. The main contraindication is acute respiratory depression. The initial dose is 5–10 mg. However, it is important to be aware that the increased prescribing of oral opioids is associated with increased deaths. Oxycodone/naloxone combinations are now available.

Codeine Codeine is the most commonly used oral opioid prodrug. Unfortunately, up to 6–10% of the Caucasian population, 2% of Asians, and 1% of Arabs have poorly functional cytochrome P450 2D6 (CYP2D6), which may render codeine largely ineffective for analgesia in these patients, although some analgesic efficacy may occur via alternate cytochrome P450 pathways.

Prescribed alone in doses as high as 120 mg, codeine has been demonstrated to be no more effective than placebo in both the adult and geriatric populations, while causing increasing gastrointestinal side effects, such as nausea, vomiting and constipation, with increasing doses [4]. It is frequently given in combination with paracetamol or aspirin.

Tramadol Tramadol is a new opioid, with novel non-opioid properties [21]. Its efficacy lies between codeine and morphine. It has a relative lack of serious side effects, such as respiratory depression, and the potential for abuse and psychological dependence is low [21]. However, other side effects, such as nausea, vomiting, dizziness and somnolence, may be troublesome and there is a risk of seizures [21,22]. Thus, it should be avoided or used with caution in patients who are taking drugs that reduce the seizure threshold, such as tricyclic antidepressants and SSRIs. Also the concomitant administration of tramadol with monoamine oxidase inhibitors, or within 2 weeks of their withdrawal, is contraindicated [21].

The role of tramadol in emergency medicine is ill defined. One review concluded that tramadol does not offer any particular benefits over existing analgesics for the majority of emergency pain relief situations [22], with oral doses having equivalent analgesic effects in mild-to-moderate severity acute pain compared with currently available analgesics [22]. Intravenous tramadol is less effective than intravenous morphine [22].

However, tramadol may be useful in certain situations: [22]

- for patients in whom codeine is not effective
- where non-steroidal anti-inflammatory drugs (NSAIDs) are contraindicated
- for the treatment of chronic pain.

Non-opioid analgesics

Simple analgesics

Non-steroidal anti-inflammatory drugs
Non-steroidal anti-inflammatory drugs are either non-selective cyclo-oxygenase (COX) inhibitors or selective inhibitors of COX-2 (COX-2 inhibitors). NSAIDs are effective analgesic agents for moderate pain, specifically when there is associated inflammation [4]. As with opioids, there are multiple routes of administration available. Unfortunately, their use in acute severe pain is limited by the length of onset time of 20–30 min. There is no clear superiority of one agent over another.

There is up to a 30% incidence of upper gastrointestinal bleeding when NSAIDs are used for over 1–2 weeks. The risk of bleeding in the elderly for short (3–5 days) acute therapy appears to be minimal [4]. NSAID use in pregnancy (especially late) is not recommended. Ibuprofen is considered the NSAID of choice in lactation.

NSAIDs have a spectrum of analgesic, anti-inflammatory and antipyretic effects and are effective analgesics in a variety of pain states [2]. Unfortunately, significant contraindications and adverse effects limit the use of NSAIDs, many of these being regulated by COX-1 [2]. NSAIDs are useful analgesic adjuncts and hence NSAIDs are therefore integral components of multimodal analgesia [2]. NSAID side effects are more common with long-term use. The main concerns are renal impairment, interference with platelet function, peptic ulceration and bronchospasm in individuals who have aspirin-exacerbated respiratory disease [2]. In general, the risk and severity of NSAID-associated side effects is increased in elderly people [2].

Caution is therefore needed in the elderly and in patients with renal disease, hypertension and heart failure, or with asthma. NSAIDs reduce renal cortical blood flow and may induce renal impairment, especially when used in patients already on diuretics. In patients with asthma, 2–20% are aspirin sensitive and there is a 50–100% cross-sensitivity with NSAIDs.

Ketorolac is a parenteral NSAID that is equipotent to opioids, with ketorolac and morphine equivalent in reducing pain. There is a benefit favouring ketorolac in terms of side effects when ketorolac is titrated intravenously for isolated limb injuries [23,24]. However, the utility of ketorolac in acute pain is limited due to a prolonged onset of action and a significant number of patients (25%) who exhibit little or no response [25]. There is also benefit to using ketorolac for acute renal colic [23,26]. A combination of morphine and ketorolac offered pain relief superior to either drug alone and was associated with a decreased requirement for rescue analgesia in patients with renal colic [27]. Rectal NSAIDs (e.g. indomethacin 100 mg) are an effective alternative to parenteral NSAIDs in the treatment of renal colic.

Paracetamol Paracetamol is an effective analgesic for acute pain [2] and has useful antipyretic activity [28]. The addition of an NSAID further improves efficacy [2]. Paracetamol inhibits prostaglandin synthetase in the hypothalamus, prevents release of spinal prostaglandin and inhibits inducible nitric oxide synthesis in macrophages [28].

Indications for paracetamol include mild pain, particularly of soft tissue and musculoskeletal origin, mild procedural pain, supplementation of opioids in the management of more severe pain allowing a reduction in opioid dosage and as an alternative to aspirin [28]. Paracetamol has no gastrointestinal side effects of note and may be prescribed safely in patients with peptic ulcer disease or gastritis [4]. Aspirin has the risk of gastrointestinal side effects, such as ulceration and bleeding. It also has an antiplatelet effect which lasts for the life of the platelet.

Paracetamol is rapidly absorbed with a peak concentration reached in 30–90 min [28]. The recommended adult dose is 1 g every 4–6 h to a generally accepted maximum of 4 g per day [28]. Paracetamol has a low adverse event profile and is an excellent analgesic, especially when used in adequate dose. Parenteral paracetamol is now available and may have additional utility, e.g. in the vomiting patient. Chronic use of paracetamol alone does not seem to cause analgesic nephropathy [28]. It can be used safely in alcoholics and patients with liver metastases [28,29].

Combination drugs Non-opioid agents, e.g. paracetamol, NSAIDs and paracetamol/codeine combinations, are all useful analgesics for mild-to-moderate pain. A systematic review found that paracetamol–codeine combinations in single dose studies produce a slightly increased analgesic effect (5%) compared with paracetamol alone [30]. However, none of the studies reviewed were based in the ED. In multidosage, paracetamol–codeine preparations have significantly increased side effects [30]. However, other reports state that the combination of paracetamol 1000 mg plus codeine 60 mg has a number needed to treat of 2.2 [2]. NSAIDs have a higher rate of serious adverse effects.

Other analgesic agents

Nitrous oxide
Nitrous oxide is an inhalational analgesic and sedative which, in a 50% mixture with oxygen

(Entonox), has equivalent potency to 10 mg morphine in an adult [7]. The Entonox delivery system uses a preferential inhalational demand arrangement for self-administration, which requires an airtight fit between the mask/mouthpiece and face. As the patient holds the mask/mouthpiece, their grip will relax if drowsiness occurs, the airtight seal will be lost and the gas flow stops, thereby avoiding overdosage.

This system requires a degree of patient involvement and cooperation and is useful for patients who have difficult intravenous access or are needle-phobic. Patients who are elderly, young, confused or uncooperative will not find the technique effective. Nitrous oxide increases the volume of a pneumothorax or any other gas-filled cavity, so is contraindicated in patients with pneumothorax or pneumoperitoneum.

Ketamine

Ketamine is an N-methyl-D-aspartate (NMDA) antagonist. It is a unique anaesthetic that induces a state of dissociation between the cortical and limbic systems to produce a state of dissociative anaesthesia, with analgesia, amnesia, mild sedation and immobilization. It does not impair protective airway reflexes and random or purposeful movements are frequently observed in patients after administration. Side effects include hypersalivation, vomiting, emergence reactions, nightmares, laryngospasm, hypertension, tachycardia and increased intracranial pressure [31,32].

There are many potential contraindications to ketamine use including upper or lower respiratory infection, procedures involving the posterior pharynx, cystic fibrosis, age younger than 3 months, head injury, increased intracranial pressure, acute glaucoma or globe penetration, uncontrolled hypertension, congestive cardiac failure, arterial aneurysm, acute intermittent porphyria and thyrotoxicosis [32]. Despite this, ketamine is used increasingly in the EDs as part of procedural sedation (see Chapter 22.3). It is also an effective analgesic at sub-dissociative doses especially for opioid resistant pain, e.g. 0.2–0.3 mg/kg bolus plus infusion at 0.2 mg/kg/h.

Pain relief in pregnancy

Non-pharmacological treatment options should be considered where possible for pain management in pregnancy, because most drugs cross the placenta [2]. Use of medications for pain in pregnancy should be guided by published recommendations [2]. Paracetamol is regarded as the analgesic of choice [2]. NSAIDs are used with caution in the last trimester of pregnancy and should be avoided after the 32nd week [2]. The use of NSAIDs is associated with increased risk of miscarriage [2]. Overall, the use of opioids to treat pain in pregnancy appears safe [2].

Non-pharmacological therapies

Although pain perception involves neuroanatomical processes, the other interrelated component of pain reaction is psychophysiological. The use of non-pharmacological techniques is therefore important. These include empathy, a compassionate approach, a calm manner and reassurance. Immobilization of fractures with splinting is effective, as is the application of ice to a wound. Other techniques, such as hypnosis, transcutaneous nerve stimulation, acupuncture and manipulation, have not been widely studied in the ED setting.

Special pain situations and non-analgesic agents

This chapter has focused on specific analgesic agents, but there are many miscellaneous agents that are effective in providing disease-specific analgesia.

Examples of these include:

- triptans for migraine
- glyceryl trinitrate and β-blockers for acute cardiac ischaemia pain
- antiviral agents for herpes zoster
- antidepressants (e.g. nortriptyline), anticonvulsants (e.g. carbamazepine) or gabapentin for neuropathic pain
- oxygen therapy for cluster headache
- calcium gluconate for hydrofluoric acid burns
- hot water (43°C) for venomous marine stings

In addition, adjuvant therapy with anxiolytics, such as midazolam, contributes to pain relief. Obtaining a definitive diagnosis allows directed therapy that contributes to pain relief. If specific treatments appear to be ineffective, then the diagnosis should be reconsidered.

Acute neuropathic pain

Acute neuropathic pain is an important issue in the ED. This may be due to conditions such as sciatica and cervical radiculopathy. In addition to agents, such as the antidepressants (e.g. nortriptylline) or anticonvulsants (e.g. carbamazepine), another option includes the use of antihyperalgesic drugs, such as gabapentin 100–300 mg per dose, repeated as necessary, titrating up to a maximum of 3600 mg per day over time. The main side effects are dizziness, somnolence and ataxia. However, there have been no ED studies of gabapentin or pregabalin and there is wide variability of response.

Chronic pain

Chronic pain 'commonly persists beyond the time of healing of an injury and frequently there may not be any clearly identifiable cause' [2]. Patients with chronic pain attend the ED with exacerbations of their chronic pain and are often taking multimodal therapies prescribed by a pain specialist. The main difference between acute and chronic pain is that, in chronic pain, central sensitization is the main underlying pathophysiology [33]. It is important to avoid a judgemental attitude to these patients as there is a risk of overlooking serious pathology.

Antihyperalgesic drugs in the setting of chronic pain, especially ketamine, are of particular value in those with poor opioid responsiveness [2]. Other antihyperalgesics may be useful for neuropathic pain, such as gabapentin and pregabalin.

Another issue with chronic pain is to be aware of adjuvant therapies for decreasing the likelihood of chronic pain developing. For example, early management of acute zoster infection may reduce the incidence of post-herpetic neuralgia [2]. Aciclovir given within 72 h of onset of the rash accelerates the resolution of pain and reduces the risk of post-herpetic neuralgia [2]. Amitriptyline 25 mg daily in patients over 60 years for 90 days, started at the onset of acute zoster, reduces pain prevalence at 6 months post-zoster infection [34].

Acute abdomen

Traditionally, it was held that pain relief masks the clinical signs of pathology in the acute abdomen. Evidence from randomized controlled trials clearly shows that the early administration of opioids in patients with an acute abdomen does not reduce the detection rate of serious pathology and may actually facilitate the diagnosis. Thus, titrated opioid analgesia should *never* be withheld, certainly not pending surgical review. The effect of analgesia on physical signs cannot be used as a diagnostic test [35–37].

Likely developments over the next 5–10 years

- Further study on the role and utility of various oral analgesics for commonly treated conditions in the ED, including new agents or formulations.
- Use of patient-controlled analgaesia.
- Alternative administration techniques, including needleless systems.
- Use of non-pharmacologic techniques, such as acupuncture.
- Better understanding of the pathophysiology of pain.

Controversies

- Development of a uniform approach to pain research in order to make meaningful comparisons between studies.
- Development of an objective measure of pain.
- The effectiveness of codeine combinations in ED patients.

References

[1] International Association for the Study of Pain. Pain terms: a list of definitions and notes on usage. Pain 1979;6:249–52.

[2] Australian and New Zealand College of Anaesthetists and Faculty of Pain Medicine. Acute pain management: scientific evidence 2nd ed. Canberra: Australian Government National Health and Medical Research Council; 2005.

[3] Bonica J. Pain management in emergency medicine. Norwalk: Appleton & Lange; 1987.

[4] Ducharme J. Emergency pain management: a Canadian Association of Emergency Physicians (CAEP) consensus document. J Emerg Med 1994;12:855–66.

[5] Loeser JD, Melzack R. Pain: an overview. Lancet 1999;353:1607–9.

[6] Paris P, Uram M, Ginsburg M. Physiological mechanisms of pain. Norwalk: Appleton & Lange; 1987.

[7] Nolan J, Baskett P. Analgesia and anaesthesia. Cambridge: Cambridge University Press; 1997.

[8] Besson JM. The neurobiology of pain. Lancet 1999;353:1610–5.

[9] Carr DB, Goudas LC. Acute pain. Lancet 1999;353:2051–8.

[10] Turk D, Melzack R. The measurement of pain and the assessment of people experiencing pain. New York: Guildford Press; 1992.

[11] Ho K, Spence J, Murphy MF. Review of pain measurement tools. Ann Emerg Med 1996;27:427–32.

[12] Turk DC, Okifuji A. Assessment of patients' reporting of pain: an integrated perspective. Lancet 1999;353:1784–8.

[13] Todd KH, Funk KG, Funk JP, et al. Clinical significance of reported changes in pain severity. Ann Emerg Med 1996;27:485–9.

[14] Fatovich D. The validity of pain scales in the emergency setting. J Emerg Med 1998;16:347.

[15] Acute Pain Management Guideline Panel. Acute pain management: operative or medical procedures and trauma: clinical practice guideline. Washington DC; 1992.

[16] McQuay H. Opioids in pain management. Lancet 1999;353:2229–32.

[17] Miller R. Analgesics. New York: Wiley; 1976.

[18] Porter J, Jick H. Addiction rare in patients treated with narcotics. N Engl J Med 1980;302:123.

[19] Barsan WG, Tomassoni AJ, Seger D, et al. Safety assessment of high-dose narcotic analgesia for emergency department procedures. Ann Emerg Med 1993;22:1444–9.

[20] Meyer D, Halfin V. Toxicity secondary to meperidine in patients on monoamine oxidase inhibitors: a case report and critical review. J Clin Psychopharmacol 1981;1:319–21.

[21] Bamigade T, Langford R. The clinical use of tramadol hydrochloride. Pain Rev 1998;5:155–82.

[22] Close BR. Tramadol: does it have a role in emergency medicine? Emerg Med Australas 2005;17:73–83.

[23] Rainer TH, Jacobs P, Ng YC, et al. Cost effectiveness analysis of intravenous ketorolac and morphine for treating pain after limb injury: double blind randomised controlled trial. Br Med J 2000;321:1247–51.

[24] Jelinek GA. Ketorolac versus morphine for severe pain. Ketorolac is more effective, cheaper, and has fewer side effects. Br Med J 2000;321:1236–7.

[25] Catapano MS. The analgesic efficacy of ketorolac for acute pain. J Emerg Med 1996;14:67–75.

[26] Holdgate A, Pollock T. Systematic review of the relative efficacy of non-steroidal anti-inflammatory drugs and opioids in the treatment of acute renal colic. Br Med J 2004;328:1401.

[27] Safdar B, Degutis LC, Landry K, et al. Intravenous morphine plus ketorolac is superior to either drug alone for treatment of acute renal colic. Ann Emerg Med 2006;48:173–81.

[28] Therapeutic Guidelines Ltd. Therapeutic guidelines: Analgesic; Version 6. North Melbourne: Therapeutic Guidelines Ltd; 2012.

[29] Dart RC, Kuffner EK, Rumack BH. Treatment of pain or fever with paracetamol (acetaminophen) in the alcoholic patient: a systematic review. Am J Ther 2000;7:123–34.

[30] de Craen AJ, Di Giulio G, Lampe-Schoenmaeckers JE. Analgesic efficacy and safety of paracetamol-codeine combinations versus paracetamol alone: a systematic review. Br Med J 1996;313:321–5.

[31] Terndrup T. Pain control, analgesia and sedation. St Louis: Mosby Year Book; 1992.

[32] Green SM, Johnson NE. Ketamine sedation for pediatric procedures: Part 2, Review and implications. Ann Emerg Med 1990;19:1033–46.

[33] Siddall PJ, Cousins MJ. Persistent pain as a disease entity: implications for clinical management. Anesth Analges 2004;99:510–20.

[34] Bowsher D. The effects of pre-emptive treatment of postherpetic neuralgia with amitriptyline: a randomized, double-blind, placebo-controlled trial. J Pain Symptom Manage 1997;13:327–31.

[35] Thomas SH, Silen W, Cheema F, et al. Effects of morphine analgesia on diagnostic accuracy in Emergency Department patients with abdominal pain: a prospective, randomized trial. J Am Coll Surg 2003;196:18–31.

[36] Attard AR, Corlett MJ, Kidner NJ, et al. Safety of early pain relief for acute abdominal pain. Br Med J 1992;305:554–6.

[37] Zoltie N, Cust MP. Analgesia in the acute abdomen. Ann Roy Coll Surg Engl 1986;68:209–10.

Further reading

Birnbaum A, Schechter C, Tufaro V, et al. Efficacy of patient-controlled analgesia for patients with acute abdominal pain in the emergency department: a randomized trial. Acad Emerg Med 2012;19:370–7.

Jao K, Taylor DMcD, Taylor SE, et al. Simple clinical targets associated with a high level of patient satisfaction with their pain management. Emerg Med Australas 2011;23:195–201.

Schug SA. Acute pain management in the opioid-tolerant patient. Pain Manage 2012;2:1–11.

Vazirani J, Knott JC. Mandatory pain scoring at triage reduces time to analgesia. Ann Emerg Med 2012;59:134–8.

22.2 Local anaesthesia

Anthony Brown • Tor NO Ercleve

ESSENTIALS

1 Local anaesthetic infiltration and nerve blocks may be used as a supplement to oral, inhaled or parenteral analgesia.

2 Or they may be the primary method of achieving analgesia, particularly where pain is localized to a digit or within a peripheral nerve distribution region.

3 Local anaesthetic toxicity may occur with inadvertent bolus intravenous injection or by exceeding the recommended maximum safe dose. Neurological and cardiovascular effects predominate and may be lethal.

4 Resuscitation equipment should always be available when using these agents. Refractory local anaesthetic systemic toxicity (LAST) with cardiovascular collapse or arrest may respond to 20% lipid emulsion therapy.

5 Intravenous regional anaesthesia with prilocaine for Bier's block is a simple, safe technique commonly used for reduction of forearm fractures, but requires two medical practitioners and specialized equipment.

6 Formal training and accreditation should occur prior to independent practice, particularly with the more complex blocks, such as Bier's and femoral nerve.

Table 22.2.1 Maximum recommended safe dose and duration of action of common local anaesthetics

Drug	Dose (mg/kg)*	Duration (h)
Lignocaine	3	0.5–1
Lignocaine with adrenaline	7	2–5
Bupivacaine	2	2–4
Prilocaine	6	0.5–1.5

*A 1% solution contains 10 mg/mL.

The duration of action of local anaesthetics is related to the degree of protein binding, vasoactivity, concentration and possibly pH, although the addition of adrenaline is the most practical way to prolong their effect. Table 22.2.1 gives standard maximum safe doses and duration of action of commonly used agents. Solutions containing adrenaline should not be injected near end arteries, such as in the fingers, toes, nose or penis, even though this well-established dogma is surprisingly not supported by the literature. Normal blood flow is restored to the digit within 60–90 min of inadvertent injection of local anaesthesia with adrenaline (epinephrine) at standard commercial dilutions, without any evidence of harm [4].

LOCAL ANAESTHESIA

Local anaesthetic infiltration and nerve blocks should be used for patients presenting to the emergency department (ED) with pain, either to supplement other analgesia or for definitive pain relief. Nerve blocks are most appropriate when the pain is localized, as in certain fractures and wounds to a digit, or within a peripheral nerve distribution region. Local anaesthesia may also be used topically, particularly in children, and prior to arterial blood gas puncture and insertion of large intravenous cannulae where, contrary to popular perception, it does not increase the likelihood of failure [1,2].

Pharmacology

Local anaesthetic agents are all weak organic bases that inactivate intracellular fast sodium channels, temporarily blocking membrane depolarization and preventing nerve impulse transmission. All are vasodilators with the exception of ropivacaine and cocaine, hence the use of adrenaline to prolong their duration of activity and to improve safety by delaying absorption and/or by administering lower effective doses.

Amino ester and amino amide local anaesthetics

Local anaesthetic agents containing an ester bond between the intermediate chain and lipophilic aromatic end (amino esters) include cocaine, procaine and amethocaine. They are poorly protein bound and undergo hydrolysis by plasma pseudocholinesterase to para-amino benzoic acid. Amide-type agents containing an amide bond between the intermediate chain and aromatic end (amino amides) include lignocaine, prilocaine, bupivacaine and ropivacaine, are highly protein bound, much more stable and undergo hepatic metabolism.

Local anaesthetics are available in single or multidose vials, with or without dilute adrenaline at 1:200 000 (containing 5 μg adrenaline per millilitre) to prolong their duration of action. Antioxidants, such as sodium bisulphite or metabisulphite, are added to adrenaline-containing solutions and preservative, such as methylparaben, to multidose vials and are implicated in some apparent allergic reactions to the local anaesthetic. True allergy to local anaesthetics is extremely rare when verified by progressive challenge testing and is usually to the amino esters [3].

Adverse effects

Systemic toxicity

Systemic toxicity occurs after unrecognized rapid intravenous injection or by exceeding the recommended safe maximum dose. Symptoms and signs of toxicity are related to plasma drug levels and progress from circumoral tingling, dizziness, tinnitus and visual disturbance to muscular twitching, confusion, convulsions, coma and apnoea. Cardiovascular effects are also seen with high plasma levels, including bradycardia, hypotension and cardiovascular collapse ultimately with ventricular fibrillation or asystole, which are all exacerbated by associated hypoxia. See Table 22.2.2 for the features of local anaesthetic toxicity related to increasing plasma levels.

The management of systemic toxicity includes immediate cessation of the drug,

Table 22.2.2 Features of systemic local anaesthetic toxicity (in order of increasing plasma levels)
Circumoral tingling
Dizziness
Tinnitus
Visual disturbance
Muscular twitching
Confusion
Convulsions
Coma
Apnoea
Cardiovascular collapse (highest plasma levels)

Table 22.2.3 Adverse reactions to local anaesthetics (other than systemic toxicity)

Allergy:
    esters >> amides
    additives, such as methylparaben, sodium
    metabisulphite

Catecholamine effects from added adrenaline
Vasovagal
Delayed wound healing
Malignant hyperthermia
Methaemoglobinaemia – prilocaine,   benzocaine

summoning help, airway maintenance, supplemental oxygen and incremental doses of an intravenous benzodiazepine, such as midazolam 0.05–0.1 mg/kg, for seizures. Major reactions may require endotracheal intubation, fluids and cautious use of vasopressors and inotropes, as high doses can impede resuscitation in toxic cardiomyopathy. Refractory arrhythmias with cardiovascular collapse from local anaesthetic systemic toxicity (LAST) may respond best to intravenous 20% lipid emulsion 1.5 mL/kg bolus followed by 0.25 mL/kg/min for roughly 10 min following recovery of vital signs [5].

As adverse reactions occur immediately or within minutes after local anaesthetic use, medical expertise, resuscitation equipment and monitoring facilities must always be available.

Other reactions

Other adverse reactions to local anaesthetics involve allergy, including anaphylaxis, predominantly to the amino esters (rarely amino amides), catecholamine effects from added adrenaline, vasovagal reactions when the patient is upright, such as during a dental procedure, cytotoxic delayed wound healing, malignant hyperthermia from amino amide use and methaemoglobinaemia due to prilocaine or benzocaine (Table 22.2.3).

Topical anaesthesia

Some agents such as EMLA (eutectic mixture of local anaesthetics including 2.5% lignocaine and 2.5% prilocaine) are used topically, particularly to decrease the pain of insertion

of cannulae or for lumbar puncture and suprapubic catheter insertion in children. EMLA takes up to 1 h for maximal effect and, paradoxically, is a venoconstrictor making vessel puncture harder. A potentially superior alternative for cannula insertion is 4% amethocaine (AnGel) as this has a quicker onset and is a vasodilator, although operator experience in cannulation is likely to be of more relevance [6].

Likewise, a mixture of 1:1000 adrenaline, 4% lignocaine and 0.5% amethocaine, with the acronym ALA (or known as LET in North America standing for lidocaine, epinephrine and tetracaine) up to 0.1 mL/kg, may be used inside small wounds instead of, or to reduce the pain of, injecting local anaesthetic prior to closure, again in children or adolescents.

SPECIFIC NERVE BLOCKS

The following nerve blocks are contraindicated in uncooperative patients, those with local sepsis in the injection zone and in the rare patient with true local anaesthetic allergy. Care must be taken not to exceed the recommended maximum local anaesthetic doses (see Table 22.2.1) and monitoring facilities, resuscitation equipment and medical expertise must be available at all times.

Formal training and accreditation should occur prior to independent practice, paticularly with the more complex blocks, such as Bier's and femoral nerve.

Digital nerve block ('ring block')

Indications
Wound debridement, suturing, drainage of infection, fracture or dislocation reduction around the nail, fingertip and distal finger or toe.

Contraindications
Local sepsis, Raynaud's phenomenon and peripheral vascular disease.

Technique
Use 2% plain lignocaine. Inject 1–1.5 mL using a 25-gauge needle into the palmar aspect of the base of the finger or toe, approaching vertically from the dorsum. Withdraw the needle until subcutaneous and rotate slightly until pointing to the extensor surface of the digit and inject a further 0.5 mL (Fig. 22.2.1). Perform the

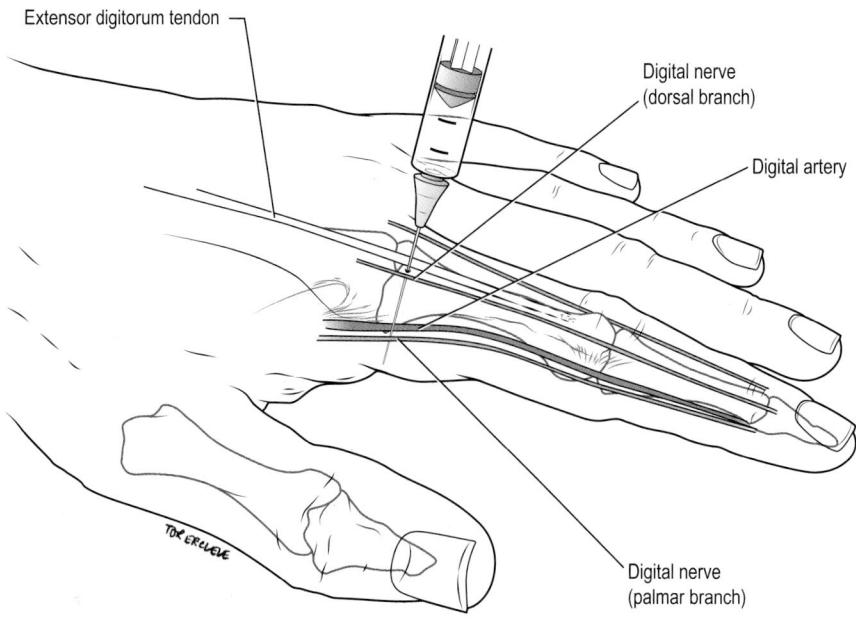

Extensor digitorum tendon

Digital nerve (dorsal branch)

Digital artery

Digital nerve (palmar branch)

Fig. 22.2.1 Digital nerve block.

same procedure on the other side of the digit. Allow at least 5 min for the block to work.

Complications

Avoid intravascular injection by aspirating prior to injection. Do not use a tourniquet or more than 4 mL total volume, to avoid impairing the circulation due to high local tissue pressures.

Nerve blocks at the wrist

These provide anaesthesia to the hand, particularly for diffuse lesions hard to infiltrate directly, such as 'gravel rash', or when the hand is swollen or burned.

Ulnar nerve wrist block (lateral approach)

Indications

Procedures on the medial border of the hand and medial 1.5 digits or combined with median and radial nerve blocks for hand anaesthesia.

Contraindications

Local sepsis, neuritis.

Technique

Identify the flexor carpi ulnaris tendon at the proximal palmar crease. Introduce a 25-gauge needle on the ulnar aspect of the tendon, directed horizontally and laterally for 1–1.5 cm

under the tendon. Inject 4 mL of 1% lignocaine. Withdraw the needle until subcutaneous then inject 5 mL of 1% lignocaine fanwise to the dorsal midline, to block superficial cutaneous branches (Fig. 22.2.2).

Median nerve wrist block

Indications

Procedures on the lateral border of the hand in the territory supplied by the median nerve, excluding the medial 1.5 digits or combined with ulnar and radial nerve blocks for hand anaesthesia.

Contraindications

Local sepsis, carpal tunnel syndrome or neuritis.

Technique

Identify the tendons of the flexor carpi radialis and palmaris longus at the proximal wrist crease. Introduce a 25-gauge needle vertically 0.5–1 cm lateral to the palmaris longus (or 0.5 cm medial to the flexor carpi radialis in the 10% of individuals lacking a palmaris longus). Inject 5 mL of 1% lignocaine when the needle gives as it penetrates the flexor retinaculum or paraesthesiae are elicited, at a depth usually of no more than 1 cm to the skin (Fig. 22.2.3). Avoid injecting into the nerve itself, as it may lie more superficial than this.

Radial nerve wrist block

Indications

Procedures on the dorsal radial aspect of the hand or combined with ulnar and median nerve blocks for hand anaesthesia.

Contraindications

Local sepsis, neuritis.

Technique

Identify the tendon of the extensor carpi radialis and infiltrate 5–10 mL of 1% lignocaine subcutaneously in a ring around the radial border of the wrist to the area overlying the radial pulse, at the level of the proximal palmar crease (Fig. 22.2.4).

Nerve blocks of the leg

Femoral nerve block

Indications

Analgesia for fractured shaft of femur, especially prior to applying dynamic splintage.

Contraindications

Local sepsis, bleeding tendency.

Technique

Palpate the femoral artery below the midpoint of the inguinal ligament, which extends from the pubic tubercle to the anterior superior iliac spine. Insert a 21-gauge needle 1 cm lateral to this point, perpendicular to the skin. Advance until paraesthesiae are elicited down the leg and withdraw slightly, aspirate to exclude intravascular placement and inject 10 mL of 0.5% bupivacaine (50 mg). Alternatively, feel for a give as the needle punctures the fascia lata, aspirate, then inject 10 mL of 0.5% bupivacaine fanwise laterally away from the artery (Fig. 22.2.5). Or preferably now use ultrasound guidance throughout. Allow up to 15–30 min for onset of maximal anaesthesia.

Complications

Puncture of femoral artery.

Foot blocks at the ankle

Indications

Where local anaesthetic infiltration of the foot is awkward or difficult because of thick sole skin or pain, or when excessive amounts of anaesthetic would otherwise be required.

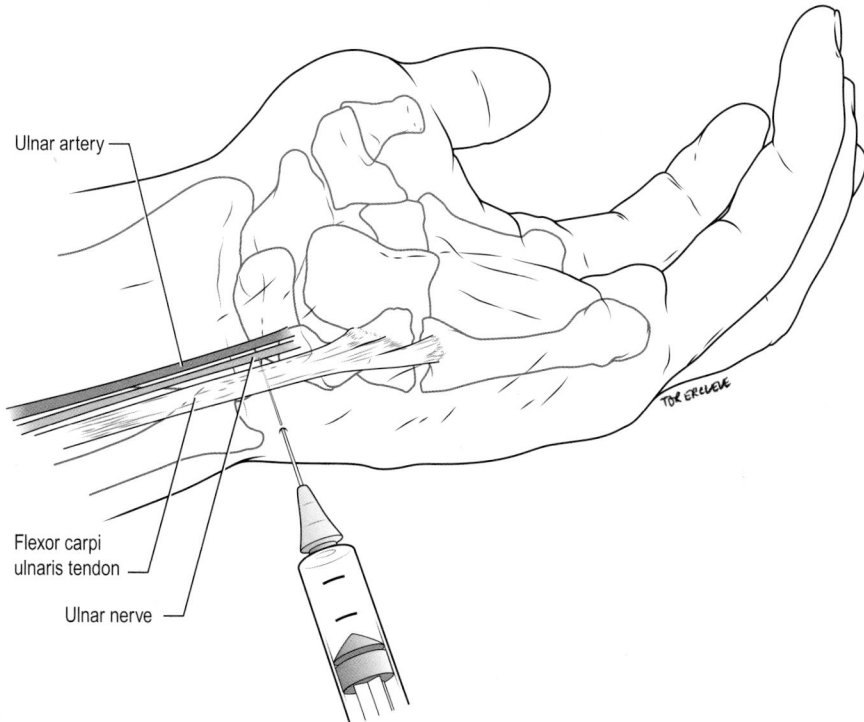

Ulnar artery

Flexor carpi ulnaris tendon

Ulnar nerve

Fig. 22.2.2 Ulnar nerve wrist block (lateral approach).

band between the extensor hallucis longus tendon and the lateral malleolus, on the anterior aspect of the ankle (see Fig. 22.2.6). This block anaesthetizes the dorsum of the foot, save for the lateral aspect (see sural nerve above) and interdigital web between the hallux and second toe (see deep peroneal nerve below).

Saphenous nerve The saphenous nerve is blocked by injecting 3–5 mL of 1% lignocaine subcutaneously above the medial malleolus, laterally until over the tibialis anterior tendon (Fig. 22.2.7). It anaesthetizes the area around the medial malleolus anteriorly and, to a lesser degree, posteriorly.

Posterior tibial nerve The posterior tibial nerve is blocked by infiltrating 3–5 mL of 1% lignocaine immediately lateral to the posterior tibial artery as it passes behind the medial malleolus, at a depth of 0.5–1 cm to the skin (see Fig. 22.2.7). It anaesthetizes the sole of the foot, excluding the posterolateral heel (see sural nerve above), via its medial and lateral plantar branches.

Deep peroneal (anterior tibial) nerve The deep peroneal (anterior tibial) nerve is blocked by infiltrating 1–2 mL of 1% lignocaine just above the base of the medial malleolus, lateral and behind the extensor hallucis longus by the dorsalis pedis pulse at a depth of 0.5 cm (see Fig. 22.2.7). It anaesthetizes the interdigital web between the hallux and second toe.

Complications

Exceeding a total volume of 20 mL of 1% lignocaine local anaesthetic (ie. 3 mg/kg) that risks systemic toxicity or poor peripheral perfusion due to raised tissue pressures.

Intravenous regional anaesthesia or Bier's block

Indications

Operative procedures, such as debridement, tendon repair and foreign body removal in the forearm and hand. Reduction of fractures and dislocations, typically Colles' fracture of the wrist.

Contraindications

Local anaesthetic sensitivity, peripheral vascular disease including Raynaud's phenomenon, sickle cell disease, cellulitis, uncooperative patients including children, hypertension with systolic blood pressure over 200 mmHg, severe liver disease, and unstable epilepsy.

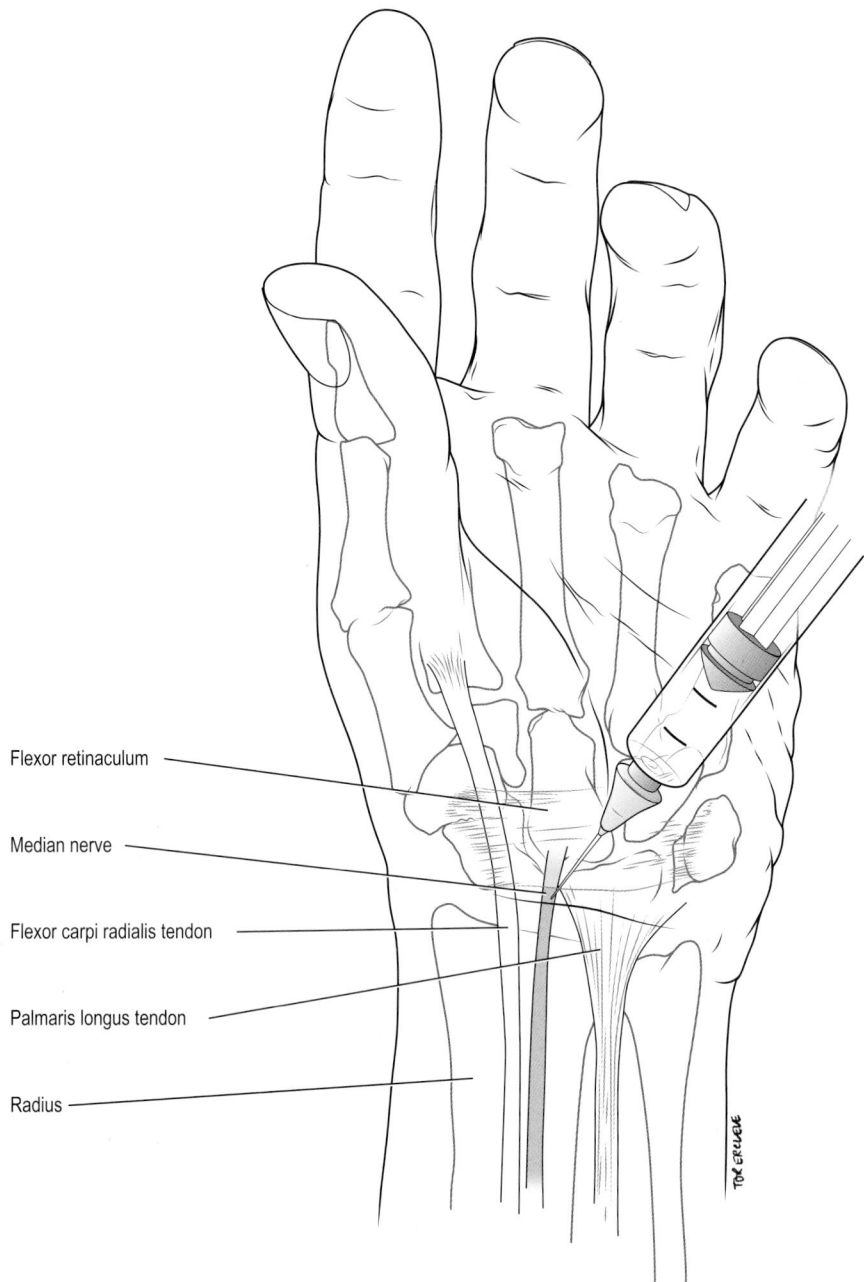

Flexor retinaculum

Median nerve

Flexor carpi radialis tendon

Palmaris longus tendon

Radius

Fig. 22.2.3 Median nerve wrist block.

Contraindications

Local sepsis, peripheral vascular disease.

Technique

Three superficial nerves, the sural, superficial peroneal and saphenous, are blocked by subcutaneous infiltration in a band around 75% of the ankle circumference. Two deeper nerves – the posterior tibial by the posterior tibial artery and the deep peroneal (anterior tibial) nerve by the dorsalis pedis artery – are blocked, usually in combinations with the superficial ones, according to the area of anaesthesia required.

Sural nerve The sural nerve is blocked by injecting 3–5 mL of 1% lignocaine subcutaneously in a band between the Achilles tendon and the lateral malleolus, 1 cm above and posterior to the malleolus (Fig. 22.2.6). It anaesthetizes a small strip on the lateral dorsum of the foot at the base of the little toe to the lateral malleolus and the posterolateral aspect of the ankle and heel.

Superficial peroneal nerves Superficial peroneal nerves are blocked by injecting 4–6 mL of 1% lignocaine subcutaneously in a

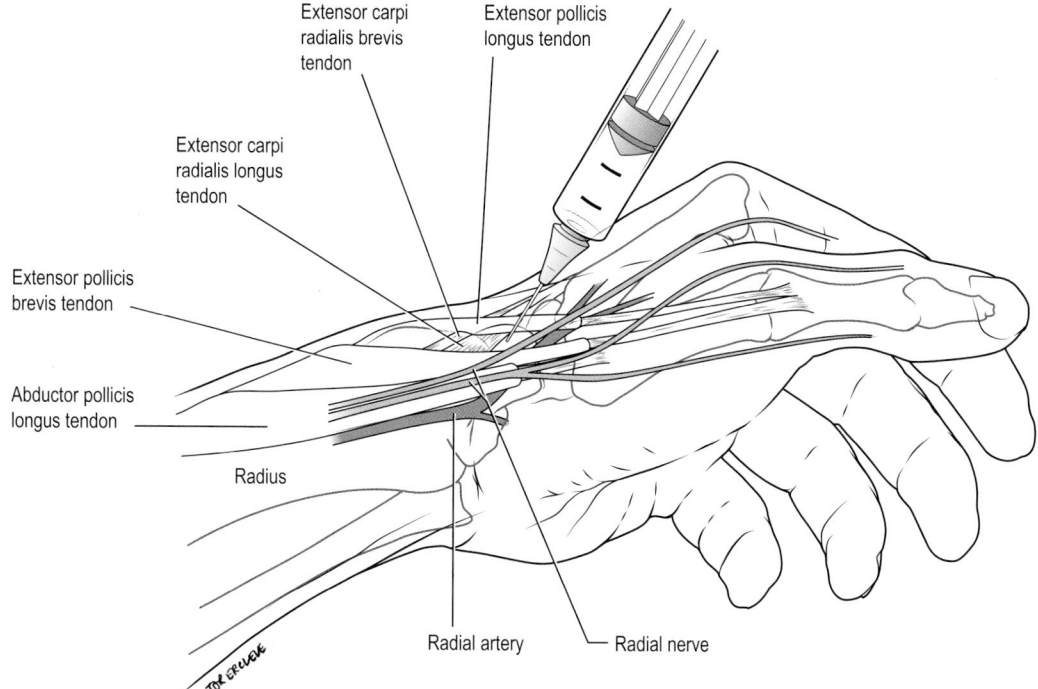

Fig. 22.2.4 Radial nerve wrist block.

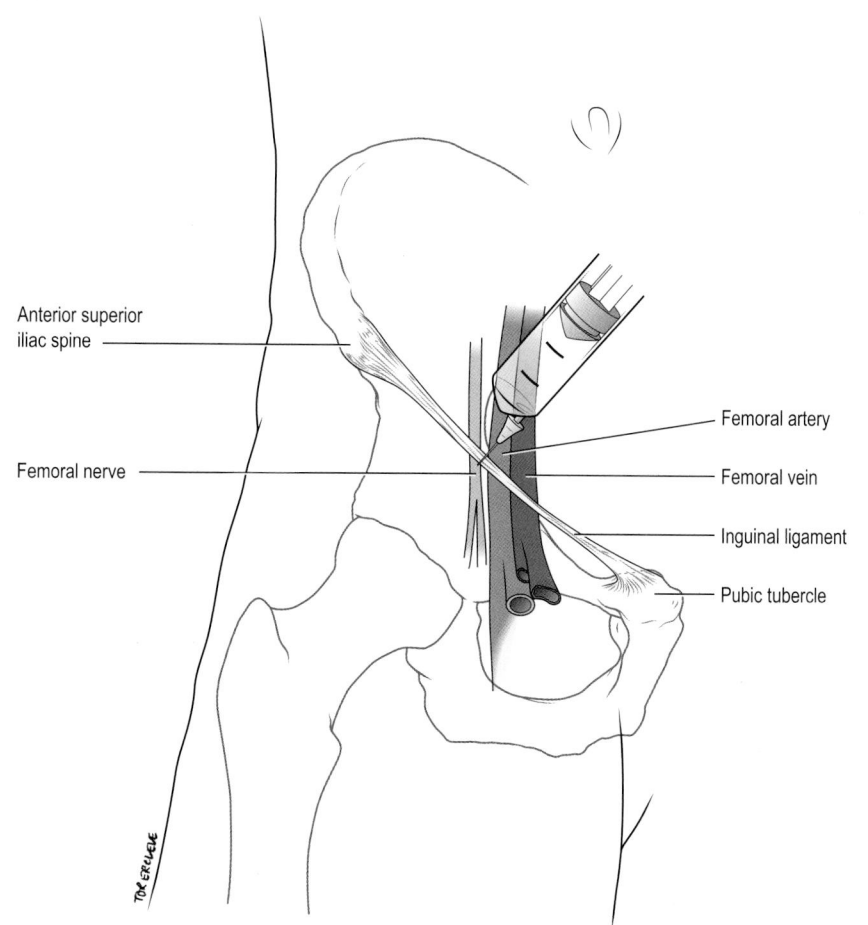

Fig. 22.2.5 Femoral nerve block.

Technique

Two doctors are required, allowing one to perform the manipulation and the other, with training in the procedure and resuscitation skills, to perform the block. Explain the procedure to the patient and obtain informed consent. Assemble and check all equipment and apply standard monitoring, including ECG, non-invasive blood pressure and pulse oximetry.

Use a specifically designed and maintained single 15 cm adult cuff, placed over cotton wool padding to the upper arm.

Double-cuff tourniquets require higher inflation pressures as they are narrower. The upper cuff is inflated first, followed by the lower cuff 15 min later, after injection of the prilocaine, thereby causing less discomfort to the patient. The upper cuff is then released. The use of a double cuff does not always reduce the ischaemia pain and predisposes to accidental wrong cuff release, so requires additional expertise and understanding.

Insert a small intravenous cannula into the dorsum of the hand of the injured limb and a second cannula in the other hand or wrist as emergency access to the central circulation. Exsanguinate the injured limb by simple elevation and direct brachial artery compression for 2–3 min, carefully supporting the limb at the site of any fracture. An Esmarch bandage may be used instead, in the absence of a painful wrist fracture.

Keep the arm elevated and inflate the cuff to 100 mmHg above systolic blood pressure. The

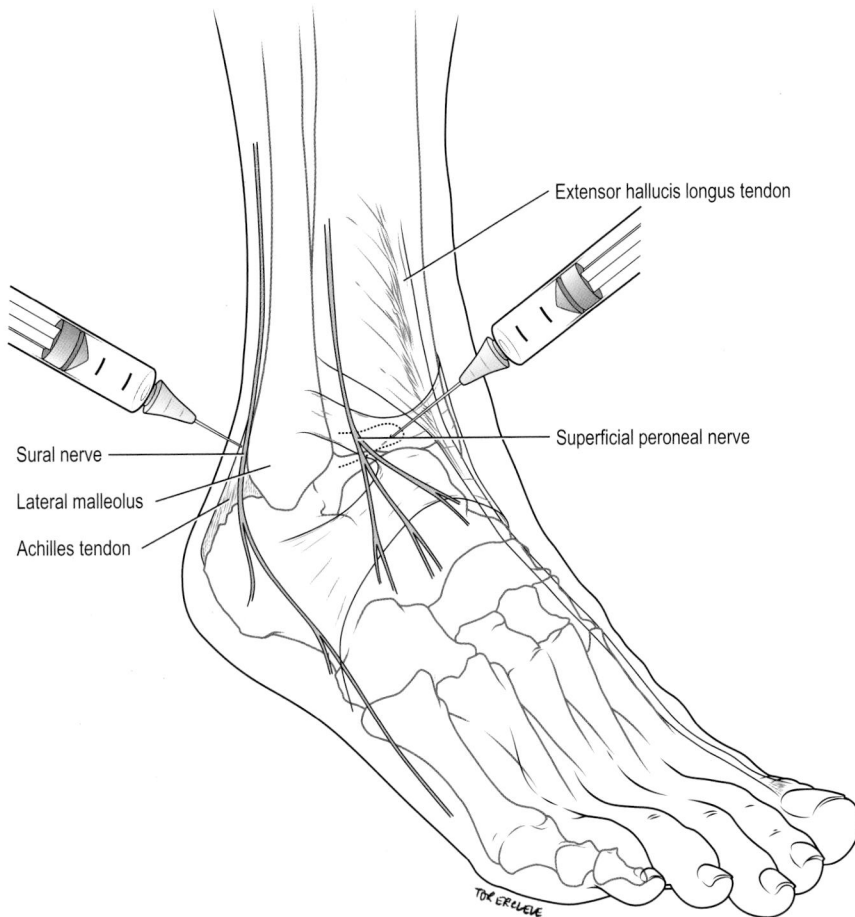

Fig. 22.2.6 Sural and superficial nerve blocks.

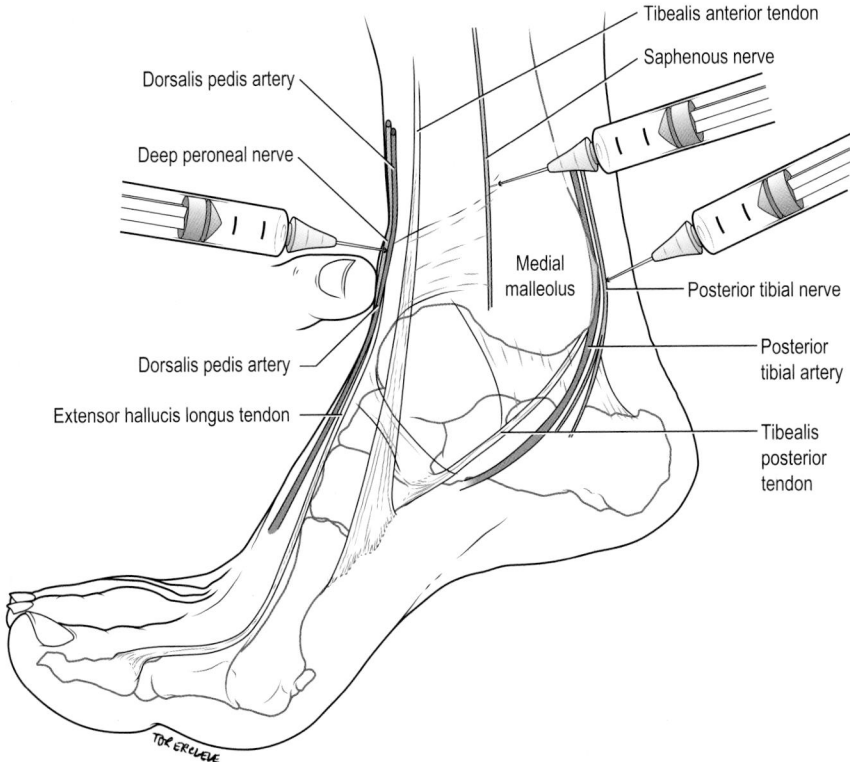

Fig. 22.2.7 Saphenous, posterior tibial and deep peroneal nerve blocks.

radial artery pulse should now be absent and the veins remain empty. If this is not the case, do not inject anaesthetic but repeat the exsanguination procedure and cuff inflation.

Lower the arm once the radial artery pulse is absent and the veins are empty, and inject 2.5 mg/kg (0.5 mL/kg) of 0.5% prilocaine slowly over 90 s and record the time.

Continuously monitor the cuff pressure and wait at least 5–10 min to confirm the adequacy of analgesia before removing the cannula on the injured limb. Perform the surgical procedure. Keep the tourniquet inflated for a minimum of 20 min and a maximum of 60 min.

Monitor the patient carefully for any signs of anaesthetic toxicity (see Table 22.2.2) over the next 15 min following cuff release, while organizing discharge from the monitored area.

Complications
No severe cardiac complications, deaths or methaemoglobinaemia have been reported using 0.5% prilocaine at the maximum dose of 2.5 mg/kg (0.5 mL/kg) [7]. Discomfort from the cuff is possible, but rarely significant.

Controversies and future directions

- There is no evidence that injecting a standard commercial preparation of local anaesthetic with adrenaline (epinephrine) into a digit is harmful.
- Lipid emulsion therapy for local anaesthetic systemic toxicity (LAST) appears well established and its use in other life-threatening lipophilic drug toxicity, such as with propranolol, verapamil and tricyclic antidepressants, is being studied.
- Need for fasting prior to a Bier's block.

References
[1] Bates D, Cutting P. Local anaesthetic and arterial puncture. Emerg Med J 2001;18:378.

[2] Murphy R, Carley S. Prior injection of local anaesthetic and the pain and success of intravenous cannulation. Emerg Med J 2000;17:406–8.

[3] Ring J, Franz R, Brockow K. Anaphylactic reactions to local anaesthetics. Chem Immunol Allerg 2010;95:190–200.

[4] Waterbrook A, Germann C, Southall J. Is epinephrine harmful when used with anesthetics for digital nerve blocks? Ann Emerg Med 2007;50:472–5.

[5] Weinberg G. Lipid emulsion infusion. Resuscitation for local anesthetic and other drug overdose. Anesthesiology 2012;117:180–7.

[6] Arendts G, Stevens M, Fry M. Topical anaesthesia and intravenous cannulation success in paediatric patients: a randomized double-blind trial. Br J Anaesth 2008;100:521–4.

[7] Lowen R, Taylor J. Bier's block – the experience of Australian emergency departments. Med J Aust 1994;60:108–11.

22.3 Procedural sedation and analgesia

Anthony J Bell • Greg Treston

ESSENTIALS

1 Emergency physicians and nurses who provide procedural sedation and analgesia in the emergency department must be trained and preferably credentialled.

2 Plan and prepare each individual procedure, with a careful risk – benefit assessment.

3 Determine the timing and nature of any recent oral intake.

4 Assess the safe limit of the targeted depth and duration of sedation.

5 Sedative agents should be titrated to clinical endpoints.

6 Sedation is a continuum. It is not always possible to predict how an individual will respond or at which point airway reflexes may become jeopardized.

7 Starting a procedure that may last 20 min or more under procedural sedation becomes a risk to the patient, if the team is likely to have competing departmental priorities. Consider deferral of the procedure until staffing is optimal and guaranteed.

Introduction/rationale

Procedural sedation and analgesia (PSA) is a core competency for the emergency physician for the performance of brief, but painful procedures and has become standard emergency medicine practice. PSA refers to the technique of administering sedatives or dissociative agents, with or without analgesics, to induce a state that allows the patient to tolerate an unpleasant or anxiety provoking therapeutic or diagnostic procedure, while maintaining cardiorespiratory function [1,2].

Significant variation exists in the practice of PSA in Australasian emergency departments (EDs) in relation to the approach, choice and combination of agent(s) given [3]. Paediatric patients in particular represent a significant challenge to the emergency physician, as children are often frightened when in pain and their presentation to the hospital disrupts family functioning [4,5]. Medical staff underestimate and undertreat pain in children [6]. Procedures may have previously been performed with inadequate sedation or 'oligoanalgesia' for fear of complications, worry about prolonged recovery time or the perception that with the procedure being brief, the child will not remember it.

Painful procedures in the ED are remembered vividly by children, parents and adult patients. Denial of relief from pain that is commensurate with the expressed need for such relief must be judged as an unjustified harm and amounts to substandard and unethical medical practice [7].

Underlying principles

Guidelines

The Australasian College for Emergency Medicine (ACEM), [8] American College of Emergency Physicians (ACEP) [2] and the Canadian Association of Emergency Physicians (CAEP) [9] have all published on the underlying principles for successful procedural sedation and analgesia within the emergency department setting. These guidelines cover pre-sedation preparation and assessment, pre-sedation fasting, physician skills, staffing, equipment and setting, patient monitoring, documentation and post-sedation care. With the gradual change in the perception accorded to PSA being performed in EDs over the last decade, regulatory approval is now in place within the USA, for example, allowing the delivery of anaesthetic agents for PSA in the ED.

The ACEM guidelines require that two medical attendants, one of whom should be a specialist or advanced trainee, be present. Nursing staff are also required and the procedure *must* be performed in a resuscitation area. Physiological monitoring is mandated during the procedure and extending into the recovery phase. Although the Australasian guidelines were developed conjointly with ANZCA, JFICM and Faculty of Pain Medicine, there is no specific recommendation as to choice of agent, despite the potentially confounding information published by ANZCA relating to the use of intravenous anaesthetic agents [10].

Depth and duration of sedation

The optimal endpoint of any sedation episode depends on the procedure being performed and the patient's characteristics. Classification of sedation state is now well established, ranging from minimal sedation (anxiolysis) through moderate sedation (formerly confusingly known as 'conscious sedation'), deep sedation to general anaesthesia. Dissociative sedation is a separate state induced by ketamine [11]. The exact characteristics of respiratory and/or airway reflex depression in relation to the depth of sedation are not well defined [1].

Titration of drug and constant verbal and tactile re-assessment of the patient reduce the risk of over-sedation [2]. Some degree of responsiveness to painful stimuli should indicate preservation of airway reflexes, decreasing the risk of aspiration if vomiting occurs [12].

Reducing the time a patient is sedated reduces the risk of airway compromise or respiratory depression (an adverse event in an obtunded patient). The duration of sedation is largely determined by the choice and dose of agent used and the procedure itself: whether this will be brief (e.g. shoulder reduction) or longer (e.g. compound scrub or manipulation of fractures), with most ED procedures taking less than 20 min.

Indications and patient selection

Patient selection is based on the need for sedation for a brief, painful procedure that will facilitate earlier discharge from the ED. These include, but are not limited to, fracture and dislocation reduction, incision and drainage of abscesses and cardioversion [13]. Inherently less painful but anxiety-provoking procedures in children will also be facilitated by the use of dissociative sedation, for example lumbar puncture, suturing, ocular or auditory canal foreign body (FB) removal or IV cannulation in an uncooperative and anxious child [11].

In Australasia, children have high numbers of laceration repairs or upper limb fractures reduced; young adults predominate with upper limb relocation and reductions; with older patients undergoing incision and drainage of abscesses, upper limb procedures or prosthetic hip relocations [3].

Departmental procedures and logistics

All departments that perform PSA should have written guidelines, a standardized data collection system and suitably trained staff. Internal processes should rapidly identify patients requiring PSA so that imaging, preparation for PSA and practitioner availability are ensured. Patient selection is informed by the pre-procedural risk assessment, departmental resources and ability to monitor and safely discharge the patient. In the context of time-based targets, patient flow patterns of this group need to be considered and systems put in place to optimize these. A recent Canadian paper highlights the inherent time challenges, resource intensity and foregone benefits if standardized processes are not adopted [14].

Pre-procedure risk assessment

Pre-procedural assessment is of critical importance before embarking upon PSA. Patient and pharmacological factors known to be associated with sedation-related events requiring a brief intervention include advancing age, deep sedation and pre-medication with or use of fentanyl in combination with either propofol or midazolam for PSA. Conversely, patient weight (within reason), procedure type and fasting status do not appear related to respiratory adverse events [15].

However, procedural failure is related to patient weight over 100 kg and certain procedure types, notably prosthetic hip reduction, digits and temporomandibular joint (TMJ) relocations. Ketamine is not only protective overall for respiratory adverse events, but has the highest procedural success rate [16]. Particular consideration should be given to:

Age

A young patient's level of anxiety and cooperation will depend upon past medical experiences, anxiety of the parent(s) and the reassurance given by medical staff [11]. Elderly patients, while mostly cooperative, may have underlying impaired cardiorespiratory reserve and are at

greater risk of peri-procedural cardiac events, respiratory depression or hypotension.

ASA classification

The American Society of Anesthesiologists (ASA) classification system [17] is used to classify patients (Table 22.3.1). ASA 1 and ASA 2 are the preferred candidates for procedural sedation in the ED. If an ASA 3 patient requires sedation out of necessity, such as for cardioversion, this should not preclude performance of the procedure. The management of respiratory depression becomes more relevant with increasing ASA class in all age groups.[18,19]

Airway assessment

An adverse past anaesthetic history and/or a focused airway assessment with attention to mouth opening, pharyngeal visualization using the Mallampatti score (Fig. 22.3.1), neck movement, thyromental distance and dentition help signal potential difficulty should active intervention be required. Table 22.3.2 contains a difficult airway predictor checklist.

Past medical history

Some conditions predispose to gastro-oesophageal reflux, such as pregnancy or hiatus hernia. Unstable acute medical/neurological conditions (with the exception of arrhythmias requiring cardioversion) may carry too high a risk to proceed with PSA. Allergies to any agent in the past precludes choosing that agent, as does egg/soy allergy as regards the use of propofol in particular [20]. A history of sleep apnoea will usually be associated with some obstructed or semiobstructed airway time during procedural sedation.

Fasting status

Fasting guidelines

Emergency department patients, particularly children [3], undergoing urgent PSA are

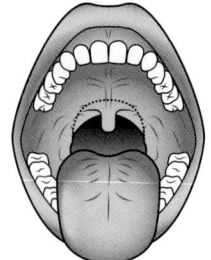 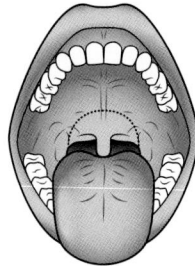

Class I: soft palate, uvula, fauces, pillars visible

No difficulty

Class II: soft palate, uvula, fauces visible

No difficulty

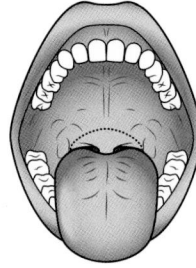 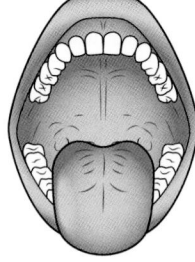

Class III: soft palate, base of uvula visible

Moderate difficulty

Class IV: hard palate only visible

Severe difficulty

Fig. 22.3.1 Mallampatti score to predict likelihood of difficulty at endotracheal intubation. Perform with the patient sitting.

Table 22.3.2 Airway assessment predictors of a difficult endotracheal intubation
● Mallampatti score III & IV
● Inability to open mouth >4 cm
● Thyromental distance <6 cm
● Limitation of neck movement
● Difficulty in protruding lower jaw
● History of difficult intubation
Mallampatti score: see Figure 22.3.1.

commonly not fasted on presentation, or at the time of the procedure. Furthermore, holding a patient for 6 h in an overcrowded ED to achieve a goal of fasting time is impractical if an urgent procedure needs to be performed. Fasting guidelines are consensus, not evidence-based. The ASA recommends by extrapolation at least 2 h and 6 h from last intake of fluid and food, respectively [17], despite a lack of evidence regarding these. There are no clinical data to support a consensus view regarding prolonged fasting prior to sedation [17,21]. In

Table 22.3.1 American Society of Anesthesiologists (ASA) classification	
Class	
1	Healthy patient, no medical problems
2	Mild systemic disease, e.g. hypertension
3	Severe systemic disease, but is not incapacitating
4	Severe systemic disease that is a constant threat to life
5	Moribund expected to live <24 h irrespective of operation

fact, prolonged pre-procedural fasting has been shown to *increase* the rate of vomiting [22,23].

Aspiration risk

The risk of aspiration is low. Fasting status is but one consideration when individualizing decisions about choice of agent, approach to dosing, desired depth of sedation or even referral for general anaesthesia (GA) instead [12,24]. PSA does not use volatile inhalational anaesthetics, which are inherently emetogenic, as may occur during GA [25]. Importantly, nor does ED PSA involve pharyngeal manipulation or instrumentation, again a potent stimulus for vomiting.

There is no association between fasting status and adverse events during procedural sedation in the ED for a range of agents that include ketamine, midazolam/fentanyl, chloral hydrate, pentobarbital [22,26,27] or nitrous oxide [20,28]. The proportion of unfasted patients in relevant studies was 53–71%. Recent data looking specifically at patients undergoing PSA with propofol with respect to fasting status showed no difference in adverse events between fasted and unfasted patients [12]. There are few reported cases of aspiration during PSA in the adult ED literature [29], with more in the paediatric literature, although the incidence is still low.

The senior ED clinician should still screen for high aspiration risk based on past history and physical characteristics, as such patients may benefit from an alternate approach or technique. The general anaesthetic literature cannot be directly extrapolated to ED PSA. Aspiration is a rare event and the decision to proceed with PSA is a pragmatic one and should be balanced against the competing harm to the patient when a procedure is unnecessarily delayed [30,31].

Post-procedure vomiting

This usually occurs well into the recovery period. Post-procedure vomiting is more common with ketamine or narcotics than it is with propofol or benzodiazepines [12,32].

A large multicentre prospective observational trial reported a vomiting incidence of 1.6% overall [15] but, as follow up occurred only during the ED phase of care, this is likely an underestimate. Oral or IV ondansetron given pre-sedation can decrease post-procedural emesis.

Procedural urgency

The endpoint of sedation in the ED should be tailored to the urgency of the procedure and

availability of appropriate staff [1,9]. Procedures may thus be regarded as [1]:

- emergency: cardioversion, fractures with neurovascular compromise needing reduction, intractable pain
- urgent: care of dirty wounds or lacerations, dislocation reduction, lumbar puncture, facilitation of neuroimaging in trauma
- semi-urgent: FB removal, care of clean wounds and lacerations
- elective.

Involvement of parents or carer

Parental cooperation is critical for the success of any procedural intervention in children. ED surveys show the vast majority of parents wish to be present for an invasive procedure performed on their child in the ED, with a small reduction with increasing invasiveness of the procedure, except for full resuscitation [33,34].

Despite this, more than one-third of parents were asked to leave the room in one study of children undergoing procedures [35]. The practice of requesting that parents leave the room when their child undergoes a procedure should be abandoned. Parental presence should instead be welcomed and, ultimately, their decision to stay or go should be supported. PSA in children should include ushering the parents to the bedside, not out of the room [33,36].

Informed consent

Informed consent must be obtained after explanation of specific risks of PSA and the procedure itself. In particular, when ketamine is used, warn parents to expect a 'staring child' with nystagmus, salivation, lacrimation, possible myoclonic jerking and vomiting in 10–15% usually after the end. This is important to parents' overall acceptance and experience of their child's procedure.

Likewise, although rare, the possibility of airway intervention beyond transient support should be raised with propofol. A practical point is that children will routinely (and adults occasionally) develop tears in their eyes. Family members should be reassured in advance that this is a drug effect, not a reaction to pain.

Documentation

A specific procedural sedation form or record is recommended. When designed in accordance with current best practice, they improve documentation and can act as the focus for educational initiatives and assist in audit, research

and quality assurance (QA) [37–39]. As well, they can act as a *de facto* protocol to ensure safety during the procedure. They also increase the chance of guideline compliance and ensure essential pre-sedation checks and monitoring are performed. A specific procedural sedation form should include provision for recording adverse events, including vomiting, aspiration or respiratory depression, as well as any intervention(s) required [12].

Choice of agent

The 'ideal' agent for PSA in the ED should have a rapid onset, short duration of action, rapid recovery profile, minimal side effects and an amnestic effect. The different classes of drugs used in PSA include sedative hypnotics, analgesics, dissociative sedatives, inhalation agents and antagonists (flumazenil and naloxone), used alone or in combination (Table 22.3.3).

Sedative hypnotics

Benzodiazepines

Midazolam Midazolam is one of the most commonly used benzodiazepines with amnestic [40], anxiolytic and sedative properties. Its side effects are dose dependent. Intravenous dosing for PSA ranges from 0.025 to 0.05 mg/kg in older children and adults, up to 0.1 mg/kg in younger children. Other routes of administration include IM and intranasal, although onset of action is slower [11] and many experienced clinicians have abandoned the use of intranasal midazolam.

Midazolam/opioid combinations

Midazolam/opioid combinations have been perceived to provide more predictable response and to have a favourable safety profile compared to propofol, owing to the potential of propofol to induce dose-related deep sedation [41]. In fact, there is additive respiratory depression with opiate and midazolam-containing combinations for PSA, with prolonged recovery times when compared to propofol [42–44]. Furthermore, patients receiving midazolam have been reported to have more recall and higher pain scores [45].

Diazepam Diazepam is less potent than midazolam, although there is little to no difference in the propensity of the two drugs to produce respiratory depression [46]. Dosing

Table 22.3.3 Choice of agent and suggested IV drug dosages (adult, 70 kg, normal BMI)

Drug	Initial bolus	Subsequent titrated IV boluses	Cumulative maximum dose
Morphine	2.5 mg	2.5 mg	10–15 mg
Fentanyl	25–50 μg	25 μg	150–200 μg
Midazolam	2 mg	1 mg	10 mg
Diazepam	5 mg	2.5 mg	10 mg
Propofol	40–50 mg	20 mg	150 mg
Ketamine	20–30 mg	10–20 mg	120 mg
Etomidate*	5–7 mg	2 mg	20 mg
'Ketafol'	6 mL	3 mL	20 mL

BMI: body mass index.
These are conservative estimates for a 70-kg adult.
Dose modification is advised where appropriate in the elderly patient (lower doses) and patients with small muscle bulk (lower doses).
'Ketafol' is made with 1 mL of 100 mg/mL ketamine made up to 10 mL with 9 mL of saline. To this add 10 mL of 10 mg/mL propofol in the same 20 mL syringe giving 5 mg:5 mg/mL, respectively.
*Etomidate is not available in Australia.

should start at 0.1–0.2 mg/kg with smaller subsequent doses. The antegrade amnestic effect of diazepam is significantly less than that of midazolam [47,48] and it causes more pain on injection but lesser early sedation [49]. The elimination half-lives of benzodiazepines do not necessarily correspond with their sedative pharmacodynamic effects and there are no clinically important sedative recovery rate differences between midazolam and diazepam [50,51].

Short-acting agents

Propofol

Propofol is a non-opioid, non-barbiturate sedative hypnotic that acts at γ-aminobutyric acid (GABA) sites within the CNS providing an amnestic effect, rapid onset <1 min and short duration (5–15 min) facilitating a rapid recovery time. It is readily titratable and has some antiemetic properties [21,52]. Hypotension is transient when propofol is titrated in a euvolaemic patient with normal cardiac function. Propofol has been shown to be safe in a wide range of settings, including PSA in the ED [2,53,54]. Propofol may cause a painful ache at the site of injection as the patient becomes sedated, which may be distressing, but is short lived.

The optimum dosing regimen for propofol in procedural sedation has yet to be defined. Options vary from single bolus [43,44,55], titration [19,56–59], bolus and infusion [42,60] or infusion alone [61–63]. Doses recommended

include 1 mg/kg initial bolus and 0.5 mg/kg subsequent boluses for PSA in the ED [44,52,64,65]. In children, initial bolus doses of 2 mg/kg have been used [66,67]. An alternative is to reduce the initial dose to 0.5–1.0 mg/kg followed by 20 mg boluses [68]. Dose reduction is also essential in those over 65 years of age [60]. Higher total mg/kg doses are used in children compared with adults [68,69].

Sedation times are shorter with propofol and the reported respiratory complication rates for propofol are equivalent to midazolam alone [42], midazolam ± flumazenil or etomidate, [43], and midazolam/fentanyl [44]. Discharge times are also earlier than with midazolam [70]. At excessive doses, propofol is associated with greater oxygen desaturation [55].

Respiratory depression is seen in up to 50% of ASA class 1 and 2 patients [57,71,72] and 61% in the critically ill [18]. Apnoea may occur in up to 22% of patients receiving propofol for PSA, but is transient [12,43,64]. Transient hypoxia has been observed in 6–44% of sedation episodes [18,19,42,43,55–57,59–61,69,71,72]. The combination of opiate and propofol results in higher levels of respiratory depression than propofol alone [73,74]. Supplemental oxygen was not routinely applied during PSA in some studies [56], although this practice is not supported. Supplemental oxygen should be applied in all ED sedations where practical, although with sedation of a young combative child it may be prudent to wait until the child is part-sedated before applying oxygen.

Etomidate

Etomidate is a non-barbiturate hypnotic currently unavailable in Australasia, although it is regularly used for RSI or procedural sedation in the UK and USA. Etomidate has a rapid onset <30 s with 5–15 min duration of action. The starting dose for PSA is up to 0.1 mg/kg with subsequent boluses of 0.05 mg/kg. It has a similar profile to propofol in terms of respiratory depression and duration of sedation when compared to midazolam, but is more cardiovascularly stable. Propofol is preferred as etomidate has a 20% rate of myoclonus plus the theoretical risk of adrenal suppression, emergence phenomena and higher vomiting rates [75–78].

Opiates

Opiates are the most commonly used analgesics before, during and after sedation, but up to half of all patients undergoing PSA receive no pre-procedural analgesia at all. Morphine is the preferred pre-procedure agent, but fentanyl is favoured intra-procedurally in a ratio of 4:1 [3]. Opiates provide analgesia but have no amnestic or anxiolytic properties.

Fentanyl

Fentanyl is the opiate of choice for ED PSA. It should be titrated up to 1 μg/kg IV, to avoid respiratory depression from a rapid push and should be combined with a pure sedative agent. It may also be delivered intranasally. Fentanyl compared to morphine has a rapid onset, a lack of histamine release and is cardiovascularly stable. Its duration of action is 30–45 min.

Despite its common use in sedation, fentanyl is linked to a higher respiratory depression event rate [77]. Some degree of respiratory depression should therefore be anticipated and actively managed if fentanyl is given. There is increasing evidence that ketamine is a safer analgesic than fentanyl for PSA [15,79].

Morphine

Morphine provides a longer duration of analgesia extending to hours and is useful after the procedure for ongoing analgesia. It may have been administered by ambulance officers pre-hospital.

Ultra-short-acting opiates

Ultra-short-acting opiates, such as remifentanil and alfentanil, play a role when combined with propofol to provide excellent sedation and analgesia enabling rapid recovery [80]. Like fentanyl, respiratory depression is to be expected and may even occur at lower levels of sedation. The higher recall rate in this scenario is a consideration [81,82]. As most patients will require some analgesia post-procedure, the logic for using ultra-short-acting narcotics in ED PSA appears more academic than practical.

Inhalational agents

Nitrous oxide

N$_2$O provides anxiolysis and mild analgesia. Entonox is a 50:50 mixture of N$_2$O and oxygen that is widely available in Australasia, delivered via a self-administered demand valve mask. It has rapid onset and offset and is safe but has little or no sedative effect. It may be useful as an anxiolytic in children and in needle-phobic individuals prior to definitive PSA.

Despite its popularly due to its convenience, N$_2$O results in poor sedation conditions. One observational convenience sample of children aged 1–17 years [83] noted that mean sedation scores (using the 7-point Children's Hospital of Wisconsin sedation scale; 6 being agitated, anxious, in pain and 0 being unresponsive to painful stimulus) were 4.4 with nitrous oxide 70% and 4.6 with nitrous oxide 50% (this case series utilized a nitrous oxide delivery and scavenging circuit not often found in emergency departments).

Another observational series [84] by the same authors examined the effect of high inhaled concentration N$_2$O on intra-procedural pain scores in children undergoing painful procedures in the ED. In just over one-third of cases the recorded pain scores actually *increased* during the procedure and, in 15.3% of cases, pain scores during the procedure compared with baseline remained unchanged. Coupled with the rate of intra-procedural emesis associated with N$_2$O use, this leaves N$_2$O as 'possibly useful' for relatively painless procedures or as adjunct sedation for a procedure performed under a Bier's block or similar.

Common side effects include vomiting and dizziness. Airway reflexes are preserved. It is contraindicated in patients with trapped gas, such as a pneumothorax.

Dissociative sedative

Ketamine

Ketamine is used with two distinct principal aims: as the primary sedative agent (that provides analgesia) or in a sub-dissociative dose as an analgesic adjunct with an alternative sedative. As a dissociative anaesthetic agent, ketamine has wide use in developing world and military applications [85]. In addition to excellent sedation and analgesia, it results in high levels of satisfaction and a lack of procedural recall [86]. Furthermore, ketamine is associated with the lowest procedural failure rate of any sedative in common use [16].

At sub-dissociative doses under 0.5 mg/kg, ketamine acts principally as an analgesic. With progressively larger amounts, dose-related 'dissociative anaesthesia', between deep sedation and general anaesthesia, occurs with doses exceeding 0.5 mg/kg. Ketamine has a rapid onset and offset with preservation of airway reflexes, although it can cause idiosyncratic laryngospasm. It is relatively contraindicated in ischaemic heart disease (IHD), due to increased sympathetic tone, or in other advanced vascular disease or uncontrolled hypertension.

Ketamine given either intravenously or intramuscularly is popular for emergency department paediatric procedural sedation. Its use is safe, with preservation of oropharyngeal reflexes and little to no respiratory depression [6,8,22,87–90]. At higher IV doses exceeding 1.5 mg/kg, subclinical respiratory depression is seen at rates similar to propofol [73], but ketamine is protective as regards the need for any actual airway intervention across the dosage spectrum [15].

There is concern about 'emergence delirium' [4,91], also known as 'emergence phenomena' [88–90,92,93]. Emergence delirium has been described as either 'patients are agitated, restless and combative and do not seem cognizant of their surroundings. Patients refuse to be comforted, even by their parents' [94], and 'combative, excited and disorientated behaviour that requires transient physical restraint' [95]. However, emergence phenomena may be as mild as an undistressing visual hallucination or a transient diplopia. Given the different definitions, the adult emergence incidence rate occurring in the recovery phase ranges from <1% to 36% [73,96–98].

Atropine as an antisialagogue with titrated IV ketamine for paediatric procedural sedation in the ED reduces hypersalivation [99] and post-procedure vomiting but, as hypersalivation rarely if ever affects the procedure, its use is optional. Hypersalivation appears less common in adults than in children.

The advantage of ketamine is its efficacy with variable routes of administration, even allowing a 'no IV cannula' sedation technique in the ED, particularly useful for pre-school-aged children.

Combinations with ketamine

Midazolam plus ketamine

Midazolam (or another benzodiazepine) has traditionally been used in combination with ketamine in an effort to decrease the incidence of 'emergence delirium', supported by studies reporting lower rates of emergence phenomena/agitation in adults who have received both ketamine and a benzodiazepine. 'Emergence phenomena' are fewer in children than in adults and the rate of emergence reactions in children is not lowered by adding a benzodiazepine [100–103], with unchanged rates of emergence agitation with midazolam added to ketamine [104–106].

Midazolam use has also been associated with higher rates of airway and respiratory compromise during procedural sedation in children [17]. Thus, use of adjunctive benzodiazepines with ketamine is not recommended. The only prospective randomized controlled trial (RCT) in adults addressing this issue showed that the prophylactic use of midazolam reduced recovery agitation by 10% [107].

Midazolam as an adjunctive medication when performing ketamine PSA has repeatedly been associated with lower rates of post-procedural emesis [104,105], yet with higher rates of airway/respiratory complications [17]. Midazolam itself as a sole sedative agent has been reported to have a rate of emergence agitation of up to 42% [108–110].

Ketamine plus propofol ('ketafol')

International RCT studies have compared 'ketafol' to propofol [111,112], 'ketafol' to midazolam/fentanyl [113] and ketamine alone [114]. All studies were small and focused on minor outcome differences. Anecdotally, there is a growing preference for the use of 'ketafol' over and above that which would be expected from the reported benefits.

The rationale for the addition of ketamine to propofol is to provide intra-procedural analgesia and sedation that has been used safely in a number of non-ED settings [115]. The combination aims to use the opposing respiratory and haemodynamic effects of each drug. Additionally, the antiemetic effect of propofol may counteract the vomiting seen with ketamine and may minimize the rate of 'emergence', although this remains unproven. Better procedural conditions and patient comfort are also suggested with the addition of ketamine [116,117].

This combination is safe in ED studies and resulted in high staff and patient satisfaction. The putative advantages in the use of 'ketafol' over propofol alone include modest dose reduction [118] and reduced respiratory depression. Recovery time remains short and there are no adverse events that altered patient disposition [114,119]. As ketamine at low doses is analgesic but not dissociative, targeted depth of sedation is important when using lower doses of propofol. The addition of ketamine to propofol has also been reported to have positive mood effects, allow earlier recovery of cognition and to reduce opiate requirement post-procedure [117,120,121].

Larger trials are still needed to compare this combination with other agents alone and to find the most synergistic ratio of ketamine to propofol [76]. Ratios of propofol:ketamine combined in the same syringe include 1:1 and 4:1 [122] or they can be titrated separately. Ketamine and propofol is a stable solution and can be safely administered from the same syringe [123].

Other drugs

Dexmedetomidine

Dexmedetomidine is a selective α-2 adrenergic agonist with sedative, anxiolytic and mild analgesic properties. Chemically, it is related to clonidine, but has a greater affinity for α-2 adrenergic receptors than α-1 receptors [124]. Dexmedetomidine acts in the CNS on vasomotor centres in the medulla, where it causes decreased sympathetic tone, which results in increased inhibitory GABA activity leading to sedation and analgesia [125]. It has been used for sedation of adults in the ICU and for paediatric sedation for non-painful radiological investigations (computed tomography [CT] and magnetic resonance imaging [MRI]) with some success. However, its utility is limited by hypotension and bradycardia mediated by the sympatholytic activity. There is minimal, if any, respiratory depression.

Current ED uses could be for decreasing agitation in a child undergoing CT or MRI scan or as a sedative agent for intubated adults in the ED. Some report that its utility as a paediatric sedation agent is restricted to sedation for CT, MRI or EEG and note that it demands a longer induction and results in a longer recovery time than propofol for similar procedures.

Preparation and monitoring

Resuscitation area

PSA should always occur in a resuscitation area, with two trained physician staff; one to perform the procedure and one to be responsible for the drugs and airway, with the assistance of an ED nurse [8]. Supplemental oxygen is given for all cases of ED PSA, except if using ketamine for paediatric PSA, when the use of supplemental oxygen by mask excessively upsets the child prior to the onset of sedation.

Equipment and monitoring

Suction, oxygen, airway adjuncts and intubation equipment should be prepared and physiological monitoring set up for pulse oximetry, non-invasive blood pressure, heart rate, ECG rhythm and respiratory rate. End-tidal carbon dioxide monitoring is recommended by some [2,12]. IV access is mandatory for all cases excluding paediatric sedation using IM ketamine or N_2O sedations. See Table 22.3.4 for essential equipment requirements.

Sedation scoring

Interactive monitoring with verbal and tactile stimulation is used constantly to assess the depth of sedation. Careful dose titration and evaluation of patient responsiveness throughout the procedure is essential [41,53]. The Ramsay sedation score [126] or motor component of the observer's assessment of alertness/sedation (OAA/S) scale [127], validated for midazolam may be used. All scales are subject to inter-observer variability and are relatively imprecise and not true objective measures of sedation. However, they require little formal training and are easily implemented (Table 22.3.5).

Bispectral EEG analysis

Bispectral (BIS) EEG analysis has been studied but is not reliably predictive of conscious state in individual patients [76]. Numerical values (0–100) are assigned to a patient's level of sedation but they are a poor measure of analgesia and ineffective when used with ketamine. Correlation with OAA/S [128,129] and Ramsay sedation scores [130,131] is poor. Lower BIS scores predict more respiratory depression (RD), but it is unclear whether BIS itself reduces the rate of RD [1,72,132]. Initial enthusiasm for BIS in ED PSA has waned as it has not proven its value over sedation scoring alone.

Capnography

Capnography can detect respiratory depression before clinical examination or oximetry, especially when on supplemental oxygen [133–136].

Table 22.3.4		Essential equipment requirements for procedural sedation 'SOAPMI'
S		Suction equipment (connected and checked)
		• Wall suction
		• Yankauer sucker and tubing
		• Paediatric suction catheters
O		Oxygen (connected and checked)
		• Supply
		• Age appropriate masks including nebulizer attachment
		• Primed bag–valve–mask
A		Airway
		• Oro- and nasopharyngeal airways
		• Laryngoscope and selection of blades (tested)
		• Appropriate selection of endotracheal tubes
		• Stylettes and bougies
		• 'Difficult airway kit' including laryngeal mask airway
P		Pharmacological agents (accessible but need not be drawn up)
		• Adrenaline and atropine
		• Naloxone and flumazenil
		• Bronchodilators
		• Drugs for rescue rapid sequence induction endotracheal intubation
M		Monitoring equipment
		• Full non-invasive physiological monitoring
		• End-tidal CO_2 tubing with transducer (if available)
I		Intravenous access trolley
		• Selection of cannulae
		• Crystalloid fluids

Table 22.3.5 Sedation scoring scales				
Score	Ramsay sedation scale	Sedation continuum	Score	OAA/S
1	Awake and alert	Minimal	5	Responds readily to name spoken in normal tone
2	Tranquil, purposeful at conversational level	Moderate		
3	Sleepy but purposeful to verbal commands at conversational level		4	Responds only after name called loudly or repeatedly
4	Sleepy and requiring louder voice or tactile stimulus to be purposeful		3	Responds only to mild prodding and shaking
5	Asleep and only purposeful to loud verbal command or harder glabellar tap	Deep	2	Does not respond to mild prodding and shaking
6	Asleep and sluggishly purposeful only to painful stimulus		1	Does not respond to painful stimulus
7	Asleep, reflex response, not purposeful			
8	Unresponsive	Anaesthetized	0	Unresponsive

OAA/S: motor component of the observer's assessment of alertness/sedation scale.

Table 22.3.6 Recommended adult discharge criteria and instructions following procedural sedation

- Patient is alert and orientated or has returned to pre-procedure state
- Patient ambulates safely or has returned to pre-procedure state
- Patient is comfortable and has discharge analgesia arranged
- Patient is discharged into care of a responsible adult
- Driving or the like is banned for a minimum of 8h
- Alcohol or other central nervous system depressants are avoided for 12–24h
- Patients are warned about the potential for post-procedure pain, unsteadiness or dizziness. Seek medical attention if significant or disabling

Capnography may even obviate the need for routine supplemental oxygen (although this is not supported by the authors of this chapter) [137]. Change in trace character or transient hypercapnoea [57,58,138] are early warning signs of hypoventilation or impending upper airway obstruction, of particular importance in children or those with reduced functional reserve [64]. Such early detection may avoid additional sedation being given and result in stimulating the patient or repositioning the airway. Only occasionally is an airway adjunct or manual (bag/valve/mask) ventilation required [12,69], and briefly 'waiting out' respiratory depression with propofol sedation in a pre-oxygenated patient is commonplace [65]. Thus, there may be a tendency to over-intervene when capnography is used as a PSA adjunct.

One Canadian study [139] noted that *capnometry* (rather than capnography) offered no advantage over pulse oximetry for the detection of respiratory depression in non-pre-oxygenated adult patients undergoing procedural sedation. The capnometric changes were poorly sensitive and a late finding in patients who developed respiratory depression undergoing orthopaedic procedures. This study reinforces the benefit of pre-oxygenation and intra-procedural supplemental oxygen during sedation when sedative agents known to cause hypoventilation (propofol, narcotics, benzodiazepines) are administered.

The 'antidote' for apnoea due to inadvertent deep sedation is a painful stimulus, in other words, to start the painful procedure which has the benefit of stimulating respiratory effort.

Post-procedure considerations

Patients should be observed until they have returned to their baseline level of functioning [2,13,17]. The exact time will depend on the patient and drugs administered with one study in children suggesting a '30-min rule' [140]. No special efforts need be made to darken the room or shield a child from the routine background visual and auditory stimuli of the busy ED.

Patients receiving propofol do not need prolonged post-procedure monitoring as re-sedation is rare [68]. Once the patient can talk, nursing staff have an 'endpoint' to cease physiological monitoring, confident that the patient is unlikely to develop any adverse event at this time (unless given further doses of narcotic).

The practice of making patients eat and drink prior to discharge after an ED sedation episode is without evidence and should be abandoned. This is supported by a recent Clinical Practice Advisory from the USA [13]. Nursing allocation should be tailored to the less intensive post-procedure monitoring requirements [141]. Discharge instructions, however, must be provided. See Table 22.3.6 for recommended adult discharge criteria.

Developments in the next 5–10 years [142]

- Standardized procedural sedation guidelines to align practice with best evidence, with optimal dosing strategies according to procedure type, patient age and depth of sedation required.
- Alternative delivery modalities, such as patient-controlled sedation or target-controlled infusions.
- Clearer understanding of the utility, or lack of, for agents, such as dexmedetomidine, alfentanil and remifentanil.
- Increasing use of and sophistication of psychological and regional techniques to augment PSA.
- Large multicentre trials with standardization of protocols, adverse event reporting and outcome measures to establish true complication rates.

Controversies

- Inadequate or oligoanalgesia still exists in emergency departments [143,144]. The degree of pre-procedural analgesia provided will impact upon the amount of sedative required.
- Additional intra-procedural narcotic analgesia increases the respiratory risk profile and is avoidable if adequate pre-procedural analgesia has been given. Whether lack of recall is a satisfactory justification for patients experiencing pain during a procedure is unclear [142].
- The relationship between practitioner skill set and complications has been described [145]. Implementation of a Paediatric Procedural Sedation (PPS) credentialling programme has resulted in significant improvements [146,147].
- Procedural success is variably defined but should encompass a lack of procedure or pain recall, adverse events, interference from the patient during the procedure and successful completion of the procedure [142].
- Whether the depth of sedation or duration of sedation places patients at greater risk for aspiration.

References

[1] Green SM, Roback MG, et al. Fasting and emergency department procedural sedation and analgesia: a consensus-based clinical practice advisory. Ann Emerg Med 2007;49:454–61.

[2] Godwin SA, Caro DA, Wolf SJ, et al. Clinical policy: procedural sedation and analgesia in the emergency department. Ann Emerg Med 2005;45:177–96.

[3] Bell A, Taylor DM, Holdgate A, et al. Procedural sedation practices in Australian emergency departments. Emerg Med Austral 2011;23:458–65.

[4] Dean A. Paediatric sedation in Australasian emergency departments. Emerg Med 1998;10:324–6.

[5] Weisman S, Bernstein B, Schechter N. Consequences of inadequate analgesia during painful procedures in children. Arch Pediatr Adolesc Med 1998;152:147–9.

[6] Wilson J, Pendleton J. Oligoanalgesia in the emergency department. Am J Emerg Med 1989;7:620–3.

[7] Walco G, Cassidy R, Schlechter N. Pain, hurt and harm – the ethics of pain control in infants and children. N Engl J Med 1994;331:541–4.

[8] Statement on clinical principles for procedural sedation. Emerg Med (Frem) 2003;15:205–6.

[9] Innes G, Murphy M, Nijssen-Jordan C, et al. Procedural sedation and analgesia in the emergency department. Canadian Consensus Guidelines. J Emerg Med 1999;17:145–56.

[10] ANZCA. Guidelines on conscious sedation for diagnostic, interventional medical and surgical procedures. 2005.

[11] Green SM, Krauss B. Procedural sedation and analgesia in children. Lancet 2006;367:766–80.

[12] Bell A, Treston G, McNabb C, et al. Profiling adverse respiratory events and vomiting when using propofol for emergency department procedural sedation. Emerg Med Australas 2007;19:411–7.

[13] Miner JR, Burton JH. Clinical practice advisory: emergency department procedural sedation with propofol. Ann Emerg Med 2007;50:182–7. 7e1.

[14] Bawden J, Villa-Roel C, Singh M, et al. Procedural sedation and analgesia in a Canadian ED: a time-in-motion study. Am J Emerg Med 29:1083–1088.

[15] Taylor DM, Bell A, Holdgate A, et al. Risk factors for sedation-related events during procedural sedation in the emergency department. Emerg Med Australas 2011;23:466–73.

[16] Holdgate A, Taylor DM, Bell A, et al. Factors associated with failure to successfully complete a procedure during emergency department sedation. Emerg Med Australas 2011;23:474–8.

[17] Practice guidelines for sedation and analgesia by non-anesthesiologists. Anesthesiology 2002;96:1004-17.

[18] Miner JR, Martel ML, Meyer M, et al. Procedural sedation of critically ill patients in the emergency department. Acad Emerg Med 2005;12:124–8.

[19] Guenther E, Pribble CG, Junkins Jr EP, et al. Propofol sedation by emergency physicians for elective pediatric outpatient procedures. Ann Emerg Med 2003;42:783–91.

[20] Hofer KN, McCarthy MW, Buck ML, et al. Possible anaphylaxis after propofol in a child with food allergy. Ann Pharmacother 2003;37:398–401.

[21] Bahn EL, Holt KR. Procedural sedation and analgesia: a review and new concepts. Emerg Med Clin N Am 2005;23:503–17.

[22] Treston G. Prolonged pre-procedure fasting time is unnecessary when using titrated intravenous ketamine for paediatric procedural sedation. Emerg Med Australas 2004;16:145–50.

[23] Green SM, Johnson NE. Ketamine sedation for pediatric procedures: Part 2, Review and implications. Ann Emerg Med 1990;19:1033–46.

[24] Green SM. Fasting is a consideration – not a necessity – for emergency department procedural sedation and analgesia. Ann Emerg Med 2003;42:647–50.

[25] Green SM, Krauss B. Pulmonary aspiration risk during emergency department procedural sedation – an examination of the role of fasting and sedation depth. Acad Emerg Med 2002;9:35–42.

[26] Agrawal D, Manzi SF, Gupta R, et al. Preprocedural fasting state and adverse events in children undergoing procedural sedation and analgesia in a pediatric emergency department. Ann Emerg Med 2003;42:636–46.

[27] Roback MG, Bajaj L, Wathen JE, et al. Preprocedural fasting and adverse events in procedural sedation and analgesia in a pediatric emergency department: are they related? Ann Emerg Med 2004;44:454–9.

[28] Babl FE, Puspitadewi A, Barnett P, et al. Preprocedural fasting state and adverse events in children receiving nitrous oxide for procedural sedation and analgesia. Pediatr Emerg Care 2005;21:736–43.

[29] Cheung KW, Watson ML, Field S, et al. Aspiration pneumonitis requiring intubation after procedural sedation and analgesia: a case report. Ann Emerg Med 2007;49:462–4.

[30] Taylor D. Pre-procedural fasting for sedation: do we need to do it? Emerg Med J 2010;27:253.

[31] Thorpe RJ, Benger J. Pre-procedural fasting in emergency sedation. Emerg Med J 2010;27:254–61.

[32] Roback MG, Wathen JE, Bajaj L, et al. Adverse events associated with procedural sedation and analgesia in a pediatric emergency department: a comparison of common parenteral drugs. Acad Emerg Med 2005;12:508–13.

[33] Isoardi J, Slabbert N, Treston G. Witnessing invasive paediatric procedures, including resuscitation, in the emergency department: a parental perspective. Emerg Med Australas 2005;17:244–8.

[34] Bauchner H, Vinci R, Waring C. Pediatric procedures: do parents want to watch? Pediatrics 1989;84:907–9.

[35] Bauchner H, Waring C, Vinci R. Parental presence during procedures in an emergency room: results from 50 observations. Pediatrics 1991;87:544–8.

[36] Ross D, Ross S. Childhood pain: the school-aged child's viewpoint. Pain 1984;20:179–91.

[37] Nicol MF. A risk management audit: are we complying with the national guidelines for sedation by non-anaesthetists? J Accid Emerg Med 1999;16:120–2.

[38] Law A, Babl F, Priestley D, et al. Pre and post implementation evaluation of a comprehensive procedural program for children in the emergency department. J Paediatr Child Hlth 2005(Suppl. 8)

[39] Swoboda TK, Munyak J. Use of a sedation-analgesia data sheet in closed shoulder reductions. J Emerg Med 2005;29:129–35.

[40] Macken E, Gevers AM, Hendrickx A, et al. Midazolam versus diazepam in lipid emulsion as conscious sedation for colonoscopy with or without reversal of sedation with flumazenil. Gastrointest Endosc 1998;47:57–61.

[41] Green SM. Propofol for emergency department procedural sedation – not yet ready for prime time. Acad Emerg Med 1999;6:975–8.

[42] Havel Jr CJ, Strait RT, Hennes H. A clinical trial of propofol vs midazolam for procedural sedation in a pediatric emergency department. Acad Emerg Med 1999;6:989–97.

[43] Coll-Vinent B, Sala X, Fernandez C, et al. Sedation for cardioversion in the emergency department: analysis of effectiveness in four protocols. Ann Emerg Med 2003;42:767–72.

[44] Taylor D, O'Brien D, Ritchie P, et al. Propofol versus midazolam/fentanyl for reduction of anterior shoulder dislocation. Acad Emerg Med 2005;12:13–19.

[45] Freeston JA, Leal A, Gray A. Procedural sedation and recall in the emergency department: the relationship between depth of sedation and patient recall and satisfaction. Emerg Med J 2012;29:670–2.

[46] Bell GD. Review article: premedication and intravenous sedation for upper gastrointestinal endoscopy. Aliment Pharmacol Ther 1990;4:103–22.

[47] Tolia V, Fleming SL, Kauffman RE. Randomized,double-blind trial of midazolam and diazepam for endoscopic sedation in children. Dev Pharmacol Ther 1990;14:141–7.

[48] Sanders LD, Davies-Evans J, Rosen M, et al. Comparison of diazepam with midazolam as i.v. sedation for outpatient gastroscopy. Br J Anaesth 1989;63:726–31.

[49] Wright SW, Chudnofsky CR, Dronen SC, et al. Comparison of midazolam and diazepam for conscious sedation in the emergency department. Ann Emerg Med 1993;22:201–5.

[50] Ariano RE, Kassum DA, Aronson KJ. Comparison of sedative recovery time after midazolam versus diazepam administration. Crit Care Med 1994;22:1492–6.

[51] Mitchell AR, Chalil S, Boodhoo L, et al. Diazepam or midazolam for external DC cardioversion (the DORM Study). Europace 2003;5:391–5.

[52] Symington L, Thakore S. A review of the use of propofol for procedural sedation in the emergency department. Emerg Med J 2006;23:89–93.

[53] Ducharme J. Propofol in the emergency department: Another interpretation of the evidence. J Can Assoc Emerg Phys 2001;3:311–2.

[54] Jackson R, Carley S. Towards evidence based emergency medicine: best BETs from the Manchester Royal Infirmary. Use of propofol for sedation in the emergency department. Emerg Med J 2001;18:378–9.

[55] Godambe SA, Elliot V, Matheny D, et al. Comparison of propofol/fentanyl versus ketamine/midazolam for brief orthopedic procedural sedation in a pediatric emergency department. Pediatrics 2003;112:116–23.

[56] Skokan EG, Pribble C, Bassett KE, et al. Use of propofol sedation in a pediatric emergency department: a prospective study. Clin Pediatr (Phila) 2001;40:663–71.

[57] Miner JR, Biros M, Krieg S, et al. Randomized clinical trial of propofol versus methohexital for procedural sedation during fracture and dislocation reduction in the emergency department. Acad Emerg Med 2003;10:931–7.

[58] Miner JR, Heegaard W, Plummer D. End-tidal carbon dioxide monitoring during procedural sedation. Acad Emerg Med 2002;9:275–80.

[59] Bassett KE, Anderson JL, Pribble CG, et al. Propofol for procedural sedation in children in the emergency department. Ann Emerg Med 2003;42:773–82.

[60] Frazee BW, Park RS, Lowery D, et al. Propofol for deep procedural sedation in the ED. Am J Emerg Med 2005;23:190–5.

[61] Swanson ER, Seaberg DC, Mathias S. The use of propofol for sedation in the emergency department. Acad Emerg Med 1996;3:234–8.

[62] Pershad J, Godambe SA. Propofol for procedural sedation in the pediatric emergency department. J Emerg Med 2004;27:11–14.

[63] Frank LR, Strote J, Hauff SR, et al. Propofol by infusion protocol for ED procedural sedation. Am J Emerg Med 2006;24:599–602.

[64] Green SM, Krauss B. Propofol in emergency medicine: pushing the sedation frontier. Ann Emerg Med 2003;42:792–7.

[65] Krauss B, Green SM. Procedural sedation and analgesia in children. 2006;(4):766–80.

[66] Sacchetti A, Cravero J. Sedation in the emergency department. Pediatr Ann 2005;34:617–22.

[67] Barnett P. Propofol for pediatric sedation. Pediatr Emerg Care 2005;21:111–4.

[68] Bell A, Treston G, Cardwell R, et al. Optimisation of propofol dose shortens procedural sedation time, prevents re-sedation and removes the requirement for post procedure physiologic monitoring. Emerg Med Australas 2007:19.

[69] Burton JH, Miner JR, Shipley ER, et al. Propofol for emergency department procedural sedation and analgesia: a tale of three centers. Acad Emerg Med 2006;13:24–30.

[70] Rahman NH, Hashim A. The use of propofol for procedural sedation and analgesia in the emergency department: a comparison with midazolam. Emerg Med J 2011;28:861–5.

[71] Miner JR, Biros MH, Heegaard W, et al. Bispectral electroencephalographic analysis of patients undergoing procedural sedation in the emergency department. Acad Emerg Med 2003;10:638–43.

[72] Miner JR, Biros MH, Seigel T, et al. The utility of the bispectral index in procedural sedation with propofol in the emergency department. Acad Emerg Med 2005;12:190–6.

[73] Miner JR, Gray RO, Bahr J, et al. Randomized clinical trial of propofol versus ketamine for procedural sedation in the emergency department. Acad Emerg Med 2010;17:604–11.

[74] Miner JR, Gray R, Delavari P, et al. Alfentanil for procedural sedation in the emergency department. Ann Emerg Med 2011;57:117–21.

[75] Falk J, Zed PJ. Etomidate for procedural sedation in the emergency department. Ann Pharmacother 2004;38:1272–7.

[76] Green SM. Research advances in procedural sedation and analgesia. Ann Emerg Med 2007;49:31–6.

[77] Van Kuelen S, Burton J. Myoclonus associated with etomidate for ED procedural sedation and analgesia. Am J Emerg Med 2003;21:556–9.

[78] Miner JR, Danahy M, Moch A, et al. Randomized clinical trial of etomidate versus propofol for procedural sedation in the emergency department. Ann Emerg Med 2007;49:15–22.

[79] Messenger DW, Murray HE, Dungey PE, et al. Subdissociative-dose ketamine versus fentanyl for analgesia during propofol procedural sedation: a randomized clinical trial. Acad Emerg Med 2008;15:877–86.

[80] Dunn MJ, Mitchell R, Souza CD, et al. Evaluation of propofol and remifentanil for intravenous sedation for reducing shoulder dislocations in the emergency department. Emerg Med J 2006;23:57–8.

[81] Miner JR, Gray RO, Stephens D, et al. Randomized clinical trial of propofol with and without alfentanil for deep procedural sedation in the emergency department. Acad Emerg Med 2009;16:825–34.

[82] Dunn MJ, Mitchell R, Desouza CI, et al. Recovery from sedation with remifentanil and propofol, compared with morphine and midazolam, for reduction in anterior shoulder dislocation. Emerg Med J 2011;28:6–10.

[83] Babl FE, Oakley E, Seaman C, et al. High-concentration nitrous oxide for procedural sedation in children: adverse events and depth of sedation. Pediatrics 2008;121:e528–32.

[84] Babl FE, Oakley E, Puspitadewi A, et al. Limited analgesic efficacy of nitrous oxide for painful procedures in children. Emerg Med J 2008;25:717–21.

[85] Guldner GT, Petinaux B, Clemens P, et al. Ketamine for procedural sedation and analgesia by nonanesthesiologists in the field: a review for military healthcare providers. Mil Med 2006;171:484–90.

[86] Sih K, Campbell SG, Tallon JM, et al. Ketamine in adult emergency medicine: controversies and recent advances. Ann Pharmacother 2011;45:1525–34.

[87] Green SM, Rothrock SG, Lynch EL, et al. Intramuscular ketamine for pediatric sedation in the emergency department: safety profile in 1,022 cases. Ann Emerg Med 1998;31:688–97.

[88] Dachs RJ, Innes GM. Intravenous ketamine sedation of pediatric patients in the emergency department. Ann Emerg Med 1997;29:146–50.

[89] McCarty EC, Mencio GA, Walker LA, et al. Ketamine sedation for the reduction of children's fractures in the emergency department. J Bone Joint Surg 2000;82A:912–8.

[90] Howes MC. Ketamine for paediatric sedation/analgesia in the emergency department. Emerg Med J 2004;21:275–80.

[91] Everitt I, Younge P, Barnett P. Paediatric sedation in emergency department: what is our practice? Emerg Med (Frem) 2002;14:62–6.

[92] Green SM, Kuppermann N, Rothrock SG, et al. Predictors of adverse events with intramuscular ketamine sedation in children. Ann Emerg Med 2000;35:35–42.

[93] Ducharme J. Ketamine. Do what is right for the patient. Emerg Med 2001;13:7–8.

[94] Wells L, Rasch D. Emergence "delirium" after sevoflurane anesthesia: a paranoid delusion? Anesth Analg 1999;88:1308–10.

[95] Uezono S, Goto T, Terui K. Emergence agitation after sevoflurane versus propofol in pediatric patients. Anesth Analg 2000;91:563–6.

[96] Newton A, Fitton L. Intravenous ketamine for adult procedural sedation in the emergency department:a prospective cohort study. Emerg Med J 2008;25:498–501.

[97] Sim TB, Seet CM. To study the effectiveness and safety of ketamine and midazolam procedural sedation in the incision and drainage of abscesses in the adult emergency department. Eur J Emerg Med 2008;15:169–72.

[98] Vardy JM, Dignon N, Mukherjee N, et al. Audit of the safety and effectiveness of ketamine for procedural sedation in the emergency department. Emerg Med J 2008;25:579–82.

[99] Heinz P, Geelhoed GC, et al. Isatropine needed with ketamine sedation? A prospective, randomised, double blind study. Emerg Med J 2006;23:206–9.

[100] Bovill J, Coppel D, Dundee J, et al. Current status of ketamine anaesthesia. Lancet 1971;297:1285–8.

[101] Coppel D, Bovill J, Dundee J. The taming of ketamine. Anaesthesia 1973;28:293–6.

[102] Cartwright P, Pingel S. Midazolam and diazepam in ketamine. Anesth Analg 1984;39:439–42.

[103] White P, Way W, Trevor A. Ketamine – its pharmacology and therapeutic uses. Anesthesiology 1982;56:119–36.

[104] Wathen JE, Roback MG, Mackenzie T, et al. Does midazolam alter the clinical effects of intravenous ketamine sedation in children? A double-blind, randomized, controlled, emergency department trial. Ann Emerg Med 2000;36:579–88.

[105] American College of Emergency Physicians. Clinical policy for procedural sedation and analgesia in the emergency department. Ann Emerg Med 1998;31:663–77.

[106] Sherwin TS, Green SM, Khan A, et al. Does adjunctive midazolam reduce recovery agitation after ketamine sedation for pediatric procedures? A randomized, double-blind, placebo-controlled trial. Ann Emerg Med 2000;35:229–38.

[107] Sener S, Eken C, Schultz CH, et al. Ketamine with and without midazolam for emergency department sedation in adults: a randomized controlled trial. Ann Emerg Med 57:109–14e2.

[108] Roelofse J, Joubert J, Roelofse G. A double blind randomised comparison of midazolam alone and midazolam combined with ketamine for sedation of pediatric dental patients. J Oral Maxillofac Surg 1996;54:838–44.

[109] Davies FC, Waters M. Oral midazolam for conscious sedation of children during minor procedures. J Accid Emerg Med 1998;15:244–8.

[110] Massanari M, Novitsky J, Reinstein L. Paradoxical reactions in children associated with midazolam use during endoscopy. Clin Pediatr 1997;36:681–4.

[111] Andolfatto G, Abu-Laban RB, Zed PJ, et al. Ketamine-propofol combination (ketofol) versus propofol alone for emergency department procedural sedation and analgesia: a randomized double-blind trial. Ann Emerg Med 59:504-12. e1-2.

[112] David H, Shipp J. A randomized controlled trial of ketamine/propofol versus propofol alone for emergency department procedural sedation. Ann Emerg Med 2011;57:435–41.

[113] Nejati A, Moharari RS, Ashraf H, et al. Ketamine/propofol versus midazolam/fentanyl for procedural sedation and analgesia in the emergency department: a randomized, prospective, double-blind trial. Acad Emerg Med 2011;18:800–6.

[114] Shah A, Mosdossy G, McLeod S, et al. A blinded, randomized controlled trial to evaluate ketamine/propofol versus ketamine alone for procedural sedation in children. Ann Emerg Med 2011;57: 425–33. e2.

[115] Loh G, Dalen D. Low-dose ketamine in addition to propofol for procedural sedation and analgesia in the emergency department. Ann Pharmacother 2007;41:485–92.

[116] Phillips W, Anderson A, Rosengreen M, et al. Propofol versus propofol/ketamine for brief painful procedures in the emergency department: clinical and bispectral index scale comparison. J Pain Palliat Care Pharmacother 2010;24:349–55.

[117] Mortero RF, Clark LD, Tolan MM, et al. The effects of small-dose ketamine on propofol sedation: respiration, postoperative mood, perception, cognition, and pain. Anesth Analg 2001;92:1465–9.

[118] Arora S. Combining ketamine and propofol ("ketofol") for emergency department procedural sedation and analgesia: a review. West J Emerg Med 2008;9:20–3.

[119] Willman EV, Andolfatto G. A prospective evaluation of "ketafol" (ketamine/propofol combination) for procedural sedation and analgesia in the emergency department. Ann Emerg Med 2007;49:23–30.

[120] Sneyd JR. Recent advances in intravenous anaesthesia. Br J Anaesth 2004;93:725–36.

[121] Badrinath S, Avramov MN, Shadrick M, et al. The use of a ketamine-propofol combination during monitored anesthesia care. Anesth Analg 2000;90:858–62.

[122] Daabiss M, Elsherbiny M, Alotibi R. Assessment of different concentration of Ketafol in procedural sedation. Br J Med Practit 2009;2:27–31.

[123] Donnelly R, Willman E, Andolfatto G. Stability of ketamine-propofol mixtures for procedural sedation and analgesia in the emrgency department. Can J Hosp Pharm 2008;61:426–30.

[124] McMorrow SP, Abramo TJ. Dexmedetomidine sedation: uses in pediatric procedural sedation outside the operating room. Pediatr Emerg Care 2012;28:292–6.

[125] Carollo DS, Nossaman BD, Ramadhyani U. Dexmedetomidine: a review of clinical applications. Curr Opin Anaesthesiol 2008;21:457–61.

[126] Habibi S, Coursin D. Assessment of sedation, analgesia, and neuromuscular blockade in the perioperative period. Int Anesthesiol Clin 1996;34:215–41.

[127] Chernik D, Gillings D. Validity and reliability of the Observer's Assessment of Alertness/Sedation Scale: study with intravenous midazolam. J Clin Psychopharm 1990;10:244–51.

[128] Fatovich DM, Gope M, Paech MJ. A pilot trial of BIS monitoring for procedural sedation in the emergency department. Emerg Med Australas 2004;16:103–7.

[129] Overly FL, Wright RO, Connor Jr FA, et al. Bispectral analysis during pediatric procedural sedation. Pediatr Emerg Care 2005;21:6–11.

[130] Gill M, Green SM, Krauss B. A study of the bispectral index monitor during procedural sedation and analgesia in the emergency department. Ann Emerg Med 2003;41:234–41.

[131] Agrawal D, Feldman HA, Krauss B, et al. Bispectral index monitoring quantifies depth of sedation during emergency department procedural sedation and analgesia in children. Ann Emerg Med 2004;43:247–55.

[132] Anesthesiologists ASA. Practice advisory for intraoperative awareness and brain function monitoring. Anesthesiology 2006;104:847–64.

[133] Burton JH, Harrah JD, Germann CA, et al. Does end-tidal carbon dioxide monitoring detect respiratory events prior to current sedation monitoring practices? Acad Emerg Med 2006;13:500–4.

[134] Anderson JL, Junkins E, Pribble C, et al. Capnography and depth of sedation during propofol sedation in children. Ann Emerg Med 2007;49:9–13.

[135] Deitch K, Chudnofsky CR, Dominici P. The utility of supplemental oxygen during emergency department procedural sedation and analgesia with midazolam and fentanyl: a randomized, controlled trial. Ann Emerg Med 2007;49:1–8.

[136] Deitch K, Chudnofsky CR, Dominici P. The utility of supplemental oxygen during emergency department procedural sedation with propofol: a randomized, controlled trial. Ann Emerg Med 2008;52:1–8.

[137] Green SM, Pershad J. Should capnographic monitoring be standard practice during emergency department procedural sedation and analgesia? Pro and con. Ann Emerg Med 2010;55:265–7.

[138] McQuillen KK, Steele DW. Capnography during sedation/analgesia in the pediatric emergency department. Pediatr Emerg Care 2000;16:401–4.

[139] Sivilotti ML, Murray HE, Messenger DW. Does end-tidal CO_2 monitoring during emergency department procedural sedation and analgesia with propofol decrease the incidence of hypoxic events? Ann Emerg Med 2010;56:702–3. (author reply 3-4).

[140] Newman DH, Azer MM, Pitetti RD, et al. When is a patient safe for discharge after procedural sedation? The timing of adverse effect events in 1367 pediatric procedural sedations. Ann Emerg Med 2003;42:627–35.

[141] Holger J, Satterlee P, Haugen S. Nursing use between 2 methods of procedural sedation: midazolam versus propofol. Am J Emerg Med 2005;23:248–52.

[142] Miner JR, Burton JH. Clinical practice advisory: emergency department procedural sedation with propofol. Ann Emerg Med 2007;50:182–7.

[143] MacLean S, Obispo J, Young KD. The gap between pediatric emergency department procedural pain management treatments available and actual practice. Pediatr Emerg Care 2007;23:87–93.

[144] Paris PM, Yealy DM. A procedural sedation and analgesia fasting consensus advisory: one small step for emergency medicine, one giant challenge remaining. Ann Emerg Med 2007;49:465–7.

[145] Cote CJ, Notterman DA, Karl HW, et al. Adverse sedation events in pediatrics: a critical incident analysis of contributing factors. Pediatrics 2000;105:805–14.

[146] Priestley S, Babl FE, Krieser D, et al. Evaluation of the impact of a paediatric procedural sedation credentialing programme on quality of care. Emerg Med Australas 2006;18:498–504.

[147] Babl F, Priestley S, Krieser D, et al. Development and implementation of an education and credentialing programme to provide safe paediatric procedural sedation in emergency departments. Emerg Med Australas 2006;18:489–97.

EMERGENCY IMAGING

Edited by **George Jelinek**

SECTION **23**

23.1 Emergency department ultrasound

James Rippey • Adrian Goudie • Andrew Haig

ESSENTIALS

1 Ultrasound examination, interpretation and clinical correlation should be available in a timely manner 24 hours a day for emergency department patients.

2 Emergency physicians providing emergency ultrasound services should possess appropriate training and hands-on experience to perform and interpret limited bedside ultrasound imaging.

3 Ultrasound imaging by emergency physicians is useful for at least the following clinical indications: traumatic haemoperitoneum, pneumothorax, abdominal aortic aneurysm, pericardial fluid, undifferentiated shock, respiratory distress, ectopic pregnancy, vascular access and other invasive procedures, hydronephrosis and biliary tract disease.

4 Continued research is required in the area of ultrasound imaging and any other known or evolving bedside imaging techniques and modalities.

5 Emergency medicine training programmes should provide instruction and experience in bedside ultrasound imaging for their trainees.

6 The Australasian College for Emergency Medicine supports the use of bedside ultrasound by emergency physicians, as does the American College of Emergency Physicians, the College of Emergency Medicine in the UK and the International Federation for Emergency Medicine.

Japan. Ultrasound is now used by many different specialties in most countries.

Clinician performed ultrasound has a different approach than formal diagnostic ultrasound, such as that performed in radiology departments. Clinician performed ultrasound is generally limited in scope and targeted to answering a specific question (such as 'is there an abdominal aortic aneurysm'), rather than providing a full assessment of an anatomical area (Table 23.1.1). In this regard, it is often viewed more as an extension of the clinical exam, than a technique that competes with other imaging techniques (including formal ultrasound).

Table 23.1.1 Current indications for emergency ultrasound
Trauma (haemoperitoneum, haemopericardium, pneumothorax)
Abdominal aortic aneurysm
Early pregnancy complications
Biliary disease
Renal stones and hydronephrosis
Echocardiography in trauma and shock
Lung ultrasound in acute dyspnoea
Proximal DVT exclusion
Procedural
Musculoskeletal

Background

Clinical ultrasound followed developments from the use of sonar, where the principle that sound waves could be used to locate objects was developed. Initially, ultrasound machines were large and cumbersome, but advances in technology have improved image quality while reducing machine size, so that today, small machines are able to produce high quality images. As a result of this improved technology, ultrasound is now available to clinicians and can be performed at the bedside of patients. There was early adoption of the technique by obstetricians and gynaecologists worldwide and later by other specialties in Europe and

The Australasian College for Emergency Medicine supports the use of bedside ultrasound by emergency physicians [1], as does the American College of Emergency Physicians, the College of Emergency Medicine in the UK and the International Federation for Emergency Medicine, where it is seen as a core skill required of all trainees. It is expected that with increasing experience the range of conditions for which ultrasound is used in emergency departments (EDs) will increase.

Basic physics of ultrasound [2]

Sound waves are mechanical waves that transmit energy through the vibration of particles. Ultrasound waves are defined as those that are above the usual range of human hearing (20–20 000 Hz). Current diagnostic ultrasound machines are based upon the pulse–echo principle, using pulses of sound waves at frequencies of 2–15 MHz which are reflected back. Processing of these reflected echoes creates the ultrasound data and image.

The ultrasound transducer converts electrical impulses into pulses of sound (via the piezoelectric effect) which are then directed into the body. As the sound wave travels through tissue, it gradually loses energy, termed attenuation. The degree of attenuation differs for different tissues and is also dependent on the frequency of the pulse wave. Upon reaching a tissue interface, some of the energy is reflected back as an echo, due to the differences in acoustic impedance (gel or other coupling material is used to minimize reflection at the probe/skin surface). This reflected echo then travels back through tissue, undergoing further attenuation, until it reaches the transducer, which converts the energy back to an electrical impulse. This returning impulse is then amplified and processed. The time taken for the pulse wave to travel to the tissue interface and back is converted into distance by using the average speed for sound in tissue. The intensity of the returning wave determines the brightness of the displayed pixel. The returning pulses from the different reflecting surfaces along the path of the ultrasound beam generate a single line of the ultrasound image. The ultrasound beam is steered across the field to generate the multiple lines of information that then form the 2D image (termed B-mode, for brightness modulation). Alternatively, if the direction of the beam is kept constant and the changing surfaces are mapped over time then an M-mode image is generated.

The degree of attenuation is dependent on the frequency of the sound wave, so higher frequency pulses undergo greater attenuation. They also have shorter wavelengths, which improve the resolution of the ultrasound beam (the ability to distinguish two separate objects close together). This leads to one of the most important trade-offs in ultrasound, between resolution and penetration. To obtain high resolution, a high frequency probe can be chosen, but these will be unable to image deep structures.

To form the image, the ultrasound machine makes certain assumptions about the ultrasound beam and sound impulse. Deviations from these behaviours will result in image artefacts, i.e. when the image does not represent the tissue accurately. There are many artefacts, most of which reduce the information available from the image. The most clinically important artefacts, however, can also be used diagnostically:

Shadowing – when all of the energy of the ultrasound pulse is reflected or absorbed at a surface (such as air or bone). In this situation, there will be no returning pulses from the tissue distal to the object. This creates a black area on the screen, known as an acoustic shadow. The presence of a shadow behind a brightly reflective surface can thus be used to diagnose a region of calcification, such as a calculus (Fig. 23.1.1). Stones and bones generally give 'clean' or black shadows, while gas gives 'dirty' or grey shadows due to the superposition of both shadow and reverberation artefact (Fig. 23.1.2).

Enhancement – when an area of interest (such as fluid in a cyst) absorbs less energy than the surrounding tissue, the pulses that have travelled through that area will have more energy than equidistant pulses that did not, resulting in a bright region deep to the area of interest on the image (Fig. 23.1.3). Enhancement is used to confirm the fluid-filled nature of lesions.

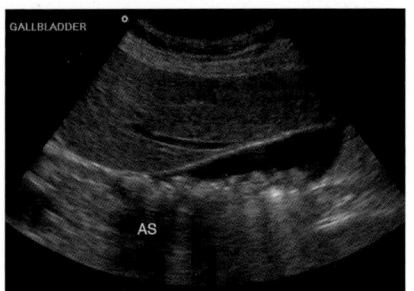

Fig. 23.1.1 Acoustic shadowing from gallstones. AS: acoustic shadow.

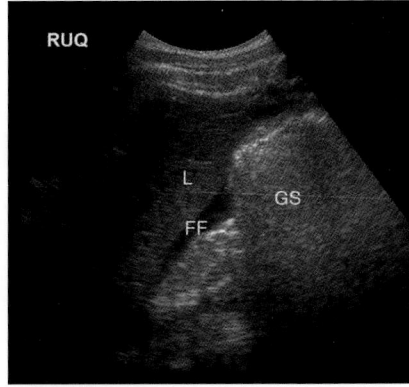

Fig. 23.1.2 Acoustic shadowing from bowel gas in a patient with free fluid. L: liver; FF: free fluid; GS: gas shadow.

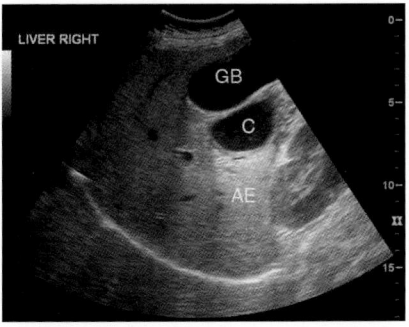

Fig. 23.1.3 Acoustic enhancement from fluid-filled structures. Acoustic enhancement is seen where the ultrasound beam passes through the gallbladder and more prominently where it passes through the gallbladder and pancreatic pseudocyst. GB: gallbladder; C: pancreatic pseudocyst; AE: acoustic enhancement.

Transducer

Different ultrasound transducers are available varying in shape, frequency and the size of the contact area (termed footprint). Transducers may have a small footprint to fit into small areas, such as between ribs, from which the beam spreads in a large arc (e.g. a sector transducer). Alternatively, they may be larger with a flat or slightly curved surface where contact can be maintained, such as a linear probe. Special transducers have been designed for use within body cavities, such as transoesophageal, endovaginal and endo-anal probes. These transducers offer the advantage of reduced distance between the transducer and area of interest, which allows higher frequencies to be used resulting in improved resolution. Very high frequency transducers have been used for intravascular and superficial ocular scanning. Appropriate choice of transducer is important in ensuring the optimal image is obtained.

The scope of emergency department ultrasound

Extended focused assessment by sonography for trauma (EFAST) [3–6]

Descriptions of the use of ultrasound by clinicians to evaluate trauma patients appeared in the European literature in the 1970s. Reports have subsequently appeared from countries around the world and the technique is now well established. Initially limited to the abdomen and pericardium (FAST), the examination is now routinely extended to include the chest (EFAST). With relatively brief training and experience, non-radiologists are able to diagnose haemoperitoneum, pericardial effusions, pleural effusions and pneumothorax with a high degree of sensitivity and specificity, although accuracy does improve with experience.

Clinical examination in abdominal trauma can be difficult and unreliable. Diagnostic peritoneal lavage (DPL), ultrasound (FAST) and computed tomography (CT) have been used to evaluate further this group of patients. In most cases, FAST has replaced diagnostic peritoneal lavage as it is non-invasive and does not interfere with subsequent interpretation of CT images. CT scanning is highly accurate for diagnosing both free fluid and solid organ injury and is slightly less accurate for hollow viscus and diaphragmatic injury.

Studies of ultrasound scanning in trauma have reported varying sensitivity. Much of this variation is due to differences in the gold standard used for comparison and definition of 'true positive'. Haemoperitoneum (on further imaging, surgical or post-mortem examination), organ injury and clinical stability have all been used in different studies. It must be remembered that the primary role of a FAST scan is to detect free fluid in the peritoneal or pericardial spaces, for which it has high sensitivity and specificity. Solid organ or retroperitoneal haemorrhage may be detected but, even in expert hands, the accuracy is much lower (with as many as two-thirds of injuries being missed). FAST has been shown to be reliable and useful in both pregnant and paediatric patients.

Technique

FAST scanning evaluates four regions for the presence of free fluid: (1) pericardial; (2) perihepatic; (3) perisplenic; and (4) pelvic (Fig. 23.1.4). The chest is then scanned to examine the pleural spaces posterolaterally for fluid and anteriorly to exclude pneumothorax. The technique is rapid, generally being completed in under 5 minutes.

Free fluid appears as an echolucent area (i.e. black) which is generally linear or triangular in shape in the most dependent area of the peritoneal or pericardial space, although blood clots may be seen as echogenic (grey) collections (Figs 23.1.5–23.1.7). While fluid is most commonly seen in the perihepatic space, all spaces should be examined before the result can be considered negative. Small amounts of fluid (<500 mL) may not to be detected.

When scanning the chest, the presence of lung sliding or lung pulse is an indication that the visceral and parietal pleura are in contact, excluding a pneumothorax at that point. The

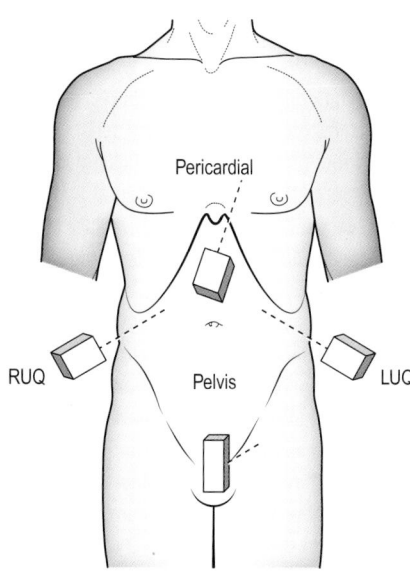

Fig. 23.1.4 Transducer placement for the four views for FAST scanning. RUQ: right upper quadrant; LUQ: left upper quadrant.

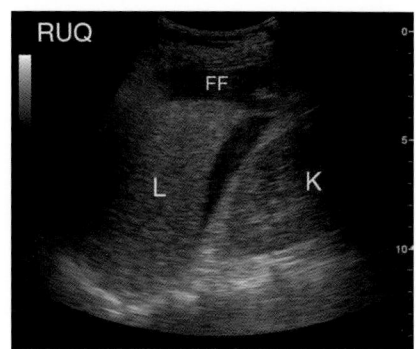

Fig. 23.1.5 Free fluid in the perihepatic view; fluid lies in Morrison's pouch between liver and right kidney. L: liver; FF: free fluid; K: kidney.

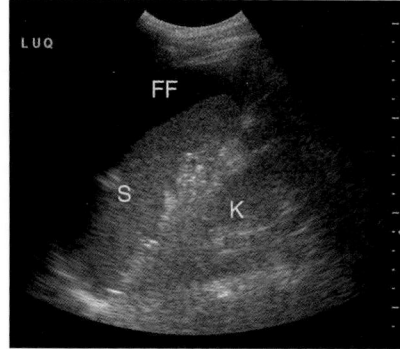

Fig. 23.1.6 Free fluid in the perisplenic view; fluid may lie anywhere around the spleen; in this case, it lies interposed between spleen and diaphragm. S: spleen; FF: free fluid; K: kidney.

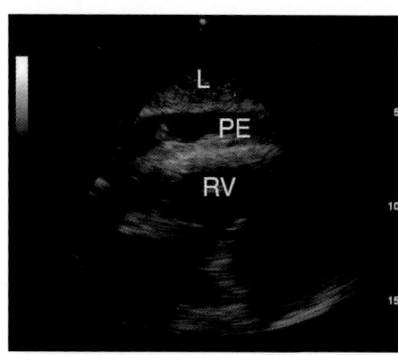

Fig. 23.1.7 Pericardial effusion with clot. L: liver; RV: right ventricle; PE: pericardial effusion with grey blood clots and black (echo free) blood.

presence of a moving transition point between areas of lung sliding and absent lung sliding (the 'lung point' sign) is diagnostic of pneumothorax.

Limitations and pitfalls

- User dependent with learning curve.
- Inadequate views occur in up to 10%, especially if the bladder is empty or with subcutaneous emphysema.
- Cannot distinguish between blood and other forms of intra-abdominal or pericardial fluid, such as ascites or pericardial effusion.
- Retroperitoneal haemorrhage may be missed.
- Solid organ, hollow viscus or diaphragmatic injuries can occur without free fluid.
- Small amounts of free fluid may not be detected.
- Small amounts of pelvic fluid may be physiological in women.
- Fluid-filled bowel can be misinterpreted as free fluid.
- Pericardial fluid may decompress into the pleural cavity.
- Loss of lung sliding may be due to causes other than pneumothorax.

Clinical implications and utility

The limitations of ultrasound in excluding all intra-abdominal injuries requiring laparotomy and the increasing use of conservative management of some injuries, even in the setting of intra-abdominal free fluid, has resulted in there being no universally accepted clinical algorithm based upon EFAST scan results. However, in this regard, EFAST scanning is no different to any other clinical, laboratory or imaging information of the trauma patient, the results of which are routinely used in combination to determine the management plan. Various algorithms incorporating EFAST scanning have been proposed, which generally incorporate haemodynamic stability and EFAST scan result, such as in Figure 23.1.8. Some algorithms incorporate a semiquantitative scoring system to estimate the amount of free fluid, with an increased volume of free fluid associated with greater need for therapeutic laparotomy. A positive abdominal EFAST scan is highly predictive of significant intra-abdominal injury and, based upon the clinical condition of the patient, generally indicates the need for CT or surgical exploration. A negative EFAST scan, stable haemodynamics and clinical observation have been shown to be highly accurate in excluding significant intra-abdominal injury. Some authors advocate serial EFAST examinations in stable patients, suggesting this can reduce the requirement for CT.

Similarly, for pneumothorax, the integration of EFAST findings with other clinical, laboratory and imaging findings will determine patient management. Conservative management of small pneumothoraces, even in the setting of positive pressure ventilation means that the ultrasound findings must be considered in the setting of the individual patient when management decisions are made.

In the Australasian setting, EFAST is generally accepted as fulfilling a complementary role to CT. Its portability and speed allow it to be used early in the evaluation of trauma patients (e.g. immediately after the primary survey) and this information is then incorporated with other clinical information to risk stratify the trauma patient to help to determine the requirement and timing for either laparotomy, thoracotomy or CT. Repeated examinations, particularly if the patient's condition changes, can be valuable. Providing the limitations of the technique are not ignored, it can rapidly provide vital information to assist with patient management.

Abdominal aortic aneurysm [7,8]

Abdominal aortic aneurysms (AAA), defined as an aortic diameter >3.0 cm, are common, occurring in 1–9% of the population. Clinical assessment of the abdominal aorta is unreliable and may be especially difficult in the obese or unstable patient with abdominal pain. Clinical presentation of ruptured abdominal aortic aneurysm can be varied, with only 50% of patients demonstrating the classic presentation of hypotension, back pain and pulsatile mass. Other presentations may include abdominal, groin or flank pain, unexplained hypotension, syncope, haematuria or cardiac failure and AAA should be considered in any of these presentations.

Ultrasound is the primary mode of investigation of the abdominal aorta. Ultrasound performed by emergency clinicians has been shown to be rapid, highly sensitive and highly specific (>95%) in assessing aortic diameter. Ultrasound may occasionally detect rupture, but it is not reliable in excluding rupture. In addition to its utility in diagnosing AAA, ED ultrasound is very beneficial in rapidly excluding AAA in the wide variety of presentations listed above.

The risk of rupture of an AAA increases with the diameter. Although the risk of rupture if the aneurysm diameter is less than 4 cm is <0.5% per year and 1.5% per year for aneurysms 4.0–4.9 cm, rupture can still occur. Approximately 10% of ruptured aneurysms measure 5 cm or less.

Technique

The aorta should be identified anterior to the vertebral body and to the left of the inferior vena cava (IVC). It should be followed from the epigastric region to its bifurcation, just above the umbilicus, remembering that, in elderly patients, it may follow an ectactic course rather than following a strictly cranial–caudal course. It must be distinguished from both the superior mesenteric artery (SMA) (which runs anterior to the aorta) and the IVC (ensuring that the venous pulsation of the IVC is not mistaken for the arterial pulse of the aorta). Measurements should be taken both proximally and distally and, if an aneurysm is present, at the widest point. Measurements from both transverse and longitudinal planes should be taken. Measurements are taken from the outer wall to outer wall, including any mural thrombus (Fig. 23.1.9). If the renal arteries or SMA origin are identifiable then the relation to the aneurysm should be noted although, in the ED setting, this may not be possible. Any retroperitoneal haematoma or peritoneal free fluid should be noted.

Limitations and pitfalls

- Pain, obesity or bowel gas may prevent adequate imaging by ultrasound.
- Mistaking the IVC or SMA for the aorta.
- Measuring the lumen without including mural thrombus.
- Attempting to exclude rupture on ultrasound.
- Forgetting that the AAA may be an incidental finding and not the primary cause of the patient's symptoms.

Clinical implications and utility

In the patient with ruptured AAA who is haemodynamically unstable, ED ultrasound allows rapid and accurate diagnosis within the resuscitation area. Rapid diagnosis of these patients

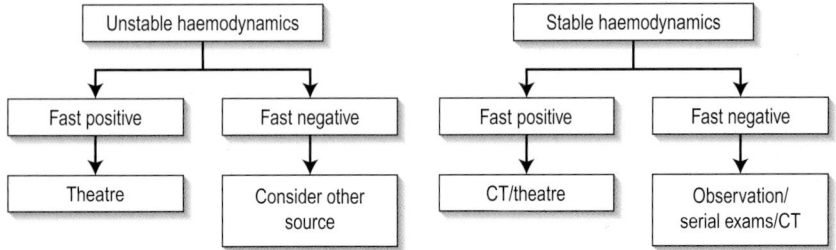

Fig. 23.1.8 Suggested algorithm using FAST results.

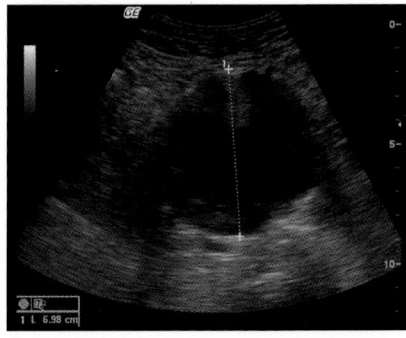

Fig. 23.1.9 Abdominal aortic aneurysm.

is essential to achieve successful treatment. In the stable patient, whose presentation may be atypical, ED ultrasound provides a rapid means of excluding the diagnosis (e.g. in the elderly patient who presents with 'renal colic'). If an AAA is detected in these patients, then further imaging will often be required to determine if the AAA is an incidental finding or the cause of the patient's symptoms. If the AAA is an incidental finding then formal follow up should be arranged.

Early pregnancy [9,10]

Ultrasound is the primary imaging modality for early pregnancy and its complications [11]. In the emergency department setting, it is most commonly used for the pregnant patient with pain or bleeding. In addition to transabdominal scanning (TAS), transvaginal scanning (TVS) can be performed with patient consent using a specifically designed probe which places the transducer close to the pelvic organs and utilizes higher frequencies to produce images of much greater detail than TAS. It does not require a full bladder and should not be a painful procedure. TAS still has an important role, as it allows a broader field of view that allows better assessment of large amounts of free intraperitoneal fluid and may diagnose other causes of pain. Emergency physician performed ultrasound for early pregnancy complications has been shown to be safe and reduce the time patients spend in emergency departments.

Technique

TAS is performed initially, preferably when the patient has a full bladder, as the pelvic organs will be better visualized. The uterus is identified and examined in both longitudinal and transverse planes (recognizing that the longitudinal axis of the uterus may not necessarily be in a strictly sagittal plane). The endometrial thickness is noted and any fluid collections or gestational sac noted. The adnexa are examined to identify the ovaries and any masses. The pelvis is scanned for free fluid. The upper abdomen can be examined to estimate the volume of free fluid if seen. The kidneys can also be examined to identify any alternate diagnoses.

TVS is performed after the procedure is explained and consent is obtained. A chaperone should be present if the sonographer is male. The patient is asked to empty their bladder and the pelvis is elevated slightly off the bed using a foam wedge or similar. The probe is covered with a sterile sheath (e.g. condom) with gel placed inside and outside the sheath. The probe is gently inserted into the vagina and advanced. The uterus and adnexa are then examined in both longitudinal and transverse planes as in TAS. After the scan is complete the probe must be cleaned and disinfected.

Limitations and pitfalls

- Confusing a corpus luteum cyst and ectopic pregnancy.
- Misinterpreting a pseudogestational sac for a gestational sac.
- Not considering heterotopic pregnancy in patients receiving fertility treatment.
- Failure to arrange follow up if an intrauterine pregnancy is not identified, even if an ectopic pregnancy is not seen.
- Failure to recognize an eccentric or low gestational sac could be an interstitial, cervical or scar ectopic.
- Assuming an empty uterus in a patient with positive BHCG is a complete miscarriage.

Clinical implications and utility

The primary aim of ultrasound in evaluating early pregnancy complications in the emergency department is to locate the gestational sac. Additional information should then be sought for the presence of free fluid, adnexal masses, embryonic size and embryonic cardiac activity (viability). The earliest ultrasound evidence of pregnancy is a small anechoic fluid collection surrounded by an echogenic ring, which can be seen on TVS at approximately 4.5 weeks. A pseudogestational sac (due to fluid within the endometrial cavity), however, can have very similar appearances. Definite signs that the sac is a true gestational sac appear at 5.5 weeks when the yolk sac can be visualized, or later when the embryo can be identified. A heartbeat may be visualized from 6.0 to 6.5 weeks onward. TAS will show the same features but 1–2 weeks later.

Pregnancies that are not identified by ultrasound are termed 'pregnancy of unknown location' (PUL). Most will either fail (miscarry or resolve spontaneously) or progress to normal pregnancy. However, 9–43% will eventually be identified as ectopic pregnancies (lower rates are seen in centres with more expert scanning ability as they have higher rates of definitively diagnosing ectopic pregnancy). Quantitative human chorionic gonadotrophin (HCG) levels have been used to determine when a gestational sac should be identifiable by ultrasound, termed the 'discriminatory zone'. For TVS, this is usually 1500 IU and for TAS 4500 IU (varying between institutions and depending on expertise and equipment). Even though a normal pregnancy may not be expected to be seen in patients with β-HCG levels below these levels, ultrasound should still be performed as it may still show diagnostic findings. In particular, ectopic pregnancies often have lower β-HCG levels than normal pregnancies of corresponding gestation and may be seen, as can the presence or absence of free fluid, which is valuable for risk stratification.

All patients with pregnancy of unknown location require close follow up with serial HCG and repeat ultrasound.

If an intrauterine pregnancy is confirmed, the risk of ectopic pregnancy is very low in spontaneously conceived pregnancies. Heterotopic pregnancy is where both an intrauterine and extrauterine pregnancy coexist and occurs in up to 1:7000 pregnancies in spontaneous conceived pregnancies, but over 1:100 pregnancies in the setting of fertility treatment. Failure to visualize an intrauterine pregnancy may be due to early dates in a normal pregnancy, failed intrauterine pregnancy (including complete miscarriage) or ectopic pregnancy. Other ultrasound findings in ectopic pregnancy include non-specific findings, such as pelvic blood and adnexal mass (Table 23.1.2) [12]. Visualization of a gestational sac (with yolk sac or embryo) outside the uterus is diagnostic, but seen only in 8–26% of ectopic pregnancies (Fig. 23.1.10).

Unusual forms of ectopic pregnancy include interstitial, cervical and scar ectopics. In these cases, a gestational sac may be seen, but not within the true uterine cavity. It is recommended that pregnancies that appear low

Table 23.1.2 Ultrasound findings of ectopic pregnancy	
Ultrasound finding	Accuracy (%)
Absent IUP	5
Any free fluid (no IUP)	50
Mod–large free fluid (no IUP)	60–85
Adnexal mass (no IUP)	75
Adnexal mass + free fluid (no IUP)	97
Ectopic pregnancy seen	100

IUP: intrauterine pregnancy.

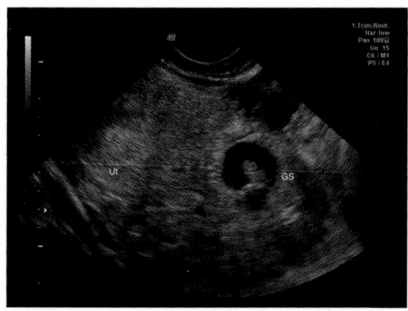

Fig. 23.1.10 Ectopic pregnancy. A gestational sac (GS) containing an embryonic pole is seen outside the uterus (Ut).

or eccentric should be reviewed by expert sonographers.

Distinguishing between miscarriage and ectopic pregnancy when no adnexal mass has been identified can be difficult on ultrasound. However, if the clinical symptoms have settled, no free fluid is identified on ultrasound and no adnexal masses have been identified, then it is safe to observe or discharge the patient for formal ultrasound review the following day and subsequent follow up with repeat ultrasound and quantitative HCG (see Chapter 19.2).

If an intrauterine pregnancy is confirmed, the gestational age can be estimated by measuring the size of the embryo. Most machines will automatically calculate gestational age based upon this measurement. Cardiac activity can usually be identified by TVS once the embryo is approximately 5 mm (9 mm by TAS). Absent cardiac activity when the embryo is 7 mm or above suggests embryonic demise. Absent yolk sac or embryo on TVS when the gestational sac is 25 mm suggests an empty sac miscarriage (also referred to as a blighted ovum) [13]. Other sonographic signs of poor prognosis for continued pregnancy exist, but they are generally beyond the scope of emergency ultrasound.

Right upper quadrant/ gallbladder [14]

Upper abdominal pain due to biliary disease is a common presenting complaint to emergency departments and includes biliary colic, choledocholithiasis, cholecystitis and ascending cholangitis. Many of the patients suspected of having acute cholecystitis will have alternate diseases and clinical examination is neither sufficiently sensitive nor specific for these patients. Ultrasound is the primary imaging modality for these patients, where it is used

to detect the presence of gallstones (see Fig. 23.1.1), other sonographic signs of cholecystitis and bile duct obstruction. It is superior to both scintigraphy and CT for these patients.

Ultrasound has a high sensitivity and specificity for the identification of stones when performed by either radiology or ED staff. Some stones may, however, be missed and false-positive results also occur. The diagnosis of cholecystitis relies upon associated findings including sonographic Murphy's sign, gallbladder wall thickening, gallbladder distension and pericholecystic fluid (Fig. 23.1.11). Gallbladder wall thickening and pericholecystic fluid are both non-specific findings and may be seen in other hepatic or generalized diseases as well as in acalculous cholecystitis. Fasting can cause gallbladder distension. The common bile duct, if visualized, should be measured and examined for stones, although this is technically more difficult and may be beyond the scope of a focused gallbladder examination.

Technique
The gallbladder (GB) is usually identified by scanning under the costal margin in a longitudinal plane. Positioning the patient in the left lateral decubitus position and/or deep inspiration may assist. The gallbladder should be scanned throughout its length in both longitudinal and transverse planes. The sonographic Murphy's sign is assessed by pressing with the ultrasound probe over the gallbladder. Wall thickness should be measured and is normally less than 3 mm. Gallstones will appear as bright, echogenic masses with posterior acoustic shadowing. Stones tend to be mobile unless impacted in the gallbladder neck or cystic duct. Stones impacted in these positions are

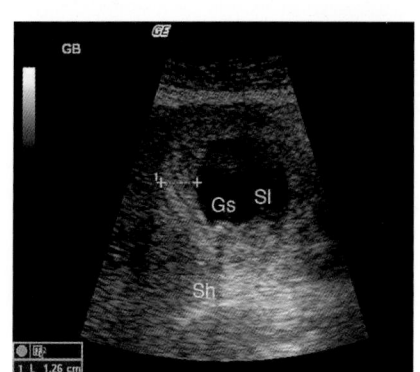

Fig. 23.1.11 Acute cholecystitis. Transverse image of a gallbladder with thickened wall and pericholecystic fluid. Within the lumen are multiple gallstones (Gs) which cast shadows (Sh).

technically more difficult to detect and may be missed if not painstakingly searched for. Sludge and polyps will also appear echogenic but will not shadow. Whenever possible, the common bile duct (CBD) should be visualized, measured and followed; when dilated, distal CBD obstruction should be considered.

Limitations and pitfalls
- Incorrectly assuming the presence of gallstones explains the patient's symptoms, when they may be an incidental finding.
- Mistaking gas in the duodenum for gallstones in the gallbladder.
- Mistaking a gallbladder that is contracted and/or full of stones for a gas- and food-filled duodenum.
- Symptomatic stones impacted in the GB neck or cystic duct are easily missed.
- Small stones (<3 mm) may not cast shadows.
- Misinterpreting sludge or polyps as stones.
- Misinterpreting other causes of GB wall thickening as cholecystitis.

Clinical implications and utility
In a patient with abdominal pain, the finding of gallstones with a positive sonographic Murphy's sign is strongly predictive of cholecystitis. The more sonographic signs of cholecystitis that are seen, the more likely the diagnosis. However, asymptomatic gallstones are common and may therefore represent an incidental finding, especially if the sonographic Murphy's sign is absent. In elderly, diabetic or critically ill patients, 5–10% of cholecystitis can be acalculous. In those patients thought to have biliary colic or cholecystitis, a negative ultrasound should prompt a search for alternative diagnoses or consideration of further imaging, either formal ultrasound or, if an alternate diagnosis is believed likely, CT.

Renal ultrasound

The primary focus of renal ultrasound in the emergency setting is the detection of hydronephrosis in the presence of acute renal failure or renal colic [15]. As experience increases, users can often detect renal calculi, particularly when located at the vesicoureteric junction (VUJ). The presence of a ureteric jet excludes complete ureteric obstruction on that side.

Technique

The kidneys are paired retroperitoneal organs lying on either side of the spine between T12 and L4. They have a convex lateral border and a concave medial border and hilum. The normal adult kidney is 9–12 cm in length, 2.5–4 cm thick and 4–6 cm wide. The kidney itself is composed of two distinct areas, the renal parenchyma and the renal sinus.

The adult kidney is scanned using a curvilinear 3.5–5 MHz transducer and a renal preset that provides the best contrast resolution and grey map for imaging the kidneys. The patient may be supine, although the kidneys are usually best seen with the patient in a lateral decubitus position. A combination of subcostal and intercostal approaches is often necessary to fully evaluate the kidneys. The kidneys should be imaged in at least two planes, including the sagittal or coronal plane and the transverse plane (Figs 23.1.12 and 23.1.13). On ultrasound, the kidney can be identified by its elliptical shape with a thin echogenic capsule. Normal renal parenchyma has slightly decreased or equal echogenicity relative to the hepatic or splenic parenchyma, although this is age dependent with it being comparatively

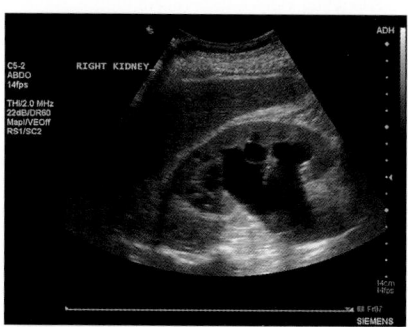

Fig. 23.1.12 Sagittal image of right kidney demonstrating moderate hydronephrosis.

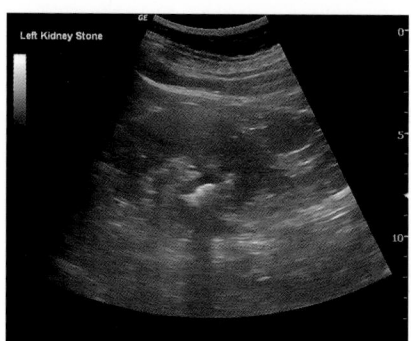

Fig. 23.1.13 Coronal image of left kidney demonstrating a calculus in the renal pelvis with acoustic shadowing.

hyperechoic in the elderly. The central renal sinus is particularly echobright due to the fat and fibrous tissue content. The renal pelvis and infundibulum are usually collapsed and not seen except in the setting of hydronephrosis when they become filled with urine, appearing anechoic. The bladder should be full and examined in both the sagittal and transverse planes to complete the study. It should be noted that an excessively full bladder may cause mild dilatation of the pelvicalyceal system, however, this will return to normal following micturition.

Ureteric jets occur when either ureter contracts propelling urine into the bladder. This occurs every 10–20 seconds in the euvolaemic patient with normal renal function and excludes complete obstruction on that side. The presence of a jet, however, does not exclude the possibility of a non-obstructive renal or ureteric calculus.

Hydronephrosis is the dilatation of the renal pelvis and calyces and may be secondary to an anatomical obstruction or may be functional in nature (such as with ureteric reflux). Obstructive hydronephrosis may be intrinsic or extrinsic. Depending on the level of obstruction, it may be unilateral or bilateral with or without associated hydroureter. When hydronephrosis is identified, the cause for the obstruction should be sought. Common intrinsic obstructive causes seen in the emergency department include obstructive or partially obstructive renal or ureteric calculi. Bladder outlet obstruction due to prostatic hypertrophy is another common cause of hydronephrosis. Extrinsic or invasive masses in the pelvis obstructing either the ureters or bladder outflow should also be considered.

Hydronephrosis may be described as mild, moderate or severe depending on the extent of dilatation of the renal collecting system:

- mild: dilatation of renal pelvis; may have some calyceal filling, however, the calyces remain cupped
- moderate: increasing dilatation extending into the pelvicalyceal system with distension and blunting of the calyces, but with preservation of cortical thickness
- severe: marked pelvicalyceal dilation with clubbed calyces and associated parenchymal cortical thinning.

Limitations and pitfalls

- Assuming hydronephrosis and obstruction are synonymous.
- Hydronephrosis takes time to develop and more so in the dehydrated patient.

- Hydronephrosis can persist transiently after obstruction is relieved.
- Mistaking an extrarenal pelvis for hydronephrosis.
- Mistaking parapelvic renal cysts for hydronephrosis.

Clinical implications and utility

Ultrasound is less sensitive than plain films or CT in detecting renal calculi. Small stones may often be obscured by the echogenic renal sinus and be hard to detect if they have a weak posterior acoustic shadow. Having said this, stones in the kidney that are greater than 5 mm in size have been shown to be detected in experienced hands with 100% sensitivity sonographically [16]. Renal stones appear as bright, echogenic foci with distal acoustic shadowing and sometimes twinkle artefact when interrogated with colour Doppler. Ureteric calculi are difficult to visualize as they are often obscured by bowel gas in their retroperitoneal position. A normal appearing kidney and the failure to visualize a calculus therefore does not exclude a ureteric calculus that is non-obstructing or where hydronephrosis has not yet developed.

Deep vein thrombosis (DVT)

The primary focus of emergency department ultrasound in the assessment of DVT is in the diagnosis or exclusion of a proximal lower limb DVT.

The clinical assessment of DVT is unreliable and inaccurate [17,18]. Positive findings on sonographic examination of only 11% have been reported for patients referred for suspected acute DVT on the basis of clinical features [19].

Technique

Ultrasound is the imaging modality of choice for assessing for DVT. The technique relies primarily on B-mode imaging with intermittent venous compression, with the main diagnostic criteria used to exclude a DVT being complete collapse of the vein with apposition of the anterior and posterior walls of the vessel.

A broadband linear array transducer with a centre frequency of about 5 MHz is used to examine the femoral, popliteal and sometimes the calf veins. In larger patients, the curved linear array transducer with a centre frequency of 3.5 MHz (as used for abdominal studies) may be substituted. The curved linear array transducer is also used to examine the iliac veins.

The machine should be configured to use the lower limb venous preset and the use of harmonic imaging may improve the contrast resolution between the vessel and surrounding tissue. Transducer compression of the interrogated vessel should be in the transverse imaging plane. Starting at the level of the groin, with the patient in a supine position, the common femoral vein is identified lying medial to the common femoral artery and the vein is compressed to demonstrate collapsibility extending distally in a stepwise fashion with the vein compressed every 2–3 cm (Fig. 23.1.14). Where thrombus is present in the vein, pressure with the transducer will not result in its collapse. The popliteal vein is best examined with the patient in a lateral or prone position with the knee slightly flexed. Colour and spectral Doppler may be used to supplement the findings of intermittent compression. Emergency physicians who had undergone standardized training to identify clot in the femoral or popliteal veins have shown an accuracy comparable to formal vascular studies [20].

Limitations and pitfalls

- Mistaking the saphenous vein for the superficial femoral vein.
- Not recognizing that the previously termed 'superficial' femoral vein is a deep vein (it is now referred to as 'femoral vein').
- Sensitivity of ultrasound for calf DVT detection is much lower than proximal DVT.
- Not recognizing a duplicated femoral or popliteal vein with one patent and one thrombosed.
- Misdiagnosing chronic clot for fresh clot.
- Not ensuring that initial ED exclusion of proximal DVT is followed up by a formal repeat scan in 7 days.

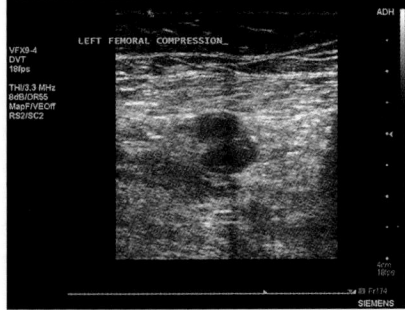

Fig. 23.1.14 Transverse image of the left femoral vein and artery with incomplete collapse of the femoral vein with compression indicating intraluminal thrombus.

Clinical implications and utility

The accuracy of compression ultrasonography is highest in symptomatic patients, with studies comparing venography with compression ultrasound demonstrating an average sensitivity of 95% and specificity of 98% [21]. For proximal lower limb DVT, this technique has demonstrated sensitivity of up to 100% [22]. The use of colour and spectral Doppler to assess for vessel filling defects and flow patterns has not been shown to increase significantly the sensitivity for proximal DVT detection in the lower limb [22–25]. It has also been suggested that an abbreviated technique, using only two compression points (the saphenofemoral junction and the lower popliteal vein) has adequate sensitivity, provided repeat examination is performed in 5–7 days [24,26,27]. The accuracy of ultrasound in detecting isolated calf DVT, especially when applied to bedside emergency ultrasound, is low with success rates as low as 40% reported [28].

Thus, the aim of focused emergency department ultrasound in the assessment of DVT is generally to confirm or exclude the presence of clot in the proximal deep veins of the lower limb. A negative compression ultrasound study of the proximal lower limb significantly reduces the likelihood of DVT and discharge from the emergency department without anticoagulation, with outpatient follow up for a definitive study can be considered [21,29–31].

Emergency echocardiography

Focused use of echocardiography in the emergency department represents one of the most valuable uses of ultrasound in emergency medicine. Applications include its use in cardiac arrest, undifferentiated hypotension, suspected pericardial effusion and tamponade, chest pain, pulmonary embolus and ultrasound guided procedures. The use of cardiac ultrasound in emergency medicine is likely to increase significantly as more emergency physicians learn the technique and look to apply it increasingly in the clinical environment.

Echocardiography provides direct structural and functional information on cardiac structures only inferred by clinical examination, which has been shown to have limited accuracy, and with greater sensitivity and specificity than indirect tests, such as ECG and chest radiography [32–34].

Technique

Modern general ultrasound machines can provide good quality transthoracic echocardiography capability. A broadband phased array transducer with a centre frequency of 2 MHz and a small footprint to improve access between the ribs should be used. Ideally, the patient should be positioned on their left side.

The full, standard echocardiographic examination includes parasternal long and short axis views obtained at the left sternal edge in the 2nd to 4th rib spaces, the apical 4-, 5-, 3- and 2- chamber views that are obtained at the cardiac apex and the subcostal views obtained from a subxiphoid position. The standard examination would involve 2-D assessment of cardiac structure and function using B-mode, supplemented by the use of colour and spectral Doppler to assess valvular function and measure chamber pressures using the windows described above.

Where an abbreviated, emergency bedside echocardiographic examination is being used to screen for the presence of tamponade, right ventricular dysfunction, left ventricular dysfunction and hypovolaemia alone, simply using B-mode and attaining the parasternal short and long axis views, the apical 4-chamber view and the subcostal view is generally enough.

In cardiac arrest, the subcostal view is used with the patient in the supine position. All preparations are made while CPR continues. During the 10-second pulse check, a loop is recorded and reviewed once CPR recommences. It is imperative that the time without CPR is minimized and echocardiography should not interfere with this.

Emergency physicians have been shown to assess accurately left ventricular function in the hypotensive patient [35].

Limitations and pitfalls

- Good views may not be obtainable in a supine patient, especially if ventilated.
- Not appreciating the limitations of focused and abbreviated emergency echocardiographic studies when compared to formal detailed echocardiographic studies.
- Focused echocardiographic examination aims to detect for tamponade, right ventricular dysfunction, left ventricular dysfunction and hypovolaemia. It does not assess for diastolic dysfunction, regional wall motion abnormality,

valvular dysfunction or aortic dissection, the detection of which generally take significantly more experience.

- Confusing pleural and pericardial effusions.
- Confusing pericardial fat pad and pericardial effusion.
- Not appreciating the fluid causing tamponade is not always anechoic, particularly when exudative, purulent or haemorrhagic.
- Not appreciating that a loculated clot or effusion may cause tamponade but not be seen, particularly in the postoperative patient
- Not appreciating a normal echo does not exclude pulmonary embolism.
- Not understanding there is difficulty distinguishing between acute pulmonary hypertension from pulmonary embolism and chronic pulmonary hypertension.
- Not appreciating that while a large, round IVC with no respiratory variation infers elevated right-sided pressures, it does not mean fluid will be futile. In tamponade and right ventricular infarction, for example, additional preload despite a 'full' IVC is often useful.

Clinical indications and utility

In cardiac arrest, the aim of echocardiography is to assess left ventricular activity as well as to exclude the presence of potentially reversible causes, particularly tamponade. In the setting of cardiac arrest, cardiac standstill on initial presenting echocardiographic assessment has important prognostic implications, irrespective of presenting electrical rhythm. Blaivas et al. demonstrated that no patients out of 136 presenting with cardiac standstill on initial echocardiographic assessment survived to leave the ED irrespective of presenting rhythm, findings supported by Salen et al. in a study of 102 patients presenting in cardiac arrest [37,38]. Having said this, several case reports have recently been written describing patients who developed return of spontaneous circulation (ROSC) after having echo-documented cardiac standstill. As is always the case, the user must integrate ultrasound findings into the clinical picture to make a final clinical decision. Cardiac standstill in the newly collapsed patient, the hypothermic patient, the young patient or the toxicological overdose should not be used as the sole criterion to cease resuscitative efforts.

Echocardiography is very useful in determining the cause of undifferentiated hypotension

and shock. The primary aim of focused emergency echocardiography in this setting is to assess for tamponade, for right ventricular (RV) dysfunction (that in the correct clinical setting would infer massive pulmonary embolism), for left ventricular systolic dysfunction and for hypovolaemia.

A pericardial effusion is seen as an anechoic collection of fluid between the visceral and parietal pericardium (Fig. 23.1.15), although an inflammatory pericardial effusion or haemopericardium may exhibit internal echoes. In differentiating between a pericardial effusion and a pleural effusion, a pericardial effusion tapers towards and anterior to the descending aorta and may extend a short distance between the aorta and left atrium, conversely, a pleural effusion will accumulate and extend behind the descending aorta. When a pericardial effusion is identified, its location and size should be documented and any evidence of tamponade looked for. The size of an effusion can be described as small, moderate or large. A small effusion is ≤1 cm in thickness and may be localized. A moderately sized effusion is between 1 and 2 cm and is generally circumferential unless loculated. A large effusion is described as being >2 cm. In a group of 515 patients at high risk for pericardial effusions (103 of whom had pericardial effusions), emergency physicians were able to detect an effusion with an overall sensitivity of 96%, specificity of 98% and accuracy of 97% [36].

The risk of tamponade is more a function of the rate of accumulation than total volume of pericardial effusion. There are a number of different echocardiographic features used to define tamponade; however, its precise echocardiographic diagnosis remains complex and controversial. The most frequently used

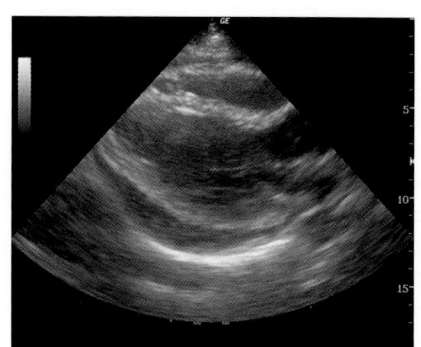

Fig. 23.1.15 Parasternal long-axis view of the heart demonstrating a moderately-sized pericardial effusion.

echocardiographic finding to support a diagnosis of tamponade is collapse of the right heart chambers during mid-to-late diastole and, specifically, right ventricular diastolic collapse. In the emergency department setting, pericardial tamponade should remain a clinical diagnosis. In a patient with signs and symptoms consistent with tamponade, the focus of emergency echocardiography is the identification of pericardial effusion. Its presence is then interpreted and acted upon in the clinical context.

Transthoracic echocardiography lacks sensitivity for diagnosing pulmonary embolism (PE). Echocardiography missed 16 of 39 patients presenting to an ED with PE, diagnosed by other modalities in a prospective observational study [39]. However, there are echocardiographic features associated with PE that, when identified and put into clinical context, can be highly suggestive or diagnostic. These include right ventricular dysfunction or dilatation, paradoxical septal motion, acute tricuspid regurgitation and the presence of clot in the right heart. While echocardiography may be a poor tool for diagnosing PE, it may be useful in assessing RV dysfunction caused by PE and may have a role in risk stratifying patients and influencing the decision to use thrombolytic therapy. RV dysfunction is associated with a significantly higher mortality [40] and thrombolysis may be considered in this setting, although the specific criteria for the use of thrombolytic therapy to treat PE remains controversial.

When the cause of shock is primarily due to pump failure, then echocardiography demonstrates a poorly functioning, often dilated left ventricle (LV) and/or atrium. Differentiating severe global left ventricular dysfunction (as occurs is cardiogenic shock) from normal LV function or the hyperdynamic LV of hypovolaemia is readily done. More precise calculations of ejection fraction and cardiac output or regional wall motion abnormality are generally beyond the scope of the emergency physician.

In shock due to hypovolaemia, echocardiography demonstrates a small left ventricular end-systolic volume with hyperdynamic left ventricular motion. The inferior vena cava also tends to be small or collapsed and demonstrates increased respiratory variation. In the spontaneously ventilating patient, inspiratory collapse of over 50%, particularly when the IVC is small, infers a high likelihood of fluid responsiveness.

The use of echocardiography for the acute assessment of chest pain is extremely useful but requires significant expertise and is generally beyond the scope of the ED user. Transthoracic echo can detect the regional wall motion abnormalities associated with cardiac ischaemia and, in expert hands, the sensitivity and specificity are relatively high. Echo too may detect the RV dilatation and dysfunction associated with PE, the pericardial effusion that may be associated with pericarditis, proximal aortic dilatation and even an intimal flap or aortic regurgitation from dissection but, for these conditions, has much lower sensitivity. Ultrasound can also detect numerous chest wall and pulmonary pathologies presenting with chest pain that may mimic cardiac pain and thoracic ultrasound is described in the next section.

Lung ultrasound

Lung ultrasound is being increasingly used by critical care clinicians and respiratory physicians to assess the patient with undifferentiated shortness of breath. It is also used to answer a diverse range of specific clinical questions, such as is there a pleural effusion, is there a pneumothorax or is there pulmonary oedema? Finally, it is used to guide pleural procedures, such as effusion drainage or biopsy.

Suggested algorithmic approaches, such as Lichtenstein's 'BLUE protocol' for the patient with acute respiratory failure, claim a diagnostic accuracy of 90.5% [41]. This protocol assesses for cardiogenic pulmonary oedema, pneumonia, decompensated chronic obstructive pulmonary disease (COPD), asthma, pulmonary embolism and pneumothorax.

It should be recalled that neither bone nor air allows the passage of ultrasound. Because of this, one cannot assess directly behind a rib where an acoustic shadow occurs, nor deep to an air interface, such as the normal pleural surface. This means that thoracic ultrasound can focus on the bony thoracic cage where fractures of ribs and the sternum can be readily detected or on the pleural space where effusions, pleural masses or free air (as in pneumothorax) can be detected and, finally on the lung itself. In aerated lung, assessment can only be made of the visceral pleural surface (and a tiny rim of lung tissue directly adjacent to this). If the lung is not aerated, as occurs with solid tumours, consolidation, collapse or infarction, the solid area of lung deeper to the surface can be explored with ultrasound.

Sonographic assessment of aerated lung relies on two things. First, movement of the lung, with the two pleural surfaces sliding against one another during ventilation and, secondly, on artefact created by reverberation of ultrasound. This reverberation occurs at the pleural surface and again within minute collections of interstitial fluid or fibrosis. Normal ventilating lung is therefore characterized by 'lung sliding' where the very slightly irregular visceral pleural surface can be seen moving to-and-fro past the parietal pleura with inspiration and expiration. Even in normal lung, tiny foci of interstitial or alveolar fluid or fibrosis create short path reverberation artefacts, which appear as bright vertical lines deep to the pleural surface. When these are short they are called comet tails and when they are long they have been termed lung rockets or 'B-lines'. When there is an increasing amount of interstitial or alveolar fluid as seen in pulmonary oedema, pneumonitis, acute respiratory distress syndrome (ARDS), lymphangitis carcinomatosis and pulmonary fibrosis the number and prominence of these vertical 'B-lines' increases dramatically. More subtle sonographic changes in the pleural surface may allow differentiation between these subgroups, however, often it is clinical correlation that makes the picture clearer.

With pneumothorax lung sliding is lost, as are the vertical comet tail and B-line artefacts. The contact or lung point can sometimes be found where the two pleural surfaces meet and allow some degree of assessment of pneumothorax size. In addition, with pneumothorax, the free air beneath the parietal pleural surface creates a smooth mirror-like effect. Long path reverberation artefacts, known as 'A-lines', occur where horizontal repetitions or reflections of the pleural surface are seen below the actual pleural surface. Lung sliding can also be absent in COPD, bullae or conditions where the lung surface is 'sticky' from inflammation of any cause.

Technique

The pleural surface is interrogated using either the curvilinear abdominal or the high frequency linear transducer. Several different methods for assessment have been described and depend on clinical suspicion, which must be used to guide and then interpret the scan. Integration of lung ultrasound and emergency echocardiography is the best approach to assessing the patient with undifferentiated acute dyspnoea.

In the absence of pleural adhesions or loculations, pneumothorax collects in the most apical portion of the thoracic cage and should be examined for there. If the patient is a supine trauma patient, assessment anteriorly along the midclavicular line from clavicle to diaphragm, with the probe in longitudinal is effective.

If considering pleural effusion or haemothorax, examining the bases and costophrenic angles from the front, side and back, usually with the patient sitting up, is best. To assess the lung parenchyma, maximizing the view of the pleura, lining the probe up in the line of the intercostal spaces and so avoiding ribs, is ideal.

For a non-trauma patient who presents in acute respiratory distress, sitting up, the author tends to examine the chest methodically:

- Anteriorly in the midclavicular line:
  - with the probe longitudinally to maximize lung sliding, explore from clavicle to diaphragm.
- Laterally in the midaxillary line:
  - initially with the probe in longitudinal position at the lung base to assess the costophrenic angle for fluid, collapse or consolidation
  - then higher with the probe aligned with the intercostal spaces to interrogate the pleural surfaces and lung higher up.
- Posteriorly just medial to the scapulae which are rotated out the way by flexing the shoulders forward:
  - initially with the probe longitudinal at the lung base to assess the costophrenic angle for pathology
  - then higher up the chest with the probe orientated along the line of the intercostal spaces (almost transverse).

Limitations and pitfalls

- Surgical emphysema, obesity or patient position may prevent adequate imaging by ultrasound.
- COPD and bullae can cause lung sliding to be minimal or absent, mimicking pneumothorax.
- Assuming lack of lung sliding is diagnostic of pneumothorax without searching for the lung point to confirm the diagnosis.
- Many pathologies can cause an increase in the number of B-lines, not just pulmonary oedema; remember to correlate clinically.
- Pericardial fat pads can be confused with consolidation.

Clinical implications and utility

ED ultrasound allows the rapid assessment of patients in acute respiratory distress at the bedside. The integration of ultrasound findings with the findings of the clinical assessment and appropriate clinical judgement can vastly expedite and improve management of these patients.

In addition to the diagnostic utility of thoracic and lung ultrasound, having access to ultrasound for procedural guidance is extremely useful. Ultrasound can be used to assess an area of opacity seen on chest X-ray, to determine whether it is solid or liquid. If a pleural effusion is confirmed, it can be further characterized as being simple or loculated and as to whether there is debris floating within it. Aspiration or tube placement can then be done after calculating the thickness of the chest wall, the depth of the effusion and the best direction from which to approach. The procedure can be done in real-time or after the patient is positioned, the skin is marked and trajectory planned.

While the benefits of lung ultrasound are clear, there is a diverse range of pathology that one can encounter and often the differences in sonographic appearance between pathologies are subtle. Appropriate education and experience are essential as is the correlation of clinical assessment with the ultrasound assessment.

Ultrasound-guided vascular access

Vascular access, both venous and arterial and central and peripheral is commonly performed in the emergency department. Widespread availability of machines and increasing familiarity and expertise among the emergency medicine community in using ultrasound to guide all forms of vascular access has had major positive implications to patients in recent years.

Traditionally, central venous access has been secured using the 'landmark technique', where surface anatomical features are used to predict the location of the internal jugular, subclavian and femoral veins. However, access using this technique has been associated with a 20% failure rate and a 10% complication rate, including inadvertent arterial puncture, excessive bleeding, vessel laceration, pneumothorax and haemothorax [42,43]. Improved success rates and decreased complication rates have been

described using ultrasound-guided central venous access, including reduction in needle puncture time, increased overall success, reduction in carotid puncture, reduction in pneumothorax and a reduction in catheter-related infection [44,45]. National guidelines from the UK [46] and the USA [47] support the use of ultrasound guidance for central venous catheter (CVC) placement.

Ultrasound guidance is also useful in aiding peripheral vascular access. The basilic, brachial and cephalic veins are frequently not visible clinically, but are readily cannulated using ultrasound guidance. Basilic vein cannulation has been shown to be very successful in the emergency department setting in patients in whom other peripheral access was difficult [48].

Technique

A medium to high frequency broad bandwidth linear array transducer is used with a centre frequency of 7.5–10 MHz. Specific presets to optimize the needle's visibility have been developed, but a musculoskeletal preset is usually adequate. The procedure is most easily performed with the ultrasound screen, the patient and operator all in line, with orientation checked and optimized. A sterile transducer cover and ultrasound gel are essential. A longer cannula is also particularly useful as the vessels being targeted are generally deep and increased length is required to reach them adequately.

Two techniques have been described, the static and dynamic techniques. The static technique may be used for very superficial or very large vessels, but is generally considered inferior to the dynamic technique. The static technique is used to locate the vessel, measure its dimensions, confirm relationships of surrounding structures and determine depth below the skin. The vessel is then centred on the screen and the skin marked at the centre of the transducer, corresponding to the vessel's subcutaneous position. This mark is then used for the puncture site without ultrasound visualization of the needle as it enters the vessel.

The dynamic technique uses real-time ultrasound guidance visualizing the needle tip as it enters the vessel. Higher success rates have been demonstrated with the dynamic technique than with the static technique [49].

Real-time ultrasound guided cannulation using both in plane and out of plane transducer orientation relative to the vessel have been described. The out of plane orientation is easier

to obtain and provides information related to adjacent structures, however, the needle tip is less clearly seen. The in plane orientation is more difficult to achieve but provides information related to vessel orientation and slope and provides visualization of the needle in its entirety as it passes through the tissues and enters the vessel.

Clinical implications and utility

In many centres, emergency staff (both medical and nursing) are gaining familiarity and expertise with ultrasound-guided vascular access of all sorts. The increased use of ultrasound to place peripheral cannulae and PICC lines has meant less trauma for our patients and, in many cases, less need for central line placement.

Miscellaneous applications

Scrotal ultrasound

Patients may present to the emergency department with scrotal or testicular pain, a scrotal mass or following scrotal trauma. Acute scrotal pain in the absence of trauma may be due to testicular torsion or epididymo-orchitis. Scrotal swelling may be due to hydrocoele, hernia or testicular mass. Scrotal trauma may be associated with testicular rupture, haematoma and testicular ischaemia. Ultrasound is the imaging modality of choice for assessing for testicular pathology and injury.

The scrotum is examined using a high-resolution linear array transducer with the patient in a supine position with the scrotum supported by a towel between the patient's legs.

In testicular torsion, the testis rotates on its axis leading to twisting of the spermatic cord with compromise of both venous drainage and arterial supply. To diagnose torsion, it is important to demonstrate normal flow within the normal testis and absent flow in the affected side [50]. However, it should be noted that flow may be very difficult to identify in normal paediatric testes and with intermittent torsion–detorsion, blood flow may appear normal or even increased in the affected testis. Partial torsion can occur with normal colour flow on ultrasound.

Epididymo-orchitis is the most common cause of scrotal pain in postpubertal men. Sonographically, the epididymis is characteristically thickened. Increased blood flow is demonstrated with colour Doppler in the epididymis or testis, or both. A reactive hydrocoele is common.

Ocular ultrasound

Ocular ultrasound has been used by ophthalmologists as an adjunct to examination for over 40 years. In the emergency setting, it is most useful to examine the eye in those patients where swelling prevents direct visualization of the eye and for disorders for which direct ophthalmoscopy has poor accuracy (particularly when performed by emergency doctors). Using a generous amount of gel, a high-frequency linear probe is gently applied to the closed eyelid and the globe examined in two planes from side to side. The posterior chamber should appear round and echo free. The optic nerve can be identified posteriorly. A retinal detachment appears as a relatively thick and echogenic membrane that may show colour flow on Doppler. In rhegmatogenous retinal detachments, the memberane undulates with eye movement (older detachments tend to move less with increasing fibrosis). Retinal detachments do not cross the optic nerve. Smaller areas of a thick elevated membrane that do not undulate may be seen with other types of detachments or other pathologies, but all of these will generally be beyond the scope of the emergency physician and require an ophthalmologist to distinguish. A vitreous detachment appears as a much thinner, avascular membrane that may only be seen when perpendicular to the beam, which also moves with globe movement. Vitreous haemorrhages appear as either dots or larger echogenic regions which move more quickly than retinal detachments. Studies have shown good accuracy when employed by emergency physicians to diagnose retinal detachment [51].

Ultrasound has also been used to diagnose globe rupture, foreign bodies and lens dislocation. Some groups have described its use in the diagnosis of intracranial hypertension, by looking at the optic nerve sheath diameter. However, while individual groups have found good accuracy, differences in technique and wide variation in the quoted normal ranges have limited the general applicability of this technique.

Appendicitis

Misdiagnosis of appendicitis on clinical assessment is associated with a negative appendectomy rate of 15%, with rates as high as 40–50% reported in some series [52]. Delays

in intervention can result in appendiceal perforation with associated increased morbidity and mortality [53]. The aim in assessing a patient with clinically suspected appendicitis is to identify adequately the appendix to confirm or refute the diagnosis, identify complications, such as perforation, or to identify other causes of the patient's presentation. The appendix is identified as a blind-ending, tubular, aperistaltic structure arising from the posteromedial caecum 1–2 cm distal to the ileocaecal junction. The patient should be examined in a supine position using a high-frequency linear array transducer to optimize image resolution. The normal appendix is compressible with a wall thickness equal to or less than 3 mm [54]. Increased wall thickness (outerwall to outerwall) of greater than 6 mm with loss of compressibility (Fig. 23.1.16), loss of definition of the mucosa, submucosa and muscularis propria and the visualization of an appendicolith support a diagnosis of appendicitis. Additionally, the detection of peri-appendiceal inflammatory changes in the presence of an abnormal appendix increases the likelihood of appendicitis [55]. Failure to identify the appendix is common and does not exclude appendicitis.

Musculoskeletal applications

There are numerous musculoskeletal applications for diagnostic ultrasound in emergency medicine. These include foreign body identification, evaluation of suspected tendon tears (Fig. 23.1.17), muscle tears and haematomas, joint effusions (Fig. 23.1.18) and fractures. Most musculoskeletal imaging is done using a broadband, high-resolution, linear array transducer with centre frequency of about 10 MHz.

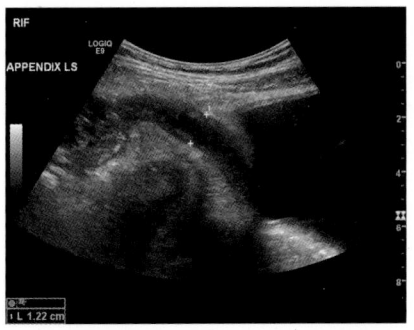

Fig. 23.1.16 Acute appendicitis. Longitudinal view of the appendix, seen originating from the caecum and draping over the iliac vessels into the pelvis where its tip lies adjacent to the bladder.

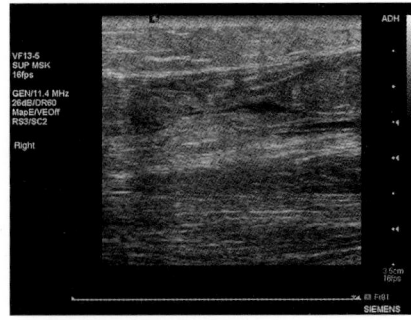

Fig. 23.1.17 Longitudinal view of the tendo Achilles showing full thickness tear at the level of the musculotendinous junction.

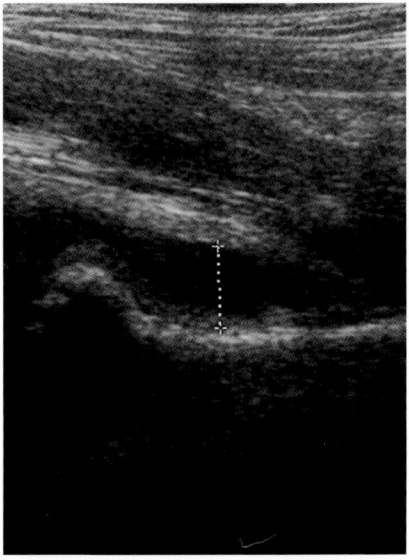

Fig. 23.1.18 Longitudinal view of right hip demonstrating joint effusion.

Ultrasound-guided procedures

Ultrasound is a useful modality for identifying fluid collections and guiding diagnostic or therapeutic aspiration, including thoracocentesis, paracentesis and arthrocentesis. It is also increasingly used by both anaesthetists and emergency physicians to guide nerve blocks.

Training and credentialling [1]

In Australasia, both the Australasian College for Emergency Medicine (ACEM) and the Australasian Society for Ultrasound in Medicine (ASUM) make recommendations and provide credentialling pathways in emergency ultrasound. ASUM provides the nationally recognized qualifications the Diploma in Diagnostic Ultrasound (DDU) and the Certificate in Clinician Performed Ultrasound (CCPU).

In 1999, ACEM proposed a policy supporting the use of ultrasound by emergency physicians for at least the detection of traumatic haemoperitoneum, abdominal aortic aneurysm, pericardial fluid, ectopic pregnancy, renal and biliary disease. The subsequently published policy document supported a credentialling process for training in FAST and AAA studies and included recommendations on training requirements. These requirements mandated a minimum of 25 FAST exams with at least five positive scans for intraperitoneal, pleural or pericardial fluid and 15 AAA exams of which five should demonstrate an aneurysm for credentialling purposes. All of these training exams should be confirmed by another study or direct supervision of a suitably qualified physician or sonographer. The requirements also included attendance at an ultrasound workshop that would cover the basic information for an emergency physician to perform and interpret FAST and AAA studies. Guidelines for the Minimum Criteria for Ultrasound Workshop were published by ACEM in 2000. These policies were reviewed in 2011, and requirements for credentialling in Basic Echo in Life Support were added.

ASUM is the recognized national training, qualifying and credentialling body in medical ultrasound. ASUM offers two qualifications to medical practitioners performing ultrasound: the Certificate in Clinician Performed Ultrasound (CCPU) and the Diploma in Diagnostic Ultrasound (DDU). Both of these qualifications are endorsed by ACEM for the purposes of training and credentialling in emergency ultrasound and describe a scope of practice that extends beyond those described by the College. Further details can be obtained from the ASUM website.

In 2005, the Royal College of Radiologists in the UK, in consultation with the clinical colleges, published a document entitled 'Ultrasound Training Recommendations for Medical & Surgical Specialties'. This document defines three levels of competency with suggested training and practice requirements for each level and has been endorsed by the College of Emergency Medicine (UK).

The 2001 American College of Emergency Physicians (ACEP) Policy Statement, Emergency Ultrasound Guidelines, reviewed the previous criteria for achievement of competency to perform focused clinical ultrasound. These recommendations included a 16-hour introductory course and a minimum of 25 ultrasound examinations for each defined primary modality.

Although the minimum training requirements for emergency physicians to become proficient in focused emergency ultrasound remains unclear, the recommendations from ACEP, ACEM, ASUM (for the CCPU) and the training recommendations of the Royal College of Radiologists (UK) for clinical ultrasound are similar and have been promulgated in a consensus document by the International Federation for Emergency Medicine.

The increasing technological sophistication, portability and affordability of ultrasound machines has led to an increasing demand for ultrasound as a diagnostic tool to be devolved to the clinician managing the patient. This is no more so than in emergency medicine where ultrasound has the potential of establishing a broad range of applications and indications that extend beyond EFAST and AAA detection as is described by the training curricula and guidelines above. The challenge now lies in developing adequate training and supervision networks to allow these skills to be learnt and maintained.

Controversies and future directions

- The scope of practice of emergency ultrasound is likely to continue to expand within EDs. Although the core uses for emergency physicians will continue to focus on unstable patients, the broad utility of ultrasound and its ability to add information to clinically challenging situations is likely to result in its application to a broader patient group.
- The major rate-limiting step is likely to be initial access and supervision of training.
- Paradoxically, skill maintenance in these so-called 'more advanced' applications of emergency ultrasound may be easier to achieve given that the majority of emergency physicians have far greater exposure to these patient groups than those with suspected haemoperitoneum in the setting of trauma or ruptured AAA.
- The amount of training required by clinicians to achieve competency and to maintain the sensitivity and specificity of an ultrasound study remains to be determined.

References

[1] ACEM. Policy on the use of bedside ultrasound by emergency physicians. Aust Coll Emerg Med 2012 Contract No.: P21.

[2] Gill R. The physics and technology of diagnositc ultrasound: a practitioner's guide. High Frequency Publishing; 2012.

[3] Rose JS. Ultrasound in abdominal trauma. Emerg Med Clin N Am 2004;22:581–99. vii.

[4] Kirkpatrick AW, Sirois M, Laupland KB, et al. Hand-held thoracic sonography for detecting post-traumatic pneumothoraces: the extended focused assessment with sonography for trauma (EFAST). J Trauma 2004;57:288–95.

[5] Scalea TM, Rodriguez A, Chiu WC, et al. Focused assessment with sonography for trauma (FAST): results from an international consensus conference. J Trauma 1999;46:466–72.

[6] Melniker LA, Leibner E, McKenney MG, et al. Randomized controlled clinical trial of point-of-care, limited ultrasonography for trauma in the emergency department: the first sonography outcomes assessment program trial. Ann Emerg Med 2006;48:227–35.

[7] Sakalihasan N, Limet R, Defawe OD. Abdominal aortic aneurysm. Lancet 2005;365:1577–89.

[8] Barkin AZ, Rosen CL. Ultrasound detection of abdominal aortic aneurysm. Emerg Med Clin N Am 2004;22:675–82.

[9] Goudie A. Ultrasound features of interstitial ectopic pregnancy: the role of the non-expert emergency medicine sonologist. Emerg Med Australas 2012;24:480–1.

[10] Condous G, Okaro E, Bourne T. Pregnancies of unknown location: diagnostic dilemmas and management. Curr Opin Obstet Gynecol 2005;17:568–73.

[11] Adhikari S, Blaivas M, Lyon M. Diagnosis and management of ectopic pregnancy using bedside transvaginal ultrasonography in the ED: a 2-year experience. Am J Emerg Med 2007;25:591–6.

[12] Brown DL, Doubilet PM. Transvaginal sonography for diagnosing ectopic pregnancy: positivity criteria and performance characteristics. J Ultrasound Med 1994;13:259–66.

[13] Abdallah Y, Daemen A, Kirk E, et al. Limitations of current definitions of miscarriage using mean gestational sac diameter and crown-rump length measurements: a multicenter observational study. Ultrasound Obstet Gynecol 2011;38:497–502.

[14] Hanbidge AE, Buckler PM, O'Malley ME, Wilson SR. From the RSNA refresher courses: imaging evaluation for acute pain in the right upper quadrant. Radiographics 2004;24:1117–35.

[15] Noble VE, Brown DF. Renal ultrasound. Emerg Med Clin N Am 2004;22:641–59.

[16] Middleton WD, Dodds WJ, Lawson TL, Foley WD. Renal calculi: sensitivity for detection with US. Radiology 1988;167:239–44.

[17] Cranley JJ, Canos AJ, Sull WJ. The diagnosis of deep venous thrombosis. Fallibility of clinical symptoms and signs. Arch Surg 1976;111:34–6.

[18] Barnes RW, Wu KK, Hoak JC. Fallibility of the clinical diagnosis of venous thrombosis. J Am Med Assoc 1975;234:605–7.

[19] Lewis BD. The peripheral veins. In: Rumack CM, WS R, Charboneau W, Jo-Ann J, editors. Diagnostic ultrasound (3rd ed.). St Louis: Elsevier Mosby; 2004.

[20] Blaivas M, Lambert MJ, Harwood RA, et al. Lower-extremity Doppler for deep venous thrombosis – can emergency physicians be accurate and fast? Acad Emerg Med 2000;7:120–6.

[21] Cronan JJ. Venous thromboembolic disease: the role of US. Radiology 1993;186:619–30.

[22] Lensing AW, Doris CI, McGrath FP, et al. A comparison of compression ultrasound with color Doppler ultrasound for the diagnosis of symptomless postoperative deep vein thrombosis. Arch Intern Med 1997;157:765–8.

[23] Trottier SJ, Todi S, Veremakis C. Validation of an inexpensive B-mode ultrasound device for detection of deep vein thrombosis. Chest 1996;110:1547–50.

[24] Poppiti R, Papanicolaou G, Perese S, Weaver FA. Limited B-mode venous imaging versus complete color-flow duplex venous scanning for detection of proximal deep venous thrombosis. J Vasc Surg 1995;22:553–7.

[25] Birdwell BG, Raskob GE, Whitsett TL, et al. The clinical validity of normal compression ultrasonography in

outpatients suspected of having deep venous thrombosis. Ann Intern Med 1998;128:1–7.

[26] Heijboer H, Buller HR, Lensing AW, et al. A comparison of real-time compression ultrasonography with impedance plethysmography for the diagnosis of deep-vein thrombosis in symptomatic outpatients. N Engl J Med 1993;329:1365–9.

[27] Cogo A, Lensing AW, Koopman MM, et al. Compression ultrasonography for diagnostic management of patients with clinically suspected deep vein thrombosis: prospective cohort study. Br Med J 1998;316:17–20.

[28] Eskandari MK, Sugimoto H, Richardson T, et al. Is color-flow duplex a good diagnostic test for detection of isolated calf vein thrombosis in high-risk patients? Angiology 2000;51:705–10.

[29] Frazee BW, Snoey ER, Levitt A. Emergency department compression ultrasound to diagnose proximal deep vein thrombosis. J Emerg Med 2001;20:107–12.

[30] Jang T, Docherty M, Aubin C, Polites G. Resident-performed compression ultrasonography for the detection of proximal deep vein thrombosis: fast and accurate. Acad Emerg Med 2004;11:319–22.

[31] Cronan JJ. Controversies in venous ultrasound. Semin Ultrasound CT MR 1997;18:33–8.

[32] Mangione S, Nieman LZ. Cardiac auscultatory skills of internal medicine and family practice trainees. A comparison of diagnostic proficiency. J Am Med Assoc 1997;278:717–22.

[33] Kontos MC, Arrowood JA, Paulsen WH, Nixon JV. Early echocardiography can predict cardiac events in emergency department patients with chest pain. Ann Emerg Med 1998;31:550–7.

[34] Thomas JT, Kelly RF, Thomas SJ, et al. Utility of history, physical examination, electrocardiogram, and chest radiograph for differentiating normal from decreased systolic function in patients with heart failure. Am J Med 2002;112:437–45.

[35] Moore CL, Rose GA, Tayal VS, et al. Determination of left ventricular function by emergency physician echocardiography of hypotensive patients. Acad Emerg Med 2002;9:186–93.

[36] Mandavia DP, Hoffner RJ, Mahaney K, Henderson SO. Bedside echocardiography by emergency physicians. Ann Emerg Med 2001;38:377–82.

[37] Blaivas M, Fox JC. Outcome in cardiac arrest patients found to have cardiac standstill on the bedside emergency department echocardiogram. Acad Emerg Med 2001;8:616–21.

[38] Salen P, O'Connor R, Sierzenski P, et al. Can cardiac sonography and capnography be used independently and in combination to predict resuscitation outcomes? Acad Emerg Med 2001;8:610–5.

[39] Jackson RE, Rudoni RR, Hauser AM, et al. Prospective evaluation of two-dimensional transthoracic echocardiography in emergency department patients with suspected pulmonary embolism. Acad Emerg Med 2000;7:994–8.

[40] Ribeiro A, Lindmarker P, Juhlin-Dannfelt A, et al. Echocardiography Doppler in pulmonary embolism: right ventricular dysfunction as a predictor of mortality rate. Am Heart J 1997;134:479–87.

[41] Lichtenstein DA, Mezière GA. Relevance of lung ultrasound in the diagnosis of acute respiratory failure: the BLUE protocol. Chest 2008;1341:117–25.

[42] Sznajder JI, Zveibil FR, Bitterman H, et al. Central vein catheterization. Failure and complication rates by three percutaneous approaches. Arch Intern Med 1986;146:259–61.

[43] Mansfield PF, Hohn DC, Fornage BD, et al. Complications and failures of subclavian-vein catheterization. N Engl J Med 1994;331:1735–8.

[44] Hudson PA, Rose JS. Real-time ultrasound guided internal jugular vein catheterization in the emergency department. Am J Emerg Med 1997;15:79–82.

[45] Karakitsos D, Labropoulos N, De Groot E, et al. Real-time ultrasound-guided catheterisation of the internal jugular vein: a prospective comparison with the landmark technique in critical care patients. Crit Care 2006;10:R162.

[46] NICE. NICE technology appraisal guidance No 49: guidance on the use of ultrasound locating devices for placing central venous catheters. London: National Institue for Clinical Excellence; 2002.

[47] Rothschild JM. Ultrasound guidance of central vein catheterization. In: Shojania KG, Duncan BW, McDonald KM, editors. Making health care safer: a critical analysis of patient safety practices evidence report/technology assessment no 43. Rockville: Agency for Healthcare Research and Quality; 2001.

[48] Keyes LE, Frazee BW, Snoey ER, et al. Ultrasound-guided brachial and basilic vein cannulation in emergency department patients with difficult intravenous access. Ann Emerg Med 1999;34:711–4.

[49] Nadig C, Leidig M, Schmiedeke T, Hoffken B. The use of ultrasound for the placement of dialysis catheters. Nephrol Dial Transplant 1998;13:978–81.

[50] Howlett DC, Marchbank ND, Sallomi DF. Pictorial review. Ultrasound of the testis. Clin Radiol 2000;55:595–601.

[51] Shinar Z, Chan L, Orlinsky M. Use of ocular ultrasound for the evaluation of retinal detachment. J Emerg Med 2011;40:53–7.

[52] Flum DR, Morris A, Koepsell T, Dellinger EP. Has misdiagnosis of appendicitis decreased over time? A population-based analysis. J Am Med Assoc 2001;286:1748–53.

[53] Wilson EB. Surgical evaluation of appendicitis in the new era of radiographic imaging. Semin Ultrasound CT MR 2003;24:65–8.

[54] Simonovsky V. Normal appendix: is there any significant difference in the maximal mural thickness at US between pediatric and adult populations? Radiology 2002;224:333–7.

[55] Vignault F, Filiatrault D, Brandt ML, et al. Acute appendicitis in children: evaluation with US. Radiology 1990;176:501–4.

23.2 CT scanning in emergency medicine

Steven J Dunjey • Swithin Song

ESSENTIALS

1 Computed tomography (CT) scans are a major diagnostic modality in modern emergency medicine.

2 Emergency physicians are ordering CTs more frequently than previously, for a variety of reasons.

3 Artefacts are occasionally encountered in CT scans and clinicians should be familiar with the more common of these artefacts.

4 CT scans are not completely benign and patients can develop reactions to contrast media and suffer from the long-term effects of radiation.

Introduction

Computed tomography (CT) was developed in 1971 by Godfrey Hounsfield and Allan Cormack and was rapidly adopted into medical practice. By the early 1980s, CT scanning was in general clinical use in the USA and, within a generation, most large emergency departments have acquired their own dedicated machines. Emergency medicine has enthusiastically embraced the utilization of this modality, which provides rapid answers to many of our diagnostic questions. It has revolutionized the approach to patients with traumatic injury, neurological emergencies, including head injuries, subarachnoid hemorrhage and strokes, abdominal pain and, more recently, chest pain. It is assuming the pre-eminent position in the investigation of patients with possible pulmonary embolism. It is cost effective, fast, less sensitive to patient movement than magnetic resonance imaging and (unless contrast is used) non-invasive. It is, however, a modality that presents some real risks to patients and clinicians need to be prudent in their use of CT. It is also an area of considerable development and, as CT scanners become faster and more accurate, more uses are being found for this modality.

Development science

CT scan machines essentially consist of a gantry around a patient, with an X-ray source on one side of the gantry and detectors on the opposite side moving in synchrony with the source. Early scanners imaged one slice at a time ('step and shoot'), with the table stationary while a static image was acquired. This produced a series of parallel slice images (tomographic images) of a region of the body. The beam produced by the source can be adjusted, producing widths from 1 to 20 mm. Traditionally, images were produced which displayed the volume of data as axial slices (transverse slices, perpendicular to the long axis of the body), but current scanners are able to display the collected information as coronal or sagittal slices which improves diagnostic yield (Figs 23.2.1–23.2.3).

Helical (spiral) CT scanners move the patient rapidly and continuously through a circular gantry opening which is equipped with

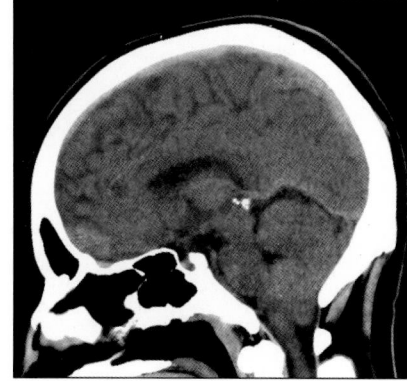
Fig. 23.2.3 Sagittal CT head.

a source and multiple detectors, which are continuously rotating and provide continued volumetric acquisition. The source describes a helical trajectory relative to the patient.

There have been considerable advances in computer technology and, in combination with the development of multislice helical CT, there has been significant improvement in the resolution and diagnostic utility of CT scanners. Helical scanners are also capable of producing a 3-dimensional image of an internal organ by digital post-processing.

Windows

The objects displayed in a scan can be differentiated from adjacent organs by their differential attenuation of the X-ray beam based on their individual density. The density of the tissues in the scan produced is measured in Hounsfield Units (HU). Water has a density of 0 and tissues that are denser than water have values greater than 0, while less dense tissues have negative values. The accepted convention

is for high-density structures to be displayed in white shades and low-density structures to be displayed in darker shades. The denser a structure, the whiter the shade displayed. The scale extends up to about +4000 for very dense metals, but cancellous bone is about +700 and dense bone about +3000. Blood is in the range of +35 to +45 and muscle about +40. At the other extreme of the scale, air is −1000, lung −700 and fat −84 (Figs 23.2.4 and 23.2.5).

Humans can only perceive a limited number of grey shades and so to highlight the tissues of interest, the full range of density values is not displayed. Instead, the display shows a narrow portion of the full range to allow clear differentiation of one tissue from another and pathological tissue from healthy tissue.

For example, bone windows are a preset that will shift the grey scale displayed to center on the range of densities which are

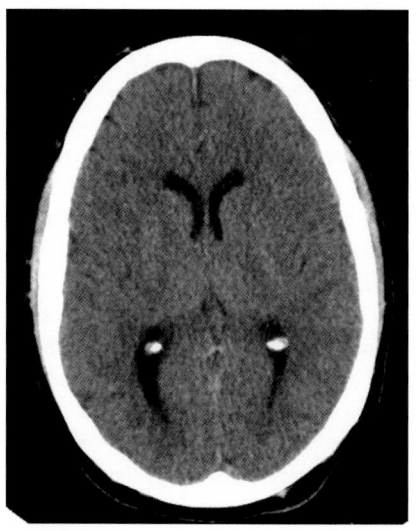
Fig. 23.2.1 Axial CT of head.

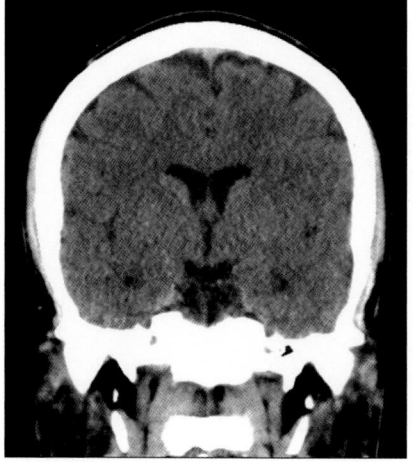
Fig. 23.2.2 Coronal CT of head.

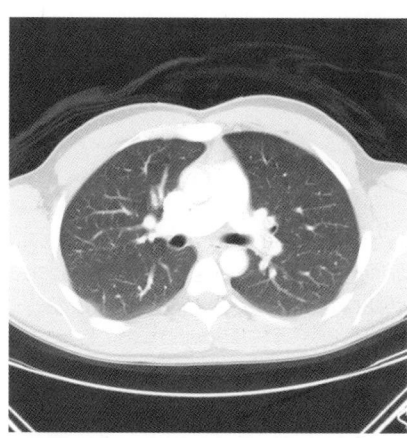
Fig. 23.2.4 Axial CT of lung using lung windows preset.

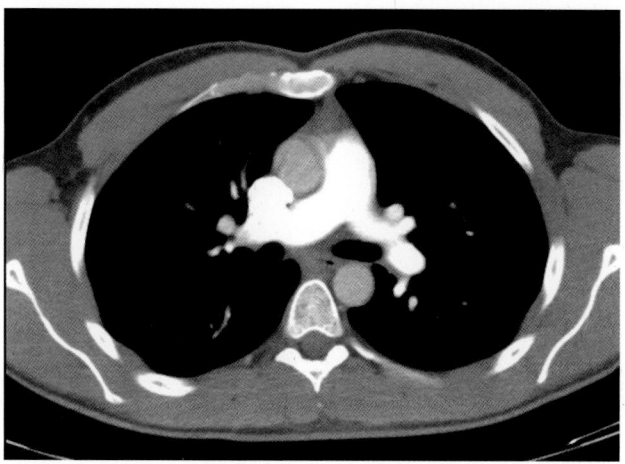
Fig. 23.2.5 Axial CT chest using preset for CT angiogram.

typical of bone and allow detection of subtle abnormalities, such as small fractures. As a consequence of focusing the display on such high-density structures, there is a marked decline in the ability to assess soft tissues on bone windows.

Display convention

The accepted convention for displaying images is for the right side of the patient to be on the left side of the image, which is best appreciated by imagining yourself standing at the feet of the CT gantry, with the patient supine.

Artefacts

There are still a number of imaging artefacts that affect the quality of the images generated and hence the diagnostic value of the scan [1]. These artefacts arise from a number of sources, classified as physics-based artefacts, patient based, scanner based and multi-section based [3]. Most emergency physicians are familiar with patient-based issues, such as patient movement (Fig. 23.2.6) or metallic objects in or around the patient (Figs 23.2.7 and 23.2.8).

Physics-based problems include beam hardening (resulting from the absorption of low-energy photons after passage through an object, leaving only high-energy photons and a higher energy beam) which can produce

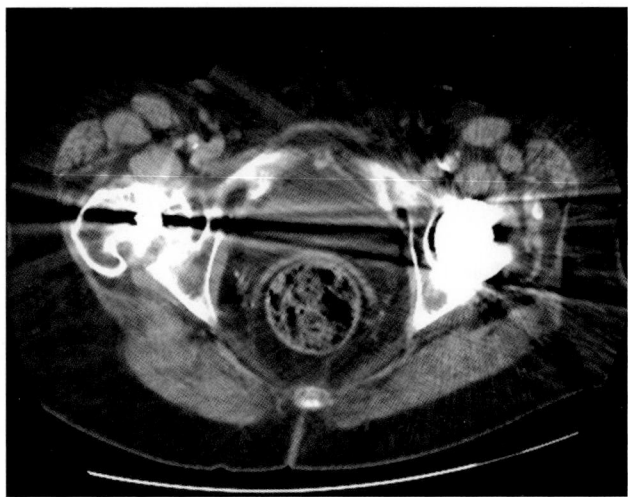

Fig. 23.2.7 Metallic artefacts from hip prostheses.

the streaks and dark bands that are sometimes seen. Undersampling is another physics-based problem, in which the distance between CT samples is large enough to create misregistration of information about small objects or sharp edges. Partial volume averaging is another common problem, in which the average of densities in a single CT is averaged rather than displaying separate individual densities. That this occurs should not be a surprise, because every CT slice displayed is a 2D representation of a finite 3D thickness of tissue [4]. Ring artefacts, a scanner-based problem, occur due to miscalibration or failure of one or more detector elements in a CT scanner (Fig. 23.2.9).

Current uses and indications

While the overall usage of CT scanning in medicine is dramatically increasing, evidence suggests a higher rate of increase in emergency medicine than elsewhere. A 2011 study showed that, in the USA between 1995 and 2007, the number of CT studies performed increased from 2.7 million to 16.2 million – nearly a sixfold increase [5].

By the end of the study period, the presenting complaints topping the list of those undergoing CT were abdominal pain, headache and chest pain. The percentage of patient visits associated with CT for all complaints increased most substantially among those who underwent CT for flank, abdominal or chest pain. Other high-use areas include shortness of breath, trauma and headache

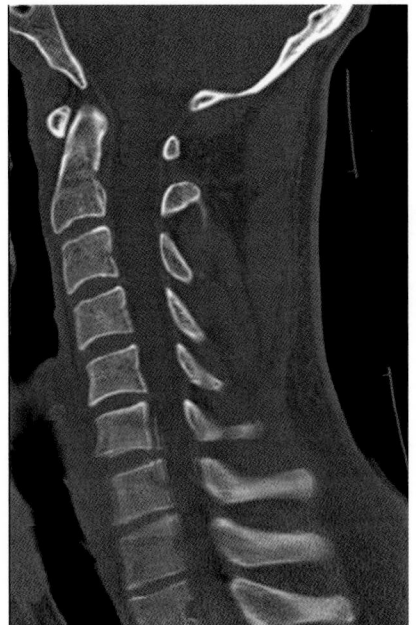

Fig. 23.2.6 Pseudofracture of C6 from patient movement.

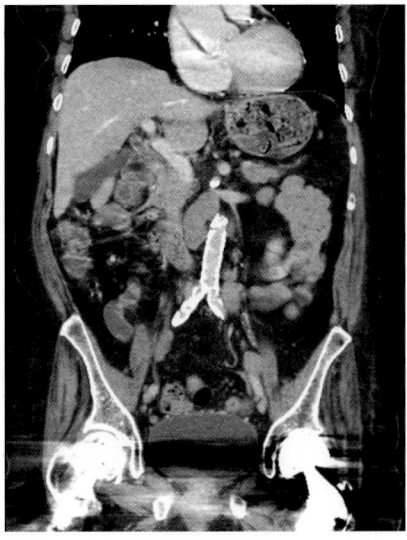

Fig. 23.2.8 Coronal CT abdomen with metallic artefact obscuring bladder.

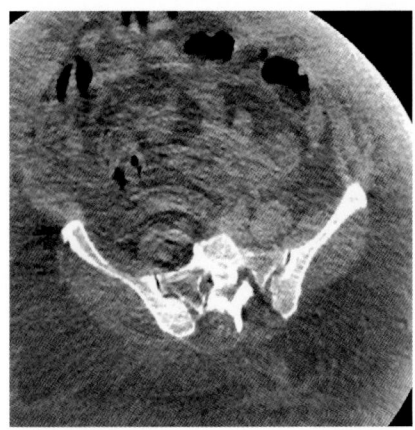

Fig. 23.2.9 Ring artefacts in a very bariatric patient.

and use is more marked in the elderly population [6].

Indications for emergency department CT scans increase every year, especially as the manifest deficiencies of plain X-rays become clearer. Examples include CT supplanting the traditional role of plain films in assessing head injury, cervical spine injury and renal colic. This era, when long-held beliefs about the accuracy of clinical examination are being challenged, acts as a force encouraging increasing reliance on good diagnostic tests. In the last decade, there has been a dramatic increase in the number of CT scanners such that even moderate-sized country hospitals now have scanners and most large urban emergency departments have their own dedicated scanners. During the same period, scanners have become faster with improved diagnostic yield. All of these factors drive the increase in scans performed and there is the promise of further developments. CT scans are likely to be used increasingly for chest pain, not just for suspected pulmonary embolism, but for suspected acute coronary syndrome, coronary artery disease and aortic dissection as well. Surgeons now wish to avoid unnecessary operations and are increasingly unwilling to take patients for exploratory laparotomies without a CT scan to provide a definitive or tentative diagnosis prior to surgical exploration.

Problems

There are some significant problems that continue to present challenges for physicians requesting CT studies.

Weight constraints

Most scanners have a weight limit, somewhere in the range of 160–200 kg depending on the unit used. Some manufacturers are developing bariatric scanners with much higher weight capabilities, but they are not in common usage at this time.

Unstable patients

A CT suite is usually limited in its provision of resuscitative care. Even with oxygen and suction outlets and full monitoring, these spaces are primarily designed for imaging not resuscitation. Most are some distance from the resuscitation area of the emergency department (ED) and from operating theatres and it represents a challenge for a team to deal with a markedly unstable patient in CT. Although current CT

scanners can perform in a short time interval, the process of manoeuvring patients into the room, off the trolley and changing over tubing and monitoring has changed little over the years. These factors are responsible for the bulk of time in the scanner and scanners that can perform a whole body scan in minutes have made surprisingly little difference to the time in the CT scan suite. Patients still die in the relative isolation of these suites and it is still important for physicians to ensure that their patients are as stable as possible prior to leaving the resuscitation area. Patients who cannot be stabilized because of the severity of their injuries should go to the operating theatre rather than be imaged.

Allergy to CT contrast media

There is significant lack of understanding in the medical community regarding reactions to contrast media. Contrast molecules are so small that that they are not capable of acting as antigens and, although they can create an allergic type reaction, it is probably not IgE mediated. Reactions range from minor skin reactions up to more severe anaphylactoid reactions (bronchospasm, angio-oedema, hypotension). IV contrast reactions are more common in atopic individuals and those with previous allergic reactions, but the most important risk factor is a previous reaction to contrast [7]. Determining the incidence of such reactions is difficult because of underreporting and because concomitant illness can produce similar symptoms in some patients. The American College of Radiologists manual on contrast media suggests rates of 0.2–0.7% overall, with the rate of serious reactions of about 1 or 2 per 10 000 [8].

Iodine is an essential element and it is not possible to be allergic to it. Although shellfish are a rich source of iodine, allergy to shellfish is due to the proteins found in the muscle of the shellfish and so the widely held belief that shellfish allergy precludes the use of contrast agents is not based on fact [7].

For patients who are at risk of a reaction, it is wise to have medication to manage a severe response easily to hand. The usefulness of prophylactic steroids for emergency patients is dubious, partly because of the time constraints imposed by the acuity of the illness and partly because of questions surrounding its efficacy. One recommendation suggests:

'Do not delay emergent studies for steroid premedication. Only lengthy 12-h premedication

protocols have shown any effect on reaction rates and this small benefit was manifested primarily by decreasing minor reactions. No steroid protocol has shown a significant benefit in decreasing severe or fatal reactions [9].

Contrast-induced nephropathy

Radiocontrast-induced nephropathy is a feared complication for those receiving IV contrast media. It has been estimated to have a mortality rate of up to 36% in hospital and a 19% 2-year survival, as well as prolonged hospitalization [10–12]. Contrast media have also been estimated to be used in approximately 50% of scans currently performed and CT scan usage is increasing at an exponential rate [13].

Under normal physiological conditions, nearly all of the contrast medium is eliminated through the kidneys. The resulting concentration in the renal tubular system is up to 100 times the concentration in plasma and approaches $\leq 30\%$ of the concentration of the injected solution [14]. With contrast concentrations of this magnitude, it is not surprising that this could be a cause of acute kidney injury.

Recent evidence suggests that some long-held beliefs about contrast-induced nephropathy (CIN) should be challenged. One of the turning points in studies in this area has been the adoption of a more uniform way of diagnosing and describing the illness (accepted basic criteria require a per cent change in the baseline creatinine of $\geq 25\%$ and/or an absolute elevation of creatinine from baseline values of 0.5 mg/dL).

The great majority of previous reports on CIN have been from observations in the cardiac catheterization laboratory. Studies focusing on contrast-enhanced CT show an overall incidence of CIN, with the current generation of non-ionic contrast media, to be in the range of about 5%. In comparison, the rates of serious outcomes generally, and CIN specifically, are much higher for cardiac catheterization. Very recent work examining contrast media away from cardiac catheterization has questioned whether the media induce CIN at all [15]. Traditionally, risks for developing CIN included renal insufficiency, age (older than 55), hypovolaemia, diabetes of longstanding and patients taking metformin among others. On the basis of recent evidence, it appears that baseline renal insufficiency is the only well-supported independent risk factor [13].

Unfortunately, there is no universally agreed threshold of serum creatinine elevation (or degree of renal dysfunction) beyond which intravascular iodinated contrast medium should not be administered.

There have been many agents used as attempted prophylaxis against development of CIN, including N-acetylcysteine (NAC), vasodilators, such as fenoldepam, calcium channel blockers, theophylline, but the only well-accepted measure for at-risk patients is adequate hydration. This position is supported by the American College of Radiology, but the ideal volume and rate of administration is not known. Isotonic fluids, such as normal saline, are preferred. Most guidelines suggest 6–12 hours of infusion prior to the procedure and for up to 4 hours afterwards [16]. Clearly these recommendations are impossible to implement for emergent patients.

Radiation

CT scanning is a source of ionizing radiation, which is capable of overcoming the binding energy of electrons and is able to knock them out of orbit, creating ions. Although X-rays can ionize DNA directly, it is the production of hydroxyl radicals from ionization of water molecules that produces strand breaks and base damage. Although there is some capacity to repair damaged DNA, unresolved damaged DNA can induce cancer. At the doses delivered in normal scanning, there is a small risk of radiation-induced carcinogenesis. This contention is supported by the historical evidence supplied by Japanese survivors of the atomic bombs dropped in 1945. The group who received low doses of radiation in the range 5–150 mSv (mean 40 mSv which approximates the organ dose from a typical CT involving two to three scans in an adult) showed a significant increase in the risk of cancer [17].

Spiral (or helical) CT is rapidly becoming the dominant type of scanner used and, under typical use (with a pitch of 1 or greater), the radiation dose is comparable to conventional CT. Slice thickness, the number of cuts obtained and the pitch affect radiation exposure. Pitch is a ratio defined as the distance the couch travels during one rotation of the radiation source divided by the section thickness [18].

In pregnancy

Radiation damages DNA and a fetus with rapidly dividing and differentiating cells is more susceptible to these effects than adults. Large doses of radiation can lead to growth retardation, birth defects, cancers, mental retardation

and even fetal death, but modern diagnostic studies are well below the threshold that would cause such catastrophic effects [19]. Exposure to less than 5 rads has not been associated with deleterious effects on a fetus [17].

In context, an abdominal X-ray exposes a fetus to about 100 mrad, a lumbar spine X-ray to 50–150 mrad, a CT of pelvis to 250 mrad and a CT of abdomen or lumbar spine to 3.5 rad.

Apart from the risks of radiation, there are often questions about the safety of contrast media. It is generally considered safe to give contrast media in all trimesters of pregnancy, although there are theoretical risks of thyroid depression in the fetus/neonate because contrast media molecules are small enough to cross the placental barrier and to be excreted in breast milk. Some centres direct pregnant or lactating women to discard breast milk for up to 24 hours after contrast administration, although this is likely not necessary [19].

In childhood

There has been a marked increase in the use of diagnostic CT scanning in the paediatric population, driven in part by the decrease in time to perform a scan, which eliminates the need for an anaesthetized child to keep them stationary [18].

The largest growth has been in the diagnosis of acute appendicitis, in which CT is cost effective and accurate, although ultrasound represents a viable and safer option in most cases [20].

The increased risk of carcinogenesis is even more marked in the paediatric population for two reasons. They are more radiosensitive and they also have more years of life in which to develop a radiation-induced cancer.

Overuse

Widespread acceptance of the use of CT scanning, the development of new indications, its speed and accuracy in diagnosis, liability issues and the improved access to scanning are among a long list of reasons why the number of scans generated by emergency departments is exploding [21].

While this change is mirrored throughout medical practice, the potential for inappropriate overuse of CT in emergency medicine is an area of concern. Unnecessary scans expose patients to radiation (particularly if there are consecutive or multiple scans done in a short period) and are financially expensive (particularly if compared with modalities like plain X-ray or ultrasound).

Some estimates have suggested a sevenfold increase in total medical radiation exposure from the 1980s to 2006 for the population of the USA. While CT scanning in that period only accounted for 17% of X-ray imaging, they were responsible for 49% of the total estimated dose [22].

In the same population, emergency medicine generates about one-third of the CT scans performed. The benefits for patients in EDs are not disputed and the American College of Radiology sponsored workshop made the following comment:

CT has proven its critical value in the detection and diagnosis of trauma patients and those with chest pain. Diagnosis and management of fatal diseases such as aortic dissection, pulmonary emboli, and others have been revolutionized with CT imaging. The mystery of the 'blackbox' of the abdomen has been revealed, improving the diagnosis of conditions such as bowel obstruction, bowel necrosis, ureteral stones, appendicitis, pancreatitis, diverticulitis, pyelonephritis, and so on. CT scans also became the principal modality for evaluating intracranial problems and, to an ever increasing extent, the diagnosis of cancers [20].

Some studies suggest that there are significant numbers of inappropriate tests ordered from emergency departments. Studdert et al. found that 70% of the emergency physicians responding to their questionnaire admitted to ordering imaging that they did not feel was clinically indicated because of the threat of medical liability [23].

Emergency physicians respond by pointing out that, although the CT radiation dose is significant (10–20 millisieverts (mSv), which is associated with a lifetime risk of fatal cancer of about one per 2000 scans), more than one in 2000 patients will have potentially life-saving information provided by a CT. To many frontline doctors, the long-term risks are theoretical and poorly quantified compared with the risk of missing significant pathology in the here-and-now [24].

One area of medicine in which CT scanning has revolutionized care is trauma management. Rapid, high-quality scanning has unequivocally led to better outcomes in many patients but, even here, questions are being asked. The pan-scan has been enthusiastically embraced and quickly become a standard of care before any chance of rigorous scientific evaluation [25].

An Australian study reported the results of a large cohort study comparing radiation exposure to trauma patients before and after the introduction of a pan-scan (whole body scan for trauma) diagnostic algorithm employing a 64-slice scanner [26]. Their findings were challenging, suggesting that patients undergoing a pan-scan, according to the calculated risk ratio, were 1.7 (95% confidence interval [CI] 1.3–2.2) times more likely to receive a radiation dose exceeding 20 mSv compared with a conventional CT work-up, but did not significantly benefit from the procedure in terms of the incidence of missed injuries (0.6% vs 0.9%).

Only one-fifth of the patients in the study fulfilled the criteria for major trauma, the major justification for a pan-scan. The authors went on to suggest that the pan-scan may be 26 times more likely to harm the patient in the long term than assist them in the acute setting.

CT scanning should not be requested in a frivolous fashion, without regard for potential long-term health risks. The speed of the investigation and the quality of the diagnostic information should always be balanced against a knowledge that the scan may harm the patient.

Clinical decision rules

Emergency physicians are responsible for ensuring that they make sensible and appropriate decisions for their patients and that their choice of CT as a modality takes account of the risks to the patient. It is unfortunately true that there has been such a proliferation of guidelines that sometimes clinicians are hard pressed to know which one to follow. There are, for example, no less than three widely accepted and well-validated decision rules for determining the need for CT in head injury (Canadian Head CT rule/New Orleans Criteria/ NEXUS II). The American College of Radiologists has developed a comprehensive list of appropriateness criteria that relate possible investigations to the presenting complaint, covering the full gamut of clinical presentations and made in conjunction with appropriate input from clinicians [27].

Diagnostic accuracy of emergency physicians

Emergency physicians are often required to interpret a CT scan. Early studies did not suggest this was done well. Many studies have examined the ability of emergency physicians (EPs) and registrars (EM residents in North America) to interpret head CT scans. In the specific clinical setting of stroke, compared to the gold standard of interpretation by neuroradiologists, EPs performed relatively poorly in recognition of both haemorrhage and early ischaemic changes (accuracy 60%), but neurologists and general radiologists only achieved a result of 80% [28–30].

A study examining EPs' abilities to assess head CT for trauma concluded that, without extra training, EPs should not be interpreting such scans [30]. While there is debate about whether the non-concordance between EPs and radiologists leads to poor clinical outcomes, there are numbers of studies that demonstrate the improvement that is possible with focused teaching [31].

There is no doubt that improvement in training must occur because, despite the advent of teleradiology, there will still be occasions when the situation dictates that an EP perform the initial interpretation of a CT scan.

Future directions

Low-dose CT scanning is an attempt to produce high-quality scans at lower doses of radiation. It is achieved by a variety of techniques, including dose modulation, noise management software (to filter out unnecessary data), lower peak voltage settings and switching off the tube at some points of its rotation and iterative dose reduction techniques. As an area of rapid development, the trade off in image quality versus radiation dose is becoming less of an issue.

References

[1] Silverman PM, Kalendar WA, Hazle JD. Common terminology for single and multislice helical CT. Am J Roetgenol 2001;176:1135–6.

[2] Broder JS. Diagnostic imaging and the emergency physician. Elsevier Saunders; 2011, p. 1–45.

[3] Barrett JF, Keat N, Artifacts in CT: recognition and avoidance. Radiographics 2004;24:1679–91.

[4] Webb WR, Brant WE, Major NM. Fundamentals of body CT. Elsevier; 2006.

[5] Larson DB, Johnson LW, Schnell BL, et al. National trends in CT use in the emergency department: 1995–2007. Radiology 2011;258:164–73.

[6] Kocker KE, Meurer WJ, Fazel R, et al. National trends in use of computed tomography in the emergency department. Ann Emerg Med 2011 published online.

[7] Bettmann MA. Frequently asked questions: iodinated contrast agents. Radiographics 2004;24:S3–10.

[8] ACR Manual on Contrast Media, Version 8, 2012. Adverse events of iodinated contrast media: 21-28.

[9] Schabelman E, Witting M. The relationship of radiocontrast, iodine, and seafood allergies: a medical myth exposed. J Emerg Med 2010;39:701–7.

[10] Neesh P, Wiebe N, Tonelli M. Prophylaxis strategies for contrast-induced nephropahthy. J Am Med Assoc 2006;295:2765–79.

[11] Gruberg L, Mehran R, Dangas G, et al. Acute renal failure requiring dialysis after percutaneous coronary interventions. Cathet Cardiovasc Intervent 2001;52:409–16.

[12] McCullough PA, Wolyn R, Rocher LL, et al. Acute renal failure after coronary intervention: incidence, risk factors and relationship to mortality. Am J Med 1997;103:368–75.

[13] Katzberg RW. Contrast-induced nephropathy in 2010. Appl Radiol Online 39 9 sept 2010.

[14] Katzberg RW. Urography into the 21st century: new contrast media, renal handling, imaging characteristics, and nephrotoxicity. Radiology 1997;204:297–312.

[15] McDonald RJ, McDonald JS, Bida S, et al. Intravenous contrast material-induced nephropathy: causal or coincident phenomenon. Radiology 267:106–18.

[16] American college of radiology manual on contrast-induced nephrotoxicity. <http://www.acr.org/~/media/ACR/ Documents/PDF/QualitySafety/Resources/Contrast%20 Manual/Contrast%20Nephrotoxicity.pdf>.

[17] Brenner DJ, Hall EJ. Computed tomography – an increasing source of radiation exposure. N Engl J Med 2007;357:2277–84.

[18] American Congress of Obstetricians and Gynecologists Committee. Opinion guidelines for diagnostic imaging during pregnancy. Number 299, September 2004, reaffirmed 2009.

[19] Christian Fox J. Clinical emergency radiology. Cambridge University Press; 2008. 399–403.

[20] Stephen AE, Segev DL, Ryan DP, et al. The diagnosis of acute appendicitis in a pediatric population: to CT or not to CT. J Pediatr Surg 2003;38:367–71.

[21] Linton O, Tenforde TS, Amis ES, et al. Summary of workshop on CT in emergency medicine: ensuring appropriate use. J Am Coll Radiol 2011;8:325–9.

[22] National council on radiation protection and measurements. Ionizing radiation exposure of the population of the United States (NCRP report no. 160). Bethesda: National Council on Radiation Protection and Measurements; 2009.

[23] Studdert DM, Mello MM, Sage WM, et al. Defensive medicine among high-risk specialist physicians in a volatile malpractice environment. J Am Med Assoc 2005;293:2609–17.

[24] Schwartz DT. Counter-point: are we really ordering too many CT scans? West J Emerg Med 2008;9:120–2.

[25] Stengel D. Rebalancing the major trauma computed tomography pan-scan between panacea and Pandora's box. Emerg Med Austral 2012;24:1–3.

[26] Asha S, Curtis KA, Grant N, et al. Comparison of radiation exposure of trauma patients from diagnostic radiology procedures before and after the introduction of a pan-scan protocol. Emerg Med Austral 2012;24:43–51.

[27] American college of radiologists appropriateness criteria. <http://www.acr.org/Quality-Safety/Appropriateness-Criteria>.

[28] Kalafut MA, Schriger DL, Saver JL, Starkman S. Detection of early CT signs of >1/3 middle cerebral artery infarctions: inter rater reliability and sensitivity of CT interpretation by physicians involved in acute stroke care. Stroke 2000;31:1667–71.

[29] Schriger DL, Kalafut M, Starkman S, et al. Cranial computed tomography interpretation in acute stroke: physician accuracy in determining eligibility for thrombolytic therapy. J Am Med Assoc 1998;279:1293–7.

[30] Boyle A, Staniclu D, Lewis S, et al. Can middle grade and consultant emergency physicians accurately interpret computed tomography scans performed for head trauma? Cross-sectional study. Emerg Med J 2009;26:583–5.

[31] Perron AD, Huff JS, Ullrich CG, et al. A multicenter study to improve emergency medicine residents' recognition of intracranial emergencies on computed tomography. Ann Emerg Med 1998;32:554–62.

23.3 Magnetic resonance imaging in emergency medicine

James Rippey

ESSENTIALS

1 Magnetic resonance imaging (MRI) is becoming more readily available in Australian hospitals and is becoming part of many imaging diagnostic algorithms.

2 The most common indication for MRI in the emergency department (ED) is suspected acute spinal cord pathology.

3 MRI is well suited to imaging soft tissues, particularly central nervous system, musculoskeletal tissues and abdominal organs.

4 Lack of ionizing radiation makes MRI a good choice for younger patients and pregnant women, although it is generally avoided in the first trimester.

5 Disadvantages for ED include the time taken for a scan and difficulties with monitoring and resuscitation in the scanner, making MRI unsuitable for most unstable patients.

Introduction

Magnetic resonance imaging (MRI), like each of the other imaging modalities, has its unique strengths and weaknesses. Emergency diagnostic imaging algorithms are complex and vary according to the clinical condition, the question being asked, patient factors, local availability and expertise. In Australasia, there are rapidly increasing numbers of MRI machines, together with appropriately trained staff. Many diagnostic algorithms are being revised to include MRI as a realistic imaging alternative. While the indications for urgent MRI are increasing, the major indication for emergency MRI remains suspected acute spinal cord pathology.

The main strength of MRI lies in its ability to image soft tissues at extremely high resolution, both spatially and with unparalleled levels of soft tissue contrast. It also has the ability to create two-dimensional slices in any plane; these multiplanar capabilities allow comparison of adjacent tissues from any angle.

Different MRI techniques allow different anatomical and pathological features to be demonstrated. MRI is particularly good at imaging the structure and pathology of brain, spinal cord and nerves, muscle, tendons and ligaments, cartilage, bone marrow and solid abdominal organs. The advent of magnetic resonance angiography (MRA) makes it an alternative to computed tomography angiography (CTA), particularly in those with contraindications to CT contrast media or those more vulnerable to ionizing radiation. Finally, the ability to perform ECG gated imaging has enabled unsurpassed dynamic non-invasive cardiac imaging.

MRI has imaging limitations in cortical bone and air-filled spaces (particularly lung) and thus tends not to be the imaging choice for assessing these tissues.

The lack of ionizing radiation makes MRI an attractive alternative to CT, particularly in younger patients, especially children and women of childbearing age. MRI's apparent safety in pregnancy is another advantage.

Currently, the main limitations of MRI lie in its lack of availability, expertise and associated high costs. From the emergency perspective, even when availability is not an issue, a major disadvantage is the time it takes to complete a scan. The patient is in an inaccessible, confined space, usually with limited monitoring for the duration of the 30–60 minute scan. MRI is therefore unsuitable for the unstable patient. If a patient is stable and intubated, specialized anaesthetic and monitoring equipment and expertise in using it, is required to ensure patient safety.

Patients with metallic foreign bodies or electronic implants are often unable to have MRI, which can also limit its use.

Technical issues

Put very simply, the steps of an MRI involve putting the patient into a powerful magnet, sending in a radiowave, turning the radiowave off, the patient then emits a signal which is received and used for reconstruction of the image.

The components

The traditional MRI suite is centred around the MRI scanner, with its mobile patient table that moves the patient in and out of the MRI tunnel (Fig. 23.3.1). Current machines have a bore (internal diameter of the tunnel) of up to 70 cm and utilize short bore architecture that allows the tunnel to be approximately half the length of that required in the previous generation of MRI scanners. The machine houses a superconductor magnet, the strength of which is measured in Tesla. Current machines operate at 1.5 or 3 Tesla. A 3 Tesla magnet creates a magnetic field around the patient 60 000 times the strength of the earth's magnetic field. As well as the magnet, there are radiofrequency transmitter and receiver coils that send and receive radiofrequency pulses. These briefly disturb the magnetic field and ultimately create the MRI image. Another three sets of gradient coils provide additional linear electromagnetic fields important for spatial information – determining the origin of the signal in the 3-dimensional space. It is these coils banging against their anchoring devices that cause the loud noises associated with MRI.

The high magnetic field generated by MRI means metallic objects within range can become projectile missiles and great care has to be taken to ensure metal objects are well secured or do not enter the room. The magnet can also interfere with electronic equipment, such as computers, monitors and medical equipment like pacemakers and these must be kept away. Finally, the receiver coils are highly sensitive and are designed to detect very minor fluctuations in returning radiowaves (which are a form of electromagnetic radiation). External radiowaves can interfere with the waves received by the coils and this noise will create artefacts interfering with image production. To

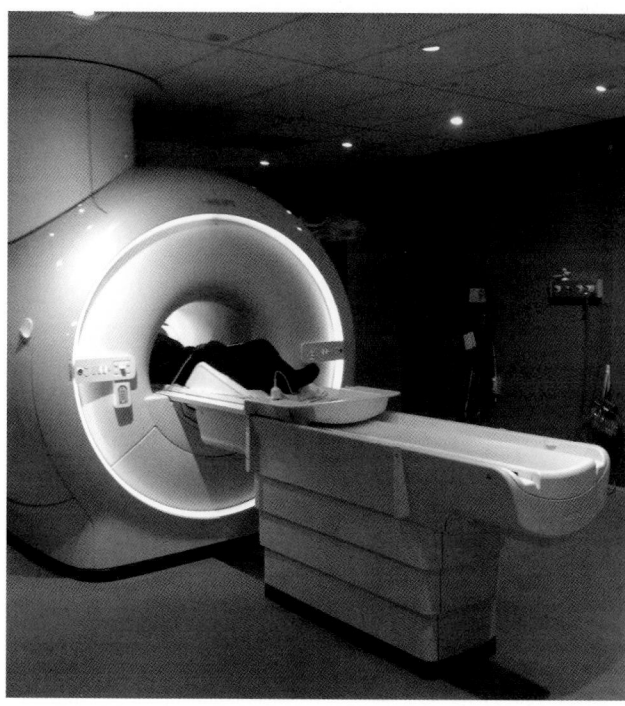

Fig. 23.3.1 Typical 3 Tesla short bore, 70 cm opening diameter MRI machine.

minimize this, the entire MRI room is secured inside a Faraday cage, whose external conducting surface blocks or markedly attenuates any outside potentially interfering radiowaves. The MRI control room and computer terminals with operating console are located immediately adjacent to, but outside the MRI room, in a similar fashion to the CT control room.

Creating an image

MRI depends on the alignment of hydrogen nuclei or positively charged protons within organic compounds in the body. Hydrogen nuclei act like tiny bar magnets. Under the influence of the external MRI magnet, mobile hydrogen ions align and spin in the orientation of the MRI magnet's field, creating a magnet of the patient's body. As well as aligning and spinning on their own axis, protons also rotate or 'precess' as would a spinning top with a slight wobble, around a central axis.

Pulses of electromagnetic energy, called radiofrequency or RF pulses, are then sent into the area being imaged. This briefly disturbs the orientation and precession of the aligned protons. A transient reduction in the longitudinal magnetic field results and a new magnetic vector in the transverse direction, called transversal magnetization, is created. Once the RF pulse is stopped, the protons relax back to their initial aligned state and the longitudinal and transverse magnetic

vectors return to their original state. The realignment rate depends on tissue characteristics and water content. As the magnetic vectors realign, electric currents are induced and the MRI signal and signal intensity created. The receiver coils receive these minute pulses of newly created electromagnetic radiation and these are interpreted to create the ultimate image.

Different MRI imaging techniques

Numerous different MRI imaging sequences and techniques have been developed to create the optimal images for varying body tissues and pathology. The following is not an exhaustive list.

T1- and T2-imaging

These are the most common MRI images with which we are familiar.

T1-weighted images (anatomical) create high definition anatomical images with optimal tissue contrast resolution. In these images, fat is white and water is black. The resultant image gives detailed representation of the internal structure of soft tissue organs. T1 is a time constant that refers to the time it takes for the changes in longitudinal magnetization induced by the RF pulse, to return toward the original state. Measuring this tends to define structural tissue proteins and fats optimally.

T2-weighted images (pathological) highlight pathological processes where there is increased water content within tissues (Fig. 23.3.2). Most pathological processes involve an element of tissue oedema and whether it be trauma, infection, infarction or neoplasia, these images highlight water. Water is seen as white in these images. T2 is a time constant that refers to the time it takes for the changes in transversal magnetization induced by the RF pulse, to return toward their initial state. Measuring this tends to highlight water optimally.

Other MRI techniques each aimed at highlighting other anatomical or pathological features are shown in Figure 23.3.3. The left image (A) is a FLAIR (fluid attenuated inversion recovery) sequence that nulls fluid and can highlight

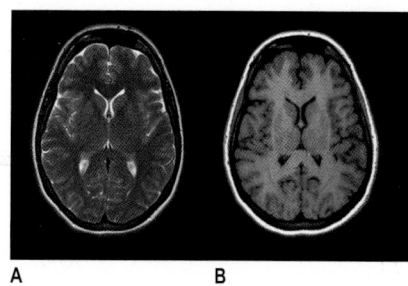

A   B

Fig. 23.3.2 Left: **(A)** T2-weighted MRI image of the brain where water is bright and pathology involving oedema is best demonstrated.
Right: **(B)** T1-weighted MRI, water is black and anatomical features are well demonstrated maximizing soft tissue contrast.

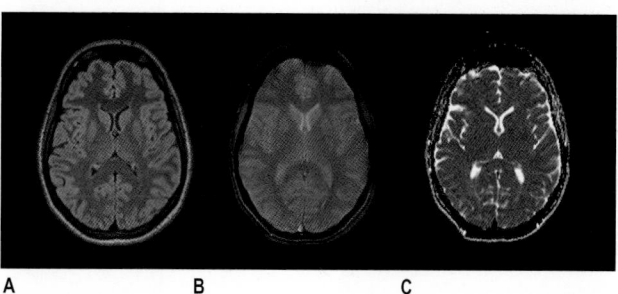

A   B   C

Fig. 23.3.3 Other MRI techniques. Left: **(A)** FLAIR (fluid attenuated inversion recovery) sequence; centre: **(B)** T2 gradient image; right: **(C)** diffusion ADC image.

periventricular demyelination; the central image **(B)** is a T2 gradient image which detects haemoglobin and its breakdown products; the right hand image **(C)** is a diffusion ADC image detecting cell injury in early stroke.

Angiography and gadolinium

Magnetic resonance angiography (MRA) can be done with or without contrast media (Fig. 23.3.4 shows non-contrast MRI). Flow itself alters the MR signal simply by moving the protons that have been exposed to the RF pulse. This can leave what is called a flow void phenomenon and, using this, the machine can create an angiographic image.

Where a contrast agent is used, the para-magnetic rare earth, gadolinium (Gd), is the agent of choice. Its use creates excellent angiographic images. In addition, gadolinium does not cross the normal blood–brain barrier. If, however, this is disrupted, as can occur in many pathological processes, gadolinium improves lesion detection and diagnostic accuracy. Gadolinium is not an iodinated contrast medium and is generally very well tolerated.

The sagittal images of the lumbar spine shown in Figure 23.3.5 demonstrate a tumour involving the L1, causing some cord compression. The left image is T1, the centre T2 and the right a T1 fat-saturated post-gadolinium image where the tumour with its abnormal vasculature is most obvious.

Diffusion and perfusion weighted imaging

MRI imaging changes occur early after stroke and can be detected prior to any visible change on CT. Diffusion weighted imaging assesses water

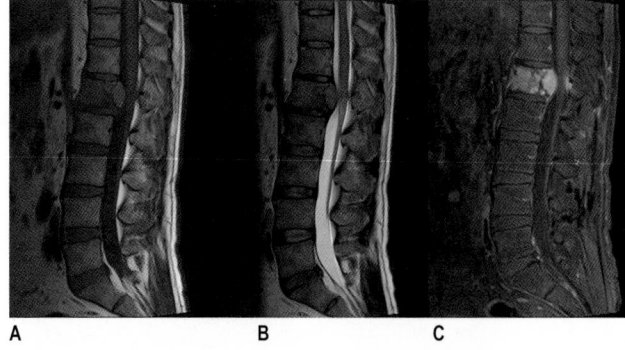

Fig. 23.3.5 Sagittal images of the lumbar spine showing tumour involving the L1, causing some cord compression. The left image **(A)** is T1, the centre **(B)** is T2 and the right **(C)** is a T1 fat-saturated post-gadolinium image where the tumour with its abnormal vasculature is most obvious.

diffusion across cell membranes. There is no water movement across cell membranes when cells are damaged. Diffusion imaging is used to define areas of newly infarcted cerebral tissue. These changes can occur as early as 10 minutes after infarction. Perfusion imaging aims to detect the potentially salvageable cerebrovascular accident 'penumbra' surrounding the non-viable ischaemic core, with a view to decision making regarding thrombolysis and revascularization.

Cardiac imaging

Cardiac imaging is done by using ECG gating and imaging the heart over several cardiac cycles. Sequentially timed images taken from separate cardiac cycles are stitched together to create an animation representative of a single cardiac cycle. The result is a very high resolution, dynamic study of heart function and blood flow within the heart (Fig. 23.3.6).

Monitoring patients in the MRI

The patient in the MRI suite is particularly vulnerable. Their physical movement is restricted while in the MRI tunnel, they are inaccessible to immediate assistance and there are particular challenges with traditional patient monitoring in the MRI environment. This makes MRI unsuitable for the unstable patient and makes those requiring sedation or general anaesthesia a far greater challenge.

As a minimum requirement, visual camera and verbal monitoring are mandated for all MRI machines, ensuring some degree of immediate communication between radiographer and patient.

If any sedation is required, it is essential the patient have oxygen saturation monitoring. There are MRI compatible units, with no ferromagnetic

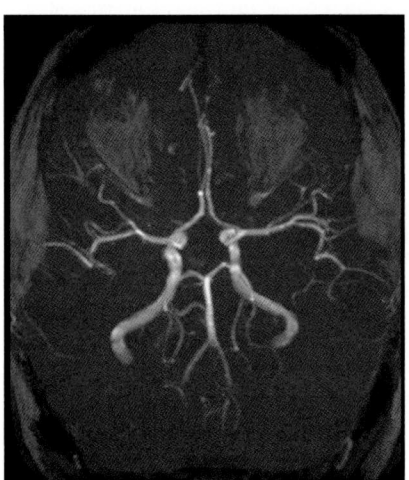

Fig. 23.3.4 Non-contrast MRI demonstrating the circle of Willis.

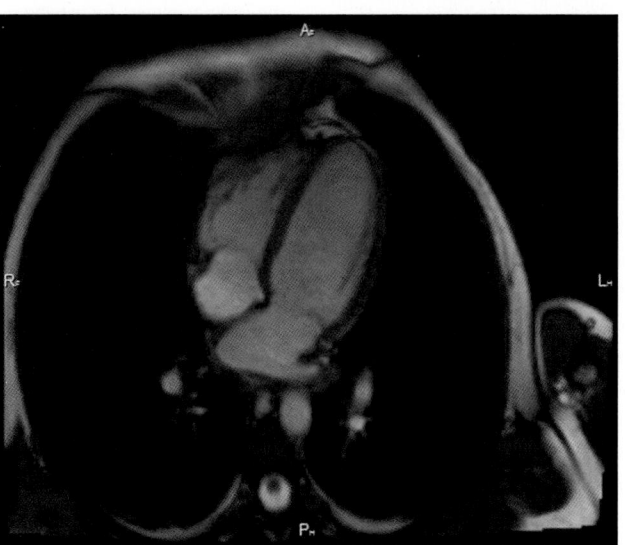

Fig. 23.3.6 MRI 4-chamber cardiac view.

components, often fibreoptic, suited to this purpose and available in most units.

Patients who are under general anaesthetic require highly specialized anaesthetic staff and equipment. This form of remote anaesthesia requires unique training and practice. MRI compatible and prepared equipment is required. This includes specially prepared ventilators and monitors. Attention to detail is required regarding all the equipment involved. Even inappropriate ECG dots and leads can heat and cause injury.

Indications for MRI

In most parts of the world, access to MRI, with its great cost and requirement for highly specialized radiography and radiology staff, is extremely limited. Australasia falls into the category where truly emergent MRI requests can usually be met by most tertiary hospitals. Arranging the scan in a public hospital generally requires consultant-to-consultant discussion and involvement of the inpatient specialty team.

Where there are reasonable imaging alternatives to MRI, diagnostic imaging guidelines have been designed to create effective alternative pathways.

Suspected acute spinal cord and cauda equina pathology

There is little argument that emergency MRI is the investigation of choice when it comes to imaging the spinal cord, spinal nerves, intervertebral discs and ligaments of the spine. Where there are long tract signs and suspicion of an acute spinal cord-threatening lesion, most would proceed directly to MRI. In the setting of trauma, a CT to define bony injury is usually performed prior to MRI.

MRI clearly defines any pathological process affecting the cord, CSF space and surrounding soft tissues. In the emergency setting, trauma with cord injury (Fig. 23.3.7) or contusion may occur and MRI gives additional information regarding spinal ligamentous injury. Other common cord-threatening pathology includes malignancy, which may originate in the vertebrae, most commonly the bodies, and extend into the spinal canal or may invade the canal through the spinal foramina. Malignant deposits, particularly metastases, may also originate within the spinal canal, involving the cord or dura. Infective processes, such as discitis and

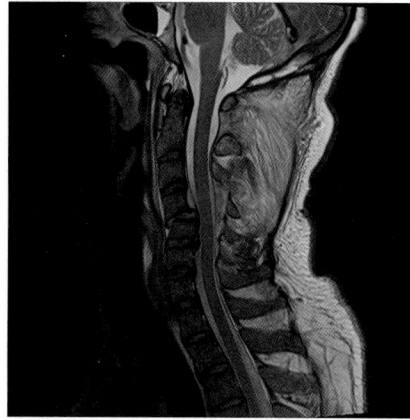

Fig 23.3.7 T2 sagittal image of an acute cervical spine injury with bifacetal dislocation and marked anterior displacement of the body of C4 on C5, with some cord oedema. The anterior and posterior longitudinal ligaments are well demonstrated.

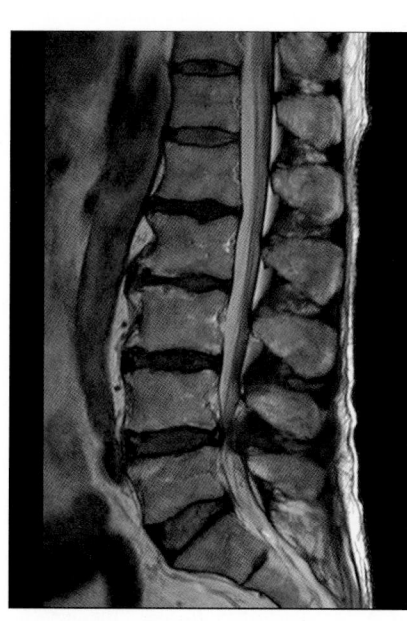

Fig. 23.3.8 T2 image shows L4/5 disc prolapse with marked narrowing of the spinal canal and cauda equina compression.

epidural abcess, are not infrequent causes of acute cord compression and are more common in IV drug users, the immunosuppressed and those who have had spinal procedures. Vascular phenomena, such as epidural haematoma, AV malformation with bleed, aneurysms and spinal cord infarction can all be defined by MRI. Degenerative conditions, such as disc prolapse (Fig. 23.3.8) and spinal canal stenosis from any cause may also threaten the cord.

Rapidly defining the cause of the spinal cord lesion enables surgical planning or, if a malignant process, consideration and planning for radiotherapy.

Stroke

MRI is an excellent modality for defining any brain pathology and stroke is no exception. As well as confirming the presence of stroke and excluding the presence of haemorrhage, MRI can detail the extent of brain injury, the vascular supply, any ischaemic penumbra and can assess for dissection or other predisposing vascular causes.

Unfortunately, even if immediately available, performing an MRI and then preparing and reporting the images often puts the patient outside the window of benefit for thrombolysis. CT is far more accessible and provides adequate information for the majority of cases and this is currently the accepted gold standard.

The exception is the posterior circulation and suspected brainstem infarction where MRI is superior to CT and generally required before interventional attempts at revascularization.

Headache

CT scan is the first choice for investigation of headache. MRI is performed where consideration for intervention for brain tumours, acoustic neuromas and pituitary tumours is being made. Where patients are young or cannot have iodinated contrast and sinus venous thrombosis is being considered, MR venography would be performed over CT venography; however, in most people, CT is adequate to define sinus venous thrombosis and other sinister causes of headache.

Angiography

MR angiography and CT angiography are considered similar in their utility for imaging blood vessels. Dissection is well imaged with either modality and factors that would swing one in favour of MRI include a young patient age (MRI avoids radiation) and allergy to CT contrast.

Occult fracture detection

In the Australasian setting, it is unusual to attain an MRI to assess for occult fracture. Hip and scaphoid fractures are the classic examples where early detection and intervention can benefit the patient. CT scan has lower sensitivity than MRI for detecting occult hip fractures, but it remains reasonable. Where concern remains, a bone scan will give the answer. Similarly, for scaphoid fractures, CT or bone scan or immobilization and delayed repeat plain films at 10 days are reasonable alternatives.

Soft-tissue musculoskeletal injury

MRI is increasingly being used to assess for soft-tissue injury when complex injuries are suspected. Requests generally come from the orthopaedic team involved in the patient's care. MRI can image injuries to muscles, tendons, ligaments, joint capsule and cartilaginous surfaces extremely well (Fig. 23.3.9). Acute shoulder and knee injuries are most commonly assessed with MRI, but complex elbow, wrist, foot and ankle injuries can also be assessed by MRI.

Where there is complex fracture/dislocation and the relationship of adjacent bones and bone fragments need defining, CT is more appropriate.

Magnetic resonance cholangiopancreatogram (MRCP)

MRI can image the liver and biliary tree well. Ultrasound is generally the first imaging modality used to investigate for biliary pathology. Where concern remains and ultrasound imaging has not been definitive, MRCP can help. This is most common with distal biliary obstruction where ultrasound has not been able to image the extreme distal common bile duct. An effective alternative is endoscopic retrograde cholangiopancreatogram (ERCP) and endoscopic ultrasound. The advantage of ERCP is that therapeutic interventions, such as stone retrieval or stenting, can be carried out at the same time.

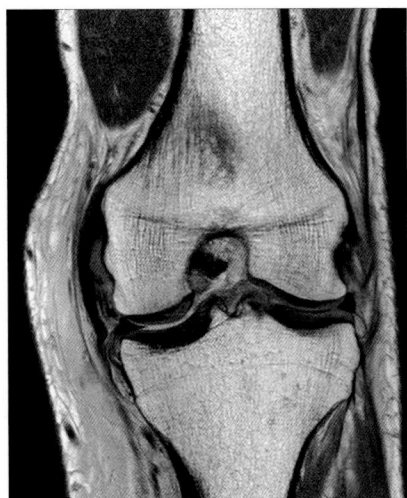

Fig. 23.3.9 Coronal knee MRI showing ACL and MCL ligamentous disruption.

Appendicitis in pregnancy

Ultrasound is the first indicated investigation. MRI may sometimes be used where there is diagnostic uncertainty.

Contraindications, precautions and limitations

There are numerous contraindications to MRI and pre-MRI safety checklists can be found at www.mrisafety.com. MRI technicians should be made aware of any implanted metallic, prosthetic, electronic or drug delivery device. The pre-MRI questionnaire also covers past medical history, particularly renal dysfunction and allergies.

Ferrous and metallic materials

The high magnetic field generated by MRI can move and heat metallic materials. While most joint and heart valve prostheses are now MRI compatible, older prostheses, implanted metallic medical devices, aneurysm clips and metallic shrapnel, especially intraocular metallic foreign bodies, are contraindications to MRI.

Metallic drug transdermal drug infusion patches often contain metal and can heat.

Some tattoos and permanent makeup contain iron oxide and can heat in the MRI environment, although this is rare.

Electronic implants

The intense magnetic field can affect electronic and magnetic equipment. Cardiac pacemakers, implantable cardioverter defibrillators, implanted nerve stimulators, cochlear implants and other electronic implants can be affected. Some are now MRI-compatible, however, most are a contraindication to MRI. The website www.mrisafety.com has lists of thousands of implants and devices that have been tested in MRI machines and is recommended by RANZCR as a resource for obtaining information on patient's implanted devices.

Noise

The MRI is very loud, with constant banging heard. Ear protection is recommended.

Pregnancy

There has been no demonstrated adverse effect from MRI or gadolinium-based contrast media to the mother or embryo/fetus. The evidence in this setting, however, is limited and, with regard to MRI exposure, the ALARA principle (as low as reasonably acceptable) is followed. MRI should only be pursued where potential benefits outweigh the risks. Generally, it is considered prudent to avoid MRI in the first trimester.

Gadolinium

Gadolinium can rarely cause nephrogenic systemic fibrosis (NSF). This disabling disease is more likely in patients with underlying renal disease. It is recommended that patients over 60, those with hypertension or diabetes, a history of renal disease (including transplant or a single kidney), those within a month of a liver transplant or those with an acute deterioration in renal function have renal function tested prior to MRI. If their renal function is not normal, further discussion and consideration of the risk benefit ratio of gadolinium should be made in conjunction with the MRI radiologists.

Weight and size limits

Different MRI machines can tolerate different patient weight and size limits. Some tolerate patients up to 250 kg. Occasionally, it is the patient diameter or shape rather than absolute weight that limits entry to the MRI tunnel.

Claustrophobia

The MRI tunnel frequently causes claustrophobia. Non-pharmaceutical management may include patient education, allowing a patient companion to accompany the patient, continuous verbal contact, headphones with audio, use of prone and or feet first positioning, use of a blindfold, fan, bright lights, aromas or other relaxation techniques or watching videos or movies via mirrors.

Despite these measures, sedation is sometimes required and should be done only with oxygen and saturation monitoring and a single dedicated and trained person responsible to supervise and monitor the sedation.

Conclusion

The increasing availability of MRI within Australasia, together with improving imaging times and a diverse range of MRI techniques, mean MRI is becoming the imaging modality of choice for an increasing number of indications.

Currently, it is generally used in conjunction with other imaging modalities, particularly if they have been unsuccessful, in imaging soft-tissue structures and pathology.

The required isolation of the patient for the duration of the scan and difficulty in monitoring and managing anaesthetized patients in the MRI, mean it is not the place for unstable critically unwell patients.

Controversies and future directions

- Although currently limited to tertiary centres, as with other expensive technologies, MRI is likely to diffuse more widely through the hospital system.
- The indications for MRI from EDs are likely to expand as scanners become more widely available.

- Scanners which can accommodate the sitting patient are being developed and these may enable wider access to MRI.

Acknowledgements

The author declares no conflict of interest.

Thanks to the MRI unit at Sir Charles Gairdner Hospital for their advice on emergency MRI and the images, particularly Dr Rohan Van den Driesen, Dr Andrew Thompson and Ms Anne Windsor.

Further reading

[1] Schild HH, MRI made easy…well almost; Originally published 1992 by Berlex Laboratories, University of Michigan. This edition supplied by Bayer.

[2] Choo EK, DeMayo RF. Magnetic resonance imaging, Chapter e299.3. In: Tintinalli JE, Stapczynski JS, Cline DM, et al. Tintinalli's emergency medicine: a comprehensive study guide, 7th ed. New York: McGraw-Hill; 2011. [Accessed June 2013].

[3] Mendelson R, Dhillon R, Bairstow P. Diagnostic imaging pathways. A clinical decision support tool and educational resource for diagnostic imaging. Government of Western Australia Department of Health. <http://www.imagingpathways.health.wa.gov.au> (Accessed May 2013).

[4] Shallock F. MRI safety.com. Your information resource for MRI safety, bioeffects and patient management. <http://www.mrisafety.com/> [Accessed June 2013].

[5] The royal australian and new zealand college of radiologists (RANCR). Policy library. Guidelines on the use of gadolinium containing contrast agents. October 2009; revised 17 May, 2013. <http://www.ranzcr.edu.au/resources/professional-documents/guidelines> [Accessed June 2013].

[6] The royal Australian and new zealand college of radiologists (RANCR). Policy library. MRI safety guidelines, April 2007. <http://www.ranzcr.edu.au/resources/professional-documents/guidelines> [Accessed June 2013].

[7] Magnetic resonance imaging. Wikipedia. <https://en.wikipedia.org/wiki/Magnetic_resonance_imaging> [Accessed May 2013].

ACADEMIC EMERGENCY MEDICINE

Edited by **George Jelinek**

24.1 Research methodology

David M Taylor

ESSENTIALS

1 Research projects should be designed and undertaken in a structured, predetermined fashion.

2 During the study design phase, assistance from a statistician is highly recommended.

3 The study protocol should be written in advance of data collection and adhered to throughout the project.

4 Most research mistakes relate to inadequate sample size calculations and selection bias in subject recruitment.

5 Research ethics issues are becoming more important, especially since the introduction of new privacy legislation. Ethics committee authorization must be sought prior to study commencement.

Introduction

One important strategy in clinical research is to compare groups of people. These might be different groups or the same group pre- and post-intervention. The methods used are mainly non-experimental, that is observational. They are based on what we can observe and compare in groups of people within populations. By comparing the characteristics (such as behaviours and exposures) and the health experiences of these groups of people, it is possible to identify associations that might be responsible for the cause of a disease.

Initiating the research project

The research question

The research question forms the basis of every research study and is the reason that it is undertaken. It is the scientific, clinical, practical or hypothetical question that, when answered, will allow the researcher to apply newly found knowledge for some useful purpose.

The research question may be generated from many sources, including questions raised by clinical observations, the published medical literature, scientific conferences, seminars and discussions or the effectiveness of currently used or new treatment.

For example:

- Is drug A better than drug B?

The study hypothesis

A hypothesis is a bold statement of what we think the answer to the research question is. Essentially, it is our best guess of what the underlying reality is. As such, it has a pivotal role in any study. The purpose of a research study is to weigh the evidence for and against the study hypothesis. Accordingly, the hypothesis is directly related to the research question.

For example:

- 'directional' hypothesis: drug A is *better* than drug B
- 'null' hypothesis: drug A is as *good as* drug B.

In expressing a hypothesis, the researcher needs to be very specific about who or what is to be observed and under what conditions. A failure to define clearly the study groups and the study endpoints often leads to sloppy research.

The study aims

The aims of a study are a description of what the researcher hopes to do in order to weigh up the evidence for and against the study hypothesis.

For example:

- We aim to determine which is the better drug, drug A or drug B.

Just as the research question begs the hypothesis, the hypothesis begs the study aims. The examples above demonstrate clearly the natural progression from research question through to the study aims. This is a simple, yet important, process and time spent defining these components will greatly assist in clarifying the study's objectives. These concepts are discussed more fully elsewhere [1,2].

Assembling the research team

Most research projects are undertaken as collaborative efforts with the co-investigators each contributing in their area of expertise. Co-investigators should meet the criteria for co-authorship of the publication reporting the study's findings [3].

Usually, the person who has developed the research question takes the role of principal investigator (team leader) for the project. Among the first tasks is to assemble the research team. Ideally, the principal investigator determines the areas of expertise required for successful completion of the project (e.g. biostatistics) and invites appropriately skilled personnel to join the team [1]. It is advisable to keep the numbers within the team to a minimum. In most cases, three or four people are adequate to provide a range of expertise without the team becoming cumbersome. It is recommended that nursing staff be invited to join the team, if this is appropriate. This may foster research interest among these staff, improve departmental morale and may greatly assist data collection and patient enrolment.

All co-investigators are expected to contribute time and effort to the project, although the extent of this contribution will vary. The temptation to include very senior staff or department heads simply to bolster the profile of the project should be avoided if possible. It is recommended that personality and track record for 'pulling one's weight' be considered when assembling the team. There is little more frustrating than having poor contributors impede the progress of a study. Assigning specific responsibilities, in writing, to each member of the team is a useful tactic in preventing this potential problem. However, care should be

taken to ensure that the timelines for assignment completion are reasonable.

The importance of good communication within the research team cannot be overemphasized. This is usually the responsibility of the principal investigator and may involve regular meetings or reports. At the risk of flooding each co-investigator with excessive or trivial communications (e.g. e-mail), selected important communications should be forwarded as they appear, for instance, notification of ethics committee approval and updates on enrolment.

Development of the study protocol

The protocol is the blue print or recipe of a research study. It is a document drawn up prior to commencement of data collection that is a complete description of the study to be undertaken [4]. Every member of the study team should be in possession of an up-to-date copy. Furthermore, an outside researcher should be able to pick up the protocol and successfully undertake the study without additional instruction.

Purpose of the study protocol

Research protocols are required:

- for the ethics committee application
- for applications for research funding
- to facilitate the smooth and efficient running of the study through the provision of well-researched and documented information
- for the basis of the Introduction and Methods sections of the final research report.

Protocol structure

The protocol should be structured largely in the style of a journal article's Introduction and Methods sections [4]. Hence, the general structure is as follows:

Introduction

- Background, including a brief summary of the literature.
- Research question.
- Hypothesis.
- Aims.
- Need for the proposed research, that is, the purpose of the study.

Methods

- Study design – a simple description of the design of the proposed study, e.g. randomized clinical trial, cohort study, cross-sectional survey.
- Study setting and period – a description of where and when the study will take place.
- Study subjects – inclusion and exclusion criteria and a description of how participants are to be recruited.
- Procedures and interventions – the nature of any interventions to be used, including information on safety, necessary precautions and rationale for the choice of dose(s).
- Study endpoints (outcome variables) – variables that are impacted upon by the factors under investigation, e.g. those that are affected by a study intervention.
- Data-collection instruments, e.g. questionnaires, proformas, equipment.
- Data-collection procedures including quality-control procedures to ensure integrity of data.
- Data management – including a description of how data will be handled, how privacy concerns will be addressed and how storage and backup of data will be undertaken.
- Bias and confounding control – sources of bias and variability and measures to be taken to address them.
- Ethical issues – subject confidentiality, safety, security and access to data.
- Statistical analysis:
  ❶ sample size: a description of calculations used to determine sample size and assumptions included in this process should be included. This should include calculations, where appropriate, to ensure that it is clear that the study can recruit a sufficient number of patients to answer the research question
  ❷ data analysis: this should include a description of the primary variables to be analysed, a specification of any *a priori* subgroup analyses and the statistical methods to be used. It is highly recommended that a statistician be consulted during protocol development and for data analysis.

This general plan should be followed in the preparation of any study protocol. However, the final protocol will vary from study to study.

Study design

Study design, in its broadest sense, is the method used to obtain data to weigh up the evidence for and against the study hypothesis. Many factors influence the decision to use a particular study design and each design has advantages and disadvantages. For a more extensive discussion on study design the reader is referred elsewhere [1,5].

Observational studies

In general, research studies examine the relationship between an exposure or risk factor (e.g. smoking, obesity, vaccination) and an outcome of interest (e.g. lung cancer, cardiac disease, protection from infection).

In observational (non-experimental) studies, the principal challenge is to find a naturally occurring experiment, i.e. a comparison of two or more populations that enables the investigator to address a hypothesis about the outcome of interest.

Cross-sectional studies

Cross-sectional studies examine the present association between two variables. For example, within a population you could take a single random sample of all persons, measure some variable of interest (e.g. lung function) and then correlate that variable with the presence or absence of lung cancer. Data are often collected in surveys and the information on exposure and outcome of interest is collected from each subject at one point in time. The main outcome measure obtained from a cross-sectional study is prevalence.

Ecological studies

Ecological studies relate the rate of an outcome of interest to an average level of exposure that is presumed to apply to all persons in the population or group under investigation. So, for example, we could determine the association between the average amount smoked per capita in different countries and the incidence of lung cancer in each country.

Cohort studies

In a cohort study, a group of individuals, in whom the personal exposures to a risk factor have been documented, are followed over time. The rate of disease that subsequently occurs is examined in relation to the individuals' exposure levels. For example, within a population you could take a sample (cohort) of healthy individuals, document their personal past and ongoing smoking history, and relate that to the subsequent occurrence of lung cancer in that same sample. Although not as powerful a study design as clinical trials (see below), cohort studies are able to provide valuable data relating to the causation of disease.

Case-control studies

Case-control studies involve a comparison between a representative sample of people with an outcome of interest (cases) and another sample of people without the outcome (controls). If an antecedent feature (exposure) is found to be more common in the cases than the controls, this suggests an association between that exposure and the development of the outcome. The frequencies of past exposures to risk factors of interest are compared in each group. Case-control studies provide only medium level evidence of an association between exposure and outcome of interest.

Case reports and case series

This study design is often employed in emergency medicine research. The clinical details (history, management, outcome) of interesting or similar patients are described. This study design provides weak evidence for an association between exposure and outcome of interest and is best employed for hypothesis generation. For example, a series of patients who all developed skin necrosis after being bitten by a certain spider would reasonably lead to the hypothesis that the venom of the spider of interest contained a particular tissue necrosis factor. However, this hypothesis would need to be proven by the isolation of the factor and experimental demonstration of its effects.

Data for case reports/series are often extracted from medical record reviews or existing databases. This is one reason for the weakness of this study design insofar as the data were most likely collected for purposes other than the research study. Accordingly, such data are often of low quality and may suffer from inaccuracies, incompleteness and measurement bias.

Experimental studies

In an experimental study, the researcher is more than a mere observer and actively manipulates the exposure of study subjects to an exposure of interest (risk) and measures the effects (outcomes) of this manipulation.

The preferred form of experimental study is currently the randomized, controlled trial, in which the intervention is randomly assigned at the level of the individual study subject. Although this is the most scientifically rigorous design, other study designs must often be used for a number of reasons including:

- the state of knowledge about a disease process
- real-world opportunities
- logistics and costs
- ethical considerations.

For ethical reasons, we cannot easily use experimental studies to study factors that are thought to increase the risk of disease in humans. For example, you could not do a study where you ask half of the group to smoke for 10 years and half of the group to remain non-smokers.

Main types of clinical trials

- Parallel group trials – these are the most common type of clinical trial and involve two or more groups of patients treated separately, but concurrently.
- Two-period crossover trials – patients are treated for two periods using a different treatment in each period. Patients are randomly allocated to the two possible orders of treatment so that half the patients receive the treatments in the sequence AB and the other half in the sequence BA.
- Pre- and post-intervention trials – these trials measure the impact of an intervention when it is introduced into the management of a patient population. For example, the introduction of nurse-initiated analgesia may improve the pain management of emergency department patients.
- Cluster-randomized, crossover trials – institutions (e.g. emergency departments) are randomized to provide certain types of care, e.g. oxygen therapy or no oxygen therapy for patients following myocardial infarction. After a pre-determined data collection period, the institutions crossover to the other form of care and data are again collected.
- Other types – factorial trials, N-of-one trials and sequential trials – are used much less frequently.

Key features of clinical trials

Randomization   This is a process by which patients are allocated to one of two or more study groups, purely by chance. Randomization prevents any manipulation by the investigators or treating doctors in the creation of the treatment groups. This prevents a situation whereby a doctor can, for example, allocate the sicker (or not so sick) patients to a new treatment. Randomization also helps to produce study groups comparable to one another with respect to known, as well as unknown, confounding variables (e.g. risk factors). The most convenient methods of randomizing patients are random number tables in statistical textbooks or computerized random-number-generating programs.

A fundamental aspect of randomization is that it must only take place after the commitment to participate has been made (enrolment has taken place). Another important principle is that randomized patients are irrevocably committed to follow up and must not be excluded from, or lost to, follow up, regardless of their subsequent compliance or progress ('intention to treat analysis').

Blinding Blinding is the most effective method of minimizing systematic error (bias) in clinical trials. In single-blinded studies, patients participating in the trial are unaware which treatment they are receiving but the investigators do know. In double-blind studies, neither the subjects nor the investigators know which patient is receiving which treatment. This type of study is usually only feasible with drug studies where it is possible to provide identically appearing medication. This is often achieved using the double dummy approach in which patients receive two medications, one active and the other placebo. The alternative treatment involves a swap-over of the active and placebo medications. Even in apparently blinded studies, there may be various indicators that allow the patient or investigator to determine which treatment they are receiving. In this circumstance, additional methods of bias control may be needed.

Concepts of methodology

Validity and repeatability of the study methods

It is essential that the study uses valid and repeatable methods, that is, measurements that measure what they purport to measure. Ideally, the validity of each of the measurements used in any study should be tested, during the design stage of the study, against another method of measuring the same thing that is known to be valid.

Two types of validity are described:

- Internal validity means that, within the confines of the study, the results appear to be accurate, the methods and analysis used bear scrutiny and the interpretation of the investigators appears supported.
- External validity is the extent to which the results of a study can be generalized to other samples or situations. Again, for all types of study, it is important that repeatable methods are used, for example measurements that are closely similar when repeated under the same circumstances. Thus, if someone is asked the same question twice about a characteristic that has not changed in the meantime (such as their height), it would be said to be repeatable if they always (or almost always) answered in the same way. Repeatability of the question should be tested during the design phase, although it is also useful to monitor it during the main study. A good example would be a haemoglobinometer that consistently measured the haemoglobin level 2 g/dL too low. Although the haemoglobin measurements would be repeatable, they would be wrong (invalid).

Response rate

Non-response is a problem for many types of observational study. Often people who participate in a study (responders) have different characteristics from those who do not (non-responders). This can introduce substantial selection bias into the prevalence estimates of a cross-sectional study. In order to minimize this bias, as large a sample as possible is required. To this end, investigators undertaking cross-sectional surveys aim for at least 70% of invited participants actually to respond. Unfortunately, a target response rate of 70% is often not met and low response rates are likely to impact significantly upon bias and validity of the study.

Study variables

A variable is a property or parameter that may vary from patient to patient. The framework for the study hypothesis is the independent variable. This variable is often the factor that is thought to affect the measurable endpoints, or dependent variables, in the study. For example, cigarette smoking causes lung cancer. In this example, cigarette smoking is the independent variable and lung cancer is the dependent variable, as its incidence and nature depends upon cigarette smoking.

Study endpoints

Study endpoints are variables that are impacted upon by the factors under investigation. It is the extent to which the endpoints are affected, as measured statistically, that will allow us to weigh up the evidence for and against the hypothesis. For example, a researcher wishes to examine the effects of a new anti-hypertensive drug. It is known that this drug has minor side effects of impotence and nightmares. A study of this new drug would have a primary endpoint of blood pressure drop and secondary endpoints of the incidence of the known side effects.

Essentially, all forms of investigation involve counting or measuring to quantify the study endpoints. In doing so, there is always the opportunity for error, either in the measurement itself or in the observer who makes the measurement. Such errors (measurement bias) can invalidate the study findings and render the conclusions worthless.

Sampling study subjects

There are several important principles in sampling study subjects:

- The sample must be representative of the study population. If the study population comprises all people living in a certain area, the study sample should include a representative sample of all members of the population. Certain groups are frequently left out (for instance the homeless, squatters, people in institutions or people with no telephone). Such groups must be thought of in advance and steps taken to ensure their inclusion. Otherwise, selection bias may be introduced.
- The sample must be derived from the population randomly. The way in which the sample is drawn from the study population is critical to how well the sample represents that population. This determines how 'generalizable' the results will be. Although there are many alternative ways to maximize sample representativeness, as a general rule, a random sample is preferred. A random sample is one in which each member of the population has an equal likelihood or probability of being selected.
- Loss to follow up. The researcher must avoid loss of members from the sample

once it has been taken, for two reasons. First, loss of subjects will effectively decrease the study sample size and may impact adversely on the power of the study to generate statistically meaningful results. Second, if subjects lost to follow up differ in important ways from subjects who remain in the study, then the study results may be affected by selection bias.

Sampling frame

This is a list of all members (for instance persons, households, businesses) of the target population that can be used as a basis for selecting a sample. For example, a sampling frame might be the electoral roll, the membership list of a club or a register of schools. It is important to ensure that the sampling frame is complete, that all known deficiencies are identified and that flaws have been considered (omissions, duplications, incorrect entries).

Sampling methodology

Probability sampling

When every member of the population has some known probability of inclusion in the sample, we have probability sampling. There are several varieties:

Simple random sampling: in this type of sampling, every element has an equal chance of being selected and every possible sample has an equal chance of being selected. This technique is simple and easy to apply when small numbers are involved, but requires a complete list of members of the target population.

Systematic sampling: this employs a fixed interval to select members from a sampling frame. For example, every twentieth member can be chosen from the sampling frame. It is often used as an alternative to simple random sampling as it is easier to apply and less likely to make mistakes. Furthermore, the cost is less, its process can be easily checked and it can increase the accuracy and decrease the standard errors of the estimate.

Stratified sampling

A stratified sample is obtained by separating the population into non-overlapping groups or strata (e.g. males and females) and then selecting a single random (or systematic) sample from each stratum. This may be done to:

- gain precision – this is possible by dividing a heterogeneous population into strata in

such a way that each stratum is internally homogeneous
- accommodate administrative convenience – field work is organized by strata, which usually results in cost savings
- obtain separate estimates for each stratum
- accommodate different sampling plans in different strata, e.g. over-sampling.

However, the strata should be designed so that they collectively include all members of the target population, each member must appear in only one stratum and the definitions or boundaries of the strata should be precise and unambiguous.

Non-probability sampling

Convenience sampling is an example of non-probability sampling. This technique is used when patients are sampled during periods convenient for the investigators. For example, patients presenting to an emergency department after midnight are much less likely to be sampled if research staff are not present. This technique is less preferred than probability sampling, as there is less confidence that a non-probability sample will be representative of the population of interest or can be generalized to it. However, it does have its uses, such as in in-depth interviews for groups difficult to find and for pilot studies.

Data-collection instruments

Surveys

Surveys are one of the most commonly used means of obtaining research data. While seemingly simple in concept, the execution of a well-designed, questionnaire-based survey can be difficult.

Designing a survey

From a practical point of view, the following points are suggested:

Before a survey
- Define the research question(s) to be answered.
- Determine the sampling strategy.
- Design, test and revise the questionnaire (validation).
- Train the data collectors.
- Determine the technique for cross-validation.
- Define the methods of data analysis.

During the survey
- Verify and cross-validate the questionnaire.
- Check timetables and budget.

After the survey
- Cross-check all the data again.
- Perform the main data analysis.
- Perform any other exploratory data analysis.
- Write the report.

If possible, incorporate commonly asked questions into your questionnaire. One good source of such questions is standard surveys (such as Australian Bureau of Statistics). There are many other sources of pre-validated questions (for instance measures on quality of life, functional ability and disease-specific symptoms). The scientific literature, accessible through MEDLINE and other databases, is a good start. This is particularly important if you want to compare the sample with other surveys or, in general, if you want to be able to compare the sample's responses to previously completed work.

Also, previously used questionnaires for similar topics are very helpful and often can be used directly. The advantage to doing this is that these questionnaires' reliability and validity are established.

The wording of a question can affect its interpretation. Attitude questions with slightly different wordings can elicit differing responses, so several questions on the same topic may be helpful to be certain that the 'true attitude' of the respondent is obtained. This technique can enhance internal validity and consistency.

Pre-testing of a questionnaire is most important. Consider the following points:

- Assess face validity of all questions.
- Is the wording clear?
- Do different people have similar interpretations of questions?
- Do closed questions have appropriate possible answers?
- Does the questionnaire give a positive impression?
- Is there any bias in the questions?

It is always worth checking with your colleagues to determine whether the questionnaire will answer the study question. Also, test the questionnaire on a cross-section of potential respondents of differing reading levels and background. There can be a few surprises and several revisions may be required before the final questionnaire is determined.

Data-collection proformas

These documents, also called case report forms, are generally used to record individual case data that are later transferred to electronic databases. These data may be obtained from the patient directly (e.g. vital sign measurements) or extracted from the medical records or similar source.

While simple in concept, careful design of a data-collection proforma should be undertaken. First, a list of the data required should be drafted and translated into data fields on the proforma. These fields should be clearly laid out and well separated. Prior to data collection, the proforma should be trialled on a small selection of subjects. In such an exercise, it is commonly found that the data fields are not adequate for the collection of the required data. Hence, revision of the proforma is often required.

Consideration should be given to the ease of data entry and extraction from the proforma. Data entry should progress logically from the top to the bottom of the document without interruption. This is particularly important for data extraction from medical records. Data extracted from the front of the record should be entered at the top of the proforma and so on. Consideration should also be given to later translation of the data to an electronic database. This should follow the same principles as described above. If possible, design a proforma that will allow data to be scanned directly into an electronic database.

Bias and confounding

Study design errors

In any study design, errors may occur. This is particularly so for observational studies. When interpreting findings from an observational study, it is essential to consider how much of the association between the exposure (risk factor) and the outcome may have resulted from errors in the design, conduct or analysis of the study [5]. The following questions should be addressed when considering the association between an exposure and outcome:

- Could the observed association be due to bias (systematic errors) in the way subjects were selected for the study or in the way information was obtained from them?
- Can the result be explained by confounding factors?
- Could the result be due to chance?

Systematic error (bias)

Bias resulting from the way a study is designed or carried out can result in an incorrect conclusion about the relationship between an exposure (risk factor) and an outcome (such as a disease) of interest [5]. Small degrees of systematic error may result in high degrees of inaccuracy. Many types of bias can be identified:

- Selection bias occurs when there is a difference between the people selected for a study (study sample) and those who are not, for instance employed versus unemployed. Only proportional representation of all groups can, in a way, indicate the absence of selection bias.
- Non-response bias is a function of two components: the non-response rate and the extent to which non-respondents systematically differ from respondents. We may need to ask why a survey question was not answered. Is it not clear? Is it too personal? Is there a negative interaction with the interviewer? Non-response bias may be a type of selection bias.
- Measurement bias may result from faulty methods to measure study endpoints. These may include poorly calibrated machines or stretched measuring tapes, for example. Strictly speaking, the following examples of bias are all types of measurement bias.
- Prevarication bias relates to subjects purposely giving incorrect answers and may result from threatening or insensitive questions.
- Interviewer bias results from the incorrect interpretations by the interviewer of the responses made by the interviewee. This is often an unconscious process, but may result if the interviewer expects, or would like, certain responses.
- Interpretation bias may result from questions that are not clear enough or that the subject does not understand. Some subjects may 'interpret' the question differently from others; for instance, does 'teeth' include 'dentures'?
- Recall bias may result when asking about events that happened a long time ago. For example, 'Were you ever vaccinated against tetanus?' Every effort to avoid historical questions should be made.

Confounding

This is not the same as bias. A confounding factor can be described as one that is associated with the exposure under study and independently affects the risk of developing the outcome [5]. Thus, it may offer an alternative explanation for an association that is found and, as such, must be taken into account when collecting and analysing the study results.

Confounding may be a very important problem in all study designs. Confounding factors themselves affect the risk of disease and, if they are unequally distributed between the groups of people being compared, a wrong conclusion about an association between a risk factor and a disease may be made. A lot of the effort put into designing non-experimental studies is in addressing potential bias and confounding. For example, in an often-cited case-control study on the relationship between coffee drinking and pancreatic cancer, the association between exposure and disease was found to be confounded by smoking. Smoking is a risk factor for pancreatic cancer; it is also known that coffee drinkers are more likely to smoke than non-coffee drinkers. These two points create a situation in which the proportion of smokers will be higher in those who drink coffee than in those who do not. The uneven distribution of smokers then creates the impression that coffee drinking is associated with an increased rate of pancreatic cancer when it is smoking (related to those who drink coffee and to pancreatic cancer) that underlies the apparent association.

Common confounders

Common confounders that need to be considered in almost every study include age, gender, ethnicity and socioeconomic status. Age is associated with increased rates of many diseases. If the age distribution in the exposure groups differs (such as where the exposed group is older than the non-exposed group) then the exposed group will appear to be at increased risk for the disease. However, this relationship would be confounded by age. Age would be the factor that underlies the apparent, observed, association between the exposure and disease. Although age is a common confounder, it is the biological and perhaps social changes that occur with age that may be the true causes that increase the rate of disease.

There are several ways to control for the effect of confounding. To control for confounding during the design of the study, there are several possible alternatives:

- Randomization – random assignment into treatment groups, the cornerstone of a randomized, controlled trial, randomly distributes potential confounding factors between the control and intervention groups.

- Restriction – restricting the participants to one level of a potentially confounding variable helps to control for confounding, for instance only enrolling patients aged 60 years or more.
- Matching – matching subjects on potential confounding variables ensures that these variables are evenly distributed between cases and controls, especially in case-control studies.

In the analysis phase of a study, one can use:

- Stratification – during the analysis phase of a study, the effect of potential confounders can be assessed within separate strata of the confounding variable.
- Statistical modelling – regression models offer the benefit of controlling for multiple confounders simultaneously.

Principles of clinical research statistics

Sample size
The sample must be sufficiently large to give adequate precision in the prevalence estimates obtained by the study for the purposes required. The most common mistake made by inexperienced researchers is to underestimate the sample size required. As a result, the sample size may be too small and not representative of the population that the sample is meant to represent. This usually leads to outcome measures that have very wide 95% confidence intervals and, hence, statistically significant differences between study groups may not be found.

To ensure that a study has adequate sample sizes to show statistically significant differences, if they are there, sample sizes should be calculated prior to the study commencement. In reality, sample size is often determined by logistic and financial considerations, that is to say a trade-off between sample size and costs.

Study power
The power of a study is the chance of correctly identifying, as statistically significant, an effect that truly exists. If we increase the sample size, we increase the power. As a general rule, the closer the power of a study is to 1.0, the better. This means that the type II error will be

small, that is there will be only a small chance of not finding a statistical difference when there really is one. Usually, a power of 0.8 or more is sufficient.

Statistical versus clinical significance
To determine statistical significance, we can obtain a P value, relative risk or some other statistical parameter that is indicative of a difference between study groups. However, a statistical difference (e.g. $P<0.05$) between groups may be found if the study is highly powered (many subjects), even though the absolute difference between the groups is very small and not a clinically significant (meaningful) difference.

This difference is important for two reasons. First, it forms the basis of sample size calculations. These calculations include consideration of what is thought to be a clinically significant difference between study groups. The resulting sample sizes adequately power the study to demonstrate a statistically and clinically significant difference between the study groups, if one exists. Second, when reviewing a research report, the absolute differences between the study groups should be compared. Whether or not these differences are statistically significant is of little importance if the difference is not clinically relevant. For example, a study might find an absolute difference in blood pressure between two groups of 3 mmHg. This difference may be statistically significant, but too small to be clinically relevant.

Databases and principles of data management
The fundamental objective of any research project is to collect information (data) to analyse statistically and, eventually, produce a result. Data can come in many forms (laboratory results, personal details) and are the raw material from which information is generated. Therefore, how data are managed is an essential part of any research project [4].

Defining data to be collected
Many a study has foundered because the wrong data were collected or important data were not collected. Generally, data fall into the following groups:

- identification data: personal information needed to link to an individual patient

- research data: provides the information that is analysed to answer the study question, i.e. endpoints
- administrative data: initials of the data collector, the study centre if a multicentred trial.

Collect only the research data that are essential to answer the study question. Collection of data that will not be of use is time-consuming, expensive and may detract from the quality of the remaining data. However, there will usually be a minimum of data that must be collected. If these data are not collected, then the remaining data may not be analysed adequately. This relates particularly to data on confounding factors.

Database design
A database is a specific collection of data that is organized in a structured fashion. In other words, database software provides us with a way of organizing the data we collect from a research project in a systematic way.

Good database design will:

- reduce repetitiveness, for instance entering in an address or age for a patient many times
- include validation
- have data in a convenient form for analysis
- be pilot tested.

Data entry
This refers to the entry of data into the electronic database, e.g. Access, Excel. Even if the study design and the data collection have been well done, the final data set may contain inaccurate data if the data-entry process is inadequate. This relates particularly to manually entered data where mistakes are bound to happen.

Data entry can be achieved in many ways:

- Manual data entry – this may be single entry undertaken by one person. Alternatively, double entry involves two independent people entering the same data. Any differences between the two are reconciled. This is a form of double checking but is clearly more time-consuming and, therefore, expensive.
- Direct data entry – this can be achieved by having database forms (proformas) on a computer screen. Direct entry of data via an Internet web page is one form of direct data entry. Alternatively, scannable forms can be fed into a scanner, avoiding the need for manual transcription.

Data validation

Effectively, this is a quality assurance process that confirms the accuracy of the data and can be done in the following ways:

- Visual review: matching data on questionnaires with medical records (source data)
- Value range checks: cholesterol levels should be >0 and <20 mmol/L (i.e. do the numbers in the database make sense?)
- Field type checks: text should not be entered into numerical fields
- Logical checks (if, then): if classed as a non-smoker, then cigarettes per day should be zero.

Research ethics

Participation in a clinical trial may involve a sacrifice by the participant of some of the privileges of normal medical care for the benefit of other individuals with the same illness. The privileges forgone might include:

- the right to have treatment decided entirely on the basis of the treating doctor's judgement rather than by random allocation
- the right to have concomitant therapy according to requirements, rather than be standardized for all trial participants.

Participation may also require the discomfort and inconvenience associated with additional investigations and the potential incursion on privacy. Without the willingness of some individuals to make these sacrifices, progress in clinical medicine would be greatly impaired. Most individuals who now expect to receive safe and effective medical care are benefiting by the sacrifices previously made by other individuals.

Some have argued, in contrast, that enrolment into clinical trials ensures the absolute best care currently available, with greater involvement and scrutiny by attending healthcare teams.

If one accepts that clinical trials are morally appropriate, then the ethical challenge is to ensure a proper balance between the degree of individual sacrifice and the extent of the community benefit. However, it is a widely accepted community standard that no individual should be asked to undergo any significant degree of risk regardless of the community benefit involved, that is, the balance of risks and benefits must be firmly biased towards an individual participant.

Because of the trade-offs required and because of the spectrum of views about the degree of personal sacrifice that might be justified by a given community benefit, it is accepted that all clinical trials should be reviewed by an ethics committee that should have as a minimum:

- sufficient technical expertise to quantify the risks and benefits involved
- adequate community representation so that any decisions are in keeping with community standards.

Scientific value

It is unethical to request individuals to undergo the risks and inconvenience of a study that is unlikely to provide a scientifically worthwhile result. It is also unethical to request sacrifices from volunteers that are out of keeping with the value of the research being undertaken. In keeping with this principle, studies that suffer from substantial design errors or are susceptible to serious bias should not be approved until these deficiencies are remedied.

It is unethical to allow scientifically invalid studies to proceed. Sample-size calculations should be scrutinized because of the ethical undesirability of including too few subjects to provide an answer or many more than is needed to provide a convincing answer. Another safeguard to ensure that the research will be valuable is that the investigator should be qualified, experienced and competent, with a good knowledge of the area of study and have adequate resources to ensure its completion.

Benefits forgone

It is unethical to require any patient to forgo proven effective treatment during the course of a trial. It follows that clinical trials should only be undertaken when each of the treatments being compared is equally likely to have the more favourable outcome.

Very commonly, however, there is an expectation before a trial is commenced that one or other treatment is the more beneficial. This may be based on results of uncontrolled studies or even on biochemical or physiological expectations. The large number of times such expectations have been proven wrong can still provide strong justification for a trial.

If such an expectation of benefits is held strongly by an individual, it is probably not ethical for that individual to participate in a study. Furthermore, it is the responsibility of an ethics committee to assess the strength of the presumptive evidence facing one or other treatment and consider whether any substantial imbalance in likely outcome exists. This must be considered in relation to the importance of the question being addressed.

Informed consent

Participants in clinical trials have a fundamental right to be fully informed about the nature of a clinical trial and to be free to choose whether or not to take part. Ethical principles also dictate that prospective participants be:

- told they are taking part in a clinical trial and have an unambiguous right to decline to participate or to withdraw at any time
- provided with a full explanation about the discomforts and inconvenience associated with the study and a description of all risks that may reasonably be considered likely to influence the decision whether or not to participate [4].

It is usual practice to provide prospective participants with a Participant Information and Consent Form that provides a simple, easy to understand account of the purposes, risks and benefits associated with participation in the study. Ethics committees are required to review these statements and confirm that they provide a reasonable account.

In practice, the procedures involved in obtaining informed consent are often problematic. Considering the dependence of sick patients on the health system, their anxiety and their desire to cooperate with their physicians, it is doubtful whether informed consent is ever freely given. When ethics committees identify situations where this scenario is likely to be a particular problem, the involvement of an independent uninvolved person to explain the study may be useful.

Controversies and future directions

- The issue of consent of patients requiring resuscitation raises serious ethical issues. In this circumstance, the patient is clearly unable to give consent and some argue that this automatically precludes their enrolment. Others disagree and note that such a position would terminate much research in this difficult area.
- In response to perceived difficulties in the passage of research through the ethical approval process, ethics

committee streamlining is occurring in most jurisdictions and standardization of application forms now exists at the national level.

- Substantial clinical research requires skilled personnel, time, funding and a supportive infrastructure. Emergency medicine in Australasia has established a respected clinical practice. However,

among its present challenges is the establishment of a culture of research with the resources to support and promote it.

References

[1] Taylor DMCD. Practical issues in the design and execution of an emergency medicine research study. Emerg Med 1999;11:167–74.

[2] Hall GM, editor. How to write a paper, 2nd edn. London: British Medical Journal Publishing; 1999.

[3] Uniform requirements for manuscripts submitted to biomedical journals. <http://www.jama.ama-assn.org/info/auinst_req.html> [Accessed Mar. 2002].

[4] Good Research Practice Committee. A guide to good research practice. Melbourne: Department of Epidemiology and Preventive Medicine, Monash University; 2001.

[5] Jekel JF, Katz DL, Elmore JG, editors. Epidemiology, biostatistics, and preventive medicine, 2nd edn. Philadelphia: WB Saunders; 2001.

24.2 Writing for publication

Anne-Maree Kelly

ESSENTIALS

1 Check and follow the journal's suggested format and length. Pay particular attention to format of abstract, text and references.

2 Make sure that the objectives, methods, results and conclusions are logically consistent.

3 Be clear and concise.

Introduction

Sharing of knowledge and experience through publication is an important way of improving clinical practice. In addition, researchers have an ethical obligation to publish their findings. Communication may be by way of an original research publication, brief report, case report or letter to the editor. Each of these has different requirements in terms of content, format and length and these requirements may vary between journals. It is useful to choose the intended journal for publication early. While impact factor may be a consideration in this choice, most authors are more concerned with publishing in a journal that has the appropriate target audience for the subject matter of the paper. It is important to check the *Instructions for Authors* for the chosen journal to ensure that your submission matches that journal's requirements. Failure to do so reduces the chances of acceptance considerably.

Although journals may have differences in format and style, all prefer clear and concise communications. In particular, it is important for the material to be arranged logically so that clear relationships can be seen between the objective of the study or communication, the evidence and any conclusions drawn.

Important principles

Authorship, acknowledgement and competing interests

Authorship can be a contentious issue, however, there are defined requirements for qualification as an author. The International Committee of Medical Journal Editors state that authorship credit should be based on:

- substantial contributions to conception and design, acquisition of data or analysis and interpretation of data
- drafting the article or revising it critically for important intellectual content and
- final approval of the version to be published.

All three conditions must be met. Contributions that do not meet these criteria can be recognized in an Acknowledgement. To avoid misunderstandings, authorship should be decided as early as possible in the research process with the outcome clearly documented.

Most journals also require authors to disclose competing interests relevant to this paper. This is to assist readers in deciding if those interests have a potential bearing on the conduct or reporting of the research. Competing interests may be financial (e.g. external research funding, support from a company for activities potentially related to the project) or personal (authorship of guidelines, editorship of the journal of submission).

Duplicate publication

Duplicate submission and duplicate publication are unacceptable. An exception is secondary publication of material with the express approval of the editors of the relevant journals. This only occurs under special circumstances.

Sometimes studies generate large amounts of data that are difficult or unsuitable for reporting as a single paper. Authors must strike a balance between including data about a large number of secondary outcomes in a single paper (potentially causing confusion about the research question and distracting from main messages) and splitting data into a large number of small papers. In principle, separation of data into meaningful groups for separate papers is acceptable but should be acknowledged in each paper.

Readability

To get your message across, it must be accessible to the reader. This is best achieved by avoiding long sentences, using simple words and avoiding jargon. Abbreviations should be kept to a minimum and always defined in the paper at their first use.

Manuscript preparation

Original research manuscripts

Original research manuscripts aim to answer a relevant research question. Defining that question, indicating why it is important, what methods were used to answer it, key findings and their interpretation is the purpose of this type of paper. An original research manuscript is usually divided into five sections: Abstract, Introduction (or Background), Methods, Results and Discussion. In addition, some journals prefer a separate concise Conclusion, although many prefer this as the last paragraph of the Discussion. Uncommonly, journals have additional section headings, such as Theoretical Concept and Limitations. It is very important to check the journal's preferred format for each section and ensure the manuscript complies. Most manuscripts also require a key word list of up to five words or phrases to assist with indexing.

Abstract

This is a very important part of the paper as it is the part that will appear in on-line indexing services. The usual word limit is 250 words under the headings 'Objectives', 'Methods', 'Results' and 'Conclusion'. There is considerable variation between journals about how the abstract section is set out. Some prefer a single paragraph without subheadings but many of the major journals require structured abstracts with particular subheadings. These are detailed under *Instructions for Authors*.

The abstract should contain all key data. In particular, the specific aims, methods, outcomes of interest, main results (with numbers) and conclusions should be clear enough to be understood without the support of the text. It is important that no data or conclusions appear in the abstract that have not been presented in the main body of the paper.

Introduction

Shorter introductions are often more effective. The aim is to convince the reader why the area of study is important, what this study adds to the body of knowledge and the specific aims of the study. A lengthy review of the literature should be avoided unless it is imperative to put the study in context. A concise review of the literature is more appropriately reported in the Discussion. The last paragraph should explicitly state the aims of the study.

Methods

The Methods sections should address a number of headings. Some journals like this done explicitly, while others are happy for it to be rolled into logical paragraphs.

- *Study design:* what type of study is it?
- *Setting:* where was it conducted? What are the special features of this setting?
- *Selection of patients:* what are the inclusion and exclusion criteria? How were patients identified? Was anything extra done to ensure that no patients were missed?
- *Data collected:* this should describe all the data collected.
- *Outcomes measures:* what was the primary outcome of interest? Were secondary outcomes also collected?
- *Sample size:* how was the number of subjects chosen? A power calculation is often helpful to justify the numbers.
- *Data analysis:* what types of analyses were used? This refers to the types of tests used rather than the name of a software program.
- *Ethics approval:* there should be a statement saying that the study was approved and by whom or whether it was deemed a quality activity.
- *Clinical trials registry registration:* many journals now require that prospective clinical studies are registered in a public trials register (e.g. www.anzctr.org.au, www.cct.cuhk.edu.hk, clinicaltrials.gov). The trial's registration number should be included in *Methods*.

Results

It is important for the results to be presented logically and for the relationships with the objectives and methods to be obvious. A useful structure is to start by describing the study population. This should include how it was derived (a summary figure such as a Consolidated Standards of Reporting Trials (CONSORT) diagram may be very effective for this) and its features such as gender, age and so on.

This should be followed by descriptions of the results with respect to stated outcomes of interest: primary outcomes first then secondary outcomes. These should align with the stated objectives. Any subgroup or other analysis should follow this. All results should give the appropriate statistics with confidence intervals (if appropriate) and the type of test used. A significant proportion of journals are moving away from P values as a way of expressing statistical significance, instead preferring effect size with confidence intervals (or similar). Avoid any comments on what the results might mean or why they might have occurred. Interpretation of the results belongs in the Discussion section.

Tables and figures can be very effective ways of communicating results. They should not repeat what can be described adequately in the text. All tables and figures should be self-explanatory, with clear descriptive headings. Tables should be constructed so that the main comparisons of interest are horizontal and left-to-right, with number of subjects clearly shown for each column. Graphs or figures should be used to convey patterns and details that cannot be succinctly conveyed in tables or text. Figures that show the distribution of data (scatterplots, box plots, etc.) are more effective than those simply summarizing data (bar graphs, pie charts, etc.). Axes must be clearly labelled. Tables and figures should be kept to the minimum number needed to convey the information, and should be numbered in the convention of the journal.

Discussion

The Discussion should be concise and to the point and can be challenging. This structure may assist:

- Summarize the principal findings.
- Comment on how it compares with other research. Where does it agree? Disagree?
- Taken together with the other available evidence, comment on possible explanations and implications, avoiding the temptation to overstate the significance of the findings.
- Discuss any other results that are worthy of comment.
- Describe any unanswered questions or directions for future research.
- Describe the limitations of the study. This is important as it is an opportunity to acknowledge limitations and give the rationale for some of these. A good limitations section adds to the quality of the paper rather than detracting from it.
- Give a summary or conclusion. This should be a few sentences only. Avoid overstating the findings. Some journals prefer this as a separate heading.

All statements throughout the Introduction, Methods and Discussion that make an assertion or refer to other evidence or methods must be referenced. Ensure that referencing is in the journal's preferred style. Selective referencing should be avoided, that is choosing references that agree with the study findings, or worse, citing mostly the authors' own work. Journal referees are likely to know the relevant literature and detect any selection bias.

In general, as long as the key elements are included, shorter is better than longer in manuscripts. If in doubt, shorten the Introduction and Discussion rather than Methods or Results. As Stephen Lock, former Editor of the British Medical Journal states: 'A good paper has a definite structure, makes its point, and then shuts up'.

An alternative to the full original research manuscript is the short report. This form has a word limit of 1000–1500 words and usually has some minor formatting differences. It is, however, indexed the same as a full original research manuscript and for many studies is a good choice of format.

Case reports

Fewer journals are accepting case reports. Those accepted for publication tend to have an exceptional element or important clinical message, either in terms of an unusual diagnosis, an innovative use of tests or treatments or an unusual adverse event. It is not enough for a case to simply be 'interesting'.

The usual structure for a case report is an abstract of about 100–150 words summarizing the case and the clinical messages, the case report itself and a discussion. The case should be described in sufficient detail for the reader to be confident of the evidence. The Discussion is the key element of a case report. It usually includes a review of the literature and uses the case to draw out important clinical messages. It needs to be logical in idea development and well referenced.

Systematic reviews and meta-analyses

A systematic review is a summary of primary studies. It aims to answer a clinical or research question by using strategies that limit bias, critically appraise and synthesize all relevant studies on a selected topic. A meta-analysis is a mathematical synthesis of the results of primary studies addressing the same question in a similar way.

A detailed description of the methods for systematic reviews and meta-analyses is beyond the scope of this chapter. That said, they share several aspects with original research including definition of a research question, development of a research protocol, literature search/review, data analysis and interpretation.

The PRISMA (Preferred Reporting Items for Systematic Reviews and Meta-Analyses; www.prisma-statement.org) checklist is an evidence-based minimum set of items aimed at assisting authors improve the quality of systematic reviews and meta-analyses. Many journals require the submission of a PRISMA checklist when review articles are submitted.

Letter to the editor

These are short communications, usually 500–600 words in length. Most often they comment on a recently published paper in the journal concerned, but they may also be used to report a case or case series, an observation or an opinion.

Manuscript submission

Most journals require online submission of manuscripts. This is good for authors as it significantly reduces turn-around time. The sites vary in the way they want material entered, so it is important to check this.

A manuscript must only be under consideration by one journal at a time. Authors will be required to attest to this and to the fact that appropriate ethics approvals were obtained.

The cover letter

Whether manuscripts are submitted electronically or in hard copy, a cover letter is usually required. This is often quite short and includes a request for consideration for publication in the journal concerned, a statement that the paper has not been published and is not under consideration by another journal, a statement regarding ethics approvals and a note of the presence or absence of author conflicts of interest.

The cover letter is also an opportunity to alert the editor to other issues that may be important. For example, if the manuscript overlaps with previously published work or another manuscript such that there might be a possibility of duplicate publication, it allows the editors to assess any overlap for themselves. Alternatively, it also provides the opportunity to identify potential reviewers that the authors believe should be avoided, usually because of actual or perceived conflicts of interest.

Feedback from journals

It is quite rare for manuscripts to be accepted 'as is'. Usually, some revision is required and, in some cases, manuscripts are rejected. Neither of these necessarily implies that the study or material is not worth publication. It may simply be that the editors consider that their journal is not appropriate for the subject matter of the paper. Seriously consider the comments given, which are often detailed, and decide whether the issues can be addressed. If so, it is important to undertake a revision and re-submit as soon as practical. If the journal requested revisions and the concerns can be addressed, re-submit to that journal, otherwise submit to another journal after notifying the initial journal that the paper will not be re-submitted to them. Reformatting as a short report or letter to the editor are sometimes alternative ways to get your findings published.

Post-acceptance issues

There are usually several actions required post-acceptance. These include completion of assignment of copyright forms and checking the proofs of the paper. The publisher will usually manage these processes.

Further reading

Committee of Publication Ethics. Guidelines on good publication practice. <http://www.publicationethics.org.uk/guidelines> [Accessed Jul. 2007].

Davidson A, Taylor DMcD, Babl FE. Review article: a primer for clinical researchers in the emergency department: Part III: how to write a scientific paper. Emerg Med Australas 2012;24:357–62.

International Committee of Medical Journal Editors. <http://www.icmje.org/urm_main.html> [Accessed Oct. 2012].

24.3 Principles of medical education

Debbie Paltridge

ACADEMIC EMERGENCY MEDICINE

ESSENTIALS

1 The emergency department (ED) provides a rich learning environment despite the constraints of service provision and time pressure.

2 Applying adult learning principles, acknowledging prior learning experiences, the need for self-evaluation, the preference for problem-based and experiential learning and the desire for feedback assists the effectiveness of the ED teacher.

3 Setting clear learning objectives at the beginning and summarizing the learning experience at its conclusion enhances any form of teaching.

4 A learner-centred approach allows the learner to determine learning objectives, actively engage in learning opportunities and participate in evaluation.

5 Characteristics of a 'good' ED teacher include providing a role model, tailoring teaching to the learner and situation, involving the learner in problem-solving, actively seeking opportunities to teach and giving timely feedback.

Introduction

George Bernard Shaw famously quipped, 'He who can, does. He who cannot, teaches'. However, the emergency physician can rarely teach without doing. The tradition for doctors to teach their colleagues and students goes back to the Hippocratic Oath, where the duties of a doctor to students are outlined: '… to teach them this art, if they want to learn it, without fee or indenture' [1].

Emergency physicians have been taking an increasing role in teaching and education, in part because of the need for all doctors to learn and refresh emergency skills, but also because emergency physicians are usually full time and hospital-based and have access to students, patients and teaching resources. In addition, they have a unique opportunity of seeing students progress in their chosen specialty and may have multiple inputs vertically over several years in a younger doctor's career. This can be very satisfying and also very motivating.

The emergency environment is one of constant new learning experiences while, at the same time, being the location for patient care and critical decision making. Barriers to teaching in hospitals in general, but applicable to emergency departments (ED), have been summarized by Lake in her 'Teaching on the Run' series as lack of time, lack of knowledge, lack of training in teaching,

criticism of teaching when given and lack of rewards, either materially or by recognition [1].

In addition, teaching in the pressure cooker environment of an ED gives further layers of difficulty, both logistically and ethically. Challenges include:

- shifts, requiring teaching at all hours of the day and night
- junior medical staff from a variety of specialties and backgrounds with varying needs
- numbers of junior medical staff and rostering affecting continuity for teacher and learner
- huge variation in workloads from shift to shift
- administration pressures to reduce waiting times
- physical restraints in many ED environments caused by overcrowding [2].

The ED is a teaching environment, not only for physicians at various levels, but also for nurses, allied health workers, paramedics and others. A significant component of ED teaching is procedural. It is suggested that most patients believe they should be informed if it is the first time a doctor is performing a procedure on them, but less than half of patients feel comfortable about themselves being the first patient ever for suturing (49%), intubation (29%) or

lumbar puncture (15%) for a resident [3]. For non-procedural medicine the evidence is that most patients enjoy being part of the teaching process, in outpatient and ambulatory settings at least, and that no extra negative effects on patients occur from teaching [4,5]

An added component of complexity in teaching in the ED is the potential for slowing patient processing by having to stop and supervise a junior. It is often so much quicker just to do it yourself. Supervising a lumbar puncture, for example, may take both the teacher and the taught away from seeing new patients for half an hour. However, as far as it has been researched, teaching in academic EDs does not appear to slow down patient care but in fact improves quality of care [6]. Doctors who are seen by their juniors as good teachers are just as likely to see as many patients per shift as those who are not [7].

ED crowding can be seen to have positive and negative effects on emergency teaching. On the one hand, if crowding is due to patients staying for longer periods of time, it may provide increased patient contact and teaching opportunities over that time. On the other hand, the emergency doctors may have less time for teaching if the crowding is due to increased throughput and production pressure is high [8].

All emergency physicians are teachers at some stage in their career at various levels and, as in Hippocrates' time, are mostly unpaid for it. Although most doctors become teachers, the majority of prevocational doctors in Australia have had no exposure to learning how to teach [9]. Here we present the principles of teaching and learning to assist emergency physicians, whether they are involved with medical students, residents, registrars or other health professionals.

Adult learning principles

Contemporary medical education needs to be couched in terms of contemporary education theory. Adult learning principles should underpin educational practice from the bedside, through the clinical skills laboratory to the seminar room. In addition, these principles are relevant to the education of the undergraduate, prevocational (first 2 years' postgraduate) and vocational registrar years, as well as the continuing professional development of the mature medical practitioner.

Malcolm Knowles first introduced the notion of andragogy or adult learning in the early 1970s [10]. He described five assumptions regarding how adults learn:

❶ As mature people they move from being dependent to being self-directing. This transition allows them to determine their own learning needs.

❷ Adults bring a wide range of experiences accumulated over their lifetime to the learning situation. These experiences provide both a context and a resource for new learning.

❸ Adults' readiness to learn (or motivation) is linked to the applicability of the learning to their current life/employment.

❹ Adults are more problem-centred, that is, they want learning relating to a problem they may encounter in everyday life.

❺ Adults are motivated to learn by internal factors, such as desire to succeed, personal goals, etc. as compared to external factors, such as rewards.

Knowles and other authors have since developed principles of adult learning that can be used to guide education activities [11–15]:

- An effective educational climate is one that allows learners to feel safe. They should be encouraged to express themselves without fear of judgement.
- Establishment of learning needs requires learner participation so that their intrinsic motivation to learn is engaged. The process of developing learning needs helps to assist learners' self-reflection and establish relevancy for them.
- Once a need has been identified, learners should be involved in determining specific learning objectives for the educational intervention.
- Designing the educational intervention should be collaborative, ensuring communication between the learner and teacher/facilitator. This will ensure that the methodology chosen will be relevant to the learner's needs.
- Learners should be encouraged to identify appropriate resources to assist their achievement of learning objectives. This will ensure that activities are learner-centred

Table 24.3.1 Application of adult learning principles and assumptions in the ED environment

Adult learners	Application to ED teaching
Have prior learning and experience	Even the most junior doctors (e.g. interns) bring experiences with them to the ED. They may have specific experience relevant to the condition that they are treating (e.g. they saw similar patients in their undergraduate course) or it may be life experience (e.g. they had relatives with that experience). Open questioning techniques (requiring a more detailed answer from the learner as opposed to a closed question requiring a yes/no answer) can be used to promote reflection on past experiences and practices. A case study with short answer questions to facilitate this reflection could be used in a small group tutorial situation. Small group discussions can also provide opportunities for learners to draw on their own experiences and to learn from each other as well as the facilitator.
Are self-directed learners	At the commencement of a rotation in the ED, junior staff should be asked as part of their orientation what it is they specifically want to get out of this rotation. This allows the identification of personal learning goals. This is relevant to new senior staff as well. Orientation is also very important for establishing expectations of both learner and facilitator and ground rules for how education will be carried out within the ED rotation. Learners should also be offered a choice of learning activities. This will allow learners to choose activities which will address their individual learning objectives and which will address their specific learning requirements and styles. For example, one intern may want to watch a lumbar puncture before performing one under supervision, another may want to practise a lumbar puncture on a manikin first before performing one.
Learn most effectively when they perceive a need for learning	The ED educator needs to help learners recognize the relevance of a learning experience. This will significantly impact on their motivation to learn. Sharing of experiences, e.g. a case example from real life, can help to establish relevancy for a learner. Additional methods may include documentation of ED presentations, participation in unit audit meetings or presentations of cases.
Prefer problem-centred approaches	ED presentations require sophisticated problem-solving techniques. The undifferentiated patient is the norm. Modelling of clinical reasoning from experienced practitioners can assist the novice to understand problem-solving approaches. Evidence suggests that the experienced practitioner does this subconsciously, however, verbalization is necessary to promote collaborative problem solving by the less experienced. Unit case-based discussions also encourage shared problem solving.
Practise self-evaluation	Adults require an opportunity for 'reflection-on-action'[1] or self-evaluation. Self-evaluation opportunities can be incorporated formally by: • use of case studies in a tutorial setting • end of shift review of cases • trolley-side reflection opportunities using open questions.
Require feedback	Opportunities for feedback on performance should be incorporated into the ED term both formally (as part of a requirement of training, e.g. mid- and end of term feedback) and informally from supervisors or peers. Written and verbal feedback can be used.
Value experiential ('hands on') learning opportunities	There are numerous opportunities for hands on experience within the ED. Educators need to involve learners in case-based discussions and problem-solving activities. However, procedural skills may need to be practised away from patients until competence is determined. Then practice under supervision will be appropriate.

[1]Schön D. The reflective practitioner. How professionals think in action. London: Temple Smith; 1983 with permission.

and self-directed as required by adult learners.
- Facilitators should assist learners to implement their learning plans so that objectives are achieved.
- Learners should be involved in evaluating their learning.

However, these principles of adult learning are irrelevant to the emergency physician educator unless they are actively applied to the education of their postgraduate charges. The question remains of how these principles are put into practice. Table 24.3.1 outlines some examples of how these principles may be incorporated into education within the ED.

Learner-centred education

Many traditional medical education experiences are teacher centred. The teacher is the expert and determines what, how, when and where much is learnt. The teacher is the active participant and the learner is the passive recipient [16]. However, a more effective approach to education is the learner-centred approach. Learner-centred education refers to educational events that place the learner in the pivotal position, responsible for determining learning objectives, actively engaging in learning opportunities and participating in evaluation [17]. This is more in line with adult learning principles.

So how does the ED physician become a learner-centred educationalist? The following suggestions are provided to assist:

- Orientation – to the unit, to the department, to the rotation. Junior medical staff require an orientation for a number of practical workplace reasons, such as awareness of policies and procedures, occupational health and safety, rostering, pay, etc. However, this is an important opportunity from an educational perspective. The orientation can allow exploration of the junior doctor's learning goals and objectives, past experiences, confidence with procedural tasks and expectations of their ED rotation. The orientation allows the educational supervisor the opportunity to establish ground rules in terms of educational interactions, when feedback will be given and how education with patients will occur. The ED supervisor can acknowledge barriers to learning which are more specific to the ED environment and discuss how these will be overcome.
- Ask the resident to select a patient to present rather than dictating which patient or topic will be discussed.
- Ask residents about past experiences to assist in determining their confidence in managing certain conditions independently. Obviously, supervision will be required until this is determined first hand, but demonstrating insertion of an intravenous (IV) cannula to an intern who has previously inserted numerous IVs may not be the most appropriate and you will not know unless you ask!
- Present junior medical staff with suggested topics for in-service education and ask them to prioritize.
- Ask junior medical staff to present a case to their peers. Let them determine the format they want to use and resources they require. Junior medical staff are not a homogeneous

group. They differ in how they learn, what they need to learn and why they want to learn. By involving learners in the planning, implementation and evaluation of their learning experiences, both relevance and motivation to learn will be facilitated.

What makes a good ED teacher?

The challenges facing the emergency physician educator, including environmental constraints, patient characteristics, administrative and production imperatives and resource availability, cannot be overstated. However, despite this, there is a consistent commitment to education by emergency physicians. What then makes a good ED teacher? Bandiera and colleagues used a qualitative research design to investigate experienced ED teachers and establish the behaviours that made them good teachers [2].

Twelve strategies were identified:

❶ Tailor teaching to the learner – taking time to get to know the learner was seen to increase the efficacy of the teaching and learning interaction.

❷ Optimize the teacher–learner interaction – this refers to making the teaching more directed and efficient by listening to the learner and using what you know about them.

❸ Tailor teaching to the situation – this relies on being adaptable to the situation and changing strategies accordingly, for example by adjusting teaching amounts, types and timing to the time of day, workload and case mix.

❹ Actively involve the learner – involve the junior doctor in problem solving, give them responsibility and some autonomy appropriate to their skill level.

❺ Actively seek opportunities to teach – sometimes it is necessary to seek out learners. The junior doctor may be busy with an administrative task when an interesting teaching case arrives. The teacher needs to recognize the potential for learning and bring this to the junior doctor's attention.

❻ Agree on expectations – this can be done at the orientation, when learning objectives and ground rules for interactions are established.

❼ Demonstrate a good teacher attitude – this is about being an approachable supervisor/teacher. The teacher's affect influences

the learner's willingness to engage in the learning activity, e.g. the teacher's positive approach to the learner, enthusiasm for teaching and openness to questioning [18].

❽ Make additional teaching resources – this may involve collecting sample cardiographs, X-rays or blood gases for a resource file. It may be writing up some interesting case-generated problems for future review or development of evidence-based clinical guidelines.

❾ Use teaching methods beyond patient care. With the advent of interest in clinical skills training and simulation there are opportunities to take the teaching away from the bedside on occasion. Use of standardized patients and role-plays may also be appropriate.

❿ Be a role model. This is about demonstrating and practising the principles that you are trying to teach. Don't underestimate the importance of role modelling appropriate professional behaviours. Junior doctor learning needs encompass aspects of professionalism that can be actively learnt through positive role models.

⓫ Provide and encourage feedback – adult learners require feedback for motivation and for learning.

⓬ Improve the environment – the competing demands within an ED environment make this difficult, but the effective teacher identifies ways in which to enhance the learning environment, e.g. by creating space and time in a crowded ED, and providing feedback away from others.

These findings are supported further in the literature with what learners want. Additional suggestions include:

- using teachable moments well
- taking the time to teach
- challenging the learner
- treating the junior doctor as a colleague [19].

The factors reported by ED teachers and ED learners reflect what is required according to adult learning theory and reinforce the applicability within the ED environment.

Types of teaching in the ED

There are a number of teaching and learning strategies available for use within the ED environment. These can include spot electronic searches on active clinical problems, formal quarantined tutorials, case discussions, demonstrations of procedures or techniques, audit meetings, self-directed learning opportunities, such as reading medical literature, online learning programmes and so on. This section deals with three strategies: 'trolley-side' teaching, teaching procedural skills which most ED physicians are familiar with and perform regularly, and simulation, which is developing an emergent role within teaching and learning in the ED.

'Trolley-side' teaching

Interactions with patients at the bedside are a crucial component for learning in medicine, the traditional apprenticeship model relying on this methodology. Bedside teaching can provide an opportunity for the experienced clinician to explain clinical reasoning and role model appropriate communication, including listening, patient questioning and respect, supervising the more junior clinicians as they practise these skills, assessing the junior clinicians' interaction with the patient and providing feedback to them [20]. However, with the numerous environmental constraints within the ED there is a need to look at bedside teaching and determine how best to conduct this activity. In addition, the care of the patient remains paramount and ensuring that this is maintained and that the junior doctor–patient relationship is not undermined is an additional challenge.

The benefits of orientation have previously been mentioned in terms of adult learning principles and learner-centred instruction. However, they are crucial to establishing the expectations from both the learner and the teacher's perspectives in regards to bedside teaching. Establishing up front how bedside teaching will be conducted, while remaining patient-centred, will enable the learner's needs to be met. Briefing the patients beforehand and getting them involved in the teaching process enhances patient comfort and participation and may provide enjoyment. Expectations of patient-based teaching may include:

❶ Number of bedside teaching opportunities per shift. The supervisor may want to ensure one bedside teaching interaction per shift, identified by either the supervisor or the learner. Alternatively, the supervisor may prefer to be less prescriptive and more opportunistic, identifying bedside opportunities as they arrive, accepting that some shifts may have none and others numerous.

❷ Type of bedside teaching. This involves discussing the types of teaching and learning the supervisor is prepared to undertake, e.g. a procedural skill or history taking or interaction with relatives.

❸ What will happen by the trolley-side? It is important to discuss what will and won't happen by the trolley-side. For example, the history and physical examination will be done at the bedside, but discussion of clinical reasoning may occur away from the patient. This is important to consider, especially if the junior doctor is to have an ongoing professional relationship with the patient. Feedback as to the resident's performance should also be conducted away from the patient. The supervisor should establish whether or not the resident will be asked questions at the bedside so that this is understood prior to the interaction at the bedside.

❹ Outline specific teaching approaches. There are a number of models of bedside teaching that can be used. Lake and Ryan [21] describe the use of set, dialogue and closure. This technique involves an introduction, outlining the objectives of the session (set), a discussion in which questioning techniques are used to elicit information from the learner and to discuss reasoning/rationales (dialogue) and a summation in which the main learning points are discussed and further learning required (closure). An alternative to this is the SNAPPS model described by Wolpaw et al. [22] in which the learner:

- summarizes the case history and their findings
- narrows the differential diagnosis usually to two or three possibilities
- analyses the different diagnoses by comparing and contrasting them
- probes the supervisor/teacher for opinions or any information on which they require clarification
- plans the patient's management
- selects an issue for self-directed learning later on.

This model was piloted and tested within the outpatient setting. However, it has relevance and application for a number of clinical settings. It would require the experienced clinician to explain and possibly model the process in the first instance.

Procedural skill teaching

Management of patients in the ED often involves the practitioner performing procedural skills. Some of these are to assist in formulating diagnoses in the undifferentiated patient, e.g. performance of bedside ultrasound, others are for treatment of patient conditions, e.g. application of a plaster to a fracture. Ideally, in this day and age, procedural skills should be practised in a clinical skills setting prior to implementation on a 'real' patient [23]. However, observation by a junior doctor of an experienced clinician performing a task is also valuable and can sometimes be overlooked in the busy ED department. Sometimes it is done before you realize you could have shown a junior doctor.

The educational theories relevant to teaching clinical skills are drawn from psychomotor theories. There are seven basic principles of the psychomotor domain [24], including:

❶ conceptualization – where the learner needs to understand the background knowledge element of the skill, that is, the cognitive components – this involves a knowledge of why the skill should be done, when to do it, precautions and contraindications, etc.

❷ visualization – where the learner needs to see the skill demonstrated to get a clear picture of what the skill looks like in real time and as a whole 'in toto'

❸ verbalization – where the learner needs to hear the steps of the skill verbalized

❹ practice – where the learner gets the chance to practise the skill

❺ correction and reinforcement – where feedback is given to reinforce performance

❻ skill mastery – where the learner can perform the skill independently in the learning environment

❼ skill autonomy – where the learner can perform the skill independently in a variety of real life situations.

Similarly, Cagne [25] describes three phases in instructional design relevant to teaching a technical skill, including a cognitive phase where the learner is developing cues from the facilitator, an associative phase where the learner is integrating the component parts and an autonomous phase where the skill has become automatic for the learner.

The issue of the relationship of the learner to the experienced clinician is further investigated within the cognitive apprenticeship model [26,27]. The emphasis in this model is on the requirement that the thinking of the expert be made visible and brought to the surface for the learner. Underpinning this model is the ability of the teacher to assess/recognize the skill level of the learner.

Another debate in the literature is around the issue of whole skill training versus part skill training. Evidence would suggest that the part skill training method be used for the more complex skills while whole skill training be used for the relatively straightforward skills. This requires the facilitator to analyse the skills to be taught and determine the level of complexity of that specific skill. Additionally, what is the whole skill? It can be argued that procedural skills do not occur in isolation. Rather, communication skills are required along with the technical expertise and should be taught together rather than in isolation to reflect the requirement in reality [28,29].

So what do these theories mean for the ED physician wanting to assist a learner in developing a procedural skill? The important requirements are:

- background knowledge is required – why, what, how?
- demonstration by, or observation of an experienced clinician is an important component of learning a psychomotor skill
- verbalization of steps – this requires breaking the skill down into steps
- feedback on performance by the expert
- opportunities for repeated practice under supervision, to allow for feedback and self-reflection
- teaching the skill in context not in isolation.

A dedicated skills area within the ED is most beneficial, as this can be used in quarantined or quieter times for supervised or independent practice (once the learner is deemed relatively competent in the skill, to avoid practising incorrect technique). Highlighting the need for practice and observation to all the experienced clinicians assists in identifying these opportunities for the learner within the ED environment.

Simulation

Simulation is an emergent teaching methodology within the ED environment. In its broadest sense, it refers to any situation in which the real situation is emulated. It may involve actors playing the role of patients, who are often described as standardized patients, or

manikins with computer-generated physiological responses [30,31].

The underpinning educational theory behind simulation comes from a number of theories, including adult learning. However, experiential learning theory is probably of most relevance. Kolb [32] describes experiential learning activities as opportunities for learners to acquire and apply knowledge, skills and attitudes in an immediate and relevant setting. A four-point continuous learning cycle is described:

❶ concrete experience
❷ observation and reflection
❸ forming abstract concepts
❹ testing in new situations.

Simulation in healthcare education is clearly an example of experiential learning. It provides the learners with a relevant and realistic patient problem to manage. Following this experience, the learners are able to observe their performance and reflect, while exploring with a facilitator hypotheses and new concepts. They can then test this experience by repeat simulations.

There are a number of ways in which ED physicians can incorporate simulation opportunities into their teaching in ED. It may be that paper-based simulations are used to explore clinical reasoning. This involves developing case scenarios and structured questions. Role-playing, using peers or expert clinicians, can be used to practise difficult communication skills, such as breaking bad news. Simple part-task trainers can be incorporated into a more complex scenario involving the practice of the skill while interacting with a patient. Kneebone and colleagues [29] describe integrating a urinary catheter manikin with an actor to ensure that the technical and communication skills are taught concurrently.

Where higher level manikins are available, whole patient scenarios can be conducted. Teams of junior medical staff can practise rarer critical situations and explore not only technical skills but non-technical skills, such as teamwork. Use of audio-visual aids to capture performance is important for providing feedback after such activities. It also allows an opportunity for reflection and peer feedback.

Not all EDs have the luxury of the highly technical simulation 'gadgetry', but this should not put them off using simulation as a teaching methodology. Determining the content areas appropriate for using simulation and how this fits into the overall curriculum will be important to ensure that resources are used rationally [33].

Feedback to learners

Feedback is a crucial requirement for learning and the importance of positive feedback for learning has been well established [34]. Feedback should provide the learner with information that offers 'insight into what he or she did as well as the consequences of his or her actions' [35]. It should allow the learner to know what went well and what could be improved or changed next time. Feedback is part of the formative assessment process that occurs throughout the learning period, rather than as a summative assessment that is to determine a grade or make a final judgment.

Effective feedback has a number of characteristics [36,37]. It should be given in a suitable environment to allow privacy and maintain confidentiality for the learner. There should be adequate time to allow the learner and the facilitator to explore the observed behaviour or skill. There should be clear goals established at the beginning of the learning so that feedback can be related to these goals. The feedback should come from direct observation of the learner's performance where possible.

Providing learners with feedback is a specific skill in itself and requires practice to develop. A structured approach to giving feedback will assist the teacher/facilitator to provide effective and useful feedback. There are many models of feedback in the literature; however, one such model from Pendleton's [38] work is suggested here to assist the ED physician:

- Ask the learner how he or she felt.
- Ask the learner what went well and why.
- Ask the facilitator/teacher to say what went well and why.
- Ask the learner what could have been done better and why.
- Ask the facilitator/teacher to say what could have been done better and why.
- Ask the facilitator/teacher to summarize the strengths and up to three things to concentrate on.

Feedback, when delivered effectively, is a strong motivator to the adult learner and encourages ongoing performance review and reflection by the learner.

Conclusion

Juggling the demands of a being a busy emergency physician requires balancing clinical, administrative and teaching duties. Time is often limited and yet the rewards of being involved in teaching are obvious. Apart from personal satisfaction gained from interacting with junior colleagues, the ability to keep up to date and the opportunity to reflect on one's own performance are enhanced. Reviewing performance as a teacher and practising education techniques to improve the effectiveness of the facilitation motivate the teacher to continue to teach and improve the satisfaction from teaching. Structuring learning experiences, considering learner needs and providing effective feedback are essential for learners in the ED environment.

Likely developments over the next 5–10 years

- Increasing numbers of medical students and junior medical staff seeking learning in the ED may lead to the need for specific emergency physician educators to orientate and supervise them in the ED.
- Expansion of scenario-based simulation and skills centres may lead to more opportunities for ED team-based interdisciplinary education.
- Increasing patient participation in decision making will necessitate more detailed consent when procedures are performed by the inexperienced.

Controversies

- Teaching procedural skills should no longer be 'see one, do one, teach one' on surprised patients, although some find it difficult to break out of this mold.

- What is the best way to teach clinical skills and ensure a patient centred approach?
- Should patients be informed of the level of experience of those providing care or performing a procedure?

References

[1] Lake FR. Teaching on the run tips: doctors as teachers. Med J Aust 2004;180:415–6.
[2] Bandiera G, Lee S, Tiberius R. Creating effective learning in today's emergency departments: how accomplished teachers get it done. Ann Emerg Med 2005;45:253–61.
[3] Santen S, Hemphill R, McDonald F, et al. Patients' willingness to allow residents to learn to practice medical procedures. Acad Med 2004;79:144–7.
[4] Simons R, Imboden E, Mattel J. Patient attitudes toward medical student participation in a general internal medicine clinic. J Gen Intern Med 1995;10:251–4.
[5] Simon S, Peters A, Christiansen C. Effect of medical student teaching on patient satisfaction in a managed care setting. J Gen Intern Med 2000;15:457–61.
[6] Berger TJ, Ander DS, Terrell ML, et al. The impact of the demand for clinical productivity on student teaching in academic emergency departments. Acad Emerg Med 2004;11:1364–7.
[7] Denninghoff KR, Moye PK. Teaching students during an emergency walk-in clinic rotation does not delay care. Acad Med 1998;73:1311.
[8] Atzema C, Bandiera G, Schull MJ. Emergency department crowding: the effect on resident education. Ann Emerg Med 2005;45:276–81.
[9] Dent AW, Crotty B, Cuddihy H, et al. Learning opportunities for Australian prevocational hospital doctors: exposure, perceived quality and desired methods of learning. Med J Aust 2006;184:436–40.
[10] Knowles M. The adult learner: a neglected species. Houston: Gulf Publishing; 1973.
[11] Cantillon P, Hutchinson L, Wood D. ABC of learning and teaching in medicine. London: British Medical Journal Publishing; 2003.
[12] Knowles M. The modern practice of adult education: from pedagogy to andragogy, 2nd edn. New York: Cambridge Books; 1980.
[13] Kaufman D, Mann K. Teaching and learning in medical education: how theory can inform practice. Edinburgh: Association for the Study of Medical Education; 2007.
[14] Peyton J. Teaching and learning in medical practice. Great Britain: Manticore Europe; 1998.
[15] Brookfield S. Understanding and facilitating adult learning. Buckingham: Open University Press; 1986.
[16] Gunderman R, Williamson K, Frank M, et al. Learner centered education. Radiology 2003;227:15–17.
[17] Weimer M. Learner centred teaching. New York: Jossey-Bass; 2002.
[18] Reeve JM, Jang H. What teachers say and do to support students' autonomy during a learning activity. J. Educ Psychol 2006;98:209
[19] Thurger L, Bandiera G, Lee S. What do emergency medicine learners want from their teachers? A multicentre focus group analysis. Acad Emerg Med 2005;12:856–61.
[20] Celenza A, Rogers I. Qualitative evaluation of a formal bedside clinical teaching programme in an emergency department. Emerg Med J 2007;23:769–73.
[21] Lake F, Ryan G. Teaching on the run tips 4: teaching with patients. Med J Aust 2004;181:158–9.
[22] Wolpaw T, Wolpaw D, Papp K. SNAPPS: a learner centred model for outpatient education. Acad Med 2003;78:893–8.
[23] De Young S. Teaching psychomotor skills Teaching strategies for nurse educators. United Kingdom: Prentice Hall Health; 2003. 201–215.
[24] George J, Doto F. A simple five-step method for teaching clinical skills. Fam Med 2001;33:577–8.
[25] Gagne R. The conditions of learning, 4th edn. New York: Holt, Rinehart & Winston; 1985.
[26] Collins A, Brown J, Newman S. Cognitive apprenticeship: teaching the crafts of reading, writing and mathematics. In: Resnick L, editor. Learning and instruction: essays in honor of Robert Glaser. New Jersey: Lawrence Erlbaum, 1989, p. 453–94.
[27] Woolley N, Jarvis Y. Situated cognition and cognitive apprenticeship: a model for teaching and learning clinical skills in a technologically rich and authentic learning environment. Nurse Educ Today 2007;27:73–9.
[28] Kneebone R, Kidd J, Nestel D, et al. An innovative model for teaching and learning clinical procedures. Med Educ 2002;36:628–34.
[29] Kneebone R, Nestel D, Yadollahi F, et al. Assessing procedural skills in context: exploring the feasibility of an integrated procedural performance instrument (IPPI). Med Educ 2006;40:1105–14.
[30] Ker J, Bradley P. Simulation in medical education. Edinburgh: Association for the Study of Medical Education; 2007.
[31] Good M. Patient simulation for training basic and advanced clinical skills. Med Educ 2003;37(suppl):14–21.
[32] Kolb D. Experiential learning. Englewood Cliffs: Prentice Hall; 1984.
[33] Binstadt E, Walls R, White B, et al. A comprehensive medical simulation education curriculum for emergency residents. Ann Emerg Med 2007;49:495–504.
[34] Kilminster S, Jolly B, van der Vleuten C. A framework for effective training for supervisors. Med Teach 2002;24:385–9.
[35] Ende J. Feedback in clinical medical education. Am Med Assoc 1983;250:777–81.
[36] Schwenk T, Whitman N. The physician as teacher. Baltimore: Williams & Wilkins; 1987.
[37] Vickery A, Lake F. Teaching on the run tips 10: giving feedback. Med J Aust 2005;183:267–8.
[38] Pendleton D, Schofield T, Tate P, et al. The consultation: an approach to teaching and learning. Oxford: Oxford University Press; 1984.

24.4 Undergraduate teaching in emergency medicine

Geoffrey A Couser

ESSENTIALS

1 Medical student teaching needs to be considered one of the core businesses of an emergency department.

2 The specialty of emergency medicine has a unique body of knowledge that can contribute much to the entire undergraduate curriculum and it is essential that emergency physicians 'own' this knowledge.

3 To be effective educators, academic emergency physicians need to adopt a strategic and comprehensive approach to curriculum development, delivery and assessment throughout all years of the medical course.

4 It is essential that goals and objectives of student education in emergency medicine be clearly defined and articulated to all staff so that a consistent and integrated curriculum is delivered.

5 The specialty is playing a critically important role in medical student education as numbers of students rapidly increase and models of healthcare continue to change.

6 Emergency physicians are ideally placed to be able to introduce new and emerging topics in healthcare and to embrace innovative teaching methods, such as simulation and mobile learning.

Table 24.4.1 Essential roles and key competencies of specialist physicians – the CanMEDS criteria [1]
Medical expert
Communicator
Collaborator
Manager
Health advocate
Scholar
Professional

Copyright © 1996 The Royal College of Physicians and Surgeons of Canada. http://www.royalcollege.ca/portal/page/portal/rc/canmeds. CanMEDS 2000 Project skills for the new millennium: Report of the societal needs working group. Reproduced with permission.

Introduction

Emergency medicine now plays a central role in medical curricula in undergraduate and postgraduate medical schools in Australia and New Zealand. This is not unexpected, as the principles and practice of the specialty have much in common with the desired features of contemporary medical education: it is problem focused, interdisciplinary and integrates many aspects of community-based and hospital-based clinical practice. Clinical practice easily integrates and builds upon the biomedical sciences traditionally taught early in the medical course. Much growth in academic emergency medicine has occurred in the last two decades, with the establishment of academic departments and dedicated university positions. However, the majority of medical student teaching is performed by emergency physicians in clinical practice in public and an increasing number of private emergency departments (EDs). This chapter will address the issues surrounding medical student teaching at the departmental and the broader faculty level.

Overview of undergraduate medical education in Australia

It is important for emergency physicians interested in teaching medical students to be aware of recent trends and developments in medical education in Australasia. The CanMEDS 2000 Project and the World Health Organization, among others, have listed the key outcomes expected of a doctor [1]. These outcomes have been adopted by many schools worldwide as a basis for reform and reorganization and are listed in Table 24.4.1. Of interest, these principles have been embraced at the early postgraduate level through the Australian Curriculum Framework for Junior Doctors [2] and at a specialty college level, such as the Australasian College for Emergency Medicine's Curriculum Revision Project [3]. Some schools have adopted problem-based learning as a tool to achieve these educational outcomes, with others using case-based and outcomes-based learning to place content in a clinical context. In 2010, the US-based Carnegie

Foundation (which published the landmark Flexner Report in 1910) published a comprehensive review of current physician education and the need for reform which should be essential reading for any prospective medical educator [4].

Curriculum reform has occurred in parallel with significant changes in the health system, with a growth in information technology, changing patient expectations and a massive increase in medical knowledge. Models of healthcare delivery are changing, with increased pressures on public hospitals, such as access block, the unsustainable increase in health spending in relation to all other public spending, declining numbers of inpatient beds and the increasing complexity of medical conditions. The shift to the home and community management of many conditions has altered the patient mix available for student teaching. University salaries have not kept pace with the growth in public and private medical salaries, which has contributed to a decline in numbers of academic faculty and core medical school functions often shifting to sometimes reluctant specialists within the public hospital system. Despite this, there has been an increasing number of medical students and medical schools, with 3770 medical students commencing study in Australia in 2011 [5].

Table 24.4.2 Benefits of medical student teaching in emergency departments

Benefits to students
- Usually an enjoyable term with unparalleled pathology and clinical experience
- Integrates theoretical knowledge with the workplace
- Learns acute care resuscitation skills
- The opportunity to see patients before anyone else in the system
- Emergency medicine is the embodiment of an equitable and accessible healthcare system

Benefits to the emergency department and hospital
- Students gain a positive view of the specialty and this may influence subsequent career choice
- May improve subsequent intern performance
- Improves the overall professionalism and reputation of the department
- Teaching is a core business of a hospital and should be embraced
- May assist with recruitment and retention of staff with an interest in teaching
- Students can assist with procedures and may improve patient flow in some circumstances

Benefits to the medical school
- Allows access to a large number of patients with a broad range of clinical conditions otherwise not available for teaching
- Allows access to a large pool of medical and nursing staff otherwise not available for teaching
- Emergency medicine can teach knowledge and skills not readily taught by other disciplines, such as resuscitation, health systems and time management

Table 24.4.3 Minimum requirements for developing student placements in emergency departments

- Nominate one person to be the term coordinator and liaison with the university
- Understand the rules and regulations which govern student placements in your hospital and at the affiliated university
- Develop a clear orientation package for students and make it clear that students will not be allowed into the department until they have received orientation
- Develop a clear curriculum statement providing a broad overview of goals and objectives for the term (see Table 24.4.4)
- Define specific learning objectives for students, e.g. 'At the end of this placement you will be able to describe the assessment of the patient presenting with chest pain'
- Consider how students will be assessed and clearly describe this prior to the commencement of the term
- Consider who will supervise the students, for this reason it is essential to engage with all levels of staff within the department and to provide them with support, training and guidance

It is in this changing environment that emergency medicine has established itself as a key part of modern medical curricula and the specialty is poised to play an even greater role in the training of future doctors. Both the need and the opportunity exist for such expansion.

The importance of medical student teaching

Many clinicians feel that the provision of clinical care is the core business of an emergency department (ED) and hence may not be initially willing to allocate resources for teaching students. Similarly, university medical schools may not be aware of the growth of emergency medicine as a specialty and hence may not be aware of what it can offer students or, indeed, may not even be aware that it is an independent specialty with its own body of knowledge. However, once established, a strong academic presence can contribute to departmental morale, quality of care, performance and the standing of the department within the hospital and community. Table 24.4.2 lists the benefits of emergency medicine teaching to students, EDs and medical schools. These points may be used to argue for an increased presence and accompanying resources within a curriculum [6]. Resources and a formal place in the curriculum often come only after years of hard work in establishing the bona fides of emergency medicine. This may require much time and effort from a dedicated individual.

Curriculum development

Undergraduate emergency medicine in the past was *ad hoc*, unstructured and highly selective, in that clinical exposure was based around what the students themselves thought was interesting and useful in the department at the time. With the growth of the specialty as an academic discipline, departments have been able to take a more active role in education, control student entry to the department, ensure appropriate orientation and attempt to take advantage of the rich and broad clinical experience on offer. As faculties have become aware of the learning opportunities on offer in EDs, as well as the teaching abilities of staff, emergency physicians have been able to negotiate a greater role in university affairs and integrate emergency medicine into the broader undergraduate curriculum. With this comes a responsibility for emergency physicians to understand the function of universities and the requirements which come with running an academic term. Table 24.4.3 provides suggestions for developing a university teaching presence.

It is essential that once a department has decided that medical student teaching should be a part of its function then a curriculum must be considered. The Australasian College for Emergency Medicine, the American College of Emergency Physicians and the International Federation of Emergency Medicine have produced documents with varying degrees of detail concerning this [7–9] and a growing number of papers are being published providing guidance to curriculum developers [10,11]. Most core curriculum statements contain elements which reflect the clinical practice of emergency medicine and an example of such a list is provided in Table 24.4.4. This provides a framework around which specific topics can then be taught. The teaching programme will need to be modified and adapted accordingly depending upon the expertise of and time available to specialists within the department, as well as the local epidemiology and patient demographics.

An often overlooked but essential component to consider is that of the 'hidden curriculum'. This is less well understood, but relates to what students learn by being exposed to the practice of medicine. It can cover aspects such as professionalism, ethics and physician behaviour. As the vanguard of a fair, accessible and equitable health system, emergency medicine can teach important attitudes to the next generation of doctors.

Methods of teaching emergency medicine

Once teaching content is decided upon, then it is worth spending time considering which format is the best way to deliver the material. Until recently, undergraduate emergency

Table 24.4.4   Suggested core curriculum topics in emergency medicine

Assessment and management of the undifferentiated patient
Key practical skills: basic life support skills and basic procedural skills
Recognition and management of the seriously ill and injured patient
The assessment and management of common clinical problems in emergency medicine
Assessment and management of the unwell child
Acute pain management
Acute mental health
Toxinology and toxicology
Health systems management
Critical thinking and clinical decision making
Safety and quality in healthcare: medical error and handover
Professional issues: teamwork, communication, time management
Care of the elderly and end-of-life issues

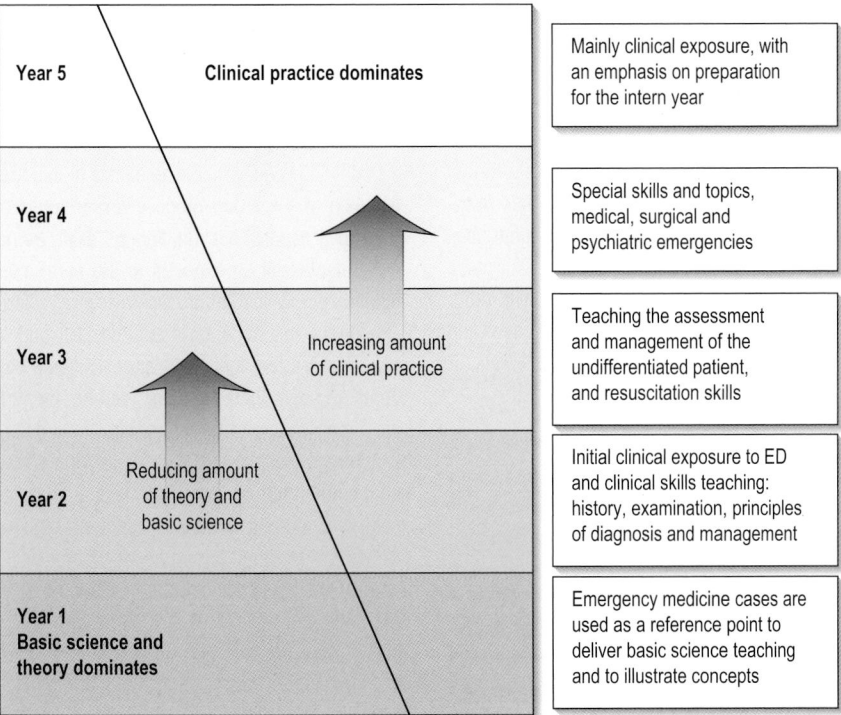

Fig. 24.4.1 A suggested overview of the progression of emergency medicine in an integrated 5-year curriculum.

medicine has largely been taught in the workplace and no other teaching options have existed. However, with the growth of the specialty and the increased need for teachers, the specialty has been able to attract resources and play a greater role in all years of the medical course in some universities. Therefore, depending upon available time and resources, different formats of teaching should be considered for different situations. For example, resuscitation skills are best taught using team-based simulation and practice to reflect the reality of the workplace, once basic concepts have been covered by lectures or online modules.

In all formats, teachers should consider the basic principles of adult learning and teach accordingly. When delivering material, teachers should remember that adults learn best when the topic is meaningful, linked to experience and pitched at the correct level and the students are motivated, have clear goals, are actively involved, receive regular feedback and have time for reflection [12]. Utilizing a range of methods means that material can be delivered in a meaningful way and optimal learning conditions can be achieved. It is essential that the physician taking responsibility for undergraduate teaching within a department takes a leadership role and provides ongoing training and support for both junior and senior colleagues in effective teaching methods.

Whichever teaching method is chosen, evaluation of the process by the participants is an essential part of the quality improvement cycle. Evaluation helps ensure teaching is meeting students' learning needs, identifies areas where teaching can be improved and provides feedback and encouragement for teachers [13]. Documenting evaluations can form part of a teaching portfolio, which can be used in academic job applications as tangible evidence of a clinician's and a department's commitment to and proficiency in teaching. Importantly, from a student's perspective, being asked to evaluate a teaching session and then seeing the comments acted upon provides a strong sense that their participation is valued and, as a result, may improve the learning process overall.

Some basic pedagogical theory should be considered when choosing and applying methods of teaching: many educators refer to Miller's triangle of clinical competence [14] and the concept of a spiral curriculum [15] when designing curricula. Figure 24.4.1 is a schematic representation of how emergency medicine as a subject could ideally progress through a 5-year course utilizing these theories of curriculum design. Most departments will only be in a position to offer clinical exposure in the final years of the course, but much progress has been made across the region in penetrating all years. The following delivery methods could be used in this framework to deliver a comprehensive and effective emergency medicine curriculum.

Lecture based

Lectures can be delivered at any stage of the medical course but, to maximize their effectiveness, they need to be developed in an integrated fashion and linked to other components of the course. Emergency medicine can be used effectively as a vehicle to illustrate biomedical science concepts to junior medical students [16]. Case-based learning is a popular method to use in this setting, as learning objectives and concepts can be illustrated in a 'real-world' setting. For example, rather than delivering a lecture on ischaemic heart disease, an emergency medicine lecture would be entitled 'I've got pain in my chest' and the lecturer would engage with students to create a genuine feel for this common emergency presentation. The content would need to be modified depending upon the seniority of students, for example, junior medical students would use the case as a reference point to illustrate anatomy and physiology, while more senior students may use the same scenario to learn about clinical decision making and evidence-based medicine.

Lectures need not be didactic and overloaded with content – a good lecture should be an efficient and entertaining means of effectively transmitting information to large groups. In general, lectures should add value. There is little point simply repeating content from a text, as students can gather the information themselves either in their own time or by using information technology during a boring lecture. In this sense, prospective lecturers should remind themselves of the qualities of an effective educator: expertise in the subject area, enthusiasm for the topic and the task, and capacity to engage the learners [17]. By utilizing these qualities, educators can turn a lecture into a valuable learning experience. Lecturers should have notes pre-prepared and available for students and be prepared for the fact that most will have mobile devices open while the lecture is taking place, will be busy annotating and linking to other resources and may not appear to be giving the lecturer their undivided attention. These are the principles of blended learning, and they will be a key part of education in the twenty-first century. Recording lectures on the university's learning management system allows for later review and discussion.

Tutorials and small-group learning

Tutorials are small group sessions, with opportunities for interaction and reflection. This model of teaching is well suited to emergency medicine, as individual cases and experiences can be presented and discussed in a comfortable and safe environment. The learners can lead the discussion and take the topics into new and previously unconsidered areas. Nevertheless, providing a structure to the tutorial will help ensure that the time is spent

Table 24.4.5 Planning a teaching episode		
Concept	Components	Example in practice
Set	Roles – trainers, learners, patients Objectives – what are they going to learn? Linkages – to other learning events Environment – seating, lighting, distractions	Gather the students in a quieter part of the department where distractions will be minimal and make it clear what the session is about: 'I'd like to talk about ways we assess headaches in the emergency department'
Dialogue	Questions — use often Understanding Eyes – two-way contact Stimulation – make it interesting Timing – finish on time	Check what the students know about the topic and ask an open question to start, e.g. 'What are the worrying signs of a headache?' Encourage discussion, use first names in the discussion
Closure	Review – ask for questions, check understanding Eyes – contact with learner Summary Termination	Summarize the discussion, check that the students have understood it, terminate with a comment (e.g. 'Thunderclap headaches are a feature of subarachnoid haemorrhage and later we'll talk about the role of a lumbar puncture')

You have just assessed a young male with a severe headache. You realize that this is an ideal teaching opportunity for the medical students present.

wisely and learning opportunities are maximized. These are usually easily implemented in a department, as they can be integrated with other departmental activities and can run independently of any broader curriculum. This is often the only way that the specialty can deliver its core curriculum in a school without a formal emergency medicine presence. Another pragmatic way to utilize the emergency patient population and promote the department as a place of learning is to work in partnership with other disciplines who can access the department and utilize the patients and the physical space for teaching.

Web-based

This is growing in popularity as schools rely more on information technology to deliver content and this is occurring at the same time that emergency physicans worldwide are taking a leading role in developing resources and promoting the role of social media and other online resources for teaching and clinical care. At a basic level, bulletin boards, web logs (blogs) and e-mail are useful ways to maintain regular communication with students and to distribute journal articles and policies and orientation manuals can be posted online [18].

However, with faster Internet connections and a new generation of students increasingly utilizing mobile learning devices, such as smartphones and tablets, new opportunities are emerging with applications, podcasts, social media and e-books playing increasingly prominent roles in education at all levels. Specific details are provided in the next chapter.

Work-based

This is the original method of medical student education: at the bedside of the patient. Medicine has been taught this way for thousands of years and reinforces the point that medical students are essentially apprentices in a trade. Emergency medicine excels in this area because of the broad range of experiences on offer in a department. Challenges exist, as not all students will be exposed to the same conditions during a rotation. Achieving a uniform experience for students is difficult [19] and so workbooks have been developed to guide students through their rotation, alerting them to the broad range of undifferentiated conditions which regularly present. Utilizing junior staff can be helpful in the education of medical students: pairing a student with a resident or registrar allows the students to see how a doctor works and it involves junior doctors in teaching at an early stage of their careers. It helps with rostering, in that students can be allocated to medical staff with a pre-existing timetable. Medical schools offer clinical academic titles to doctors involved in teaching and all staff should be encouraged to apply for such titles.

Teaching by the bedside is an important activity and opportunities abound for clinical teaching. Clinicians being aware of a broader curriculum can be of assistance, as it can be difficult to think on the spot when confronted with a 'teachable moment'. Some guidelines exist to maximize the value of bedside teaching and the well-developed principles of 'set, dialogue and closure' [20] are explained and listed with an example in Table 24.4.5.

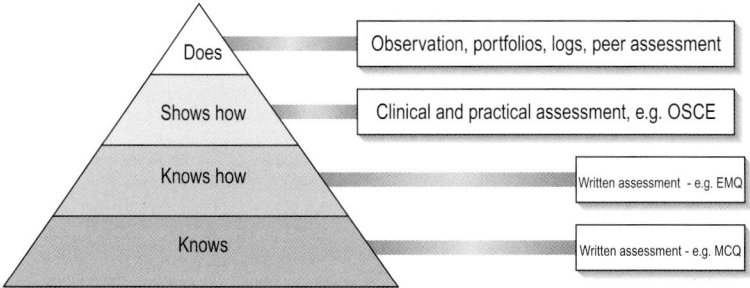

Fig. 24.4.2 The learning assessment pyramid. OSCE: objective structured clinical examination. (Lake F, Hamdorf J. Teaching on the run tips 5: teaching a skill. Medical Journal Association 2004;181(6):327-8 with permission.) [21]

Simulation

Simulation is a growing field which has been embraced by emergency physicians and the Australasian College for Emergency Medicine. A large knowledge base has been developed and, as such, it will not be discussed at length here. However, the main barrier to utilizing simulation for undergraduate teaching is cost and the available time of emergency physicians. Fortunately, universities are starting to recognize the value of this method of teaching and opportunities are being created, with simulation utilizing people factors and the principles of interprofessional learning being integrated into curricula at all levels.

Clinical skills teaching

Emergency medicine has long had a reputation among students for 'being the place where you get to do useful things'. While proponents of the specialty as an academic discipline are keen to promote the other features of emergency medicine in an educational setting, this statement is still undoubtedly true. Many skills can be taught in the ED or a skills laboratory and emergency physicians are ideally placed to teach them. Whether it is junior medical students examining patients for the first time or learning practical skills, such as venesection and suturing, emergency physicians have a lot to offer in this regard. Like most teaching, there are useful techniques that can be employed to improve learning [21].

Assessment principles

Assessment should be considered as a tool which drives learning and should be developed in parallel with the curriculum rather than considered at the end. It is essential that the appropriate form of assessment be matched to the subject matter. Assessment tools selected should be valid, reliable and practical and have an appropriate impact on student learning [22]. For instance, when assessing competency in advanced cardiac life support, it would be more valid to use a practical-based assessment process, such as an observed objective structured clinical examination (OSCE) rather than a written examination. Figure 24.4.2 provides a graphical representation of matching assessment processes to skills and knowledge. A large number of assessment methods exist and educators should possess at least a basic understanding of their use and application. It is essential to understand that all universities have rules which govern the assessment of students and failure to adhere strictly to these rules exposes a department to academic appeals and complaints of unfairness and bias. Emergency physicians need to become intimately involved in examination processes throughout the course so that the speciality is taken seriously by students and to ensure that appropriate and realistic emergency conditions and scenarios are presented.

Likely developments over the next 5–10 years

Emergency medicine will continue to play a significant role in medical student education and is poised to make greater contributions in coming years. This will occur both by design and necessity: as described, the increase in student numbers is coinciding with the growth and maturation of the specialty in Australia and New Zealand. Emergency medicine will continue to expand throughout medical curricula rather than being the practice-based pre-intern term it currently occupies in the latter years of most medical courses. A recent shift in focus in the tertiary sector towards teaching ability rather than purely a research output will create opportunities for emergency medicine to gain a stronger foothold in universities. Teaching programmes will expand to deliver material, not just unique to emergency medicine, but the specialty will be opportunistic and be called upon to teach where significant gaps exist at an undergraduate level. In many universities, there is no academic presence in surgical subspecialties, such as ear, nose and throat, ophthalmology and orthopaedics. It will be left to emergency physicians to teach students the basics of these specialties, just as we currently manage many common acute conditions in these areas without specialist input.

It is now time for the specialty to move beyond just the provision of training in acute medicine as envisaged by the landmark Macy report in 1994 [23]. The specialty is developing its own body of knowledge and curriculum in important but under-represented areas of medical education, such as clinical decision making, toxicology, medical error and health systems design and management. The management of elderly patients and end-of-life decision making is becoming a significant part of most emergency physicians' practice. Hence, emergency physicians need to take a leading role in the development and delivery of curricula in these areas. There is much to suggest that the increased sub-specialization of medicine has led to fragmentation of the health system, with the subsequent inability of society to achieve coherent and sustainable outcomes in health policy. Emergency medicine as a specialty has the opportunity to take a leading role in training doctors and other health professionals capable of understanding the key challenges facing the health system in the 21st century.

Controversies

- There is much debate about the effectiveness of current methods of medical student training, but emergency medicine as an academic specialty is adaptable and capable of working within any number of curricular styles.
- EDs will struggle to handle increased numbers of students without additional dedicated support from universities and may need to consider withholding access until appropriate sustainable resources can be provided.
- Emergency physicians still have much to do in creating a coordinated

undergraduate curriculum that is vertically integrated with prevocational and specialist training in the specialty.

- It is inevitable that more academic departments of emergency medicine will be created but first the specialty must clearly define its core curriculum and its role in the health education system.
- Changes in the health workforce with a re-definition of the role of the doctor and an evolution of the other health professions will necessitate that the specialty apply its knowledge base to broader health science training, including that of evolving positions such as physician assistants.

References

[1] The Royal College of Physicians and Surgeons of Canada. Can MEDS 2000 Project skills for the new millennium: Report of the societal needs working group. Ontario; 1996.

[2] Confederation of Postgraduate Medical Education Councils Australia: Australian curriculum framework for junior doctors November 2012 <http://curriculum.cpmec.org.au/index.cfm> [Accessed Feb. 2013].

[3] Australasian College for Emergency Medicine curriculum revision project. <http://www.acem.org.au/education.aspx?docId=1197> [Accessed Feb. 2013].

[4] Cooke M, Irby D, O'Brien B. The Carnegie Foundation for the advancement of teaching: educating physicians: a call for reform of medical school and residency. San Francisco: Jossey-Bass; 2010.

[5] Australian Institute of Health and Welfare. Medical workforce 2011. National health workforce series no. 3. Cat. no. HWL 49. Canberra: AIHW; 2013.

[6] Russi CS, Hamilton GC. A case for emergency medicine in the undergraduate medical school curriculum. Acad Emerg Med 2005;12:994–8.

[7] Australasian College for Emergency Medicine. Policy on the emergency medicine component of the undergraduate medical curriculum. <http://www.acem.org.au> [Accessed Feb. 2013].

[8] ACEP Academic Affairs Committee. Guidelines for undergraduate education in emergency medicine. <http://www.acep.org/Clinical-Practice-Management/Guidelines-for-Undergraduate-Education-in-Emergency-Medicine/> [Accessed Feb. 2013].

[9] International Federation for Emergency Medicine. International Federation for Emergency Medicine model curriculum for medical student education in emergency medicine. Int J Emerg Med 2010;3:1–7.

[10] Task Force on National Fourth Year Medical Student Emergency Medicine Curriculum Guide. Report of the task force on national fourth year medical student emergency

medicine curriculum guide. Ann Emerg Med 2006;47:E1–E7.

[11] Pacella CB. Advanced opportunities for student education in emergency medicine. Acad Emerg Med 2004;11:9–12.

[12] Lake F, Ryan G. Teaching on the run tips 2: educational guides for teaching in a clinical setting. Med J Assoc 2004;180:527–8.

[13] Morrison J. ABC of learning and teaching in medicine: evaluation. Br Med J 2003;326:385–7.

[14] Miller GE. The assessment of clinical skills/competence/performance. Acad Med J 1990;65:563–7.

[15] Harden RM, Stamper N. What is a spiral curriculum? Med Teach 1999;21:141–3.

[16] Walls J, Couser GA, Gennat H, et al. Clinical cases in emergency medicine: a physiological approach. Sydney: McGraw-Hill; 2006.

[17] Arnold R. The theory and principles of psychodynamic pedagogy. Forum Educ 1994;49:2.

[18] McKimm J, Jollie C, Cantillon P. ABC of learning and teaching: web based learning. Br Med J 2003;326:870–3.

[19] Coates WC, Gendy MS, Gill AM. Emergency medicine subinternship: can we provide a standard clinical experience? Acad Emerg Med 2003;10:1138–41.

[20] Lake F, Ryan G. Teaching on the run tips 3: planning a teaching episode. Med J Assoc 2004;180:643–4.

[21] Lake F, Hamdorf J. Teaching on the run tips 5: teaching a skill. Med J Assoc 2004;181:327–8.

[22] Shumway JM, Harden RM. AMEE guide no. 25: the assessment of learning outcomes for the competent and reflective physician. Med Teach 2003;25:569–84.

[23] Josiah Macy Jr Foundation. The role of emergency medicine in the future of American medical care. Ann Emerg Med 1995;25:230–3.

24.5 Postgraduate emergency medicine teaching and simulation

Victoria Brazil

ESSENTIALS

1 Emergency medicine training programmes need explicit curricular objectives, effective clinical teaching and contemporary assessment methods.

2 Technology and online collaboration are affecting the way trainees in emergency medicine learn and access information and they have enormous further potential.

3 Simulation offers learning opportunities in procedural skills, teamwork and communication, but requires expert application for good educational outcomes.

Introduction

Emergency departments (EDs) are fertile learning environments for postgraduate doctors. The varied clinical case mix, procedural practice and enthusiastic teaching by emergency physicians have made emergency medicine an important experience for new medical graduates [1]. Many of these same factors attract doctors to vocational training in emergency medicine.

Postgraduate training in this field, like most other specialties, traditionally followed an apprenticeship model. It was assumed that patient care experience and opportunistic bedside teaching from clinical experts provided all the knowledge, skills and attitudes requisite for emergency medicine practice. However, this approach has been changing over the last 15–20 years. Contemporary emergency medicine practice requires new knowledge and skills and encompasses different expectations from patients and healthcare systems. Emergency medicine educators need to recognize these changes in practice and employ contemporary educational approaches in developing the relevant knowledge and skills in trainee emergency physicians.

The governance of emergency medicine training, certification and credentialling varies internationally. In Australasia, training and assessment is by the Australasian College for Emergency Medicine (www.acem.org), in conjunction with hospitals and health services. Formal specialist recognition is granted by the Medical Boards of Australia (MBA) or New Zealand (MBNZ). Some 'non-specialist' training in emergency medicine is provided by the Australian College of Rural and Remote Medicine (ACRRM).

Other governance models of specialist training exist internationally and include oversight by universities (Malaysia), government organizations (UK Deaneries) or cross-specialty professional associations (Royal College of Physicians and Surgeons of Canada).

Curricular trends in emergency medicine

There has been a global trend in postgraduate medical education toward 'outcomes based' curricular models. This has resulted in a shift from curricula defining a knowledge base to be acquired, to 'outcome' concepts of roles and competencies for specialist physicians.

The CanMEDS model, developed in Canada and adopted by the Australasian College for Emergency Medicine (ACEM), requires training be orientated toward preparing emergency physicians (and other specialist trainees) for their roles as medical expert, communicator, collaborator, manager, health advocate, scholar and professional [2].

Integral to this curricular trend has been increased recognition of communication and professional domains of practice. Concepts of teamwork, leadership, patient safety, quality improvement and communication with patients and peers have been specified in recent curricula [3]. New domains of learning, such as medical informatics and evidence-based medicine, have become explicit curricular content.

Teaching methods in emergency medicine

Bedside teaching, or 'teaching on the floor', remains the foundation of most ED trainees' educational experience. It provides the opportunity to reflect upon clinical and professional aspects of emergency medicine practice in an integrated manner. It should be facilitated by a graduated increase in patient care responsibility during training. However, the quality of this experience is dependent on the availability and skill of clinical supervisors and on time constraints in busy EDs. In this environment, clinical teaching can be 'education by random opportunity' and learners may not encounter important conditions or procedures and may not reflect usefully on the experiences they do have.

Didactic elements of specialist training vary in format but most programmes or institutions provide a structured element of training that consists of trainee- and supervisor-delivered presentations, procedural skill sessions, journal clubs and lectures by visitors or outside specialists. Following the trend towards competency-based curricular models, there is a general trend toward these teaching activities

Table 24.5.1	Examples of popular emergency medicine blogs and podcasts		
Life in the Fast Lane	www.lifeinthefastlane.com	Emergency medicine	Australia
Academic Life in Emergency Medicine	www.academiclifeinem. blogspot.com	Emergency, research, education	USA
EMcrit	www.emcrit.org	Emergency, critical care, podcast	USA
EDExam	www.edexam.com.au	Emergency, clinical	Australia
St Emlyns	www.stemlynsblog.org/blog/	Emergency, research	UK
ResusME	Resus.me/	Emergency critical care, podcast	
The Poison Review	www.thepoisonreview.com	Toxicology	USA
Ultrasound Podcast	www.ultrasoundpodcast.com	Emergency ultrasound	
iTeachEM	www.iteachem.net	Emergency, education	USA, Australia

More detailed listing available at EMCC Blogs, www.lifeinthelastlane.com [7].

becoming more standardized and structured and supported by online content.

Reflective practice is an important learning skill for postgraduate trainees. Clinical audit and portfolios [4] can facilitate this and most training programmes also encourage participation in critical incident review, trauma review meetings and morbidity and mortality rounds.

There is a trend toward interprofessional and team-based learning, recognizing the team approach required for effective clinical practice. This includes multidisciplinary formal educational sessions and team-based simulation experiences [5]. These activities are focused on communication and professional domains of competence and provide trainees with a broader perspective on systems-based practice in emergency medicine.

Technology for learning in emergency medicine

Technological advances offer many potential teaching and learning applications in emergency medicine. Content-based technological adjuncts, such as textbooks and CD ROMs, are now more likely to be accessed online or in e-book formats, making published references more available and more easily updated. Electronic formats allow replication of high quality images and videos.

More significant is the change toward accessing web-based content for emergency medicine training and for continuing medical education. Websites, podcasts and blogs

on emergency medicine topics number in the thousands (Table 24.5.1). As a result, the emergency medicine trainee requires effective information retrieval and quality analysis skills. Public access search engines, such as Google, have replaced traditional Medline database searches as the preferred method of information retrieval by trainees, although not always with effective results [6].

The use of social media such as Twitter (San Francisco, CA, USA) and global collaboration to 'collate and curate' these resources [7] offers unparalleled access to educational materials and online discussions, as well as opportunities for informal peer review.

Procedural skill training has been enhanced by the use of manikins, part trainers and virtual reality systems, reducing the use of animal labs and cadavers. Video-based instruction of procedures allows demonstration of procedural performance under ideal conditions, with rehearsed teaching scripts. Many of these are now available on personal digital assistants for 'just-in-time learning' for trainees.

Clinical decision support software provides educational opportunities in conjunction with solutions to clinical problems. Many are in 'app' format (e.g. Medcalc) for mobile access and have extensive embedded resource materials that can be utilized in clinical practice or for primarily educational purposes.

Videoconferencing, webinars and tele-education have sought to answer the challenges of distance in emergency medicine education. Improvements in technology (including 'retail' platforms such as Skype (Luxembourg),

Google Hangouts, etc.) and bandwidth promise greater opportunities in this regard. It may help to relieve the teaching workload in smaller or more remote EDs.

Simulation-based learning

Medical simulation encompasses any kind of simulated clinical encounter. Simulations employ a range of possible modalities including simple part task trainers, such as an intravenous cannulation arm, simulated patients (SPs) or actors with a role-play script, high fidelity mannequin simulators, virtual-reality-based procedural skill trainers or combinations of modalities.

Effective simulation-based learning for emergency medicine requires clear educational objectives. These may include knowledge acquisition, procedural skill proficiency, applied physiology and pharmacology or complex teamwork skills and behaviours inherent in crisis resource management. The educational objective should then determine the nature of the equipment used, scenario design, the level of fidelity required and the approach to debriefing.

Simulators, equipment and fidelity

Mannequin technology continues to improve. The most technologically complex full body simulators operate via detailed physiological modelling software and can manifest pulses, breathing, blinking and vocalization, together with an ability to alter lung mechanics and compliance and cardiovascular parameters. Less complex simulators can manifest most of these features, but with the benefit of lower cost and increased portability.

Learner perceptions of fidelity of the simulation experience are variable. Individual learning styles, the authenticity of the scenario presented, the realism of the team composition and the physical environment all appear to be more important than the complexity of a mannequin to the learners' perception of fidelity and the learning outcomes achieved.

'Hybrid' simulation – combining simple part task trainers with standardized patients – has been successfully used to integrate a procedural skill with communication performance, e.g. an actor wearing a synthetic skin pad with a laceration interacts with a doctor suturing the wound.

Teamwork and communication skills training using medical simulation

Crisis resource management (CRM) training in emergency medicine using human patient simulation draws on parallels between acute patient care and the aviation and military industries, where it has been recognized that human factors are crucial to team performance [8].

A typical scenario might involve a team of medical and nursing participants managing a patient with chest pain, complicated by a life-threatening arrhythmia. Participants would be expected to identify and manage clinical issues, while engaging in the communication, teamwork and leadership activities inherent in real clinical practice. The scenario is then followed by video-assisted, expert debriefing to reflect upon individual and team performance. This experiential learning approach enables cross-domain training in which cognitive, procedural and affective domains of practice are authentically integrated. The interprofessional nature of the learning experience provides a unique opportunity for increased understanding of the role of other healthcare disciplines.

Educational benefits

Simulation enables 'efficient' learning through standardized exposure to clinical challenges which may be infrequent in clinical practice. It allows practice and failure in a safe environment, without risk to patients.

Advanced mannequin and audiovisual technology, together with logistic expertise, mean that these learning experiences can be provided *in situ* – in clinicians' own EDs. The use of the authentic work environment allows high levels of fidelity to be achieved. The usual work team can engage in learning together and review their everyday systems and processes, without the cost and logistical barriers of travelling to a synthetic environment. Provision of simulation-based experience and group debriefing via videoconferencing and remote control of equipment is at the boundary of present technological capacity.

In addition to their role in learning, human patient simulators can be used for competency assessment, which is made reliable by standardized challenges. However, it is important that assessment activities are clearly distinguished from those whose objective is learning, as key differences in simulation performance are observed. This reproducibility of challenges also provides opportunities to study the effect

of fatigue or expertise level on emergency physician or trainee performance and for testing new medical equipment or clinical systems.

Evidence for clinical practice improvement resulting from simulation-based learning is currently lacking, despite intuitive appeal. There are methodological challenges in the reliable measurement of teamwork and communication performance and attribution issues involved in any demonstration of patient outcome improvement. Features of simulations that lead to effective learning are better understood [9].

There are limitations to simulation-based training. There are significant costs in equipment and trained personnel to run programmes. Critical care situations, especially cardiac and airway emergencies can be simulated with a high degree of fidelity, but many other emergency medicine clinical challenges are not suitable. Negative training is a recognized risk, i.e. allowing participants not to wear gloves or lead aprons or simulating overly positive clinical outcomes can allow poor behaviour patterns to develop or train learners to have unrealistic expectations in the real clinical environment.

Training for providers of simulation-based learning

Educators using simulation-based modalities require proficiency in technological issues, experiential learning principles and small group process. Training for providers of simulation-based emergency medicine education is varied. Short courses exist at many simulation centres and most providers run their own 'in-house' quality assurance process to ensure a standardized approach to scenario design, delivery and group debriefing. In Australia, Health Workforce Australia (HWA) is currently working on a national approach to provider training through the National Health Education and Training in Simulation (NHET-Sim) programme.

Assessment and performance appraisal for emergency medicine training

Assessment in medical education is a complex issue [10]. No single assessment format can adequately measure performance across all domains of emergency medicine practice. Within the specialty there is considerable international variation in the domains of performance formally assessed, the definition of 'professional competence' required and in the standardization of assessment processes undertaken.

In-training assessment by clinical supervisors is a core element in most programmes, but this may be provided by one designated supervisor of training or many clinical supervisors in a group-based assessment. Literature suggests that in-training assessment is a valid tool (i.e. measures the right thing), but the potentially subjective nature of supervisor assessments and recall bias can decrease the reliability of assessment [11].

Most training programmes also have formal examination components, generally developed and administered externally by a national training body. A variety of formats exists, including multiple-choice questions, written tests, structured interviews and clinical examination vivas.

Workplace-based assessment (WBA) is becoming more prevalent. This includes formats such as mini-CEX (clinical evaluation exercise) and DOPS (direct observation of procedural skills) in which trainees are directly observed and assessed in a clinical encounter and given immediate feedback. WBAs are valid and reliable if sufficient assessments are undertaken, but resource-intensive and challenging in implementation [12].

Other contemporary assessment tools include clinical simulations, portfolios, standardized patients and multisource '360 degree' feedback assessment. Patient care quality outcomes have been suggested as an assessment tool [13]. These formats support the trend toward specific assessment of communication and professionalism domains, which mirror contemporary shifts in curricular content.

Faculty development in emergency medicine

Many emergency physicians are enthusiastic clinical teachers. However, clinician educators also require specific skills and preparation for their teaching role. Training for educators in emergency medicine might include Masters

level courses, short workshops or institution-based group professional development activities. These courses typically cover topics such as curriculum development, teaching and learning processes and assessment and feedback skills.

Programmes are more formally developed in the USA, where a number of teaching fellowships exist in emergency medicine and where the Society for Academic Emergency Medicine (SAEM) has published a *Faculty Development Handbook* [14]. These initiatives have been reinforced by the emergence of 'clinician educator tracks' in academic institutions to provide an academic career structure for clinical teachers.

Continuing medical education (CME)

There is a societal expectation in developed countries that physicians maintain their skills and competence to practice. Australasian emergency physicians are required by the Medical Boards of Australia and New Zealand to demonstrate participation in a continuing professional development programme accredited by the Australian Medical Council. Internationally, the nature of CME requirements vary, but most require periodic assimilation of a portfolio of attendance at conferences and workshops, together with demonstration of participation in clinical practice, teaching, quality assurance activities, research and other special interests. Some jurisdictions require update examinations.

Controversies and future directions

- Technology and online collaboration will continue to challenge traditional learning and assessment methods for emergency medicine practitioners at all levels.
- The involvement of professional educators in postgraduate emergency medicine training is likely to bring more contemporary approaches to curriculum design, teaching and assessment.

- Training programmes will need flexibility to match changes in contemporary healthcare delivery. Changing workforce roles – with challenges to traditional emergency physician scope of practice from nurse practitioners, physician assistants and others – need to be reflected in curricular objectives.
- An international medical workforce shortage, plus a doubling of medical graduate numbers in Australia will increase pressure to produce qualified specialist practitioners, including emergency physicians, in a shorter time and with a more 'work ready' focus.

References

[1] AMA position statement. Core terms for internship 2007. Australian Medical Association. <http://www.ama.com.au/node/2712> [Accessed Mar. 2010].
[2] CanMEDS: better standards, better physicians, better care. <http://www.royalcollege.ca/portal/page/portal/rc/resources/aboutcanmeds> [Accessed Dec. 2012].
[3] Kelly JJ, Thallner E, Broida RI, et al. Emergency medicine quality improvement and patient safety curriculum. Acad Emerg Med 2010;17:e110–29.
[4] O'Sullivan P, Greene C. Portfolios: possibilities for addressing emergency medicine resident competencies. Acad Emerg Med 2002;9:1305–9.
[5] Shapiro MJ, Morey JC, Small SD, et al. Simulation based teamwork training for emergency department staff: does it improve clinical team performance when added to an existing didactic teamwork curriculum? Qual Safety Hlth Care 2004;13:417–21.
[6] Krause R, Moscati R, Halpern S, et al. Can emergency medicine residents reliably use the internet to answer clinical questions? West J Emerg Med 2011;12:442–7.
[7] Cadogan M. Life in the Fast Lane EMCC Blogs. <http://lifeinthefastlane.com/resources/emergency-medicine-blogs/> [Accessed Jan. 2013].
[8] Carne B, Kennedy M, Gray T. Review article: crisis resource management in emergency medicine. Emerg Med Australas 2012;24:7–13.
[9] Issenberg SB, McGaghie WC, et al. Features and uses of high-fidelity medical simulations that lead to effective learning: a BEME systematic review. Med Teach 2005;27:10–28.
[10] Epstein RM. Assessment in medical education. N Engl J Med 2007;356:387–96.
[11] Wilkinson TJ, Wade WB. Problems with using a supervisor's report as a form of summative assessment. Postgrad Med J 2007;83:504–6.
[12] Crossley J, Jolly B. Making sense of work-based assessment: ask the right questions, in the right way, about the right things, of the right people. Med Educ 2012;46:28–37.
[13] Swing SR, Schneider S, Bizovi K, et al. Using patient care quality measures to assess educational outcomes. Acad Emerg Med 2007;14:463–73.
[14] Gallagher EJ, Martin M. Faculty development handbook. Society for Academic Emergency Medicine; 2011. <http://www.saem.org/faculty-development-handbook> [Accessed Jan. 2013].

EMERGENCY MEDICINE AND THE LAW

Edited by **George Jelinek**

25.1 Mental health and the law: the Australasian and UK perspectives

Georgina Phillips • Suzanne Mason • Simon Baston

ESSENTIALS

1 The emergency department is frequently the point of access to the mental health system.

2 Emergency physicians need to be able to distinguish between patients with physical and those with psychiatric illness.

3 Patients should only be committed involuntarily to an approved hospital if they have a mental illness requiring immediate treatment for their own health or safety or the protection of others and if adequate treatment cannot be obtained in a less restrictive manner.

4 Emergency physicians need to have a sound working knowledge of mental health legislation as it relates to their practice and to the jurisdiction in which they work.

5 Recent mental health legislative reform across Australasia emphasizes autonomy and self-determination within a human rights framework and is moving towards minimizing restrictive practices, increasing safeguards and transparency and enhancing independent oversight.

Introduction

The emergency department (ED) is frequently the interface between the community and the mental health system. In recent years, changes in health policy have resulted in 'mainstreaming' of mental health services, so that stand-alone psychiatric services are less common and services are more likely to be provided in a general hospital setting. Linked to this has been a move away from managing long-term psychiatric patients in institutional settings, so that many of these former patients are now living in the community with or without support from mental health services.

Traditionally, by virtue of their accessibility, EDs have been a point of access to mental health services for persons with acute psychiatric illness, whether this be self- or family referral or by referral from ambulance, police or outside medical practitioners. An important function of an ED is to differentiate between those who require psychiatric care for a psychiatric illness and those who present with a psychiatric manifestation of a physical illness and who require medical care. Admission of a patient with a psychiatric manifestation of a physical illness to a psychiatric unit may result in further harm to or death of the patient.

In the UK and Australasia, doctors in general are empowered by legislation to detain a mentally ill person who is in need of treatment. Mental illness, particularly its manifestation as self-harm, is a common ED presentation (in the UK, making up around 1–2% of new patient attendances and up to 5% of attendances in Australasia) and emergency physicians require not only the clinical skills to distinguish between those who require psychiatric or medical intervention, but also a sound working knowledge of the mental health legislation and services relevant to the state where they practise. This ensures that patients with psychiatric illness are managed in the most appropriate way, with optimal utilization of mental health resources and with the best interests and rights of the patient and the community taken into consideration.

While there are variations in mental health legislation between the UK, Australia and New Zealand, all legislation recognizes fundamental common principles that respect individual autonomy and employ least restrictive management practices. The World Health Organization (WHO) advises 10 basic principles of mental healthcare law, including enshrining geographical, cultural and economic equity of access to mental health care, acceptable standards of clinical assessment, facilitating self-determination, minimizing restrictive treatment and enshrining regular and impartial decision making and review of care [1]. These themes are all present in Australasian and UK law and awareness of such principles aids the clinician in delivering humane and ethical treatment for mentally unwell patients who seek emergency care.

Variations in practice

Mental health legislation in England and Wales

The National Service Framework for Mental Health

The National Service Framework for Mental Health produced by the Department of Health in the UK (1999) is aimed at improving quality and addresses the mental health needs of working age adults up to 65 years. It states as one of its standards that:

Any individual with a common mental health problem should be able to make contact round the clock with the local services necessary to meet their needs and receive adequate care.

Although EDs do not provide the ideal environment for a mental health assessment, they are likely to continue to provide an entry point for people with mental health problems. Easy access to the ED can lead to individuals with acute mental health problems seeking help directly, making up to perhaps 5% of ED attenders.

Two pieces of legislation cover the care and treatment of patients with disorders of the brain or mind. The Mental Health Act (1983) deals with compulsory assessment and treatment of people with mental illnesses, while the Mental Capacity Act (2005) deals with people who are unable to make decisions about their medical treatment for themselves for various reasons.

Mental Health Act

Definition of mentally ill or mental illness According to the 1983 Mental Health Act, mental illness is undefined. However, in practice it includes conditions such as schizophrenia, bipolar disorder, depression, psychosis and organic brain syndromes. Mental impairment is defined as: 'a state of arrested or incomplete development of mind which includes significant impairment of intelligence and social functioning and is associated with abnormally aggressive or seriously irresponsible conduct on the part of the person concerned'. A psychopathic disorder is defined as 'a persistent disorder or disability of mind which results in abnormally aggressive or seriously irresponsible conduct on the part of the person concerned'. The Act does not cover promiscuity or other immoral conduct or sexual deviancy which, in the past, could result in incarceration in psychiatric hospitals or dependence on drugs or alcohol.

Detention of patients with mental illness The Mental Health Act 1983 provides legislation with regard to the management of patients with a mental illness unwilling to be admitted or detained in hospital voluntarily, where this would be in the best interests of the health and safety of patients and others. For the purposes of the Act, patients in the ED are not considered inpatients until they are admitted to a ward. In order for legislation to be imposed, it is necessary for two conditions to be satisfied: the patient must be suffering from a mental illness and emergency hospital admission is required because the patient is considered to be a danger to themselves or others.

Detention under the Mental Health Act does not permit treatment for psychiatric or physical illness. Treatment can be given under common law where the patient is considered to pose a serious threat to themselves or others. Otherwise all treatment must be with the patient's consent.

Section 2 of the Mental Health Act facilitates compulsory admission to hospital for assessment and treatment for up to 28 days. The application is usually made by an approved social worker or the patient's nearest relative and requires two medical recommendations, usually from the patient's general practitioner and the duty senior psychiatrist (who is approved under Section 12 of the Mental Health Act). In the ED, the responsibility for coordinating the procedure often lies with the emergency physician.

Section 3 of the Mental Health Act covers compulsory admission for treatment. Once again, recommendations must be made by two doctors, one of whom is usually the general practitioner and the other a psychiatrist approved under Section 12 of the Act. The application is usually made by an approved social worker or the patient's nearest relative. Detention is for up to 6 months but can be renewed.

Section 4 of the Mental Health Act covers emergency admission for assessment and attempts to avoid delay in emergency situations when obtaining a second recommendation could be dangerous. It requires the recommendation of only one doctor, who may be any registered medical practitioner who must have seen the patient within the previous 24h. The order lasts for 72h. Application can be made by the patient's nearest relative or an approved social worker. In practice, the application of Section 4 of the Mental Health Act rarely happens. Usually Section 2 or 3 is the preferred option.

Section 5(2) – doctors holding power and Section 5(4) – nurses holding power of the Act allow the detention of patients who are already admitted to hospital until a more formal Mental Health Act assessment can take place. Unfortunately, presence in the ED is not considered to constitute admission to hospital and this section is, therefore, not applicable to the ED.

A new draft Mental Health Bill, published in 2002, was opposed by professional and patient groups alike. It aimed to introduce a new legal framework for the compulsory treatment of people with mental disorders in hospitals and the community. The new procedure involved a single pathway in three stages: a preliminary examination, a period of formal assessment lasting up to 28 days and treatment under a Mental Health Act order. In order for the compulsory process to be used, four conditions needed to be satisfied: the patient must have a mental disorder, the disorder must warrant medical treatment, treatment must be necessary for the health and safety of the patient or others, and an appropriate treatment for the disorder must be available. The draft Bill made provision for treatment without consent as it is justified under the European Convention on Human Rights Article 8(2) in the interests of public safety or to protect health or moral standards.

The resulting debate saw much of the draft Bill being scrapped in favour of amendments being made to the existing Mental Health Act. This included the creation of community treatment orders and a broader definition of mental disorder.

Police powers

Section 136 of the Act authorizes the police to remove patients who are believed to be mentally disordered and causing a public disturbance to a place of safety. The place of safety referred to in the Act is defined in Section 135 as 'residential accommodation provided by a local authority under Part III of the National Assistance Act 1948, or under Paragraph 2, Schedule 8 of the National Health Service Act 1977, a hospital as defined by this Act, a police station, a mental nursing home or residential home for mentally disordered persons or any other suitable place, the occupier of which is willing temporarily to receive the patient'. In practice, the police often transport these patients to local EDs. The patient must be assessed by an approved social worker and a registered doctor. The order lasts for 72 h.

Section 135 allows the police to enter premises to remove a patient believed to be suffering from a mental disorder to a place of safety for up to 72 h. The patient is then assessed as above.

Mental Capacity Act

The Mental Capacity Act relates to decision making, for those whose mental capacity is in doubt, on any issue from what to wear to the more difficult issues of medical treatment, personal finance and housing.

Lack of capacity can occur in two distinct ways. First, that capacity is never achieved – for example someone with a severe learning difficulty. Secondly, capacity can be lost either as a result of long-term conditions, such as dementia, or for a short period because of a temporary factor, such as intoxication, shock, pain or emotional distress.

It is also important that decision making is task specific. An individual may be able to make decisions about simple matters, such as what to eat or wear, but may be unable to make more complex decisions, for example about medical care.

Assessment of capacity   To have capacity about a decision, the patient should be able to comply with the following four steps:

- understand the information relevant to the decision
- retain the information for the period of decision making
- use or weigh that information as part of the process of making a decision
- communicate their decisions.

Every effort needs to be made to enable people to make their own decisions.

The Act points out that people should be allowed to make 'eccentric' or 'unwise' decisions, as it is their ability to decide that is the issue not the decision itself.

Advance directives   The Act makes provision for advance directives to be made at a time when the patient has capacity. These directives need to make specific reference to the medical treatments involved and include the statement 'even if life is at risk'. The validity of any advance decision needs to be clearly documented.

Advocates   Although family and friends have no legal powers (unless specified in advance) to make decisions for the incapacitated patient, the Act recognizes their role in acting as an advocate. An independent mental capacity advocate is available to represent those with no close family or friends.

Emergency treatment   Treatment can be given to patients who lack capacity but several factors need to be considered:

- any action must be in the best interest of the patient
- anything done must be the least restrictive of the patient's rights and freedoms
- where time can be afforded, every effort should be made to enable the patient to make his or her own decision
- treatment should not be delayed while attempts are made to establish the validity of any advance decision
- medical staff have a duty of care to the incapacitated patient.

Use of sedation or physical restraint

This is covered in detail elsewhere (Chapters 20.6 and 21.5). From the perspective of the mental health legislation, there are occasions where physical or pharmacological restraint is needed. Sedation or restraint must be the minimum that is necessary to prevent the patient from self-harming or harming others. Generally, a patient committed involuntarily is subject to treatment necessary for their care and control and this may reasonably include the administration of sedative or antipsychotic medication as emergency treatment. Transporting these patients to a mental health service should be done by suitably trained medical or ambulance staff and not delegated to police officers or other persons acting alone.

Mental health legislation in Australasia

In Australia, mental health legislation is a state jurisdiction and, among the various states and territories, there is considerable variation in the scope of mental health acts and between definitions and applications of the various sections. Since the National Mental Health Strategy in 1992, there has been an effort in Australia to adopt a consistent approach between jurisdictions, with an emphasis on ensuring legislated review mechanisms and a broad spectrum of treatment modalities [2]. In 2009, this national strategic approach was reaffirmed by all the States and Territories of Australia with the release of a National Mental Health Plan, focusing on promoting mental health and preventing mental disorders, minimizing the impact of mental illness across the whole community and protecting the rights of people with mental illness.

Several Australian states and territories have recently initiated mental health law reform, all within a human rights framework. Generally, there is an increased recognition of autonomous and supported decision making with a particular focus on enhancing informed consent through advance directives or involving a nominated support person. Increased transparency of and limitations around restrictive practices will affect activities within EDs. Community visitors and mental health tribunals are introduced to ensure frequent independent oversight and review and it is now mandatory in several jurisdictions to give patients and carers written copies of involuntary orders made about them, as well as a statement of their rights. Despite these common themes, key differences apply between mental health acts and therefore specific issues should be referred to the Act relevant to the emergency physician's practice location.

The Australian and New Zealand mental health acts and related documents referred to in this chapter are the following:

ACT – Mental Health (Treatment and Care) Act 1994, amendments 2007 and current review documents 2012

New South Wales – Mental Health Act 2007 and the NSW Mental Health for Emergency Departments: Reference Guide 2009

New Zealand – Mental Health (Compulsory Assessment and Treatment) Act 1992, 1999 Amendment and the Second New Zealand Mental Health and Addiction Plan 2005 (Te Tahuhu, Improving Mental Health 2005–2015) Northern Territory – Mental Health and Related Services Act 1998, amendments 2005 and as in force October 2012
Queensland – Mental Health Act 2000
South Australia – Mental Health Act 2009, Clinicians Guide and Code of Practice (Mental Health Act 2009 SA), SA Mental Health and Emergency Services Memorandum of Understanding 2010
Tasmania – Mental Health Act 1996 and the new Mental Health Bill introduced 2012
Victoria – Mental Health Act 1986 and incorporating amendments as at 1 July 2007 and A New Mental Health Act for Victoria; Summary of Proposed Reforms 2012
Western Australia – Mental Health Act 1996 and the New Mental Health Bill (draft for public comment) 2012.

Sections of the various mental health acts relevant to emergency medicine include those dealing with:

- the definition of mentally ill
- indigenous and cultural acknowledgement
- the effects of drugs or alcohol
- criteria for detention and admission as an involuntary patient
- involuntary admission
- persons unable to recommend a patient for involuntary admission
- physical restraint and sedation
- emergency treatment
- powers of police
- prisoners with mental illness
- offences in relation to documents
- information and patient transfer between jurisdictions
- deaths.

Definition of mentally ill or mental illness

For the purposes of their respective mental health acts, New Zealand and all the Australian states and territories define mental illness or disorder as follows.

Australian Capital Territory

The Australian Capital Territory (ACT) Act defines a psychiatric illness as a condition that seriously impairs (either temporarily or permanently) the mental functioning of a person

and is characterized by the presence in the person of any of the following symptoms: delusions, hallucinations, serious disorder of thought form, a severe disturbance of mood or sustained or repeated irrational behaviour indicating the presence of these symptoms.

The ACT Mental Health Act also defines 'mental dysfunction' as a 'disturbance or defect, to a substantially disabling degree, of perceptual interpretation, comprehension, reasoning, learning, judgement, memory, motivation or emotion'.

New South Wales

The New South Wales Act defines mental illness in the same way as the ACT but, in addition, distinguishes between a mentally ill person and a mentally disordered person, chiefly for the purposes of determining need for involuntary admission and treatment.

A person (whether or not the person is suffering from mental illness) is mentally disordered if the person's behaviour for the time being is so irrational as to justify conclusion on reasonable grounds that temporary care, treatment or control of the person is necessary for the person's own protection from serious physical harm or for the protection of others from serious physical harm.

New Zealand

In New Zealand, the Mental Health Act defines a mentally disordered person as possessing an abnormal state of mind, whether continuous or intermittent, characterized by delusions or by disorders of mood, perception, volition or cognition to such a degree that it poses a danger to the health or safety of the person or others, or seriously diminishes the capacity of the person to take care of themselves.

Northern Territory

In the Northern Territory, mental illness means a condition that seriously impairs, either temporarily or permanently, the mental functioning of a person in one or more of the areas of thought, mood, volition, perception, orientation or memory and is characterized by the presence of at least one of the following symptoms: delusions, hallucinations, serious disorders of the stream of thought, serious disorders of thought form or serious disturbances of mood. A mental illness is also characterized by sustained or repeated irrational behaviour that may be taken to indicate the presence of at least one of the symptoms mentioned above. The

Northern Territory Act goes further to specify that the determination of mental illness is only to be made in accordance with internationally accepted clinical standards.

Similar to the New South Wales Act, there is a provision in the Northern Territory for those who are 'mentally disturbed', which means behaviour of a person that is so irrational as to justify the person being temporarily detained under the Act. The Northern Territory also has provisions for people with complex cognitive impairment who require involuntary treatment.

Queensland

The Queensland Act defines mental illness in a similar way to Victoria, in that it is a condition characterized by a clinically significant disturbance of thought, mood, perception or memory, in accordance with internationally acceptable standards.

South Australia

In the South Australian Act, mental illness means any illness or disorder of the mind.

Tasmania

A person is taken to have a mental illness if they experience temporarily, repeatedly or continuously, a serious impairment of thought (which may include delusions) or a serious impairment of mood, volition, perception or cognition.

Victoria

A person is mentally ill if they have a mental illness, being a medical condition characterized by a significant disturbance of thought, mood, perception or memory.

Western Australia

Persons have a mental illness if they suffer from a disturbance of thought, mood, volition, perception, orientation or memory that impairs judgement or behaviour to a significant extent.

Indigenous and cultural acknowledgement

Cultural differences in the understanding and experiences of mental illness can impact greatly on the ability to provide adequate care. While there are some cursory references to acknowledging special cultural and linguistic needs when interpreting the various mental health acts, only the Northern Territory and South Australia in Australia and the New Zealand Mental Health Acts make specific mention of indigenous people, who are known to be a particularly vulnerable group [3]. Recent legislative reform in some Australian states incorporates recognition of the needs of Aboriginal and Torres Strait Islander and other culturally diverse peoples within a general statement of principles.

The Northern Territory Act states that there are fundamental principles to be taken into account when caring for Aborigines and Torres Strait Islanders. Treatment and care needs to be appropriate to the cultural beliefs and practices of the person, their family and community and involuntary treatment for an Aborigine is to be provided in collaboration with an Aboriginal health worker.

New Zealand stipulates that powers are to be exercised in relation to the Mental Health Act with proper respect for cultural identity and personal beliefs and with proper recognition of the importance and significance to the persons of their ties with family, whanau, hapu, iwi and family group. Interpreters are to be provided if the first or preferred language is not English, with special mention of Maori and New Zealand Sign Language.

Safeguards against prejudice

New Zealand and all Australian states include a number of criteria that, alone, cannot be used to determine that a person has a mental illness and requires involuntary admission. These generally include the expression of or refusal to express particular religious, political and philosophical beliefs; cultural or racial origin; sexual promiscuity or preference; intellectual disability; drug or alcohol taking; economic or social status; immoral or indecent conduct; illegal conduct; and antisocial behaviour. The Northern Territory, Western Australia and Queensland also include past treatment for mental illness and past involuntary admission under these criteria.

Effects of drugs or alcohol

In most Australian states and New Zealand, the taking of drugs or alcohol cannot, of itself, be taken as an indication of mental illness. However, the mental health acts of New South Wales, South Australia, Tasmania, Western Australia and Victoria specify that this does not prevent the serious temporary or permanent physiological, biochemical or psychological effects of alcohol or drug taking from being regarded as an indication that a person is mentally ill. The Queensland Act acknowledges that a person may have a mental illness caused by taking drugs or alcohol.

The remaining states do not specifically exclude the temporary or permanent effects of drugs or alcohol but use definitions of mental or psychiatric illness that are broad enough to cover this. Generally, when a person is so mentally and behaviourally disordered as a result of drug or alcohol use that adequate assessment is impossible and risk of harm to self or others is high, then detaining them for the purposes of assessment and treatment is possible under all Australian and New Zealand mental health acts.

Criteria for admission and detention as an involuntary patient

All states require that an involuntary patient has a mental illness that requires urgent treatment while detained in an inpatient setting for the health (mental or physical) and safety of that patient or for the protection of others. Most states also require that the patient has refused or is unable to consent to voluntary admission. It is also emphasized that appropriate treatment must be available and cannot be given in a less restrictive setting. In New South Wales, the effects of chronicity and the likely deterioration of the person's condition should be taken into account when determining need for involuntary admission.

Western Australia includes the protection of the patient from self-inflicted harm to the patient's reputation, relationships or finances as grounds for involuntary admission, although future legislation is likely to remove this criterion.

In New Zealand, the doctor must have reasonable grounds for believing that the person may be mentally disordered and that it is desirable, in the interests of the person, or of any other person or of the public, that assessment, examination and treatment of the person are conducted as a matter of urgency.

Involuntary admission

The process of involuntary admission varies quite markedly across the states. It is variously known as recommendation, certification or committal. All jurisdictions require doctors to examine patients and carefully document on prescribed forms the date and time of examination as well as the particular reasons why the doctor believes that the person has a mental illness that requires involuntary treatment. In addition, patients or their advocates are to be informed of the decisions made about them and their rights under the law at all stages of the involuntary admission process. Increasingly,

clinicians are required to give copies of formal orders and printed information about their rights to patients and guardians.

ACT

In the ACT, a medical or police officer is able to apprehend a mentally ill person who requires involuntary admission and is able to use reasonable force and enter premises in order to do so. The officer is required, as soon as possible, to provide a written statement to the person in charge of the mental health facility giving patient details and the reasons for taking the action.

A doctor employed by the mental health facility must examine the patient within 4 h of arrival and may authorize detention for up to 3 days. The doctor must inform the Community Advocate and Mental Health Tribunal of the patient's admission within 12 h and the patient must receive a physical and psychiatric examination within 24 h of detention.

New South Wales

The Mental Health Act in New South Wales allows for a patient requiring involuntary admission to be detained in a declared mental health facility (which includes EDs) on the certificate of a doctor (or trained 'accredited person') who has personally examined the patient immediately or shortly before completing the certificate.

For a mentally ill patient, the certificate is valid for 5 days from the time of writing, whereas for a mentally disordered patient, the certificate is valid for 1 day. Mentally disordered patients cannot be detained on the grounds of being mentally disordered on more than three occasions in any 1 month.

Part of the certificate, if completed, directs the police to apprehend and bring the patient to hospital and also enables them to enter premises without a warrant.

An involuntary patient must be examined by an authorized medical officer (including emergency doctors) as soon as practicable, but within 12 h of admission. The patient cannot be detained unless further certified mentally ill or disordered. This doctor cannot be the same doctor who requested admission or certified the patient. After their own examination, the medical officer must arrange for a second examination as soon as practicable, this time by a psychiatrist. If neither doctor thinks that the person is mentally ill or disordered, then the person must be released from the hospital.

A patient who has been certified as mentally disordered, but not subsequently found to be mentally ill, cannot be detained for more than 3 days and must be examined by an authorized medical officer at least once every 24h and discharged if no longer mentally ill or disordered or if appropriate and less restrictive care is available. New South Wales legislation involves several checks and balances, including timely and regular Mental Health Review Tribunal assessment for all patients recommended for involuntary care.

New Zealand

In New Zealand, a person aged 18 years or over may request an assessment by the area mental health service if it has seen the person within the last 3 days and believes the person to be suffering from a mental disorder. The request may be accompanied by a certificate from a doctor who has examined the 'proposed patient' within the preceding 3 days and who believes that the person requires compulsory assessment and treatment. The medical certificate must state the reasons for the opinion and that the patient is not a relative. The area mental health service must then arrange an assessment examination by a psychiatrist or other suitable person forthwith. If the assessing doctor considers that the patient requires compulsory treatment, the patient may be detained in the 'first period' for up to 5 days. Subsequent assessment may result in detention for a 'second period' of up to 14 more days, after which a 'compulsory treatment order' must be issued by a family court judge.

Northern Territory

Any person with a genuine interest in or concern for the welfare of another person may request an assessment by any medical practitioner to determine if that person is in need of treatment under the Northern Territory Mental Health Act. The assessment must then occur as soon as practicable and a subsequent recommendation for psychiatric examination made if the doctor believes that the person fulfils the criteria for involuntary admission on the grounds of mental illness or mental disturbance. The person may then be detained by police, ambulance officers or the doctor making the recommendation and taken to an approved treatment facility, where the person may be held for up to 12h. The Northern Territory Act acknowledges that delays in this process are likely and enshrines a process to

account for this, including the use of interactive video conferencing. A psychiatrist must examine and assess the recommended person at the approved treatment facility and must either admit as an involuntary patient or release the patient if the criteria for involuntary admission are not fulfilled.

A patient admitted on the grounds of mental illness may be detained for 24h or 7 days if the recommending doctor was also a psychiatrist. Patients admitted on the grounds of mental disturbance may be detained for 72h or have that extended by 7 days if two examining psychiatrists believe that the person still requires involuntary treatment and cannot or will not consent. Frequent psychiatric reassessment of detained and admitted patients is required to either extend admission or release patients who do not fulfil involuntary criteria.

Queensland

In Queensland, the recommendation for involuntary assessment of a patient must be made by a doctor who has personally examined the patient within the preceding 3 days and is valid for 7 days from the time the recommendation was made. The recommendation needs to be accompanied by an 'application' for assessment made by a person over the age of 18 years who has seen the patient within 3 days. The person making the application cannot be the doctor making the recommendation or be a relative or employee of the doctor. The recommendation enables the health practitioner, ambulance officer or police, if necessary, to take the patient to a mental health service or public hospital for assessment. Once there, or if the recommendation was made at a hospital, the assessment period lasts for no longer than 24h.

The patient must be assessed by a psychiatrist (who cannot be the recommending doctor) as soon as practicable and, if the treatment criteria apply, will have the involuntary status upheld through an involuntary treatment order. The assessment period can be extended up to 72h by the psychiatrist after regular review.

South Australia

In South Australia, a doctor or trained authorized health professional (who may be a nurse, allied or aboriginal health worker) who considers that a patient requires involuntary admission authorizes a Level 1 Detention and Treatment Order, which is valid for 7 days. A psychiatrist or authorized medical practitioner

(senior psychiatry registrar) must examine the person within 24h or as soon as practicable.

In recognition of the difficulties in accessing appropriate care for people in remote and rural environments, the South Australian Mental Health Act allows for audiovisual conferencing and a range of community and inpatient based treatment orders. A wider range of health professionals can authorize treatment orders so that early access to care in the least restrictive environment can occur.

Tasmania

In Tasmania, an application for involuntary admission of a person may be made by a close relative or guardians or an 'authorized officer.' A medical practitioner must then assess the person and, if satisfied that the criteria are met, make an order for admission and detention as an involuntary patient in an approved hospital. This initial 'assessment order' is valid for 72h and gives authority for the patient to be taken to the hospital and detained, whereupon a psychiatric assessment must be carried out within 24h and the assessment order extended for up to 72h or discharged. A 'treatment order' for the continuing detention of a person as an involuntary patient can only be made by application (including an individualized treatment plan) through an independent tribunal.

Victoria

A person may be admitted to and detained in an approved mental health service once the 'request' and the 'recommendation' have been completed. The request can be completed by any person over 18 years of age, including relatives of the patient, but cannot be completed by the recommending doctor. The recommendation is valid for 3 days after completion and the recommending doctor must have personally examined or observed the patient.

The request and recommendation are sufficient authority for the medical practitioner, police officer or ambulance officer to take the person to a mental health service or to enter premises without a warrant and to use reasonable force or restraint in order to take the person to a mental health service. Prescribed medical practitioners (psychiatrists, forensic physicians, doctors employed by a mental health service, the head of an ED of a general hospital or the regular treating doctor in a remote area) are also enabled to use sedation or restraint to enable a person to be taken safely to a mental health service.

Once admitted, the patient must be seen by a medical practitioner employed by the mental health service as soon as possible, but must be seen by a registered psychiatrist within 24 h of admission. The admitting doctor must make an involuntary treatment order, which allows for the detention of the patient until psychiatrist review and the urgent administration of medication if needed. The psychiatrist can then either authorize further detention, a community treatment order or discharge the patient.

Western Australia

In Western Australia, a person who requires involuntary admission is referred, in writing, for examination by a psychiatrist in an authorized hospital. The referring doctor or authorized mental health practitioner must have personally examined the person within the previous 48 h and may also make a detention and/or transport order which allows safe transport involving the police or ambulance personnel if required. These orders are valid for up to 72 h, although there are provisions for time extensions outside the metropolitan area.

The referral for assessment is valid for 72 h (although this can also be extended); however, the patient must be examined by a psychiatrist within 24 h of admission and cannot be detained further if not examined. The patient can be detained for further assessment for up to 72 h after initial admission on the order of the psychiatrist, after which time the patient is formally admitted as an involuntary patient, discharged on a community treatment order or released.

Persons unable to recommend a patient for involuntary admission

New Zealand and most states, except for the ACT, specify that certain relationships prevent a doctor from requesting or recommending a patient for involuntary admission.

The recommending doctor cannot be a relative (by blood or marriage) or guardian of the patient and, in addition, in the Northern Territory, Queensland, Tasmania and Western Australia, the doctor cannot be a business partner or assistant of the patient. In Queensland and Tasmania, the recommending doctor cannot be in receipt of payments for the maintenance of the patient.

In New South Wales, the doctor must declare, on the schedule, any direct or indirect pecuniary interest, or those of their relatives, partners or assistants, in a private mental

health facility. In Western Australia, the doctor cannot hold a licence from or have a family or financial relationship with the licence holder of a private hospital in which the patient will be treated, nor can the doctor be a board member of a public hospital treating the patient.

Use of sedation or physical restraint

From time to time a patient may need to be sedated or even restrained. The various mental health acts vary considerably in dealing with this issue and accepted clinical practice has evolved differently in each jurisdiction and does not necessarily reflect subtleties within the legislation.

Generally, patients committed involuntarily are subject to treatment necessary for their care and control and this may reasonably include the administration of sedative or antipsychotic medication as emergency treatment. In general, sedation or restraint must be the minimum that is necessary to prevent the patient from self-harming or harming others and careful documentation of the reasons for restraint and the types of restraint is required. While restrained, access to clothing, sustenance, toilet facilities and other basic comforts must be assured.

Patients who are physically or pharmacologically restrained must be closely supervised and not left alone or in the care of persons not trained or equipped to deal with the potential complications of these procedures. Transporting these patients to a mental health service should be done by suitably trained medical or ambulance staff and not delegated to police officers or other persons acting alone.

The ACT specifies that sedation may be used to prevent harm, whereas Western Australia specifies that sedation can be used for emergency treatment without consent and that the details must be recorded in a report to the Mental Health Review Board. Queensland allows a doctor to administer medication for recommended patients without consent to ensure safety during transport to a health facility.

Victoria specifically permits the administration of sedative medication by a 'prescribed medical practitioner' to allow for the safe transport of a patient to a mental health service. There is a schedule to complete if this is undertaken. The South Australian law stipulates that medication can only be used for therapeutic purposes and that chemical, physical restraint and seclusion is to be used as a last resort for

safety reasons and not as a punishment or for the convenience of others.

The legislation is more specific with regard to the use of physical restraint or seclusion. In the ACT, this can be done to prevent an immediate and substantial risk of harm to the patient or others or to keep the patient in custody.

Queensland requires that restraint used for the protection of the patient or others can only be done on an 'order' but is permissible for the purposes of treatment if it is clinically appropriate. Victoria permits the restraint of involuntary patients for the purposes of medical treatment and the prevention of injury or persistent property destruction. Victoria also allows the use of restraint by ambulance officers, police or doctors in order to safely transport the patient to a mental health service, but this must be documented in the recommendation schedule. Tasmania differentiates between chemical restraint and chemical treatment and allows for both chemical and physical restraint as emergency short-term interventions to prevent harm, damage or interference, break up an affray or facilitate transport. The Chief Civil Psychiatrist is required to develop standing orders for clinical use regarding these issues.

Both the Northern Territory and Western Australia permit the use of restraint for the purposes of medical treatment and for the protection of the patient, other persons or property. In Western Australia, this authorization must be in writing and must be notified to the senior psychiatrist as soon as possible, while in the Northern Territory, it must be approved by a psychiatrist or the senior nurse on duty in the case of an emergency.

The New Zealand Mental Health Act makes minimal specific reference to restraint or sedation but enables any urgent treatment to protect the patient or others and allows hospitals and police to take all reasonable steps to detain patients for assessment and treatment. Authority is given to administer sedative drugs if necessary, but the Act mandates a record of this for the area mental health service.

New South Wales has a Reference Guide specifically for mental health issues in the ED which covers sedation and restraint issues. The law permits the use of involuntary sedation for acute behavioural disturbance in an emergency situation in order to prevent individual death or serious danger to the health of others under the common law principle of 'Duty of Care'. The same applies for children, although consent should be sought from both children or adolescents and their parents or guardians. For the use of physical restraints, although acknowledged as a clinical decision, four pre-conditions must be met:

- the person has a medical or psychiatric condition requiring care
- the person is at the time incapable of responding to reasonable requests from health staff to cooperate and other self-control measures are impractical or have failed
- the person's behaviour is putting themselves or others at serious risk
- less restrictive alternatives are not appropriate.

Emergency treatment and surgery

On occasions, involuntary patients may require emergency medical or surgical treatment. New Zealand and most states, except for Queensland, make provision for this in their legislation, in that patients can undergo emergency treatment without consent, but usually only with the approval of the relevant mental health authorities or treating psychiatrist. In New Zealand, treatment that is immediately necessary to save life, prevent serious damage to health or prevent injury to the person or others can be undertaken without consent.

Victoria has the most specific reference to this treatment by making special allowance for a patient requiring treatment that is life sustaining or preventing serious physical deterioration to be admitted as an involuntary patient to a general hospital or ED for the purposes of receiving treatment. The patient is deemed to be on leave from the mental health service and all the other provisions of the Act apply.

Apprehension of absent involuntary patients

Involuntary patients who escape from custody or who fail to return from 'leave' are considered in most state mental health acts to be 'absent without leave' (AWOL) or 'unlawfully at large'. Authorized persons, including ambulance officers, mental health workers and police, have the same powers of entry and apprehension as for other persons to whom a recommendation or certificate relates.

In New Zealand, any compulsory patient who becomes AWOL may be 'retaken' by any person and taken to any hospital within 3 months of becoming absent. If not returned after 3

months the patient is deemed to be released from compulsory status.

Powers of the police

The police in all states and New Zealand have powers in relation to mentally ill persons who may or may not have been assessed by a doctor. For someone who is not already an involuntary patient and who is reasonably believed to be mentally ill, a risk to self or others and requiring care, police are able to enter premises and apprehend, without a warrant, and to use reasonable force if necessary, in order to remove the person to a 'place of safety'. Generally, this means taking the person to a medical practitioner or a mental health service for examination without undue delay.

South Australia and Queensland specifically include ambulance or other authorized officers within this legislation and acknowledge that they often work together with police to detain and transport people for mental health assessment. In Tasmania, people may only be held in protective custody for the purposes of medical assessment for no longer than 4 h and then released if no involuntary assessment order has been made. The ACT law is moving towards replacing police with ambulance paramedics in the role of emergency apprehension and transport to hospital for assessment.

Some states (ACT, New South Wales and Victoria) make special mention of a threatened or actual suicide attempt as justification for police apprehension and transfer to a health facility. New South Wales allows police discretion after a person who appears mentally disordered has committed an offence (including attempted murder), to determine whether it is beneficial to their welfare to be detained under the mental health act rather than under other criminal law. The Victorian and South Australian Acts, in contrast, acknowledge that police do not need clinical judgement about mental illness but may exercise their powers based on their own perception of a person's appearance and behaviour that may be suggestive of mental illness.

In New Zealand, detention by police is limited to 6 h, by which time a medical examination should have taken place. Ideally, police should not enter premises without a warrant, if it is reasonably practicable to obtain one.

The same powers apply to involuntary patients who abscond or are absent without leave, although some states have specific schedules or orders to complete for this to be done. In general, once police become aware of

the patient they are obliged to make attempts to find and return them to what can be viewed as lawful custody.

Prisoners with mental illness

Mental illness among people in prison is extremely prevalent, either as a cause or as a result of incarceration. New Zealand and most Australian states and territories include provisions for prisoners with mental illness within their mental health legislation. While the healthcare of prisoners is generally managed within regional forensic systems, EDs in rural and less-well-resourced areas can become a site of care for prisoners with acute psychiatric illness.

The New Zealand Act states that prisoners with mental illness who require acute care can be transferred to a general hospital for involuntary psychiatric treatment if the prison is unable to provide that care. Australian Acts in New South Wales, the Northern Territory and Victoria all include similar specific provisions for mentally ill prisoners to be able to access involuntary care in public hospitals if needed. New South Wales has separate legislation specifically dealing with mental illness in the forensic setting (NSW Mental Health [Forensic Provisions] Act 1990), while the Tasmanian Act includes a large section involving the admission, custody, treatment and management of forensic patients within secure mental health units. The Victorian Act has some detail in this matter although, in practice, rarely relies on public hospitals due to the development of a stand alone forensic psychiatric hospital. Both Queensland and Western Australia enshrine the same principle of allowing prisoners access to general psychiatric treatment, although their legislation is less specific, while the South Australian Act does not mention prisoners at all. The ACT will incorporate care for prisoners with mental illness in their new Act, emphasizing concern for the community who may be affected by prisoners with mental illness, improving communication between forensic and health services and allowing prisoners with mental illness access to appropriate healthcare. In all jurisdictions, there is significant overlap with other laws such as Crimes and Prisons Acts, which also mention health needs of prisoners.

Offences in relation to certificates

Most states and New Zealand specify in their respective mental health acts that it is an offence to make wilfully a false or misleading statement in regard to the certification of an involuntary patient.

Some states (New South Wales, South Australia, the Northern Territory and Victoria), except in certain circumstances, also regard failure personally to examine or observe the patient as an offence.

Protection from suit or liability

New Zealand and all Australian states specify in their Mental Health Acts that legal proceedings cannot be brought against doctors acting in good faith and with reasonable care within the provisions of the Mental Health Act relevant to their practice.

Information and patient transfer between jurisdictions

All Australian states and territories include special provisions for the apprehension, treatment and transfer of mentally ill patients from other jurisdictions. State governments can enter into agreements to recognize warrants or orders made under 'corresponding law' in other states or territories, as long as appropriate conditions are met within their own law. Thus, a patient under an involuntary detention or community treatment order in another state can be apprehended and treated under the corresponding law in a different jurisdiction. Authority is given to police and doctors to detain such patients and information to facilitate assessment and treatment can be shared between states.

Deaths

Involuntary patients should be considered to be held in lawful custody, whether in an ED, as an inpatient in a general hospital or psychiatric hospital or as an AWOL. As such, the death of such a patient must be referred for a coroner's investigation.

Controversies and future directions

United Kingdom

- The provision of mental health services to EDs varies widely across the UK. Responsiveness of services remains an issue of contention, particularly in light of national 4 h targets for treatment in EDs. Representatives of the various Royal Colleges are currently writing a national strategy, which aims to set standards for what they describe as 'emergency psychiatry'.
- In the UK, the most commonly used places of safety for individuals deemed to be a danger to themselves or the public are EDs, police stations and psychiatric units. Concern exists about the suitability of EDs for acting as places of safety. The Royal College of Psychiatrists jointly with the British Association for Emergency Medicine stated in 1996 that EDs were inappropriately staffed and equipped to supervise such individuals. However, the National Service Framework on Mental Health states that hospitals should be used in preference to police stations. To date, there has been no national consensus on the future use of the ED as a place of safety. Currently, individual departments are entering into local policy agreements with other agencies on their use.
- As the specialty of emergency medicine expands, health professionals, such as emergency nurse practitioners and paramedics, are increasingly making clinical decisions about patients. This presents a challenge to the specialty in ensuring that all are appropriately trained and informed of the law relating to patients with mental health problems. It is vital that training and education continue to be central to delivering an appropriate service in often difficult circumstances.
- In 2004, the National Institute for Health and Clinical Excellence (NICE) published a guideline on the treatment and prevention of self-harm focusing on care in the ED. It stressed the importance of staff attitudes towards these patients. Patients who have self-harmed reported frequently being treated not only with a lack of respect, as 'time wasters', but at times receiving punitive treatment at the hands of ED staff.

Australasia

- Greater uniformity between the mental health legislation of Australian states and territories is desirable from both a patient's and a healthcare provider's perspective. While there has been some move towards commonality with recognition of 'corresponding laws', great disparity still exists in some areas between jurisdictions. These differences could be overcome without compromising the fundamental principles of mental health legislation in the Australasian region.
- More legal recognition of cultural and language difference is required as Australia and New Zealand become home to increasingly diverse populations. In particular, refugees and people from areas exposed to warfare and torture have specific mental health needs that should be accounted for within progressive legislation. Better acknowledgement of indigenous mental health issues is also an area requiring legislative improvement.
- Police are given great powers within Australasian laws to apprehend and detain mentally unwell people, yet lack a sophisticated knowledge of mental illness. Greater education and collaborative work between police and healthcare providers, especially those working in EDs, should lead to more humane and patient-focused provision of care.
- Governments and the community are taking increasing interest in what actually happens within EDs, particularly in regard to practices of chemical sedation and physical restraint for patients with mental illness and acute behavioural disturbance. Increased clarity, uniformity and transparency around criteria for the use of chemical and physical restraints will benefit clinicians, patients and external observers from a both a clinical quality and safety perspective. A human rights framework that enshrines least restrictive practices is recommended.
- With an increased legislative focus on recognition of individual human rights and elevation of autonomous decision making, recognition of advanced directives may shape future emergency care for patients with mental illness and acute behavioural disturbance.

References

[1] World Health Organization. Mental health care law: ten basic principles. Geneva: World Health Organization, Division of Mental Health and Prevention of Substance Abuse; 1996.

[2] Forrester K, Griffiths D. Essentials of law for health professionals, 2nd edn. Sydney: Elsevier; 2005.

[3] Australian Human Rights and Equal Opportunity Commission. Human rights and mental illness. Report of the national inquiry into the human rights of people with mental illness. Canberra: Australian Government Publishing Service; 1993.

Further reading

Jones R. Mental Health Act manual, 8th edn. London: Sweet and Maxwell; 2002.

Jones R. Mental Capacity Act manual, 2nd edn. London: Sweet and Maxwell; 2007.

Mental Capacity Act. <http://www.opsi.gov.uk/acts/acts2005/20050009.html>; 2005.

Wallace M. Health care and the law, 2nd edn. Sydney: The Law Book Company Ltd; 1995.

WHO. Resource book on mental health, human rights and legislation. Geneva: World Health Organization; 2005.

25.2 The coroner: the Australasian and UK perspectives

Robyn Parker • Jane Terris

AUSTRALASIA

ESSENTIALS

1 The function of the coroner is to investigate and report on a person's death. Where possible, the coroner must determine the identity of the deceased, the medical cause of death and, where relevant, the circumstances surrounding the death. As part of the investigation, the coroner may hold an inquest into the death and may recommend ways to prevent similar deaths in the future. The coroner may also comment on matters of public health and safety.

2 Each jurisdiction has a number of defined circumstances in which the coroner must be notified of a death. A death is considered as being notifiable if it was sudden or unexpected, appears to have been caused by violent, unnatural or accidental means or where the circumstances are not readily apparent. Further investigation may also occur if there is a request by the next of kin to investigate the death.

3 Preparation for a coronial investigation starts as soon as someone dies in reportable circumstances. The body, medical notes and details of all investigations and procedures undertaken in the period leading up to the death may be required by the coroner. Accurate and complete medical notes are an essential part of this process.

4 A coronial inquest is a public inquiry into a death to which a medical practitioner may be subpoenaed. The doctor may be required to give evidence regarding the circumstances of the death or may act as an expert witness.

5 The findings of a coronial inquest in which the performance of an emergency physician or department has been examined should be carefully scrutinized. They may contain important statements regarding the practice of the emergency physician, the functioning of the emergency department and the emergency medical system as a whole.

6 Coronial findings may be used constructively to effect positive change within a department, institution or system. Coronial findings are released for public perusal at the conclusion of the investigation and are sent to the institutions which may be interested in the findings, such as specialist medical colleges and nursing associations.

Introduction

The function of the coroner is to investigate and report the circumstances surrounding a person's death. A coronial inquest is a public inquiry into one or more deaths conducted by a coroner within a court of law. Legislation in each Australian state and territory defines the powers of this office and the obligations of medical practitioners and the public towards it. The process effectively puts details concerning a death on the public record and is being increasingly used to provide information and recommendations for future injury prevention.

As many people die each year either in an emergency department (ED) or having attended an ED during their last illness, it is almost inevitable that emergency physicians will become involved in the coronial process at some stage during their career. Such involvement may be brief, such as the discharge of a legal obligation by reporting a death, or may extend further to providing statements to the coroner regarding deaths of which they have some direct knowledge. Later, the coroner may require them to appear at an inquest to give evidence regarding the facts of the case and, possibly, their opinion. Occasionally, the coroner requires a suitably experienced emergency physician to provide an expert opinion regarding aspects of a patient's emergency care.

Although the inquisitorial nature of the coronial process is sometimes threatening to medical practitioners, their involvement is a valuable community service. In addition, they may obtain important information regarding aspects of a patient's clinical diagnoses and emergency care which may improve the provision of emergency care to future patients.

Legislation

The office of the coroner and its functions, procedures and powers is created by state and territory legislation. The legislation also creates obligations on medical practitioners to notify the coroner of reportable deaths and to cooperate with the coroner by providing certain information in the course of an inquiry. The normal constraints of obtaining consent for the provision of clinical information to a third party do not apply in these circumstances.

The coroner is vested with wide-ranging powers to assist in obtaining information. In practice, the police are most commonly used to conduct the investigation. Under the various Coroners Acts they have the power to enter and inspect buildings or places, take possession of and copy documents or other articles, take statements and subpoena people to appear in court. The coroner has control of a body whose death has been reported and may direct that an autopsy be performed.

As each Australian state and territory legislation is different, emergency physicians must be familiar with the details in their particular jurisdiction. The current legislation in each state and territory is the following:

Australian Capital Territory – Coroners Act 1997
New South Wales – Coroners Act 2009
New Zealand – Coroners Act 2006
Northern Territory – Coroners Act 2011
Queensland – Coroners Act 2003
South Australia – Coroners Act 2003
Tasmania – Coroners Act 1995
Western Australia – Coroners Act 1996
Victoria – Coroners Act 2008.

Reportable deaths

Most deaths that occur in the community are not reported to a coroner and, consequently, are not investigated. The coroner has no power to initiate an investigation unless a death is reported, but may choose to investigate the death at the request of a next of kin or a person who registers themselves as an interested party. If a medical practitioner is able to issue

a medical certificate of the cause of death, the Registrars-General of that state or territory may issue a death certificate and the body of the deceased may be lawfully disposed of without coronial involvement.

In general, to issue a certificate of the cause of death, a doctor must have attended the deceased during the last illness and the death must not be encompassed by that jurisdiction's definition of a reportable death. It is essential that every medical practitioner has a precise knowledge of what constitutes a reportable death within the jurisdiction.

It is uncommon for a doctor who is working in an ED to have had prior contact with a patient during the last illness. Therefore, even if sure of the reason why the patient died, the doctor is often unable to complete a medical certificate of the cause of death. It is quite permissible, and even desirable, under these circumstances, to contact the patient's treating doctor to inquire as to whether that doctor is able to complete the certificate. This process reduces the number of deaths that must be reported and assists families who may be distressed about coronial involvement.

All Australian Coroners Acts contain a definition of the deaths that must be reported. Although the precise terminology varies, there are many similarities between them. In general, each Act has provisions for inquiring into deaths that are of unknown cause or that appear to have been caused by violent, unnatural or accidental means. Many acts also refer to deaths that occur in suspicious circumstances and some specifically mention killing, drowning, dependence on non-therapeutic drugs and deaths occurring while under anaesthesia. The Tasmanian Act goes further to specify deaths that occur under sedation.

As an example, the Victorian Coroners Act 2008 defines a reportable death as a death that is unexpected, unnatural or violent or resulting from an accident or injury. The definition has also been widened to include a death during or after a medical procedure where a doctor would not reasonably have expected the person to die. 'Medical procedure' is defined broadly to include 'imaging, internal examination and surgical procedure'. A reportable death under the Act of 2008 is also the death of a person placed in custody, including deaths involving police or prison officers attempting to take a person into custody.

Despite the seemingly straightforward definitions given in the various acts, there are many

instances where it may not be clear whether a death is reportable or not. Emergency physicians are often faced with situations where there is a paucity of information regarding the circumstances of an event and where the cause of death may be difficult to deduce. Correlation between the clinical diagnoses recorded on death certificates and subsequent autopsies has been consistently shown to be poor. What exactly constitutes unexpected, unnatural or unknown is open to debate and may require some judgement. In all cases, the coroner expects the doctor to act with common sense and integrity. If at all in doubt it is wise to discuss the circumstances with the coroner or assistant and to seek advice. This conversation and the advice given must be recorded in the medical notes.

The process of reporting a death is generally a matter of speaking to the coroner's assistants (often referred to as coroner's clerks), who will record pertinent details and, if necessary, investigate. The report should be made as soon as practicable after the death. A medical practitioner who does not report a reportable death is liable to a penalty.

Even though coroners' offices and the police work closely together, reporting a death to the coroner is not necessarily equivalent to reporting an event to the police. If it is possible that a person has died or been seriously injured in suspicious circumstances, then it is prudent to ensure that the police are also notified.

A coronial investigation

After a death has been reported, the coroner or designated assistant may initiate an investigation. This is most commonly conducted by the police assisting the coroner, with an autopsy conducted by a forensic pathologist.

The body, once certified dead, becomes part of that investigation and should be left as far as possible in the condition at death. If the body is to be viewed by relatives immediately, it is often necessary to make it presentable. This must be done carefully, so as to not remove or change anything that may be of importance to the coroner. If a resuscitation was attempted all cannulae, endotracheal tubes and catheters should be left *in situ*. All clothing and objects that were on (or in) the deceased should be collected, bagged and labelled. All medical and nursing notes, radiographs, electrocardiographs and blood tests should accompany the body if it is to be transported to a place as directed by the coroner.

Medical notes taken during or soon after the activity of a busy resuscitation are often incomplete. It is not easy to recall accurately procedures, times and events when the main task is to prevent someone from dying. Similarly, after death there are many urgent tasks, such as talking to relatives, notifying treating or referring doctors and debriefing staff. It is essential, however, that the documentation is completed as accurately and thoroughly as possible. The notes must contain a date and time and clearly specify the identity of the author. If points are recalled after completing the notes, these may be added at the end of the previous notes, again with a time and a date added. Do not under any circumstances change or add to the body of the previous notes.

In addition to completing the medical notes, a medical practitioner may be requested to provide a statement to the coroner regarding the doctor's involvement with the deceased and an opinion on certain matters. Such a statement should be carefully prepared from the original notes and written in a structured fashion, using non-medical terminology where possible. The statement often gives the opportunity for the medical practitioner to give further information to the coroner regarding medical qualifications and experience, the position fulfilled in the department at the time of the death and a more detailed interpretation of the events. If a statement is requested from junior ED staff, it is strongly advisable for these to be read by someone both clinically and medicolegally experienced.

Providing honest, accurate and expeditious information to relatives when a death occurs assists in preventing misunderstandings and serious issues arising in the course of a coronial investigation. Relatives vary enormously in the quantity and depth of medical information they request or can assimilate after an unexpected death. It is wise not only to talk to the relatives present at the death but also to offer to meet later with selected family members. Clarification with the family of what actually occurred, what diagnoses were entertained and what investigations and procedures were performed is not only good medical practice but can allay concerns regarding management. Such communication, as well as aiding in the grieving process for relatives of the deceased, may avert an unnecessary coronial investigation initiated by relatives seeking answers about the death by contacting the coroner.

If a significant diagnosis was missed or inappropriate or an inadequate treatment given, or a serious complication of an investigation or procedure occurred, assistance and advice from the hospital insurers and medical defence organizations should be sought before talking to the family. However difficult it may be, it is far better that the family is aware of any adverse occurrences before the inquest than for them to harbour suspicions or to get a feeling something is being covered up. Such a conversation should be part of an open disclosure approach to patient care, involving open communication with a patient or family following an adverse or unexpected event. The coroner is far more likely to be sympathetic to a genuine mistake or omission when it has been discussed with the family and the hospital has taken steps to prevent a recurrence.

Expert opinion

Having gathered all the available information regarding a death, the coroner may decide that expert opinion is necessary on one or more points. Commonly, this involves the standard of care afforded to the deceased. It may, however, also include issues such as the seniority of doctors involved, the use of appropriate investigations, the interpretation of investigations and the occurrence of complications of a procedure. The coroner relies heavily on such opinions for the findings and the selection of an appropriate expert is essential.

The person selected by the coroner to give this opinion should possess postgraduate specialist medical qualifications and be broadly experienced in the relevant medical specialty. For events occurring in the ED, a senior emergency physician with over 5 years of experience is usually most appropriate. The specialist medical colleges may be requested to nominate such a person.

The emergency physician requested to give expert opinion must be able to review all of the available relevant information. Such persons must also consider themselves adequately qualified and experienced to provide an opinion and to answer any specific questions the coroner may have requested to be addressed. The doctor must have the time and ability to provide a comprehensive statement and to appear as a witness at the inquest if requested and to act impartially. The doctor should decline involvement if an interest in the outcome of

the case could be implied or if there is a close relationship between the expert witness and any doctors or other personnel who are being investigated as part of the coronial process. Because of the close-knit nature of the medical community, an expert witness is often sought from a location remote from where the death occurred, such as interstate.

A coronial inquest

A coronial inquest is a public inquiry into one or more deaths. Deaths may be grouped together if they occurred in the same instance or in apparently similar circumstances. The purpose of the inquest is to put findings on the public record. These may include the identity of the deceased, the circumstances surrounding the death, the medical cause of death and the identity of any person who contributed to the death. The coroner may also make comments and recommendations concerning matters of health and safety. In some jurisdictions these are termed 'riders'. In addition, as His Honour BR Thorley pointed out, the inquest serves to:

…include the satisfaction of legitimate concerns of relatives, the concern of the public in the proper administration of institutions and matters of public and private interest…

The inquest does not serve to commit people for trial or to provide information for a subsequent criminal investigation.

With broad terms of reference and the ability to admit testimony that may not be allowed in criminal courts, inquests interest many people, not only those who may have been directly involved. They are often highly publicized media events and may provoke political comment, especially where government bodies are involved. A medical practitioner served a subpoena to attend should prepare carefully, both individually and in conjunction with the hospital, and should ensure that he or she has legal representation, either individually or through the hospital insurers. Where the doctor subpoenaed is being provided legal counsel by the hospital, it is vital to ensure that the hospital administrators support the actions of the doctor in relation to the death. It is advised that, in the event of being subpoenaed to a coronial inquest, the doctor seek advice immediately from the appropriate medical defence agency.

Preparation for an inquest begins at the time of the death. Complete and accurate medical notes, together with a carefully considered statement, provide a solid foundation for giving evidence and handling any subsequent issues. Statements containing complex medical terminology, ambiguities or omissions only serve to create confusion. Discuss the case with colleagues who are not directly involved and have the hospital lawyers read the statement before it is submitted.

Appearing at an inquest can be a stressful event, especially if, on a review of the circumstances, a doctor's actions or judgement may be called into question. Professional peer support, as well as legal advice, should be offered to all medical staff. Simple actions, such as a briefing on court procedures and some advice on how to deal with cross-examination, can be of immense value.

A coroner's court is conducted with a mix of 'inquisitorial' and 'adversarial' legal styles. It is inquisitorial in that the coroner may take part in direct proceedings and can question witnesses and appoint court advisers. It is adversarial in that parties with a legitimate interest can be represented in proceedings and can challenge and test witnesses' evidence, especially where it differs from what they would like presented. Interested parties generally attend court and can ask any questions of the doctor through their own legal representative or through the police counsel to the coroner. The 'rules of evidence' are more relaxed in the coroner's court than in a criminal court. Hearsay evidence – that is, evidence of what someone else said to a witness – is generally admissible. Despite these differences, it is important to remember that it is no less a court than a criminal court and demands the same degree of respect and professional conduct one would accord to the latter.

Coronial findings

At the conclusion of an inquest, the coroner makes a number of findings directed at satisfying the aims of that inquest. These findings are made public and are often of interest to those who are directly involved, as well as to a wider audience.

The findings of an inquest in which the conduct of a particular emergency physician, ED or hospital has been scrutinized will be of particular interest. Although it is always pleasing to have either positive or a lack of negative comment delivered in the finding, criticism of some aspect of the conduct of an individual, department, hospital or the medical system in general is not uncommon. Unfortunately, it is often this criticism that attracts the most public attention and, somewhat unfairly, the public perception of our acute healthcare system is shaped by the media's attention to coronial findings.

In the recent past, coroners have commented on inadequate training, experience and supervision of junior doctors, inadequate systems of organization within departments and poor communication between doctors and family members.

Although adverse or critical findings have no legal weight or penalties attached to them, they are in many respects a considered community response to a situation in which the wider population has a vested interest. Used constructively, they can be extremely useful in convincing hospital management that a problem exists and beginning a process for effecting positive change within a department or institution.

THE UK

ESSENTIALS

1 A coroner is an independent judicial officer who may be a lawyer or, sometimes, both a lawyer and a doctor. The coroner, or procurator fiscal in Scotland, is responsible for the investigation of circumstances surrounding death in particular situations. The purposes of the coroner/procurator fiscal service include minimizing the risk of undetected homicide or other crime and reducing public dangers to life and health.

2 Emergency physicians should be familiar with the types of death that require referral to the coroner/procurator fiscal. Less than 50% of deaths are reported to the coroner including deaths potentially due to any trauma, poisoning or other unnatural causes, deaths related to medical procedures and from the effects of an anaesthetic and deaths whose cause is unknown. Deaths that occur while in medical or legal custody should also be reported.

3 The Coroners and Justice Act 2009 introduced changes to the coroner system in the UK, including reforms to the training, structure, appointment and governance of the coronial system. Death certification in the UK, which previously went to a non-medically qualified registrar for permission for burial, must now go through a medically qualified medical examiner attached to a primary care trust for scrutiny and investigation if required.

4 Concise documentation of the clinical circumstances surrounding a death may direct the pathologist towards a detailed external physical and internal examination of the relevant organ or system and acts as a solid basis for the emergency physician to aid preparation of a subsequent statement and examination at inquest.

5 Post-mortem imaging has, in recent years, been used as an adjunct, or sometimes as an alternative, to autopsy, although the scope and indications for its use are still controversial.

6 Emergency physicians should seek assistance from senior colleagues and may require legal advice when asked to prepare a statement for the coroner or procurator fiscal or attend an inquest.

Introduction

The investigation into the circumstances surrounding a death is an important part of a civilized society. Accurate recording of the cause of death serves many purposes, including accurate disease surveillance, the detection of secret homicide and the detection of potentially avoidable factors that have contributed to a death. Various death investigation systems exist around the world. The UK uses the coronial system, Scotland the procurator fiscal. By virtue of the patient population encountered by emergency physicians and the types of deaths that are subject to investigation, emergency physicians may expect to find themselves in contact with either the coroner or the procurator fiscal system during their working lives, thus necessitating an understanding of the workings of these systems.

History of the coroner

The history of the coroner's office is an interesting reflection of events that shaped our civilization and is in constant evolution. The Shipman Inquiry (2003) and the Fundamental review of Death Certification and Investigation (2003) identified problems within the services available to bereaved families and the process of death certification and led to a reform of the system in the UK in the form of the Coroners and Justice Act 2009.

The office of the coroner was established in 1194 and its primary function then was that of protection of the crown's pecuniary interests in criminal proceedings. The coroner was involved when a death was sudden or unexpected or a body was found in the open; however, aside from the duty to ensure the arrest of anyone involved in homicide, the coroner held a significant role in the collection of the deceased's chattels and collection of various fines [1].

Introduction of the Births and Deaths Registration Act in 1836, mandated registration of all deaths before burial could legally occur. This may have arisen out of concern regarding accurate statistical information concerning deaths, but also concern about hidden homicide. Another act introduced the same year enabled coroners to order a medical practitioner to attend an inquest and perform an autopsy in equivocal cases. The Coroners Act of 1887 saw a shift of emphasis from protection of financial interests to the emphasis that remains today, namely the medical cause of

Table 25.2.1 Reasons for an inquest (according to the Broderick committee)

- To determine the medical cause of death
- To allay rumours or suspicion
- To draw attention to the existence of circumstances which, if unremedied, might lead to further deaths
- To advance medical knowledge
- To preserve the legal interests of the deceased person's family, heirs or other interested parties [2]

death and its surrounding circumstances with eventual community benefit in mind.

The Broderick committee was appointed in 1965 to review death certification in response to adverse publicity about inquests and pressures to improve death certification. Their report published in 1971 contained 114 recommendations, many of which were enacted. Table 25.2.1 lists the reasons the Broderick Committee considered the purpose of an inquest [2].

The Coroners Act (1988) states that a coroner shall hold an inquest into a death when there is:

…*reasonable cause to suspect that the deceased has died a violent or unnatural death, has died a sudden death of which the cause is unknown, or has died in prison or in such a place or circumstances as to require an inquest under any Act [3].*

The Coroners and Justice Act 2009 introduced changes to the structure and appointment system for coroners, more flexibility between working areas of coroners and the mandate for all coroners to have held a legal qualification for 5 years, which was intended to standardize practice and ensure sufficient legal understanding for coroners. The new appointment of a chief coroner, with a senior legal background, and with annual reporting to the government, was recommended to be responsible for establishing national training and governance standards and developing a charter for improving services to bereaved families. The death certification system under the Act was modified to provide consistency whether the body is buried or cremated and to ensure that adequate scrutiny of the circumstances around the death happens and is documented. The introduction of a medical examiner attached to a primary care trust to scrutinize all death certificates prior to burial or cremation replaced the previously medically unqualified registrar.

Structure of the coroner system in the UK

Coroners are independent judicial officers who have a legal background, including having been a qualified barrister or solicitor for at least 5 years and, in addition, some may also have a medical background. They are responsible to the Chief Coroner, a senior legal practitioner who must have previously held the position of high court or circuit judge and, ultimately, is responsible to the Crown through the Lord Chancellor. They must work within the laws and regulations that apply to them: The Coroners and Justice Act 2009 replaced the previous framework as described in The Coroners Act 1988, Coroners Rules 1984 and the Model Coroners Charter. There are approximately 148 coroner's districts throughout England and Wales and each district has a coroner and a deputy and possibly several assistant deputy coroners. Coroners are assisted in their duties by coroner's officers, who are frequently police officers or ex-police officers and whose work is dedicated solely to coronial matters. This follows long-established practice and has probably arisen because of the significant proportion of cases in which police are the notifying agent. The nature of a coronial investigation requires a person to possess knowledge about legal matters and skill in information gathering. From a practical viewpoint, the coroner's assistants may be responsible for performing such duties as attending the scene of a death, arranging transport of the body to the mortuary, notification of the next of kin and obtaining statements from relevant parties. Clearly, variation in the structure of the service between regions is inevitable and reflects the size, composition and workload within the district [4].

The 2009 reforms to the coronial process

The UK coronial system underwent fundamental changes following the Coroners and Justice Act 2009, which constituted the first major reforms of the existing system for over 100 years. It included changes to the investigation process for certain deaths previously governed by the Coroners Act 1988. There were also reforms of the certification and registration of deaths. The need for reform was galvanized by several landmark cases including the Shipman Inquiry (2003), in which the system had not identified and isolated a pattern of criminal activities spanning years by the UK

Table 25.2.2 Circumstances in which a death should be reported to the coroner

- The cause of death is unknown
- The deceased was not seen by the certifying doctor either after death or within the 14 days before the death
- The death was violent, unnatural or suspicious (including accident or suicide)
- The death occurred in custody or state detention
- The death may be due to self-neglect or neglect by others, or the result of a medical mishap
- The death may be due to an industrial disease or related to the deceased's employment
- The death may be due to an abortion
- The death occurred during an operation or before recovery from the effects of an anaesthetic
- The death may be a suicide
- The death occurred during or shortly after detention in police or prison custody

Table 25.2.3 Circumstances in which a death should be reported to the procurator fiscal in Scotland

- Deaths that occur unexpectedly involving fault or neglect on the part of another
- Some deaths of children including foster children, newborns, suffocation
- Deaths that are violent, suspicious, unexplained or due to poisoning
- Possible or suspected suicide
- Deaths that are apparently associated with lack of medical care
- Deaths as a result of a medical mishap or as a result of treatment, or absence thereof, including during the actual administration of general or local anaesthetic or which may be due to an anaesthetic
- Any death at work, whether or not due to an accident, or due to occupation or industrial disease
- Any death due to notifiable infectious disease including food poisoning
- Any death in legal custody
- Any death by drowning

GP Dr Harold Shipman, and the Fundamental Review of death Certification and Investigation (2003) which revealed a number of problems and inconsistencies in the process of death certification and the services available to bereaved relatives. Other findings prompting reforms included a lack of leadership and training for coroners and a perceived deficiency of medical knowledge within the system. The structure, training and appointment systems for coroners were changed to include a Chief Coroner, improved training and guidance for coroners, who have to be legally qualified, and powers allowing evidence to be obtained, with search and entry where necessary. Changes to the process for issuing a death certificate include the replacement of a non-medically qualified registrar with a Medical Examiner, reporting to a Chief Medical examiner, who scrutinizes and, if necessary, recommends investigation, following the issuing of the death certificate.

Outline of the coronial system

Upon notification of a death, the coroner makes initial inquiries and may direct a pathologist, who is generally a specialist forensic pathologist, to perform a post-mortem autopsy. Sometimes it becomes clear at this early point that the death is a natural one and does not fall within the Coroners Act, thus no further investigation is required and a death certificate is issued. In other circumstances, further

investigations occur and relevant information is gathered. If the coroner is subsequently satisfied that the death is natural, again no inquest is required. In other cases, or in certain prescribed circumstances, an inquest is held. At the conclusion of an inquest, a finding or verdict is delivered. This verdict must not be framed in a way that implies civil or criminal liability.

Reportable deaths

As opposed to the Australasian situation, there is no statutory obligation in the UK for a doctor or any member of the public to report certain deaths to the coroner, however, an ethical responsibility exists and it is recognized practice to do so in particular circumstances. A 1996 letter from the Deputy Chief Medical Statistician to all doctors outlined these circumstances (Table 25.2.2) [5].

Each booklet of medical death certificates also contains a reminder of the deaths that a coroner needs to consider. The list is not exhaustive.

Scotland

In Scotland, the role of death investigation is undertaken by the procurator fiscal's office, which is also responsible for the investigation and prosecution of crime and also has responsibility for any treasure found within the district! The registrar of births and deaths in Scotland

has a statutory duty to report certain deaths, for example, those due to industrial disease and those occurring during surgery, to the procurator fiscal. The spectrum of deaths investigated is essentially the same as in England and Wales; however, more specific guidelines regarding deaths possibly related to medical mismanagement are provided (Table 25.2.3).

How to report a death

Having determined that a death is reportable, the emergency physician should contact the district coroner's office and notify the details of the deceased. Where doubt exists about the necessity or otherwise to report a death, a doctor should contact that office to discuss the matter further. The discussion and subsequent decision should be recorded in the patient's clinical notes. A death certificate should not be written at this stage.

Handling the body

There appear to be no official guidelines in place regarding handling of the body once death has been reported to the coroner; however, this aspect may be an important component of the subsequent investigation. Any therapeutic and monitoring devices, such as endotracheal tubes, intercostal catheters and intravascular catheters, should be left *in situ*, as determination of their correct placement or otherwise may be relevant to the death investigation. Similarly, it may be important to isolate any equipment (e.g. intravenous infusion pump devices) suspected of being faulty and contributing to the death. In circumstances of suspicious or violent deaths in particular, the body should be not be handled unnecessarily, nor should the body be washed. Important trace evidence that may be crucial for subsequent criminal proceedings could conceivably be lost. For example, in deaths involving firearms, it may be useful for a forensic scientist to swab the deceased's hands for gunshot residue to help confirm or refute the notion of a self-inflicted injury.

Clothing removed from the deceased during resuscitation efforts should be set aside and preferably placed into individual paper bags. Any remaining clothing on the deceased should be left *in situ* [6]. Blood taken during resuscitation attempts, regardless of whether it was processed or not, should not be discarded, but kept refrigerated and its existence indicated to the coroner. The examination of ante-mortem blood samples can provide valuable information, particularly with respect to electrolyte and glucose concentrations, drug concentrations and, in deaths possibly attributable to anaphylaxis, tryptase assay [7].

Documentation

The clinical record of the deceased will usually accompany the body to the mortuary and is scrutinized by the pathologist. Clinical information is crucial in consideration of the cause of death and may help direct the pathologist towards an appropriately detailed examination of the relevant system or organ. The guidelines for appropriate documentation in reportable cases are the same as those that apply to medical record-keeping in general. They should be made contemporaneously or as close to as is possible in a resuscitation environment. Each entry should be dated and the time recorded. They must be legible, objective and the sources of information identified. Any errors made should be crossed out, dated and signed. Likewise, if information comes to hand or is recalled at a later date, that entry should be dated and timed. Finally, the author's name and designation should be clear and all entries signed.

The medical certificate of cause of death (MCCD) is usually written by the medical practitioner who cared for the deceased during their last illness and then passed to a medical examiner attached to the relevant primary care department for scrutiny and investigation if required. The medical examiner may then, if satisfied, authorize burial or cremation or may request further investigation.

Information for families

The 2009 Coroners and Justice Act sought to create a charter of rights for bereaved families in response to perceptions of non-uniform and sometimes inadequate, care and information given to relatives. The next-of-kin of the deceased must be informed that the death has been reported to the coroner and the requirement or reasons for doing so. It is important to inform them that police may be involved in the investigation of the death on behalf of the coroner, but that this does not imply a criminal wrongdoing. Many coroners have a process for meeting with bereaved families to share information and answer questions about the subsequent process. An information leaflet explaining the coroner's work and rights of the next-of-kin is available from the Home Office [8] and should be available in every ED to pass on to bereaved families. Another useful publication written for bereaved families provides information regarding post-mortems and is available from the Royal College of Pathologists [9].

Post-mortems

The coroner may decide upon the initial report of a death that a post-mortem is necessary in order to determine the cause of death or resolve an issue relevant to a coronial inquiry. In 2010, post-mortem examinations were conducted in approximately 22% of cases by the coroner or procurator fiscal, which may still be a relatively high number but represents a steady downward trend in the proportion of post-mortems conducted [10]. Having decided upon the necessity for a post-mortem, the coroner directs a pathologist to conduct a post-mortem. The Coroners Act states that, in fact, the coroner may 'direct any legally qualified medical practitioner' to conduct the post-mortem; however, the Coroners Rules 1984 direct that they should be performed 'whenever practicable by a pathologist with suitable qualifications and experience' and, in practice, most are conducted by Home Office accredited forensic pathologists. Clearly, if the standard of medical care provided by the hospital in which the death occurred is in question, it is inappropriate for a pathologist employed by that hospital to conduct the post-mortem.

Consent from relatives to conduct the post-mortem is not required in coroner's cases. In the event that relatives object to the post-mortem examination, the coroner may delay it to allow them time to obtain legal advice. The adjunct, and sometimes alternative, to autopsy of post-mortem imaging may be seen as more acceptable if the refusal for autopsy is made on religious grounds; however, if the death does fall within the coroner's jurisdiction and a post-mortem is deemed to be necessary, their objection would be over-ridden. Relatives may request a second post-mortem, although this seldom occurs in practice.

The coroner must, in theory, notify certain persons, including the usual medical attendant of the deceased or the hospital in which the death occurred, of the time and date of the post-mortem (Rule 7, The Coroners Rules 1984). In practice, this tends to occur when a desire to be represented at the examination has been expressed to the coroner and, in that instance, a nominated, medically qualified representative (not a doctor whose practice may be in question) may be present to observe the post-mortem.

The issue of tissue retention at autopsy has received worldwide attention. The Human Tissue Act 2004 laid down guidelines around the process of tissue and organ removal and the need for informed consent by relatives. Guidelines issued by The Royal College of Pathologists [11] recommend that, in coroner's cases, clear protocols between the coroner and the pathologist should exist and retention of tissues outside of the above-mentioned context should occur with the agreement of both the relatives of the deceased and the coroner.

Preparing a statement for the coroner

The coroner may request a statement from a doctor involved in the care of the deceased and, while there is no obligation to comply with this request, it is generally in the doctor's interest to do so. The coroner, otherwise, has no option but to compel the doctor to attend court and answer questions. A statement, therefore, that has been carefully prepared with due thought to any issues identified may, indeed, avert the need for an inquest or at least can act as a solid base upon which the examination in court will occur. It is important that the doctor writing the statement understands the circumstances of the death; thus, access to the post-mortem report is often vital and is allowable under Rule 57 of the Coroners Rules. It is generally advisable, except perhaps in circumstances where it is clear that simple, factual background information only is required, to seek legal advice early when requested to provide a statement or attend an inquest.

The statement should be typewritten and contain the author's qualifications, work experience and current employment post. The sources from which the report is prepared, including clinical notes and pathology reports, should be acknowledged and it should be set out in a logical manner, in chronological order. Technical terms should be qualified with an explanation readily understood by a layperson.

It is advisable to have a senior colleague review the statement before submission to the legal representative for final review. The final statement should be dated and signed and a copy kept for future reference.

Inquest

An inquest is a public hearing at which the identity of the deceased and how, when and where the deceased came by his/her death are to be determined. In 2010, only around 10% of reported deaths proceeded to inquest, the remainder being examined 'in chambers'. Inquests (or fatal accident inquiries in Scotland) are mandatory in certain prescribed circumstances, including deaths in prison or police custody and deaths resulting from workplace incidents. In certain unusual circumstances, inquests are held with a jury that is responsible for the final verdict.

The inquest is inquisitorial in nature, where the truth surrounding the circumstances of the death is sought, rather than adversarial, where two or more parties have a particular claim to prove. As with the preparation of a statement for the coroner, it is wise for a medical witness to seek legal advice and possibly representation prior to attendance at an inquest. The legal arena in which they are held is unfamiliar territory to most doctors and they frequently attract intense media scrutiny; thus, involvement in an inquest may be a daunting and stressful experience requiring support from colleagues and friends.

Controversies and future directions

- The coronial system in the UK was seen to be outdated, but took many years to revise. The Coroners and Justice Act 2009, the first major reform of the coroner's service in over 100 years, made changes to the structure, training and governance of the coronial system.
- Post-mortem imaging is emerging as a possible, although controversial, non-invasive alternative to ascertaining cause of death either instead of, or sometimes as an adjunct to, autopsy [12].
- There are ongoing reviews and discussions around the number of coroner autopsies performed, with debates around whether too many autopsies, with too few standard indications, are being performed [13].

References

[1] Knapman P, Powers M. The law and practice on coroners. Chichester: Barry Rose; 1985.
[2] Cordner S, Loff B. 800 years of coroners: have they a future? Lancet 1994;344:799–801.
[3] Coroners Act. 1988 (c.13). <www.hmso.gov.uk>.
[4] Tarling R. Coroner service survey: a research and statistics directorate report. London: Home Office; 1998.
[5] Dorries C. Coroner's courts–a guide to law and practice. Chichester: Wiley; 1999.
[6] Dimond B. Death in accident and emergency. Accid Emerg Nurs 1995;3:38–41.
[7] Burton J, Rutty G. The hospital autopsy, 2nd edn. London: Arnold; 2001.
[8] Home Office. When sudden death occurs–coroners and inquests. London: Home Office; 2002.
[9] The Royal College of Pathologists. Examination of the body after death–information about post-mortem examination for relatives. London: The Royal College of Pathologists; 2000. <www.rcpath.org>.
[10] Allen R. Deaths reported to coroners England and Wales 2000. London: Home Office Research Development and Statistics Directorate; 2000.
[11] The Royal College of Pathologists. Guidelines for the retention of tissues and organs at post-mortem examination. London: The Royal College of Pathologists; 2000. <www.rcpath.org>.
[12] Underwood J. Post-mortem imaging and autopsy: rivals or allies? Lancet 2012;379:100–102.
[13] Pounder D, Jones M, Peschel H. How can we reduce the number of coroner autopsies? Lessons from Scotland and the Dundee initiative. J R Soc Med 2011;104:19–24.

Further reading

National Confidential Enquiry into Patient Outcome and Death. The coroner's autopsy: do we deserve better? <http://www.ncepod.org.uk/2006Report/Downloads/Coronial%20Autopsy%20Report%20 2006.pdf>; 2006 [Accessed Apr. 2013].
The Coroners and Justice Act 2009. <www.opsi.gov.uk>.

25.3 Consent and competence – the Australasian and UK perspectives

Jane Terris • Edward Brentnall

ESSENTIALS

1 Informed consent is an essential process for medical treatment that has ethical, legal and administrative elements. Complexities of the practical situation may result in deviation from the theoretical ideal.

2 Consent may be implied, verbal or written and should always be clearly documented.

3 Consent must be informed, specific and freely given and must cover that which is actually done.

4 The patient must be competent, or have the capacity, to give or to refuse the consent and the default assumption, until proven otherwise, should be that an adult patient has capacity. Patients who are minors or have serious mental health problems or impaired consciousness are examples of those who may not have capacity to consent, although these are not absolute and exceptions may apply.

5 In life-threatening situations, it is often necessary to give treatment without waiting for consent, in which case the emergency physician must be able to demonstrate and document that they were acting in the patient's best interests.

6 The emergency department (ED) environment has unique challenges for the determination of capacity, including lack of privacy and time, lack of a pre-existing relationship with the patient and often lack of knowledge of the various factors that may influence patient choice.

7 Capacity is decision specific. A patient may be deemed competent to consent to one procedure but may not fully understand the implications of another.

8 Assessing capacity and obtaining informed consent for ED treatment are core skills within emergency medicine and should not be delegated to non-ED colleagues although, in complex situations, a supporting psychiatric opinion may be useful.

9 Informed consent discussions must cover the diagnosis, proposed and alternative treatments, no treatment option and the risks and benefits of each.

10 The informed consent process should be driven by the desire to enable and support appropriate treatment choice by a patient, rather than the fear of litigation.

Introduction

Consent is necessary for any clinical intervention performed on a patient and the higher standard of informed consent has become accepted.

Consent is an essential basis for any medical intervention and has ethical, legal and administrative elements [1].

Historically, the need for consent may have been applied more variably than today. The American physician, Oliver Wendell Jones said in 1871 to his students: 'your patient has no more right to all the truth than he has to all the medicine in your saddle bags and should get only so much as is good for him' [2]. Self-determination was addressed in 1914 by Justice Cardozo who said: 'every human being of adult years and sound mind has a right to determine what shall be done with his own body' [3]. The pendulum has recently swung in the direction of patient autonomy and informed choice to the extent that clinicians now need to go to extensive efforts to ensure that enough specific information is given to the patient prior to consent being obtained and the threat of successful litigation, although rare, serves as a potent stimulus to this.

Respect for patient autonomy is enshrined within consent law and to impose care or treatment on patients without respecting their wishes is illegal and unethical.

Consent serves to protect the patient from assault and battery, namely unwanted medical interventions. The more exacting standard of informed consent requires that the patient be given and understand adequate and appropriate information specific to the procedure or intervention to be performed. There is debate around what defines reasonable consent practice in different clinical circumstances. There is also debate around the ethical and legal interpretations of the principles underpinning informed consent, which may vary according to local jurisdiction, subjective interpretation and may, in practice, deviate from the theoretical ideal.

Legally, informed consent protects the patient from assault and protects the clinician from an allegation of assault. On an ethical level, the clinician should aim to facilitate autonomous decision making around treatment goals as jointly agreed with the patient. From an administrative point of view, consent documentation serves as proof of a systematic check that the patient received information concerning, and agreed to, the procedure undertaken. The consent form is only the documentation of consent having been obtained and should not be seen as equivalent to or a substitute for the consent process.

Consent

All medical treatment is based on legal and ethical principles. The four basic ethical principles in medicine are:

- Beneficence: the duty to do the best for the patient.
- Non-maleficence: the duty to do no harm to the patient.

- Autonomy: the right of individuals to make decisions on their own behalf.
- Justice: the fair distribution of resources, incorporating the notion of responsibility to the wider community.

Resources may need to be rationed to ensure fair and equitable distribution and no patient has the right to demand treatment not felt to be indicated by the treating clinician.

There is a requirement that patients consent to the specific interventions proposed, provided they have sufficient information to make an informed choice and are competent to do so. It is the job of the emergency physician to ensure that the patient is sufficiently well informed to make the choices that best meet their own needs in the context of patient-centred care. Legal judgements have centred around the nature of the relevant material risks disclosed and whether the patient was actually given sufficient specific information to make an informed choice, in addition to the determination of whether a particular patient has competence in a specific situation.

The term 'informed decision making' is preferred by some to informed consent as it reflects consideration of patient autonomy [4]. Consent should be considered as a two-way process in emergency medicine, with an exchange of adequate and relevant knowledge between a patient and the emergency physician, or nurse in some circumstances, and the end goal should be to share the aims of treatment, although it has been suggested that the means of getting to the shared end could reasonably be guided by the clinician, if acting in the patient's best interests. Failure to obtain informed consent can lead to prosecution. The risk of litigation is related to patient dissatisfaction due to perceived lack of clinician communication or rapport [5], therefore this should serve to build in good communication skills as an essential part of the consent process.

Consent requires the clinician to take an active role in giving information and choice, while respecting the patient's wishes [6]. The concepts of competence, provision of adequate information and the voluntariness with which consent is given are crucial in the consideration of obtaining valid consent or seeking an informed decision. Treatment without consent may be considered an assault, although the law is generally pragmatic if the clinician is able to demonstrate that they gave the information that most reasonable patients would wish to know and acted in the best interests of the patient, in a manner that most reasonable professionals of similar clinical background and seniority would have done. Judgements may take into account whether the treatment was carried out in an emergency rather than an elective situation and documentation should aim to demonstrate the circumstances under which the decision was taken at the time. There has been debate in both Australian and UK law around what constitutes the reasonable standard of care around consent practices and whether the standard should be that which is thought to be reasonable by a responsible body of professional opinion, known as the Bolam standard [7]. The Bolam ruling was challenged in the Bolitho case [8] which ruled that even expert clinical opinion may be challenged if it was felt to be illogical and not to stand up to analysis. Legal discussion has also centred around precisely what information most patients in a particular situation would want or need to know in order to be considered adequately informed. This principle was the deciding factor in Rogers vs Whittaker [9], in which consent given by the patient was held to be invalid on the grounds of a ruling that insufficiently detailed disclosure by the surgeon did not allow the consent to be informed. Judgements are likely to be subject to location specific jurisprudence and to consideration of the urgency of the situation; however, it should be emphasized that there is a strong need to demonstrate, and to document, that the decision around gaining consent was taken in good faith, with the available evidence at the time, in the patient's best interests.

The patient has the right to self-determination. Consent lies at the heart of the medical contract between the clinician and the patient. Medical investigation and treatment are essentially voluntary acts, which the patient consents to the clinician performing.

Consent may be given in several ways: implied, verbal or written. If the patient voluntarily presents to the emergency department then some degree of consent is implied, although consent must be specific to the intervention proposed. Simply presenting to the emergency department (ED) with a severe headache does not automatically imply consent to lumbar puncture, for example. Such a procedure would usually need sufficient explanation in order that the patient understood what was to be done and the potential consequences of not doing the procedure, before the consent was given. If a doctor says 'put your arm out straight because I need to take some blood for a test' then this may be taken as implied consent for venesection. Written consent is generally sought before more invasive, potentially complex or prolonged procedures, such as procedural sedation for hip relocation in ED and surgery under general anaesthetic. Written consent is not more valid than verbal consent that is documented, but is easier to prove.

Adjuncts to written consent may serve to strengthen both the patient's understanding of the procedure and to protect the clinician. These may include procedure-specific consent forms and patient information leaflets detailing what to expect after local anaesthetic or recovery from procedural sedation.

Consent must be sought after full and relevant explanation of what is to be done and the expected results, risks and the consequences if it is not done. The explanation should, as much as possible, be balanced and realistic in describing the advantages and disadvantages of each option. To present only a one-sided option may be seen as a form of coercion. There is, however, much potential for debate on ethical and legal points of what defines full, relevant and expected. This is not surprising as the literature around informed consent comes from multiple disciplines including clinical, legal and ethical cases and judgements are open to unique interpretation.

In some ways, written consent is the most difficult to establish. It is impossible to cover every outcome and to establish statistical likelihood of those outcomes occurring in every patient. The difficulties lie with the sometimes discordant medical and legal definitions of being specific and of the patient being adequately informed. For simpler procedures, it may be better to have implied or verbal consent, rather than written consent, although every effort must be taken to record in writing details of the discussion surrounding implied and verbal consent. Consent must be informed, specific and freely given and must cover that which is actually done. Informed consent or decision making requires that clear, accurate and relevant information must be given to the patient. Legal judgements have defined the importance of considering what may be material or significant to that particular individual when disclosing information. Essentially, the patient should be provided with information regarding: (1) treatment options; (2) the foreseeable consequences and side effects of any proposed treatment or intervention; and (3) the consequences of not proceeding with the advised treatment. This information should be conveyed in unambiguous terms and in a manner that is likely to be understood by the patient. Language and other communication needs must be met and there must be an opportunity for the patient to ask questions and to reflect on the information given.

The information should be given by the clinician responsible for the intervention or a delegate who is suitably qualified and has sufficient knowledge of the proposed intervention. It is appropriate for a doctor to give advice as to the best clinical options and for the reasons for this professional opinion. Such an opinion is frequently expected and desired by patients and cannot be considered as coercive unless the information has been presented in a manipulative fashion in order to elicit a particular choice. It is important to avoid subtle forms of information bias, for instance, presenting the patient with only the benefits of having a fracture reduced on an operative list under general anaesthetic in order to minimize workflow disruption in ED, without the relevant statistics of complications of general anaesthetic versus those of procedural sedation in the ED.

In Australia, it is common practice for hospitals to assist staff in making their communications contextual and understanding the unique needs and preferences of indigenous patients.

In New Zealand, the Treaty of Waitangi [10] creates a particular specification in relation to Maori, whereupon doctors may be expected to include the extended family in decision making and to allow the family to be present with the patient. There are other cultures that may have similar expectations within the multicultural environments of both Australasia and the UK.

Competence

The terms 'competence' and 'capacity' are often used interchangeably in the context of informed consent. The patient must be competent to give the consent or to refuse.

For consent to be valid, it must be given by a person who has the capacity to make that decision which, generally, will be the patient. The default assumption should be that the adult patient has capacity unless clinical assessment clearly finds otherwise [11]. Indicators that the patient may not have intact capacity and may need a more detailed assessment of

capacity, include decisions at odds with the treatment advice without a rational explanation, decisions that change with no clear justification and decisions taken on the background of failure to understand the discussion around treatment options for any reason. Capacity may fluctuate in either direction, for instance, in a patient with altered cognition due to alcohol or recreational drugs, and it may be necessary to reassess capacity prior to performing the procedure. The assessment of the competence or capacity of adults to make decisions on their own behalf is a functional one that requires more than cognitive testing with a tool such as the mini-mental status examination, although this should be performed and documented as part of the assessment process. Assessment of competence should be sought and conducted by the doctor proposing the treatment or investigation and should not be delegated to other colleagues, although in complex situations of impaired capacity, a psychiatric opinion may be helpful and legally advisable.

The essential elements required to demonstrate competence are:

- the ability to maintain and communicate a choice
- the ability to understand the relevant information
- the ability to appreciate the situation and its consequences
- the ability to weigh the information in a rational fashion.

Questions that may be of assistance in assessing capacity are listed in Table 25.3.1. Third parties, such as relatives, are unable legally to provide consent, although it is frequently assumed that they are; however, it is a long-established practice and frequently a useful exercise to involve relatives in the process

of determining what the patient would have wanted in a particular circumstance. They may also provide valuable information during the process of competence assessment regarding a person's set of values and beliefs, cultural considerations and usual behaviour.

Patients may make an advance statement or living will detailing their wishes for medical treatment should they become incapacitated at a later date in the form of a written document or witnessed oral statement. This is legally binding provided the patient is an adult and was competent at the time made and the statement can be proven to be legally valid and applicable to the current circumstances. This is often difficult to validate in an emergency situation and, if doubt exists about validity, a court ruling should be sought.

Patients who may be incompetent to consent (Table 25.3.2)

Children and adolescents

The legal age of consent in Australasia has changed in the last quarter of a century from 21 to 18 years and, in some circumstances, to 16 years or less. This has occurred against a background of differing ages at which persons may vote, buy tobacco or alcohol, drive cars or engage in sexual activity. There is ongoing debate in both Australia and the UK around the age at which a child may be considered competent to consent, as tested in the cases of Gillick [12] in the UK and Marion's case [13] in Australia (Table 25.3.3). In the UK, the principle of decision making by a proxy grants a parent or guardian, or a designated person or local authority, the right to give consent. If the proxy is unavailable in an emergency, the principle of

Table 25.3.1	Questions for determining competence
Parameter	**Questions**
Comprehension	What is your present condition? What treatment choices have been suggested?
Belief	What do you think is wrong with you? Do you believe that you need treatment? What do you think the treatment will achieve? What do you think will happen if you have no treatment? Why has the doctor recommended this particular treatment for you?
Weighing	How did you reach the treatment decision that you have chosen and what factors helped you make that decision?
Choice	Have you decided whether to accept the treatment choice that was recommended for you? Have you made any other decision about your treatment?

necessity justifies treatment provided it can be demonstrated that any decision is taken in the best interests of the patient.

The most important factor to be considered is the competence of the patient to understand what is wrong and what the treatment entails. This has more to do with intellectual and emotional maturity than chronological age. It would be reasonable for a 14-year-old girl to consent to appendicectomy, but quite unreasonable to expect the same person to understand the consequences of hysterectomy. In a genuine emergency, the care of the patient is the most important factor and the absence of a parent or guardian is not a bar to an emergency procedure. Should treatment of a minor be required and valid consent not obtainable, the steps taken to obtain consent and the reason why the treatment must be carried out must be clearly documented. If at all possible, the opinion of a second equally or more senior clinician should

be documented. Many hospitals require that, in such circumstances, the hospital medical director or delegate give approval. This is simply a means of ensuring that the hospital is aware of the situation and accepts responsibility.

A special situation occurs for children whose parents hold religious beliefs that proscribe the administration of blood products. This creates a situation where the child is incompetent and the parents do not consent. There is now almost standard legislation that allows the attending doctors to certify that blood transfusion is required to sustain life and to then administer the treatment despite opposition from the parents in the best interests of the patient.

Intellectually impaired

For consent to be valid, the patient must be able to understand the nature of the condition, the options available and the treatment being

recommended, plus the material risks and the possible outcome of any potential treatments.

The mildly intellectually impaired patient may be able to satisfy these criteria, but the more severely disabled will not be in a position to give valid consent. In the latter situation, in Australia, the guardian or regional Guardianship Board would have to be involved in all but the most urgent cases and there is legislation that covers the protection and administration of incompetent patients. The Board is available to give timely help and has the authority to conduct hearings, receive evidence and make decisions on behalf of incompetent persons. This provides protection for the patient and the doctor. Emergency physicians should ensure that they are aware of how to contact their local Board, both in and out of working hours.

Mentally ill

A diagnosis of mental illness does not automatically preclude a patient from giving consent. The attending doctor must decide on the competence of the patient to consent. The attending psychiatrist may be in a position to assist. If the patient is not competent then the relevant mental health legislation must be considered. Within Australia, the regional Guardianship Boards should be consulted. In the UK, The Mental Capacity Act Deprivation of Liberty Safeguards protects patients in hospitals or care homes from harm.

In an emergency where life or quality of life is seriously threatened and time is of the essence, the facts should be recorded and

Table 25.3.2 Examples of patients who may not be able to give consent and who may consent for them	
Patient	Proxy consent
Children	Parent, guardian, guardianship board, local authority
Serious mental illness	Parent, guardian, guardianship board
Toxic impairment (drugs and alcohol)	Patient when competent, guardianship board, medical director
Intellectual impairment	Guardian, guardianship board, local authority
Emergency situations	Patient, guardian, medical director, local authority

Table 25.3.3 Examples of relevant landmark legal rulings		
Case	Australia	UK
Bolam, 1957 Patient undergoing ECT was not given any muscle relaxant and sustained fractures. Not warned of this risk by psychiatrist		Ruling that the psychiatrist acted in accordance with a reasonable body of psychiatric opinion in not disclosing small risks of injury. Concept became known as the Bolam test of what a reasonable professional opinion would do or say.
Bolitho, 1997 Case of whether a 2-year-old boy with respiratory problems who died should have been intubated		Bolam test challenged. Ruling that decisions had to stand up to logical scrutiny, whether or not other similar professionals would have taken that decision
Gillick, 1986 Mother of five girls brought case in UK to prevent contraceptive advice being given to under 16s without parental knowledge	Principles of Gillick case were accepted as part of common law in Australia	Some forms of medical treatment (contraceptives in original case) could be prescribed to under 16s without parental consent or knowledge if the child had sufficient maturity and understanding. Ambiguity around what sufficient meant
Marion's case, 1992 Request for sterilization of a girl with intellectual impairment	Recognition of the requirement to respect the autonomy and bodily integrity of the individual	
Rogers vs Whittaker, 1992	Consent deemed invalid on grounds that surgeon had given insufficient detail to inform. View that courts rather than medical professionals, should determine the relevant standard of care. Overturned Bolam standard	

treatment commenced. A sound knowledge of the mental health and guardianship legislation relevant to the region is essential.

Patient disabled by drugs or alcohol

When a patient is temporarily disabled by drugs or alcohol, the situation is less clear. Legal and medical opinions do not always agree, especially in respect of capacity and blood alcohol readings. The absolute legal position is unclear as to whether an intoxicated person can give consent, but there is no doubt that any clinician who acts in the best interest of the patient will always be on solid ground in the event of legal challenge.

Restraint may be justified in order to prevent patients taking their own discharge with adverse consequences. In these complex situations, it is worth considering whether it is better to be sued for assault and wrongful imprisonment or to be sued for the damage that followed to a patient who was allowed to leave. It may be possible to ask the regional Guardianship Board for help in Australia and the hospital medical director for advice in both Australia and the UK, but there will be occasions in which immediate decisions must be taken and the best rule is to do whatever would be the best for the patient in the longer term. Again, documentation at the time and the signatures of witnesses will help if the court is involved.

The emergency patient

There has been little written about the patient who requires emergency care but is temporarily incapable of providing consent. The overriding principle, however, is one of the duty of care owed by the clinician to the patient. There is also an obligation to explain to the patient what has been done as early as is reasonable in the recovery phase.

The emergency physician must know the essentials of consent and the differences between implied, verbal and written consent. A sound knowledge of regional mental health and guardianship legislation is required. There must be adequate and contemporaneous documentation of decisions. If it is clear that the clinician was acting in the best interests of the patient and that the processes followed were deemed

to have been logical and necessary in an emergency situation, it increases the chance that the law will be applied pragmatically.

Emergency physicians work in an environment of multiple simultaneous demands. With respect to critically ill and injured patients, detailed information regarding presentation, past history, cultural considerations and usual level of functioning is often lacking and may, in fact, be wrong. A clinician may have little time to make a detailed assessment before a treatment decision is required. Similarly, the information available at a point in time may be lacking or may change later. Emergency physicians often make complex decisions at short notice with little background information. In situations where decisions have been made on behalf of a patient who is felt to be incompetent, it is important to document carefully the information available at the time and the differential diagnosis and reasons for the course taken. It is good practice also to seek the assistance and advice of a senior colleague where the competence of a patient is in doubt and significant interventions are deemed necessary.

The informed consent process should be driven by the desire to enable and support an appropriate treatment choice by a patient, rather than the fear of litigation and is a core skill within emergency medicine.

Controversies and future directions

- English medical law was influenced by the introduction of the Human Rights Act 1998, with courts having to take into consideration case law of the European Court of Human Rights. Decisions are made on a case-by-case basis and established precedents may not always guide future judgements. There is debate around the importance of medical expert opinion versus the logical legal argument.

- Case law on the issue of what is considered appropriate information to give to patients regarding treatment options points to the need to be as

specific as possible during consent discussions.

- Computerized decision support tools have been suggested as an aid to improve patient understanding.

- The concept of what constitutes a minor, and in what situations, is changing with increased emphasis on the autonomy of the child in some situations.

References

[1] Hall D, Prochazka A, Fink A. Informed consent for clinical treatment. Can Med Assoc J 2012;184(5)

[2] Ted Jr. Oliver Wendell Holmes on telling the patient the whole truth. Pediatrics 1982;69:528.

[3] Schloendorff vs Society of New York Hospital, vol. 211, NY 125, 1914.

[4] Skene L, Nisselle P. High Court warns of the retrospectoscope in informed consent cases: Rosenberg v. Percival. Med Today 2001;October:79–82.

[5] Hickson GB, Federspiel CF, Pichert JW, et al. Patient complaints and malpractice risk. J Am Med Assoc 2002;287:2951–7.

[6] Code of ethics for emergency physicians. Ann Emerg Med 2008;52:581–90.

[7] Bolam vs Friern Hospital, House of Lords, UK, 1957.

[8] Bolitho vs City and Hackney Health Authority, 1997, House of Lords, UK.

[9] Rogers vs Whittaker, High Court of Australia, 1992.

[10] The Treaty of Waitangi, 1840, New Zealand.

[11] Consent – the Basics. Medical Protection Society, UK, April 2012.

[12] Gillick vs West Norfolk and Wisbech Health Authority, House of Lords, UK, 1986.

[13] Secretary, Dept of Health and Community Services V JWB and JMB, High court of Australia, 1992 (Marion's case).

Further reading

Beauchamp TL, Childress JF. Principles of biomedical ethics. 5th ed. New York: Oxford University Press; 2001.

Biegler P, Stewart C. Assessing treatment. Med J Aust 2001;174:522–5.

Braun A, Skene A, Merry F. Informed consent for anaesthesia in Australia and New Zealand. Anaesth Intens Care 2010;38:809–22.

GMC. Consent: patients and doctors making decisions together. General Medical Council, UK. <www.gmc-uk.org/guidance> [Accessed Nov. 2012].

Magauran BG. Risk management for the emergency physician: competency and decision-making capacity, informed consent, and refusal of care against medical advice. Emerg Med Clin N Am 2009;27:605–14.

Medical Practitioners Board of Victoria. Medico-Legal Guidelines. Medical Practitioners Board of Victoria; Melbourne.

Savulescu J, Kerridge I. Competence and consent. Med J Aust 2001;175:313–5.

Stewart C, Kerridge I, Parker M. The Australian medico-legal handbook. Sydney: Elsevier; 2008.

The Mental Capacity Act Code of Practice. <www.opsi.gov.uk>.

World Medical Association. Declaration on the Rights of the Patient. <www.wma.net/e/policy> [Accessed Nov. 2012].

World Medical Association. International Code of Medical Ethics. <www.wma.net/e/policy> [Accessed Nov. 2012].

25.4 Privacy and confidentiality

Allen Yuen • Biswadev Mitra

ESSENTIALS

1 Privacy and confidentiality issues can be related to the physical environment in which care is given or to the personal health information involved in the patient's care.

2 Breaching confidentiality of personal health information now breaks Australian and New Zealand legislation.

Introduction

An individual's right to privacy and confidentiality has gained increasing recognition over the past decade. In an emergency setting, where patients are more vulnerable because of illness or injury, staff are often provided with confidential family and legal information, which would otherwise not be divulged, trusting that this will only be used to assist in the care of the patient. The law preserving confidentiality in public and private hospitals, day procedure centres and community health centres (called 'relevant health services' in the Act) is to be found in the relevant sections of individual state and territory Health Services Acts [1–3]. The section applies to the health service itself, the board of the service or a person who is or was a member of the board, a delegate to a board, a proprietor of such a service or engaged or employed in a service or performing work for it. These people are generally prohibited from disclosing information that could directly or indirectly identify a patient. In addition, the individual state or territory's health records act and the Privacy Act 1988 (Commonwealth) confer statutory privacy rights on patients, whether they are treated in a public or private facility. Both Acts set up complaint procedures for patients who believe confidential information about them has been unlawfully disclosed to a third party. New Zealand has similar legislation [4].

Physical privacy

Emergency departments (EDs) are necessarily designed in an open plan to increase efficiency, observation and communication, but these requirements do intrude on privacy, particularly if cubicles are separated by curtains rather than solid walls. Consultations may be overheard during history taking and when discussing patients with other medical staff or specialists, either directly or by telephone.

Patient privacy incidents occur frequently in an ED, risk factors being length of stay and absence of a walled cubicle. Patients who have their conversations overheard are more likely to withhold information and less likely to have their expectations of privacy met [5]. Privacy and confidentiality are challenged by physical design, crowding, visitors, film crews, communication and other factors [6].

Prior permission should be obtained from the patient to allow students, nurses, other medical officers to be present during history taking, examination and procedures. This applies both in public and private hospitals. Some aspects of privacy in healthcare in the ED relate to confidentiality while being assessed (being overheard, being seen, being exposed and being embarrassed), which relate to ED design, staff awareness, sensitivity and care. ED staff may be unaware how their routine behaviour may infringe on patient privacy [7].

Staff bays are now often enclosed by glass screens to prevent others from hearing details on a patient's history or to prevent patients from becoming unnecessarily alarmed by discussion of serious differential diagnoses, which may need to be excluded. Inappropriate or unprofessional comments by staff may also be heard [8].

When the patient is an adolescent, privacy needs may exclude communication with a parent. An understanding of the relevant informed consent law relating to minors is required [9]. The federal Privacy Act does not specify an age at which a child is considered of sufficient maturity to make his or her own privacy decisions. Doctors need to address each case individually, having regard to the child's maturity, degree of autonomy, understanding of the circumstances and the sensitivity of the information being sought [3].

It is only within the last 5 years that the almost universal 'whiteboard' has virtually disappeared. This was a popular and useful management tool in EDs, displaying the patients' names, working diagnoses, locations and management plans. They were easily visible to anyone who came into the department. To preserve privacy and confidentiality, it was inevitable that they were withdrawn despite strong opposition from ED staff, claiming that this would lead to disruptions in patient care, coordination and flow. These problems did occur during the change-over period, but staff adapted well and the advent of patient-tracking computer systems means that each monitor now provides more clinical information than the whiteboard ever did.

Well-known people (VIPs, politicians, media personalities and sports stars) need even more privacy than others, since they may be accompanied by support staff and, perhaps, a bevy of reporters who may be difficult to control, armed with video cameras and portable recorders. They cannot be restricted until the patient is actually inside the hospital building, after which security is in charge. Even when outside the building, most will accept advice to remain in a provided access zone where they may use their cameras or microphones without intruding on the privacy of other patients or their subject of interest. Hospital staff involved in the care of such patients may also wish to have their own privacy protected. Most hospitals now have media relations officers to take on the role of providing regular updated bulletins.

Healthcare providers

There is also the important matter of privacy for health providers. Whether full names should be displayed on identity badges is debatable. Details of contact numbers and home addresses of consultants, medical staff and nurses must be kept confidential, as there are cases of disgruntled or psychotic patients harassing and stalking clinical staff. Even if the request for contact details is innocent, it is an invasion of a healthcare worker's privacy for that information to be released without consent. In addition to the statutory offences of breaching confidentiality, doctors and other healthcare providers may be sued at common law if they divulge confidential information without a patient's consent. The patient may sue for breach of contract or because the doctor has been negligent in disclosing the information. It should be noted that it is lawful for a health professional to disclose information if:

- some other law requires disclosure
- it can be argued that the person has provided express or implied consent for the disclosure
- it may be in the public interest for the information to be disclosed.

Mandatory reporting

Mandatory reporting overrides privacy laws where they are for the purpose of protection of the health of individuals or communities. Examples are:

- revealing to police or a court the presence of alcohol or any other drug in the breath or blood of a car driver after a motor vehicle accident
- reporting a reportable death or a reviewable death to the coroner
- notification of communicable infectious diseases [10]
- child abuse
- elder abuse
- domestic violence.

This becomes more difficult when there is merely a suspicion, but doctors are protected if they report on this basis only. The laws vary between jurisdictions.

Police

Assistance must be given to the police when a criminal offence has been committed. In such cases, patient name, date of birth, address, nature of incident, description of injuries and conscious state may be released. An opinion of causation must not be stated.

If an injured patient is suspected of being a crime victim or perpetrator and may be a

danger to that patient's or another's life, it is the doctor's civic duty to inform police of the circumstances [11].

If a police enquiry is made by telephone, record the name, station, contact number and request and advise that the information will be obtained and provided. The given contact number must be checked to ensure if it is genuine before providing information, heeding the principles of confidentiality.

With police statements, the doctor should state credentials and experience before giving details of alleged history and physical findings. It is important to be objective and to avoid venturing opinions outside a doctor's area of expertise. It is preferable for all police statements to be written by the ED director, so that a confidential record is kept of all statements issued.

Assistance is also given to help police identify missing or deceased persons.

Blood samples may need to be collected by law for drug or alcohol screening for patients involved in motor vehicle accidents. These are provided to police for testing.

Forensic issues

All deaths from unknown, unexpected, unnatural, accidental, violent or suspicious causes must be reported to the state coroner. This also includes cases of unknown identity, during or after surgery, in custody, a ward of the state, requested by next of kin or where unable to issue a death certificate.

Patient health information

Privacy of patients' health information refers to:

- their medical and social conditions
- their medical records
- any images (still, video or diagnostic imaging)
- results of investigations
- their treatments
- their treating doctors
- specialist and medicolegal reports.

Legislation

Confidentiality of health information has been the focus of legislation over recent years.

The Privacy Act 1988 [1] applied only to the Australian Commonwealth public sector,

but steps were taken early on to introduce it to the private sector, resulting in the Privacy Amendment (Private Sector) Act 2000 becoming law to cover the private (and public) health sector in December 2001 [2]. Patients who have been treated in public hospitals are able to gain access to their medical records by means of the relevant state or territory freedom of information act, e.g. Freedom of Information Act 1982 (Vic). Patients treated in a private hospital, by a private doctor or other private health professional, have a right to gain access under the relevant state or territory health records act, e.g. Health Records Act 2001 (Vic) and also under the Privacy Act 1988 (Commonwealth).

In New Zealand, the Privacy Act was enacted in 1993 and was used to develop the Health Network Code of Practice and Health Information Privacy Code 1994, which was further modified by the Health Information Standards Organization in 2005 [5].

Australian privacy principles [12]

The 13 Australian Privacy Principles (APPs) replace the National Privacy Principles (NPPs) for organizations from 12 March 2014. The APPs are found in the Privacy Amendment (Enhancing Privacy Protection) Act 2012 (Commonwealth). The amendments to the Privacy Act introduce the concept of a 'permitted general situation' and a 'permitted health situation'. The existence of a permitted general situation or permitted health situation is an exception to various obligations in the APPs. A new section 16A outlines seven permitted general situations, where the collection, use or disclosure of personal information about an individual, or of a government-related identifier, will not be a breach of certain APP obligations.

New section 16B outlines five permitted health situations, where the collection, use or disclosure of certain health information or genetic information, will not be a breach of certain APP obligations.

APP1

APP1 requires hospitals or healthcare agencies to have ongoing practices and policies in place to ensure that they manage personal information in an open and transparent way. APP1 introduces a new requirement for agencies to have a clearly expressed and up-to-date policy about the management of personal information by the agency. APP1 specifies the minimum information that should be included in the agency's APP privacy policy. An agency needs to take reasonable steps to make its APP privacy policy available free of charge and in an appropriate form. The agency must take reasonable steps to provide the policy in a particular form if requested by an individual or body. APP1 also requires an agency to take reasonable steps to implement practices, procedures and systems that will ensure compliance with the APPs and any registered APP codes and enable the agency to deal with inquiries and complaints by individuals.

APP2

APP2 deals with anonymity and pseudonymity and allows individuals to interact with agencies while not identifying themselves or by using a pseudonym. Both requirements are subject to certain limited exceptions, including where it is impracticable for the agency to deal with individuals who have not identified themselves or where the law or a court/tribunal order requires or authorizes the agency to deal with individuals who have identified themselves.

APP3

APP3 outlines when and how an agency may collect personal and sensitive information that it solicits from an individual or another entity. An agency must not collect personal information (other than sensitive information) unless the information is reasonably necessary for, or directly related to, one or more of the agency's functions or activities. The APPs impose obligations on agencies regarding sensitive information for the first time. APP3 deals with the collection of sensitive information by agencies, which is not permissible unless certain exceptions apply. An agency must only collect personal information from the individual, unless an exception applies. In EDs, it is sometimes difficult to obtain an accurate history, due to the patients' anxiety about their presenting symptoms. More accurate information may become available after they have had a chance to collect their thoughts, or to affirm areas of their history with family or other witnesses. It is useful to recheck details that may not fit a working diagnosis.

Medication histories are often also inaccurate, since the patient may not be responsible for self-administration or may obtain tablets from a prepackaged dispensing system. Computerized GP letters often have all medications ever prescribed for that patient by the GP practice and, to be accurate, every medication should be checked with the patient or carer to ensure their currency. Patients are not obliged to give their reason for requesting access. Patients do not have immediate right to investigation results. The doctor ordering the tests must be given the opportunity to assess and discuss the results; otherwise there is the risk of misinterpretation.

APP4

APP4 introduces new obligations for agencies in relation to unsolicited personal information. Where an agency receives unsolicited personal information, it must determine whether it would have been permitted to collect the information under APP3. If so, APPs 5 to 13 will apply to that information. If the information could not have been collected under APP3 and the information is not contained in a Commonwealth record, the agency must destroy or de-identify that information as soon as practicable, but only if it is lawful and reasonable to do so.

Computerized patient data must only be accessible to authorized personnel by password-protected access [10].

APP5

APP5 specifies certain matters about which an agency must generally make an individual aware at the time of, or as soon as practicable after, the agency collects their personal information. Patients do have a right to access opinion as well as factual material, including a specialist's report, whether or not the report states that it is not to be shown to the patient without the patient's consent [3].

APP6

APP6 outlines the circumstances in which an agency may use or disclose the personal information that it holds about an individual. If an agency collected personal information for a particular purpose, it must not use that information for any other purpose unless:

- the individual has consented to the use for another purpose
- the purpose is directly related to the purpose for which the information was obtained.

In addition, disclosure is allowed if:

- the agency believes that the use or disclosure is necessary to prevent or lessen a serious and imminent threat to the life or health of the individual or another person
- the use or disclosure is required or authorized by or under law, e.g. the Road Traffic Act requiring disclosure of blood alcohol results
- the use or disclosure is reasonably necessary for enforcement of the criminal law or of a law imposing a pecuniary penalty, or for the protection of the public revenue
- if an agency uses or discloses the information for this purpose, a note of this should be made on the record
- the agency has reason to suspect that unlawful activity or misconduct of a serious nature that relates to the agency's functions or activities has been, is being, or may be engaged in and the agency reasonably believes that the use or disclosure is necessary in order for an agency to take appropriate action in relation to the matter
- the agency reasonably believes that it is necessary to assist any APP entity, body or person to locate a missing person and the use or disclosure complies with rules made by the Commissioner
- it is reasonably necessary for the establishment, exercise or defence of a legal or equitable claim
- it is reasonably necessary for the purpose of a confidential alternative dispute resolution process
- the agency reasonably believes that it is necessary for the agency's diplomatic or consular functions or activities.

APP7

APP7 regulates the use and disclosure of personal information by organizations for the purpose of direct marketing.

APP8

APP8 introduces an accountability approach in relation to an agency's cross-border disclosures of personal information. Before an agency discloses personal information to an overseas recipient, the agency must take reasonable steps to ensure that the overseas recipient does not breach the APPs (other than APP1) in relation to that information. In some circumstances, an act done, or a practice engaged in, by the overseas recipient that would breach the APPs, is taken to be a breach of the APPs by the agency. Hospitals may transfer health information to countries where similar privacy laws exist. Consent needs to be obtained from the patient when in doubt or when sending to countries where no such protection exists.

APP9

APP9 prohibits an organization from adopting, using or disclosing a government-related identifier unless an exception applies. In some settings, such as counselling in HIV/AIDS or sexual health, there are instances where anonymity is requested and granted. In the case of public or private hospital EDs, for providing a safe health service and for billing and rebate purposes, doctors are required to record the identity of the patient [3].

APP10

Under APP10, an agency must take reasonable steps to ensure that the personal information it collects is accurate, up-to-date and complete. An agency must also ensure that the personal information that it uses or discloses is accurate, up-to-date and complete and relevant, having regard to the purpose of the use or disclosure.

APP11

APP11 requires an agency to take reasonable steps to protect the personal information it holds from interference, in addition to misuse and loss and unauthorized access, modification and disclosure. APP11 imposes a new requirement on agencies to take reasonable steps to destroy or de-identify information if the agency no longer needs the information for any authorized purpose, unless:

- it is contained in a Commonwealth record, or
- the agency is required by or law or a court/ tribunal order to retain the information.

APP12

APP12 requires an agency to give an individual access to the personal information that it holds about that individual, unless the agency is required or authorized to refuse to give access by or under the Freedom of Information Act 1982 or any other Commonwealth or Norfolk Island legislation that provides for access by persons to documents. Agencies must respond to requests for access within 30 days. Agencies must give access in the manner requested by the individual if it is reasonable and practicable to do so and must not charge for this access.

APP13

APP13 requires an agency to take reasonable steps to correct personal information to ensure that, having regard to a purpose for which it is held, it is accurate, up-to-date, complete, relevant and not misleading.

New Zealand

New Zealand implemented its Privacy Act in 1993, with 12 principles that are similar to the Australian NPPs [4]. The Privacy Act has 12 information privacy principles:

Principles 1–4 govern the collection of personal information. This includes the reasons why personal information may be collected, where it may be collected from and how it is collected.

Principle 5 governs the way personal information is stored. It is designed to protect personal information from unauthorized use or disclosure.

Principle 6 gives individuals the right to access information about themselves.

Principle 7 gives individuals the right to correct information about themselves.

Principles 8–11 place restrictions on how people and organizations can use or disclose personal information. These include ensuring information is accurate and up to date and that it is not improperly disclosed.

Principle 12 governs how 'unique identifiers' (such as IRD numbers, bank client numbers, driver's licence and passport numbers) can be used.

In 2005, the Ministry of Health released the Health Information Strategy for New Zealand [4], with an emphasis on security of electronic data and maintenance of trust in and integrity of, communication. They developed a Privacy, Authentication and Security (PAS) guide, which brought all the existing relevant documents together [15].

Implementation

Most hospitals now provide brochures to patients on arrival outlining these privacy issues. These are important whether the hospital is public or private [16,17]. ED staff must be aware that some patients will require more detailed explanation before they are prepared to reveal all relevant information and a sensitive approach is needed. Complaints about alleged breaches of privacy may be made

and, if necessary, may be referred to the state health ombudsman or the state or federal privacy commissioner.

Communications

In this electronic era, sending information by facsimile, e-mail or telephone messaging can breach security and ED staff need to take great care to ensure that there is a responsible person receiving the data or that with telephone messages, only the caller's contact details are left. Health details should only be discussed directly with the patient, or parent in the case of a minor.

Medicolegal reports

Medical reports can be provided to lawyers or police officers acting on behalf of a prosecution or defending lawyer, after written consent is obtained from the patient. Such reports are the intellectual property of the doctor writing the report. While a patient has a right to view them, there is no right for a copy to be supplied, unless an appropriate fee for preparation of the report is paid.

Where a lawyer requests copies of medical records, rather than a report, the doctor must check the records to ensure that information collected is not sensitive information and does not contain information about others. Payment may be requested for the costs of reviewing and photocopying.

Research and quality assurance

Patients must be asked for consent before participating in research or quality assurance studies and must be de-identified in any reports. They must be fully informed of the reasons for and the possible side effects of the study.

Complaints and non-compliance

Doctors are advised to obtain their own independent legal advice and notify their medical indemnity/insurance company if they are investigated by the privacy commissioner as the result of a complaint that privacy may have been breached. Monetary fines or imprisonment may result from non-compliance [18].

Controversies

- Release of information on adolescents to parents is a difficult and controversial area.
- Protection of staff privacy is also an issue – should full names be displayed on identity badges?
- There is debate about the extent to which information may be provided to the police or other authorities. Many clinicians feel uncomfortable about providing information to police when pressured.
- Controversy exists about whether reporting of elder and domestic abuse should be mandatory in all regions.
- The security on current computer systems may not be sufficient to protect personal health information.

References

[1] Office of the Federal Privacy Commissioner. National Privacy Principles. The Privacy Act 1988. <http://www.oaic.gov.au/privacy/privacy-act/the-privacy-act>.

[2] Office of the Federal Privacy Commissioner. Guidelines on privacy in the private health sector, Nov 2001. <http://www.oaic.gov.au/privacy/privacy-resources/privacy-guides/privacy-in-the-private-health-sector-november-2001> [Accessed Dec. 2013].

[3] Phelps K, Mudge T. Privacy resource handbook. Canberra: Australian Medical Association; 2002.

[4] Health Information Standards Organisation. Health information strategy for New Zealand. 2005. <http://www.health.govt.nz/system/files/documents/publications/health-information-strategy.pdf>.

[5] Karro J, Dent AW, Farish S. Patient perceptions of privacy infringements in an emergency department. Emerg Med Australas 2005;17:117–23.

[6] Geiderman JM, Moskop JC, Derse AR. Privacy and confidentiality in emergency medicine: obligations and challenges. Emerg Med Clin N Am 2006;24:633–56.

[7] Knopp RK, Satterlee PA. Confidentiality in the ED. Emerg Med Clin N Am 1999;17:385–96.

[8] Olsen JC, Sabin BR. ED patient perceptions of privacy and confidentiality. J Emerg Med 2003;25:329–33.

[9] Baren JM. Ethical dilemmas in the care of minors in the ED. Emerg Clin N Am 2006;24:619–31.

[10] Notifying infectious diseases and blood lead within Victoria. <http://ideas.health.vic.gov.au/notifying.asp>.

[11] Frampton A. Some legal and ethical issues surrounding breaking patient confidentiality. Emerg Med J 2005;22:84–6.

[12] Schedule 1 of the Privacy Amendment (Enhancing Privacy Protection) Act 2012 (Cth) <http://www.comlaw.gov.au/Details/C2012A00197>.

[13] Otlowski MFA. Disclosure of genetic information to at-risk relatives. Med J Aust 2007;187:398–9.

[14] Skene L. Patient's rights or family responsibilities? Two approaches to genetic testing. Med Law Rev 1998;6:1–41.

[15] Information Privacy Bill, March 2007. Western Australia Legislative Assembly.

[16] Treatment of Patient Information at Epworth Hospital, 2001.

[17] Know your rights and responsibilities: private patients hospital charter. Commonwealth of Australia, 2006.

[18] Data breach notification — A guide to handling personal information security breaches. Available from: <http://www.oaic.gov.au/privacy/privacy-resources/privacy-guides/data-breach-notification-a-guide-to-handling-personal-information-security-breaches>. [Accessed Feb. 2014].

[19] Health Records and Information Privacy Act. Office of the New South Wales Privacy Commissioner; 2002.

[20] Information to private health service providers. Health Services Commissioner, Victoria. <http://www.health.vic.gov.au/hsc/resources/phsp.htm> [Accessed Dec. 2013].

[21] Queensland Government Information Standard (IS42A). Queensland Department of Health; Sep 2001.

[22] Code of Fair Information Practice. South Australian Department of Health. <http://www.health.sa.gov.au/Portals/0/Health-Code-July04.pdf> [Accessed Dec. 2013].

[23] Personal Information and Protection Act 2004. Tasmanian Ombudsman. <http://www.austlii.edu.au/au/legis/tas/consol_act/pipa2004361/> [Accessed Dec. 2013].

[24] Northern Territory Government. Health information privacy website: <http://www.health.nt.gov.au/Agency/Freedom_of_Information_and_Privacy/index.aspx> [Accessed Dec. 2012].

[25] Health Records (Privacy and Access) Act 1997. Australian Capital Territory.

[26] The Privacy, Authentication and Security Guide. Ministry of Health, New Zealand; 2005.

25.5 Ethics in emergency medicine

Mike W Ardagh

ESSENTIALS

1 Ethics is about doing the right thing for the patient.

2 The morality of the doctor and the morality of the patient will influence decision making.

3 The two most common ethical dilemmas in emergency medicine concern treating patients who do not consent and stopping resuscitation.

4 When addressing these dilemmas, the application of pragmatic tools assists ethical decision making.

5 The first tool considers the four principles of Beauchamp and Childress, but specifically respect for patient autonomy and the benefits and harms of the treatment options.

6 The second tool helps to determine whether the patient's expressed decision is autonomous by asking three questions:
  a Does the patient know enough?
  b Can the patient think enough?
  c Is the patient free enough?

7 The third tool explores patient competence (can the patient think enough?) by asking if the patient understands:
  a the problem
  b the options for treating the problem
  c the pros and cons of each of the options.

8 Subsequent tools reassure that the ultimate decision is the patient's true autonomous wish.

9 Resuscitation, like any other medical intervention, requires consent to proceed. Presumed consent using professional substituted judgement is a model which may be the best for honouring respect for patient autonomy.

Introduction

To be ethical in emergency medicine is to do the right thing for the patient. However, this can be challenging in the context of urgency, uncertainty and impaired patient competence.

How do we know if we should let the intoxicated head-injured patient leave the emergency department (ED) without being fully assessed? How do we decide if the decision of the elderly lady with the fractured neck of femur not to have surgery should be honoured? How could we possibly know what the unconscious cardiac arrest patient wants?

Briefly, decisions about such cases can be guided by a number of tools for clinicians who work among the ethical complexities of emergency medicine. This approach is based on current, popular bioethics. Although it is reasonably generic, there will be places and times when it fits less well. In emergency medicine, standardized processes are popular and the toolkit below suggests a standardized approach to ethics. However, in practice, ethics must be individualized to the patient in front of us. Good clinicians need to superimpose their own morality and understanding of the patient and the patient's context. This involves a unique interaction with the person the patient is. Ultimately, the aim is to facilitate a process whereby the patient's true autonomous wishes are honoured. The nature of emergency medicine makes this challenging, but not impossible.

Ethics and law

The ethics methodology described here is a relatively simple approach, to be applied in specific cases, taking into account the peculiarities of the patient's medical condition and the patient's 'world view'. However, this methodology, and ethics in general, struggle to arrive at an indisputable, definitive answer. The law, however, intends to arrive at a definitive answer so that a determination can be made regarding the lawfulness of what was done. The law uses a combination of statute (written law) and precedents (previous interpretation of written law in specific cases) to come to this determination. It is a complex methodology which is best applied retrospectively once all the facts are known. In emergency medicine, ethics is an easier model to use as it can be applied prospectively while there is still uncertainty. However, it is the law which is called upon, from time to time, to determine the 'rightness' of medical decision making. Good ethics, well documented, should see the law get behind the medical decision making. However, the decisions of emergency physicians need to be consistent with local law. In reality, this places the emergency physician in a difficult situation, being required to act in keeping with the law, yet with an incomplete knowledge of the law and, at the time of decision making, dealing with many unknowns. Generally, the law is sufficiently consistent to apply ethics with confidence but there are some local differences, particularly regarding how consent might be obtained and who might give it (particularly the acceptance of proxy consent – that is consent from relatives), which should be well known in relevant emergency departments.

Ethical decision making – influences and processes

The words 'ethics' and 'morals' have origins in different languages but their origins have similar meanings – 'the done thing' or 'the right thing to do'. The use of the words in the English language generally has morals or morality as qualities of an individual and ethics as a description or study of those qualities. However, they both relate to 'doing the right thing'.

What encourages us to do the right thing?

An individual's morality is a manifestation of the interactions of many influences, including belief, upbringing, culture, societal influences and professional obligations. Some of these are internal drivers of behaviour (for example, religious or other beliefs), others are 'internalized' (for example, societal codes of conduct which are learnt and become habit) and some are 'external' (for example laws and professional codes which are obeyed for fear of the consequences if not). The relative contribution of these influences varies from person to person and from context to context. Whatever that mix in an individual doctor, it is a prerequisite for ethical practice that the doctor is of good moral character.

The method of decision making we employ might be 'utilitarian' or 'deontological' [1]. A utilitarian approach considers the outcomes of actions and values the positive balance of good over bad (or benefit over harm) that ensues. A deontological approach values actions that adhere to overriding moral principles.

Considering the influences on morality and the methods of decision making we might, for example, be nice to our patients because we are nice people (internal morality), we have learnt that being nice is the right thing to do (internalized morality), the code of ethics of our professional body instructs us to be nice (external morality), we believe that being nice is a governing principle of behaviour (deontology) or we think that being nice means patients are less likely to complain about us (utilitarianism). Of course, these are not mutually exclusive and, in practice, there is a mix of all of these influencing our behaviour.

In addition to the clinician's mix of morality and decision-making methodologies, patients' choices will be influenced by their own morality and 'world view'. Some individuals are influenced considerably by spirituality or religion and some cultures have a predominance of such individuals. A deontological approach has appeal in this context. Some individuals have no such influence and instead are influenced by a rational consideration of utility. Some cultures champion the individual's freedom to determine his or her own destiny. Other cultures consider a group, often a family group, as appropriate to make decisions on behalf of the individual. In some cultures, there is a relatively high level of respect for authority (power differential), so there might be a reluctance to question those of perceived authority, such as doctors. In other cultures, there is less of a barrier to questioning authority, potentially allowing a better exchange of information.

These three dimensions help define the context in which the patient considers ethical decisions: 'belief' versus 'rationality'; 'individualism' versus 'collectivism'; and 'high power differential' versus 'low power differential'. Popular medical ethics of this time tends to come from a Western context of rationality, individualism and relatively low power differential. It is appreciated that this context is not applicable to all. Of most importance, the individual patients we manage have varying positions on each of these three dimensions. Just as one model does not fit all contexts, in the same ED, one model does not fit all patients. One of the challenges we face is to welcome the patient's perspective (context, values, world view) into the process of decision making.

The contributions to our morality and our processes of ethical decision making are a complex and variable mix, but that does not mean we cannot employ a standardized process for decision making. A song varies in sound depending on who sings it – the music does not

---

Box 25.5.1   An ethics toolkit for the ED

- Tool 1: the four principles (of Beauchamp and Childress)
- Tool 2: respecting autonomy
- Tool 3: assessing competence
- Tool 4: reassurance about competence
- Tool 5: confirmation the decision is the right one
- Tool 6: stopping resuscitation

Box 25.5.2   Tool 1: the four principles

1 Respect for patient autonomy
2 Beneficence
3 Non-maleficence
4 Justice

---

change, it is the quality of the voice that makes the difference. So, with the 'tools' that follow – it is the quality of the individual's morality that makes these tools work to best effect.

An ethics toolkit for the emergency department

In emergency medicine there are many aspects of ethics relevant to our practice, including research ethics, professional ethics, ethical issues in resource allocation and so on which, although relevant, are not peculiar to the ED. However, there are two dilemmas which are common in EDs:

❶ treating people who express a desire not to be treated (for example the elderly lady with the fractured neck of femur who refuses surgery and the intoxicated head-injured patient who seeks to take his own discharge)

❷ deciding to stop resuscitation efforts (such as the man in cardiac arrest).

The following 'tools' in ethical deliberation provide a structure for decisions in these two areas (Box 25.5.1).

Tool 1: the four principles (Box 25.5.2)

Beauchamp and Childress [2] combined the traditional principles of Hippocrates (try to help and try not to harm) with a consideration of the rights of the individual to determine their own destiny and the rights of others who might be affected. In so doing, they described four principles that offer a pragmatic structure for deliberation. Although the 'Principlism' of Beauchamp and Childress has attracted criticism, it remains a popular and useful starting point.

Autonomy describes the patient's right to determine his or her own destiny. However, there are occasions in emergency medicine when respecting autonomy is difficult because the patient's competence is impaired or there are other influences undermining his or her autonomy.

Beneficence is the principle of acting in a way that benefits the patient. Non-maleficence, or the principle of avoiding harm, is attributed to Hippocrates. All medical interventions have the capacity to harm and it is unrealistic to expect to 'do no harm'. Instead, we proceed if the benefit/harm balance is acceptable to the patient. When the benefits and harms are determined by the doctor without due consideration of, or in contradiction to, the patient's perception of benefits and harms, the action is termed 'paternalistic' (as a father might treat a child), although 'parentalistic' might be a more appropriate, less sexist term.

Ideally, the benefits and harms of our interventions are reasonably clear before we proceed. For example, the performance of gastric lavage on a non-consenting patient after a trivial overdose several hours earlier is ethically unjustifiable, as there is insufficient benefit to override the principles of respect for autonomy and non-maleficence. Research is an ethical necessity to provide the evidence of benefit and harm, upon which to base decisions.

Justice, or the concept of fairness, is best addressed by questioning whether there are others who might be adversely affected by a particular action. Usually, it does not offer much to the deliberations when considering interventions for an individual in an emergency, but there are exceptions. For example, in a mass casualty incident, the performance of a hopeless resuscitation might be unjust, in addition to harming the patient, if it deprives another person with a greater chance of survival. Or, if the intoxicated head-injured young man were to leave the ED with car keys in his hand and an intention to drive, then there is a potential injustice to other road users, possibly sufficient to override his intention to leave.

In addition, there might be questions about the cost of life-sustaining and other emergency care in comparison to other care, such as hip replacements or immunizations. Although such considerations of 'distributive justice' are important, it is not appropriate for the clinician managing an individual patient to be influenced by such concerns at that time. However, it is very appropriate for clinicians to contribute to debate regarding healthcare funding and policy, but in a meeting room rather than a resuscitation room.

In applying this tool, it is necessary to discuss with the patient the clinical utility (the beneficence and maleficence, benefits and harms, pros and cons) of the therapeutic options and identify the preferred option or options. The patient is allowed the opportunity, as circumstances permit, to deliberate, discuss with others and then express a decision. Urgency and impaired patient competence might limit how much information can be provided to the patient but these barriers should not be used as a reason not to try. Patients should receive the maximum information circumstances allow. In many cases in EDs, the urgency is related to pressures of work rather than real clinical urgency.

Allowing, even encouraging, a discussion with an interchange of questions and answers will enhance the opportunity for the patient to understand what is available. For the patient, the belief that he or she has been able to maintain control, to take time, to say what he or she thinks and to be listened to, is immensely fulfilling. Independent of the clinical outcome, this belief enhances patient satisfaction.

It is inevitable, and appropriate, that clinicians have a preferred option, based on their understanding of the utility of the interventions and their experience of what the average patient in similar circumstances, and the average clinician in similar circumstances, would choose.

The clinicians' preferred option should not be stated 'up front', but may be offered during conversation. The patient might ask what the clinician thinks is best or the clinician may offer it if the patient appears to be struggling to make a decision ('would you like me to tell you what I think would be best?').

If the decision the patient has made is concordant with the clinician's preferred option, then it is appropriate to proceed with that option. If the patient has been given the best chance possible to make a considered, free and informed choice and that choice is the same as the clinicians' preferred option, then it is reasonable to assume a true autonomous choice has been made and to get on with it. If the decision the patient has made is discordant with the clinician's preferred option (as might be the case with the elderly lady who refused surgery for her fractured neck of femur), then it is sensible to proceed to the next tool.

Some would argue that accepting a decision because it is concordant with the clinician's is a thinly veiled parentalism. However, it is unlikely a concordant decision is a wrong one, it is likely that such a decision will lead to ongoing treatment (thereby keeping the options open) and the practicalities of emergency clinicians in an emergency context unravelling the complexity of such a scenario relegate this concern to fine print.

Although a discordant patient choice may well be a true autonomous choice and, therefore, should be honoured, the discordance with the preferred choice is a trigger for a higher degree of scrutiny. The higher degree of scrutiny continues with the next tool.

However, prior to proceeding to that tool it is important to explore (as part of the continuing interaction started above) the reasons for the patient's decision. There might be 'cons' or 'harms' of the preferred choice which can be addressed to the patient's satisfaction, thereby allowing the patient a chance to choose again with a new perception of pros and cons. The clinician should not be coercive in content nor in manner, however, if there are possibilities which would influence the patient's decision, they should be offered. An interaction such as this is permissive, not coercive; 'That's OK and we will respect your decision, but is there any particular reason you are against the operation?' 'OK, I see what you mean. Is there anything we can do so that this is less of an issue for you?'

For example, if it transpires that the elderly woman's main reason for declining surgery for her fractured neck of femur is an intense concept of privacy, with anticipated unbearable embarrassment associated with being in a multibed room, having to use a bed pan and being examined by multiple people, then offering a single room and enforcing a rule of no medical or other students may give her a new balance of pros and cons which changes her decision.

Tool 2: respecting autonomy (Box 25.5.3)

We have arrived at Tool 2, because at Tool 1 the patient's expressed choice was discordant

Box 25.5.3   Tool 2: respecting autonomy

1   Does the patient know enough? (information)

2   Can the patient think enough? (competence)

3   Is the patient free enough? (free from coercion)

with the preferred option of the clinicians. The expressed choice of the elderly lady who refuses to consent to surgery is explicit. The expressed choice of the drunk young man taking his own discharge is not articulated as clearly, but his violent and offensive behaviour and his self-initiated discharge represents a 'discordance' with the choice of the clinicians.

As part of Tool 1, the reasons for the patient's decision have been explored (as opportunity allowed) and any possibilities of mitigating the 'cons' of the preferred option have been explored and the options reconsidered. The patient's decision remains discordant.

There are two questions for the clinicians to consider at this point:

❶ Is this decision a truly autonomous decision?

If the answer to this question is 'no' then the next question is:

❷ Would the patient's truly autonomous decision be different?

If the answer to this question is 'yes', then respecting the patient's autonomy means disregarding the expressed wish of the patient and honouring the truly autonomous wish. It is an important concept that overriding the expressed wishes of a patient (which on the surface appears parentalistic) is done to honour the truly autonomous wishes of the patient (which have not been expressed due to influences undermining autonomy).

To answer the first question ('is this decision a truly autonomous decision?'), it is necessary to consider the elements of autonomy – information, competence and freedom – by asking three questions. See Table 25.5.3, which describes Tool 2. Respecting Autonomy.

The first component of an autonomous decision is sufficient information to make the decision. A patient is at liberty to decline to be informed and to make a decision based on whatever information they consider sufficient.

However, if a lack of information is clearly leading to a decision the patient would not make if sufficiently informed then the decision is non-autonomous.

The second component of an autonomous decision is the ability to deliberate and express a decision. Some refer to this as competence, or decision-making capacity (although both of these terms may have wider definitions). For this chapter, the term competence is used. Is the patient cognitively impaired, thus impairing his or her competence and, if he or she were competent, is it likely he or she would make a different decision? Determining the patient's competence is challenging and is covered more fully in Chapter 25.3. However, a simple approach is outlined in Tool 3.

Are there coercive influences leading the patient to make a decision he or she would not make if free from the influence? In the ED, the most common coercive influence is suicidal ideation secondary to depression. Occasionally, other influences, from family or friends, may be present. The presumption in the ED is that someone who has attempted suicide has a depressive illness which is reversible and that their true autonomous wish (if the coercive influence of depression were reversed) would be to receive treatment to preserve their life. This presumption is not always correct as some suicides might be considered to be 'rational,' 'autonomous' decisions (for instance, the patient with advanced incurable neurological disease). Determining that the patient's choice is free from a reversible coercive influence is very difficult for an emergency department clinician, in the emergency department and in a hurry. In this context, the most senior and qualified assessment should be called upon (the emergency physician or the psychiatrist, for example). However, if unavailable or still uncertain, then it is appropriate to default to the presumption that the patient's suicidality is reversible and that the truly autonomous wish would be to receive treatment to preserve life. This default keeps options open and allows further specialist assessment of psychiatric illness. As such, it is the lesser of two possible errors.

Tool 3: assessing competence (Box 25.5.4)

Tool 3 comes into play because it is believed that the patient's discordant decision might not be their truly autonomous one and the reason relates to possible impaired competence.

The initial test of competence in this step might or might not be definitive. If it is clear the patient 'knows what they are doing,' or it is clear they do not, decision making might be finished at this point. Otherwise, and if there is any doubt, reassurance might be required, as discussed in Tool 4.

Competence mostly is about understanding. An initial assessment of competence can be made by asking if the patient displays understanding of three things. See Table 25.5.4 which describes Tool 3. Assessing Competence.

Does the patient display understanding of the illness or injury, the therapeutic options and the perceived or estimated benefits and harms of the various therapeutic options? If it is clear that they do, then competence can be assumed. If it is clear they do not, then competence can be assumed to be absent. If it is unclear if they understand or not, reassurance can be gained as described below.

Box 25.5.4 Tool 3: assessing competence

Does the patient display understanding of:
1 The problem they have?
2 The options to address the problem?
3 The pros and cons of the options?

Box 25.5.5 Tool 4: reassurance about competence

Does the patient have the capacity for understanding?
- Indications the patient might not have the capacity to understand:
  - low level of consciousness (GCS)
  - intoxication (clinical assessment and/or levels)
  - repetition (perseveration) suggesting short term memory impairment.
- Indications the patient probably does have the capacity to understand:
  - listening, hearing, thinking and expressing a view
  - reason behind the decision.

Box 25.5.6 Tool 5a: respecting the patient's refusal of treatment

Although the patient's refusal of treatment is discordant with our preferred choice, the refusal should be respected, because:
- there are not good beneficent or non-maleficent justifications to override the patient's decision
  OR
- the patient's choice to decline treatment seems to be their truly autonomous wish (the patient appears to know enough, think enough and is free enough)
  OR
- we are reasonably confident that *if* he or she knew enough, *could* think enough and *were* free enough, he or she would most likely give the same answer he or she is giving now.

Tool 4: reassurance about competence (Box 25.5.5)

Competence mostly is about understanding, but there will be supporting information concerning the patient's capacity to understand, which this tool explores.

Observations regarding the Glasgow coma scale (GCS) and intoxication are important, as they provide 'hard data' in the clinical notes (and should be recorded there). However, they are not absolute as they indicate capacity to understand and not actual understanding. A GCS of less than 9 (indicating the patient is not interacting with his or her environment, except non-communicative responses to painful stimuli) will clearly indicate impaired competence as no decision can be made nor expressed. However, a GCS of 14 out of 15 (or even 13 or 12) does not necessarily mean the patient does not understand. The head-injured man who wishes to take his own discharge might be drunk with an initial GCS of 14. This suggests competence might be impaired but does not define incompetence. Incompetence must be proven by a determination that understanding is impaired, by reapplying Tool 3.

Similarly, an early, humane and judicious dose of intravenous morphine for a painful condition (such as for the elderly lady with a fractured neck of femur) does not necessarily render the patient incompetent. If she still indicates understanding then competence should be assumed.

Perseveration is common in mild/moderate head injuries, often manifesting as repeating the same questions over and over ('Hey doc, what happened to me?' 'Why am I here?' etc.). If new information is not being stored, then competence to make important treatment decisions is unlikely to be present.

If the decision the patient makes is discordant with the preferred option, then we have already challenged his or her understanding: 'OK, we well respect your decision but can I please, for my own reassurance, ask you a few questions so that I am sure you understand the decision you are making? Can you tell me what you understand about what has happened to you? Can you tell me what you understand about the operation? Can you tell me what you understand about what will happen if you do not have the operation?' Then, the first part of Tool 4 has asked us to note some potential indicators of impaired capacity to understand. Now, the second part of Tool 4 asks about 'reason', as an indicator of the capacity to understand. Reason (I am making this decision because…) is a powerful indicator of a competent decision. The intoxicated head-injured patient might be asked why he wants to leave. He might answer 'I left my girlfriend at the nightclub with a bloke she fancies. I'm worried about what she's up to.'

Although we might challenge his reason (and counsel him that, if his girlfriend is cavorting while he is in hospital she's not the girl for him), he has displayed reason and it is not our place to challenge 'what makes people tick' (their context, their values, their world view). Instead, we have the task of ensuring patients are making the right choice for them – their truly autonomous choice. Reason in a decision suggests the choice is a competent one and, consequently, probably an autonomous one.

Tool 5: confirmation the decision is the right one (Boxes 25.5.6 and 25.5.7)

At this stage, one of two possible decisions about the patient's discordant decision has been made. A final confirmation for each of these decisions follows.

Box 25.5.6 describes Tool 5a. Respecting the patient's refusal of care. It is important to emphasize that any of these three prove the case. In other words, the presence of any of these three disallows the clinician overriding of the patient's refusal of care.

Box 25.5.7   Tool 5b: overruling the patient's refusal of treatment

Despite the patient's expressed refusal of treatment, we believe the patient's truly autonomous wish is to receive treatment, because:

- There are good beneficent or non-maleficent justifications to treat them

  and
- The patient is non-autonomous because he or she doesn't know enough, can't think enough or isn't free enough

  and
- It is believed that the patient's true autonomous wish is to be treated (*if* he or she knew enough, *could* think enough and *were* free enough).

Box 25.5.8   Tool 6: stopping resuscitation

Presumed consent using professional substituted judgment:

Knowing what I know about the benefits and harms of this resuscitation

and

knowing what I know about the patient and their possible/likely wishes

and

if I could pause the resuscitation, sit the patient up and calmly talk to them, would they consent to resuscitation?

- If the answer is 'yes' then resuscitation proceeds.
- If the answer is 'no' then resuscitation stops.
- If the answer is uncertain, then resuscitation should usually continue (a 'trial of treatment') and the question repeated as resuscitation brings or fails to bring improvement, or more information about the patient's likely wishes is forthcoming.
- As soon as the answer becomes a clear 'no', resuscitation must stop.

Box 25.5.8 describes Tool 5b. Overruling the patient's refusal of treatment. It is important to emphasize that all three are needed to justify treating a patient against expressed wishes. In this case, the truly autonomous wishes of the patient (to be treated) are being honoured.

In the case of the elderly lady who refused an operation for her fractured neck of femur, discussion might reveal that she had understanding of the consequences of her (discordant) decision. Further discussion might confirm the reasons (intense sense of privacy). Both understanding and reason refute any allegation that she has impaired competence. Her decision is a truly autonomous one and should be honoured. However, there is the possibility of mitigating her reasons (redefining the pros and cons) by arranging greater privacy as suggested earlier. Then her truly autonomous choice and the preferred option of the clinicians may become concordant.

The drunk young man became offensive and disruptive and then left the department. Was his refusal of care a truly autonomous one? If not, would his truly autonomous decision be to accept care? Applying Tool 1, there might be concern that his worsening aggression in the context of a violent blow to the side of his head, represents a deterioration consistent with an expanding extradural haematoma needing urgent attention (beneficence and non-maleficence) and that his discordant decision may be non-autonomous. Applying Tool 2, there might be concern that he 'wasn't thinking enough' (had impaired patient competence). Applying Tools 3 and 4 might reveal that he didn't know what day it was, he seemed to need reorientation about where he was and what had happened and, when asked if he understood how serious his injury might be and why he was refusing to cooperate with treatment, he was irrational and incoherent. A decision is made that his refusal of care should be overruled and if reassurance, persuasion, bargaining and threats do not allow treatment to proceed, then the clinical staff should consider the use of drugs and restraint to provide treatment. Tool 5 is used for confirmation that this decision is the right one. Finally, and of great importance, the clinicians must document carefully their reasons for intervention (beneficence and non-maleficence) and how they respected his autonomy (the evidence of incompetence and a belief that his true autonomous wish would be to receive treatment).

Tool 6: stopping resuscitation (Box 25.5.8)

When considering whether to stop a resuscitation, the tools listed above are relevant. But, if the patient is unconscious, there is no expressed indication of his or her autonomous wishes. Respect for autonomy and consent may appear irrelevant, but consent should be obtained for resuscitation, like all other medical interventions.

There is an assumption that resuscitation offers hope of a good outcome (which is true), but does not cause harm (which is false). Resuscitation is often provided with this 'no harm in trying' belief, but without due consideration of the harms of resuscitation nor how the patient would percieve the balance of benefits and harms. The benefits of resuscitation include the avoidance of death and the restoration of good health. However, resuscitation can cause unnecessary discomfort, indignity, false hope, a lingering death, financial and opportunity costs and survival with a poor quality of life [3]. If patients undergoing resuscitation were able to consider the potential benefits and harms of the resuscitation intervention recieved in a calm and rational state, just as a patient might when consenting for elective surgery, then it would not be suprising to find a number declining consent.

Consent, in relation to resuscitation, attempts to determine what the patient would want if able to consider the benefits and harms of resuscitation. Informed consent, as is appropriate for elective surgery, might be inappropriate during resuscitation owing to the urgency of the treatment and impaired competence of the patient. However, if informed consent is not relevant, other forms of consent still are [4]. The two most common forms of consent used in resuscitation scenarios, where there is both urgency and impaired patient competence, are presumed consent and proxy consent.

Presumed consent uses the concept that a reasonable patient under similar circumstances – or this patient if he or she were able to – would consent to the resuscitation endeavours proposed. This form of consent has merit and is commonly employed but, occasionally, attracts criticism as being a form of medical parentalism, in that it may be perceived to be respecting the principle of beneficence, as the resuscitators perceive it rather than as the patient would perceive it.

Proxy consent involves obtaining consent for resuscitation from a family member or other person, who is perceived to be able to speak on behalf of the patient. Proxy consent avoids the criticism of medical parentalism as the decision is taken out of the physician's hands, but it suffers as a model as the decision maker may be unable adequately to receive information, understand it and deliberate during a hurried and rapidly evolving resuscitation.

In addition, the proxy might not reflect the views of the patient. There might be occasional circumstances where the proxy declines resuscitation because of some financial or other benefit that would accrue from the patient's death. More commonly, proxies have a tendency to demand more resuscitation than the patient would have wanted [5,6].

A modification of proxy consent that better addresses the issue of respect for patient autonomy is proxy consent with substituted judgement. This involves not asking what the proxy would want done for the patient, but instead what the proxy thinks the patient would want done. In other words, it attempts to see the resuscitation from the patient's perspective, as the proxy understands it.

Similarly, a modification to presumed consent is presumed consent with professional substituted judgement [7]. In this model, the resuscitators gather as much information about the patient as they possibly can to attempt to understand how the patient would view this decision. This usually involves speaking with the patient's loved ones. Then, with some knowledge of the likely outcome of the resuscitation proposed, based on previous experience and a knowledge of the medical literature, they can exercise their moral imagination by asking *'If I could pause the resuscitation, sit the patient up, talk to him and ask if he wants this resuscitation, what would he say?'* In this way, the patient's autonomy is respected as best it can be under difficult circumstances, by combining a knowledge of the harms and benefits

of the resuscitation with an appreciation of this balance from the patient's perspective, as best the resuscitators can appreciate it.

For example, in a cardiac arrest, the patient's primary care doctor might relay details of the conversation he had with the patient during which the patient expressed a desire not to be resuscitated from cardiac arrest. With that information known, asking the question above would bring a clear *'No, I do not want this resuscitation'*. With that response, the resuscitators have an obligation to stop.

The resuscitation should not proceed if presumed consent using professional substituted judgement is employed and the answer to the question is *'No'*. To resuscitate without regard for the patient's explicit or perceived wishes is a harmful disrespect for his or her autonomy.

Often, and appropriately, a decision to proceed will be made on the basis of a perceived balance of benefit over harm and an uncertainty about what this patient would want. In this case, a 'trial of treatment' keeps options open (by keeping the patient alive) and it allows time to gather a clearer view of the likely benefits and harms of resuscitation (as the patient responds or not to the resuscitation) and the likely desires of the patient (as information about the patient comes from relatives or others). The question is asked again, (*'If I could pause the resuscitation, sit the patient up, talk to him and ask if he wants this resuscitation, what would he say?'*), until a clear *'Yes'* or *'No'* is apparent.

The resuscitators should recognize when the balance of benefit and harm becomes unfavourable from the patient's perspective, by employing professional substituted judgement. When it is clear that the patient would say *'No'* to ongoing resuscitation, the resuscitators have a moral obligation to withdraw resuscitation as they can no longer presume the patient's consent.

The consent model used in resuscitation (proxy or presumed, with or without substituted judgement) will be influenced by the moral dimensions above (especially individualism versus collectivism) and by the legal jurisdiction in which the decision is being made (some may favour a stronger role of proxies in decision

making). The law, like ethics, has the objective of ensuring the right things are done for the patient. Presumed consent using professional substituted judgement aims to achieve this, but clinicians should ensure the model they use is consistent with local law.

Summary

To be ethical in emergency medicine is to do the right thing for the patient. The right thing is what the patient would choose if given the ideal circumstances to exercise autonomy. The difficulty we have is determining what the right thing is. The clinician's morality and methods of weighing ethical issues form a platform for this determination. From this platform the clinician can then apply pragmatic tools, including the four principles, the three questions about autonomy and then the three questions about competence. Further consideration can reassure the clinician about competence and about decisions to treat, or not treat, patients without their consent. In the setting of the unconscious patient undergoing resuscitation, a presumption of consent using professional substituted judgement has the greatest potential to reflect the patient's truly autonomous wishes.

Having made a good ethical decision, the final task is to document it well. Considerations of the benefits and harms of interventions and how the patient's autonomy was respected should be well documented and should be concordant with the events that transpired.

References

[1] Beauchamp TL. Philosophical ethics. An introduction to moral philosophy, 3rd edn. New York: McGraw-Hill College; 2001.

[2] Beauchamp TL, Childress JF. Principles of biomedical ethics, 5th edn. Oxford University Press; 2001.

[3] Ardagh M. Preventing harm in resuscitation medicine. NZ Med J 1997;110:113–5.

[4] Ardagh M. May we practise endotracheal intubation on the newly dead? J Med Ethics 1997;23:289–94.

[5] Mead GE, Turnball LJ. Cardiopulmonary resuscitation in the elderly: patients' and relatives' views. J Med Ethics 1995;21:39–44.

[6] Hauswald M, Tanberg D. Out-of-hospital cardiac arrest resuscitation preferences of emergency health care workers. Am J Emerg Med 1993;11:221–4.

[7] Ardagh M. Resurrecting autonomy during resuscitation – the concept of professional substituted judgement. J Med Ethics 1999;25:375–8.

EMERGENCY AND MEDICAL SYSTEMS

Edited by George Jelinek

26.1 Pre-hospital emergency medicine

Stephen A Bernard • Paul A Jennings

ESSENTIALS

1 Ambulance dispatch is increasingly becoming computerized and this allows for medical determination of response speed and skill set, as well as telephone instructions for cardiopulmonary resuscitation and first aid.

2 Paramedic care of the critically ill or injured patient is similar to initial evaluation and management by an emergency physician.

3 The role of advanced life-support measures, such as endotracheal intubation and intravenous fluid therapy, in patients with severe trauma or cardiac arrest is uncertain.

4 Patients with chest pain and ST segment elevation on 12-lead electrocardiogram should be triaged to a centre with facilities for percutaneous cardiological intervention. If this transfer cannot be achieved with 1 hour, then pre-hospital thrombolysis should be considered.

5 Paramedics have effective treatment for other medical emergencies including cardiac arrhythmias, acute pulmonary oedema, narcotic drug overdose, seizures, hypoglycaemia and anaphylaxis.

Introduction

Ambulance services have the primary role of providing rapid stretcher transport of patients to an emergency department (ED). Increasingly, paramedics are also trained to provide emergency medical care prior to hospital arrival in a wide range of life-threatening illnesses with the expectation that earlier treatment will improve patient outcomes.

Dispatch

Many countries have a single telephone number for immediate access to the ambulance service in cases of emergency, such as 911 in North America, 999 in the United Kingdom and 000 in Australasia. However, the accurate dispatch of the correct ambulance skill set in the optimal time frame is complex. It is inappropriate to dispatch all ambulances on a 'code 1' (lights and sirens) response, since this entails some level of risk to the paramedics and other road users. On the other hand, it may be difficult to identify accurately life-threatening illnesses or injuries using information gained from telephone communication alone, especially from bystanders. Also, it may be inappropriate to dispatch paramedics with advanced life-support training to routine cases where these skills are not required since they then become unavailable for a subsequent call.

In order to have consistent, accurate dispatch of the appropriate skill set in the optimal time frame, many ambulance services are now using computer-aided dispatch programs. These computer programs have structured questions for use by call-takers with limited medical training. Pivotal to accurate telephone dispatch is identification of the chief complaint, followed by subsequent structured questions to determine the severity of the illness. The answers to these questions allow the computerized system to recommend the optimal paramedic skill set and priority of response. This computer algorithm is medically determined according to local protocols and practices and provides consistency of dispatch.

Most ambulance services generally have at least four dispatch codes. A code 1 (or local equivalent terminology) is used for conditions that are considered immediately life threatening. For these, emergency warning devices (lights and sirens) are routinely used.

The possibility of life-saving therapy arriving as soon as possible is judged as outweighing the potential hazard of a rapid response. In a code 2 (or equivalent) response, the condition is regarded as being urgent and emergency warning devices may be used only when traffic is heavy. In a code 3 response, an attendance by ambulance within an hour is deemed medically appropriate. Finally, a non-emergency or 'booked' call is a transport arranged at a designated time negotiated by the caller and the ambulance service.

Despite continuous developments in computer algorithms, accurate telephone identification of life-threatening conditions may be difficult. For example, identification of patients who are deceased (beyond resuscitation) [1], in cardiac arrest [2], or suffering acute coronary syndrome [3] has been shown to lack the very high sensitivity and specificity that might be expected.

The dispatch centre also has a role for telephone instructions on bystander cardiopulmonary resuscitation [4] and first aid. For conditions that are regarded as non-urgent, the dispatch centre may transfer the call to a 'referral service' for the provision of a medical response other than an emergency ambulance. This might include dispatch of a district nurse for a home visit or the provision of simple medical advice with instructions to see a family physician or attend an emergency department if symptoms persist.

Clinical skills

Ambulance treatment protocols vary considerably around the world. Since there are few randomized, controlled trials to provide high quality evidence-based guidance for pre-hospital care, there is still much controversy and considerable variation in the ambulance skill set in different ambulance services.

Many ambulance services provide a number of varying levels of skill set, dispatching ambulance officers trained in basic life support (including defibrillation) to non-emergency or urgent cases (ambulance paramedics) and more highly trained officers (designated as advanced life-support paramedics or intensive-care paramedics) to patients with an immediately life-threatening condition for which advanced life-support skills may be appropriate [5]. In addition, ambulance services may co-respond with other emergency services

(such as fire fighters) to provide rapid-response defibrillation.

The evidence for some of the more common pre-hospital interventions is outlined in the following sections.

Trauma care

Pre-hospital trauma care may be considered as either basic trauma life support (clearing of the airway, assisted ventilation with a bag/mask, administration of supplemental oxygen, control of external haemorrhage, spinal immobilization, splinting of fractures and the administration of inhaled analgesics) or advanced trauma life support (ATLS) including intubation of the trachea, intravenous (IV) fluid therapy, decompression of tension pneumothorax and the administration of intravenous analgesia.

Basic trauma life support

On arrival at the scene of the patient with suspected major trauma, paramedics are trained to perform an initial 'DR-ABCDE' evaluation which is similar to the approach that has been developed for physicians, namely consideration of dangers, response, airway, breathing, circulation, disability and exposure. Of particular importance in the pre-hospital trauma setting are dangers to paramedics from passing traffic, fallen electrical wires and fire from spillage of fuel.

The initial assessment of the airway and breathing includes the application of cervical immobilization in patients who have a mechanism of injury that suggests a risk of spinal column instability. Although decision instruments have been developed to identify patients in the emergency department who require radiographic imaging [6], the accuracy of these guidelines in the pre-hospital setting is uncertain. Spinal immobilization of many patients with minimal risk of spinal cord injury is uncomfortable and may lead to unnecessary radiographic studies [7]. Therefore, the recommendation to immobilize the neck in all cases of suspected spinal-column injury based on mechanism of injury alone is currently being challenged [8]. On the other hand, if spinal cord injury is suspected, patients should be transported with full spine immobilization [9].

Accurate triage of major trauma patients is an important component of trauma care in cities with designated major trauma centres. Triage tools based on vital signs, injuries

and modifying factors, such as age, co-morbidities and mechanism of injury, are used [10]. Paramedic judgement may also have a role, although some injuries, such as occult intra-abdominal injuries, are difficult to detect on clinical grounds [11].

Advanced trauma life support

The role of ATLS by paramedics, particularly intubation of the trachea in comatose patients and intravenous cannulation for fluid therapy in hypotensive patients, is controversial. Although these interventions are routinely used in critically injured patients after hospital admission, studies to date indicate that the provision of ATLS provided by paramedics may not improve outcomes [5,12]. On the other hand, few studies conducted to date have been sufficiently rigorous to allow definitive conclusions and many were conducted in an urban setting with predominantly penetrating trauma rather than blunt trauma. Therefore, many ambulance services continue to authorize advanced airway management and intravenous fluid resuscitation in selected trauma patients, particularly those who are injured some distance from a trauma service.

Intubation

Following severe head injury, many unconscious patients have decreased oxygenation and ventilation during pre-hospital care and this secondary brain injury is associated with worse neurological outcome [13]. In addition, a depressed gag or cough reflex may lead to aspiration of vomit and this may cause a pneumonitis, which may be fatal or result in a prolonged stay in an intensive care unit. To prevent these complications of severe head injury, endotracheal intubation may be performed. This facilitates control of oxygen and carbon dioxide, provides airway protection and is routinely performed in patients with Glasgow coma score <9 following severe head injury after hospital arrival [14].

Most patients with severe head injury maintain a gag or cough reflex and successful intubation requires the use of drugs to facilitate laryngoscopy and placement of the endotracheal tube. The usual approach in the emergency department involves rapid sequence intubation (RSI), which is the administration of both a sedative drug and a rapidly acting muscle-relaxant, such as suxamethonium. It is unclear from the literature as to whether RSI should be performed pre-hospital by paramedics or, alternatively, be performed in an emergency department by appropriately trained physicians.

Pre-hospital RSI performed by paramedics has been reported in numerous studies as having a high success rate [15]. However, it is uncertain whether this procedure is associated with improved outcomes [16]. Recently, a prospective, randomized, trial in adult patients with severe traumatic brain injury reported that paramedic RSI increased the rate of favourable neurological outcome at 6 months when compared to intubation in the hospital by physicians [17]. On the other hand, this study also showed a relatively high incidence of cardiac arrest in the patients who underwent paramedic RSI. Therefore, some uncertainty remains as to the efficacy of this procedure.

Intravenous fluid

Intravenous fluid resuscitation has been shown to worsen outcome in patients with penetrating trauma and hypotension [18]. However, most major trauma in Australasia and Europe is blunt rather than penetrating and few patients require urgent surgical control of haemorrhage. Therefore, the issue of pre-hospital IV fluid for the treatment of hypotension remains the subject of debate.

Supporters of pre-hospital IV fluid therapy suggest that this treatment is intuitively beneficial and that any delay of this therapy increases the adverse effects of prolonged hypotension, which may result in end-organ ischaemia, leading to multiorgan system failure and increased morbidity and mortality. On the other hand, opponents of pre-hospital IV fluid therapy suggest that this therapy prior to surgical control in patients with uncontrolled bleeding increases blood loss due to increased blood pressure, dilution coagulopathy and hypothermia from large volumes of unwarmed IV fluid. Any additional blood loss would increase transfusion requirements and could be associated with increased morbidity and mortality.

There is no evidence from clinical trials for benefit of the administration of IV fluid to bleeding patients in the pre-hospital setting. A meta-analysis of the studies to date suggests that pre-hospital IV fluid does not improve outcomes [5]. Nevertheless, if intravenous fluid is given to patients with hypotension and severe head injury, crystalloid rather than colloid should be given, particularly in hypotensive patients with severe traumatic brain injury [19].

Analgesia

The administration of effective analgesia in the pre-hospital setting for traumatic pain remains a difficult issue for ambulance services. Many paramedics are not trained to administer IV therapy and treatment options are, therefore, limited to inhaled therapy.

Inhaled analgesic treatments include methoxyflurane and oxygen/nitrous oxide. However, while the former is reasonably effective [20], there are concerns with the administration of this agent in an enclosed space, such as the rear of an ambulance, because of the perceived risk of repeated exposures of these analgesics to the paramedics.

Alternatively, the training of paramedics in the insertion of an IV cannula and administration of small increments of IV morphine is increasingly regarded as a feasible alternative to inhalation analgesia. Alternative routes of narcotic administration, such as intranasal administration, are the subject of current studies. For example, the use of intranasal fentanyl has been shown to be equivalent to intravenous morphine [21].

An alternative analgesic agent for paramedic use is ketamine. Ketamine, in addition to morphine, has been shown to be superior to morphine alone for traumatic pain. In a randomized, controlled trial, adult patients with moderate to severe traumatic pain were randomized to receive either 5 mg of morphine followed by ketamine, or morphine alone [22]. Those who received morphine and ketamine reported a significant pain score reduction compared to those who received morphine alone. However, the rate of adverse effects, such as nausea and dysphoria, was higher following ketamine compared with morphine.

Cardiac care

Cardiac arrest

In 1966, external defibrillation was introduced into pre-hospital care and this led to the development of 'mobile coronary care units' in many countries for the delivery of advanced cardiac care for the patient with suspected myocardial ischaemia [23]. This approach was subsequently extended to rapid response for defibrillation of patients in cardiac arrest. Protocols for the management of pre-hospital cardiac arrest are based on the concept of the 'chain of survival', which includes an immediate call to the ambulance service, the initiation of bystander CPR, early defibrillation and advanced cardiac life support (intubation and drug therapy).

The patient in cardiac arrest represents the most time-critical patient attended by ambulance services. For the patient with ventricular fibrillation, each minute increase from time of collapse to defibrillation is associated with an increase in mortality of approximately 10%. However, most ambulance services have urban response times that average 8–9 minutes. Since there may be 2 minutes between collapse and dispatch and 1 minute between arrival at the scene to delivery of the first defibrillation, total time from collapse to defibrillation would usually be approximately 12 minutes. Therefore, current survival rates for witnessed cardiac arrest in urban areas are low [24] and there are even fewer survivors in rural areas [25].

The most effective strategy to improve outcomes would be to decrease ambulance response times. However, this would require very significant increases in ambulance resources and would be an expensive strategy in terms of cost per life saved. Alternatively, response times to cardiac arrest patients may be reduced with the use of co-response by first responders equipped with defibrillators. Such a first responder programme has been introduced in Melbourne, Australia with promising results [26].

The role of advanced cardiac life support (ACLS) during cardiac arrest remains controversial [27]. For example, in a randomized, controlled trial comparing a basic life-support approach with an advanced life-support approach, the rate of survival to hospital discharge was 10.5% for the ACLS group compared with 9.2% for the no ACLS group ($P = 0.61$) [28]. This finding of a lack of efficacy of ACLS during cardiac arrest remained after adjustment for underlying differences between the groups in the rates of ventricular fibrillation, response interval, witnessed arrest or arrest in a public location.

Therapeutic hypothermia after resuscitation from cardiac arrest is used in many hospitals, particularly when the initial cardiac arrest rhythm is ventricular fibrillation. A number of clinical trials have tested whether therapeutic hypothermia should be initiated by paramedics after resuscitation using a bolus of cold IV fluid [29,30] or intranasal cooling [31]; however, the results of these studies do not currently support this therapy prior to hospital arrival.

Acute coronary syndromes

Most ambulance services have protocols for the management of the patient with chest pain where the cause is suspected as an acute coronary syndrome. These protocols usually include administration of aspirin and sublingual trinitrates followed by rapid transfer to an emergency department for definitive diagnosis and management. In addition, pain relief using intravenous morphine may be given by advanced life-support paramedics. The role of supplemental oxygen in patients with ST segment elevation myocardial ischaemia (STEMI) but without hypoxia remains uncertain [32].

While these interventions may decrease symptoms, more recent strategies to improve overall outcomes involve triage by paramedics of patients with STEMI using 12-lead electrocardiography to centres for interventional cardiology [33]. For patients with STEMI who are greater than 1 hour to a cardiac catheterization laboratory (i.e. rural patients), pre-hospital thrombolysis may be considered. In a recent European trial, patients with STEMI who presented within 3 hours after symptom onset but who were unable to undergo primary percutaneous coronary intervention (PCI) within 1 hour were assigned to undergo either primary PCI or fibrinolytic therapy [34]. The primary endpoint of death, shock, congestive heart failure or reinfarction occurred in 12.4% of patients in the pre-hospital fibrinolysis group and in 14.3% of patients in the primary PCI group (relative risk in the fibrinolysis group, 0.86; 95% confidence interval, 0.68 to 1.09; $P = 0.21$). The rates of intracranial bleeding were similar in the two groups (after the dose of fibrinolysis was halved in the over 75 years patients). These data suggest that pre-hospital thrombolytic therapy is appropriate if there is a delay of greater than 1 hour in transport to a definitive centre for PCI.

Cardiac arrhythmias

Some patients with an acute coronary syndrome develop a cardiac arrhythmia during ambulance care. Pulseless ventricular tachycardia is treated with immediate defibrillation and amiodarone by slow IV infusion is recommended for ventricular tachycardia where a pulse is palpable and the patient is alert [35]. However, the pre-hospital drug treatment of supraventricular tachycardia is more controversial. While the use of verapamil or adenosine appears to be equivalent in efficacy [36], many ambulance services require the patient to be transported for 12-lead electrocardiography and management of the supraventricular tachyarrhythmia in an emergency department.

Pulmonary oedema

During myocardial ischaemia, the patient may develop pulmonary oedema and, in these patients, the use of oxygen and glyceryl trinitrates is regarded as useful [37]. Despite common use of non-invasive ventilation (NIV) in the emergency department for patients with acute pulmonarty oedema, pre-hospital continuous positive airway pressure for this indication has not been widely adopted, since the equipment is expensive and oxygen consumption is high. Nevertheless, there is some evidence that continuous positive airway pressure is feasible in the pre-hospital setting, may reduce the need for intubation and may reduce short-term morbidity [38].

Other medical emergencies

Stroke

Early identification and effective management of stroke aims to promote optimal recovery. The ambulance plays an important role in stroke management by triaging patients with suspected stroke to an appropriate hospital. Use of a validated stroke screen tool has been shown to increase diagnostic accuracy in identifying stoke and thus facilitate transfer to a stroke centre. There are a number of published stroke screening tools for paramedic use such as the Los Angeles Motor Score (LAMS) [39] and the Melbourne Ambulance Stroke Score [40] that have been shown to be effective in accurately identifying stroke. Patients suspected to be suffering from a stroke should be preferentially transported to a facility with stroke expertise.

Hypoglycaemia

The patient with hypoglycaemia due to relative excess of exogenous injected insulin will suffer neurological injury unless the blood glucose level is promptly corrected. Treatment of the conscious patient involves orally administered dextrose. For unconscious patients, intravenous 20% dextrose should be administered. For paramedics who are not trained to insert IV cannulae or where IV access is not possible, the administration of intramuscular glucagon is also effective, although this is associated with an increase in the time to full consciousness [41].

Patients who respond to treatment may refuse transport to hospital since they feel they have recovered. However, patients on oral hypoglycaemic agents may later develop recurrent hypoglycaemia [42]. Therefore, transport to hospital in this patient group is recommended.

Narcotic overdose

Patients who inject narcotic drugs may suffer coma and respiratory depression which is readily reversed by naloxone. However, the administration of IV naloxone by paramedics is somewhat problematic, since IV access may be difficult and the half-life of IV naloxone (approximately 20 minutes) may be shorter than the injected narcotic. If the patient awakens and leaves medical care, there may also be a recurrence of sedation. Therefore, many ambulance services administer naloxone via the intramuscular or subcutaneous route. While the absorption via this route may be slower, overall, the time to return of normal respirations is equivalent. To avoid the use of needles, naloxone may also be administered via the intranasal route and this has an equivalent onset time to intramuscular naloxone [43].

Anaphylaxis

Many patients with known severe anaphylaxis are prescribed adrenaline (epinephrine) by their physician for self-administration. The use of intramuscular adrenaline (epinephrine) by paramedics is a safe and effective pre-hospital therapy [44]. Generally, a dose of adrenaline 0.3 mg IM together with IV fluid therapy is recommended as first-line therapy for anaphylaxis with intravenous adrenaline reserved for patients who become severely hypotensive.

Seizures

Out-of-hospital status epilepticus is also regarded as a time-critical medical emergency. The first-line treatment of status epilepticus is usually a benzodiazepine. For many years, this was provided using the IV or rectal route of administration. More recently, there are supportive data that intramuscular midazolam is equally effective to intravenous benzodiazepine [45]. Many ambulance services therefore now authorize midazolam 0.1 mg/kg in the adult patient with seizure, with a half dose considered in older patients.

Controversies and future directions

- Computer-aided dispatch algorithms require further improvement to increase the sensitivity and specificity for the detection of life-threatening emergencies.

- Advanced life support, including intubation and intravenous fluid therapy, by ambulance paramedics for the severe trauma and cardiac arrest patient is unproven and expensive. Further randomized, controlled trials are required to justify these interventions.

- Patients with chest pain and ST segment elevation myocardial ischaemia should be identified with 12-lead electrocardiography and triaged to a centre with facilities for interventional cardiology. There is a possible role for pre-hospital thrombolysis if time to a cardiac catheterization exceeds 1 hour.

- Routine application of cervical spine immobilization interventions on the basis of mechanism of injury alone is being challenged. The utility of clinical examination and decision support tools to identify accurately those at increased risk of spinal injury requires further research.

References

[1] Harvey L, Woollard M. Outcome of patients identified as dead (beyond resuscitation) at the point of the emergency call. Emerg Med J 2004;21:367–9.

[2] Flynn J, Archer F, Morgans A. Sensitivity and specificity of the medical priority dispatch system in detecting cardiac arrest emergency calls in Melbourne. Prehosp Disaster Med 2006;21:72–6.

[3] Deakin CD, Sherwood DM, Smith A, Cassidy M. Does telephone triage of emergency (999) calls using advanced medical priority dispatch (AMPDS) with Department of Health (DH) call prioritisation effectively identify patients with an acute coronary syndrome? An audit of 42,657 emergency calls to Hampshire Ambulance Service NHS Trust. Emerg Med J 2006;23:232–5.

[4] Lerner EB, Rea TD, Bobrow BJ, et al. American Heart Association Emergency Cardiovascular Care Committee; Council on Cardiopulmonary, Critical Care, Perioperative and Resuscitation. Emergency medical service dispatch cardiopulmonary resuscitation prearrival instructions to improve survival from out-of-hospital cardiac arrest: a scientific statement from the American Heart Association. Circulation 2012;125:648–55.

[5] Ryynänen OP, Iirola T, Reitala J, et al. Is advanced life support better than basic life support in prehospital care? A systematic review. Scand J Trauma Resusc Emerg Med 2010;18:62–5.

[6] Hoffman JR, Mower WR, Wolfson AB, et al. Validity of a set of clinical criteria to rule out injury to the cervical spine in patients with blunt trauma. National Emergency X-Radiography Utilization study (NEXUS) Group. N Engl J Med 2000;343:94–9.

[7] Armstrong BP, Simpson HK, Crouch R, Deakin CD. Prehospital clearance of the cervical spine: does it need to be a pain in the neck? Emerg Med J 2007;24:501–3.

[8] Haut ER, Kalish BT, Efron DT, et al. Spine immobilization in penetrating trauma: more harm than good? J Trauma 2010;68:115–20.

[9] Ahn H, Singh J, Nathens A, et al. Pre-hospital care management of a potential spinal cord injured patient: a systematic review of the literature and evidence-based guidelines. J Neurotrauma 2011;28:1341–61.

[10] Sartorius D, Le Manach Y, David JS, et al. Mechanism, Glasgow coma scale, age, and arterial pressure (MGAP): a new simple prehospital triage score to predict mortality in trauma patients. Crit Care Med 2010;38:831–7.

[11] Mulholland SA, Gabbe BJ, Cameron P, Victorian State Trauma Outcomes Registry and Monitoring Group (VSTORM). Is paramedic judgement useful in prehospital trauma triage? Injury 2005;36:1298–305.

[12] Seamon MJ, Doane SM, Gaughan JP, et al. Prehospital interventions for penetrating trauma victims: a prospective comparison between advanced life support and basic life support. Injury 4 Feb. 2013 [Epub ahead of print.]

[13] Chi JH, Knudson MM, Vassar MJ, et al. Prehospital hypoxia affects outcome in patients with traumatic brain injury: a prospective multicenter study. J Trauma 2006;61:1134–41.

[14] <https://www.braintrauma.org/coma-guidelines> [Accessed Mar. 2013].

[15] Hubble MW, Brown L, Wilfong DA, et al. A meta-analysis of prehospital airway control techniques part I: orotracheal and nasotracheal intubation success rates. Prehosp Emerg Care 2010;14:377–401.

[16] Bernard SA. Paramedic intubation of patients with severe head injury: a review of current Australian practice and recommendations for change. Emerg Med Australas 2006;18:221–8.

[17] Bernard SA, Nguyen V, Cameron P, et al. Prehospital rapid sequence intubation improves functional outcome for patients with severe traumatic brain injury: a randomized controlled trial. Ann Surg 2010;252:959–65.

[18] Bickell W, Pepe P, Mattox K, et al. Immediate versus delayed fluid resuscitation for hypotensive patients with penetrating torso injuries. N Engl J Med 1994;331:1105–8.

[19] Cooper DJ, Myburgh J, Heritier S, et al. Albumin resuscitation for traumatic brain injury: is intracranial hypertension the cause of increased mortality? J Neurotrauma 21 Mar. 2013. [Epub ahead of print.]

[20] Buntine P, Thom O, Babl F, et al. Prehospital analgesia in adults using inhaled methoxyflurane. Emerg Med Australas 2007;19:509–14.

[21] Rickard C, O'Meara P, McGrail M, et al. A randomized controlled trial of intranasal fentanyl vs intravenous morphine for analgesia in the prehospital setting. Am J Emerg Med 2007;25:911–7.

[22] Jennings P, Cameron P, Bernard SA, Fitzgerald M. Morphine and ketamine is superior to morphine alone for prehospital trauma analgesia: a randomized controlled trial. Ann Emerg Med 2012;59:497–503.

[23] Eisenberg MS. The C. J. Shanaberger lecture: the evolution of prehospital cardiac care: 1966–2006 and beyond. Prehosp Emerg Care 2006;10:411–7.

[24] Fridman M, Barnes V, Whyman A, et al. A model of survival following pre-hospital cardiac arrest based on the Victorian Ambulance Cardiac Arrest Register. Resuscitation 2007;75:311–22.

[25] Jennings PA, Cameron P, Walker T, et al. Out-of-hospital cardiac arrest in Victoria: rural and urban outcomes. Med J Aust 2006;185:135–9.

[26] Smith KL, McNeill JJ, the Emergency Medical Response Steering Committee. Cardiac arrests treated by ambulance paramedics and fire fighters. Med J Aust 2002;177:305–9.

[27] Stiell IG, Wells GA, Field B, et al. Advanced cardiac life support in out-of-hospital cardiac arrest. N Engl J Med 2004;351:647–56.

[28] Olasveengen TM, Sunde K, Brunborg C, et al. Intravenous drug administration during out-of-hospital cardiac arrest: a randomized trial. J Am Med Assoc 2009;302:2222–9.

[29] Bernard SA, Smith K, Cameron P, Rapid Infusion of Cold Hartmanns (RICH) Investigators. Induction of therapeutic hypothermia by paramedics after resuscitation from out-of-hospital ventricular fibrillation cardiac arrest. A randomized controlled trial. Circulation 2010;122:737–42.

[30] Bernard SA, Smith K, Cameron P, Rapid Infusion of Cold Hartmanns (RICH) Investigators. Induction of therapeutic hypothermia by paramedics after resuscitation from out-of-hospital non-ventricular fibrillation cardiac arrest. Crit Care Med 2012;40:747–53.

[31] Castrén M, Nordberg P, Svensson L. Intra-arrest transnasal evaporative cooling: a randomized, prehospital, multicenter study (PRINCE: Pre-ROSC IntraNasal Cooling Effectiveness). Circulation 2010;122:729–36.

[32] Stub D, Smith K, Bernard S, AVOID Investigators. A randomised controlled trial of air verses oxygen in myocardial infarction study (AVOID Study). Am Heart J 2012;163:339–45.

[33] Le May MR, Davies RF, Dionne R, et al. Comparison of early mortality of paramedic-diagnosed ST-segment elevation myocardial infarction with immediate transport to a designated primary percutaneous coronary intervention center to that of similar patients transported to the nearest hospital. Am J Cardiol 2006;98:1329–33.

[34] Armstrong PW, Gershlick AH. Fibrinolysis or primary PCI in ST-segment elevation myocardial infarction. N Engl J Med 2013. http://dx.doi.org/10.1056/NEJMoa1301092.

[35] Neumar RW, Otto CW, Link MS, et al. American heart association guidelines for cardiopulmonary resuscitation and emergency cardiovascular care part 8: adult advanced cardiovascular life support. Circulation 2010;122:S729–67.

[36] Delaney B, Loy J, Kelly AM. The relative efficacy of adenosine versus verapamil for the treatment of stable paroxysmal supraventricular tachycardia in adults: a meta-analysis. Eur J Emerg Med 2011;18:148–52.

[37] Stiell IG, Spaite DW, Field B, et al. Advanced life support for out-of-hospital respiratory distress. N Engl J Med 2007;356:2156–64.

[38] Plaisance P, Pirracchio R, Berton C, et al. A randomized study of out-of-hospital continuous positive airway pressure for acute cardiogenic pulmonary oedema: physiology and clinical effects. Eur Heart J 2007;28:2895–901.

[39] Nazliel B, Starkman S, Liebeskind DS, et al. A brief prehospital stroke severity scale identifies ischemic stroke patients harboring persisting large arterial occlusions. Stroke 2008;39:2264–7.

[40] Bray JE, Coughlan K, Barger B, Bladin C. Paramedic diagnosis of stroke: examining long-term use of the Melbourne Ambulance Stroke Screen (MASS) in the field. Stroke 2010;41:1363–6.

[41] Howell MA, Guly HR. A comparison of glucagon and glucose in prehospital hypoglycaemia. J Accid Emerg Med 1997;14:30–2.

[42] Fitzpatrick D, Duncan EA. Improving post-hypoglycaemic patient safety in the prehospital environment: a systematic review. Emerg Med J 2009;26:472–8.

[43] Kelly AM, Kerr D, Dietze P, et al. Randomised trial of intranasal versus intramuscular naloxone in prehospital treatment for suspected opioid overdose. Med J Aust 2005;182:24–7.

[44] Jacobsen RC, Millin MG. The use of epinephrine for out-of-hospital treatment of anaphylaxis: resource document for the National Association of EMS Physicians position statement. Prehosp Emerg Care 2011;15:570–6.

[45] Silbergleit R, Durkalski V, Lowenstein D, NETT Investigators. Intramuscular versus intravenous therapy for prehospital status epilepticus. N Engl J Med 2012;366:591–600.

26.2 Retrieval

Marcus Kennedy

ESSENTIALS

1 Mature retrieval systems act as a single point of entry for the referrer, preferably providing services by initiation of a single call to a system-wide phone number.

2 Retrieved patients are often unstable, at the margin of physiological compensation and in need of specialized investigation and intervention. They are often at that phase of an emergency presentation where diagnosis is incomplete, treatment is problem-focused and risk is high. This setting therefore requires special expertise, risk-averse processes and fail-safe systems characterized by anticipation, redundancy, rapid response and reliability.

3 The retrieval environment poses particular risk and technical training regarding platforms, procedures, relevant legislation, communication methods, rescue and escape procedures and equipment performance characteristics is needed.

4 Retrieval crew members must be trained to critical care standard. The skill set they provide must meet the clinical needs of the patient.

5 It is likely that the most complex patients receiving the highest levels of support are also the most likely to be exposed to in-transit critical incidents or equipment failure. Clinical practice in this setting requires the anticipation of such events, vigilance to detect them and rehearsed and standardized problem-solving algorithms to rectify them.

Retrieval systems

The definition of retrieval varies by jurisdiction, however, it includes the interhospital transfer of critical patients using specialized clinical staff, transport platforms and equipment. In most regions, this definition extends to the pre-hospital environment when medical staff crewing is deployed and, in this setting, is termed primary retrieval. In various systems, staff may include medical, nursing, advanced life support (ALS) paramedic or intensive care paramedic (or equivalents) in a range of combinations or crew-mix. Retrieval generally involves the transfer of patients with critical illness or life-threatening injury: situations where the patient requires the highest levels of clinical care and vigilance. Retrieved patients are often unstable, at the margin of physiological compensation and in need of specialized investigation and intervention. They are often at that phase of an emergency presentation where diagnosis is incomplete, treatment is problem-focused and risk is high. This setting therefore requires special expertise, risk-averse processes and fail-safe systems characterized by anticipation, redundancy, rapid response and reliability.

Retrieval is a coordinated process that provides specialized assessment and management, prior to and during transfer of critically ill patients from situations where resources or services are inadequate, to a destination where definitive care can be provided. It aims to deliver the same or higher level of clinical care as that available at the point of referral, thus ensuring that the patient is not exposed to any reduction in the quality of clinical care, despite the inherent risks of the transport environment.

The need for retrieval is related to the limitations of health facilities and the geography of populations. It is a reasonable premise that rural communities have a right to equitable and timely access to critical care medicine; however, it is recognized that there is often an urban/rural divide in regard to the accessibility of healthcare generally and to specialized critical care in particular. Key clinical 'gap' areas exist at both urban and rural and regional levels in regard to trauma, neurosurgery, cardiac and neonatal and paediatric critical care. Advances in medicine and technology are inevitably (at least initially) usually concentrated in major metropolitan centres, thus increasing the need for critical patient transport (e.g. coronary percutaneous procedures, interventional radiology, such as angio-embolization, major trauma centres and paediatric tertiary and quaternary care hospitals. Given that such divides exist and that critical-care transfer is inevitable, retrieval medicine aims to ensure quality of care in transfer in distinction to the somewhat *ad hoc* approach to irregular critical-care transfers that otherwise may be the case in less systematized approaches.

Retrieval systems are often a product of their geography and some services have evolved due to their unique environment. Examples include Nordic systems and alpine systems that have emerged from the demands of challenging altitude and temperature extremes, urban trauma service (such as HEMS London) and systems driven by the tyranny of distance, such as the Queensland retrieval system.

Retrieval systems vary by state and internationally. There are no uniform system designs or standards and, consequently, services vary in their use of transport platforms and crew types (nurse, paramedic, doctor). Staff may be employed by a health department, ambulance service, by contract with a private provider or a retrieval service may utilize hospital personnel. A state service may incorporate several retrieval service providers with central coordination; alternately, systems exist with local governance and responsibility at a district or area level. Transport platforms are generally state owned and operated or contracted; however, non-government-owned helicopters may be part of a state system (and have historically received both benevolent and state funding). In the past, such services were the mainstay of retrieval practice and were often initiated by passionate volunteers, being funded by community donations, corporate sponsorship and government grants. Governance systems for such services and their coordination and performance responsibilities were typically variable. Consequently, retrieval systems have evolved, leading to increased systematization and corporate and clinical governance, aiming at reduction in variation, greater accountability and increased reliability at the system level.

Most countries have progressively moved towards centralized state systems. These are characterized by central coordination centres that use nurses, paramedics and doctors who work together utilizing their complementary skills and experience. Neonatal, paediatric, perinatal and adult retrieval services may be integrated, co-located or separate; however, the trend of recent years is to co-locate these services with common governance, to allow synergies to be realized in regard to operational processes, infrastructure, management, education, research, response platforms and clinical staff.

Most retrieval services have developed similar systems for management of the generic operational processes of: patient referral, case coordination, response and logistics, clinical intervention, and destination determination (Table 26.2.1). In addition, these are usually supported by a formal array of governance elements (Table 26.2.2).

In addition, states may legislate [1] or learned and academic bodies may publish guidelines and standards to promote safe systems of patient transfer, particularly in the critical-care sector [2].

Retrieval processes

Retrieval coordination

Case coordination is at the heart of all retrieval systems. As a process it commences with the initiation of contact from a referral site. It is important for referrers to understand

Table 26.2.1 Elements of operational management of retrieval services
Programme guidelines
Quality reporting
Reporting to Medical Standards Committee
Management guidelines
Data management
Organizational structure
Contracts and memoranda of understanding
Budget and financial system
Annual and strategic planning
Management and data reports

Table 26.2.2 Elements of clinical governance of retrieval services
Guidelines for coordinators
Guidelines for retrieval clinicians
Support staff guidelines
Equipment management systems
Orientation and training
Professional development
Clinical documentation
Case follow up and feedback
Case review and audit
Incident management
Indicator measurement
Credentialling
Performance management

the indications for retrieval and to have clear guidelines (both system and local) to encourage early referral and good decision making. Statewide trauma systems and neonatal paediatric care systems often have well established transfer criteria; however, processes for other clinical groups are often less developed and may be *ad hoc*. Mature retrieval systems act as a single point of entry for the referrer, preferably providing services by initiation of a single call to a system-wide phone number. Coordination staff are appropriately qualified senior clinicians, with specialized training and knowledge. Case coordination fundamentally answers: what are the needs of the referrer and their patient? Are the needs for clinical advice, for organization of transport and crew or for assistance in obtaining an appropriate destination for a critical patient? The coordinator must determine quickly and efficiently the planning and intervention priorities for each case. These may be for immediate care or advice, immediate response, destination planning or consideration of complex decisions involving logistics, crew or transport platforms. Coordinators need to display leadership while at all times taking a systems perspective and avoiding tunnel vision or task fixation.

Coordination must be provided through high performance organizations and, typically, utilizes sophisticated communication technologies, such as multiparty conference calls, telehealth videoconferencing, case recording and comprehensive data management systems.

Coordination of retrieval also implies an ongoing process of communication and feedback with the referrer of case progress, estimated response times and knowledge of patient status changes. During the response and transfer phase the coordination centre maintains communication with response teams, providing logistic support and mission oversight.

Transport platforms

Retrieval services generally use road, rotary wing (helicopter), or fixed wing aircraft response and transport platforms. For international retrieval missions, commercial larger jet transport is used and, in uncommon settings, aquatic transport platforms may be used. In consideration of platform selection for a mission, clinical factors must be factored first; these will include need for pressurization, need for space for specialized crew or equipment and patient size. Further to these factors, urgency (of response or return leg or both outbound and return components), distance to referral hospital, availability of helipads at referral and destination hospitals and need to minimize the out-of-hospital time for the patient. Heightened risk for patients in transit is experienced during platform transfers (from bed to trolley to ambulance to aircraft stretcher and so on) and, in general terms, in the out-of-hospital setting. Minimization of number of patient transfers and the out-of-hospital time for the critical care retrieval patient are important principles.

Road transport platforms should be specifically designed and fitted out for retrieval purposes to minimize variation (improving crew performance and safety) and the risk of *ad hoc* unsecured equipment placement. Use of helicopters (with crews of appropriate skill mix) in retrieval response has been demonstrated to improve patient outcomes [3,4], particularly patients with severe trauma and others with a need for time-critical interventions. In general, helicopter transfer is considered for retrieval of patients approximately 75–175 km from base, with road response used for shorter transfers and fixed wing for longer. These broad recommendations vary depending on road, geography and climatic conditions and on the performance characteristics and landing options for individual aircraft. Fixed wing transfers have the advantage of providing a (usually) pressurized aircraft, greater speed and comfort, more space and a controlled temperature. Rotary wing aircraft have advantages of door-to-door transfer where helipads exist at referral and destination sites, the primary response capability and the potential to avoid road transport legs, and multiple patient transfers. Road transfer offers spatial flexibility, door-to-door transfer and cost efficiency (Fig. 26.2.1).

Crew

Staff selected for roles in retrieval must meet required professional and personal standards. Critical-care capability is essential and medical staff specialist training in a critical-care specialty is desirable. Similarly, nursing and paramedic staff must be trained to intensive care practitioner level. In addition, all staff must have specific training in management of the retrieval environment, clinical care in transport settings and personal and crew behaviours.

The retrieval environment poses particular risk and technical training regarding platforms, procedures, relevant legislation, communication methods, rescue and escape procedures and equipment performance characteristics is needed. Training in clinical care during retrieval needs to ensure capability in management of the complete range of critical care, trauma and intensive care scenarios and an ability to apply depth of clinical knowledge to the relatively compact window of patient care that the retrieval mission represents. Practitioners need to understand in a retrieval setting that an intervention may be possible and ideal while also being inappropriate and inefficient or, that an intervention may be desirable but not be possible or practical. Compromise and pragmatism have a role in pre- and interhospital transfer particularly where priority exists for

reaching a definitive care destination. Training in personal and crew behaviours is necessary to optimize the cohesiveness and functionality of the retrieval team – formal exposure to crisis resource management tools is a standard component of aeromedical and road-based retrieval education [5]. In interaction with referring practitioners and primary responders, the retrieval team needs to exhibit empathy, listening skills and professional behaviours – avoiding arrogance, premature conclusions or judgemental behaviour. The training and knowledge base required is significant, therefore training processes must be formalized and must be supported by ongoing professional development and regular credentialling in addition to compliance with relevant regulations.

Crew safety is paramount, so personal protective equipment and clothing which meets aviation and ambulance service standards is mandatory. Safety risk arises also in long and overnight missions and crewing must be adequate to allow sharing of clinical vigilance duties and patient interventions at times of fatigue and to allow for adequate breaks and rest.

Retrieval services play a major role in disaster response and management and generally provide a significant component of the early response to such incidents. Retrieval services and, in particular, their coordination processes are also key to the distribution and reception phase of the disaster response – providing system overview of capability and capacity of health services to receive victims. Retrieval staff must therefore be trained to expert status in this discipline [2,6].

Skill sets

Retrieval medicine and primary response aeromedical settings provide the most challenging of all clinical environments and, therefore, choice of staff skill sets and professional team makeup is fundamental to optimizing clinical outcomes. The central tenets of this clinical environment are that a critical-care retrieval team must consist of (at least) two professionals [6]. They must be trained to critical-care standard and work within their core scope of practice. The skill set they provide must meet the clinical needs of the patient. In most national and international jurisdictions, blended medical practitioner and paramedic or nursing crews satisfy these tenets. Significant literature supports the role of medical practitioners in this environment due to the additional diagnostic capability, procedural range, extent of knowledge and depth of clinical understanding they contribute [7]. Such skills are complemented by the skill set of critical-care-trained nursing staff. Paramedic staff contribute substantial critical-care capability (depending on individual jurisdictional training levels) together with expertise in the transport and pre-hospital scene environments. Crews comprised of paramedic or nursing staff paired in various combinations and without a medical crew member are appropriate for lower risk critical-care transfers, or for non-critical-care retrieval. Skill set needs to match the requirements of the patient in the basic dimensions of clinical complexity and physiological stability; the more unstable and complex patient clearly requiring a higher skill mix in the retrieval team. In rare situations, and where life-saving intervention may be possible, the transport of highly specialized clinical staff to the patient may be appropriate and should be considered, for example, transporting a surgeon to perform an infield amputation on an entrapped patient (Fig. 26.2.2).

Equipment

Within a retrieval service, equipment should be standardized as far as possible. Response kits and platform layouts will then be familiar to all practitioners at all times, including at night and during uncontrolled clinical emergencies. Equipment must meet the needs of the patient population or therapeutic interventions and must consider the operating environment, mission duration, availability of electrical power in transport platforms, oxygen consumption and standard oxygen supplies available in vehicles.

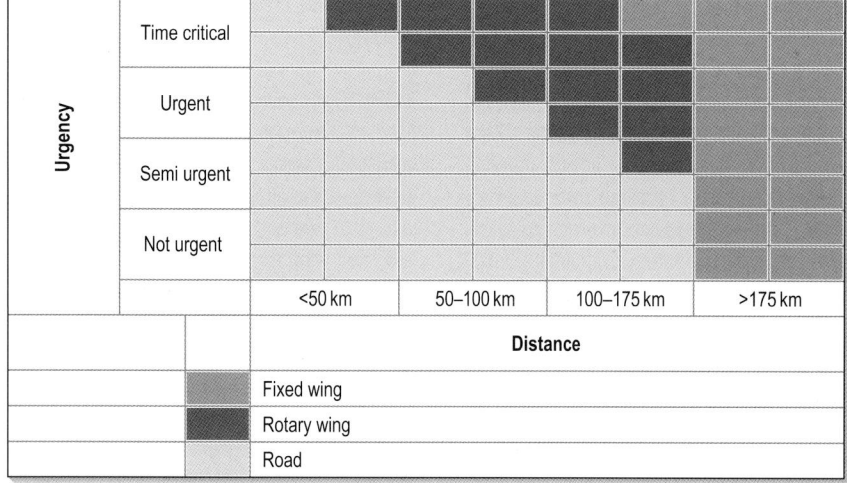

Fig. 26.2.1 Retrieval transport platform allocation grid for fixed wing, helicopter and road transport based on distance vs transport urgency of either the response leg or the patient transfer leg of the retrieval mission.

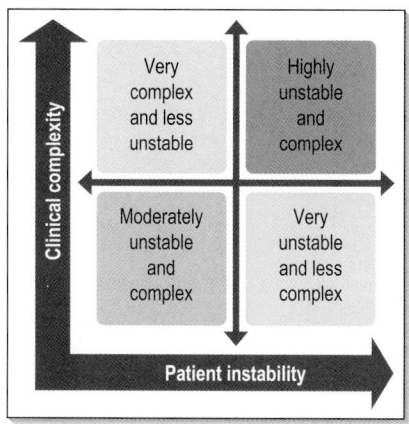

Fig. 26.2.2 Crew skill set matches the clinical requirements of the patient.

Stretchers and equipment bridges must meet aviation engineering standards, as must all electrical equipment that may be used in aircraft.

On all missions, the retrieval practitioner must have access to the complete range of airway management equipment including a difficult airway kit, cardiac monitor defibrillator pacer, multiple infusion pumps appropriate for inotrope infusions, a transport ventilator capable of complex respiratory support, invasive pressure monitoring, temperature monitoring, capnography and oximetry. All equipment must be maintained to the highest level of biomedical support and be fitted with appropriate auditory and visual alert systems. A comprehensive range of drugs is necessary to cover the spectrum of clinical presentations and scenarios encountered in the retrieval setting. These should be maintained in sealed drug kits, with attention paid to expiry dates and to temperature control where relevant. The retrievalist will also require access to antivenoms, thrombolytics, blood and blood products and other specialized agents at times – systems must be in place to ensure timely access to uncommonly used pharmacological agents.

Clinical principles in retrieval and pre-hospital medicine

Preparation for transport

In many cases, the referral of a patient for retrieval is an uncommon event that may occur at one site perhaps once or twice each month and which may involve individual staff members only once or twice per year. Therefore,

clear understanding and communication of the needs of the critical-care patient for transfer must be in place. Common dilemmas are faced:

- Does the patient require intubation for transfer?
- If so, should the patient be intubated now, later or wait for the retrieval team to arrive to intubate?
- What IV access does the patient require? CVC? Arterial line?
- Drug and equipment compatibility – what will the retrieval team expect? What will they want to take with them?
- What if the patient's clinical status changes?

Airway management is perhaps the greatest risk in the critical-care retrieval setting. The need for intubation for transfer should be discussed between the retrieval coordinator, referring staff and the retrieval team. In general terms, the patient should be intubated if needed for respiratory failure or, if significantly aggressive, agitated or obtunded, or if their clinical condition makes it likely that they will deteriorate *en route*, e.g. large intracranial haemorrhage, complete cervical cord injury, or if they have threatened airway obstruction, e.g. burns, epiglottitis which would present a high risk in-transit intubation.

The general principles that should be applied systematically in the preparation of patients for retrieval are given in Box 26.2.1.

Monitoring

Monitoring equipment used in transport should be in accordance with recommended jurisdictional standards. Most patients require at least continuous ECG, pulse oximetry and blood pressure monitoring. In addition, capnography, invasive pressure monitoring, temperature, ventilation and other monitoring may be required. Equipment must be selected carefully and, where possible, be integrated. Sophisticated light, transport-specific, multimodal monitoring units are now available which include the above components plus defibrillation and external pacing capability. Display screens must be visible in daylight and battery life must be appropriate for duration of transport. Equipment alarms must be clearly visible as auditory alarms are difficult or impossible to hear in moving vehicles, especially aircraft. A major component of any monitoring system is the observer and, in the retrieval setting, the need for vigilance is paramount; at all times at least one of the retrieval crew members must

be absolutely focused on the patient and monitors, continually scanning measured parameters and clinical status (including temperature, peripheral circulation, urine output, conscious state and respiratory oscillation).

Environmental impacts

Transport environments are usually confined and limited in space, which may present hazards for all staff, the patient and equipment. Care, deliberate planned actions and vigilance are important as is the need to ensure all equipment is secured (and equipment that is needed is accessible). Planned exercise, movement, nourishment, breaks and fatigue avoidance must be considered, depending on the mission characteristics. Aircraft retrieval presents particular challenges [8]. Altitude results in reduction in barometric pressure and associated reduction in partial pressure of oxygen and expansion of gas within enclosed spaces. Expansion of gas (such as in an undrained pneumothorax or in a distended bowel) may result in pain or significant worsening of underlying pathology. In a normal person with sea level SpO_2 of 98% and without supplemental oxygen, SpO_2 decreases to about 90% at 3000 m altitude (10 000 ft). Most passenger jet aircraft are routinely pressurized to around 8000 ft; however, some aeromedical platforms may be able to be pressurized to sea level, while some (including most helicopters) cannot be pressurized at all. In patients with respiratory and cardiac disease, impacts are felt at lower altitudes. During descent, trapped gas will occupy less space causing contraction of flexible tissues, such as membranes and mucosal surfaces – this may cause pain, for example when middle ear or sinus space pressures cannot be equalized with the rising external atmospheric pressure. Air transport of patients with decompression sickness requires particular planning and care, since the condition may be significantly worsened at altitude as gas solubility in blood decreases with altitude (due to reduced barometric pressure) and dissolved gas comes out of solution in the circulation, forming nitrogen bubbles with devastating consequences.

Other impacts of flight include those due to noise, vibration, humidity, gravity, acceleration and deceleration, third space effects (swelling) and fatigue.

Critical incidents

It is likely that the most complex patients receiving the highest levels of support are also

Box 26.2.1   General principles to be applied in preparation of patients for retrieval

Airway
1. Assess airway stability for all patients, particularly those with compromise in conscious state or risk of deterioration
2. If an endotracheal tube is in place, record laryngoscopic grade during intubation, note any intubation difficulties and record ETT size and lip length
3. Secure endotracheal tube
4. Insert an orogastric tube unless there is a major contraindication
5. Perform a CXR to confirm position of endotracheal tube

Breathing
1. Observe respiratory rate and character
2. Measure SpO_2 and $ETCO_2$
3. Administer oxygen using the correct delivery device
4. Check ABGs if indicated/possible
5. Secure intercostal catheters if present

Circulation
1. Insert two peripheral IV lines
2. Secure all lines – ensure injection ports are accessible
3. Prepare drug infusions in 50 mL syringes (or other standard as used by the regional retrieval or ambulance service)
4. For advice on standard infusion concentrations discuss with the retrieval coordinator
5. Record all IV fluids and consider insertion of a urinary catheter (mandatory in intubated patients)
6. Transduce all arterial and central lines

Documentation
1. Complete standard referral forms if available
2. Provide copies of all patient charts
3. Investigation results – pathology & ECG
4. Imaging – films/scan/MRI
5. Advise any 'limitation of treatment' orders
6. Notify any infectious disease risk/contagious disease risk or exposure

Other priorities
1. Monitor and maintain body temperature
2. Empty drainage bags prior to transport
3. Administer antiemetic in conscious patients
4. Maintain spinal precautions if indicated
5. Splints and pressure care
6. Remove possible contaminants, such as glass, dirt, etc.
7. Notify significant deterioration in conscious state, blood pressure, heart rate, respiratory status, oxygenation; or any major clinical developments, such as significantly abnormal diagnostic tests, new clinical signs or the need for major interventions prior to the retrieval team arriving (e.g. intubation, surgery)

most likely to be exposed to in-transit critical incidents or equipment failure. A component of clinical practice in this setting is therefore the anticipation of such events, vigilance to detect them and rehearsed and standardized problem-solving algorithms to rectify them (Fig. 26.2.3). Examples include ventilator failure, unexpected hypoxia, high airway pressures, cardiac arrest in flight, etc. Such approaches are routine in the aviation industry, from which retrieval and pre-hospital medicine draws much at a cultural level, and have been applied commonly in anaesthesia [9].

Respiratory support
Provision of appropriate oxygen therapy via correct delivery systems will be required for most retrieval patients. Oxygen supplies vary on different patient transport platforms and these must be checked prior to transport. Assisted ventilation is a frequent intervention in critical-care retrieval and must be approached with discipline. A reliable and capable transport ventilator will provide suitable ventilation mode options including intermittent positive pressure ventilation (IPPV), synchronized intermittent mandatory ventilation (SIMV)

and pressure support. Non-invasive ventilation (NIV) methods are not commonly utilized in air transport; however, may be valuable in road transfer and in retrieval of patients in whom intubation and assisted ventilation may be undesirable or contraindicated or in patients for whom short-term assisted ventilation is indicated. Ventilators are almost universally power dependent so back-up ventilation systems (manual self-inflating bag/valve system) must be available at all times in the patient cabin to allow management of power, gas or mechanical failure.

EXTUBATION IN TRANSIT

Recognition

- Tube out
- Sound of air leak
- Falling CO2
- Ventilator alarm: low MVe
- Dropping sats

- Differential
  - Isolated cuff leak:
    check pressure, reinflate
  - Circuit disconnection / kink

Communication

- Stop ambulance (consider urgent landing or diversion)
- Notify pilot
- Notify coordinator, Med ONE status

Action

- If isolated cuff leak (as long as oxygenation is okay): leave it in
- Rescue: bag-mask ventilation
- Attempt re-intubation
- Consider
  - LMA
  - Surgical airway

- Systems issues / risk avoidance
  - Secure ETT, circuit and ensure cuff working before moving
  - Controlled patient movements

Fig. 26.2.3 Example of a critical incident algorithmic prompt card.

Circulatory support and infusions

Intravenous infusions are best delivered using simple and compact syringe drivers. These are available in various sizes and configurations, including banks of multiple syringes. Each retrieval service and, preferably the jurisdiction in which it operates, should maintain standard infusion protocols for preparation, labelling and administration of therapeutic agents and, in particular, inotropes. Use of syringe systems that have error reducing software and programs integrated in them reduces risk of adverse events and patient harm. The retrieval environment is dynamic and attention must be paid to maintenance of infusion rates during transfer and power interruption. Critical patients are often highly dependent on inotropic support and brief periods of interruption of infusions may be associated with catastrophic circulatory collapse. Adequate fluid volumes and spare syringes which are pre-prepared for longer transfers must be planned for, as must the availability of blood and blood products which may need significant coordination.

Infectious risk

The proximity of the retrieval environment means that patients with infectious diseases may present hazards to medical crew, flight crew including pilots and other patients or passengers. Clearly, the application of universal precautions against infectious diseases is applicable as in all clinical settings; however, other measures may be important, such as use of ventilator expiratory filters, avoidance of use of nebulizers which may, for instance, aerosolize influenza, use of prophylactic medications, such as rifampicin, after prolonged exposure to meningococcal disease, barrier precautions in patients with vancomycin-resistant enterococci (VRE) and so on.

Highly-specialized retrieval

Neonatal, obstetric and paediatric specialized retrieval systems have been a part of many health systems for decades. While the clinical demands of these systems require particular sets of knowledge, the retrieval frameworks required are complementary and intersect with the larger and higher volume world of adult retrieval and pre-hospital care. Consequently, blending, collocating or integrating retrieval services is seen as a sustainable model and has become more common. Technical advances in critical care, such as increased use of extracorporeal membrane oxygenation (ECMO) support in severe respiratory failure for example in influenza, have promoted the development of specialized retrieval systems to manage these highly fragile patients [10]. Interestingly, in response to these needs, technology has evolved rapidly to offer lighter, smaller, less invasive and simpler ECMO systems.

Controversies/emerging issues

- Increased centralization is a consistent feature in Australian retrieval (and internationally). Where states and regions previously may have had multiple systems for retrieval, it is more common now to see single coordinated systems with improved governance.
  In addition, there is a nationally progressing movement for co-location of adult and paediatric services, integration of these services and for the increased formalization of the role of retrieval and pre-hospital medical services in disaster medicine.

- Building economy and efficiency from such commonality in systems is a driver for these developments; however, such benefits and advantages often require cultural and system readjustment and therefore may remain unrealized while change is managed.
- Building on relevant interfaces which are a strong part of retrieval work is a common theme so that movement of retrieval services into management of critical and acute care bed flow and access management, outreach and support, telehealth and education is being seen.
- Retrieval and pre-hospital medicine in Australia is moving progressively to specialist status within academic colleges and has fully reached this point in some countries [11]. Formal training systems and qualifications are evolving in both the tertiary education sector and in specialist medical college settings.

References

[1] Hedges JR, Newgard CD, Mullins RJ. Emergency medical treatment and active labor act and trauma triage. Prehosp Emerg Care 2006;10:332–9.
[2] Australasian College for Emergency Medicine, Joint faculty of Intensive Care Medicine, Australian and New Zealand College of Anaesthetists. Minimum standards for transport of critically ill patients. <http://www.acem.org.au/media/policies_and_guidelines/min_standard_crit_ill.pdf>; 2003 [Accessed Nov. 2012].
[3] Brown JB, Stassen NA, Bankey PE, et al. J Trauma Injury Infect Crit Care 2011;70:310–4.
[4] Brown JB, Stassen NA, Bankey PE, et al. Helicopters and the civilian trauma system: national utilization patterns demonstrate improved outcomes after traumatic injury. J Trauma Injury Infect Crit Care 2010;69:1030–6.
[5] Carne B, Kennedy M, Gray T. Crisis resource management in emergency medicine. Emerg Med Australas 2012;24:7–13.
[6] Intensive Care Society UK. Guidelines for the transport of the critically ill adult, 3rd ed. <http://www.ics.ac.uk/professional/standards_and_guidelines/transport_of_the_critically_ill_adult>; 2011 [Accessed Nov. 2012].
[7] Garner A. The role of physician staffing of helicopter emergency medical services in prehospital trauma response. Emerg Med Australas 2004;16:318–23.
[8] Martin T. Clinical considerations in transport of the sick and injured Aeromedical transportation – a clinical guide, 2nd edn. Aldershot: Ashgate; 2006.
[9] Runciman W, Merry A. Crises in clinical care: an approach to management. Qual Saf Hlth Care 2005;14:156–63.
[10] Forrest P, Ratchford J, Burns B, et al. Retrieval of critically ill adults using ECMO: an Australian experience. Intens Care Med 2011;37:824–30.
[11] Intercollegiate Board for Training in Pre-hospital Emergency Medicine. Subspecialty training in prehospital and retrieval medicine – a guide for trainees, trainers, local education providers, employers and deaneries. London: College of Emergency Medicine; 2012.

Further reading

Ellis D, Hooper M. Cases in pre-hospital and retrieval medicine. Sydney: Elsevier; 2010.
Martin T. Aeromedical transportation – a clinical guide, 2nd edn. Aldershot: Ashgate; 2006.

EMERGENCY AND MEDICAL SYSTEMS

26.3 Medical issues in disasters

Richard J Brennan • David A Bradt • Jonathan Abrahams

ESSENTIALS

1 The incidence of natural and technological disasters has increased exponentially from 1960 to the present.

2 Disaster deaths steadily declined over the last half of the 20th century, but numbers of disaster-affected populations continue to rise, encompassing 40% of the world's population over the last decade.

3 Economic damage from natural disasters commonly surpasses $US100 b/yr.

4 Effective disaster planning requires knowledge of a community's major hazards, vulnerabilities and capabilities, disaster history and disaster-associated patterns of morbidity and mortality. Disaster management is 80% generic for all hazards, 15% hazard-specific and 5% unique to the event.

5 Public health interventions are high priorities following disasters that disrupt environmental health infrastructure (e.g. water supply, sewerage), disasters that result in significant population displacement (e.g. conflict), disasters associated with epidemics and pandemics and disasters that involve the unintentional or deliberate release of chemical, biological or radiological agents.

6 Emergency physicians and other health professionals have a vital role in disaster management including prevention, mitigation, preparedness, response and recovery operations.

7 Continuing disaster losses have led to calls for community resilience as a cornerstone of national disaster management strategies.

8 The disasters most likely to confront emergency physicians are domestic transportation disasters associated with trauma-associated multiple casualties.

9 Effective management of mass casualty incidents requires knowledge of local and regional disaster response plans, scene assessment issues, site management, communications, casualty flow plans, field triage and the clinical management of hazard-specific conditions, such as crush injury and blast injury.

Introduction

Disaster management involves a complex, multidisciplinary process of which emergency medicine comprises one component. Domestically, fire fighters, law enforcement, ambulance services, civil defence, State Emergency Services, Red Cross national society, defence forces and other aid organizations commonly play major roles. Internationally, governmental and non-governmental organizations, International Federation of the Red Cross and Red Crescent Societies and United Nations agencies are frequently involved. The health and medical management of disasters can also cut across healthcare disciplines, requiring contributions from emergency medicine, public health, primary care, surgery, anaesthetics and intensive care.

From the health perspective, certain types of disasters are usually associated with well-described patterns of morbidity and mortality. The clinical and public health needs of an affected community therefore also vary according to the type and extent of disaster. Emergency physicians should understand the public health and medical consequences of the various types of disasters in order to determine their own roles in preparedness and response.

In practice, emergency physicians are most actively involved in the response to an acute-onset disaster that involves multiple casualties, such as a transportation incident. Several other types of disasters, including floods and cyclones, are generally associated with few, if any, casualties. The health and medical needs in these settings usually involve augmenting public health and primary care services.

Emergency physicians should be familiar with disaster epidemiology and disaster management arrangements and understand the medical response to a disaster involving multiple casualties.

The differential effects of disasters on communities in all countries are associated with risk factors which make some communities and subpopulations more vulnerable and less capable of dealing with the risks than others. Apart from health and medical issues, the impact of disasters is often widespread and long term. Disasters can cause significant social, economic and environmental losses that may have devastating effects on the general well-being of the affected community. They may set back years of development progress in poorer countries, including disruption of health systems, such as the Pakistan floods of 2010. Their effects may be felt well beyond the borders of the first affected country. Epidemics, for example, may be prone to widespread international spread, with a broad range economic and sociopolitical consequences, for example, the H1N1 pandemic of 2009.

Definitions and classification

There is no internationally agreed definition of disaster or disaster classification. There are increasingly consistent uses of disaster terms among stakeholder organizations. Common to most definitions is the concept that, following a disaster, the capacity of the impacted community to respond is exceeded and there is, therefore, a need for external assistance.

The United Nations Office for Disaster Risk Reduction (UNISDR), defines a disaster as: 'a serious disruption of the functioning of a community or a society causing widespread human, material, economic or environmental losses which exceed the ability of the affected community or society to cope using its own resources' [1]. This definition is also one of several recognized by the World Health Organization (WHO).

The Australian Emergency Management Glossary defines disaster as: 'a serious disruption to community life which threatens or causes death or injury in that community and/or damage to property which is beyond the day-to-day capacity of the prescribed statutory authorities and which requires special mobilization and organization of resources other than those normally available to those authorities' [2].

The Center for Research on the Epidemiology of Disasters (CRED), which compiles the data behind the annual World Disasters Report of the International Federation of Red Cross and Red Crescent Societies, stipulates a quantitative surveillance definition involving one of the following: 10 or more people killed; 100 or more people affected; declaration of state of emergency; or an appeal for international assistance [3].

Disaster risk management is the range of activities designed to establish and maintain control over disaster and emergency situations and to provide a framework for helping at-risk populations avoid or recover from the impact of a disaster. It addresses a much broader array of issues than health alone, including a multisectoral approach to hazard identification, vulnerability analysis, risk assessment, risk evaluation and risk treatments [4].

Disaster medicine can be defined as the study and application of clinical care, public health, mental health and disaster management to the prevention, preparedness, response and recovery from the health problems arising from disasters [5]. This must be achieved in cooperation with other agencies and disciplines involved in comprehensive disaster management. In practice, emergency medicine and public health are the two specialties most intimately involved in disaster medicine.

A mass casualty incident is an event causing illness or injury among multiple patients simultaneously through a similar mechanism, such as a major vehicular crash, structural collapse, explosion or exposure to a hazardous material. A complex disaster is a disaster complicated by civil conflict, government instability, macroeconomic collapse, population migration and an elusive political solution.

Disasters are commonly classified as natural versus technological/human-generated (Box 26.3.1) [3]. Disasters may also be classified according to other characteristics, including sudden versus slow onset, short versus long duration, unifocal versus multifocal distribution and primary versus secondary. Classifications of disaster magnitude exist for selected natural hazards, such as earthquakes and hurricanes/cyclones; however, there is currently no standard classification of severity of disaster impact.

Box 26.3.1 Classification of disasters

Natural	Technological/ human-generated
Hydrological Floods (waves and surges) Wet mass movements	**Technological** *Industrial accidents:* Chemical spills Building collapses Explosions Fires Gas leaks Poisoning Radiation
Meteorological Storms Climatological Extreme temperatures Wildfires Droughts	
Geophysical Earthquakes Tsunamis Volcanic eruptions Dry mass movements	*Transportation accidents:* Air Rail Road Water
Biological Insect/pest infestations Epidemics	*Miscellaneous accidents:* Domestic building collapses, fires and explosions **War/terrorism/ complex emergencies**

Epidemiology

Globally, the types of disasters associated with the greatest numbers of deaths are complex emergencies (CEs). These are crises characterized by political instability, armed conflict, large population displacements, food shortages and collapse of public health infrastructure. Because of insecurity and poor access to the affected population, aggregate epidemiological data for CEs are somewhat limited. However, between 1998 and 2007 in the Democratic Republic of Congo, it is estimated that 5.4 million people lost their lives due to the consequences of the major humanitarian crisis afflicting that country [6]. This was four times the UNISDR estimate of deaths globally due to natural and technological disasters during the 20 years between 1992 and 2012.

According to information compiled by the International Federation of the Red Cross, there has been a significant increase in the total number of natural and technological disasters worldwide during the past 50 years. From 1960 to 2010, the annual number of disasters rose from 50 per year to approximately 700 per year peaking at 810 in 2005. While the total number of people killed by natural and technological disasters is currently approximately 150 000 per year, there is a wide annual range (17 660 in 2009 to 304 476 in 2010 due to the Haiti earthquake and the Russian heatwave). Moreover, the total number affected has almost quadrupled over the past three decades. It is estimated that approximately 200 million people are directly affected on an annual basis. Selected data are presented in Figures 26.3.1 and 26.3.2 [3].

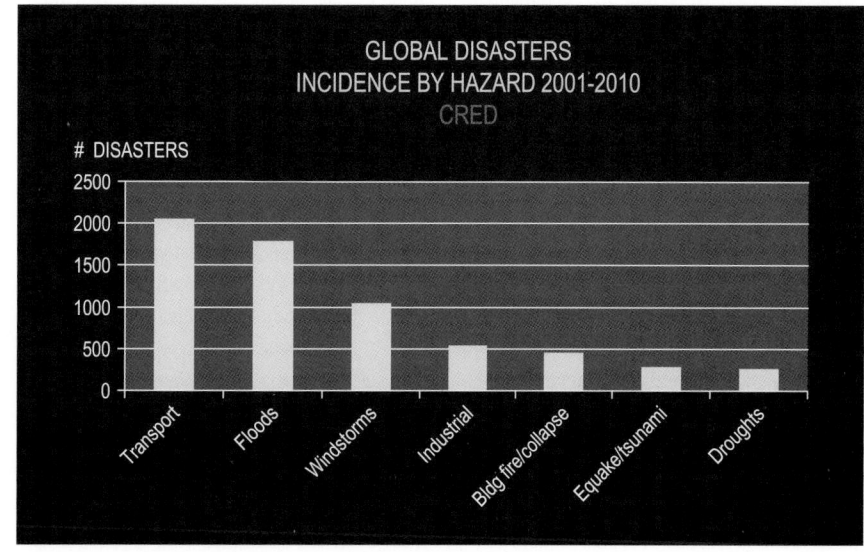

Fig. 26.3.1 Global disasters incidence by hazard 2001–2010 [3].

EMERGENCY AND MEDICAL SYSTEMS

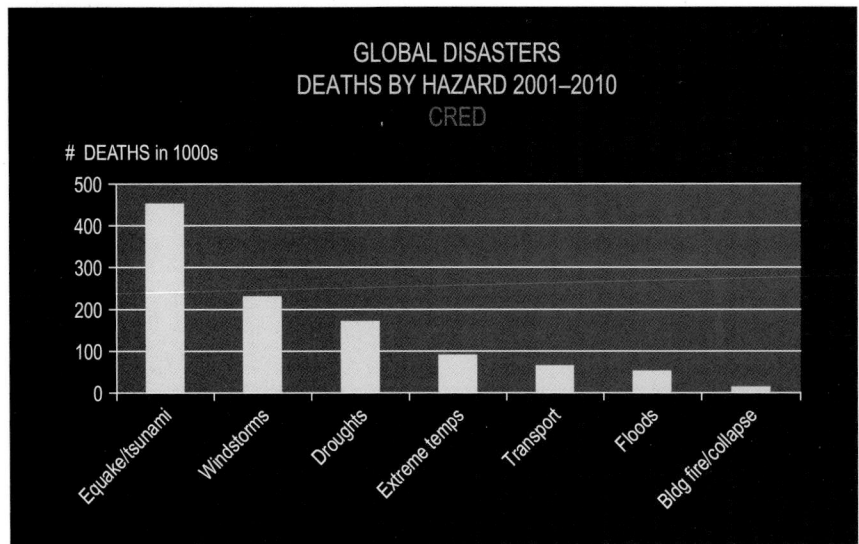

Fig. 26.3.2 Global disasters death by hazard 2001–2010 [3].

The commonest types of disasters across the globe are: transportation incidents, floods, windstorms, industrial incidents, building collapses, droughts, and earthquakes/tsunamis (see Fig. 26.3.1). Asia is the region of the world most prone to natural and technological disasters, recording 41% of such incidents between 2001 and 2010. It is followed by Africa (24%), the Americas (19%), Europe (14%) and Oceania (2%). Compared with other regions of the world, Australasia and Oceania have a relatively low incidence of disasters. Nonetheless, the World Risk Index (WRI) Report of 2012 included Vanuatu, Tonga and the Solomon Islands among the 10 countries most at risk to natural hazards [7].

Over the past 10 years, the commonest causes of disasters in Australia have been severe storms, including hail, transportation events and bushfires. Historically, the leading cause of death from natural disasters in Australia have been heatwaves (438 killed in 1939, 404 killed in 2009), followed by cyclone and bushfire. Human-generated disasters resulting in multiple casualties have occurred more frequently in Australia in recent years. The commonest causes of mass casualty incidents have been bus crashes, structural fires, mining incidents, aviation incidents and train crashes.

The impact of disasters has been less in New Zealand, where only 75 lives were lost among 307 000 persons affected over the period 2001–2010. However, 2011 brought the Christchurch earthquake with 185 deaths surpassing the death toll of the previous decade.

The incidence of disasters also differs, with the commonest major events being transportation disasters, industrial disasters and earthquakes. Data reporting on the incidence of armed conflict is complicated by varying and changing definitions and political motivations of the reporting agencies. The Uppsala Conflict Database Program identified 37 on-going conflicts on five continents in 2011 [8].

The regions recording the highest number of terrorist attacks over the past decade have been Afghanistan and Iraq. Excluding those countries, the number of terrorist attacks worldwide resulting in the death of at least 10 persons, has ranged between 193 and 353 events per year [9]. Overall, this is just a very small fraction of the total number deaths attributed to natural and technological disasters and complex emergencies.

Disaster epidemiology globally, including the Australasian region, is being affected by climate change. Global warming has already been associated with an increase in the frequency, severity, and unpredictability of weather-related disasters, such as heatwaves, floods and droughts. Rising temperatures have been implicated in the spread of infectious disease, such as malaria and dengue, through increases in vector populations, such as mosquitoes. Other important diseases are also sensitive to changing temperatures and rainfall, including malnutrition and diarrhoea. The health-related and other impacts of climate change will not be evenly distributed. Disasters associated with global warming are particularly likely to threaten the lives and livelihoods of coastal communities, those living in low-lying islands (e.g. due to rising sea levels) and in arid and high mountain zones.

Socioeconomic impact

Disasters have the potential for major socioeconomic impact of direct damages plus economic losses, costing the host countries and international community billions of dollars annually. In developing countries, years of development work and investment can be devastated by a single disaster. During the decade 2000–2010, disasters caused a global average of approximately $US107 billion damage per year. Windstorms were the costliest disaster over the decade accounting for 49% of disaster-associated costs led by Hurricane Katrina with over $200 billion in damage. Terrorist attacks on major financial centres, such as the World Trade Center in New York, have demonstrated the potential for tens of billions of direct economic impact, enormous social consequences and political repercussions. These figures may be overshadowed by pandemic disease, such as from avian influenza, for which economic cost estimates range to upwards of $US1 trillion [10].

In Australia over the past 30 years, floods, storms, then cyclones have caused the greatest disaster-related economic losses with an average of approximately $AUS1 billion annually. The most economically costly disaster was the 2010–2011 Queensland floods exceeding $A7 billion in damages and losses.

Economic estimates, of course, are unable to reflect the true scale of human suffering associated with disasters. While we can often document the mortality, morbidity and financial losses associated with disasters, it is impossible to quantify the associated personal, psychological, social, cultural and political losses.

Disaster management/ emergency management

As emergency physicians play a vital role in the medical aspects of disaster management, they should be familiar with the underlying concepts on which these arrangements are based [11].

Integrated approach

The basis for the Australian system for managing disasters is a partnership between the

Commonwealth, State/Territory local governments, the private sector and the community. Under legislation, State and Territory governments have the primary responsibility for coordinating disaster-management activities and maintain government and statutory agencies that provide emergency services to the community. Local governments play an active role in risk assessments, land-use planning, public education and awareness, local emergency planning and providing local resources in emergency relief and recovery. The major roles of the Australian Federal Government are to support State and Territory governments in coordinating national strategic policy, to assist with disaster information and knowledge management (e.g. meteorological and geological data to support risk assessments and early warnings), to provide financial resources on a cost-sharing basis with States and Territories and to provide operational support in the event that a disaster exceeds the affected State or Territory's response capability [12]. Federal assistance in the area of health would most likely be medical resources provided by the Australian Defence Force (ADF). The ADF also has special expertise in the management of incidents involving chemical and biological agents.

Comprehensive approach

The comprehensive approach to disaster management encompasses prevention, preparedness, response and recovery. The traditional view is that health and medical professionals contribute most significantly to disaster preparedness and response. A broader appreciation of the factors that enable communities to be more disaster resilient would further recognize the role of the health sector in prevention and mitigation – specifically, by improving overall health, immunization rates and nutritional status of individuals, as measures to reduce vulnerabilities and strengthen resilience. The disaster equivalent of primary prevention activities includes regulatory and physical measures that prevent or mitigate the effects of hazards and to reduce community exposure to these hazards. Preparedness involves arrangements to ensure that resources and services that may be needed can be rapidly mobilized and deployed. Response activities are those actions taken during and immediately after impact to ensure that the disaster's effects are minimized. Recovery involves strategies and services that support

affected communities in reconstructing their physical infrastructure and restoration of their social, economic, physical and emotional well-being.

All-hazards approach

Different types of disasters can cause similar problems. Therefore, disaster management plans are based on a core set of arrangements and measures that can be applied to all hazards. Many risks, however, including acts of terrorism, also require specific prevention, preparedness, response and recovery measures.

The prepared community

The prepared community is the foundation of Australia's disaster management arrangements. Local governments, voluntary organizations and individuals all play a critical role in this area. Individuals can reduce their own risks by being aware of the local hazards and taking appropriate precautions. Experience has demonstrated that individual and community self-help can often provide the most immediate, decisive and effective relief following a disaster, as it cannot be assumed that assistance from external sources always arrives promptly, particularly in remote area communities.

Risk management

From 1996, following the endorsement of the National Emergency Management Committee, the principles and processes of the joint Australian and New Zealand Standard for Risk Management have been adopted by the Australian emergency management community. The risk management methodology embraces the key approaches identified above and ensures a greater focus on reducing vulnerability of communities, as well as hazard prevention, emergency response and recovery measures [13].

Disaster resilience

Against the background of disasters, climate change and a myriad of social, economic and environmental factors, the Council of Australian Governments adopted the National Strategy for Disaster Resilience in 2011. The Strategy emphasizes the shared responsibility of individuals, households, community organizations, businesses and governments to enhance Australia's capacity to prepare for, withstand and recover from disasters. According to the Strategy, a disaster-resilient community has the characteristics of: functioning well while under stress, successful adaptation, self-reliance and social capacity.

The Strategy provides high-level direction and guidance on how to achieve disaster-resilient communities through a long-term commitment to a broad range of measures including understanding risks, communicating and educating about risks, reducing risks and supporting capacities for resilience [14].

Disaster response planning

Disaster response planning is the process by which a community develops a comprehensive strategy effectively to manage and respond to disasters. It is a collaborative effort that requires cooperation among government agencies, community services and private organizations. The objectives of the planning process include identification of the main hazards facing the community; clarification of the capabilities, roles and responsibilities of responding agencies; and the strengthening of emergency networks. Other operational issues, such as emergency communications and public warning systems, should also be addressed.

All-hazards planning for response and recovery remains fundamental to disaster preparedness. To that end, disaster experience to date reveals a generic set of issues that disaster planners must address in the management of any hazard. These include risk assessment, incident management, on-scene and overall disaster command, control and coordination, relief operations, risk communication and media management, reconstruction, and community recovery. By contrast, the nature of the hazard imposes specific implications for epidemiology, search and rescue, medical care and consequences of contamination and communicable diseases. To this end, governments have elaborated all hazards disaster response planning including hazard-specific disaster subplans (e.g. mass casualty management for burns).

Finally, the circumstances of time, place, climate, geography, politics and security are unique for each disaster and challenge disaster planners to anticipate the issues arising from those specific circumstances.

Several high-profile terrorist events (e.g. World Trade Center attack in New York City) and important gatherings (e.g. London Olympic Games) have highlighted the need for specific planning for terrorist events. Such planning frequently involves collaboration with relevant military, security and intelligence agencies and a consideration of the tactics used by terrorists.

EMERGENCY AND MEDICAL SYSTEMS

855

The majority of terrorist attacks have employed conventional weapons, including explosives and small arms. Other terrorist tactics include assassinations, hijacking and kidnapping. Unconventional attacks, including those using jet airliners as weapons of mass destruction, or chemical, biological and radiological weapons have constituted only a tiny fraction of international terrorist attacks.

Disaster exercises must be conducted regularly to test the response and recovery aspects of the plan. Exercises range from desktop simulations to realistic scenarios with moulaged patients in the field. If conducted appropriately, they demonstrate strengths and weaknesses of the plan and highlight any need for an updating of response procedures. They are also considered to provide the most practice-based form of disaster response training. Disaster planning is a continuous process and plans need to be regularly reviewed and updated.

Planning and responding for international disasters has become more relevant for Australasian health professionals in light of the terrorist attacks in Bali (2002 and 2005), the Indian Ocean tsunami (2004), the earthquake in Pakistan and India (2005) and the Pakistan floods (2010), including through the deployment of Australian medical response teams (AusMATs) [15]. Such planning and response can be advised by the internationally-recognized Sphere Minimum Standards in Disaster Response [16] and in collaboration with important international agencies, such as the United Nation's Office for Coordination of Humanitarian Affairs. Sphere specifies standards in six sectors of disaster response: water and sanitation, food security, food aid, nutrition, shelter and health services. These standards are relevant for all disasters and represent an extremely useful reference to guide planning and response for domestic incidents as well.

A major reform of the international humanitarian system was initiated at the end of 2011 under the leadership of the UN's Office for Coordination of Humanitarian Assistance (OCHA) and involving all major relief agencies through the UN's Inter-agency Standing Committee (IASC). This reform process, known as the IASC Transformative Agenda, includes a broad range of policy and procedural measures to improve the leadership, coordination, predictability and effectiveness of international disaster response. It also aims to increase the accountability of responding agencies, especially to the affected populations.

Domestic disaster response activities

Disaster management is increasingly seen as a cardinal sign of good governance in civil society. Healthcare systems have become mandated to undertake a range of health emergency and disaster risk management actions, with a focus on disaster preparedness, including disaster planning, training and exercises and response. Specific to emergency medicine, mass casualty management is the subject of well-developed training packages, such as Emergotrain, Major Incident Medical Management and Support (MIMMS), Basic Disaster Life Support (BDLS) and Advanced Disaster Life Support (ADLS).

Incident management

Scene assessment and stabilization

The initial scene assessment is conducted by first responders, such as police, fire or ambulance personnel. It is important for the first medical responder, generally an ambulance officer, rapidly to report findings to the Ambulance Communications Centre. An accurate, timely assessment is critical to initiating an appropriate and effective response. Key information that should be relayed from the scene includes the nature and magnitude of the disaster, the presence of ongoing hazards, the estimated number of deaths and injuries, the need for further assistance and the most appropriate routes of access to the scene. In large-scale disasters that affect entire populations, such as cyclone or earthquake, a rapid multisectoral assessment followed by broader epidemiological assessments is required, including an evaluation of the impact on the health infrastructure, health services, public utilities and shelter.

Site security and safety procedures must be observed to ensure that rescuers and bystanders do not become victims. This is particularly relevant in chemical and radiological incidents or when a terrorist incident is suspected, because of the threats posed by a secondary attack on responders or the potential use of weapons of mass destruction. The police should establish a perimeter around the scene of a multiple casualty incident and allow access only to authorized personnel. If a hazardous material is involved, rescuers may be required to wear specialized personal protective equipment (PPE) to protect their airways, eyes and skin. Electrical hazards, fires, explosions, leaking gases and unstable structures may all pose significant threats to rescue personnel. These hazards must be eliminated or controlled prior to initiating rescue operations.

Hazard-specific issues

While the all-hazards approach remains fundamental to disaster management, a unifying approach for undifferentiated hazards has been developed for the management of incidents involving chemical, biological or radiological agents. Basic principles of awareness include: recognition of potential terrorist events; avoidance of the affected area; isolation of the affected area; and notification of proper authorities. Basic principles for first responders include the four don'ts: don't become a victim, don't rush in, don't TEST (taste, eat, smell, touch) anything, and don't assume anything. Only properly trained and equipped hazardous material personnel should be in contaminated areas.

Site arrangements

Regardless of the nature of the incident, a Forward Command Post should be set up at or near the disaster site at the beginning of the emergency operation. The Command Post has representatives from the major responding services and reports back to the regional or State Emergency Operations Centre. The function of the Command Post is to coordinate the activities of the various services during the rescue operations. It also provides a central point for the submission of requests for assistance by each of the responding services. Medical and ambulance commanders are located at the Command Post to direct and coordinate medical care to victims at the scene, patient transportation, hospital communications, provision of medical supplies and medical air operations.

Communications

Good communications are vital to ensure appropriate command, control and coordination during a disaster. Communication problems are often cited as a major cause of suboptimal disaster response. There are many factors that may contribute to poor communications at the scene. Damaged equipment and overloaded telephone systems indicate the need for back-up systems, including reserved cellular phone lines. The use of different radio frequencies by different agencies may lead to poor coordination and an inability to communicate vital information. Compatible frequencies need to be identified and utilized. Megaphones may be required to overcome noise at the scene due to heavy extrication equipment, helicopters and general rescue activities. Information overload may also hamper the rescue effort. Radio and telephone reports should be kept brief, relevant and succinct. Professional jargon is frequently misunderstood or misinterpreted by other agencies and is best avoided.

Hospitals must also have reliable communications systems. Designated phone lines, cellular phones and back-up radio networks may augment the existing system during a disaster. It is essential for hospitals to remain in regular contact with the incident medical director, to provide information regarding medical capabilities, bed capacity and bed availability.

Medical management

Personnel

Provider roles in disasters continue to evolve. Dedicated disaster medical response teams have been extensively studied [17]. These teams form an integral part of national response plans in many developed countries notwithstanding lack of data attesting to any reduction in disaster-associated mortality associated with their deployments [18]. At international level, standards and procedures for foreign medical teams are currently being developed, after the poor experiences with many clinical teams following the Haiti earthquake in 2010.

Emergency responders generally respond best when their disaster roles are similar to their daily professional practice. Medical and nursing personnel are best suited to staffing emergency rooms and hospitals, where they have the advantage of working in a familiar, more stable environment. Ambulance personnel have more experience in pre-hospital settings and are usually responsible for conducting the initial on-site medical assessment and triage. In situations where there are multiple casualties, it may be appropriate to send a hospital team to the scene of a disaster, where their main functions are to perform primary and secondary triage and to provide medical care at the Patient Treatment Post. The science and practice of disaster medicine has progressed substantially. Therefore, only doctors and nurses specifically trained to work in the field environment and familiar with the relevant best practices and standards should be deployed to the disaster scene, as inexperienced personnel may well hinder the medical response.

Pre-hospital mass casualty management

Disaster epidemiology has refined the expectations of casualty flow plans. Current epidemiological evidence indicates that 50–80% of people acutely injured in a mass casualty disaster arrive at the closest medical facilities generally within 90 minutes after the event [19]. Moreover, the vast majority of disaster-affected patients self-evacuate without benefit of pre-hospital triage, transport or decontamination. A casualty-flow plan remains crucial to optimize patient care and transportation of those remaining at the scene.

A Casualty Collection Area should be established at a site that is close enough to the disaster scene to allow easy access, but far enough away to ensure protection from potential hazards. Patients are assembled and triaged here prior to transfer to a nearby Patient Treatment Post, where they are once again triaged and basic medical care provided. An Ambulance Loading Point and Ambulance Holding Point also need to be clearly marked so that patient transportation is conducted efficiently and to ensure that scene convergence and congestion is minimized. Landing zones for helicopters are established away from the incident site for safety reasons, to limit noise and to reduce downwash from rotor blades. A temporary morgue may need to be established in a nearby area when many fatalities have occurred.

Triage

The aim of triage is to allocate medical resources, including personnel, supplies and facilities, in a manner that provides the greatest good to the greatest number of patients. The emphasis is not on providing optimal care to each individual patient, but rather on directing limited medical resources to those who are most likely to benefit. Triage is the single most important medical activity at the disaster site. It is a dynamic, ongoing process that occurs at every stage of patient management, from the disaster site, to the Casualty Collection Area, Patient Treatment Post and again at the hospital. Patients are rapidly assessed and categorized according to priority of treatment and transport. The condition of patients frequently changes and repeated examinations are required so that patients may be moved up or down in the order of priority. Triage is a learned skill and should be conducted by the most experienced medical or ambulance officer at the scene.

Different triage systems have emerged in different parts of the world. In British and Australasian health systems, 'sieve and sort' triage processes have become the preferred approach through MIMMS training courses [20]. In North America, 'start and save' triage processes have become incorporated into the National Disaster Medical System [21]. More recently, a National Disaster Life Support Consortium in the USA has promulgated a triage approach based on 'move, assess, sort and send' [22]. These different systems rely on different assessment approaches with different vital sign thresholds to assign triage priority.

In general, most systems recognize that there are categories of patients who require immediate care, delayed care, minimal care and those that are expectant or unsalvageable. Patients requiring immediate care are individuals in critical condition, but to whom simple life-saving procedures may be successfully applied, such as the manual clearing of the airway. Patients classified as requiring delayed care may have significant injuries, such as major fractures, but are likely to survive if treatment is postponed for several hours. Minimal care patients are generally ambulatory and their treatment may be delayed until other patients have been appropriately treated. Expectant or unsalvageable patients are those that have acutely life-threatening injuries requiring advanced resuscitation, or those that have non-survivable injuries, such as massive head trauma. Advanced life support measures, such as cardiopulmonary resuscitation, are rarely indicated at a scene with multiple casualties. Instead, these patients generally receive palliative care, but only after patients in the immediate category have received appropriate treatment.

Stabilization

Following triage of the affected patients, rapid stabilization of airway, breathing and circulation is provided to those with the greatest potential for survival. Definitive care is not generally provided at the scene. On-scene medical care concentrates on securing the airway, administration of oxygen, external pressure to control haemorrhage and insertion of intravenous catheters for volume expansion prior to hospital transportation. Medical care should generally be provided at the Patient Treatment Post but, during prolonged rescues, resuscitative procedures may be required prior to extrication. Appropriate use of analgesia, including parenteral narcotics and regional nerve blocks, may assist with the extrication of trapped individuals. Special on-scene procedures are sometimes required for those with crush injury, blast injury, burns or hypothermia. Amputation of a mangled limb, although rarely indicated, may be a life-saving procedure for an entrapped patient.

Decontamination

Chemical, biological, radiological and nuclear (CBRN) agents have the potential to contaminate individuals, property and the general environment. In practice, industrial accidents represent by far the most common cause of exposure to hazardous materials that may require decontamination. A small number of high-profile chemical–biological terrorist incidents over the past 20 years have also prompted medical as well as lay attention to this potential threat. Regardless of the cause, the principles guiding the process of decontamination remain consistent.

Decontamination is the process of removing or neutralizing a hazard from the victim or environment. Detailed management protocols exist for these hazards [23–25]. Fundamental principles involve:

❶ staff and site preparation with establishment of hot/warm/cold zones
❷ casualty, staff and crowd protection
❸ decontamination procedures
❹ clinical treatment of contaminated patients and transport to definitive care
❺ recovery of environment.

Removal of contaminated clothes should be conducted as a matter of urgency. Rapid decontamination of the skin is especially necessary following exposure to the liquid or aerosolized form of an agent. It is most useful when conducted within 1 minute of exposure but, in practice, this is rarely possible. When indicated, decontamination should be conducted close to the scene (i.e. in the 'warm zone') and, ideally, prior to transportation. Commonly used agents for decontamination include soap and water and hypochlorite (household bleach) in concentrations of 0.5–2.0%. Steps must be taken to ensure that emergency responders, health personnel and other patients are not at risk of secondary exposure to the chemical agent. Decontamination after exposure to a biological agent is less important, as most biological agents are not dermally active. But decontamination may be an effective way to limit the spread of the agent from potential secondary aerosolization.

Transportation

Efficient and rational transportation of patients to appropriate health facilities is dependent on good communications between hospitals and the incident Transport Officer. Capabilities of the affected community's hospitals should be identified and documented in the regional disaster plan. Hospitals are required regularly to update the Incident Commander and Transport Officer of their bed availability status. The closest hospitals may be flooded by 'walking wounded' who have made their own way from the scene and by victims transported by well-meaning civilians. This has the potential of overwhelming local emergency departments and the Transport Officer must take this into consideration when determining the appropriate distribution of patients. It is essential that the disaster scene not be relocated to the nearest hospitals.

A number of factors need to be considered when determining the most appropriate hospital for a particular patient, including the patient's triage category, the hospital's capabilities (e.g. trauma, burns), transportation times, distance from the scene and the available transportation modalities. Medical helicopters may be able to transport patients to more distant hospitals, to relieve pressure on nearby facilities.

Health facility management

Guidance on hospital planning for disaster management has become widely available from the World Health Organization [26] as well as domestic stakeholders [27]. Emergency physicians are expected to be familiar with their own hospital disaster plan and have contributed significantly to its development. The plan should address both internal and external disasters. Surge strategies for hospitals and emergency departments have become well elaborated [28].

The emergency department needs to be cleared of non-critical patients and steps taken to expedite appropriate discharge of stable ward patients, so that bed capacity may be optimized. The emergency department should be well stocked with supplies and have arrangements with suppliers for rapid replenishment. A recall system for additional medical and nursing staff mobilized in a disaster needs to be incorporated into the plan. Extra security staff should be on standby to assist with the management of patients, families, friends, onlookers and the media.

Patients require re-triage by a senior medical officer as they arrive at the emergency department. Those with acutely life-threatening injuries are immediately resuscitated. Less severely injured patients need to be regularly reviewed while awaiting definitive care, to monitor for a potential deterioration in their condition. Expectant, unsalvageable patients are provided appropriate palliative care and their condition clearly explained to their relatives. Documentation is kept succinct and should generally be limited to the essential points about each patient's condition and treatment. Any forensic investigations are likely to require the cooperation of emergency physicians and other health personnel. Cultural and religious needs associated with the management of dead bodies and in communication with relatives should be respected at all times.

Urban search and rescue

Urban search and rescue (USAR) is the science of locating, reaching, treating and safely extricating survivors who remain trapped following a structural collapse. Search and rescue response capabilities have increased significantly, due to advances in rescue technology and in emergency services.

In the period immediately following a structural collapse, many survivors are rescued by uninjured bystanders. Those who remain trapped generally require the assistance of specially trained and equipped units from fire, ambulance or police services in order to be safely extricated. Medical members of search and rescue teams are tasked to provide medical care to the victims and medical support to the rescuers. They are not usually involved in the actual extrication process. Potential hazards to victims and rescuers are numerous and scene safety is of critical importance. The identification and extrication of victims following a major structural collapse is one of the most physically and emotionally challenging tasks of any rescue operation. The shock of dealing with scenes of carnage and mutilation may render some rescue personnel ineffective. These teams must therefore be trained and prepared to deal with the emotional strains of working in such a demanding environment.

Mental health

It is easy to overlook the mental health needs of affected individuals during the emergency response, when rescue and life-saving interventions receive top priority. Emergency physicians should be aware of the significant psychological impact of disasters on victims, families and rescue personnel. Psychological support is recommended as first-level assistance to disaster-affected communities and personnel [29]. Mental health consequences, such as depression, anxiety states and post-traumatic stress syndrome, are well described following disasters and need to be considered when developing the disaster plan. Crisis counselling may play an important role in the overall medical care provided to patients following a disaster. In addition, rescue personnel may well suffer psychological consequences from their own involvement in the disaster response and should therefore be provided with access to appropriate support and services.

Mass gatherings

Social and cultural events can result in the gathering of many people in one place at a particular time, sometimes over several days. Common examples include religious events, music festivals, sporting events, fairs and parades. The organization of medical services for mass gatherings is generally designed to address minor medical needs, but must also take into consideration medical emergencies, such as cardiac arrests, and disaster planning, for incidents such as extreme weather, fire, structural collapse or terrorism. Medical services developed for the mass gathering must be linked to local emergency medical systems. Public health and occupational health regulations, including food safety and environmental health measures, must be observed.

Public health issues in disasters

Public health professionals are involved in all phases of disaster risk management and it is important for emergency physicians to understand the role of public health in disaster medicine and disaster risk management. Epidemiological studies that have identified risk factors for illness and injury following disasters have contributed greatly to disaster risk assessments, prevention, mitigation, preparedness (including planning), response and recovery. These investigations have been central to the development of the science of disaster medicine. They have led to key strategies that

have been effective in reducing disaster-related morbidity and mortality.

Public health interventions become high priorities following disasters that disrupt the social infrastructure (for instance, cyclone, flooding, earthquake) and disasters that result in significant population displacement (such as complex emergencies). Priorities for the affected population include the provision of adequate water quantity and quality, sanitation, food, shelter, infectious disease control and disease surveillance. The role of public health following a mass casualty incident includes injury control, occupational health and safety measures for responders and injury surveillance.

The interface between emergency medicine and public health becomes increasingly important following technological disasters or terrorist events involving biological, chemical or nuclear agents. The terrorist attacks with anthrax in the USA during 2001 and their aftermath demonstrated the vital importance of key public health tools, such as disease surveillance and outbreak investigation and control. Following incidents with chemical or radiological agents, public health officials may be required to provide guidance on issues, such as evacuation of the public, mass decontamination and the mass distribution of iodine. Emergency physicians should become more familiar with the skills, roles and responsibilities of their public health colleagues, especially as they relate to disaster management and infectious disease control.

Conclusion

State-of-the-art in contemporary disaster management emerges from interdisciplinary, interagency and international best practices. Curative medical skills and public health skills are both fundamental to the comprehensive management of a community affected by a disaster. Emergency physicians contribute most significantly to the preparedness and response aspects of disaster management. Emergency physicians should plan and build capacities for disasters based on an assessment of the major risks that their communities face and those which are most likely to result in multiple casualties. These include the risks associated with natural, technological, biological and societal hazards. The increased risks posed by climate change and terrorists require the continuing review and revision of disaster risk-assessment processes and disaster planning. Disasters

associated with multiple casualties provide unique challenges to the health and medical communities. Short courses in disaster management are widely available and should be part of every emergency physician's training.

Likely developments

- Increasing frequency, severity and unpredictability of natural disasters.
- Increasing standardization in international response mechanisms, including foreign medical teams.
- Increasing accountability of health factors for disaster clinical interventions and their outcomes.
- Strengthened mechanisms for the leadership, coordination and effectiveness of international disaster response, in line with recent reform measures.

Controversies and future directions

- The fields of disaster management and disaster medicine continue to professionalize. There are updated standards, best practices and trainings for most aspects of disaster response. There has also been significant progress in managing the risks posed by various hazards prior to disasters striking. Emergency physicians should familiarize themselves with these developments so that they are better able to respond to both small- and large-scale disasters.
- Disaster planning and preparedness must address the most common hazards and vulnerabilities within a community, while still including a prudent approach to high profile events that have low probability and high consequences, such as terrorist attacks with CBRN agents. The all-hazards approach provides appropriate guiding principles for such planning.
- The threat of pandemic influenza and other potential epidemics must also be considered in disaster planning and preparedness. Emergency physicians should increase their familiarity with important concepts, such as infectious disease surveillance, case detection and outbreak investigation and response. They

should also become more familiar with the skills, roles and responsibilities of their public health colleagues, especially as they relate to disaster management and infectious disease control.

• The recently developed Australian medical response teams (AusMATs) and the Australian Civilian Corps provide opportunities for civilian specialists, including emergency physicians, to be deployed to countries experiencing or emerging from natural disaster or conflict. Opportunities also exist with a range of non-governmental organizations and UN agencies. Emergency physicians wishing to take advantage of these opportunities need to be familiar with specific clinical and public health issues, security considerations and international disaster response architecture and procedures.

References

[1] International Strategy for Disaster Reduction. UNISDR terminology on disaster risk reduction. Geneva: UNISDR; 2009.

[2] Australian Government Attorney-General's Department. Australian emergency management handbook series. Disaster health handbook, vol. 1. Barton, ACT: Australian Emergency Management Institute; 2011.

[3] International Federation of Red Cross and Red Crescent Societies. World disasters report. Geneva: International Federation of Red Cross and Red Crescent Societies; 2011. p. 203.

[4] Keim MJ, Abrahams J. Health and disaster. In: Wisner B, Gaillard JC, Kelman I, editors. The Routledge handbook of hazards and disaster risk reduction. Oxford/New York: Routledge; 2012.

[5] Murray V, Clifford J, Seynaeve G, Fisher J. Disaster health education and training: a pilot questionnaire to understand current status. Prehosp Disast Med 2006;21:156–67.

[6] International Rescue Committee. Mortality in the democratic republic of Congo: an ongoing crisis. New York: International Rescue Committee; 2007.

[7] Alliance Development Works, United Nations University Institute for Environment and Human Security (UNU-EHS), The Nature Conservancy Trust. World Risk Report 2012. Berlin: Bündnis Entwicklung Hilft (Alliance Development Works); 2012.

[8] Uppsala Conflict Data Program. Uppsala Conflict Data Program. <http://www.pcr.uu.se/research/ucdp/> [Accessed Dec. 2012].

[9] US Department of State, National Counterterrorism Center: Annex of Statistical Information. Country reports on terrorism 2011. <http://www.state.gov/j/ct/rls/crt/2011/195555.htm> [Accessed Nov. 2012].

[10] Brahmbhatt M. Avian influenza: economic and social impacts. <http://web.worldbank.org/WBSITE/EXTERNAL/NEWS/0,contentMDK:20663668~pagePK:34370~piPK:42770~theSitePK:4607,00.html> [Accessed Jan. 2012].

[11] Australian Government Australian Emergency Manuals. Principles and reference series. Emergency management concepts and principles. Canberra: Emergency Management Australia; 2004.

[12] Australian Government Attorney General's Department. Australian emergency management arrangements. Canberra: Australian Attorney-General's Department; 2009.

[13] Australian Government Australian Emergency Manuals. Principles and reference series . Emergency risk management applications guide, 2nd edn. Canberra: Emergency Management Australia; 2004.

[14] Council of Australian Governments. National strategy for disaster resilience: building the resilience of our nation to disasters. Canberra: Commonwealth of Australia; 2011.

[15] National Critical Care and Trauma Response Centre. <http://www.nationaltraumacentre.nt.gov.au/disaster> [Accessed Feb. 2013].

[16] Sphere Project. Humanitarian charter and minimum standards in humanitarian response. Rugby, United Kingdom: Practical Action Publishing; 2011.

[17] Anton Breil Centre for Public Health and Tropical Medicine, James Cook University. Disaster Medical Assistance Teams: a literature review; 2006. Available from the Health Protection Group, Department of Health, Western Australia, Australia.

[18] Bradt DA. Site management of health issues in the 2001 World Trade Center disaster. Acad Emerg Med 2003;10:650–60.

[19] US Centers for Disease Control and Prevention. Mass trauma casualty predictor. <http://www.bt.cdc.gov/masscasualties/predictor.asp> [Accessed Feb. 2013].

[20] Advanced Life Support Group. Major incident medical management and support – the practical approach, 3rd edn. UK: John Wiley & Sons; 2012.

[21] Benson M, Koenig KL, Schultz CH. Disaster triage: START, then SAVE – a new method of dynamic triage for victims of a catastrophic earthquake. Prehosp Disaster Med 1996;11:117–24.

[22] American Medical Association. Basic disaster life support provider manual (Ver 2.6). American Medical Association; 2007.

[23] US Department of Health and Human Services Public Health Service Agency for Toxic Substances and Disease Registry Hospital Emergency Departments: a planning guide for the management of contaminated patients (Volume 2). December 2012. CreateSpace Independent Publishing Platform. <http://www.atsdr.cdc.gov>.

[24] US Army Medical Research Institute of Infectious Diseases. Medical management of biological casualties handbook, 7th edn. September 2011. <http://www.usamriid.army.mil/education/bluebookpdf/USAMRIID%20BlueBook%207th%20Edition%20-%20Sep%202011.pdf> [Accessed Feb. 2013].

[25] US Army Medical Research Institute of Chemical Defense. Medical management of chemical casualties handbook, 4th edn. February 2007. <http://www.globalsecurity.org/wmd/library/policy/army/other/mmcc-hbk_4th-ed.pdf> [Accessed Feb. 2013].

[26] World Health Organization Western Pacific Region. Field manual for capacity assessment of health facilities in responding to emergencies, 2006. Available from the WHO Western Pacific Regional Publications Office, WHO Regional Office for the Western Pacific.

[27] Qureshi K, Gebbie KM, Gebbie EN. Public Health Incident Command System: a guide for the management of emergencies or other unusual incidents within public health agencies, Volumes 1 & 2. August 2006. <http://www.ualbanycphp.org/pinata/phics/default.cfm>.

[28] Bradt DA, Aitken P, Fitzgerald G, et al. Augmentation of hospital emergency department surge capacity: recommendations of the Australasian Surge Strategy Working Group. Acad Emerg Med 2009;16:1350–8.

[29] Interagency Standing Committee. IASC guidelines on mental health and psychosocial support in emergency settings. Geneva: IASC; 2007.

26.4 Triage

Drew Richardson

ESSENTIALS

1 Triage is the ongoing process of sorting patients on the basis of the urgency of their need for medical care.

2 Urgency is distinct from both severity and complexity.

3 Triage categorization has been found to relate strongly to both resource use and patient outcome in the near term.

4 The 5-level Australasian Triage Scale (ATS) forms the basis of emergency department triage in Australasia.

5 The ATS is also used in case mix funding models and important performance measures.

6 The 'treatment strategy' by which the next patient to be seen is chosen from the various treatment queues continues to evolve in the face of increasing demand and 'streaming' according to likely therapeutic need.

7 Similar triage scales have been developed and adopted in other jurisdictions.

Introduction

Provision of high-availability quality medical care is expensive and has been traditionally limited to the very wealthy or to situations of great demand, such as the military in battle. Even today, well-organized emergency medical systems are concentrated in societies sufficiently affluent to spend 5% or more of GDP on health. Some form of rationing is required whenever an expensive resource is coupled with fluctuating demand. Price, queuing and denial are all used in different areas of medicine. Simple application of any of these methods in emergency medicine would not be efficient nor equitable, so the majority of emergency medical systems use a triage process to sort patients into a number of queues.

Triage, the sorting of patients on the basis of urgency, is an ongoing process that nevertheless requires formal structures at different points within the continuum of care. In the emergency department (ED) setting there is considerable evidence that urgency can be assigned reliably and distinctly on a five level scale and that this categorization is applicable

and useful beyond the concept of 'urgency' into other aspects of hospital care.

Origins of triage

The word 'triage', arising from the French 'trier' meaning 'to sort' has its origins in Latin. It has entered English at least three times: from the 18th century wood industry, the 19th century coffee industry and from 20th century emergency medicine. The process understood today as triage was first described by Baron Dominique Jean-Larrey (1766–1842) [1], the surgeon to Napoleon, who also developed the ambulance volante, the first field ambulance. This delivered large numbers of injured but salvageable cases to medical units, mandating a more efficient system than treatment in order of military rank. Jean-Larrey's 'order of dressing and arrangement' by urgency was also in keeping with the egalitarian spirit of the French revolution, although there is no evidence that he actually used the word triage. His concept was embraced and refined by military surgeons over the next 150 years, usually with the primary intent of returning soldiers to battle in the most efficient manner.

Civilian triage developments

There was certainly some sorting of patients from the moment 'casual wards' opened in 19th century hospitals, but the first systematic description in civilian medicine was by E. Richard Weinerman in Baltimore in 1966 [2]. Since that time, there has been a huge growth in emergency medicine as a specialty and a number of workers have undertaken formal investigation of triage, particularly in Australasia. The Australasian experience formed the basis of ED triage development in Canada and the UK, while some other jurisdictions have developed systems independently.

Process of triage

The underlying principles of triage are those of equity (or justice) and efficiency. EDs experience potentially overwhelming demand from patients with an enormous range of conditions. Equity demands that the distribution of resources for treatment is fair in the broadest sense. The concept of urgency is well understood by the population who generally accept that it is fair to treat those in the greatest need ahead of those who arrived before them. Efficiency demands that best use is made of available resources. In the setting of ED, cost and resource pressures prevent all demand being satisfied simultaneously. The overall philosophy of 'doing the greatest good for the greatest number' requires resource allocation on the basis of need which, in turn, requires a process to identify and prioritize the needs of the presenting population.

In the ED, urgency is distinct from severity, prognosis, complexity and case mix, although a correlation exists. Some urgent problems (for example, upper airway obstruction) have a poor outcome without rapid intervention but are not severe in the sense of requiring long-term care, other severe problems (for example, life-threatening malignancy) may not require any treatment in the ED time frame. Complexity is reflected in the number of interventions, such as investigations or consultations required, whereas case mix is an indication of the resources required to provide care.

Triage is an ongoing process that may change in response to alterations in patient status and resource availability, but it is efficient to undertake a formal process once, early in the patient's encounter, and then review only as necessary. ED triage is normally undertaken by trained nursing staff at the time of arrival and the assigned urgency is then used to guide treatment order. 'Triage', used as a noun, is now regarded as the first point of patient contact in EDs.

The overall efficiency and effectiveness of such a system depends not only on the allocated priority but also on the treatment strategy, that is, the way in which the next patient is chosen from the different queues. A more urgent case should wait less time than a less urgent case but, when resources become available to treat the next patient, choice may still be required between a new arrival and a slightly less urgent patient who has already been waiting for some time. It may also be a more efficient strategy in terms of both waiting time and patient care time to 'stream' particular patients to particular providers, for example uncomplicated muscular injuries to a physiotherapist.

Australasian triage development

The first Australasian description was of the Box Hill Triage Scale by Pink and Brentnall in 1977 [3]. They used verbal descriptions without time consideration and classified patients into five categories: immediate, urgent, prompt, non-urgent and routine. Fitzgerald modified this scale in 1989 [4], to produce the Ipswich Triage Scale. This used five colours to categorize patients according to the question: 'This patient should under optimal circumstances be seen within…'. The five categories were seconds, minutes, an hour, hours and days. Fitzgerald found his triage scale to have good interobserver reliability on formal testing and to be a practical predictor of ED outcome and length of ICU stay, but a relatively poor predictor of outcome at hospital discharge.

Jelinek [5] investigated the relationship between the Ipswich Triage Scale and case mix, observing a strong correlation between triage categorization and overall use of

resources in the ED and validated possible funding models. He proposed two possible case mix classifications: urgency and disposition groups (UDGs – 12 groups) and urgency related groups (URGs – 73 groups) based on urgency, disposition and diagnosis. After trimming for outliers, these were found to account for 47% and 58% of the cost variance in large hospitals.

In 1994, the Australasian College for Emergency Medicine formalized the National Triage Scale [6], derived from the Ipswich Triage Scale. This used colours, names or numerical categories to represent five groups, based on the answer to the question 'This patient should wait for medical care no longer than…'. The categories were: immediate, 10 minutes, 30 minutes, 1 hour and 2 hours. The definition document also proposed Jelinek's concept [5] of performance indicators based on the proportion of patients whose care fell within the desired time threshold and audit by means of admission rates and sentinel diagnoses. It influenced treatment strategies by indicating the need to achieve performance indicators in a high proportion of patients in every category (higher in the more urgent) and it clearly established the need for EDs to employ systematic, accountable and audited triage processes.

Over the next few years, the National Triage Scale was widely accepted and recognized by all Australian State Governments as an appropriate measure of access to emergency care. It was also adopted in the performance indicators promulgated by the Australian Council on Healthcare Standards [7]. Research repeated the findings of Fitzgerald and Jelinek with reference to the new 5-point scale and investigated many more of the subtleties of triage scale use.

The Australasian Triage Scale

The Australasian Triage Scale (ATS) [8] is the current refinement of the National Triage Scale (NTS). It has been jointly developed by the Australasian College for Emergency Medicine, emergency nursing organizations and other interested parties. For practical purposes, the scale concept itself is unchanged, but the ATS uses numeric classification only, better defines waiting time and includes associated implementation guidelines and educational material, partly derived from work on the NTS in areas such as mental health triage [9]. Further training packages have subsequently been

developed [10], secondary to concerns about variation in triage training [11].

The ATS categorizes patients presenting to EDs in response to the question: 'This patient should wait for medical assessment and treatment no longer than…' (Table 26.4.1)

Other triage scales

The concept of desirable waiting time must include some subjective component but has, nevertheless, been found to be reliable and reproducible. Achievement of ATS waiting times has proven to be a useful performance indicator, but remains a measure of process rather than ED outcome. Concerns have been expressed in some jurisdictions about the medicolegal implications of a time-based threshold which will not always be met and other systems have taken different approaches in development of their own ED triage systems. Nevertheless, most have developed five-level triage systems along the Australasian model. Major validated triage scales include:

- the Canadian Emergency Department Triage and Acuity Scale (CTAS) [12]: derived from the ATS but using a 15-minute threshold in category 2
- the Manchester Triage Scale [13]: uses an algorithmic approach to the UK Triage scale, similar to the ATS but with longer thresholds in the lower acuity categories
- the ESI Triage Algorithm [14]: developed in the USA without any time thresholds, but using a simple approach to classifying urgency.

Use beyond waiting time

Triage is based on a brief assessment and an individual triage categorization can reflect only

Table 26.4.1 The ATS categorization of patients presenting to EDs	
ATS category	Treatment acuity (maximum waiting time)
ATS 1	Immediate
ATS 2	10 minutes
ATS 3	30 minutes
ATS 4	60 minutes
ATS 5	120 minutes

the probability of certain outcomes. Large populations of triaged patients, however, exhibit predictable patterns. There is a very strong, almost linear relationship between triage category and total rate of admission, transfer or death, ranging from 80–100% in ATS 1 to 0–20% in ATS 5 [15]. This pattern is repeated across hospitals of different size and different patient mix. Admission rates by triage category follow the pattern of overall admission rates in relation to age, giving a flattened 'U-shaped' distribution. The inter-rater reliability studies performed using the Ipswich Triage Scale have been repeated using the NTS/ATS, which has been found to be slightly better [16]. Further, admission rates by triage category have been shown to be constant over time in individual institutions [17].

The NTS/ATS has been extensively studied as a case-mix tool. ED outcome (admission/transfer/death versus discharge) accounts for the largest variance in cost, but triage categorization comes a close second, with age third. The mean cost of care for a category 1 patient is approximately 10 times that of a category 5 patient. Urgency and Disposition Groups (UDGs), described by Jelinek using the Ipswich Triage Scale, have been validated using the National Triage Scale on large samples [18]. Age has been included to derive urgency, disposition and age groups (UDAGs – 32 groups), which account for 51% of the cost variance and are not susceptible to different diagnostic approaches [19]. The relativities derived in these studies should no longer be considered valid in the era of overcrowding and access block, because staff costs for admitted patients reflect length of time in the ED, which may now be driven by outside factors. Further, the costs for discharged patients are becoming skewed by increased pressure to keep complex patients out of hospital.

Triage categorization is a very strong predictor of ED outcome and a good predictor of utilization of critical care resources. However, it is a relatively poor predictor of outcome at hospital discharge [20,21]. Many patients with chronic or subacute conditions that frequently cause death are triaged to less urgent categories because there is no benefit from earlier treatment within the time scales available in the ED.

Attainment of performance indicators for patients seen within triage thresholds has been shown to be a measure of resource allocation within the ED. A longitudinal comparative study

has demonstrated a significant improvement with an increase in ED staff and funding [22].

Triage staff are well able to assess complexity [23] and so initial triage is also the appropriate point to start streaming decisions, for example to a 'fast track' area for low-complexity patients [24]. Although streaming can be seen as decreasing equity because the less urgent patients achieve shorter waiting times than more urgent, in practice, this is compensated by the gain in overall efficiency [25–27]. Like the triage process itself, changes to the treatment strategy, such as streaming, can and should be ongoing, reflecting not the urgency of the patients, but the best distribution of the resources available at that moment.

Structure and function of a triage system

The exact requirements for triage vary with the role, location and size of the hospital, but effective systems share a number of important features, mostly derived from experience:

- A single point in the ED near the entrance where triage is undertaken so that all patients will be exposed to the nurse(s) undertaking triage.
- Appropriate facilities for undertaking brief assessment and limited treatment (first aid) including relevant equipment and washing facilities for staff and patients.
- A balance between competing concerns of accessibility, confidentiality and security.
- A means of recording assessment and triage categorization that will 'follow' the patient through their time in the ED and be available for review afterwards. In most departments, this is now a computerized information system.
- Contemporary data on the state of the ED and the expected patients, such as the information system and ambulance and police radio systems.

Pre-hospital triage

The principle of making best use of available resources to maximize patient outcome remains the basis of triage in any setting. Relatively less therapeutic options are available to pre-hospital providers and patient disposition is generally limited to transport and sometimes choice of hospitals. The initial pre-hospital

phase, the travel to the patient, must be undertaken on the basis of minimal information. Most pre-hospital systems are strongly protocol driven and tend towards three or four level assessment: rapid response (lights and sirens), immediate response, routine response or no transport. Once the patient is assessed in the field, there is patient benefit in triaging to the most appropriate hospital for tertiary-level conditions, such as major trauma [28] or ST-elevation myocardial infarction [29].

Military and disaster triage

In situations of overwhelming imbalance between resources and demand, triage remains critical in ensuring that available resources are used to achieve the greatest good. The principles of rapid assessment, documentation and multiple queues for care remain the same, but competing demands on resources may mean triaging cases to receive minimal or no care or treating first those who can return to work or duty. The need for both human and physical resources for more important tasks may profoundly limit individual patient care.

Military and disaster triage require seniority and experience (which by definition is rarely available), the ability to make and defend rapid decisions and a successful liaison with other players outside the medical or nursing hierarchy. Senior personnel with significant experience and preferably with additional training should be chosen for this role if possible. Formal triage and documentation must be brief and will use different scales from those appropriate in the ED.

Controversies and future directions

- The research base undertaken on the National Triage Scale has shown it to be relatively reliable and reproducible, but identified some areas for improvement. The Australasian Triage Scale and its associated guidelines and educational materials were designed to address some of the recognized problems with the NTS, but revision and improvement of the Scale will continue. Further study is required on issues including:
  - variation in implementation between sites, particularly hospitals of different role delineation

- the most appropriate 'treatment strategy', that is, how the next patient to be treated is chosen from the various queues, in both normal and overcrowded conditions
- variation associated with activity or overcrowding – there is evidence of consistency in some hospitals but changes in others
- variation in approach to paediatric triage, especially between mixed and paediatric EDs and to psychiatric triage
- whether the ATS has any role outside its design base of EDs with 24-hour medical staffing, for example in smaller hospitals and pre-hospital settings.

References

[1] Larrey DJ. Surgical memoirs of the campaigns in Russia, Germany, and France. Translated Mercer JC. Philadelphia: Carey and Lea; 1832. Cited in Winslow G. Triage and justice. University of California Press.

[2] Weinerman ER, Rateen RS, Robbins A. Yale studies in ambulatory care V. Determinants of use of hospital emergency services. Am J Publ Hlth Nations Hlth 1966;56:1037–56.

[3] Pink N. Triage in the accident and emergency department. Aust Nurses J 1977;6:35–6.

[4] Fitzgerald GJ. Emergency department triage. Doctor of Medicine Thesis. University of Queensland; 1989.

[5] Jelinek GA. Casemix classification of patients attending hospital emergency departments in Perth, Western Australia. Doctor of Medicine Thesis. University of Western Australia; 1995.

[6] Australasian College for Emergency Medicine: National Triage Scale. Emerg Med (Aust) 1994; 6:145–46.

[7] Australian Council on Healthcare Standards. Clinical indicators – a user's manual. Zetland NSW: ACHS; 1996.

[8] Australasian College for Emergency Medicine: Australasian Triage Scale. Emerg Med (Aust) 2002; 14:335–36.

[9] Smart D, Pollard C, Walpole B. Mental health triage in emergency medicine. Aust NZ J Psychiatr 1999;33:57–66.

[10] Gerdtz MF, Considine J, Sands N, et al. Emergency triage education kit. Australian Commonwealth Department of Health Ageing. Canberra: Commonwealth Government of Australia, 2007, p. 10–15.

[11] Kelly AM, Richardson D. Training for the role of triage in Australasia. Emerg Med (Aust) 2001;13:230–2.

[12] Beveridge R, Ducharme J, James L, et al. Reliability of the Canadian Emergency Department Triage and acuity scale: interrater agreement. Ann Emerg Med 1999;34:155–9.

[13] Manchester Triage Group. Emergency triage. London: Publishing Group; 1997.

[14] Wuerz RC, Milne LW, Eitel DR, et al. Reliability and validity of a new five-level triage instrument. Acad Emerg Med 2000;7:236–42.

[15] Whitby S, Leraci S, Johnson D, Mohsin M. Analysis of the process of triage: the use and outcome of the National Triage Scale. Liverpool NSW: Liverpool Health Service; 1997.

[16] Jelinek GA, Little M. Inter-rater reliability of the National Triage Scale over 11,500 simulated occasions of triage. Emerg Med (Aust) 1996;8:226–30.

[17] Richardson DB. No relationship between emergency department activity and triage categorization. Acad Emerg Med 1998;5:141–5.

[18] Erwich MA, Bond MJ, Phillips DG, Baggoley CJ. The identification of costs associated with Emergency Department attendances. Emerg Med (Aust) 1997; 9:181–7.

[19] Erwich MA, Bond MJ, Baggoley CJ. Costings in the emergency department. Report to the Commonwealth Department of Health and Human Services (Australia); 1996.

[20] Dent A, Rofe G, Sansom G. Which triage category patients die in hospital after being admitted through emergency departments? A study in one teaching hospital. Emerg Med (Aust) 1999;11:68–71.

[21] Doherty SR, Hore CT, Curran SW. Inpatient mortality as related to triage category in three New South Wales regional base hospitals. Emerg Med (Aust) 2003;15:334–40.

[22] Rogers IR, Evans L, Jelinek GA. Using clinical indicators in emergency medicine: documenting performance improvements to justify increased resource allocation. J Accid Emerg Med 1999;16:319–21.

[23] Vance J, Sprivulis P. Triage nurses validly and reliably estimate emergency department patient complexity. Emerg Med Australas 2005;17:382–6.

[24] King DL, Ben-Tovim DI, Bassham J. Redesigning emergency department patient flows: application of Lean Thinking to health care. Emerg Med Australas 2006;18:391–7.

[25] O'Brien D, Williams A, Blondell K, Jelinek GA. Impact of streaming 'fast track' emergency department patients. Aust Hlth Rev 2006;30:525–32.

[26] Kwa P, Blake D. Fast track: has it changed patient care in the emergency department? Emerg Med Australas 2008;20:10–15.

[27] Shetty A, Gunja N, Byth K, Vukasovic M. Senior streaming assessment further evaluation after triage zone: a novel model of care encompassing various emergency department throughput measures. Emerg Med Australas 2012;24:374–82.

[28] Cox S, Currell A, Harriss L, et al. Evaluation of the Victorian state adult pre-hospital trauma triage criteria. Injury 2012;43:573–81.

[29] Carstensen S, Nelson GC, Hansen PS, et al. Field triage to primary angioplasty combined with emergency department bypass reduces treatment delays and is associated with improved outcome. Eur Heart J 2007;28:2313–9.

26.5 Emergency care in a humanitarian crisis

Angela Jackson • Mark Little

ESSENTIALS

1 The worldwide problem of displaced persons is massive and likely to increase. Millions more are displaced within their own countries compared to those refugees who have crossed international borders.

2 Overall responsibility for displaced persons lies with the United Nations High Commission for Refugees (UNHCR), although numerous other organizations also assist.

3 When people are displaced, they often establish alternate homes, usually tented, which increases the risks of disease, violence and social dislocation.

4 The UN has introduced the cluster system to improve communication and coordination of the humanitarian crisis. Involvement of the local community and displaced leaders is essential.

5 The basics of nutrition, shelter, clean water and sanitation are always the most important. Minimum standards (Sphere handbook) exist for the provision of care provided.

6 The four major health threats in a humanitarian crisis are malaria, measles, diarrhoeal illness and respiratory tract infections.

7 For those displaced, the durable solutions are resettlement in their country of origin, integration into the new host country or resettlement into a third country.

8 The ultimate solution to solving the problem of the world's displaced population is political.

Introduction

Increasingly over the past few years, Australian health professionals, including emergency medicine staff, have responded to humanitarian crises due to conflict or natural disasters within our region. Caring for displaced persons is not a new problem. Since World War II up to 100 million civilians have been forced to flee their homes due to unrest. The major factors that cause people to flee their country include conflict, political repression and persecution, and are as old as humanity. In 1573, the term 'refugee' was first used for Calvinists fleeing political repression in the Spanish-controlled Netherlands.

The modern response to refugees started at the end of World War II and, in 1946, the International Refugee Organisation (IRO) was created. The United Nations High Commissioner for Refugees (UNHCR) replaced the IRO in 1951 and the *Convention Relating to the Status of*

Refugees, came into being. This key legal document defines who is a refugee and sets out the rights of those who are granted asylum and the legal obligations of nations that grant it. It has been widely ratified to date and, notably, was signed by the President of Nauru, Marcus Stephen on 17 June 2011. With some fine-tuning over the years it remains the cornerstone of International Refugee Law. It defines a refugee as:

A person who owing to a well-founded fear of being persecuted for reasons of race, religion, nationality, membership of a particular social group or political opinion, is outside the country of his nationality and is unable or, owing to such fear, is unwilling to avail himself of the protection of that country; or who, not having a nationality and being outside the country of his former habitual residence as a result of such events, is unable or, owing to such fear, is unwilling to return to it...

The UNHCR encourages countries to receive refugees and to provide them with assistance and protection. One of the major points of the Convention is the principle of 'non-refoulement', which means that refugees cannot be forcibly returned to their countries of origin if to do so would threaten their life or freedom.

Perhaps of more concern to the humanitarian community are the large numbers of Internally Displaced Persons (IDPs). IDPs are people displaced from their home but who have not crossed an international border. They are commonly fleeing situations such as internal armed conflict, communal violence and other human rights violations. Although the national government has a responsibility to care and protect IDPs, in many instances, state authorities may not only be the cause of displacement but may lack the will or capacity to address the IDPs' needs which include, not only humanitarian relief assistance, but also protection. Where a state lacks capacity, it can request humanitarian relief assistance from UNHCR. Since 1992, UNHCR has been focusing more efforts to the protection of IDPs and, since 2007, has taken the lead in complex emergencies.

In 2011, according to UNHCR, there were 42.5 million people displaced worldwide. Of these, 15.2 million were refugees and 26.4 million were internally displaced persons (IDPs); 25.9 million were living under protection of the UNHCR mandate. Pakistan was hosting 1.7 million refugees. Up to 93% of all refugees were being hosted within the region of the country they had fled. The major sources of refugees in 2011 were Afghanistan (2.66 million), Iraq (1.43 million) and Somalia (1.07 million). Of all these refugees, 46% are less than 18 years of age.

There were 2.9 million newly displaced persons in 2011. The largest numbers of IDPs are found in the Democratic Republic of the Congo (DRC) 0.83 million and Pakistan 0.62 million. At the height of the crises in 2010, the floods in Pakistan saw 20 million people displaced. The worldwide problem is clearly significant.

The solution to any displacement problem is ultimately non-medical as the problem is commonly based on political instability. Even in the acute phases of refugee movement, the most important needs are basic and are commonly food, shelter and clean water. Physicians, however, can play a considerable role in relief efforts, particularly where they are adaptable and able to use simple, cheap and effective solutions to problems. Of particular importance, however, is that at all stages of relief assistance, the displaced population, sometimes referred to as 'the beneficiaries', must be actively involved in planning and delivery of aid. Affected communities themselves know what they need, who their leaders are and they speak the local language.

Emergency physicians need to have an understanding of the issues and possible solutions for those displaced, including links to appropriate organizations and information where necessary.

Responsibility for refugee care

Until the end of the World War I, the response to refugees was from philanthropic sections of the community. The formation of the League of Nations began the process of the international community assuming responsibility for refugees. In 1921, a High Commission for Refugees was established with a mandate to look after refugees fleeing the Russian and Armenian wars. Its first Commissioner was Fridtjof Nansen, who established a special identity document, the 'Nansen Passport', as refugees frequently had no means of identification.

In the wake of World War II, the United Nations (UN) established the International Refugee Organisation to assist the millions of displaced persons in Europe. Between 1947 and 1951, it helped 1.6 million people, mainly Germans and Austrians.

Coordination in a humanitarian crisis

Overcoming problems of poor planning and coordination has been the major thrust of more recent developments. After the Great Lakes Disaster in the early 1990s, it was decided in 1997 to establish a set of minimum standards and rights to which refugees were entitled. The collaborative project, called Sphere, was initiated in 1997 by a group of humanitarian non-government organizations (NGOs) and

the International Red Cross and Red Crescent Movement with the overall aim of improving the quality of their actions and accountability during disaster response. The Sphere Project produced a manual that is available free from the website www.sphereproject.org. The Sphere Handbook is widely known and sets out common principles and universal minimum standards for humanitarian response. The Sphere Handbook was first published in 2000 with the most recent revision in 2010. Other organizations, such as Médecins Sans Frontières (MSF), UNHCR and the World Health Organization (WHO), also have several excellent manuals describing in detail the approach to humanitarian emergencies.

The Office for the Coordination of Humanitarian Affairs (OCHA) is the UN agency responsible for mobilizing and coordinating effective and principled humanitarian action in partnership with national and international factors. In 2005, realizing the need for improved coordination to humanitarian crises, OCHA initiated a review of its processes. This resulted in the introduction of the UN clusters with the aim of building sufficient response capacity, improving humanitarian coordination and leadership and building effective partnerships. Organizational leaders are responsible for nine themed clusters at both field and global level coordination. Table 26.5.1 shows the current clusters and their lead agencies.

Global cluster leaders develop partnerships, humanitarian preparedness and set standards and policy. At a field level, the cluster lead ensures collaboration and coordination and is accountable to the senior UN person in the country coordinating the response, referred to as the Humanitarian Coordinator. The cluster lead is also the 'provider of last resort', which means they must do their utmost to ensure an adequate response and, if lacking resources, seek assistance to receive these resources from others higher up in the UN chain (such as the Humanitarian Coordinator). Any organization responding to a humanitarian crisis and working in a specified area of response (e.g. health) is welcome to attend any relevant cluster meeting.

Funding is another important issue. In 2006, the UN General Assembly established the Central Emergency Response Fund (CERF) to provide funds rapidly for the immediate assistance to a humanitarian crisis. It has a grant facility of $US450 M and a loan facility of $US30 M.

Table 26.5.1 Clusters and cluster lead agencies

Technical clusters	
Nutrition	UNICEF
WASH	UNICEF
Health	WHO
Shelter (conflict/IDP)	UNHCR
Shelter (natural disaster)	IFRC 'convener'
Cross-cutting clusters	
Camp coord & mgmt (conflict/IDP)	UNHCR
Camp coord & mgmt (natural disaster)	IOM
Protection (conflict/IDP & affected)	UNHCR
Protection (natural disaster)	UNHCR/ OHCHR/UNICEF
Early recovery	UNDP
Common service clusters	
Logistics	WFP
Telecommunications	OCHA/UNICEF/ WFP
Sector	*Organization*
Refugees	UNHCR FAO
Agriculture*	UNICEF/SCF UK
Education*	WFP
Food	

UNICEF: United Nations International Children's Emergency Fund; WHO: World Health Organization; UNHCR: UN High Commissioner for Refugees; IFRC: International Federation of Red Cross; IOM: International Organization of Migration; OHCHR: Office of the High Commissioner for Human Rights; UNDP: UN Development Program; WFP : World Food Program; FAO: Food & Agriculture Organization; SCF UK: Save the Children Fund UK.
*Agriculture and education were the newer clusters established.

Before you go

The Internet and electronic media are increasingly being used in innovative ways by humanitarian agencies. It is now possible to follow evolving disasters on several websites, such as UN affiliated sites, Red Cross sites, major NGOs and MSF sites and explore what each particular organization is doing. OCHA has an excellent website called Reliefweb (www.reliefweb.int) which gives regular updates on all crises. Relevant data can also be sourced from gapminder (www.gapminder.org). In most humanitarian crises, the health issues are predictable (e.g. orthopaedic injuries with earthquakes). It is important to be aware of the literature and to scan previous reports of health issues within the region where you are intending to travel. As soon as clusters are operational, they will report recent data for the affected region, as will the local Ministry of Health. Where possible, it is preferable to be in contact with these organizations prior to departure. WHO publish on the Internet some excellent manuals on diagnosing and managing cases in humanitarian crises and have prepacked medical kits (Interagency Emergency Medical Kits). The Sphere guidelines are an essential resource and the Australian Medical Assistance Team training manual is also helpful.

Personal attributes

Working under difficult conditions imposed by a humanitarian crisis demands special qualities. It is certainly not glamorous and often much of what has been learned from training and practice in the West is either irrelevant or needs modification to suit local conditions and resources. In general the main requirements are:

- flexibility, versatility and ability to improvise
- appropriate qualifications and sufficient experience along with the ability to work independently in extreme conditions
- cultural awareness and sensitivity
- good interpersonal and communication skills and the personality to get along with all types of people
- willingness to follow leadership and direction
- good pre-deployment preparation, including appropriate vaccinations and insurance arrangements
- acceptance of security and health risks both by the individual and their family.

Camps for refugees and IDPs

Persons fleeing war or persecution escape in a variety of ways. They may be integrated within the local community or be accommodated by friends and relatives. Typical, however, is the mass movement of populations either across a country or a border into temporary accommodations or camps. It is under these circumstances that the displaced are most at risk, as they are not accommodated in isolation. There are generally interactions with a local population, which are not necessarily cordial. There may also be important political and ethnic factors within the displaced population themselves, which can lead to tensions or even violence within the camps. This scenario was tragically demonstrated in the post-Rwandan holocaust camps in 1994. Camps themselves can sustain conflict in some areas, for example, the West Bank and the camps on the Thai–Cambodian border which were used as refuges by Khmer Rouge and became a platform from which they could carry on the war.

Responding to a crisis

Emergency phase
As a result of a crisis, due either to war or acts of nature, large populations can be displaced from their normal environment. This often results in large numbers of people, with minimal or no basic life needs, descending upon a region and where they stop is generally where a camp evolves. Most population movements into such camps occur in developing countries that already have limited resources with which to deal with such issues. Preplanning by the UN, aid agencies and host governments is essential to ensure a rapid and well-coordinated humanitarian response. Considerable expertise in responding to refugee emergencies has been gained and the main priorities are now well recognized. In accordance with Sphere guidelines the main priorities are as follows.

Initial assessment
A rapid assessment of the population structure, their medical and other needs, is essential in the very early stages to prioritize planning and allocate resources appropriately. It is essential to involve local leaders and population in assessing needs and planning priorities.

Measles immunization
Conditions in refugee camps can facilitate large-scale measles epidemics which, in an at-risk population, can have devastating consequences. In 2011, the UNHCR reported that in one of the Dollo Ado camps in Ethiopia – host to mainly Somali refugees – up to 10 children per day were dying, mainly due to measles and malnutrition. Combined with malnutrition, measles can have a case fatality rate as high as 33%. The detection of one case of measles in a camp is a public health emergency and requires urgent intervention. Mass vaccination of all children from 6 months to 15 years is essential and should be done as soon as possible. To increase vaccination efficacy, WHO recommend combining measles vaccination with the administration of vitamin A. According to WHO, vitamin A has been shown to reduce the burden of disease mortality and morbidity, particularly in children less than 5 years, by improving immune response. The dosing schedule for vitamin A administration is available from the WHO website and is age specific.

Water and sanitation
Poor water supply and sanitation play a major role in the spread of diarrhoeal diseases. Well-defined standards that can be checked with simple kits now exist for acceptable water quality. The Sphere guidelines stipulate minimum quantities of water in the emergency phase of a disaster are 5 L/person/day initially and rising to 15 L/person/day when possible. Sphere also set standards for the location, type and number of latrines and washing facilities per person in camp situations.

Food and nutrition
Malnutrition is common in refugee populations and particularly in the at-risk young and elderly groups. The initial food ration recommended is 2100 kcal/person/day. It is also important to undertake surveys to assess for specific micronutrient deficiencies, such as scurvy or pellagra, and treat accordingly. Measurement of mid-upper arm circumference (MUAC) in children between 6 months and 5 years is a common quick way to asses the overall nutritional status of a population.

Assessment of nutrition in the population is an ongoing process and special feeding programmes may need to be set up for at-risk groups. Generally, there are specific agencies, such as the UN World Food Program, which specialize in this area. It is therefore important that adverse findings are reported to the health cluster to determine who will be responsible for targeting the at-risk population.

Shelter and site planning
Proper shelter and adequate clothing are essential early priorities. Overcrowding can lead to or worsen disease outbreaks and may affect the mental health of the camp population. Protection from the elements is

essential for well-being and particularly so in extreme climates. When planning camps, it is important to consider the size, terrain, security, access in and out, nearby water supply, distance to host community, etc. Again, well-defined standards for living space and shelter construction exist.

General healthcare
Organizing a system to deal with the health needs of a population is essential. Medical needs of a population are rapidly assessed and endemic diseases taken into account. There may be numerous organizations involved in health delivery activities. To avoid duplication and the waste of valuable resources, it is important for all providers to participate in ongoing communication and health planning. In disaster situations, this is best achieved by reporting to the health cluster, which has overall responsibility to coordinate the health response. Accurate data collection and reporting is necessary to monitor response progress. There are manuals and guidelines available to assist and WHO have created medical kits intended to cover the needs per 1000 refugees for a 3-month period.

Control of infectious disease
The four most frequent infectious diseases in the emergency phase are diarrhoea, malaria, respiratory infections and measles. Providing good basic living conditions will help ward off these and other illnesses; however, if an outbreak occurs, there is potential for high mortality rates. Aggressive treatment and decisive public health interventions are therefore essential. As diarrhoea is a major cause of death, the early establishment of oral rehydration centres is essential.

Public health surveillance
Collecting epidemiological data on a daily basis provides essential information to those in charge of a camp so that interventions can be planned and disease outbreaks rapidly recognized. The most useful health indicator is the daily crude mortality rate (CMR), which is normally expressed as deaths/10 000 population/day. The Sphere manual gives baseline CMRs for different regions worldwide. Double the baseline CMR is an indication the emergency threshold has been reached. If the baseline CMR is unknown then a CMR of over 1/10 000/day for adults (or 2/10 000/day for children less than 5 years) is an indicator of an emergency situation. Disease-specific mortality rates may also be useful.

Human resources and training
Administering a refugee camp is complex and requires a variety of skilled personnel who include doctors, nurses, water/sanitation experts, nutritionists, logisticians and others. The need for different types of personnel should be determined followed by appointment of the appropriate personnel – ideally from the local population where possible.

Post-emergency phase
This phase begins when the basic needs of the population are met (food, shelter, water and so on) and the CMR is either back to the baseline or less than 1 per day/10 000 for the adult population and 2 per day/10 000 for the under 5 year olds. The situation in the post-emergency phase is complex and fluid. Some of the displaced persons may become quite settled and start to work locally or farm some land. The health and nutritional status of refugees may even surpass those of the local population because of the availability of overseas aid. This may lead to resentment. Complex political issues may arise. Where a large population remains in place, descent back to the emergency phase is an ongoing possibility and may occur with epidemic outbreaks or fresh influxes of newly displaced people. In general, however, the post-emergency phase is concerned with consolidating earlier achievements, preparation for possible new emergencies and future sustainability. The continuation of water quality monitoring, public health surveillance and nutritional status assessment is important for early detection and intervention.

Healthcare delivery in the post-emergency phase is complex. Some issues that warrant consideration for planning purposes include:

- standardization of training, supervision and delivery of health services
- curative healthcare services
- reproductive healthcare, including antenatal and delivery, postnatal and family planning, sexually transmitted infections (STIs) and HIV/AIDS
- child health activities, such as expanded programmes of immunization (EPIs)
- specific HIV/AIDS/STI programmes
- tuberculosis programmes
- addressing psychosocial and mental health issues.

Permanent 'durable' solutions
There are three possible solutions to any displaced situation – repatriation, integration or resettlement in another country. Many displaced populations reside in countries neighbouring their own country and are thereby the responsibility of the UNHCR. Repatriation is the preferred option but is often quite complex. In 2011, UNHCR reported that 532 000 refugees were voluntarily repatriated. This will generally only occur where there is a solution to the problem that caused the refugees to leave initially. This can take years. People returning need a lot of extra support in order to rebuild their lives. At the time of repatriation, some families have lived in refugee camps for years and children and grandchildren have been born in camps in the host country. The newborns may have no link to the original country they fled and have more of a relationship with the host country and hence, some refugees remain in the host countries and integrate into local communities. In the past, integration into the host community was commonplace in African nations but, more recently, has become increasingly difficult, particularly when African governments see their Western counterparts' increasing reluctance to accept refugees.

The minority of refugees who cannot return are resettled in third (mostly Western) countries. Many countries have quotas and will only admit those refugees determined by UNHCR as having a valid claim. In 2011, the UNHCR reported 80 000 refugees were resettled. Of these, the USA took 51 500, Canada took 12 900 and Australia received 9200.

Past problems
In the past, there have been important problems with the response to a refugee crisis. Often these have their root in poor coordination between agencies responding to a particular crisis. It is well documented that poor coordination has in the past led to inappropriate interventions and even frank competition. Often, in a dramatic disaster, such as an earthquake which has considerable media coverage, there is a frenzy of intervention as agencies attempt to get their image across to international viewers to assist in fundraising. In the 2001 earthquake in Gujarat province, India, it was estimated that there were as many as 200 different

government and non-government agencies in the field. There is no doubt that such competition has resulted in unnecessary death, most notably in the great lakes region of Africa following the Rwandan genocide.

Controversies and future directions

- There is often a lack of coordination and communication between agencies involved in responding to a humanitarian crisis. The challenge is to coordinate the response and maximize efficiencies and outcomes.
- Since the Haiti earthquake of 2010, there has been a call for the standardization and registration of foreign medical teams responding to humanitarian crises, the aim being to improve the quality and appropriateness of medical care.

- Developing durable solutions for the world's displaced population that stands at 42.5 million is challenging. Part of the challenge is to change the attitude of many developed countries towards accepting these people for resettlement.
- Instead of spending millions of dollars each year on international staff to assist in humanitarian crises, would this money be better spent if given directly to those affected by the crisis?
- Although the UN cluster system has been established, there is a need to build resilience in this system.
- Disaster risk reduction and mitigation is probably more important than humanitarian response and, in the long term, will be more effective. Unfortunately, this is an area that needs more support and planning, although there has recently been an increase in effort in this area.

Further reading

Emergency Relief Items. Vols 1 & 2. United Nations Development Program; 2000.
Hospitals for War Wounded 1998 International Committee of the Red Cross. <www.icrc.org/eng/assets/files/other/icrc_002_0714.pdf> This is the entry point into the UN agencies, such as OCHA and its various branches. Also publishes situation reports of evolving disasters.
International Committee of the Red Cross site. <www.icrc.org>. This is more concerned with war zones.
International Federation of Red Cross and Red Crescent societies. <www.ifrc.org>.
Médecins Sans Frontières (MSF) <www.msf.org>. The MSF website is a very useful resource with several free publications on refugee healthcare.
Médecins Sans Frontières. Refugee health, an approach to emergency situations. McMillan Education Ltd; 1997. This and many other invaluable MSF texts on treatment protocols, basic kits are all available free on the MSF website <www.msf.org>.
Oxfam. <www.oxfam.org>.
Relief Web. <www.reliefweb.int>. A UN website with information on humanitarian relief organizations. Information in what is happening in recent crises as well as job availability.
The Sphere Project. <www.sphereproject.org>. The Sphere handbook and related resources.
UNHCR. <www.unhcr.int>. Refugee facts, figures and histories.
World Health Organisation. <www.who.int>. Health topics, data and programmes. Good information and publications.

26.6 Emergency department observation wards

Jessamine Soderstrom

ESSENTIALS

1 Observation wards play a key role in modern emergency departments.

2 They have an increasing role in improving patient flow while maintaining quality of care and safety in the era of National Emergency Access Target (NEAT).

3 Staffing is ideally by emergency department staff with defined admission criteria and a plan for disposition usually within 24 hours.

4 They offer time-limited intensive treatment with clear treatment and follow-up guidelines.

5 Observation wards reduce length of stay and cost compared to inpatient ward admissions.

defined by the following general characteristics [1–4]:

- discrete wards with 4–20 beds, located adjacent to or in close proximity to the main body of the ED
- capacity to care for approximately 5–10% of the total ED volume
- staffed and run by ED personnel
- provide an area for patients who require further treatment or diagnostics before being safely discharged
- the average length of stay is 10 hours and 80% of patients are discharged home.

Acute care hospitals are facing enormous pressures to improve patient access and flow while maintaining quality of care and patient satisfaction without increasing costs. In the era of improved patient flow and time targets (e.g. 4-hour rule or National Emergency Access Target [NEAT]), the observation ward provides a degree of control and flexibility to emergency physicians to extend investigation and care beyond the 4-hour targets.

Introduction

The observation ward is an essential part of an emergency department (ED) that has evolved over time to service changing needs. Its growth is a response to the emergency

physician's desire not to be forced into a dichotomous decision to admit or discharge patients. It provides a third option for medically complex patients who require more diagnostic testing and therapeutic intervention in a short time frame. Observation wards are

The benefits of having an observation ward adjacent to the emergency department include [1–4]:

- allowing patients to access investigations before leaving the emergency department, ensuring accurate diagnosis and formulation of a discharge plan
- admission to the correct inpatient service once an accurate diagnosis has been made
- provides an alternative to inpatient hospital admission as a way to improve efficiency, clinical care and patient satisfaction, while minimizing the costs [1,3]
- reducing inpatient admissions [1,3]
- temporary holding areas for access blocked patients
- temporary accommodation for patients (e.g. elderly or those with acute situational crisis) where discharge at an antisocial hour would be inappropriate
- safeguard for junior medical staff who require assistance with disposition plans
- shorter length of stay and cost compared to inpatient stay (Table 26.6.1) [1].

Observation ward policies and protocols

The overall function of the observation ward varies depending on the needs of the individual department. There are some common requirements essential to the smooth functioning of the ward [1–4].

Admission process

There must be clear medical governance and responsibility for the patient at all times. This will vary between institutions based on the functionality of the observation ward. Minimizing the number of handovers during the patient's journey through the observation ward reduces medical errors. As an example, if the observation ward functions primarily as a clinical decision unit to await investigations, then the care should remain with the primary physician. The aim is to have a senior clinician making key decisions, minimizing handovers and ensuring nursing staff are aware of who to contact in the event of patient deterioration. All patients must have a treatment plan, defined objectives for admission and conditions to be met prior to discharge.

Admission criteria

Admission criteria need to be clear. Suitable patients require time limited intensive treatment or have single system problems with clear treatment and follow-up guidelines. It is useful to have pre-negotiated referral pathways to other inpatient teams in the event of failed discharge planning. The general principle of admission to the observation ward is an expectation by the admitting doctor that the patient will be discharged within a set time limit (usually within 24 hours). This will vary depending on the available resources of each department. Some examples of conditions that may be treated in an observation ward include the following [1–9]:

Time-limited intensive treatment:

- renal colic
- mild to moderate asthma
- gastroenteritis
- migraines
- analgesia and mobilization after soft-tissue injuries
- commencement of therapy that will be continued out of hospital by hospital in the home services, general practitioners or home care nurses (e.g. intravenous antibiotics for cellulitis).

Patients requiring a longer ED stay before a disposition decision can be made:

- requiring investigations before disposition planning (e.g. clinical decision unit)
- post-procedure observation (e.g. lumbar puncture or Bier's block)
- alcohol and drug intoxication
- minor head injury with normal Glasgow coma scale (GCS) for neurological observation
- envenoming requiring a period of investigation and treatment.

Patients requiring input from allied health (e.g. physiotherapy, occupational therapy or social work), psychiatric services or where discharge after hours is not appropriate:

- elderly or other vulnerable patients to ensure safety for discharge, or where after hours discharge is inappropriate
- acute situational crisis where patients would benefit from psychiatric input.

Other uses of an observation ward

- A 'holding bay' as a means of decanting access-blocked patients. This can be a useful means of decongesting the ED but can also impair the function of the observation ward (reducing capacity of the observation ward to accept observation ward patients)
- Chest pain assessment unit – for low-risk chest pain patients [10–12]
- Toxicology unit – providing care for envenomed patients, acutely poisoned patients not requiring intensive care procedures and after intensive care (ICU) admission. Such units may be run by clinical toxicologists where present and have been demonstrated to be efficient, particularly in post-ICU care, reducing length of stay in the ICU [13].

Exclusion criteria

Exclusion criteria will vary between institutions. There are some general themes [2]:

Patients who clearly require >24-hour admission:

- patients who have more than one or complex medical problems, especially the elderly
- patients without clear treatment plans or who will not meet conditions for discharge in a timely fashion.

Table 26.6.1 Cost and LOS comparisons for observation ward vs inpatient care

Diagnosis	Observation ward cost (A$)	Inpatient cost of care (A$)	EDOU LOS (h)	Inpatient LOS (h)	References
Chest pain	844	987			2
Chest pain	1450	1989	33	45	3
Chest pain (UK)	450	638			4
Asthma	1141	2133			5
TIA	820	1451	26	61	6
Croup	1259	1599	21	27	7
Infections	1506	2643	44	88	8

EDOU: Emergency department observation units; LOS: length of stay; TIA: transient ischaemic attack.
Adapted from Baugh C, Venkatesh A, Bohan J. Emergency department observation units: a clinical and financial benefit from hospitals. Hlth Care Manag Rev 2011;36:28-37 [1] with permission.

Patients who require intensive nursing care:

- patients who are a heavy nursing load, e.g. those who are immobile, requiring full care with all their activities of daily living (ADLs)
- patients who are violent, psychotic or disruptive.

Some patients are admitted to the observation ward pending review and opinions from inpatient teams where the expectation is that the patient will be discharged. It is important that inpatient treatment is not delayed unnecessarily.

Efficiency of patient care

The observation ward is an area of rapid patient turnover within a defined time frame. There are a number of factors that assist with the efficient running of the ward [1–4]:

- Senior clinician input is required for rapid decision making and referral as necessary. Ward rounds and presence of the senior decision maker is not affected by weekends or public holidays (as may be the case with other inpatient teams).
- Defined clinical pathways and referral process to facilitate patient disposition. This improves and streamlines the referral process. As an example, the management of renal colic should be a straightforward process with analgesia, imaging and referral to urology as required [7]. Efficiencies can be gained by negotiation with radiology for a streamlined process for appropriate imaging and admission, discharge and follow-up criteria with urology. These pathways need to be negotiated at a departmental level and this improves efficiency by streamlining the process and removing any inconsistencies in management.
- Access to allied health staff. In many hospitals, allied health teams have been established within the emergency department to reduce the number of admissions and expedite care in the community, especially in the elderly age group. They are an invaluable part of the team; this includes physiotherapist, social workers, discharge coordinators, occupational therapist, drug and alcohol counsellors and psychiatry liaison nurses.
- Ten to 20% of patients in the observation ward will be further referred to inpatient teams for admission. This is a key performance indicator in most departments. For this group

of patients, it is important to negotiate priority admission to inpatient wards so as not to impact on the efficiency of the ward.

Staffing

Observation wards are staffed by ED personnel. It is important to have defined medical governance. This means that there is a specified senior clinician who is responsible for the patients at all times. The precise detail varies between departments. The nursing staff usually rotate between the emergency department and the observation ward.

Audit and feedback

As the function of the observation ward evolves and matures, it is important to have some form of monitoring and auditing process. Some key performance indicators have been established. Examples of these include:

- number of observation ward patients transferred to the care of inpatient teams (internationally 10–20% is acceptable)
- occupancy rates
- length of stay
- discharge to home rate
- representation rates within 48 hours
- adverse events and outcomes
- complaints.

Conclusions

The emergency observation unit is an integral extension of the emergency department. Its value is in improved clinical decision making and improved flow, especially in the overcrowded emergency department. There is increasing evidence for various discrete conditions where the role of the observation unit reduces hospital admission rates and length of stay.

As the emergency observation unit matures in some institutions, it has taken on the role as a defined diagnostic and therapeutic unit. It will be interesting to see how the emergency observation unit interacts with other short-stay units in the future. The role of the emergency physician in the care of patients beyond 24 hours is slowly expanding, with an increasing number developing an interest in short-stay medicine. This can only be a positive move, allowing emergency physicians to expand their interests, for job satisfaction and professional longevity, while meeting increasing demands for improved flow and throughput.

Controversies

The latest controversies relate to funding. With the introduction of activity-based funding and the 4-hour rule or NEAT:

- What is the definition of an admission? There is now a separate category of short-stay admission (with length of stay less than 8 hours) and an observation unit observation (with length of stay greater than 8 hours).
- There is a blurring of boundaries between acute assessment units, chest pain assessment units and observation medicine.
- What is the true financial benefit of an observation ward: do such wards change emergency physicians' behaviour by reducing the number of discharges? [3]

References

[1] Baugh C, Venkatesh A, Bohan J. Emergency department observation units: a clinical and financial benefit from hospitals. Hlth Care Manage Rev 2011;36:28–37.
[2] Williams A, Jelinek GA, Rogers IR. The effect of establishment of an observation ward on hospital admission profiles. Med J Aust 2000;173:411–4.
[3] Ventakesh AK, Geisler BP, Gibson Chambers JJ, et al. Use of observation care in US emergency departments, 2001–2 to 9. PLos ONE 2011;6:e24326.
[4] Jagminas L, Partridge R. A comparison of emergency department versus in hospital chest pain observation units. Am J Emerg Med 2005;2:111–3.
[5] Wiler J, Ross MA, Ginde AA. National study of emergency department observation services. Acad Emerg Med 2011;18:959–65.
[6] McDermott MF, Murphy DG, Zalenski RJ, et al. A comparison of emergency department observation units between emergency diagnostic and treatment unit and in-patient care in the management of acute asthma. Arch Intern Med 1997;157:2055–62.
[7] Ross MA, Compton S, Medado P, et al. An emergency department diagnostic protocol for patients with transient ischemic attack: a randomized controlled trial. Ann Emerg Med 2007;50:109–19.
[8] Greenberg RA, Dudley NC, Rittichier KK. A reduction in hospitalization, length of stay, and hospital charges for croup with the institution of pediatric observation unit. Am J Emerg Med 2006;7:818–21.
[9] Schrock JW, Rezvikova S, Weller S. The effect of an observation unit on the rate of ED admission and discharge for pyelonephritis. Am J Emerg Med 2010;28:682–8.
[10] Grossman S, Shapiro N, et al. Is telemetry useful in evaluation chest pain patients in an observation unit. Intern Emerg Med 2011;6:545–6.
[11] Roberts RR, Zalenski RJ, Mensah EK, et al. Costs of an emergency department-based accelerated diagnostic protocol vs. hospitalization in patients with chest pain: a randomized controlled trial. J Am Med Assoc 1997;278:1670–6.
[12] Goodacre S, Nicholl J, Dixon S, et al. Randomized controlled trial and economic evaluation of a chest pain observation unit compared with routine care. Br Med J 2004;328:254.
[13] Western Australia Toxicology Service (Royal Perth Hospital data) 2009–2012.

26.7 Overcrowding

Drew Richardson

ESSENTIALS

1 Overcrowding is the situation where emergency department (ED) function is impeded primarily by the excessive number of patients needing or receiving care.

2 Access block is excessive delay in accessing appropriate inpatient beds and, in Australasia, is defined as the proportion of patients with longer than 8 hours total ED time.

3 Access block is the principal cause of overcrowding but overall demand is also increasing.

4 Although multiple different definitions have been used in studying overcrowding and access block, there is clear evidence that both are associated with diminished quality of care and worse patient outcomes including mortality.

5 Changes to ED structure and function including senior staffing, increased size, fast-track observation units and multidisciplinary discharge procedures can to some extent improve the function of the ED in the face of overcrowding, but do not address the underlying causes and are easily overwhelmed by increasing access block.

6 The causes of overcrowding and hence the solutions lie largely outside the ED, especially in managing hospital bedstock in such a way that inpatient beds remain available.

Introduction

Wherever human beings gather there are fluctuations in number and, without outside control, numbers occasionally exceed the efficient maximum for a given purpose. Emergency departments (EDs) are designed largely for ongoing flow of patients rather than gathering, but even in systems designed purely for flow (such as roads) there are peaks and troughs of activity and occupancy sometimes exceeds the number able to move safely and smoothly.

Overcrowding to the point of dysfunction has gradually become the norm in Australasian EDs since the mid-1990s. The greatest contributing factor has been access block, the inability of patients requiring inpatient admission to access appropriate beds in a timely fashion, a phenomenon which is generally called 'boarding' in North America. There has additionally been some increase in demand on EDs in both number and complexity of patients resulting from the enlarging, ageing population and the growth in diagnostic and therapeutic choices. This has not been matched by growth in

other services, especially outside office hours, increasing the burden on EDs.

Theoretical basis of overcrowding

Queuing theory indicates that the length of a queue and hence the waiting time to treatment is determined by the arrival rate, the treatment rate and the baulk rate (did not wait to be seen rate, which is usually dependent on the length of the queue). An individual patient's access to emergency care is dependent first on their urgency (assuming the patient is triaged to the correct queue), secondly on the number of similar patients already waiting ahead and thirdly, on the rate and strategy of treatment. Treatment rate is dependent on staffing and on the number of patients already being treated (occupancy), which determines physical availability of resources and the competing demands on staff. On a daily basis, patient flow is significantly dependent on occupancy because even a small decrease in treatment rate has a cumulative

effect: it further increases the number waiting ahead of each new arrival.

EDs can be considered as overcrowded when treatment is dysfunctional, that is, the treatment rate is reduced or the treatment quality suffers. Some authorities believe that an ED can be purely overcrowded with patients waiting to be seen while the treatment function remains optimal, others regard this situation as a 'surge' – a subset of disaster medicine, rather than an overcrowding problem.

Definition of overcrowding

The Australasian College for Emergency Medicine (ACEM) defines ED overcrowding [1] as the situation where ED function is impeded primarily because the number of patients waiting to be seen, undergoing assessment and treatment or waiting for departure exceeds either the physical or the staffing capacity of the ED. Access block is quantified as the proportion of admissions to hospital, transfers to other hospitals and deaths that have a total ED time of greater than 8 hours [1].

The American College of Emergency Physicians defines crowding [2] as occurring when the identified need for emergency services exceeds available resources for patient care in the ED, hospital, or both, a definition deliberately closer in spirit to that of disaster medicine. Most research on the subject, however, is concerned with the balance between daily fluctuations and ED occupancy, rather than the response to mass-casualty surges.

'Crowding' might be the more descriptive term, but 'overcrowding' is in common use and researchers have used multiple definitions in attempts to quantify the phenomenon. All major recognized definitions incorporate occupancy with patients under treatment, but many also include subjective factors and outcomes, such as ambulance bypass, which are not applicable to all EDs.

Retrospectively identified episodes of overcrowding tend to be reliable for research but are of only strategic significance in ED management. Real-time assessments may be correlated with patient service (number of patients waiting correlates well with waiting time for new arrivals) but are only useful if there is a managerial commitment to intervening. Predictive algorithms based on the number being treated suffer from false positives and again are only justified if interventions exist to prevent deterioration in flow.

Although there are multiple scales proposed and used to define overcrowding [3,4], recent research indicates that overcrowding to some extent is a local problem: variation in ED performance metrics between apparently similar departments cannot be easily explained in terms of routinely collected data [5]. Validation studies are difficult and many rely on ambulance diversion as an outcome measure, which is only suitable for multi-ED urban centres. The few Australasian studies have not shown US-derived scales to be clinically useful in real time [6].

Causes of overcrowding

The single most important factor affecting ED overcrowding is the availability of inpatient beds [7–9]. Bed availability depends not only on the number of physical beds but also on the way the bedstock is managed. Modelling of extensive hospital datasets has identified the importance of discharge practice [10], patient complexity [11] and even admission practice at off-peak times [12] to ED flow at peak times. ED overcrowding is best seen as a marker of whole-of-hospital dysfunction which requires a whole-of-hospital response [13].

Hospitals providing a local service in areas of significant demographic change, such as a large ageing cohort or rapid growth, may experience ED overcrowding simply through the pressure of presenting numbers exceeding appropriate ED changes. Although locally hospitals may rarely close when demand falls, overall ED demand continues to increase worldwide at rates well above population growth [14,15], reflecting both changing patient expectations and demographics. This will likely be exacerbated among Western cohorts with a large ageing 'baby boomer' population.

Development and adoption of new diagnostic and therapeutic approaches and therapies has contributed to increases in total ED time in some groups. Chest pain 'rule-out' protocols using delayed marker measurements and increasing use of computed tomography (CT) scans for conditions such as abdominal pain are two examples. These are only partly mitigated by shorter, protocol-driven care of other conditions, for example routine CT for minor head injury with immediate discharge after a normal result rather than observation. Substitution of hospital admission by longer ED stays is likely contributing to an increase in ED 'practice intensity' but admission numbers are rising as well [15].

Consequences of overcrowding

Adverse effects of hospital overcrowding have been described since the birth of modern medicine and ED overcrowding had been seen as undesirable since before the recognition of emergency medicine as a specialty. In Australasia, access block was recognized as a quality issue from 1998 [16], first shown to be associated with decreased ED function in 2000 [17] and defined by the ACEM from 2002 [1]. Worldwide, properly conducted research started in 2001 and, since that time, multiple studies in different centres have found an association between overcrowding and reduced access to care [17–19], decreased quality measures [19–22] and lesser outcomes [23–25]. This relationship is robust and applies both to patients who experience delay in obtaining an inpatient bed and to those who present to, or are unlucky enough to already be in, an overcrowded department.

The most important studies are those linking overcrowding with excess patient mortality. The first well-controlled studies were Australian [26,27] and they have been followed by multiple, large, well-designed international studies linking mortality with ED overcrowding in specific disease processes [28,29], patients who 'board' in ED [30], admissions [31], discharges [32] and in populations served by potentially overcrowded EDs [33,34]. Demonstration of the link with quality measures, widespread similar results and a dose–response effect have removed any doubt that the relationship between overcrowding and mortality is causative.

Strategies to deal with overcrowding

EDs have an obligation to reduce overcrowding and to mitigate its effects. Multiple successful strategies have been described at an individual ED level, although systematic reviews have tended to be critical of the quality of the evidence [35]. There is no doubt that overcrowding can be reduced, but single interventions may not be easily transferred between different EDs.

As noted, any reduction in overcrowding will be largely achieved through whole-of-hospital changes. Long time series suggest that, in the absence of hospital-wide changes, access block tends to continue to increase even after mitigation efforts within the ED [36]. However, long-term, jurisdiction-wide reports make it clear that overcrowding can be reduced by increasing hospital resources and provision of appropriate incentives [37–39].

Increases in the number and seniority of ED staff are associated with improvements in process measures [40,41] and are a widely used initial response to overcrowding. Physical rebuilding is used to increase patient care spaces but changes in flow dynamics are highly dependent on the rest of the hospital [42]. Analysis of flow and system redesign can allow better use of existing resources [43]. Use of senior medical staff earlier in the patient's journey (at triage) [44], triage nurse ordering of investigations [45] and streaming of selected patients through a rapid assessment ('fast track') area [46] are all effective interventions in the ED. None of these responses can be used indefinitely if access block keeps increasing.

Mandated time targets for ED patients associated with appropriate hospital-wide incentives are effective at reducing overcrowding. Evidence from the British and Western Australian experience with a '4-hour rule' has not shown a negative effect on quality, safety or use of tests [47]. There are early suggestions that patient mortality may be reduced with study ongoing [39]. It is worth noting that hospital commitment to aiming at such a target appears to have beneficial effects on ED function even if the target is not fully achieved.

Evidence is accumulating in favour of hospital enforced 'overcapacity protocols' which distribute the overcrowding burden between ED and inpatient areas [48]. Major success has been reported in Alberta, Canada, again without apparent detrimental effects on patient care [49].

Discretionary, low-complexity presentations by patients who might reasonably be managed elsewhere, often incorrectly called 'GP-type' patients, constitute a significant number but an insignificant workload in most EDs [50]. Such presentations have a short assessment and treatment time and do not need fixed capacity spaces, such as resuscitation rooms, so their contribution to occupancy with patients under treatment is low. However, being of lower triage urgency their contribution to the number waiting at any given time is relatively high. Use of Primary Care professionals in ED to provide non-urgent care has not been shown to be beneficial [51].

Telephone advice services have not been shown to reduce ED workload in Australasia [52,53] but are highly regarded by the public. Dedicated ED fast-track areas [46] address the management of low-complexity patients in an efficient manner and thus tend to improve overall waiting time performance and staff and patient satisfaction. Their contribution to reducing occupancy with patients under treatment, and hence improving ambulance offload, is low.

EDs also themselves have a small but significant role in reducing hospital occupancy. Observation medicine within the ED is a useful adjunct or alternative to formal inpatient admission [54]. Multidisciplinary assessment and discharge is effective at reducing representation at least in the elderly [55].

Conclusions

Overcrowding has changed the nature of emergency medicine practice. Access block represents a useful simple description of overcrowding because the fundamental issue is the availability of inpatient beds. There is a causal relationship between overcrowding and worse patient outcomes including mortality. Emergency physicians have a role to play in maintaining patient care function in the face of overcrowding, but most of the solutions lie outside the ED.

Future research

The relationship between overcrowding and adverse outcomes is accepted to be causal. Large, well-designed studies of hospital- or system-wide interventions to reduce overcrowding, with adequate follow up to detect improvements in outcome, especially mortality, are now being undertaken and will assist in clarifying barriers and enablers in improving ED overcrowding.

Controversies/future directions

There are medicopolitical, financial and ethical controversies related to ED overcrowding.

- Political dimension: ED overcrowding is the product of hospital overcrowding, that is lack of available inpatient beds. Hospital overcrowding is likely to continue while hospital funding schemes favour elective surgery over emergency cases and utilization over efficiency. Politically driven funding incentives can improve this situation but sufficiently robust change is not yet widespread.
- Financial dimension: demand for healthcare is effectively unlimited, but demand for current levels of care will grow as the cohort of 'baby boomers' age, meaning significant rationing is inevitable if health spending remains contained. Although EDs have a role to play in reducing admissions, the major change needs to be in increasing early discharges, as the inpatient bed-day is the largest driver of acute hospital costs.
- Ethical dimension: emergency physicians are comfortable with rationing on the basis of need – it is the foundation of the triage system. However, rationing by queuing becomes fundamentally inefficient once the time in the queue starts to approach the time course of the disease. The current institutional culture of the majority of hospital units does not accept rationing of care to ward inpatients even when other patients with clearly greater medical needs are waiting for immediate access. These differences partly reflect ethical conflict between the principles of justice for all patients and beneficence for individual patients.

References

[1] Australasian College for Emergency Medicine. Policy document–standard terminology. Emerg Med (Aust) 2002;14:337–40.
[2] American College of Emergency Physicians. Crowding. Ann Emerg Med 2006;47:585.
[3] Hwang U, Concato J. Care in the emergency department: how crowded is overcrowded? Acad Emerg Med 2004;11:1097–101.
[4] Jones SS, Allen TL, Flottemesch TJ, et al. An independent evaluation of four quantitative emergency department crowding scales. Acad Emerg Med 2006;13:1204–11.
[5] Pines JM, Decker SL, Hu T. Exogenous predictors of national performance measures for emergency department crowding. Ann Emerg Med 2012;60:293–8.
[6] Raj K, Baker K, Brierley S, et al. National emergency department overcrowding study tool is not useful in an Australian emergency department. Emerg Med Australas 2006;18:282–8.
[7] Hostetler MA, Mace S, Brown K, et al. Subcommittee on Emergency Department Overcrowding and Children, Section of Pediatric Emergency Medicine, American College of Emergency Physicians. Emergency department overcrowding and children. Pediatr Emerg Care 2007;23:507–15.
[8] Trzeciak S, Rivers EP. Emergency department overcrowding in the United States: an emerging threat to patient safety and public health. Emerg Med J 2003;20:402–5.
[9] Crilly J, Keijzers G, Krahn D, et al. The impact of a temporary medical ward closure on emergency department and hospital service delivery outcomes. Qual Manag Hlth Care 2011;20:322–33.
[10] Khanna S, Boyle J, Good N, Lind J. Unravelling relationships: hospital occupancy levels, discharge timing and emergency department access block. Emerg Med Australas 2012;24:510–7.
[11] Rathlev NK, Obendorfer D, White LF, et al. Time series analysis of emergency department length of stay per 8-hour shift. West J Emerg Med 2012;13:163–8.
[12] Luo W, Cao J, Gallagher M, Wiles J. Estimating the intensity of ward admission and its effect on emergency department access block. Stat Med 2012. http://dx.doi.org/10.1002/sim.5684.
[13] Richardson DB. Reducing patient time in the emergency department. Med J Aust 2003;179:516–7.
[14] Pitts SR, Pines JM, Handrigan MT, Kellermann AL. National trends in emergency department occupancy, 2001 to 2008: effect of inpatient admissions versus emergency department practice intensity. Ann Emerg Med 2012;60:679–86.
[15] FitzGerald G, Toloo S, Rego J, et al. Demand for public hospital emergency department services in Australia: 2000–2001 to 2009–2010. Emerg Med Australas 2012;24:72–8.
[16] Baggoley C. President's message. Emerg Med (Aust) 1998;10:169–71.
[17] Richardson DB. Quantifying the effects of access block [abstract]. Emerg Med (Aust) 2001;13:A10.
[18] Fatovich DM, Nagree Y, Sprivulis P. Access block causes emergency department overcrowding and ambulance diversion in Perth, Western Australia. Emerg Med J 2005;22:351–4.
[19] Vieth TL, Rhodes KV. The effect of crowding on access and quality in an academic ED. Am J Emerg Med 2006;24:787–94.
[20] Dunn R. Reduced access block causes shorter emergency department waiting times: an historical control observational study. Emerg Med (Aust) 2003;15:232–8.
[21] Schull MJ, Vermeulen MJ, Slaughter G, et al. Emergency department crowding and thrombolysis delays in acute myocardial infarction. Ann Emerg Med 2004;44:577–85. Erratum in Ann Emerg Med 2005; 45:84.
[22] Fee C, Weber EJ, Maak CA, et al. Effect of emergency department crowding on time to antibiotics in patients admitted with community-acquired pneumonia. Ann Emerg Med 2007;50 501–9, 509.e1.
[23] Carr BG, Kaye AJ, Wiebe DJ, et al. Emergency department length of stay: a major risk factor for pneumonia in intubated blunt trauma patients. J Trauma 2007;63:9–12.
[24] Liew D, Liew D, Kennedy MP. Emergency department length of stay independently predicts excess inpatient length of stay. Med J Aust 2003;179:524–6.
[25] Chalfin DB, Trzeciak S, Likourezos A, et al. DELAY-ED study group. Impact of delayed transfer of critically ill patients from the emergency department to the intensive care unit. Crit Care Med 2007;35:1477–83.
[26] Sprivulis PC, Da Silva JA, Jacobs IG, et al. The association between hospital overcrowding and mortality among patients admitted via Western Australian emergency departments. Med J Aust 2006;184:208–12.
[27] Richardson DB. Increase in patient mortality at 10 days associated with emergency department overcrowding. Med J Aust 2006;184:213–6.
[28] Hong YC, Chou MH, Liu EH, et al. The effect of prolonged ED stay on outcome in patients with necrotising fasciitis. Am J Emerg Med 2009;27:385–90.

[29] Jo S, Kim K, Lee JH, et al. Emergency department crowding is associated with 28-day mortality in community-acquired pneumonia patients. J Infect 2012;64:268–75.

[30] Singer AJ, Thode Jr HC, Viccellio P, Pines JM. The association between length of emergency department boarding and mortality. Acad Emerg Med 2011;18:1324–9.

[31] Sun BC, Hsia RY, Weiss RE, et al. Effect of emergency department crowding on outcomes of admitted patients. Ann Emerg Med 2012;5 S0196-0644(12)01699-X.

[32] Guttmann A, Schull MJ, Vermeulen MJ, Stukel TA. Association between waiting times and short term mortality and hospital admission after departure from emergency department: population based cohort study from Ontario, Canada. Br Med J 2011;342:d2983.

[33] Shenoi RP, Ma L, Jones J, et al. Ambulance diversion as a proxy for emergency department crowding: the effect on pediatric mortality in a metropolitan area. Acad Emerg Med 2009;16:116–23.

[34] Shen Y, Hsia RY. Association between ambulance diversion and survival among patients with acute myocardial infarction. J Am Med Assoc 2011;305:2440–7.

[35] Morris ZS, Boyle A, Beniuk K, Robinson S. Emergency department crowding: towards an agenda for evidence-based intervention. Emerg Med J 2012;29:460–6.

[36] Richardson DB. Responses to access block in Australia: Australian Capital Territory. Med J Aust 2003;178:103–4.

[37] Weber EJ, Mason S, Carter A, Hew RL. Emptying the corridors of shame: organizational lessons from England's 4-hour emergency throughput target. Ann Emerg Med 2011;57:79–88. e1.

[38] Richardson DB, Kelly A-M, Kerr D. Prevalence of access block in Australia 2004–8. Emerg Med Australas 2009;21:472–8.

[39] Geelhoed GC, de Klerk NH. Emergency department overcrowding, mortality and the 4-hour rule in Western Australia. Med J Aust 2012;196:122–6.

[40] Rogers IR, Evans L, Jelinek GA, et al. Using clinical indicators in emergency medicine: documenting performance improvements to justify increased resource allocation. J Accid Emerg Med 1999;16:319–21.

[41] Cardin S, Afilalo M, Lang E, et al. Intervention to decrease emergency department crowding: does it have an effect on return visits and hospital readmissions? Ann Emerg Med 2003;41:173–85.

[42] Han JH, Zhou C, France DJ, et al. The effect of emergency department expansion on emergency department overcrowding. Acad Emerg Med 2007;14:338–43.

[43] King DL, Ben-Tovim DI, Bassham J. Redesigning emergency department patient flows: application of Lean Thinking to health care. Emerg Med Australas 2006;18:391–7.

[44] Rowe BH, Guo X, Villa-Roel C, et al. The role of triage liaison physicians on mitigating overcrowding in emergency departments: a systematic review. Acad Emerg Med 2011;18:111–20.

[45] Rowe BH, Villa-Roel C, Guo X, et al. The role of triage nurse ordering on mitigating overcrowding in emergency departments: a systematic review. Acad Emerg Med 2011;18:1349–57.

[46] Bullard MJ, Villa-Roel C, Guo X, et al. The role of a rapid assessment zone/pod on reducing overcrowding in emergency departments: a systematic review. Emerg Med J 2012;29:372–8.

[47] Weber EJ, Mason S, Freeman JV, Coster J. Implications of England's four-hour target for quality of care and resource use in the emergency department. Ann Emerg Med 2012;60:699–706.

[48] Villa-Roel C, Guo X, Holroyd BR, et al. The role of full capacity protocols on mitigating overcrowding in EDs. Am J Emerg Med 2012;30:412–20.

[49] Innes G, McRae A, Holroyd B, et al. Policy-driven improvements in crowding: system-level changes introduced by a provincial health authority and its impact on emergency department operations in 15 centers. [abstract]. Acad Emerg Med 2012;19:s14.

[50] Sprivulis P, Grainger S, Nagree Y. Ambulance diversion is not associated with low acuity patients attending Perth metropolitan emergency departments. Emerg Med Australas 2005;17:11–15.

[51] Khangura JK, Flodgren G, Perera R, et al. Primary care professionals providing non-urgent care in hospital emergency departments. Cochrane Database Syst Rev 2012:11.

[52] Graber DJ, Ardagh MW, O'Donovan P, et al. A telephone advice line does not decrease the number of presentations to Christchurch Emergency Department, but does decrease the number of phone callers seeking advice. NZ Med J 2003;116:U495.

[53] Sprivulis P, Carey M, Rouse I. Compliance with advice and appropriateness of emergency presentation following contact with the HealthDirect telephone triage service. Emerg Med Australas 2004;16:35–40.

[54] Williams AG, Jelinek GA, Rogers IR, et al. The effect on hospital admission profiles of establishing an emergency department observation ward. Med J Aust 2000;173:411–4.

[55] Caplan GA, Williams AJ, Daly BA. Randomized controlled trial of comprehensive geriatric assessment and multidisciplinary intervention after discharge of elderly from the emergency department – the DEED II study. J Am Geriatr Soc 2004;52:1417–23.

26.8 Rapid response systems and the emergency department

Daryl A Jones • Julie Considine

ESSENTIALS

1 Up to 17% of hospitalized ward patients suffer serious adverse events (SAEs), including cardiac arrest.

2 These events are often preceded by signs of physiological derangement for up to 24 hours prior to the event.

3 Rapid response systems (RRSs) are designed to review ward patients in the early phases of such deterioration.

4 There is increasing, but conflicting evidence supporting the effectiveness of RRSs in reducing cardiac arrests and unplanned intensive care unit (ICU) admissions in ward patients.

5 Increasing literature suggests that patients in the emergency department (ED) can experience clinical instability which predicts subsequent development of adverse events.

6 Single centre studies suggest that implementing a rapid response system into an ED is feasible.

7 Future research needs to validate activation criteria and response for an ED-specific RRS and to assess the potential benefits of such a system for deteriorating patients in the ED.

Introduction and definitions

Rapid response teams (RRTs) are composed of staff who review acutely unwell hospital ward patients in an attempt to reduce cardiac arrests and other serious adverse events (SAEs) [1]. When the team leader is a doctor, the RRT is called a medical emergency team (MET). A MET should have a number of competencies, including abilities in the following areas [1]:

- prescription of therapies
- advanced airway management skills
- insertion of invasive vascular lines
- commencement of intensive care level of care at the bedside.

The term 'rapid response system' (RRS) has been proposed to represent an entire system that provides both an 'afferent' component to identify patient deterioration and an 'efferent' component to assess and treat the patient. Other types of review team include the rapid response team and critical-care outreach team

(CCO), which differ in their staff composition, skill set and mechanism of activation [1]. The remainder of this chapter will focus on the MET, which is the predominant model in hospitals in Australia and New Zealand.

Additional components of the RRS include quality improvement and clinical governance arms, which permit audit and evaluation of SAEs and implementation of hospital-wide strategies to prevent recurrence [1].

Epidemiology and principles underlying the MET

Several principles underpin the MET and RRS. In summary, SAEs are common in hospitalized patients and are often preceded by a period of instability of up to 24 h. The MET is summoned to review patients in the early phases of deterioration in an attempt to prevent further deterioration, morbidity and mortality.

SAEs are common in hospitalized patients

Studies in Australia [2], New Zealand [3,4], England [5] and Canada [6] have assessed the incidence of SAEs in hospitalized patients. These studies defined an SAE as 'unintended injury or complication resulting from medical management rather than the underlying disease process'. They reported an incidence of SAEs ranging between 7.5% and 16.6% and suggested that 36.9–51% were preventable.

A single-centre study in an Australian hospital [7] found that 16.9% of 1125 patients undergoing major surgery suffered at least one of 11 predefined SAEs (which included myocardial infarction, stroke, arrest and respiratory failure).

SAEs are preceded by signs of clinical instability

At least four studies [8–11] have demonstrated that patients suffering SAEs develop new complaints, deterioration of commonly measured vital signs or derangement in laboratory investigations in up to 84% of cases prior to the event. It is for this reason that common triggers for MET activation are based on derangements in vital signs. More importantly, three studies [12–14] have confirmed that patients who develop vital signs that satisfy MET criteria are at increased risk of death.

Deterioration of the MET patient is typically gradual

Unexpected out-of-hospital cardiac arrest is usually sudden and due to cardiac arrhythmias, pulmonary embolism or major vascular catastrophe. In contrast, progression to in-hospital cardiac arrests and other SAEs is typically gradual [8]. This allows sufficient time for intervention and, potentially, prevention of the event.

Early intervention improves outcome

One of the tenets underlying the MET principle is that early intervention in the course of critical illness is associated with improved outcome. This observation has been made in patients suffering trauma [15,16], myocardial infarction [17] and in resuscitation of patients presenting to the emergency department (ED) with sepsis [18].

Skilled staff already exist in the hospital

METs are usually composed of critical-care staff with skills in advanced airway management, insertion of invasive vascular lines and with knowledge of therapies commonly used in acute care medicine (Table 26.8.1). Staff need to be available 24 hours per day, 7 days a week to manage acutely unwell patients anywhere in the hospital [19].

How MET services and RRSs work

Different roles of the MET

The MET was originally described in 1995 when Lee and coworkers reported the introduction of a MET service into Liverpool Hospital in Sydney, Australia [19]. The MET superseded the existing cardiac arrest team and was modelled on rapid detection and correction of abnormal vital signs indicative of trauma teams. In this model, the MET is merely an expansion of the existing cardiac arrest team and reviews all medical emergencies including arrests.

In other hospitals [20,21], two separate RRTs operate: a cardiac arrest team to review patients who have suffered cardiorespiratory arrest and a MET that reviews all medical emergencies other than cardiac arrest.

Activation of the MET – the afferent arm

The MET service is activated when one or more predefined criteria are reached. Typical criteria involve derangement of commonly measured vital signs (Table 26.8.2). Other criteria include conditions such as uncontrolled seizures or chest pain. Finally, some hospital MET criteria contain a 'staff member worried' criterion to permit activation of the MET service for any possible medical emergency.

Composition of the MET – the effector arm

The precise composition of each MET varies between hospitals. Each member has a predefined role (see Table 26.8.1) and simulation or mock sessions may be held as part of training [22]. The teams typically bring their own equipment to the MET call, either on a trolley or in a carry bag, which includes equipment needed for endotracheal intubation, invasive vascular access and medicines and fluids used in advanced resuscitation.

Table 26.8.1 MET staff members and their roles	
Staff member	*Roles*
Intensive care registrar	• Knowledge of acute care medicine and physiological basis of acute deterioration • Skills in advanced resuscitation and insertion of invasive vascular lines • Skills in airway management and advanced cardiac life support
Intensive care nurse	• Knowledge of delivering advanced resuscitation • Provision of ongoing information and advice to ward nurses for patients remaining on the ward following MET call • Liaising with intensive care unit regarding potential for patient admission
Medical registrar	• Skill in diagnosis and management of underlying aetiology of medical condition • Follow up and ongoing management of patients remaining on ward following MET call
Ward nurses and doctors	• Knowledge of patient's nursing issues since admission and leading up to MET call

Table 26.8.2 Commonly used MET calling criteria

System	Criteria
Airway	Stridor Threatened airway
Breathing	Acute change in RR <8 or >30 breaths/min Acute change in saturation <90% despite oxygen Difficulty breathing Noisy breathing
Circulation	Acute change in heart rate <40 or >130 bpm Acute change in systolic BP <90 mmHg Uncontrolled chest pain
Neurology	Acute change in conscious state Agitation or delirium
Other	Staff member is worried about the patient Acute change in UO to <50 mL in 4 h

RR: respiratory rate; BP: blood pressure; UO: urine output.

Table 26.8.3 Relative frequency (%) of MET triggers leading to MET calls

Criteria	Bellomo et al. (2003) [21] (n = 99)	Buist et al. (2004) [13] (n = 564)	Jones et al. (2006) [23] (n = 400)
Hypoxia	37	51	41
Respiratory rate	19	≈7	14
Hypotension	35	17.3	28
Tachycardia	20	≈7	19
Altered conscious state	28	≈7	23
Oliguria	2	Not assessed	8
Worried	46	Not assessed	Not assessed

Table 26.8.4 A to G approach to management of a hypoxic MET call

Step of A to G approach	Approach for hypoxic MET call
Ask	How can I help? Why was the MET called?
Assess for aetiology	Pulmonary oedema, atelectasis, pneumonia, asthma, sepsis and pulmonary embolism

Begin:
  Basic investigations
  Basic resuscitation
	Chest X-ray, sepsis screen, ECG and cardiac enzymes and arterial blood gas; consider V/Q scan
	Apply oxygen and monitor arterial saturation
	CCF – loop diuretic, morphine, nitrates, oxygen and upright posture
	COAD – bronchodilators, hydrocortisone and non-invasive ventilation
	Atelectasis – chest physiotherapy and humidified oxygen
	Pulmonary embolism – anticoagulation or thrombolysis

Call for help (if needed)	SaO₂ <90% despite 10L inspired oxygen Respiratory rate >40, elevated PaCO₂, altered conscious state
Discuss	With parent unit, patient and next of kin, intensive care consultant
Decide	Where the patient is most appropriately managed
Document	If limitations of therapy should be instituted The cause, management and follow up of the call
Explain	To the patient, nursing and junior medical staff The cause, management and follow up of the call
Follow up	Clearly indicate who will follow up the patient and when this will occur
Graciously thank the staff	

MET: medical emergency team; ECG: electrocardiogram; CCF: congestive cardiac failure; COAD: chronic obstructive airways disease.

Clinical features of MET patients

Characteristics of triggers leading to MET activation

A number of studies [13,21,23] have reported the relative frequency of MET call criteria leading to MET calls (Table 26.8.3). Variations between hospitals are likely to represent differences in the limits of the criteria as well as differences in local case mix. Hypoxaemia, hypotension and altered conscious state were the commonest causes of MET calls in these studies.

Medical conditions leading to MET calls

The clinical cause of MET calls has also been assessed in a number of studies and the concept of 'MET syndromes' (e.g. the 'hypoxic MET syndrome') has recently been raised [23,24]. Again, variations in case mix and MET calling criteria are likely to account for these differences. In the original description of the MET, Lee and coworkers reported that acute respiratory failure, status epilepticus, coma and pulmonary oedema were the most common causes of MET calls [19]. In a district general hospital, Daly and coworkers reported that chest pain, respiratory distress, seizures and cardiopulmonary arrest caused most MET calls [25]. Finally, a study of 400 MET calls at the Austin hospital [23] revealed that infections, pulmonary oedema and arrhythmias caused 53% of MET calls.

Management of MET call patients

One of the most underinvestigated aspects of the MET system is the details of the management undertaken by the staff during a MET call. De Vita and coworkers have recently reported that use of a detailed curriculum and a computerized human patient simulator resulted in increased task completion rate and improved survival of the simulated patient [22].

An analysis of the MET syndromes associated with 400 MET calls and an approach to their management has been reported [23]. The 'A to G' approach described can be used to manage any possible medical emergency and can be used in the management of specific MET syndromes (Table 26.8.4).

The MET and the ED

Hospital-wide MET services that involve ED staff and patients

In the original description of the MET system, the ED was one of the hospital areas serviced by the MET and, in fact, was the area that attracted the highest number of MET activations [19]. This approach involves review of ED patients by intensive care unit (ICU) staff and is most appropriate during periods when there are limited senior emergency medical staff, particularly out of hours. In contrast, Daly and coworkers described a MET model for a district general hospital in which staff from the ED formed the core of the MET and reviewed patients in the general wards when the MET service was activated [25].

The MET philosophy in the ED

The MET involves a coordinated multidisciplinary approach to the management of acute deterioration of hospital ward patients [1]. As outlined above (see Table 26.8.1), each member has a designated role coordinated by the team leader. This is similar to the team-based approach to trauma management seen in most EDs and trauma centres (Table 26.8.5).

The MET system principle is equally applicable in the ED as it is on the hospital ward. For example, a multidisciplinary programme was shown to reduce the hospital mortality rate of patients presenting to a community hospital with non-traumatic shock [26]. Coordinated team work is required for the management of acute myocardial ischaemia, severe sepsis, intracranial haemorrhage and ischaemic stroke. These are discrete clinical entities where the clinical diagnosis is rapidly determined and algorithmic- or guideline-based therapies exist.

How often do patients in ED develop clinical instability?

The epidemiology of deterioration in the ED is poorly understood. Unplanned ICU admission is a well documented largely preventable serious adverse event in general ward patients and is associated with up to a 10-fold increase in mortality [27,28]. It may be argued that there are ED patients in whom ICU admission is unplanned as these patients appear stable on ED arrival (indicated by allocation to lower acuity triage categories) but, subsequently, require ICU admission following clinical deterioration [29]. Australian data can be used to explore the prevalence of ICU admissions of ED patients. Of 6.2 million patients attending Australian EDs annually [30], more than 24 500 patients require ICU admission directly from the ED and over 2700 die [31]. Victorian Government data from 2010–11 show that of the 7220 (0.5%) admissions directly from ED to ICU, 70% (5088) were recognized as critically ill or injured on arrival to the ED (triage category 1 or 2). However, 30% (2132) were assessed as moderate or low acuity (triage category 3, 4 or 5) on ED arrival hence may have suffered an unplanned ICU admission [32].

There is even less information about early deterioration in ED patients. Recent single site pilot studies from Victoria, Australia suggest that approximately 1% of general ED patients (excluding patients in resuscitation areas) Fulfilled organizational MET criteria [33] and 1.5% of ED patients suffered clinical deterioration significant enough to warrant activation of a local ED rapid response system [34].

Clinical instability in ED predicts subsequent adverse outcomes

There is a body of evidence related to the predictors of deterioration in ED patients, the use of modified early warning score (MEWS) in ED and prediction of critical care or ICU admission in ED patients that may be used to inform a standardized approach to deteriorating ED patients. In a study of medical ED patients, Burch et al. [35] found systolic blood pressure ≤ 100 mmHg, pulse rate ≥ 130 per minute, respiratory rate ≥ 30 breaths per minute, temperature $\geq 38.5°C$ and decreased conscious state on ED arrival were independent predictors of hospital admission. Further, systolic blood pressure ≤ 100 mmHg or ≥ 200 mmHg, respiratory rate ≥ 30 breaths per minute and decreased conscious state on ED arrival were independent predictors of in-hospital death [35]. In this same study, an increased MEWS score was associated with higher rates of hospital admission in medical patients, so MEWS may be used to identify medical patients who require hospital admission and who are at increased risk of hospital death [35]. Similarly, Groarke et al. [36] examined the predictive value of an EWS calculated on hospital presentation in medical patients. For each increase in score category, there was increased risk of ICU admission, CCU admission, death and hospital length of stay [36]. Groarke et al. concluded that early warning score is a potential triage tool for ED medical patients and that improved serial EWS within 4 hours of hospital presentation may be used to predict clinical outcomes.

Known predictors of unplanned ICU admission in patients admitted to hospital via the ED are older age, male gender, higher acuity triage category and a history of co-morbid conditions [37]. Further, diagnostic groups associated with higher incidence of unplanned ICU admission included sepsis, acute renal failure, lymphatic–haematopoietic tissue neoplasms, pneumonia, chronic obstructive pulmonary disease and bowel obstruction [37]. Clinical factors evident on ED arrival predictive of critical care admission (ICU and coronary care unit) in patients triaged as low to moderate acuity were chief complaint of nausea, vomiting and diarrhoea on ED arrival; heart rate or temperature abnormalities at triage; and respiratory rate or heart rate abnormalities at first ED nursing assessment [38]. Hypotension during ED care significantly increases risk of in-hospital death in both trauma [39] and non-trauma patients [40]. The results of these studies demonstrate relationships between mortality and morbidity and ED patient characteristics; physiological abnormalities present on ED arrival; or physiological abnormalities that occur during ED care [37–40] and may be used to inform ED systems for

Table 26.8.5 Similarities and differences between MET services and trauma teams		
Variable	Trauma team	MET service
Location of patient	Emergency department or trauma centre	Hospital ward
Team leader	Typically emergency department doctor	Typically intensive care unit registrar
Patient profile	Young with few co-morbidities	Elderly with multiple co-morbidities
Presenting problem	Trauma	Hypoxia, hypotension and tachycardia
Need for early intervention	Concept of 'golden hour'	Shown for sepsis, myocardial ischaemia, stroke

recognition of, and response to deteriorating ED patients. Further, parameters currently absent from inpatient MET criteria, such as advanced age and temperature abnormalities, have been linked to critical-care admission and death and therefore may have a place in increasing recognition of deteriorating ED patients and warrant further investigation [38,41].

Existing studies describing RRS in EDs

There are a number of studies describing RRS in EDs. A review of EWS from the UK showed that high EWS triggered review by senior ED staff in 71% of patients and critical-care input in 44% of patients [42]. However, there are no details of whether a structured approach to escalating care was used or the outcomes of patients not reviewed by senior clinicians or critical-care referral despite high EWS. One recently reported Australian model is a single trigger approach with escalation of care to the emergency physician and nurse in charge to ensure timely review of the patient by senior personnel and mobilization of ED resources as required by personnel who have a global overview of ED activity [34]. This model resulted in two to three early warning system activations per day so did not overburden ED clinicians and simple interventions, such as intravenous fluids and supplemental oxygen, restored physiological normality in most patients within 1 hour [34]. This same model also showed that nurses were well placed to identify deteriorating patients and rapidly escalate care within 5 minutes [34].

The ideal response to deteriorating ED patients is unknown and for many deteriorating patients, the ED response will be appropriate, albeit *ad hoc*. However, the advantages of a structured and consistent approach to escalation of care include further development of already positive multidisciplinary relationships and enhanced inter-professional communication, particularly for new or transient ED staff [43]. A systematic and ED-led approach to recognizing and responding to deteriorating ED patients is a logical progression, building on other patient safety systems, such as triage and systematized approaches to ED care of critically ill or injured patients. There is a need to develop and test ED-specific approaches to improve the sequential detection, recognition and timely escalation of care for ED patients who have deteriorated after initial triage and assessment [43].

Likely future developments

Despite the absence of level 1 evidence of the effectiveness of MET services, RRSs have been introduced into thousands of hospitals worldwide to manage deteriorating ward patients. RRSs are a key component of the Institute of Health Improvement's 100k campaign, which aims to save 100 000 lives across American hospitals [44]. RRSs are also an integral component of The Australian National Safety and Quality Health Service Standards [45]. For these reasons, it is unlikely that further randomized trials will be conducted to assess the effectiveness of METs in improving the outcome of acutely unwell hospitalized patients.

The most important questions that need addressing regarding rapid response systems for ward patients in the near future include:

❶ Why do patients need MET calls? – clinical, disease state and system factors.

❷ What is the outcome of MET calls?

❸ What are barriers to MET activation?

❹ How can MET be most effectively used to review patients most likely to benefit from MET service intervention?

❺ In the cases of RRSs in the ED, there is a need to better quantify the point prevalence and consequences of clinical instability and to validate activation criteria.

Controversies

The MET service and deskilling of ward staff

The increasing use of MET services to manage acutely unwell hospital ward patients has the potential to deskill ward nursing and medical staff [46]. However, in a survey conducted in hospitals with a well-established MET service, most of the nurses questioned stated that the MET actually taught them how better to manage sick ward patients [47,48].

Improved outcome is demonstrated only in single-centre studies

Reduction in cardiac arrests, unplanned ICU admission and other SAEs following introduction of MET services and RRSs has been shown in a number of single-centre studies [20,21,49–51]. A cluster randomized trial of 23 Australian hospitals was recently reported in which 12 hospitals introduced a MET system and 11 continued with usual care [52]. The study did not demonstrate that introduction of a MET service reduced the incidence of cardiac arrests, unplanned ICU admissions or unexpected deaths. While this finding may suggest that MET services do not improve the outcome of acutely unwell ward patients, the negative result is at least in part due to other factors. First, the education period preceding introduction of the MET was brief (4 months) and the subsequent call rate was only 8.3 calls/1000 admissions [52]. At the Austin hospital, a 1-year education period resulted in a progressive increase in the use of the MET to a call rate of >40 calls/1000 admissions [53].

Most importantly, only 30% of the patients admitted to the ICU who had MET criteria actually received a MET call [52]. Combined, these findings suggest that the negative result of the MERIT study was at least in part due to a failure of MET use as opposed to a failure of the process of MET review.

Other controversies

A number of other problems with the MET service have been proposed [46,54] including inappropriate patient management because the MET is unfamiliar with the patient, diversion of attention away from adequate ward staffing and development of other strategies that might benefit acutely ill ward patients, diversion of critical care staff from their usual duties and conflict between MET staff and the ward staff caring for the patient.

References

[1] Devita MA, Bellomo R, Hillman K, et al. Findings of the first consensus conference on medical emergency teams. Crit Care Med 2006;34:2463–78.

[2] Wilson RM, Runciman WB, Gibberd RW, et al. The quality in Australian health care study. Med J Aust 1995;163:458–71.

[3] Davis P, Lay-Yee R, Briant R, et al. Adverse events in New Zealand public hospitals I: occurrence and impact. NZ Med J 2002;115:U271.

[4] Davis P, Lay-Yee R, Briant R, et al. Adverse events in New Zealand public hospitals II: preventability and clinical context. NZ Med J 2003;116:U624.

[5] Vincent C, Neale G, Woloshynowych M. Adverse events in British hospitals: preliminary retrospective record review. Br Med J 2001;322:517–9.

[6] Baker GR, Norton PG, Flintoft V, et al. The Canadian Adverse Events Study: the incidence of adverse events among hospital patients in Canada. Can Med Assoc J 2004;170:1678–86.

[7] Bellomo R, Goldsmith D, Russell S, et al. Postoperative serious adverse events in a teaching hospital: a prospective study. Med J Aust 2002;176:216–8.

[8] Buist MD, Jarmolowski E, Burton PR, et al. Recognising clinical instability in hospital patients before cardiac arrest or unplanned admission to intensive care. A pilot study in a tertiary-care hospital. Med J Aust 1999;171:22–5.

[9] Hodgetts TJ, Kenward G, Vlackonikolis I, et al. Incidence, location and reasons for avoidable in-hospital cardiac arrest in a district general hospital. Resuscitation 2002;54:115–23.

[10] Nurmi J, Harjola VP, Nolan J, et al. Observations and warning signs prior to cardiac arrest. Should a medical emergency team intervene earlier? Acta Anaesthesiol Scand 2005;49:702–6.

[11] Schein RM, Hazday N, Pena M, et al. Clinical antecedents to in-hospital cardiopulmonary arrest. Chest 1990;98: 1388–92.

[12] Bell MB, Konrad D, Granath F, et al. Prevalence and sensitivity of MET-criteria in a Scandinavian University Hospital. Resuscitation 2006;70:66–73.

[13] Buist M, Bernard S, Nguyen TV. Association between clinically abnormal observations and subsequent inhospital mortality: a prospective study. Resuscitation 2004;62:137–41.

[14] Goldhill DR, White SA, Sumner A. Physiological values and procedures in the 24 h before ICU admission from the ward. Anaesthesia 1999;54:529–34.

[15] Hedges J, Adams A. Gunnels M. ATLS practices and survival at rural level trauma hospitals, 1995–1999. Prehosp Emerg Care 2002;6:299–305.

[16] Nardi G, Riccioni L, Cerchiari E, et al. Impact of an integrated treatment approach to the severely injured patients (ISS >16) on hospital mortality and quality of care. Minerva Anesthesiol 2002;68:25–35.

[17] Fresco C, Carinci F, Maggioni AP, et al. Very early assessment of risk for in-hospital death among 11,483 patients with acute myocardial infarction. GISSI investigators. Am Heart J 1999;138:1058–64.

[18] Rivers E, Nguyen B, Havstad S, et al. Early goal-directed therapy in the treatment of severe sepsis and septic shock. N Engl J Med 2001;345:1368–77.

[19] Lee A, Bishop G, Hillman KM. The medical emergency team. Anaesth Intens Care 1995;23:183–6.

[20] Bellomo R, Goldsmith D, Uchino S, et al. Prospective controlled trial of effect of medical emergency team on postoperative morbidity and mortality rates. Crit Care Med 2004;32:916–21.

[21] Bellomo R, Goldsmith D, Uchino S, et al. A prospective before-and-after trial of a medical emergency team. Med J Aust 2003;179:283–7.

[22] De Vita M, Schaefer J, Lutz J, et al. Improving medical emergency team (MET) performance using a novel curriculum and a computerized human simulator. Qual Safe Hlth Care 2005;14:326–31.

[23] Jones D, Duke G, Green J, et al. Medical emergency team syndromes and an approach to their management. Crit Care 2006;10:R30.

[24] DeVita M. Medical emergency teams: deciphering clues to crises in hospitals. Crit Care 2005;9:325–6.

[25] Daly FF, Sidney KL, Fatovich DM. The medical emergency team (MET): a model for the district general hospital. Aust NZ J Med 1998;28:795–8.

[26] Sebat F, Johnson D, Musthafa A, et al. A multidisciplinary community hospital program for early and rapid resuscitation of shock in non-trauma patients. Chest 2005;127:1729–43.

[27] Haller G, Myles PS, Wolfe R, et al. Validity of unplanned admission to an intensive care unit as a measure of patient safety in surgical patients. Anesthesiology 2005;103:1121–9.

[28] Bristow P, Hillman K, Chey T, et al. Rates of in-hospital arrests, deaths and intensive care admissions: the effect of a medical emergency team. Med J Aust 2000;173:236–40.

[29] Kennedy M, Joyce N, Howell MD, et al. Identifying infected emergency department patients admitted to the hospital ward at risk of clinical deterioration and intensive care unit transfer. Acad Emerg Med 2010;17:1080–5.

[30] Australian Institute of Health and Welfare. Australian hospital statistics 2010–11: emergency department care and elective surgery waiting times. Canberra: Australian Institute of Health and Welfare. Health services series no. 41. Cat. no. HSE 115. Retrieved January 2012 from <http://www.aihw. gov.au/publication-detail/?id=6442472405>; 2011.

[31] Drennan K, Hart G, Hicks P. Intensive care resources & activity: Australia and New Zealand 2006/2007. Carlton, Victoria Australia and New Zealand Intensive Care Society. Retrieved March 2011 from <http://www.anzics.com.au/ core/reports>; 2009.

[32] Victorian Health Information Reporting System. Victorian Emergency Department data, Victorian Government Department of Health 2010:2011.

[33] Hosking J, Considine J, Sands N. Recognising clinical deterioration in the emergency department: point prevalence of emergency department patients fulfilling MET criteria and patient outcomes. In Tenth international conference for emergency nurses, Hotel Grand Chancellor: Hobart, Australia; October 2012.

[34] Considine J, Lucas E, Wunderlich B. The uptake of an early warning system in one Australian emergency department: a pilot study. Crit Care Resus 2012;14:135–41.

[35] Burch VC, Tarr G, Morroni C. Modified early warning score predicts the need for hospital admission and inhospital mortality. Emerg Med J 2008;25:674–8.

[36] Groarke JD, Gallagher J, Stack J, et al. Use of an admission early warning score to predict patient morbidity and mortality and treatment success. Emerg Med J 2008;25:803–6.

[37] Frost SA, Alexandrou E, Bogdanovski T, et al. Unplanned admission to intensive care after emergency hospitalisation: risk factors and development of a nomogram for individualising risk. resuscitation 2009;80:224–30.

[38] Considine J, Thomas S, Potter R. Predictors of critical care admission in emergency department patients triaged as low to moderate urgency. J Adv Nurs 2009;65:818–27.

[39] Sikorski TJ, Black L, Ho E, Mills T. Survival in posttraumatic hypotension. Ann Emerg Med 2004;44:S128–9.

[40] Jones AE, Yiannibas V, Johnson C, Kline JA. Emergency department hypotension predicts sudden unexpected in-hospital mortality: a prospective cohort study. Chest 2006;130:941–6.

[41] Smith GB, Prytherch DR, Schmidt PE, et al. Should age be included as a component of track and trigger systems used to identify sick adult patients? Resuscitation 2008;78:109–15.

[42] Griffiths JR, Kidney EM. Current use of early warning scores in UK emergency departments. Emerg Med J 2012;29:65–6.

[43] Considine J, Jones DA, Bellomo R, Emergency Department Rapid Response Systems: The case for a standardised approach to deteriorating patients. Eur J Emerg Med. 2013;20:375–381.

[44] Overview of the 100,000 Lives Campaign. <http://www.ihi. org/IHI/Programs/Campaign/100kCampaignOverviewArchive. htm> [Accessed Jan. 2007].

[45] Australian Commission on Safety and Quality in Health Care. National consensus statement: essential elements for recognising and responding to clinical deterioration. Sydney: ACSQHC, 2010. <http://www.safetyandquality. gov.au/internet/safety/publishing.nsf/Content/ F329E60CC4149933CA2577740009229C/$File/national_ consensus_statement.pdf> [Accessed Nov. 2012].

[46] Brown D, Bellomo R. Are medical emergency teams worth the cost? In: DeVita MA, Hillman K, Bellomo R, editors. Medical emergency teams: a guide to implementation and outcome measurement. New York: Springer; 2006.

[47] Jones D, Baldwin I, McIntryre T, et al. Nurses' attitudes to a medical emergency team service in a teaching hospital. Qual Safe Hlth Care 2006;15:427–32.

[48] Bagshaw SM, Mondor EE, Scouten C, Capital Health Medical Emergency Team Investigators. A survey of nurses' beliefs about the medical emergency team system in a Canadian tertiary hospital. Am J Crit Care 2010;19:74–83.

[49] Bristow PJ, Hillman KM, Chey T, et al. Rates of inhospital arrests, deaths and intensive care admissions: the effect of a medical emergency team. Med J Aust 2000;173: 236–40.

[50] Buist MD, Moore GE, Bernard SA, et al. Effects of a medical emergency team on reduction of incidence and mortality from unexpected cardiac arrests in hospital: preliminary study. Br Med J 2002;324:387–90.

[51] DeVita MA, Braithwaite RS, Mahidhara R, et al. Use of medical emergency team responses to reduce hospital cardiopulmonary arrests. Qual Safe Hlth Care 2004;13:251–4.

[52] Hillman K, Chen J, Cretikos M, et al. Introduction of the medical emergency team (MET) system: a cluster randomised controlled trial. Lancet 2005;365:2091–7.

[53] Jones D, Bates S, Warrillow S, et al. Effect of an education programme on the utilization of a medical emergency team in a teaching hospital. Intern Med J 2006;36:231–6.

[54] Joyce C, McArthur C. Rapid response systems: have we MET the need? Crit Care Resus 2007;9:127–8.

26.9 Public health and emergency medicine

Diana Egerton-Warburton • Jennie Hutton • Peter Aitken • Hilary Tyler

ESSENTIALS

1 Public health is a key component of a sustainable health system.

2 Emergency medicine has a mandate to advocate for public health initiatives.

3 Acute healthcare has limited opportunity to affect healthcare outcomes compared to public health.

4 Screening, brief intervention and referral for treatment (SBIRT) are the cornerstone of emergency department (ED) prevention.

5 Disease and injury surveillance is an important function for emergency departments including identification of emerging infectious diseases.

6 Emergency medicine can take a leadership role in highlighting and addressing socially determined health inequalities, particularly the healthcare gap of indigenous and other vulnerable populations.

Introduction

Public health (PH) is an organized attempt by society to ensure a healthy population. It is recognized as key to a sustainable and effective healthcare system. The UN Universal Declaration of Human Rights (1948) states that all people are equally entitled to good health and decent living conditions and it is this humanistic ideal that drives much of public health.

Emergency medicine (EM) is an important but under recognized and utilized player in public health. While at first glance it may appear an anathema to the practice of EM, PH and EM interact over a number of domains. These include: diseases surveillance, healthcare access, disease and injury prevention and advocacy. The International Federation for Emergency Medicine provides a clear mandate for public health in its definition of EM as: 'A field of practice based on the knowledge and skills required for the prevention, diagnosis and management of acute and urgent aspects of illness and injury'.

Emergency departments (EDs) Australasia-wide see over 7 million attendances annually. This population is receptive to PH intervention in a concept described as the 'teachable moment'. This has been described as a brief opportunity to intervene to change behaviour. This is particularly pertinent when patients present as a consequence of risky health behaviour. While patients are open to PH messages, providing them in the ED setting is challenging. EDs have limited resources and strive to provide safe and timely acute care. PH roles may be seen as simply adding to the burden. However, many emergency physicians (EP) see PH as part of their role as a healthcare advocate. This has been inculcated by the Australasian College for Emergency Medicine (ACEM) adopting the CanMEDS competency framework, which includes the role of health advocate.

A number of barriers exist to the introduction of PH measures into EDs. Lack of time and resources are almost universally cited and it is recognized that additional resources will be required for widespread adoption. PH roles within the ED are performed by a wide range of clinical and non-clinical staff members.

Increasingly, the social determinants of health affect individuals' opportunity to have a healthy life. Examples include access to safe and affordable housing, education and exposure to violence. This is particularly the case in indigenous populations. Many ED patients have poor social determinants and limited access to alternate healthcare options. EM should, through its surveillance and advocacy role, help to highlight and address these issues at a community and policy level. Social and environmental factors can be influenced by advocacy both at a local and national level. EP and ACEM are credible and persuasive healthcare advocates to provide effective public health messages.

Disease and injury surveillance

Emergency departments play an ongoing and pivotal role in injury prevention through surveillance. ED surveillance plays an important role in injury campaigns, such as child drowning and road safety. In regards to road traffic accidents, EM has advocated for changes to seatbelt and helmet legislation.

Based upon figures from the World Health Organization (WHO), the health profile of many countries is changing. The burden of non-communicable diseases has risen and will increase further with ageing populations. Non-communicable diseases, mainly cardiovascular diseases, diabetes and cancers, were responsible for 63% of the 57 million deaths that occurred worldwide in 2008.

According to the Australian Institute of Health and Welfare, coronary heart disease, anxiety and depression and type II diabetes are the largest specific contributors to overall burden of disease. Within 15 years, type II diabetes and obesity will be the leading cause.

A small number of unhealthy lifestyle choices, described in Table 26.9.1, account for much of this disease burden. From an Australian perspective, while smoking rates are comparatively low, rates of drinking alcohol, obesity and sedentary lifestyles are relatively high.

Potentially avoidable diseases account for at least 20% of healthcare expenditure. While Australia spent 8.7% of GDP on health in 2008, the Organization for Economic Cooperation and Development estimated that health spending will increase by 78% over the next four decades, partly due to the rise in preventable conditions. In response to this looming health

Table 26.9.1 Health impact of main risk factors for non-communicable disease

	Tobacco	Alcohol	Obesity	Insufficient exercise
WHO estimate of annual lives lost worldwide	6.0 million	2.3 million	2.8 million	3.2 million
Global and/or OECD average	OECD (2008) 21% of those aged 15 years and over are daily smokers	OECD (2008) 9.6 L of pure alcohol per person (aged 15 years and over) per year	Global (2008) Aged 20 and over 35% overweight + 11% obese OECD (2008) 17% obese	Global (2008) 31% of those >15 years insufficient physical activity
Australia average	2008 17% of those aged 15 years and over are daily smokers Smoking kills about 15 000 Australians each year and costs Australia $31.5 billion each year	2008 For those aged 15 years and over 10.3 L of pure alcohol per person per year This is 2.2 standard drinks per day per person 13% of people at long-term risk from alcohol consumption >813 000 people hospitalized for alcohol-related injury and disease 1996–2005	2008 25% obese 2010 More than 60% of Australians aged over 18 years are overweight or obese	2008 38% of those >15 years insufficient physical activity
Australian trend	Decreasing tobacco use	Stable alcohol use	Increasing obesity	Increasing inactivity

burden, the WHO and many nations are working to endorse international strategies for health promotion and protection.

Emerging infectious diseases (EID) are increasing and becoming a significant burden on global economies and health [1]. The Institute of Medicine defines EID as: 'infections whose incidence in humans has increased within the past two decades or whose incidence threatens to increase in the near future'. These may be new pathogens, such as sudden acute respiratory syndrome (SARS) or bat viruses; old pathogens expanding in range and incidence, such as dengue or ebola; and multidrug resistant tuberculosis strains. The majority of EID originates in wildlife and is correlated with socioeconomic, environmental and ecological factors [1]. Increasing temperatures, associated with climate change, may contribute to malaria and dengue extending to more temperate zones [2].

Increased global travel, coupled with the incubation periods of some diseases, such as SARS (2–10 days) or avian influenza (2–10 days), also means travellers may not become ill until returning home. Monitoring increases in ED visits for key 'chief complaints' has been shown to provide timely indicators for outbreaks and ED staff should be aware of EIDs and what tests to request. They should be suspected in patients: aged up to 49 years; with life-threatening illness of potentially infectious aetiology; and with no cause for illness identified by preliminary testing [3].

Both screening and diagnostic tests are needed. Screening tests help detect a disease early, often in relatively asymptomatic patients. They are sensitive but often less specific. Screening tests correctly identify those individuals who may have a given disease but often require more specific diagnostic testing to confirm or exclude this. Because screening tests are also performed on larger patient numbers, they should be cheap and simple to perform.

The ED is part of a system with integrated management and communication strategies needed rapidly to identify EID. Collaboration needs to occur locally, regionally, nationally and globally as well as between ED and multiple disciplines.

Disease prevention and control

The role of delivering preventive care may seem at first glance at odds with the normally very pragmatic function of an ED. In the current climate, where EDs are overcrowded and resources scarce, we are challenged to deliver the principal role of acute care. However, ED patients are often those that most need to be targeted for preventive measures and are least able to access it by other means. These populations include: the homeless, people on low incomes, people living with a disability, mental illness, refugees, migrants and indigenous populations. These populations have poor health literacy and limited health access.

There is a growing body of evidence that can guide us as to the optimum way to target our time and resources in the ED setting to deliver effective, efficient preventive care. Bernstein suggests that any intervention would be approached by asking the following questions [4]. Is the public health purpose clear? Is the screening appropriate and accurate? Will the intervention be effective and is this the best approach? Also the intervention needs to be assessed long term and an appropriate endpoint reached.

Prevention in the ED setting can be divided into primary, secondary and tertiary measures. Primary prevention involves intervention in a population prior to illness occurring. In the ED, this would include the routine vaccination of patients with the tetanus immunization and post-exposure prophylaxis for diseases such as rabies, hepatitis and HIV.

Secondary prevention involves an intervention in an at-risk population, early in the course of the disease. A good example in the emergency setting is that of screening for chlamydia. A further example would be a brief intervention for smoking cessation in a patient presenting for an unrelated issue.

Tertiary prevention involves an intervention in a population that is at risk and has experienced a resulting illness. This is treating an established disease which is core EM practice.

Screening, brief intervention and referral for treatment (SBIRT)

SBIRT has been described as the cornerstone of EM preventive care. There is some evidence that supports the use of SBIRT in the ED in family violence, risky alcohol use and smoking cessation. Much of this evidence comes from North America [5].

The methods that traditionally can be utilized for SBIRT include paper-based, computer questionnaire, video and a computer-based intervention. Innovations including the use of new technology and social media will provide many opportunities.

SBIRT need not be resource intensive for EDs, but additional resources are required to make them sustainable [5]. It also requires dedicated time for planning interventions and in measuring outcomes. Both the setting and the provider of the prevention activity may vary. It can occur at any opportune time in the patient's journey though the ED and by all health workers in the ED.

The cost to Australian society of alcohol, tobacco and other drug misuse in 2004–05 was estimated at $56.1 billion, including costs to the health and hospital system, lost workplace productivity, road crashes and crime. Of this, tobacco accounted for $31.5 billion (56.2%), alcohol accounted for $15.3 billion (27.3%) and illegal drugs $8.2 billion (14.6%) [6].

The act of quitting smoking involves five stages of which a number can occur in an ED. A single physician encounter results in 2% of patients quitting. Routine physician screening and counselling may increase cessation from 3% (usual care) to 8–11% at 6–12 months [7]. Smoking cessation interventions are more cost-effective than other interventions, such as treatment of blood pressure or cholesterol and Pap smears. In one investigation, it was found that EPs were likely to gather information about smoking but not to counsel or educate patients to quit; 56% of discussions with current smokers contained advice to quit, 16% an assessment of readiness to quit and only 13% a referral to quit. Smoking was more likely to be discussed when the patient presented with a smoking-associated condition [7]. Smoking interventions in the ED, even if low efficiency, will have high reach due to the absolute number of smokers attending. This results in a high impact intervention, which is cost-effective.

Over 800 000 Australians aged 15 years or over were hospitalized for alcohol attributable disease or injury in the 10-year period up to 2006 and it is likely that this figure will increase in the following decade [6]. The risk of sustaining an injury increases with the quantity of alcohol consumed and that risk is significantly higher for women.

EDs are well placed to recognize patients with both binge and chronic drinking problems. Validated screening tools can be used. The general efficacy of brief alcohol interventions in these settings has been recognized, although the evidence has been mixed [2]. The effectiveness of brief interventions varies with patient populations and treatment contexts [2]. Some trials have demonstrated small effect sizes, but this may be the result of lack of a true control arm, which typically received more than current standard care.

Many ED-based SBIRT are disease or risk behaviour focused rather that patient centred. They fail to recognize that many risk behaviours interact and are synergistic. They also have limited capacity to consider health literacy and social and cultural determinants of health. Thus, paradoxically, the most vulnerable populations may be least likely to benefit from them. For example, a smoking intervention is not likely to be effective in a person with low health literacy and alcohol dependence. While a role exists for simple effective interventions, future research should be patient centred and take into consideration the social and cultural context. More rigorous multicentred research is required in the Australasian context to determine the effective of SBIRT before widespread introduction can be recommended.

Health of indigenous people and cultural safety

The first peoples of Australia and New Zealand have not fared well from the respective colonization of their countries and this is apparent in the health status of these people. Australia's Aboriginal and Torres Strait Islander people have poor health outcomes, resulting from limited access to resources, such as adequate housing, education, employment, municipal infrastructure, health services and an enforced dismantling of cultural practice and community governance.

Many chronic diseases are the direct result of overcrowding and poverty. Post-streptococcal glomerulonephritis (PSGN) resulting in end-stage renal disease and high rates of type II diabetes are two striking examples of poverty-related disease. Recurrent streptococcal skin infections resulting in renal disease occurring at an early age is the direct result of poor living conditions. The risk and severity of type II diabetes is a consequence of limited access to affordable healthy food. Issues of alcoholism can be linked to dislocation, homelessness, experiences of racism and despair.

Aboriginal people living in poverty often access healthcare infrequently. Although many co-morbidities may appear to be peripheral to the prime reason for attendance, an opportunistic approach with this group of people and liaison with allied health services, including Aboriginal liaison officers and Aboriginal health services where available, can have long-term health benefits.

New Zealand's Indigenous Maori have had very similar health issues to combat but there are encouraging signs of improvement in their general health status, although poverty and associated health issues continue in many communities, particularly rural.

Addressing issues of cultural safety and competency in EDs in Australia and New Zealand has the potential to improve healthcare and thus outcomes.

Australian Indigenous Aboriginal and Torres Strait Islanders

According to the Australian Bureau of Statistics in 2011, the median age of death for Australian indigenous men and women is around 20 years less than for non-indigenous Australians. Mortality from coronary artery disease is significantly higher in indigenous people. The overall incidence rate of end-stage renal disease is higher in Aboriginal and Torres Strait Islander people, with an age-standardized notification rate almost 10 times that of non-indigenous Australians. The mortality rate from respiratory disease in those aged 35–44 is 20 times that of other Australians. Infectious diseases, such as tuberculosis, hepatitis, sexually transmitted diseases including HIV/AIDS, *Haemophilus influenzae* type b and pneumococcal and meningococcal disease are common. The adjusted mortality rate from diabetes is almost seven times the rate for other Australians. These health outcomes are based upon figures from the Australian Institute of Health and Welfare.

Suicide is the third leading cause of death for indigenous males. Significant stressors, such as family death, unemployment, alcohol, trouble with police, overcrowding and discrimination, are common. Assault is the commonest cause of injury and the leading causes of death from injury are intentional self-harm and transport accidents. Overall, fewer Aboriginal and Torres Strait Island people drink alcohol than non-Aboriginal people; however, of those who do drink, more drink at harmful levels [8].

New Zealand's indigenous Maori people

Even though life expectancy of Maori people has improved, it is still not level with non-Maori in New Zealand. Cardiovascular disease is the leading cause of mortality for Maori, with rates 2.5 times those of non-Maori. Maori and non-Maori have similar self-reported diabetes prevalence, but there are disparities in developing complications, such as renal failure and lower limb amputation. Maori female breast cancer registrations are 1.3 times that of non-Maori and breast cancer mortality is 1.8 times higher than that of non-Maori. Smoking rates are higher in this population with an estimated 50% of Maori female adults smoking.

New Zealand has moved to a focus on reducing inequality across all ethnicities by addressing the issues and barriers and by placing training in cultural safety high in health workforce priorities. Sir Mason Durie [9] gives wise guidance on the three principles that can be gained from the New Zealand experience and applied in Australia, these being integrated solutions, indigenous pathways and empowering relationships.

Cultural safety and cultural competency

To be able to have a positive impact on health status, practitioners working in Australasian EDs must be able to work in a culturally safe manner. This requires an understanding of the social, political, historical and cultural influences on the health of indigenous people.

While indigenous cultures are diverse, themes, such as the importance of customary law, the extended family and kinship obligations, the notion of reciprocity and a differing worldview are common. Identity is complex and it is essential that ED staff do not perpetuate notions of racial percentage and skin colour as determinants of someone's identity.

It is critical for health professionals to understand and acknowledge the existence of racism and how it has affected the health of indigenous people. Institutional racism [10] relates to the systems, policies and processes that disadvantage indigenous people.

Cultural competence is 'a set of behaviours and attitudes and a culture within business or system that respects and takes into account the person's cultural background, cultural beliefs and their values and incorporates them in the way healthcare is delivered to that individual' [11].

Similarly, cultural safety is defined as a way of practising in which the health professional undertakes a process of reflection on their own cultural identity and recognizes the impact of that culture on their professional practice. Unsafe cultural practice is any action which diminishes, demeans or disempowers the cultural identity and well-being of an individual [12]. A culturally safe health professional is one who knows what culture is, values their own culture, reflects on the interface between power and practice and acts to change unequal power relationships.

Acknowledgements

Hilary Tyler wishes to thank her colleagues, the members of the Indigenous Health Subcommittee.

Controversies/emerging issues

- New technologies and social media provide new opportunities in preventive health initiatives in the ED.

- SBIRT should be rigorously evaluated prior to widespread introduction.
- PH interventions in the ED will require additional resources in order to be effective and sustainable.
- Smoking cessation and addressing risky alcohol use are priorities for EM.
- Developing cultural competency and practising in a cultural safe manner is important for EPs.

References

[1] Jones KE, Patel NG, Levy MA, et al. Trends in emerging infectious diseases. Nature 2008;451:990–3.

[2] Saniotis A, Bi P. Global warming and public health: reasons to be concerned. Aust Hlth Rev 2009;33:611–7.

[3] Perkins BA, Flood JM, Danila R, et al. Unexplained deaths due to possibly infectious causes in the United States: defining the problem and designing surveillance and laboratory approaches. The Unexplained Deaths Working Group. Emerg Infect Dis 1996;2:47–53.

[4] Bernstein J, Haukoos J. Public health, prevention and emergency medicine: a critical juxtaposition. Acad Emerg Med 2008;15:190–3.

[5] Bernstein E, Bernstein J, Stein J. SBIRT in emergency care setting: are we ready to take the scale? Acad Emerg Med 2009;16:1072–7.

[6] National Drug Strategy. Ministerial council on drug strategy. Australian Government; 2010–2015. <http://www.nationaldrugstrategy.gov.au/> [Accessed Jan. 2013].

[7] Vokes N, Bailey J, Rhodes K. 'Should I give you my smoking lecture now or later?' Characterizing emergency physician smoking discussions and cesssation counseling. Ann Emerg Med 2006;48:406–14.

[8] Wilson M, Stearne A, Gray D, Saggers S. The harmful use of alcohol amongst indigenous Australians; 2010. <http://www.healthinfonet.ecu.edu.au/alcoholuse_review> [Accessed Jan. 2013].

[9] Durie M. Indigenous health: the New Zealand experience. Med J Aust 2012;197:10–11.

[10] Henry BR, Houston S, Mooney GH. Institutional racism in Australian healthcare: a plea for decency. Med J Aust 2004;180:517–20.

[11] Betancourt. In: Thomson N. Cultural respect and related concepts: a brief summary of the literature. Aust Indig Hlth Bull 2005;5:1–11.

[12] Te Kaunihera Tapuhi o Aotearoa Nursing Council of New Zealand. Guidelines for cultural safety, the Treaty of Waitangi and Maori health in nursing education and practice. Nursing Council of New Zealand. 2011; <http://www.nursingcouncil.org.nz/download/97/cultural-safety11.pdf> [Accessed Jan. 2013].

ADMINISTRATION

Edited by **George Jelinek**

27.1 Emergency department staffing

Sue Ieraci • Julie Considine

ESSENTIALS

1 An ED staff that is appropriate in numbers and skill mix is required to provide high-quality and timely clinical care, while maintaining sustainable working conditions for staff.

2 Senior medical and nursing staff have clinical roles that include direct patient care, as well as supervision and teaching of junior staff, coordination of patient flow and liaison with other clinicians.

3 The senior clinical staff profile should provide protected time for administrative, educational and research roles.

4 In calculating staff numbers required, it is essential to consider not only the hours of extent of senior cover required, but also the volume of the clinical and non-clinical workload.

5 Precise numbers and types of staff required depend on individual and institutional work practices and hospital roles.

General principles

Patients requiring emergency care have the right to timely care by skilled staff. The aim of staffing an emergency department is ultimately to provide care in an acceptable time according to the patient's clinical urgency (triage category). Staff working in the emergency department also have the right to safe and manageable working conditions and reasonable job satisfaction.

As the activity of an emergency department fluctuates in both volume and acuity, a threshold level of staffing and resources is required in order to be prepared for likely influxes of patients. In addition, the staffing number and mix needs to take account of the important teaching role of emergency departments.

The precise numbers and designation of medical, nursing, allied health and other staff employed will be determined by the local work practices (what tasks are carried out and by whom). This chapter discusses staffing requirements under the current Australasian model of emergency department work practices. This includes a major supervisory and teaching role for consultants and a significant proportion of specialist trainees and junior medical staff in the medical workforce, with a range of tasks, including venepuncture, test requisitioning and written documentation. In addition, roles are expanding into wider realms, such as toxicology, ultrasound and academic and observation medicine. Nursing roles range from bedside monitoring, physical care and treatment to advanced practice roles, including the initiation of tests and treatment.

Estimating medical workload

Emergency department (ED) case mix and costing studies have sought to measure the medical time commitment for various clinical conditions. Table 27.1.1 describes the approximate average medical time commitment for each of the Australasian Triage Scale categories [1]:

- The direct clinical workload can then be calculated from census data (number of presentations by triage category).
- Additional staffing will need to be added to cover the requirements of short-stay units or other services.
- The workforce should be resourced and organized so that patients are treated within the benchmark times for their clinical acuity (triage category). The Australasian College

Table 27.1.1	Australasian Triage Scale categories
NTS category	Medical time (min)
Category 1	160
Category 2	80
Category 3	60
Category 4	40
Category 5	20

Table 27.1.2 Benchmarks for waiting time by triage category	Category 1	Category 2	Category 3	Category 4	Category 5
Treatment acuity	Immediate	Within 10 min	Within 30 min	Within 60 min	Within 120 min
Benchmark performance (%)	98	95	90	90	85

for Emergency Medicine (ACEM) has defined benchmarks for waiting time by triage category (Table 27.1.2) [2].

- Staffing should be adequate to achieve benchmark clinical performance, as well as providing for the various clinical and non-clinical medical roles that supplement direct patient care.

Structure of medical staff

The medical workforce of Australasian emergency departments currently includes the following categories:

- consultants (specialist emergency physicians), including a medical director
- registrars (specialist trainees)
- senior non-specialist staff: experienced hospital medical officers
- junior medical staff: interns and resident medical officers who have not yet started specialty training.

The specialist practice of emergency medicine includes non-clinical roles (including departmental management and administration, planning, education, research and medicopolitical activities) as well as clinical roles. The non-clinical workload of an individual department varies with its size and role, the structure of its staffing and the other management systems within the institution. For senior staff, clinical work generally includes coordination of patient flow, bed management and supervision and bedside teaching of junior staff, in addition to direct patient care. Some emergency physicians may have other particular roles, such as retrieval and hyperbaric medicine or toxicology services. The increasing number of academic staff may have major research and teaching commitments.

To cover these roles, the ACEM recommends a minimum of 30% non-clinical time for consultants (more for directors of departments and directors of emergency medicine training) and 15% non-clinical time for registrars.

Throughout Australasia, EDs are experiencing increasing levels of activity. The calculation of medical staff numbers required for a particular department must include not only the extent of consultant cover required, but also the clinical workload and performance, local work practices and the nature of clinical and non-clinical roles. Because of variations in roles and work practices between sites, it is not possible to devise a staffing profile that is universally appropriate. Other recent changes in staffing patterns include employment across a network, increasing part-time work and sessional contract arrangements. Many emergency physicians are diversifying their practice profile to achieve a balanced and sustainable career, combining salaried and contract work, different types of hospitals and part-time work with a range of other interests.

Estimating nursing workload

Australian models for calculating ED nursing workload include the Emergency Care Workload Unit [3] (based on triage category and admission status) and the Victorian Nurse-to-Patient Ratio model [4] (using patient dependencies). Additionally, a minimum skill mix is required to manage the acute and complex workload. In addition to the bedside nursing workload, there are requirements to provide for education and training, patient flow and both clinical and departmental administrative roles. Larger departments require clinical managers on every shift.

Nurse staffing structure

In Australia, there are three levels of nurses registered with the Australian Health Professionals Regulation Agency (AHPRA):

- enrolled nurses
- registered nurses
- nurse practitioners.

Enrolled nurses work under the supervision of registered nurses and their scope of practice is generally limited to general adult or paediatric areas. One of the major changes to enrolled nurse scope of practice in recent years is their ability to administer medications and, depending on their level of education and registration notation, they may administer oral or parenteral (including intravenous) medications.

The majority of nurses working in emergency departments are registered nurses who have completed a 3-year bachelor degree typically followed by a 12-month graduate nurse programmme. In many states, 6–12 month transition programmes to specialty practice in emergency nursing are offered to novice nurses wishing to pursue a career in emergency nursing and are often a precursor to postgraduate studies in emergency nursing. Australian emergency nurses have one of the highest standards of education worldwide with the majority holding a graduate certificate or graduate diploma in emergency nursing. Postgraduate qualifications are considered by many as the industry standard for complex emergency nursing roles, such as resuscitation and triage. Triage assessment is a nursing role in Australia and emergency nurses are often responsible for advanced patient assessment, initiation of investigations and symptom relief care prior to medical assessment. Emergency nurses are also primarily responsible for ongoing surveillance and escalation of care in the event of deterioration. Advanced emergency nursing roles for postgraduate qualified emergency nurses are widespread in Australia and nurse initiated pathology, X-rays and analgesia are among common examples. There are also a number of Masters and PhD prepared emergency nurses in Australia working in various advanced clinical roles, joint clinical–academic appointments, nursing education and nursing management.

At the time of writing, there were over 700 endorsed nurse practitioners in Australia and emergency nursing has the largest cohort of nurse practitioners. In Australia, to be endorsed as a nurse practitioner, nurses must complete a clinically based master's degree or a specific nurse practitioner master's degree, demonstrate experience in advanced nursing practice in a clinical leadership role in emergency nursing and have undertaken an approved course of study for prescribing scheduled medicines as determined by the NMBA. Nurse practitioners form a key workforce strategy in managing demand for emergency care and are able independently to manage specific patient groups within their defined scope of practice, including prescribing medications, ordering diagnostic tests, referring to specialists and discharging patients home. Published research shows that emergency nurse practitioners can provide safe, efficient and timely care and are a valuable member of the emergency department team [5,6].

Allied health, clerical and other support staff

Allied health, clerical and other ancillary staff are essential to the efficient provision of emergency department services. They should be specifically trained and experienced for emergency department work. Clerical staff have a crucial role, encompassing reception, registration, data entry and communications within and outside the department, as well as maintenance of medical records. Dedicated paramedical staff, including therapists and social workers, are important in providing thorough assessment and management of patients, including participating in disposition decisions and discharge support. Other staff, such as porters and ward assistants, play an important role in releasing clinical staff from non-clinical roles as well as movement of patients within and beyond the emergency department.

Optimizing work practices

Traditional hospital work practices involve systems and tasks that are inefficient for the smooth running of modern, busy emergency departments. In a work environment with a rapid patient throughput and large numbers of staff, efficient work practices are crucial in optimizing clinical performance as well as job satisfaction. A review of staff numbers and seniority cannot provide maximum benefit without consideration of the way the work is done, what tasks are done and by whom.

A review of emergency department work practices can encompass the following principles:

- re-allocation or deletion of inefficient tasks
- optimal use of the specific skills of all staff
- use of communication technology and data systems.

As the emergency department workforce develops greater seniority and specialization and the demands of patient care increase, it is no longer possible to justify outdated work practices. Local research has shown that it is possible to improve clinical service provision by reorganizing roles and tasks in a sustainable way [7]. The opportunity exists to create a work environment that both delivers good clinical service and is rewarding and satisfying for staff.

Controversies and future directions

- The role of junior medical staff in Australasian EDs continues to evolve in the effort to balance clinical care and service provision with teaching and training. The ratio of senior to junior staff is crucial to maintaining safety and performance.
- Many urban and rural EDs rely on experienced doctors who have not completed specialist training in emergency medicine. As trained specialists begin to be employed in these EDs, hospitals should also aim to retain the expertise of other senior doctors.
- There are moves to increase numbers of enrolled nurses and introduce a third level of healthcare worker, such as assistants in nursing or patient care attendants in emergency departments. Any redesign of the emergency nursing workforce needs to be evidence-based and take into account the needs of patients seeking emergency care and the key role emergency nurses play in patient safety. There is debate regarding the utility and safety of enrolled nurses within the ED. Recognizing that ED patients are becoming more complex, it is essential that team members have the widest possible scope of practice.

References

[1] Bond MJ, Erwich-Nijout MA, Phillips D, Baggoley C. Urgency, disposition and age groups: a casemix model for emergency medicine. Emerg Med 1998;10:103–10.
[2] Australasian College for Emergency Medicine Policy P06, March 2006.
[3] Emergency care workload units: a novel tool to compare emergency department activity. Bond University ePublications@bond.
[4] Gertz MF, Nelson S. 5–20: a model of minimum nurse-to-patient ratios in Victoria, Australia. J Nurs Manag 2007;15:64–71.
[5] Considine J, Martin R, Smit D, et al. Defining the scope of practice of the emergency nurse practitioner role in a metropolitan emergency department. Int J Nurs Pract 2006;12:205–13.
[6] Considine J, Martin R, Smit D, et al. Emergency nurse practitioner care and emergency department patient flow: a case control study. Emerg Med Australas 2006;18:385–90.
[7] Morris J, Ieraci S, Bauman A, Mohsin M. Emergency department workpractice review project: introduction of workpractice model and development of clinical documentation system specifications. EDWPR Project. May 2001.

27.2 Emergency department layout

Matthew WG Chu

ESSENTIALS

1 The layout of the emergency department should promote efficient patient flow and maximize access to every space with the minimum of cross-traffic.

2 The triage location should enable staff directly to observe and gain access to both the ambulance entry and the patient waiting areas.

3 The acute treatment area should be open, with all spaces directly observable from the staff station.

4 Supporting areas, such as the clean and dirty utilities, the medication room and equipment stores, should be centrally located.

5 Areas often poorly planned include office, clinical support area, clinical spaces and tutorial rooms. The number of data and telephone entry points and the amount of storage space required are often underestimated.

6 Planning should consider the implications on night staffing when minimal staff are on duty.

7 The security of staff and patients is paramount in planning an emergency department.

Introduction

The emergency department (ED) is a core clinical unit within a hospital. The experience and satisfaction of patients attending the ED are significant contributors to the public image of the hospital. Its primary function is to receive, triage, stabilize and provide emergency care to patients who present with a wide range of undifferentiated conditions which may be critical to semi-urgent in nature. The ED may contribute between 15 and 75% of a hospital's total number of admissions. It plays an important role in the hospital's response to major incidents and trauma and in the reception and management of disaster victims. To optimize its core function, the department should be purpose-built, providing a safe environment for patients, their carers and staff. The physical environment includes an effective communication system, appropriate signposting, adequate ambulance access and clear observation of relevant areas from the triage area. There should be easy access to the resuscitation area and quiet and private areas should cater for patients and their relatives. Adequate staff facilities and tutorial areas should be available. Clean and dirty utilities and storage areas are also required.

Design considerations

The design of the department should promote rapid access to every area with the minimum of cross-traffic. There must be proximity between the resuscitation and the acute treatment areas for non-ambulant patients. Supporting areas, such as clean and dirty utilities, the pharmacy room and equipment stores, should be centrally located to prevent staff traversing long distances. The main aggregation of clinical staff will be at the staff station in the acute treatment area. This is the focus around which the other clinical areas should be grouped.

Lighting should conform to national standards and clinical care areas should have exposure to daylight whenever possible to minimize patient disorientation. Climate control is essential for the comfort of both patients and staff. Each clinical area needs to be serviced with medical gases, suction, scavenging units and power outlets. The minimum suggested configuration for each type of clinical area is outlined in Table 27.2.1.

Medical gases should be internally piped to all patient care areas and adequate cabling should ensure the availability of power outlets to all clinical and non-clinical areas. Although patient and emergency call facilities are often considered, there is often inadequate provision for telephone and information technology ports. The availability of wireless technology to support equipment, such as computer on wheels (COWS), is desirable. Emergency power must be available to all lighting and power outlets in the resuscitation and acute treatment areas. All computer terminals in the department should have access to emergency power and emergency lighting should be available in all other areas. The electricity supply should be surge protected to protect electronic and computer equipment, physiological monitoring areas should be cardiac protected and other patient care areas should be body protected.

Approximately 35–45% of the total area of the department is circulation space. An example of this would be the provision of corridors wide enough to allow the easy passage of two hospital beds with attached intravenous fluids. Although circulation space should be kept to a minimum, functionality, fire safety and occupational health and safety requirements also need to be considered. The floor covering in all patient care areas should be durable and non-slip, easy to clean, impermeable to water and body fluids and with properties that reduce sound transmission and absorb shocks. Areas accommodating the administrative functions, interview and counselling and support of distressed relatives should be carpeted.

Size and composition of the emergency department

The appropriate size of the ED depends on a number of factors: the census, patient mix and acuity, the admission rate, the defined performance levels manifested in waiting times, the length of stay of patients in the ED and the role delineation of the department. Departments of inadequate size are uncomfortable for patients, often function inefficiently and may significantly impair patient care. Overcrowding of patients increases mortality and morbidity with the risk of infectious disease transmission and increases harmful cognitive stimulation for patients with mental disturbance. For the average Australasian ED with an admission rate of approximately

Table 27.2.1 Configurations for clinical areas				
	Resuscitation	Acute treatment	Specialty plaster/ procedure	Consultation room
Oxygen outlets	3	2	2	1
Medical air outlets	2	1	1	–
Suction outlets	3	2	1	1
Nitrous oxide	1	1	1	–
Scavenging unit	1	1	1	–
Power outlets	16	8	8	4

25–35%, its total internal area (excluding departmental radiological imaging facilities and observation/holding ward) should be approximately 50 m^2/1000 yearly attendances. The total number of patient treatment areas (excluding interview, plaster and procedure rooms) should be at least 1/1100 yearly attendances and the number of resuscitation areas should be at least one for every 15 000 yearly attendances. It is recommended that, for departments with average patient acuity, at least half the total number of treatment areas should have physiological monitoring available.

Clinical areas

Individual treatment areas

The design of individual treatment areas should be determined by their specific functions. Adequate space should be allowed around the bed for patient transfer, assessment, performance of procedures and storage of commonly used items. The use of modular storage bins or other materials employing a similar design concept should be considered.

To prevent transmission of confidential information, each area should be separated by solid partitions that extend from floor to ceiling. The entrance to each area should be able to be closed by a movable partition or curtain.

Each acute treatment bed should have access to a physiological monitor. Central monitoring is recommended and monitors should ideally be of the modular type, with recording and print capabilities. The minimum monitored physiological parameters should include oxygen saturation (SpO_2), non-invasive blood pressure (NIBP), electrocardiogram (ECG) and temperature. Monitors may be mounted adjacent to the bed on an appropriate pivoting bracket or be movable.

All patient care areas, including toilets and bathrooms, require individual patient call facilities and emergency call facilities, so urgent assistance can be summoned when required. In addition, an examination light, a sphygmomanometer, ophthalmoscope and otoscope, waste disposal unit should all be immediately available. Hand washing facilities should be easily accessible.

Resuscitation area

This area is used for the resuscitation and treatment of critically ill or injured patients. It must be large enough to fit a standard resuscitation bed, allow access to all parts of the patient and allow movement of staff and equipment around the work area. As space must also be provided for equipment, monitors, storage, wash-up and disposal facilities, the minimum suitable size for such a room is usually 35 m^2 (including storage area) or 25 m^2 (excluding storage area) for each bed space in a multi-bedded room. The area should also have visual and auditory privacy for both the occupants of the room and for other patients, their carers and relatives. The resuscitation area should be easily accessible from the ambulance entrance and the staff station and be separate from the patient circulation areas. In addition to standard physiological monitoring, invasive pressure, capnography and temperature probe monitoring should be available. Other desirable features include a ceiling-mounted operating theatre light, a radiolucent resuscitation trolley with cassette trays, overhead X-ray and lead lining of walls and partitions between beds.

Acute treatment area

This area is used for the assessment, treatment and observation of patients with acute medical or surgical illnesses. Each bed space must be large enough to fit a standard mobile bed, with adequate storage and circulation space. The recommended minimum space between beds is 2.4 m and each treatment area should be at least 12 m^2. All of these beds should be positioned to enable direct observation from the staff station and easy access to the clean and dirty utility rooms, procedure room, pharmacy room and patient shower and toilet.

Single rooms

These rooms should be used for the management of patients who require isolation, privacy or who are a source of visual, olfactory or auditory distress to others. Deceased patients may also be placed there for the convenience of grieving relatives. These rooms must be completely enclosed by floor-to-ceiling partitions but allow controlled visual access and have a solid door. Each department should have at least two such rooms. The isolation room is used to treat potentially infectious patients. The isolation room should be located in an area which does not allow cross infection to other patients in the emergency department. Each isolation room should have negative-pressure ventilation, an ante room with change and scrub facilities and be self-contained with en-suite facilities. A decontamination area should be available for patients contaminated with toxic substances. In addition to the design requirements of an isolation room, this room must have a floor drain and contaminated water trap. The decontamination area should be directly accessible from the ambulance bay and be located in an area which will prevent the ED from being contaminated in the event of a chemical or biological incident. Single rooms should otherwise have the same requirements as acute treatment area bed spaces.

Acute mental health area

This is a specialty area designed specifically for the assessment, protection and containment of patients with actual or potential behavioural disturbances. Ideally, each unit comprises two separate but adjacent rooms allowing for interview, behavioural assessment and treatment functions. Each room should have two doors large enough to allow a patient to be carried through and must be lockable only from the outside. One of the doors may be of the 'barn door' type, enabling the lower section to be closed while the upper section remains open. This allows direct observation of and communication with the patient without requiring staff to enter the room. Each room should be squarely configured and be at least 16 m^2 in size to enable a restraint team of five members to contain a patient without the potential of injury to a staff member. The examination/treatment room will facilitate physical examination or chemical restraint when indicated. The unit should be shielded from external noise, located as far away as possible from external sources of stimulation (e.g. noise, traffic) and must be designed in such a way that direct observation of the patient by staff outside the room is possible at all times. Services, such as electricity, medical gases and air vents or hanging points, should not be accessible to the patient. It is preferable that furniture be made of material which would prevent it being used as a weapon or inflicting self-harm. A smoke detector should be fitted and closed-circuit television may be considered as an adjunct to direct visual monitoring. Psychiatric Emergency Care Centres (PECC) have been introduced in some hospitals. They are located within or adjacent to an ED and consist of 4–6 rooms with the configurations previously mentioned. Governance is dictated by the local operational policies.

Consultation area

Consultation rooms are provided for the examination and treatment of ambulant patients who are not suffering a major or serious illness. These rooms have similar space requirements to acute treatment area bed spaces. In addition, they are equipped with office furniture with a computer terminal, a radiological viewing panel and a basin for hand washing. Consultation rooms may be adapted and equipped to serve specific functions, such as ENT or ophthalmology treatment, or as part of a fast track area to treat patients with non-complex single system diseases. When the fast track model of care is adopted, the provision of an adjacent subwaiting area for patients waiting for the results of investigations will promote the efficient use of the available floor space.

Plaster room

The plaster room allows for the application of splints, plaster of Paris and for the closed reduction of displaced fractures or dislocations and should be at least 20 m^2 in size. Physiological equipment to monitor the patient undergoing procedural sedation or regional anaesthesia is required. Specific features of such a room include a storage area for plaster, splints and bandages; X-ray viewing panel/

digital imaging systems facility; provision of oxygen and suction; a nitrous oxide delivery system; a trolley with plaster supplies and equipment; and a sink and drainer with a plaster trap. Ideally, a splint and crutch store should be directly accessible in the plaster room.

Procedure room

A procedure room(s) may be required to undertake procedures, such as lumbar puncture, tube thoracostomy, thoracocentesis, peritoneal lavage, bladder catheterization or suturing. It requires noise insulation and should be at least 20 m^2 in size excluding a storage area for minor equipment and supporting sterile supplies. Physiological equipment to monitor the patient undergoing procedures, a ceiling mounted operating theatre light, X-ray viewing panel/digital imaging systems facility, provision of oxygen and suction, a nitrous oxide delivery system, a waste disposal unit and hand washing facilities should all be available.

Staff station

A single central staff area is recommended for staff servicing the different treatment areas, as this enables better communication between, and coordination of, staff members. The staff station in the acute treatment area should be the major staff area within the department. The staff area should be of an 'arena' or 'semi-arena' design, whereby the main areas of clinical activity are directly observable. The station may be raised in order to give uninterrupted vision of patients and should be centrally located. In larger departments, interlocking pods each involving a centrally located staff station overseeing an acute treatment area may be arranged to ensure patient visibility is maximized. The staff station should be constructed to ensure that confidential information can be conveyed without breach of privacy. Sliding windows and adjustable blinds may be used to modulate external stimuli and a separate write-up area may be considered. Sufficient space should be available to house an adequate number of telephones, computer terminals, printers and data outlets and X-ray viewing panels/digital imaging systems, dangerous drug/medication cupboards, emergency and patient call displays, under-desk duress alarm, valuables storage area, police blood alcohol sample safe, photocopier and stationery store, and write-up areas and workbenches. Direct telephone lines, bypassing the

hospital switchboard, should be available to allow staff to receive admitting requests from outside medical practitioners or to participate in internal or external emergencies when the need arises. A dedicated line to the ambulance and police service is essential, as is the provision of a facsimile line. A pneumatic tube system for the transport of specimens to pathology, drugs from pharmacy and the transfer of medical records and imaging requests may also be located in this area.

Short-stay unit

Many EDs possess a short-stay unit, i.e. emergency medical unit (EMU) which is managed under its governance and operates as an extension of the department. The purpose of these units is to manage patients who would benefit from extended observation and treatment but have an expected length of stay of less than 24 hours. It is considered that the minimum functional unit size is eight beds. It is configured along similar lines to a hospital ward with its own staff station. The capacity is calculated to be 1 bed per 4000 attendances per year and its size will be influenced by its function and case mix. As short-stay units are usually high volume users of mental health, social work, physiotherapy, drug and alcohol and community support services, appropriate space should be allocated to allow these services to operate effectively.

Medical assessment and planning unit

A medical assessment and planning unit (MAPU) or medical assessment unit (MAU) is an inpatient hospital unit which may either be co-located or built near an ED. It is managed by the inpatient medical service. The purpose is to facilitate the assessment and treatment of patients who require intensive coordinated multidisciplinary team interventions to minimize the length of stay and optimize health outcomes. The expected length of stay of patients utilizing this type of unit tends to be less than 72 hours. Its configuration and function is determined by case mix and local operational policies. It is usually configured up to 30 beds along similar lines to a hospital ward.

Clinical support areas

The clean utility area requires sufficient space for the storage of clean and sterile supplies and procedural equipment and bench tops to prepare procedure trays. The dirty utility should have sufficient space to house a stainless steel bench top with sink and drainer, pan and bottle rack, bowl and basin rack, utensil washer, pan/ bowl washer/sanitizer and slop hopper and storage space for testing equipment (such as for urinalysis). A separate store room may be used for the storage of equipment and disposable medical supplies. A common design fault is to underestimate the amount of storage space required for a modern department. A pharmacy/medication room may be used for the storage of medications and vaccines used by the department and should be accessible to all clinical areas. Entry should be secure with a self-closing door and the area should have sufficient space to house a refrigerator for the storage of heat-sensitive drugs and vaccines. Other design features should include spaces for a linen trolley, mobile radiology equipment, patient trolleys and wheelchairs. Beverage-making facilities for patients and relatives, a blanket-warming cupboard, disaster equipment store, a cleaners' room and shower and toilet facilities also need to be accommodated. An interview room allows for the interviewing or counselling of patients, carers and relatives in private. It should be acoustically treated and removed from the main clinical area of the department. A distressed relatives' room should be provided for the relatives of seriously ill or deceased patients. Consideration for the provision of two rooms should be given in larger departments to allow the separation of relatives of patients who have been protagonists in violent incidents or clashes. They should be acoustically insulated and have access to beverage-making facilities, a toilet and telephones. A single-room treatment area should be in close proximity to these rooms to enable relatives to be with dying patients and should be of a size appropriate to local cultural practices.

Non-clinical areas

Waiting area
The waiting area should provide sufficient space for waiting patients as well as relatives or carers and should be open and easily observed from the triage and reception areas. Seating should be comfortable and adequate space should be allowed for wheelchairs, prams, walking aids and patients being assisted. There should be an area where children may play and support facilities, such as television, should be available. Easy access from the waiting room to the triage and reception area, toilets and baby change rooms and light refreshment should be possible. Public telephones should be accessible and dedicated telephones with direct lines to taxi firms should be encouraged. The area should be monitored to safeguard security and patient well-being and it is desirable to have a separate waiting area for children. The waiting area should be at least 5 m^2/1000 yearly attendances and should contain at least one seat per 1000 yearly attendances.

Reception/triage area
The department should be accessed by two separate entrances: one for ambulance patients and the other for ambulant patients. It is recommended that each contain a separate foyer that can be sealed by the remote activation of security doors. Access to treatment areas should also be restricted by the use of security doors. Both entrances should direct the patient flow towards the reception/ triage area, which should have clear vision to the waiting room and the ambulance entrance. The triage area should have access to a vital signs monitor, computer terminal, hand basin, examination light, telephones, chairs and desk and patient weighing scales. There should be adequate storage space nearby for bandages, minor medical equipment and stationery.

Reception/clerical office
Staff at the reception counter receive patients arriving for treatment and direct them to the triage area. After triage assessment, patients or relatives will generally be directed back to the reception/clerical area, where clerical staff will conduct registration interviews, collate the medical record and print identification labels. Clerks may interview patients or relatives at the bedside but return to the reception area to finalize the administrative details. The counter should provide seating and be partitioned for privacy for interviews. There should be the ability for direct communication between the reception/triage area and the staff station in the acute treatment area to occur. The design should take due consideration for staff safety. This area should have access to an adequate number of telephones, computer terminals, printers, facsimile machines and the photocopier. It should also have sufficient storage space for stationery and medical records.

Tutorial room
This room provides facilities for formal undergraduate and postgraduate education and meetings. It should be in a quiet, non-clinical area near the staff room and offices. Provision should be made to accommodate webcasting, webconferencing, simulation and procedural skills training as well as local lectures and small group teaching. Technological support systems integrating computer, screen projection facilities, broadband access to capitalize on advances in web technology, electronic picture archiving and communication systems are essential. Equipment to support traditional teaching methods utilizing whiteboard, tube X-ray viewer system and examination couch must also be available.

Telemedicine area
Telemedicine is becoming increasing important, particularly for EDs in hospitals which are either remotely located or have limited access to subspecialty support. In these EDs, the telemedicine equipment may be located in the resuscitation area or in a dedicated room where patient encounters, such as mental health assessments, may be undertaken or the transmission of images, such as burns or digital X-rays, expedited. A dedicated facility with appropriate power and communications cabling is necessary. For facilities that receive the telemedicine transmissions, the room should be of a suitable size to allow simultaneous interactions by members of the consulting service teams. It should be in close proximity to the staff station.

Offices
Offices provide space for the administrative, managerial, quality improvement activities, teaching and research roles of the ED. The number of offices required will be determined by the number and type of staff. In a large department, offices may be needed for the director, deputy director, nurse manager, academic staff, specialists, registrars, nurse consultants/practitioners, nurse educator, secretary, social worker/mental health crisis worker, information support officer, research and projects officers and clerical supervisor. Larger departments will require the incorporation of a meeting room into the office area.

Staff facilities
A room should be provided within the department to allow staff a break and to relax from

ADMINISTRATION

the intensity of their clinical work. Food and drink should be able to be prepared and stored and appropriate table and seating arrangements should be provided in bright and attractive surroundings. It should be located away from patient care areas and have access to natural lighting and appropriate floor and wall coverings. A staff change area with lockers, toilets and shower facilities should also be provided.

Likely developments over the next 5–10 years

Over the last 20 years, EDs have been facing significant challenges. There has been a never-ending increase in demand. The work environment has become increasingly pressured. This has been compounded by resource constraints and the introduction of electronic information management technology. The provision of care has been increasingly complex. Changes in technology have enabled the management of greater numbers of patients in the community who would previously have required hospitalization. As financial pressures on hospitals have also increased, the importance of the ED has grown considerably and modern departments have significantly expanded facilities. Future design considerations are likely to centre on advances in the areas of information technology, telecommunications and newer non-invasive diagnostic modalities. In addition to these technologically driven changes, a greater emphasis will be placed on developing ED design configurations which will support redefined service delivery models to maximize efficient work practices aimed to minimize the number of patient moves, to ensure patients receive timely definitive care and to allow time-critical interventions to be delivered. Computerized patient tracking systems using electronic tags and built-in sensors will provide additional information that may further improve operational efficiency. The electronic medical record will make detailed medical information immediately available and will greatly facilitate the provision of timely care, quality improvement and research activities. Digital radiography, personal communication devices, voice recognition systems, wireless technology and portable computers and expanded telemedicine facilities will make the ED of the future as reliant on electricity and cabling as it is on oxygen and suction.

The increasing age of the population needs also to be considered when designing an ED.

Older patients have multiple co-morbidities leading to impaired mobility, vision and balance as well as being at increased risk of delirium due to underlying disease or hospitalization. They are likely to require greater space for the use of mobility aids and require greater shielding from sources of cognitive overstimulation than other patients. Standard hospital trolleys may pose a falls risk and contribute to the development of pressure areas. Strategies, such as the use of alternative hospital beds with pressure relieving mattresses and more comfortable 'reclining lounge chair' style seating, should be adopted for this subset of patients. Adequate lighting, the availability of natural lighting and the maintenance of a normal diurnal 'night–day' light pattern should be considered in the design to cater for the elderly patients who may spend prolonged periods of time in the emergency department.

Controversies

- Expert opinion significantly differs in the design of security features. Some experts argue that the use of physical barriers, such as that which are commonly seen in the reception/triage areas, to isolate potentially violent people may cause further aggravation to those people and this may have the paradoxical effect of increasing the incidence of violence. Others argue that protective physical features are of significant benefit, as staff may feel less vulnerable to physical attack and are, therefore, better able to diffuse potentially violent situations.
- Another area of debate relates to how patient privacy can be protected while still maintaining the ability to monitor closely patients within the department. Advocates of the direct observation of all patients believe that the resultant loss of privacy is a small price to pay to prevent the deterioration of a small number of patients with unrecognized severe illness. Opponents of this view believe that a significant number of patients in emergency departments do not require constant observation and that 'open-plan' departments inhibit good communication and create a noisy and distressing environment. A

satisfactory solution that meets the requirements of each group can be obtained by the use of solid partitions between treatment areas while leaving the entrance to each area open. Ceiling baffles installed in the staff station significantly reduces noise transmission. If the treatment areas are also arranged in such a way that they surround the staff base, direct observation of each area is still possible.

Further reading

A look at our new emergency department series. J Emerg Nurs 1992–6.

American Institute of Architects/Facilities Guidelines Institute. Guidelines for design and construction of health care facilities; 2006.

Australasian Health Infrastructure Alliance. Australasian Health Facility Guidelines. Health planning units; 2010. <http://www.healthfacilityguidelines.com.au/AusHFG_Documents/Guidelines/aushfg_schedules_accommodation%284%29.pdf> [Accessed Nov. 2012].

Bentley F. Emergency department investment blueprint–strategic forecast and capital planning guidance. The Advisory Board Company; 2007.

Christie C. Waiting for health–strategies and evidence for emergency waiting areas, inform ED Program; 2005.

Emergency Unit Design Guidelines. Health Department of Western Australia Facilities Unit; 1995.

Exadaktylos A, et al. Strategic emergency department design: an approach to capacity planning in healthcare provision in overcrowded emergency rooms. J Trauma Manag Outcomes 2008;2:11.

Guidelines on Emergency Department Design. Australasian College for Emergency Medicine; 2007. <http://www.acem.org.au/media/policies_and_guidelines/G15_ED_Design.pdf> [Accessed Nov. 2012].

Huddy J. Emergency department design–a practical guide to planning for the future. American College of Emergency Physicians; 2002.

Huddy J, McKay JI. The top 25 problems to avoid when planning your new emergency department. J Emerg Nurs 1996;22:296–301.

McKay JI. Building the emergency department of the future: philosophical, operational and physical dimensions. Nurs Clin N Am 2002;37:111–22, vii.

New South Wales Ministry of Health. Emergency department models of care; 2012 <http://www.ecinsw.com.au/sites/default/files/field/file/Emergency%20Department%20Models%20of%20Care%20July%202012.pdf> [Accessed Nov. 2012].

New South Wales Ministry of Health. Emergency department senior assessment and streaming model of care and toolkit; 2012. <http://www.ecinsw.com.au/sites/default/files/field/file/Emergency%20Department%20Senior%20Assessment%20and%20Streaming%20Model%20of%20Care%20and%20Toolkit.pdf> [Accessed Nov. 2012].

<http://www.aia.org/searchresults/index.htm?Ntt=emergency + department&Nty = 1&Ntx = mode%2Bmatchallpartial&Ntk= Main_Search> [Accessed Nov. 2012].

<http://www.designcouncil.org.uk/AEtoolkit/> [Accessed Nov. 2012].

<http://www.epmonthly.com/archives/features/building-a-better-emergency-department-an-architects-perspective/> [Accessed Nov. 2012].

<http://www.healthcaredesignmagazine.com/search/apachesolr_search/emergency%20department%20design> [Accessed Nov. 2012].

<http://www.aihi.unsw.edu.au/search/node/emergency%20department> [Accessed Nov. 2012].

27.3 Quality assurance/quality improvement

Diane King

ESSENTIALS

1 Quality management plays a pivotal role in the running of an emergency department.

2 The quality cycle of 'plan, do, study, act' requires accessible data and measures.

3 Major domains of quality are patient centredness, efficiency, effectiveness, safety, equity and access.

4 Keys to success in quality improvement activities are leadership, engagement of all staff, effective governance and change management.

Introduction

A primary role of the emergency department (ED) is to deliver the best possible care to all presenting patients. In order to deliver optimal care, a system of quality management must be part of the culture for all staff and be applied to all functions of the department. A quality framework provides the structure for the wide-ranging aspects of practice that are involved. Quality management requires effective leadership and commitment to improving processes and systems through analysis of data, change of processes and practice, staff engagement accountability and communication. Quality management is a continuous cycle, with measurement and monitoring required to establish that improvement is required in a practice or process, planning of the change, implementation, with re-evaluation and monitoring to ensure the change has the desired effect. Consumer involvement is a fundamental part of quality management. In the emergency setting, consumers include patients, families and carers, staff and the other clinical and hospital staff who interface with the ED.

History

The traditional approach of quality assurance involves a number of retrospective attempts to police various activities of the ED. The types of tools used in this approach are pathology result checking, missed fractures, medical record reviews, death audits and patient complaints.

The role of quality improvement in healthcare has evolved from the 1990s as it became evident that healthcare is prone to significant error and that, despite medical advances and escalating costs, the delivery of safe, acceptable and effective care is frequently lacking. Most industries adopted the quality improvement model to improve safety, reliability and efficiency. The implementation in the healthcare environment is noteworthy for the complexity of its systems, difficulty measuring clinical outcomes and competing priorities [1]. A modern quality system provides a framework that includes monitoring, audit and improvement of the clinical aspects of care, processes and structure, competence of staff, including education and training, and has clear governance and accountability [2].

Definitions

- Quality–'doing those things necessary to meet the needs and reasonable expectations of those we service and doing those things right every time' [3].
- Quality assurance (QA)–'a system used to establish standards for patient care, to monitor how well standards of care are met, and to correct unwarranted deviations from the standards' [4]. This implies intervention to correct deficiencies and is often externally driven.
- Quality improvement (QI)–raising quality performance to ever increasing levels.
- Continuous quality improvement (CQI)–a management approach that focuses

on providing a service that meets the 'customers' needs in such a fashion that the process itself leads to continuous improvement. This uses data collection, statistical tools and team dynamics to develop quality processes.

- Total quality management (TQM)–uses the management approach of continuous quality improvement and implies the commitment of the whole organization to the implementation of a quality plan. This involves the crossing of boundaries and traditional spheres of activity.
- Clinical indicators–measures of the clinical outcomes of care. They are population-based screens that help point to potential problems. They also allow comparative data to be collected nationally and benchmarking to occur.
- Clinical guidelines–are reference tools that help guide clinical practice. They provide a focus for standardization and a reference point for peer review.
- Benchmarking–comparing performance with others and the use of the best practices in a field to act as a marker and goal for improvement.
- Credentialling–a formal process to recognize and verify an individual's qualifications to enable a view of their capacity to perform safely in relation to a particular field or task.

Continuous quality improvement

The Deming cycle (described by WE Deming) is a fundamental tool for the approach to quality in any system. The PDSA (plan, do, study, act) cycle should incorporate the important sequential steps of planning, staff engagement, implementation, measurement, re-measurement and re-evaluation, followed by an improved plan and so on.

A QI system covers a number of dimensions. These are variously described, but include:

- access and equity, e.g. waiting times and access to inpatient beds

- safety: do no harm–this may relate to medication errors, adverse events or body fluid exposure, for example
- acceptability or patient centredness, e.g. complaint rates, patient satisfaction surveys
- effectiveness: this is the interface of quality management with evidence-based medicine, e.g. time to thrombolysis, appropriate antibiotic prescribing, following best practice standard guidelines
- efficiency: cost-effectiveness and value, e.g. appropriate imaging, avoiding waste.

There are a number of vital characteristics of a CQI programme that are necessary for its successful operation. A CQI programme:

- requires leadership (management) commitment and strategic planning
- is 'customer' focused. Customers include patients primarily, but also relatives, staff, other departments within the hospital, students, ambulance personnel and anyone who is involved with the functioning of the ED
- is performance-based. This requires accurate and relevant data and performance measures, monitoring and benchmarking. The availability of electronic, reliable and usable data is important.
- focuses around clear governance structures and accountability
- has effective communication and change management
- focuses on systems first and individuals second. This acknowledges the fact that a perfect world does not exist, but that quality can always be improved within a system (improving the norm) and takes the emphasis away from apportioning blame
- incorporates a risk management framework, with risk analysis and monitoring, risk mitigation and where possible risk avoidance
- includes sound credentialling processes.

A more detailed outline of TQM is beyond the scope of this book, however, the recent literature abounds with discussion on the various tools used, pitfalls in introduction and so on [5–8].

National bodies

The quality agenda has been facilitated by various bodies, including The Australian Council on Healthcare Standards (ACHS), that, in 1997, introduced its Evaluation and Quality Improvement Programme (EQuIP) as a framework for hospitals to establish quality processes. This is a requirement for accreditation with the ACHS. In 2006, the Australian Commission for Safety and Quality of Health Care was established to oversee improvements in the Australian context (previously the Australian Council for Safety and Quality). In the USA, the Joint Commission on Accreditation of Healthcare Organizations (JCAHO) and the Institute for Healthcare Improvement have led the way in the move from QA to QI [9,10].

The Australasian College for Emergency Medicine, the American College of Emergency Physicians and the UK College of Emergency Medicine are facilitating the process of QI by their training role, introduction of clinical indicators, policy development and standards for EDs. In addition, the International Federation for Emergency Medicine (IFEM) has developed a consensus document outlining a framework for measuring quality in 2012 available on the IFEM website.

Quality in the ED

The ED is a complex environment, which involves close interaction with the rest of the hospital and the community. The inputs are uncontrollable and unregulated and the 'customers' are under a high level of stress because of the nature of their problems, the unfamiliarity of the environment and the lack of control they perceive at a time when they are feeling personally vulnerable.

The ED is dealing simultaneously with life-threatening illness and minor complaints. It is an area under a high level of scrutiny from all quarters: the patients, the families and friends, the other departments in the hospital and the wider community–both medical and non-medical. This in itself is error prone and is compounded by the fact that many of the staff working in the ED are rotating through the department for relatively short periods of time, are often relatively junior and are undergoing training themselves. This training role is of critical importance in most EDs and must not be forgotten in any process dealing with quality issues. All these aspects of an ED make the maintenance of quality difficult and all the more imperative. In order to establish a system where quality care can be delivered with any degree of reliability, it is important that all staff are committed to the process and that management provides appropriate leadership and resources. The delivery of quality involves a continuing process of data collection (performance measures), analysis, feedback and introduction of strategies to improve the system, followed by re-analysis of the performance measures (the quality cycle).

Common quality measures in ED

The following are not exhaustive but are commonly used measures:

- time to thrombolysis or percutaneous coronary intervention (PCI)
- waiting time by triage category
- 'did not wait' rates
- death audits–and morbidity or adverse event reviews
- flow measures: 4 hour total ED times, times to inpatient bed
- chart audits for specific complaints, e.g. management of headache, abdominal pain, etc.
- time to analgesia: generally and for specific conditions, such as abdominal pain or fractures
- time to antibiotic for sentinel diagnoses, such as febrile neutropaenia or pneumonia
- trauma audits–missed cervical fractures, delay in craniotomy
- registries–such as trauma
- patient satisfaction surveys
- staff satisfaction surveys
- X-ray and pathology report follow up
- patient complaints audits
- equipment functioning and supply
- safety of the working environment including, for example, electrical safety or violent incidents
- staff retention or sick leave
- discharge communication.

It is clear from the list that the measures are potentially innumerable, that local factors must dictate those areas of special interest and that this will vary from hospital to hospital. In deciding which areas should be measured, it is important to focus on areas critical for patient or staff safety, that are strategically aligned or have been targeted as requiring improvements with which staff engage.

All EDs have common areas where there is high potential for problems to develop and these areas should be routinely monitored. The mechanism for doing this will vary from institution to institution.

Another aspect of the measuring of performance is that the process is one in evolution.

Not only should the quality of the service improve as the measures are improved and re-assessed, but the areas for attention can change and develop with the whole system. Peeling off layers as problems are addressed, exposes new things to improve. Again, this process must be internally driven to be effective. There is little point in collecting an enormous amount of data, unless the process is useful to the improved functioning of the whole system. Those best able to make those improvements should be an integral part of the system.

Likely developments over the next 5–10 years

- Credentialling, continuous professional development and re-credentialling for

practice are likely to become key areas of focus.
- Practice is likely to be increasingly standardized. Standardization is the platform from which quality care is delivered.
- Patient safety will be a growing priority. There will be a national focus on aspects such as accreditation standards and priority areas.
- There will be increasing professional accountability and public access to performance measure and benchmarks.
- Information technology, particularly the electronic health record, will be used to support quality and safety.

References

[1] Graff L, Stevens C, Spaite D, Foody J. Measuring and improving quality in emergency medicine. Acad Emerg Med 2002;9:11.

[2] Australasian College for Emergency Medicine Policy Document. Policy On a Quality Framework for Emergency Departments. April 2012: 28.

[3] Mayer TA. Industrial models of continuous quality improvement. Implications for emergency medicine. Emerg Med Clin N Am 1992;10:523–47.

[4] American College of Emergency Physicians. Quality assurance manual for emergency medicine. Dallas: American College of Emergency Physicians; 1986.

[5] Kaissier JP. The quality of care and the quality of measuring it. N Engl J Med 1993;329:1263–4.

[6] Berwick DM. Quality comes home. Ann Intern Med 1996;125:839–43.

[7] Kennedy MP, Cleaton PGA, Harrington AP, et al. Quality assurance to continuous quality improvement: development of an emergency department system. Emerg Med 1997;9:247–53.

[8] Berwick DM. The science of improvement. J Am Med Assoc 2008;299:10.

[9] Institute for Healthcare Improvement. <http://www.ihi.org>.

[10] The Australian Council on Healthcare Standards Clinical Indicators. Emergency medicine indicators, version 5. Indicator Report 2004–2011; October 2012.

27.4 Business planning

Richard H Ashby

ESSENTIALS

1 The business plan is an important multipurpose document, developed annually by the emergency department (ED) management group, to inform the organization about the agreed performance dimensions of revenue and expenditure, activity, efficiency and quality of services proposed for the next financial year.

2 The basic content of the business plan should include a projection and analysis of the current year's performance, together with proposed budget, activity, efficiency and quality targets and indicators for the next financial year. Additional issues which may require inclusion are capital expenditure, information and communication technology and special projects.

3 Once approved by the hospital executive, the ED management group should regularly monitor actual outcomes against the targets and take remedial action where necessary.

Introduction

Emergency departments (EDs) in public sector health services in Australasia are typically mid-sized clinical units within the organizational structures of hospitals. Staff numbers may range from 30 to over 200 and expenditure budgets from $3 m to over $30 m per annum. ED efficiency directly affects the global efficiency of the healthcare process in the hospital and purchasers are therefore increasingly interested in the value and performance of emergency medicine services. ED managers are being required to report on the dimensions of cost, output, quality and efficiency through a business planning process and other reporting mechanisms in order to justify their level of resourcing.

Types of plans

ED plans are relatively low in the hierarchy of planning instruments that begin with national and state health policy, health departments' strategic and corporate plans, regional and hospital strategic and business plans and, finally, the business and project plans of individual clinical units and departments. Strategic plans describe how organizations propose to respond to changing technology, altered demographics, shifting paradigms of care and industrial and regulatory reform, as well as issues associated with the cost, quality and accessibility of healthcare. These plans typically look 5–10 years into the future and the ED should reasonably expect to have input at a variety of levels into the strategic planning process.

Project plans, on the other hand, are highly focused on a particular objective outcome to be achieved within a given time frame and with a specified level of resources. Project plans may need to be created by an ED for the implementation of a new and significant piece of technology, major refurbishment or redevelopment or some types of clinical process redesign.

However, the most important planning instrument for an ED is its annual business plan.

The business plan

The business plan is an important multipurpose document that needs to be developed by the ED management group, in consultation with hospital management, on an annual basis. At one level, the business plan represents a management contract between the executive of the hospital and the ED. At another level, the business plan provides information to the staff of the department about the agreed targets for revenue and expenditure, activity, efficiency and quality of services to be provided in the next financial year.

Planning process

The plan should be developed by the medical director, business manager and nurse manager of the ED informed by consultation with the wider staff group. It is often useful to include a representative from the hospital's financial services department early in the process, so that there is a clear understanding of the financial framework for the plan. It is vitally important that the process be informed with as many useful data as possible, including accurate and up-to-date financial and activity statistics and quality and efficiency indicators. The premises, or context, of the business plan needs to be established. Unless there are specific reasons for change, it can usually be assumed that hospital managers will require that the business plan be based on management of the same level of activity at a similar quality to the previous year. In some years, there may be a requirement for a productivity dividend where management expects the same output from a reduced budget or improved performance from the same budget. Other assumptions, relating to estimated wages growth, non-labour cost escalations, leave requirements and so on, should be stated.

The timing of business plan development depends on the government budget cycle for public sector EDs and the timing of the financial year for private sector EDs. In most jurisdictions, this process needs to commence in early January, with the draft business plan available for the hospital executive by the end of February. The process may need to begin much earlier if significant additional or special

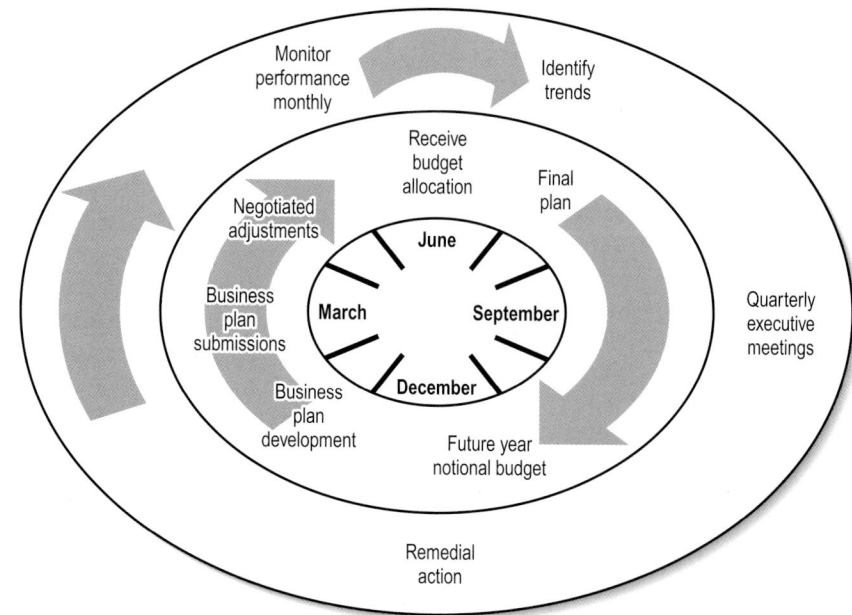

Fig. 27.4.1 Business plan cycle.

funding is being sought. Such requests are best handled as separate submissions, which will then need to pass through the various evaluation and approval steps. It is uncommon for special projects requiring substantial funds to be approved and funded within one budget cycle.

A typical business planning cycle is illustrated in Figure 27.4.1.

Business plan content

The ED business plan must address, as a minimum, each of the dimensions of performance, that is, revenue, expenditure, activity, quality and efficiency. A typical index is illustrated in Table 27.4.1. Some hospitals may require that their own format be used.

The introduction to the business plan should be brief. It is often useful to re-state the role and objectives of the ED and of any of its sub-units. The executive summary should present an overview of the business plan, including a general perspective on the integrity of the budget and activity targets for the current year and outlining any premises used in the creation of the current plan. Special issues may be highlighted.

Budget

The projected financial outcomes for the current financial year should have been carefully estimated. This projected end-of-year position should be shown in a tabular format against the

agreed targets from the previous year's business plan, as well as the actual outcomes of the previous year. In government organizations, adherence to budget is the highest priority and, therefore, the budget details should be presented first. The management group should have a detailed understanding of every variance from the budget that has occurred in the current year and a note of explanation of variance on every line item should be provided. Because the high fixed costs associated with operating an ED are related to the labour intensity of the service, it is useful to include a section tracking paid full-time equivalent staff, by month, for the current year compared to the previous financial year. This is especially important if there has been an overrun in the labour budget, as the hospital executive will wish to be reassured that this is not due to the employment of excess staff or excessive overtime.

In some jurisdictions, hospitals are funded based on activity, including ED activity, and it is incumbent on the ED to gather accurately and completely all necessary information to optimize this revenue. Similarly, privately insured patients must be identified as well as individuals for whom special funding or revenue premiums apply. Such expectations should be discussed with the finance department.

Activity

The activity of the ED may be shown as total attendances and attendances by category of the Australasian Triage Scale. The admission rate by triage category should also be shown and all values should be tabulated against the previous year's activity levels. Where an ED operates a short-stay ward or observation unit, the top 20 diagnosis-related groups by volume should be shown, together with the number of total separations, weighted separations and the case-mix index. This information should be available from the finance department. Again, the data should be benchmarked to the previous year. Additional relevant activity data, such as inter-hospital transfers, retrievals and so on, should be included.

Quality and efficiency
Waiting time by triage category is the key quality and efficiency indicator for an ED. The average waiting time per patient in each triage category should be shown, together with the percentage of patients in each triage category who are seen within the timeframe specified by the Australasian Triage Scale. In addition, the percentage of all ED patients seen and admitted, discharged or transferred within 4 hours (Australia-National Emergency Access Target) must be reported against target. These data should be benchmarked against the previous year's performance and, ideally, also against benchmarking data from similar hospitals elsewhere. Performance against clinical indicators recommended or required by government and other central agencies should also be reported. Additional access indicators include the frequency and duration of ambulance bypass, patient off-stretcher time and admission access block (percentage of total admitted patients spending longer than 8 hours in the ED) should be provided. EDs need to have a complete understanding of the Key Performance Indicators (KPIs) that are applicable to their services and have clear plans to achieve these. Dashboard displays of KPI achievement should be regularly published to both managers and staff.

It is appropriate in the section on 'quality' that research and educational achievements and plans should be succinctly reported, together with any innovative projects.

Projections
Having summarized the current year's performance, the remainder of the business plan should be used to present the ED's projections and estimates for the next financial year. Again, the projected budget should be presented first. This is best done in a tabular format and compared to the previous year's budget and projected actual expenditure. Any premises, assumptions or caveats related to the projected budget should be included as footnotes to the table. The most common premise relates to the volume and quality of services to be provided and the usual approach is iso-volume/iso-quality; this should not be varied in the business plan unless previously agreed by the hospital executive. Periodically, circumstances will dictate that a hospital vary the desired quality of services, perhaps as part of a strategic initiative to develop the ED or the volume of services in response to changing demographic projections. Apart from anticipated wages growth, it is important for the management group to make reasonable enquiries about predictable leave (such as sabbaticals or long-service leave) and these should be appropriately costed. In the non-labour budget, possible variations in the cost of overseas-sourced clinical supplies or pharmaceuticals due to revaluation of the currency should be considered although, in some jurisdictions, non-labour increments are specified, for budget purposes, across the whole of government. Particular attention should be paid to high-cost areas of pathology, radiology and pharmacy with evidence-based utilization being regularly assessed.

Realistically, most hospital executives will reject a budget proposal that exceeds the previous year's expenditure, escalated by projected wages growth, unless there are special mitigating factors or a source of funds for the predicted additional expenditure has been identified. For this reason, it is often useful to have three additional sections in the business plan addressing equipment needs, facility maintenance needs and a projects summary.

Equipment
The ED management group should canvass widely among the staff about perceived equipment needs. It is important that the totality of clinical and non-clinical equipment needs is understood and equitably prioritized in order to optimize the efficiency of the whole department. Most hospitals require that equipment requests be stratified according to cost, with items less than $5000 typically being met from a global allocation to the department. Apart from tabulating the need for this lower-priced equipment, a few lines of narrative about each item often assists the executive in ensuring the reasonableness of the request. The table should indicate whether the equipment is new or replacement. New high-cost equipment (e.g. ultrasound machines, computed tomography scanners or arterial blood gas machines) or large-scale renovations or new builds usually require the presentation of a full business case in line with government procurement instructions. The replacement of old, high-cost equipment should be part of a pre-planned hospital programme.

Facility maintenance
All but the newest departments will require some expenditure on maintenance each year. Again, it is useful for the ED management group to undertake a focused tour of all areas of the department to establish an inventory of maintenance needs. Reasonably accurate costings can be obtained from hospital engineering services or external contractors.

Projects

This final section can be used to describe and cost small or large projects to enhance the ED facilities, infrastructure or services. For example, there may be a proposal to establish a 10-bed short-stay unit adjacent to the ED, involving facility redevelopment, the acquisition of clinical and non-clinical equipment (including information systems), staff resourcing and clinical process redesign. This is best presented in a project format, including a clear description of the business need (supported by all available, relevant data), a business case outlining all the costs and benefits and, if possible, additional material, such as architects' sketches and a project implementation plan, including a project timetable. Professional advice in preparing this documentation is essential.

Private EDs

The overview of business planning presented above is equally relevant to EDs in private hospitals. However, private EDs also need to develop a more robust revenue budget and marketing plan appropriate to their circumstances. The marketing plan will usually be a part of the hospital's overall arrangements, but the ED should be in a position to report on any changes in referral pattern or on any opportunities to expand the business.

Business plan implementation and monitoring

Soon after the hospital receives its global budget, activity targets and KPIs from government, a short process of negotiation between the hospital executive and the ED management group should take place. This will fine-tune the business plan and, ultimately, permit authorization of the plan and the appropriate delegation for its implementation.

The ED management group should meet at least monthly to review actual performance against the outcomes predicted by the plan. Any variance from the budget in particular should be studied and understood. Remedial action should be taken wherever possible to maintain budget integrity. In many places, the ED management group would meet with the hospital executive at least quarterly to review department performance and to deal with any variation that may have occurred.

27.5 Accreditation, specialist training and recognition in Australasia

James Collier • Allen Yuen

ESSENTIALS

1 Specialist training in emergency medicine (EM) in Australia and New Zealand is the responsibility of the Australasian College for Emergency Medicine (ACEM).

2 International medical graduates with specialist qualifications or overseas-trained specialists (OTS) also require recognition from either the Australian Medical Council or the Medical Council of New Zealand.

3 OTS must undergo an assessment by the ACEM in order to be recognized as specialist emergency physicians in either country.

4 Specialist training in EM under the ACEM occurs in three phases: basic, provisional and advanced training. Provisional trainees must complete the ACEM Primary Examination and advanced trainees, the Fellowship Examination. Advanced trainees must complete a minimum paediatric requirement, as well as a research component.

5 ACEM training accreditation is awarded to hospitals if they satisfy minimum threshold criteria and the criteria that are set for the minimum level of accreditation.

6 There are three levels of accreditation which pertain to the maximum amount of advanced training that a trainee can complete in these departments: 6 months, 12 months and 24 months.

7 Accreditation criteria are set by the ACEM in the form of transparent comprehensive guidelines.

8 Hospitals are inspected at regular 5-year intervals to determine whether standards are being maintained to allow continuation of accreditation. This is supplemented by mandatory on-line trainee feedback on each training rotation.

9 Following an accreditation inspection, recommendations are made and fed back to the hospital and emergency department. The accreditation process is an important component in improving ACEM specialist training performance.

Specialist recognition and registration

Specialist recognition in New Zealand and Australia is handled by the respective medical councils in each country–the Medical Council of New Zealand (MCNZ) and the Australian Medical Council (AMC). In New Zealand, MCNZ handles both specialist recognition (termed vocational registration) and general medical registration. In Australia, the AMC has responsibility for the assessment of International Medical Graduates (IMG) seeking registration to practise medicine in Australia, including specialist recognition of overseas-trained specialists (OTS) and the accreditation of specialist medical colleges. Medical registration (both general and specialist where applicable) is the responsibility of the Medical Board of Australia, which is supported in this role by the Australian Health Practitioner Regulation Agency (AHPRA). Medical registration is required to undertake specialist training. All IMG must be both recognized by the AMC and registered with the Medical Board of Australia. There are three pathways to registration that are available to IMG: Competent Authority Pathway, Specialist Pathway and the Standard Pathway.

Specialist training in emergency medicine

Specialist medical training is the responsibility of the various specialist medical colleges. Most of these organizations cover both Australia and New Zealand. They are accredited by the AMC. Specialist training in emergency medicine (EM) is covered by the ACEM.

The college provides the framework, standards and supervision for specialist training in EM and successful trainees are granted Fellowship of the ACEM (FACEM).

Training occurs in hospitals and rotations approved by the ACEM for training. Each accredited emergency department (ED) is required to have an appointed Director of Emergency Medicine Training (DEMT). This is the college Fellow with the responsibility of facilitating the delivery of the training programme in that department and hospital. The description below of the training programme reflects the situation in November 2012 [1]. The training programme undergoes regular review and revision.

Specialist training in EM is divided into three phases:

- basic training
- provisional training
- advanced training.

Basic training

This usually consists of the pre-registration year of practice (internship in Australia or postgraduate year 1 [PGY 1] in New Zealand) and the second year of practice following a doctor's primary medical degree. It must occur in a variety of clinical rotations and be signed off by the administration of the employing institution.

Provisional training

This usually occurs in the third postgraduate year or beyond. There are three requirements of provisional training:

- Completion of 12 months of training in approved rotations. At least 6 months of this must be in EM. Each term, of 2 months' minimum duration, is assessed and signed off at its completion by the DEMT or local supervisor for non-ED rotations. Trainees, at the conclusion of each term, complete mandatory, on-line, de-identified feedback describing their experience.
- Successful completion of the ACEM primary examination. The ACEM primary examination is a basic science examination covering four subjects: anatomy, pathology, physiology and pharmacology. From mid-2013, the exam will involve a 90-minute multiple-choice examination (MCE) for each subject. Once all subject MCEs are successfully completed an integrated viva-voce examination can be undertaken. The examination is conducted twice a year in a number of locations across Australia and New Zealand. Each subject MCE and the integrated viva-voce examination may be attempted multiple times until successfully passed.
- Provision of three structured references and completion of the trainee selection process. Each trainee must obtain three structured references, as supplied by the ACEM, from their DEMT and two other Fellows who have supervised 6 months of their ED provisional training time. These assess the trainee's potential for a career in EM and are reviewed by the Trainee Selection Committee.

Advanced training

Advanced training occurs once the trainee has completed all the requirements of provisional training. The ACEM has a detailed curriculum outlining the knowledge and skills required by the completion of advanced training. The main elements are ED training, non-ED training, the minimum paediatric requirement, a research component and completion of the fellowship examination.

ED training

Trainees must complete 30 months of training in accredited EDs. Each accredited ED is allowed to provide training for an individual trainee up to a specified maximum amount of time (6, 12 or 24 months). Training must be in a minimum of 3-month terms. Each term is assessed and signed-off at its completion by the DEMT. As per provisional training, trainee feedback is required at the conclusion of each term.

Hospitals are also assigned a role delineation (major referral, urban district, rural/regional) when they are inspected for training accreditation. Trainees must complete at least 6 months in a major referral hospital and either an urban district or rural/regional hospital.

Non-ED training

Trainees must complete 18 months of training in approved non-ED rotations. These are usually in hospitals accredited for training by the respective college for that specialty. It is required that at least 6 months be spent in critical-care rotations (anaesthesia and/or intensive care). Experience can also be gained in the ACEM accredited special skills terms, such as pre-hospital and retrieval, trauma, toxicology, rural/remote health, ultrasound, research, medical education, simulation, safety and quality and medical administration.

Minimum paediatric requirement

This can be gained by two pathways: completion of a 6-month term in an accredited paediatric emergency department or via completion of a paediatric logbook. With respect to the logbook, this can be utilized during ED and non-ED advanced training involving paediatric (aged 15 years and under) patients. Trainees must log at least 400 substantive encounters with paediatric patients, of which 200 must occur within an ED setting and 100 of these must be from Australasian Triage Scale categories 1, 2 or 3. EDs are given specific accreditation for the use of a paediatric logbook.

Research component

The mandatory learning objectives of the research requirement of training can be met by publishing or presenting a research project to the satisfaction of the ACEM Trainee Research Committee or by successful completion of a minimum of two approved postgraduate subjects from the same course at an Australasian Univeristy.

Fellowship examination

Trainees may attempt the fellowship examination when they are within 1 year of completion of their training. The examination consists of three written sections (multiple choice, short-answer questions and visual aid questions) and three clinical sections (long case, short cases and structured clinical examination). It is run twice a year in various locations across Australia and New Zealand.

Variations to training

Recognition of prior learning can be applied for in line with regulations and upon registration. Up to 2 years of advanced training (up to 1 year of which can be in EM) can be gained overseas, with the prior approval of the ACEM.

Training can also be completed on a part-time basis (at least 50% of the time and conditions of a full-time post) and can be suspended for up to 2 years. All requirements of the training programme must be completed within 12 years of commencement of provisional training.

Dual training

Dual training programmes in paediatric EM (in conjunction with the Royal Australasian College of Physicians) and intensive care medicine (in conjunction with the College of Intensive Care Medicine) are operational.

Recognition of specialist training obtained outside of the ACEM

OTS in EM must apply for specialist recognition from either AMC or MCNZ. In both cases, once the documentation and English language status have been confirmed, the OTS is referred to the ACEM for assessment. The ACEM reviews the applicant's training, qualifications and experience on paper. If these appear potentially substantially comparable, the ACEM conducts a structured interview for further clarification. The three senior FACEMs on the interview panel review the applicant's qualifications and experience and determine their level of confidence in the following areas: undergraduate training,

basic training, advanced training, postgraduate experience, research and publication profile, education and training experience and administration. Additionally, three topical issues are discussed.

The ACEM then makes a recommendation to the AMC or MCNZ for specialist recognition, further supervision or further training.

The ACEM has a comprehensive website (http://www.acem.org.au) that provides up-to-date information on all aspects of training and other college matters. The AMC (http://www.amc.org.au) and MCNZ (http://www.mcnz.org.nz) also have websites with useful information for overseas-trained doctors wishing to work in either country.

Accreditation

Hospitals seeking accreditation for defined purposes, such as service provision or training, must comply with set standards determined by external institutions which oversee the criteria applicable to such hospitals.

In the case of hospitals overall, the Australian Council on Healthcare Standards (ACHS) determines the service standards of patient care provided by a hospital and its individual departments [2]. The ACHS has included the 10 National Safety and Quality Health Service Standards within its framework and integrated these with standards concerning service delivery, provision of care, workforce planning and management, information management and corporate systems and safety.

The learned colleges, including the ACEM, separately accredit hospitals for their ability to provide postgraduate training, taking the above criteria into account, but placing greater emphasis on the quality of experience, education and supervision for trainees. The items that the ACEM considers and takes into account in any accreditation decision are outlined in the following list from the ACEM guidelines [3]:

- The level and numbers of emergency physicians and senior staff capable of providing adequate and appropriate supervision for trainees of all levels of experience and at all times.
- An appropriate number and case mix of emergency patients to provide adequate clinical experience and with trainees having an adequate and appropriate level of involvement at an assessment, procedural and management level.

- An adequate specialist workforce. In considering the adequacy of the specialist workforce, regard will be given to the appropriateness of rosters, safe hours, access to leave, overall department performance and benchmarks.
- Compliance with the ACEM Continuing Professional Development Programme by the FACEM staff.
- Appropriate levels of staffing with respect to medical, nursing, secretarial and other personnel.
- Design and equipment of the department appropriate to the provision of emergency care and training.
- An appropriate range and level of support services.
- An appropriate education programme, including lectures, case presentations, mortality and morbidity review, discussions, audit and review. There should be a strong emphasis on activities that encourage adult learning, reflection, self-evaluation, discussion and collaborative learning. There should be emphasis placed on interactive teaching. There should be appropriate provisions in the education programme to meet the needs of trainees sitting the primary or fellowship examination.
- The opportunity for trainee research and the infrastructure supporting this.
- Accreditation of an appropriate range of specialties within the hospital by their respective colleges and the opportunity for rotations which will provide relevant clinical experience for EM.
- Evaluation of ED function and level of access block so as to determine how this may impact on training and trainee well-being.
- The ACEM Statement document–Emergency Department Role Delineation.

Accreditation guidelines

Transparent comprehensive ACEM guidelines for mixed and adult EDs seeking training accreditation can be viewed on the ACEM website [3].

The minimum threshold criteria that must be met before an ED can be considered for ACEM training accreditation is 2.5 full time equivalent (FTE) total FACEMs inclusive of the Director and DEMT [3]. The rationale for the minimum threshold relates to the minimum number of specialists required to provide a combination of leadership, mentorship, off-floor training, feedback and assessment and on-floor clinical supervision and feedback.

In addition to this minimum threshold, departments must meet mandatory criteria as outlined below before any level of accreditation can be considered [3]:

- appropriate and acceptable standards of patient care
- documented management, admission, discharge and referral policies
- a functional electronic patient information management system
- a formal system of quality management; trainees are expected to participate in these activities
- a formal orientation programme for new staff
- educational programmes for all grades of medical and nursing staff
- adequate EM textbooks, journals, management guidelines and protocols available on site; there should also be access to electronic sources of medical information
- access to advice or information which facilitates trainees seeking mentorship if they wish to do so.

College procedure

The ACEM conducts regular (at least 5-yearly) inspections of ACEM training-accredited EDs, to ensure that standards are maintained and that the various criteria for accreditation are met [4,5,6].

In the intervening period, the Accreditation Committee conducts annual reviews of a department's aggregated Trainee Feedback Reports. Identified issues require clarification, explanation or resolution by departments.

With respect to an accreditation inspection, the completed hospital information questionnaire, ED criteria checklist and any accompanying documents supplied to the inspection team before the inspection are carefully studied. Interviews with administration, department heads, specialists, trainees, nurse managers and educators contribute significantly to the decisions made.

The ED criteria checklist is a checklist against the minimum threshold, mandatory criteria and a number of specific criteria per level of accreditation currently held or desired in the future. An example of these specific criteria for a 24-month department is illustrated below [3]:

Minimum criteria:

- There should be at least 30 000 presentations per year to the ED, which are primarily attended to by ED staff.

- The ED should have a comprehensive case mix, which may include major trauma, critically ill patients, a broad range of complex patients and acute cardiology. It is important to ensure that, with increasing experience, trainees are able to provide immediate care and assume increased responsibility for these patients, while at the same time receiving appropriate levels of supervision.
- The ED should have an admission rate of >25%.
- The ED should have one FTE Nurse Unit Manager, or equivalent, who is supernumerary to the clinical staffing needs of the department.
- The ED should have at least one FTE Nurse Educator.
- The ED should display a willingness and capacity to host or co-host the fellowship clinical examinations and to contribute invigilators for the primary and fellowship examinations.

With respect to the level of supervision of trainees, the ED requires:

- One FTE position for the Director of Emergency Medicine which should ideally be supernumerary to the clinical staffing needs of the department. If this is not possible, the position should be provided with at least 50% clinical support time. This position may be undertaken by a single FACEM or two FACEMs (i.e. within a Co-DEM structure)
- Director(s) of Emergency Medicine Training (DEMT). The DEMT will be a FACEM who is required to be employed at a minimum of 0.5 FTE and undertake clinical work within the emergency department. The DEMT should be at least 3 years post-fellowship (within a Co-DEMT model, this is mandatory for at least one of the DEMT). With reference to provisional and advanced trainees within an emergency department roster, the following should be approximated with respect to the amount of clinical support time required within an emergency department for DEMT duties:
  - 1 hour DEMT clinical support time/ trainee/week.
  With the following minimum also applying:
  - 20 hours/week.
  - The clinical support time required within an emergency department for DEMT duties can be utilized by a single DEMT

or by a co-DEMT model. A maximum of two DEMTs may be appointed within a co-DEMT model. The division of an emergency department's clinical support time for DEMT duties between the two co-DEMTs may occur in any ratio.

- A minimum of eight FTE FACEMs within the department (inclusive of the DEM and DEMT positions). Each FACEM (exclusive of the DEM and DEMT positions) should ideally be provided with at least 25% non-clinical time for approved teaching, research or administrative activities.
- The presence of a FACEM exclusively rostered to clinical duties for at least 98 hours of every week.
- A minimum of 60% of trainee time to be under the direct clinical supervision of a FACEM.

With respect to the structure of the training programme, the ED requires:

- An educational programme, which includes access to teaching for both the primary and fellowship examination. For EDs seeking a continuation of accreditation, there should be demonstrated proven performance in (1) assisting trainees to pass both the primary and fellowship examination and (2) the development of highly regarded emergency physicians who practise good clinical care.
- There must be protected teaching time for trainees of 4 hours per week. Additional non-clinical time should be provided to allow trainees to complete other non-clinical duties specified by the department.
- Formal arrangements for the rotation of trainees to other specialty areas. Adult-only departments should be able to demonstrate that they can offer assistance to trainees wishing to access appropriate paediatric terms, either emergency or ward-based.
- There should be at least one FACEM formally responsible for the provision of advice, supervision and support of trainees undertaking the research component of their training (i.e. a trainee research project or approved university subjects). If applicable, they should also be responsible for providing critical review of the trainee's final manuscript to ensure it is suitable for adjudication by the Trainee Research Committee.

These specific criteria are repeated for 6- and 12-month accreditation but the numbers or threshold for each criterion are devised such as to be appropriate to these lower levels of accreditation [3].

Prior to the inspection, the department does a self-assessment on the relevant ED criteria checklist and indicates which criteria it meets, partially meets or does not meet. At the end of an inspection, the inspection team revisits the checklist and performs its own criteria assessment. Any variance between the department's assessment and the inspectors' assessment can then be discussed to clarify items of confusion, error or misunderstanding.

Levels of accreditation

There are three levels of accreditation awarded: 6 months, 12 months or 2 years. These periods refer to the amount of accredited time recognized as a part of a trainee's advanced EM training in that particular ED. The trainee may spend more time in the department, but the extra time will not count towards training requirements. The trainee may spend more time within the same hospital accruing non-ED time in accredited rotations in other specialties relevant to EM.

Since the period of advanced training is 4 years, the above periods of accreditation ensure that trainees rotate through at least two hospitals, benefiting from the particular strengths of each.

Rationale for the accreditation criteria

The Accreditation Committee has discretion on how the criteria are applied. This is for a number of reasons. First, the criteria are not comprehensive and factors not listed in the criteria may weigh positively or negatively on the outcome. Not all criteria necessarily need to be met as great strengths in some criteria may outweigh concerns of not meeting another; however, criteria concerning education, supervision and trainee welfare are a priority. Any criteria that are clearly not met are at least fed back as an issue.

The rationales for the mandatory criteria are fairly self-explanatory. Standards required for acceptable patient care and well-being of staff are paramount. The ACEM would not wish to put a trainee at risk in an environment where this was jeopardized.

Access to a mentoring system is also mandatory and is an AMC requirement of colleges. Trainees need to have the opportunity to seek a mentor, although it is not an obligation of the department to have a mentor for each trainee. Some departments run a supervisor system to aid the DEMT but, as supervisors participate in assessment, these are different from mentor systems.

With regard to specific criteria per level of accreditation, adequate senior staffing with emergency physicians is essential. Trainees must be well supervised, particularly after-hours and during busy evening and weekend periods. As the level of accreditation increases FACEM minimum numbers and the overlap of FACEMs working directly on the floor with trainees increases also. The number of FACEM FTE required increases from 2.5 to 5 to 8, the hours of the week of FACEM clinical presence increases from 50 hours to 80 hours to 98 hours, and the minimum percentage of trainee time under the direct supervision of a FACEM increases from 30% to 40% to 60%; respectively per 6-, 12- and 24-month level of accreditation criteria.

At the same time, trainees need to be given increasing levels of responsibility, including administrative, as they advance in their training, as some may be appointed to director positions at smaller hospitals soon after attaining their specialist qualification [6,7].

Excellent leadership is a requirement for a well-functioning department and training environment, hence the FACEM Director requirement and, as clinical leadership in the ED goes hand in hand with nursing leadership, the nurse unit manager requirement. The ability to utilize a Co-DEM management structure provides larger departments the ability to share an increasing administrative workload and smaller, in particular regional rural departments, the flexibility to use fractional appointees within the role.

Educators are of course an absolute requirement and medical and nursing education should be closely linked. Nurses can be a great source of trainee education and trainees can gain experience by participating in nurse education. Inspectors take note of the interaction between medical and nursing staff education and it becomes easily apparent whether these are well-integrated or separate entities.

The use of a Co-DEMT model is widespread as departments strive to meet the needs of an increasing number of trainees. The use of a DEMT to trainee ratio to determine the clinical support time for DEMT duties within a department applies equally across all levels of accreditation to the benefit of trainees.

Education programmes, particularly for 24-month accredited departments, must show the full spectrum of education. These should include on-floor clinical teaching; fellowship exam-specific programmes; primary exam-specific programmes; and departmental general education sessions. These programmes may be shared between a network of hospitals (ACEM accredited Emergency Medicine Training Network) and trainees must be provided with protected teaching time to allow them to attend education sessions. The culture for education and training can also be demonstrated by the quality and standard of resident and undergraduate education programmes, as well as FACEM university academic appointments. It is expected that the registrars, as advanced trainees, will be involved in student and resident teaching. Access to simulation training is becoming more widespread and available. FACEM commitment to assisting in college exam processes is a requirement for higher levels of accreditation and, again, is a marker of enthusiasm and educational culture.

The ability of a hospital to provide rotations for EM trainees to terms such as medicine, surgery, cardiology, anaesthesia, intensive care, paediatrics and psychiatry enhances a hospital's chances of attaining accreditation.

Research and quality assurance projects provide a framework for improving performance and the College examines the department's commitment to research [8]. Smaller 6-month departments may not have significant research infrastructure, but 24-month accredited departments must have at least an individual or a few individuals to assist trainees in their research component.

Case mix and attendance can, of course, ultimately limit or maximize a training experience and this also varies in stipulation per level of accreditation.

Recommendations

Following an accreditation inspection, a detailed report is forwarded to the College's Accreditation Committee for discussion.

Recommendations are then made regarding level of accreditation, suitability for paediatric logbook status, the number of trainee positions the particular ED can sustain and the role delineation of the hospital. Identified issues are also listed and it is expected the hospital will address these over the course of the next accreditation cycle, with regional Accreditation Committee members reviewing progress annually. Significant concerns require written correspondence to the Chair of Accreditation describing satisfactory resolution of issues. If standards for the level of existing accreditation are not met, departments receive 12-months' notice that the accreditation status may be reduced to a lower level. A further inspection in 12-months' time is conducted to determine the outcome. If any hospital at inspection fails to meet the minimum threshold criteria, accreditation is immediately lost without any notice period. The ACEM Board of Education and Council ratify accreditation decisions made by the Committee.

Implications

The accreditation process is comprehensive, fair and important, but it can also be intimidating [9]. Hospitals will retain their accreditation as long as they maintain the desired standards. Inspections by the College can highlight a department's or hospital's shortcomings to administrators, so that attention can be paid to correcting the deficiencies.

There has historically been little disagreement from EDs and hospitals with the recommendations made.

Loss of accreditation can occur at any time if departments fall below the minimum threshold. Losing accreditation can have adverse long-term consequences in terms of loss of reputation and lack of good applicants for positions in these departments.

In order to protect the trainees at an institution that loses accreditation, or has a reduction in accreditation status, trainees are allowed to continue having training accredited up to the end point of the current employment contract or change in training year [4].

Success with accreditation ensures a continuation or upgrading of an ED's reputation and makes that hospital more attractive for prospective trainees and staff specialists. Hospitals therefore have strong incentives to maintain high standards in their EDs.

Accreditation of paediatric-only departments

Accreditation guidelines for paediatric-only departments were jointly developed by the ACEM and the RACP (Royal Australian College of Physicians) through the Joint Training Committee in Paediatric EM. They follow a very similar format and structure to the adult and mixed guidelines but have a paediatric-specific theme.

Accreditation of overseas rotations

ACEM regulations are relatively flexible and trainees are encouraged to work in a variety of hospitals, both in Australia and New Zealand as well as overseas. Overseas terms are preferably in centres with respective college specialist training accreditation and prior approval needs to be sought from the ACEM. So far, most of these overseas accredited terms have been in the UK [10,11].

Accreditation in the future

The Australian Health Ministers' Advisory Council and the Health Workforce Principal Committee is conducting the Accreditation of Specialist Medical Training Sites Project. In consultation with the learned colleges and jurisdictions, the project is considering opportunities to streamline, improve efficiency and eliminate duplication in regard to accreditation practices across all colleges and disciplines. To date the proposed deliverables of the project are as follows:

- develop overarching accreditation principles
- develop a generic demographic dataset
- develop generic standards with craft specific criteria
- explore the use of other modalities, apart from site visits, in the accreditation process
- explore the feasibility of an ongoing quality assurance process
- explore the possibility with the National Health Performance Authority to include key performance indicators for teaching and training.

The criteria that are utilized to determine the role delineation of a hospital are being reviewed within the College and are likely to transition to describe the role delineation of EDs as opposed to hospitals.

In line with these initiatives and the ACEM Curriculum Revision Project (CRP), the ACEM accreditation guidelines are under review. Rising ED attendances, increasing staffing numbers and changing models of care in EDs have seen certain criteria now unable to be used to differentiate across the levels of accreditation. Similarly, the advent of trauma, cardiac and stroke systems across regions has resulted in a narrowing of where trainees can access certain patient cohorts and also blur the historic definition of a 'tertiary' facility. With respect to the CRP, the development of learning outcomes for the stages of training and the potential incorporation of specific formative

assessment processes within the work place will allow for the creation of more objective criteria concerning the delivery of education within departments. The recent move towards providing options by which departments can meet accreditation criteria (e.g. Co-DEM and Co-DEMT models and formally accrediting training networks) is likely to continue as the College seeks to meet AMC recommendations to explore strategies by which training opportunities can be optimized in smaller facilities, in particular in regional and rural locations.

Overall, the development of a new accreditation framework that meets national requirements, incorporates new criteria from the ACEM CRP and modifies current criteria to reflect better the realities of the modern emergency medicine environment should result in new, more objective accreditation guidelines that focus on education delivery and the associated required resources, clinical supervision and trainee welfare.

Controversies

- Collection of information and reviewing of practices and standards that are under the remit of the ACHS accreditation process results in duplication and potentially distracts the ACEM accreditation process from focusing on education and training.
- The ongoing pressure to have trainees rotate to rural regional areas needs to be reconciled with the ability of such facilities to meet the accreditation criteria and thus provide a beneficial education and training experience. Potentially, new criteria will assist these facilities to meet the requirements for accreditation, while the option of forming Emergency Medicine Training Networks provides them with an ability to optimize training opportunities.
- The evolving models of care within health regions, hospitals and EDs are potentially changing what has been defined as a tertiary hospital experience for trainees. Defining the patient cohorts trainees require exposure to may better delineate which facilities trainees need to work in, rather than simply to mandate tertiary and non-tertiary time.
- There continues to be some debate over whether a fair accreditation assessment

can be made on the basis of a single inspection. Many argue that a single snapshot of an ED in time cannot adequately represent the complex pattern of functions and activities going on within that department and that a longer inspection over a period of time may be necessary. This has to be balanced against the drain on college resources this would entail. The trainee feedback reporting system and the follow up of issues, identified at inspection, over the ensuing accreditation cycle provide some compromise.

- The development of generic accreditation processes covering all medical colleges will need to be balanced against the ability of colleges to continue to set and accredit against craft-specific criteria for their specialist training programmes.

References

[1] Australasian College for Emergency Medicine. Training and Examination Handbook; 2012. <http://www.acem.org.au>.

[2] Australian Council on Healthcare Standards. The EQuIPNational Standards, Guidelines and Program; 2012.

[3] Australasian College for Emergency Medicine. AC01 Minimum Requirements: Accreditation of Adult and Mixed Emergency Departments; 2012. <http://www.acem.org.au>.

[4] Australasian College for Emergency Medicine. AC94 Accreditation Information–Emergency Departments; 2012. <http://www.acem.org.au> .

[5] Yuen A. A review of Australasian College for Emergency Medicine accreditation: 1986–1995. Emerg Med 1996;8:152–62.

[6] Gaudry PL. Did you pass accreditation? Emerg Med 1992;4:29.

[7] Baggoley C. Emergency medicine. Where to from here? The College. Emerg Med 1999;11:234–7.

[8] O'Leary DS, O'Leary MR. From quality assurance to quality improvement. The Joint Commission on Accreditation of Healthcare Organizations and Emergency Care. Emerg Med Clin N Am 1992;10:477–92.

[9] Taylor DM, Jelinek GA. A comparison of Australasian and United Sates emergency medicine training programmes. Emerg Med 1999;11:49–56.

[10] Hamilton G. Emergency medicine: where to from here? Overseas viewpoint. Emerg Med 1999;11:229–33.

[11] Vinen J. Accreditation–was it worth it? Emerg Med 1992;4:30.

27.6 Specialist training and recognition in emergency medicine in the United Kingdom

Kevin Reynard

ESSENTIALS

1 Postgraduate medical training in the UK has become increasingly regulated and controlled by the General Medical Council (GMC).

2 Changes to immigration rules have occurred in response to insufficient training opportunities for UK and European graduates. This has produced a deficit in the number of doctors in training in EM. Nevertheless, it is relatively easy for graduates from Australia, New Zealand, Hong Kong, Singapore, South Africa and the West Indies to undertake postgraduate training in the UK.

3 The GMC sets standards for the curricula and training programmes of the royal colleges and faculties.

4 The route to specialist recognition in the UK is by completing a full GMC-approved programme of training or for relevant College and GMC approval of training, qualifications and experience gained elsewhere.

5 EM training lasts for 6 years comprising a 3-year core training programme, successful completion of which results in Membership of the College of Emergency Medicine (CEM) at examination, followed by a 3-year specialist training programme leading to Fellowship of the CEM by exit examination.

Introduction

The changing landscape of postgraduate medical training in all specialties in the UK that occurred within the past decade is set to continue. The changes to the structure of training and recruitment have become embedded, during which time large-scale changes to the regulatory systems occurred. The system to fund, control and manage postgraduate medical education is in the process of large-scale change following recent legislation relating to health and social care in England. These systems have developed differently in Scotland, Wales and Northern Ireland.

An understanding of UK training in emergency medicine (EM) requires some knowledge of the regulatory bodies and systems that have been put in place since 2003, relating to the regulation of training, the shape of training and the content of training.

Regulation of training

General Medical Council (GMC)

Anyone who wishes to practise medicine in the UK must be registered with the General Medical Council. The GMC introduced a new registration framework in October 2007. This framework simplifies registration to either 'full' or 'provisional'. Provisional registration allows newly qualified doctors to undertake general clinical training in the UK as a Foundation Year 1 doctor (see below) in posts specifically approved for this purpose. Full registration allows doctors to undertake unsupervised medical practice.

Those new to full registration, or those who have been away from UK practice for 5 years or more, must work for 1 year in an 'approved practice setting'. A list of these placements can be found on the GMC website. They meet defined standards for training, support and management of doctors.

For either provisional or full registration, non-European Economic Area (EAA) applicants need to demonstrate to the GMC that they:

- hold an acceptable primary medical qualification
- have the requisite knowledge and skills for registration
- have no impairment to their fitness to practise
- have the necessary knowledge of English.

This can be done by:

- a pass in the PLAB test (Professional and Linguistic Assessments Board)*
- sponsorship by a medical royal college (or other approved sponsoring body)
- an acceptable postgraduate qualification
- eligibility for entry to the specialist or GP register.

Doctors applying for full registration must also supply evidence that they have had a period of postgraduate experience equivalent to the general clinical training of the Foundation Year 1.

Detailed guidance is available at www. gmc-uk.org.

The GMC has taken over the role of independent regulator of postgraduate medical education, responsible for approval of curricula, training programmes and certification of completion of training.

Approval of curricula

The GMC has approved the curriculum for training in emergency medicine in the UK. The curriculum includes the syllabus, assessment methodology (including workplace based assessment and examinations) and the required training programme. There is also an approved curriculum for subspeciality training in paediatric emergency medicine. The GMC has approved speciality training programmes in intensive care medicine and pre-hospital emergency medicine, making the training period for those doctors who wish to achieve dual training in EM and one of these specialties longer than previously.

Specialist registration

Doctors who are fully registered with the GMC and who wish to practise as a substantive consultant or GP in the NHS must be on the specialist or GP register. The usual route for registration is to complete a full approved programme of training. Such doctors may then apply via their royal college for a Certificate of Completion of Training (CCT).

A second route, Certification of Eligibility for Specialist Registration (CESR), is available to doctors who have not completed a full approved training programme but who wish their training, qualifications and experience, wherever gained, to be considered for eligibility to be entered on to the specialist or GP register. Application forms, portfolios and other documentary evidence of what the doctor has achieved are sent by GMC to the relevant college for consideration and for a recommendation to be made with regard to registration. It is important to note that GMC is not bound by that recommendation.

If successful, such doctors are issued with a Certificate of Eligibility for Specialist Registration (CESR) which entitles them to apply for inclusion on the UK register but does not confer EEA registration privileges. The process tends to be slow and an application currently costs £1500. Fees to be included on the Medical Register are in addition to this.

Immigration rules

Immigration rules restrict access to UK postgraduate medical education (PGME) for international medical graduates (IMGs). This was driven by the concern that there may be insufficient training opportunities for UK and EEA graduates. A points-based system has been introduced to control immigration. Emergency medicine is currently a 'shortage occupation' in the UK. Hence, applicants who meet the requirements for registration with the GMC are highly likely to achieve the points total required under a tier 2 application for a visa for consultant posts or non-training junior doctor posts. It is possible that specialist training posts in emergency medicine will be included on the shortage occupation list. Further details and up to date information is available at www.ukba.homeoffice.gov.uk/visas-immigration.

Medical training initiative (MTI)

EM training in the UK for non-EAA doctors is also available for a period of 6–24 months under the medical training initiative. At the end of this period, trainees must return to their home country. Trainees are sponsored by the College of Emergency Medicine under a Government authorized exchange programme. Successful applicants are exempted from the PLAB test (but are excluded from applying if they have previously failed this test).

To be eligible for sponsorship the doctor must be one of the following:

❶ a current trainee in a non-UK emergency medicine training programme, with the support of the training programme director for the plan to spend a period of time training in the UK

❷ a consultant who has completed a specialist training programme in emergency medicine, with the support of the employer for the plan to spend a period of time training in the UK

❸ a consultant who has trained in a specialty other than emergency medicine with at least 12 months experience in emergency medicine with the support of the employer for the plan to spend a period of time training in the UK.

The individual requirements for the MTI are that the doctor must:

- not (normally) hold EEA citizenship or EEA rights of residency
- hold a primary medical qualification acceptable to the GMC for full registration
- be able to provide certificates of good standing (CGS) from all licensing and regulatory bodies which have been registered within the last 5 years. The GMC requires that doctors must provide a CGS from the country in which they obtained their primary medical qualification and each of the countries they have worked in during the 5 years immediately preceding an application for registration
- have completed at least 3 years postgraduate training, including an internship

- have an institutional sponsor in their home country specifying the post to which they will return
- provide evidence of satisfactory progression through training. Acceptable evidence would be documentation of passing any required postgraduate exam, a logbook or training portfolio (if applicable), evidence of clinical governance activity, or appraisal documentation. Evidence should cover both generic emergency medicine and acute specialties. Any evidence should be validated by the overseas sponsor
- be certified in at least one life support course–ATLS, APLS/PALS or ALS
- have achieved a score of 7.0 in each section (speaking, listening, reading and writing) of the academic module of the International English Language Testing System (IELTS). If the doctor is practising in a country where the first language is English, they may apply to the GMC for exemption from IELTS.

Postgraduate training in the UK

Following graduation, doctors enter a 2-year Foundation programme that delivers general clinical training, a broader experience and the acquisition and verification of generic competencies. Thereafter, those who have successfully completed such programmes and those doctors from other countries who can provide evidence of equivalent experience and competence (and who satisfy immigration rules) can apply for specialist training programmes. These programmes vary in their duration and pattern according to the specialty but lead to the award of a CCT.

Training in EM in the UK

The EM training programme in the UK lasts for 6 years. Acute care common stem (ACCS) training plus a further year in emergency medicine form the first 3 years (core training). During ACCS trainees undertake posts in EM, acute medicine, anaesthesia and intensive care medicine. This is followed by a year working in EM, with a particular focus on gaining paediatric competences and the non-technical skills to be able to lead and supervise others as a registrar. During this period, trainees must pass the diploma of Membership of the College of Emergency Medicine. This is followed by a 3-year specialist training programme leading to fellowship of the CEM to those successful in the

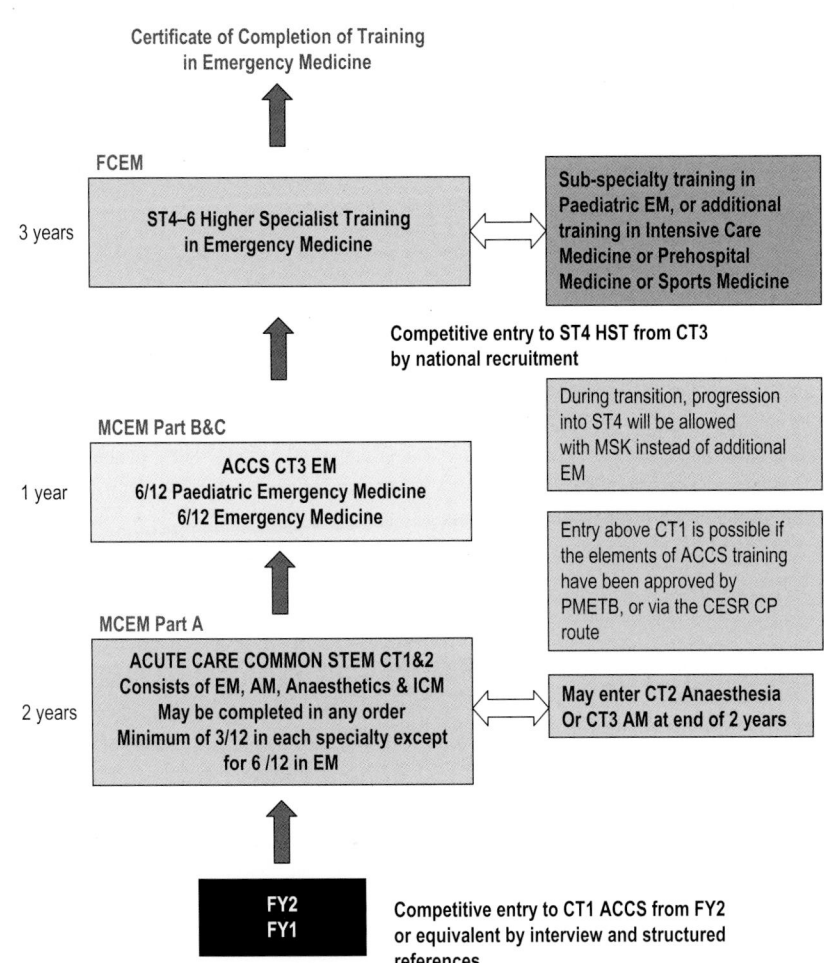

Emergency Medicine Training Programme Flow Chart

Fig. 27.6.1 Emergency medicine training programme flow chart *(from Curriculum June 2010, revised May 2012 from College of Emergency Medicine with permission).*

exit examination. Transition from core to specialist training is by competition (Fig. 27.6.1).

Specialty training (ST) years 4–6 are spent in a series of EDs. Year-to-year progression is dependent on satisfactory assessment and appraisals, mostly conducted in the workplace. In the final year of training, candidates who are supported by their local programme are eligible to sit for the FCEM examination, successful completion of which is necessary for eligibility for a CCT.

Many higher training posts are unfilled. The reasons for this are widely debated, but include the unsocial nature of the work, the intensity of work, terms and conditions of service compared to elective specialties and primary care, the change in the specialty as a consequence of the emergency care standard ('4-hour target') and changes in immigration rules. Currently, these

pressures are not adequately compensated for by the rich and rewarding aspects of the work. CEM, in conjunction with other bodies, is striving to correct this imbalance.

It is anticipated that, in the future, trainees will be eligible to move from other training programmes, with recognition of transferable competencies allowing entry at an appropriate point, rather than starting at the beginning of ACCS.

Subspecialty training

Paediatric EM is a recognized CCT subspecialty of both EM and of paediatrics. EM trainees who hold a CCT may undertake additional training in the care of children. The format and content of this training has been agreed by CEM and the Royal College of Paediatrics and Child Health (RCPCH) and lasts for at least 1 year.

Conclusion

The training programme has been through a period of marked transition as a result of forces from within and outside the specialty. There has been a period of stability upon which further refinement, rather than wholesale change, will be likely. ACCS is very popular with trainees with significant competition for places. There is much less competition for higher training posts. Anyone interested in EM training in the UK is advised to make frequent visits to the websites of CEM, GMC and the UK Border Agency.

Controversies and future directions

- Today's junior doctors are not attracted to working in emergency medicine in the UK in high enough numbers. There are major steps being taken to address the imbalance of work and reward. The future success of EM is dependent on continuing to attract and retain doctors of the highest quality.

- EM has always been a broad church. Constraining EM training in the UK to a single core training programme has resulted in many benefits, but has limited the diversity of additional skills within the consultant workforce. The introduction of alternative routes of training within EM in the UK may be helpful to reverse this trend.

27.7 Complaints

Peter Garrett

ESSENTIALS

1 Complaints occur in every emergency department. They can be considered useful feedback.

2 An immediate, supportive, open, even-handed approach reduces future stress and workload.

3 The majority of complaints are at least partly justified when properly investigated.

4 An acknowledgement, apology, commitment to investigate and truthful response are expected.

5 Resolution is by conveying the facts, any corrective actions done and expressing regret.

6 Staff should be supported throughout and confidentiality upheld.

7 Lessons learnt should be integrated into risk management and quality improvement processes.

Table 27.7.1 Contributing factors and reasons for complaints
Unpredictability of case mix and case load
Variation in attendance rates
Long waiting times
Insufficient staffing for unexpected peaks
Junior staff with variable experience and supervision
Deficiencies in treatment (real or perceived)
Inadequate assessment and missed diagnosis (real or perceived)
Poor attitudes, lack of professionalism
Poor communication, lack of information or consent
Interruptions, multiple concurrent tasks
Delays in investigations, consultations
Access block to inpatient beds
No appropriate follow up
Inappropriate or premature discharge
Unmet expectations
Invasion of privacy
Fees in private hospital EDs
Litigation for compensation

Introduction

Complaints are inevitable in the setting of busy emergency departments (EDs) and high patient expectations. Senior ED staff are well aware of what constitutes optimal care. Unfortunately, EDs are areas where there is little control over the cases presenting or the timing and volume of new arrivals; that combined with a mixture of staff with different levels of experience, long waits and multiple other reasons (Table 27.7.1) means that complaints are common.

Improvements in clinical care resulting from advances in emergency medicine (EM) and nursing have set new standards with which the public has become familiar through the media. Patients and their relatives have much higher expectations of EDs than previously. They are better informed, more litigious and encouraged by marketing from legal firms. Nevertheless, most patients who may have legitimate cause for complaint do not formally complain. The frequency of complaints is not an accurate gauge of patient satisfaction.

Incidence

Complaint rates about ED care vary from 0.26 to 3.8 complaints/1000 patients [1,2]. Some hospitals only record written complaints, while others also include verbal complaints in their data. Often the complaints refer to more than one issue. More complaints relate to paediatric patients and more are made by the literate.

In a Victorian study of 2419 ED-related complaints from 36 hospitals over 5 years, 37% were made by the patient while 48% were from relatives. Friends accounted for 3% and the rest included GPs, specialists, government representatives and lawyers. ED complaints were 14.3% of the total 16 901 hospital complaints [1].

Reasons

In this study, there were four main categories for complaint: problems relating to care (inadequate treatment, diagnosis or follow up–33%), communication (relaying information, rudeness and discourtesy–31%), access (26%) and administrative deficiencies (incorrect documentation, inability to obtain previous records, lack of privacy or confidentiality and loss of property–7%) [1]. In most other studies, communication is far and away the highest category [2]. In private hospitals, fees are an increasing source of complaint.

The two commonest motivations behind complaints are either the seeking of compensation or threatening litigation due to inadequate clinical care or seeking assurance that corrective measures will be made to ensure that no one else has a similarly unpleasant experience for a variety of reasons [3].

Clinical care

About 50% of complaints claiming inadequate medical assessment and treatment are substantiated [2]. Inadequate physical examination followed by a missed or delayed diagnosis is a frequent complaint and can only be refuted if relevant positives and negatives found at the initial visit are documented accurately.

Medicine is not an exact science and early clinical features may be atypical or overlap with other causes which seem unlikely at initial presentation. Explaining this to the anxious patient who wants a quick diagnosis and symptom relief can pose difficulties for a busy doctor.

Missed fractures are the most frequent 'misdiagnosis'. Some 'misdiagnoses' as perceived by patients result from poor communication, with lack of explanation by the treating doctor of the possible causes or what to do if there is no improvement [2].

Lack of treatment includes insufficient or no analgesia, lack of X-rays, blood tests, urine culture or antibiotics (where an initial presentation, particularly in a child, may have suggested a viral illness with eventual progression to

a bacterial infection) and lack of a splint for a 'soft-tissue injury', which is subsequently diagnosed as a fracture.

Rough, unskilled or incompetent treatment still occurs despite advances in training of both doctors and nurses. A heavy workload is not an acceptable excuse. With the reduction in allowable weekly labour hours for hospital-employed doctors, EDs may rely to some extent on junior staff and locums under variable levels of senior supervision on some rosters.

Unprofessional conduct and refusal to refer to a specialist or to a previous treating doctor are unacceptable causes of complaint. Cases of sexual misconduct are very rare in EDs and would be referred to a medical board.

Communication

Failures of communication feature prominently in most complaints [4]. Failure of doctors to introduce themselves and to explain the reasons for examination, investigations, treatment, admission or discharge, referrals or delays are all avoidable causes of complaints.

Abruptness, rudeness, discourtesy, insensitivity, absence of caring and other aspects of poor attitude used to be the main reason for complaints but, perhaps as standards in general society have changed, this is no longer the case. However, in EDs, when people are rightfully anxious about their medical condition, such attitudes should not be tolerated. Lack of formality, addressing older patients by their given name, casual dress standards and missing identification have become the accepted norm in many Australasian hospitals, but may still upset some of our senior citizens and immigrants.

Failure to obtain consent in the case of minors or to gain informed consent for procedures and to warn about risks occurs commonly in EDs, where it is assumed that attendance implies consent, but this can be challenged if the patient is brought to hospital by ambulance or other means.

Doctors may miss significant clues if they ignore aspects of a patient's history which do not fit with a presumptive diagnosis. This may also occur if the history is rushed and overly brief. Incorrect documentation and poor clinical handover is a common source of complaint, particularly when it results in the wrong treatment.

Reliance on referring letters or ambulance sheets without interviewing the patient can result in transcribing incorrect past history, medication charts and allergies. It cannot be

assumed that referral details or old case histories are correct. Objective evidence of diagnoses should be sought.

It can be difficult to identify a 'source of truth', when people do not have a regular physician. This can be compounded by 'doctor-shopping', where patients attend the most convenient bulk-billing family medicine clinic, where their past history is unknown, hoping for a quick cure for acute problems, while reserving attendances at their usual general practitioner for more complicated ongoing illnesses.

Clinical staff in EDs are commonly faced with excessive communication loads. The combination of interruptions and multiple concurrent tasks resulted in 36 communication events an hour in one study and this may produce clinical errors by disrupting memory processes [5].

Delays

Difficulty with access to healthcare is a worldwide problem, even in first world countries, where economic rationalism and changing government policies have resulted in closure of hospital beds, mental health institutions and community resources. Lifestyle and industrial issues have decreased the numbers of medical and nursing staff in hospitals, particularly after hours.

Diminished outpatient services may mean that patients need to be referred to private consultants' rooms where appointments may not be readily available. Fewer general practices open in the evenings or weekends. Some patients want a one-stop service for their medical consultation, their laboratory tests and their radiology. These social reasons make unnecessary use of scarce resources, despite strategies, such as telephone triage services and hospital-run after hours GP clinics. All the above have contributed somewhat to increased ED attendances.

Delays in triage, time seen by doctor, treatment, investigations, consultations, admission or discharge may therefore occur. Measures to decrease these are only partially successful because there is generally no excess of staff or resources to call upon when there are unexpected peaks in workload. Steps to improve waiting times, increase throughput of short-stay patients and decrease misdiagnosis of fractures have resulted in fewer complaints [6].

Particularly in the case of children and distressed patients, long delays cannot be easily tolerated and a significant number 'walk out' without being seen. The majority of these do not generate a complaint, but some progress to increased morbidity [8]. The elderly are less likely to complain, but suffer in silence, such that any pain they have may be unrecognized and untreated until late in the management [9].

Administration

Incorrect documentation by clerical, nursing or medical staff, lack of privacy or confidentiality, loss of valuables, poor cleaning or other environmental issues and queries regarding billing in private hospitals comprise the majority of administrative complaints [1,2].

Errors can be made by doctors in giving advice regarding a patient's right to claim compensation, since the full circumstances cannot easily be ascertained at the time of consultation. Doctors should not advise patients regarding entitlements to worker's or traffic accident compensation, but should complete the necessary documentation objectively.

Poor department design, lack of an accessible staff room or little adherence to departmental policy may cause complaints about staff socializing, eating or drinking. Their laughter may be seen by some patients as inappropriate, but by others as a sign of good staff morale.

The Federal Privacy Act 1988 was recently amended and became effective in December 2001 and resulted in removal of prominent whiteboards detailing patient information viewable by other patients and visitors [7,10]. Computers are now used in most departments, but even these may be visible to passers-by.

The Federal Privacy Act gives patients a general right of access to information held about them (see Chapter 25.4 Privacy and confidentiality). While patients have right of access, they must obtain consent from the doctors for further reproduction of the material, as the doctor still has ownership of clinical notes and specialists have legal rights over their reports. Relevant material must be made available to another doctor. Refusal of access must be based on reasonable grounds, such as that access would pose a serious threat to the life or health of any person. Conversely, information held by the doctor on the patient must not be divulged to third parties without patient consent, unless compelled by law, such as with mandatory reporting of child abuse [7].

Unmet expectations

Patient satisfaction surveys have ranked waiting times, symptom relief, a caring and concerned attitude and correct diagnosis as priorities when attending an ED. However, there is a mismatch when compared with staff who agree with the priorities but rank waiting time fourth [11].

Patients expect ED doctors to identify serious or dangerous conditions and to treat these appropriately. Explanation and reassurance are needed. Patients expect investigations and admission as indicated [3].

Responding to a complaint

Effectively responding to a complaint minimizes the likelihood of adversity and escalation. An effective response is early, supportive, open, even-handed and constructive. It should be backed up by a clear, accountable and outcome driven complaints management process that is supported by hospital administration (Table 27.7.2).

The immediate response

When a verbal complaint is made, the person to whom it is made has a responsibility to respond at the time as well as notify the appropriate manager of the service. This response should be immediate, genuine and supportive of the complainant's right to raise issues. The more immediate and active the response the less likely that the complainant will feel alienated or aggrieved and the more likely that anger will be rapidly defused [12]. If a consultation is not going well or there appears to be

Table 27.7.2 Suggested procedure for response to complaints
Accept the complaint
Apologize for the complainant's dissatisfaction
Defuse any anger
Record the details
Undertake to investigate
Arrange follow up
Investigate
Discuss with staff
Inform administration
Consider legal implications
Follow up with complainant
Resolve complaint
Lessons to be learnt

dissatisfaction brewing, rather than avoid the issue and escape from the situation, it can help to ask if there is anything on the patient's mind or ask a colleague or senior to assist by consulting. In both the public and private sectors, most unsatisfied patients may not complain immediately, but will spread their disapproval more widely via contacts or media, which can ultimately have an adverse effect on staff morale and future interactions.

Diffusing dissatisfaction and conflict

A genuine empathic response to a complaint will be more likely to lead to a successful outcome [13]. The person should be interviewed in a private place or office away from distractions and listened to in an open and supportive way, without interruption, and avoiding defensive postures and interjections. This is similar to how doctors listen to the medical 'complaint' and using the same principles helps. Early excuses, uninformed speculation or a defensive response without appearing to look into the matter will be seen through easily and regarded as dismissive and arrogant. If the person is rude or abusive, it is wise not to mirror this or terminate the meeting prematurely, but state that one still wants to help, understands that they are upset, in the knowledge that showing anger will make it harder to work together to get an appropriate outcome. If an 'independent' support person is available, such as a social worker, interpreter (or even a neighbour), for emotional, psychological or other support, this can help both doctor and patient.

Support of the complainant

The person has a right to alert the doctor of their concerns and be heard and to receive reassurance that they will be taken seriously. It helps to let the patient know what the doctor intends to do with their complaint, what the patient's rights are and that they have alternative routes to raise issues. Some experienced doctors are confident enough to thank the person for their complaint, on the basis that it provides an opportunity to improve services. A person who cares enough to report a problem in a department has great potential later to become a satisfied client. If some complaints may seem trivial, any underlying reasons or causes should be explored, as failure to address their underlying concern may perpetuate the correspondence. It can help to encourage the patient to bring their support person as the presence of a less emotional witness improves recall and can moderate the experience.

Expressing regret

An expression of regret acknowledges the complaint and does not admit error or that the complainant is correct. The more serious the issue being complained about, the more relevant the apology is to establishing empathy and creating an open and honest relationship with the person [15].

Documenting and investigating

As part of receiving the complaint, it is important to document clearly the complainant's perception of the issues, as well as the name, relationship to patient and correct contact details. At the end of the meeting it is a good exercise to summarize their perception of the issues, outline what actions will be next and the timelines for response.

In the information gathering process it pays to cross-check facts meticulously as any sloppiness in this phase will damage the process later. Take the time to interview involved staff, check medical records and do not be surprised if early assumptions are incorrect.

Determining the issues

Determining what the person wants may not be straightforward, as they may not have crystallized it yet, or be willing to articulate it. People would reasonably expect respect, an understanding of point of view, an immediate investigation of the true facts, early feedback and/or resolution and assurance that the problem will not recur to them or others. These are reasonable and deliverable aspirations and any department should have a system that supports this.

Some complainants want 'someone' to be reprimanded or punished (particularly if rudeness or lack of compassion featured) and some may feel they need some financial recompense. The desire for censure can be mitigated by a genuine apology for their experience by the involved staff or by their senior and, if relevant, explanation that contributing systemic issues were involved and will be addressed. If a complaint about unprofessional conduct is upheld, the option of escalating the complaint to a professional body should be available. There may be some scope in private hospitals to renegotiate costs if these contribute to a complaint.

Supporting staff and confidentiality

Most doctors and nurses are devastated when a complaint is made and might feel the need to justify what the patient perceived, disagree with recall and may feel anger towards the complainant. It should be sensitively explained that any complainant is voicing dissatisfaction with a perception and that everyone's views are being sought to investigate the facts fairly and openly and it may have value in improving the service.

It helps to reassure all that the principles of natural justice will be upheld and confidentiality of the staff and patient will be maintained.

If staff are distressed by the process, support and counselling should be offered, as many doctors and nurses have left the profession as a result of complaints, even though they were not directly responsible for the outcome [14]. Most jurisdictions now operate a 'systems approach' to what we used to call 'human error' and part of this is accepting personal fallibility (it's normal to be human) and concentrating on identifying what systems issues require action. Any competence or conduct issue should be addressed by the director of training or supervisors and may form part of a regular 'performance appraisal' [15].

Resolution

Once the facts have been established, ideally, corrective actions are identified that will prevent the event that provoked the complaint from recurring. Assess what the most appropriate resolution approach to take is. Facts laid out in a non-judgemental way, any corrective actions proposed and perhaps a repeat of the expression of regret form the basis of the follow-up interview or letter. Address all the issues raised. Rarely, it is advisable to refer to an external investigator or mediator and there should be hospital policy available on this.

In the Victorian study, most complaints (75%) were satisfactorily resolved by explanation of facts and/or apology [1]. Changes in policy occurred in 2% and remedial action took place in 5%. Very few complaints went to the legal system (<1%). The remainder were not upheld, not pursued or found to be frivolous. This is similar to the experience of the state health complaints commissions or ombudsmen where most complaints are resolved by free and open investigation, explanation and conciliation, and very few are seeking censure.

Integrating with risk management

An effective complaints handling process can integrate well with risk management processes, by identifying areas for improvement. A complaint may highlight unusual patterns of practice, deficiencies in protocols and guidelines, areas for further training and even provide the objective evidence needed for development of an ED business case. Complaints and compliments should be included in the risk management discussion of any senior staff meeting.

If the complaint has medicolegal or adverse publicity implications, the Medical Director and/or Executive Officers need to be informed to allow a considered response. Systems might exist that facilitate or enforce this, such as incident monitoring systems, sentinel event monitoring or the formal open disclosure process.

Prevention

System design

A well-equipped ED with adequate numbers of senior medical and nursing staff supervising junior staff, all aware of their scope of practice, will likely have fewer complaints. The department's design can enhance safety, with good waiting area and resuscitation area visibility, patient privacy maintained, temperature and noise levels comfortable, provide sufficient space, easy access to rest rooms and refreshment and education areas for staff close by [6]. Pain or X-ray protocols should be considered and prioritizing pathology requests.

Verbal and printed information on the frequently complained about areas of triage system, assessment and investigation turn around times, can be provided to waiting patients. High-risk groups that poorly tolerate prolonged waits, like children and psychiatric patients, can be triaged to be seen earlier.

Systems and procedures to follow up abnormal pathology and imaging results should exist and be audited, as 1 in 6 missed diagnoses are related to follow-up processes. Clinical handover, the effective transfer of information and responsibility, is now a major initiative of the Australasian College for Emergency Medicine (ACEM) and Australian Council for Safety and Quality in Health Care (ACHQS) and each department should support a protected and formalized handover process.

People

A polite well-groomed doctor who introduces him- or herself, makes eye contact, shakes hands and uses the person's title and surname can help to avert complaints. Talking out loud any examination findings as they conduct the examination can minimize accusations of inadequate examination, as stressed patients have poor recall and distorted perception of the interaction.

Adequate documentation of the encounter may provide the only means of refuting or resolving a complaint and while complaint-specific proforma, computerized decision support and discharge instructions can help documentation, preserving time to complete documentation is still important. Records must not be altered after a complaint.

A pro-active approach to complaints handling as part of a wider incident reporting system can result in higher patient and staff satisfaction. Specific training on how to relate to people in the pressured ED environment and how to handle complaints effectively should be incorporated into orientation and undergraduate education for nurses and doctors.

Managing specific aspects

Written formal complaints

Acknowledging the notification as immediately as possible, ideally within 3 days, together with an apology that they have experienced dissatisfaction is an expectation in many jurisdictions. This early response, along with the commitment to investigate and act on any findings may be satisfactory for many complainants. If the matter is clinically significant or may escalate, an early phone call in advance of the written response, perhaps to invite more information or, better, a managed face-to-face meeting. The Australian Council for Safety and Quality in Health Care has published examples of letters and responses [15].

Catastrophic adverse events

If the complaint is about a serious adverse event, such as a deterioration or death, many hospitals advocate the Open Disclosure model, an initiative of the former Australian Council for Safety and Quality in Health Care. The elements of open disclosure are an expression of regret, a factual explanation of what happened, the potential consequences and the steps being taken to manage the event and prevent

recurrence. There is an early informal phase where the treating clinician informs the patient of what has occurred and expresses regret for the harm caused or adverse outcome, with follow up in the form of formal open disclosure, which is about facilitating more consistent and effective communication between the patient, the senior clinician and the organization using a *trained* team in response to the most serious adverse events [15,16].

Grief reactions

Manifestations of grief and the desire to know all the circumstances should be respected but avoiding unverified explanation. Sometimes, a need to blame is part of the grieving process. Again, it is useful to offer support [11] (pastoral care, social worker, external counsellors or psychologists) and some Open Disclosure systems approve financial support to facilitate supportive acts (transport for a family member to come, accommodation close by).

Unreasonable requests or expectations

While the ultimate outcome may be a negative, it can help to start with a positive assertion and try to establish a working relationship: 'Yes, I can see that this needs to be sorted out. Let me enquire what resources are available to your GP to assist us in this'. A two-way communication allows the complainant to vent and prevents missing any important information. 'Yes, I can see why you are worried about taking John home. Let's talk through what the problems are and the early and longer term solutions to this.'

'Pests' or persistent complainants

A small number of complainants are unwilling to accept decisions, continue to demand further action, insist on outcomes that are clearly not appropriate or demand things they are not entitled to. They may constantly change the complaints, complain about the process, complain to multiple bodies simultaneously or make inappropriate freedom of information (FOI) requests. While it is tempting to pass them quickly up the chain, this can reinforce their behaviour and create more work. Try to own the complaint, manage their expectations early of what is going to happen and what is possible. Focus your attention on the conduct, not the person and, similarly, separate the conduct from the complaint. Be firm and clear

about what is not going to happen, that some complaints have no further avenues and that re-raising the complaint will not be responded to [17].

Delays

Frequent and realistic communication by all staff can help, explaining what delays are occurring, that triage times are revised, why repeated consultations occur, why tests are being done and what the likely outcome of the wait is. It is useful to avoid unrealistic promises like 'I'll be back in a minute' or 'they said they'd be down from theatre straight away'.

Summary

Complaints are a source of stress and concern for both emergency physicians and their patients. They are inevitable, part of our responsibility and should not be avoided. An understanding of the public's expectations from their attendance will assist in prevention of complaints [17].

Poor complaints management can damage a department. A good complaints management process can help by saving time, avoiding escalation, restoring the trust and confidence of patients, improving the safety and quality of the service and creating a more satisfactory working environment for staff.

Good complaints management can be easily learnt, but it sometimes requires a change in attitude; the most influential factor in changing attitudes and culture in an organization is senior leadership.

Controversies

Areas where clinicians vary in their acceptance of best practice as proposed by complaints and conflict experts include:

- The first person to field a complaint has a responsibility to acknowledge and respond to the issue.
- An expression of regret or an apology is not an admission of liability.
- Staff members should be notified of complaints against them to allow a right of reply/natural justice.
- A vexatious, time wasting or 'difficult' complainant who is avoided or 'passed up the chain' is encouraged in this behaviour.

References

[1] Taylor DMcD, Wolfe R, Cameron PA. Complaints from emergency department patients largely result from treatment and communication problems. Emerg Med 2002;14:43–9.

[2] Anderson K, Allan D, Finucane P. A 30-month study of patient complaints at a major Australian hospital. J Qual Clin Pract 2001;21:109–11.

[3] Bartley B, Cameron PA. QUEST: questionnaire relating to patients' understanding and expectations of their symptoms and treatment. Emerg Med 2000;12:123–7.

[4] Wilson B. Using complaints constructively. Aust J Emerg Care 1998;5:269.

[5] Coiera A, Jayasuriya R, Hardy J, et al. Communication loads on clinical staff in the emergency department. Med J Austral 2002;176:415–8.

[6] Jelinek GA, Mountain D, O'Brien D, et al. Re-engineering an Australian emergency department. J Qual Clin Pract 1999;19:133–8.

[7] Federal Privacy Commissioner. Guidelines on privacy in the private health sector. 8 November 2001.

[8] Hanson R, Clifton-Smith B, Fasher B, et al. Patient dissatisfaction in a paediatric accident and emergency department. J Qual Clin Pract; 14:137–43.

[9] Nerney M, Chin M, Jin L, et al. Factors associated with older patients' satisfaction with care in an inner-city emergency department. Ann Emerg Med 2001;38:140–5.

[10] Burton P. Privacy an ongoing concern. Austral Med 2002:10.

[11] Holden D, Smart D. Adding value to the patient experience in emergency medicine: what features of the emergency department visit are most important to patients? Emerg Med 1999;11:3–8.

[12] Doig G. Responding to formal complaints about the emergency department. Emerg Med Australas 2004;16:353–60.

[13] Bryce G. Complaints–How to deal with them. J Accid Emerg Med 1998;14:63–4.

[14] Valent P. Treating helper stresses and illnesses. In: Valent P, editor. Trauma and fulfillment therapy. Brunner/Mazel; 1998, p. 153–6.

[15] Complaints Management Handbook For Health Care Services. Australian Council For Safety And Quality In Health Care–July 2005.

[16] Nisselle P. Crisis management: honest and open disclosure. Aust Med 2002:9.

[17] Managing unreasonable complainant conduct–practice manual. Commonwealth Ombudsman; 2009 <www.ombudsman.gov.au>.

27.8 Patient safety

Peter Sprivulis

ESSENTIALS

1 Approximately 1 in 10 hospital patients experiences an adverse event, of which half may be attributed to clinical error and one-third results in significant harm or death.

2 Emergency medicine faces particular challenges to safe patient care due to the undifferentiated and potentially unstable patient case mix, high staff turnover, staff inexperience and fatigue and distractions, noise and overcrowding in the clinical care environment.

3 Clinical errors in emergency medicine may include errors of patient identification, hospital-acquired infections due to poor procedure asepsis and patient isolation procedures, medication errors, misdiagnosis and failure of follow up of investigation and imaging abnormalities, communication errors, physical care errors and mis-triage.

4 Improving patient safety in emergency departments (EDs) requires an understanding of the ED environment and a methodical stepwise approach to improving safety based upon:

   a. fostering reporting of clinical incidents, including 'near misses'

   b. evaluating reported incidents using accepted methodologies such as root cause analysis

   c. treating the risk: this is rarely achieved by exhorting staff to 'try harder' or removing the offending individual. Rather, risk reduction usually requires process redesign to make the 'right' thing easier to do and an error less likely.

5 Patient safety should be monitored proactively in order to ascertain risks and assist assessment and refinement of interventions to improve patient safety.

6 An open, communicative culture that promotes reporting and minimizes blame supports patient safety improvement.

Introduction

Patient safety, or the freedom from accidental injury due to medical care or from medical error, is increasingly being recognized as a critical consideration in the delivery of acute and emergency healthcare [1]. Several OECD countries have examined the proportion of acute care admissions during which an adverse event (an unexpected medical problem that happens during treatment with a drug or other therapy) is identifiable using a standard medical chart review. They typically report that 1 in 10 admitted patients experiences an adverse event, of which half are considered preventable with the current state of medical knowledge (i.e. are due to medical error) [1]. Typically, one-third of adverse events leads to moderate or greater disability or death [1]. An important consideration for the emergency care of admitted patients is that the day of greatest risk of an adverse event is usually the first day of admission to hospital. This is when knowledge of the patient's clinical condition is often incomplete, the clinical condition is least stable and when most patients experience the greatest number of procedures and interventions [2].

Specific emergency department factors that may compromise patient safety

Safe patient care is challenged by several specific emergency department (ED) factors that include:

- *Staff factors*: ED staffing profiles, particularly in public EDs, typically include a high proportion of junior medical and nursing staff who are still in training. Safety improves with experience. In addition, there is usually a scheduled high turnover of staff, as staff are rotated between alternate training positions. These high levels of rotation can corrode 'memory' of safe and desirable processes and systems of care. ED staff are usually rostered to work shifts spanning 24 h a day. Poorly designed rosters may contribute to fatigue [3,4].
- *Clinical factors*: ED patients have an inherently high severity of illness, placing them at greater risk of serious adverse sequelae if a medical error occurs. In addition, the undifferentiated nature of illness and injuries cared for, often coupled with the incomplete clinical information, creates clinical uncertainty, increasing risk [4,5].
- *Physical environment*: EDs are noisy, busy work spaces, with frequent intrusions from alarms, pages, telephone calls and personal consultations, all of which create distractions, increasing the risk of error [6].
- *Linkages to other care systems*: emergency care is reliant upon a complex set of relationships between the ED, referring practitioners, pre-hospital carers, other hospital services and other services responsible for aftercare or following up after discharge from the ED. Poor linkages or communication between the ED and any of these other services can result in errors or omissions in information transfer that compromise patient safety [7].
- *Overcrowding*: EDs have little control over patient attendance and, increasingly, suffer overcrowding as a consequence of poor access to beds downstream of the ED for admitted patients. This is associated with overcrowding and increased mortality, most likely due to a combination of resource effects (incorrect or insufficient resources or attempting procedures or monitoring in inappropriate locations) and delays in time to critical care [4,8].

Common safety problems encountered in emergency departments

The factors described above interact to create a wide range of risks to patients needing emergency care [4]. Some of the errors observed in the emergency setting include:

- *Patient identification errors*: errors in patient identification, incorrect labelling of laboratory requests and mislabelled samples may result in delays, misdiagnosis and incorrect treatment, such as transfusion errors.
- *Hospital-acquired infection*: the conduct of simple procedures, such as peripheral intravenous line insertion, by inexperienced staff using suboptimal asepsis techniques in inappropriate or crowded locations, increases the risk of hospital-acquired infection. Poor screening or compromise of isolation procedures due to overcrowding can pose genuine life threats to other patients.
- *Incorrect interpretation or failure to follow up pending imaging or laboratory investigations*: incorrect interpretation of radiographs or failure to check for a pending laboratory result can result in incorrect or delayed diagnosis.
- *Medication errors*: illegible, incomplete and verbal drug prescriptions, dosing errors (particularly in children) and compromise of medication administration procedures increase the risk of adverse drug events.
- *Communication errors*: omissions in the handover of care between clinicians within the ED at the change of shift, upon transfer to inpatient teams or upon discharge/transfer may cause serious delays in both diagnosis and the follow up of urgently needed investigations or treatment.
- *Physical care errors*: the care of elderly patients for extended periods in a bright, noisy environment, in the era of access block, increases the risk of confusion and falls.
- *Triage errors*: triage is known to be an imperfect art, however, in the era of overcrowding, which may result in significant delays in care for low-priority patients, a triage error may result in significant delays in diagnosis or initiation of treatment.

Improving safety in the emergency department

Specific actions to improve patient safety should be undertaken in the context of a comprehensive organizational framework for clinical governance and quality improvement [1]. The development of a programme of safety improvement for an ED should be undertaken methodically, in accordance with existing Australasian and international standards that usually encompass the following process elements:

- *Understand the environment*: initially, it is essential that the specific environment of emergency care, including the characteristics of EDs and emergency patients that impair safety and the types of errors encountered in emergency care, are fully understood.
- *Identify specific risks*: risk identification is usually undertaken with the aid of clinical incident reporting systems that encourage the structured reporting of clinical incidents that resulted, or could have resulted, in unexpected harm to the patient (e.g. the Australian Incident Monitoring System). These reports are usually collated both at the ED level and also at the hospital or organization level and even at the jurisdictional or national level.
- For every thousand prevented or no-harm incidents there may be a hundred of the same type that cause minor to moderate harm, 10 that cause severe harm and 1 that causes death. Therefore, it is important to learn from the prevented or no harm incidents to reduce the chance of the single death incident happening. Often, employees are more willing to report near misses. The importance of including near misses in the incident reporting systems cannot be overemphasized [1].
- *Analyse and evaluate the risks*: risk analysis should be undertaken using an accepted methodology with the support of staff trained in its use. Two common forms of analysis are root cause analysis and failure modes and effects analysis. Root cause analysis is conducted 'after the event' and aims to identify what happened, why and what can be done to prevent it in the future by attempting to identify systems problems that contributed to the clinical event. Failure modes and effects analysis can be conducted in the absence of specific clinical

events. It uses a proactive and systematic approach to evaluate common clinical processes in order to identify where and how they might fail and to assess the relative impact of different failures in order to identify the parts of the process that are most in need of change. This approach is particularly useful in evaluating a new process prior to implementation and in assessing the impact of a proposed change to an existing process.

- *Treat the risks*: two common preconceptions that can stand in the way of an effective remedy include the 'perfection myth'–if we try hard enough we will not make any errors–and the 'punishment myth'–if we punish people when they make errors they will make fewer of them. In reality, at least 80% of errors may be attributed to poorly designed care systems and processes that fail to account for human fallibility. Unfortunately, the mere publication of a new clinical guideline rarely results in a sustained change in practice. For these reasons, the preferred approach to reducing risk is to use the principles of reliability engineering and process redesign that substitute clumsy, unreliable and dangerous processes or systems with standardized and sustainable processes that make errors more difficult to perform, make the 'right' thing to do the easiest thing to do and aid the detection and correction of errors if they do occur (e.g. replacement of vials of similar appearing drugs with well-labelled, prefilled syringes on a resuscitation trolley) [1].

At all times:

- *Monitor and review*: the improvement of patient safety is a continuous process and information concerning safety should be collated systematically and routinely and evaluated at scheduled intervals in order to detect changes in patient safety trends as early as possible. Additionally, the impact of any changes to processes to improve patient safety should be monitored and evaluated in order to determine the effectiveness of the changes in reducing errors and to identify any unintended consequences that necessitate further refinement.

- *Communicate and consult*: patient safety is a team activity that requires communication of the approach to improving safety and its high priority to all members of an ED's staff. An open and fair culture, rather than a blame culture, must be promoted in order to yield the benefits of reporting systems. Participation in wider hospital and regional or national reporting systems offers the opportunity to learn from the mistakes of others. Expert help should be sought in attempting to evaluate patient risks or design interventions to improve safety. In the event of an adverse event, being open and honest with patients and with other staff improves the prospect of learning and the prevention of further errors.

Conclusion

Patients seeking emergency care are at significant risk of harm, in part due to their clinical situation and in part due to the challenges of delivery of emergency care itself. Improving patient safety in the ED requires a systematic approach to risk identification, risk analysis and evaluation and the implementation of safer processes of care. Monitoring is an essential component of patient safety improvement. An open, communicative culture that promotes reporting and minimizes blame supports patient safety improvement.

References

[1] Botwinick L, Bisognano M, Haraden C. Leadership guide to patient safety. Cambridge, MA: Institute for Healthcare Improvement; 2006.

[2] Weissman J, Rothschild J, Bendavid E, et al. Hospital workload and adverse events. Med Care 2007;45:448–55.

[3] Feddock CA, Hoellein AR, Wilson JF, et al. Do pressure and fatigue influence resident job performance? Med Teach 2007;29:495–7.

[4] Croskerry P, Sinclair D. Emergency medicine: a practice prone to error? Can J Emerg Med 2001;3:271–6.

[5] Brown AF. Do we realize when we do not know? Recognizing uncertainty in clinical medicine. Emerg Med Australas 2005;17:413–5.

[6] Brixey JJ, Tang Z, Robinson DJ, et al. Interruptions in a level one trauma center: a case study. Int J Med Inform 2007;77:235–41.

[7] Bomba DT, Prakash R. A description of handover processes in an Australian public hospital. Aust Hlth Rev 2005;29:68–79.

[8] Sprivulis PC, Da Silva JA, Jacobs IG, et al. The association between hospital overcrowding and mortality among patients admitted via Western Australian emergency departments. Med J Aust 2006;184:208–12.

ENVIRONMENTAL EMERGENCIES

Edited by **Mark Little**

28.1 Heat-related illness

Ian Rogers

ESSENTIALS

1 Exercise-associated collapse is the most common heat- and exercise-related illness. It is due to an impaired compensation for the drop in blood pressure that occurs when muscle pumping ceases and venous return drops at the cessation of exercise. It responds rapidly to supine posture followed by rest and oral fluids.

2 Heatstroke is a true medical emergency, where rapid cooling using tepid spraying, fanning and ice packs is essential to minimize morbidity and mortality.

3 Water immersion may cool patients more rapidly but is not always practical in an emergency department setting. Its major role is in the pre-hospital setting.

4 Patients with drug-related hyperthermia die from the complications of the high temperature, not from direct drug toxicity. Early and aggressive treatment of hyperthermia before complications occur is vital.

Introduction

Heat-related disorders have a broad range of potential aetiologies and manifestations. In some, the primary disorder is a failure of thermal homoeostasis whereas, in others, the hyperthermia is secondary to other processes. The major heat-related illnesses to consider are exercise-associated collapse (EAC), heatstroke, neuroleptic malignant syndrome, serotonin toxicity and malignant hyperthermia. Although of different aetiologies, the latter four, all associated with significantly elevated core temperatures, share much common ground with regard to complications and treatment.

Epidemiology and pathophysiology

EAC is the most common heat-related illness presenting either to medical tents at sporting events or to emergency departments. EAC manifests at the end of a race when muscle pump enhanced venous return ceases and cardiac output drops. This leads to collapse, often with a brief loss of consciousness. Despite the claims of the advocates of fluid loading and sports drinks in exercise, the primary mechanism is a failure of prompt baroreceptor responses and not haemodynamically significant dehydration. Severe heat-related dehydration is rare.

The other, more serious, heat-related disorders are all associated with, or the potential for, significant hyperthermia which, if not treated promptly, results in similar pathophysiology at a cellular and organ system level. A core body temperature around or greater than 41.5°C results in progressive denaturing of a number of vital cellular proteins, failure of vital energy-producing processes and loss of cell membrane function. At a cellular level, the exact mechanisms leading to loss of cell membrane function and cell death in heat illness remain uncertain. At an organ system level, these changes may manifest as rhabdomyolysis, acute pulmonary oedema, disseminated intravascular coagulation, cardiovascular dysfunction, electrolyte disturbance, renal failure, liver failure and permanent neurological damage [1,2]. Any or all of these complications must be expected in severe heat illness.

The hallmark of heatstroke is failure of the hypothalamic thermostat, leading to hyperthermia and the associated additional pathophysiological features described above. Clinically, heatstroke can be divided into 'exertional heatstroke' due to exercise in a thermally stressful environment, and 'classic heatstroke', which occurs in patients with impaired thermostatic mechanisms. Common risk factors for heatstroke are listed in Table 28.1.1.

Certain drugs produce hyperthermia by mechanisms in addition to interference with thermostatic function. In severe serotonin toxicity and neuroleptic malignant syndrome,

915

Table 28.1.1 Heatstroke risk factors
Behavioural
Army recruits
Athletes
Exertion
Inappropriate clothing
Elderly
Inappropriate exposure
Babies left in cars
Manual workers
Pilgrims
Drugs
Anticholinergics
Diuretics
Phenothiazines
Salicylates
Stimulants/hallucinogens
Illness
Delirium tremens
Dystonias
Infections
Seizures

Table 28.1.2 Drugs causing severe serotonin toxicity
Antidepressants
Monoamine oxidase inhibitors (MAOIs)
Selective serotonin reuptake inhibitors (SSRIs)
Selective serotonin and noradrenaline reuptake inhibitors (SSNRIs)
St John's wort
Tricyclics
Analgesics
Pethidine
Tramadol
Recreational drugs
Amphetamines
Methylenedioxymethamphetamine (MDMA, 'ecstasy')

Table 28.1.3 Risk factors for neuroleptic malignant syndrome
Patient factors
Agitation
Dehydration
Male sex (male:female = 2:1)
Organic brain disease
Drug dosing factors
Depot neuroleptics
High initial neuroleptic dose
High-potency neuroleptic (e.g. haloperidol)
Rapid dosage increase
NB: Duration of drug exposure and toxic overdose are not related to risk of developing NMS.

increased motor activity and central resetting of the hypothalamic thermostat combine to produce hyperthermia. In the case of serotonin toxicity, these effects are a consequence of a relative excess of central nervous system serotonin whereas, in neuroleptic malignant syndrome, dopamine depletion or dopamine receptor blockade is responsible.

The elevation of central nervous system serotonin in serotonin toxicity is usually associated with combinations of serotoninergically active drugs, taken either therapeutically or in overdose. The incidence of serotonin toxicity when such combinations are taken is not known, but is low and there is much individual variation in susceptibility [3]. Less often the syndrome is precipitated by a single serotoninergic agent. Drugs associated with the serotonin syndrome are listed in Table 28.1.2. The most commonly implicated are combinations of serotinergically active drugs, such as selective serotonin reuptake inhibitors (SSRIs), lithium, pethidine, monoamine oxidase inhibitors (MAOIs) and amphetamines.

Neuroleptic malignant syndrome (NMS) is a rare idiosyncratic reaction to neuroleptic agents with an incidence of between 0.02% and 3.0%, depending on the diagnostic criteria used. It occurs in response to a single agent, usually at therapeutic dosage. In individuals, the occurrence may be dose related. Certain at-risk groups have been identified and are listed in Table 28.1.3.

Malignant hyperthermia is a genetically inherited disorder in which triggering agents cause a release of sarcoplasmic Ca^{2+} stores.

The resulting elevation of myoplasmic Ca^{2+} stimulates many intercellular processes, including glycolysis, muscle contraction and an uncoupling of oxidative phosphorylation. This leads to hyperthermia that, in contrast to neuroleptic malignant and serotonin syndromes, is purely peripheral in origin.

Prevention

Prevention of exertional heatstroke should focus on the education of at-risk groups. Dehydration is not as important aetiologically in heatstroke as once thought. Exertional heatstroke is most often reported in shorter, high intensity exercise where marked dehydration is unlikely. So, although adequate fluid intake is needed for prolonged exercise, it is not a key factor in heatstroke prevention. As high ambient temperatures and high humidity predispose to exertional heatstroke, exertion in these environments should be limited.

Clinical features

Exercise-associated collapse

The clinical presentation of EAC will be familiar to all emergency practitioners as it mirrors that of poor cerebral perfusion from any other cause. Patients complain of nausea, vomiting, malaise and dizziness. There may be a history of collapse and there is likely to be a tachycardia and (orthostatic) hypotension. The orthostatic hypotension may manifest at the end of physical exertion by collapse with brief loss of consciousness that is typical of EAC. In this syndrome, and in distinction to heatstroke, the core temperature will be less than 40°C and neurological function will rapidly return to normal once the patient is lying down.

Heatstroke

The classic clinical features of heatstroke are neurological dysfunction, core temperature above 41.5°C and hot, dry skin. However, relying on this classic triad to make the diagnosis will result in a number of cases being missed. Loss of consciousness is a constant feature of heatstroke [1] but, by the time of ED presentation, conscious state may be improving, although some neurological abnormality will persist. Temperature readings may be misleadingly low, due either to effective pre-hospital care or to measurements at inappropriate sites, such as the oral cavity or axilla. Profuse sweating is a much more common feature than previously thought [1]. Other clinical features may include tachycardia, hyperventilation, seizures, vomiting and hypotension.

Serotonin toxicity

Serotonin syndrome is characterized by CNS, autonomic and motor dysfunction (Table 28.1.4). It is a clinical diagnosis. It develops after a latent period, which is normally a few hours, but may be as long as several days. The spectrum of illness produced is broad. Most patients are only mildly affected and may escape clinical detection. Only the most serious develop hyperthermia (usually in the setting of muscular rigidity) severe enough to produce the complications of rhabdomyolysis, disseminated intravascular coagulation and renal failure. Most cases will resolve within 24–48h once the precipitating agents are withdrawn. Even in severe cases, the underlying biochemical abnormality rapidly improves, usually with the institution of muscular paralysis. The morbidity and mortality in

Table 28.1.4 Features of the serotonin toxicity

Central nervous system
Agitation
Anxiety
Confusion
Decreased level of consciousness
Seizures

Motor
Clonus
Hyperreflexia
Hypertonia
Incoordination
Myoclonus
Tremor

Autonomic
Diaphoresis
Diarrhoea
Hypertension
Hyperthermia
Tachycardia

these cases is caused by the complications that develop while the syndrome is active.

Neuroleptic malignant syndrome

This syndrome manifests in patients who have recently been started on neuroleptic treatment or in whom the dose of a neuroleptic agent has been increased. It has been associated with almost all antipsychotics (both first and second generation) and has also been reported in patients in whom a dopaminergic agent has been rapidly withdrawn (e.g. in parkinsonism). There is a latent period of many hours to several days. Characteristically, there are four classic signs: fever, rigidity, altered mental state and autonomic instability. In practice, it may be difficult to distinguish clinically from serotonin toxicity unless a good drug history is obtained. As in serotonin toxicity, the spectrum of illness is very broad, with only the more severe cases developing hyperthermia and its complications [5].

Malignant hyperthermia

This occurs when a triggering agent is given to a susceptible individual, usually in the context of an anaesthetic. Triggering agents identified include inhalational anaesthetic agents, such as halothane, isoflurane and enflurane, as well as succinylcholine and ketamine. The first signs are failure to achieve muscle relaxation following succinylcholine, tachypnoea and tachycardia. If not recognized and treated, acidosis, rhabdomyolysis and hyperthermia will ensue. In some cases, signs and symptoms may be delayed or even reappear after apparently successful treatment, so that malignant

hyperthermia may even present as a postoperative fever. Untreated, the mortality is as high as 70%, but this can be reduced tenfold by appropriate management.

Clinical investigations

Diagnosis of the hyperthermic disorders is based on the history, clinical picture and exclusion of alternative diagnoses. Investigations are thus directed towards excluding other possible causes of temperature elevation (e.g. infection, metabolic disorders) and evaluation of the specific complications of hyperthermia.

Patients with a presumed clinical diagnosis of EAC should still have serum electrolytes and creatine kinase measured to exclude exercise associated hyponatraemia and rhabdomyolysis, respectively. Should mental state not rapidly normalize with supine posture, then an urgent finger prick or serum glucose estimation is needed. Collapsed athletes should also have an ECG to identify unrecognized cardiac abnormalities.

All other heat disorders warrant a far more extensive laboratory and radiological work-up, as multiorgan system dysfunction is the rule [2,6]. Tests must include an ECG , serum electrolytes, disseminated intravascular coagulation (DIC) screen, liver function tests, muscle enzyme assays, renal function and urinalysis, serum glucose and a chest X-ray.

Treatment

Exercise-associated collapse

EAC responds rapidly to supine posture (ideally with the legs elevated), rest and oral fluids. Intravenous normal saline is rarely required as few athletes will be profoundly dehydrated. The use of 'routine' IV normal saline in collapsed athletes should be actively discouraged as it will worsen exercise associated hyponatraemia where there are persistent, inappropriate antidiuretic hormone levels.

Heatstroke

This is a true medical emergency. Early recognition and aggressive therapy in the field and in hospital can prevent substantial morbidity and mortality. The key management is aggressive cooling. Cooling rates of at least 0.1°C/min should be achievable. Several cooling methods have been proposed, including evaporative cooling, iced water immersion, ice slush, cool

water immersion, iced peritoneal lavage and pharmacological methods [7]. A combination of methods is most widely used in EDs. All of the patient's clothing should be removed and the patient sprayed with a fine mist of tepid water while gentle fanning is commenced (a ceiling fan is ideal). At the same time, areas with vascular beds close to the surface (neck, axillae and groins) should be packed with ice bags. This technique facilitates patient access and monitoring when compared to methods, such as ice-bath immersion even though an iced bath may offer more rapid cooling. Although ice-cold IV fluids can also aid in rapid cooling (as used in therapeutic hypothermia post-cardiac arrest), fluid requirements in heatstroke can be difficult to estimate and balance.

In hospital, shivering, seizures and muscle activity may need to be controlled with pharmacological agents, such as chlorpromazine, benzodiazepines and paralysing agents. Aspirin and paracetamol are ineffective and should be avoided. Intravenous fluids need to be used cautiously and may need titrating to central venous or pulmonary capillary wedge pressures. Maintain adequate oxygenation but avoid hyperoxia. Ventilatory support may be required. Urine flow needs to be maintained with initial volume loading, and later with mannitol or furosemide, to prevent secondary renal injury, especially from rhabdomyolysis. Electrolyte, acid–base and clotting disturbances should be closely monitored and treated by standard measures.

Serotonin toxicity

Treatment of the drug-related hyperthermia involves both specific pharmacological therapy and full supportive and cooling measures, as described above. The objective is to recognize and treat before serious complications occur. In mild cases of the serotonin syndrome, no treatment or small doses of benzodiazepines may be all that is required while awaiting spontaneous resolution. In severe cases, neuromuscular paralysis should be considered early, especially in cases of markedly altered mental state. The duration of treatment used is partly judged on the half-life of the presumed causative agents [4]. Specific antiserotoninergic drugs that can be used include chlorpromazine (12.5–50 mg IM/IV) and cyproheptadine (4–8 mg orally 8-hourly).

Neuroleptic malignant syndrome

Again, early recognition and full supportive care, combined with specific therapy, is the mainstay of treatment. Dopamine agonists, such as bromocriptine, may reduce the duration of the syndrome. It can be administered orally or by nasogastric tube at an initial dose of 2.5–10 mg tds.

Malignant hyperthermia

Dantrolene acts by inhibiting the release of calcium from the sarcoplasmic reticulum and is the specific agent used in the treatment of malignant hyperthermia. It should be given in addition to full supportive care and discontinuing the triggering agents. The dose is 2.5 mg/kg IV initially, repeated every 15 min up to a maximum of 30 mg/kg if needed.

Prognosis and disposition

In heatstroke, both the maximum core temperature and the duration of temperature elevation are predictors of outcome. Prolonged coma and oliguric renal failure are poor prognostic signs [1]. Mortality is still of the order of 10%, but most survivors will not suffer long-term sequelae [1,2]. Any patient with suspected heatstroke should routinely be referred to the intensive care unit for ongoing care. Most cases of EAC will be suitable for short-stay ED treatment or, indeed, simply for treatment on-site in an event medical tent.

Prognosis in the drug-related group of hyperthermia is dependent largely on the degree to which the complications have progressed before definitive and aggressive treatment is begun. Again, early referral to intensive care is indicated. Even with appropriate treatment, mortality for malignant hyperthermia approaches 7%. After recovery, the patient's medication regimen will need to be reassessed although, in the case of neuroleptic malignant syndrome, it may be possible slowly to reintroduce a neuroleptic agent at a lower dose. With malignant hyperthermia, future anaesthesia will need to be modified to avoid precipitating agents. In addition, family members should be tested for susceptibility.

Controversies

- Although debate is likely to continue about the most effective cooling therapy in heatstroke, this is largely of academic interest as all methods seem to achieve the desired outcome of rapid temperature drop. Of more interest will be research that focuses on the cellular mechanisms of the damage seen with hyperthermia. Such research may lead to the development of pharmacological agents that can prevent or treat heatstroke.

- There are still no prospective trials comparing the various antiserotoninergic drugs available for the treatment of serotonin toxicity, so treatment is still based on case reports and clinical experience.

- The long-standing dogma that vigorous hydration prevents heat illness is now challenged. A greater concern now is to highlight the risks of promotion of aggressive hydration strategies in sport.

References

[1] Shapiro Y, Seidman DS. Field and clinical observations of exertional heat stroke patients. Med Sci Sports Exer 1990;22:6–14.
[2] Sithinamsuwan P, Piyavechviratana K, Kittiaweesin T, et al. Exertional heatstroke: early recognition and outcome with aggressive combined cooling–a 12 year experience. Milit Med 2009;174:496–502.
[3] Isbister GK, Buckley NA, Whyte IM. Serotonin toxicity: a practical approach to diagnosis and treatment. Med J Aust 2007;187:361–5.
[4] Toxicology and Wilderness Expert Group. Serotonin toxicity. In: Therapeutic guidelines: toxicology and wilderness, Version 2. Melbourne: Therapeutic Guidelines Limited; 2012.
[5] Bristow MF, Kohen D. How malignant is the neuroleptic malignant syndrome? Br Med J 1993;307:1223–4.
[6] Dematte JE, O'Mara K, Buescher J, et al. Near fatal heat stroke during the 1995 heat wave in Chicago. Ann Intern Med 1998;130:173–81.
[7] Smith JE. Cooling methods used in the treatment of exertional heat illness. Brit J Sports Med 2005;39:503–7.

Further reading

Brearley M, Norton I, Trewin T, Mitchel C. Fire fighter cooling in tropical field conditions. National Critical Care and Trauma Response Centre 2011. <http://www.nationaltraumacentre.nt.gov.au/sites/default/files/publications/Fire%20Fighters%20Report%20Final.pdf> [Accessed Dec. 2012].
This study showed temperate water immersion (25°C paddling pool) was more effective at lowering core body temperature than shade, crushed ice or use of misting fans in the resting cycles of firefighters.

28.2 Hypothermia

Ian Rogers

ESSENTIALS

1 Hypothermia is categorized into mild (32–35°C), moderate (29–32°C) and severe (<29°C) on the basis of a rectal or other core temperature reading.

2 Moderate-to-severe hypothermia produces progressive delirium and coma, hypotension, bradycardia and failure of thermogenesis.

3 The electrocardiograph will often show slow atrial fibrillation and an extra positive deflection in the QRS (the J or Osborn wave) in leads II and V3–V6 with worsening hypothermia.

4 Endotracheal intubation is safe in hypothermia. Ventilation and acid–base status should be manipulated to maintain uncorrected blood gases within the normal range.

5 Endogenous rewarming should form part of all rewarming protocols. In most cases of moderate-to-severe hypothermia, rewarming can be achieved with forced-air rewarming blankets without the need to resort to more aggressive techniques.

6 In the arrested hypothermic patient, rewarming should be with cardiopulmonary bypass or warm left pleural lavage.

Table 28.2.1 Hypothermia aetiologies	
Environmental	Cold, wet, windy ambient conditions Cold water immersion Exhaustion
Trauma	Multitrauma (entrapment, resuscitation, head injury) Minor trauma and immobility (e.g. #NOF, #NOH) Major burns
Drugs	Ethanol Sedatives (e.g. benzodiazepines) in overdose Phenothiazines (impaired shivering)
Neurological	CVA Paraplegia Parkinson's disease
Endocrine	Hypoglycaemia Hypothyroidism Hypoadrenalism
Systemic illness	Sepsis Malnutrition

Introduction

Hypothermia is defined as a core temperature of less than 35°C. This can be measured at a number of sites (including oesophageal, right heart, tympanic and bladder). Rectal remains the routine in most emergency departments (EDs), despite concerns at how rapidly it equilibrates to and reflects true core temperature. Conventionally, hypothermia is divided into three groups: mild (32–35°C), moderate (29–32°C) and severe (<29°C) on the basis of measured core temperature. In a field setting, where core temperature measurements may not be possible, moderate and severe are often grouped together as they typically share the clinical features of absence of shivering and altered mental state. These categorization systems can be used both out of and in hospital as a guide to selecting rewarming therapies and prognosis. Mild hypothermia is considered the stage where thermogenesis is still possible; moderate is characterized by a progressive failure of thermogenesis; and severe by adoption of the temperature of the surrounding environment (poikilothermia) and an increasing risk of malignant cardiac arrhythmia. Nevertheless, there are substantial differences between individuals in their response to hypothermia.

Epidemiology and pathophysiology

Hypothermia may occur in any setting or season [1]. True environmental hypothermia occurring in a healthy patient in an adverse physical environment is less common in clinical practice than that secondary to an underlying disorder. Common precipitants include injury, systemic illness, drug overdose and immersion and are outlined in more detail in Table 28.2.1. The elderly are at greater risk of hypothermia because of reduced metabolic heat production and impaired responses to a cold environment. Alcohol is a common aetiological factor and probably acts by a number of mechanisms, including cutaneous vasodilatation, altered behavioural responses, impaired shivering and hypothalamic dysfunction. Hypothermia in the ED setting is often associated with underlying infection [2].

Clinical features

Despite substantial individual variations, it is still possible to describe the typical patient in each category of hypothermia. The clinical manifestations of hypothermia also depend on the features of the underlying aetiology.

Mild hypothermia manifests clinically as shivering, apathy, ataxia, dysarthria and tachycardia. Moderate hypothermia is typically marked by a loss of shivering, altered mental state, muscular rigidity, bradycardia and hypotension. In severe hypothermia, signs of life may become almost undetectable, with coma, fixed and dilated pupils, areflexia and profound bradycardia and hypotension. The typical cardiac rhythm of severe hypothermia is slow atrial fibrillation. This may degenerate spontaneously, or with rough handling, into ventricular fibrillation or asystole. In the field, moderate and severe hypothermia are often grouped together, with the key clinical feature of absent shivering suggesting the loss of the ability to rewarm without medical intervention.

Many complications may also manifest as part of a hypothermia presentation, although at times it may be difficult to separate cause from effect. These include cardiac arrhythmias, thromboembolism, rhabdomyolysis, renal failure, disseminated intravascular coagulation and pancreatitis.

Clinical investigations

Mild hypothermia with shivering and without apparent underlying illness needs no investigation in the ED.

Moderate or severe hypothermia mandates a comprehensive work-up to seek common precipitants and complications that may not be clinically apparent.

Biochemical and haematological abnormalities are frequently associated with hypothermia [1], although there is no consistent pattern. Blood tests that are indicated include sodium, potassium, glucose, renal function, calcium, phosphate, magnesium, amylase, creatine kinase, ethanol, full blood count and clotting profile. Arterial blood gases, if taken, should be accepted at face value, rather than adjusting for the patient's temperature.

Impaired ciliary function, stasis of respiratory secretions or aspiration may be expected in moderate-to-severe hypothermia, so chest radiography should be routine. Other radiology may be indicated if a trauma-related aetiology is suspected.

A 12-lead electrocardiograph and continuous ECG monitoring should be routine in moderate-to-severe hypothermia. The typical appearance is slow atrial fibrillation, with J or Osborn waves most prominent in leads II and V3–V6 (Fig. 28.2.1). The J wave is the extra positive deflection after the normal S wave and is more obvious and more commonly seen with increasing severity of hypothermia.

Treatment

General

The general and supportive management of hypothermia victims largely follows that of other critically ill patients. However, some syndrome-specific issues demand careful attention.

Muscle glycogen is the substrate preferentially used by the body to generate heat by shivering. All hypothermics, therefore, need glucose. In mild cases, this can be given orally as sweetened drinks or easily palatable food. With more severe hypothermia, gastric stasis and ileus are common and glucose should be given intravenously: 5% dextrose can be infused at 200 mL/h. Additional volume resuscitation with normal saline or colloid should be gentle, bearing in mind the contracted intravascular space in severe hypothermia and that hypotension that would be classified as severe at a core temperature of 37°C is a normal physiological state at 27°C. All intravenous fluids should be warmed to minimize ongoing cooling. Endotracheal intubation by a skilled operator is safe in severe hypothermia. Intubation is indicated as in any other clinical condition to provide airway protection or to assist in ventilation.

Ventilatory support and, where necessary, manipulation of acid–base status, should be titrated to maintain uncorrected blood gas pH and PCO_2 within the normal range.

The slow atrial fibrillation so common in more severe hypothermia is a benign rhythm and requires no chemical or electrical correction. It will revert spontaneously with rewarming. Pulseless ventricular tachycardia and ventricular fibrillation should largely be managed along conventional lines. However, if initial DC shocks are unsuccessful, then others are unlikely to be so until the patient is warmer. Repeat countershocks are generally reapplied with every 1°C increase in core temperature. Magnesium may be the antiarrhythmic drug of choice in hypothermia.

The pharmacokinetics and dynamics of most drugs are substantially altered at low body core temperatures. Indeed, for many of the common drugs used in an ED they are unknown. Insulin is known to be inactive at <30°C. Hyperglycaemia, due in part to loss of insulin activity, is common in hypothermia, but should probably be managed expectantly until sufficient rewarming has occurred to ensure full endogenous insulin activity.

Rewarming therapies

Strategies for rewarming in hypothermia have only a limited evidence base on which to base recommendations. Although more invasive and rapid techniques are advocated for more severe hypothermia, there is little evidence to support this advice. The traditional concern of afterdrop (a paradoxical initial drop in core temperature with rewarming) is probably of little or no relevance in a clinical setting [3].

Rewarming therapies are broadly divided into three groups: endogenous rewarming,

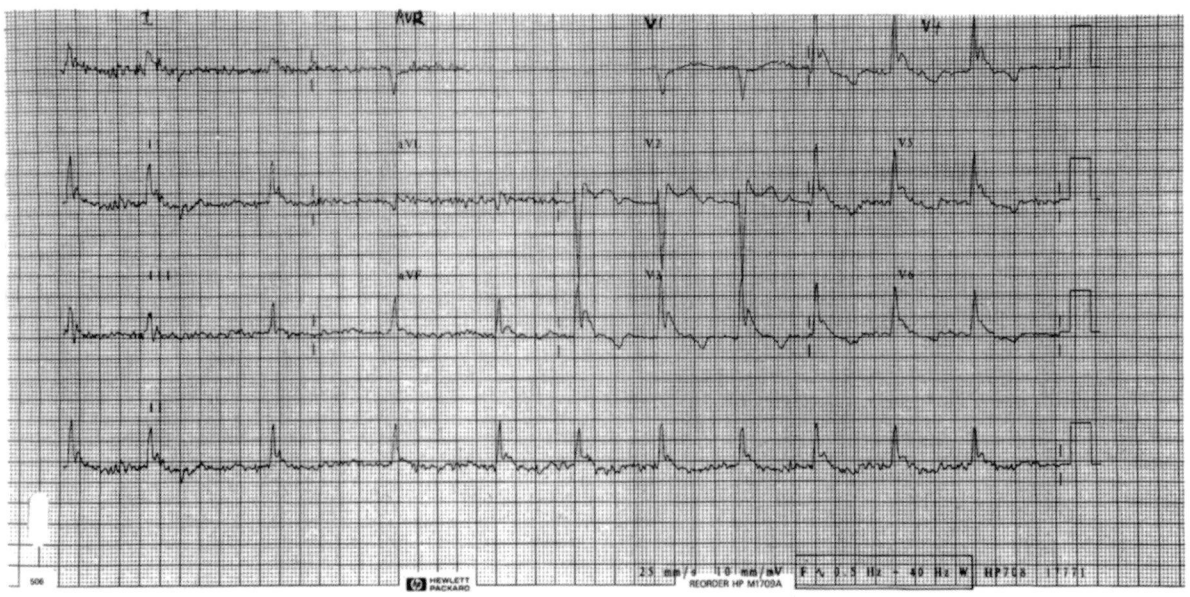

Fig. 28.2.1 ECG in hypothermia: slow atrial fibrillation and J waves in leads II, V3–V6 in a patient with a core temperature of 23.9°C.

ENVIRONMENTAL EMERGENCIES

Table 28.2.2	Rewarming therapy classification
Endogenous rewarming	Warm, dry, wind-free environment Warmed intravenous fluids (to prevent cooling)
External exogenous rewarming	Hot bath immersion Forced-air blankets Heat packs Body-to-body contact
Core exogenous rewarming	Warmed, humidified inhalation Left pleural cavity lavage Extracorporeal circulation

which is allowing the body to rewarm by its own endogenous heat production; external exogenous rewarming, which is supplying heat to the outside of the body; and core exogenous rewarming, which is applying the heat centrally. The classification of the commonly utilized rewarming therapies is outlined in Table 28.2.2.

Endogenous rewarming is a mandatory component of any emergency rewarming protocol. It consists of drying the patient, covering them with blankets, placing them in a warm and wind-free environment and warming any intravenous or oral fluids that are administered. Endogenous rewarming alone can be expected to rewarm at a rate of about 0.75°C/h. For most patients above 32°C (the level at which shivering thermogenesis is typically preserved), endogenous rewarming is the only therapy required. The exception is the exhausted patient in whom shivering has ceased at a core temperature higher than expected. Although more sophisticated techniques, such as bath immersion, will more rapidly rewarm a mildly hypothermic patient, there is no evidence that an increased rewarming rate improves prognosis in this group.

In moderate hypothermia, endogenous heat production is likely to fail progressively and more aggressive exogenous rewarming therapies are indicated. Hot-bath immersion has the theoretical disadvantage of causing peripheral vasodilatation, with shunting of cool blood to the core and convective heat loss. This might be expected to increase core afterdrop and produce circulatory collapse. In fact, rewarming rates of at least 2.5°C/h with minimal afterdrop have been achieved using baths

at 43°C [4]. Nevertheless, substantial practical difficulties are obvious with monitoring a more seriously ill patient immersed in a bath. This method of rewarming can only be recommended for otherwise healthy patients who are expected to make a rapid recovery from accidental environmental hypothermia (e.g. immersion in very cold water).

The two therapies that have been best studied and are widely used in moderate hypothermia are forced-air rewarming and warm humidified inhalation [5]. Forced-air rewarming is achieved by covering the patient with a blanket filled with air at 43°C. These devices direct a continuous current of air over the patient's skin through a series of slits in the patient surface of the blanket. This method produces minimal, if any, afterdrop is apparently without complication and, combined with warm humidified inhalation, should produce rewarming at about 2.5°C/h. The value of warm humidified inhalation is probably by preventing ongoing respiratory heat loss. Given its widespread availability and lack of complications, it seems reasonable to combine it with forced-air rewarming in moderate hypothermia [6]. Body-to-body contact and chemical heat packs are often recommended as field treatments for all degrees of hypothermia. In mild hypothermia, it seems that the benefit of any heat they deliver is negated by an inhibition of shivering thermogenesis. In more severe cases, where shivering is absent, it may be that even the small amount of exogenous heat they deliver is beneficial, but this remains unproven.

In severe hypothermia, more aggressive exogenous rewarming therapies may be indicated in order rapidly to achieve core temperature above 30°C, the threshold below which malignant cardiac arrhythmias may occur spontaneously. Bladder, gastric or peritoneal lavage with warm fluids are all relatively ineffective methods of heat transfer and, as such, are not recommended for use in emergency situations. When available, full cardiopulmonary bypass achieves rewarming rates of about 7.5°C/h without core afterdrop. Pleural lavage using large volumes of fluid warmed to 40–45°C through an intercostal catheter may be nearly as effective. Both techniques have the advantage of delivering heat to the heart which acts as a heat pump to distribute rewarming to key core organs, but are clearly invasive and carry associated risks. These risks are certainly acceptable in a hypothermic arrest but, in the non-arrested patient, a slower rate of

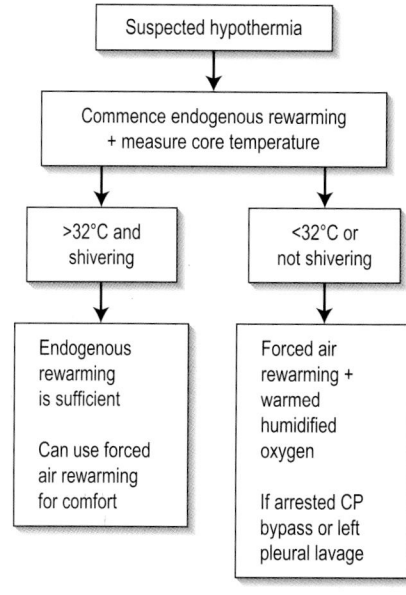

Fig. 28.2.2 A recommended rewarming algorithm in hypothermia.

rewarming using forced-air and warm humidified inhalation may be more appropriate.

A suggested rewarming algorithm based on the evidence available to date is shown in Figure 28.2.2.

Prognosis and disposition

Attempts at developing a valid outcome prediction model for hypothermia are likely to be frustrated by its multifactorial aetiology. Recovery with appropriate treatment is likely from accidental environmental hypothermia when there is no associated trauma. To date, the coldest patient to survive accidental hypothermia neurologically intact had an initial measured temperature of 13.7°C [7]. Although increasing severity of hypothermia does worsen prognosis, the major determinant of outcome is the precipitating illness or injury. Reported mortality rates vary from 0 to 85%.

Mild hypothermics without associated illness or injury can be safely managed at home in the care of a responsible adult. Moderate hypothermia may be treatable in a short-stay observation ward, but often requires a longer inpatient stay to manage underlying illness or injury. Severe hypothermics are at risk of multiorgan system complications and should be considered for admission to an intensive care unit.

Controversies

- The question of which rewarming therapy to use will only be answered when the focus moves to randomized clinical trials measuring clinically relevant outcomes, such as morbidity and mortality, rather than surrogate markers such as rewarming rate and core afterdrop.
- Future research may confirm the expanding clinical use of induced mild hypothermia for more conditions other than that already shown post-cardiac arrest [8–10].

References

[1] Danzl DF, Pozos RS, Auerbach PS, et al. Multicentre hypothermia survey. Ann Emerg Med 1987;16: 1042–55.
[2] Delaney KA, Vasallo SU, Larkin GL, Goldfrank LR. Rewarming rates in urban patients with hypothermia: prediction of underlying infection. Acad Emerg Med 2006;13:913–21.
[3] Rogers IR. Which rewarming therapy in hypothermia? A review of the randomised trials. Emerg Med Australas 1997;9:213–20.
[4] Hoskin RW, Melinshyn MG, Romet TT, Goode RC. Bath rewarming from immersion hypothermia. J Appl Physiol 1986;61:1518–22.
[5] Steele MT, Nelson MJ, Sessler DI, et al. Forced air speeds rewarming in accidental hypothermia. Ann Emerg Med 1996;27:479–84.
[6] Giesbrecht GG. Emergency treatment of hypothermia. Emerg Med Australas 2001;13:9–16.
[7] Gilbert M, Busund R, Skogseth A, et al. Resuscitation from accidental hypothermia of 13°C with circulatory arrest. Lancet 2000;355:375–6.
[8] Alzaga AG, Cerdan M, Varon J. Therapeutic hypothermia. Resuscitation 2006;70:369–80.
[9] Bernard SA, Gray TW, Buist M, et al. Treatment of comatose survivors of out-of-hospital cardiac arrest with induced hypothermia. N Engl J Med 2002;346: 557–63.
[10] The hypothermia after cardiac arrest study group. Mild therapeutic hypothermia to improve neurologic outcome after cardiac arrest. N Engl J Med 2002;346: 549–555.

28.3 Dysbarism

David R Smart

ESSENTIALS

1 Dysbarism is the term given to medical complications of exposure to gases at higher than normal atmospheric pressure. It includes barotrauma and decompression illness.

2 An understanding of the pathophysiology of dysbarism requires an understanding of the gas laws.

3 Barotrauma occurs as a consequence of excessive expansion or contraction of gas within enclosed body cavities. It principally affects the middle ear, the sinuses and the lungs. Lung barotrauma may result in pneumomediastinum, pneumothorax or gas embolism. Inner-ear barotrauma is rare but serious and may mimic vestibular decompression illness.

4 Decompression illness occurs when gas bubbles develop within the body. This may occur as a complication of pulmonary barotrauma or when a diver whose tissues are supersaturated with nitrogen ascends too rapidly.

5 The clinical manifestations of decompression illness may affect many body systems and are extremely variable in nature and severity. Loss of consciousness or neurological symptoms and signs (including cognitive dysfunction) indicate serious decompression illness.

6 If a diver becomes unwell during or after diving, then diving is the likely cause of the illness, until proven otherwise. Early consultation with a diving medicine specialist is mandatory, especially where retrieval to a recompression facility may be necessary.

7 The seriously injured diver should be managed lying flat and urgently referred for recompression treatment. The diver should not exceed 300 m altitude during retrieval for recompression treatment.

8 Non-diving causes of dysbarism include caisson work, altitude decompression, recreational use of compressed gases (nitrous oxide and helium) causing pulmonary barotrauma and gas embolism and medical adverse events where gas enters the circulation. These cases are likely to benefit from early recompression with hyperbaric oxygen.

Introduction

This chapter focuses on medical problems that develop secondary to breathing gases at higher than normal atmospheric pressure (dysbarism). This usually occurs in the context of scuba (self-contained underwater breathing apparatus) diving, a popular recreational activity in Australasia. Diving is generally very safe and serious decompression incidents occur approximately 1:10 000 dives. However, because of a high participation rate, between 200 and 300 cases of decompression illness are treated in Australia each year. It is estimated that 10 times that number of divers experience less serious health problems after diving. Emergency physicians are often the first medical staff to assess the diver after a diving accident and it is essential they understand the risks and potential injuries.

Diving physics and physiology

An understanding of pressure and some gas laws is essential to understand the pathophysiology of diving injuries. The air pressure at sea level is 1 atmosphere absolute (ATA). Multiple units are used to measure pressure (Table 28.3.1). For every 10 m a diver descends in sea-water, the pressure increases by 1 ATA. This pressure change impacts on gas spaces within the body according to Boyle's law.

Table 28.3.1 Atmospheric pressure at sea level in various units

1 Atmosphere absolute (ATA)
101.3 kPa (SI units)
1.013 Bar
10 m of sea water (MSW)
760 mm of mercury (mmHg)
14.7 pounds per square inch (PSI)

Table 28.3.2 Depth vs pressure and gas volume (Boyle's law)

Depth (m)	Absolute pressure (ATA)	Gas volume (%)
0	1	100
10	2	50
20	3	33
30	4	25
40	5	20

Boyle's law states that, at a constant temperature, the volume of a gas varies inversely to the pressure acting on it:

$$PV = k$$

where P = pressure, V = volume and k = constant.

The proportionate change in volume is greatest near the surface (Table 28.3.2).

Dalton's law states that the total pressure (P_t) exerted by a mixture of gases is equal to the sum of the pressures of the constituent gases (P_x, P_y, P_z):

$$P_t = P_x + P_y + P_z$$

Therefore, as divers breathe air at increasing atmospheric pressure, the partial pressures of nitrogen and oxygen increase:

Surface = 1 ATA
      = 0.8 ATA N_2 + 0.2 ATA O_2
10 m = 2 ATA
      = 1.6 ATA N_2 + 0.4 ATA O_2
40 m = 5 ATA
      = 4.0 ATA N_2 + 1.0 ATA O_2

A diver breathing air at 40 m is inhaling a gas with a partial pressure of oxygen equivalent to breathing 100% oxygen at the surface. At partial pressures above 3 ATA, the PN_2 affects coordination and judgement ('nitrogen narcosis'). Oxygen may also become toxic at partial pressures greater than 1 ATA. Recreational scuba diving generally has a limit of 40 m because of these effects.

Henry's law states that at a constant temperature the amount of a gas that will dissolve in a liquid is proportional to the partial pressure of the gas in contact with the liquid:

$$Q = kP_{gas}$$

where Q = volume of gas dissolved in a liquid, k = constant and P_{gas} = partial pressure of the gas.

Henry's law is relevant in diving illness because it is the basis of decompression illness (DCI). As the ambient pressure increases, the diver is exposed to increasing partial pressures of nitrogen, which dissolves in bodily fluids. The amount of nitrogen absorbed depends on both the depth (which determines the partial pressure of nitrogen) and the duration of the dive. Tissues also take up nitrogen at different rates depending on their blood supply and permeability. Eventually, the tissues become saturated with nitrogen and no further absorption occurs. As the diver ascends and ambient pressure decreases, the partial pressure of nitrogen in some tissues will exceed ambient pressure, resulting in tissue supersaturation. If the diver ascends slowly enough, nitrogen diffuses out of the tissues and is transported, safely dissolved in the blood, to the lungs for elimination. This is known as 'off-gassing'.

If the diver ascends too rapidly, sufficient nitrogen bubbles will form in their body to cause decompression illness. Oxygen does not cause problems because it is rapidly metabolized by the tissues.

Barotrauma

Barotrauma occurs when changes in ambient pressure lead to expansion or contraction of gas within enclosed body cavities. The change in gas volume distorts or tears adjacent tissue. Injury by this mechanism may occur to the middle ear, inner ear, sinuses, lungs, eyes (via the diver's mask) and, rarely, the gut. Different injury patterns occur in breath-hold divers (snorkellers) compared to those breathing compressed air. Both breath-hold and scuba divers may experience injury of the middle and inner ear, sinuses and eyes if they do not equalize pressures in the gas spaces as they descend. Breath-hold divers are unlikely to injure their lungs as their lung volumes reduce as they descend and return to their original volume as they ascend to the surface by the increasing ambient pressure.

Middle-ear barotrauma

Pathophysiology
Middle-ear barotrauma (MEBT), the most common medical disorder of diving, usually occurs during descent. Increased ambient pressure results in a reduction of middle-ear volume. If equalization of the volume via the eustachian tube is inadequate, a series of pathological changes results. The tympanic membrane (TM) is deformed inwards, causing inflammation and haemorrhage. Middle-ear mucosal oedema is followed by vascular engorgement, effusion, haemorrhage and, rarely, TM rupture.

Clinical features
Symptoms of middle-ear barotraumas include ear pain, tinnitus and conductive hearing loss. Mild vertigo may also be experienced. More severe vertigo and pain occur if water passes through a perforated TM. Severe vertigo and significant sensorineural hearing loss should alert the emergency physician to possible inner-ear barotrauma (IEBT) (see below). MEBT severity is graded by visual inspection of the TM (Table 28.3.3). An audiogram is useful to document any hearing loss.

Treatment
Treatment of MEBT consists of analgesia, decongestants and ear, nose and throat (ENT) referral if there is TM perforation or suspected IEBT. Antibiotics are indicated for TM

Table 28.3.3 Grading of severity of middle-ear barotrauma

Grade 0	Symptoms without signs
Grade 1	Injection of TM along handle of malleus
Grade 2	Slight haemorrhage within the TM
Grade 3	Gross haemorrhage within the TM
Grade 4	Free blood in middle ear
Grade 5	Perforation of TM

TM: tympanic membrane.

rupture because of potential contamination with water. The patient should not dive again until symptoms and signs have resolved, any TM perforation has healed, and the eustachian tube is patent.

Inner-ear barotrauma

Pathophysiology
Sudden pressure changes between the middle and inner ears can cause rupture of the round or oval windows or a tear of Reissner's membrane. This usually occurs during rapid descent without equalizing or forceful Valsalva manoeuvres.

Clinical features
Symptoms include sudden onset of tinnitus, vertigo, nausea and vomiting, vestibular symptoms and profound sensorineural hearing loss, which may not be apparent until the diver has left the water. Onset of symptoms after the dive while performing an activity that increases intracranial pressure (e.g. heavy lifting) suggests IEBT. Coexistent middle-ear barotrauma is absent in about one-third of cases.

The main differential diagnosis is DCI involving the inner ear or vestibular apparatus. Inner-ear DCI usually occurs on deep dives using helium and oxygen mixtures (heliox) and is typically accompanied by other symptoms or signs of DCI. Frequently it is difficult to distinguish between IEBT and vestibular DCI. Isolated inner-ear DCI has been reported in sports divers breathing air.

Treatment
Treatment of IEBT consists of avoidance of activities that increase intracranial pressure and urgent (same day) ENT referral for more detailed assessment and audiometry. Surgical repair may be undertaken when vertiginous symptoms are severe. Vomiting should be treated with antiemetics and the diver kept supine with their head on a pillow. If DCI is excluded, then a 45° semirecumbent position is preferred. If DCI cannot be excluded the diver should have a trial of recompression. In one series, exposure to pressure did not worsen the diver's condition. The benefit of steroids in IEBT has not been confirmed.

It was thought that further diving was contraindicated after IEBT, but recent case data suggest that diving might be possible following full recovery of hearing.

External ear barotrauma

Ear-canal barotrauma is very rare and only occurs if there is a complete obstruction of the canal (usually by wax or ear plugs), creating a non-communicating gas cavity between the obstruction and the TM. Treatment is symptomatic. ENT specialist referral may be necessary if the TM cannot be visualized.

Sinus barotrauma

Pathophysiology
Mucosal swelling and haemorrhage occur if the communication of the sinuses with the nasopharynx is blocked and equalization of sinus pressure is not possible during descent. The frontal sinuses are most commonly involved.

Clinical features
Sinus pain usually develops during descent. Maxillary sinus involvement can refer pain to the upper teeth or cheek. There may be resolution of the pain at depth, due to mucosal oedema and blood filling the volume deficit left by gas compression. Pain and epistaxis may occur as the diver ascends. The pain usually persists after diving. Tenderness will be noted over the affected sinus. In doubtful cases, a sinus CT (computed tomography) scan will assist the diagnosis.

Treatment
Treatment includes analgesia, decongestants and recommendations to avoid diving until asymptomatic. Antibiotics may be required if secondary infection occurs.

Mask squeeze

If divers fail to exhale air into their masks on descent, the reduced volume inside the mask can cause pain, petechiae and conjunctival haemorrhage. In assessing these divers, it is important to confirm that they have normal visual acuity and fundi are normal. Treatment is with analgesia alone.

Gastrointestinal barotrauma

Expansion of gas within the gastrointestinal tract on ascent can occasionally cause colicky abdominal pain. Rupture of the stomach is rare but has occurred where panic or equipment failure has led to air swallowing and rapid ascent. Presentation is with abdominal pain and distension. Shoulder pain may be due to diaphragmatic irritation or coexisting DCI.

Sub-diaphragmatic free air may be visible on an erect chest X-ray. The differential diagnosis includes pulmonary barotrauma, because air can enter the peritoneum via the mediastinum and oesophageal or aortic openings in the diaphragm. The diagnosis is confirmed with endoscopy and surgical repair is necessary.

Dental barotrauma

Severe tooth pain may occur with descent or ascent if air is trapped under a decaying tooth or recent filling. Percussion of the involved tooth is painful. Treatment is with analgesia and dental repair.

Pulmonary barotrauma

Pathophysiology
Breathing compressed air at depth, the diver's lungs contain greater amounts of gas than they would on the surface. Divers are trained to breathe continuously during ascent or to exhale continuously if they have lost their air supply. Pulmonary barotrauma results when a diver ascends without exhaling adequately and the expanding gas in the lungs exceeds the lung's elasticity, tearing alveoli. This occurs most commonly when a diver runs out of air, panics and ascends too rapidly. The change in pressure over 1 m near the surface is sufficient to cause lung barotrauma. It has been reported in student divers training in swimming pools and in helicopter escape training. It can also occur with a normal ascent if there is a localized area of lung that does not empty properly, as is possible in divers with asthma, reduced pulmonary compliance or air trapping.

The resultant clinical syndromes depend on the sites at which the air escapes and include arterial gas embolism (AGE), pneumomediastinum and pneumothorax.

Clinical features
Onset of symptoms is usually rapid. If pneumomediastinum or pneumothorax is detected after diving, it is essential to look for features consistent with associated gas embolism. These include impairment or loss of consciousness, cognition impairment including loss of memory, or neurological abnormalities. Sometimes the abnormalities are subtle and tests of cognition and memory should be performed in addition to a detailed history and thorough examination.

Treatment
If AGE is suspected, then the affected individual should be kept supine and urgent

recompression treatment is required. Management of AGE is discussed under the heading of decompression illness. Lung barotrauma is regarded as the cause of AGE, however, in early studies, only about 5% of divers with AGE had radiographic evidence of a pneumothorax on plain chest X-ray. Subtle signs of extra-alveolar air suggesting pulmonary barotrauma are present in nearly half with more sophisticated imaging, such as CT.

The reverse also applies. If divers present with a pneumomediastinum or pneumothorax, then they may have up to 50% chance of AGE. The signs of AGE in these circumstances may be subtle with only a brief period of loss of memory or dizziness.

Pneumomediastinum and subcutaneous emphysema can usually be managed conservatively. If symptoms are severe, 100% oxygen can accelerate resolution of the trapped gas. If recompression is required for coexistent AGE, then the pneumomediastinum does not require any specific additional management unless a pneumothorax is present.

Isolated pneumothorax resulting from pulmonary barotrauma is very uncommon. Pneumothorax from pulmonary barotrauma should be managed in the same way as non-diving-related causes and recompression is not necessary. If recompression is required for coexisting AGE, a chest tube with a Heimlich valve should be placed before commencing treatment, because the size of any remaining pneumothorax will increase markedly on depressurization.

Once the acute management of pneumomediastinum and pneumothorax has occurred, the divers should be referred to a diving medical specialist for long-term follow up, because the conditions will impact upon their future diving fitness.

Decompression illness

Classification and criteria for diagnosis

Diving accidents involving bubbles were traditionally divided into *decompression sickness* (DCS; due to nitrogen bubbles coming out of tissue) and *arterial gas embolism* (AGE; due to pulmonary barotrauma releasing air into the circulation). DCS is then classified as type I or II. Type I DCS involves the joints or skin only; type II involves all other pain, neurological injury, vestibular and pulmonary symptoms.

In the 1990s, the term 'decompression illness' (DCI) was proposed to include both DCS and AGE, for the following reasons:

- It can be difficult to distinguish clinically between cerebral arterial gas embolism (CAGE) and neurological DCS
- AGE can be caused by arterialization of venous bubbles released from tissues
- Pre-hospital and emergency management prior to recompression is identical
- The division of DCS into type I and type II is inadequate for research purposes and divers classified as type I have been found to have subtle subclinical neurological manifestations
- Symptomatic classification is adequate to guide management.

The current classification system describes DCI in terms of four components:

❶ onset (acute/chronic)
❷ evolution of symptoms (spontaneously resolving/static/progressive/relapsing)
❸ body system affected (musculoskeletal/ cutaneous/lymphatic/neurological/ vestibular/cardiorespiratory)
❹ presence/absence of barotrauma.

For example, a diver may be classified as having acute progressive neurological DCI with no evidence of barotrauma. The classification has been generally adopted in Australia and New Zealand, but not in North America. DCI is a satisfactory term from a management perspective but, from a scientific perspective, it does not describe differing aetiologies and pathophysiology.

Pathophysiology

DCI occurs if excessive nitrogen comes out of solution to form bubbles which gain access to the venous and lymphatic systems or if bubbles form within tissues themselves. The formation of bubbles requires tissues to be super-saturated with nitrogen and for ascent to be excessively rapid. As bubbles form in tissues, they distort tissue architecture, which results in impaired function, pain and inflammation and is probably responsible for most musculoskeletal symptoms.

Many bubbles entering the venous system do not cause symptoms. In fact, using ultrasonic detection methods, intravascular microbubbles are detected after approximately 60% of routine dives. It appears that these bubbles are safely filtered by the lung and diffuse into the alveoli.

Bubbles entering the arterial system are more likely to cause serious problems. This can occur under several circumstances. Large volumes of bubbles may overwhelm the pulmonary filter and arterialize. Bubbles may also bypass the lungs via a right-to-left shunt. Up to one-quarter of the population may have a patent foramen ovale (PFO). Under normal circumstances, the valve over the foramen is kept closed by the pressure difference between the left and right atria. However, during diving, the pressure differential may reverse during a Valsalva manoeuvre or with acute increases in right-sided pressures associated with a large pulmonary gas load.

Alternatively, gas can enter the circulation following pulmonary barotrauma. Air entering the pulmonary arterial system is carried to the pulmonary capillaries where it is trapped and reabsorbed by the alveoli. Air entering the pulmonary venous system, however, will pass through the heart and result in AGE.

Gas bubbles entering the circulation (either from tissues or barotrauma) cause both mechanical and biochemical abnormalities. Trapping in the pulmonary circulation may result in elevation of right heart and pulmonary pressures, leading to increased venous pressures, reduced cardiac output and impairment of tissue microcirculation. Arterial bubbles can cause end-organ ischaemia, although most pass through the capillaries and into the venous system. Most of the deleterious effects are a consequence of secondary inflammation of the vascular endothelium.

Bubble–endothelial interaction activates complement, kinin and coagulation systems and precipitates leucocyte adherence. This results in increased vascular permeability, interstitial oedema and microvascular sludging. The end result is ischaemia and haemoconcentration. Increased vascular permeability of the cerebral circulation will produce cerebral oedema. Vasospasm and reduced flow occurs approximately 1–2 h after bubbles have passed through the arterial tree. This explains the commonly observed clinical course of a diver with a cerebral AGE experiencing an initial deterioration (bubble emboli), followed by spontaneous improvement (bubbles pass through the cerebral capillaries) and then a subsequent secondary deterioration. Animal studies have demonstrated that bubbles travel against arterial flow because of their buoyancy and lodge in

Prevention

A number of dive tables and computer algorithms have been developed in an attempt to avoid nitrogen supersaturation of tissues and improve diver safety. Limits are placed on depth, time and ascent rates to allow safe decompression after diving. However, as with all mathematical models which attempt to predict biological behaviour, the dive tables are far from perfect. One series has shown that 39% of DCI cases were within the limits of the table they were using and 24% within the limits of the conservative Canadian Defence and Civil Institute of Environmental Medicine (DCIEM) tables. Historically, it was assumed that DCI could not occur after dives shallower than 10 m, but it is now known that this can occur, particularly if there has been more than one dive per day or multiple ascents. The occurrence of DCI is a probabilistic event where risk increases with increasing depth, time, numbers of dives, numbers of ascents and rates of ascent.

Flying after diving can precipitate DCI. Even if there are no bubbles at the end of the dive, excess nitrogen remains in the tissues and is slowly off-gassed. Further reduction in ambient pressure at altitude can cause bubbles or enlarge pre-existing asymptomatic ones. Current guidelines advise against flying for 12 h after a single short no-decompression dive and 24 h following multiple or decompression dives.

Clinical features

Onset of any symptoms during or in the hours after diving should be regarded as DCI until proven otherwise. Failure to recognize and treat milder cases can lead to permanent morbidity because the disease can progress as the bubble load increases with time. Early onset of symptoms or signs (up to 1 h), especially those that are neurological in nature, indicates a serious decompression emergency and recompression is a time-critical treatment. Milder syndromes of decompression illness may develop up to 24 h after a dive or even later if there is a precipitant, such as heavy exercise or ascent to altitude (e.g. flying).

In general, pulmonary barotrauma that results in AGE has a dramatic clinical presentation and the onset of major neurological symptoms and signs occurs within seconds to minutes after the dive. DCI caused by intravascular bubbles from barotrauma can be rapidly fatal and has a mortality of 5% in sport divers who reach a recompression chamber alive. In Australia, it is the second most common cause of diving-related death after drowning. The brain is the organ most commonly affected, probably because of the vertical positioning of the diver on ascent. Cerebral gas emboli can cause sudden loss of consciousness, convulsions, visual disturbances, deafness, cranial nerve palsies, memory disturbance and asymmetric multiplegias. Hemiplegia is much less common than asymmetric multiplegias. Symptoms almost always begin within 10 min of surfacing. Sudden loss of consciousness on surfacing should be assumed to be due to cerebral gas emboli. Spontaneous improvement may occur with first aid measures, but relapse is common.

Coronary arterial emboli rarely may present as acute myocardial infarction or arrhythmia. Abdominal organs and skin may also be embolized. Elevation of serum creatine kinase (predominantly from skeletal muscle), serum transaminase and lactate dehydrogenase levels in divers with AGE suggests that emboli are distributed more extensively than previously recognized. Peak creatine kinase (CK) may be a marker of the degree and severity of AGE.

Onset of DCI due to gas bubbles coming out of solution can be equally as dramatic (especially after rapid ascents from deep dives), but frequently evolves over hours post-dive. DCI caused by bubbles released from tissues usually causes symptoms within 1 h of completing a dive and 90% of cases have symptoms within 6 h. Neurological symptoms occurring around 30 min after a dive have been associated with PFO. Common symptoms include profound fatigue, myalgia, periarticular pain and headache. Shoulders and elbows are the joints most commonly involved. The pain is usually a dull ache, which may initially be intermittent and migrate from joint to joint, but later becomes constant. Movement aggravates the pain, but local pressure with an inflated sphygmomanometer cuff may improve it. Paraesthesia and numbness may accompany the pain suggesting concomitant neurological disease.

Neurological DCI may present as personality change, headache, memory loss, visual defects, convulsions, confusion and altered level of consciousness. A flat affect may be the only symptom. The vestibular system can also be involved, with dizziness, vertigo, vomiting, nystagmus and ataxia.

Spinal-cord involvement occurs in up to 60% of cases of neurological DCI. The exact cause of spinal DCI is still debated. It may be a result of venous infarction of the cord due to obstruction of the epidural vertebral venous plexus. Other explanations include ischaemia and inflammation from bubble emboli or the formation of local bubbles within the spinal cord (autochthonous bubbles). Symptoms include back pain, paraesthesia and paraplegia, with bowel and bladder involvement. It is potentially disastrous to misdiagnose back pain coming on a few minutes after a dive as musculoskeletal pain and not consider spinal cord DCI.

If the bubble load overwhelms the pulmonary filter, a diver can present with a syndrome known as pulmonary DCI or 'the chokes'. The symptoms of this syndrome include dyspnoea, pleuritic substernal chest pain, cough, pink frothy sputum, cyanosis and haemoptysis. It indicates the diver has sustained a large intravascular gas load, so a careful inquiry about other symptoms of DCI is mandatory and, if present, recompression is advised. Diving-related pulmonary oedema and salt-water aspiration syndrome are the major differential diagnoses.

A variety of rashes may be caused by cutaneous bubbles; however, these syndromes affect less than 10% of divers. The most common presentations are pruritus with no rash, a scarlatinaform rash with pruritus and *cutis marmorata*. Cutis marmorata begins as a spreading erythema but subsequently develops a marbled appearance of pale areas surrounded by cyanotic mottling.

Assessment of the injured diver

The injured diver requires simultaneous assessment and treatment. One hundred per cent oxygen treatment should be continued during the assessment. If the history suggests AGE, the patient should be kept in the horizontal position to avoid re-embolization. If symptoms are progressing rapidly, the examination should be brief but thorough so as to ensure rapid access to recompression. In serious cases, some of the historical information may be obtained once the diver is receiving treatment in the recompression chamber.

The diagnosis of DCI is made on history and examination. A full dive history must be obtained, in addition to the medical history. Important details include the number of dives over recent days, depth, bottom time (the time from beginning descent to beginning direct ascent), performance of any decompression or safety stops, dive complications, such as rapid ascents, surface interval between dives and the time interval between completing the dive and onset of symptoms. Previous dive experience, equipment used and gases breathed should also be recorded. A history of using surface supply equipment (the 'Hookah' apparatus) should alert the examining physician to the possibility of carbon monoxide poisoning and carboxyhaemoglobin measurement is required. Cold water, hard exercise during the dive, increasing age, multiple ascents and repetitive dives are predisposing factors in the development of DCI. Any exposure to altitude (>300 m) or heavy exercise post-dive should be recorded.

A thorough examination, particularly of the neurological system, to detect subtle abnormalities is required. It is also helpful to perform basic tests of cognitive function, such as the mini-mental state examination. For milder static DCI syndromes with delayed presentation, the sharpened Romberg test provides useful information. It is performed by asking the patient to stand heel-to-toe with open palms on opposite shoulders. The patient is stable. They are then asked to close their eyes and timed until they lose balance or achieve 60 s. A score of less than 60 s is suggestive of DCI in an injured diver. This test should not be performed if the history was suggestive of AGE or if there are neurological symptoms or signs.

Clinical investigations

Recompression should only be delayed for investigations if they will directly alter management. A full blood count and electrolytes are useful in that intravascular fluid depletion is common in severe DCI and the degree of haemoconcentration may correlate with eventual neurological outcome. Serum CK and liver function tests (LFTs) may be indicators of gas embolism; however, these do not influence clinical management. The blood glucose level should be checked in divers with impaired consciousness. A chest X-ray is indicated if pulmonary barotrauma is suspected, because a pneumothorax requires treatment before recompression. A dilemma occurs if the diver has a neurological presentation, because they should not be moved from the horizontal position until they are recompressed. If CAGE is suspected and CT is available, a supine CT scan of the thorax is preferable to a chest X-ray to diagnose pneumothorax or pneumomediastinum. Ultrasound in emergency may also be used to confirm a pneumothorax. Magnetic resonance imaging has no role in the acute investigation of DCI.

Treatment

First aid

One hundred per cent oxygen provides the maximum gradient for diffusion of nitrogen out of the bubbles. A large consecutive comparative series involving over 2000 divers has demonstrated that first aid oxygen significantly improves outcomes for divers with decompression illness. It should be administered in the pre-hospital setting and continue until and during recompression. Failure to improve on oxygen does not rule out DCI. Conversely, complete improvement on oxygen does not obviate the need for recompression. The diver should be supine or in the left lateral position if unable to protect their airway. Traditionally, the Trendelenburg position was advocated to reduce bubble embolization to the brain, but is now thought to increase the risk of cerebral oedema and should only be used if required to maintain blood pressure. The diver should be prevented from sitting or standing up, to avoid bubbles redistributing from the left ventricle to the brain. Initial resuscitation is along standard basic and advanced life support protocols. If intubation is required, the endotracheal tube cuff should be filled with saline prior to recompression to avoid a change in volume and a tube leak as ambient pressure increases.

Intravenous isotonic crystalloids should be commenced and titrated to response. Glucose-containing fluids are to be avoided because they may exacerbate CNS injury. Divers who present after several days with mild symptoms may be adequately managed with oral fluids. A urinary catheter should be inserted for spinal cord DCI with bladder involvement. Hypothermia should be corrected.

Retrieval

Long-distance retrieval can either be by air transport pressurized to 1 ATA or by portable recompression chambers. There is little debate that the longer the delay in recompression of severe DCI, the worse the outcome. However, Australian experience suggests that the number of cases where a portable chamber would have made a difference is so small that their use is unwarranted, largely because of the time required to prepare and transport portable chambers. Commercial aircraft are pressurized to 0.74 ATA (2440 m) and not appropriate to retrieve DCI patients, unless arrangements can be made to fly lower and pressurize to sea level. Road retrieval is not suitable over great distances or where an altitude of 300 m will be exceeded. Consultation with a hyperbaric physician should occur if retrieval is difficult.

Recompression

Recompression in a hyperbaric chamber is indicated even if the diver becomes asymptomatic with first aid, because otherwise many will relapse. The relapse may be more severe than the original presentation, due to the pathophysiological changes already initiated by bubbles in the microvasculature and tissues or redistribution of bubbles. Response to recompression is determined by time to recompression and the initial severity of injury. Recompression should always occur as soon as possible. It is particularly urgent for severe cases where treatment commenced later than 4 h after injury is associated with a poor response. Mild cases often respond despite longer delays to recompression.

Two types of hyperbaric chamber are available to administer recompression treatment:

- *Multiplace* chambers can accommodate more than one person, including a clinician attendant and are compressed on air while the patient breathes 100% oxygen via a head hood, demand regulator or endotracheal tube. Air breaks to lessen the risks of oxygen toxicity are provided by removing the head hood in a multiplace chamber. Full monitoring and mechanical ventilation are possible. All hyperbaric facilities in Australasia use multiplace chambers.
- *Monoplace* chambers accommodate one patient only and are usually compressed with 100% oxygen. These are more frequently used to treat non-diving medical illness; however, in other countries, they may be used for definitive treatment of divers.

Hyperbaric oxygen has the following beneficial effects:

- Reduction in bubble size in accordance with Boyle's law. Increased pressure also increases the partial pressure of nitrogen within the bubble. There is no nitrogen outside the bubble because of the 100% oxygen. This markedly increases the outward diffusion gradient for nitrogen. This relieves the obstruction caused by intravascular bubbles and the tissue distortion of extravascular bubbles.

- Reduction of endothelial inflammation caused by the bubbles.
- Relief of ischaemia and hypoxia.

There are no published randomized trials comparing recompression protocols and hence no international agreement on how to manage DCI. The general consensus is that initial treatments should begin with a standard 18 m (2.8 ATA) table breathing 100% oxygen. Some studies have suggested a benefit from initially recompressing deeper, however, this procedure is not universally accepted and subject to considerable debate.

The identical Royal Navy 62 (RN62) and US Navy 6 recompression tables have become the standard of care for initial treatment of diving accidents in Australia and New Zealand. These are 18 m tables, lasting 4.75 h to 7.25 h (Fig. 28.3.1). Recompression is followed by gradual decompression. A response to treatment is usually evident by the second air break. If there is a partial response then there is the option of extending the table at 18 m. If there is minimal or no response and there is no doubt about the diagnosis, then it is reasonable to proceed to a deeper table (most units use the Comex 30 table). Because of the risks of oxygen toxicity at greater than 18 m, a combination of helium and oxygen (heliox) is used. Anecdotal evidence suggests that this technique is particularly effective for severe spinal cord DCI. In-water recompression is dangerous and difficult and should only be considered if retrieval is impossible. Hypothermia and oxygen toxicity pose serious risks during treatment and supervision by an experienced hyperbaric physician is essential.

Adverse effects of hyperbaric oxygen

Adverse effects of hyperbaric oxygen are uncommon. Even in non-divers, significant middle-ear barotrauma interrupting treatment occurs in 1/170 treatments. Claustrophobia is even rarer at 1/910 treatments.

The most serious adverse effect is oxygen toxicity and the attendant must continually watch for signs of its development. Toxicity is due to the formation of oxygen free radicals, which overwhelm the body's antioxidants. It can affect the brain and the lung.

Cerebral oxygen toxicity can occur with brief exposures to 2 ATA oxygen and pulmonary toxicity may occur with prolonged exposure to 0.5 ATA or higher. The most common presentation of cerebral oxygen toxicity is muscle twitching, particularly of the lips and face. Other possible symptoms include apprehension, vertigo, visual disturbance, nausea, confusion and dizziness. If the oxygen is removed at this stage, progression to generalized convulsions may be avoided. Convulsions can, however, occur without premonitory symptoms. Treatment is as for any generalized convulsion, although removal of the oxygen will almost always stop it. Decompression should not be attempted during the convulsion as this may cause pulmonary barotrauma. Oxygen can be safely reinstituted 15 min after all symptoms have resolved. Predisposing factors to cerebral oxygen toxicity include fever, steroids, a past history of epilepsy and carbon monoxide poisoning. Incidence is directly proportional to time of exposure and inspired oxygen partial pressure. The incidence of convulsions in divers treated at 2.8 ATA on the RN62 is 0.56%.

Pulmonary oxygen toxicity manifests initially as an asymptomatic reduction in vital capacity, followed by cough and retrosternal pain. The symptoms usually abate when treatment is completed. Up to 10% reduction in vital capacity has been measured during extended treatments, which reverses within 24 h of completing treatment.

Adjuvant therapies for DCI

Recent research in the use of lignocaine infusions in patients undergoing open-heart surgery has demonstrated a significant benefit for the lignocaine group in terms of the incidence of postoperative neuropsychiatric abnormalities. The mechanism of injury in open-heart surgery is likely to be gas emboli and therefore provides a useful model for divers with AGE. There is now sufficient evidence to recommend a 48-h lignocaine infusion at standard antiarrhythmic doses to divers with unequivocal CAGE. A randomized clinical trial has demonstrated a reduction in symptoms after treatment for decompression illness if tenoxicam was administered to divers in the recovery phase. There was a reduction in total recompression requirements.

Prognosis after treatment

Relapses may occur after initial recompression and all neurological cases should be observed in hospital to allow immediate recompression if deterioration occurs. Further daily recompression is carried out until the patient stops improving or becomes asymptomatic and then one additional treatment is performed. Follow-up treatments are usually at 18 m, using either the RN61 table (18 m for 45 min, ascent to 9 m over 30 min, 9 m for 30 min then ascent over 30 min) or the 18:60:30 table (18 m for 60 min then ascent over 30 min).

Residual symptoms occur in up to 30% of cases and are more likely where recompression is delayed. Delays to treatment are not unusual with a mean time to recompression of 68 h in one series. There is no clear time interval after diving that recompression becomes

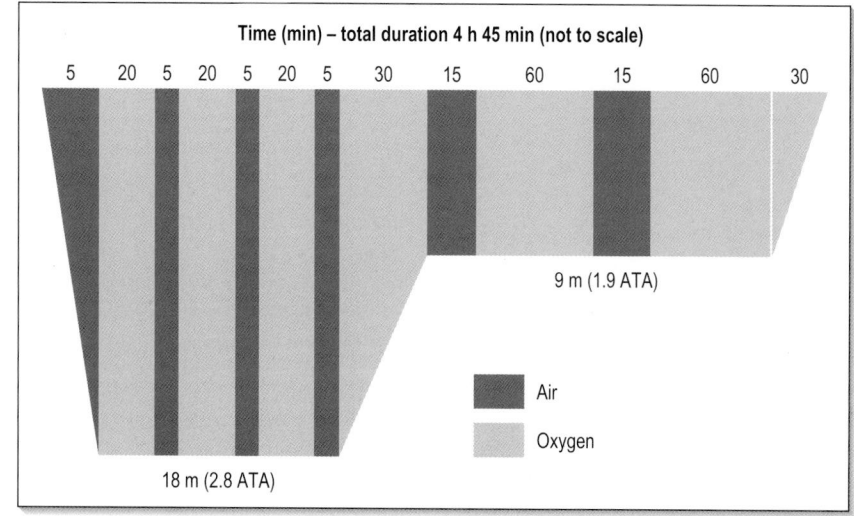

Fig. 28.3.1 US Navy treatment table 6.

ineffective. Many divers with DCI still respond to treatment even when delayed for 7–10 days and, therefore, any diver with unexplained symptoms after diving should be referred to a diving medicine specialist.

Flying after treatment and return to diving

Recommendations for flying and diving after treatment for DCI vary greatly and are not evidence based. Flying should be avoided for at least 1 week after treatment to avoid relapse. It is reasonable to permit resumption of diving after 4 weeks if there are no residual symptoms or signs. Because of the risk of recurrence, further diving is contraindicated if the DCI is thought to be due to pulmonary barotrauma, or where there are residual neurological signs or symptoms.

Other issues

Vertigo and headache in divers

These two symptom complexes are challenging to assess and diagnose. There are several possible causes of vertigo in divers. Vertigo developing while the diver is underwater is extremely dangerous: it can induce panic and lead to a rapid ascent. It can disorientate the diver so that they do not know which way the surface is and is often associated with vomiting.

The most common cause, alternobaric vertigo, begins just as divers commence their ascent and is caused by a unilateral pressure difference between the middle and inner ears. It usually lasts only a few minutes. Middle-ear barotrauma can also cause mild vertigo. Other causes include inner-ear DCI, inner-ear barotrauma and TM rupture. Any persistent vertiginous symptoms may indicate a more serious cause, such as neurological decompression illness or inner-ear barotrauma. Headache occurring during or after diving has a number of possible diving-related causes, such as sinus and mask squeeze, carbon dioxide accumulation, carbon monoxide toxicity, decompression illness, patent foramen ovale, ill-fitting wetsuits and marine envenomation. It is recommended that for all divers presenting with vertigo or headache, there is early consultation with a diving medicine specialist.

Oxygen toxicity

Cerebral oxygen toxicity in the diver underwater causes the same problems as in the hyperbaric chamber. Divers are more likely to develop toxicity underwater than in the chamber because immersion, exercise and carbon-dioxide retention increase the risk. The use of oxygen-enriched gases, such as nitrox, may increase the risk of cerebral oxygen toxicity. Enriched-air divers should ensure they stay at depths that maintain an oxygen partial pressure of less than 1.4 ATA.

Nitrogen narcosis

Described by Jacques Cousteau as 'rapture of the deep', nitrogen narcosis is due to the anaesthetic effect of nitrogen dissolved in lipid membranes. Symptoms are similar to those of alcohol intoxication. Some divers experience it at 30 m and almost all by 50. Loss of consciousness occurs at 90 m. This condition will not present to the emergency department because it is immediately reversible on ascent. However, it may result in other diving accidents, such as rapid ascent or near drowning. Divers planning to dive deeper than 50 m should use an alternative to air, such as heliox.

Gas contamination

Contaminants may be in the air before compression, added during compression or already in the tanks. Common contaminants include carbon dioxide, carbon monoxide and oil. Increasing partial pressures of the contaminant gases at depth may result in toxicity. Contamination is rare but must always be included in the differential diagnosis of injured divers, particularly those presenting with headache, shortness of breath or loss of consciousness at depth.

Diving-related pulmonary oedema

Pulmonary oedema in the diver may be caused by DCI, near drowning or immersion itself. Preexisting cardiovascular disease, increasing age (>40), hypertension and beta blockade appear to be risk factors for immersion-induced pulmonary oedema. Symptoms often begin while the diver is still at depth, distinguishing it from DCI. There may also be episodes occurring when immersed but not diving (e.g. swimming). Treatment is supportive and recompression is not required provided DCI can be excluded. However, if detected, the occurrence of pulmonary oedema as a result of diving has long-term ramifications for future diving fitness.

Controversies

- *What position is best for managing the injured diver?* There are no controlled trials assessing the best position to manage an injured diver. The current recommendation is to maintain a supine position for all suspected or confirmed neurological presentations, based on expert opinion and known pathophysiology.
- *Should intravenous or oral fluids be administered?* Based on expert consensus and known pathophysiology, the injured diver is usually dehydrated. Fluid management is regarded as an important adjunct to recompression. In an acute diving accident <12 h, where consciousness or airway reflexes are impaired or where there is nausea and vomiting, IV salt-based crystalloids should be administered, due to the need for 100% oxygen and the possible risk of oxygen toxicity during the initial treatment phase at 2.8 ATA. In the less acute presentation of static DCI, oral fluids may be acceptable, although there are some risks if an oxygen toxicity seizure occurs during treatment at 2.8 ATA.
- *Should we compress divers deeper than 2.8 ATA during treatment?* This is very controversial, with reports of deep tables being used successfully in Hawaii. To date, there are no completed randomized controlled trials comparing outcomes of different treatment pressures.

Important phone numbers

24-h services offering advice on management, retrieval and location of the nearest hyperbaric facility:

Australia

Divers Alert Network 1800 088 200
+61 8 8212 9242 (outside Australia)

New Zealand

Diver Alert Network 0800 4337 111

USA

Diving Accident Network (DAN) (919) 6849111

UK

Aberdeen Royal Infirmary 07831 151523

Diving Diseases Research Centre, Plymouth
01752 209999

Institute of Naval Medicine, Hampshire 023
9276 8170

Further reading

Banham ND. Oxygen toxicity seizures: 20 years' experience from a single hyperbaric unit. Diving Hyperb Med 2011;4:202–10.

Bennett M, Mitchell S, Dominquez A. Adjunctive treatment of decompression illness with a non-steroidal antiiflammatory drug (tenoxicam) reduces recompression requirement. Undersea Hyperb Med 2003;30:195–205.

Billinger M, Zbinden R, Mordasini R, et al. Patent foramen ovale closure in recreational divers: effect on decompression illness and ischaemic brain lesions during long-term follow-up. Heart 2011;97:1932–7.

Edmonds C. Inner ear barotrauma: a retrospective clinical series of 50 cases. S Pacif Underwater Med Soc J 2004;34:11–14.

Edmonds C, Lowry C, Pennefather J, et al. Diving and subaquatic medicine, 4th ed. London: Arnold Publishers; 2002.

Francis J. Pulmonary barotrauma: a new look at mechanisms. S Pacif Underwater Med Soc J 1997;27:205–18.

Francis TJR, Mitchell SJ. Manifestations of decompression disorders. In: Brubakk AO, Neuman TS, editors. Bennett and Elliott's physiology and medicine of diving (5th ed.). London: Harcourt Publishers; 2003. p. 578–99.

Hampson NB, Dunford RG. Pulmonary edema of scuba divers. Undersea Hyperb Med 1997;24:29–33.

Longphre JM, Denoble PJ, Moon RE, et al. First-aid normobaric oxygen for the treatment of recreational diving injuries. Undersea Hyperb Med 2007;34:43–9.

Smerz RW, Overlock RK, Nakayama H. Hawaiian deep treatments: efficacy and outcomes 1983–2003. Undersea Hyperb Med 2005;32:363–73.

Standards Australia. Occupational diving operations. Part 1. Standard operational practice AS/NZS 2299.1; 2007.

Tetzlaff K, Beuter B, Leplow B, et al. Risk factors for pulmonary barotrauma in divers. Chest 1997;112:654–9.

28.4 Radiation incidents

Paul D Mark

ESSENTIALS

1 Radiation accidents are rare but require well-planned protocols for successful management. The principal challenge will be managing anxious patients who are potentially contaminated with radioactive particulate material.

2 Effective triage is based on early clinical symptoms and lymphocyte counts.

3 The management of life-threatening illness or injury always takes precedence over the radiation aspects of the patient's condition.

4 The principles of contamination control are little different from those dealing with patients contaminated with chemical or biological material.

5 Contamination with radioactive material should be distinguished from exposure to ionizing radiation. Except in nuclear detonations or reactor accidents, it is very uncommon for both to occur in the same victim.

6 Removing the patient's clothing and washing exposed skin and hair can reduce the level of external contamination by up to 90%.

7 The risks to hospital personnel are minimal provided appropriate precautions are taken.

8 The presence of a qualified radiation physicist with appropriate radiation monitoring equipment is invaluable when dealing with (potentially) contaminated patients.

9 Following whole-body irradiation, survival is likely only from the haemopoietic and milder gastrointestinal syndromes.

10 Blocking and chelating agents can successfully reduce the incorporation of radioactive substances into body tissues if they are given early.

11 The advent of bone marrow transplant can increase the survival rates of more severely affected patients but resources around the nation are limited.

Introduction

In August 1945, the first atomic fission bombs were detonated above the Japanese cities of Hiroshima and Nagasaki with devastating effects. Most radiation incidents, however, have been accidental with the most serious occurring in 1986 at Chernobyl in the former Soviet Union when a nuclear reactor unit exploded, dispersing radioactive material over a wide area. One hundred and thirty six people developed the acute radiation syndrome, of which 28 died. A dramatic increase in thyroid cancers was observed among those who were either very young or *in utero*. The majority of incidents, however, have involved small numbers of people and many have occurred as a result of deliberate bypassing of safety procedures.

There were no deaths from exposure to radiation or cases of radiation sickness following the 2011 Fukushima accident but over 160 000 people had to be evacuated from their homes to ensure this.

Much of our knowledge of the long-term effects of ionizing radiation comes from the study of people who survived the Chernobyl incident and the atomic detonations over Japan.

In Australia, the Australian Radiation Incidence Registry records all accidents where exposures occur that are not 'within the limits known to be normal for the particular source of radiation and for the particular use being made of it'. Very few accidents are recorded in which individuals received exposure or contamination significant enough to cause health concerns [1]. Strict licensing and control systems, coupled with improving technology and training, have helped to minimize the number of Australian radiation incidents.

The advent of terrorism might increase the risk of multiple casualty incidents, particularly from the use of radiation dispersal devices. Significant acute irradiation from such a device is unlikely, but victims may present with a variety of clinical syndromes and their management requires a multidisciplinary approach and close liaison between clinical staff and health physicists [2].

Decontamination is essential for all patients to avoid the delayed effects of continuing low-dose radiation.

Radiation sources and incidents

Worldwide, the most common radiation sources are:

- X-ray equipment: used for medical diagnosis and treatment, industrial and commercial inspections, quality control techniques, irradiations and research.
- Accelerators: used for medical treatments, industrial irradiation, the production of radioisotopes and research.
- Radioactive materials: used for medical diagnosis and treatment, industrial radiography, quality control and tracing techniques, soil density and moisture tests, and research. Radioactive material may be unsealed or contained within sealed containers.
- Nuclear processing and reactor plants: used for processing uranium and plutonium for fuel purposes and nuclear weapons, power production and research.

With X-ray equipment and accelerators, the victim may be exposed to radiation but this does not make the tissues radioactive. These patients pose no threat to others, including medical attendants.

Unsealed radioactive material has the potential to cause radioactive contamination. This may be external on clothing or skin or internal following inhalation, ingestion or absorption through body orifices, mucous membranes and wounds. Following internal contamination, radioactive material may become incorporated into the patient's tissues.

Other than for accidents involving nuclear processing and reactor plants, accidents usually lead to either exposure or contamination. Contaminated patients rarely suffer significant radiation exposure and exposed patients are seldom contaminated [1].

There are no nuclear reactors in Australia except for the occasional visiting nuclear powered warship. These vessels are closely monitored while in Australian ports.

The Fukushima reactors closed down when the earthquake struck in March 2011, however, the subsequent tsunami disabled the cooling systems. Following the approved release of a quantity of radioactively contaminated water, some seafood in the immediate vicinity of the power station has been found to exceed regulatory limits. The hydrogen explosion resulted in the release of a gaseous plume, which contaminated some milk and vegetable produce. The government enacted measures to prevent the distribution and sale of several foodstuffs and fish.

Terrorism

The most likely means for terrorist organizations to deploy radiation is a radiation dispersal device (RDD) or 'dirty bomb'. These weapons use conventional explosives, such as trinitrotoluene, ammonium nitrate or other explosive material, to spread radioactive substances. A variety of substances could be used including americium, caesium, cobalt, iodine, phosphorus, plutonium, strontium, tritium and uranium. Only some of these are available in Australia.

RDDs are sometimes called 'weapons of mass disruption' because of the fear they engender in the population, multiple casualties, contamination of widespread areas and the economic cost [5]. Immediate injuries are generally the result of blast or thermal effects. Few contain sufficient material to cause acute radiation injury. Only those trapped near the site of detonation run this risk. However, radioactive material will be spread over a large area and many people might be exposed to the risks of low-dose radiation. Hospital staff treating the victims of RDD explosions are at negligible risk provided they wear appropriate protective equipment. Unlike surface burst nuclear weapons, RDDs do not cause fallout downwind of the detonation.

Radioactive material without the explosive component may constitute a radiation exposure device (RED) and could potentially be hidden in a crowded space, such as a theatre, where it could cause occult irradiation. Industrial sources are the most prevalent REDs in the civilian sector. An improvised nuclear device (IND), like a small nuclear weapon, produces blast, thermal and radiation energy; exposing people to high dose external radiation, inhalation of radioactive materials, particulate contamination and ingestion of radioactive materials in the food chain.

Measuring radioactivity

Radioactivity of an isotope is expressed as the average number of atoms that disintegrate per second. The Becquerel (Bq) is the SI unit for one nuclear disintegration per second. The activity of a given mass of a radioactive substance with a short half-life will decrease with time.

Ionization in air can be measured by portable dosimeters to give an estimate of the levels of radioactivity at the site of an incident. This is used to calculate the exposure level of a patient with acute radiation illness. The units used are Roentgens. Dosimeters are also used in hospitals to measure the level of radiation to which staff members have been exposed or to monitor patients during decontamination.

The absorbed dose of radiation is the amount of ionization energy deposited in matter by ionizing radiation. One Gray (Gy) is equivalent to one joule per kilogram. The effect of a given dose of radiation depends on the type of radiation emitted and the tissue type irradiated.

Type of radiation emitted

Different types of ionizing radiation transfer energy to tissue at different rates. The Sievert (Sv) is the international unit of effective radiation dose and is obtained by multiplying the absorbed dose measured in Gray (Gy) by a quality factor to reflect the different effects of each radiation type and their potential biological damage. For beta and gamma radiation $1\,Sv = 1\,Gy$. Alpha and neutron radiation deposit more energy in tissue so the quality factor is higher.

Alpha particles, composed of two protons and two neutrons, do not penetrate the dermis but may cause local damage if ingested, inhaled or absorbed through open wounds. Beta radiation, consisting of electron-like particles, travels about a metre through the air and is stopped by clothing. It often causes radiation injury to exposed skin. Gamma particles have no mass and are similar to X-rays, penetrating the body freely and causing the acute radiation syndrome if the trunk is involved. Neutrons are produced only during nuclear detonations and, while they can technically make an irradiated victim emit radiation, this is not clinically significant.

Grays are the preferred measure for determining acute effects while Sieverts are more useful in predicting chronic effects.

The average natural background radiation is 2 mSV per annum in Australia. The Australian

National Occupational Health and Safety Commission's standard for a worker is a maximum effective dose of 50 mSv in any year (or 20 mSv per year averaged over 5 years).

Pathophysiology

Radiation damages tissue both directly and indirectly by the production of free radicals from water molecules. Direct damage to cell membranes may cause changes in permeability and the release of lysosomes. Germinal, haemopoietic and gastrointestinal epithelial cells are relatively radiosensitive. The cells of bone, liver, kidney, cartilage, muscle and nerve tissue are relatively radioresistant. The delayed effects of radiation depend on whether the dose is lethal or sublethal to the tissue involved.

Lethal (deterministic) injuries are threshold dependent. Cells are killed when they receive a radiation dose, which varies with different tissues. Clinical expression occurs when the amount of cell killing cannot be compensated for by proliferation of viable cells. The acute and chronic radiation syndromes are deterministic. The earliest delayed effect of acute radiation injury, cataract formation at about 10 months, is an example of this type of injury.

For sublethal (stochastic) injuries there is no threshold level of radiation and the consequence is based on statistical probability. Sublethal injury to chromosomes is the most important effect of ionizing radiation. Double-strand breaks are not easily reparable, especially if the damage occurs simultaneously to both strands. This results in broken chromosomes with no template for repair. The exposed ends of chromosome fragments may join up at random, resulting in morphological chromosomal abnormalities. Sublethal damage to chromosomes is implicated in the development of tumours. Children are more prone to radiation-induced carcinogenesis. Although the incidence of malignancy in adults is increased by radiation exposure, the age at which malignancies are clinically expressed does not change. The estimated increase in lifetime risk of fatal cancer is 0.008% per millisievert of gamma radiation exposure [4]. Therefore, an individual who is exposed to 100 milligrays (twice the acceptable Australian occupational annual exposure) has a 0.8% increase in the lifetime risk of fatal cancer.

Radiation exposure to the gonads may produce temporary or permanent infertility in men depending on the dose. With temporary infertility, there is preservation of the secondary sexual characteristics. In the female, however, all ova are present at birth and larger radiation doses are required to produce sterility. Radiation-induced infertility in females is associated with premature menopause. Unlike animals, in humans, gonadal exposure to radiation does not affect future generations [8].

The fetus may receive less radiation than the mother when exposed to external radiation. However, when internal contamination occurs, it is possible for the fetus to receive a higher dose as material excreted in the urine collects in the maternal bladder. Exposures during organogenesis (weeks 3 to 7) may cause malformations. Exposure during weeks 8 to 25 causes decreasing IQ with increasing dose. There is a small increased risk of childhood cancers and possibly leukaemia.

Chronic radiation exposure

Chronic radiation exposure was first described in Russia following the exposure of workers in the plutonium enrichment programme to excessive doses of radiation over a period of time. Persons at risk have been exposed to radiation well above occupational health and safety standards for at least 3 years and have received a dose of 1 Gy or more to the bone marrow. Symptoms include sleep and appetite disturbance, easy fatiguability, impaired concentration and memory, vertigo, ataxia, paraesthesia, bone pain and hot flushes. Clinical findings include localized bone and muscle tenderness, tremor, hyperreflexia and underdeveloped secondary sexual characteristics. Investigations may reveal pancytopaenia and bone dysplasia. Following cessation of exposure, symptoms may slowly resolve.

Acute radiation exposure

Radiation exposure accidents usually involve penetrating radiation, such as high-energy X-rays or gamma rays. The effects are primarily due to the loss of cells in the body. Acute exposure is more dangerous than chronic, as it does not allow time for cell replacement or tissue recovery. Clinically, radiation exposure may produce a generalized acute radiation syndrome or a localized irradiation injury.

The acute radiation syndrome

The acute radiation syndrome refers to the effects of radiation on one or more body systems. The haemopoietic tissue alone is affected at doses of 1–4 Gy and produces pancytopaenia with its consequent risks of infection, bleeding and anaemia. Above 6 Gy, gastrointestinal effects are also manifest and the prognosis is poorer. The neurovascular syndrome occurs with doses above 20 Gy and is manifest by leaky capillaries, hypotension and a progressive decline in mental function with eventual death in weeks to months. The symptoms depend on the part of the body irradiated, the dose and the time over which it is delivered.

Clinical features

The course of the illness can be divided into four phases. The higher the dose, the shorter the duration of each phase and the more severe the symptoms:

- the prodromal phase, which generally lasts up to 48 h
- a latent period, lasting hours to weeks
- the manifest illness period
- death or recovery; the latter may take up to 10 weeks.

The prodromal symptoms are due to the effects of radiation on cell membranes and the release of vasoactive amines. The symptoms are non-specific, with anorexia, nausea, vomiting, weakness, fever, conjunctivitis, erythema and hyperaesthesia. The time to emesis, presence of diarrhoea and duration of symptoms are markers of the severity of the exposure [5]. Vomiting, however, may be psychogenic.

The phase of manifest illness corresponds to the loss of cells. The haemopoietic syndrome occurs alone with whole-body radiation doses of between 1 and 4 Gy. It is due to loss of stem cells in the bone marrow. At these doses, some stem cells survive and recovery is therefore possible. The latent period lasts from 2 to 20 days and is followed by a rapid fall in the number of white blood cells and platelets. Recovery commences about 30 days after exposure, regardless of the exact dose.

The gastrointestinal syndrome predominates with radiation doses greater than 6 Gy. The prodromal symptoms are more severe. Early bloody diarrhoea suggests death within 2 weeks. The gastrointestinal symptoms recur during the manifest illness phase and can be very severe leading to dehydration and electrolyte imbalance. This syndrome is due to the loss of stem cells in the intestinal mucosal crypts. It is superimposed upon the haemopoietic syndrome with both occurring after a short latent period of under a week.

The neurovascular syndrome occurs with doses of greater than 20 Gy and is characterized by leakage of fluid into tissues and hypotension. The latent period is just a few days. Leakage into the brain causes neurological symptoms. These effects are superimposed on those due to gastrointestinal and haemopoietic damage. At very high doses, greater than 30 Gy, there is incapacitation usually within the first few minutes and certainly within 40 min. The effects are largely due to disruption of cell membranes and electrochemical inactivation of neurons. Death can be anticipated within hours. In a nuclear detonation, however, death from other injuries is more likely in those close enough to receive this level of exposure.

Whole body irradiation also produces visible changes in the skin. Hair epilation occurs at 3 Gy, erythema at 6 Gy, dry desquamation at 10 Gy and wet desquamation at 20 Gy. The erythema may come and go and occurs earlier with higher doses but rarely within 24 h.

Patients presenting after definite or presumed exposure to ionizing radiation can be triaged based on symptoms and lymphocyte counts. Less than 10% of people vomit if the radiation dose is less than 1 Gy, whereas most vomit if the dose is more than 2 Gy. Onset of emesis in less than 2 h suggests a dose of at least 3 Gy.

Treatment

The threshold for admission on initial presentation will depend on the number of casualties but, in general, patients who do not vomit within 6 h can be managed as outpatients. A useful triage tool for patients without other injuries or chronic illnesses utilizes a combination of the neutrophil/lymphocyte count and the presence of emesis at 4 or more hours post-exposure:

T = N/L + E, where E = 0 if no emesis and E = 2 if emesis.

If T is >3.7, the patient requires admission for further evaluation as the radiation dose is likely >1 Gy.

Supportive treatment includes maintenance of fluid and electrolyte balance, nutritional supplementation, antiemetics, such as ondansetron or granisetron, and antidiarrhoeals. Colony stimulating factors should be commenced as soon as possible if the radiation dose was >3 Gy and be continued until the lymphocyte count reaches 1000/mm^3. Control of infection

commences in the prodromal phase, with identification and aggressive treatment of any potential infection, so that the patient is in optimal condition to survive a period of manifest haemopoietic depression. To reduce the infection risk, patients may be kept home during the latent period and admitted to hospital when neutropaenia develops. Hospital management involves strict isolation and laminar airflow units. The prophylactic administration of antibacterial, antiviral, antifungal and antihelminthic therapy is reserved for the most severely neutropaenic. Non-absorbable agents are commonly used to sterilize the gastrointestinal tract. Anaerobic agents should be included if there is gut injury.

Management of neutropaenia follows the principles established in the management of bone marrow suppression secondary to chemotherapeutic agents. Fever is investigated and managed with empirical therapy in the first instance. If as many as 10% of the stem cells remain intact, the blood cells will repopulate. Platelet transfusion must be commenced early, especially if surgical procedures are required. The role of stem cell transplantation is evolving. Early reintroduction of enteral nutrition is important to maintain gastric acidity and prevent infectious organisms spreading from the gut to the respiratory system. Gastric acidity is maintained by avoiding antacids, H$_2$ blockers and proton pump inhibitors: sucralfate is used for stress ulcer prophylaxis. Povodine-iodine or chlorhexidine is use for skin disinfection and shampoo. Meticulous oral hygiene must be maintained.

Clinical investigations

Acute radiation exposure is confirmed by laboratory investigation. A lymphocyte count of 1000/mm^3 at 24 h suggests a dose of at least 2 Gy and the eventual development of the haemopoietic syndrome. A count of 500/mm^3 suggests a radiation dose of 6 Gy and the subsequent development of both the gastrointestinal and haemopoietic syndromes. If lymphocytes disappear within 6 h, the dose is likely to be fatal.

Lymphocyte counts every 6–12 h for 48 h are useful for admitted patients further to refine the likely dose and clinical course [6].

- No symptoms and lymphocytes >1500/mm^3 after 48 h–unlikely to require clinical support but should be observed periodically.

- Nausea, vomiting, erythema and lymphocytes between 800 and 1500/mm^3 at 48 h–probable serious injury, which will require clinical support.
- Pronounced nausea, vomiting, diarrhoea, erythema and lymphocytes between 100 and 800/mm^3 at 48 h–probable life-threatening injury, which will require maximal clinical support.
- Early vomiting and bloody diarrhoea, erythema and lymphocytes <100/mm^3 at 48 h–lethal injury.

The lymphocyte count may be less useful if there is significant concomitant trauma or at low levels of exposure. A dose-dependent increase in serum amylase is evident after 24 h.

Cytogenetic studies using blood collected at 48 h in a lithium heparin tube examine the number and structure of chromosomes. Radiation dose is reflected in the number of excess acentric and dicentric forms. T lymphocytes are relatively long-lived and reliable dose estimates can be made up to 5 weeks after collection of the sample. A newer method involves electron spin resonance of tooth enamel and can detect very low doses (0.1 Gy).

Prognosis

The LD$_{50/60}$ is the dose at which half the victims succumb within 60 days. Without treatment, the LD$_{50/60}$ is 4 Gy. With supportive care, antibiotics and colony stimulating factors, the LD$_{50/60}$ is almost doubled up to around 7 Gy. Bone marrow transplantation may be used in patients exposed to 8–10 Gy.

Survival from the cardiovascular and neurovascular syndromes does not occur.

Combined injuries

Combined injury occurs when there is additional trauma, either physical or thermal, in addition to the radiation injury. The effects of the radiation exposure may become apparent earlier and may be more severe when other injuries are present. Healing of tissues, including callus formation at fracture sites, will be delayed even with subclinical radiation doses. Radiation exposure increases the probability of mortality when combined with other injuries or pre-existing conditions that result in immunosuppression, blood loss and danger of infectious complications. All administered blood products should be irradiated to remove the T-cell population and minimize graft-versus-host reactions. Platelets should be transfused if the platelet count falls below 20×10^9/L and, if surgery is anticipated, it should be maintained higher than 75×10^9/L. Emergency surgery, including the excision of dead tissue and the closure of wounds, should be completed within 48 h while some white blood cells remain. For thermal burns, early excision of potentially septic tissue and skin grafting are indicated. Wound closure is an important means of reducing vulnerability to infection. Non-urgent surgery should wait until any bone marrow suppression resolves.

Radiation pneumonitis may develop some time following the exposure and be confused with acute respiratory distress syndrome (ARDS).

Local irradiation injuries

The majority of local irradiation injuries occur when operators of X-ray diffraction units inadvertently place their fingers or hands in the direct X-ray beam. Other accidents have occurred when radioactive sources, often from industrial radiography equipment, are detached and then picked up and placed in the pockets of workers. There have been misadministrations of radiation to patients undergoing radiotherapy. The higher the dose, the greater the severity and the earlier the onset of the local injury. The smaller the area irradiated, the higher the dose required to produce a particular change.

Clinical features

Symptoms may include tenderness, itching, tingling and a changed sensitivity to heat and cold. Skin changes include epilation, erythema, dry desquamation, wet desquamation, blisters and radionecrotic lesions. If the area irradiated includes the epigastrium, nausea and vomiting may also occur. The degree of radiosensitivity of the skin depends on the thickness of the epidermis. The most sensitive areas are those that are also moist and subject to friction, such as the axillae, groins and skin folds. The least sensitive areas are the nape of the neck, scalp, palms and soles.

Erythema may not appear for some days. If it occurs within 48 h, the lesion will probably progress to ulceration. If irradiated skin appears normal at 72 h, the lesion is likely to be less severe but may still ulcerate in 1 or 2 weeks. Erythema may be delayed for up to 30 days. Pain is minimal unless ulceration occurs or the dose is extreme. Magnetic resonance imaging (MRI) and Doppler studies may help define the extent of the damage. Late effects include progressive tissue atrophy, fibrosis and chronic radiodermatitis with tissue breakdown. There may be stiffness and tenderness and decreased sensitivity to temperature change.

Treatment

Mild injuries may be simply observed. An effort should be made to protect the area from additional trauma. Topical corticosteroids may help. For more severe injuries, particularly with pain, local debridement and skin grafting may be necessary but should be delayed until the full extent of the lesion is known. Ideally, surgeons experienced in managing chronic vascular disease should be consulted. Amputation is reserved for gangrene. Skin grafts are indicated for areas of exposed cartilage or bone or for severe scarring. Topical antibiotics are often prescribed in an attempt to reduce infection. Vascular therapy with hyperbaric oxygen and pentoxifylline may be useful. In the long term, the irradiated area must be watched for the possible development of neoplastic change.

Occult radiation exposure

Occult exposure to radiation without an explosion might result in unsuspecting patients presenting with delayed symptoms. It should be in the differential diagnosis of the following, especially if associated with a 2- to 3-week prior history of nausea and vomiting:

- unexplained bone marrow suppression (neutropaenia, lymphopaenia and thrombocytopaenia)
- immunological dysfunction with secondary infections
- an unexplained tendency to bleeding
- acute onset of alopecia
- thermal burn-like skin changes or desquamation with no history of thermal injury.

Contamination with radioactive material

The care of individuals who are contaminated with radioactive material requires similar preparation and precautions as for those contaminated with hazardous chemicals. Radioactive contamination has the advantage that it can be readily detected by instruments when on the skin. With the exception of Chernobyl, survivors of radiation accidents have not been sufficiently contaminated so as to pose a threat to emergency or hospital personnel using appropriate precautions and procedures.

Prevention

All staff using shielded or unshielded radiation sources in their daily work must be thoroughly trained in their safe use. Facilities using unshielded radioactive material must have procedures in place to deal with spillage and other accidents and all workers must be adequately trained in emergency procedures.

Preparedness

Emergency equipment must include appropriate monitors for detecting ionizing radiation or contamination, facilities for decontaminating victims and plastic bags for biological and other samples. Appropriate blocking or chelating agents should be stocked at the facility. Emergency planning must include early warning of the receiving hospital so that adequate preparations can be made prior to the arrival of patients.

Scene management

For incidents involving small numbers of patients, members of the rescue team should put on the protective clothing normally used by personnel working with radioactive material at that site. This includes gloves, facemask and cap. Gowns may be covered with large plastic aprons to make them waterproof. Additional measures, such as taping plastic bags over shoes, may be used if the normal protective clothing is judged inadequate. The implementation of life-saving procedures may make it necessary to forgo some of this protection. Contamination of the rescuer will be low and decontamination can be carried out later.

Serious illness or injury is not due to radiation *per se* and should be treated on its own merits. Unless the patient's condition is serious, external decontamination begins at the scene so as to minimize internal contamination and incorporation of the radionuclide into the body tissues and to reduce the risk of contaminating other persons and the hospital environment. As much as 80% of contaminating material may be on the clothing [7]. Accordingly, the victim's outer clothing should be removed at the earliest practicable stage. If monitoring is not available, it should be assumed that all outer clothing is contaminated. Clothing is cut from head to toe and down the sleeves, folded back over itself as it is cut and then rolled up. The person removing the contaminated clothing must wear protective clothing and limit contact with the outside of the victim's clothing. The victim is then wrapped in plain sheets and transferred to hospital. If small contamination spots on the skin cannot be easily removed at the scene, they should be dressed and the victim transported to hospital.

At larger incidents, it may also be necessary to establish a controlled area, the periphery of which is located just beyond the region where contamination is detected above background levels. Rescue team members should wear the maximum level of personal protective equipment available. This should be removed at the perimeter of this area prior to both patient and rescuers leaving. Monitoring of all personnel leaving the area should be undertaken if facilities are available.

Portable vacuum units with high efficiency particulate air filters have reportedly been used to facilitate rapid decontamination outdoors.

Emergency department

The elements of planning for the management of radiation accident patients are similar to those for other types of emergencies, namely prevention, preparedness, response and recovery.

Facilities using unsealed radioactive sources should be identified in advance. These include nuclear medicine departments, scientific laboratories and nuclear facilities. An emergency department (ED) response plan should be developed and emergency response team membership designated. Equipment for monitoring, decontamination and contamination control should be in place. Regular practice is essential [8].

A decontamination area must be designated and be itself capable of adequate decontamination. Ambulant patients and lower acuity stretcher bound patients should be decontaminated outside the ED. Waste water may be legally discharged into normal draining systems if it does not exceed specified limits. In the clinical setting of a few patients, this is unlikely. Incidents involving contaminated or possibly contaminated patients rapidly deplete a receiving hospital's emergency response. If multiple patients with possible contamination are being managed, the hospital may need to defer where possible the arrival of other patients.

Hospital protocols should include plans for dealing with relatives, the press and the public. The timely release of appropriate information is important. Persons issuing this information should be well versed in radiation medicine, as the avoidance of questions and confusion in answers may generate public uncertainty and panic. Security personnel will be required to restrict the entry of unauthorized persons to the treatment area.

Decontamination process

Life-saving procedures resulting from trauma or burns should take priority over consideration of the radiation aspects of the patient's condition, even if preparations to minimize the spread of contamination have not been completed. A radiation physicist with appropriate monitoring equipment should be present in the ED. However, if patients arrive before monitoring is available, treatment of severe injury should proceed immediately and subsequent decisions regarding decontamination should be based on the patient's likely exposure.

In the ideal situation, all patients should be monitored at triage and, if found to be contaminated, those without severe injury should be showered and re-monitored prior to admission to the ED. This is especially so if whole-body contamination has occurred, for example from a gaseous plume from a reactor accident [1]. Washing starts with the hair and works downwards. Patients should bend forward while washing their hair so that any contamination is not washed into their eyes, nose or mouth. Wounds should be covered with a waterproof dressing before showering to avoid washing contaminated water into them.

Because some patients with severe injury will require immediate admission to the ED, adequate preparations are necessary. The floor of the entry and some treatment cubicles should be covered with plastic and any non-essential items removed. Access to this controlled area must be strictly supervised and there should preferably be a buffer zone. Disposable fluid-repellent gowns are ideal but surgical gowns covered by plastic aprons are satisfactory. Lead aprons as used in X-ray departments are not satisfactory; these prevent exposure but not contamination and are heavy and hot to wear. Plastic bags are taped over the shoes and the cuffs of overalls should be taped and secured to the outsides of overshoes. Facemasks are required to protect against airborne contamination but they do not protect the face from being touched by contaminated hands. N95 masks may be superior to standard surgical masks [9]. Trauma masks with clear plastic visors are the best option. Two pairs of gloves should be worn. The inner ones should be surgical gloves taped to the sleeves. The outer gloves are not taped down and should be changed frequently. Hair cover is desirable. Rubbish bins lined with garbage bags serve as waste receptacles and should be emptied promptly to minimize the amount of radiation in the department.

Once the patient is in the controlled area, all clothing should be removed and other medical conditions assessed and treated. Blocking agents can be administered if they have not already been given. All mucosal surfaces should be swabbed to aid in the assessment of likely internal contamination. These include nostrils and ears, the mouth and rectum. The swabs should be placed in sealed labelled plastic bags and sent for radiation assessment and identification of the chemicals involved. Blood samples should be drawn for a baseline complete blood count, differential and absolute lymphocyte counts and later cytogenic analysis. A serum amylase is also important as the parotid is very sensitive to radiation.

External decontamination utilizes the principles of barrier nursing and contamination control. Staff should stand back from the patient except when actually examining them or performing procedures. Radiation exposure is inversely proportional to the distance from the source squared. Hospital personnel should be rotated during the decontamination procedure to minimize the perceived risk to any one individual. Pregnant staff should not be involved. Each staff member should shower following completion of their turn in decontamination.

The priority areas for external decontamination are wounds and orifices, as it is through these that the risk of subsequent internal contamination is greatest. Other priority areas include the hands, face and head, as early contamination removal reduces spread. Decontamination of intact skin is the last priority.

Wounds are decontaminated in the same manner as when removing dirt or bacteria. Deeper wounds should be opened up and thoroughly irrigated. Burnt areas also should be carefully irrigated. Metal fragments should be removed with forceps. Deep debridement and excision of a wound is rarely necessary in extreme cases where highly toxic material is embedded in the tissues. Decontamination efforts should continue until the radiation level is at background levels or there is minimal reduction with further washing.

The mouth is decontaminated by gentle irrigation and frequent rinsing with 30%

hydrogen peroxide solution. Brushing of the teeth with toothpaste is helpful, as toothpaste contains chelating agents. External ear canals should be irrigated and nasal douches can be effective. The eyes are rinsed by directing a stream of water or saline from the inner canthus to the outer canthus, so that material is not forced into the lacrimal duct. Hair should be shampooed several times with the head deflected backwards over a basin to keep water from the eyes and ears. A hair dryer is used to dry the hair. Clipping of hair may occasionally be necessary.

The skin is washed initially with warm water and mild soap. If this is ineffective, 0.5% hypochlorite or stronger detergents can be used. If the skin becomes damaged or red and sore, cleansing should be discontinued. If contamination is only discovered after patients are admitted to an ED, the entire area through which they have passed should be taped off, surveyed with the help of a radiation physicist and, if necessary, decontaminated. Staff should put on protective clothing and remove nearby patients so as to create a spacious treatment area. Following a radiation incident, all equipment, instruments and work areas used in treating contaminated patients must be thoroughly cleaned.

Monitoring decontamination

Radiation physicists should check the background level of radiation in the ED from time to time so that they have a baseline from which to assess each patient's exposure. Scanning should occur slowly to avoid missing radiation. Headphones should be used or the sound turned off to avoid alarming patients.

Internal contamination

Internal contamination causes no acute clinical effects and it is usually not feasible to confirm its presence before commencing treatment directed at the reduction of absorption, prevention of incorporation into tissues and promotion of elimination. Significant internal contamination has traditionally occurred through wounds or body orifices in small-scale accidents. It could readily occur on a wider scale following the explosion of an RDD, a reactor accident or a nuclear detonation. Absorption would be by inhalation of contaminated air and/or ingestion of foodstuffs contaminated by fallout. Radionuclides which have short effective half-lives, such as technetium used in nuclear medicine ($t_{1/2} = 5\,h$), pose no danger. For isotopes with effective half-lives measured in days, the decision to treat will depend on the likely intake especially via the lungs, whether the drug is concentrated in tissue, such as iodine in the thyroid or uranium or americium in bone, whether the emission is high energy as with cobalt and whether the chemical itself is toxic. The effective half-life combines radioactive and chemical properties and describes the rate of elimination without decontamination.

Table 28.4.1 describes the radioisotopes most likely to be available in Australia, their common uses, emissions, toxicity, effective half-life and treatment.

To assist in the determination of the extent of internal contamination a 24-h urine sample should be collected. If gastrointestinal contamination is suspected a 24-h stool sample should also be collected.

Selection of the appropriate technique or drug depends on knowledge of the radionuclide involved and its physical form [10]. For example, uranium is found in order of increasing radioactivity in depleted uranium used in artillery shells, natural uranium, fuel rods and weapons grade enriched uranium. The first two are not significant radiation hazards but the latter two can emit significant levels of gamma radiation if sufficient quantity is present.

Uptake by the various organs can be reduced by the use of blocking agents, dilution techniques or chelating agents.

Administration of stable iodine in the form of potassium iodate or potassium iodide tablets will reduce uptake by the thyroid gland by up to 90% if given less than 2 h after intake and by about 50% if in less than 3 h. Chelating agents and mobilizing agents may be useful for up to 2 weeks. Mobilizing agents, such as antithyroid drugs, increase the natural rate of turnover of a biological molecule and thereby increase excretion. Gastrointestinal decontamination is unusual but an enema might be used to empty the bowel. In the absence of external contamination, this would be the only circumstance in which internal contamination posed any risk to hospital staff.

Table 28.4.1	Isotopes likely to cause internal contamination in Australia						
Element	Emissions	Primary toxicity	Effective $t_{1/2}$[a]	Common use	Detection[b]	Absorption	Treatment
Americium[241]	Alpha Gamma	Marrow suppression	Years	Smoke detector	Yes	Lung, skin	DTPA or EDTA IV
Caesium[137]	Beta Gamma	Whole body irradiation	70 days	Medical radiology	Yes	Lung. GI tract, wounds	Prussian blue orally
Cobalt[60]	Gamma Beta	Whole body irradiation	10 days	Medical radiology Commercial food irradiation	Yes	Lung	Penicillamine orally
Iodine[131]	Beta Some gamma	Thyroid	8 days	Nuclear medicine therapy	Yes	Lung	Iodine orally[c]
Tritium[3]	Beta	No significant hazard	12 days	Signs	No	Lung[d]	Increase fluids
Uranium[235/238]	Alpha	Kidney	Can be permanent in bone	Fuel rods for reactors[e]	Yes	Lung	NaHCO$_3$ Tubular diuretics

[a]Effective half-life combines radioactive and chemical properties and describes rates of elimination without decontamination.
[b]Detection by standard radiation detection equipment.
[c]Iodine dose in adults 130 mg daily.
[d]Tritium is not a significant radiation hazard except perhaps in closed spaces.
[e]Natural and depleted uranium are not serious irradiation threats. GI: gastrointestinal.

Likely developments over the next 5–10 years

- The cumulative effects on patients of low-dose radiation from repeated diagnostic examinations is receiving much attention in the medical literature as they are by far the largest source of radiation exposure from human activity. Critically appraising the need for complex and repeated examinations and utilizing imaging algorithms to select the most appropriate modality are increasingly important.

- Just as much was learnt about the effects of radiation from studies of the survivors on the Chernobyl accident and Japanese atomic bombs, more will no doubt be learnt by following the survivors of the Fukushima nuclear accident. The high incidence of non-radiation related death following the evacuations requires further analysis.

- Biodosimetry using multiple parameters, such as percentage of patients who develop emesis, median onset of emesis, the absolute lymphocyte count as a percentage of normal in the first 24 hours, relative increase in amylase day 1 and the number of dicentrics per 50 metaphases, can improve the estimate of radiation dose. Cytogenic dosimetry using multiple chromosomal parameters takes time, although automated machines can speed the process. Dose estimates can also be calculated from cytokinesis block micronucleus assays which are quicker to perform; premature chromosome condensation which is better when higher radiation doses are involved; electron paramagnetic resonance of teeth the effectiveness of which has been well demonstrated; and a range of molecular markers which offer exciting possibilities to expand multiparametric assays.

- Dose reconstruction from a small source is the gamma constant multiplied by the activity of the source, times the amount of time spent near the source divided by the square of the person's distance from the source in metres. Dose reconstruction from a larger source utilizes computer modelling to predict exposure rates at various places combined with real time environmental radiation measurements to determine each person's likely exposure.

- The specialists most used to managing inpatients with acute radiation illness are oncologists and haematologists. Advances in care in these specialties are likely to improve the treatment available when the number of patients is low.

- The most effective life-saving opportunity in the first 60 min following a nuclear explosion will be to shelter people safely in possible fallout areas in the nearest basement or in the middle of buildings, but not in cars. This is called sheltering in place. In most cases, effective self-decontamination can be performed if straightforward instructions are provided.

- The most important isotopes in relation to terrorism and industrial accidents are:
  - the University seven: H-3 (tritium), C^{14}, P^{32}, Co^{60}, I^{125}, I^{131} and Cf^{252}
  - industrial three: Ir^{192}, Cs^{137} and Co^{60}
  - military four: tritium, U^{235}, Pu^{239} and Am^{241}.

References

[1] Swindon T. Manual on the medical management of individuals involved in radiation accidents. Australian Radiation Laboratory; 1991.

[2] Ricks RC. Guidance for radiation accident management. Radiation Emergency Assistance Centre/Training Site (REAC/TS) Oak Ridge Institute for Science and Education; 2002.

[3] Levi M, Kelly H. Weapons of mass disruption. Sci Am 2002;287:77–81.

[4] Beir V. National Research Council Health effects of exposure to low levels of ionizing radiation. Washington, DC: National Academy Press; 1990.

[5] Berger M, Christensen D, Lowry P, et al. Medical management of radiation injuries: current approaches. Occupat Med 2006;56:162–72.

[6] Anno GH, Baum SJ, Withers HR, et al. Symptomatology of acute radiation effects in humans after exposure to doses of 0.5–30 Gray. Hlth Phys 1989;56:821–38.

[7] Hugner KF, Fry SA, editors. The medical basis for radiation accident preparedness. New York: Elsevier; 1980.

[8] Fong F, Schrader DC. Radiation disasters and emergency department preparedness. Emerg Med Clin N Am 1996;14:349–70.

[9] Sansom G. Emergency department personal protective equipment requirements following out-of-hospital chemical, biological or radiological events in Australasia. Emerg Med Australas 2007;19:86–95.

[10] Zarzycki W, Zonenberg A, Telejko B, et al. Iodide prophylaxis in the aftermath of the Chernobyl accident in the area of Senjy in north-eastern Poland. Hormone Metabol Res 1994;26:293–6.

Further reading

Armed Forces Radiobiology Research Institute. Medical management of radiological casualties, 3rd ed. Bethesda, MD: 2010. <http://www.afrri.usuhs.mil>.

Daly F, Inglis T, Mark P, Robertson A. Protocols for the hospital management of chemical, biological, radiological and explosive incidents. Perth: Western Australian Department of Health; 2010.

Radiation Emergency Action Centre/Training Site. <www.orau.gov/reacts>.

US Centre for Disease Control and Prevention. <www.bt.cdc.gov/radiation>.

US Department of Health & Human Services. Radiation emergency medical management. Guidance on diagnosis and treatment for health care providers. <http://www.remm.nlm.gov/>.

US Department of Homeland Security. Planning guidance for response to a nuclear detonation, 2nd ed. Federal Emergency Management Agency; 2010. <http://www.usuhs.edu/afrri/outreach/pdf/planning-guidance2010.pdf>.

ENVIRONMENTAL EMERGENCIES

28.5 Drowning

David Mountain

ESSENTIALS

1 The incidence of non-fatal drowning requiring medical assessment is estimated to be 2 to 20 times greater than fatal drowning.

2 The highest rates of drowning occur in children from 1 to 4 years of age and young adult males. Alcohol or intoxicants are associated with many adult deaths.

3 10–20% of fatal drownings have minimal aspiration with asphyxia probably due to laryngospasm, shunting and mucus plug formation. Experimental differences between fresh- and salt-water drowning have been demonstrated but are unimportant for management.

4 Hypothermia following warm-water (>10°C) drowning carries a very poor prognosis. Hypothermia following cold-water (<5 (<10)°C) drowning sometimes allows intact neurological outcome even after very prolonged resuscitation.

5 Initiation of good-quality CPR, with assisted ventilation being the essential component (e.g. aBc), within 10 min of witnessed drowning or any attempts at breathing before hospital arrival are associated with better outcomes. Initial management on the side for airway drainage is recommended in the spontaneously breathing but active lung drainage procedures and the Heimlich manoeuvre are contraindicated.

6 Positive end-expiratory pressure/continuous positive airway pressure are useful therapies in hospital. Newer therapies, such as artificial surfactant and inhaled nitric oxide, have so far shown equivocal results. Therapeutic hypothermia is recommended after arrests and extracorporeal membrane oxygenation is being used more frequently for severe lung injury.

Introduction

Australia, the driest inhabited continent, has one of the highest reported incidences of drowning in the developed world. It is a major cause of death in those under 30 years of age with peaks in young children and young adult males. Nomenclature and definitions are now generally agreed with all respiratory distress (of any level, e.g. cough, wheeze, etc.) from immersion or submersion defined as drowning (fatal or non-fatal).

Good outcomes are mainly determined by pre-hospital factors, particularly witnessed drowning, early cardiopulmonary resuscitation (CPR) (and patient response to CPR) and early access to emergency services. However, an accurate history, well-run resuscitation and informed judgement on prognosis will optimize outcomes, resource use and aid management of the patient and their family. Patients with spontaneous respiration and/or neurological responsiveness on arrival in the emergency department (ED) are expected to recover unless severe lung injury/acute respiratory distress syndrome (ARDS) supervenes. Treatment after recovering from a non-fatal drowning is mainly supportive, although therapeutic hypothermia and possibly extracoporeal membrane oxygenation (ECMO) may potentially improve outcomes in the future.

In many groups/regions, preventative and educative measures have reduced fatality rates dramatically in the last 20 years. Emergency physicians should be strong advocates of these initiatives.

Epidemiology

Overall, there is a marked preponderance of male over female deaths from drowning and, in adults, the ratio has been reported as high as 9:1. This ratio seems to have declined in recent years with fewer male deaths and drownings being reported. Groups with high rates of drowning include: infants (particularly males), young adult males (15–30 years), epileptics (up to 20 × higher), overseas visitors, the mentally retarded and those from deprived/underresourced communities with poor public health initiatives. In young adult males, bravado, inexperience and alcohol lead to many deaths. Alcohol is found in 14–50% of adult drownings and the majority of male adult drownings are related to recreational activities in some series. In the elderly, underlying medical illnesses and suicide attempts are common causative factors. Most of these factors (except age) are associated with worse outcomes. Cold water is associated with worse outcomes overall (shorter time to submersion in icy waters), although some younger patients may survive very prolonged immersions when they rapidly cool their brains.

The ratio of those who initially survive (but require medical attention) to fatal drownings is not accurately known because of differences in nomenclature, definitions and the inability to collect all attendances related to drowning, but is estimated at between 2 and 20:1. In a well-conducted observational study from the Netherlands, the ratio of patients admitted to the intensive care unit (ICU) following drowning compared to those who died before admission was 2:1.

Prevention

Prevention of drowning is a major area for ongoing research and it is important that emergency physicians act as advocates for preventative strategies of proven benefit.

Patrolled beaches and early, good quality CPR with early assisted breathing are associated with better outcomes. Important public educational initiatives include early swimming lessons/survival techniques, beach safety and patrolled water areas and beaches, CPR training, protective fencing, parental supervision of children, raising public awareness of the dangers of mixing alcohol and water activities and wearing of life vests and appropriate safety equipment. Enforcement of alcohol laws on the water and safety regulations pertaining to providers of water activities are also important.

Definitions and terminology

Much confusion has been caused in research and management by imprecise drowning definitions. Phrases commonly used have been near-drowning, dry, wet, active, passive or silent, late or secondary drowning, immersion, submersion, suffocation and asphyxia. Modell historically gave succinct definitions with drowning defined as death due to suffocation (asphyxia) after submersion in a liquid medium then further divided into 'dry' or 'wet', depending on the presence or absence of aspirated fluid in the lungs. Near-drowning was defined as survival of any length after suffocation (asphyxia) due to submersion in a liquid medium.

In 2002, ILCOR (International Liaison Committee on Resuscitation) provided updated and internationally agreed Utstein style nomenclature for drowning. The system simplifies the definition of drowning to '… a process resulting in primary respiratory impairment from submersion/immersion in a liquid medium'. Implicit in this definition is that a liquid/air interface is present at the entrance of the victim's airway, preventing the victim from freely breathing.

The distinction between 'near-drowning' and 'drowning' is redundant as all are drowning events, irrespective of the outcome Similarly, there is no distinction between 'wet' and 'dry' drownings; all drowning is wet by definition and just have differing degrees of aspiration. Descriptions of 'active' and 'passive' or 'silent' drowning (determined by bystander descriptions of activity) have been replaced by 'witnessed' and 'unwitnessed' drowning, defined according to whether or not entry to the water was observed. The term 'secondary drowning' was used to describe both problems causing drowning (e.g. intoxication, injury, illness, etc.) or death after drowning due to secondary problems (e.g. lung problems, hypoxic encephalopathy, etc.) and this description was inherently confusing. Therefore, associated precipitating factors and sequelae should be specifically described as such. Immersion describes any situation when the patient is unable to maintain a fluid-free air interface while submersion implies the whole airway is underwater.

Pathophysiology

The sequential pathophysiology of drowning is well described:

- Initial submersion or significant immersion leads to voluntary apnoea except where drowning is due to initial loss of consciousness, e.g. congenital prolonged QT syndrome or other catastrophic illness. Unless submersion is voluntary, most adult victims panic and struggle, with spitting or expulsion of fluid from nasal and oral cavities with associated increases in blood pressure (BP) and pulse rate (PR). Slow PR may occur secondary to primitive dive reflexes or cold-induced reflex bradyarrhythmias, particularly in children or adults affected by alcohol and particularly so in cold water and late in drownings.

- After an interval dependent on presubmersion oxygenation, intoxication, injuries, illness, fitness and the degree of panic and struggle, synergistic hypercapnia and hypoxia lead to an involuntary breath known as the 'breaking point', which is normally reached in under a minute. During this stage, large quantities of water are often swallowed. If an individual hyperventilates before diving, plasma CO_2 concentrations may remain so low that unconsciousness from hypoxia occurs before the breaking point is reached.

- The initial inhalation of fluid causes sudden increases in airway pressures, bronchoconstriction, pulmonary hypertension and shunting. In 10–20% laryngospasm reduces further aspiration, with a mucus and foam plug forming (previously called 'dry drowning').

- Secondary apnoea occurs and is closely followed by loss of consciousness.

- Involuntary gasping respirations lead to flooding of the lungs and alveolar injury, surfactant loss, increased ventilation/perfusion (V/Q) mismatch, shunting and hypoxia. Vomiting of swallowed fluid is common and frequently results in pulmonary aspiration.

- Hypoxia causes marked bradycardia, hypotension and irreversible brain injury within 3–10 min (except occasionally in icy water induced rapid hypothermia) culminating in cardiorespiratory arrest. In fatal drownings, the average fluid quantity retrieved is 3–4 mL/kg, less than 10% of total lung volume. However, the effect on the lungs is dramatic. Experimentally, fresh water and sea water cause alveolar injury by different mechanisms. Fresh water denatures surfactant and damages the alveolar cells. Sea water tends to draw in fluid, wash out surfactant and cause foam formation. The aspiration of vomitus and/or chemicals further complicates the clinical picture. Soap and chlorine in water do not appear to affect outcome. Clinically, the type of fluid inhaled rarely makes a difference, unless grossly polluted. Electrolyte disturbances are normally minimal and transient except in prolonged arrests, owing to the small volumes aspirated (more than 20 mL/kg are required for major disturbances).

Clinical features and organ-specific effects

Lungs/airways

The major features are intense laryngospasm, bronchospasm, pulmonary hypertension and marked V/Q mismatch with physiological shunt. Even in patients without overt respiratory embarrassment after near drowning, shunts of up to 70% may occur and take up to a week to resolve. In the alveoli, there is surfactant loss, formation of protein-rich exudate and alveolar cell injury, often exacerbated by pneumonitis from gastric aspiration, chemicals and secondary infection (seen in up to 15% of intubated patients). These changes markedly reduce pulmonary compliance and oxygen transfer. The importance of the pulmonary insult in determining outcomes are seen by the fact that level of lung involvement from full cardiopulmonary arrest through different amounts of respiratory distress, down to cough or asymptomatic patients clearly stratify death and morbidity (Table 28.5.1).

Brain

The major effects on the brain are secondary to hypoxia and are the major cause of death in drownings. Cerebral oedema, convulsions and persistent vegetative states are all observed all too frequently. The possibility of trauma or an underlying medical complaint should be considered in the differential diagnosis of an altered mental state especially in unwitnessed events, drowning involving water transport or motor vehicles, the intoxicated and the elderly.

Table 28.5.1 Grading of drowning severity–pre-hospital based on cardiorespiratory status

Drowning grade	Dead	Grade 6	Grade 5	Grade 4	Grade 3	Grade 2	Grade 1	Rescue
Submersion time	>1 h/unknown	<1 h						
Signs at scene/ rescue	Clearly dead	No pulse No breaths	Pulse No breaths	Rales–all fields Hypotension	Rales–all fields BP normal	Rales–some BP normal	Cough only	No signs
Mortality rate (%)	100	88–93	31–44	18–22	4–5	1	0	0%
Management	Transport	CPR–ABC resus	Rescue ventilation	O₂–prob ETT	O₂–poss ETT	O₂	Check nil other probs	Nil required
Expected level of care	Forensic	ICU	ICU	ICU	HDU–ICU	ED review	Scene first aid	Nil required

CPR: cardiopulmonary resuscitation; ICU: intensive care unit; ETT: ; HDU: high-dependency unit.
Modified from Szpilman D, Bierens JJLM, Handley AJ, Orlowski JP. Drowning. N Engl J Med 2012;366:2102–10 with permission.

Table 28.5.2 Modell/Conn classification of mental status following drowning

Grade	Description of mental status	Equivalent GCS	Expected Likelihood of good outcome (neurologically intact) (%)
A	Awake/alert	14–15	100
B	Blunted	8–13	100
C	Comatose	6–7	>90
C1	Decerebrate	5	>90
C2	Decorticate	4	>90
C3/4	Flaccid coma or arrest	3	<20

GCS: Glasgow coma scale.

The severity of hypoxic brain injury is a major determinant predicting survival from out of hospital arrest from drowning (Table 28.5.2).

Cardiovascular

Most drowning patients are haemodynamically stable after resuscitation. Hypothermic patients may develop any arrhythmia and should be gently handled and aggressively rewarmed (see Chapter 28.2 Hypothermia). In older patients, underlying ischaemic heart disease should be considered. Congenital long QT syndrome may be associated with arrhythmia in some cold-water immersions.

Haematological

Haemolysis occurs occasionally in fresh-water drownings [8].

Renal

Acute tubular necrosis or tubular injury from hypoxia may occur. Electrolyte disturbances are rarely significant.

Gastrointestinal

Vomiting is frequently observed (up to 80% in some series). It is secondary to ingestion of large volumes of water, potentially aggravated by poor resuscitation techniques and positioning, often leading to aspiration. Diarrhoea is less frequent except with grossly polluted water. Hypoxic gut injury may contribute to late multiorgan failure, ARDS and potential sepsis.

Orthopaedic

Cervical spine injury should always be considered and excluded in drownings related to diving injuries. Coexistent trauma may complicate recreational drowning particularly if alcohol, water sports or boating related.

Treatment

Pre-hospital

Hypoxia (particularly brain hypoxia) is the major cause of almost all early mortality and

morbidity and many late problems. Rapid institution of effective pre-hospital care, particularly supplemented (or exhaled responder) breathing/oxygenation (potentially in water if expert providers, e.g. surf lifesavers) and rapid emergency service activation are the most important factors in determining good outcome following drowning. All patients seen alive within 1 h of removal from cold water (<5–10°C) should be transported for definitive care. The level of pre-hospital care varies with the clinical severity of the case (see Table 25.8.1), ranging from asymptomatic (the majority) to cardiopulmonary arrest. Initial assessment of the ABCs may be done with the patient on their side to assist airway fluid drainage followed by institution of cardiopulmonary resuscitation (with an ABC emphasis) if respirations or pulse are absent. There is little role for in-water resuscitation except in deepwater retrievals on patrolled beaches with properly equipped expert retrievers who can get to shore easily. Lung drainage procedures (e.g. abdominal compressions) and the Heimlich manoeuvre are dangerous as they increase gastric aspiration. The Heimlich manoeuvre is only indicated for removal of a clearly inhaled foreign body and has no real place in drownings. The priority in drowning is to re-initiate breathing and, in drowning arrests, A and B are priorities. In particular, rescue breathing (or bagging if available) are obligatory (2 breaths with good chest movement before CPR). Additional breaths, up to 5, may be required if there is initial inadequate chest movement because of poor lung compliance with large fluid aspiration. Victims often vomit upon resumption of spontaneous respiration and obtunded, spontaneously breathing patients should be transported on their side to minimize the risk of aspiration. Wet clothing should be removed and the patient wrapped/ covered to minimize further heat loss. If associated neck trauma is likely, the cervical spine should be immobilized. All symptomatic patients should be given supplemental high-flow oxygen. Early access to emergency medical systems is essential to minimize time to definitive care. A person with knowledge of the patient or witness to the drowning should be encouraged to go directly to the hospital or travel in the ambulance and, if not, a clear history taken and documented from bystanders.

Emergency department

History

Important factors in the history of arrested drowning include, environment of drowning and potential associated factors, e.g. water temperature, duration of submersion (or the time since last seen), time to institution of CPR, quality of CPR and response to first assisted breaths and/or CPR, time of first spontaneous breath or return of spontaneous cardiac output, initial Glasgow coma scale (GCS) and GCS after resuscitation recorded in Utstein style if possible. A collateral history regarding previous health problems (including psychiatric issues), use of alcohol and drugs, occurrence of vomiting and likelihood of associated trauma is also useful.

Initial resuscitation

Initial assessment and resuscitation, continuing the priorities established in the pre-hospital setting, is directed towards the assessment and maintenance of ABCs. Monitoring should include oximetry, capnometry, cardiac rhythm, blood pressure (BP) and core temperature (urinary or rectal probes are fine).

Airway management may initially simply involve clearing and positioning the airway and the provision of supplemental oxygen via a non-rebreathing mask. Endotracheal intubation is indicated if respiration is ineffective, saturations poor or lung fields are full of rales or the patient is comatose. Patients who cannot maintain a PaO_2 greater than 90 mmHg on a non-rebreathing mask should be considered for early intubation, although continuous positive airway pressure (CPAP) ventilation is a potential alternative in the cooperative patient. Persistent rales in significant portions of the lung fields are a marker of a high risk for later severe respiratory compromise and potential

ARDS. Patients with bronchospasm should be treated with nebulized β-agonists, with the use of steroids controversial unless the patient is a known asthmatic. In the unconscious patient, a nasogastric tube should be placed early after intubation to minimize the risk of pulmonary aspiration. All intubated patients require early positive end-expiratory pressure (PEEP) and end-tidal CO_2 monitoring.

Cardiac complications should be managed according to standard treatment regimens except in patients with core temperatures less than 33°C. Hypothermic patients (see Chapter 28.2 Hypothermia) must be handled gently and antiarrhythmic drugs avoided if possible until rewarming has occurred. All rhythms without output require CPR. In general, asystole following drowning has the same dire prognosis as from other causes, particularly if still present after adequate resuscitation in the field. However, cold-water arrests (particularly in younger patients) do have occasional very good outcomes after very prolonged (60+ min) resuscitations. Hypotension is managed with early inotropes and judicious (e.g. small bolus) fluids, together with invasive monitoring if required. This is particularly important in patients with pulmonary oedema.

The management of hypothermia is described elsewhere in this book (see Chapter 28.2). Where cervical spine injury is a distinct possibility (especially following diving and water/motor vehicle accidents), cervical spine immobilization should be maintained until the injury can be excluded radiologically or clinically.

Ongoing management

Patients who require intubation, especially if pulmonary changes are present on chest X-ray, should be given PEEP. Commence with low pressures (5–7.5 cm H_2O) and then increase until adequate oxygenation is achieved or hypotension or high airway pressures prevent further increases. Pressure-controlled ventilation may be added but may increase barotrauma and alveolar injury. Use should be discussed with the intensive care unit (ICU) that will be managing the ongoing care. These modalities improve outcome for near-drowning patients with secondary lung injury. Ventilatory weaning should begin as soon as possible after 24 h in order to minimize the risk of barotrauma. Maintenance of normoglycaemia, normovolaemia, normocarbia, seizure control and avoiding hyperthermia, hypoxia and hypotension are important in optimizing cerebral

outcomes. Dehydration and prolonged hyperventilation are dangerous. Induced hypothermia post-arrest from drowning has been an area of some controversy (see below), but is recommended by expert consensus.

Experimental therapies

A number of other therapeutic modalities have been trialled in an effort to improve the outcome of lung and brain injuries caused by near-drowning. These include the following:

- Induced hypothermia. Popularized by Conn, this therapy offers the theoretical advantage of cerebral protection. Unfortunately, drowning patients were actively excluded from trials of therapeutic hypothermia, ironically because this group had shown the most likely benefit already from environmental hypothermia! Induced hypothermia trials after cardiac arrest from ventricular fibrillation (VF) have renewed interest in this area with induced hypothermia being a Level 1A recommendation. As drownings tend to both be primarily asystolic/PEA arrests and with little prospective trial data, current recommendations are expert consensus only but *do* recommend therapeutic hypothermia in resuscitated drowning arrests (after initial rewarming if hypothermic).
- Pharmacological cerebral protection. Barbiturate infusions, steroids, magnesium and chlorpromazine have all been trialled. None has been shown to be of benefit and all may have deleterious effects.
- Intracranial pressure monitoring. Its use is controversial and lacking in outcome data and depends on which ICU cares for the patient.
- Prophylactic antibiotics. These are of no value except following drowning in grossly polluted water. In such cases, a second-generation cephalosporin is recommended. Drownings in hot spas and tubs may require anti-pseudomonal cover.
- Hyperbaric oxygen therapy and nitric oxide therapy are of unproven benefit.
- Exogenous surfactant therapy. Has no proven benefit and some animal research has suggested it may increase lung injury.
- Extracorporeal oxygenation. Has been used successfully in some centres for severe lung injury, particularly in hypothermic children. It may be used to bridge drowning related ARDS which should be more reversible than inflammatory ARDS.

Clinical investigations

Ordering of investigations in the ED is guided by the clinical status of the patient, in particular, mental and cardiorespiratory status. All patients require continuous pulse oximtery and a chest X-ray which should be repeated at 4–6 h. Using the Modell/Conn classification of mental status (see Table 28.5.2), patients in group A only require a chest X-ray and oximetry. Patients in group B may also require a full blood count, electrolytes and creatinine, blood sugar, arterial blood gases and an ECG. If they do not improve rapidly after arrival and supplemental oxygen, they should be investigated and managed like group C patients. Patients in group C should also have liver function tests, creatine kinase and troponin at 6 h, coagulation profile, alcohol levels and possibly a drug screen, urine dipstick and microscopy, along with a computed tomography (CT) scan and possibly other imaging of the head if coma persists. Cervical spine X-rays and other trauma films are indicated if trauma is likely. Intracranial pressure monitoring, EEGs, MRI and brain injury markers are not really part of ED care and should be left to ICU discretion.

Prognosis

Mortality rates of 15–30% and persistent severe neurological deficit rates of up to 25% are reported in series of patients admitted to hospital following drowning events (but these studies are highly selected). Patients with prolonged cardiac arrests and poor initial response have a very high rate of mortality and persistent vegetative states (see Tables 28.5.1 and 28.5.2). Patients with relatively good GCS but with persistent hypoxia, early recovery from arrest and/or persistent rales are at high risk of secondary lung injury and multiorgan failure and have relatively high mortality rates (persistent rales 4–5%–recovered arrest 40%).

Potential prognostic features in drowning have been extensively evaluated in an effort to reduce the number of neurovegetative survivors, avoid prolonged CPR and to provide relatives and medical personnel with early accurate prognostic information. The most useful predictors of neurological outcome relate to the initial resuscitation (field predictors). Factors associated with good outcome include witnessed drowning, time to retrieval of less than 5 min, good-quality CPR provided within 10 min, a first spontaneous breath within 30 min of retrieval from the water and early return of spontaneous circulation before arrival at hospital. The last two are often associated with good neurological outcome, provided secondary lung injury does not supervene. Pre-hospital factors associated with poor outcome include male sex, unwitnessed or prolonged submersion, prolonged arrests (particularly asystole), fresh-water drownings, cold-water submersions and prolonged resuscitation before arrival at hospital. However, absolute field predictors of poor outcome have not been identified and all patients who arrive in the ED following drowning deserve full resuscitation efforts, short of clear signs of prolonged death (e.g. lividity, rigor) or clearly unsurvivable combination of prognostic features.

Emergency department prognostic factors have also been identified, but again no combination of factors reliably predicts all patients who will do badly. Features suggesting good outcomes in ED are pupillary response on arrival, perfusing cardiac rhythm on arrival or any motor response to pain on arrival. Asystole (particularly if the initial rhythm in the field and a significant pre-hospital time) is predictive of very poor outcome and, except in paediatric/young adults in ice-water drownings, should lead to early cessation of CPR in the ED. Hypothermia *per se*, has been described as a favourable prognostic indicator but is debatable. Although this may be true following near drowning of children or younger adults in ice-cold water with shorter immersion times (e.g. rapid brain cooling has occurred), hypothermia is generally a marker of prolonged submersion and, as such, is associated with a poor prognosis in most cases.

In-hospital factors associated with poor outcome include Glasgow coma score less than 5 on transfer to intensive care (less than 20% intact survival–see Table 28.5.2), fixed dilated pupils at 24 h (if not hypothermic) and any abnormality on CT scan in the first 36 h. However, a normal CT scan is of no prognostic value.

Disposition

All drowning victims requiring ED assessment should be carefully observed for a minimum of 6 h. Monitoring during that time should include pulse oximetry. Any patient with an abnormal chest X-ray or widespread respiratory rales or significant hypoxaemia after 6 h should be admitted with strong consideration for HDU/ICU environments. Those requiring intubation, with a history of cardiorespiratory arrest, persistently altered mental status or significant hypoxaemia require intensive care. Truly asymptomatic patients or non-progressive rales with stable oximetry, may be discharged home after 6 h of observation, but should be instructed to return to hospital if they develop worsening respiratory symptoms.

Further reading

Australian Resuscitation Council, Guideline 8.7 resuscitation of the drowning victim. <http://www.resus.org.au/public/ guidelines/section_8/resuscitation_of_drowning_victim. htm> [Accessed Sept. 2007].

Conn AW, Montes JE, Barker GA, et al. Cerebral salvage in near-drowning following neurological classification by triage. Can Anaesth Soc J 1980;27:211–21.

Driscoll TR, Harrison JA, Steenkamp M. Review of the role of alcohol in drowning associated with recreational aquatic activity. Inj Prev 2004;10:107–13.

Hoek TLV, Morrison LJ, Shuster M, et al. Part 12: cardiac arrest in special situations. 2010 American heart association guidelines for cardiopulmonary resuscitation and emergency cardiovascular care. Circulation 2010;122 (18 suppl 3):S829–61.

Idris AH, Berg RA, Bierens JJ, et al. Recommended guidelines for uniform reporting of data from drowning. Circulation 2003;108:2565–74.

Modell JH, Graves SA, Kuck EJ. Near-drowning: correlation of level of consciousness and survival. Can Anaesth Soc J 1980; 27:211–5.

Quan L, Kinder D. Paediatric submersions: prehospital predictors of outcome. Pediatrics 1992;90:909–13.

Report of the new South wales chief health officer 2006: injury and poisoning; drowning deaths and hospitalizations. <http://www.health.nsw.gov.au/public->.

Szpilman D, Bierens JJLM, Handley AJ, Orlowski JP. Drowning. N Engl J Med 2012;366:2102–10.

Szpilman D. Near-drowning and drowning classification: a proposal to stratify mortality based on the analysis of 1831 cases. Chest 1997;112:660–5.

Topjian AA, Berg RA, Bierens JJLM, et al. Brain resuscitation in the drowning victim. Neurocrit Care 2012;17:441–67.

WHO. A new definition of drowning: towards documentation and prevention of a global public health problem [Internet]. WHO. [cited 2012 Dec 31]. <http://www.who.int/bulletin/ volumes/83/11/vanbeeck1105abstract/en/>.

28.6 Electric shock and lightning injury

Daniel Fatovich

ESSENTIALS

1 Death from electric shock is due to ventricular fibrillation, the lethal arrhythmia occurring at the time of the exposure. Routine admission for ECG monitoring is unnecessary.

2 Most deaths are caused by low-voltage (<1000V) exposures.

3 The amount of current passing through the body is determined mainly by tissue resistance, which is dramatically reduced by moisture.

4 Electrical injury resembles a crush injury more than a burn. The tissue damage below skin level is invariably more severe than the cutaneous wound would suggest.

5 There is a diversity of clinical manifestations seen with electrical injury.

6 Lightning injury is different from high-voltage electrical injury and has a unique range of clinical features. The management is predominantly expectant.

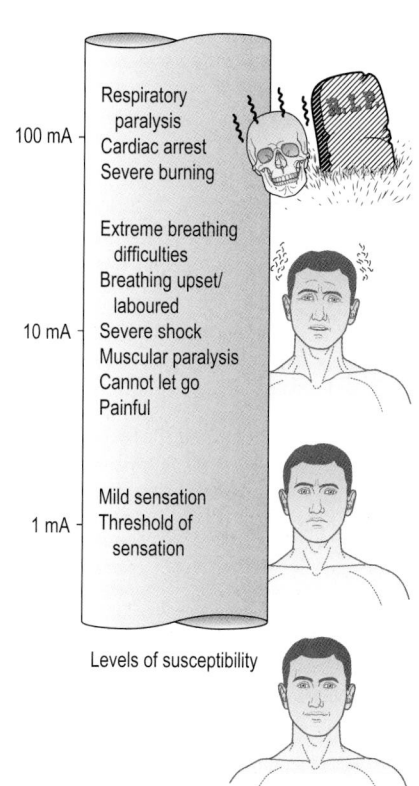

Fig. 28.6.1 The levels of electric shock and their effects.

ELECTRIC SHOCK

Introduction and epidemiology

Electricity is an integral part of our everyday world and electric shock is common. Patients may present to the emergency department (ED) with resulting injuries that range from trivial to fatal (termed electrocution). Although permanent disability can occur, it is reassuring to note that if the initial exposure is survived, subsequent death is unlikely. For each death caused by electricity, there are two serious injuries and 36 reported electric shocks.

There are approximately 20–30 electrical fatalities each year in Australia. Victims are predominantly male and relatively young. Death is just as likely to occur at home as in the workplace, most often in summer. Electricians and linesmen are most at risk. The ratio of low-to-high-voltage deaths ranges from 3:1 to 7:1. The presence of water is associated with fatality. Electrical burns represent 3–5% of admissions to burns units.

Physics of electricity and pathophysiology of electrical injury

Electrical current passing through the body can cause damage in two ways:

❶ thermal injury
❷ physiological change.

The threshold for perception of an electrical current is 1 mA, which results in a tingling sensation. Current greater than 10 mA can induce muscular tetany and prevent the patient letting go of the current source. Paralysis of respiratory muscles occurs at 20 mA. The threshold for ventricular fibrillation is 100 mA (Fig. 28.6.1). Cardiac standstill and internal organ damage occurs at 2A. The maximum 'safe' current tolerable for 1 s is 50 mA.

Ohm's law is fundamental to the understanding of the physics of electricity. This states that:

The amount of current passing through the body is directly proportional to voltage and inversely proportional to resistance (current [amperes] = voltage [volts]/resistance [ohms]).

Factors that determine the effects of an electrical current passing through the body are:

- type of current
- voltage
- tissue resistance
- current path
- contact duration.

Type of current

The vast majority of serious electrical injuries result from alternating current (AC), which is approximately three times as dangerous as direct current (DC). Alternating current can produce tetanic contraction of muscle such that the victim may not be able to let go of the current source. This is not a feature of direct current shock.

Human muscular tissue is sensitive to frequencies between 40 and 150 Hz. As the frequency increases beyond 150 Hz, the response decreases and the current is less dangerous. In Australia, a frequency of 50 Hz is used for household current because this is optimal for the transmission and use of electricity and also has advantages in terms of generation. As such, household current lies directly within the dangerous frequency range. It also spans the vulnerable period of the cardiac electrical potential and is thus capable of causing ventricular fibrillation.

Voltage

Voltage is the electromotive force in the system. In general terms, the greater the voltage the more extensive the injury, but it must be remembered that the amount of current passing through the body will also be determined by resistance (Ohm's law). High voltage is defined as greater than 1000 V. Household voltage in Australia is 240 V. Voltages less than 50 V (50 Hz) have not been proved hazardous. Survival has been reported following shocks of greater than 50 000 V.

Resistance

Different tissues provide differing resistances to the passage of electrical current. Bone has the highest resistance, followed by, in decreasing order, fat, tendon, skin, muscle, blood vessels and nerves. Importantly, however, skin resistance varies greatly according to moisture, cleanliness, thickness and vascularity. Moist skin may have a resistance of 1000 Ω and dry, thick, calloused skin a resistance of 100 000 Ω. By Ohm's law, dry skin resistance to a contact with a 240 V potential results in a current of about 2.4 mA, which is just above the threshold for perception. However, the resistance of wet or sweat-soaked skin drops to 1000 Ω, increasing the current flow to 240 mA, which is easily enough to induce ventricular fibrillation. Not surprisingly, moisture has been identified as a key factor in over half of electrocutions.

Current path

Prediction of injuries from knowledge of the current path is unreliable. Mortalities of 60% for hand-to-hand (transthoracic) and 20% for head-to-foot passage of current are quoted, but have not been verified. When current passes hand-to-hand (or hand-to-foot), only about 5% of the total current passes through the heart. If current passes leg-to-leg, no current traverses the heart.

Contact duration

The longer the duration of contact, the greater the potential for injury. Fortunately, most contacts are brief and frequently result in the victim being thrown back from the current source. This may result in a secondary injury, especially if the victim falls from a height.

Unfortunately, exposures to more than 10 mA of alternating current can induce sweating. Moisture decreases skin resistance and increases current flow, thereby reducing the ability to release the current source. This can progress to a fatal exposure.

Prevention

All members of the community must be encouraged to treat electricity with respect and to practise electrical safety. Licensed electrical contractors should be used to carry out any electrical repairs or installations. Water and electricity should never be mixed.

Residual current devices are useful in providing an additional level of personal protection from electric shock. These devices continuously compare current flow in both active and neutral conductors of an electrical circuit. If current flow becomes sufficiently unbalanced, then some of the current in the active conductor is not returned through the neutral conductor and leaks to earth. These devices operate within 10–50 ms and disconnect the electricity supply when they sense harmful leakage, typically 30 mA.

Clinical features

Electrical injury resembles a crush injury more than a burn. Invariably, the damage below skin level is more severe than the cutaneous wound suggests. The current passing through low-resistance structures produces massive necrosis of muscles, vessels, nerves and subcutaneous tissues.

The clinical manifestations differ from thermal burns in the following ways:

- there are direct effects on the heart and nervous system
- electrical injury classically involves deep structures
- the small entry and exit wounds do not accurately indicate the extent or depth of tissue damage
- a diversity of clinical manifestations is seen with electrical injury.

Burns

As electricity traverses the skin, energy is converted to heat. The smaller the area of contact, the greater the current density, heat production and the consequent skin and adjacent tissue destruction.

Electrothermal burns are best characterized by arc burns, which result from the external passage of current from the contact point to the ground. These may be associated with extensive damage to skin and underlying tissue. Secondary flame burns may occur when the current arc ignites clothing or nearby combustibles.

Electrical burns may range from first degree to third degree. The typical appearance is of a central depressed charred black area surrounded by oedema and erythema. Single or multiple exit wounds may be present.

Cardiac

Ventricular fibrillation is the usual cause of immediate death from electric shock and occurs at the time of the shock. Delayed arrhythmia resulting in death is exceptionally rare. Sinus tachycardia is common and non-specific ST- and T-wave changes may be observed. Atrial fibrillation occurs infrequently and usually resolves spontaneously. Acute myocardial infarction following electric shock has been reported.

Nervous system

Both acute and delayed neurological sequelae have been described following electric shock. Acute complications include respiratory arrest, seizures, altered mental state, amnesia, coma, expressive dysphasia and motor deficits. Reported delayed complications include spinal cord injury (myelopathy) with local amyotrophy and long tract signs, and reflex sympathetic dystrophy.

Peripheral nerve injury is usually associated with significant soft-tissue injury. It has also been reported in the absence of soft-tissue injury and such cases appear to have a good prognosis.

Renal

Acute renal failure may occur secondary to myoglobinuria. Electric shock results in disruption of muscle cells with the release of myoglobin and creatine phosphokinase, similar to a crush injury. Transient oliguria, albuminuria, haemoglobinuria and renal casts are common and there have been reports of high-output renal failure.

Vascular

Large and small vessel arterial and venous thrombosis are responsible for the tissue damage in electrical injury. Vascular complications have included immediate and delayed major vessel haemorrhage, arterial thrombosis and deep vein thrombosis.

Musculoskeletal

Tetanic muscle contractures can result in compression fractures of vertebral bodies, fractures of long bones and dislocations of joints. Injuries may also result from a secondary fall, rather than from the electric shock.

Other

Numerous complications involving other systems, including the eye (especially cataracts) have been reported following electric shock.

Electric shock in pregnancy

Reports of electric shock in pregnancy are rare and the true incidence is unknown. A high mortality has been reported in the literature. However, this may represent publication bias and a prospective cohort study concluded that, in most cases, accidental electric shocks during pregnancy do not pose a major fetal risk.

If there was an immediate problem, the mother may notice a sudden cessation of fetal movements. However, there is no preventative action possible in the ED. Other reported fetal complications of electric shock include intrauterine growth retardation, oligohydramnios and abortion.

Fortunately, therapeutic electric shocks, such as DC cardioversion and electroconvulsive therapy, are known to be safe in pregnancy. The critical factor is current path: accidental electric shocks include the uterus, whereas therapeutic shocks do not.

Treatment

Pre-hospital

Everyone should be aware of the pre-hospital management of electric shock. Most importantly, the rescuer should avoid becoming a further victim. The victim can be separated from the electrical source by using rubber, a wooden handle, a mat or any other non-conductive substance or, if possible, by turning off the electricity supply. Cardiopulmonary resuscitation

(CPR) should begin immediately, if indicated, and help summoned. CPR may need to be prolonged. Ventricular fibrillation is the most common lethal arrhythmia after electric shock and early defibrillation provides the greatest chance for survival.

Emergency department

The majority of patients who present to the ED after electric shock are relatively well. Following appropriate assessment to exclude primary or secondary injury, an ECG should be performed. Cardiac monitoring is not indicated if the patient is asymptomatic and has a normal ECG. Most patients are able to be reassured and discharged directly from the ED. Measurement of creatine phosphokinase levels is not required. It should be remembered that exposure to an electric shock is an unpleasant experience and this should be acknowledged. Tetanus status should be checked.

Many patients have a degree of muscle pain following electric shock owing to the tetanic nature of alternating current. Simple analgesia is appropriate. Any secondary injury, such as fractures or loss of consciousness, should be treated as dictated by the injury.

If an arrhythmia is present it will usually resolve spontaneously and not require specific treatment. Delayed lethal arrhythmias have not been reported in patients without initial arrhythmias.

Severe electrical injury with extensive soft-tissue damage should be managed as a crush injury. This is more likely following high-voltage exposure, which results in a large exudation and sequestration of fluids in the damaged area. Emergency management includes adequate volume replacement and treatment of acidosis and myoglobinuria.

Emergency physicians should be aware of the low potential for fetal harm following electric shock in pregnancy. Publication bias suggests that apparently minor exposures can have profound effects. It would be prudent to adopt a conservative approach of performing a fetal heart Doppler assessment with obstetric follow up including ultrasound.

Prognosis

The prognosis for the majority of patients surviving the initial shock is excellent. Those with significant soft-tissue injury or secondary injury may be left with long-term deficits.

Disposition

The majority of patients presenting to the ED following an electric shock will be suitable for discharge home following assessment and reassurance as detailed above. Those suffering muscle pain secondary to tetanic contractions should be given simple analgesia and instructed to follow up with their general practitioner.

Patients with cardiac arrhythmias require admission for observation until the arrhythmia resolves. Those with evidence of neuropathy should be referred to a neurologist, as nerve conduction studies may be required.

Severe electrical injuries with extensive soft-tissue damage require admission to hospital and, sometimes, to an intensive care unit. All patients with electrical burns should be reviewed by a burns specialist and referral to a specialist burns unit may be indicated. Minor burns may be suitable for elective review.

Secondary injuries, such as loss of consciousness or fractures, should be admitted or referred on their merits.

The Taser

The Taser is a development of the stun gun. It is used by the police service to fill the operational gap between the baton and the gun for controlling potentially dangerous and violent suspects. 'tasered' victims are occasionally brought to the ED for assessment.

The device is a battery operated unit resembling a hand gun that fires two barbed electrodes on 7 m long copper wires at 60 m/s. The barbs attach to the subject's skin or clothing and deliver up to 50 000 V of electricity in rapid pulses over 5 s. The current can cross up to 5 cm of clothing.

Electricity delivered by a taser is neither pure AC nor pure DC and is probably akin to rapid-fire low-amplitude DC shocks. The output is believed to stay near the surface of the body in the skin and muscles and does not penetrate into the internal organs. There is no evidence to date that this form of electrical delivery interfered with cardiac or neurological function in the 30 000 volunteers or in the reported operational uses.

One author concluded that the pre-existing injuries and toxic conditions leading to the patient being tasered are the most important problems requiring medical treatment after Taser use. It seems that the device is essentially safe on healthy people. However, there is limited evidence to base recommendations for the assessment and management of patients that are brought to the ED after being 'tasered'. Suggestions for management of these patients attending EDs are:

- Most healthy subjects may be safely discharged after barb removal and a clinical assessment. It may be appropriate to consider a bedside blood sugar level (BSL), ECG and a venous blood gas.
- High-risk patients are those with known cardiac disease including implanted pacemaker or defibrillator, pregnancy, drug or alcohol intoxication, bizarre behaviour at the time of arrest, other psychiatric disturbance or coincidental medical problems. Often the coexistent condition (e.g. intoxication or mental health issue) will need to be addressed.
- Any patient with chest pain or abnormal ECG should be assessed as per routine clinical practice.
- Pregnant women >24 weeks' gestation should be considered for cardiotocograpic monitoring.
- Look closely for direct injury from the barbs or indirect injury from falls. Barb injuries should be approached as a potential penetrating injury and managed accordingly. There are likely to be small puncture wounds and minor burns at the barb sites. On occasion, medical intervention will be required if the barbs are not easily removed, if the barb tip breaks off in the skin or if the barbs have struck vulnerable areas (e.g. mouth, eyes, neck and groin).
- Most patients will complain of muscle aches and anxiety.

It is clear that, properly used as a method of restraining violent people, Tasers are less likely than guns to cause injury and death of the target (and of the police officer). They are also generally more effective than other methods of restraint. The deaths that have followed taser use have occurred in people who were out of control and who had taken potentially fatal drugs. It is likely that the deaths would have occurred whether or not the Taser was used. However, the medical effects of multiple shocks on such persons is unknown.

LIGHTNING INJURY

Introduction and epidemiology

There are several deaths each year in Australia from lightning. For each death, there are five injuries. These events are always prominent and emergency physicians should be familiar with the pathophysiology. In addition, about 60 people each year report injuries caused by lightning surges while using the telephone during thunderstorms.

Many myths surround lightning injury; they include:

- Lightning strike is invariably fatal. In fact, the mortality is 30%. In addition, the probability of long-term impairment after recovery is low.
- A victim of lightning is charged and dangerous to touch. This false notion has led to the withholding of CPR, with fatal results.
- Lightning should be treated in the same way as high-voltage electrical injury. This is incorrect.

Physics

Lightning occurs most commonly during thunderstorms. Particles moving up and down in a thunderstorm create static electricity, with a large negative charge building up at the bottom of clouds. Electrical discharge (lightning) occurs as a result of the great charge difference between the negatively-charged thundercloud underside and the positively charged ground. The duration of the lightning stroke is between 1 and 100 ms.

Lightning strike is very different from high-voltage electric shock (Table 28.6.1) and produces different clinical effects, requiring a different management approach.

An interesting phenomenon called 'flashover' seems to save many victims from death by lightning. Current passes around and over, but not through the body. The victim's clothing and shoes may be blasted apart. Only cutaneous flame-type burns result.

Clinical features

Immediate

- Cardiac arrest. This takes the form of asystole, as opposed to the ventricular fibrillation of high-voltage electrical injury. The heart is thought to undergo massive depolarization. Although primary lightning-induced arrest may revert quickly, it can be followed by secondary hypoxic arrest.
- Chest pain and muscle aches.
- Neurological deficits. A person struck by lightning may be rendered unconscious. On first regaining consciousness, they may be mute and unable to move. This is transient and usually resolves within minutes, but may take up to 24 h.
- Contusions from shock waves.
- Tympanic membrane rupture.

Delayed

- Keraunoparalysis. Lightning-induced limb paralysis is extremely common. Flaccidity and complete loss of sensation of the affected limb are observed. Peripheral pulses are generally impalpable and the affected limb takes on a mottled, pale, blue appearance. The mechanism is unclear, but may be lightning-induced vasospasm. The condition is self-limiting and resolves within 1–6 h.
- 'Feathery' cutaneous burns (Lichtenberg flowers). These burns, pathognomonic of lightning injury, may appear immediately but more often become visible a few hours after injury. Burns may be severe but heal remarkably easily.

Table 28.6.1 Lightning versus high-voltage injury		
Factor	Lightning	High voltage
Time of exposure	Brief instantaneous	Prolonged tetanic
Energy level	100 million V 200 000 A	Usually much lower
Type of current	Direct	Alternating
Shock wave	Yes	No
Flashover	Yes	No

Adapted from Cooper MA. Lightning injuries. In: Auerbach P, et al (eds). Management of wilderness and environmental emergencies. New York: Macmillan; 1983: 500–21.

- Cataracts. Occur more commonly than following electrical injuries.
- Myoglobinuria and haemoglobinuria are rare.

Other
- Sensorineural deafness.
- Vestibular dysfunction.
- Retinal detachment.
- Optic nerve damage.

Reports of lightning strike in pregnancy reveal a high rate of fetal death *in utero*, despite maternal survival.

Treatment

Pre-hospital
The important principle is that those who appear dead should be resuscitated first. Immediate institution of basic cardiopulmonary resuscitation in the field for those in asystole prevents secondary hypoxic cardiac arrest during the interval until cardiac function resumes spontaneously. Fixed dilated pupils should not be taken as an indicator of death after lightning strike.

Emergency department
Most lightning strikes are unwitnessed and diagnosis may be difficult in the unconscious or confused patient. The diagnosis should be considered where such patients were found outdoors in stormy weather. The presence of multiple victims, exploded clothing, linear or punctuate burns, keraunic markings or tympanic membrane rupture all add weight to the diagnosis. The differential diagnosis includes cerebrovascular event, seizure disorder, spinal cord injury, closed-head injury, Stokes–Adams attack, myocardial infarction and toxin effects.

Standard trauma resuscitation measures should be adopted. Examination of the ears for tympanic rupture and eyes for lens/corneal defects, retinal detachment and optic nerve injury is especially important. If the conscious state deteriorates after arrival, cranial computed tomography scan is indicated. Examination of the cardiovascular system should include an ECG.

Burns are rarely more than superficial and are managed expectantly using standard treatments. Tetanus prophylaxis should be arranged.

Treatment of lightning-induced limb paralysis is expectant. If it does not resolve within a few hours, other causes should be considered. Fasciotomy is unnecessary.

Standard therapy for ocular complications, such as retinal detachment or cataracts, is indicated. Baseline visual acuity should be documented for future reference.

Prognosis and disposition

For survivors of the initial strike the prognosis is excellent unless significant secondary injury has occurred. Admission for observation is indicated for those with abnormal mental status or ECG, or with significant burns or traumatic complications. The burns usually heal well and grafting is rarely required. For those with ocular complications, long-term ophthalmic follow up is necessary.

Controversies
- Timing and extent of development of tissue necrosis associated with electrical injury.

Further reading

Andrews CJ, Darveniza M, Mackerras D. Lightning injury–a review of clinical aspects, pathophysiology and treatment. Adv Trauma 1989;4:241–88.

Bleetman A, Steyn R, Lee C. Introduction of the Taser into British policing. Implications for UK emergency departments: an overview of electronic weaponry. Emerg Med J 2004;21:136–40.

Bruner JMR, Leonard PF. Electricity, safety and the patient. Chicago: Yearbook Medical Publishers; 1989.

Dixon GF. The evaluation and management of electrical injuries. Crit Care Med 1983;11:384–7.

Einarson A, Bailey B, Inocencion G, et al. Accidental electric shock in pregnancy: a prospective cohort study. Am J Obstet Gynecol 1997;176:678–81.

Fatovich D. Delayed lethal arrhythmia after an electrical injury. Emerg Med J 2007;24:743.

Fatovich DM, Lee KY. Household electric shocks: who should be monitored? Med J Aust 1991;155:301–3.

Fish RM, Geddes LA. Conduction of electrical current to and through the human body: a review. Eplasty 2009;9:e44.

Fish RM. Electric injury, part III: cardiac monitoring indications, the pregnant patient, and lightning. J Emerg Med 2000;18:181–7.

Kobernick M. Electrical injuries: pathophysiology and emergency management. Ann Emerg Med 1982;11: 633–8.

Robb M, Close B, Furyk J, Aitken P. Review article: Emergency department implications of the TASER. Emerg Med Australas 2009;21:250–8.

Spies C, Trohman RG. Narrative review: electrocution and life threatening electrical injuries. Ann Intern Med 2006;145:531–7.

28.7 Altitude illness

Ian Rogers

ESSENTIALS

1 The high-altitude syndromes–acute mountain sickness (AMS), high-altitude cerebral oedema (HACE) and high-altitude pulmonary oedema (HAPE)–are all clinical diagnoses, where management may need to be undertaken without access to diagnostic testing.

2 AMS and HACE represent stages along a continuum owing to cerebral vasodilatation and cerebral oedema while, in HAPE, the oedema manifests in the lungs.

3 Descent is the single best treatment for AMS, HACE and HAPE; however, milder cases in selected settings may be able to be managed with rest and/or oxygen.

4 Additional drug treatments may be used in the treatment of established altitude illness. The most often employed therapies are dexamethasone for AMS/HACE and nifedipine for HAPE.

5 Prevention is best achieved by controlled ascent, with adequate time for acclimatization.

6 Low-dose acetazolamide provides effective prophylaxis against AMS.

Introduction

Altitude illness comprises a number of syndromes that can occur on exposure to the hypobaric hypoxic environment of high altitude. At any altitude, the partial pressure of inspired oxygen (P_iO_2) is equal to 0.21 times the barometric pressure minus water vapour pressure of 47 mmHg. At an altitude of 5500 m, barometric pressure is halved. On the summit of Mount Everest (8850 m), the P_iO_2 is only 43 mmHg and a typical climber without oxygen can be expected to have a PaO_2 of <30 mmHg and a $PaCO_2$ of about 13 mmHg [1]. In addition to the hypoxic stress of altitude, a subject may also be exposed to cold, low humidity, fatigue, poor diet and increased ultraviolet radiation. For the emergency physician, the unique feature of altitude illness is that it requires recognition and treatment in the field, frequently without access to sophisticated diagnostic and imaging techniques and often without access to rapid evacuation.

Epidemiology and pathophysiology

The human body has the capacity to acclimatize to hypoxic environments. This is principally achieved by increasing ventilation (the hypoxic ventilatory response effected by the carotid body), increasing numbers of red blood cells (via stimulation of erythropoietin), increasing the diffusing capacity of the lungs (resulting from increased lung volume and pulmonary capillary blood volume), increasing vascularity of the tissues and increasing the tissues' ability to use oxygen (possibly owing to increased numbers of mitochondria and oxidative enzyme systems).

In some individuals, exposure to low PO_2 initiates a sequence of pathophysiological changes, which result in oedema formation in the brain and lungs. The altitude illness syndromes, acute mountain sickness (AMS), high-altitude cerebral oedema (HACE) and high-altitude pulmonary oedema (HAPE), are the result of this oedema formation. The exact mechanism of these pathophysiological changes is still debated but vasodilatation is a key part.

In the brain, the development of oedema causes intracranial pressure (ICP) to rise. Initially, this is partially compensated for by displacement of cerebrospinal fluid (CSF) into the spinal space and adjustment of the balance between production and absorption of CSF. However, once these compensatory mechanisms are overwhelmed, ICP can rise beyond the cerebral perfusion pressure. Without intervention, cerebral blood flow ceases and the patient dies.

In the lung, non-cardiogenic pulmonary oedema develops. A significant rise in pulmonary artery pressure appears to be a crucial pathophysiological factor [2]. Impaired sodium driven clearance of alveolar fluid may contribute to HAPE [3]. It has been postulated that uneven pulmonary vasoconstriction increases the filtration pressure in non-vasoconstricted lung areas, worsening the interstitial and alveolar oedema.

The tendency to develop altitude illness is idiosyncratic. The major predisposing factors are the rate of ascent and the altitude reached. It is not related to physical fitness or gender. Individuals vary in their ability to compensate for changes in ICP and in their pressor responses to hypoxia. This may explain the reproducibility of AMS, HACE and HAPE in susceptible individuals and why some, and not others, develop symptoms at the same altitude. The risk is higher in those who have an impaired ventilatory response to hypoxia in normobaric conditions and with dehydration, vigorous exercise and the use of depressant drugs.

Prevention

The best form of prevention is gradual ascent to allow sufficient time for acclimatization. Although individuals vary in how quickly they acclimatize, a sensible recommendation is sleeping no more than 500 m higher than the previous day once above 2500 m. Keeping warm, avoiding alcohol, maintaining hydration and eating a high-carbohydrate diet to improve the respiratory quotient, may all decrease the incidence of altitude illness. Modest exercise on acclimatization days should be encouraged.

Acclimatization is not always practical or possible and so pharmacological agents may be required [4]. Acetazolamide reduces the incidence and severity of AMS/HACE when used prophylactically in subjects experiencing rapid ascent [5]. Doses recommended have decreased as a result of ongoing research [6].

Chemoprophylaxis can be achieved with 125 mg bd, starting the day before ascent and continued for 2 days after reaching high altitude. Dexamethasone 4 mg bd may be equally effective and may be more so when a rapid onset is required, such as in unacclimatized personnel involved in high-altitude rescue missions.

Nifedipine 20 mg slow-release tds or 30 mg bd provides protection against HAPE in susceptible individuals. More recent research suggests that other drugs, such as sildenafil, tadalafil and salmeterol, may have a role in HAPE prevention, but it is generally advised that vasodilators not be combined.

Clinical features

AMS is common, occurring in about 30% of subjects exposed to moderate altitude (3500 m). HACE and HAPE are less common, but a study in pilgrims at 4300 m reported AMS in 68%, HACE in 31% and HAPE in 5% of subjects [7]. The diagnosis is usually made purely on clinical assessment.

Acute mountain sickness

AMS is primarily a neurological syndrome, associated with some degree of respiratory compromise. The onset is usually 6–24 h after arrival at high altitude. The majority of patients present in the early stages when the symptoms are like those of a hangover and include headache, nausea, anorexia, weakness and lassitude. In the early stage of AMS, there are no abnormalities on physical examination and the oxygen saturation, if measured, should be no lower than that expected for a given altitude. Mild AMS is usually benign and self-limiting.

If the illness progresses, the more severe form of AMS is characterized by dyspnoea at rest, nausea and vomiting, altered mental state, headache and ataxia. Ataxia is the most useful sign of progression to serious illness. Left untreated, severe AMS may progress to life-threatening HACE or HAPE.

AMS can be scored using the Lake Louise AMS score [8]. This consists of five symptom groups: headache, gastrointestinal distress, fatigue or weakness, dizziness or light headedness and difficulty sleeping. Each symptom is scored on a scale from 0 (not present) to 3 (severe or incapacitating) and the totals of the five symptom groups are summed. A total score of 3 or more is considered diagnostic of AMS.

High-altitude cerebral oedema

HACE is the progression of neurological signs and symptoms in the setting of AMS. There is a progressive decline in mental status and truncal ataxia is a prominent physical finding. Focal neurological signs, such as third and sixth cranial nerve palsies, may develop as a result of raised intracranial pressure. Unrecognized and untreated, there may be rapid progression to coma and death due to raised intracranial pressure.

High-altitude pulmonary oedema

HAPE occurs in susceptible individuals who may have no underlying pulmonary or cardiac disease. It most commonly manifests on the second night at high altitude. In the early stages, the oedema is interstitial and the patient may only have a dry cough and decreased exercise tolerance. Few abnormalities will be seen on examination at this stage. As more fluid accumulates, the patient develops tachycardia, increasing dyspnoea, marked weakness, cough productive of frothy sputum and cyanosis. Pulse oximetry, if available, confirms profound hypoxia. A chest X-ray will demonstrate widespread interstitial and alveolar infiltrates. It may occur in conjunction with AMS/HACE or as an isolated clinical syndrome.

Treatment

Early recognition is an essential component of the management of all acute altitude syndromes. Developing symptoms in a party member may have substantial impact on route planning choices, particularly whether to halt ascent or descend. The goal is to stop the pathophysiological process with the key interventions summarized in Table 28.7.1.

Table 28.7.1 Key treatments in severe altitude syndromes	
HACE/severe AMS	*HAPE*
Descent	Descent
Oxygen	Oxygen
Simulated descent (e.g. Gamow bag)	Simulated descent (e.g. Gamow bag)
Dexamethasone 8 mg stat then 4 mg 6-hourly	Nifedipine SR 20 mg 8-hourly

HACE: high-altitude cerebral oedema; AMS: acute mountain sickness; HAPE: high-altitude pulmonary oedema; SR: slow release.

Acute mountain sickness and high-altitude cerebral oedema

A patient presenting with symptoms of mild AMS should be advised to halt ascent to allow time for acclimatization. They should rest, as physical exertion aggravates symptoms, and take simple analgesics and antiemetics if desired. It is important that the patient be closely observed for progression of symptoms.

With moderate symptoms, the management is the same as for mild AMS, with the addition of oxygen 2–4 L/min and, possibly, pharmacological agents. Acetazolamide, a carbonic anhydrase inhibitor, aids the normal process of ventilatory acclimatization by reducing the renal reabsorption of bicarbonate, resulting in metabolic acidosis and compensatory hyperventilation. It relieves symptoms, improves arterial oxygenation and prevents further impairment of pulmonary gas exchange. It also helps to maintain cerebral blood flow despite hypocapnia and opposes the fluid retention of AMS. The recommended treatment dose is 250 mg orally bd. Acetazolamide is a sulpha drug and contraindicated in those with known allergy. Dexamethasone is also an effective agent in this condition [9], presumably by reducing capillary permeability and ICP. It does not aid in acclimatization. It may be given as an alternative, or in addition to, acetazolamide. The recommended dose is 8 mg stat then 4 mg every 6 h.

If a patient shows signs of severe AMS progressing to HACE, then rapid and controlled descent is the highest priority. Oxygen 2–4 L/min should be administered. Additional therapy may be required if the illness is severe, the patient's condition must be improved to allow descent or where immediate descent is not possible. Additional therapeutic options include dexamethasone 8 mg stat then 4 g every 6 hours and hyperbaric therapy using a portable fabric hyperbaric chamber (e.g. Gamow bag) [4]. The bags are expensive and need to be pumped continuously, but have the advantage of using air rather than oxygen.

High-altitude pulmonary oedema

Rapid and controlled descent, with oxygen, is the mainstay of management in a patient suffering from HAPE, although milder cases may be managed with oxygen without altitude change. In a large proportion of cases this is sufficient. Oxygen flow should be titrated to maintain adequate oxygen saturation. Continuous positive airway pressure may be

949

required. The patient should be rested and kept warm, as cold may further increase pulmonary hypertension through sympathetic stimulation.

Nifedipine should be considered as adjunctive therapy to oxygen and descent. It lowers the raised pulmonary artery pressure that characterizes HAPE and results in clinical improvement, better oxygenation and progressive clearing of alveolar oedema on chest X-ray. The recommended dosage is 20 mg of the slow release formulation 8-hourly or 30 mg 12-hourly [4].

Controversies

- The effectiveness of acetazolamide and dexamethasone in AMS prophylaxis is now generally well accepted but, which agent is more effective and in which circumstances they should be used, is less clear. The side effects of acetazolamide at recommended doses can mimic AMS and, conversely, the euphoriant effects of dexamethasone can interfere with a subject's ability accurately to report symptoms. Dexamethasone and acetazolamide appear to differ in their effectiveness when trialled in field conditions compared to simulated conditions in hypobaric chambers. The dose of each drug used is not the same across trials. The rate of ascent appears to influence the effectiveness of pharmacological prophylaxis. Further research may clarify their respective roles.
- Further research is required to clarify the role of newer preventive strategies, such as ibuprofen, sildenafil and salmeterol, for both AMS and HAPE.
- Although descent is a mainstay of altitude illness treatment, a greater understanding of its pathophysiology and spectrum of illness will allow more patients to be effectively treated at altitude when appropriate facilities are available.

References

[1] Grocott PW, Martin DS, Levett DZH, et al. Arterial blood gases and oxygen content in climbers on Mount Everest. N Engl J Med 2009;360:140–9.

[2] Bartsch P. High altitude pulmonary edema. Respiration 1997;64:435–43.

[3] Sartori C, Allemann Y, Duplain H, et al. Salmeterol for the prevention of high altitude pulmonary edema. N Engl J Med 2002;346:1631–6.

[4] Luks AM, McIntosh SE, Grissom CK, et al. Wilderness Medical Society consensus guidelines for the prevention and treatment of acute altitude illness. Wild Environ Med 2010;21:146–55.

[5] Hackett PH, Rennie D. The incidence, importance, and prophylaxis of acute mountain sickness. Lancet 1976;2:1149–55.

[6] Basnyat B, Gerstsch JH, Holck PS, et al. Acetazolamide 125 mg BD is not significantly different from 375 mg BD in the prevention of acute mountain sickness: the prophylactic acetazolamide dosage comparison for efficacy (PACE) trial. High Alt Med Biol 2006;7:17–27.

[7] Basnyat B, Subedi D, Sleggs J, et al. Disorientated and ataxic pilgrims: an epidemiological study of acute mountain sickness and high altitude cerebral edema at a sacred lake at 4300 m in the Nepal Himalayas. Wild Environ Med 2000;11:89–93.

[8] Roach RC, Bartsch P, Hackett PH, Oelz O. (Lake Louise AMS Scoring Consensus Committee.) The Lake Louise acute mountain sickness scoring system. In: Sutton JR, Houston CS, Coates G, editors. Hypoxia and molecular medicine. Burlington, VT: Queen City: Printers; 1993, p. 272–4.

[9] Ferrazzini G, Maggiorini M, Kriemler S, et al. Successful treatment of acute mountain sickness with dexamethasone. Br Med J 1997;294:1380–2.

TOXICOLOGY EMERGENCIES

Edited by **Mark Little**

29.1 Approach to the poisoned patient

Lindsay Murray

ESSENTIALS

1 Self-poisoning is a manifestation of an underlying psychiatric, drug and alcohol or social disorder.

2 A wide range of clinical manifestations of toxicity may be observed following drug overdose.

3 An accurate risk assessment predicts the likely clinical course and informs planning for subsequent investigation, management and disposition.

4 The mainstay of management is timely institution of an appropriate level of supportive care.

5 The role of gastrointestinal decontamination is controversial. Except in select cases, it is unlikely that these procedures have a significant impact on clinical outcome when performed more than 1 h following ingestion.

6 Specific antidotes and techniques of enhanced elimination are rarely indicated, but their timely use may be life saving in specific instances.

Introduction

Drug overdose in adults usually occurs in the context of self-poisoning, which may be either recreational or an act of deliberate self-harm.

Deliberate self-poisoning accounts for 1–5% of all public hospital admissions in Australia [1,2]. The bulk of the medical management of cases presenting to hospital is carried out in the emergency department (ED) and the emergency physician is expected to be expert in the field. Although the management must vary considerably according to the nature and severity of the poisoning, some general principles apply.

Above all, it must be remembered that the acute overdose presentation is only a discrete time-limited event in the course of the underlying condition, which is usually psychiatric or social in origin.

Pathophysiology and clinical features

The effects of ingestion of pharmaceuticals or illicit drugs range from the non-toxic to the life threatening and may involve any system. Poisoning is a dynamic presentation and the patient may present at varying points in the time course of the poisoning. Consequently, rapid clinical deterioration or improvement may be observed after the initial presentation and assessment.

Acute morbidity and mortality from poisoning is usually a consequence of the cardiovascular,

Table 29.1.1 Toxic causes of respiratory failure

Central nervous system depression
Alcohols
Anticonvulsants
Antidepressants
Antihistamines
Barbiturates
Baclofen
Clonidine
Opioids
Phenothiazines
Sedative hypnotics

Weakness of ventilatory muscles
Botulism
Carbamate pesticides
Muscle relaxants
Organophosphorus pesticides and warfare agents
Snakebite
Strychnine

Pulmonary
ARDS
Cardiogenic pulmonary oedema
Non-cardiogenic pulmonary oedema
Pulmonary aspiration and pneumonitis
• Activated charcoal
• Gastric contents
• Hydrocarbons
Paraquat

ARDS: acute respiratory distress syndrome.

Table 29.1.2 Cardiovascular effects of poisoning

Tachycardia
Anticholinergics
• Antihistamines
• Benztropine
• Phenothiazines
Quetiapine
• Tricyclic antidepressants
Reflex response to hypotension
Sympathomimetics
• Amphetamines
• Caffeine
• Cocaine
• Theophylline

Bradycardia (includes AV block)
β-Blockers
Calcium channel blockers
Clonidine
Digoxin

Hypotension
Fluid loss/third spacing
Myocardial depressants
• β-Blockers
• Calcium channel blockers
Peripheral vasodilators

Hypertension
Anticholinergics
Sympathomimetics
• Amphetamines
• Cocaine
• MAO inhibitors

Rhythm/ECG abnormalities
QRS prolongation (fast sodium channel blockade)
• Class 1a and 1c antiarrhythmics
• Thioridazine
• Tricyclic antidepressants
• Propranolol
QT prolongation/torsades de pointes
• Amisulpride
• Chloroquine
• Citalopram
• Quinine
• Thioridazine
• Tricyclic antidepressants
Ventricular tachycardia/fibrillation
• Amphetamines
• Chloral hydrate
• Cocaine
• Digoxin
• Theophylline
• Tricyclic antidepressants

Ischaemia/infarction
Cocaine
Complication of hypoxia or hypotension

Table 29.1.3 Toxic causes of agitation or delirium

Alcohol

Anticholinergic syndrome

Antidepressants
• Bupropion
• Venlafaxine

Atypical antipsychotic agents
• Olanzapine

Benzodiazepines and other sedative hypnotics

Cannabis

Hallucinogenic agents

Serotonin syndrome

Sympathomimetic syndrome
• Amphetamines
• Cocaine

Theophylline

Withdrawal syndromes

respiratory or central nervous system (CNS) complications of the poisoning. Less commonly, hepatic, renal or metabolic effects are potentially life threatening.

The most frequent life-threatening respiratory complication of poisoning is ventilatory failure, which is usually a consequence of CNS depression. Less commonly, it is secondary to ventilatory muscle paralysis. The frequency and depth of respirations are reduced. Respiratory failure may also be caused by direct pulmonary toxicity or complications, such as pulmonary aspiration or non-cardiogenic pulmonary oedema (Table 29.1.1).

Cardiovascular manifestations of poisoning include tachycardia, bradycardia, hypertension, hypotension, conduction defects and arrhythmias (Table 29.1.2). Bradycardia is relatively rarely observed and is associated with a number of potentially life-threatening ingestions. Tachycardia is commonly observed and is usually benign. It may be due to intrinsic sympathomimetic or anticholinergic effects of a drug or a reflex response to hypotension or hypoxia. Hypotension is also commonly observed and may be due to a number of

different causes (Table 29.1.2). Hypertension is unusual. Severe hypertension is usually associated with illicit drug use and is important because it may produce complications such as intracerebral haemorrhage.

CNS manifestations of poisoning include decreased level of consciousness, agitation or delirium, seizures and disordered temperature regulation. A decreased level of consciousness is a common presentation of poisoning and is associated with many drugs, some of which are listed in Table 29.1.1. Although usually a direct drug effect, CNS depression is occasionally secondary to hypoglycaemia, hypoxia or hypotension. Common causes of agitation or delirium following overdose are listed in Table 29.1.3. Toxic seizures are potentially life threatening and important causes are listed in Table 29.1.4.

Hypothermia is usually a complication of environmental exposure secondary to a decreased level of consciousness or altered behaviour. Hyperthermia is a direct toxic effect and causes are listed in Table 29.1.5. Severe hyperthermia is rapidly lethal if not corrected.

Metabolic and other manifestations of poisoning include hyper- and hypoglycaemia, hyper- and hyponatraemia, acidosis and alkalosis and hepatic failure.

Acute poisoning is distinguished from many other forms of acute illness in that, given appropriate supportive care over a relatively short period, a full recovery can usually be expected. A small number of potentially fatal poisonings may demonstrate progressive toxicity despite full supportive care. These are the

Table 29.1.4 Toxic causes of seizures
Amphetamines
Bupropion
Carbamazepine
Chloroquine
Cocaine
Isoniazid
Mefanamic acid
Theophylline
Tramadol
Tricyclic antidepressants
Venlafaxine

Table 29.1.5 Toxic causes of hyperthermia
Amphetamines
Anticholinergics
Cocaine
MAO inhibitors
Salicylates
Serotonin syndrome

Table 29.1.6 Risk assessment-based approach to poisoning

Resuscitation
• Airway
• Breathing
• Circulation
• Detect and correct:
   hypoglycaemia
   seizures
   hyper-/hypothermia
• Emergency antidote administration

Risk assessment • Agent • Dose • Time since ingestion • Clinical features and course • Patient factors
Supportive care and monitoring
Investigations • Screening: 12-lead ECG, paracetamol • Specific
Decontamination
Enhanced elimination
Antidotes
Disposition

Reproduced from Murray L, Daly F, Little M, Cadogan M. Toxicology handbook, 2nd edn. Sydney: Elsevier; 2011.

so-called cellular toxins and include colchicine, iron, salicylate, cyanide, paracetamol, theophylline and digoxin. In some of these cases, early aggressive gastrointestinal decontamination, timely administration of antidotes or the institution of techniques of enhanced elimination may be life saving.

Mortality or morbidity may also result from specific complications of a poisoning. These include trauma, pulmonary aspiration, adult respiratory distress syndrome, rhabdomyolysis, renal failure and hypoxic encephalopathy. These complications usually occur prior to arrival in the ED.

Pulmonary aspiration frequently complicates a period of decreased level of consciousness or a seizure. It is a leading cause of in-hospital morbidity and mortality following overdose. This complication is characterized by rapid onset of dyspnoea, cough, fever, wheeze and cyanosis.

Rhabdomyolysis occurs as a direct toxic effect (rare) or secondary to excessive muscular hyperactivity, seizures, hyperthermia or prolonged coma with direct muscle compression. The urine is dark and acute renal failure can develop secondary to tubular deposition of myoglobin.

Assessment

Risk assessment

A risk assessment should be made as soon as possible in the management of the poisoned patient. Only resuscitation is a greater priority (Table 29.1.6). Risk assessment is a distinct quantitative cognitive step through which the clinician attempts to predict the likely clinical course and potential complications for the individual patient at that particular presentation [3]. An accurate risk assessment allows informed decision making in regard to all subsequent management steps including duration and intensity of supportive care and monitoring, screening and specialized testing, decontamination, enhanced elimination, antidotes and disposition. Factors that are taken into account when formulating this risk assessment include: the agent(s), the dose, the time since ingestion, the clinical features present and patient factors (Table 29.1.6). Specialized testing may refine

risk assessment. Access to specialized poisons information in the form of a poisons information centre or in-house databases is often necessary to formulate an accurate risk assessment.

History

Every effort should be made to obtain information as to the type and dose of drug ingested, the time of ingestion and the progression of symptoms since ingestion. History provided by the patient, if they are awake, is usually reliable and should not be dismissed.

Physical examination

The focused physical examination of the poisoned patient aims to:

- identify any immediate threats to life and the need for intervention
- establish a baseline clinical status
- corroborate the history
- identify intoxication syndromes
- identify possible alternative diagnoses
- identify any complications of the poisoning.

The initial physical examination of the overdose patient in many ways parallels the primary survey of the trauma patient. The airway, breathing and circulation are assessed and stabilized as necessary. The level of consciousness should be assessed, the presence of seizure activity noted and the blood glucose and temperature measured.

A more complete examination is carried out when the patient is stable. This should include a full neurological examination, including assessment of the level of consciousness and mental status, pupil size, muscle tone and movements and the presence or absence of focal neurological signs. Poisoning normally causes global CNS depression and focal signs suggest an alternative diagnosis or a CNS complication, such as cerebral haemorrhage.

Other features that should be specifically sought are any evidence of associated trauma, the state of hydration, the condition of the skin, in particular the presence of pressure areas, the presence or absence of bowel sounds and the condition of the urine.

Several toxic autonomic syndromes, or 'toxidromes', have been described in relation to poisoning. The principal ones are listed in Table 29.1.7. Identification of these syndromes may narrow the differential diagnosis in cases of unknown poisoning.

Table 29.1.7 Toxic autonomic syndromes or 'toxidromes'

Toxidrome	Features	Common causes
Anticholinergic	Agitated delirium Tachycardia Hyperthermia Dilated pupils Dry flushed skin Urinary retention Ileus	Antihistamines Benztropine Carbamazepine Phenothiazines Plant poisonings Tricyclic antidepressants
Mixed cholinergic	Brady- or tachycardia Hypo- or hypertension Miosis or mydriasis Sweating Increased bronchial secretion Gastrointestinal hyperactivity Muscle weakness Fasciculations	Organophosphates Carbamates
Mixed α- and β-adrenergic	Hypertension Tachycardia Mydriasis Agitation	Amphetamines Cocaine
β-Adrenergic	Hypotension Tachycardia Hypokalaemia Hyperglycaemia	Caffeine Salbutamol Theophylline
Serotonin	Altered mental status Autonomic dysfunction Fever Hypertension Sweating Tachycardia Motor dysfunction Hyperreflexia Hypertonia (esp. lower limbs) Myoclonus	Amphetamines Antihistamines Monoamine oxidase inhibitors NSSRIs SSRIs Tricyclic antidepressants (Usually combined overdose)

NSSRI: non-selective serotonin re-uptake inhibitor; SSRI: selective serotonin re-uptake inhibitor.

Table 29.1.8 Supportive care measures for the poisoned patient

Airway	Endotracheal intubation
Breathing	Supplemental oxygen Ventilation
Circulation	Intravenous fluids Inotropes Antihypertensives Antiarrhythmics Defibrillation/cardioversion Cardiac pacing Cardiopulmonary bypass
Metabolic	Hypertonic dextrose Hypertonic saline Insulin/dextrose Calcium salts Sodium bicarbonate
Agitation/ delirium	Benzodiazepines Butyrophenones
Seizures	Benzodiazepines Barbiturates
Body	External rewarming
Temperature	External cooling
Impaired renal function	Rehydration Haemodialysis

Poisons information

Information on the clinical course and toxic doses of specific pharmaceutical and non-pharmaceutical poisons is available on a 24 h basis throughout Australia by telephoning 131126. The poison information centres are staffed by trained poisons information specialists and are also able to refer cases to clinical toxicologists for consultation.

Treatment

The management of poisoning should be approached in a systematic way. Following initial resuscitation, further treatment is informed by the risk assessment (see Table 29.1.6).

Resuscitation, supportive care and monitoring

Supportive care is the key element in the management of poisoning. The vast majority of poisonings result in temporary dysfunction of one or more of the body systems. If appropriate support of the system in question is instituted in a timely fashion and continued until the toxic substance is metabolized or excreted, a good outcome can be anticipated. In severe poisonings, supportive care may be very aggressive and possible interventions are listed in Table 29.1.8.

The specific supportive management of a number of manifestations or complications of poisoning warrants further mention insofar as it may differ from the standard management of such conditions with other aetiologies.

Cardiopulmonary arrest from poisoning should be aggressively resuscitated. Direct current cardioversion is rarely successful in terminating toxic arrhythmias and should not take precedence over establishing adequate ventilation and oxygenation, cardiac compressions, correction of acidosis or hypovolaemia and the administration of specific antidotes. Resuscitative efforts should be continued beyond the usual time frame. In cardiac arrest due to drugs with direct cardiac toxicity, the use of cardiopulmonary bypass or extracorporeal membrane oxygenation (ECMO) until the drug is metabolized may be life saving.

In general, intravenous benzodiazepines are the drugs of choice for control of toxic seizures. Large doses may be required. Hypoxia and hypoglycaemia must be corrected if they are contributory factors. Patients with toxic seizures do not generally need long-term anticonvulsant therapy. Isoniazid-induced seizures are difficult to control without administration of an adequate dose of the specific antidote, pyridoxine.

The management of pulmonary aspiration is essentially supportive, with supplemental oxygenation and intubation and mechanical ventilation if necessary. Neither prophylactic antibiotics nor corticosteroids have been shown to be helpful in the management of this condition, which is essentially a chemical pneumonitis.

Toxic hypertension rarely requires specific therapy. Most cases are mild and simple observation is sufficient. Agitation or delirium is a feature of many intoxications associated with hypertension and adequate sedation with benzodiazepines usually lowers the blood pressure.

Severe toxic hypertension is most likely in toxicity from cocaine or amphetamine-type drugs and treatment may be indicated to avoid complications, such as cardiac failure or intracerebral haemorrhage. The drug of choice in this situation is sodium nitroprusside by intravenous infusion. The extremely short duration of action of this vasodilator allows accurate control of hypertension during the toxic phase and avoids the development of hypotension once toxicity begins to wear off.

Management of rhabdomyolysis consists of treatment of the causative factors, fluid resuscitation and careful monitoring of fluids and electrolytes. The role of mannitol and urinary alkalinization in reducing the risk of renal failure is not clear. Established acute renal failure requires haemodialysis, often for up to 6 weeks.

Decontamination

The aim of decontamination of the gastrointestinal tract is to bind or remove ingested material before it is absorbed into the circulation and able to exert its toxic effects. This is a very attractive concept and has long been considered one of the fundamental interventions in management of the overdose patient.

However, gastrointestinal decontamination should not be regarded as a routine procedure in the management of the patient presenting to the ED following an overdose. The decision to perform gastrointestinal decontamination and the choice of method should be based on an assessment of the likely benefit, the likely risk and the resources required. Gastrointestinal decontamination should only be considered where there is likely to be a significant amount of a significantly toxic material remaining in the gut. It is never indicated when the risk assessment predicts a benign course. Efforts at decontamination technique should never take precedence over the institution of appropriate supportive care.

Three basic approaches to gastrointestinal decontamination are available: gastric emptying, administration of an adsorbent and catharsis.

Gastric emptying can be attempted by the administration of an emetic, most commonly syrup of ipecac, or by gastric lavage. In volunteer studies, both of these techniques removed highly variable amounts of marker substances from the stomach even if performed immediately after ingestion and the effect diminished rapidly with time to the point of being negligible after 1 hour [4,5]. Clinical outcome trials have

failed to demonstrate improved outcome as a result of routine gastric emptying in addition to administration of activated charcoal, except, perhaps, in patients presenting unconscious within 1 h of ingestion [6–8].

The principal adsorbent available to clinicians is activated charcoal (AC), which effectively binds most pharmaceuticals and chemicals, and is currently the decontamination method of choice for most poisonings. Materials that do not bind well to charcoal are listed in Table 29.1.9.

Charcoal is 'activated' by treatment in acid and steam at high temperature. This process removes impurities and greatly increases the surface area available for binding. Activated charcoal (AC) is packaged as a 50 g dose premixed with water or sorbitol, which is likely to be sufficient for the majority of ingestions. Adult patients are usually able to drink AC slurry from a cup. If the level of consciousness is too impaired to allow this, they should be intubated first. Administration of AC is absolutely contraindicated unless the patient has an intact or protected airway.

Volunteer studies demonstrate that the effect of AC diminishes rapidly with time and that the greatest benefit occurs if it is administered within 1 h. There is as yet no evidence that AC improves clinical outcome [9].

There is no evidence to suggest that the addition of a cathartic, such as sorbitol, to AC improves clinical outcome [10].

Apart from rarely employed endoscopic and surgical techniques, whole-bowel irrigation (WBI) is the most aggressive form of gastrointestinal decontamination. Polyethylene

glycol solution (Golytely is administered via a nasogastric tube at a rate of 2 L/h until a clear rectal effluent is produced. This usually takes about 6 h and requires one-to-one nursing. In volunteer studies, this technique reduced the absorption of slow-release pharmaceuticals and so may be of benefit in life-threatening overdoses of these agents. Again, clinical benefit has not yet been conclusively demonstrated [11]. The use of WBI has also been reported in the management of potentially toxic ingestions of iron, lead and packets of illicit drugs. Whole-bowel irrigation is contraindicated if there is evidence of ileus or bowel obstruction and in patients who have an unprotected airway or haemodynamic compromise.

Enhanced elimination

A number of techniques are available to enhance the elimination of toxins from the body. Their use is rarely indicated, as only a very few drugs capable of causing severe poisoning have pharmacokinetic parameters that render them amenable to these techniques (Table 29.1.10).

Multiple-dose AC (25–50 g every 3–4 h) may enhance drug elimination by interrupting the enterohepatic circulation or by 'gastrointestinal dialysis'. Gastrointestinal dialysis is the movement of a toxin across the gastrointestinal wall from the circulation into the gut down a concentration gradient that is maintained by charcoal binding. For this technique to be effective, a drug must undergo considerable enterohepatic circulation or, in the case of

Table 29.1.9 Materials that do not bind well to activated charcoal

Alcohols
- Ethanol
- Ethylene glycol
- Isopropanol
- Methanol

Corrosives
- Acids
- Alkalis

Hydrocarbons

Metals and their salts
- Arsenic
- Iron
- Lead
- Lithium
- Mercury
- Potassium

Table 29.1.10 Techniques of enhanced elimination

Technique	Suitable toxin
Multiple-dose activated charcoal	Carbamazepine Dapsone Phenobarbitone Phenytoin Theophylline
Urinary alkalinization	Phenobarbitone Salicylate
Haemodialysis	Ethylene glycol Lithium Metformin lactic acidosis Methanol Salicylate Theophylline Valproic acid
Charcoal haemoperfusion	Theophylline

'gastrointestinal dialysis', have a small volume of distribution, small molecular weight, low protein binding, slow endogenous elimination and bind to charcoal [12]. The advantages of this technique are that it is non-invasive and simple to carry out.

Alkalinization of the urine enhances urinary excretion of drugs that are filtered at the glomerulus and are unable to be reabsorbed across the tubular epithelium when in an ionized form at alkaline pH. For elimination to be effectively enhanced by this method, the drug must be predominantly eliminated by the kidneys in the unchanged form, have a low pKa, be distributed mainly to the extracellular fluid compartment and be minimally protein bound.

Haemodialysis (HD) and haemoperfusion (HP) are both very invasive techniques and for that reason are reserved for potentially life-threatening intoxications. Only a small number of drugs that have small volumes of distribution, slow endogenous clearance rates, small molecular weights (HD) and bind to charcoal (HP) will have their rates of elimination significantly enhanced by these procedures.

Antidotes

Very few drugs have effective antidotes. Occasionally, however, timely use of an antidote may be life saving or substantially reduce morbidity, time in hospital or resource requirements. Antidotes that may be indicated in the ED setting are listed in Table 29.1.11. However, it must be remembered that antidotes are also drugs and are frequently associated with adverse effects of their own. An antidote should only be used where a specific indication exists and then only at the correct dose, by the correct route and with appropriate monitoring. Because many antidotes are so infrequently used, obtaining sufficient supplies when the need arises can be difficult. Every ED must review its stocking of antidotes and have a plan for obtaining further supplies should the need arise.

Differential diagnosis

It is essential to exclude important non-toxic diagnoses in the patient presenting with coma or altered mental status presumed to be due to drug overdose. These diagnoses include head injury, intracerebral haemorrhage or infarction, CNS infection, hyponatraemia, hypoglycaemia,

Table 29.1.11 Useful emergency antidotes	
Poisoning	*Antidote*
Atropine	Physostigmine
Benzodiazepines	Flumazenil
Cyanide	Dicobalt edetate, hydroxocobalamin
Digoxin	Digoxin-specific Fab fragments
Insulin	Dextrose
Iron	Desferoxamine
Isoniazid	Pyridoxine
Methaemoglobinaemia	Methylene blue
Methanol and ethylene glycol	Ethanol, fomepizole
Organophosphates and carbamates	Atropine, oximes
Opioids	Naloxone
Paracetamol	N-acetyl cysteine
Sulphonylureas	Dextrose, octreotide
Tricyclic antidepressants	Sodium bicarbonate
Warfarin, brodifacoum	Vitamin K

hypo- or hyperthermia, post-ictal states and psychiatric disorders.

Clinical investigations

Investigations should only be performed if they are likely to affect the management of the patient. They are employed as either screening tests or for specific purposes.

In poisoning, screening tests aim to identify occult toxic ingestions for which early specific treatment might improve outcome. The recommended screening tests for acute poisoning are the 12-lead ECG and the serum paracetamol level. The ECG is used to exclude conduction defects which may predict potentially life-threatening cardiotoxicity. The serum paracetamol is useful to ensure that paracetamol poisoning is diagnosed within the time available for effective antidotal treatment.

Other specific investigations may be indicated to exclude important differential diagnoses, confirm a specific poisoning for which significant complications might be anticipated, assess the severity of intoxication, assess response to

Table 29.1.12 Drug levels that may be helpful in the management of selected cases of overdose
Carbamazepine
Digoxin
Dilantin
Lithium
Iron
Paracetamol
Phenobarbitone
Salicylate
Theophylline
Valproate

Table 29.1.13 Drug levels that are not helpful in the management of overdose	
CNS drugs	*Cardiovascular drugs*
Antidepressants	ACE inhibitors
Benzodiazepines	β-Blockers
Benztropine	Calcium channel blockers
Cocaine	Clonidine
Newer antipsychotics	
Opiates	
Phenothiazines	

treatment or assess the need for a specific antidote or enhanced elimination technique.

The patient with only minor manifestations of poisoning may require no other blood tests apart from a screening paracetamol level. Pregnancy should be excluded in women of childbearing age by serum or urine β-HCG if necessary. More seriously ill patients may require electrolyte, renal and liver function tests and a full blood count, creatine kinase and arterial blood gases. Urinalysis reveals myoglobinuria in significant rhabdomyolysis.

Routine qualitative drug screening of urine or blood in the overdose patient is rarely useful in planning management.

Measurement of serum drug concentrations is only useful if this provides important diagnostic or prognostic information or assists in planning management. Some drug levels that may be useful are listed in Table 29.1.12.

For most cases, drug overdose management is guided by clinical findings and not by drug levels. Some drugs commonly taken in overdose for which serum concentrations are of no value in planning management are listed in Table 29.1.13.

Radiology has a limited role in the management of overdose. A chest X-ray is indicated in any patient with a significantly decreased level of consciousness, seizures or hypoxia. It may show evidence of pulmonary aspiration. A computed tomography scan of the head may be indicated to exclude other intracranial pathology in the patient with an altered mental status. The abdominal X-ray is useful in evaluating overdose of radiopaque metals including iron, lithium, potassium, lead and arsenic.

Disposition

Both the medical and the psychiatric disposition of the overdose patient must be considered. A good risk assessment is essential to determining timely and safe disposition.

The majority of overdose patients who remain stable at 4–6 h after the ingestion do not need further close monitoring and may be admitted to a non-monitored bed until manifestations of toxicity completely resolve. An emergency observation ward is ideal for this purpose.

Any patient who develops clinical manifestations of intoxication severe enough to require the institution of specific supportive care measures requires admission to an intensive care environment. A few patients will require admission for prolonged monitoring based on the history of the ingestion. For example, anyone with a history of ingestion of colchicine, organophosphates, slow-release theophylline or slow-release calcium channel blockers requires admission because of the possibility of delayed onset of severe toxicity.

Psychiatric evaluation of deliberate self-poisoning cases is indicated as soon as the patient's medical condition permits. All such patients must be continuously supervised until the psychiatric evaluation has taken place.

Controversies

- The role of, choice of method and indications for gastric decontamination remain controversial. These procedures are no longer regarded as routine, but there are likely to be subgroups of overdose patients who may derive clinical benefit from gastrointestinal decontamination. These groups have not yet been precisely identified.

- The clinical and economic utility of establishing specialized toxicology treatment centres.

References

[1] McGrath J. A survey of deliberate self-poisoning. Med J Aust 1989;150:317–22.
[2] Pond SM. Prescription for poisoning. Med J Aust 1995;162:174–5.
[3] Murray L, Daly F, Little M, Cadogan M, editors. Toxicology handbook (2nd ed.). Sydney: Elsevier Australia; 2011.
[4] American Academy of Clinical Toxicology European Association of Poisons Centres and Clinical Toxicologists. Position paper: ipecac syrup. J Toxicol Clin Toxicol 2004;42:133–43.
[5] American Academy of Clinical Toxicology European Association of Poison Centres and Clinical Toxicologists. Position paper: gastric lavage. J Toxicol Clin Toxicol 2004;42:933–43.
[6] Kulig K, Bar-Or D, Kantrill SV, et al. Management of acutely poisoned patients without gastric emptying. Ann Emerg Med 1990;14:562–7.
[7] Merigian KS, Woodard M, Hedges JR, et al. Prospective evaluation of gastric emptying in the self-poisoned patient. Am J Emerg Med 1990;8:479–83.
[8] Pond SM, Lewis-Driver DJ, Williams G, et al. Gastric emptying in acute overdose: a prospective randomised controlled trial. Med J Aust 1995;163:345–9.
[9] American Academy of Clinical Toxicology European Association of Poisons Centres and Clinical Toxicologists. Position paper: single-dose activated charcoal. J Toxicol Clin Toxicol 2005;43:61–87.
[10] American Academy of Clinical Toxicology European Association of Poisons Centres and Clinical Toxicologists. Position paper: cathartics. J Toxicol Clinl Toxicol 2004;42:243–53.
[11] American Academy of Clinical Toxicology European Association of Poisons Centres and Clinical Toxicologists. Position paper: whole bowel irrigation. J Toxicol Clin Toxicol 2004;24:843–54.
[12] Chyka PA. Multiple-dose activated charcoal and enhancement of systemic drug clearance: summary of studies in animals and human volunteers. Clin Toxicol 1995;33:399–405.

29.2 Cardiovascular drugs

Betty Shuk Han Chan • Angela Chiew

ESSENTIALS

1 Calcium channel blockers, β-blockers, digoxin and sodium channel blocker poisonings are associated with potentially life-threatening toxicity.

2 The key to the management of calcium channel blocker and β-blocker toxicity rests with aggressive supportive care of the circulation including early use of hyperinsulinaemia euglycaemic therapy.

3 The onset of toxicity following overdose with slow-release formulations of calcium channel blockers may be delayed.

4 Early aggressive decontamination with whole-bowel irrigation is important in the management of slow-release calcium channel blocker overdose.

5 The key to management of sodium channel blockers is sodium bicarbonate therapy and hyperventilation.

6 Early identification of patients presenting with potentially severe digoxin toxicity and appropriate use of the specific Fab fragment antibody is life saving.

7 The management of clonidine poisoning is largely supportive.

8 Intravenous lipid emulsion therapy should be reserved for the treatment of severe local anaesthetic toxicity. It is not standard treatment in other overdoses.

CALCIUM CHANNEL BLOCKERS AND β-BLOCKERS

Introduction

The calcium channel blockers (CCBs) and β-blockers are widely prescribed in the community. In overdose, they present with similar clinical pictures of potentially life-threatening impairment of cardiac function. The management of both types of overdose is similar and they are discussed together.

Pharmacokinetics

Standard CCB preparations are rapidly absorbed from the gastrointestinal tract, with onset of action occurring within 30 min. Pharmacokinetic parameters are shown in Table 29.2.1. Verapamil and diltiazem undergo significant first-pass hepatic clearance. Verapamil is metabolized to norverapamil, which possesses 15–20% of verapamil's pharmacological activity and is renally excreted. Diltiazem is metabolized

to deacetyldiltiazem, which has half the potency of the parent compound and undergoes biliary excretion. The elimination half-lives of all CCBs may be prolonged following massive overdose. Amlodipine has a longer plasma half-life (30–50 h) than other CCBs.

Importantly, slow-release preparations of both verapamil and diltiazem are widely prescribed and are associated with much longer times to peak plasma concentration and clinical effect.

Absorption of β-blockers is rapid, with peak clinical effects occurring within 1–4 h. Pharmacokinetic parameters of the principal β-blockers are detailed in Table 29.2.2. Agents with high lipid solubility, such as propranolol, penetrate the blood–brain barrier better than the water-soluble agents and hence cause greater central nervous system (CNS) toxicity.

Pathophysiology

CCBs antagonize the entry of extracellular calcium into cardiac and smooth muscle, but not skeletal muscle. Upon entry into cells, calcium

participates in mechanical, electrical and biochemical reactions. It is involved in excitation–contraction of cardiac and smooth muscles, as well as phase 0 depolarization in the sinus and atrioventricular (AV) nodes by calcium influx through channels. CCBs affect myocardial contractility and slow conduction through the sinus and AV nodes. Contraction of smooth muscle is mediated by calcium influx, which is inhibited by CCBs. This results in vasodilatation and secondary reflex tachycardia from an increase in sympathetic activity.

The different classes of CCB have somewhat different pharmacological and toxic effects, as a consequence of their different binding characteristics to the dihydropyridine (DHP) receptors. Verapamil, a phenylalkylamine, produces more profound cardiac conduction defects and equal reductions in systemic vascular resistance when compared with other CCBs on a mg/kg basis. Verapamil is more likely to produce symptomatic decreases in blood pressure, heart rate and cardiac output than diltiazem, a benzothiazepine. The DHPs, which include amlodipine, felodipine, lercanidipine, nifedipine and nimodipine, preferentially bind to vascular smooth muscle and predominantly decrease systemic and coronary vascular resistance. With the exception of felodipine, they also produce a reflex tachycardia by the unloading of baroreceptors.

β-Blockers prevent the binding of catecholamines to β-receptors (β₁, β₂). β₁-Receptors are located in the myocardium, kidney and eye and β₂-receptors in adipose tissue, pancreas, liver and both smooth and skeletal muscle. β₁-Stimulation produces increased chronotropy and inotropy in the heart, increased renin secretion in the kidney and increased aqueous humor production. β₂-Stimulation relaxes smooth muscle in the blood vessels, bronchial tree, intestinal tract and uterus.

Blockade of β-receptors results in blunting of the metabolic, chronotropic and inotropic effects of catecholamines. Some β-blockers, especially propranolol, may also impede sodium entry via myocardial fast inward sodium channels, thus slowing phase 0 of the action potential. This results in a prolonged QRS duration on the electrocardiogram and produces cardiotoxicity in overdose similar to that of the tricyclic antidepressants.

The different β-blockers have slightly differing pharmacological properties, including selectivity for β-adrenoreceptors, intrinsic sympathomimetic activity and membrane-stabilizing activity. The relative affinity for β-adrenoreceptors may influence expression of toxicity. Atenolol, esmolol and metoprolol are β₁-selective agents and therapeutic use of

these drugs is less likely to produce the peripheral vasoconstriction, bronchospasm and disturbances in glucose homoeostasis that result from β₂ inhibition. However, pharmacological specificity decreases with increasing dose. Several β-blockers have partial agonist activity such that, although they block the β-receptor to catecholamines, they also weakly stimulate the receptor. This partial agonist activity may have a protective effect in overdose.

Clinical features

Calcium channel blockers

The severity of toxicity is determined by a number of factors, including the amount and characteristics of the drug ingested, the underlying health of the patient, co-ingestants and delay until treatment. The majority of serious cases and deaths result from the ingestion of verapamil or diltiazem, the most toxic of the CCBs. Ingestion of as few as 10 tablets of the higher dose formulation of verapamil or diltiazem can cause severe toxicity. Elderly patients and those with congestive cardiac failure may develop toxicity with ingestions of two to three times their normal daily dose. The principal clinical features are shown in Table 29.2.3. Ingestion of toxic amounts of standard preparations typically produces symptoms within 2 h, although maximal toxicity may not occur for up to 6–8 h. The slow-release preparations can produce significant toxicity with onset of symptoms more than 6 h post-ingestion. The major threats to life are myocardial depression and hypotension. Overdose of DHPs often produces tachycardia with normal blood pressure during the first 30 min, followed later by hypotension and bradycardia in large ingestions (>10 mg/kg). Even though amlodipine has been reported to be less toxic than verapamil and diltiazem, it can cause severe shock in large overdoses. With verapamil and diltiazem poisoning, nausea, vomiting, hyperglycaemia and metabolic acidosis can develop. All CCBs can cause

Table 29.2.1 Pharmacological profiles of the calcium channel blockers

Class	Phenylalkylamines	Benzothiazepines	Dihydropyridines
Prototype	Verapamil	Diltiazem	Nifedipine
Hours to peak plasma concentration (NR/SR)	1.5/5–7	2.3/5–11	0.5/5
Half-life (h)	3–7/10–12	3–5/6–7	2–5–5–7
Half-life in massive overdose (h)	10–12	8–9	7–8
Absorption (%)	>90	>90	>90
Vd (L/kg)	4	5	1.2
Protein binding (%)	90	80–90	90
Predominant excretion route	(1) Hepatic; (2) renal	Hepatic	Renal
Active metabolite	Yes (20%)	Yes (25–50%)	No
Heart rate (%)	−10	−15	+10
Systemic vascular resistance (%)	−10	−10	−20
AV node conduction velocity (%)	−20	−25	+10

Adapted from Kerns W II, Kline J, Ford MD. β-Blocker and calcium channel blocker toxicity. Emerg Med Clin N Am 1994;12:365–89 with permission.
NR: normal release; SR: slow release.

Table 29.2.2 Pharmacological profiles of the β-blockers

Agent	β₁-selective	Membrane stabilization	Absorption (%)	Protein binding (%)	Volume of distribution (L/kg)	Elimination/half-life (h)	Lipophilic
Atenolol	Yes	No	50	<5	0.6–1.1	Renal/6–9	Weak
Carvedilol	No	Yes	25	98	2	Hepatic/6	Weak
Esmolol	Yes	No	NA	55	3.4	Blood esterase 9 min	Weak
Labetalol	No	No	90	50	5.1–9.4	Hepatic/3–4	Weak
Metoprolol	Yes	No	90	12	5.6	Hepatic/3–4	Moderate
Oxyprenolol	No	Yes	90	80	1.2	Hepatic/2–3	Moderate
Pindolol	No	Yes	90	57	1.2–2	Renal/3–4	Moderate
Propranolol	No	Yes	90	93	3.4–6	Hepatic/3–4	High
Sotalol	No	No	70	0	0.23–0.7	Renal/9–10	Weak
Timolol	No	No	90	10	1.3–3.6	Renal/4–5	Weak

Adapted from Kerns W II, Kline J, Ford MD. β-Blocker and calcium channel blocker toxicity. Emerg Med Clin N Am 1994;12:365–89 with permission.

Table 29.2.3   Clinical features of CCB overdose

Central nervous system
- Lethargy, slurred speech, confusion, coma
- Respiratory arrest
- Coma

Gastrointestinal
- Nausea, vomiting

Cardiovascular
- Hypotension
- Bradycardia and other arrhythmias
- Sinus bradycardia
- Accelerated AV nodal rhythm
- 2° AV block
- 3° AV block with AV nodal or ventricular escape rhythm
- Sinus arrest with AV nodal escape rhythm
- Asystole

Metabolic
- Hyperglycaemia
- Lactic acidosis

Table 29.2.4   Useful drugs in the management of CCB and β-blocker toxicity

	CCBs	β-Blockers
Calcium	Calcium gluconate 10% 30 mL (child 0.6 mL/kg) IV over 10 min OR calcium chloride 10% 10 mL (child 0.2 mL/kg) IV over 10 min. Repeat every 5 min as required. Further administration guided by serum calcium concentrations	
Catecholamines	Adrenaline (epinephrine) infusion started at 1 µg/kg/min and titrate to maintain organ perfusion	Isoprenaline or adrenaline (epinephrine) infusion titrated to maintain organ perfusion
Sodium bicarbonate	A bolus dose of sodium bicarbonate 8.4% 1–2 mmol/kg, every 3–5 min, to correct severe metabolic acidosis to a pH greater than 7.3	A bolus dose of sodium bicarbonate 8.4% 1–2 mmol/kg, every 3–5 min, titrated to a narrowing of the QRS complex, resolution of arrhythmias
Hyperinsulinaemia euglycaemia	Actrapid 1 U/kg IV bolus followed by an infusion starting at 1 U/kg/h. Give with 50% dextrose 50 mL followed by infusion to maintain euglycaemia	Actrapid 1 U/kg IV bolus followed by an infusion commencing at 1 U/kg/h. Give with 50% dextrose 50 mL followed by infusion to maintain euglycaemia

symptoms of cerebral hypoperfusion, such as syncope, lethargy, lightheadedness, dizziness, altered mental status, seizures and coma.

β-Blockers

In one large series of patients with β-blocker overdose, 30–40% of patients remained asymptomatic and only 20% developed severe toxicity. Most of the life-threatening presentations or deaths that have been reported in the literature are due to overdosage of propranolol or sototol. Significant toxicity is more likely to develop in patient ingestions with these β-blockers, in patients with pre-existing cardiac disease or where there is co-ingestion of other drugs with effects on the cardiovascular system, especially CCBs and cyclic antidepressants. Ingestion of more than 1.5 g propranolol is associated with severe toxicity. If β-blocker toxicity is to develop, it is usually observed within 6 h of ingestion.

Sinus node suppression, conduction abnormalities and decreased contractility are typical. First-degree AV block, AV dissociation, right bundle branch block and intraventricular conduction delay have been reported.

Propranolol in overdose, has sodium channel blocking effect, that is characterized by cardiotoxicity including prolongation of the QRS interval and ventricular arrhythmias that more closely resemble tricyclic antidepressant overdose. Sotalol has both β-blocker activity and class 3 antiarrhythmic properties. Class 3 drugs lengthen the duration of the QT interval owing to prolongation of the action potential in His–Purkinje tissue. Therefore, ventricular

arrhythmias, such as torsades de pointes, are more common with sotalol.

Hypotension occurs as a result of negative inotropic effect. In addition, CNS effects, such as depressed conscious level and seizures, can occur, especially with the more lipid-soluble and membrane-depressant agents, such as propranolol. Hypoglycaemia is reported following atenolol overdose.

Clinical investigation

The ECG is essential in evaluating and monitoring toxic conduction defects. Serum drug levels are unhelpful in management. Patients with severe toxicity require monitoring of serum electrolytes and glucose. Serum calcium must be closely monitored if calcium salts are administered therapeutically.

Treatment

The primary aim in both β-blocker and CCB toxicity is to restore perfusion to vital organs by increasing cardiac output and the methods used are similar.

Supportive management may include airway and ventilatory support, intravenous fluid administration, early implemenation of hyperinsulinaemia euglycaemic therapy and administration of inotropes. Transcutaneous or transvenous pacing may be tried in cases with profound bradycardia, but often is of limited benefit. Severe cases may require studies on

cardiac output and peripheral vascular resistance using either Swan–Ganz catheter or pulse contour cardiac output monitoring (PiCCO) and invasive blood pressure monitoring.

If safe to do so, oral-activated charcoal should be administered as soon as practicable to all those presenting after ingestion of slow-release preparations and may be considered for other β-blocker ingestions. More aggressive decontamination, with whole-bowel irrigation, is indicated following overdose with slow-release CCBs.

A number of drugs play a role in the management of significant CCB or β-blocker poisoning, although none is a completely effective antidote. Suggested doses are shown in Table 29.2.4.

Calcium, an inotropic agent, is the initial drug of choice for CCB toxicity and has also been used successfully for β-blocker poisoning. Administration must be closely monitored, with ionized calcium measured 30 min after commencing the infusion and then second-hourly. Catecholamines are useful in attempting to restore adequate tissue perfusion.

Hyperinsulinaemic euglycaemia therapy (HIET) is increasingly advocated as therapy for hypotension unresponsive to fluids and calcium salts, with many toxicologists using HIET early in the management of these poisonings if inotropes are being considered. This therapy is supported by animal work and multiple human case reports, but a randomized controlled trial is lacking. Insulin administration switches cardiac cell metabolism from fatty acids to carbohydrates. It restores calcium fluxes and improves myocardial contractility. The recommended initial dose of actrapid is 1 U/kg IV followed by an infusion commencing at 1 U/kg/h. Although the optimal dose is still to be determined, there are some human case reports suggesting increasing doses up to 10 U/kg/h. This should be accompanied by an initial bolus dose of 50 mL 50% dextrose followed by an infusion of dextrose to maintain euglycaemia. Case reports often describe patients needing no more than 25 g/h of dextrose while poisoned (i.e. 50 mL/h of 50% dextrose).

The use of glucagon is supported only by case reports and some animal studies. There are no clinical trials supporting its efficacy in either calcium channel or β-blocker poisoning. Due to the significant doses often required, it is frequently difficult to source adequate stocks of glucagon for use as an inotropic agent. As such, its use in the treatment of calcium channel or β-blocker poisoning is not routinely recommended.

Severe propranolol toxicity is usually due to sodium channel blockade and treatment is similar to tricyclic antidepressant poisoning, including intubation, ventilation and sodium bicarbonate.

There are no clinically effective methods of enhancing the elimination of CCBs or β-blockers. When all else fails, extra-corporeal life support has been shown to allow organ perfusion until reversal of cardiac dysfunction and elimination of the drugs.

Disposition

Following overdose of β-blockers or standard CCBs, patients should be observed in a monitored environment for at least 6 h. Overdoses of slow-release CCBs require monitoring for at least 16 h from the time of ingestion. All symptomatic patients should be admitted to a monitored environment until toxicity resolves.

DIGOXIN

Introduction

Both acute and chronic digoxin toxicity are potentially life-threatening presentations to the emergency department (ED). Early recognition and administration of the specific Fab fragment antidote, if indicated, usually results in a good outcome.

Pharmacokinetics

Digoxin is moderately well absorbed following oral administration, with a bioavailability in the range of 50–80%. The initial volume of distribution is relatively small, but it is then slowly redistributed, predominantly to skeletal muscle, to give a relatively large volume of distribution of approximately 7 L/kg. Digoxin is excreted predominantly unchanged by the kidney, with an elimination half-life of about 36 h.

Pathophysiology

At a subcellular level, digoxin inhibits the function of Na–K ATPase, which leads to intracellular depletion of potassium and accumulation of sodium and calcium ions. Alteration of ionic fluxes affects cell membrane conduction. At toxic concentrations of digoxin, the effects on the cardiac conducting system produce decreased conduction velocity throughout the system, increased refractoriness at the AV node and enhanced automaticity of the Purkinje fibres. Vagal tone is also enhanced. In acute digoxin poisoning, the sudden loss of Na–K ATPase function produces hyperkalaemia.

Clinical features

Two distinct clinical presentations of digoxin toxicity are observed: acute and chronic. Both are characterized by cardiac arrhythmias and virtually all types of arrhythmia have been reported in the context of digoxin toxicity.

Acute digoxin overdose in adults is usually intentional. The therapeutic margin for digoxin is relatively narrow and any ingestion with suicidal intent is regarded as potentially life threatening.

The non-cardiac manifestations of toxicity are nausea and vomiting and hyperkalaemia. Nausea and vomiting occur early and may be the presenting complaint. The most common cardiac manifestations are sinus bradycardia, increased ventricular ectopy, sinoatrial node arrest and first-, second- or third-degree heart block. Ventricular tachycardia and fibrillation may occur. In significant acute overdose, progressive worsening of the conduction disturbance over a period of hours is usually observed.

Chronic digoxin toxicity may be precipitated by therapeutic errors, intercurrent illnesses that decrease renal elimination of digoxin or by drug interactions. Common drug interactions include those with quinidine, CCBs, amiodarone and indomethacin. The patient is commonly elderly. Reduced muscle mass and reduced renal function in the elderly mean that both the volume of distribution and rate of elimination of digoxin may be substantially reduced.

Nausea and vomiting are also common manifestations of chronic digoxin toxicity and are frequent presenting symptoms. Neurological manifestations are characteristic of chronic toxicity and include visual disturbances, weakness and fatigue. The most common cardiovascular manifestations of chronic digoxin toxicity are arrhythmias and these may be sinus bradycardia, atrial fibrillation with slowed ventricular response or a junctional escape rhythm, atrial tachycardia with block and ventricular tachycardia and fibrillation.

Death from digoxin toxicity results from pump failure, severe cardiac conduction impairment or ventricular arrhythmia.

Clinical investigations

The most important investigations are the ECG, serum electrolytes and creatinine and serum digoxin concentration.

The ECG is invaluable in documenting the type and severity of any cardiac conduction defect. Serial ECGs may demonstrate worsening of the cardiac conduction defects as toxicity progresses.

In acute poisoning, the serum potassium rises as Na–K ATPase function is progressively impaired. Hyperkalaemia denotes significant acute digoxin toxicity. Prior to the availability of a specific antidote for digoxin poisoning, a serum potassium concentration >5.5 mEq/L was associated with a high probability of lethal outcome. Hyperkalaemia seldom occurs in chronic digoxin poisoning, unless patient has acute renal failure. In fact, these patients are frequently hypokalaemic and hypomagnesaemic secondary to chronic diuretic use. Both these electrolyte disorders are important as they exacerbate digoxin toxicity.

Serum digoxin levels taken at 6 hours post ingestion are useful in assessing and confirming toxicity, but must be carefully interpreted in the context of the clinical presentation. They do not accurately correlate with clinical toxicity. Therapeutic concentrations are usually quoted as 0.6–1.0 nmol/L (0.5–0.8 mcg/L). Significant chronic toxicity may be associated with 0.6–1.0 nmol/L (0.5–0.8 mcg/L) elevations of the serum digoxin concentration. This is particularly the case in the presence of pre-existing cardiac disease, hypokalaemia or hypomagnesaemia. Following acute overdose, the serum digoxin concentration is relatively high compared to tissue concentrations, until distribution is completed by 6–12 h post-ingestion. However, early concentrations greater than 15 nmol/L indicate serious poisoning.

Treatment

The best outcome is associated with early recognition of digoxin toxicity.

For chronic toxicity with minimal symptoms, management may involve no more than observation, cessation of digoxin administration, correction of hypokalaemia and hypomagnesaemia and appropriate management of any factors that contributed to the development of toxicity. However, the presence of any cardiovascular system effects, particularly in elderly patients, is an indication for the administration of Fab fragments of digoxin-specific antibodies. Apart from brady-tachy arrhythmias that are associated with haemodynamic instability, patients who have increased automaticies with cardiac or gastrointestinal symptoms may be considered for digoxin specific antibody. This is especially for patients who have renal failure with a Creatinine clearance <30 ml/min. From an economic viewpoint, the potential reduction in length of stay of 1-2 days as a result of treatment with digoxin specific antibody needs to take into consieration of the increase in the cost of 1 vial of digoxin Fab to A$850 per 40 mg vial.

Following acute overdose, the patient should be initially managed in a monitored area with full resuscitative equipment available. Immediate attention to the airway, breathing and circulation may be required. Intravenous access should be established and blood sent for urgent electrolytes and serum digoxin concentration. Although digoxin is well bound by charcoal, administration is usually difficult because of repetitive vomiting and attempts should not detract from other interventions.

The specific antidote to digoxin poisoning is Fab fragments of digoxin-specific antibodies, which should be administered as soon as possible in any potentially life-threatening digoxin intoxication. Commonly accepted indications for the administration of Fab fragments are listed in Table 29.2.5.

Fab fragments of digoxin-specific antibodies

These are derived from IgG antidigoxin antibodies produced in sheep. Removal of the Fc fragments of the antibodies greatly reduces the

Table 29.2.5 Indications for administration of fab fragments of digoxin-specific antibodies following acute overdose

Hyperkalaemia (K >5.5 mmol/L) associated with digoxin toxicity
History of ingestion of more than 10 mg of digoxin
Haemodynamically unstable cardiac arrhythmia
Cardiac arrest from digoxin toxicity
Serum digoxin concentration greater than 15 nmol/L

potential for hypersensitivity reactions and contributes to the remarkable safety profile of the product. Intravenously administered Fab fragments bind digoxin in the intravascular space on a mole-for-mole basis. As binding continues, digoxin moves down a concentration gradient from the tissue compartments to the intravascular compartment. Bound digoxin is inactive. A clinical response is usually observed within 20–30 min of administration. The Fab–digoxin complexes are excreted in the urine.

The extraordinary clinical efficacy of digoxin-specific fragments has been well documented in a few multicentre studies. These studies demonstrated the safety of the product, with the adverse reactions reported being hypokalaemia (4%), rapid atrial fibrillation or worsening of congestive cardiac failure (3%) and allergic reaction (0.8%).

The correct dose of Fab fragments may be calculated on the basis that 40 mg (one vial) will bind 0.5 mg of digoxin. If the dose ingested is unknown and/or a steady-state serum digoxin concentration is not available, dosing of Fab fragments must be empiric. A reasonable empiric dosing is to give 2 vials initially and then check for a clinical response. Further digoxin specific antibody may be given to neutralise half of the body burden once digoxin concentration is available. If the digoxin ingested dose or serum concentration is known, give half of the equimolar dose is adequate to stablise patient with severe digoxin toxiicty. In cardiac arrest, give a bolus dose (5 vials), and this dose can be repeated after 30 to 60 minutes if there has been no clinical response. Smaller doses (two vials) are usually sufficient to reverse the effects of chronic toxicity.

It is important that ED staff are aware of the amount and location of supplies of Fab fragments within their own institution and know the most rapid way to acquire further stocks should the need arise.

Serum digoxin concentrations will be extremely high following the administration of Fab fragments because most assays measure both bound and unbound digoxin.

Disposition

Patients with mild, chronic digoxin toxicity (gastrointestinal symptoms only) may be discharged after cessation of digoxin therapy provided there are no significant electrolyte disturbances, renal failure or other precipitating medical conditions. Following administration of Fab fragments, cases of chronic toxicity with conduction defects usually require medical admission for observation and treatment of intercurrent illness.

Acute overdoses require close observation for at least 12 h. Those that develop toxicity require admission and an appropriate level of monitoring. Following successful administration of digoxin-specific Fab fragments, patients must be carefully monitored for hypokalaemia and worsening of any underlying medical conditions for which digoxin may have been prescribed therapeutically. All intentional ingestions require psychiatric evaluation prior to medical discharge.

CLONIDINE

Introduction

Clonidine, an imidazoline derivative, is a central α_2-adrenergic agonist. It was first developed in the 1960s as a nasal decongestant. It is currently used for the management of hypertension, attention deficit hyperactivity disorder (ADHD) as well as withdrawal symptoms from drug and alcohol addiction, tobacco withdrawal and Tourette's syndrome. Clonidine toxicity often mimics that of opioids.

Pharmacokinetics

Clonidine is well absorbed with a bioavailability of almost 100%. The peak concentration in plasma and effect is observed within 1–3 h. The elimination half-life is 6–24 h with a mean half-life of 12 h. Half of the administered dose is excreted unchanged by the kidney.

Pathophysiology

Clonidine activates central α_2-receptors. This results in a reduction in CNS sympathetic

Table 29.2.6 Drugs highly associated with QRS widening and sodium channel blockade

Antidepressants	Tricyclic antidepressants Venlafaxine
Antiepileptic drugs	Carbamazepine
Antihistamines	Diphenhydramine
Antipsychotics*	Chlorpromazine
Cardiovascular drugs	Flecainide Propranolol
Local anaesthetics	Bupivacaine Ropivacaine
Others	Bupropion Chloroquine, hydroxychloroquine and quinine Cocaine Dextropropoxyphene Dolasetron Orphenadrine

*Antipsychotic drugs are not highly associated with QRS widening, but are commonly taken in overdose.
Reproduced with permission from Toxicology and Wilderness Expert Group. Drugs highly associated with QRS widening and sodium channel blockade (Table 17.1) [revised 2011 June]. In: Therapeutic guidelines eTG complete [Internet]. Melbourne: Therapeutic Guidelines Limited; 2012 Nov.

outflow at the vasomotor centre in the medulla oblongata. Clonidine is thought to reduce blood pressure through a reduction in cardiac output as well as its weak peripheral α-adrenergic antagonist properties. Clonidine also stimulates parasympathetic outflow and this may contribute to the slowing of heart rate as a consequence of increased vagal tone. Paradoxically, clonidine overdose can result in an initial hypertension from its partial α_1-adrenergic agonist effect. It is suggested that clonidine's inhibition of sympathetic outflow is mediated through endogenous opiate release.

Clinical features

Clonidine can cause transient hypertension from initial vasoconstriction with parenteral administration followed by hypotension. In addition to bradycardia and conduction defects, it can cause a central chlorpromazine-like effect with sedation. Other CNS symptoms include coma, seizure, miosis, reduced respiration and hypothermia. The median onset of symptoms following clonidine ingestion is 30 min and patients are usually symptomatic on arrival at the ED. Symptoms usually resolve by 24 h.

Investigations

The ECG is essential in evaluating and monitoring for bradycardia and conduction defects.

Treatment

The management of clonidine poisoning is primarily supportive. Hypotension usually responds to intravenous fluids. Atropine has been shown to abolish bradycardia in some case reports. Occasionally, inotropes may be required to maintain haemodynamic stability. Hypertension is usually short lived and rarely requires treatment. Patients are usually symptomatic on arrival and the benefits of administering activated charcoal are unlikely to outweigh the risk of aspiration.

Disposition

Patients should be observed in hospital until they are asymptomatic and bradycardia has resolved. They do not require ongoing cardiac monitoring for a stable sinus bradycardia.

CLASS 1C ANTIARRHYTHMICS

Introduction

Apart from the class one antiarrhythmics, many drugs in overdose cause sodium channel blockade. Drugs highly associated with sodium channel blockade and QRS widening are shown in Table 29.2.6. Overdose with class 1c antiarrhythmic drugs is among the most serious ingestions and is associated with a high morbidity and mortality. Overdoses with these agents are rare but they may be rapidly lethal with profound cardiovascular collapse. Drugs in this class include flecainide and propafenone; they are used for the treatment of SVT and ventricular arrhythmias. Class 1c antiarrhythmics block the fast inward sodium channel during phase 0 of the action potential. They have slow offset kinetics and cause complete blockade of sodium channel for a much longer duration than class 1a and 1b antiarrhythmics.

Pharmacokinetics

Flecainide has a high oral bioavailability and a rapid onset of action of 30 to 60 min. It has a long elimination half-life of 7–23 h. In adults, ingestions of 800 mg or more should be considered as life threatening. Similarly, propafenone has a long elimination half-life.

Clinical Features

In overdose, they have a rapid onset of clinical symptoms, typically with 30 min to 2 h. Overdose symptoms include nausea, vomiting, hypotension, bradycardia, varying degrees of atrioventricular block and tachyarrhythmia. In severe cases, coma and seizures may occur. Severe intoxication is frequently fatal because of the rapid onset of hypotension and ventricular arrhythmias.

Investigations

The ECG is essential in evaluating and monitoring the QRS duration, conduction defects and QT interval. The most common and important ECG change in overdose is QRS widening (more than 120 ms). Although QT prolongation occurs in flecainide overdose, torsades de pointes is rare.

Treatment

The mainstay of management of class 1c overdose is good supportive care including inotropic support, gastrointestinal decontamination and early and repeated doses of sodium bicarbonate to treat any broad complex arrhythmias and hypotension. Treatment is similar to other sodium channel blocking agents, such as the tricyclic antidepressants and includes plasma alkalinization to a pH of 7.5 with hyperventilation and repeated boluses of sodium bicarbonate. The use of antiarrhythmic drugs is problematic and are generally contraindicated

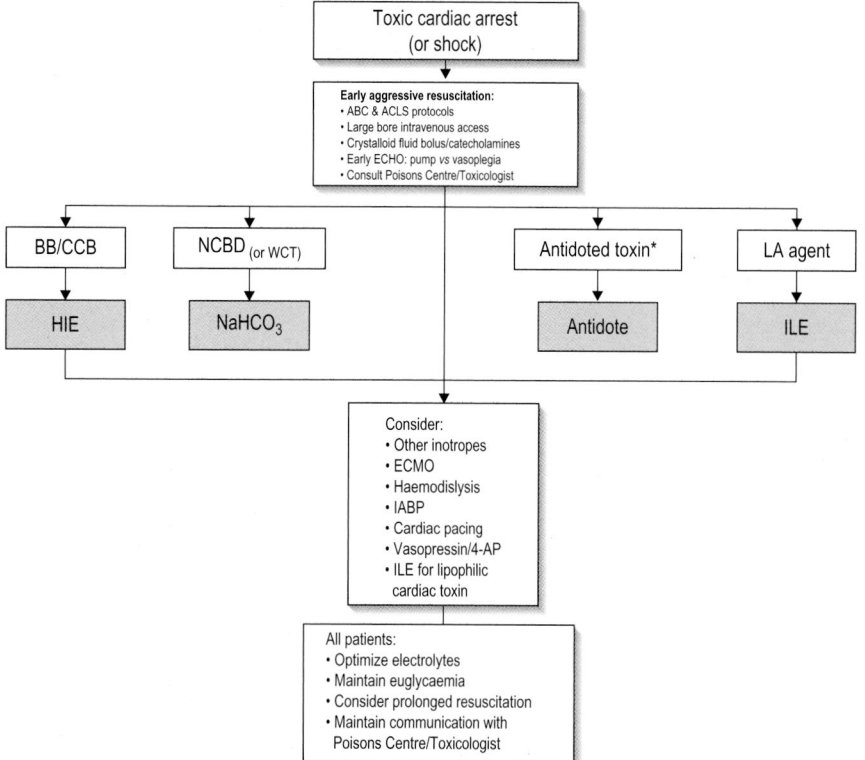

Fig. 29.2.1 Flow chart management of cardiac arrest following poisonings. *Toxin with available antidote, e.g. natural toxin, digoxin, organophosphates; 4-AP: 4-aminopyridine; BB: β-blocker; CCB: calcium channel blocker; ECMO: extracorporeal membrane oxygenation; HIE: high-dose insulin euglycaemia; IABP: intra-aortic balloon pump; ILE: intravenous lipid emulsion; LA: local anaesthetic; NACB: sodium channel blocker; WCT: wide complex tachycardia. *(From Gunja N, Graudins A. Management of cardiac arrest following poisoning. Emerg Med Australas 2011; 23:16–22, with permission.)*

and sufficient amounts of sodium bicarbonate should be used first.

Disposition

Asymptomatic patients with a normal ECG 4 h after ingestion of flecainide are unlikely to develop toxicity. Patients who are symptomatic should be admitted to a monitored area.

CARDIAC ARREST DUE TO CARDIOVASCULARLY ACTIVE DRUGS

It is important for clinicians to be aware that cardiac arrest due to overdose of cardiovascularly active drugs may necessitate prolonged CPR and resuscitative manoeuvres and consideration of heroic measures, such as cardiopulmonary bypass (Fig. 29.2.1). Consultation with a clinical toxicologist is always recommended prior to cessation of resuscitative efforts in these cases.

Controversies

- The advantages of glucagon over other inotropic agents in the management of CCB and β-blocker overdose are questionable. It is now rarely used as a first-line agent.
- The indications for initiation of hyperinsulinaemia euglycaemia therapy in CCB and β-blocker overdose are not well defined. This therapy is being advocated as first-line therapy for toxic hypotension.
- There are case reports of the successful use of cardiopulmonary bypass to maintain an adequate cardiac output following severe CCB, β-blocker and sodium channel blocker overdoses. Techniques such as this and extracorporeal membrane oxygenation may play a role in the management of otherwise fatal cases of cardiovascular collapse.
- The dosing regime of digoxin specific antibody is likely to be lower than the full equimolar dose that was previously advocated. It is proposed that giving half of the equimolar dose is adequate to stabilise patients with severe digoxin toxicity. The cost of the digoxin antibody should be weighed against the costs of additional in-hospital care that may be incurred if they are withheld.
- A clinical response to naloxone may occur in up to 31% of cases of clonidine toxicity but the clinical value of this intervention is doubtful.

Further reading

Antman EM, Stone PH, Muller JE, et al. Calcium channel blocking agents in the treatment of cardiovascular diseases: Part E basic and clinical electrophysiological effects. Ann Intern Med 1980;93:875–85.

Antman EM, Wenger FL, Butler VP, et al. Treatment of 150 cases of life threatening digitalis intoxication with digoxin specific Fab antibody fragments: final report of multicenter study. Circulation 1990;81:1744–52.

Auzinger GM, Scheinkestel CD. Successful extracorporeal life support in a case of severe flecainide intoxication. Crit Care Med 2001;29:887–90.

Bateman DN. Digoxin-specific antibody fragments: how much and when? Toxicological reviews. 2004;3:135–43.

Baud FJ, et al. Clinical review: aggressive management and extracorporeal support for drug-induced cardiotoxicity. Crit Care 2007;11:207.

Buckley N, Dawson AH, Howarth D, et al. Slow release verapamil poisoning. Use of polyethylene glycol whole bowel lavage and high dose calcium. Med J Aust 1993;158:202.

Engebretsen KM, Kaczmarek KM, Morgan J, Holger J. High-dose insulin therapy in beta-blocker and calcium channel blocker poisoning. Clintox 2011;49:277–83.

Gunja N, Graudins A. Management of cardiac arrest following poisoning. Emerg Med Australas 2011;23:16–22.

Holger JS, Engerbretsen KM, Fritzlar SJ, et al. Insulin versus vasopressin and epinephrine to treat β-blocker toxicity. Clin Toxicol 2007;45:396–401.

Kolecki PF, Curry SC. Poisoning by sodium channel blocking agents. Crit Care Clin 1997;13:829–48.

Love J, Howell JM, Litovitz TL, et al. Acute beta blocker overdose: factors associated with the development of cardiovascular morbidity. J Toxicol Clin Toxicol 2000;38:275–81.

Seger D. Clonidine toxicity revisited. Clin Toxicol 2002;40:145–55.

29.3 Antipsychotic drugs

Dino Druda • Shaun Greene

ESSENTIALS

1 Antipsychotics can cause numerous adverse effects at therapeutic doses, which may limit compliance and require changes to treatment regimens.

2 Extrapyramidal effects are less pronounced with the newer agents.

3 Clozapine is associated with agranulocytosis and myocarditis with therapeutic use and requires strict surveillance.

4 Following overdose, antipsychotics predominantly cause CNS depression and cardiovascular effects.

5 Amisulpride can cause significant QT prolongation which may result in torsades de pointes.

6 The mainstay of management of antipsychotic overdose is supportive.

7 Neuroleptic malignant syndrome is a rare, idiosyncratic adverse reaction which may be lethal without timely diagnosis and treatment.

Table 29.3.1 Typical and atypical antipsychotic drugs

Typical	Atypical
Chlorpromazine	Clozapine
Prochlorperazine	Olanzapine
Fluphenazine	Quetiapine
Haloperidol	Risperidone
Droperidol	Paliperidone
Flupenthixol	Amisulpride
Zuclopenthixol	Ziprasidone Aripiprazole

Introduction

The antipsychotics form a heterogeneous group of medications that has evolved since chlorpromazine was first used to treat schizophrenia in the 1950s. The first-generation or so-called 'typical' antipsychotics caused many adverse effects, especially movement disorders such as extrapyramidal symptoms (EPS) and tardive dyskinesia (TD). They also have very little efficacy in treating the negative symptoms of schizophrenia (social withdrawal, anhedonia, poverty of speech, etc.). This led to the development and marketing of the second-generation, or atypical, antipsychotics in the late 1980s. In general, these drugs have fewer tendencies to cause movement disorders and have efficacy in managing the negative symptoms of schizophrenia, while maintaining efficacy in the management of acute psychosis. For this reason, they have largely replaced the older antipsychotic as first-line therapy in the treatment of schizophrenia and psychotic disorders.

Pharmacology

There are numerous ways of classifying the antipsychotic drugs; typical or atypical as described above (Table 29.3.1), by their chemical structure or according to neuroreceptor binding affinity.

All antipsychotic drugs produce their beneficial therapeutic effects by antagonizing the dopamine D_2 receptors in the mesolimbic system. The first-generation antipsychotics were classified as high or low potency depending on their affinity for the D_2 receptor. However, antagonism of the other D_2 receptors leads to many of the adverse clinical effects. Antagonism of D_2 receptors in the nigrostriatal pathway leads to movement disorders (EPS, akathisia, TD), antagonism of the D_2 receptors in the mesocortical area can contribute to the negative symptoms and antagonism of D_2 receptors in the anterior pituitary stimulates prolactin secretion which can lead to gynaecomastia and galactorrhoea. Blockade of D_2 receptors in the anterior hypothalamus is associated with alterations in temperature regulation, which can lead to hypo- or hyperthermia and may be involved in the development of neuroleptic malignant syndrome, which is discussed later. The antiemetic effect of some of the antipsychotics is due to antagonism of the D_2 receptors in the chemoreceptor trigger zone in the medulla.

The newer atypical antipsychotics also derive therapeutic efficacy from affinity and antagonism at various serotonin (5-HT) receptors. Antagonism at the $5-HT_{2A}$ receptor is implicated both in increasing the efficacy of treating the negative symptoms of schizophrenia and also in reducing the incidence of EPS.

Agents with high antagonism of muscarinic M_1 and M_2 receptors (e.g. olanzapine, quetiapine) can cause an agitated delirium and peripheral features characteristic of anticholinergic toxicity (flushing, dry skin, tachycardia, urinary retention, etc.). Drugs that have a higher anticholinergic activity than dopaminergic tend to cause fewer extrapyramidal effects. High relative antagonism of histamine H_1 receptors leads to sedation and, to a lesser extent, hypotension. Antagonism at the α_1-adrenergic receptor can result in hypotension (e.g. quetiapine, clozapine) and clozapine also antagonizes the α_2-receptor, although the clinical significance of this is uncertain.

Several first-generation antipsychotics can block voltage-gated fast sodium channels which, in overdose, can lead to slowing of cardiac conduction thus prolonging the QRS complex and impairing myocardial contractility. Blockade of the delayed rectifier potassium channel causes delayed repolarization and leads to prolongation of the QT interval.

Despite the heterogeneous nature of the antipsychotics, in general, they share similar pharmacokinetic properties. They are well absorbed after oral administration, with peak serum concentrations usually occurring within 2–6 hours of ingestion. This may be delayed following overdose of agents with significant anticholinergic properties. They are lipophilic, have large volumes of distribution and the majority of the agents are highly protein bound. They are extensively metabolized in the liver, with some having active metabolites.

Clinical effects

Adverse effects

Adverse effects at therapeutic doses may be dose related or idiosyncratic.

Extrapyramidal syndromes

These are a heterogeneous group of disorders characterized by abnormal neuromuscular activity. They can be particularly distressing to patients and may lead to difficulties with compliance and cessation of treatment. There are four well-recognized syndromes–acute dystonia, akathisia, parkinsonism and tardive dyskinesia. Of these, the first three are usually reversible, whereas tardive dyskinesia is irreversible, but occurs late, usually after months to years of treatment.

EPS are more common among the first-generation typical antipsychotics, especially those with high potency, such as haloperidol. Atypical antipsychotics are associated with a lower incidence of EPS, although it must be appreciated that EPS can occur with the use of any antipsychotic. Reactions are usually idiosyncratic, although can occur following overdose.

Acute dystonia is characterized by sustained involuntary muscle contraction, which commonly involves the face, head and neck, but can also involve the extremities. Rarely, the larynx can be involved, which may be life threatening. Risk factors for developing dystonia include male gender, young age and previous history of dystonic reaction. Onset is usually within a few hours of exposure, but may be delayed for several days.

Akathisia is characterized by an unpleasant sensation of restlessness or unease and, often, the patient is unable to remain still. It can be difficult to diagnose and can often be attributed to the underlying psychiatric condition rather than to the treatment.

Drug-induced parkinsonism is similar to idiopathic Parkinson's disease, with rigidity and bradykinesia, although the characteristic tremor may be less pronounced. It is more common in older patients and patients on high potency agents.

Tardive dyskinesia is characterized by repetitive, involuntary, purposeless movements, classically involving the muscles of the face

and mouth, although the limbs and trunk may be involved. It usually appears after months or years of therapy with antipsychotic medication and is usually resistant to treatment.

Cardiovascular effects

Cardiovascular effects of antipsychotics with therapeutic use include tachycardia, postural hypotension and ECG changes. Postural hypotension may be multifactorial, with α_1-adrenergic blockade and direct myocardial depression playing a role. ECG changes may be diverse, with QRS prolongation, QT prolongation and non-specific ST-segment and T-wave changes being reported.

Seizures

All antipsychotics can lower the seizure threshold. However, seizures rarely complicate therapeutic use of antipsychotics, unless the patient has underlying risk factors, such as organic brain disease or epilepsy.

Metabolic syndromes

Chronic use of many of the antipsychotics is associated with the development of a metabolic syndrome, which can lead to weight gain, dyslipidaemia, hypertension and impaired glucose tolerance. These can be distressing and also contribute to the development of cardiovascular disease and type II diabetes. The development of these adverse effects can affect compliance with treatment. Metabolic affects are particularly associated with the use of olanzapine and clozapine.

Neuroleptic malignant syndrome (NMS)

NMS is a rare idiosyncratic adverse reaction, which can occur with any of the antipsychotic medications. Risk factors, diagnosis and management of NMS are described later in this chapter.

Clozapine

Clozapine is associated with a number of idiosyncratic effects that can occur with therapeutic use and requires more vigilant surveillance. These include agranulocytosis and myocarditis. These should be considered in the differential diagnosis if a patient on clozapine presents unwell.

Overdose

Following overdose of antipsychotics, the most common and significant manifestations involve the CNS and cardiovascular system.

Dose-dependent CNS depression occurs, ranging from lethargy and somnolence to coma and seizures. Airway protective reflexes may be impaired, requiring intensive care. Many of the agents can cause significant anticholinergic delirium with associated peripheral effects, such as urinary retention, flushed skin and reduction in sweat and saliva secretion.

The most common cardiovascular effects are tachycardia and hypotension. Tachycardia may be due to anticholinergic effects and also as a response to hypotension. Hypotension often occurs as a result of peripheral α_1-receptor blockade, leading to vasodilatation.

ECG changes are often present after overdose and can include QRS prolongation and QT interval prolongation. Significant arrhythmias are uncommon, apart from following overdose with amisulpride, which can cause torsades des pointes.

Some of the specific clinical features following overdose of individual agents are described below.

Amisulpride

Overdose of amisulpride commonly causes QT prolongation, bradycardia and hypotension. Episodes of torsades de pointes have been reported and so amisulpride is considered to be particularly cardiotoxic. Onset of cardiotoxicity may be delayed for greater than 12 hours and QT prolongation can persist for many hours, with the potential to develop torsades de pointes abruptly. Ingestions greater than 4 g have been associated with development of prolonged QT and ingestions greater than 8 g can cause significant sedation and hypotension.

Chlorpromazine

Ingestions of greater than 15 mg/kg of chlorpromazine in children are associated with significant toxicity. Large overdoses >5 g, especially in drug-naïve patients, may lead to significant CNS depression, which may require intubation and intensive care due to loss of airway protective reflexes. Significant hypotension also occurs following overdose.

Clozapine

Acute overdose of clozapine leads to CNS depression, which is more pronounced in clozapine-naïve patients, who may require intubation. Seizures are reported in overdose. Despite the known anticholinergic properties of clozapine, hypersalivation is common. Miosis is classically described, but mydriasis can also occur. Agranulocytosis does not occur after a single overdose.

Haloperidol

Sedation and EPS are common following overdose of haloperidol. Haloperidol has also been associated with QT prolongation and arrhythmias following large ingestions or intravenous administration.

Olanzapine

Onset of clinical features following overdose is within 6 hours. Sedation and anticholinergic effects are the most common manifestations, leading to a combination of agitation and drowsiness, which may require intubation. Miosis may be noted. Tachycardia is common, but significant ECG abnormalities are rare.

Quetiapine

Quetiapine is available in immediate and extended release preparations. Overdose causes dose-related CNS depression and tachycardia. Hypotension and seizures are also reported after larger ingestions. Ingested doses of greater than 3 g are associated with increased length of stay and ICU admission. QTc prolongation is often reported, although the clinical significance of this is unclear, as there have been no reported cases of torsades de pointes. It may be that the prolongation of the QTc is as a result of overcorrection for tachycardia rather than intrinsic cardiotoxicity.

Risperidone

Risperidone is relatively benign following overdose, with tachycardia and dystonia being the most common effects. Onset of dystonia may be delayed and may recur after treatment.

Ziprasidone

Ziprasidone is associated with QT prolongation, both with therapeutic use and following overdose. Torsades de pointes has been reported after ziprasidone overdose with co-ingestants, but not in isolation.

Investigations

Antipsychotic toxicity is primarily diagnosed on history and examination for typical clinical features. Serum drug concentrations are not usually available in a clinically useful time frame or helpful in the management of acute overdose. In the case of patients on clozapine who present unwell to hospital, then a clozapine concentration can be measured. For these patients, a WCC is helpful when looking for agranulocytosis and troponin may be elevated in cases of clozapine-induced myocarditis. If this is suspected, then ECG and echocardiography may also be required.

Initial ECG evaluation should occur for all patients following antipsychotic overdose and any abnormality of the QRS or QT intervals warrants continuous cardiac monitoring. If initial ECG is normal, then it should be repeated after 6 hours in asymptomatic patients. More prolonged cardiac monitoring is required for patients following overdose with amisulpride or ziprasidone.

Treatment

The management of antipsychotic toxicity is primarily supportive. Attention to initial resuscitation should occur initially. Mild sedation requires no specific treatment. Patients with significantly decreased conscious state with loss of airway protective reflexes will require intubation, ventilation and intensive care.

Decontamination with activated charcoal can be considered if the presentation is within an hour and there is no clinical sign of CNS depression. Otherwise, administration of activated charcoal should be delayed until after the airway has been secured with intubation. There is no evidence for any benefit from enhanced elimination techniques, either with multidose activated charcoal or extracorporeal techniques and so they are not indicated.

Hypotension should initially be treated with an appropriate bolus of crystalloid solution. If there is no response to initial fluid bolus, then vasopressors may be required. There have been reports of worsening hypotension following the administration of adrenaline to patients who are hypotensive following quetiapine overdose, so noradrenaline is the preferred initial vasopressor. Patients with ventricular arrhythmias or with prolonged QRS should be managed with sodium bicarbonate in a similar fashion to patients with significant tricyclic antidepressant (TCA) toxicity. Intravenous bicarbonate 8.4% (1 mL = 1 mmol) 1–2 mmol/kg boluses should be administered to obtain an arterial pH of 7.50–7.55. The pH may then be maintained in this range using hyperventilation in intubated patients. QT prolongation requires no specific management other than cardiac monitoring and correction of any potential contributing electrolyte abnormalities, such as hypokalaemia or hypomagnesaemia. Should torsades de pointes develop, it should be treated in the first instance with IV magnesium sulphate 50% 2–4 mL (1–2 g or 4–8 mmol) infusion over 10 minutes. Chemical or electrical overdrive pacing may also be required to avoid further instances.

Seizures are often self-limiting and require no treatment. However, should intervention be necessary, benzodiazepines should be used first line. Barbiturates and/or general anaesthesia are used for refractory seizures or status. There is no role for other anticonvulsants, such as phenytoin, in the management of drug-induced seizures.

Anticholinergic delirium should be managed initially with non-pharmacological measures, such as nursing in a quiet area and limiting stimulation. Urinary retention should be sought and relieved with a urinary catheter, as the distress caused by this may contribute to any agitation. Should medication be required, titrated doses of benzodiazepines (e.g. diazepam) should be used, although it must be appreciated that benzodiazepines may contribute to any CNS depressant effects of the ingested antipsychotic.

Acute dystonia is managed with an anticholinergic agent, such as benztropine (1–2 mg given IV or IM). Benzodiazepines may also be used. Repeat dosing may be required as the dystonia can recur.

Disposition

Patients should be observed for 6 hours after overdose of most antipsychotics. If they remain asymptomatic and have a normal ECG at this time, then they can be medically cleared for discharge. This observation period should be extended for 12 hours following significant ingestion of extended release preparations of quetiapine, ingestions of >4 g amisulpride and ingestions of ziprasidone.

Patients with significant symptoms should be admitted for observation until symptoms are resolving. Intensive care admission is required for patients requiring intubation and ventilation. In the event of any concerning ECG abnormalities, such as QT prolongation, then admission for cardiac monitoring is recommended until these changes are resolving.

Neuroleptic malignant syndrome

Neuroleptic malignant syndrome is a rare, idiosyncratic, potentially life-threatening adverse reaction that has been reported to occur with all the antipsychotics. There is a large variation in reported incidence, but recent pooled data suggest an incidence of 0.01–0.2%. The pathophysiology of NMS is not completely understood, but is thought to be due to central dopamine blockade, especially in the nigrostriatal and hypothalamic pathways. Risk factors for the development of NMS include male gender, young age, use of high potency antipsychotics, recent increase in dose, parenteral administration, dehydration and organic brain disease.

Clinical features

The onset of NMS occurs typically over 1–3 days. The typical clinical features are a combination of altered mental status, hyperthermia (temperature >38°C), autonomic dysfunction and muscular rigidity ('lead pipe' rigidity). The altered mental status ranges from delirium and confusion to stupor and coma. Autonomic dysfunction can manifest as tachycardia, cardiac arrhythmias, respiratory irregularities and hypo- or hypertension. The muscular rigidity is classically described as 'lead-pipe' rigidity, with increased tone and resistance to passive movement. There may be superimposed tremor leading to cogwheeling. Other neuromuscular abnormalities include bradykinesia, dystonia, mutism and dysarthria.

Differential diagnosis

There have been numerous diagnostic criteria proposed for NMS, but none are universally accepted. Alternate diagnoses must be considered and excluded, particularly CNS infection. Other conditions to be considered in the differential include heatstroke, thyrotoxicosis, serotonin toxicity, anticholinergic syndrome, malignant catatonia, non-convulsive status epilepticus, phaeochromocytoma and drug intoxication (MAOIs, sympathomimetics).

However, NMS must be considered in any patient on antipsychotic medication who is unwell, particularly when there is altered mental status, fever or muscle rigidity, especially if there has been a recent change in the antipsychotic regimen.

Investigations

There is no diagnostic test for NMS, although there are characteristic laboratory abnormalities in some cases. Increased muscle enzymes (CK, LDH, AST) are often present in cases of NMS. Leucocytosis is also frequently observed. There may be other electrolyte disturbance, metabolic acidosis and coagulation abnormalities.

Investigations to rule out alternate diagnoses need to be carried out, including CT scan of the brain and lumbar puncture to rule out CNS infection.

Treatment

Once NMS is diagnosed, it is essential to institute aggressive supportive care. The offending drug must be immediately withdrawn. Patients are often dehydrated, so fluid resuscitation should be commenced. Hyperthermia must be managed aggressively with passive and active cooling. If the temperature is >39.5°C, then intubation and neuromuscular paralysis should be considered. There is increased risk of thromboembolism, so prophylaxis should be commenced.

Benzodiazepines are often used early in the treatment of NMS and they may be effective in ameliorating symptoms in milder cases. Bromocriptine is a centrally acting dopamine agonist that can only be administered orally or via NG tube. The starting dose is 2.5 mg three times daily, increased to a daily maximum of 40 mg. It needs to be continued for 1–2 weeks, as premature discontinuation can lead to rebound symptoms. Potential adverse effects include vomiting and worsening of psychosis.

Dantrolene interferes with calcium release in skeletal muscle cells and therefore reduces skeletal muscle activity. It may be useful in cases of NMS with prominent hyperthermia and muscle rigidity. It can be given by IV infusion at 2–3 mg/kg/day. However, there are conflicting reports regarding the efficacy and outcome benefit of dantrolene in the management of NMS. Electroconvulsive therapy (ECT) has been advocated for cases of NMS refractory to pharmacological treatments, although its efficacy is unclear.

Controversies

- The clinical significance of QTc prolongation following quetiapine overdose is unclear. It is thought to be due to overcorrection of the QT for tachycardia and, as yet, there have been no reported cases of torsades de pointes.
- The optimum time for cardiac monitoring following significant amisulpride or ziprasidone overdose is yet to be clearly defined.
- Many antipsychotics are highly lipophilic and there have been case reports of lipid rescue therapy being used to treat significant toxicity. However, evidence for definite outcome benefit is lacking.
- The efficacy of specific therapies for NMS, such as dantrolene, bromocriptine and ECT, is controversial and evidence of outcome benefit is lacking.

Further reading

Balit CR, Isbister GK, Hackett LP, Whyte IM. Quetiapine poisoning: a case series. Ann Emerg Med 2003;42:751–8.

Burns MJ. The pharmacology and toxicology of atypical antipsychotic agents. Clin Toxicol 2001;39:1–14.

Hawkins DJ, Unwin P. Paradoxical and severe hypotension in response to adrenaline infusions in massive quetiapine overdose. Crit Care Resusc 2008;10:320–2.

Isbister GK, Balit CR, Kilham HA. Antipsychotic poisoning in young children. Drug Safety 2005;28:1029–34.

Isbister GK, Balit CR, Macleod D, Duffull SB. Amisulpride overdose is frequently associated with QT prolongation and torsades de pointes. J Clin Psychopharmacol 2010;30:391–5.

Juurlink DN. Antipsychotics. In: Nelson LS, Levin NA, Howland MA, editors. Goldfrank's toxicologic emergencies (9th ed.). New York: McGraw-Hill; 2010, p. 1003–15.

Levine M, Ruhn A-M. Overdose of atypical antipsychotics: clinical presentation, mechanisms of toxicity and management. CNS Drugs 2012;26:601–11.

Minns AB, Clark RF. Toxicology and overdose of atypical antipsychotics. J Emerg Med 2012;43:906–13.

Morgan M, Hackett LP, Isbister GK. Olanzapine overdose: a series of analytically confirmed cases. Internatl Clin Psychopharmacol 2007;22:183–6.

Page CB, Calver LA, Isbiter GK. Risperidone overdose causes extrapyramidal effects but not cardiac toxicity. J Clinic Psychopharmacol 2010;30:387–90.

Reulbach U, Dutsch C, Biermann T, et al. Managing an effective treatment of neuroleptic malignant syndrome. Crit Care 2007;11:R4.

Strawn JR, Keck PE, Caroff SN. Neuroleptic malignant syndrome. Am J Psychiatr 2007;164:870–6.

29.4 Antidepressant drugs

Shaun Greene • Dino Druda

ESSENTIALS

1 Tricyclic antidepressant (TCA) overdose is associated with severe cardiovascular toxicity, seizures, coma and death.

2 Sodium bicarbonate is the specific treatment of TCA cardiotoxicity.

3 Overdose of extended-release bupropion is associated with dose-related delayed onset of seizures.

4 Selective serotonin reuptake inhibitors generally produce relatively mild toxicity, however, citalopram and escitalopram are associated with QT prolongation and torsades des pointes.

5 Selective serotonin reuptake inhibitors are associated with serotonin toxicity in overdose and following interactions with other serotonergic drugs.

6 Selective noradrenaline reuptake inhibitors produce a sympathomimetic toxidrome and delayed onset of seizures.

7 Serotonin toxicity may be life threatening and can occur following administration of multiple serotonergic agents or serotonergic drug overdose. Treatment is supportive with cessation of serotonergic drugs and administration of a serotonin receptor antagonist in selected cases.

Table 29.4.1 Tricyclic antidepressants available in Australia

| Amitriptyline |
| Clomipramine |
| Dothiepin |
| Doxepin |
| Imipramine |
| Nortriptyline |
| Trimipramine |

- Binding to inactivated cardiac sodium channels producing rate-dependent inhibition of sodium conductance leading to membrane stabilizing effects, QRS prolongation and potentially lethal arrhythmias and impaired myocardial contractility.
- Stimulation of central postsynaptic histamine receptors producing CNS depression, sedation and coma.
- Antagonism of muscarinic acetylcholine receptors producing anticholinergic effects including tachycardia, agitation and urinary retention.
- Antagonism of peripheral α_1-adrenergic receptors producing peripheral vasodilatation.
- Varying degrees of antagonism at potassium, chloride and γ-aminobutyric acid (GABA) receptors.

Tricyclic antidepressants are well absorbed following ingestion, undergo extensive first pass metabolism, are hepatically metabolized (often producing active metabolites), are highly protein bound and are lipophilic and therefore widely distributed throughout the body. Half-lives are relatively long (10–81 hours) and often observed to be longer following OD.

Introduction

Severity of clinical toxicity following overdose (OD) of antidepressant drugs available in Australia varies according to the class of drug. Toxicity is dose dependent and produces clinical manifestations affecting multiple organ systems. Cardiovascular and neurological features can be life threatening. Early risk assessment and aggressive supportive care are essential in ensuring a good outcome.

TRICYCLIC ANTIDEPRESSANTS

Although efficacious in treating depression, tricyclic antidepressants (TCAs) are relatively more toxic than other classes of antidepressants in OD. Significant toxicity including death is associated with ingested doses of more than 10 mg/kg in adults and 5 mg/kg in children. Of the tricyclic antidepressants available in Australia (Table 29.4.1), dothiepin is associated with the greatest toxicity. Cardiovascular system dysfunction and coma typically manifest rapidly following significant ingestion. Good outcome is dependent on aggressive airway management, utilization of sodium bicarbonate and provision of supportive care in a critical care environment.

Pharmacology

The tertiary amine structure of TCAs nonselectively interacts with multiple receptors throughout the body, most of which are not implicated in positive antidepressant effects. Pharmacodynamic interactions include:

- Inhibition of central nervous system (CNS) serotonin and noradrenaline reuptake and modulation of genetic expression of serotonin, β-adrenergic and other CNS receptors contribute to antidepressant effects. This pharmacodynamic property does not contribute significantly to classical TCA toxicity, but is likely responsible for TCA-related serotonin toxicity (described later in this chapter).

Clinical features

The most common clinical features of significant TCA overdose are CNS depression (varying from agitated delirium to coma) and sinus tachycardia; these manifest rapidly within 1–2

Table 29.4.2   Tricyclic antidepressants: dose-related risk assessment and clinical effects

Dose	Effect
<5 mg/kg	Minimal symptoms
5–10 mg/kg	Anticholinergic effects, mild sedation Major toxicity not expected
>10 mg/kg	Significant clinical toxicity likely to occur within 2–4 hours of ingestion Anticholinergic effects Coma, myoclonic jerks, seizures (early in course, 3–4% of cases) Sinus tachycardia, supraventricular tachycardia, torsades de pointes, ventricular fibrillation, idioventricular rhythm, 2nd/3rd degree heart block, asystole, hypotension (myocardial dysfunction + peripheral vasodilation)
>20 mg/kg	Coma, hypotension, potential for seizures and arrhythmias. Duration toxicity potentially >24 hours

hours of exposure. Risk assessment based on dose ingested and associated anticholinergic, CNS and cardiovascular clinical effects are described in Table 29.4.2. Agitated delirium secondary to anticholinergic receptor agonism is not always evident in more severe cases as coma predominates. Sodium channel blockade and α-receptor mediated peripheral vasodilatation lead to supraventricular and ventricular arrhythmias, hypotension and asystole in a dose-dependent manner. Anticholinergic features may become more apparent during the recovery phase as histamine receptor-induced sedation resolves.

Clinical investigations

A 12-lead ECG is the most valuable prognostic investigation following TCA overdose. A terminal 40 ms axis between 120 and 270 degrees is a sensitive indicator of TCA presence but this is difficult to measure at the bedside. Measurement of maximal limb lead QRS duration is a useful predictor of toxicity. Prolongation of greater than 100 ms is associated with an increased incidence of coma, need for intubation, seizures, hypotension and arrhythmias. One study demonstrated no seizures or arrhythmias in patients with a QRS duration that remained <100 ms. Ventricular arrhythmias were predicted in one study by a QRS duration >160 ms. The finding of a positive R wave of greater than 3 mm in amplitude in lead aVR or a ratio of >0.7 between the amplitude of R and S waves in aVR are sensitive markers for seizures and arrhythmias. A rightward frontal plane QRS vector (indicated by an S wave in lead I and an R wave in aVR)

is associated with TCA toxicity. Although QT prolongation is observed in TCA therapy and toxicity, this finding is not predictive of clinical toxicity.

TCA blood concentrations can be measured, but are poorly correlated with degree of clinical toxicity.

Treatment

Patients with significant clinical toxicity or those with a recent (previous 3–4 hours) reported ingestion of a potentially toxic amount of a TCA receive aggressive supportive care in a resuscitation area. Early securing of the airway via endotracheal intubation is indicated when there is any decrease in conscious state. Poor respiratory function and secondary hypoxia potentially worsen TCA toxicity.

Administration of activated charcoal should be considered within 1 hour of ingestion, provided facilities exist to protect the airway if decreased consciousness or seizures occur. Activated charcoal may reduce TCA absorption if administered to intubated patients via a nasogastric tube up to 4 hours post-ingestion.

Early aggressive use of sodium bicarbonate in conjunction with hyperventilation is indicated where there is any cardiovascular dysfunction in conjunction with QRS prolongation (>100 ms), hypotension unresponsive to initial intravenous fluid (see further discussion below) or in the presence of any arrhythmia. Intravenous bicarbonate 8.4% (1 mL = 1 mmol) 1–2 mmol/kg boluses should be administered to obtain an arterial pH of 7.50–7.55. pH should then be maintained in this range using hyperventilation. Sodium bicarbonate provides

hypertonic sodium, competitively overcoming sodium channel blockade. Alkalization improves sodium channel function and reduces the free concentration of TCA available to produce toxicity. Acid–base manipulation using sodium bicarbonate is more effective than hyperventilation alone in TCA toxicity. Sodium bicarbonate may be prophylactically beneficial in cases where there is a significant history of TCA ingestion and a QRS duration of >100 ms.

Other therapies, including concentrated hypertonic saline (3% sodium chloride) and lignocaine, may be beneficial in treating resistant arrhythmias. Class 1a antiarrhythmics, including procainamide, quinidine and phenytoin, are contraindicated.

Hypotension is treated with intravenous crystalloid (up to 20–30 mL/kg). Administration of sodium bicarbonate is indicated if hypotension persists. Inotropes are indicated for resistant hypotension despite intravenous fluid administration and normalization of acid–base status.

Disposition

Patients who are well with no CNS depression and a normal ECG 6 hours post-reported TCA ingestion are safe for medical discharge. Those with any signs of significant toxicity require admission to a critical care environment.

BUPROPION

Pharmacology

Bupropion is a drug with a unicyclic structure used as a smoking cessation aid in Australia and as an antidepressant in a number of other countries. It has a structure similar to amphetamine and inhibits reuptake of dopamine, with a lesser effect on noradrenaline and serotonin. Bupropion is licensed for use as an antidepressant in some countries. It is only available as an extended release preparation in Australia. Bupropion and its active metabolite hydroxyl-bupropion have half-lives of approximately 20 hours. Both are relatively highly protein bound (84% and 77%). Bupropion has a volume of distribution of 2000 L. Mild anticholinergic properties may be evident following OD. Bupropion OD is characterized by a high risk of seizures; studies suggest hydroxyl-bupropion is responsible, although the exact mechanism is unclear.

Clinical features

Bupropion is only available as a modified release preparation in Australia. In therapeutic doses, bupropion may cause mild hypertension, postural hypotension in sporadic cases, headache, agitation, seizures and gastrointestinal irritation. Cardiac conduction abnormalities are not reported in therapeutic dosing.

Tachycardia, hypertension, nausea, vomiting, tremor and hallucinations may be observed following bupropion OD; however, severe agitation and seizures are the most significant clinical features; seizures are typically delayed up to 6–8 hours (in some cases up 16 hours) post-exposure and are dose dependent. In a series of 59 patients presenting following OD of modified release bupropion, seizures occurred in 30% of those ingesting <4.5 g, 50% with 4.5–9 g ingested and 100% of individuals who ingested >9 g.

QT and QRS prolongation, arrhythmias and hypotension have been reported following ingestions of >9 g of bupropion. QT prolongation is likely to be related to coexisting tachycardia. A QT nomogram should be utilized in the risk assessment of any measured QT prolongation related to bupropion toxicity. Deaths have been reported following massive ingestions.

Treatment

Provision of meticulous supportive care is the mainstay of management following bupropion OD. Patients should be managed in a monitored area with resuscitation facilities available in case of seizures or cardiovascular deteriorations. Activated charcoal should be considered in patients who are cooperative and not agitated within 4 hours of ingestion. Intravenous benzodiazepines should be administered in incremental doses to control agitation at an early stage as they may increase the threshold for seizure activity. Resistant agitation may require sedation and intubation. Seizures are managed using benzodiazepines.

Hypotension is initially treated with intravenous crystalloid. QRS prolongation is treated with intravenous sodium bicarbonate (see tricyclic antidepressant section).

Disposition

Patients who are well with a normal ECG and no agitation or seizures 16 hours post-bupropion exposure are safe for medial discharge. Patients with significant agitation, ongoing seizures, or CVS instability require admission to a critical care environment.

MONOAMINE OXIDASE INHIBITORS

Pharmacology

Monoamine oxidase inhibitors (MAOIs) either reversibly or irreversibly inhibit function of the enzymes monoamine oxidase A and B (MAO-A, MAO-B), leading to increased CNS concentrations of adrenaline, noradrenaline, serotonin and dopamine. The pharmacodynamic effects of non-selective irreversible MAOIs (including phenelzine and tranylcypromine) are not overcome until MAO is resynthesized, resulting in dose-dependent toxicity that may last for days. Moclobemide, a selective reversible inhibitor of MAO-A is more benign in OD, but may cause severe serotonin toxicity when combined with other serotonergic agents.

The MAOIs are well absorbed orally, undergo extensive first-pass metabolism, readily cross the blood–brain barrier and have moderate volumes of distribution. Peak concentrations occur within 2 or 3 hours of ingestion. Metabolites are renally eliminated.

Clinical features

Overdose of irreversible MAOIs is characterized initially by peripheral sympathomimetic stimulation and central nervous system excitation. Symptoms do not usually manifest until 6–12 hours post-overdose. Initial symptoms include tachycardia, agitation, restlessness, hyperreflexia and voluntary movements. As toxicity progresses, there is progressive muscle rigidity, respiratory failure, decreasing conscious state, hyperthermia, rhabdomyolysis, coma and cardiovascular collapse. Clinical toxicity may last for days.

Lone overdose of the reversible selective MAOI moclobemide generally produces only mild symptoms including tachycardia, nausea and anxiety. Overdose of moclobemide with another serotonergic agent may lead to significant serotonin toxicity.

MAOI adverse effects in therapeutic doses include the development of serotonin toxicity when combined with other serotonergic agents. The tyramine reaction may occur following ingestion of tyramine-containing foods. Tyramine is an indirect acting sympathomimetic. MAOI inhibition of tyramine metabolism can lead to a hyperadrenergic crisis with severe hypertension, intracranial haemorrhage, renal failure, disseminated intravascular coagulopathy (DIC) and rhabdomyolysis.

Treatment

Management of MAOI toxicity is primarily supportive. Asymptomatic patients presenting within 2 hours of ingestion of tranylcypromine or phenelzine may benefit from administration of activated charcoal. Patients with evidence of severe toxicity are managed in a resuscitation area with particular attention to supporting organ function and limiting complications. Hypertension is initially treated using titrated doses of intravenous benzodiazepines. Refractory hypotension requires treatment with intravenous nitrates, sodium nitroprusside or phentolamine. Beta-adrenergic blockers are contraindicated; unopposed α-receptor stimulation may worsen toxicity. Hypothermia unresponsive to sedation with benzodiazepines must be treated aggressively along conventional lines. Serotonin toxicity requires specific care as outlined below. Moclobemide toxicity usually only requires basic supportive care.

Disposition

Patients who remain clinically well 6 hours post-ingestion of moclobemide or 12 hours post-ingestion of phenelzine or tranylcypromine are safe for medical discharge. Patients who are symptomatic following overdose of an irreversible MAOI require admission to an intensive care unit.

SELECTIVE SEROTONIN REUPTAKE INHIBITORS

Selective serotonin reuptake inhibitors (SRRIs) are associated with fewer adverse effects both in therapeutic use and OD compared to TCAs. They are utilized in treating depression, obsessive–compulsive disorder, panic/anxiety disorders, eating disorders and chronic pain syndromes. Table 29.4.3 lists SSRIs available in Australia.

Table 29.4.3 Serotonin reuptake inhibitors available in Australia
Selective serotonin reuptake inhibitors (SSRIs)
Citalopram, escitalopram, fluoxetine, fluvoxamine, paroxetine, sertraline
Combined selective serotonin and noradrenaline reuptake inhibitors (SNRIs)
Venlafaxine, desvenlafaxine, duloxetine, reboxetine
Serotonin reuptake inhibition with α-adrenergic antagonism
Mirtazepine

Pharmacology

SSRIs increase synaptic concentrations of serotonin in the CNS via interaction with G-protein coupled serotonin receptors (14 different receptors have been described currently). With extended use, downregulation of serotonin inhibitory autoreceptors occurs, leading to increased serotonin synthesis and decreased reuptake.

SSRIs are well absorbed post-ingestion. SSRIs and metabolites are substrates for and inhibitors of numerous hepatic microsomal enzymes, the most important being CYP2D6. Hepatic metabolism produces various metabolites; many are active and capable of prolonging therapeutic effect and also increasing the probability of adverse drug interactions.

Clinical features

Therapeutic use of SSRIs is associated with headache, insomnia, sexual dysfunction, gastrointestinal symptoms, dizziness and fatigue. Serotonin toxicity can occur in therapeutic use if exposure to another serotonergic agent occurs.

OD is rarely associated with severe adverse effects. Mild CNS depression may occur, but is not severe. Nausea, vomiting, tachycardia, diaphoresis and dizziness are reported, but are generally mild and self-limiting.

QT prolongation and torsades des pointes have been reported following citalopram and escitalopram OD. Fluoxetine, citalopram and escitalopram may cause mild bradycardia.

Treatment

Activated charcoal is only indicated following massive ingestion of an SSRI within the previous hour. There is evidence that cardiovascular toxicity may be limited if activated charcoal is administered to patients who have taken >300 mg escitalopram or >600 mg citalopram within the previous 4 hours.

Treatment is primarily supportive. Regular ECGs and cardiac monitoring are indicated following ingestion >1000 mg citalopram (or 600 mg if activated charcoal has not been given within 4 hours of ingestion) or >400 mg escitalopram (or 400 mg if activated charcoal has not been given within 4 hours of ingestion). Cardiac monitoring is continued for at least 13 hours post-exposure in these cases or until the QT interval has normalized.

COMBINED SEROTONIN AND NORADRENALINE REUPTAKE INHIBITORS

Duloxetine, reboxetine, venlafaxine and desvenlafaxine are the combined selective serotonin and noradrenaline reuptake inhibitor antidepressants available in Australia.

Pharmacology

Selective serotonin and noradrenaline reuptake inhibitor (SNRIs) inhibit both serotonin and noradrenaline reuptake in the CNS. Rapid downregulation of β-adrenergic receptors may increase the speed of onset of therapeutic effect compared to SSRIs.

SNRIs are rapidly absorbed after oral administration and are hepatically metabolized. Desvenlafaxine and venlafaxine are only available in Australia in modified release formulations.

Clinical features

Overdose produces a noradrenergic mediated sympathomimetic toxidrome characterized by tachycardia, tremor, nausea, vomiting, dizziness and agitation. Venlafaxine is associated with seizures following ingestions of >5 g. Increasing agitation may herald onset of seizures. Hyperthermia and rhabdomyolysis may occur with large ingestions. Cardiovascular toxicity may occur following ingestions of >8 g of venlafaxine. QRS prolongation, QT prolongation, ventricular arrhythmias and hypotension have been reported. Desvenlafaxine is more potent than venlafaxine therapeutically (50 mg desvenlafaxine is equivalent to 75 mg venlafaxine) and therefore thresholds for toxic effects are likely to be lower with desvenlafaxine.

Treatment

Following large ingestions of SNRIs, patients should be managed in an area equipped with cardiac monitoring and facilities to manage seizures. Activated charcoal may be beneficial if administered within an hour of a large ingestion. Intubation and administration of activated charcoal within 4 hours of ingestion of >5 g of venlafaxine should be considered.

Agitation should be controlled using incremental doses of benzodiazepines. Seizures are normally self-limiting, but may require treatment with intravenous benzodiazepines.

Hypotension is treated initially with intravenous fluid. Arrhythmias associated with QRS prolongation should be treated with sodium bicarbonate (see TCA section).

Disposition

Patients should be observed for at least 6 hours post-ingestion of standard release preparations and 16 hours post-ingestion of modified release preparations or until clinically well. Cardiac monitoring is indicated following large ingestions (>5 g venlafaxine). Ingestion of >5 g of venlafaxine mandates 24 hours of observation due to the risk of delayed seizures.

MIRTAZAPINE

Mirtazapine is a unique antidepressant; in addition to blocking the reuptake of serotonin, mirtazapine is a centrally acting $α_2$-antagonist (increasing concentrations of serotonin and noradrenaline) and serotonin receptor (5-HT2 and 5-HT3) agonist.

Overdose of mirtazapine typically only causes minor effects including minor sedation. Tachycardia, more significant CNS sedation and seizures have been reported following large ingestions. Treatment is supportive.

Table 29.4.4 Selected drugs associated with serotonin toxicity

Increased serotonin production and release
Tryptophan, lysergic acid diethylamide (LSD)

Increased release of stored serotonin
Amphetamines (including MDMA), cocaine, lithium, mirtazapine

Impaired reuptake of serotonin into presynaptic nerve
SSRIs (fluoxetine, citalopram, sertraline, fluvoxamine, paroxetine), bupropion, fentanyl, cocaine, tramadol, venlafaxine

Inhibition of serotonin metabolism
Monoamine oxidase inhibitors (moclobemide, phenelzine, tranylcypromine), methylene blue, linezolid

SEROTONIN TOXICITY

Pharmacology

Serotonin toxicity (traditionally described as serotonin syndrome) is a consequence of excess serotonin acting at CNS and peripheral receptor sites. Table 29.4.4 lists drugs associated with serotonin toxicity. Although the exact pathophysiological mechanism is not fully elucidated, 5-HT1A and 5-HT2A receptors appear to be predominantly involved.

Although serotonin toxicity may occur following lone therapeutic or excess exposure to a serotonergic agent, it most commonly occurs in the context of combination use of serotonergic drugs or in instances where there has been an inadequate 'wash-out' time between substitution of one serotonergic agent for another.

Clinical features

Serotonin toxicity normally develops within hours of exposure to the offending agent or agents. A number of diagnostic criteria have been suggested, but none widely validated. Most commonly, the diagnosis has been defined as the presence of clinical findings affecting three distinct systems (in the context of exposure to a serotonergic agent):

- autonomic system: tachycardia, flushing, diaphoresis, mydriasis, hyperthermia, tachypnoea, diarrhoea
- central nervous system: altered conscious state, elevated mood, akathesia, insomnia, agitation, anxiety, confusion, seizures
- neuromuscular: hyperreflexia, clonus (inducible or spontaneous), hypertonia (lower limbs > upper limbs), myoclonus, tremor, rigors, rigidity, incoordination.

Toxicity is seen along a spectrum and varies from subclinical non-specific feelings of anxiety and apprehension, through to life-threatening hyperthermia, autonomic instability, cardiovascular dysfunction, multiorgan failure, seizures and rigidity. Most patients recover, but deaths have been reported. The variety and variable severity of symptoms may make the diagnosis challenging and it is not uncommon for the differential diagnosis to include neuromuscular malignant syndrome (NMS). Distinguishing features include the slower onset of NMS and the typical associated 'bradykinetic' clinical picture and severe muscle rigidity. Serotonergic toxicity is characterized by hyperexcitability with hyperreflexia and clonus. Other differential diagnoses include CNS infection, anticholinergic syndrome, sympathomimetic syndrome, acute dystonia, malignant hyperthermia and non-convulsive seizures. Blood concentrations of serotonergic drugs do not correlate with clinical toxicity.

Treatment

Cessation of the serotonergic agents implicated in toxicity and avoidance of further serotonergic agents are mandatory in all cases. Benzodiazepines are first-line treatment to reduce muscle rigidity or to treat seizures. Cases of severe hyperthermia or muscle rigidity should be treated aggressively: sedation with neuromuscular paralysis and admission to a critical care environment.

The use of a number of antidotes known to antagonize 5-HT1 and 5-HT2 receptors has been reported. No clinical trials have examined the safety or efficacy of these drugs. They include cyproheptadine, olanzapine, chlorpromazine and propranolol. Of these, cyproheptadine appears to be the most widely utilized. The dose is 12 mg orally (via a nasogastric tube in the intubated patient) as a single dose followed by 4–8 mg orally 8-hourly. Chlorpromazine may be useful in cases where additional sedation is required, but the possibility of dehydration may combine with the peripheral vasodilating effects of chlorpromazine to produce significant hypotension.

Controversies

- The role of sodium bicarbonate in preventing development of neurological and cardiovascular toxicity following TCA ingestion is not well defined.
- Many TCAs are highly lipophilic and there have been case reports of lipid rescue therapy being used to treat significant toxicity. However, evidence for definite outcome benefit is lacking.
- Diagnostic criteria for serotonin toxicity have not been widely validated.
- The efficacy of serotonin receptor antagonists in treating serotonin toxicity has not been well studied.
- Indications for administration of serotonin antagonists in the treatment of serotonin toxicity are poorly defined.

Further reading

Balit CR, Lynch CN, Isbister GK. Bupropion poisoning: a case series. Med J Aust 2003;178:61–3.
Bateman ND. Tricyclic antidepressant poisoning: central nervous system effects and management. Toxicol Rev 2005;24:181–6.
Boyer EW, Shannon M. The serotonin syndrome. N Engl J Med 2005;352:1112–20.
Bradberry SM, Thanacoody HKR, Watt BE, et al. Management of the cardiovascular complications of tricyclic antidepressant toxicity: role of sodium bicarbonate. Toxicol Rev 2005;24:195–204.
Dunkley EJ, Isister GK, Sibbritt D, et al. The hunter serotonin toxicity criteria: simple and accurate diagnostic decision rules for serotonin toxicity. Q J Med 2003;96:635–42.
Isbister GK. Electrocardiogram changes and arrhythmias in venlafaxine overdose. Br J Clin Pharmacol 2009;67:572–6.
Isbister GK, Bowe SJ, Dawson A, et al. Relative toxicity of selective serotonin re-uptake inhibitors (SSRIs) in overdose. Clin Toxicol 2004;42:277–85.
Isbister GK, Hackett LP, Dawson AH, et al. Moclobemide poisoning: toxicokinetics and occurrence of serotonin toxicity. Br J Clin Pharmacol 2003;56:441–50.
Liebelt EL, Francis PD, Woolf AD. ECG lead aR versus QRS interval in predicting seizures and arrhythmias in acute tricyclic antidepressant toxicity. Ann Emerg Med 1995;26:195–201.
Mills KC. Monoamine oxidase inhibitor toxicity. Emerg Med 1993;15:58–71.
Thanacoody HKR, Thomas SHL. Tricyclic antidepressant poisoning–cardiovascular toxicity. Toxicol Rev 2005;24:205–14.
Whyte IM, Dawson AH, Buckley NA. Relative toxicity of venlafaxine and selective serotonin reuptake inhibitors in overdose compared to tricyclic antidepressants. Q J Med 2003;96:369–74.

29.5 Lithium

Mark Monaghan

ESSENTIALS

1 Chronic lithium toxicity is associated with significant morbidity and mortality, especially where diagnosis and treatment are delayed. Acute lithium overdose, unless massive, has a more benign course.

2 Chronic lithium poisoning presents with neurological dysfunction. Acute lithium overdose presents with gastrointestinal dysfunction.

3 Consider the diagnosis of lithium intoxication and check a serum lithium concentration in any patient on lithium therapy who presents unwell.

4 Chronic lithium intoxication usually develops because of impaired lithium excretion. The underlying factors must be identified and corrected.

5 Serum lithium levels correlate with central nervous system (CNS) levels and clinical severity in chronic but not acute intoxication.

6 Haemodialysis effectively enhances lithium elimination but is rarely required in patients with normal renal function. This intervention is more likely to be necessary in chronic intoxication than acute overdose.

Introduction

Lithium, the metal with the lowest molecular weight, is usually dispensed as the carbonate salt. It is widely used in the therapy of bipolar disorder and a number of other conditions. Both immediate-release and sustained-release preparations are available. This drug has a relatively narrow therapeutic index and chronic intoxication develops relatively frequently. Acute overdose is less common.

Pharmacokinetics

Standard lithium preparations are rapidly and completely absorbed after oral administration with peak serum levels occurring at 2–4 h. Absorption and time to peak level is delayed after administration of sustained-release preparations and following overdose. Once absorbed, lithium is slowly redistributed from the intravascular space to the total body water. Lithium is not metabolized and its elimination is almost exclusively renal. Lithium is freely filtered at the glomerulus but, under normal circumstances, approximately 80% of filtered ions are reabsorbed in the proximal tubule and only 20% are excreted in the urine. Under these circumstances, renal clearance of lithium is approximately 10–40 mL/min and its elimination half-life is 20–24 h. The renal elimination of lithium is greatly affected by sodium and water balance and by the presence of drugs that affect renal tubular reabsorption of sodium. In the early stages following acute overdose, renal elimination is much greater because lithium is relatively concentrated in the intravascular compartment and available for filtration at the glomerulus.

Clinical features

Acute lithium overdose

Patients who take a significant overdose of lithium carbonate as with any other metal salt, develop rapid onset of gastrointestinal toxicity characterized by nausea, vomiting, abdominal pain and diarrhoea. This gastrointestinal disturbance can be very severe and may result in significant fluid and electrolyte losses. It is usually observed where more than 25 g are ingested, but can occur following smaller doses. Gastrointestinal upset is not a prominent feature of chronic lithium toxicity.

Acute lithium overdose is much less likely to result in significant neurotoxicity than is chronic lithium toxicity. Neurotoxicity can develop following massive acute overdose if renal clearance is sufficiently impaired so as to allow redistribution of sufficient lithium from the intravascular compartment to tissue compartments before it could be excreted. This situation may develop if there is pre-existing renal failure or if inadequate fluid resuscitation leads to dehydration, sodium depletion or renal impairment as a consequence of the fluid losses from gastrointestinal toxicity.

Chronic lithium toxicity

Chronic lithium toxicity may develop in association with prolonged excessive dosing or, more commonly, as a result of impaired lithium excretion due to intercurrent illness or a drug interaction. Lithium excretion is impaired in renal failure and congestive cardiac failure because of reduced filtration at the glomerulus and also in water or sodium depletion states because of increased reabsorption of sodium (and lithium) in the proximal tubule. A number of drugs including non-steroidal anti-inflammatory drugs (NSAIDs), selective serotonin reuptake inhibitors (SSRIs), neuroleptics, angiotesin converting enzyme (ACE) inhibitors, thiazide diuretics and topiramate may either impair lithium excretion or exacerbate toxicity.

The clinical features of chronic lithium toxicity are almost exclusively neurological and the following severity grading system is widely used:

- Grade I (mild): nausea, vomiting, tremor, hyperreflexia, agitation, muscle weakness, ataxia
- Grade II (serious): stupor, rigidity, hypotonia, hypotension
- Grade III (life threatening): coma, seizures, myoclonia, cardiovascular collapse.

The differential diagnosis for this presentation is broad and includes non-convulsive status epilepticus, serotonin and neuroleptic malignant syndromes, electrolyte abnormalities and CNS pathologies, such as sepsis.

While minor benign ECG changes may be observed, Lithium toxicity is generally not associated with significant cardiovascular effects, although delayed bradycardia has been reported.

Chronic lithium therapy is also associated with nephrogenic diabetes insipidus and thyroid dysfunction, which may complicate the clinical presentation of toxicity.

Clinical investigations

Essential laboratory investigations in the assessment of lithium toxicity are serum electrolytes, renal function and serum lithium concentration. Serial serum lithium concentrations are often required. Other investigations are performed as indicated to evaluate and manage intercurrent disease processes and to exclude important differential diagnoses.

Therapeutic serum lithium concentrations are generally quoted as 0.6–1.2 mEq/L, although clinical evidence of lithium toxicity can be observed at concentrations within this range, particularly in the elderly. More commonly in cases of chronic intoxication, mild toxicity is observed at lithium concentrations of 1.5–2.5 mEq/L, severe toxicity at concentrations of 2.5–3.5 mEq/L and life-threatening toxicity at concentrations >3.5 mEq/L. Following acute overdose, serum lithium concentrations do not correlate with clinical severity as they do not reflect CNS concentrations; however, when performed serially, they are useful in guiding management. Peak serum lithium concentrations >4.0 mEq/L are frequently observed following acute overdose in patients who do not go on to develop neurotoxicity. Seum levels in chronic toxicity are more equilibrated with and therefore more accurately reflect CNS levels.

Treatment

Acute lithium overdose

The vast majority of acute poisonings can be managed solely with good supportive care. Intravenous access should be established and infusion of normal saline commenced during the initial assessment. Administration should be sufficient to correct any sodium or water deficits arising as a result of the toxic gastroenteritis and to ensure a good urine output. Excessive administration of normal saline or attempts at forced diuresis do not further enhance lithium excretion. A serum lithium concentration, renal function and electrolytes should be performed as part of the initial assessment and repeated as necessary to guide further management. In particular, the serum lithium should be followed until falling and <2 mEq/L.

Activated charcoal does not bind lithium well and need not be administered unless there has

been a significant co-ingestion. On the basis of a single volunteer study, whole-bowel irrigation has been recommended for overdose of extended-release preparations but the gastrointestinal upset renders this intervention technically difficult in patients with large ingestions. Sodium polystyrene sulphonate has been proposed as an effective alternative absorbent, which may also enhance elimination of lithium. At this stage, this agent is not widely used and repeated administration can cause hypokalaemia.

Haemodialysis is rarely indicated following acute overdose in the patient with normal renal function who receives good supportive care. It may be necessary in the presence of renal failure or in the patient post-massive ingestion who goes on to develop neurotoxicity in the presence of a slowly falling serum lithium concentration.

Chronic lithium toxicity

The diagnosis of lithium toxicity should be considered in any individual on lithium therapy who presents to the emergency department unwell, in particular with evidence of neurological dysfunction. The diagnosis should be confirmed or excluded by ordering a serum lithium concentration as part of the initial work-up. A precipitating illness that has resulted in impaired lithium excretion will usually be present and require assessment and treatment on its own merits.

Appropriate supportive care measures should be instituted on arrival. Once the diagnosis of chronic lithium toxicity is confirmed, further care is orientated towards management of the precipitating medical condition and enhancing lithium excretion by optimizing renal function and correcting any water or sodium deficits with intravenous normal saline. Therapy with lithium carbonate and any drugs contributing to lithium toxicity should be immediately discontinued.

Enhanced elimination of lithium by haemodialysis may be attempted in severe or worsening chronic lithium neurotoxicity. The aim of this intervention is to minimize the duration of neurological dysfunction and avoid permanent neurological sequelae. Lithium has physico-chemical and pharmacokinetic properties that render it very suitable for enhancing elimination by haemodialysis: low molecular weight, high water solubility, small volume of distribution, no plasma protein binding and an endogenous renal clearance rate much lower than that achieved by haemodialysis. There is, however, no evidence that haemodialysis improves clinical outcome or survival rates.

The indications for haemodialysis are difficult to define. It should be considered in any patient with an elevated serum lithium concentration and severe or life-threatening neurotoxicity. It may be considered in the patient with less severe toxicity in whom adequate renal function and a falling lithium concentration are unable to be established with initial fluid resuscitation. Once instituted, haemodialysis should be continued until the serum lithium is <1 mEq/L. Some rebound in serum lithium may be noted after intermittent haemodialysis is discontinued, which may be avoided if prolonged intermittent renal replacement therapy is used or continuous arteriovenous (AV) or venovenous (VV) haemodiafiltration (HDF) is sustained for >16 h. The combination of haemodialysis followed by CVVHDF is recommended by some authors. The decision to dialyse can usually be made some 8–12 h after admission.

Disposition and prognosis

Patients with chronic lithium intoxication require admission for management of their fluid and electrolyte status, monitoring of renal function and serum lithium concentration and management of intercurrent illnesses. Ideally, admission should be to an institution with a capacity to perform haemodialysis where toxicity is moderate or severe. Following haemodialysis, neurological recovery may be delayed well beyond the removal of lithium and permanent neurological deficits are reported.

Acute lithium overdose usually has an excellent outcome with good supportive care and may be admitted to a non-monitored setting for intravenous fluids and monitoring of fluid and electrolytes and lithium concentrations. The asymptomatic patient with normal renal function and lithium level falling to below 2 mEq/L is fit for medical discharge. This usually occurs within 24 h. Psychiatric evaluation is mandatory and may take place while waiting for lithium levels to fall.

Controversies

- The indications for and preferred method of gastrointestinal decontamination following acute lithium overdose remain undefined.
- Precise criteria for haemodialysis in chronic lithium intoxication remain undefined.

- Continuous arterio- or venovenous haemofiltration have been proposed as alternatives to haemodialyis for enhancement of lithium elimination. Although lower clearances are achieved with these methods, they are often easier to institute and may minimize rapid transcellular fluid and electrolyte shifts. At the moment they can only be recommended where haemodialysis is not available.

Further reading

Bailey AR, Sathianathan VJ, Chiew AL, et al. Comparison of intermittent haemodialysis, prolonged intermittent renal replacement therapy and continuous renal replacement haemofiltration for lithium toxicity: a case report. Crit Care Resusc 2011;13:120–2.

Eyer F, Pfab R, Felgenhauer N, et al. Lithium poisoning: pharmacokinetics and clearance during different therapeutic measures. J Clin Psychopharmacol 2006;26:325–30.

Hansen HE, Amdisen A. Lithium intoxication. Q J Med 1978;47:123–44.

Jaeger A, Saunder P, Kopferschmidt J, et al. When should dialysis be performed in lithium poisoning? A kinetic study in 14 cases of lithium poisoning. Clin Toxicol 1993;31:429–47.

Meertens JH, Jagernath DR, Eleveld DJ, et al. Haemodialysis followed by continuous veno-venous haemodiafiltration in lithium intoxication; a model and a case. Eur J Intern Med 2009;20:e70–3.

Netto I, Phutane VH. Reversible ithium neurotoxicity: review of the literature. Prim Care Companion CNS Disord 2012;14:1.

Oakley PW, Whyte IM, Carter GL. Lithium toxicity: an iatrogenic problem in susceptible individuals. Aust NZ J Psychiatr 2001;35:833–40.

Shou M. Long lasting neurological sequelae after lithium intoxication. Acta Psychiatr Scand 1984;70:594.

Strayhorn JM, Nash JL. Severe neurotoxicity despite 'therapeutic' serum lithium levels. Dis Nerv Syst 1977;38:107–11.

Waring WS. Management of lithium toxicity. Toxicol Rev 2006;25:221–30.

Waring WS. Delayed cardiotoxicity in chronic lithium poisoning: discrepancy between serum lithium concentrations and clinical status. Basic Clin Pharmacol Toxicol 2007;100: 353–5.

29.6 Antihistamine and anticholinergic poisoning

Naren Gunja • Andis Graudins

ESSENTIALS

1 Anticholinergic toxicity is a relatively common and often unrecognized toxicological problem in the emergency department.

2 Many common psychotropic medications may cause antimuscarinic effects, such as neuroleptics and tricyclic antidepressants.

3 H_1-receptor antagonists are readily accessible and a common cause of anticholinergic poisoning.

4 Significant central nervous system and cardiovascular toxicity may infrequently complicate large ingestions of first-generation H_1-receptor antagonists.

5 H_2-receptor antagonist overdose rarely produces any significant clinical effects.

Introduction

Anticholinergic toxicity is a common side effect of many pharmaceutical agents, natural remedies and plants, both in therapeutic dosing and in overdose (Table 29.6.1). Symptoms and signs may range from mild manifestations of the syndrome (e.g. dry mouth and blurred vision) to severe anticholinergic delirium with agitation, hallucinations and aggressive behaviour.

The antihistamine agents are a diverse group of drugs that can be broadly classified, based upon receptor specificity, into H_1- and H_2-receptor antagonists. The H_1-receptor antagonists are widely used in the treatment of allergic conditions, nasal congestion, and as over-the-counter sleep aids. This group can be further divided into the 'first-generation' agents, which tend to be more lipophilic and are more sedating, and the 'second-generation' or non-sedating agents. The H_2-receptor antagonists are primarily used in the treatment of peptic ulcer disease and gastro-oesophageal reflux, but may also be used in conjunction with H_1-antagonists in the treatment of severe allergic reactions.

Antihistamine agents are relatively easy to obtain and frequently ingested in overdose or abused recreationally for their sedating and anticholinergic effects. The incidence of antihistamine poisoning and abuse in Australia is not well characterized. Other prescription drugs may also result in anticholinergic toxicity both in therapeutic dosing and in overdose. These may also be intentionally abused for their anticholinergic effects. Chinese and traditional herbal medicines may result in anticholinergic toxicity, either directly from the herbal agent ingested or as a result of contamination with anticholinergic agents, such as atropine or scopolamine. The intentional abuse of botanicals (e.g. *Datura* spp.) may also present with anticholinergic toxicity. In view of the easy availability of many of these pharmaceutical and herbal agents, the emergency physician should include a detailed drug history in the evaluation of any patient presenting with evidence of mental status change and anticholinergic symptoms or signs. In particular, polypharmacy and drug interactions between multiple agents with the potential for anticholinergic effects should be included in the differential diagnosis of elderly patients presenting with mental status changes.

Pharmacodynamics and pharmacokinetics

The H_1-antagonists are a diverse group of agents that reversibly block the action of histamine at H_1-receptors. High lipid solubility results in good central nervous system (CNS) penetration and sedation. The first-generation agents also block muscarinic, α-adrenergic and serotonergic receptors. Local anaesthetic effects due to sodium channel blockade may

Table 29.6.1 Anticholinergic agents

Pharmaceuticals

Anticholinergic agents
Atropine
Benzhexol
Benztropine
Oxybutynin
Scopolamine

Antipsychotic agents
Clozapine
Olanzapine
Phenothiazines
Quetiapine
Risperidone

Cyclic antidepressants
Amitriptyline
Chlormipramine
Dothiepin
Doxepin
Imipramine
Nortriptyline

First-generation H$_1$-receptor blockers
Chlorpheniramine
Cyproheptadine
Dexchlorpheniramine
Diphenhydramine
Doxylamine
Orphenadrine
Pheniramine
Promethazine

Others
Amantadine
Carbamazepine

Botanicals
Datura spp. (Jimson weed or thorn apple)
Brugmansia spp. (Angel's trumpet)
Atropa belladona (deadly nightshade)

mimic the antiarrhythmic properties of class 1a antiarrhythmic agents. Diphenhydramine, dimenhydrinate and cyproheptadine, in particular, may prolong the cardiac muscle cell action potential duration by this mechanism. The second-generation H$_1$-antagonists (fexofenadine, loratadine) have much less CNS penetration and are more histamine-receptor specific with little or no effect at other receptor subtypes.

All the H$_1$-antagonists are well absorbed orally with peak serum concentrations occurring within 2–4 h. Absorption may be delayed in overdose due to anticholinergic effects seen with the first-generation agents. Bioavailability is limited by significant first-pass metabolism. Some agents may be converted to active metabolites (e.g. hydroxyzine). Volume of distribution and protein binding are generally high. Elimination half-lives for the first-generation agents are between 2 and 6 h. The second-generation agents generally have longer half-lives (e.g. loratadine 8.3 h).

The H$_2$-antagonist agents are generally well tolerated with few side effects with therapeutic dosing. Cimetidine inhibits hepatic microsomal enzyme metabolism and reduces the metabolism of drugs eliminated by this pathway. This may result in increased serum concentrations and clinical effects of co-ingested medications.

All drugs with anticholinergic side effects have the potential to slow gastric emptying and produce gastrointestinal ileus when taken in overdose. As a result, absorption of these agents may be slowed and result in the potential for prolonged toxicity.

Clinical features

The anticholinergic toxidrome is usually manifest by a combination of peripheral and central muscarinic cholinergic receptor blockade. Peripheral effects may include sinus tachycardia, cutaneous vasodilatation and flushing, low-grade temperature, warm dry skin with an absence of axillary sweat, dry mucous membranes, gastrointestinal ileus and urinary retention. CNS effects include mydriasis with blurred vision due to the inhibition of visual accommodation, delirium, confusion, visual hallucinations, incoherent speech, agitation, combativeness, aggression and coma. Patients presenting with anticholinergic syndrome will often have an impaired perception of their environment which may result in behaviour that could injure the patient. Anticholinergic symptoms and signs may be prominent with ingestion of first-generation antihistamines. Over half of patients ingesting >1 g of promethazine are likely to develop delirium. Even therapeutic doses of some of the H$_1$-antagonist agents may be sufficient to produce an anticholinergic delirium in susceptible individuals (especially the elderly and children). Topical use of these agents, particularly on broken skin surfaces, may also result in anticholinergic delirium.

In patients who present to hospital several hours following poisoning with an anticholinergic agent, the peripheral features of the toxidrome may be absent. This may also occur in elderly people with mild-to-moderate anticholinergic delirium resulting from the side effects of therapeutic drug administration.

Other manifestations of H$_1$-antagonist toxicity may include CNS and cardiovascular effects and rhabdomyolysis. Overdose of first-generation agents commonly produces sedation, confusion, agitation and ataxia. Large ingestions may result in coma and seizures. Pheniramine, a commonly abused antihistamine in Australia, appears to be more proconvulsant than other agents following overdose, with a reported incidence of seizures of 30%. Seizures have been reported with other first-generation H$_1$-antagonists, such as orphenadrine and diphenhydramine. Fatal doses of diphenhydramine in adults range from 20 to 40 mg/kg. Doxylamine poisoning may result in non-traumatic rhabdomyolysis. Hypotension, due to α-receptor blockade, can occur following large ingestions of first-generation agents. Conduction defects are infrequent following poisoning with first-generation H$_1$-antagonists. Orphenadrine, diphenhydramine and dimenhydrinate poisoning can result in QRS-interval prolongation, broad-complex tachycardia and ventricular arrhythmias similar to that seen in cyclic antidepressant poisoning. Promethazine does not appear to cause seizures or arrhythmias.

Overdose with H$_2$-antagonists, such as cimetidine, usually results in little or no evidence of toxicity. Doses of up to 15 g have failed to produce clinical toxicity.

Clinical investigations

A 12-lead electrocardiograph should be performed to check for the presence of sinus tachycardia, QRS and QT-interval duration. Bedside blood glucose testing is indicated in all patients with altered mental status. Blood for serum electrolytes and paracetamol level should be collected. In patients with mental status changes not easily explained by drug intoxication, other organic causes for cognitive impairment should be ruled out. Serum antihistamine levels are not readily available and do not influence patient management. Standard 'drugs-of-abuse' urine screens do not detect antihistamines or most other agents with anticholinergic toxicity. Bedside bladder scan should be performed to rule out urinary retention, a common finding in anticholinergic poisoning.

Treatment

The mainstay of therapy for poisoning with anticholinergic agents is supportive care in a safe environment. Comatose or hypoventilating patients should have appropriate airway intervention and ventilatory support. Hypotension should be treated initially with intravenous crystalloid boluses. Hypotension refractory to fluids may necessitate the use of pressor agents, such as noradrenaline. Agitation and seizures can be controlled using parenteral benzodiazepines in the first instance. Barbiturates (thiopentone, phenobarbitone) may be considered in refractory seizures. Bladder catheterization should be performed in cases of urinary retention.

Gastrointestinal decontamination, if indicated, should be performed with a single-dose of oral activated charcoal. Charcoal given within 2 h has been shown to reduce the risk of promethazine-induced delirium. The benefit of activated charcoal in patients presenting with minimal or no signs of toxicity more than 2 h following ingestion is doubtful. Methods of enhancing elimination of antihistamines are ineffective because of their large volumes of distribution and high protein binding.

The reversible acetylcholinesterase inhibitor physostigmine has been used in the diagnosis and management of anticholinergic agitation and delirium. Physostigmine rapidly reverses the effects of anticholinergic delirium and may prevent the need for escalating doses of benzodiazepines to control agitation. Physostigmine may decrease the need for other interventions, such as cerebral computed tomography scanning and lumbar puncture in patients with suspected anticholinergic delirium.

When using physostigmine, an initial test dose 0.5 mg IV is followed by 1.0–2.0 mg over the following 3–5 min in an adult. A partial response may necessitate further 0.5–1.0 mg boluses. Clinical effects may last from 30 to 120 min. Caution should be exercised in using physostigmine in patients with suspected antihistamine or cyclic antidepressant poisoning with ECG evidence of cardiac conduction delay because of the risk of precipitating cardiac asystole.

Broad-complex tachycardia resulting from severe poisoning with orphenadrine, diphenhydramine or dimenhydrinate should be treated with serum alkalinization with intravenous sodium bicarbonate boluses (1.0–2.0 mmol/kg) as for severe cyclic antidepressant poisoning. Symptomatic bradycardia and high degree atrioventricular block should be initially treated with atropine. Unresponsive cases may need cardiac pacing or inotropic support.

Disposition

Patients who present with minimal or no signs of toxicity require 4–6 h of observation and monitoring. They may be medically cleared if, at the end of this period, they are alert with a normal ECG and no signs of delirium or urinary retention. Patients with persistent mental status changes require further observation but, if the ECG is normal, do not require further cardiac monitoring. The duration of anticholinergic delirium may be from 12 h to several days depending on the agent and dose ingested. Severe toxicity, if it is to develop, will be evident within 2–3 h of ingestion. Those patients with poisoning complicated by coma, seizures or cardiovascular system toxicity require admission and observation in an intensive care or high-dependency setting.

All patients with intentional ingestions or suspicion of self-harm require psychiatric assessment prior to discharge.

Controversies

- The precise indications, contraindications and timing of physostigmine continue to be controversial in the management of anticholinergic delirium.

Further reading

Beaver KM, Gavin TJ. Treatment of acute anticholinergic poisoning with physostigmine. Am J Emerg Med 1998;16:505–7.

Burns MJ, Linden CH, Graudins A, et al. A comparison of physostigmine and benzodiazepines for the treatment of anticholinergic poisoning. Ann Emerg Med 2000;35:374–81.

Clark RF, Vance MV. Massive diphenhydramine poisoning resulting in a wide-complex tachycardia: successful treatment with sodium bicarbonate. Ann Emerg Med 1992;21:318–21.

Farrell M, Heinrichs M, Tilelli JA. Response of life threatening dimenhydrinate intoxication to sodium bicarbonate administration. J Toxicol Clin Toxicol 1991;29:527–35.

Feinberg M. The problems of anticholinergic adverse effects in older patients. Drugs Aging 1993;3:335–48.

Koppel C, Ibe K, Tenczer J. Clinical symptomatology of diphenhydramine overdose: an evaluation of 136 cases in 1982 to 1985. J Toxicol Clin Toxicol 1987;25:53–70.

Koppel C, Tenczer J, Ibe K. Poisoning with over-the-counter doxylamine preparations: an evaluation of 109 cases. Hum Toxicol 1987;6:355–9.

Page CB, Duffull SB, Whyte IM, et al. Promethazine overdose: clinical effects, predicting delirium and the effect of charcoal. Q J Med 2009;102:123–31.

Pentel P, Peterson CD. Asystole complicating physostigmine treatment of tricyclic antidepressant overdose. Ann Emerg Med 1980;9:588–90.

Rimmer SJ, Church MK. The pharmacology and mechanism of action of histamine H1 antagonists. Clin Exp Allerg 1990;20:3–17.

Schneir AB, Offerman SR, Ly BT, et al. Complications of diagnostic physostigmine administration to emergency department patients. Ann Emerg Med 2003;42:14–19.

Suchard JR. Assessing physostigmine's contraindication in cyclic antidepressant ingestions. J Emerg Med 2003;25:185–91.

29.7 Paracetamol

Andis Graudins

ESSENTIALS

1 Paracetamol poisoning is one of the most common toxicological presentations to Australasian emergency departments.

2 The decision to treat patients with antidotal therapy following acute single ingestions should be made using the paracetamol treatment nomogram.

3 N-acetylcysteine (NAC) prevents liver toxicity, however, this effect decreases with delay to treatment. Patients presenting more than 8 h post-ingestion should have NAC commenced while waiting for the return of serum paracetamol concentrations and liver function tests.

4 The paracetamol treatment nomogram cannot be used to assess the risk of hepatotoxicity following repeated supratherapeutic ingestions.

5 Paracetamol overdose should be excluded in all patients with suspected deliberate self-poisoning, especially when presenting with impaired conscious state and in anyone with evidence of unexplained hepatic impairment on liver function studies.

6 Extended-release formulations of paracetamol are available in Australia and should be sought when taking the drug history.

7 The routinely recommended dose of NAC infusion may not be sufficient to prevent development of hepatotoxicity following massive ingestion of paracetamol (>50 g). Clinical toxicologist advice is recommended.

8 In patients where timing of paracetamol ingestion or history of exposure cannot be reliably elicited to make a risk assessment, treatment with NAC should be commenced until the infusion is completed or the clinical scenario can be clarified and there is no biochemical evidence of liver toxicity.

Introduction

Poisoning with paracetamol is common in Australia, as well as other Western countries. In the USA, over 100 000 potential paracetamol poisonings are reported annually to the American Association of Poison Control Centers. In the UK, paracetamol poisoning accounts for up to 43% of poisoning exposures presenting to emergency departments.

Pharmacokinetics and pathophysiology

Paracetamol (N-acetyl para-aminophenol, acetaminophen) is rapidly absorbed from the gastrointestinal (GI) tract in therapeutic doses with peak plasma concentrations occurring within 30–60 min with tablet formulations and less than 30 min with liquid preparations. Bioavailability increases with size of the dose, ranging from 68% following 500 mg to 90% following 1–2 g orally. Time to peak plasma concentration may be delayed in the presence of co-ingestants that delay gastric emptying, such as opioids, antihistamines and anticholinergic agents. The volume of distribution for paracetamol is approximately 1 L/kg, with around 50% plasma protein binding. Metabolism occurs primarily in the liver with small amounts also metabolized renally. Metabolites are renally excreted with less than 4% excreted unchanged in the urine. Elimination half-life is approximately 1.5–2.5 h following therapeutic dosing. Paracetamol is metabolized by three mechanisms. With therapeutic dosing, approximately 60% is conjugated to glucuronide metabolites and 35% to sulphate metabolites. Less than 5% of paracetamol is metabolized by microsomal enzymes. CYP2E1 is the major isoenzyme but CYP2A and CYP1A2 are also significant. Microsomal metabolism produces a reactive intermediary metabolite, N-acetyl-para-benzoquinoneimine (NAPQI). This is rapidly conjugated with glutathione to produce non-toxic mercapturic acid and cysteine metabolites that are renally excreted. Elimination half-life is the same for adults, children and elderly patients but may be slightly elevated in neonates.

In overdose, glucuronidation and sulphation pathways are rapidly saturated, resulting in increased metabolism of paracetamol by the microsomal enzyme pathway. When glutathione stores are depleted by more than 70%, NAPQI accumulates in the liver and binds to hepatocytes, resulting in cell death and predominantly centrilobular hepatic necrosis.

Microsomal metabolism of paracetamol may be enhanced by barbiturates, carbamazepine, oral contraceptives, chronic alcohol ingestion or starvation. Inhibition of microsomal metabolism may occur in the presence of acute alcohol ingestion and with the administration of 4-methylpyrazole. Therapeutic doses of cimetidine do not decrease excretion of mercapturate metabolites of paracetamol following therapeutic doses in humans. There are no human studies to support the use of cimetidine in prevention of hepatotoxicity following paracetamol poisoning.

A sustained-release formulation of paracetamol (Panadol Osteo) has been on the market in Australia for the management of arthritis pain since 2002. This formulation contains 665 mg of paracetamol in a bilayer tablet with one-third being immediate-release and two-thirds sustained-release. It has been designed to release paracetamol slowly and maintain a therapeutic concentration for up to 8 h. Human volunteer data in simulated overdose suggests a delay to, and reduction in, peak paracetamol concentration. Comparison with immediate-release paracetamol at similar doses showed reduction in peak paracetamol concentration and area under the curve by more than 50% and delay to peak paracetamol concentration from 1 to 3 h. Pharmacokinetic data following deliberate self-poisoning with this formulation suggests that there may be a delay in peak serum concentration which may go undetected with a single 4-hour serum paracetamol estimation. Panadol Osteo overdose may also be associated prolonged absorption and detectable paracetamol concentrations beyond the duration of the standard 20 h N-acetylcysteine treatment protocol. Massive ingestions of immediate-release paracetamol (>50 g), particularly with co-ingestants that slow GI motility (opioids, antihistamines, anticholinergic agents), can also be associated with delayed peak and prolonged elevation of serum paracetamol concentrations.

An isolated small rise in INR has been observed in patients with paracetamol poisoning in the absence of hepatic impairment. Mild elevations in INR and reduced levels of functional Factor VII occurred in 66% of patients with an extrapolated 4-hour paracetamol concentration greater or equal to 1000 µmol/L (150 mg/L). This effect appears to be related to inhibition of vitamin K-dependent activation of coagulation factors.

Clinical features

The clinical features of early paracetamol poisoning are non-specific and do not permit diagnosis on clinical grounds. Classically, untreated poisoning progresses through four stages of toxicity. Stage 1 lasts about 24 h and is a subclinical period where the patient may exhibit only mild nausea, vomiting and malaise. During this period, paracetamol is being metabolized, glutathione stores are being depleted and hepatotoxicity is in its early stages. In severe poisoning, mild elevations of hepatic aminotranferases may be apparent as early as 16 h post-ingestion. In stage 2, nausea and vomiting resolve. Patients may develop right upper quadrant pain and hepatic tenderness 24–48 h post-ingestion. Liver function begins to deteriorate, with increasing aminotransferases, bilirubin and prothrombin time. Stage 3 is essentially a continuum of the above between 72 and 96 h post-ingestion. Hepatic function deteriorates and chemical hepatitis, jaundice and encephalopathy may develop. Peak aminotransferases are seen around 72 h post-ingestion. Stage 4 is either the stage of

resolution with a fall in aminotransferase concentrations or, less commonly, the development of fulminant hepatic failure. Renal failure may also develop as a consequence of paracetamol toxicity. This may either be independent of hepatoxicity with direct renal toxicity from renal microsomal enzymatic metabolism of paracetamol to NAPQI or as a consequence of liver failure induced hepatorenal syndrome.

Other manifestations of acute paracetamol poisoning may include coma, lactic acidaemia and myocardial damage. Coma results from massive ingestion of paracetamol and is independent of any hepatic impairment. Serum paracetamol concentrations greater than 6500 µmol/L (1000 mg/L) may present with coma. Similarly, massive overdose may result in cardiac changes, such as ST–T-wave changes, bundle-branch block and sinus bradycardia.

In general, most patients recover from paracetamol toxicity. The overall untreated mortality is less than 1% and that of untreated patients with hepatotoxicity around 3.5%.

There are a number of 'over-the-counter' cough and cold preparations containing paracetamol in combination with other agents. These include sympathomimetics, such as pseudoephedrine, antihistamines, such as diphenhydramine, or cough suppressants, such as dextromethorphan. Patients may present with symptoms and signs of an acute toxidrome from one or more of these agents. Compound analgesics may also be ingested. These may result in the development of associated salicylate, opioid or caffeine (Panadol Extra) toxicity.

Assessment of risk of hepatotoxicity

The risk of hepatotoxicity following acute ingestion of paracetamol is dose dependent. In healthy adults, hepatotoxicity may result from ingestion of more than 200 mg/kg or 10 g, whichever is the least. In children less than 6 years old, ingestion of more than 200 mg/kg may result in toxic serum concentrations. The threshold for toxicity may be less in patients with underlying hepatic impairment (e.g. chronic alcoholic liver disease, chronic active hepatitis), severe malnutrition or in the presence of microsomal enzyme-inducing agents.

The paracetamol-treatment nomogram shows a clear relationship between the serum paracetamol concentration and the potential for subsequent hepatotoxicity following a single ingestion of immediate-release paracetamol. The nomogram begins at 4 h post-ingestion to allow for absorption and distribution of paracetamol. Serum concentrations taken less than 4 h post-ingestion may be unreliable in predicting the potential for hepatotoxicity.

The risk of hepatotoxicity from untreated acute paracetamol ingestion can be estimated from the nomogram. Patients with a serum concentration falling above a line from 1300 µmol/L (200 mg/L) at 4 h post-ingestion to 170 µmol/L (25 mg/L) at 16 h post-ingestion (the 'probable toxicity' line) will have a 60% chance of developing hepatotoxicity (AST >1000 IU/L) if left untreated. This risk increases to 87% in untreated patients with paracetamol concentrations above 2000 µmol/L (300 mg/L) 4 h post-ingestion.

The current 'treatment line' in Australasia is the 'possible hepatotoxicity' line, 1000 µmol/L (150 mg/L) at 4 h post-ingestion to 125 µmol/L (16 mg/L) at 16 h post-ingestion. This was adopted to allow for errors in calculation of the time of ingestion. The safety of treatment decisions to commence NAC based upon this 1000 µmol/L at 4 h nomogram line has been demonstrated in the USA in over 11 000 patients, where no patients treated with NAC within 15 h of ingestion died. In contrast, use of the higher line (1300 µmol/L at 4 h) has been associated with isolated reports of untreated patients who subsequently developed acute hepatic failure or suffered a fatal outcome with concentrations below this line.

With the recognition that there are numerous 'at-risk' groups that may have a lower threshold for hepatotoxicity, it has previously been recommended that the treatment line be dropped by 50% of the 'probable toxicity line'. It must be noted that lowering of the treatment threshold is purely empiric in these cases and there have been no studies to confirm this approach.

As a result, Australasian treatment guidelines for paracetamol poisoning utilize a single-nomogram line approach to the management of paracetamol poisoning. The current nomogram (Fig. 29.7.1) starts at 1000 µmol/L (150 mg/L at 4 h) and parallels the treatment approach practised in North America. This provides an additional margin of safety

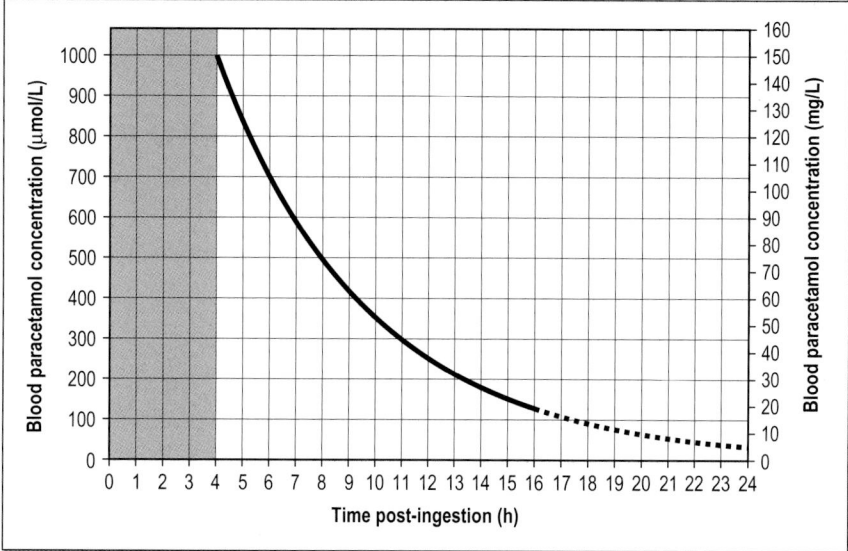

Fig. 29.7.1 Paracetamol treatment nomogram. For use in the risk assessment of acute paracetamol ingestion at a single point in time.

for patients who may possess risk factors, provides a margin of error for estimation of time of ingestion and removes the need for potentially confusing additional lines.

Repeated supratherapeutic dosing with paracetamol is associated with a risk of hepatotoxicity, particularly in those with the hepatic risk factors. Liver failure has been reported in retrospective case series with chronic use of as little as 4 g a day in patients with underlying acute illnesses with associated decreased oral intake. However, prospective evaluation of the risk of liver failure with therapeutic doses of paracetamol in chronic alcoholics does not provide an indication that there is an increased susceptibility to liver failure in this subset of patients. It is important to note that the paracetamol-treatment nomogram is not useful in the assessment of hepatotoxic risk in these patients. In alcoholic patients, raised hepatic aminotransferases into the thousands are suggestive of a toxin-induced hepatitis as seen with paracetamol. Both alcoholic hepatitis and viral hepatitis rarely produce aminotransferase that rises above 1000 IU/L.

Antidotal therapy with N-acetylcysteine

N-acetylcysteine (NAC) is effective at preventing the development of hepatotoxicity.

(AST >1000 IU/L) following paracetamol poisoning. It is metabolized to cysteine in the liver and is a precursor to glutathione, necessary for the inactivation of the toxic metabolite NAPQI. Additionally, NAC may act as a substrate for hepatic sulphation, thus reducing the amount of paracetamol being shunted to the microsomal pathway of metabolism. In Australia, NAC is administered according to the 20-h intravenous protocol described by Prescott (150 mg/kg over 15 min, 50 mg/kg over 4 h, 100 mg/kg over 16 h). There is no need empirically to commence NAC therapy in patients presenting within 8 h of acute ingestion. The incidence of any hepatotoxicity following institution of therapy within 8 h of ingestion is very low (1–6%) and independent of the route of dosing (IV versus oral). The incidence of hepatotoxicity increases to 40% if NAC is delayed from 10 to 16 h following ingestion and may be as high as 87% if delayed from 16 to 24 h in patients treated with the 20 h intravenous protocol. However, NAC probably limits the degree of hepatic damage even in late presenting patients. In addition, the dose of NAC may need to be increased or prolonged beyond the standard 20 h regimen in cases of massive ingestion of immediate-release or extended-release paracetamol (>50 g) or where serum concentration of paracetamol remains persistently elevated. Clinical toxicologist advice is recommended in these settings.

Adverse reactions to intravenous NAC are either anaphylactoid, allergy-like, phenomena (urticaria, bronchospasm, hypotension) usually occurring during or soon after the administration of the intravenous loading dose or gastrointestinal reactions (nausea, vomiting) related to sulphydryl groups on the molecule. Adverse reactions may also be seen following administration of oral NAC. Anaphylactoid reactions are not IgE-mediated but related to direct histamine release from mast cells. They are dose dependent in nature and usually respond to slowing or cessation of the infusion for a short period. Occasionally, administration of antihistamines and/or adrenaline may be necessary. The incidence of anaphylactoid reactions may be as high as 20%. A prospective study varying the rate of infusion of the NAC loading dose found a small, non-significant difference in the incidence of anaphylactoid reactions between the standard 15 min loading-dose rate to a 1 h loading-dose rate (18 vs 14%, respectively). Many local dosing guidelines now recommend a 1-h infusion rate for the NAC loading dose. The history of a previous adverse reaction to NAC does not preclude its use in the event of subsequent presentations for paracetamol poisoning. Life-threatening reactions are rare but have uncommonly been reported in patients with pre-existing asthma.

Treatment

Management of paracetamol poisoning is tailored according to the specific clinical scenario.

Acute overdose presenting within 8 h of ingestion

GI decontamination with activated charcoal (AC) should be considered in cooperative patients presenting within 1–2 h of ingestion. Early administration of AC may reduce the risk of reaching a toxic 4-h paracetamol concentration and the need for subsequent antidotal therapy. Administration of AC more than 2 h post-ingestion is unlikely to affect serum paracetamol concentrations. Antidotal therapy with NAC is commenced if the serum paracetamol concentration falls above the paracetamol-nomogram line. Clinically well patients treated within 8 h of ingestion do not require blood tests at the end of their 20-h NAC infusion if they remain well (no nausea, vomiting, anorexia, abdominal pain or tenderness) and do not fall into one of the at risk groups that may require prolonged NAC therapy.

Pregnant patients are treated in a similar fashion to other patients. Paracetamol crosses the placenta and in overdose may result in an increased risk of spontaneous abortion. Cord blood samples taken from newborns of mothers being treated with NAC for paracetamol poisoning have shown that therapeutic serum NAC concentrations occur in the fetal circulation. There are reports of neonates being overdosed with paracetamol (after birth) being successfully treated with IV NAC.

Acute overdose presenting 8–24 h post-ingestion

In view of the increased incidence of hepatotoxicity with delayed antidote administration, NAC therapy should be commenced on presentation. Blood is then taken for serum paracetamol concentration and liver function tests (LFTs). Antidotal treatment may be ceased if the paracetamol level is non-toxic and liver function normal. Otherwise, a full 20-h course of NAC is administered. Prolonged NAC infusion, usually at the 16-h bag (100 mg/kg), is indicated if repeat LFTs indicate rising aminotransferases prior to the end of 20-h course.

Acute overdose presenting more than 24 h post-ingestion

Patients presenting more than 24 h following paracetamol ingestion may still benefit from antidotal therapy with NAC. Therapy should be commenced if the patient has a detectable serum paracetamol level, there is evidence of aminotransferase elevation suggesting paracetamol hepatic injury or there is clinical evidence of paracetamol hepatotoxicity (nausea, vomiting, right upper quadrant pain). Patients may benefit from prolonged duration of NAC therapy if serum aminotransferases and/or prothrombin-time/INR continue to rise after 24 h of therapy. NAC should be continued at a rate of 100 mg/kg/12 h until prothrombin-time/INR and liver function begins to normalize or the patient requires liver transplantation.

Table 29.7.1 Paracetamol dosing associated with hepatic injury in adults and children over 6 years of age	
Acute single ingestion	>200 mg/kg or 10 g (whichever is lower) over a period of <8 h
Repeated supratherapeutic ingestion (RSI)	>200 mg/kg or 10 g (whichever is lower) over a single 24-h period >150 mg/kg or 6 g (whichever is lower) per 24-h period for the preceding 48 h >100 mg/kg or 4 g/day (whichever is less) in patients with predisposing risk factors (see text)

Adapted from Dart RC, et al. Acetaminophen poisoning: an evidence-based consensus guideline for out-of-hospital management. Clin Toxicol 2006;44:1–18.

Acute overdose with unknown time of ingestion

The time of ingestion of a single overdose of paracetamol may be unknown. This may especially occur in patients with altered mental status from co-ingestants or other causes. In view of the relative safety of NAC as an antidote, it should be commenced empirically in these patients to avoid delayed therapy using the standard 20-h NAC protocol. Serum paracetamol, LFTs and prothrombin-time/INR are collected. A more accurate history of overdose may be elicited when the patient is awake. Treatment may be ceased if accurate history is subsequently elicited or if aminotransferase enzymes are normal at the end of 20 h of NAC therapy.

The staggered acute overdose

In patients presenting with a history of more than one paracetamol overdose over several hours, a worse case scenario can be adopted. An assumption is made that the total dose of paracetamol has been ingested as a single-dose at the earliest possible time and is greater than 200 mg/kg. The serum paracetamol concentration is plotted on the nomogram based on this time point. Treatment is initiated if it is above the nomogram line.

Repeated supratherapeutic ingestion

Current consensus guidelines suggest that in adults and children over 6 years of age with normal liver function, the risk of hepatic injury may be increased if more than 200 mg/kg or 10 g (whichever is the least) are ingested over 24 h, or more than 150 mg/kg or 6 g are ingested per 24 h for the preceding 48 h or, in patients with underlying liver impairment, more than 100 mg/kg or 4 g a day is ingested per 24 h (Table 29.7.1). In these groups, a biochemical risk assessment should be made. If serum paracetamol is less than 70 μmol/L (10 mg/L) and serum aminotransferases are less than 50 IU/L, no treatment is required. If either assay is elevated, NAC should be commenced and LFTs reassessed 8 h later. If these are not rising and the patient is well, NAC therapy may be ceased. Otherwise, the full 20-h course should be administered or continued further until aminotransferases begin to fall. Static aminotransferases suggest an alternative cause for hepatic pathology. The reason for analgesic overuse should also be sought.

Paracetamol-induced hepatic failure

The development of hepatic failure is uncommon following paracetamol poisoning. The risk is greater in late presenting patients. Patients with evidence of developing fulminant hepatic failure following paracetamol poisoning exhibit clinical signs of encephalopathy and liver failure. Poorer prognosis is associated with an INR more than 2 at 24 h or more than 3 at 48 h, INR increasing between days 3 and 4, serum creatinine greater than 200 μmol/L, pH <7.3 despite fluid resuscitation, or rising serum lactate. Patients may benefit from prolonged NAC therapy along with supportive care in a specialized liver unit. A lower mortality is reported in patients with hepatic failure treated with NAC. Early consultation with a liver transplantation unit should be sought.

Sustained-release paracetamol ingestion

Delayed peak serum paracetamol concentration and delayed crossing of the nomogram line is possible following overdose with extended-release paracetamol (Panadol Osteo). The administration of NAC more than 20 h post-ingestion may be of benefit in view of the sustained-release nature of this product. To avoid delays in N-acetylcysteine treatment, this should be commenced if the reported ingested dose is greater than 200 mg/kg or 10 g (whichever is the least). Serum paracetamol concentration should be estimated 4 or more hours post-ingestion and a second estimation collected 4 h after the first. If both concentrations fall below the nomogram line, treatment may be discontinued, otherwise NAC should be administered for the full 20-h dose. Large ingestions (>30 g) of this formulation have the potential to result in prolonged paracetamol absorption. Serial paracetamol estimations are useful in this setting to ascertain when the concentration is falling to an insignificant level. If paracetamol concentration is detectable prior to completion of the 20-h infusion or if LFTs suggest developing hepatotoxicity, treatment with NAC should continue with the 100 mg/kg/16-h infusion.

Massive ingestions of paracetamol

This may be suspected in two situations: (1) in patients with history of large ingestions of paracetamol (>500 mg/kg or >50 g); (2) where serum paracetamol concentration is very high and suggests a massive ingestion (>3000 μmol/L or 450 mg/L). In these cases, the standard N-acetylcysteine dosing regimen may not be adequate to prevent hepatotoxicity developing. Clinical toxicologist advice is recommended. Consideration should be given to increasing the dose of NAC, particularly in the 16-h maintenance infusion. An empiric doubling of the 16-h infusion dose to 200 mg/kg/16 h has been suggested in these cases as it provides more NAC to mitigate hepatotoxicity. Serum paracetamol concentrations should be followed serially. If these remain detectable prior to cessation of the 20-h regimen, NAC treatment should be continued beyond this period, repeating the 16-h infusion dose, until paracetamol concentration is undetectable and there is no evidence of hepatotoxicity.

Controversies

- The optimal duration of and dose regimen for N-acetylcysteine treatment in atypical paracetamol poisoning presentations, such as supratherapeutic ingestions, massive overdoses and extended-release paracetamol poisoning.
- The clinical significance of suggested 'risk factors' for the development of hepatotoxicity. Most of the suggested factors are theoretical and have never been validated. Current treatment guidelines should be able to be applied without taking these factors into account.

- Variations in international recommendations on the threshold for treatment of acute paracetamol poisoning utilizing different nomogram cut-offs for toxicity.

Further reading

Buckley NA, Whyte IM, O'Connell DL, Dawson AH. Activated charcoal reduces the need for N-acetylcysteine treatment after acetaminophen (paracetamol) overdose. J Toxicol Clin Toxicol 1999;37:753–7.

Chiew A, Day P, Salonikas C, et al. The comparative pharmacokinetics of modified-release and immediate-release paracetamol in a simulated overdose model. Emerg Med Australas 2010;22:548–55.

Daly FFS, Fountain J, Graudins A, et al. Consensus statement: new guidelines for the management of paracetamol (Acetaminophen) poisoning in Australia and New Zealand–explanation and elaboration. Med J Aust 2008;188:296–301.

Flanagan RJ, Mant TG. Coma and metabolic acidosis early in severe acute paracetamol poisoning. Hum Toxicol 1986;5:179–82.

Graudins A, Chiew A, Chan B. Overdose with modified-release paracetamol results in delayed and prolonged absorption of paracetamol. Intern Med J 2010;40:72–6.

Green TJ, Sivilotti MLA, Langmann C, et al. When do the aminotransferases rise after acute acetaminophen overdose? Clin Toxicol (Phila) 2010;48:787–92.

Keays R, Harrison PM, Wendon JA, et al. Intravenous acetylcysteine in paracetamol induced fulminant hepatic failure: a prospective controlled trial. Br Med J 1991;303:1026–9.

Kerr F, Dawson AH, Whyte IM, et al. The Australasian clinical toxicology investigators collaboration randomized trial of different loading infusion rates of N-acetylcysteine. Ann Emerg Med 2005;45:402–8.

Prescott LF, Illingworth RN, Critchley JA, et al. Intravenous N-acetylcysteine: the treatment of choice for paracetamol poisoning. Br Med J 1979;2:1097–100.

Sivilotti MLA, Green TJ, Langmann C, et al. Multiplying the serum aminotransferase by the acetaminophen concentration to predict toxicity following overdose. Clin Toxicol (Phila) 2010;48:793–9.

Waring WS, Stephen AF, Robinson OD, et al. Lower incidence of anaphylactoid reactions to N-acetylcysteine in patients with high acetaminophen concentrations after overdose. Clin Toxicol (Phila) 2008;46:496–500.

Whyte IM, Buckley NA, Reith DM, et al. Acetaminophen causes an increased international normalized ratio by reducing functional factor VII. Ther Drug Monitor 2000;22:742–8.

29.8 Salicylate

Digby Green • Andis Graudins

ESSENTIALS

1 Salicylate pharmacokinetics become complex and alter markedly following overdose.

2 Therapeutic serum salicylate concentrations range from 1.1 to 2.2 mmol/L (15–30 mg/dL).

3 Treatment and disposition decisions cannot be made on the basis of a single serum salicylate concentration.

4 The Done nomogram is unreliable and should not be used in the management of salicylate poisoning.

5 Urinary alkalinization is an effective method of enhanced elimination of salicylate. Haemodialysis is rarely indicated.

6 Chronic salicylate poisoning is an insidious condition, mostly seen in the elderly, manifested by an unexplained metabolic acidosis that may be incorrectly attributed to another medical condition.

Introduction

Salicylate is a plant-derived compound, now pharmaceutically manufactured and widely used in a variety of pharmaceutical preparations and over-the-counter herbal products, cough and cold remedies, ointments and topical rubefacients. Despite this, salicylate poisoning is an infrequent presentation to Australian emergency departments, due largely to the preference of paracetamol as the over-the-counter analgesic of choice. Acute deliberate self-poisoning with salicylate results in a well-recognized constellation of symptoms and signs that are dose related. Emergency physicians have a number of treatment modalities available to manage this condition. Chronic intoxication, in contrast, occurs more commonly in the elderly with multiple co-morbidities and is more likely to require haemodialysis. Chronic intoxication is associated with significant morbidity and mortality. Children rarely ingest sufficient amounts to cause toxicity, but ingestion of small amounts (>5 mL) of topical agents containing methyl salicylate can result in severe toxicity in children under 5 years of age. Attention should be given to the quoted units of measurement,

standard or SI, to avoid incorrect interpretation of serum drug concentration.

Pharmacology and pathophysiology

Aspirin (acetylsalicylic acid, ASA) is rapidly absorbed in the acid medium of the upper gastrointestinal (GI) tract and undergoes rapid hydrolysis to form salicylic acid. Peak serum salicylate concentrations are reached within 2 h of therapeutic dosing. Absorption is erratic and delayed following overdose partly due to pylorospasm and pharmacobezoar formation. Overdose with sustained-release or enteric-coated preparations may delay peak serum concentrations for up to 24 h.

Salicylic acid has a pKa of 3.0 and exists predominantly in the unionized form at a pH of 7.4. It is highly protein bound (85–90%) following therapeutic doses with a very small apparent volume of distribution (0.1–0.2 L/kg). Plasma protein binding becomes saturated and free salicylate concentration rises in overdose. As pH falls, a greater proportion of salicylate exists in the unionized form and movement into the extravascular compartments, including the central

nervous system (CNS), is enhanced with resulting increases in the volume of distribution and tissue toxicity.

Salicylic acid is metabolized in the liver and kidney to form salicyluric acid, glycine, glucuronic, acyl and salicyl phenolic conjugates. These conjugates are excreted renally along with small amounts of free salicylate. The elimination half-life following therapeutic dosing is around 4 h. Salicylate metabolism is saturated when plasma salicylate concentration rises above the therapeutic range. Elimination kinetics change from first-order to zero-order, dramatically increasing the elimination half-life. Urinary excretion of unchanged salicylate is minimal when the urine pH is acidic. As urine pH increases, a greater proportion of filtered salicylate is in an ionized state and is unavailable for reabsorption in the proximal convoluted tubule. An increase in urine pH from 5.0 to 8.0 results in up to 1000-fold increase in ionized salicylate excretion.

At therapeutic doses, salicylate acts as an analgesic, antipyretic, antiplatelet and anti-inflammatory agent primarily by way of its inhibitory effects on prostaglandin synthesis mediated by irreversible inhibition of cyclo-oxygenase enzymes one and two (COX-1 and COX-2). Overdose results in toxic effects on the CNS, acid–base balance, cellular metabolism, coagulation, lungs and the GI tract. CNS effects include an initial direct stimulation of the medullary respiratory centre producing an increase in rate and depth of respiration and a corresponding primary respiratory alkalosis, tinnitus, deafness and confusion. In severe poisoning, where systemic acidaemia enhances cerebral penetration of unionized salicylate, coma, convulsions and cerebral oedema occur.

Metabolic effects include direct uncoupling of oxidative phosphorylation and inhibition of Krebs cycle enzymes leading to systemic acidaemia, hyperglycaemia, hyperthermia, derangement of carbohydrate, amino acid and lipid metabolism. Increased oxygen consumption and carbon dioxide production are also apparent. Dehydration results from increased insensible respiratory and cutaneous fluid

Table 29.8.1 Dose-related effect of aspirin toxicity

Dose	Effect
<150 mg/kg	Minimal symptoms
150–300 mg/kg	Mild to moderate toxicity Salicylism with hyperpnoea, tinnitus and vomiting
>300 mg/kg	Severe toxicity Hyperpyrexia, metabolic acidosis, altered mental status, seizures
>500 mg/kg	Potentially fatal

losses, as well as from nausea and vomiting from GI irritation. Inhibition of platelet aggregation as well as vitamin-K-sensitive clotting factor function may produce a mild coagulopathy. Haemorrhage rarely occurs in humans or animals following severe salicylate poisoning. Salicylate-induced non-cardiogenic pulmonary oedema is also reported in association with severe poisoning.

Clinical features

The degree of toxicity following acute ingestion of salicylate is dose related (Table 29.8.1). The most useful features in risk assessment are the clinical signs and symptoms, the acid–base status and serum salicylate concentration and the reported dose ingested.

The diagnosis of chronic salicylate poisoning is often missed. Recurrent dosing with aspirin, usually in the context of a viral illness or chronic pain, results in accumulation of plasma salicylate and prolongation of the elimination half-life. Patients may present with non-specific symptoms or signs suggesting inflammatory or infective aetiology, such as confusion, delirium, fever, dehydration or hyperglycaemia. The history of excessive salicylate ingestion may not be elicited and the clinical findings erroneously attributed to other conditions, such as septicaemia, cardiogenic pulmonary oedema, cerebrovascular accidents or diabetic ketoacidosis. The presence of an unexplained metabolic acidosis may be the vital clue leading to the diagnosis. Delay in the diagnosis of chronic salicylate poisoning is associated with an increased morbidity and mortality.

Clinical investigations

Salicylate intoxication should be suspected in any patient with clinical signs suggestive of poisoning, an unexplained respiratory alkalaemia or metabolic acidosis. Patients in whom the diagnosis is suspected should have blood drawn for serum electrolytes, urea, creatinine, blood glucose, prothrombin time and paracetamol and salicylate concentration. An arterial or venous blood gas is necessary to assess acid–base status and urine pH should be checked.

Patients with mild or early poisoning may present with a pure respiratory alkalosis due to respiratory centre stimulation and hypokalaemia. Urine pH may initially be alkaline as a response to hyperventilation. Adult patients with moderate-to-severe poisoning may present with a mixed acid–base disturbance of respiratory alkalosis and metabolic acidosis. Urine pH is commonly acidic in this setting due to increased excretion of hydrogen ions. A metabolic acidosis with normal or falling serum pH signifies development of potentially severe salicylate poisoning. Co-ingestion of sedatives may depress respiratory drive leading to loss of respiratory compensation for the metabolic acidosis and an earlier deterioration in acid–base status.

The Done nomogram was developed in 1960 to relate peak serum salicylate concentration to clinical severity of salicylate poisoning. This nomogram cannot be relied upon in the risk assessment of salicylate toxicity. The combined use of serial clinical observation, blood-gas estimations and serial salicylate measurements to monitor for ongoing absorption of aspirin will give the best indication of the degree of toxicity and response to treatment.

Treatment

Patients presenting following salicylate ingestion should have intravenous access established, blood drawn for serum salicylate estimation, electrolytes and blood sugar level. In moderate-to-severe poisoning these should be repeated every 3–4 h in view of the potential erratic salicylate absorption. Intravenous rehydration is often necessary in view of the increased insensible fluid losses due to hyperventilation and pyrexia and vomiting from GI irritation. Attention to fluid balance is particularly important in the very young, elderly or those with cardiac disease. Central venous and arterial pressure monitoring may be necessary in severe cases as well as urinary catheterization and hourly urine measurement.

Gastrointestinal decontamination with activated charcoal should be performed on presentation and in patients who present several hours following ingestion in view of the potential for delayed aspirin absorption. Whole-bowel irrigation with polyethylene glycol-electrolyte solution may be considered in patients with ingestion of large amounts of sustained-release formulation aspirin. Repeat-dose activated charcoal may be of benefit where there is ongoing absorption of salicylate evidenced by rising serial serum levels. Multiple-dose activated charcoal does not enhance salicylate elimination but may inhibit ongoing GI absorption from pharmacobezoars or aspirin concretions.

Pulmonary oedema should be treated with continuous positive pressure ventilation by mask or endotracheal intubation. Salicylate poisoning results in high minute volumes and respiratory alkalosis. Ventilation strategies are aimed at providing appropriate positive ventilation and preventing respiratory acidaemia. Seizures should be treated with parenteral benzodiazepines.

Urinary salicylate excretion can be enhanced by urinary alkalinization which may reduce salicylate elimination half-life from 20 to 5 h. The aim of urinary alkalinization is to increase urine pH above 7.5 to enhance the trapping of ionized salicylate in the urine. Indications include the presence of symptoms, acid–base abnormalities or serum salicylate levels greater than 2.2 mmol/L (30 mg/dL). Patients with clinical symptoms and signs of salicylate toxicity should have urinary alkalinization commenced while awaiting the results of drug assays and electrolyte concentrations. Urinary alkalinization is accomplished by an initial loading dose of intravenous sodium bicarbonate (0.5–1.0 mmol/kg) followed by an infusion of 100–150 mmol of sodium bicarbonate in 1 L of 5% dextrose solution at a rate of 100–250 mL/h adjusted to urine pH. Urine output should be maintained between 1 and 2 mL/kg/h. Serum potassium should be maintained within normal limits by the addition of supplemental potassium to the bicarbonate infusion (40 mmol per bag). In the presence of systemic hypokalaemia, the potassium ions are retained in the renal tubules in preference to hydrogen. This makes it extremely difficult to achieve urinary alkalinization. Serial serum electrolytes, salicylate concentrations and urinary pH should be measured every 3–4 h. The endpoint for therapy is a serum salicylate concentration

Table 29.8.2   Indications for haemodialysis in salicylate poisoning

Metabolic acidosis refractory to optimal supportive care and urinary alkalinization
Evidence of end-organ injury (i.e. cerebral oedema, seizures, rhabdomyolysis, pulmonary oedema)
Renal failure and fluid overload
Serum aspirin concentration >6.0 mmol/L or 100 mg/dL in acute poisoning
Serum aspirin concentration >4.0 mmol/L or 60 mg/dL in chronic poisoning

Note: in elderly patients, with chronic salicylate toxicity, the suggested serum threshold for haemodialysis is lower at 2.2–4.4 mmol/L (30–60 mg/dL).

within the therapeutic range (1.1–2.2 mmol/L or 15–30 mg/dL), resolution of clinical signs of toxicity and normalization of acid–base status.

Extracorporeal removal of salicylate is infrequently required and the accepted clinical indications are listed in Table 29.8.2. Intermittent high-flow haemodialysis (HD) is the preferred option as it can rapidly normalize acid–base, fluid balance and electrolyte abnormalities as well as remove salicylate from the blood.

Severe cases of salicylate intoxication may require endotracheal intubation and ventilation as a direct result of toxicity or co-ingestants. Importantly, minute volume should be large to maintain the hyperventilation. However, in such circumstances, urinary alkalinization, followed by haemodialysis is essential to prevent a worsening metabolic acidosis as ventilatory manipulation is often insufficient to maintain alkalaemia.

Disposition

In view of the potential for delayed and erratic salicylate absorption, patients require serial salicylate concentrations and observation for a minimum of 12 h. Salicylate estimations earlier than 6 h post-ingestion do not usually reflect peak serum concentrations following overdose.

Patients without clinical evidence of salicylate toxicity may be medically cleared in the presence of normal arterial or venous blood gas and two falling serum salicylate levels in the therapeutic range (1.1–2.2 mmol/L; 15–30 mg/dL) 3–4 h apart. Patients with evidence of acid–base abnormalities, end-organ dysfunction or requiring urinary alkalinization should be admitted to a high-dependency or intensive care unit. Transfer to a tertiary referral centre with facilities for haemodialysis should be considered if criteria for severe toxicity are present.

Controversies

- The threshold for initiating urinary alkalinization is not well defined. Many clinicians now prefer to alkalinize any symptomatic patient with a view to minimizing the duration of medical admission.

- Although there is minimal case-controlled evidence supporting the use of continuous arteriovenous or venovenous haemodialysis in severe salicylate poisoning, newer high-flow continuous venovenous haemodialysis units may be able to remove significant amounts of salicylate and provide an alternative to intermittent high-flow dialysis in selected cases.

Further reading

Chalasani N, Roman J, Jurado RL. Systemic inflammatory response syndrome caused by chronic salicylate intoxication. South Med J 1996;89:479–82.

Dargan PI, Wallace CI, Jones AL. An evidence based flowchart to guide the management of acute salicylate (aspirin) overdose. Emerg Med J 2002;19:206–9.

Dugandzic RM, Tierney MG, Dickinson GE, et al. Evaluation of the validity of the Done nomogram in the management of acute salicylate intoxication. Ann Emerg Med 1989;18:1186–90.

Herres J, Ryan D, Salzman M. Delayed salicylate toxicity with undetectable initial levels after large-dose aspirin ingestion. Am J Emerg Med 2009;27(1173):e1–3.

Jacobsen D, Wiik-Larsen E, Bredesen JE. Haemodialysis or haemoperfusion in severe salicylate poisoning? Hum Toxicol 1998;7:161–3.

Mayer AL, Sitar DS, Tenenbein M. Multiple-dose charcoal and whole-bowel irrigation do not increase clearance of absorbed salicylate. Arch Intern Med 1992;152:393–6.

Notarianni L. A reassessment of the treatment of salicylate poisoning. Drug Safe 1992;7:292–303.

O'Malley GF. Emergency department management of the salicylate-poisoned patient. Emerg Med Clin N Am 2007;25:333–46.

Pearlman BL, Gambhir R. Salicylate intoxication; a clinical review. Postgrad Med 2009;121:162–8.

Thisted B, Krantz T, Strom J, et al. Acute salicylate self-poisoning in 177 consecutive patients treated in ICU. Acta Anaesthesiol Scand 1987;31:312–6.

Wortzman DJ, Grunfeld A. Delayed absorption following enteric-coated aspirin overdose. Ann Emerg Med 1987;16:434–6.

Wrathall G, Sinclair R, Moore A, Pogson D. Three case reports of the use of haemodiafiltration in the treatment of salicylate overdose. Hum Exp Toxicol 2001;20:491–5.

29.9 Antidiabetic drugs

Jason Armstrong

ESSENTIALS

1 Deliberate self-poisoning with insulin or sulphonylureas may lead to life-threatening hypoglycaemia requiring prolonged observation and treatment over several days.

2 Octreotide blocks endogenous insulin secretion and is indicated in the management of symptomatic sulphonylurea toxicity.

3 Central venous access is often required following deliberate insulin overdose to facilitate treatment with concentrated glucose solutions.

4 Metformin is associated with life-threatening lactic acidosis. It does not cause significant hypoglycaemia in overdose.

Introduction

Diabetes mellitus (DM) is a chronic metabolic condition caused by an absolute (type I) or relative (type II) lack of insulin. In Australia, over one million people have diabetes and 100 000 people are diagnosed every year with the condition. Aboriginal and Maori populations in Australasia have some of the highest rates of type II diabetes in the world [1]. For these reasons, antidiabetic medications are readily available and frequently taken in overdose by both diabetic and non-diabetic individuals.

The three major groups of antidiabetic medications are insulin, sulphonylureas and biguanides, all of which have been used for over 50 years. Toxicity can result from intentional overdose, but also from decreased clearance of the medication at therapeutic dosing, due to underlying hepatic or renal disease.

A number of new agents for type II DM have been developed recently, including dipeptidyl peptidase-IV (DPP-IV) inhibitors, incretin mimetics, thiazolidinediones, alpha-glucosidase inhibitors and glinides. Overdose with these medications is less likely to cause significant clinical effects.

INSULIN

Pharmacology and pathophysiology

Insulin is synthesized by the pancreatic β islet cells as a pro-hormone packaged inside secretory vesicles. It is secreted primarily in response to elevated serum glucose levels and becomes metabolically active when pro-insulin is cleaved by serum proteases to form insulin and C-peptide. Exogenous insulin, administered therapeutically in the management of type I and II DM, does not contain C-peptide.

Insulin is eliminated by hepatic metabolism (60%) and renal clearance (40%). A number of preparations are available and these have varying durations of action. However, following overdose, the usual pharmacokinetic properties of insulin may be altered because the injected dose forms a subcutaneous or intramuscular depot. Slow and erratic release of insulin from the depot can result in a markedly extended duration of action (up to several days) even with short-acting preparations [2].

Insulin promotes the intracellular movement of glucose, potassium, magnesium and phosphate, as well as decreasing ketone production from the breakdown of fatty acids. It inhibits the breakdown of fat and protein to release glucose (gluconeogenesis) and stimulates the synthesis of glycogen, protein and triglycerides.

In overdose, the principal effect of clinical significance is hypoglycaemia, which may be prolonged and profound following self-administration of large doses subcutaneously or intramuscularly. Hypoglycaemia tends to be more profound and prolonged in non-diabetic patients [3]. Insulin toxicity also causes electrolyte abnormalities, the most important of which is hypokalaemia, secondary to intracellular shift of potassium. Hypophosphataemia and hypomagnesaemia are also reported.

Clinical features

The clinical features of insulin toxicity are the neuropsychiatric and autonomic manifestations of hypoglycaemia. Autonomic symptoms and signs include diaphoresis, tremor, nausea, palpitations and tachycardia; neuropsychiatric features are confusion, agitation, seizures, coma and focal neurological deficits. These manifestations are usually evident within hours of self-administration of an insulin overdose and the patient frequently presents in coma. The suspicion of deliberate overdose is entertained when recurrent profound hypoglycaemia occurs following an initial response to dextrose administration. If the history of deliberate overdose is known at the time of presentation, then profound prolonged hypoglycaemia should be anticipated.

Prolonged severe hypoglycaemia can cause permanent neurological sequelae or death.

Clinical investigations

Serial measurement of blood glucose concentrations, usually at the bedside, allows titration of dextrose administration. Serial measurements of electrolytes are necessary to monitor hypokalaemia and potassium replacement. Serum magnesium and phosphate levels may also be affected.

If surreptitious or malicious administration is suspected, assays of insulin and C-peptide levels can be useful to provide objective evidence of the presence of exogenous insulin, as endogenous insulin levels should always be suppressed in the presence of hypoglycaemia unless an insulinoma is present.

Treatment

Management of insulin overdose is essentially supportive and requires administration of sufficient concentrated dextrose solution to maintain euglycaemia until all the insulin is absorbed from the depot site and its hypoglycaemic action terminated. After initial correction of hypoglycaemia with 50% dextrose, a 10% dextrose infusion should be commenced at 100 mL/h and blood sugar levels followed closely. Further boluses of dextrose and titration of the infusion rate are implemented as necessary. Very large dose of dextrose may be required, sometimes over days [2,3]. Frequently, it is necessary to administer a 50% dextrose infusion to maintain euglycaemia and this usually requires placement of a central venous line because concentrated dextrose solutions can cause sclerosing thrombophlebitis in peripheral veins.

Hypokalaemia due to intracellular shifts should be anticipated and supplemental K+ administered (e.g. 10–40 mmol/h IV in adults), guided by serial monitoring. Excessive K+ administration should be avoided. Hyponatraemia and volume overload are other complications of hypertonic dextrose therapy.

Disposition

Patients who report an overdose of insulin should be admitted and observed with bedside blood glucose assays for at least 8 h after self-administration. They are medically fit for discharge if they remain asymptomatic and euglycaemic at this stage. Those who develop hypoglycaemia requiring dextrose therapy should be admitted to a high-dependency or intensive care unit for ongoing dextrose infusion, potassium supplementation and close monitoring of blood sugar and electrolytes.

The duration of therapy required is variable. Dextrose therapy may be withdrawn by halving the rate of infusion every 2–4 h once hyperglycaemia develops, guided by regular bedside assessments of serum glucose. This minimizes the risk of precipitous hypoglycaemia. It may be particularly difficult to wean dextrose infusions in non-diabetic patients, as the large load of infused dextrose tends to stimulate endogenous insulin secretion after the effects of the initial overdose have worn off. In these cases, a slower weaning regimen may be required to prevent hypoglycaemia. It is sensible to avoid withdrawing dextrose infusions overnight when clinical features of hypoglycaemia are less easily recognized.

Patients are medically fit for discharge if they remain asymptomatic and euglycaemic 6 h after dextrose therapy is ceased. All intentional overdoses require psychiatric assessment once their medical condition has stabilized.

SULPHONYLUREAS

Pharmacology and pathophysiology

Sulphonylureas are the most commonly prescribed oral hypoglycaemics in Australasia. Currently available agents include glibenclamide, gliclazide, glimepiride and glipizide. These agents bind to and block outgoing K+ channels on the pancreatic β cells leading to depolarization of the cell membrane, which opens voltage-gated Ca^{2+} channels and causes insulin release secondary to Ca^{2+} influx [4]. The result is a hyperinsulinaemic state. Although in therapeutic dose the duration of action is usually from 12 to 24 h, this can be markedly prolonged following overdose. Sulphonylureas undergo hepatic metabolism and have a combination of active and inactive metabolites, which are excreted renally. An exaggerated therapeutic effect can therefore occur when these agents accumulate in patients with coexistent hepatic or renal disease.

Clinical features

Sulphonylurea-induced hypoglycaemia may occur as a complication of therapy, inadvertent administration to a non-diabetic patient or as a consequence of deliberate self-poisoning. The hypoglycaemia after intentional ingestion is likely to be particularly profound and prolonged.

Treatment

Hypoglycaemia should be corrected immediately once identified with bedside blood glucose testing or suspected on clinical grounds. An initial bolus of 50 mL 50% dextrose followed by an infusion of 10% dextrose at 100 mL/h is appropriate for hypoglycaemia secondary to deliberate self-poisoning with sulphonylureas. However, hypoglycaemia is frequently refractory to dextrose supplementation in this setting and early use of octreotide is then indicated to maintain euglycaemia (see below).

Activated charcoal can be administered to patients who present within a few hours of intentional ingestion of sulphonylureas (especially with extended-release preparations) but does not take precedence over resuscitation and correction of hypoglycaemia.

Elderly patients with sulphonylurea-induced hypoglycaemia often have intercurrent medical illnesses that require treatment. Euglycaemia

may be relatively easy to maintain with intravenous or oral dextrose supplementation, but octreotide may also have a role in therapeutic management (see below).

OCTREOTIDE

Octreotide is a synthetic octapeptide analogue of the naturally occurring foregut hormone somatostatin. It suppresses insulin release from pancreatic β cells by binding to Ca^{2+} channels on the cell membrane, inhibiting Ca^{2+} influx and subsequent insulin release.

Octreotide is now seen as first-line antidotal therapy in patients with hypoglycaemia secondary to sulphonylurea overdose. Early administration of octreotide may greatly reduce or abolish the dextrose requirement, obviate the need for central venous access and greatly simplify subsequent management and disposition. Therapy can be initiated with an initial bolus of 50 μg IV followed by an infusion of 25 μg/h. An alternative dosing regimen is 100 μg by intramuscular or subcutaneous injection every 6 h. Once initiated, octreotide therapy should be continued for at least 24 h before withdrawal is attempted. Octreotide is well tolerated, with nausea and vomiting only occasionally reported [4,5].

For the treatment of hypoglycaemia due to therapeutic accumulation of sulphonylurea agents, a single dose of octreotide 25–50 μg subcutaneously may be adequate to prevent recurrent hypoglycaemia during in-patient management.

Disposition

Patients with a history of sulphonylurea overdose should be admitted and observed with bedside blood glucose assays for at least 8 h after ingestion or up to 12 h if a slow-release preparation. They are medically fit for discharge if they remain asymptomatic and euglycaemic at this stage.

Patients who require treatment for hypoglycaemia need admission, usually for several days. Discharge can occur once they are tolerating a normal diet and their blood glucose level remains normal 6 h after cessation of glucose and/or octreotide therapy.

Patients who develop hypoglycaemia on therapeutic doses of sulphonylureas should be admitted for at least 24 h to monitor serum glucose and to review their medication regimen.

In all cases of sulphonylurea overdose or toxicity, discharge should not occur at night, due to the increased risk of occult hypoglycaemia.

METFORMIN

Pharmacology and pathophysiology

Metformin is the only biguanide currently available in Australasia. It is rapidly absorbed from the gastrointestinal tract, minimally metabolized and excreted almost entirely by the kidneys. The major antidiabetic effect is to inhibit gluconeogenesis, as well as to increase tissue sensitivity to insulin, thereby improving HbA1c control. It does not cause hypoglycaemia at therapeutic doses and, even following massive overdose, clinically significant hypoglycaemia is rarely observed. However, metformin is associated with life-threatening lactic acidosis because it blocks intracellular oxidative pathways leading to increased anaerobic metabolism. Metformin-associated lactic acidosis can occur during therapeutic dosing when impaired renal function leads to drug accumulation or when intercurrent illness leads to tissue hypoperfusion. It is also reported after massive overdose, even in non-diabetic patients. The threshold for this effect is not well established but is probably over 10 g [6]. The risk of toxicity from an acute ingestion will be exacerbated by other agents that cause hypotension or decreased renal perfusion.

Clinical features

The majority of metformin overdoses are associated with only minor symptoms. In particular, hypoglycaemia is not a feature of the presentation. Paediatric ingestions are unlikely to cause significant toxicity, provided that co-ingestion of sulphonylureas can confidently be excluded [7]. Where the clinical course is complicated by lactic acidosis, the insidious onset of non-specific symptoms, such as nausea, malaise and lethargy, may be observed. As lactate levels rise, the patient's condition will deteriorate with progressive tachypnoea, cardiovascular instability and altered mental state [8]. Patients who develop progressive lactic acidosis while on therapeutic metformin may present severely unwell.

Metformin-associated lactic acidosis carries a significant mortality risk if it is not recognized and treated effectively [9].

Clinical investigation

Urgent electrolytes, renal function and lactate levels are indicated in any patient on metformin therapy who presents unwell or in any patient who becomes symptomatic while being observed following deliberate self-poisoning with metformin.

Treatment

Most cases of metformin overdose can be managed supportively. Maintenance of euvolaemia is imperative and IV crystalloid should be given to ensure effective renal perfusion and clearance. If lactate levels are elevated, serial estimations of pH and lactate must be performed until they return to the normal range. If lactate rises above 10 mmol/L or worsening acidosis, renal dysfunction and clinical deterioration occur, immediate treatment with lactate-free haemodialysis is indicated. This not only corrects the acid–base disturbance, but also rapidly removes metformin from the circulation. Either intermittent or continuous dialysis techniques can be used, as long as flow rates are adequate to ensure effective clearance [8].

Temporary improvement in acidosis can be achieved by infusion of $NaHCO_3$ while organizing dialysis, but this does not address ongoing metformin toxicity and progressive deterioration is likely without definitive therapy.

Disposition

Patients can be discharged following metformin overdose if they remain clinically well with normal haemodynamic parameters and acid–base status. Those who develop significant lactic acidosis require intensive care admission and consideration for haemodialysis. All patients on therapeutic metformin who develop lactic acidosis require admission for close clinical and biochemical monitoring and consideration for haemodialysis.

OTHER AGENTS

Dipeptidyl peptidase-IV (DPP-IV) inhibitors ('gliptins', e.g. sitagliptin) prevent hydrolysis of the endogenous foregut incretin hormones, glucagon-like peptide-1 (GLP-1) and glucose dependent insulinotropic polypeptide (GIP). This results in increased insulin release and a decrease in endogenous glucagon activity. There is a possibility of gliptin-induced hypoglycaemia as a consequence of therapy or overdose [10].

Exanetide, an incretin analogue, is a synthetic, long-acting polypeptide derived from the saliva of the Gila monster (*Heloderma suspectum*). It is administered by subcutaneous injection and adverse effects include significant vomiting. As with gliptin toxicity, drug-induced hypoglycaemia is likely to be mild, transient and readily responsive to supplemental dextrose [11].

Thiazolidinediones ('glitazones', e.g. pioglitazone) are used in type II DM. They improve insulin sensitivity in skeletal muscle and adipose tissue via the receptor peroxisome proliferator-activated receptor gamma (PPAR-γ) and also inhibit hepatic gluconeogenesis. They improve insulin resistance and thereby act to decrease circulating insulin levels. They do not stimulate insulin secretion and are not associated with hypoglycaemia

Alpha-glucosidase inhibitors (acarbose) are oligosaccharide agents that inhibit the activity of enzymes in the GI endoluminal brush border. Their action decreases the breakdown of complex sugars to monosaccharides, thereby decreasing the postprandial rise in blood glucose levels. They are not absorbed to any significant degree and do not cause hypoglycaemia or other systemic effects in overdose.

Glinides (e.g. repaglinide) are not commonly available in Australasia, but are prescribed more frequently in other countries. Their mode of action is to stimulate insulin secretion from the pancreas, but via a different part of the membrane receptor than sulphonylurea agents [12]. There are limited data available on overdose presentations, but there is potential for hypoglycaemia requiring therapy with IV dextrose. Because of the short half-life of glinides in comparison to sulphonylureas, prolonged toxicity is unlikely to result.

Controversies

- Glucagon is sometimes given pre-hospital for symptomatic hypoglycaemia. It can raise serum glucose due to enhanced breakdown of hepatic glycogen stores, but this effect is short lived and unreliable. It does not have a role in the in-patient management of deliberate self-poisoning with insulin or sulphonylureas.

- Surgical excision of insulin depot stores has been attempted but is not indicated as medical management is effective in dealing with all clinical manifestations of insulin overdose.
- The optimal dose and route of administration of octreotide in sulphonylurea overdose is not well defined. Recommendations are empiric. Greater doses than those quoted above might be necessary following massive overdose of sulphonylureas in non-diabetic patients.

- The role of insulin assays in determining ongoing requirement for octreotide therapy in sulphonylurea toxicity could be explored. Currently, insulin levels are not routinely monitored in this setting.

References

[1] AusDiab Report. International Diabetes Institute, Melbourne. <http://www.diabetes.com.au> [Accessed Feb. 2008].
[2] Samuels MH, Eckel RH. Massive insulin overdose: detailed studies of free insulin levels and glucose requirements. Clin Toxicol 1989;27:157–68.
[3] Haskell RJ, Stapczynski JS. Duration of hypoglycaemia and need for intravenous glucose following intentional overdoses of insulin. Ann Emerg Med 1984;13:505–11.
[4] McLaughlin SA, Crandall CS, McKinney PE. Octreotide: an antidote for sulphonylurea induced hypoglycaemia. Ann Emerg Med 2000;36:133–8.
[5] Glatstein M, Scolnik D, Bentur Y. Octreotide for the treatment of sulfonylurea poisoning. Clin Toxicol 2012;50:795–804.
[6] Wills BK, Bryant SM, Bucley P, Seo B. Can acute overdose of metformin lead to lactic acidosis? Am J Emerg Med 2010;28:857–61.
[7] Spiller HA, Weber JA, Winter ML, et al. Multicenter case series of pediatric metformin ingestion. Ann Pharmacother 2000;34:1385–8.
[8] Dell'Aglio DM, Perino LJ, Todino JD, et al. Metformin overdose with a resultant serum pH of 6.59: survival without sequelae. J Emerg Med 2010;39:77–80.
[9] Bailey CJ, Turner RC. Metformin. N Engl J Med 1996;334:574–9.
[10] Karagiannis T, Paschos P, Paletas K, et al. Dipeptidyl peptidase-4 inhibitors for treatment of type 2 diabetes mellitus in the clinical setting: systematic review and meta-analysis. Br Med J 2012;344:e1369.
[11] Lovshin JA, Drucker DJ. Incretin-based therapies for type 2 diabetes mellitus. Nat Rev Endocrinol 2009;5:262–9.
[12] Frandsen KB, Tambascia MA. Repaglinide and prandial glucose regulation: the rational approach to therapy in type 2 diabetes? Arquiv Brasil Endocrinol Metabol 1999;43:325–35.

29.10 Colchicine

Lindsay Murray

ESSENTIALS

1 All deliberate self-poisonings with colchicine should be regarded as potentially life threatening.

2 May present asymptomatically or with gastrointestinal symptoms only.

3 Consider the diagnosis in patients presenting with gastrointestinal symptoms followed by development of multiorgan failure, especially bone marrow failure.

4 The key points in management are early recognition of the potential severity of this intoxication, early gastrointestinal decontamination and aggressive supportive care.

Introduction

Colchicine is an alkaloid extracted from the plants, *Colchicum autumnale* (Autumn Crocus) or *Gloriosa superba* (Glory Lily). It has traditionally been widely used in the treatment of acute gout but has also been prescribed for conditions including familial Mediterranean fever, scleroderma, primary biliary cirrhosis and recurrent pericarditis.

Colchicine poisoning is relatively rare, most commonly occurring in the context of deliberate self-poisoning or therapeutic overdose. Severe toxicity from therapeutic administration of oral colchicine is unusual, but can occur in the elderly or patients with renal or hepatic disease. In this situation, the appearance of gastrointestinal symptoms usually acts as a safety mechanism and results in discontinuation of the drug before the appearance of more severe symptoms. Poisoning is also reported from ingestion of *Colchicum autumnale* itself.

It is important for the emergency physician to be familiar with the recognition and management of colchicine poisoning because it is associated with high mortality and the potential seriousness of the intoxication is often underestimated at initial presentation.

Toxicokinetics

Colchicine is rapidly absorbed following oral administration, with peak levels occurring from 0.5 to 2 h post-ingestion. Absorption is not significantly delayed following overdose. Bioavailability following oral administration ranges from 25 to 40% because of extensive first-pass hepatic metabolism. Following absorption, colchicine rapidly distributes from plasma to tissues, where it binds with high affinity to intracellular binding sites. The distribution half-life is from 45 to 90 min and the apparent volume of distribution is 21 L/kg in patients with toxicity. Terminal elimination half-lives in toxic patients range from 10.6 to 31.7 h, elimination being via renal excretion, hepatic metabolism via CYP3a4 and enterohepatic circulation. Drug clearance is significantly reduced in patients with renal and hepatic insufficiency.

Pathophysiology

Colchicine binds to tubulin and prevents its polymerization to form microtubules [1]. Microtubules are not only essential components of the cell cytoskeleton during mitosis, but are also integral to other cellular processes, such as endocytosis, exocytosis, phagocytosis, cell motility and protein assembly in the Golgi apparatus. In toxic doses, colchicine causes mitosis to arrest in metaphase with serious consequences for the rapidly dividing

Table 29.10.1	Clinical stages of significant colchicine toxicity
Stage 1: Gastrointestinal phase Time of onset: 2–24 h post-ingestion	Nausea, vomiting, diarrhoea, abdominal pain Intravascular volume depletion Peripheral leucocytosis
Stage 2: Multiorgan failure phase Time of onset: 24–72 h post-ingestion	Adult respiratory distress syndrome Bone marrow suppression Cardiac arrhythmias, failure, arrest Consumptive coagulopathy Fever Hypomagnesaemia Hyponatraemia Hypocalcaemia Hypophosphataemia Ileus Metabolic acidosis Mental status changes Neuromuscular abnormalities Oliguric renal failure Secondary sepsis Seizures
Stage 3: Recovery phase Time of onset: 6–8 days post-ingestion	Resolution of organ system derangements Rebound leucocytosis Alopecia

cells of the gut mucosa and bone marrow. As colchicine-induced microtubular disruption continues, it affects cell shape, intracellular transport and the secretion of hormones, enzymes and neurotransmitters, resulting in toxicity to virtually every cell in the body [2].

Clinical features

Severe colchicine poisoning presents as a relatively distinct clinical syndrome characterized by early onset of gastrointestinal symptoms followed by delayed onset of multiorgan toxicity and a high incidence of mortality.

In the largest reported series of colchicine poisoning (69 cases), ingestions estimated at <0.5 mg/kg were associated with gastrointestinal symptoms and coagulation disturbances only and a mortality of 0%. Ingestions of 0.5–0.8 mg/kg were associated with bone-marrow aplasia and a mortality of 10% and ingestions >0.8 mg/kg with cardiovascular collapse and 100% mortality at 72 h [3]. However, a number of fatalities have been reported following ingestions of doses <0.5 mg/kg, therefore, any overdose of colchicine should be regarded as potentially serious. The highest reported overdose that survived with aggressive supportive care is 1.38 mg/kg [4].

It is convenient to divide the clinical course of colchicine toxicity into three sequential (and usually overlapping) stages (Table 29.10.1). Less severe cases may not progress beyond the first stage. The most severe cases die during the second stage.

Following a significant acute oral overdose the patient may remain asymptomatic for between 2 and 24 h. The toxic patient then develops severe nausea, vomiting, diarrhoea and abdominal pain. This symptomatology corresponds to gastrointestinal mucosal damage and impairment of secretion of normal mucosal enzymes [5]. During this stage, fluid losses from vomiting and diarrhoea may be significant enough to result in hypovolaemic shock.

Multisystem organ failure is characteristic of the second stage, with onset from 24 to 72 h following ingestion. Respiratory, neurological, renal, haematological and cardiovascular involvement is typical. Acute adult respiratory distress syndrome may be a consequence of hypovolaemic shock or sepsis or occur as a result of direct damage to the pulmonary vasculature [6]. Bone marrow suppression is heralded by lymphopaenia, followed by granulocytopaenia, reticulocytopaenia and thrombocytopaenia, reaching a nadir at 4–8 days following ingestion.

Sepsis may complicate this stage of toxicity [3]. Disseminated intravascular coagulopathy was noted to be a frequent complication in one large series of patients with colchicine toxicity [3]. Fever occurs commonly and may be a direct drug effect or a sign of complicating infection. Shock, frequently observed during this phase, is cardiogenic and/or hypovolaemic in origin and is strongly associated with death [7]. Cardiac rhythm disturbances, including sinus bradycardia and sinus arrest, complete atrioventricular block and sudden cardiac arrest have been reported. Renal failure in acute colchicine toxicity is multifactorial and related to prolonged hypotension, hypoxia, sepsis and rhabdomyolysis. Metabolic derangements described include metabolic acidosis, hyperglycaemia, hypokalaemia, hypocalcaemia, hypophosphataemia and hypomagnesaemia [8]. Neurological disturbances include delirium, coma, seizures, transverse myelitis and ascending paralysis. Death is common during this period and usually occurs as a result of profound cardiogenic shock, sudden cardiac arrest or sepsis. Cardiac arrest has been observed as early as 36 h following acute colchicine ingestion.

In those who survive stage two, a rebound leucocytosis occurs at 7 or more days after initial symptoms and corresponds to the recovery of bone-marrow function. Alopecia commonly occurs at about this time. Complete recovery is the rule in patients surviving stage two.

Differential diagnosis

The diagnosis of colchicine poisoning is usually evident when the history and clinical features are taken into account. Difficulties and delayed diagnosis occur when the history of ingestion of colchicine or colchicine-containing plant material is not obtained. In the absence of such a history, colchicine poisoning has been misdiagnosed as gastroenteritis, sepsis or an acute abdomen requiring laparotomy. Colchicine poisoning should be considered whenever progressive multiple organ dysfunction, especially with bone marrow depression, develops following predominantly gastrointestinal symptoms.

Clinical investigations

Given the potential for severe multisystem organ failure as described above, extensive baseline laboratory studies should be performed upon presentation. These include electrolytes, full blood count, coagulation profile, renal function tests, liver function tests, electrocardiography and chest radiography. These studies need to be repeated during a hospital admission at intervals dictated by the patient's clinical course. Although colchicine concentrations in biological fluids can be measured, they are not readily available and not useful in the management of colchicine poisoning.

Treatment

The key points in the management of acute colchicine toxicity are early recognition of the potential severity of this intoxication, early gastrointestinal decontamination and aggressive supportive care.

Decontamination of the gut by the administration of oral-activated charcoal is the management priority for the patient presenting in the first (asymptomatic) stage of colchicine intoxication; prevention of absorption of even small amounts may favourably affect the severity of the intoxication and the ultimate outcome. In patients who present later (during the second stage), resuscitative efforts take precedence over gastrointestinal decontamination.

Careful monitoring of vital signs and cardiac rhythm should be instituted upon arrival. An IV cannula should be placed and IV fluid therapy commenced in any symptomatic patient. In those patients who present with substantial delay, immediate resuscitative measures may be required. Baseline laboratory studies as outlined above should be performed.

All patients with colchicine overdose require admission to hospital for a minimum of 24 h observation. Careful monitoring, not only of vital signs and cardiac rhythm but also of fluid and electrolyte status and blood cell counts, is mandatory. Further supportive therapy is dictated by clinical status and may include intravenous crystalloid rehydration, plasma expansion, inotropes, artificial ventilation, correction of electrolyte and acid–base disturbances, correction of coagulation disorders and antibiotic treatment of infectious complications.

Because of colchicine's large volume of distribution and high affinity to intracellular binding sites, attempts to enhance elimination by repeat-dose activated charcoal, haemodialysis or haemoperfusion are unlikely to be effective.

Disposition

All patients in whom colchicine toxicity is diagnosed or even suspected require admission. The asymptomatic patient should be observed for a minimum of 24 h. If no symptoms of intoxication (diarrhoea, vomiting or abdominal pain) are evident at the end of that period, colchicine toxicity may be confidently excluded and the patient discharged. The symptomatic patient should be admitted to an intensive care unit for careful monitoring and supportive care as outlined above.

Prognosis

As noted above, a relatively high mortality is associated with colchicine overdose. Prognosis is to a large extent determined by the dose ingested. Early resuscitation and provision of excellent supportive care improve prognosis. Patients who present late, in whom the diagnosis is delayed or where the potential seriousness of the presentation is underestimated initially do worse. In patients who survive stage two, a complete recovery can be anticipated. The alopecia observed during the recovery phase is not permanent, with hair growth commencing after the first month.

Controversies

- The bone-marrow suppression associated with colchicine toxicity has been reported to respond to the administration of granulocyte colony-stimulating factor [9]. However, it is unclear whether these reports represent a true therapeutic response or the natural course of recovery.

- Colchicine-specific Fab fragments have been produced in goats immunized with a conjugate of colchicine and serum albumin and effectively reverse colchicine toxicity in mice [10]. When administered to a patient with severe colchicine toxicity, rapid improvement in haemodynamic parameters and ultimate survival were observed [11]. Unfortunately, colchicine-specific Fab fragments are not yet commercially available.

References

[1] Borizy GG, Taylor EW. The mechanism of action of colchicine: binding of colchicine-H^3 to cellular protein. J Cell Biol 1967;34:525–33.
[2] Stapczynski JS, Rothstein RJ, Gaye WA, et al. Colchicine overdose: report of two cases and a review of the literature. Ann Emerg Med 1981;10:364–9.
[3] Bismuth C, Gautier M, Conso F. Aplasie médullaire après intoxication aiguë à la colchicine. Nouv Presse Med 1977;6:1625–9.
[4] Iosfina I, Lan J, Chin C, et al. Massive colchicine overdose with recovery. Case Rep Nephrol Urol 2012;2:20–4.
[5] Stemmermann GN, Hayashi T. Colchicine intoxication. A reappraisal of its pathology based on a study of three fatal cases. Hum Pathol 1971;2:321–32.
[6] Heaney D, Derghazarian CB, Pineo GF, et al. Massive colchicine overdose: report on the toxicity. Am J Med Sci 1976;271:233–8.
[7] Sauder P, Kopferschmitt J, Jaeger A, et al. Haemodynamic studies in eight cases of acute colchicines poisoning. Hum Toxicol 1983;2:169–79.
[8] Putterman C, Ben-Cherit E, Caraco Y, Levy M. Colchicine intoxication: clinical pharmacology, risk factors, features and management. Semin Arthritis Rheum 1991;3:143–55.
[9] Harris R, Marx G, Gillett M, Kark A. Colchicine-induced bone marrow suppression: treatment with granulocyte colony-stimulating factor. J Emerg Med 2000;18:435–40.
[10] Sabouraud A, Urtizberea M, Grandgeorge M, et al. Dose-dependent reversal of acute murine colchicine poisoning by goat colchicine-specific Fab fragments. Toxicology 1991;68:121–32.
[11] Baud FJ, Sabouraud A, Vicaut E, et al. Brief report: treatment of severe colchicine overdose with colchicine-specific Fab fragments. N Engl J Med 1995;332:642–5.

Further reading

Finkelstein Y, Aks SE, Hutson JE, et al. Colchicine poisoning: the dark side of an ancient drug. Clin Toxicol 2010;48:407–14.

29.11 Theophylline

Lindsay Murray

ESSENTIALS

1 Theophylline toxicity is associated with life-threatening seizures and cardiac arrhythmias.

2 Serum theophylline levels are useful in assessing and managing acute theophylline toxicity.

3 Onset of maximal toxicity may be significantly delayed following overdose of sustained-release preparations.

4 Techniques of enhancing drug elimination play an important role in the management of severe theophylline toxicity.

5 Early identification of high-risk patients allows the institution of enhanced elimination techniques before life-threatening complications develop.

Introduction

Theophylline, a methylxanthine derivative related to caffeine, has long been used in the treatment of asthma and chronic airflow limitation. Although the use of the drug has declined, both acute and chronic theophylline toxicity continue to result in potentially life-threatening presentations to the emergency department (ED).

Therapeutic blood concentrations of theophylline are generally regarded as being between 55 and 110 μmol/L (10 and 20 mg/L). A single ingestion of more than 10 mg/kg of theophylline by an adult is capable of producing a blood concentration above this range.

Pharmacokinetics

Theophylline is well absorbed orally, with a bioavailability of almost 100%. The rate of absorption depends on the pharmaceutical formulation. The most commonly prescribed preparations are sustained-release and, following overdose of these preparations, peak absorption may be delayed up to 15 h.

Once absorbed, theophylline is rapidly distributed with a relatively small volume of distribution (0.3–0.7 L/kg). Theophylline is metabolized via the cytochrome P450 system to produce active and inactive metabolites. Only about 10% of absorbed theophylline is excreted unchanged in the urine. The rate of metabolism is extremely variable and decreases with time. Theophylline metabolism exhibits saturable kinetics. At higher doses of theophylline, relatively small increments in dose are associated with disproportionate increases in serum concentration. In cases of severe intoxication, endogenous elimination of theophylline is very slow.

Pathophysiology

The precise mechanisms of toxicity of theophylline are unknown. Proposed mechanisms include inhibition of phosphodiesterase leading to elevated concentrations of intracellular cAMP, augmented plasma catecholamine activity, competitive antagonism of adenosine and changes in intracellular calcium transport.

Clinical features

Two different clinical syndromes of theophylline poisoning are recognized: acute and chronic. Both are potentially life threatening, although the chronic form is associated with greater morbidity and mortality.

Chronic intoxication is the most common clinical presentation and occurs when excessive doses of theophylline are administered repeatedly or where intercurrent illness or drug interaction interferes with hepatic metabolism.

Theophylline has a notoriously narrow therapeutic index and up to 15% of patients with a serum theophylline concentration in the therapeutic range have clinical manifestations of toxicity.

Acute intoxication is usually the result of deliberate overdose with suicidal intent, but is occasionally observed following inadvertent iatrogenic overdose. Toxicity is anticipated following a single acute ingestion of >10 mg/kg and life-threatening toxicity is anticipated with >50 mg/kg.

The clinical manifestations of theophylline intoxication are numerous and principally affect the gastrointestinal, cardiovascular, central nervous, musculoskeletal and metabolic systems.

The gastrointestinal tract is particularly sensitive to theophylline toxicity, the most prominent symptom being vomiting. This is usually severe and frequently refractory to treatment with antiemetics.

Sinus tachycardia is an almost universal manifestation of theophylline toxicity. However, severe intoxication is also associated with more unstable rhythms, including supraventricular tachycardia, atrial fibrillation, atrial flutter, multifocal atrial tachycardia and ventricular tachycardia [1]. Refractory hypotension may occur in severe toxicity as a result of β_2-mediated peripheral vasodilatation.

Central nervous system manifestations most commonly consist of anxiety and insomnia. With more severe intoxication, tachypnoea from respiratory centre stimulation and seizures occur. Seizures can develop suddenly, may be repetitive, are difficult to treat and are associated with poor outcome.

Metabolic complications of theophylline poisoning include hypokalaemia, hypophosphataemia, hypomagnesaemia, hyperglycaemia and metabolic acidosis [2]. Hypokalaemia is frequent following acute overdose, occurs early and is a consequence of intracellular shift of potassium secondary to catecholamine excess [3,4]. Musculoskeletal manifestations include muscle aches, increased muscle tone and myoclonus.

Chronic intoxication usually occurs in elderly patients and is associated with vomiting and tachycardia. The metabolic abnormalities are less frequently observed. Seizures and cardiac arrhythmias occur more frequently and at much lower serum theophylline concentrations than in acute intoxication [5,6].

Following acute overdose, especially where sustained-release preparations are involved, the clinical manifestations of severe toxicity may be delayed up to 12 h. These patients usually present with severe vomiting before the onset of more severe toxicity, including seizures and arrhythmias.

Clinical investigations

The diagnosis of theophylline toxicity is suspected on history and clinical presentation and confirmed by documentation of a significant serum theophylline concentration. The serum theophylline concentration is also invaluable in the assessment of severity and ongoing management of theophylline poisoning. Although theophylline is readily measured, it is not detected on routine drug screens.

Patients with acute theophylline overdose generally exhibit signs of minor toxicity at serum concentrations from 110 to 220 μmol/L (20–40 mg/L), moderate toxicity with concentrations from 220 to 440 μmol/L (40–80 mg/L) and severe toxicity with concentrations greater than 440 μmol/L (80 mg/L). Serum theophylline concentrations of greater than 550 μmol/L (100 mg/L) are frequently fatal [7]. After an acute overdose, serum theophylline should be measured every 3 h or so until a falling concentration is documented.

In chronic theophylline poisoning, serious toxicity is observed at lower serum concentrations and the measured concentration is not predictive of the severity of poisoning [8]. Seizures, arrhythmias and fatalities can occur at concentrations as low as 220–330 μmol/L (20–30 mg/L). In these patients, the best predictor of poor outcome is age over 60 years [9].

Other useful laboratory studies include electrolytes and creatinine, glucose, liver function tests (LFTs) and electrocardiogram (ECG).

Treatment

The initial management of theophylline poisoning follows the principles of general supportive care. Specific attention may need to be directed towards control of the airway, hypotension, tachyarrhythmias and seizures.

Hypotension usually responds to intravenous fluid administration. A noradrenaline (norepinephrine) infusion may be necessary in resistant cases. Supraventricular arrhythmias can be treated with a β-blocker, such as propranolol or esmolol, intravenously but this may induce bronchospasm in susceptible individuals. Seizures must be treated aggressively with high-dose benzodiazepines. If this fails, phenobarbitone and even general anaesthesia may be required. Phenytoin is ineffective and contraindicated. Metabolic disturbances do not generally require specific therapy. Severe hypokalaemia should be corrected with potassium supplementation.

Following acute overdose, oral-activated charcoal should be administered, even if presentation is delayed. Antiemetics are usually required for successful administration.

The pharmacokinetic properties of theophylline, especially the small volume of distribution, lend themselves to methods of enhanced elimination. Theophylline is relatively efficiently removed by haemodialysis, charcoal haemoperfusion and administration of repeat-dose activated charcoal [10].

Theophylline clearance rates of 100 mL/min have been reported with multiple-dose activated charcoal [10]. Again, aggressive antiemetic therapy may be necessary if this non-invasive method of enhancing drug elimination is to be effective. Administration of a selective serotonin antagonist, such as ondansetron, has proved particularly effective in this setting.

Both charcoal haemoperfusion and haemodialysis greatly increase the elimination of theophylline and are highly effective in achieving a good clinical outcome [11]. Such invasive methods are only indicated in potentially life-threatening theophylline toxicity. Commonly accepted indications include acute intoxication, where the serum theophylline is greater than 550 μmol/L; chronic intoxication, where it is greater than 220–330 μmol/L or in any patient with intractable hypotension, ventricular ectopy or resistant seizures [5,7]. Ideally, patients at greatest risk of developing arrhythmias or seizures should be identified early and haemodialysis or haemoperfusion instituted before these complications develop. Continuous venovenous haemofiltration has been successfully used as an alternative to standard intermittent haemodialysis in the treatment of severe theophylline poisoning with a reduction in the elimination half-life to 5.87 h reported [12].

Disposition

All patients with symptomatic theophylline toxicity require admission to hospital. Patients with acute overdose of sustained-release preparations should be admitted for monitoring and serial serum theophylline concentrations. Patients with moderate-to-severe theophylline toxicity require admission to a monitored bed.

Controversies

- Although charcoal haemoperfusion has been recommended as the most effective way to enhance theophylline elimination, it has not yet been shown to be associated with any additional improvement in clinical outcome compared to haemodialysis.

- Continuous renal replacement therapies offer a number of advantages over standard intermittent dialysis as a method of enhancing theophylline elimination. They are easily set up and run in most intensive care units and can be run 24 h a day. However, clearance rates are slower and these techniques are not currently recommended except where standard dialysis is not available or unfeasible because of haemodynamic instability.

References

[1] Bender PR, Brent J, Kulig K. Cardiac arrhythmias during theophylline toxicity. Chest 1991;100:884–6.
[2] Hall KW, Dobson KE, Dalton JG, et al. Metabolic abnormalities associated with intentional theophylline overdose. Ann Intern Med 1984;101:457–62.
[3] Amitai Y, Lovejoy FH. Hypokalaemia in acute theophylline poisoning. Am J Emerg Med 1988;6:214–8.
[4] Shannon M, Lovejoy FH. Hypokalemia after theophylline intoxication. The effects of acute vs chronic poisoning. Arch Intern Med 1989;149:2725–9.
[5] Olson KR, Benowitz NL, Woo OF, Pond SM. Theophylline overdose: acute single ingestion versus chronic repeated overmedication. Am J Emerg Med 1984;3:386–94.
[6] Shannon M. Life-threatening events after theophylline overdose: a 10-year prospective analysis. Arch Intern Med 1999;159:989–94.
[7] Sessler C. Theophylline toxicity: clinical features of 116 consecutive cases. Am J Med 1990;88:567–76.
[8] Shannon M, Lovejoy F. Effect of acute versus chronic intoxication on clinical features of theophylline poisoning in children. J Pediatr 1992;121:125.
[9] Shannon M. Predictors of major toxicity after theophylline overdose. Ann Intern Med 1993;119:1161–7.
[10] Kulig KW, Bar-Or D, Rumack BH. Intravenous theophylline poisoning and multiple-dose charcoal in an animal model. Ann Emerg Med 1987;16:842.
[11] Heath A, Knudsen K. Role of extracorporeal drug removal in acute theophylline poisoning–a review. Med Toxicol 1987;2:294.
[12] Henderson JH, McKenzie CA, Hilton PJ, Leach RM. Continuous venovenous haemofiltration for the treatment of theophylline toxicity. Thorax 2001;56:242–3.

29.12 Iron

Zeff Koutsogiannis

ESSENTIALS

1 Acute iron poisoning is a potentially life-threatening condition.

2 The risk of severe toxicity is determined by the dose of elemental iron ingested not the weight of the iron salt.

3 Iron poisoning has both local (gastrointestinal) and systemic effects.

4 Early effective gastrointestinal decontamination with whole-bowel irrigation is important in the management of high-risk cases.

5 Chelation therapy with intravenous desferrioxamine is the definitive treatment for severe poisoning.

6 Generally, most patients recover, although presence of shock or coma indicates a poor prognosis.

7 Long-term sequelae are gastrointestinal scarring and obstruction but this is uncommon.

Introduction

The majority of exposures to iron occur in preschool children, but significant iron ingestions also occur in adults as a result of deliberate self-poisoning. It is also one of the most commonly ingested agents in self-poisoning during pregnancy as a result of its ready availability to obstetric patients. Iron supplements are often considered by patients and parents to be innocuous dietary supplements, leading to careless storage and handling and delays in seeking medical care following ingestions.

Due to education, different packaging, smaller dosages and toxicovigilance by poisons centres, iron toxicity has declined in the past decade, but significant poisonings still occur.

Pathophysiology

Iron is an essential element in red blood cell production, haemoglobin and myoglobin oxygenation and cytochrome function. The body cannot directly excrete iron so body stores are finely regulated by controlling absorption of iron from the gastrointestinal (GI) tract. After absorption across the GI mucosa in the ferrous form (Fe^{2+}), iron is oxidized to the ferric state (Fe^{3+}) and then stored bound to ferritin or transported across the cell membrane into the blood, where it binds to transferrin. Iron is

extracted from transferrin in the bone marrow and used for haemoglobin synthesis. It is also removed from transferrin by the reticuloendothelial system and hepatocytes and stored as haemosiderin and ferritin. Total iron binding capacity (TIBC) is a measurement of the total amount of iron that transferrin can bind and normally exceeds serum iron by two- to threefold.

Ferritin is a large storage protein that reversibly binds to iron. When an iron deficit exists, iron is transported from ferritin and the GI tract. If the body's iron requirements have been met, iron remains stored in the intestinal cell rather than bound to transferrin. Eventually, the intestinal cell dies and sloughs off into the lumen for elimination. This is the main mechanism limiting excessive iron absorption and the mechanism by which the body regulates iron balance.

Iron rarely exists as an unbound or 'free' element. It is free iron that is toxic to cellular processes. As a result, iron toxicity results from direct local (GI) effects and cellular toxicity (systemic effects).

Local effects

Iron preparations, like other metal salts, have a direct corrosive effect on the GI mucosa. In overdose, this can lead to irritation, ulceration, bleeding, ischaemia, infarction and perforation.

Associated profound fluid losses can result in hypotension, shock and lactate formation leading to metabolic acidosis. The long-term sequelae of this corrosive action include GI scarring and obstruction. As the mucosal surface is disrupted, iron is absorbed passively down concentration gradients.

Systemic effects

When the absorbed iron exceeds the protein binding capacity, the free iron causes cellular dysfunction and death. Free iron is an intracellular toxin localizing to the mitochondria, forming free radicals and disrupting oxidative phosphorylation. The resultant mitochondrial dysfunction and destruction lead to cell death and can occur in any organ. Other systemic findings of iron poisoning include cardiovascular collapse, anion-gap metabolic acidosis, coagulopathy and encephalopathy. Metabolic acidosis persisting after correction of hypovolaemia and hypoperfusion is probably a result of mitochondrial toxicity. Coagulopathy developing early in iron poisoning results from inhibition of serum proteases while, in the later stages, it is due to hepatic dysfunction.

Toxic dose

In general, the risk of developing iron toxicity can be predicted from the dose of elemental iron ingested per kilogram body weight (Table 29.12.1). It is essential to calculate the dose of elemental iron rather than dose of iron salt. If the formulation of the iron salt is not known, then assume a worst-case scenario and calculate 105 mg of elemental iron per tablet.

Table 29.12.1 Risk assessment based on dose of elemental iron ingested

Risk assessment	Dose ingested (mg/kg)
Asymptomatic	<20
Local (GI) symptoms only	20–60
Risk of systemic toxicity	60–120
Potentially lethal	>120

Prevention

Iron poisoning is a major cause of unintentional poisoning death in young children making up almost one-third of all toxicological deaths in that age group in the 1980s to the 1990s. However, there has been a decrease in the incidence of non-intentional ingestion by young children and decreased mortality following the introduction of unit-dose packaging. This, together with education may further decrease the incidence of toxicity and late presentations.

Clinical features

The clinical course of iron poisoning is traditionally described as comprising five stages. Not all patients will experience all stages; they can die at any stage; can present at any stage and the time frames for each stage are imprecise and may overlap.

A more practical approach is to consider iron poisoning as comprising two clinical stages with a pathophysiological basis: GI toxicity and systemic toxicity.

Stage 1 (0–6 h)

This stage is dominated by symptoms and signs of GI injury particularly vomiting, but also abdominal pain, diarrhoea and GI bleeding. In severe cases, hypovolaemic shock secondary to GI losses can develop. The failure to develop any GI symptoms within 6 h of ingestion effectively excludes significant iron poisoning.

Stage 2 (2–24 h)

Also known as the 'latent' or 'quiescent' phase, this stage represents the period between resolution of GI symptoms and appearance of overt systemic toxicity. It is not a true quiescent phase as ongoing cellular toxicity occurs. Although clinicians should be wary of GI symptom resolution, most patients have in fact recovered and do not progress to Stage 3. Those with significant poisoning remain clinically ill with subtle signs (but should be easily identifiable) and progress to Stage 3.

Stage 3 (6–48 h)

This is the stage of systemic toxicity characterized by shock and multiorgan system failure. By definition, it represents severe toxicity. The shock is multifactorial arising from hypovolaemia, vasodilation and poor cardiac output with evidence of poor peripheral perfusion, worsening acidosis and acute renal failure. A coagulopathy may develop and lead to recurrent GI bleeding. Central nervous system effects include lethargy, coma and convulsions.

Stage 4 (2–5 days)

This is the hepatic phase of iron toxicity and is relatively uncommon. It is characterized by acute hepatic failure with jaundice, hepatic coma, hypoglycaemia, coagulopathy and elevated transaminase and ammonia levels. It has a high mortality.

Stage 5 (2–6 weeks)

This stage is relatively rare and represents the delayed sequelae from the corrosive effects of iron resulting in GI scarring. This results in gastric outlet (pyloric stricture) and small bowel obstructions.

Clinical investigations

Acute iron poisoning is a clinical diagnosis and all significantly symptomatic patients require treatment regardless of the iron level or results of other tests. However, serum iron levels, abdominal X-rays and other tests do play a role in determining management.

Serum iron concentration

Normal serum iron concentrations are between 10 and 30 μmol/L. Peak iron levels usually occur between 2 and 6 h after overdose, although they may sometimes be delayed. Frequent levels may need to be taken to determine the true peak. Repeat levels should be determined at 8–12 hours to rule out delayed absorption from sustained release preparations or bezoar formation. Although iron poisoning is a clinical diagnosis, iron levels have been used to determine toxicity and direct management. A serum iron concentration greater than 90 μmol/L at 4–6 h after an overdose is associated with a greater risk of subsequently developing systemic iron toxicity. However, it is intracellular and not serum iron that is responsible for systemic toxicity and, thus, during Stages 2 or 3, the iron level may be decreasing or even normal while the patient deteriorates. In the presence of desferrioxamine, the serum iron level is artificially lowered.

The TIBC is falsely elevated in the presence of high iron concentrations or desferrioxamine and is no longer regarded as useful in the assessment of iron poisoning.

Plain abdominal X-rays

Most iron preparations are radiopaque and an early abdominal X-ray is useful in confirming ingestion of iron and in subsequently guiding gastric decontamination. A negative X-ray does not exclude iron ingestion as the tablets may have disintegrated or not be radiopaque. Liquid preparations or chewable tablets are typically not radiopaque.

Other laboratory tests

Although leucocytosis and hyperglycaemia are frequently observed in iron poisoning, they are not useful in terms of diagnosis or management. The presence of an anion-gap metabolic acidosis is a useful marker of systemic iron poisoning and, as such, a low serum bicarbonate concentration is a good surrogate marker of systemic iron poisoning in places where serum iron levels are not readily available.

Other tests that are useful in managing patients with established iron poisoning include serum electrolytes, renal function, liver function, blood gases and clotting profile.

However, if the white cell count, blood glucose, radiographic findings are normal and there are no GI symptoms, serious toxicity is unlikely.

Differential diagnosis

Usually, the diagnosis is self-evident from the history of exposure, but iron poisoning needs consideration in the undifferentiated poisoning with an anion-gap metabolic acidosis and GI symptoms.

Treatment

The approach to management of a patient presenting following an iron overdose is determined by the initial risk assessment. This is based on the dose ingested and the presence or absence of GI and/or systemic features of iron poisoning. For most patients, a period of observation and good supportive care, often including intravenous fluids, will be sufficient. In those patients at risk of systemic poisoning or who present with established iron poisoning, aggressive decontamination measures and chelation therapy may be necessary to achieve a good outcome. The aim is to prevent the development of systemic toxicity.

Observation and supportive care

All patients demonstrating signs and symptoms consistent with clinical toxicity of Stages 1, 2 or 3 warrant further treatment. Aggressive fluid replacement with isotonic fluid is essential. An initial bolus of 20 mL/kg should be given, followed by boluses as needed to replace fluid losses and maintain urine output. Patients with established iron poisoning may require more advanced supportive care, including inotropic support, blood transfusions, correction of coagulopathy with fresh frozen plasma and correction of acidosis.

Any lethargic patient who is likely to deteriorate should be promptly intubated to facilitate safe decontamination.

Gastrointestinal decontamination

Iron is not well adsorbed to activated charcoal. Other modalities designed to reduce iron absorption from the GI tract, including oral bicarbonate, phosphate, magnesium hydroxide, oral calcium disodium EDTA and sodium polystyrene sulphonate, are equally ineffective. Thus, alternative methods of GI decontamination must be considered in patients who present following ingestion of more than 60 mg/kg of elemental iron, especially where unabsorbed iron is evident on abdominal X-ray.

Inducing emesis with syrup of ipecac is not recommended because it may mask the symptoms produced by iron, aggravate the GI irritation and can lead to an underestimation of the severity of the toxicity. Gastric lavage may be a useful option if performed early, but is often technically difficult in that the tablets tend to clump together, form pharmacobezoars and attach to the gastric mucosa. Endoscopy has been used to remove large iron loads, but this is also technically difficult. Surgical removal has been reported.

Whole-bowel irrigation (WBI) is widely advocated as the GI decontamination method of choice in the setting of iron poisoning, although there are no controlled trials. It should be initiated in any patient who has ingested more than 60 mg/kg of elemental iron and still has large number of iron tablets present in the GI tract on X-ray. The procedure is continued until there is a clear rectal effluent and no visible iron on X-ray. As iron has a direct corrosive effect on the GI mucosa, caution is therefore advised with the use of WBI in late presenters who may have sustained mucosal damage.

Chelation therapy

Desferrioxamine is the parenteral chelating agent of choice for iron poisoning. It binds Fe^{3+} to form ferrioxamine which is water soluble,

red-to-orange in colour and renally excreted. Desferrioxamine binds free iron and iron in transit between transferrin and ferritin thus effecting a redistribution of iron from tissue sites back into plasma. It does not chelate iron bound to transferrin, haemoglobin, myoglobin or cytochrome enzymes.

Chelation therapy is indicated in any patient with established systemic iron toxicity or at risk of developing such toxicity. Thus, the indications are:

- systemic toxicity (shock, metabolic acidosis, altered mental status) irrespective of iron levels
- serum iron levels greater than 60 μmol/L and symptomatic
- serum iron levels greater than 90 μmol/L are generally regarded as being predictive of subsequent systemic toxicity and an indication to commence chelation therapy even if asymptomatic.

Ferrioxamine's red-to-orange colour is responsible for the classically described vin rose urine in patients given desferrioxamine but this colour change is an insensitive marker of the presence of free iron and the desferrioxamine intramuscular challenge test is no longer used.

Desferrioxamine is given as a continuous intravenous infusion starting slowly and aiming for a rate of 15 mg/kg/h. Administration rate may be limited by hypotension, the principal adverse effect. Intramuscular administration is not recommended as it is painful, requires multiple injections, has erratic absorption and higher side-effect profile. The precise endpoints for chelation therapy are unclear but therapy can be safely discontinued once the serum iron level is normal or low, the patient is clinically well and the anion-gap metabolic acidosis has resolved. Except under exceptional circumstances, desferrioxamine should not be continued for longer than 24 h or exceed 80 mg/kg/24 h because of the risk of pulmonary toxicity and acute respiratory distress syndrome (ARDS). Treatment duration of 6 h is usually sufficient.

Expert advice from a clinical toxicologist should be sought if using desferrioxamine therapy.

The approach to iron poisoning is not altered in the pregnant patient. Symptomatic iron overdose in pregnancy is associated with preterm labour, spontaneous abortion and maternal death. Desferrioxamine does not cause perinatal complications or fetal toxicity and is potentially

life saving. It is therefore indicated in iron intoxication in pregnancy with clinical evidence of moderate to severe toxicity. The dose is based on the pre-pregnancy weight of the patient.

Enhanced elimination

Haemodialysis and haemoperfusion are not effective at removing iron but may be necessary to remove the ferrioxamine complex in patients with renal failure.

Exchange transfusion has been used in massive paediatric ingestions but it is of questionable value.

Disposition

Patients who have ingested less than 60 mg/kg of elemental iron and remain asymptomatic at 6 h may be medically discharged. Those with GI symptoms or requiring WBI because of large ingestion require admission for supportive care and ongoing observation and monitoring. Those with systemic toxicity and/or requiring chelation therapy require intensive care admission. All patients where deliberate self-poisoning is suspected require psychosocial assessment.

Prognosis

Most patients with iron overdose remain asymptomatic or develop minor GI toxicity only and do well with supportive care. Those with large ingestions should have an excellent outcome if recognized early and appropriate and timely decontamination and/or chelation therapy is instituted. Patients presenting late with established severe systemic toxicity have a poorer prognosis. Gastrointestinal stricture formation is a potential long-term sequela.

Controversies

- N-acetylcysteine may protect against iron-induced hepatotoxicity.
- New oral chelating agents, such as deferiprone (effective in patients with chronic iron overload states such as thalassaemia) and the hexadentate phenolic aminocarboxylate iron chelator sodium N, N″-bis(2-hydroxybenzyl) ethylenediamine-N, N″-diacetic acid (HBED) ligand have been shown to improve survival and enhance iron excretion in animal studies, but no human data are as yet available.

- Modifications of desferrioxamine, such as conjugation with dextran or hydroxyethyl starch, have shown the potential for enhanced efficacy and improved patient tolerability. Additional research must be conducted to determine the role of these agents.
- Diazepam has been shown in animal studies to reduce mortality without chelation.

Further reading

Banner W, Tong TG. Iron poisoning. Pediatr Clin N Am 1986;33:393–409.

Chang T, Rangan C. Iron poisoning: a literature-based review of epidemiology, diagnosis and management. Pediatr Emerg Care 2011;27:978–85.

Finch CA, Huebers H. Perspectives in iron metabolism. N Engl J Med 1982;306:1520.

Henretig FM, Temple AR. Acute iron poisoning in children. Emerg Med Clin N Am 1984;2:121.

Iron. In: WikiTox: open source clinical toxicology curriculum. <http://curriculum.toxicology.wikispaces.net/2.1.9.6+Iron>

Jacobs J, Greene H. Acute iron intoxication. N Engl J Med 1965;273:1124–7.

Manoguerra AS, Booze LL, Scharman EJ, et al. Iron ingestion: an evidence-based consensus guideline for out of hospital management. Clin Toxicol 2005;43:553–70.

Mills KC, Curry SC. Acute iron poisoning. Emerg Med Clin N Am 1994;12:397–413.

Perrone J. Iron. In: Nelson LS, Levin NA, Howland MA, editors. Goldfrank's toxicologic emergencies (9th ed.). New York: McGraw-Hill; 2010, p. 629–38.

Tenenbein M. Position statement: whole bowel irrigation. American academy of clinical toxicology; European association of poisons centres and clinical toxicologists. J Toxicol Clin Toxicol 1993;35:753–62.

Tenenbein M. Benefits of parenteral deferoxamine for acute iron poisoning. J Toxicol Clin Toxicol 1996;34:485–9.

Tenenbein M, Littman C, Stimpson RE, et al. Gastrointestinal pathology in adult iron overdose. J Toxicol Clin Toxicol 1990;28:311–20.

29.13 Drugs of abuse

Kerry A Hoggett

ESSENTIALS

1 The diagnosis of intoxication with drugs of abuse is clinical. Good supportive care ensures optimal outcome in the majority of cases.

2 Predisposing factors for heroin overdose include co-ingestion of CNS depressant drugs, poor tolerance, high purity and reluctance to seek medical care. Naloxone is a useful adjunct in the management of airway and ventilation in opiate overdose.

3 Benzodiazepines are important in the management of the central nervous system and cardiovascular manifestations of amphetamine intoxication. Hyperthermia, decreased conscious state, headache, neurological signs or chest pain suggest life-threatening complications and warrant aggressive management and investigation.

4 Cocaine use is associated with both cardiac and non-cardiac toxicity and may be life threatening. Toxicity may be difficult to distinguish clinically from amphetamines, although it tends to be of shorter duration. Aggressive investigation and management is required for hyperthermia, seizures, chest pain and ventricular cardiac arrhythmias.

5 Gamma hydroxybutyric acid is a sedative-hypnotic drug causing CNS depression. Management is supportive.

6 Newer synthetic psychoactive agents (stimulants, hallucinogens and depressants) are becoming widely available, with evolving structural modifications and variable effects. Management is supportive.

7 Presentation to the emergency department following overdose provides an opportunity for intervention. Education to avoid future overdoses and referral to agencies specializing in detoxification and rehabilitation is appropriate.

Introduction

Australian data report 37.3% of people aged over 14 years have used illicit drugs at least once during their lifetime. In 2010, the most commonly used illicit drugs included ecstasy (10.3%), hallucinogens (8.8%), cocaine (7.3%) and methamphetamines (7.0%). Novel synthetic psychoactive drugs have become widely available from street vendors and Internet sources. The ongoing emergence of new 'legal highs' has been challenging for health professionals and law makers alike. For all agents, the complications of illicit drug abuse are classified into three groups: primary toxic effect, complications of intoxication and complications of administration/injection technique. Trauma must be considered in all intoxicated patients.

OPIATES

Opiates are derivatives of the opium poppy, *Papaver somniferum*, which contains approximately 20 alkaloids, including morphine and codeine.

Aetiology, pharmacology and pathogenesis

Opiates are agonists, partial agonists or antagonists at μ (mu), δ (delta) and κ (kappa) receptors in the brain and spinal cord. The principal effects of opiates on the CNS are due to their action on μ receptors. Most opiates are well absorbed across mucous membranes and from subcutaneous and intramuscular sites. Oral opiates undergo extensive first-pass metabolism by glucuronidation (morphine), demethylation and oxidative metabolism. Metabolites are excreted in the urine and may accumulate in renal failure.

Morphine and heroin (diacetylmorphine) taken parenterally reach peak clinical effect within minutes and have a short half-life of 3 h. In contrast, methadone, slow-release oral morphine preparations and ingested transdermal patches have slow and erratic absorption, reach peak plasma concentrations after several hours and have long durations of effect. Transdermal fentanyl patches applied to the skin result in a subcutaneous depot of opiate from which absorption continues after patch removal.

Epidemiology

Opiate overdose is common among Australian heroin users. Factors that contribute to non-fatal and fatal opiate overdose include the co-ingestion of other central nervous system (CNS) depressant drugs, poor tolerance, high street purity and reluctance to seek medical care.

Clinical features

The diagnosis of opioid intoxication is clinical, based on history and examination. The clinical signs of opiate intoxication are related to their effect on the CNS and may be modified by co-ingested alcohol, drugs, trauma or medical complications. A Glasgow coma scale (GCS) less than 12 associated with respirations of 12 breaths/min or less, miotic pupils or circumstantial evidence of drug use is suggestive. 'Track marks' are not always evident. With increasing dose, analgesia, euphoria, miosis, sedation, coma, respiratory depression and apnoea occur. Hypoxia, hypercarbia and acidaemia lead to tachycardia, hypertension and variable pupillary responses, followed by bradycardia, hypotension and cardiac arrest as terminal events.

Respiratory depression may lead to hypoxic encephalopathy. Dependent areas suffer peripheral neuropathy, compartment syndrome or rhabdomyolysis which may combine with hypovolaemia and hypoxia to produce renal failure and hyperkalaemia. Hypothermia or hyperthermia can occur. Non-cardiogenic pulmonary oedema is an infrequent complication of opiate overdose, recognized in the context of resuscitation from apnoea, when hypoxia and other metabolic derangements are present. Symptoms usually develop within 4 h of presentation and only a minority require mechanical ventilation.

Complications of poor injection technique include cellulitis, thrombophlebitis, intra-arterial injection and embolization, mycotic aneurysm, endocarditis, anaerobic infection and blood-borne virus infection. A high index of suspicion is required. In addition, the purity of heroin

varies and the drug is 'cut' with agents which have their own clinical effects.

Differential diagnosis

The differential diagnosis is that of any patient with an altered level of consciousness and includes toxicological and metabolic causes, sepsis, neurotrauma, stroke and post-ictal state. Clonidine ingestion may present with low GCS and miosis and may show partial response to naloxone. Toxicity from paracetamol or ibuprofen in co-formulation with opiates should be considered. The presence of fever without localizing symptoms and signs should raise the suspicion of bacteraemia secondary to parenteral drug abuse.

Clinical investigations

Thorough physical examination is usually adequate to exclude complications, such as aspiration, non-cardiogenic pulmonary oedema and compartment syndrome. Further investigations are directed at confirming or excluding alternative diagnoses and complications.

Treatment

Initial care is directed at the resuscitation and immediate life threats. All patients should have bedside blood glucose measurement. Patients with an altered level of consciousness should be closely monitored in a resuscitation area, positioned to minimize the probability of aspiration and moved frequently to prevent dependent injuries.

Naloxone is a short-acting opioid antagonist active at μ receptors, useful as an adjunct to support airway and ventilation. It may be given via the intravenous, intramuscular, subcutaneous or endotracheal routes. Naloxone is safe and rarely associated with serious complications. Bolus therapy (e.g. 0.4–2.0 mg intravenously or intramuscularly in an adult; 0.01 mg/kg in a child) reverses the respiratory depression of opioid intoxication, but may be complicated by rapid wakening, agitation and an acute withdrawal state in opioid-dependent patients. An alternative approach is the use of small intravenous doses (e.g. 0.04 mg) titrated to achieve airway control and ventilation while avoiding abrupt emergence. Intravenous doses of naloxone are effective within a few minutes. The duration of effect of naloxone (20–90

minutes) is less than that of most opioids, therefore, patients must be carefully monitored for resedation. Naloxone infusions may be useful in carefully selected patients who are intoxicated by long-acting opioids, to prevent airway compromise or need for intubation. However, absorption and elimination of opioids may be unpredictable and undulating CNS depression may persist despite continuous naloxone infusion. Intubation is a safe alternative to prolonged infusion for large ingestions.

The duration of observation in the emergency department (ED) and the need for admission depends on the opioid involved, route of administration, co-ingested drugs and the presence of co-morbidity or complications. Long-acting or slow-release opioids require observation for at least 12 hours. Following overdose with short-acting agents, patients can be safely discharged when they are ambulant and alert, have normal vital signs and oxygen saturation and at least 4–6 h have passed since naloxone administration. Discharge should not occur at night.

Other issues

Children and the elderly are more susceptible to opiate toxicity. In children, delayed onset of toxicity and prolonged effects are commonly seen. Co-morbid conditions and physiological changes in the elderly may result in prolonged intoxication. Prolonged observation may be required.

Heroin overdose indicates ongoing hazard and presentation to the ED provides an opportunity for intervention. Patients should be counselled regarding strategies to avoid future overdose and early activation of emergency medical services. If willing, the patient should be referred to agencies specializing in drug detoxification and rehabilitation.

Opioid withdrawal syndrome

The development of physiological dependence with repeated doses of opioid agonists leads to an abstinence or withdrawal syndrome when opioids are ceased. The symptoms represent the reverse of the central and peripheral effects of opioid administration, including anxiety, insomnia, apprehension, hyperventilation, mydriasis, nausea, vomiting, diarrhoea and abdominal pain. Symptoms usually occur 12 h after the last dose of morphine or heroin, peak at approximately 2 days and abate after 5 days. Seizures do not occur and the prognosis is good, even without medical intervention.

After exclusion of concomitant pathology, management should include treatment of dehydration, symptomatic care and referral to drug and alcohol services. Clonidine, an α_2-receptor adrenergic agonist, is used to decrease autonomic symptoms. An initial dose of 1–2 µ/kg, 2–3 times per day, can be increased depending on side effects, such as orthostatic hypotension.

AMPHETAMINES

Pharmacology and pathophysiology

Amphetamines refer to a broad group of related derivatives of β-phenylisopropylamine characterized clinically by CNS stimulatory and peripheral sympathomimetic responses. Amphetamines are structurally related to ephedrine and resemble the catecholamines. Substitutions on the basic structure of β-phenylisopropylamine include methamphetamine ('ice', 'speed'), 3,4-methylenedioxymethamphetamine (MDMA, 'ecstasy', 'Adam' or 'E'), 3,4-methylenedioxyethamphetamine (MDEA, 'Eve') and 3,4-methylenedioxyamphetamine (MDA, 'love drug') and paramethoxyamphetamine (PMA).

Amphetamines may be ingested, smoked, insufflated or injected. All are absorbed from the gastrointestinal (GI) system, with peak serum levels within 3 h. They are weak bases, 20% bound to plasma proteins and have large volumes of distribution. Half-lives vary from 8 to 30 h. Hepatic transformation is the major route of elimination, however, up to 30% of amphetamine and metamphetamine may be eliminated in the urine.

Amphetamines enhance the release of catecholamines and block their reuptake causing increased stimulation of central and peripheral adrenergic receptors leading to CNS excitation and a sympathomimetic syndrome. Higher doses lead to central serotonin release. Substitutions alter the hallucinogenic, behavioural and cardiovascular effects of the drugs at low doses. In overdose, it may be impossible to distinguish the exact amphetamine derivative involved as effects are more uniform.

Epidemiology

The use of amphetamine as a drug of abuse has been prevalent since its introduction in 1932. The 2010 National Drug Strategy Household Survey found 7% of Australians over 14 years reported using amphetamine or methamphetamine in their lifetime. 3,4-Methylenedioxymethamphetamine (MDMA, ecstasy) use was also common, with 10% of people over age 14 years reporting use in their lifetime.

Clinical features

The diagnosis of amphetamine intoxication is clinical. The predominant symptoms are those of CNS excitation and peripheral sympathomimetic response. Euphoria, apprehension and agitation are common. Tachypnoea, mydriasis, tremor, diaphoresis and hyperpyrexia may also be seen. After acute intoxication or binges, psychosis may occur with visual and tactile hallucinations, severe agitation and paranoia resembling paranoid schizophrenia. Myocardial infarction, aortic dissection, rhabdomyolysis, acidosis, acute cardiomyopathy, shock, renal failure and coagulopathy are documented. Symptoms may persist for several days. Death is secondary to hyperpyrexia, seizures, arrhythmia or intracerebral haemorrhage.

Hyponatraemia with cerebral oedema is reported following MDMA use and may be fatal, presenting initially as altered consciousness and seizures. Mechanisms contributing to hyponatraemia include psychogenic polydipsia and inappropriate secretion of antidiuretic hormone.

Complications of injection technique include cellulitis, thrombophlebitis, intra-arterial injection and embolization, mycotic aneurysm, staphylococcal pneumonia, endocarditis, anaerobic clostridial infection and blood-borne viral infections. In addition, chronic abuse of amphetamines may be complicated by a necrotizing vasculitis which may involve multiple organ systems and lead to renal failure, myocardial ischaemia and cerebrovascular disease.

Amphetamine dependence and withdrawal is recognized. Withdrawal is characterized by neurasthenic symptoms, including somnolence and intense cravings for amphetamines. Management is supportive.

Differential diagnosis

Intoxication by an amphetamine derivative may not be discernible clinically from cocaine, except for the increased psychotic features and longer duration of action. The differential diagnosis includes cocaine intoxication, anticholinergic delirium, serotonin syndrome, monoamine oxidase inhibitors, alcohol and benzodiazepine withdrawal, sepsis, hypoglycaemia, thyrotoxicosis and phaeochromocytoma.

Clinical investigations

Physical examination and investigations should be directed at excluding complications and alternative diagnoses. Seizures or coma should prompt investigation for complications, such as intracerebral haemorrhage or electrolyte disturbance.

Treatment

Initial attention must be directed at resuscitation and immediate threats to airway, breathing and circulation. All patients should receive oxygen and have a bedside blood glucose measurement. Close monitoring of the patient in a quiet area away from excessive stimulation may be advantageous. Patients exhibiting psychomotor acceleration or psychosis should be managed with an intravenous benzodiazepine titrated to achieve adequate sedation.

Hyperthermia and seizures should be managed aggressively. Hyperthermia is an important contributing factor to morbidity and mortality. Core temperature should be measured in all patients and continuous monitoring is recommended if the temperature is elevated. Mild-to-moderate hyperthermia (<39°C) usually responds to benzodiazepine sedation and fluid resuscitation. If this is unsuccessful, intubation and paralysis are indicated. There is no evidence that dantrolene has a role in the management of hyperthermia associated with psychostimulants. Benzodiazepines are first-line therapy for seizures, followed by barbiturates, then general anaesthesia and paralysis. Seizures in the context of acute hyponatraemia require initial rapid sodium replacement.

Following resolution of the acute intoxication phase, patients with persistent psychotic features may respond to an antipsychotic agent.

Disposition

The duration of observation in the ED and the need for admission will depend on the severity of intoxication, the influence of co-ingested drugs and the presence of co-morbidity or complications. Patients with mild intoxication (without hyperthermia or chest pain) may be observed in the ED and discharged when vital signs and mental status have returned to normal. The long half-lives of the amphetamines may dictate inpatient care if symptoms or abnormal vital signs do not resolve within a few hours.

Presentation to an ED provides an opportunity for preventative intervention. Patients should be counselled and offered strategies to avoid future toxicity or overdose or referred to drug detoxification services.

COCAINE

Pharmacology and pathophysiology

Coca leaves have been chewed by the natives of the South American Andes for approximately 1200 years and were first exported to Europe in 1580. Cocaine hydrochloride, or benzoylmethylecgonine hydrochloride, is a white powder prepared from the leaves of the *Erythroxylon coca* plant. 'Freebase' cocaine is an alkaloid prepared by mixing cocaine hydrochloride, water and baking soda and separating the precipitate. If the solvent is allowed to evaporate, pure cocaine crystals remain, known as 'rock' or 'crack'. Cocaine reaches the cerebral circulation within seconds after smoking or insufflation. Gastrointestinal absorption may not peak for 90 min. Cocaine is hydrolysed by plasma and liver cholinesterase to an active metabolite. In animal models, cocaine is metabolized in the presence of ethanol to ethylecgonine. This is a myocardial depressant more potent than the sum of the depressant effects of cocaine and ethanol alone. Five to ten per cent of cocaine is excreted in the urine unchanged with a half-life of 60–90 min.

The pathophysiology of cocaine is complex. It is a CNS stimulant acting via enhanced release of noradrenaline, plus blockade of noradrenaline, dopamine and serotonin reuptake. With increasing doses, euphoria is followed by dysphoria, agitation, seizures and coma. Cocaine stimulates the medullary vasomotor centre resulting in hypertension and tachycardia. Small doses may produce transient bradycardia. At high levels, the medullary centre may be depressed, leading to respiratory depression.

Peripherally, cocaine inhibits the reuptake of adrenaline and noradrenaline and stimulates the presynaptic release of noradrenaline. This leads to a sympathomimetic response mediated through both α- and β-adrenoreceptors, leading to tachycardia, diaphoresis, vasoconstriction and hypertension. Increased psychomotor activity, vasoconstriction and direct hypothalamic toxicity, possibly mediated by dopamine receptors, contribute to hyperpyrexia.

Cocaine is an ester-type local anaesthetic that blocks fast sodium channels. In severe toxicity, hypotension may occur due to a direct toxic effect on the myocardium. Wide complex tachyarrhythmias are observed with cocaine toxicity. Sodium channel and potassium channel blockade occur, in addition to sympathomimetic, ischaemic and cardiomyopathic effects. Arrhythmias are related to multiple factors including dose, co-exposures, acid–base and electrolyte imbalance and genetic variability. Transient arrhythmias may account for syncope not attributable to seizures.

Epidemiology

In Australia, the prevalence of cocaine use is increasing, with 7.3% of the population aged over 14 years reporting cocaine use in their lifetime in 2010.

Clinical features

The predominant symptoms are those of CNS excitation and peripheral sympathomimetic response. CNS manifestations include agitation, altered mental state, seizures, dyspnoea, transient focal neurological signs, intracranial haemorrhage and coma. Cerebral infarction, transient ischaemic attacks, subarachnoid haemorrhage, cerebral vasculitis and migraine-like headache are described. Contributing mechanisms include hypertension, vasoconstriction, vasculitis, increased coagulability, altered cerebrovascular autoregulation and embolization of particulate matter.

Cardiovascular manifestations include tachycardia, hypertension, supraventricular or ventricular tachydysrrhythmias and syncope. Chest pain may be due to musculoskeletal, pulmonary or cardiovascular causes.

Cocaine-induced myocardial ischaemia and infarction is multifactorial, due to increased myocardial oxygen demand, immediate or delayed coronary artery vasospasm, increased platelet aggregation, impaired thrombolysis, accelerated atherosclerosis and dilated cardiomyopathy. Aortic dissection associated with cocaine use is reported. A retrospective study of patients intoxicated with cocaine presenting with chest pain consistent with ischaemia found 6% suffered acute myocardial infarction.

Smoking cocaine may lead to respiratory complications including thermal airway injury, pneumothorax and pneumomediastinum, non-cardiac pulmonary oedema, interstitial pneumonitis and bronchiolitis obliterans. Tachypnoea, mydriasis, tremor, diaphoresis and hyperpyrexia may also be seen. Mesenteric vasoconstriction and vasculitis may lead to bowel ischaemia and infarction. Rhabdomyolysis complicated by renal failure and hyperkalaemia is reported.

Differential diagnosis

The differential diagnosis includes intoxication with other sympathomimetic agents, hallucinogenic agents, anticholinergic delirium, serotonin syndrome, monoamine oxidase inhibitors, alcohol and benzodiazepine withdrawal, sepsis, hypoglycaemia, thyrotoxicosis and phaeochromocytoma.

Clinical investigations

The diagnosis is clinical, based on history, sympathomimetic symptoms and signs and the exclusion of other conditions. Physical examination and investigations are directed at excluding complications and alternative diagnoses. All patients with altered vital signs should have a 12-lead ECG and continuous ECG monitoring.

Treatment

Initial care is directed towards the resuscitation and immediate threats to airway, breathing and circulation. Patients exhibiting CNS agitation or sympathomimetic cardiovascular effects should receive an intravenous benzodiazepine titrated to achieve sedation. This will control manifestations of cocaine toxicity in the majority of patients. Hyperthermia and seizures require aggressive resuscitation (as for amphetamines) to prevent a poor outcome. Seizures should be managed with benzodiazepines and barbiturates, escalating to general anaesthesia if required.

Atrial tachycardia and hypertension usually respond to sedation with benzodiazepines. Atrial tachyarrhythmias are usually benign and rarely require specific treatment. Vasodilators, such as nitrates or phentolamine, are recommended for hypertension not responding to benzodiazepines. Ventricular arrhythmias should be treated according to advanced cardiac life support guidelines. In addition to defibrillation or cardioversion, immediate intravenous bolus bicarbonate (1–2 mEq/kg) and benzodiazepine sedation are used. Lignocaine may be an acceptable alternative. The use of β-adrenergic receptor blockers and class 1a and 1c antiarrhythmics in cocaine intoxication is contraindicated.

If myocardial ischaemia or infarction is suspected, investigation should be as for ischaemic chest pain of non-toxicological aetiology. Benzodiazepine sedation, nitrates and verapamil are recommended to decrease heart rate, reduce hypertension and reduce cocaine-induced coronary vasoconstriction. Primary angioplasty is considered the treatment of choice for cocaine-induced acute myocardial infarction. Thrombolytic therapy may be considered if angioplasty is not available, maximal medical management has failed, hypertension has been controlled and there is no evidence of intracranial haemorrhage. Ventricular arrhythmias occurring after the acute phase are presumed to be secondary to myocardial ischaemia and should therefore be treated in a standard manner. In patients with non-diagnostic electrocardiograms, short-term admission may be required to exclude myocardial infarction.

Disposition

The duration of observation in the ED and the need for admission depend on the severity of toxicity, co-ingested drugs and the presence of co-morbidity or complications. Patients with mild intoxication (without hyperthermia or ischaemic chest pain) may be observed in the ED and discharged when the patient is asymptomatic with normal vital signs and mental status.

Presentation to an ED provides an opportunity for preventative intervention. Patients should be counselled and offered strategies to avoid future toxicity or overdose or, if willing, referred to agencies specializing in drug detoxification and rehabilitation.

GAMMA-HYDROXYBUTYRIC ACID

Pharmacology and pathophysiology

Gamma-hydroxybutyric acid (GHB) (4-hydroxybutanoate; sodium oxybate) is a sedative-hypnotic agent causing sedation and psychotropic effects. GHB is a short-chain fatty acid that acts as a neurotransmitter. It is one of the metabolites of gamma-aminobutyric acid (GABA). The mechanism by which GHB causes its effects is unclear, but is probably mediated by specific GHB and GABA-B receptors. It also has dopaminergic activity, increases acetylcholine and serotonin levels and may interact with endogenous opioids. GHB was developed as a short-acting anaesthetic agent, but lost favour due to poor analgesic properties and a propensity to cause seizure-like activity at the onset of coma.

GHB is ingested as a liquid and is rapidly absorbed, peaking within 15–45 min. It is metabolized by alcohol dehydrogenase to succinate, which enters the Krebs cycle. The average half-life is 20–50 min.

Epidemiology

GHB ('grievous bodily harm', 'fantasy', 'scoop', 'liquid X', 'liquid E') and its congeners gamma-butyrolactone (GBL) and 1,4-butanediol, have been advocated for body building, euphoria, sleep enhancement and sexual stimulation. Recreational use of GHB in Australia is uncommon, but increasing. The 2010 National Drug Strategy Household Survey reported that 0.8% of Australians over 14 years reported using GHB in their lifetime.

Clinical features

Most patients present to the ED following acute GHB intoxication. CNS effects with increasing dose include euphoria, then agitation followed rapidly by sedation and coma. Respiratory depression and apnoea may occur, but this is usually reported in the context of co-ingestants. Profound coma may occur but the patient may resist instrumentation of the airway or rouse when stimulated, only to relapse again when the stimulus is removed. Abrupt resolution of coma within 2–3 h of presentation is characteristic of GHB intoxication. However, co-ingested agents may cloud the clinical picture.

Agitation, myoclonus and generalized seizures are reported. 'Seizures' commonly represent myoclonic movements or may be generalized due to hypoxia or a co-ingested agent. Agitation is common on emergence from coma and patients may rapidly change from unresponsive to agitated and combative. Altered conscious state is associated with mild bradycardia and/or hypotension which rarely requires intervention. Chronic users may develop a withdrawal syndrome that mimics alcohol or sedative–hypnotic withdrawal.

Differential diagnosis

The differential diagnosis is that of any patient with an altered level of consciousness and includes toxicological and metabolic causes, sepsis, neurotrauma, stroke and post-ictal state. Persistent CNS depression beyond 6 h should prompt a search for alternative causes.

Investigations

The diagnosis of GHB intoxication is clinical. A thorough physical examination is usually adequate to exclude complications. Investigations are directed at excluding alternative diagnoses and complications.

Treatment

Management is supportive. Initial care is directed at resuscitation and immediate threats to airway, breathing and circulation. All patients should receive oxygen and have a bedside blood glucose measurement. Patients with an altered level of consciousness should be closely monitored in a resuscitation area, positioned to minimize the probability of aspiration and moved frequently to prevent dependent injuries. Intubation may required if the airway is threatened due to vomiting or prolonged coma due to co-ingested agents or complications. There is no specific antidote for GHB.

Disposition

The duration of observation will depend on the need for intubation, co-ingested agents or the presence of complications. Most patients recover within a few hours and may be safely discharged from the ED when they are ambulant and orientated.

Presentation to an ED also provides an opportunity for preventative intervention. Patients should be counselled regarding strategies to avoid future overdose. In addition, the patient may be referred to agencies specializing in drug detoxification and rehabilitation.

EMERGING DRUGS OF ABUSE–'LEGAL HIGHS'

Introduction and epidemiology

Novel agents derived from synthetic chemicals, plants or fungal matter have recently come into use as alternatives to controlled drugs of abuse. These agents are structural analogues of endogenous neurotransmitters (especially serotonin, noradrenaline and dopamine) resulting in similar effects. There is a lack of data surrounding the pharmacology, toxicology, prevalence and effects of most of these agents. Most are sold as benign substances, such as 'bath salts' or 'incense' and labelled 'not for human consumption'. Understanding of the effects of these agents is difficult given misleading packaging, unpredictable consistency and continual emergence of structural analogues. Caffeine is commonly added to the product, altering the observed clinical effects. There are three main groups of 'legal highs':

- stimulants (cathinones, synthetic cocaine, pipradols, piperazines)
- hallucinogens (cannabinoid receptor agonists, piperazines, methoxetamine)
- depressants (GBL, novel opioids).

Cathinones, piperazines, synthetic cannabinoid receptor agonists and methoxetamine are most well studied and will be considered here.

Stimulants: synthetic cathinones

Pharmacology and pathophysiology

Cathinone is a beta-ketone amphetamine analogue present in young leaves of the *Catha edulis* plant. Khat leaf chewing causes sympathomimetic effects similar to amphetamine,

including tachycardia, hypertension, euphoria and increased alertness. Numerous synthetic phenylalkylamines have been derived, including mephedrone ('meow-meow', 'MCAT'), methcathinone, methylone and methylenedioxypyrovalerone (MDPV; 'bath salts', 'ivory wave'). Most cause sympathomimetic effects by increased release and reduced synaptic clearance of noradrenaline, dopamine and serotonin via monoamine uptake transporters. They are presented as a powder or pill which is insufflated, ingested or injected. The pharmacology of these agents in humans has not been well established. Reported onset of action after ingestion is 15–45 min with effects lasting 2–7 h.

Clinical features

Increased energy from ingestion of cathinones is reported by users to be better and longer lasting than cocaine. Twenty per cent report adverse symptoms including palpitations, GI upset and mental disturbance. Cardiac, neurological and psychiatric derangement is common, with agitation, sometimes severe and requiring restraint, being most common. A sympathomimetic toxidrome with chest pain, diaphoresis, tachycardia and hypertension may occur. Psychosis, anxiety, hallucinations and delusions are common, abnormal liver and renal function, rhabdomyolysis and hyponatraemia with seizures and death have been reported. Addiction potential and withdrawal symptoms are considered probable but are uncharacterized.

Clinical investigations

Diagnosis of intoxication is clinical, although cathinone levels can be obtained for forensic purposes.

Treatment

There are no data to suggest the optimal management of patients with cathinone toxicity. Routine decontamination and enhanced elimination are unlikely to be effective and there is no specific antidote. Management is supportive and has been extrapolated from that of other sympathomimetic agents, using benzodiazepine sedation as first line for agitation, seizures, psychosis, tachycardia and hypertension. Hyperthermia is treated aggressively with cooling measures and benzodiazepines, escalating to intubation and paralysis for fever with severe muscle rigidity. Treatment of hyponatraemia follows standard protocols depending on severity and clinical features.

Stimulants/hallucinogens: piperazines

Pharmacology and pathophysiology

Benzylpiperazine (BZP, 'herbal party pills', 'BenzoFury') is most well known among this group of agents, however, other agents, such as trifluoromethylphenylpiperazine (TFMPP), are commonly available. BZP is a dopamine reuptake inhibitor and increases dopamine release. BZP increases peripheral catecholamine release, causing sympathomimetic stimulation.

TFMPP is a direct serotonin agonist at 5HT-1 and 5HT-2 receptors and inhibits serotonin reuptake. Piperazines are metabolized by cytochrome P450 and may inhibit these enzymes, leading to drug interactions.

Clinical features

BZP and TFMPP are often combined to mimic closely the effects of MDMA. Effects depend on agent and dose administered, with stimulant effects predominant at lower doses and hallucinogenic effects (TFMPP) at higher doses; however, there is significant inter-individual variability. A sympathomimetic-type toxidrome is common with sinus tachycardia, hypertension, agitation, anxiety, confusion and gastrointestinal upset being reported. More severe effects include seizures, hyperthermia and related complications, movement disorders, chest pain/myocardial toxicity and hyponatraemia (rare). Effects are reported to last 6–8 h, however, lethargy, insomnia, anxiety, paranoia and mood disorders may persist for several days.

Clinical investigations

Diagnosis is clinical based on history and clinical features. While levels are available for forensic reasons, they do not correlate well with toxicity and are not clinically useful. Further investigation may be required to exclude complications or co-morbid conditions.

Treatment

Management is symptomatic and supportive. Routine gastrointestinal decontamination and enhanced elimination are unlikely to be of benefit. There is no specific antidote. Initial management is aimed at resuscitation and immediate life threats of airway, breathing, circulation and seizures along normal pathways. Intravenous benzodiazepine sedation may be required for seizures, agitation or generalized muscle rigidity and is adequate to control symptoms for most cases. Hyperthermia should be treated aggressively with cooling measures and titrated benzodiazepines with escalation to intubation and paralysis if necessary.

Hallucinogens: synthetic cannabinoid receptor agonists

Pharmacology and pathophysiology

Synthetic cannabinoid receptor agonists ('kronic', 'spice', 'k2', 'chill out', 'chaos') act at cannabinoid receptors CB1 and CB2, as well as NMDA receptors. There are seven structural groups of agents (JWH, CP and HU compounds) which are added to herbal mixes and smoked. These agents have a higher affinity for the cannabinoid receptors than tetrahydrocannabinol (THC). Pharmacokinetic properties have not been characterized.

Clinical features

Case series suggest psychiatric effects predominate including anxiety and paranoia, agitation and delusions. Tachycardia and diaphoresis are common. Seizures have been reported with some compounds. A withdrawal syndrome has been reported in habitual users.

Clinical investigations

Diagnosis is clinical based on history and examination findings. Further investigations are aimed at excluding complications and alternative diagnoses. Levels are not readily available within a clinically significant time frame, but can be obtained for occupational and forensic reasons.

Treatment

There is no specific antidote for cannabinoid receptor antagonists. Management is symptomatic and supportive. Benzodiazepine sedation may be required for agitation, hallucinations and seizures.

Hallucinogens: methoxetamine

Pharmacology and pathophysiology

Methoxetamine is a ketamine analogue/phencyclidine derivative which is an antagonist at

NMDA receptors and inhibits dopamine reuptake from the synapse. It is absorbed by oral, nasal, rectal and intramuscular routes with rapid onset and short duration of symptoms.

Clinical features

Effects are similar to those of ketamine, with euphoria and perceptual disturbances. Severe nausea and vomiting, diarrhoea, anxiety and paranoia have been reported. Tachycardia and nystagmus are common. Respiratory depression may occur.

Treatment

Diagnosis is clinical. Management is symptomatic and supportive. Benzodiazepines, antiemetics and intravenous fluid are likely to be required. Respiratory support may be needed.

'BODY-PACKERS', 'BODY-STUFFERS'

Epidemiology

Body-packers and body-stuffers conceal illicit drugs within body cavities. Patients may ingest many times a lethal dose but appear asymptomatic at presentation. A body-packer conceals a large quantity of an illicit drug inside a body cavity, usually the GI tract, in an attempt to smuggle it across international borders. Up to 1 kg of drugs may be carefully packaged in 50–150 packages and layered with wax to prevent leaking. A body-stuffer ingests smaller quantities of drugs before apprehension by the authorities. The package is usually poorly constructed and is more likely to leak. Time from ingestion to hospital arrival is usually short. The vagina and rectum are alternative sites for drug concealment in the body-stuffer. Heroin, cocaine, amphetamine derivatives, MDMA and cannabis are all reported in body-packers and -stuffers.

History may be misleading, especially if taken in the presence of law enforcement officers. Ideally, a detailed history should be obtained noting the type and amount of drug ingested, the method of packaging, symptoms of drug intoxication and any factors that may increase the likelihood of bowel obstruction or ileus. A thorough physical examination should include examination of the vagina and rectum and a search for any signs of drug intoxication.

Clinical investigations

There is a paucity of data regarding optimal imaging modality, decontamination and treatment. Imaging of the potential body-packer is controversial. Abdominal radiographs are often positive in body-packers, where multiple package–air interfaces may be seen. The sensitivity and specificity of plain abdominal films in large series is reported to be 85–90%. Importantly, negative plain radiographs do not exclude the diagnosis. Abdominal computed tomography (CT) scanning with oral contrast has been recommended, although sensitivity is not 100%. Qualitative urine drug screens do not change management and are not routinely indicated. In the presence of signs of intoxication, investigations for complications and co-morbidities may be appropriate.

Treatment

In view of the potential sudden lethality of both these practices, patients should receive a high triage priority and be managed in a resuscitation setting with secure IV access regardless of presenting symptoms or signs. Evidence of drug intoxication, either at presentation or during decontamination, represents a medical emergency and requires aggressive management. Initial care is directed at assessment and resuscitation of immediate threats to airway, breathing, circulation and the control of seizures as required.

Gastrointestinal decontamination of body-packers and body-stuffers is controversial and should be considered on a case-by-case basis. If cooperative, patients should receive activated charcoal to adsorb intraluminal drug. Whole bowel irrigation with polyethylene glycol at 2 L/h via nasogastric tube until all packages are passed has been recommended. However, a conservative approach to asymptomatic patients has recently been advocated with observation, laxatives and light diet until all packets are retrieved. The risk of late-onset drug intoxication, bowel obstruction, laparotomy or death is less than 5% with this approach. Surgical exploration is indicated if there is gastric outflow or bowel obstruction, concretion formation, ileus or perforation. If a cocaine or amphetamine body-packer exhibits toxicity, immediate surgical exploration to remove all packages has been advocated. Surgery is probably not necessary in the opiate body-packer as adequate resuscitation, supportive care and antidote therapy should ensure a favourable outcome. Body-stuffers with a single package located in the stomach may be amenable to endoscopic removal, especially if there is failure to progress.

All body-packers should remain in a closely monitored environment in the ED, observation unit or intensive care unit until all packages have been retrieved. Staff should be aware of potential signs of intoxication and be available to intervene in the event of complications. Patients are observed until all packages have been accounted for and there have been three normal package-free stools. Repeat radiology is performed to confirm clearance before discharge.

Controversies

- Optimal sedation regimen for cocaine and amphetamine-intoxicated patients.
- Intubation vs expectant management for patients with GHB intoxication.
- Optimal management of patients using synthetic agents or 'legal highs'.
- Optimal imaging and gastrointestinal decontamination in body-packers.

Further reading

Fatovich DM, Bartu A, Davis G, et al. Morbidity associated with heroin overdose presentations to an emergency department: a 10 year record linkage study. Emerg Med Australas 2010;22:240–5.

Glauser J, Queen JR. An overview of non-cardiac cocaine toxicity. J Emerg Med 2007;32:181–6.

Greene S, Kerr F, Braitberg G. Review article: amphetamines and related drugs of abuse. Emerg Med Australas 2008;20:391–402.

Hoffman RS. Treatment of patients with cocaine-induced arrhythmias: bringing the bench to the bedside. Br J Clin Pharmacol 2010;69:448–57.

Lange RA, Hillis LD. Medical progress: cardiovascular complications of cocaine use. N Engl J Med 2001;345:351–8.

Mason PE, Kerns WP. Gamma hydroxybutyric acid (GHB) intoxication. Acad Emerg Med 2002;9:730–9.

Prosser JM, Nelson LS. The toxicology of bath salts: a review of synthetic cathinones. J Med Toxicol 2012;8:33–42.

Rosenbaum CD, Carreiro SP, Babu KM. Here today, gone tomorrow…and back again? A review of herbal marijuana alternatives (K2, spice). Synthetic cathinones (bath salts), kratom, Salvia divinorum, methoxetamine and piperazines. J Med Toxicol 2012;8:15–32.

Schep LJ, Slaughter RJ, Vale JA, et al. The clinical toxicology of the designer "party pills" benzylpiperazine and trifluoromethylphenylpiperazine. Clin Toxicol 2011;49: 131–41.

Sporer KA. Acute heroin overdose. Ann Intern Med 1999;130: 584–90.

Traub SJ, Hoffman RS, Nelson LS. Body packing–the internal concealment of drugs. N Engl J Med 2003;349:2519–26.

29.14 Methaemoglobinaemia

Robert Edwards

ESSENTIALS

1 Consider the diagnosis of methaemoglobinaemia in patients with cyanosis unresponsive to oxygen.

2 Multiple presentations can occur following incidents involving contamination of food or water. Early clinical recognition allows institution of treatment and prevention of further cases.

3 Pulse oximetry is misleading in methaemoglobinaemia. Readings do not usually fall below 85%.

4 Administer methylene blue to symptomatic patients with elevated methaemoglobin levels and to unstable patients with a history of exposure to an agent known to cause methaemoglobinaemia.

5 Methylene blue can cause haemolysis and methaemoglobinaemia if given to patients who do not have methaemoglobinaemia or who are G6PD deficient or if more than 5 mg/kg is used.

6 Failure to respond to methylene blue may result from too small or too large a dose, congenital enzyme or haemoglobin defects or an incorrect diagnosis.

Introduction

Although it is an uncommon presentation, the emergency physician must be able to diagnose methaemoglobinaemia because it is potentially fatal and can be readily treated with the antidote, methylene blue.

Aetiology and pathophysiology

Under normal conditions, methaemoglobin is continuously produced from haemoglobin by the oxidation of the iron molecule from the ferrous (Fe^{2+}) to the ferric (Fe^{3+}) state. In the normal physiological state, less than 1% of haemoglobin is methaemoglobin because it is continuously being reduced, predominantly by the enzyme NADH methaemoglobin reductase.

Excessive methaemoglobinaemia causes tissue hypoxia because methaemoglobin is incapable of carrying oxygen and causes a shift of the oxygen haemoglobin dissociation curve to the left.

Methaemoglobinaemia may be acquired or congenital. Congenital methaemoglobinaemia is due either to a deficiency of the enzyme NADH methaemoglobin reductase (a rare autosomal recessive condition) or the haemoglobinopathy, haemoglobin M (Milwaukee). The latter is transmitted with an autosomal inheritance. Homozygotes usually do not survive and heterozygotes live with a methaemoglobin level of around 15–30%. Patients with glucose-6-phosphate dehydrogenase (G6PD) deficiency are at increased risk of developing methaemoglobinaemia when exposed to an oxidizing agent, due to low levels of NADPH.

Acquired methaemoglobinaemia in adults arises as a consequence of accidental or intentional exposure to a therapeutic drug or other oxidizing agent. Oxidants that commonly result in excessive methaemoglobin production are listed in Table 29.14.1.

Table 29.14.1 Agents causing acquired methaemoglobinaemia

Nitrites
- Amyl nitrite
- Isobutyl nitrite

Nitrates
- Glyceryl trinitrate
- Nitrate food preservatives
- Silver nitrate burns treatments
- Sodium nitrate
- Water contaminated with nitrates

Local anaesthetics (including topical)
- Benzocaine
- Lidocaine
- Prilocaine

Aniline dyes and related compounds
- Aniline
- Nitroethane
- Toluidine
- Nitrobenzene (used in manufacture of dyes, rubber chemicals)

Antimicrobial agents
- Dapsone
- Quinones (chloroquine, primaquine)
- Sulphonamides

Others
- Cetrimide
- Chlorates
- Combustion products
- Nitric oxide
- Copper sulphates
- Methylene blue
- Naphthalene
- Chemotherapy agents: 3 amino-pyridine 2 carboxaldehyde
- Cocaine

Edwards RJ, Ujma J. Extreme methaemoglobinaemia secondary to recreational use of amyl nitrite. Journal of Accident and Emergency Medicine 1995;12:138–42 with permission.

Nitrates, nitrites and local anaesthetics are the culprits most commonly reported in the medical literature. Recreational use of amyl, butyl or isobutyl nitrite can cause severe methaemoglobinaemia. Transdermal absorption of industrial nitrate solutions, ingestion of food and water contaminated with nitrates and the intravenous use or inhalation of nitrates may all cause methaemoglobinaemia. Sodium nitrite is commonly used commercially as a food preservative, colouring agent or corrosion inhibitor. In 2006, a total of five patients suffering methaemoglobinaemia (ranging from 21 to 57%) presented to a Sydney emergency department in two separate clusters due to Asian food being prepared with an additive containing 100% sodium nitrite bought in Asian grocery stores.

Therapeutic use of glyceryl trinitrate (GTN) has been reported to increase methaemoglobin levels up to 38%, but it is more likely to cause severe hypotension before methaemoglobinaemia develops. Prolonged use of high doses of GTN ($>10\,\mu g/kg/min$) and the presence of renal or hepatic dysfunction make this complication more likely.

Local anaesthetics, prilocaine and benzocaine in particular, can cause methaemoglobinaemia even when applied topically and administered in standard doses.

Risk factors for the development of methaemoglobinaemia from topically applied local anaesthetics include excessive dosing, a break in the mucosal barrier and a partial deficiency of the enzyme NADH methaemoglobin reductase.

Dapsone therapy can cause both haemolytic anaemia and methaemoglobinaemia.

Aniline (aminobenzene) and its major metabolite, phenyl hydroxylamine, are potent methaemoglobin-forming agents, even after transdermal exposure. Aniline and related compounds, such as nitrobenzene, are used widely in industry, especially the chemical and rubber industries.

In more recent times, the widespread availability of drugs over the Internet has seen further reports of methaemoglobinaemia. This includes a report of two men who took a small amount of what they believed to be the recreational psychoactive drug 2C-E (a member of the phenethylamine family) produced in China which was later found to be pure aniline.

Clinical features

The symptoms and signs of methaemoglobinaemia are attributable to the effects of cellular hypoxia on the CNS and the heart. At levels between 25% and 40%, headache, weakness, anxiety, lethargy, syncope, tachycardia and dyspnoea are observed. Further elevations are associated with decreasing level of consciousness (45–55%) leading to coma, seizures, arrhythmias and cardiac conduction disturbances (55–70%). Levels above 70% are associated with mortality, but deaths can occur at lower levels.

With accidental exposures (either ingestion or cutaneous), multiple presentations of either family members or co-workers can be encountered after common exposure to the offending agent. It is not unusual in these circumstances for the relationship between the toxic substance and the presentations to be unclear initially.

The hallmark of methaemoglobinaemia is a deep cyanosis that is unresponsive to oxygen therapy. The cyanosis may be so deep that it is more brown than blue and has been termed chocolate cyanosis. A useful diagnostic clue is the classic chocolate brown appearance of the patient's blood. This may be observed at methaemoglobin levels as low as 15–20%.

Clinical investigations

The diagnosis of methaemoglobinaemia is confirmed by spectrophotometric measurement of methaemoglobin. The result is expressed as a percentage of the total haemoglobin level. Analysis of the sample should be performed as soon as possible because methaemoglobin levels fall with time. The indications for spectrophotometry are:

- cyanosis unresponsive to oxygen
- tachypnoea or other features of hypoxia and history of exposure to methaemoglobin-inducing agents
- normal or raised PaO_2 and low SpO_2 on pulse oximetry
- chocolate brown appearance of arterial blood.

Arterial blood gas analysis often demonstrates a metabolic acidosis with a normal oxygen tension. Other important investigations include a chest X-ray to exclude pulmonary pathology that might contribute to hypoxia and an ECG to assess cardiac rhythm and look for evidence of myocardial ischaemia or infarction. A full blood count to check haemoglobin (oxidizing agents, such as aniline and their metabolites, can cause a chemical-induced haemolytic anaemia) and electrolytes, urea, creatinine and liver function tests should also be performed. Consider a G6PD level if methylene blue fails to work.

Pulse oximetry

Methaemoglobin interferes with the accuracy of pulse oximetry. With increasing levels of methaemoglobin, pulse oximetry readings approach 85% (at around 30% methaemoglobin) and remain in the mid-eighties range. Methaemoglobin has a maximal light absorption at a wavelength similar to that of oxyhaemoglobin (660 nm) and is therefore not differentiated from oxyhaemoglobin.

Pulse co-oximeters which measure more than the standard two wavelengths of light, can distinguish not only methaemoglobin but also carboxyhaemoglobin and, if available, can confirm the diagnosis of methaemoglobin by direct transcutaneous measurement.

Treatment

Initial management includes assessment of the airway, breathing and circulation and institution of appropriate measures of care. Administration of oxygen therapy is often not associated with any clinical benefit but the presence of cyanosis not responsive to oxygen is a diagnostic clue.

Decontamination of the gastrointestinal (GI) tract or skin may be indicated.

Antidote

Methylene blue (tetramethyl thionine), 1–2 mg/kg IV, is a specific antidote for methaemoglobinaemia. Normally, 95% of methaemoglobin is reduced by the NADH methaemoglobin reductase system, a greater proportion is reduced by a second enzyme system, NADPH methaemoglobin reductase when methylene blue is present acting as a cofactor to methaemoglobin reductase.

NADPH is produced by the Embden–Myerhoff pathway and requires adequate G6PD activity. Thus, in states of G6PD deficiency, methylene blue may not be as effective.

Methylene blue is indicated for symptomatic patients with an elevated methaemoglobin level. Patients who are blue but asymptomatic do not require methylene blue. Symptoms can normally be expected in patients with levels greater than 15%, less if the patient is anaemic.

The dose of methylene blue is 1–2 mg/kg intravenously over 5 min. Unstable patients with cyanosis unresponsive to high flow oxygen and a history of oxidant exposure or 'chocolate brown' blood should be given methylene blue even if the methaemoglobin level is not available. A reduction in the methaemoglobin level and accompanying clinical improvement usually occur over 30–60 min. A further dose of 1 mg/kg can be given after 1 h if the methaemoglobin level remains elevated. Factors that may result in failure to respond are listed in Table 29.14.2.

The side effects of methylene blue include dyspnoea, a feeling of pressure on the chest, restlessness, apprehension, tremor, nausea and vomiting. Paradoxically, methylene blue itself can oxidize haemoglobin to methaemoglobin if given in high doses (>5–7 mg/kg). Adverse effects are minimized if the correct dose is

Table 29.14.2   Reasons for failure of methaemoglobinaemia to respond to methylene blue (MB)

Excessive oxidant
- Ongoing exposure
- Inadequate decontamination

Insufficient methylene blue
- Inadequate dose
- Shorter half-life of MB compared to oxidizing substance (e.g. dapsone)

Excessive methylene blue
- Excessive methylene blue acts as an oxidant in high doses (>7 mg/kg)

Methylene blue ineffective
- G6PD deficiency
- NADPH metHb reductase deficiency
- Haemoglobin M

Incorrect diagnosis
- Sulphaemoglobinaemia
- Carbon monoxide poisoning
- Cyanosis unresponsive to oxygen: cardiac shunt

used. Methylene blue occasionally causes persistent blue discoloration of the patient or haemolytic anaemia. G6PD-deficient patients should not be given methylene blue as it may precipitate massive haemoloysis.

Continuous infusion of methylene blue has been used to treat prolonged methaemoglobinaemia formation associated with dapsone. Methylene blue has a short half-life, there may be delayed increase in methaemoglobin level up to 12 h after the administration of methylene blue. Therefore, serial monitoring of methaemoglobin level may be indicated. Aniline dye-induced methaemoglobinaemia may be resistant to treatment as its metabolite (phenylhydroxylamine) blocks uptake of methylene blue.

Other therapies

Exchange transfusion

Exchange transfusion is indicated for patients with G6PD deficiency or where there is failure to respond to methylene blue or where there is significant haemolysis and methylene blue relatively contraindicated.

N-acetylcysteine

N-acetylcysteine (NAC) has been proposed and used in case reports as a supplemental reducing substance in methaemoglobinaemia. It contains a reduced sulphydryl group. However, small *in vitro* and *in vivo* studies have not shown an improvement in methaemoglobin levels and its effectiveness has not been proven.

Controversies

- Treatment with hyperbaric oxygen has been recommended as an adjuvant treatment to methylene blue. Realistically, it should only be considered where there has been an inadequate response to methylene blue. The partial pressure of oxygen can be increased to such a degree so as to ensure adequate oxygen transport in the absence of functioning haemoglobin.
- Adjuvant treatment with ascorbic acid (vitamin C) has been recommended. It has a direct effect in reducing methaemoglobin, but this effect is too slow for it to be used as a primary treatment. The dose is 0.5–1.0 g 6-hourly, either orally or intravenously.

Further reading

Berlin G, Brod AB, Hilden JO, et al. Acute dapsone intoxication: a case treated with continuous infusion of methylene blue, forced diuresis and plasma exchange. Clin Toxicol 1984;22:537–48.

Center for Disease Control. Severe methemoglobinemia and hemolytic anemia from aniline purchased as 2C-E (4-ethyl2,5-dimethoxyphenethylamine), a recreational drug, on the Internet. MMWR 2012;61:88–91.

Curry S. Methemoglobinemia. Ann Emerg Med 1982;11:214–21.

Edwards RJ, Ujma J. Extreme methaemoglobinaemia secondary to recreational use of amyl nitrite. J Accid Emerg Med 1995;12:134–7.

Goluboff N, Wheaton R. Methylene blue induced cyanosis and acute haemolytic anaemia complicating treatment of methaemoglobinaemia. J Paediatr 1961;58:86–90.

Hunter L, Gordge L, Dargan PI. Methaemoglobinaemia associated with the use of cocaine and volatile nitrites as recreational drugs: a review. Br J Clin Pharmacol 2011;7291:18–26.

Kellet PB, Copeland CS. Methemoglobinemia associated with benzocaine containing lubricant. Anesthesiology 1983;59:463–4.

Maric P, Sayed SA, Heron LG, et al. Methaemoglobinaemia following ingestion of a commonly available food additive. Med J Am 2008;188:156–8.

Reider HU, Frei FJ, Zbinden AM, Thomson DA. Pulse oximetry in methaemoglobinaemia. Failure to detect low oxygen saturation. Anaesthesia 1989;44:326–7.

Rosen PL, Johnson C, McGehee WG. Failure of methylene blue in toxic methaemoglobinaemia. Association with glucose-6-phosphate dehydrogenase deficiency. Ann Intern Med 1971;75:83–6.

Skold A, Cosco DL, Klein R. Methemoglobinemia: pathogenesis, diagnosis and management. South Med J 2011;104:757–61.

Stucke AG, Riess ML, Connolly LA. Hemoglobin M (Milwaukee) affects arterial oxygen saturation and makes pulse oximetry unreliable. Anesthesiology 2006;104:887–8.

29.15 Cyanide

George Braitberg

ESSENTIALS

1 Cyanide is a metabolic poison associated with a high mortality.

2 Cyanide toxicity is characterized by rapid onset of central nervous, respiratory and cardiovascular effects and by metabolic acidosis.

3 Cyanide exposure correlates well with serum lactate levels.

4 Prompt resuscitative efforts with high flow oxygen and administration of antidotes may be life saving; a number of alternative agents are available.

5 Cyanide poisoning from smoke inhalation is often overlooked and treatment is complicated by the potential coexistence of carboxy- and methaemoglobinaemia.

Introduction and epidemiology

Cyanide is used in a variety of commercial processes including metal extraction (especially gold) and recovery, metal hardening and in the production of agricultural and horticultural pest control compounds. Exposure can also occur to hydrogen cyanide (HCN) gas, produced when inorganic cyanide comes in contact with mineral acids as in electroplating, or accidentally when cyanide solutions are poured into acid waste containers. Cyanide off-gassing in house fires is well documented.

Death from cyanide poisoning is one of the most rapid and dramatic seen in medicine and antidotal therapy must be given early to alter outcome. Having said that, there is a number of case reports where patients with lethal cyanide blood levels have survived with good supportive care. A dose of 200 mg of ingested cyanide, or 3 min exposure to HCN gas, is potentially lethal.

Fortunately, serious acute cyanide poisoning is rare. However, the incidence of cyanide poisoning may be significantly underestimated. Blood cyanide concentrations greater than the toxic level of 40 μmol/L were found in 74% of victims found dead at the scenes of fires.

Cyanide is considered a likely agent of terrorism because it possesses attributes of the ideal chemical weapon. It is plentiful, available and, because of its use in industry and research laboratories, is widely distributed making it susceptible to theft, hijacking attempts and other terrorist acts. Cyanide does not require special knowledge to use and it is capable of causing mass incapacitation and casualties. It can be released in the atmosphere as a gaseous weapon or introduced into pharmaceuticals, the food supply and is considered a primary threat to water supplies. In Australia, cyanide has been used to adulterate medications.

Toxicokinetics and pathophysiology

The uptake of cyanide into cells is rapid and follows a first-order kinetic simple diffusion process. The half-life of cyanide is from 2 to 3 h.

While the precise *in vivo* action of cyanide is yet to be determined, it is thought that its major effect is due to binding with the ferric ion (Fe^{3+}) of cytochrome oxidase, the last cytochrome in the respiratory chain. This results in inhibition of oxidative phosphorylation, halting electron transport, oxygen consumption and ATP formation. This leads to a net accumulation of hydrogen ions, a change in the NAD:NADH ratio and greatly increased lactic acid production. Other enzymatic processes, involving antioxidant enzymes, catalase, superoxide dismutase and glutathione, may contribute to toxicity. Cyanide is also a potent stimulator of neurotransmitter release in both the central and the peripheral nervous systems. Humans detoxify cyanide by transferring sulphane sulphur, R–Sx–SH, to cyanide to form thiocyanate (SCN). The availability of R–Sx–SH is the rate-limiting step.

Clinical features

Any acute cyanide exposure is potentially lethal. Onset of symptoms is usually rapid and can be within seconds to minutes for inhalation and within an hour for oral exposure. The 'classical' presentation is rapid onset of coma, seizures, shock and profound lactic acidosis.

Cyanide toxicity is characterized by effects on the central nervous system (CNS), respiratory and cardiovascular systems and by a marked metabolic acidosis.

CNS manifestations, in order of increasing severity of cyanide exposure, are headache, anxiety, disorientation, lethargy, seizures, respiratory depression, CNS depression and cerebral death. An initial tachypnoea gives way to respiratory depression as CNS depression develops.

Cardiovascular manifestations include hypertension followed by hypotension, tachycardia followed by bradycardia, arrhythmias, atrioventricular block and increased cardiac output followed by myocardial depression and cardiovascular collapse. Cyanide poisoning can shorten the QT interval to the point of 'T on R' phenomenon. The classic finding of bright red skin due to poor tissue oxygen (secondary to a decreased arteriovenous oxygen gradient) is not observed if significant myocardial, respiratory or CNS depression has already occurred, in which case the patient may appear cyanotic.

Clinical investigations

Arterial blood gas analysis and serum lactate measurements reveal metabolic acidosis with a raised lactate. Concentration decay curves suggest that serum lactate concentration is closely correlated to blood cyanide concentration. In smoke-inhalation victims without severe burns, plasma lactate concentrations above 10 mmol/L correlate with blood cyanide concentrations above 40 μmol/L, with a sensitivity of 87%, a specificity of 94% and a positive predictive value of 95%.

Cyanide is concentrated 10-fold by erythrocytes and whole-blood cyanide concentrations are used as the benchmark when comparing levels. A level of 40 μmol/L is considered toxic and a level of 100 μmol/L potentially lethal. Symptomatic intoxication starts at levels of about 20 μmol/L. Cyanide levels are usually not available in a clinically significant time frame.

A semiquantitative bedside test for cyanide in blood has been used but is not readily available.

Treatment

Resuscitation

Attention to airway, breathing, circulation and other resuscitative measures must be instituted immediately. Patients should be ventilated with 100% O_2. Patients must be removed from enclosed or confined spaces with high airborne concentrations of cyanide. Rescuers, likewise, must not enter such areas without full protective clothing and proper respirators or self-contained breathing apparatus. Mouth-to-mouth breathing should never be done.

Decontamination

Exposed skin and eyes should be copiously flushed with water or normal saline in an attempt to decontaminate the patient. All clothes should be removed and bagged. Activated charcoal is given only after the airway is secured.

Antidote treatment principles

In a recent review for the Australian Resuscitation Council, Reade et al. concluded that:

Cardiorespiratory collapse, combined with either a high blood cyanide level or obvious evidence of cyanide poisoning, is a clear indication for use of an antidote. Under these circumstances, the use of antidotes with even narrow therapeutic indices would appear reasonable. However, the indication for use of a cyanide antidote is less clear when smaller quantities are ingested, in patients without cardiorespiratory collapse, or where the diagnosis is unclear. Under these circumstances, it is logical to avoid the more toxic antidotes and this is reflected in the TGA-approved product information for dicobaltedetate. Hydroxocobalamin and sodium thiosulphate have few adverse effects, justifying their use in lesser degrees of cyanide poisoning.

There is uncertainty about the prevalence and clinical significance of cyanide poisoning from smoke inhalation. Yeoh and Braitberg found 11 of 138 patients with fire-related

deaths had potentially fatal blood cyanide levels. They suggested that in patients with severe burns, elevated lactate or carboxy-haemoglobin greater than 10%, the use of a safe antidote should be considered.

Therapeutic endpoints in treatment are improvement in conscious state, haemodynamic stability and improvement in metabolic acidosis.

Specific cyanide antidotes

Hydroxocobalamin (*Cyanokit* [package insert] Columbia, MD: Meridian Technologies, Inc., 2009)

A recent systematic review of cyanide poisoning management for the Australian Resuscitation Council has recommended this as the initial antidote for the management of adults with suspected severe cyanide poisoning.

Hydroxocobalamin (vitamin B12A) is the cyanide antidote most widely used in Europe. It complexes with cyanide, on a mole-for-mole ratio to form cyanocobalamin. Antidotal doses of hydroxocobalamin are approximately 5000 times the physiological dose.

Hydroxocobalamin and cyanocobalamin are excreted by the kidney. The half-life of hydroxocobalamin in cyanide-exposed patients is 26.2 h. As the half-life of cyanide in smoke inhalation victims is calculated to be between 1.2 and 3.0 h, it is suggested that hydroxocobalamin can be satisfactorily used as single-dose therapy. The amount of cyanocobalamin formed after a dose of 5 g hydroxocobalamin correlates linearly until a blood cyanide level of 40 μmol/L is reached. At higher blood cyanide concentrations, there is little further rise in plasma cyanocobalamin and it is suggested that the rate-limiting step in the formation of cyanocobalamin is the availability of antidote, not the absence of cyanide ions. In cases of ingestion of cyanide with suicidal intent (where blood cyanide levels may be >150 μmol/L or plasma lactate concentrations >20 μmol/L), the usual dose of 5–10 g may be insufficient.

Extensive research has demonstrated the safety of this drug. In healthy adult smokers, 5 g of IV hydroxocobalamin is associated with a transient reddish discoloration of the skin, mucous membranes and urine and a mean elevation in systolic blood pressure of 14%, with a concomitant 16% decrease in heart rate.

No other clinical adverse effects are noted and allergic reactions are rare. There is substantial experimental evidence to support the efficacy of hydroxocobalamin at lower levels of toxicity Hydroxocobalamin has been shown to be safe and efficacious in mild-to-moderate cyanide poisonings with levels up to 150 μmol/L and has been given successfully to patients with severe cyanide toxicity.

There are no data comparing the efficacy of hydroxocobalamin with other antidotes, so it is not possible to make any definitive conclusion about which antidote is best. However, in the emergency situation hydroxocobalamin appears to offer a greater margin of safety.

Hydroxocobalamin is a strong red chromophore with absorption maxima at 274 nm and 351 nm and no absorption above 600 nm. Interference with co-oximetric and colorimetric laboratory measurements has been reported. Carlsson et al. found some clinically important result errors that might lead to misdiagnoses and incorrect treatment, including a falsely lowered carboxyhaemoglobin and a falsely elevated lactate. Depending on the pathology system used a positive bias on methaemoglobin measurements may occur.

Hydroxocobalamin has a reasonably long shelf life, but is expensive. Hydroxocobalamin has also been recommended as the treatment of choice for mass casualty chemical disasters where cyanide poisoning is suspected.

Cyanide antidote kit

Administration of sodium nitrite followed by sodium thiosulphate is a long-accepted antidote for cyanide poisoning. The Cyanide Antidote kit was originally introduced in 1970 (under the pharmaceutical name *Eli Lilly Cyanide kit*) and contains:

- amyl nitrite perles*
- sodium nitrite 10 mL (30 mg/mL)
- sodium thiosulphate 50 mL (250 mg/mL).

The kit is based upon the premise that humans can tolerate up to 30% methaemoglobinaemia. Conversion of haemoglobin to methaemoglobin promotes the movement of cyanide out of the cytochrome system; 4 mg/kg of sodium nitrite takes 30 min to achieve 7–10.5% methaemoglobin. The

---

*Commercial kits such as *Nithiodote* are now available that omit amyl nitrite (*Nithiodote* [sodium nitrite injection and sodium thiosulphate injection] package insert. Scottsdale, AZ: Hope Pharmaceuticals; 2011).

formation of sodium thiocyanate allows for the reformation of Hb^{2+}, restoring the oxygen-carrying capacity of haemoglobin. Cellular respiration can continue as normal with cyanide removed from the respiratory chain. The observation that dramatic improvements in symptoms have occurred well before methaemoglobin levels have peaked has led many authors to suggest different mechanisms of action, such as vasodilatation and extracellular redistribution of cyanide. In smoke inhalation victims with suspected combined carbon monoxide and cyanide poisoning, the addition of 10% methaemoglobin may have clinically significant synergistic detrimental effects on the oxyhaemoglobin dissociation curve; in this setting, methaemoglobin inducers should be avoided.

Amyl nitrite alone in the management of per-hospital mass casualty cyanide poisoning has been reviewed recently. Evidence for its use is limited to animal studies and its role in the management of human case reports relative to the other treatments administered (e.g. life support, sodium nitrite and sodium thiosulphate) is unclear. Amyl nitrite has significant adverse effects (hypotension, syncope, excessive methaemoglobinaemia and haemolysis in glucose-6-phosphate dehydrogenase [G6PD] deficient patients). On balance, its use is not recommended in the pre-hospital or hospital setting.

Thiosulphate on its own can function as a slow sulphur donor, converting cyanide to thiocyanate. Thiosulphate is relatively non-toxic, although nausea and vomiting may occur following treatment. When hydroxocobalamin is not available, given its relatively favourable adverse-effect profile, it should be given to all patients with suspected cyanide toxicity, including those with smoke inhalation. It has been effective in the treatment of toxicity due to sodium nitroprusside therapy.

Dicobalt edetate (Kelocyanor)

This inorganic cobalt salt was introduced as a cyanide antidote in the late 1950s. It complexes with cyanide to form cobalt cyanide, thus removing cyanide from the circulation and reducing toxicity. However, unless cyanide is forced into the extracellular fluid, tissue levels are minimally affected.

Adverse effects are considerable and may be life threatening. Severe hypotension, cardiac arrhythmias, convulsions and gross oedema are reported. These effects are exacerbated when the drug is administered to an individual who is not cyanide poisoned. The treating physician therefore faces a significant dilemma when presented with a critically ill patient in whom the history of exposure is unclear. The use of this antidote is only for confirmed cyanide poisoning cases where the patient has lost consciousness and safer antidotes are not available.

The recommended initial dose of dicobaltedetate is 300 mg IV. Further doses may be required.

Other therapies

Hyperbaric oxygen (HBO) has been proposed as a treatment in cyanide poisoning but remains controversial with conflicting animal data. In most published human reports, HBO is offered after a combination of modalities and it is not possible to determine the treatment effect specific to each.

Experimental antidotes, such as nano alpha-ketoglutarate and trimethoprim derivatives, are currently being studied.

Recommended antidotal regimen

The regimen below is recommended if available:

- 5–15 g of hydroxocobalamin IV over 30 min (but may be given as IV push if needed). Repeat if needed.
- Plus (as an adjunct to the treatment of severe cyanide poisoning following failure to respond to hydroxycobalamin).
- 12.5 g sodium thiosulphate (or 0.5 g/kg IV for paediatric patients up to the adult dose) as a bolus injection or infused over 10–30 min. One half of the initial dose can be administered 2 h later if toxicity reappears.

Consultation with a toxicologist is recommended for all suspected cases of cyanide poisoning.

Controversies

- The effectiveness of any antidote to treat cyanide poisoning is based on case reports and animal data. Hydroxocobalamin is more commonly recommended as the choice of antidote in cyanide poisoning. Data on human exposure are limited. The current TGA approved product in Australia, dicobalt edetate, Kelocyanor, is not recommended because of its substantial risk profile. There is little indication for the use of methaemoglobin inducers (e.g. amyl nitrite) of the cyanide antidote kit in the pre-hospital or the hospital setting.
- Initiation of treatment for cyanide poisoning will be based upon clinical presentation and indirect laboratory results. There may be a greater importance of good resuscitation efforts without the use of antidotes in some cases.

Further reading

Baud FJ, Barriot P, Toffis V, et al. Elevated blood cyanide levels in victims of smoke inhalation. N Engl J Med 1991;325:1761–6.

Baud FJ, Borron SW, Bavoux E, et al. Relationship between plasma lactate and blood cyanide concentrations in acute poisoning. Br Med J 1996;312:26–7.

Carlsson CJ, Hansen HE, Hilsted L, Malm J. An evaluation of the interference of hydroxycobalamin with chemistry and co-oximetry tests on nine commonly used instruments. Scand J Clin Lab Invest 2011;71:378–86.

Eckstein M. Enhancing public health preparedness for a terrorist attack involving cyanide. J Emerg Med 2008;35:59–65.

Forsyth JC, Mueller PD, Becker CE, et al. Hydroxocobalamin as a cyanide antidote: safety, efficacy and pharamacokinetics in heavily smoking normal volunteers. J Toxicol Clin Toxicol 1993;31:277–94.

Hart GB, Strauss MB, Lennon PA, et al. Treatment of smoke inhalation by hyperbaric oxygen. J Emerg Med 1985;3:111.

Houeto P, Hoffman JR, Imbert M, et al. Relation of blood cyanide to plasma cyanocobalamin concentration after a fixed dose of hydroxocobalamin in cyanide poisoning. Lancet 1995;346:605–8.

Lavon O, Bentur Y. Does amyl nitrite have a role in the management of pre-hospital mass casualty cyanide poisoning? Clin Toxicol 2010;48:477–84.

Marraffa JM, Howland MA. Antidotes for toxicological emergencies: a practical review. Am J Hlth Syst Pharm 2012;89:199–212.

Reade MC, Davies SR, Morley PT, et al. Review article: management of cyanide poisoning. Emerg Med Australas 2012;24:225–38.

Singh P, Kaur M. CN-scavenger: a leap towards development of a CN-antidote. Chem Commun 2011;47:9122–4.

Yeoh MJ, Braitberg G. Carbon monoxide and cyanide poisoning in fire related deaths in Victoria, Australia. J Toxicol Clin Toxicol 2004;42:855–63.

29.16 Corrosive ingestion

Robert Dowsett

ESSENTIALS

1 Symptomatic patients may have burns to the airway or supraglottic tissues.

2 Decontamination has limited utility; care should be taken not to make patients vomit and no attempt should be made to neutralize corrosives.

3 Serious injuries to the oesophagus or stomach may occur in the absence of visible burns to the lips, mouth or throat.

4 Admit all symptomatic patients.

5 The major acute complications are perforation and necrosis.

6 The major long-term complication is oesophageal stricture.

Table 29.16.1   Approximate pH of some common solutions

Solution	pH
Battery acid (1% solution)	1.4
Domestic toilet cleaner (1%)	2.0
Bleach (1% solution)	9.5–10.2
Automatic dishwasher detergents	10.4–13
Laundry detergents	11.6–12.6
Domestic ammonium cleaners	11.9–12.4
Drain cleaner (containing NaOH, KOH)	13.3–14

Table 29.16.2   pKa of some common corrosives

Chemical	pKa	Highly corrosive?
Hydrochloric acid	–3	Yes
Bromic acid	<1	Yes
Nitric acid	<1	Yes
Sulphuric acid	1.9	
Arsenic acid	2.3	
Nitrous acid	3.3	
Hydrofluoric acid	3.4	
Ammonia	9.3	
Ammonium hydroxide	9.3	
Magnesium hydroxide	10	
Zinc hydroxide	11	
Calcium hydroxide	11.6	
Lithium hydroxide	>14	Yes
Potassium hydroxide	>14	Yes
Sodium hydroxide	>14	Yes
Calcium oxide	>14	Yes
Sodium carbonate	>14	Yes
Potassium carbonate	>14	Yes
Sodium hypochlorite	>14	Yes

Introduction

Strong corrosives capable of causing significant injury are those with a pH in solution of less than 2 or greater than 12 (Table 29.16.1). The pH of a solution is dependent on the concentration and dissociation constant (pK_a) of the chemical. Strong acids have a pK_a <0 and strong alkalis have a pK_a >14 (Table 29.16.2). The extent of injury also depends on the volume ingested, contact time and viscosity.

Domestic bleaches, automatic dishwasher detergents, toilet bowel cleaners and drain cleaners are the commonest substances ingested, but severe injury generally does not occur unless large amounts are swallowed [1]. Deaths result mainly from the ingestion of acid-containing drain or toilet cleaners continuing a trend over the last 20 years with a decline in fatalities from alkali drain cleaners [2].

Pathophysiology

Acid–base reactions cause injury by disrupting organic macromolecules. Heat generation may cause thermal burns. Chemical reactions may also result in the production of other compounds that can cause additional injury to the gastrointestinal (GI) tract and lungs (Table 29.16.3).

Alkalis cause 'liquefactive' necrosis, a process that involves saponification of fats, dissolution of proteins and emulsification of lipid membranes. Acids cause 'coagulative' necrosis, a process that involves denaturation of protein.

In both settings, tissue injury can continue for several hours. Granulation tissue develops after 3–4 days, but collagen deposition may not begin until the second week, making the tissue extremely fragile during this period. Complete repair of the epithelium may take weeks. From the third week, newly deposited collagen begins to contract and may produce strictures of the oesophagus, stomach and affected bowel.

Hydrocarbon compounds can produce injury by dissolving lipids and coagulating proteins. Other chemicals can injure tissues by redox reactions and alkylation.

Narrowings in the GI tract are most at risk from corrosive ingestion: the cricopharyngeal area, the diaphragmatic oesophagus, antrum and pylorus [2]. Alkalis are more likely to produce oesophageal injury than are acids, which typically injure the stomach [2–4]. Solid corrosives are more likely to affect the mouth, pharynx and upper oesophagus and to cause deeper burns.

The main acute complications of corrosive ingestion are haemorrhage, perforation and fistula formation. These result from severe burns causing full-thickness necrosis. Tissue inflammation, necrosis and infection can result in hypovolaemia, acidosis and organ failure.

Full-thickness necrosis of the stomach may be associated with injury to the transverse colon, pancreas, spleen, small bowel, liver

Table 29.16.3 Chemical reactions resulting in the production of further toxic chemicals

Chemical	Plus	Produces
Chlorine	Water	Hydrochloric acid Hypochlorous acid Oxygen radicals Heat
Ammonia	Water	Ammonium hydroxide Heat
Nitrogen dioxide	Water	Nitric acid Nitrous acid
Ammonia	Hypochlorite	Chloramine gas (NH_2Cl and $NHCl_2$)
Hypochlorite	Acid	Chlorine gas Hydrogen Sulphide
Sulphur compounds (e.g. plaster casts)	Acid	Sulphur oxide

and kidneys. Perforation of the upper anterior oesophagus may lead to the formation of a tracheo-oesophageal fistula. Formation of a tracheo-oesophago-aortic fistula is a rapidly lethal complication.

Clinical features

Symptoms and signs associated with significant alkali ingestion include oropharyngeal pain, drooling, pain on swallowing, vomiting, abdominal pain and haematemesis [4]. If the larynx is involved, local oedema may produce respiratory distress, stridor and a hoarse voice [5].

Extensive tissue injury may be associated with fever, tachycardia, hypotension and tachypnoea.

Inspection of the oropharynx may reveal areas of mucosal burn. The absence of visible burns does not imply an absence of significant burns to the oesophagus [3,4,6].

Symptoms and signs associated with the life-threatening complications of oesophageal perforation and mediastinitis include chest pain, dyspnoea, fever, subcutaneous emphysema of the chest or neck and a pleural rub. Perforation of the abdominal oesophagus or stomach is associated with the clinical features of chemical peritonitis, including abdominal pain, fever and ileus [3].

The systemic effects of large acid ingestion include hypotension, metabolic acidosis, haemolysis, haemoglobinuria, nephrotoxicity, pulmonary oedema and hypotension. Systemic toxicity can result from the ingestion of arsenic, cyanide and other heavy metal salts, fluoride, ammonia, hydrazine, hydrochloric acid, nitrates,

sulphuric acid and phosphoric acid. Ingestion of ammonia can cause coma, hypotension, acidosis, pulmonary oedema, liver dysfunction and coagulopathy. Systemic effects of phenol and related compounds include haemolysis and renal failure.

Long-term complications

The major late complication of corrosive ingestion is the development of an oesophageal stricture. All patients with full-thickness necrosis of the oesophageal wall develop strictures, as do 70% of those with deep ulceration [3]. Symptoms of oesophageal narrowing (principally dysphagia) may develop within 2 weeks; 80% occur within the first 2 months. Early onset of symptoms is associated with a more rapidly progressive and severe obstruction. Strictures do not develop in areas of superficial mucosal ulceration [7–9]. Strictures can also affect the mouth, pharynx and stomach. Only 40% of gastric outlet strictures become symptomatic [3]. A very late complication of alkali ingestion is the development of oesophageal carcinoma, reported to develop 22–81 years after exposure.

Clinical investigations

Initial investigations in symptomatic patients should include an ECG, arterial blood gas, blood count, type and cross-match, coagulation profile, serum electrolytes, blood glucose and liver and renal function.

Chest and upright abdominal X-rays should be assessed for evidence of mediastinal widening, pleural effusions and free air.

All patients who are symptomatic or have visible oropharyngeal burns should be considered for upper GI endoscopy within 24 hours. The entire upper GI tract may be safely examined with a small-diameter flexible endoscope, provided it is not retroflexed or forced through areas of narrowing [2,3]. It is not necessary to terminate the examination at the first circumferential or full-thickness lesion. The cricopharynx should be assessed initially to identify any laryngeal burns. If laryngeal oedema or ulceration is encountered, endotracheal intubation may be necessary before continuing with endoscopy.

A retrospective case series of 49 patients with caustic ingestion underwent computed tomography (CT) scanning and upper GI endoscopy to assess the degree of damage to the oesophagus and adjacent tissues [10]. In this small study, CT scanning was shown to be more sensitive and specific than endoscopy, although this was not statistically significant. Contrast oesophagography with a water-soluble contrast agent is useful for the detection of perforation, but is less sensitive than endoscopy in evaluating ulceration.

Oesophageal burns can be graded according to the depth of ulceration and the presence of necrosis (Table 29.16.4). Injuries can be divided into three main groups:

- Mucosal inflammation or superficial ulceration only. These injuries will heal completely and are not at risk of stricture formation.
- Areas of deep ulceration or discrete areas of necrosis or circumferential ulceration of any depth. Stricture formation may occur.
- Deep circumferential burns or extensive areas of necrosis. These patients are at high risk of perforation and stricture formation.

Treatment

Patients should initially be assessed for the presence of any symptomatic airway burns or respiratory distress. The need for urgent intubation should be considered in any patient with stridor or hypoxia.

Efforts at decontamination must not induce vomiting, as this may exacerbate the oesophageal injury. The mouth should be rinsed thoroughly with water. Dilution of an ingested solid chemical by drinking 250 mL of water or milk is recommended. Patients should otherwise be given nothing by mouth. Neutralization,

Table 29.16.4   Classification of gastrointestinal corrosive burns

Grade I	First-degree
Mucosal inflammation	Mucosal inflammation, oedema or superficial sloughing
Grade IIA	**Second-degree**
Haemorrhages, erosions and superficial ulceration	Damage extends to all layers of, but not through, the oesophagus
Grade IIB	
Isolated discrete or circumferential superficial ulceration	
Grade IIIA	**Third-degree**
Small scattered areas of necrosis	Ulceration through to perioesophageal tissues
Grade IIIB	
Extensive necrosis involving the whole oesophagus	

aspiration and administration of activated charcoal are all contraindicated.

Patients with persistent symptoms should be admitted for observation and undergo endoscopy 12–24 hours later. Further management is dictated by the findings at endoscopy.

Patients with endoscopic evidence of superficial injury can be managed on a general medical ward with supportive care only. Patients with deep discrete ulceration, circumferential ulceration or isolated areas of necrosis should be admitted to high-dependency or the intensive care unit and kept nil by mouth. Intravenous fluid replacement, accurate fluid and electrolyte balance and symptom control are the mainstays of therapy. These patients may require prolonged IV access and parenteral feeding and central venous access should be considered.

If perforation or penetration is suspected clinically or documented by endoscopy or contrast radiography, urgent laparotomy with or without thoracotomy must be considered. Early excision of areas with extensive full-thickness necrosis has been proposed, but this needs to be weighed against mortality rates of 40–50% for patients undergoing such emergency surgery.

Prophylactic broad-spectrum antibiotics are only indicated where there is evidence of GI tract perforation.

Strictures are dilated by endoscopy 3–4 weeks after ingestion. Reconstructive surgery may be required if the oesophageal lumen becomes completely obstructed or if perforation occurs.

Disposition

Asymptomatic patients can be discharged after observation and do not require investigation. They should be instructed to return if they develop pain, respiratory symptoms or difficulty swallowing. Symptomatic patients should be admitted for endoscopy with subsequent disposition dependent on the findings, as detailed above.

Controversies

- The value of administering oral fluids following ingestion of a liquid corrosive is controversial but probably of little value.
- The use of corticosteroids to prevent oesophageal strictures following corrosive ingestion is controversial.

Clinical trials show contradictory results but the balance of available evidence and current opinion would suggest a lack of efficacy [7,11,12]. However, in all studies steroids were commenced after endoscopy. If they are to be effective steroids should be commenced on presentation. There is no role for continuing steroids in patients with Grade III injuries as they may increase the risk of perforation.

- CT scanning may be a less invasive approach to the assessment of corrosive ingestions but further studies are needed before it can be recommended.

References

[1] Bronstein AC, Spyker DA, Cantilena LR, et al. 2011 Annual Report of the American Association of Poison Control Centers' National Poison Data System (NPDS): 29th Annual Report. Clin Toxicol 2012;50:911–1164.

[2] Sugawa C, Lucas CE. Caustic injury of the upper gastrointestinal tract in adults: a clinical and endoscopic study. Surgery 1989;106:802–6.

[3] Zargar SA, Kochhar R, Mehta S, et al. The role of fiberoptic endoscopy in the management of corrosive ingestion and modified endoscopic classification of burns. Gastrointest Endosc 1991;37:165–9.

[4] Gorman RL, Khin-Maung-Gyi MT, Klein-Schwartz W, et al. Initial symptoms as predictors of esophageal injury in alkaline corrosive ingestions. Am J Emerg Med 1992;10:189–94.

[5] Moulin D, Bertrand JM, Buts JP, et al. Upper airway lesions in children after accidental ingestion of caustic substances. J Pediatr 1985;106:408–10.

[6] Crain EF, Gershel JC, Mezey AP. Caustic ingestions: symptoms as predictors of esophageal injury. Am J Dis Child 1984;138:863–5.

[7] Anderson KD, Rouse TM, Randolph JG. A controlled trial of corticosteroids in children with corrosive injury of the esophagus. N Engl J Med 1990;323:637–40.

[8] Webb WR, Koutras P, Eckker RR, et al. An evaluation of steroids and antibiotics in caustic burns of the esophagus. Ann Thorac Surg 1970;9:95–102.

[9] Cannon S, Chandler JR. Corrosive burns of the esophagus: analysis of 100 patients. Eye Ear Nose Throat Month 1963;42:35–44.

[10] Ryu HH, Jeung KW, Lee BK, et al. Caustic injury: can CT grading system enable prediction of esophageal stricture? Clin Toxicol 2010;48:137–42.

[11] Howell JM, Dalsey WC, Hartsell FW, et al. Steroids for the treatment of corrosive esophageal injury: a statistical analysis of past studies. Am J Emerg Med 1992;10:421–5.

[12] Fulton JA, Hoffman RS. Steroids in second degree caustic burns of the esophagus: a systematic pooled analysis of fifty years of human data: 1956–2006. Clin Toxicol 2007;45:402–8.

TOXICOLOGY EMERGENCIES

29.17 Hydrofluoric acid

Sam Alfred • Andis Graudins

ESSENTIALS

1 Patients and medical staff are often unaware of the presence of hydrofluoric acid (HF) in household cleaning products.

2 Topical HF exposures may result in the gradual onset of severe local pain out of proportion to any clinical signs evident on presentation.

3 Patients may not relate their dermal symptoms to HF exposure due to the delay in onset of pain that occurs with domestic low concentration preparations.

4 Systemic toxicity may be life threatening and is expected following dermal burns caused by high concentration solutions or involving body surface areas of greater than 5% and following significant inhalations or ingestions.

5 Systemic toxicity is typically manifest as severe hypocalcaemia, hypomagnesaemia, hyperkalaemia and ventricular arrhythmias.

6 Ingestion and inhalation of HF may also result in significant gastrointestinal or respiratory injury.

Introduction

The inorganic acid of fluoride, hydrofluoric acid (HF), is a moderately corrosive chemical widely used in industry for the etching of glass, metal and stone and in the preparation of silicon computer chips. HF is also a common constituent of rust and scale removers, car wheel cleaners, brick cleaners and solder flux mixtures. These products may be for either commercial or home use and are often found in containers with inadequate labelling in regard to the potential toxicity. Concentrations of commercially available HF may vary from 50 to 100%. Products containing HF for domestic use generally have a concentration of less than 10%, but higher concentration products may be obtained illicitly for home use.

The most common route of accidental exposure to HF is topical [1–3]. This may occur when high-concentration HF leaks through damaged gloves in the industrial setting or when HF products are used in the home without gloves. Massive topical HF exposure and inhalational exposure to HF may also occur in the industrial setting. Finally, ingestion of HF products may occur accidentally in the home in the paediatric age group or as a result of deliberate self-harm in adults.

Pathophysiology

HF is a relatively weak acid with less corrosive effects than other stronger acids, such as hydrochloric or sulphuric. In particular, low concentrations of HF (<20%) may result in little or no perceptible corrosive injury to the skin immediately following exposure. This is due to the relatively low dissociation constant ($pK_a = 3.8$), which limits the concentration of free hydrogen ions on the skin surface [2–4]. As HF tends to remain in an undissociated neutral state, its ability to penetrate through the skin into deeper tissues is enhanced. Gradual dissociation of HF producing free fluoride ions in the tissues leads to local tissue injury characterized by liquefactive necrosis rather than the coagulative necrosis more commonly associated with acid burns [2,3]. As the concentration of HF increases so does the potential for corrosive injury [3,5]. Nevertheless, chemical burns may result from exposures to dilute (<5%) solutions of HF and fatal systemic poisoning has resulted from relatively small (<5% total body surface area [BSA]) burns caused by more concentrated solutions [6].

The primary mechanism of tissue damage resulting from exposure to HF is related to fluoride toxicity following on from dissociation of the acid in exposed tissues [2,3]. A number of pathological mechanisms may be involved in both local and systemic fluoride poisoning. Fluoride binds divalent cations, especially calcium and magnesium, to form insoluble fluoride salts. The resulting hypocalcaemia and hypomagnesaemia may have profound local and systemic effects on cellular and organ functions. Fluoride is a cellular poison. It inhibits both aerobic and anaerobic metabolic enzyme systems and interferes with cellular respiration [6]. Fluoride also interferes with Na^+/K^+ ATPase activity and opens calcium-dependent potassium channels in cell membranes, resulting in the leak of potassium into the extracellular space with the potential for systemic hyperkalaemia [1,7]. Precipitation of calcium may also interfere with calcium-dependent clotting factors, resulting in coagulopathy. Finally, exposure to HF may produce direct corrosive injury.

Fatal systemic fluoride poisonings have also been reported following inhalational and gastrointestinal (GI) exposures [6]. Once absorbed, fluoride ions are distributed to virtually every tissue and organ resulting in widespread disruption of organ function. Fluoride is slowly eliminated in the urine and elevations of urinary fluoride excretion can be detected following exposure to HF, although these do not correlate with clinical toxicity [3].

Clinical features

Exposure to HF in the industrial setting is usually recognized as such and patients will often have been decontaminated and had topical therapy applied prior to arrival at hospital. They are also likely to be in possession of appropriate information in the form of material safety data sheets. Acute dermal exposures in the domestic setting may present a more difficult diagnostic dilemma. Domestic product labels may be incomplete and offer no advice regarding the use of protective apparel such as gloves. Additionally, the onset of the signs and symptoms of HF injury may be delayed after exposure to low concentration domestic products and the patient may not recognize that the symptoms are related to chemical exposure [3].

Highly concentrated (>70%) HF contains enough free hydrogen ions to produce a burning sensation on the skin providing some degree of warning of an acute exposure with symptom onset within 1–2 h [1,5]. However, low concentrations of HF (<10%), found in products, such as over-the-counter rust removers, often produce no symptoms at the time of contact and patients can present with gradually increasing pain from 6 to 12 h following exposure [1].

The primary presenting complaint of acute topical HF injury is pain out of all proportion to any physical signs. HF exposure should always be considered in this situation. The pain is usually described as a tingling sensation that progresses to a burning pain and then to a typical deep, throbbing and severe pain [1,5,8]. This means there is often a delay of some hours to onset of significant symptoms and presentation.

Visible evidence of HF burns also follows a fairly common pattern. Initially, the burn site is erythematous and may be oedematous. As tissue injury progresses, the site becomes pale and blanched, progressing to a classical silvery grey appearance [2]. Local vesiculation and frank tissue necrosis may ensue. This process can progress over several days in untreated patients, resulting in the development of deep ulceration and extensive tissue loss.

Dermal exposure to HF commonly occurs on the hands or feet with relatively small areas of the skin being exposed. Systemic fluoride poisoning is rarely a problem under these circumstances. The risk of systemic toxicity increases with the percentage of BSA exposed to HF and the concentration of HF [3]. In general, if more than 3–5% BSA has been exposed to HF, there is a risk of hypocalcaemia [3]. Systemic fluoride toxicity is more likely following large dermal exposures, ingestion or inhalation of HF [3].

Systemic fluoride toxicity is manifest by various effects, the most lethal of which are the severe electrolyte abnormalities produced by direct interaction with fluoride or effects on cell membranes and cellular enzyme systems [3,6,7]. Hypocalcaemia is due to the complexing of calcium by fluoride ions. Hypomagnesaemia may also occur. However, the primary cause of the lethal arrhythmias (refractory ventricular tachycardia, ventricular fibrillation and pulseless idioventricular rhythm) is the development of hyperkalaemia [4,7]. Patients with systemic fluoride poisoning

also develop a significant metabolic acidosis [3,4]. This is the result of fluoride interference with intracellular metabolism. The systemic manifestations of significant hypocalcaemia include carpopedal spasm, hyperreflexia, tetany and coagulopathy. Headache, paraesthesiae and visual complaints may be noted. In severe cases, coma, seizures, shock and dysrhythmias often precede death.

Fluoride inhalation is associated with pulmonary injury, including the development of non-cardiogenic pulmonary oedema, adult respiratory distress syndrome (ARDS) and the potential for systemic fluoride toxicity [3].

Clinical investigations

No investigations are necessary following dermal exposures to dilute domestic preparations involving less than 5% of BSA. Following significant dermal exposures to HF or any ingestion or inhalational exposure, serum electrolytes including magnesium and calcium, baseline coagulation studies and a 12-lead ECG (looking for evidence of hypocalcaemia or hyperkalaemia) are indicated. A chest radiograph should be performed in any patient with respiratory symptoms or severe systemic toxicity.

Treatment

All patients with significant dermal HF exposures (>5% BSA, exposure to concentrated industrial preparations) or any ingestion or inhalation exposures should have continuous cardiac monitoring and intravenous access established on arrival.

The initial management of an acute topical HF exposure is thorough skin decontamination with generous water irrigation. This ideally should be performed as a first-aid measure as soon as possible following the exposure as the delayed presentation of most patients makes it unlikely that significant amounts of HF still remain on the surface of the skin. Despite experimental evidence of enhanced decontamination with hexafluorine preparations, clinical experience suggests hexafluorine preparations offer no benefit in terms of local burn minimization or prevention of systemic toxicity when compared to water irrigation of exposed surfaces [9,10]. Other first-aid measures in the work place for known or suspected HF burns include topical treatments, such as

calcium gluconate gel (2.5–10%) or soaks with quaternary ammonium salts, such as benzalkonium or benzethonium chloride. Topical therapies are intended to form insoluble complexes with any surface fluoride ion thus preventing tissue penetration and minimizing deeper injury. Topical therapy is probably of little value once fluoride ions penetrate to deeper tissues but should be initiated on presentation to the emergency department (ED). Calcium gluconate gel can be applied to the hand in a rubber glove. It may provide relief to some patients with low concentration HF exposures to the digits. In most cases, topical therapy is a temporizing measure until more invasive methods of calcium administration can be employed. If calcium gluconate gel is not readily available, a 4.8% preparation can be rapidly prepared by mixing one ampoule of calcium gluconate in 10 g of KY jelly.

The definitive treatment of dermal HF burns involves the administration of calcium gluconate into the tissues affected by the exposure [1–3,5,8]. This may be achieved by a number of methods: direct tissue infiltration, regional intravenous infusion using a Bier's block technique and intra-arterial infusion [1–3,5,8]. The choice of method depends upon the site and concentration of HF involved.

Direct injection of approximately 0.5 mL/cm^2 of 10% calcium gluconate solution at the burn site can be considered in areas with little skin tension, such as the trunk, forearms and legs. A small needle (25 gauge) should be used to minimize discomfort and care should be taken to infiltrate into, around and beneath the burn area as completely as possible. Only calcium gluconate should be used for local infiltration as calcium chloride produces direct injury when injected into tissues [3].

HF burns to the hands are relatively common. In view of the lack of loose tissues in the digits, direct dermal injection may be extremely painful and only small amounts of calcium gluconate may be injected. Additionally, the introduction of hyperosmolar calcium solutions to these limited tissue spaces may exacerbate oedema and result in vascular compromise [1,2]. HF may also penetrate beneath the fingernails. In the past, removal of fingernails was advocated to allow for injection of calcium gluconate into the nail bed. Fortunately the advent of focused, parenteral calcium administration techniques to the affected limb have meant that nail removal is less frequently required.

Two techniques are available for direct injection of calcium gluconate into digital HF burns. The first is intra-arterial infusion of calcium gluconate. This technique involves inserting an arterial cannula into the radial (for burns of the thumb, index and middle fingers) or brachial artery (for more extensive hand involvement) and slowly infusing a dilute solution of calcium gluconate utilizing an infusion pump. This allows the calcium to be delivered to the affected tissues through the vascular supply and avoids the pain and tissue distension associated with direct injection [8]. A typical dose is 10–20 mL of 10% calcium gluconate in 50–100 mL of 5% dextrose infused over 4 h and repeated as necessary. The endpoint for therapy is the absence of pain. The number of intra-arterial infusions required for pain relief may vary from one to four or five and depends on the concentration of HF to which exposure occurred. There is case report level evidence for the use of continuous infusions [11].

Regional intravenous calcium gluconate infusion using a Bier's block technique has also been employed in the treatment of HF burns to the limbs [5]. Success has been observed for digital, hand and forearm exposures as well as for exposures to the leg [5]. The technique is similar to that described by Bier for regional limb anaesthesia and has the advantages of relative simplicity and of not requiring arterial cannulation. An intravenous cannula is inserted in the dorsum of the hand of the affected limb and the arm is raised to exsanguinate the superficial venous system. A pneumatic tourniquet is applied to the upper arm and inflated to a pressure 100 mmHg above systolic blood pressure. Ten to 15 mL of 10% calcium gluconate is diluted to a total volume of 50 mL with normal saline and injected via the cannula into the ischaemic arm. The tourniquet is sequentially released after 20 to 25 min [5]. Pain relief is usually apparent within 30 min of tourniquet release.

There have been no controlled studies comparing any of these techniques in the treatment of HF burns. However, intra-arterial calcium infusion appears to be a better technique for distal digital exposures, particularly in cases where exposure has been to high concentrations (>20%) or where multiple digits are involved [5]. Intra-arterial infusion of calcium has the advantages of more focal provision of calcium to the site of digital exposures and the potential for multiple infusions

in patients with ongoing pain. If the intravenous route is selected as the primary therapy and is unsuccessful following one treatment, intra-arterial calcium infusion should then be used. The use of intra-arterial magnesium sulphate in place of calcium gluconate has resulted in tissue necrosis requiring surgical debridement in a small case series and cannot be recommended.

It is sometimes difficult to determine whether ongoing pain at the exposure site is due to continued tissue destruction from fluoride still present in the tissues or established tissue damage. This is particularly the case with patients who have had digital exposures to high concentrations of HF and received multiple infusions of intra-arterial calcium which do not seem to produce further pain relief. It also applies to patients who present more than 24 h post-exposure with ongoing pain despite calcium therapy. In both instances, failure to achieve pain relief with repeated infusions of calcium gluconate suggests that pain may be related to established tissue damage rather than ongoing tissue destruction.

Ocular HF exposures can result in serious consequences if left untreated. Patients should be treated as for other chemical exposures to the eye with copious saline irrigation and local anaesthetic drops for pain relief. Calcium gluconate (10–20 mL/L) may be added to saline irrigation fluid, although animal studies suggest that calcium gluconate eye drops are no better than copious irrigation with normal saline and may, in fact, result in delayed corneal healing [12]. In contrast, clinical case reports of calcium gluconate eye drop use suggest that this treatment is not harmful, but controlled studies are lacking.

Systemic fluoride poisoning resulting from HF ingestion, inhalation or significant dermal exposures is potentially life threatening. Patients with HF ingestion should receive rapid GI decontamination. Aspiration of HF through a small bore nasogastric tube may limit absorption if the patient presents within an hour of ingestion. Calcium or magnesium-containing antacids can complex intragastric HF and prevent some systemic absorption of fluoride ions, although any benefit is likely to be marginal at best. Endoscopy should be performed following HF ingestion as soon as the patient is clinically stable to assess the extent of any upper GI corrosive injury [1]. Nebulized calcium gluconate has been administered acutely

to patients following HF inhalation. Serum calcium, magnesium and potassium levels should be closely monitored. Intravenous calcium and magnesium replacement should be commenced prior to any fall in serum Ca^{2+} or Mg^{2+} concentrations and replacement doses may be guided by the calculated dose of fluoride ingested. Large amounts of calcium (200–300 mmol) have been used in severe cases of systemic HF poisoning with hypocalcaemia [3,4]. Hyperkalaemia may be recognized on the 12-lead ECG, but close monitoring of serum potassium levels is warranted. Hyperkalaemia in systemic fluoride poisoning may be resistant to standard measures of potassium reduction, such as insulin, glucose and bicarbonate infusions. Ventricular arrhythmias associated with systemic fluoride poisoning may be refractory to cardioversion and defibrillation and may not respond to antiarrhythmic agents [7]. Haemodialysis is indicated for severe or refractory hypocalcaemia, hyperkalaemia or clinical toxicity (e.g. arrhythmias) and may be useful for the removal of fluoride ions [3]. Calcium and magnesium monitoring and replacement should continue during this procedure.

Disposition

Patients with minor dermal exposures in whom ED treatment produces complete resolution of symptoms may be discharged home with follow up arranged within 24 h or should pain return. Those patients in whom tissue damage is evident require referral to a plastic or hand surgeon.

Patients at risk of systemic fluoride poisoning (exposure to high concentration solutions, greater than 5% BSA burns, inhalations and ingestions) require admission to an intensive care unit for ongoing monitoring and management of the electrolyte disturbances and other complications of systemic toxicity.

All patients with eye exposures require early ophthalmological referral.

Controversies

- Relative value of intra-arterial versus regional intravenous calcium gluconate administration.
- Role of hexafluorine preparations in decontamination.

References

[1] Salzman M, O'Malley RN. Updates on the evaluation and management of caustic exposures. Emerg Med Clin N Am 2007;25:459–76.

[2] Burd A. Hydrofluoric acid-revisited. Burns 2004;30:720–2.

[3] Dunser MW, Ohlbauer M, Rieder J, et al. Critical care management of major hydrofluoric acid burns: a case report, review of the literature, and recommendations for therapy. Burns 2004;30:391–8.

[4] Chan BS, Duggin GG. Survival after a massive hydrofluoric acid ingestion. J Toxicol Clin Toxicol 1997;35:307–9.

[5] Graudins A, Burns MJ, Aaron CK. Regional intravenous infusion of calcium gluconate for hydrofluoric acid burns of the upper extremity. Ann Emerg Med 1997;30:604–7.

[6] Caravati EM. Acute hydrofluoric acid exposure. Am J Emerg Med 1988;6:143–50.

[7] Cummings CC, McIvor ME. Fluoride-induced hyperkalemia: the role of Ca++ dependent K+ channels. Am J Emerg Med 1988;6:1.

[8] Vance MV, Curry SC, Kunkel DB, et al. Digital hydrofluoric acid burns: treatment with intra arterial calcium infusion. Ann Emerg Med 1986;15:890–6.

[9] Hojer J, Personne M, Hulten P, Ludwigs U. Topical treatments for hydrofluoric acid burns: a blind controlled experimental study. J Toxicol Clini Toxicol 2002;40:861–6.

[10] Hulten P, Hojer J, Ludwigs U, Janson A. Hexafluorine vs standard decontamination to reduce systemic toxicity after dermal exposure to hydrofluoric acid. J Toxicol Clin Toxicol 2004;42:355–61.

[11] Lin TM, Tsai CC, Lin SD, Lai CS. Continuous intra-arterial infusion therapy in hydrofluoric acid burns. J Occupat Environ Med 2000;42:892–7.

[12] Beiran I, Miller B, Bentur Y. The efficacy of calcium gluconate in ocular hydrofluoric acid burns. Hum Exp Toxicol 1997;16:223–8.

29.18 Pesticides

Darren M Roberts

ESSENTIALS

1 Acute pesticide poisoning is an important cause of morbidity and mortality worldwide.

2 Existing systems for classifying the toxicity of pesticides are imperfect. The toxicity of even 'slightly hazardous' pesticides is sometimes significant. Moderate-to-highly toxic pesticides may have a case-fatality rate of between 5 and 70% in patients with self-poisoning.

3 In addition to the pesticide constituent, other components of the formulation can also contribute to its toxicity. For example, concentrated formulations, inclusion of certain salts, solvents or surfactants can lead to worse outcomes.

4 Many pesticides have a delayed onset of poisoning. All patients with oral exposure should be monitored for a minimum of 6–12 h post-ingestion.

5 Resuscitation and supportive care are priorities in management of acute pesticide poisoning. Patients manifesting significant poisoning require prolonged admission, preferably in an intensive care unit.

6 The specific antidotes for anticholinesterase pesticide poisoning are atropine and, possibly, pralidoxime. These should be administered as soon as possible and titrated to effect.

7 The mortality from acute paraquat poisoning is high and due to multiorgan failure or progressive pulmonary fibrosis. Ingestion of as little as 20 mL of 20% w/v solution is sufficient to cause death. No satisfactory treatments have been confirmed to date.

8 The toxic component of glyphosate-containing herbicides appears to be the surfactant and potentially the isopropylamine salt. The mechanism of toxicity is not confirmed, but severe poisoning is associated with multiorgan toxicity and metabolic acidosis. Treatment is supportive.

Introduction

Pesticide poisoning occurs worldwide. Poisoning may occur due to either acute (intentional self-poisoning) or chronic (such as occupational) exposures. Acute poisoning is of more importance to the emergency physician and is the focus of this chapter.

A pesticide is any chemical used for the control of a plant or animal, which encompasses hundreds of chemicals. They can be subclassified in terms of their intended target, the most common being insecticides, herbicides (selective or non-selective), fungicides, rodenticides and nematocides. Other methods for classification that have been used include toxicity to animal species (LD$_{50}$; dose that kills 50% of animal subjects), mechanism of action and chemical structure.

Worldwide, pesticides are the most common cause of death from acute self-poisoning. As with pharmaceutical poisoning, the toxicity of pesticides varies between individual compounds but, in general, pesticides are intrinsically more toxic than pharmaceuticals. However, not all pesticide exposures lead to clinically significant poisoning. In Australasia, most acute pesticide exposures are accidental and the majority of patients do not require admission to hospital.

An accurate risk assessment is necessary in each patient with acute pesticide poisoning. This considers the dose ingested, time since ingestion, clinical features, patient factors and available medical facilities. An understanding of the clinical toxicology of a pesticide in the context of the exposure allows for the likely complications to be anticipated and, with appropriate treatment, these may be prevented. If a patient presents to a facility that is unable to provide sufficient medical and nursing care or does not have ready access to necessary antidotes, then arrangements should be made to transport the patient rapidly and safely to a healthcare facility where this is available.

Due to the low incidence, pesticide poisoning is not always considered in the differential diagnosis. A number of case reports from Australia have described a delay in the diagnosis of significant pesticide poisoning because it was not considered initially. These delays did not appear to affect adversely patient outcomes, but they highlight the importance for clinicians to be familiar with the clinical features of pesticide poisoning.

This chapter primarily focuses on agrochemicals used in Australasia, in particular insecticides (organophosphorus pesticides [OPs] and carbamates) and herbicides (glyphosate and paraquat).

Aetiology, pathogenesis and pathology

Acute intentional self-poisoning with pesticides commonly requires admission to hospital and ongoing care. However, significant poisoning may also occur with accidental (e.g. storage of a pesticide in a milk carton) or criminal exposures.

The pathophysiology of acute pesticide poisoning and, therefore, the clinical manifestations vary widely between individual compounds. Many pesticides induce multisystem toxicity due to interactions with a number of physiological systems. Where known, the mechanism of toxicity in humans is discussed for each pesticide; often this bears little relation to the mechanism of action in the target pest. For many pesticides, the mechanism of toxicity is poorly described so less information is available to guide management of these exposures.

It should be noted that proprietary pesticide products contain co-formulants, in particular hydrocarbon-based solvents. Herbicide products also contain surfactants to enhance herbicide penetration into the plant. These co-formulants can contribute to the toxicity of a pesticide product and, in some cases, are more toxic than the active pesiticide constituent.

Epidemiology

Acute pesticide poisoning is a major issue in developing countries of the Asia-Pacific region and OPs are considered the most important cause of death from acute poisoning worldwide. In developed countries, however, the incidence of severe pesticide poisoning is relatively low. In rural areas, the incidence of severe pesticide poisoning may be higher compared to urban regions due to ready access, including concentrated formulations.

Prevention

Primary exposures

Regulatory restrictions to the availability of the more toxic pesticides may contribute to a decrease in mortality from pesticide self-poisoning. In Australia, for example, pesticides with a high case fatality, such as paraquat, organochlorines and parathion, are heavily regulated so poison exposures are increasingly rare. Proper storage, handling and use of pesticides can prevent accidental exposures and associated health consequences.

Secondary exposures or nosocomial poisoning

Secondary exposure refers to staff and family members being exposed to patients with acute pesticide poisoning, predisposing them to nosocomial poisoning. Few cases of nosocomial poisoning, if any, have been confirmed by abnormal cholinesterase activities. While mild symptoms, such as nausea, dizziness, weakness and headache, have been reported, these resolved after exposure to fresh air and were probably due to inhalation of the hydrocarbon solvent. Universal precautions including nitrile gloves are most likely to provide sufficient protection for staff members. Dermal decontamination is performed by washing spilt pesticide off the patient with soap and water and removing and discarding contaminated clothes.

ANTICHOLINESTERASE PESTICIDES

Anticholinesterase pesticides are among the most widely used pesticides and include organophosphorus (organophosphate, OP, OGP) and carbamate compounds. In Australasia, the most commonly encountered anticholinesterase compounds are chlorpyrifos, dimethoate, fenthion, malathion (maldison), diazinon and propoxur (carbamate).

The relationship between exposure and clinical toxicity is poorly defined and therefore all exposures should be treated as significant. Deliberate self-poisoning by ingestion is the scenario most likely to result in severe toxicity, reflecting the larger exposure. Carbamates appear to be less toxic and induce poisoning of a shorter duration than OPs, although notable exceptions include carbofuran and carbosulfan which are associated with severe toxicity and death.

Mechanism of toxicity

The effects of anticholinesterase compounds on human physiology are multiple, complex and incompletely described. Inhibition of acetylcholinesterase (AChE), thus preventing the hydrolysis of acetylcholine, is considered the most important mechanism. Accumulation of acetylcholine at cholinergic synapses causes excessive stimulation of postsynaptic receptors. This interferes with systemic nervous function, producing a range of clinical manifestations which are known as the acute cholinergic crisis (Table 29.18.1).

Inhibition of other esterases also contributes to the clinical manifestations of acute poisoning. Inhibition of neuropathy target esterase leads to organophosphorus-induced delayed polyneuropathy (see Table 29.18.1).

Enzyme inhibition by an anticholinesterase compound is potentially reversible using an oxime, particularly when treatment is initiated early post-exposure. In the case of OP-inhibited AChE, in the absence of reactivation, a large proportion of inhibited AChE undergoes irreversible inhibition ('ageing') and enzyme resynthesis is required for restoration of nervous function. The rate of these competing reactions varies between individual OPs which also influences the clinical manifestations and response to oximes. Carbamates are structurally different to OPs such that there is spontaneous reactivation of carbamate-inhibited AChE and ageing does not occur.

Marked differences in the clinical manifestations of acute anticholinergic poisoning from different compounds are observed. This may reflect the variability in potency of enzyme inhibition, physiological adaptations following prolonged stimulation, pharmacokinetic factors, additional mechanisms of toxicity such as oxidative stress, inter-patient differences and/or other unknown factors.

Clinical features

The initial and prominent manifestation of acute anticholinesterase poisoning is the acute cholinergic crisis (see Table 29.18.1). The duration and manifestations of the acute cholinergic crisis vary between individual anticholinesterase compounds, as mentioned above.

Gastrointestinal symptoms are most prevalent following oral exposures, probably a result of high pesticide concentrations in the gut prior to absorption and the hydrocarbon solvent. Tachycardia does not consistently correlate with hypotension or pneumonitis, but can be secondary to catecholamine release from the adrenal medulla under nicotinic stimulation.

Table 29.18.1 Clinical manifestations and treatment of acute anticholinesterase poisoning

Clinical manifestations		Specific treatments for the routine management of acute anticholinesterase poisoning	Endpoints for titration
Acute cholinergic crisis	Markers of significant poisoning[1]		
• Muscarinic features: diarrhoea, urinary frequency, miosis, bradycardia, bronchorrhoea and bronchoconstriction, emesis, lacrimation, salivation (DUMBELS) and hypotension. Cardiac arrhythmias have also been reported	Bradycardia, bronchorrhoea or bronchospasm, hypotension	Atropine. Initially 1–3 mg IV for adults. If endpoints are not achieved by 3–5 min, double the dose IV. Continue to double the dose every 3–5 min until atropinization has been achieved. Large doses (hundreds of mg) may be required with massive poisoning. Maintain atropinization by infusion, commencing with 10–20% of the loading dose every hour	Clear chest on auscultation with resolution of bronchorrhea[2] and heart rate >80/min. Regular clinical observations are necessary to ensure that atropinization is achieved without toxicity (delirium, hyperthermia and/or ileus)
• Nicotinic features: fasciculations and muscle weakness which may progress to paralysis and respiratory failure[3], mydriasis, tachycardia, and hypertension	Muscle weakness, e.g. difficulty mobilizing or a decrease in forced vital capacity, progressing to respiratory failure requiring ventilatory support	Intubation and ventilation, oximes (for OPs only). The usual oxime used in Australasia for acute OP poisoning is pralidoxime and its indications and dosing regimen are controversial, see text for details	If oximes are administered, continue until recovery (12 h after atropine ceased or once BChE is noted to increase)
• Central nervous system: altered level of consciousness, respiratory failure[3] and seizures; the relative contributions of cholinergic and other neurotransmitters are not well characterized	Altered mental status, respiratory failure and seizures	Intubation and ventilation (avoid suxamethonium, if possible) and benzodiazepines. Administer IV as required for agitation or seizures, e.g. 5–10 mg diazepam, lorazepam 2–4 mg or midazolam 5–10 mg	Termination of agitation and/or seizures
• OP-induced delayed polyneuropathy: characterized by demyelination of long nerves, where 1–3 weeks after an acute exposure there is neurological dysfunction, particularly motor but also sensory, which may be chronic or recurrent		Supportive care and rehabilitation	Return to independent function

IV: intravenously; BchE: butyrylcholinesterase; OP: organophosphorus pesticides.
[1]A guide for identifying patients with a significant exposure and to guide clinical management in terms of who requires close observation and specific treatments, rather than for prognostication.
[2]Focal crepitations and/or wheeze may be noted when there has been pulmonary aspiration.
[3]Respiratory failure occurs due to centrally- and/or peripherally-mediated mechanisms. It may manifest either during the acute cholinergic crisis (type I paralysis) or suddenly during an apparent recovery phase (intermediate syndrome, or type II paralysis). Weakness of neck flexors is an early sign of significant muscle weakness. Intermediate syndrome is noted in approximately 5% of patients in various series.

Differential diagnosis

In situations where the history is not forthcoming, the differential diagnosis is broad and includes other toxins (clonidine, opioids, dopamine antagonists, such as chlorpromazine or haloperidol), funnel web spider envenoming and pontine haemorrhage.

Clinical investigations

The diagnosis and management of acute anticholinesterase poisoning is primarily clinical but measurement of cholinesterase activity can assist. The reference ranges are wide due to the large inter-individual variability in baseline AChE and butyrylcholinesterase (BChE, plasma cholinesterase, pseudocholinesterase) activities. Cholinesterase inhibition is generally noted prior to clinical effects. AChE and BChE are generally depressed within 6 h, although enzyme inhibition may progress until 12–24 h post-ingestion. AChE or BChE activity that is less than 80% of the lower reference range is consistent with significant anticholinesterase exposure. Patients in whom cholinesterase activity is higher than this might still have been exposed, but to a minimal degree only.

Erythrocyte AChE is structurally similar to synaptic AChE and their activities decrease in a similar manner following exposure to anticholinesterase compounds. The degree of AChE inhibition is considered the most useful biomarker of severity because it appears to correlate with severity of OP poisoning. In severe poisoning due to an anticholinesterase agent, the erythrocyte AChE activity is less than 20% of normal. Serial measurements of erythrocyte AChE activity can be useful for confirming reactivation of the enzyme by an oxime. For example, if AChE activity normalizes following initiation of oxime therapy, then this suggests that ageing has not occurred and that the dose of oximes is sufficient.

BChE inhibition is a sensitive biomarker of anticholinesterase exposure but has no relation to the severity of poisoning because the affinity of anticholinesterase compounds for BChE is highly variable and differs to that of AChE. Serial measurements of BChE cannot be used for measuring the effect of oximes because there is rapid ageing. However, these may be useful for confirming systemic elimination of the anticholinesterase compounds. Here, once BChE activity starts to increase (the rate of this depends on hepatic function) this suggests that the plasma concentration of the anticholinesterase compound is negligible.

Cholinesterase mixing tests have been used in the management of patients with acute OP poisoning to titrate the oxime regimen. In one method, the patient's plasma is mixed with an equal volume of non-poisoned donor (control) plasma. If BChE activity in the mixed sample is less than the mean of the samples from the patient and control, it suggests that free anticholinesterase compounds are present. It has been suggested that a decrease in cholinesterase activity in mixing studies is an indication to increase the dose of oximes, although the AChE response to oximes is probably a more useful parameter to guide oxime dosing. Despite being widely used, neither of these approaches to monitor therapy has been confirmed to improve outcome.

Blood gases and routine blood laboratory analyses are recommended for measuring metabolic and respiratory derangements; hypokalaemia secondary to vomiting and diarrhoea is not uncommon.

Criteria for diagnosis

Acute anticholinesterase poisoning is diagnosed on the basis of a history of exposure and development of characteristic clinical features (see Table 29.18.1). Therefore, a high index of clinical suspicion is necessary. Since the correlation between intent, dose and severity of toxicity appears to be poor and the clinical manifestations between individual compounds differ, each patient with an anticholinesterase exposure requires a thorough review.

The onset of cholinergic toxicity is variable, however, the majority of patients who develop severe poisoning are symptomatic within 6 h. Patients remaining asymptomatic for 12 h post-ingestion are unlikely to develop significant clinical toxicity. A possible exception is highly lipophilic compounds, such as fenthion. These may produce only subtle cholinergic features initially but then go on to cause progressive muscle weakness over a number of days, including respiratory failure, requiring ventilatory support.

Where there is doubt regarding the diagnosis or significance of an OP exposure, quantification of BChE or AChE activity is helpful (if available). BChE is particularly useful because it is more widely available and a sensitive marker of exposure.

Treatment

Resuscitation and early considerations

As with all acute poisonings, initial management begins with immediate assessment and management of disturbances in airway,

breathing and circulation. Because suxamethonium is metabolized by BChE, this agent should not be used for intubation of patients with acute anticholinesterase poisoning because the duration of paralysis will be prolonged by many hours. Continuous clinical monitoring, including pulse oximetry, cardiac monitoring and blood pressure are required. Hypotension not responding to intravenous fluid loading may be due in part to OP-induced decrease in systemic vascular resistance which requires intravenous vasopressors.

Although the volume ingested as per history appears to be a poor predictor of the amount absorbed, all patients with intentional poisoning who are symptomatic should be managed in a centre with access to intensive care facilities due to the potential for severe poisoning to develop. Gastrointestinal decontamination with oral activated charcoal can be given to patients presenting within 1–2 h of ingestion if the airway is protected, although this was not shown to be useful in a randomized controlled trial.

During the immediate assessment and resuscitation of the patient, all patients should undergo some degree of dermal decontamination (discussed above).

Subsequent interventions depend on changes to the clinical observations while the patient is monitored. Antidotal therapy should be administered rapidly, as outlined in Table 29.18.1. Muscarinic features of the acute cholinergic syndrome should be reversible with adequate doses of atropine. Oximes, such as pralidoxime, are claimed to reverse muscle weakness if administered promptly, although clinical studies confirming this are lacking (discussed later). Established OP-induced delayed polyneuropathy (OPIDP) does not respond to antidotes; instead supportive care is the priority.

Mild poisoning and dermal exposures

Patients who present with a history of accidental poisoning who are asymptomatic or minimally symptomatic (limited to mild gastrointestinal symptoms) often do not require hospital admission. Management priorities for these patients are rapid triage, a detailed risk assessment and consideration of forensic implications. If the exposure is trivial, the patient does not need medical review and can be observed at home or in the workplace. Other patients should be decontaminated and monitored clinically for a minimum of 6–12 h. If available, cholinesterase activity should be

measured to exclude a significant exposure. A normal cholinesterase activity at 6 h postexposure may be sufficient to exclude a significant oral exposure, although more research is required to confirm this observation.

Patients with a single acute dermal exposure rarely develop significant clinical effects and probably do not require medical assessment. Volunteer studies document that the risk of poisoning from a dermal exposure is far below that of an oral exposure. Although the rate of anticholinesterase absorption across the skin is slower than across the gut, patients who are asymptomatic at 12 h are unlikely to develop significant poisoning. Such patients should be given instructions to present for medical review if there is a significant worsening of symptoms. If there is significant concern regarding a dermal exposure, testing for changes in cholinesterase activity is recommended.

Moderate-to-severe poisoning

Patients with moderate-to-severe anticholinesterase poisoning experience prolonged and complicated hospital admissions. Close observation is required to monitor for a rapid clinical deterioration, even if there is an apparent recovery from the acute cholinergic crisis. Therefore, following resuscitation, these patients require ongoing management in an intensive care unit (ICU). Priorities post-admission to ICU include careful titration of antidotes and supportive care, including ventilation and inotropes/vasopressors.

Antidotes

The three most widely used antidotes for anticholinesterase poisoning are muscarinic antagonists (usually atropine), oximes (usually pralidoxime in Australasia) and benzodiazepines. The indications and dosing regimen of these specific antidotes are described in Table 29.18.1.

Antimuscarinic agents

Atropine is the most widely used antimuscarinic agent. It is carefully titrated to reverse muscarinic effects and has no effect on the neuromuscular features.

Oximes

Oximes are used to reverse neuromuscular blockade by reactivating the inhibited AChE before ageing occurs and should therefore be administered as early as possible. In general, oximes are more effective in poisoning due to diethyl OPs (e.g. chlorpyrifos, diazinon) than dimethyl OPs (e.g. dimethoate, fenthion, malathion), due in part to slower ageing of inhibited AChE by diethyl OPs.

Evidence supporting the indications for oxime therapy, their efficacy and the optimal dosing regimen is lacking and controversial. The earlier clinical studies reported either no effect or harm from oximes. However, these conclusions were limited by inadequacies in study design and also because the commonly used oxime dosing regimen was 1 g every 6 h which was less than that advocated by the WHO at the time. This prompted further research.

Two subsequent randomized controlled trials (RCTs) are worthy of mention. One RCT (n = 200 patients in India) concluded efficacy from higher doses of pralidoxime iodide: pralidoxime iodide 2 g loading dose in all patients, followed by either 24 g/day for 48 h, then 1 g every 4 h until recovery (higher dose) or the 1 g every 4 h (lower dose) until recovery. AChE activity was not measured in this study. The other RCT (n = 235 patients in Sri Lanka) reported no benefit from pralidoxime dosed according to a WHO recommended regimen: pralidoxime chloride 2 g loading dose, followed by a constant infusion of 0.5 g/h for up to 7 days; this was compared to saline. AChE was measured at multiple points in this study, confirming severe poisoning on arrival and an appropriate response to pralidoxime therapy. A concern in the latter study was the higher mortality in the intervention group, although this was not statistically significant. However, because the study was terminated early due to slow recruitment, the importance of this observation cannot be determined. Regarding dose equivalents, 1 g of pralidoxime iodide is equivalent to 650 mg of pralidoxime chloride. Both of these RCTs acknowledged limitations in their study designs and/or patient cohort and recommended further studies.

Because carbamate-inhibited AChE does not undergo ageing, the role for oximes appears limited. However, it remains controversial given that data have been presented to suggest that oximes may increase the reactivation of carbamate-inhibited AChE, although not consistently. Oximes appear to increase carbaryl toxicity for reasons that are not understood.

In summary, the efficacy of oximes in anticholinesterase poisoning is not confirmed. Due to limitations in the existing literature, studies exploring differing dosing regimens, types of oximes (obidoxime may be more effective) and

selection criteria are required. Until that time, it is reasonable to conclude that oximes are not a standard of care in the treatment of anticholinesterase poisoning. However, it is not unreasonable to administer obidoxime or lower doses of pralidoxime (e.g. 1 g pralidoxime chloride every 6 h) to patients with significant anticholinesterase poisoning, in particular by diethyl OPs, and monitor for reactivation of AChE.

Benzodiazepines

Benzodiazepines are recommended for use in patients with agitation or seizures. It is proposed that early use of benzodiazepines may prevent cognitive deficits or improve the central control of respiration preventing the need for intubation, however, this has not yet been sufficiently studied.

Prognosis

The mortality in patients with anticholinesterase poisoning is variable, which may reflect differences in degree of exposure, reporting, resources, genetics or the types of compounds encountered. However, the mortality can exceed 10%, compared to a mortality of less than 0.5% for pharmaceuticals.

Various tools are proposed to classify the severity of OP poisoning, but few have been widely adopted or validated. Generalized approaches to prognostication in OP poisoning are difficult given that individual compounds vary markedly in the onset, severity and manifestations of clinical toxicity. Further, they are not often useful for guiding management.

In the case of dermal exposures, prognosis appears favourable.

PARAQUAT (BIPYRIDYL HERBICIDES)

Paraquat is a non-selective contact herbicide and is considered one of the most toxic pesticides available. The mortality from acute poisoning is high, varying between 50 and 90%. Fortunately, cases of acute paraquat poisoning are increasingly rare in a number of countries due to restrictions in availability. However, paraquat continues to be an important cause of death in a number of countries in Asia, where it is widely used in subsistence farming.

Diquat is another bipyridyl herbicide that is more widely available in Australasia.

Mechanism of toxicity

Oral exposures to paraquat are most likely to lead to poisoning. Because paraquat formulations are highly irritating (and potentially corrosive), gastrointestinal toxicity occurs with all oral exposures.

Paraquat is rapidly absorbed (although the bioavailability is low) and distributed to all tissues. Free oxygen radicals are generated and non-specifically damage the lipid membrane of cells, inducing cellular toxicity and death. The free oxygen radicals produced by paraquat require oxygen for generation so supplemental inspired oxygen may exacerbate pulmonary injury.

The extent of dysfunction depends on the concentration of paraquat at the cellular level and the efficiency of protective mechanisms, such as intracellular glutathione, which is a free radical scavenger. Following an exposure of only 10–20 mL of the 20% w/v solution, these protective mechanisms can be overwhelmed leading to multisystem toxicity and death within 24–48 h.

Paraquat displays specific toxicity in the lung and kidney due to active uptake in type II pneumocytes and renal tubular cells. Because paraquat concentrates in these cells, they are more susceptible to injury than other cells. Therefore, in the event of a smaller exposure where multisystem toxicity does not occur, kidney and lung injury may occur. Kidney injury decreases the excretion of paraquat which increases systemic exposure. Pneumonitis can be followed by progressive pulmonary fibrosis and these are associated with impaired oxygenation.

Diquat does not concentrate in the pneumocytes as readily as paraquat. Therefore, if the patient survives the acute phase of multiorgan dysfunction, delayed pulmonary fibrosis is less likely to occur.

Clinical features

Severe gastrointestinal toxicity including vomiting and diarrhoea is the initial manifestation of acute paraquat poisoning. Necrosis of the oral mucosa is often noted about 12 h post-ingestion; it has been reported in patients who drink the paraquat solution without swallowing, despite the brief contact time. Oesophageal perforation with extensive subcutaneous emphysema may also occur due to the corrosive effects of the formulation.

Patients ingesting more than 20 mL are likely to develop severe poisoning with multisystem toxicity. This manifests as pneumonitis, hypotension, hepatitis, acute kidney injury and severe diarrhoea. Death within 48 h of ingestion is expected.

Patients ingesting less than 20 mL are still at risk of death, but this is more likely to be delayed by weeks or months post-ingestion. The primary mechanism of death is respiratory failure attributed to pulmonary fibrosis following increasing dyspnoea and hypoxaemia. This is associated with various degrees of hepatic and kidney impairment; kidney injury recovers within approximately 2–3 weeks in survivors.

Differential diagnosis

Acute paraquat poisoning may resemble sepsis or poisoning with another cellular poison, such as phosphine (aluminium or zinc phosphides), colchicine or iron. Oropharyngeal necrosis is more marked in paraquat poisoning.

Clinical investigations

A range of investigations has been proposed and tested in patients with acute paraquat poisoning. Because outcomes from paraquat poisoning are generally poor, their principal role is to define prognosis.

It is useful to confirm that an exposure to paraquat is significant because this will guide subsequent management. The easiest method to do this is by the dithionite urine test which involves the addition of 1 g of sodium dithionite solution and 1 g of sodium bicarbonate (or 1–2 mL of 1% sodium dithionite in 1–2 M sodium hydroxide) to 10 mL of urine. A blue colour change indicates paraquat ingestion and green colour change indicates diquat ingestion. The darker the colour change, the higher the concentration. If the test is negative on urine passed 6 h after ingestion, a significant exposure is unlikely.

The concentration of paraquat can be quantified in plasma to estimate prognosis, as discussed later. Unfortunately, it is often difficult to locate laboratories that are able to measure paraquat concentrations in a clinically useful time frame, thereby limiting its use.

Other investigations are useful to determine the evolution of toxicity to other organ systems, in particular serial measurements of serum electrolytes, kidney and liver function.

A raised admission creatinine concentration is associated with worse outcomes. If the rate of increase in plasma creatinine concentration exceeds 4.3 μmol/L/h over 12 h then death is more likely. Serial blood gas measurements and chest X-rays demonstrate progression of pulmonary injury.

Criteria for diagnosis

The diagnosis of paraquat poisoning is made on the basis of a history of exposure and the clinical symptoms, so a high index of clinical suspicion is required. The urinary dithionite test is a simple and quick method for confirming (or hopefully excluding) paraquat poisoning.

Treatment

Because death is reported following ingestion of as little as 10–20 mL, all exposures should be treated as significant and observed in hospital for 6–12 h post-ingestion. This allows for the dithionite urinary test to be conducted and to evaluate for changes in plasma creatinine concentration. Patients should be treated symptomatically, including intravenous fluids and analgesia according to usual guidelines.

Systemic exposure to paraquat may be decreased by either reducing absorption or increasing clearance. Both Fuller's earth and activated charcoal have been advocated to decrease absorption, but Fuller's earth is of limited availability and activated charcoal has not been demonstrated to improve outcomes.

Adequate hydration is required for optimal renal function which promotes paraquat clearance. Extracorporeal methods for increasing paraquat clearance have been largely disappointing. Haemoperfusion reduces lethality in dogs if commenced within a few hours of ingestion. Increasing data published in non-English language journals suggest clinical benefits from early haemoperfusion (possibly up to 12 hours post-ingestion). So, despite limitations in the reporting and design of these studies, an effect of haemoperfusion is not currently ruled out.

Antioxidants (e.g. vitamin C, vitamin E, acetylcysteine) and anti-inflammatories (corticosteroids, salicylates) are proposed therapies but are inadequately studied. Enthusiasm for immunosuppression with cyclophosphamide and corticosteroids followed positive findings in a couple of small studies, but limitations in study design rendered these findings inconclusive.

A larger randomized controlled trial was recently completed and reported no mortality benefit from immunosuppression with cyclophosphamide, methylprednisolone and dexamethasone. The role of other forms of immunosuppression, anti-inflammatories and antioxidants in the treatment of acute paraquat poisoning requires more research.

Despite these gaps in the data, it is obvious that, in the absence of treatment, the majority of patients will die. This has led some clinicians to treat patients with a number of treatments concurrently (e.g. activated charcoal, acetylcysteine, vitamins C and E, immunosuppression and either haemodialysis or haemoperfusion) in the hope that there will be a favourable outcome. The choice of whether to commence this treatment is largely a personal one and requires discussion with the patient and family. Such a treatment regimen is probably reasonable in patients with a faintly positive dithionite urinary test. However, it is unlikely to be of assistance to patients in whom this test is strongly positive or those with evolving multiorgan dysfunction. Instead, palliation should be the priority, including oxygen for hypoxia and morphine for dyspnoea and oropharyngeal or abdominal pain.

Prognosis

Mortality is higher in patients who experience a peripheral burning sensation than those who do not.

Much research has focused on the evaluation of markers of prognosis in patients with acute paraquat poisoning. Two predictors of death are well established: the dose ingested or the plasma concentration of paraquat, relative to the time of poisoning. When the plasma concentration of paraquat is available within a timely manner, this can be used with the time since ingestion to predict prognosis using either a nomogram or the calculated severity index of paraquat poisoning (SIPP). A number of nomograms have been developed and they perform similarly. The SIPP is calculated by multiplying the paraquat plasma concentration (mg/L) by the time since ingestion (hours): SIPP <10 predicts survival, SIPP 10–50 predicts death from lung fibrosis, and SIPP >50 predicts death from circulatory failure.

Direct markers of paraquat-induced organ toxicity that allow earlier prognostication might assist with determining which patients should be treated, palliated or discharged with confidence that harm will not occur.

Alternative markers of prognosis have also been explored, although few have been validated. These include measurement of the respiratory index, temporal changes in haematological or biochemical measures, such as creatinine (discussed above), or lactic acidosis and pulmonary surfactants.

GLYPHOSATE

Glyphosate is a non-selective herbicide that acts by inhibiting the enzymatic synthesis of aromatic amino acids in plants. This target enzyme is not present in humans. Both ready-to-use ($\approx$1–5%) and concentrated ($\approx$30–50%) formulations requiring dilution are available.

Glyphosate is absorbed from the gastrointestinal tract and does not penetrate the skin to a significant extent. Respiratory, ocular and dermal symptoms may occur following occupational use but are usually of minor severity. Ingestion is the most significant route of exposure in clinical toxicology.

Mechanism of toxicity

The mechanism of toxicity of glyphosate-containing herbicides in humans is inadequately described. Experimentally, there appears to be minimal (if any) mammalian toxicity from glyphosate itself. Toxicity has been largely attributed to surfactant co-formulants and potentially the type of glyphosate salt. Polyoxyethyleneamine (POEA; tallow amine) is the most common surfactant formulated in these products.

Poisoning is more severe following ingestion of concentrated formulations. This may reflect either the total dose ingested or direct effects of the highly irritating/corrosive compounds present in these products.

Patients with severe poisoning manifest multisystem effects. This suggests that glyphosate-containing herbicides may be non-specific in their action or that they interfere with physiological functions that are common to a number of systems. Proposed mechanisms include disruption of cellular membranes and uncoupling of oxidative phosphorylation, although these may be inter-related.

Clinical features

Abdominal pain with nausea, vomiting and/or diarrhoea are the most common manifestations of acute poisoning. These may be mild and self-resolving but, in severe poisoning (particularly due to the concentrated solutions), there may be inflammation, ulceration, haemorrhage or infarction of the gastrointestinal tract. Severe diarrhoea may also occur and vomiting may be recurrent, leading to dehydration.

Multiorgan dysfunction is noted with severe poisoning, including hypotension, kidney or liver dysfunction, pulmonary oedema or pneumonitis, altered level of consciousness and/or metabolic acidosis. It is not understood which of these clinical features reflect primary or secondary toxic effects of the glyphosate-containing herbicides. These effects may be transient or severe, progressing over 12–72 h to shock and death. Some patients who subsequently died demonstrated only mild symptoms at the time of admission.

Differential diagnosis

The differential diagnoses are wide, including any poisoning or medical condition associated with gastrointestinal symptomatology and progressive multisystem toxicity.

Clinical investigations

There are no specific clinical investigations to guide management.

Targeted laboratory and radiological investigations should be conducted in patients demonstrating anything more than mild gastrointestinal symptoms. Serial blood gases may be useful for detection of metabolic disequilibria. Hyperkalaemia is reported with products where glyphosate is formulated as the potassium salt.

Although glyphosate plasma concentrations appear to correlate with outcomes, this assay is not available for clinical use.

Endoscopy can identify erosions or ulceration of the gastrointestinal tract, but this investigation is associated with a risk of viscus rupture.

Criteria for diagnosis

The principal criterion for diagnosis of acute poisoning with a glyphosate-containing herbicide is a history of exposure. Therefore, a high index of suspicion is necessary for diagnosis. A number of clinical criteria for the classification of severity have been suggested, but none has been validated.

Treatment

All patients presenting with a history of acute ingestion should be observed for a minimum of 6 h. Patients reporting a history of intentional ingestion and gastrointestinal symptoms should be observed for at least 24 h given that the severity of poisoning may progress.

Treatment of acute poisoning with glyphosate-containing herbicides is empiric. All patients should receive prompt resuscitation and supportive care. Activated charcoal may be given orally if the patient presents within 1–2 h of ingestion, although a randomized controlled trial did not support its efficacy for pesticides in general. Intravenous fluids should be administered to replace gastrointestinal losses. Because the aetiology of hypotension may be multifactorial, including fluid losses or a decrease in cardiac output and/or peripheral resistance, haemodynamic monitoring is recommended to guide treatment of hypotension not responding to routine volumes of intravenous fluids. Biochemical and acid–base abnormalities should be corrected where possible.

No specific antidote has been proposed or tested for the treatment of acute poisoning with glyphosate-containing herbicides. This relates largely to the unknown mechanism of toxicity of these products.

The literature is conflicting regarding the role of haemodialysis outside of the more common indications (resistant acidaemia, hyperkalaemia or fluid overload in the context of kidney injury). If it is to be used, it is anticipated that early initiation would optimize outcomes.

Prognosis

All intentional exposures should be considered significant. A correlation between increasing dose and glyphosate plasma concentration, increasing age and delayed presentation to hospital with severe poisoning and death has been suggested.

Mortality from acute poisoning with glyphosate-containing herbicides varies between studies (reflecting various biases) but may be as high as 30%. The mortality was 3.2% in a prospective multicentre study in rural hospitals in Sri Lanka with limited medical resources.

Tools for estimating prognosis in acute poisoning with glyphosate-containing herbicides have not been described in detail. Patients developing marked multiorgan dysfunction, including kidney injury, hypotension, pulmonary oedema, sedation, arrhythmias) are more likely to die. Patients with more extensive erosions of the upper GI tract developed more severe systemic poisoning and required prolonged admission.

Controversies

- Anticholinesterase pesticides:
  - significance of other potential mechanisms of toxicity
  - role of oximes including dose and indications and the relative efficacy of individual oximes
  - role of other proposed antidotes and treatments including α_2-adrenergic receptor agonists (e.g. clonidine), BChE replacement therapy, gastric lavage, extracorporeal blood purification, magnesium sulphate, organophosphorus hydrolases and

blood alkalinization with sodium bicarbonate
  - importance of regulatory restrictions on 'highly toxic' anticholinesterase agents in decreasing mortality.
- Paraquat:
  - efficacy of anti-inflammatories, antioxidants and enhanced elimination on clinical outcomes.
- Glyphosate:
  - the relative importance of glyphosate, its salt and other co-formulants on the severity of poisoning
  - clinical and analytical predictors of the development of significant poisoning.

Further reading

Bradberry SM, Proudfoot AT, Vale JA. Glyphosate poisoning. Toxicol Rev 2004;23:159–67.
Buckley NA, Eddleston M, Li Y, Bevan M, Robertson J. Oximes for acute organophosphate pesticide poisoning. Cochrane Database Syst Rev 2011;2:CD005085.

Eddleston M, Buckley NA, Eyer P, Dawson AH. Management of acute organophosphorus pesticide poisoning. Lancet 2008;371:597–607.
Eddleston M, Eyer P, Worek F, et al. Differences between organophosphorus insecticides in human self-poisoning: a prospective cohort study. Lancet 2005;366:1452–9.
Eddleston M, Eyer P, Worek F, et al. Pralidoxime in acute organophosphorus insecticide poisoning–a randomised controlled trial. PLoS Med 2009;6:e1000104.
Eddleston M, Juszczak E, Buckley NA, et al. Randomised controlled trial multiple dose activated charcoal in acute self-poisoning. Lancet 2008;371:579–87.
Eddleston M, Phillips MR. Self poisoning with pesticides. Br Med J 2004;328:42–4.
Gawarammana IB, Buckley NA. Medical management of paraquat ingestion. Br J Clin Pharmacol 2011;72:745–57.
Li LR, Sydenham E, Chaudhary B, You C. Glucocorticoid with cyclophosphamide for paraquat-induced lung fibrosis. Cochrane Database Syst Rev 2012;7:CD008084.
Pawar KS, Bhoite RR, Pillay CP, et al. Continuous pralidoxime infusion versus repeated bolus injection to treat organophosphorus pesticide poisoning: a randomised controlled trial. Lancet 2006;368:2136–41.
Roberts DM, Aaron CK. Management of acute organophosphorus pesticide poisoning. Br Med J 2007;334:629–34.
Roberts DM, Buckley NA, Mohamed F, et al. A prospective observational study of the clinical toxicology of glyphosate-containing herbicides in adults with acute self-poisoning. Clin Toxicol 2010;48:129–36.
Senarathna L, Eddleston M, Wilks MF, et al. Prediction of outcome after paraquat poisoning by measurement of the plasma paraquat concentration. Q J Med 2009;102:251–9.

29.19 Ethanol and other 'toxic' alcohols

David McCoubrie

ESSENTIALS

1 Ethanol is a major cause of morbidity, mortality and emergency department (ED) presentation in most Western societies. Presentations may result from acute intoxication, withdrawal or medical complications of chronic ethanol ingestion.

2 Ethanol causes central nervous system (CNS) depression that can be synergistic with other CNS depressants and can be life threatening without supportive care.

3 Ethanol withdrawal is encountered commonly in the emergency department and has a mortality of up to 5% without medical therapy.

4 Wernicke's encephalopathy (W/E) is under diagnosed. The raised likelihood of W/E in patients with altered mental status and a suspected history of prolonged alcohol abuse should prompt early treatment with parenteral thiamine.

5 Methanol and ethylene glycol, the toxic alcohols, are potentially lethal when ingested even in relatively small volumes.

6 They exert toxic effects through the production of organic acid metabolites and dialysis is the recommended treatment.

7 An elevated anion-gap metabolic acidosis and a raised osmolar gap are associated with increased mortality in toxic alcohol ingestions.

8 Osmolar gap has a poor sensitivity and is incapable of excluding toxic alcohol ingestion.

Introduction

Alcohols are hydrocarbons that contain a hydroxyl (OH) group. Ethanol, a two-carbon primary alcohol, is the most commonly used recreational drug in Australasia and elsewhere in the Western world. Ethanol misuse is a major cause of mortality and morbidity both directly and indirectly and emergency departments (EDs) deal with the results on a daily basis. It was estimated that, in 1997, 3290 Australians died from injury due to high-risk drinking and there were 72 302 hospitalizations. In excess of 30% of all ED presentations are deemed to be ethanol related.

The complications of chronic alcohol consumption contribute to the development of a number of medical and surgical emergencies, many of which are dealt with elsewhere in this text. This chapter confines its discussion to acute ethanol intoxication, ethanol withdrawal and two other important ethanol specific emergency presentations—Wernicke's encephalopathy and alcoholic ketoacidosis.

A number of other alcohols, although far less frequently implicated in ED presentation than ethanol, are metabolized to form toxic organic acids and produce life-threatening clinical syndromes. These alcohols include methanol and ethylene glycol and are termed 'toxic alcohols'. Early recognition and intervention can prevent significant morbidity and mortality.

ETHANOL

Pharmacology

Ethanol is a small molecule that is rapidly and almost completely absorbed from the stomach and small intestine. Ethanol is both water and lipid soluble and rapidly crosses lipid membranes to distribute uniformly throughout the total body water. Ethanol is principally eliminated by hepatic metabolism with smaller amounts (5–10%) excreted unchanged by the kidneys, lungs and in sweat.

Ethanol is oxidized by cytosolic and microsomal cytochrome P450 (2EI and 1A2) alcohol dehydrogenases (ADH) to acetaldehyde which, in turn, is metabolized by aldehyde dehydrogenase to acetate. Acetate is converted to acetyl-CoA and enters the Krebs cycle to be finally metabolized to carbon dioxide and water. Entry of acetyl-CoA in the Krebs cycle is dependent on adequate thiamine stores. Importantly, the ADH system is saturated at relatively low blood ethanol concentrations, which results in blood ethanol elimination moving from first-order to zero-order kinetics. The rate of ethanol metabolism in non-tolerant adults is approximately 10 g/h and blood ethanol levels fall by about 0.02 g/dL/h. An alternative pathway for ethanol metabolism is via the microsomal ethanol oxidizing system, the activity of which increases in response to chronic alcohol exposure. Metabolism by this route is relatively important at very high blood ethanol concentrations and in chronic alcoholics.

The mechanism of action of ethanol is poorly understood. However, ethanol acts as a central nervous system (CNS) depressant, at least partially by enhancing the effect of γ-aminobutyric acid (GABA) at GABA$_A$ receptors. Tolerance to the CNS depressant effect develops with chronic exposure.

Clinical presentation

Acute ethanol intoxication

The clinical features associated with acute ethanol intoxication predominantly relate to the CNS and progress with increasing blood alcohol level, although there is remarkable inter-individual variation, most commonly as a function of tolerance. Initial features include a sense of well-being, increased self-confidence and disinhibition. With increasing blood concentrations, impaired judgement, impaired coordination and emotional lability develop. At very high concentrations, ethanol can cause coma, respiratory depression, loss of airway protective reflexes and even death.

Presentation to the ED is usually as a result of the social and behavioural consequences of the alteration in higher CNS functions. Ethanol is frequently implicated in trauma, drowning, violence, self-harm, domestic and sexual abuse and other acute social and psychiatric emergencies. Ethanol is a common co-ingestant in deliberate self-poisoning.

Many other important medical and surgical conditions that cause altered mental status may be incorrectly ascribed to ethanol intoxication or coexist with ethanol intoxication. Table 29.19.1 lists an example differential diagnosis.

In the absence of a clear history, the diagnosis of ethanol intoxication is only confirmed upon determination of a breath or blood ethanol concentration. Because ethanol consumption is so ubiquitous, a positive reading does not exclude coexisting pathology.

Table 29.19.1 Differential diagnosis of acute ethanol intoxication
Encephalopathy • Hepatic • Wernicke's
Head injury
Hypo-/hyperthermia
Intracranial infarction or haemorrhage
Metabolic • Hypoglycaemia • Hyponatraemia • Hypoxia • Hypocarbia
Overdose or other toxin
Post-ictal state
Psychosis
Sepsis

Ethanol withdrawal syndrome

A withdrawal syndrome usually develops within 6–24 h of cessation or reduction in ethanol consumption in dependent individuals. Symptoms can begin any time after the blood ethanol concentration begins to fall and blood ethanol is frequently still measurable in withdrawing patients. The duration of the syndrome may be from 2 to 7 days. Although the pathophysiology is not well understood, the syndrome presents as unopposed sympathetic and CNS stimulation. It is associated with a mortality of 5% and early clinical recognition of this syndrome is important.

Patients may present to the ED already in withdrawal after deliberately abstaining from alcohol or after stopping drinking due to intercurrent illness or lack of funds to buy alcohol. Alternatively, ethanol-dependent patients may begin to withdraw while being treated in the ED, particularly where their stay is prolonged.

Clinical features of mild ethanol withdrawal are those of mild autonomic hyperactivity and include nausea, anorexia, coarse tremor, tachycardia, hypertension, hyperreflexia, insomnia and anxiety. In more severe cases, the patient goes on to develop more pronounced anxiety, insomnia, irritability, tremor, tachycardia, hyperreflexia, hypertension, fever, visual hallucinations, seizures and delirium. Symptoms usually peak by 50 h. Delirium tremens represents the extreme end of the spectrum of ethanol withdrawal. It is an uncommon but potentially lethal complication.

Wernicke's encephalopathy

This is an acute neuropsychiatric syndrome that develops in certain alcohol-dependent individuals as a result of thiamine deficiency. It is a spectrum disorder that is classically described as a triad of:

- oculomotor disturbance (usually nystagmus and ocular palsies)
- abnormal mentation (usually confusion)
- ataxia.

In up to 20% of cases, the signs and symptoms of the classic triad are not evident at presentation. Less common presentations include stupor, hypothermia, cardiovascular instability, seizures, visual disturbances, hallucinations and alterations in behaviour. In extremis, the condition may present with hyperthermia, hypertonia, spastic paresis, dyskinesias and coma.

Wernicke's encephalopathy is a clinical diagnosis and constitutes a medical emergency with significant morbidity and a mortality of 10–20 % if left untreated. For this reason, the emergency physician must maintain a high index of suspicion in any patient with altered mental status and a suspicion of prolonged heavy ethanol intake.

Alcoholic ketoacidosis

Alcoholic ketoacidosis (AKA), also termed alcoholic acidosis, is an often unrecognized potentially life-threatening medical condition that develops in the alcoholic patient in response to starvation. The normal response to starvation is increased gluconeogenesis from pyruvate. In the alcoholic patient, pyruvate is preferentially converted to lactate. In response, fatty-acid metabolism is increased as an alternative source of energy, resulting in the production of acetyl-CoA and acetoacetate which, in turn, is reduced to β-hydroxybutyrate (BOHB), producing the ketoacidotic state.

Patients with AKA usually present with a history of prolonged heavy alcohol misuse preceding a bout of particularly excessive intake, which has been terminated several days earlier by nausea, severe vomiting and abdominal pain. There may be a history of previous episodes requiring brief admissions with labels of 'query pancreatitis' or 'alcoholic gastritis'. Examination usually reveals tachypnoea, tachycardia, hypotension and diffuse epigastric tenderness on palpation. In contrast to patients with diabetic ketoacidosis, mental status is usually normal. The presence of an altered mental state should prompt consideration of other causes, especially hypoglycaemia and acute ethanol intoxication.

Toxic alcohol poisoning is an important differential diagnosis. Toxic alcohol acidosis does not produce ketosis and, in contrast, does cause significant alteration to conscious state, visual symptoms (methanol) and renal failure/crystalluria (ethylene glycol).

Clinical investigations

The excretion of ethanol by the lungs, although relatively unimportant in terms of ethanol elimination, obeys Henry's law, i.e. the ratio between the concentration of ethanol in the alveolar air and blood is constant. This allows breath sampling of ethanol to estimate reliably blood ethanol concentration.

Most non-tolerant adults would be expected to develop some impairment of higher functions at blood ethanol concentrations in the range of 0.025–0.05 mg/dL (5–11 mmol/L) and to develop significant CNS depression in the range of 0.25–0.4 mg/L (55–88 mmol/L).

In a patient presenting with acute intoxication, no investigations may be necessary; however, blood or breath ethanol levels (BAL) are frequently useful to confirm the diagnosis. A BAL of zero is highly significant in a patient with an altered level of consciousness, as ethanol intoxication is excluded and other diagnoses need to be considered. A positive blood ethanol level does not exclude alternative diagnoses.

Other investigations should be performed as clinically indicated in an effort to exclude coexisting pathologies and alternative diagnoses as detailed above.

In the patient with AKA, bedside investigations reveal a low/normal glucose, low or absent breath ethanol and urinary ketones (these may be low or absent due to the inability of bedside assays to detect all ketone moieties, especially BOHB). Laboratory investigation will reveal an anion-gap (AG) acidosis (this may be severe with AG >30) and mild hyperlactaemia insufficient to account for the AG.

Treatment

Acute ethanol intoxication

Severe ethanol intoxication with CNS depression is life threatening but a good outcome is assured by timely institution of supportive care. In particular, attention may need to be given to the airway and ventilation. Hypotension generally responds to intravenous crystalloid infusion. The blood sugar level must be checked and normoglycaemia maintained. Intravenous thiamine should be administered, particularly to those with chronic ethanol abuse. There is no specific antidote to ethanol intoxication.

Less severe ethanol intoxication presents a management challenge to the emergency physician when it results in a combative or violent patient threatening harm to self or staff or threatening to discharge against medical advice. Such patients frequently require chemical sedation with titrated doses of intravenous benzodiazepines or butyrophenones in order to facilitate assessment and observation, ensure safety for patient and staff and prevent unsafe discharge.

Ethanol withdrawal

The key to management of this condition is early recognition and institution of adequate dosing of benzodiazepines. Large doses of benzodiazepines may be required to control symptoms. The risk and likely severity of ethanol withdrawal can usually be anticipated if an accurate history of alcohol intake and previous withdrawals is obtained. Coexisting conditions should be managed on their own merits. It is important to exclude hypoglycaemia and correct if present. Thiamine 200 mg (preferably intravenously) should be immediately given to any chronic alcoholic patient who presents with or develops an altered mental status (see Wernicke's encephalopathy below). Benzodiazepines are first-line therapy for seizures resulting from ethanol withdrawal. Phenytoin is not effective in treating or preventing withdrawal seizures.

The management of ethanol withdrawal in the ED or observation ward is greatly facilitated by the use of ethanol withdrawal charts. These charts facilitate recognition of the first signs of ethanol withdrawal and timely administration of benzodiazepines in adequate doses. An example of such a chart is shown in Figure 29.19.1. Benzodiazepine, usually diazepam, administration is titrated to the clinical features of withdrawal. The total dose required to manage withdrawal is highly variable. Benzodiazepines are usually given orally but can be administered intravenously to the uncooperative or severely withdrawing patient. With extreme withdrawal, refractory to benzodiazepines, small aliquots of ethanol may be effective in controlling severe symptoms.

Wernicke's encephalopathy

As Wernicke's encephalopathy is a clinical diagnosis with high mortality if untreated, any known or suspected alcoholic patient who presents with altered mental status should receive thiamine 200 mg IV during the initial assessment. Recommendations for thiamine dosing in patients with suspected Wernicke's vary between 200 and 500 mg tds, although there is less evidence supporting the 500 mg dose. These doses ought to be continued until conscious state clears or alternative diagnosis is determined. Parenteral administration is vital as thiamine is variably absorbed orally with low bioavailablility. An example of an emergency department thiamine administration guideline is found in Figure 29.19.2. If dextrose

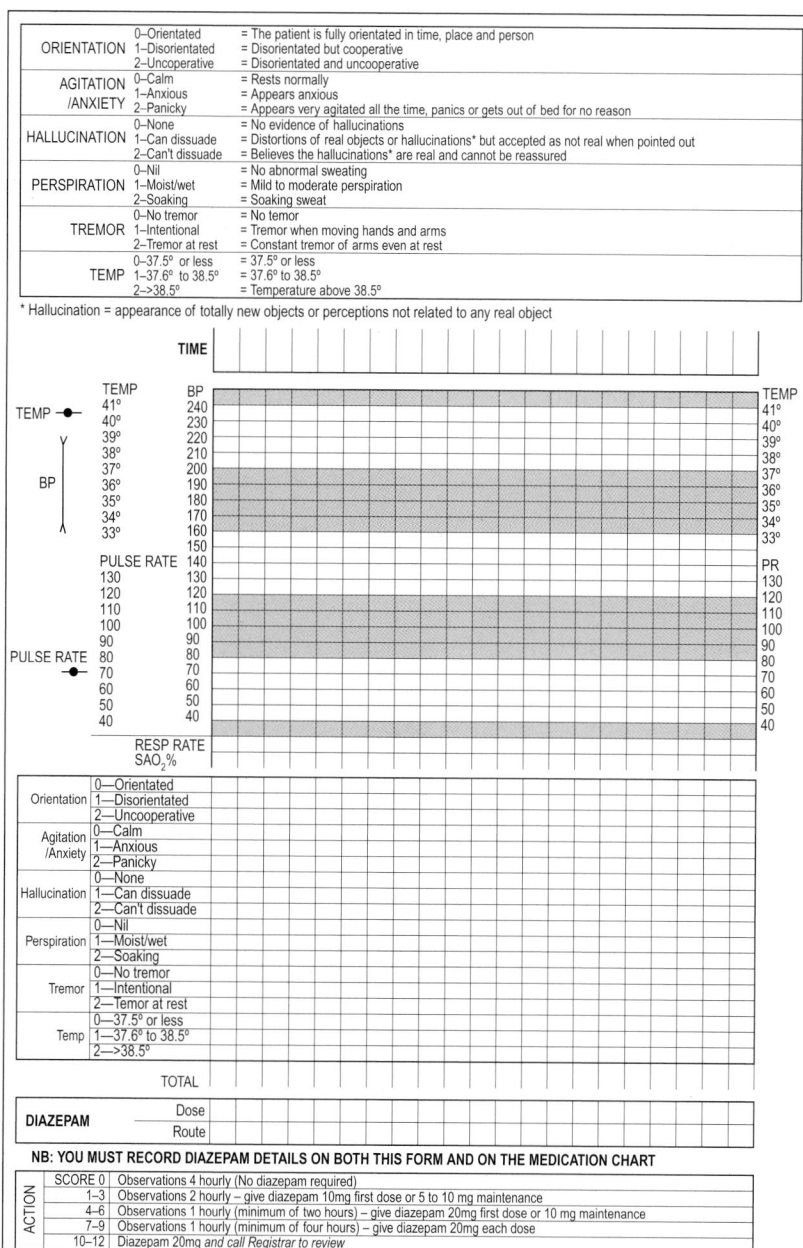

ORIENTATION	0—Orientated	= The patient is fully orientated in time, place and person		
	1—Disoriented	= Disorientated but cooperative		
	2—Uncooperative	= Disorientated and uncooperative		
AGITATION /ANXIETY	0—Calm	= Rests normally		
	1—Anxious	= Appears anxious		
	2—Panicky	= Appears very agitated all the time, panics or gets out of bed for no reason		
HALLUCINATION	0—None	= No evidence of hallucinations		
	1—Can dissuade	= Distortions of real objects or hallucinations* but accepted as not real when pointed out		
	2—Can't dissuade	= Believes the hallucinations* are real and cannot be reassured		
PERSPIRATION	0—Nil	= No abnormal sweating		
	1—Moist/wet	= Mild to moderate perspiration		
	2—Soaking	= Soaking sweat		
TREMOR	0—No tremor	= No temor		
	1—Intentional	= Tremor when moving hands and arms		
	2—Tremor at rest	= Constant tremor of arms even at rest		
TEMP	0—37.5° or less	= 37.5° or less		
	1—37.6° to 38.5°	= 37.6° to 38.5°		
	2—>38.5°	= Temperature above 38.5°		

* Hallucination = appearance of totally new objects or perceptions not related to any real object

Fig. 29.19.1 An example of an alcohol withdrawal chart.

administration is required, it must follow thiamine replacement as it may acutely worsen the neurological status of the thiamine-deficient patient. Magnesium is a co-factor for thiamine-dependent transketolase and so any magnesium deficiency should be corrected.

Alcoholic ketoacidosis

Initial resuscitation should include administration of adequate volumes of crystalloids to treat hypovolaemia followed by parenteral thiamine and infusion of dextrose-containing fluids. Potassium and magnesium supplementation should be given according to serum electrolyte results. Administration of dextrose, usually an infusion of 5% dextrose, is essential as it stimulates insulin release, inhibits glucagon release and so inhibits fatty-acid oxidation. Thiamine facilitates entry of pyruvate into the Krebs cycle. Administration of insulin or bicarbonate is not necessary.

Fluid, electrolyte and acid–base status should be closely monitored and further therapy tailored to the clinical response. Careful evaluation and treatment of the coexisting medical disorders is essential.

Disposition

The disposition of many ethanol-intoxicated patients presenting to the ED is determined by the associated medical, surgical, psychiatric or social issues. Ethanol-intoxicated patients should only be discharged from the ED when their subsequent safety can be ensured. Discharge into the care of a competent relative or friend is sometimes appropriate. Other patients, particularly if aggressive or neurologically impaired, require admission to a safe environment until such time as the intoxication resolves and they can be reassessed. An observation ward attached to the ED may be the most appropriate place if available. More severely intoxicated patients requiring airway control and support of ventilation should be admitted to the intensive care unit.

Patients in ethanol withdrawal may require admission for management of the precipitating medical or surgical illness. For those patients who wish to complete withdrawal with a view to abstinence, the remainder of the withdrawal may be managed in a general medical ward, specialized medical or non-medical detoxification centre or at home. Medical detoxification is mandatory where a severe withdrawal syndrome is anticipated. In any case, ongoing psychosocial support will be required and it is important for EDs to have a good knowledge of the locally available drug and alcohol services to ensure appropriate referral.

Patients with Wernicke's encephalopathy should be admitted for ongoing care and thiamine and magnesium supplementation. The ophthalmoplegia and nystagmus usually have a good response to thiamine within hours to days. Ataxia and mental changes improve more slowly if at all and have a poorer prognosis. Up to 50% of cases will show no response despite thiamine therapy.

Patients with ethanol-induced ketoacidosis also require admission for ongoing dextrose and thiamine, monitoring of fluids and electrolytes and management of the precipitating medical condition. Mortality from ethanol-induced ketoacidosis *per se* is rare with early recognition and treatment, but death may occur as a result of the underlying medical condition, particularly if unrecognized.

Ideally, any patient with an ethanol-related presentation should be offered referral to drug and alcohol rehabilitation services for counselling.

TOXICOLOGY EMERGENCIES

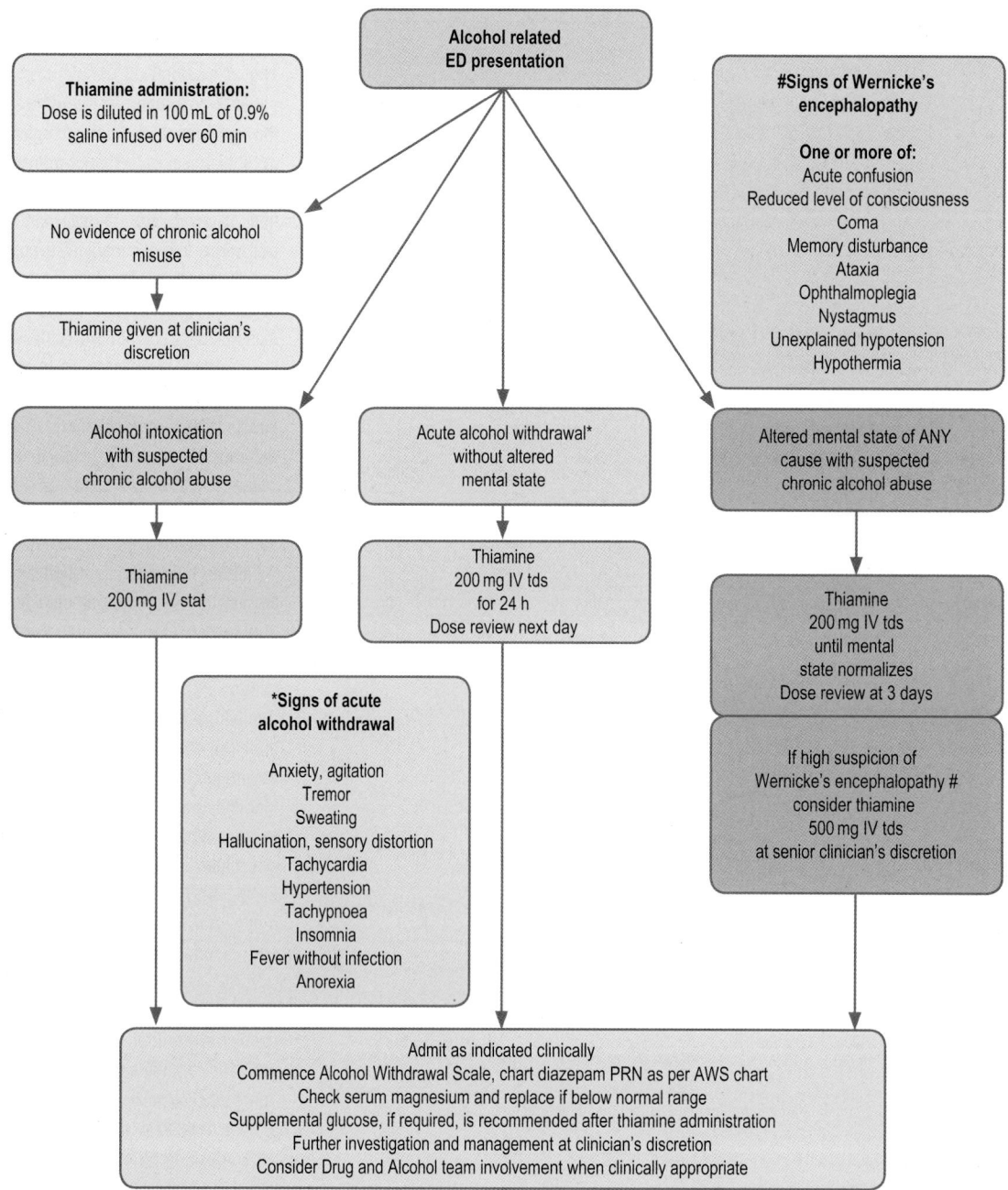

Fig. 29.19.2 Guideline for thiamine administration in the emergency department. *(Prepared by Dr Kerry Hoggett, ED Consultant and Clinical Toxicology Fellow, November 2011. On behalf of the Thiamine Working Party, RPH and FH, Government of Western Australia Department for Health.)*

TOXIC ALCOHOLS

Epidemiology

Both methanol and ethylene glycol poisoning are extremely rare in Australasia. This is primarily due to their limited availability.

Methanol is found in model aeroplane fuel and laboratory solvents. There is no methanol in 'methylated spirits' sold in Australia (this is, in fact, pure ethanol with bittering agents to minimize palatability). Methanol is more freely available in other countries where it is found in household cleaning agents and windshield de-icer. Incorrect distillation of ethanol for human consumption, usually from home-made stills, has resulted in mass poisoning incidents with severe toxicity and fatalities.

Ethylene glycol is most commonly encountered as a constituent of radiator antifreeze or coolant. It is also found in hydraulic fluids and solvent preparations. Significant poisoning in Australasia almost always occurs following deliberate ingestion.

Toxicology

Methanol and ethylene glycol are both small molecules that are rapidly absorbed from the gastrointestinal (GI) tract with a volume of distribution that approximates total body water (0.6 L/kg). Toxic alcohols are oxidized initially by hepatic cytosolic and microsomal alcohol dehydrogenases (ADH) and then further metabolized by aldehyde dehydrogenase into acidic moieties. Methanol is metabolized initially to form formaldehyde and then to formic acid. Ethylene glycol is metabolized to glycoaldehyde and then to glycolate, glyoxylate and oxylate. The plasma half-lives of the toxic alcohols are appreciably increased in the presence of ethanol because ethanol has a much higher affinity for ADH: four times that of methanol and eight times that of ethylene glycol. As a result, the presence of ethanol greatly delays the onset of clinical and biochemical features of toxicity.

Methanol toxicity is mediated through the formation of formic acid. Formic acid binds to cytochrome oxidase resulting in impairment of cellular respiration. Its half-life is prolonged (up to 20 h) and its metabolism is dependent on the presence of tetrahydrofolate. The presence of systemic acidosis enhances the movement of formic acid intracellularly. The initial acidosis is secondary to formic acid, however, as cellular respiration is disturbed and toxicity progresses, a concurrent lactic acidosis is usually evident. Accumulation of formic acid manifests as increasing AG acidosis, gastrointestinal and neurological toxicities.

Ethylene glycol itself is a direct irritant to the GI tract and has CNS depressant effects similar to those of ethanol. The major toxicity is mediated through the acid metabolites, glycolate and oxylate. Oxalate complexes with calcium, leading to crystal deposition chiefly in the renal tubules and the CNS. Myocardium and lungs can also be affected. In addition, these acids appear to be inherently toxic. Complexing with calcium produces systemic hypocalcaemia and may manifest with prolongation of the QT interval. A profound AG acidosis develops and is principally attributed to glycolic acid accumulation although a concurrent lactic acidosis (type B) also contributes.

Predictors of toxicity

Toxic dose

The lethal dose of methanol is conservatively estimated as 0.5–1.0 mL/kg of a 100% solution. Clinical toxicity and visual sequelae may be seen with smaller doses, perhaps as little as 0.25 mL/kg.

The lethal dose of ethylene glycol is thought to be in the order of 1.0 mL/kg of a 100% solution.

Biochemical markers

Biochemical predictors of mortality in toxic alcohol ingestions are an elevated anion-gap metabolic acidosis and a raised osmolar gap.

When available, serum level of methanol and ethylene glycol greater than 50 mg/dL are associated with severe toxicity.

Clinical features

Methanol

Initially, mild CNS depression typical of ethanol intoxication is evident. A latent period (6–24 h) is classically observed during which time the patient may appear asymptomatic. Progressive ophthalmic, GI and CNS symptoms may then develop. Hyperpnoea is usually observed secondary to the metabolic acidosis. Progressive obtundation leading to coma and seizures heralds the onset of cerebral oedema and signifies poorer prognosis. Those who recover from serious CNS toxicity can display extrapyramidal movement disorders. Retinal toxicity may be irreversible in up to one-third of cases.

Ethylene glycol

The progression of clinical features following ingestion of ethylene glycol is described in three stages: neurological, cardiopulmonary and renal. These stages are artificial and toxicity may progress in a rapid manner with concurrent toxicities being observed. Initially, an intoxication syndrome analogous to ethanol occurs along with nausea and vomiting due to mucosal irritation. A progressively severe AG acidosis with renal failure and hypocalcaemia is characteristic. Crystalluria may be observed. With severe poisoning, renal failure progresses rapidly. Central nervous system depression is observed with severe manifestations including seizures, coma and cerebral oedema. Hyperpnoea occurs secondary to the metabolic acidosis.

Clinical investigations

Direct assay of methanol or ethylene glycol concentrations in serum is rarely readily available. In the absence of direct assays, the ability to exclude a potentially lethal toxic alcohol ingestion at presentation is limited. The combination of an osmolar gap (OG) and a wide AG acidosis is highly suggestive of either methanol or ethylene glycol

intoxication. However, a normal OG does not exclude toxic alcohol ingestion. In the presence of a profound acidotic state, it is possible that a toxic alcohol has been largely metabolized and thus no longer sufficiently present to raise the OG. Additionally, baseline OGs may vary from −14 to +10 between individuals and so a 'normal' OG may mask a large occult increase representing a potentially lethal ingestion. Similarly, a normal AG at presentation is not sufficient to exclude toxic alcohol ingestion. Early in the clinical course an AG may be normal, only to develop rapidly as metabolism progresses. This is particularly so in the presence of ethanol where the onset of an AG acidosis will be delayed until the ethanol itself has been preferentially metabolized.

Falls in serum bicarbonate and arterial pH correlate well with levels of toxic organic acid metabolites in the circulation and, in the absence of direct assays, are their chief surrogate markers. In this context, it is common practice to exclude toxic ingestion where there is a normal venous bicarbonate (>20) 8 h after the serum or breath ethanol has been documented as undetectable.

When available in a clinically useful time frame, direct assays may shorten hospital assessment times especially with accidental exposures. The interpretation of serum methanol and ethylene glycol concentrations requires consideration of time since ingestion, ethanol co-ingestion and acid–base status.

Treatment

The definitive care for methanol and ethylene glycol ingestions is dialysis with concurrent ADH blockade therapy. All cases of deliberate self-poisonings with a toxic alcohol need to be managed in a facility with easy access to dialysis if clinical intoxication becomes apparent. ADH blockade therapy can impede the progression of clinical toxicity and permit safe transfer to an appropriate facility.

Alcohol dehydrogenase blockade

Blockade of ADH can be achieved by the administration of either ethanol or the specific ADH antagonist fomepizole (not currently available in Australasia). These agents prevent metabolism of toxic alcohols and the accumulation of their organic acid metabolites. ADH blockade significantly increases the half-life of parent toxic alcohols. In the presence of

Table 29.19.2 Indications for haemodialysis in toxic alcohol poisoning
Severe metabolic acidosis (pH <7.25)
Renal failure (ethylene glycol)
History of a large toxic alcohol ingestion and osmolar gap >10 mmol/L
Visual symptoms (methanol)
Ethylene glycol or methanol levels >50 mg/dL (if available)

Table 29.19.3 Endpoints for haemodialysis in toxic alcohol poisoning
Correction of acidosis
Osmolar gap <10 mmol/L
Ethylene glycol or methanol level <20 mg/dL (if available)

ethanol, half-life may increase to about 50 h for methanol and for ethylene glycol up to 20 h. ADH blockade with ethanol, although an essential element of care, is not definitive in most circumstances owing to the practical difficulty maintaining prolonged elevated blood ethanol concentration and obtaining serial toxic alcohol levels. However, where serial levels are available, there is evidence that fomepizole can be used in isolation to treat toxic alcohol ingestions.

Ethanol therapy can be initiated with a loading dose of 8 mL/kg of 10% ethanol intravenously or 1.8 mL/kg of 43% ethanol orally (equivalent to 3 × 40 mL shots of vodka in a 70 kg adult). Maintenance therapy requires an infusion of 1–2 mL/h of 10% ethanol or 0.2–0.4 mL/h of 43% ethanol orally (equivalent to one 40 mL shot of vodka each hour in a 70 kg adult). The ethanol concentration should be maintained in the range of 100–150 mg/dL (22–33 mmol/L) by careful titration of maintenance administration guided by frequent blood ethanol concentrations.

Haemodialysis

Haemodialysis represents definitive care for confirmed toxic alcohol ingestions. It effectively removes parent toxic alcohols and their acidic metabolites. Lactate free and bicarbonate buffered dialysates may assist the correction of acidaemia. Commonly accepted indications for haemodialysis are listed in Table 29.19.2. Endpoints for haemodialysis are listed in Table 29.19.3. Ethanol is also rapidly cleared by dialysis and ethanol infusion rates need to be increased (usually doubled) during haemodialysis.

Supportive care and co-factor therapy

Folinic or folic acid administration is recommended in methanol poisoning (folinic acid 2 mg/kg IV qid) to aid in endogenous metabolism of formic acid. Pyridoxine and thiamine supplementation is recommended in ethylene glycol poisoning when the patient is thought to be deplete (e.g. alcoholics), again to aid endogenous metabolism of the pathogenic acids.

In methanol poisoning, systemic acidaemia enhances the movement of formic acid into the intracellular compartment. Correction with intravenous bicarbonate if pH <7.3 is recommended.

Calcium replacement in ethylene glycol poisoning is contentious given that it may promote calcium oxalate crystal formation. Consequentially, calcium should only be replaced if there is symptomatic hypocalcaemia (including prolongation of the QT interval) or intractable seizures.

Prognosis

Prompt ADH blockade therapy and dialysis ensures an excellent outcome in toxic ingestions who present before the development of established end-organ toxicity. Delayed diagnosis and treatment is associated with death and permanent neurological and renal sequelae, including blindness in the case of methanol poisoning.

Controversies

- It has been suggested that EDs could play a pivotal role in reducing ethanol-related morbidity by adopting procedures to detect and refer individuals who misuse ethanol. A number of centres have successfully done trial screening and brief intervention strategies for hazardous ethanol consumption.
- It is unclear whether fomepizole provides sufficient advantages over ethanol as an ADH blocker in toxic alcohol poisoning so as to justify the expense of importing and stocking it in Australasia.
- Co-factor therapy in toxic alcohol poisoning is of unproven efficacy, however, there are few contraindications to their administration.

Further reading

Barceloux DG, Bond GR, Krenzelok EP, et al. American academy of clinical toxicology ad hoc committee on the treatment guidelines for methanol poisoning. American Academy of Clinical Toxicology practice guidelines on the treatment of methanol poisoning. J Toxicol Clin Toxicol 2002;40:415–46.

Barceloux DG, Krenzelok EK, Olson K, et al. American Academy of Clinical Toxicology practice guidelines on the treatment of ethylene glycol poisoning. J Toxicol Clin Toxicol 1999;37:537–60.

Coulter CV, et al. Methanol and ethylene glycol acute poisonings–predictors of mortality. Clin Toxicol 2011;49:900–6.

Fulop M. Alcoholic ketoacidosis. Endocrinol Metabol Clin N Am 1993;22:209–19.

Galvin R, et al. EFNS guidelines for diagnosis, therapy, and prevention of Wernicke encephalopathy. Eur J Neurol 2010:1408–18.

Hoffman RS, Smilkstein MJ, Howland MA, et al. Osmol gaps revisited: normal values and limitations. J Toxicol Clin Toxicol 1993;31:81–93.

Hungerford DW, Pollock DA, Todd KT. Acceptability of emergency department-based screening and brief intervention for alcohol problems. Acad Emerg Med 2000;7:1383–92.

McGuire LC, Cruickshank AM, Munro PT. Alcoholic ketoacidosis. Emerg Med J 2006;23:417–20.

Mégarbane B, Borron SW, Baud FJ. Current recommendations for treatment of severe toxic alcohol poisonings. Intens Care Med 2005;31:189–95.

Sechi G, Serra A. Wernicke's encephalopathy: new clinical settings and recent advances in diagnosis and management. Lancet Neurol 2007;6:442–55.

Turner RC, Lichstein PR, Peden JG, et al. Alcohol withdrawal syndromes: a review of pathophysiology, clinical presentation and treatment. J Gen Intern Med 1989;4:432–44.

Zuburan C, Fernandes JG, Rodnight R, et al. Wernicke-Korsakoff syndrome. Postgrad Med J 1997;73:27.

29.20 Carbon monoxide

Nicholas Buckley

ESSENTIALS

1 Carbon monoxide is the commonest agent used in completed suicides by poisoning in Australia and the UK.

2 Carbon monoxide is produced by incomplete combustion and is found in car exhaust, faulty heaters, fires and in industrial settings.

3 Carbon monoxide poisoning may result in significant long-term neuropsychological sequelae.

4 Oxygen increases the elimination of carbon monoxide—and the extent of increase is proportional to the inspired oxygen pressure.

5 The optimal mode of oxygen delivery to improve clinical outcomes remains controversial.

Introduction

Carbon monoxide (CO) poisoning is an important cause of mortality and morbidity from poisoning. Immediate resuscitation including 100% oxygen therapy is essential and the long-term results of most patients will be good with this simple intervention. It is unclear whether any additional intervention will reduce the low but important risk of serious long-term neurological damage.

Aetiology, pathophysiology and pathology

Carbon monoxide is a colourless, odourless, tasteless and non-irritant gas, produced by incomplete combustion of hydrocarbons [1]. Small amounts are also produced endogenously by normal metabolic processes. The most common sources of significant exposure are car exhausts, cigarette smoke, fires and faulty home heaters and barbecues. Catalytic converters reduce the production of carbon monoxide and are in all cars manufactured in the last decade or two. Carboxyhaemoglobin (COHb) concentrations in cigarette smokers range as high as 10%.

The pathophysiology of CO exposure is complex and incompletely understood. Upon exposure, CO binds to haemoglobin with an affinity 210 times that of oxygen, thereby decreasing the oxygen-carrying capacity of blood. CO can also produce injury by several other mechanisms, including direct disruption of cellular oxidative processes, binding to myoglobin and cytochrome oxidases and causing peroxidation of brain lipids [1]. However, the end result is tissue hypoxia, leading to varying degrees of end-organ damage and eventually death. The severity of poisoning is a function of the duration of exposure, the ambient concentration of CO and the underlying health status of the exposed individual. Although useful for diagnosis when detected, the initial COHb level correlates poorly with outcome [2].

Epidemiology

Poisoning with CO is an important cause of unintentional and intentional injury worldwide. In the USA alone, an estimated 1000–2000 accidental deaths due to CO exposure occur each year, resulting from an estimated 40 000 exposures [3]. In Australia and the UK, it is the most common agent in completed suicide by poisoning.

Prevention

Prevention of environmental or occupational exposure is possible by use of CO air monitors. COHb concentrations are increased for any given inspired CO concentration if the person is exercising or at high altitudes (increased breathing rate and pulmonary blood flow). These considerations are relevant to acceptable levels of exposure.

The introduction of catalytic converters has reduced CO production in vehicle exhaust and this, in turn, appears to be leading to a reduction in fatal suicidal poisoning in some countries [4,5].

Clinical features

The signs and symptoms of acute carbon monoxide poisoning are shown in Table 29.20.1 [6] and severity broadly correlates with maximum COHb concentration. Initial symptoms are non-specific and probably predominantly due to compensatory mechanisms to maintain tissue oxygen delivery to vital organs (e.g. tachycardia, headache, dizziness, gastrointestinal symptoms). Signs with more severe toxicity directly reflect tissue hypoxia with central nervous and cardiovascular toxicity being the most critical manifestations. Death results rapidly when impaired oxygenation of the heart prevents the compensatory increase in cardiac output. The skin is classically cherry pink, although severely ill patients are often pale or cyanosed. Pre-existing cerebral or cardiovascular disease, anaemia and volume depletion or cardiac failure increase toxicity (for a given COHb). These people all have a reduced ability to compensate by increasing cardiac output or redistributing blood supply to vital organs. Cardiac toxicity is common in moderate to severe poisoning. Screening with cardiac enzymes with further testing with echocardiography or SPECT have been suggested [7,8]. Abnormal troponin has also been linked to greater long-term mortality [9].

Due to low oxygen pressures, the high affinity of fetal haemoglobin for CO and the much longer half-life of CO in the fetal circulation, the fetus is particularly susceptible to CO poisoning. The outcome of significant CO poisoning in the mother is often fetal death or neurological damage.

Delayed or persistent neuropsychiatric sequelae occur, largely confined to those who have prolonged loss of consciousness at some stage [10]. Long-term follow up is necessary as more subtle defects can develop or

Table 29.20.1 Typical clinical symptoms and signs relative to COHb (normal = 0.5%) [6]

COHb (%)	Symptoms and signs
<10	Nil (commonly found in smokers)
10–20	Nil or vague non-descript symptoms
30–40	Headache, tachycardia, confusion, weakness, nausea, vomiting, collapse
50–60	Coma, convulsions, Cheyne–Stokes breathing, arrhythmias, ECG changes
70–80	Circulatory and ventilatory failure, cardiac arrest, death

Buckley NA, Dawson AH, Whyte IM. Hypertox. Assessment and treatment of poisoning. www.hypertox. com www.wikitox.com; 2012 with permission.

become apparent over a few weeks to months. The most common problems encountered are depressed mood (even in those accidentally exposed) and difficulty with higher intellectual functions (especially short-term memory and concentration) [11,12]. More severe problems include parkinsonism and speech problems. Neuropsychological testing may detect subtle defects not apparent on crude mini-mental state testing. The incidence of sequelae depends on the definition used–major deficits are relatively uncommon but neuropsychiatric complaints related to memory or concentration may occur in as many as 25–50% of patients with a loss of consciousness [11,12].

Differential diagnosis

In suicide attempts, the diagnosis of CO poisoning is generally apparent from the circumstances when the person is found. The major diagnostic issue is whether there is some other deliberate self-poisoning as this is extremely common. In unconscious patients, the ECG, paracetamol concentration and electrolytes should be reviewed with this possibility in mind [6].

A large proportion of victims of smoke inhalation also have cyanide poisoning. This rarely leads to a change in management (due to problems with administering the cyanide antidotes in this setting) but should be suspected when CNS effects are out of proportion with COHb concentrations and if there is a marked lactic acidosis.

Clinical investigations

Blood gases and oximetry

Most pulse oximeters do not attempt to measure COHb but merely the ratio of oxyHb to deoxyHb. Even those that have co-oximeters are not sufficiently accurate to use for either screening or quantification in a hospital setting [13]. Blood gases with a co-oximeter are required to quantify COHb. COHb concentrations (plus or minus a back calculation based on estimated half-life since removal) provide a rough guide to the extent of exposure. However, it is difficult to estimate accurately the oxygen dose received pre-hospital and therefore the half-life. There is also substantial variability between individuals in the extent they are able to compensate for high COHb. Therefore, the correlation with acute and long-term clinical effects is not good. COHb may confirm (or possibly exclude) the diagnosis but should not be used to estimate long-term prognosis.

ECG

Patients should have a baseline ECG (electrocardiogram), repeated 6 h later and ECG monitoring for at least 24 h and cardiac enzymes if the initial ECG is abnormal. The most important signs seen are those of cardiac ischaemia and these are identical to those seen in coronary artery disease.

Biochemistry

Cardiac enzymes should be measured when there is severe clinical toxicity or ECG changes. Metabolic acidosis, predominantly due to lactate will provide an indication of tissue hypoxia. Electrolytes (sodium, potassium, magnesium) should be measured as low concentrations of any of these may exacerbate cardiac toxicity. S100B concentrations (an astroglial structural protein), indicating acute neurological injury, have the potential to be useful in estimating neurological damage as early elevation correlates with long-term morbidity [14–16].

Criteria for diagnosis

A high COHb (>15%) with typical symptoms or signs confirms the diagnosis of acute CO poisoning.

In some parts of the world, it is common to attribute many non-specific presentations to chronic carbon monoxide exposure, often despite COHb concentrations that are normal or within the range of those seen in 'healthy' smokers. There are no agreed on criteria for making a diagnosis of chronic carbon monoxide poisoning, but the diagnosis should not be seriously entertained without confirmation of high ambient CO concentrations in the proposed environmental source.

Treatment

Initial management is directed towards securing the airway and stabilizing respiration and circulation. If there is impaired consciousness, ensure the airway is maintained with intubation if necessary. The comatose patient should be placed on a cardiac monitor, a 12-lead ECG performed, an intravenous line inserted and blood drawn for full blood count, electrolytes, lactate, COHb, blood sugar and cardiac enzymes. If awake, the patient should be reassured and discouraged from activity, for muscle activity will increase oxygen demand [6].

Metabolic acidosis should not be treated directly unless the acidosis itself contributes to toxicity (pH <7.0). It should respond to improved oxygenation and ventilation and the net effect of acidosis on oxygen delivery is probably beneficial.

Oxygen

This decreases the biological half-life substantially from 4 h in ambient air to approximately 40 min in a 100% oxygen atmosphere (Fig. 29.20.1) [6]. One hundred per cent oxygen should be administered with mechanically assisted ventilation if necessary. In patients able to tolerate it, continuous positive airway pressure by mask may allow 100% oxygen delivery without intubation. Four to 6 h of 100% normobaric oxygen will remove over 90% of the carbon monoxide. If the only available oxygen delivery device is a Hudson mask, it should be remembered that at a flow rate of 15 L/min no more than 60% oxygen is delivered. At these concentrations the half-life of CO is still around 90 min and a longer period of oxygen may be required for severe poisonings (Fig. 29.20.1). Oxygen toxicity is unlikely with less than 24 h treatment but the risk increases with increasing exposure.

When immediately available, hyperbaric oxygen (HBO) should be considered for patients

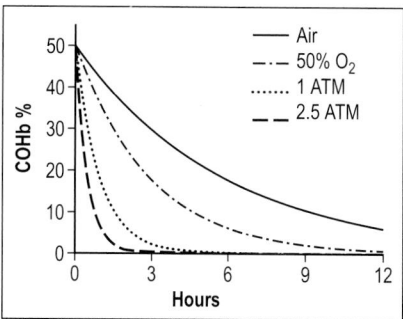

Fig. 29.20.1 Approximate decline in COHb from 50% according to the inspired oxygen concentration and pressure.

with serious CO poisoning. Oxygen at 2–3 atmospheres will further reduce the half-life of COHb to about 20 min (see Fig. 29.20.1) but, more importantly, it causes very rapid reversal of tissue hypoxia due to oxygenation of tissue from oxygen dissolved in the plasma.

Controversy exists on the benefits, risks and indications for HBO (see Controversies below). Indications for HBO commonly used by hyperbaric facilities are simply those factors that indicate a higher risk of long-term neuropsychiatric sequelae [11,12]. These include:

- loss of consciousness at anytime during or following exposure
- abnormal neuropsychiatric testing or neurological signs
- pregnancy.

Complications of HBO therapy [11,12] include:

- decompression sickness
- rupture of tympanic membranes
- damaged sinuses
- oxygen toxicity
- problems due to lack of monitoring.

Follow up

As well as psychiatric follow up for all patients who have been poisoned with CO due to self-harm, patients should have a neuropsychiatric follow up at 1–2 months to evaluate any long-term neuropsychiatric injury.

Other treatments

Animal models suggest possible benefits from use of allopurinol and N-acetylcysteine to protect against oxidative damage during hypoxic/

reperfusion injury [17]. Numerous experimental (i.e. never used in humans) agents have also been suggested. Their use cannot be recommended outside of clinical trials; however, they may be a more logical treatment to prevent neurological damage from reactive oxygen species than hyperbaric oxygen.

Controversies

- The major controversy is about the benefits, risks and indications for HBO—and resolving this 'clinical uncertainty' with further trials will likely be frustrated by some extremely certain HBO clinicians [18]. There have been eight HBO randomized clinical trials (RCTs) reporting very conflicting outcomes. Some have concluded that HBO is harmful [19,20] and others that it is beneficial [21]. Systematic reviews have found no evidence for benefit from combined analysis of the trials [11,12]. They also find empiric evidence of multiple biases that operated to inflate the benefit of HBO in two positive trials. In contrast, the interpretation of negative trials was hampered by low rates of follow up, unusual interventions for control patients and inclusion of less severely poisoned patients.
- In centres with a chamber, the use of HBO, when it can be given rapidly and safely, may be justifiable based on the biological rationale that it is the most efficient means of rapidly increasing oxygen delivery and removing carbon monoxide. However, transferring patients between hospitals for delayed use of HBO, particularly over long distances, is not justifiable on current evidence from RCTs, animal studies [22,23] or the known pathophysiology of CO.
- The use of measuring S110B protein in the assessment of prognosis of these patients.

References

[1] Weaver LK. Carbon monoxide poisoning. Crit Care Clin 1999;15:297–317.
[2] Seger D, Welch L. Carbon monoxide controversies: neuropsychologic testing, mechanism of toxicity, and hyperbaric oxygen. Ann Emerg Med 1994;24:242–8.
[3] Hampson NB. Emergency department visits for carbon monoxide poisoning in the Pacific Northwest. J Emerg Med 1998;16:695–8.
[4] Amos T, Appleby L, Kiernan K. Changes in rates of suicide by car exhaust asphyxiation in England and Wales. Psychol Med 2001;31:935–9.
[5] Mott JA, Wolfe MI, Alverson CJ, et al. National vehicle emissions policies and practices and declining US carbon monoxide-related mortality. J Am Med Assoc 2002;288:988–95.
[6] Buckley, NA, Dawson AH, Whyte IM. Hypertox. Assessment and treatment of poisoning. <www.hypertox.comwww.wikitox.com>; 2012. [Accessed Aug. 2012].
[7] Lippi G, Rastelli G, Meschi T, et al. Pathophysiology, clinics, diagnosis and treatment of carbon monoxide poisoning. Clin Biochem 2012;45:1278–85.
[8] Ahn KT, Park JH, Kim MS, et al. Prevalence and clinical outcomes of left ventricular systolic dysfunction after carbon monoxide exposure. Int J Cardiol 2011;153:108–10.
[9] Henry CR, Satran D, Lindgren B, et al. Myocardial injury and long-term mortality following moderate to severe carbon monoxide poisoning. J Am Med Assoc 2006;295:398–402.
[10] Pepe G, Castelli M, Nazerian P, et al. Delayed neuropsychological sequelae after carbon monoxide poisoning: predictive risk factors in the Emergency Department. A retrospective study. Scand J Trauma Resusc Emerg Med 2011;19:16.
[11] Buckley NA, Isbister GK, Stokes B, Juurlink DN. Hyperbaric oxygen for carbon monoxide poisoning: a systematic review and critical analysis of the evidence. Toxicol Rev 2005;24:75–92.
[12] Buckley NA, Juurlink DN, Isbister G, et al. Hyperbaric oxygen for carbon monoxide poisoning. Cochrane Database Syst Rev 2011:CD002041.
[13] Touger M, Birnbaum A, Wang J, et al. Performance of the RAD-57 pulse co-oximeter compared with standard laboratory carboxyhemoglobin measurement. Ann Emerg Med 2010;56:382–8.
[14] Park E, Ahn J, Min YG, et al. The usefulness of the serum s100b protein for predicting delayed neurological sequelae in acute carbon monoxide poisoning. Clin Toxicol (Phila) 2012;50:183–8.
[15] Ide T, Kamijo Y, Ide A, et al. Elevated S100B level in cerebrospinal fluid could predict poor outcome of carbon monoxide poisoning. Am J Emerg Med 2012;30:222–5.
[16] Brvar M, Mozina H, Osredkar J, et al. S100B protein in carbon monoxide poisoning: a pilot study. Resuscitation 2004;61:357–60.
[17] Omaye ST. Metabolic modulation of carbon monoxide toxicity. Toxicology 2002;180:139–50.
[18] Buckley NA, Isbister GK, Juurlink DN. Hyperbaric oxygen for carbon monoxide poisoning: evidence versus opinion. Toxicol Rev 2005;24:159–60.
[19] Scheinkestel CD, Bailey M, Myles PS, et al. Hyperbaric or normobaric oxygen for acute carbon monoxide poisoning: a randomised controlled clinical trial. Med J Aust 1999;170:203–10.
[20] Annane D, Chadda K, Gajdos P, et al. Hyperbaric oxygen therapy for acute domestic carbon monoxide poisoning: two randomized controlled trials. Intens Care Med 2011;37:486–92.
[21] Weaver LK, Hopkins RO, Chan KJ, et al. Hyperbaric oxygen for acute carbon monoxide poisoning. N Engl J Med 2002;347:1057–67.
[22] Bunc M, Luzar B, Finderle Z, et al. Immediate oxygen therapy prevents brain cell injury in carbon monoxide poisoned rats without loss of consciousness. Toxicology 2006;225:138–41.
[23] Brvar M, Finderle Z, Suput D, Bunc M. S100B protein in conscious carbon monoxide-poisoned rats treated with normobaric or hyperbaric oxygen. Crit Care Med 2006;34:2228–30.

30.1 Snakebite

Geoffrey Isbister

ESSENTIALS

1 Australia has a number of medically important venomous snakes. All are elapids (front-fanged). New Zealand has no snakes of medical importance.

2 All patients giving a history of possible snakebite should be assessed and observed for at least 12 h to rule out envenoming.

3 Most fatalities occur within hours of the bite from initial cardiac arrest and multiorgan failure. Delayed deaths are now uncommon and mainly due to major haemorrhage from the venom-induced consumption coagulopathy.

4 Pressure bandaging and immobilization (PBI) is the recommended first aid and should be applied early.

5 Australian snakes are difficult to identify and treatment should be guided by the possible snakes based on geography and the clinical syndrome and expert snake identification if available. Snake venom detection kit is used to identify which antivenom to use and results should not over-rule clinical judgement.

6 Antivenom is indicated for all patients with clinical or laboratory evidence of envenoming. CSL Ltd makes antivenoms against all important terrestrial snakes, as well as a polyvalent antivenom containing antivenoms to all five.

7 Antivenom should be given early and then sufficient time allowed for recovery, especially venom-induced consumption coagulopathy which takes 6–18 h to show recovery.

8 The dose of all snake antivenoms is one vial and repeat doses are never required. Further laboratory testing is only required to determine when patients have recovered and can be discharged.

9 CSL antivenom contains horse-derived F(ab′)$_2$ antibodies and is associated with systemic hypersensitivity reactions in about 20% of cases, although severe anaphylaxis occurs in less than 5%. Premedication is not recommended but adrenaline should be immediately available for treatment of anaphylaxis.

Introduction

Australia has a number of venomous snakes with some of the most potent venoms in the world. All the medically important snakes are elapids (front-fanged), although bites rarely occur from colubrids and non-venomous snakes. New Zealand has no snakes of medical importance. The risk of significant coagulopathy and uncommonly death, even after apparently trivial contact with Australian snakes, remains and must be appreciated by healthcare workers [1].

Epidemiology

It is thought that approximately 3000 suspected snakebites occur annually in Australia, but this figure is difficult to estimate and depends on how many suspected bites, non-venomous bites and non-envenomed cases are included. The number of envenomed cases is far less and probably in the order of 100–200 each year; the majority of which occur in rural and regional areas. Snakebite deaths continue to occur (about 1–5 per year) and are usually a result of early cardiac arrest in brown snakebites or major haemorrhage in coagulopathic patients [1].

Table 30.1.1   Clinical syndromes associated with the major venomous Australian snakes and the recommended antivenom

Snake	Coagulopathy	Neurotoxicity	Myotoxicity	Systemic symptoms	Thrombotic microangiopathy	Cardiovascular effects	Antivenom
Brown snake	VICC[1]	Rare and mild	–	<50%	10%	Collapse (25%) Cardiac arrest (5%)	Brown snake
Tiger snake group							
Tiger snake	VICC	Uncommon	Uncommon	Common	5%	Rare	Tiger snake
Rough-scale snake	VICC	Uncommon	Uncommon	Common	<5%	Rare	Tiger snake
Hoplocephalus spp.[2]	VICC	–	–	<50%	–	–	Tiger or brown snake
Black snakes							
Mulga snake	Anticoagulant	–	Common	Common	–	–	Black snake[3]
Red-bellied black snake	Anticoagulant	–	Uncommon	Common	–	–	Tiger snake[4]
Death adder	–	Common	–	Common	–	–	Death Adder[3]
Taipan	VICC	Common	Rare	Common	5%	Uncommon	Taipan[3]

[1]VICC: venom-induced consumption coagulopathy;
[2]The Hoplocephalus genus/group includes Stephen's banded snake (H. stephensi), the broad headed snake (H. bungaroides) and the pale-headed snake (H. bitorquatus);
[3]Polyvalent antivenom can be substituted for these large volume monovalent antivenom with no increase in risk or cost;
[4]Polyvalent or tiger snake antivenom cannot be used for sea snake envenoming.

The commonest clinical manifestation is coagulopathy which occurs in about three-quarters of envenomed cases, the majority in brown snake bites [2]. Neurotoxicity and myotoxicity are now uncommon and mechanical ventilation is rarely required for treatment [2]. The types of snakes causing major envenoming differ across Australia. Bites in snake handlers remain an important problem with about 10% of all bites being in snake handlers. However, they are almost all bites from Australian snakes, albeit the more uncommon and interesting snakes and exotic snakebite is very rare [3]. Although snake handlers often want to avoid antivenom, they should be treated like anyone else because there is little evidence to support they are at higher risk of antivenom reactions. Snake handlers and people working with snake venoms can develop systemic hypersensitivity reactions to venom itself, so venom anaphylaxis must be a differential diagnosis in these patients [3].

Prevention

Most snakebites are preventable and result from snake handling or interference with snakes in the wild, sometimes in the setting of alcohol consumption. Ideally, snakes should be left alone and those working with or keeping snakes should have appropriate training and licences. Simple precautions, such as wearing thick long pants and boots when walking in the bush or when working with snakes, can prevent most bites due to the short length of Australian elapid fangs. Snake handlers should carry and maintain first-aid kits that include at least four broad elastic bandages (15 cm; e.g. Ace) and have practised applying the bandage. If exotic snakes are being held, including Australasian snakes out of their geographical distribution, appropriate antivenoms should be available.

Clinical features

Systemic envenoming results when venom is injected subcutaneously and reaches the systemic circulation. Whether or not a snakebite results in systemic envenoming depends on a number of factors including fang length, average venom yield of the snake, effectiveness of the bite and bite site. Recent studies have suggested that only a small amount of the injected venom actually reaches the systemic circulation [1,4]. Most snakebites do not result in envenoming because either insufficient venom reaches the systemic circulation or the snake is non-venomous.

Envenoming is characterized by local and systemic effects, although Australasian elapids rarely cause major local effects, such as necrosis and local haemorrhage. The clinical features of envenoming depend on the particular toxins present in each snake's venom but non-specific systemic symptoms (nausea, vomiting, headache, abdominal pain, diarrhoea and diaphoresis) occur in many cases. The major clinical syndromes are coagulopathy, neurotoxicity, myotoxicity and acute kidney injury [2]. Severe envenoming can result in early collapse associated with dizziness, loss of consciousness, apnoea and hypotension [1]. In the majority of cases, there is spontaneous recovery over 5–15 min but, in some case, this does not occur and multiorgan failure and death ensue if resuscitation is delayed [1].

The medically important Australian snakes and their associated clinical effects are listed in Table 30.1.1.

Coagulopathy

Venom-induced consumption coagulopathy (VICC)

This is the commonest and most important clinical effect in Australian snake envenoming. Venom-induced consumption coagulopathy (VICC) results from a prothrombin activator in the snake venom converting prothrombin (Factor II) to thrombin which leads to consumption of Factors V, VIII and fibrinogen, associated with a massive increase in fibrinogen degradation products [5]. Most dangerous Australian snakes contain such a prothrombin activator including brown snakes, snakes in the tiger snake group and taipans [5]. VICC develops rapidly within 15–60 min and the onset may coincide with the initial collapse seen with major envenoming by brown snakes and taipans [1]. Recovery usually takes 12–18 h [5].

Anticoagulant coagulopathy

Anticoagulant coagulopathy occurs in black snake envenoming, including mulga and red-bellied black snakes and is characterized by an abnormal activated partial thromboplastin time (aPTT) [6,7]. It is unlikely to result in haemorrhage and of itself is rarely of clinical importance. However, anticoagulant coagulopathy is a useful marker of envenoming and is rapidly reversed with antivenom [6].

Neurotoxicity

Paralysis is a classic effect of snakebite and is due to mainly presynaptic neurotoxins that occur in almost all Australian elapids. Presynaptic neurotoxins disrupt neurotransmitter release from the terminal axon and are associated with cellular damage. This type of neurotoxicity does not respond to antivenom treatment and may take days to weeks to resolve in severe cases. Neurotoxic envenoming manifests as a progressive descending flaccid paralysis. The first sign is usually ptosis followed by facial and bulbar involvement and progressing to paralysis of the extraocular muscles, respiratory muscles and peripheral weakness in severe cases.

Myotoxicity

Some Australian snakes contain myotoxins that cause damage to skeletal muscles resulting in local and/or generalized muscle pain, tenderness and weakness, associated with a rapidly rising creatine kinase and myoglobinuria. In rare severe cases, secondary renal impairment can occur.

Renal toxicity

Renal impairment or acute kidney injury can occur in association with thrombotic microangiopathy, secondary to severe myolysis or, more rarely and to a minor degree, in isolation with brown snake envenoming. Thrombotic microangiopathy occurs in snakebites associated with VICC and is characterized by severe thrombocytopaenia worse 3–4 days after the bite,

acute renal failure that may last 2–8 weeks and require dialysis and microangiopathic haemolytic anaemia [8]. It is most common with brown snake envenoming, but also reported with all snakes that cause VICC.

Local effects

Local effects vary from minimal effects with brown snakebites to local pain, swelling and, occasionally, tissue injury following black and tiger snakebites.

Most fatalities occur within hours of the bite from initial cardiac arrest and multiorgan failure [1]. Delayed deaths are now uncommon and mainly due to major haemorrhage from VICC in brown snake, tiger snake group or taipan envenoming. Respiratory failure from neurotoxicity remains a problem in Papua New Guinea where there continue to be large numbers of cases, mainly taipan bites, and a shortage of both antivenom and resources for mechanical ventilation.

Treatment

First aid

Australian snake venoms appear to be absorbed via the lymphatic system so absorption is likely to be increased by movement and exercise. The aim of first aid is to minimize movement of venom to the systemic circulation. This is achieved by a pressure bandage (elastic bandage, such as ACE) being applied over the bite site and then covering the whole limb with a similar pressure to that used for a limb sprain. The bitten limb must be immobilized as well as the whole patient or the first aid is ineffective. Immobilization consists of splinting and complete prevention of movement or exercise of the bitten part. It has been shown that movement of all limbs, not just the affected one, needs to be minimized for optimal effect [9]. Transport should be brought to the patient and walking must be avoided. Pressure bandaging is clearly impractical for bites that are not on the limbs but direct pressure with a pad and immobilization may be useful.

First aid must eventually be removed but this should take place in a resuscitation area of a facility with the means definitively to treat envenoming. The first aid is removed when:

- thorough clinical and laboratory assessment fail to demonstrate any evidence of envenoming. In these patients, further clinical and laboratory evaluation for

suspected envenoming is needed following removal of the bandage
- there is definite clinical or laboratory evidence of envenoming. The bandage is removed after the completion of treatment with intravenous antivenom.

Initial assessment and treatment

Figure 30.1.1 provides a simple approach to the management of suspected and envenomed snakebite patients. The patient is managed in an area with full resuscitation facilities. Assessment and management proceed simultaneously. The airway, breathing and circulation are assessed and stabilized. The majority of patients are not critically unwell and can have a focused neurological examination for early signs of paralysis (e.g. ptosis, drooling), examination of draining lymph nodes and general examination for signs of bleeding (oozing from the bite site, gum bleeds). Intravenous access should be established and intravenous fluids commenced.

Further management

Two major diagnostic and risk assessment issues exist for snakebite:

- whether or not the patient is envenomed
- in patients with envenoming, which snake is responsible and therefore which antivenom should be administered.

The majority of patients are not envenomed, but all patients must initially be assessed as if they are potentially envenomed. Asymptomatic patients, particularly those seen early after a brown snakebite, may still be severely envenomed with VICC. The diagnosis of envenoming is made on history, examination and the clinical investigations listed below. Although systemic envenoming can be ambiguous in patients with mild envenoming, the following definitions are useful for determining whether patients require antivenom:

- VICC is defined as an elevated international normalized ratio (INR) or prothrombin time (PT) associated with an elevated D-dimer. A low or unrecordable fibrinogen will also occur but is not required for the diagnosis. In the majority of cases, there is complete consumption with unrecordable PT/INR, aPTT and undetectable fibrinogen and the decision to give antivenom is straightforward. Milder forms of coagulopathy may occur with elevated D-dimer and only minimally elevated INR.

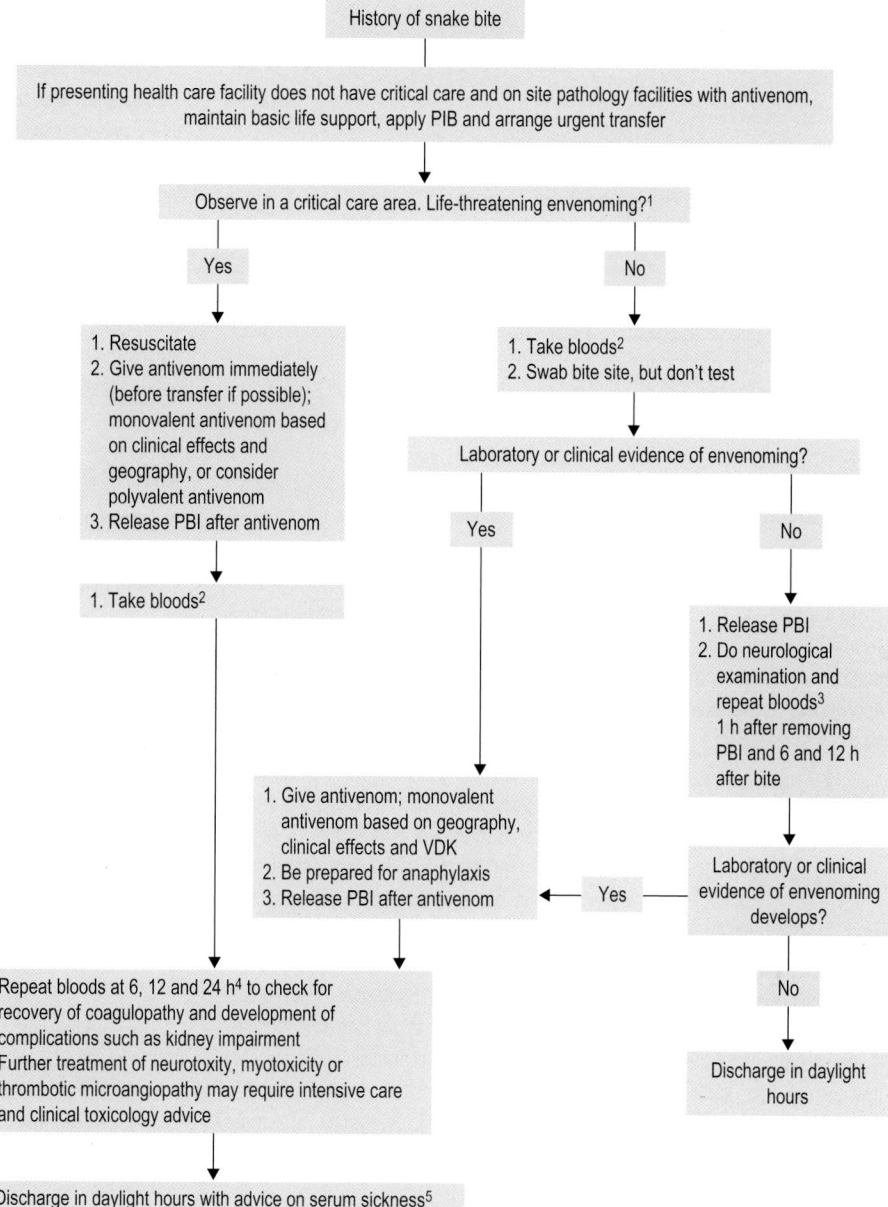

Fig. 30.1.1 Early management of snakebite *(from Therapeutic Guidelines Emergency Medicine, July 2012 with permission)* . [1]A toxicologist can be contacted at anytime via the Poison Information Centre 131126. [2]Cardiac arrest, respiratory failure secondary to paralysis or major haemorrhage (intracranial, major gastrointestinal or other life-threatening bleeding). [3]Blood tests include: coagulation tests (INR/PT, aPTT, D-dimer, fibrinogen), FBC and blood film for fragments red cells, EUC, CK and LDH. [4]Any improvement in coagulation studies, such as measurable but still abnormal aPTT or PT after 6 h, is sufficient evidence of resolving coagulopathy. Neurotoxicity and myotoxicity are usually irreversible and further antivenom is unlikely to help. [5]Any patient given antivenom needs advice on discharge about possibility of serum sickness occurring 4 to 14 days later. PBI: pressure bandaging immobilization; INR: international normalized ratio; ED: emergency department.

Antivenom is still indicated in most cases but these can be discussed with a clinical toxicologist.

- Neurotoxicity is defined as at least ptosis, but may progress without antivenom to include bulbar palsy, extraocular ophthalmoplegia, respiratory muscle paralysis and limb paralysis.
- Myotoxicity is defined as local or generalized myalgia and/or muscle weakness in association with an elevated creatine kinase (CK >1000 IU).
- Non-specific symptoms include nausea, vomiting, abdominal pain, diarrhoea, diaphoresis and headache and may, in some cases, be an indication for antivenom depending on the type of snake.

Table 30.1.2 provides a list of relative and absolute contraindications for antivenom which can be discussed with a clinical toxicologist if there is any doubt. If there is no evidence of envenoming after clinical assessment and initial laboratory testing, the first-aid bandage can be removed. The patient requires ongoing close observation including repeated investigations 1 h after bandage removal and at 6 and 12 h after the bite (see Fig. 30.1.1).

If the patient is envenomed, then management must proceed with antivenom. A small

Table 30.1.2 Absolute and relative indications for antivenom
Absolute indications
History of sudden collapse, cardiac arrest or seizure An abnormal INR Evidence of paralysis with ptosis and/or ophthalmoplegia being the earliest signs
Relative indications: (suggest consultation with clinical toxicologist)
Systemic symptoms (vomiting, headache, abdominal pain) Abnormal aPTT Creatinine kinase >1000 U/L Leucocytosis/lymphopaenia

number of patients present in extremis, usually following collapse and in cardiac arrest and should have antivenom administered immediately as part of advanced life support.

The next step is to determine the snake group responsible for envenoming in order to allow the administration of the appropriate monovalent antivenom. This is done taking into account:

- local geographical information on the potential snake species that could be responsible
- clinical syndrome (see Table 30.1.1).

In the majority of cases, a combination of these two factors allows determination of the correct monovalent snake antivenom required. In some cases, an expert may be available to identify the snake. If the snake type cannot be determined based on geography and clinical syndrome, a snake venom detection kit (SVDK) may assist in identifying the snake. However, the results of an SVDK cannot be used in isolation from the geography, expert snake identification or clinical syndrome. If it is unclear which snake is involved then one vial of polyvalent antivenom should be administered or two vials of monovalent in regions (e.g. Victoria) where this will cover all medically important snakes – most commonly brown and tiger snake antivenoms. In Tasmania, only tiger snake antivenom is required.

Administration of antivenom

Snake antivenom should be administered by the intravenous route after being diluted 1 in 10 with normal saline and administered over 15 min. In patients with cardiac arrest or life-threatening effects, undiluted antivenom may be administered as a slow intravenous bolus. The dose of antivenom is one vial for all Australian snakes and the dose for children is the same as adults. Recovery is determined by the reversibility of effects and the time it takes for recovery once venom is neutralized. Repeat doses of antivenom are never required. Although there has been controversy over the dose of antivenom, recent studies have demonstrated that previously recommended large doses are not required [1,10].

Premedication for snake antivenom administration has previously been controversial but is no longer recommended in Australia. A recent randomized controlled trial has suggested that adrenaline is an effective premedication for snake antivenom [11], but this is more appropriate in resource poor settings where the risk of reactions is higher. Systemic hypersensitivity reactions occur in about one-fifth of antivenom administrations in Australia, but are only severe (mainly hypotension) in less than 5% of administrations [2,3]. Reactions are more common with tiger snake antivenom and polyvalent antivenom compared to brown snake antivenom [2,3]. Antivenom should always be administered in a critical care area with readily available adrenaline, intravenous fluids and resuscitation equipment.

The frequency of delayed-type reactions to antivenom or serum sickness is probably higher than acute reactions and likely to depend on the amount of horse protein administered. All patients given antivenom should be warned of serum sickness. There is no evidence for the prophylactic use of a course of oral steroids but they should be used for treatment in patients who present with serum sickness (prednisolone 50 mg/day for 5–7 days).

Other treatments

Tetanus prophylaxis should be given as appropriate but local wound care is rarely required with Australasian snakes due to minimal local effects.

A recent randomized controlled trial has shown that the use of fresh frozen plasma (FFP) appears to speed the recovery of VICC [12], but whether the decreased risk of bleeding is large enough to balance the risk of blood products remains unclear. The study also suggested that use of FFP within 6 h of the bite may be associated with a poor response to FFP. Until larger studies are undertaken, FFP should be reserved for patients with coagulopathy and active bleeding.

Clinical investigations

Assessment of the potentially envenomed requires the following investigations to be performed, usually serially:

- coagulation profile: PT or INR, aPTT, cross-linked fibrinogen degradation products or D-dimers and fibrinogen
- full blood count including a blood film looking for fragments, red cells and evidence of haemolysis
- urea, creatinine, electrolytes, creatine kinase (CK) and lactate dehydrogenase
- blood group and cross-match
- snake venom detection kit: a swab should be taken from the bite site
- urinalysis.

Repeat laboratory testing, particularly coagulation studies, should not be used to determine if sufficient antivenom has been given because one vial is sufficient in all cases. Such serial testing should be used to determine when the patient has recovered and can be discharged.

Snake venom detection kit

The SVDK is designed to confirm which major snake group is responsible and therefore which antivenom to give. It does not confirm or exclude envenoming and should only be included in the assessment of envenomed patients after considering geography and clinical/laboratory effects. It is best done by laboratory staff. In non-envenomed patients, the SVDK has a high false-positive rate, especially in the brown snake well and is problematic in regions where brown snakes are uncommon (e.g. Victoria) [10]. A positive SVDK on urine does not indicate systemic toxicity and, in asymptomatic patients with normal laboratory studies, it is a false-positive result. The test should not be done on blood.

Disposition

Patients with suspected snakebite but no evidence of envenoming 1 h after the removal of first aid may be admitted to an observation area. Blood tests including coagulation studies and a CK should be repeated at 1 h after first aid is removed, and 6 and 12 h post-bite and be observed for 12 h or overnight (see Fig. 30.1.1). Envenomed patients requiring ventilatory support should have continued management in ICU, but patients with coagulopathy only are commonly managed in ED observation wards.

Controversies

- Indications for early antivenom therapy to prevent myotoxicity and neurotoxicity.

- Factor replacement appears to speed the recovery of VICC, but whether the decreased risk of bleeding is large enough to balance the risk of blood products remains unclear.

References

[1] Allen GE, Brown SG, Buckley NA, et al. Clinical effects and antivenom dosing in brown snake (*Pseudonaja* spp.) envenoming – Australian Snakebite Project (ASP-14). PLoS One 2012;7:e53188.
[2] Isbister GK, Brown SG, MacDonald E, et al. Current use of Australian snake antivenoms and frequency of immediate-type hypersensitivity reactions and anaphylaxis. Med J Aust 2008;188:473–6.
[3] Isbister GK, Brown SG. Bites in Australian snake handlers – Australian snakebite project (ASP-15). Q J Med 2012;105:1089–95.
[4] Isbister GK, O'Leary MA, Schneider JJ, et al. Efficacy of antivenom against the procoagulant effect of Australian brown snake (*Pseudonaja* sp.) venom: in vivo and in vitro studies. Toxicon 2007;49:57–67.
[5] Isbister GK, Scorgie FE, O'Leary MA, et al. Factor deficiencies in venom-induced consumption coagulopathy resulting from Australian elapid envenomation: Australian Snakebite Project (ASP-10). J Thromb Haemost 2010;8:2504–13.
[6] Churchman A, O'Leary MA, Buckley NA, et al. Clinical effects of red-bellied black snake (*Pseudechis porphyriacus*) envenoming and correlation with venom concentrations: Australian Snakebite Project (ASP-11). Med J Aust 2010;193:696–700.
[7] Johnston CI, Brown SGA, O'Leary MA, et al. Mulga snake (*Pseudechis australis*) envenoming: a spectrum of myotoxicity, anticoagulant coagulopathy, haemolysis and the role of early antivenom therapy – Australian Snakebite Project (ASP-19). Clin Toxicol. Jun 2013;51(5):417–24.
[8] Isbister GK. Snakebite doesn't cause disseminated intravascular coagulation: coagulopathy and thrombotic microangiopathy in snake envenoming. Semin Thromb Hemost 2010;36:444–51.
[9] Howarth DM, Southee AE, Whyte IM. Lymphatic flow rates and first-aid in simulated peripheral snake or spider envenomation. Med J Aust 1994;161:695–700.
[10] Isbister GK, O'Leary MA, Elliott M, et al. Tiger snake (*Notechis* spp) envenoming: Australian Snakebite Project (ASP-13). Med J Aust 2012;197:173–7.
[11] de Silva HA, Pathmeswaran A, Ranasinha CD, et al. Low-dose adrenaline, promethazine, and hydrocortisone in the prevention of acute adverse reactions to antivenom following snakebite: a randomised, double-blind, placebo-controlled trial. PLoS Med 2011;8:e1000435.
[12] Isbister GK, Buckley NA, Page CB, et al. A randomised controlled trial of fresh frozen plasma for treating venom induced consumption coagulopathy in Australian snakebite (ASP-18). J Thromb Haemost. Jul 2013;11(7):1310–8.

30.2 Exotic snakebite

Julian White

ESSENTIALS

1 Exotic snakebite is a growing issue worldwide, especially with the growth in illegally held snakes.

2 Symptoms and signs may be different to those seen in Australian snakebites

3 As many overseas snakes, especially the vipers, cause local tissue destruction and damage, pressure bandage immobilization (PBI) is not recommended

4 Expert advice is available and recommended in managing these cases and helping locate antivenom.

5 Often there is a higher rate of allergic reaction due to overseas antivenom compared to Australian antivenom.

Introduction

The snakebite chapter of this edition is targeted principally at the Australian snakebite experience, but snakebite is a global phenomenon, arguably with >2.5 million cases, >100 000 deaths and >400 000 amputations every year, so Australia accounts for only a tiny fraction of this impact.

Exotic snakebite is a worldwide problem, with increasing seizures by customs of illegally imported snakes and seizures of illegal collections by authorities in countries. Some think that the trade in exotic animals is second only to the illegal trade of drugs and weapons.

Exotic snakebite in Australia is either where an Australian snake species bites a person in a region where this snake is not usually found (e.g. pet taipan bites owner in Hobart), or where a snake, not native to Australia, bites someone in Australia. This chapter will focus on this second scenario.

This topic is vast and beyond the scope of this chapter, but similar management principles may apply. Table 30.2.1 provides a list of selected genera/species, with distribution, clinical effects and major modes of treatment.

Bites by captive non-native (exotic) venomous snakes

At least in 'Western' countries, there is an increasing number and diversity of exotic venomous snakes being kept in captivity, especially in private collections, either legally or often illegally (in Australia only registered zoos can legally keep exotic venomous snakes).

These exotic snakes may cause quite different patterns of envenoming compared to native snakes and, if any antivenom is available, it will be different to local products and may be difficult to obtain. Doctors will likely have no training in how to manage such bites. The person bitten may have limited knowledge of the risks, appropriate first aid and, if the snakes are illegally kept, may be reluctant to seek medical attention, so delayed presentation with resultant more severe

Table 30.2.1 Selected exotic snakes; overview of clinical effects and management

Snake	Distribution[†]	Clinical effects[‡]	Treatment[§]
Family 'Colubridae'[#]			
Boomslang (*Dispholidus typus*)	SSaf	CC, NF, BH, HF	AV, BP, IV, NC
Bird/vine/twig snakes (*Thelotornis* spp.)	SSaf	CC, NF, BH, HF	BP, IV, NC
Keelback & yamakagashi (*Rhabdophis* spp.)	SEAs, EAs	CC, BH, HF	AV, IV, BP
Family Elapidae			
PNG small eyed snake (*Micropechis ikaheka*)	PNG (New Guinea)	PU, M, AC, NF	AV, IV, NC, ST
Bolo (*Ogmodon vitianus*)	PNG (Fiji)	?LS	IV, ST
Bougainville coral snake (*Parapistocalamas hedigeri*)	PNG (Bougainville)	?LS	IV, ST
Solomons coral snake (*Salomonelaps par*)	PNG (Solomon Islands)	?LS	IV, ST
PNG forest snakes (*Toxicocalamus* spp.)	PNG (New Guinea)	?LS	IV, ST
Asian coral snakes (*Calliophis* spp.)	SEAs	PU, RF	IV, ST, AC
Asian spitting cobras (*Naja* spp.)	SEAs, EAs, Ind	PN, SO, LI, HF	AV, IV, LC, AC
Asian cobras (*Naja* spp.)	SEAs, EAs, Ind, As	PN, RF, LI (some)	AV, IV, LC, AC
King cobra (*Ophiophagus hannah*)	SEAs, Ind	PN, RF, LI, HF	AV, IV, LC, AC, ST
Kraits (*Bungarus* spp.)	SEAs, EAs, Ind	PP, PN, RF, M	AV, IV, ST
Desert black snake (*Walterinnesia aegyptia*)	ME, NtAf	PN, RF	ST, IV, ?AV[1]
Water cobras (*Naja* (ex *Boulengerina*) spp.)	SSAf	PN, RF	ST, IV
African spitting cobras (*Naja* spp.)	SSAf, NtAf, ME	SO, LI, PN, HF	AV, IV, LC
African cobras (*Naja* spp.)	SSAf, NtAf, ME	PN, RF, LI (some)	AV, IV, LC, ST, AC?
Mambas (*Dendroaspis* spp.)	SSAf	PD, RF, LI (some)	AV, IV, ST, LC
Rinkhals (*Hemachatus haemachatus*)	SSAf	LI, PN	AV, IV, LC, ST
African coral snakes (*Aspidelaps* spp.)	SSAf	PN, RF	IV, ST, AC?
African garter snakes (*Elapsoidea* spp.)	SSAf	LS	IV, ST
Tree cobras (*Pseudohaje* spp.)	SSAf	LS	IV, ST
Spotted harlequin snakes (*Homoroselaps* spp.)	SSAf	?LS	IV, ST
Burrowing cobra (*Paranaja* spp.)	SSAf	LS	IV, ST
American coral snakes (*Micrurus*, *Leptomicrurus* spp.)	NtAm, CeAm, StAm	PN, PP (some), M, RF	AV, IV, ST
US coral snake (*Micruroides euryxanthus*)	NTAm	PN, RF	IV, ST
Sea snakes (many species)	Indo-Pacific	PN, RF, M, NF	AV, IV, ST, AC, NC
Family Viperidae (Viperinae; old world, non-pit-vipers/adders)			
Russell's vipers (*Daboia* spp.)	SEAs, EAs, Ind	CC, BH, BD, BS, NF, HF, LI, PU, RF, M	AV, IV, ST, LC, NC, BP
Saw scaled vipers (*Echis* spp.)	Ind, WAs, ME, NtAf, SSAf	CC, BH, BD, NF, HF, LI	AV, IV, ST, LC, NC, BP
Horned vipers (*Pseudocerastes* spp.)	ME, WAs	LS, PU?	IV, ST
Horned vipers (*Cerastes* spp.)	ME, NtAf	LI, CC, BH, NF, HF	AV, IV, ST, LC, NC, BP
Puff & Gaboon adders (*Bitis* spp.)	SSAf, NtAf	LI, HF, BD	AV, IV, ST, LC
Berg adders (*Bitis atropos*, etc.)	SSAf	LI, HF, PU, RF	IV, ST, LC
Night adders (*Causus* spp.)	SSAf, NtAf	LS, PU	IV, ST, LC

(Continued)

Table 30.2.1 (Continued)

Snake	Distribution[†]	Clinical effects[‡]	Treatment[§]
Bush vipers (*Atheris*, *Montatheris*, *Proatheris* spp.)	SSAf	LS, CC, HF	AV[2], IV, ST, LC, BP
McMahon's viper (*Eristocophis mcmahoni*)	WAs, ME	LI, HF, PU?	IV, ST, LC
Barbour's bush viper (*Adenorhinos barbouri*)	SSAf	LS	IV, ST
Fea's viper (*Azemiops feae*)	EAs, SEAs, As	LS	IV, ST
European adders (*Vipera*, *Macrovipera* spp.)	NtAf, EU, ME, As	LI, CC, HF, BD, PU	AV, IV, ST, LC, BP
Family Viperidae (Crotalinae; pit vipers)			
Copperhead, cottonmouth, cantils (*Agkistrodon* spp.)	NtAm, CeAm	LI, CC, HF, BD, NF	AV, IV, ST, LC
Jumping vipers (*Atropoides* spp.)	CeAm	LS, HF	IV, ST, LC
Lancehead vipers (*Bothrops* spp.)	StAm, CeAm	LI, HF, CC, BD, NF, LA, RF, DV (Caribbean spp.)	AV, IV, ST, LC, NC
Palm pit vipers (*Bothriechis* spp.)	CeAm	LI, HF, BD	AV, IV, ST, LC, NC
Malayan pit viper (*Calloselasma rhodostoma*)	SEAs	LI, HF, CC, BH, BD, NF	AV, IV, ST, LC, NC
Montane pit vipers (*Cerriphidion* spp.)	CeAm	LI, HF, BD	AV, IV, ST, LC, NC
North American rattlesnakes (*Crotalus* spp.)	NtAm	LI, HF, CC, BH, BD, NF, PP & RF (few spp.)	AV, IV, ST, LC, NC, BP
South American rattlesnakes (*Crotalus* spp.)	CeAm, StAm	CC, BH, M, PP, RF, NF	AV, IV, ST, NC
Hundred pace viper (*Deinagkistrodon acutus*)	EAs	LI, HF, BD, NF	AV, IV, ST, LC, NC
Mamushis, etc (*Gloydius* spp.)	EAs, SEAs	LI, HF, CC, BD, PU, RF, M, NF	AV, IV, ST, LC, NC
Hump nosed vipers (*Hypnale* spp.)	Ind	LI, HF, CC, BH, NF	IV, ST, LC, NC
Bushmaster (*Lachesis* spp.)	CeAm, StAm	LI, HF, CC, BH, BD	AV, IV, ST, LC
Horned pit viper (*Ophryacus* spp.)	CeAm	LI, HF	IV, ST, LC
Montane pit vipers (*Porthidium* spp.)	CeAm	LI, HF	IV, ST, LC
Habus (*Protobothrops* spp.)	EAs, Ind	LI, HF, CC, BH, BD	AV, IV, ST, LC, NC
Pygmy rattlesnakes (*Sistrurus* spp.)	NtAm	LI, HF, CC, BD	AV, IV, ST, LC
Green tree vipers (*Trimeresurus* spp. incorporating spp. variously assigned to the genera *Ovophis*, *Crypteletrops*, *Popeia*, *Parias*, *Viridovipera*, *Himalayophis*, *Peltopelor*)	SEAs, EAs, Ind	(varies significantly between species) LI, HF, CC, BH, BD, NF	AV, IV, ST, LC, NC, BP
Temple pit vipers (*Tropidolaemus* spp.)	SEAs, Ind	LI, HF	IV, ST, LC
Mount Mang pit viper (*Protobothrops* (ex *Zhaoermia*) *mangshanensis*)	EAs	LI, HF	IV, ST, LC

The Australian snake fauna is not listed here (see previous chapter).

#The former snake family 'Colubridae' is actually an assemblage of several distinct families, some members of which have glands producing toxins (arguably 'venom' in some cases) and some of these have enlarged teeth ('fangs' in some cases), usually towards the rear of the mouth ('back-fanged' or, more correctly, 'non-front-fanged').

[1]No specific antivenom available, but some report South African Vaccine Producers polyvalent may be helpful in severe *Walterinnesia* bites.

[2]No specific antivenom available, but some report South African Vaccine Producers anti-*Echis* may be helpful in severe *Atheris* bites.

[†]Key to distribution: (Note: distribution is based on region and does not imply a given snake is either common or is found throughout the region; it may have limited distribution within the region.) NtAm: North America; CeAm: Central America; StAm: South America; SSAf: Sub-Saharan Africa; NtAf: North Africa; Eur: Europe; ME: Middle East; Ind: Indian region; SEAs: South East Asia; EAs: Eastern Asia (China, Japan, Korea, etc.); PNG: New Guinea & adjacent Pacific; Aus: Australia; WAs: Western Asia; As: rest of Asia.

[‡]Key to clinical effects: (Note: listed clinical effects are based on best available information but, in some cases, very little information is available and, for these snakes, it should be considered a 'best guess' to guide care, not definitive.) PP: presynaptic flaccid paralysis; PN: postsynaptic flaccid paralysis; PD: pre- & postsynaptic synergistic paralysis & fasciculation (mambas); PU: flaccid paralysis, unspecified toxin types; RF: respiratory failure; M: myolysis; CC: consumptive coagulopathy; AC: anticoagulant coagulopathy; DV: thrombosis & DVTs, etc.; BH: coagulopathy-based bleeding; BD: haemorrhagin-based bleeding; BS: anterior pituitary infarction/hypopituitarism; NF: renal damage/failure; HF: haemodynamic problems, shock; SO: venom spit ophthalmia; LI: local tissue injury/necrosis; LS: local swelling, not necrosis; LA: local abscess formation.

[§]Key to treatment: AV: antivenom available (for details of available antivenoms see www.toxinology.com); LC: local wound care essential (necrosis or abscess potential); BP: consider blood products as replacement in consumptive coagulopathy – if antivenom available ensure adequate antivenom given first; IV: ensure adequate IV fluid hydration, watch for & treat shock (mostly hypovolaemic); NC: particular risk of renal damage; ensure good hydration, renal output, strict fluid balance charting; AC: postsynaptic only flaccid paralysis may respond to neostigmine + atropine, if antivenom delayed or unavailable; ST: supportive treatment; may include intubation & ventilation for respiratory paralysis.

complications is common. In contrast, bites occurring in legal collections, such as in zoos, are likely to present early, with correct first aid and appropriate antivenom immediately available.

Exotic venom activity

The mix of venom toxins and corresponding clinical effects varies with species of snake, but can include one or more of: (1) paralytic neurotoxins (pre- and/or postsynaptic); (2) myotoxins (local or systemic); (3) toxins decreasing blood coagulability (many mechanisms; procoagulant, fibrin(ogen)olytic, anticoagulant, antiplatelet, etc); (4) toxins promoting clotting (cause deep vein thromboses [DVTs], etc; notably selected Caribbean pit-vipers); (5) haemorrhagins (damage vascular endothelium, promote bleeding); (6) nephrotoxins; (7) cardiotoxins; (8) local necrotoxins (cause severe local tissue injury/necrosis).

First aid

Many non-Australian venomous snakes can cause moderate to severe local effects around the bite site, including blistering, swelling, bleeding and skin necrosis (many vipers and pit-vipers, some cobras, especially spitting species) and, for these, the Australian pressure bandage and immobilization (PBI) is not recommended as it may worsen local tissue injury. Simple immobilization of the bitten limb is recommended.

For those snakes which do not cause significant local tissue injury (sea snakes, kraits, some mambas, coral snakes, South American rattlesnakes, a few other pit-vipers), the Australian PBI first aid is recommended.

Venom spit ophthalmia

Some African and Asian cobras can accurately spit venom over several metres and commonly aim for the eye. This can cause severe eye pain, corneal damage and potentially permanent blindness, but systemic envenoming does not occur. Treatment is copious irrigation of the eye, slit-lamp examination for corneal injury, standard treatment for non-infective corneal ulceration (if present) and analgesia. Topical adrenaline drops are reported as effective analgesia if standard treatments prove inadequate. Antivenom is not recommended.

Approach to hospital management

All cases should be managed as high priority and early expert clinical toxinologist advice sought (in Australia, the Toxinology Unit, Women's & Children's Hospital, Adelaide or the Australian Poisons Information Centres on ph: 131126). Provide early IV hydration, particularly important in bites by necrosis-causing species where massive fluid shifts into the bitten limb can cause shock and secondary renal failure.

Urgently assess for coagulation status, renal function, myolysis, flaccid paralysis (ptosis common early sign), haemodynamic status (beware hypovolaemic shock) and active major bleeding.

Antivenom use

The use of and dose of antivenom will vary depending on snake species, extent of envenoming and other patient-specific factors. Providing details of which antivenoms to use for bites by particular snakes is beyond the scope of this chapter (www.toxinology.com provides information on antivenoms for particular species).

A snake keeper at risk of future bites should not be given antivenom for minor envenoming, in most cases, as it may needlessly sensitize them, but this concern should never inhibit antivenom use if major envenoming is developing, because the earlier antivenom is given, once indicated, the more likely it will be effective.

All snake antivenoms should be given IV, preferably diluted. Adrenaline and resuscitation should be immediately available in case of adverse reactions. If an adverse reaction occurs, stop the antivenom infusion, control the reaction using a standard anaphylaxis protocol and then consider cautiously restarting the antivenom, as it is likely still needed.

Some antivenoms suggest in their PI that a pretreatment skin sensitivity test be performed. This is an outdated, useless and dangerous test and should not be performed.

Non-antivenom treatments

Some species capable of causing severe envenoming have no suitable antivenom available, so treatment must be supportive and secondary only. An example is certain 'colubrid' rear-fanged snakes that can cause lethal consumptive coagulopathy, where haemodynamic support and, in selected cases, use of blood products may be required. In general, antivenom is preferred to blood products in treating major coagulopathy but, if there is active severe bleeding, then blood products may be appropriate once adequate antivenom has been given (where available), otherwise blood product use is determined on a case-by-case basis based on clinical circumstances.

For some species causing postsynaptic only flaccid paralysis, if antivenom is unavailable or delayed, consider using neostigmine (+ atropine) to temper the severity of paralysis, as a short-term measure (does not replace antivenom); may be helpful in selected sea snake and cobra bites, but applicability to other neurotoxic species is less certain. This treatment will not work for predominantly presynaptic paralysis.

For species causing local tissue injury in the bitten limb, in addition to preventing shock and controlling bleeding, good wound care is important. Swelling and pain may be severe and suggest compartment syndrome, but beware of injudicious fasciotomy as this can cause long-term loss of function, severe bleeding and a risk of secondary infection. Only perform fasciotomy as a last resort in cases where compartment syndrome is confirmed by pressure measurement (commonly for pressures exceeding 35–40 mm/Hg). The role of limited digit fasciotomy for bites to fingers is unclear, but some experts suggest it may reduce incidence of later digit amputation; this is currently unproven.

Further Reading

Clinical Toxicology Resources Website. <www.toxinology.com>.
Dart RC, editor. Medical toxicology (3rd ed.). Philadelphia: Lippincott Williams &Wilkins; 2004.
Guidelines for the prevention and clinical management of snakebite in Africa. Brazzaville: World Health Organization ROA; 2010.
Meier J, White J, editors. Handbook of clinical toxicology of animal venoms and poisons. Boca Raton: CRC Press; 1995.
Warrell DA. Guidelines for the management of snakebites (in South East Asia). Bangkok: World Health Organization SEARO; 2010.

30.3 Spider bite

Geoffrey Isbister

ESSENTIALS

1 Australasia has a number of venomous spiders but the majority of bites cause only minor problems.

2 Fatalities have been recorded in Australia after bites by the redback and the funnel-web spiders (FWS).

3 Redback spider (a widow spider) bite is the most common cause of medically significant human envenoming in Australia. It can cause severe and persistent pain and, less often, systemic effects.

4 Australia appears to have the highest rate of widow spider envenoming (latrodectism) in the world.

5 Funnel-web spider bite can cause life-threatening neurotoxic envenoming.

6 Redback antivenom is a horse-derived F(ab′)$_2$ antivenom and causes relatively few allergic reactions (5%). The antivenom can be given intramuscularly or intravenously and the initial dose should be two vials.

7 Antivenom to the FWS is rabbit serum based and so less antigenic. No premedication is necessary and it is given intravenously.

Introduction

Australasia is home to a large variety of arachnids including spiders, scorpions and ticks. Spiders are the most medically important arachnids in Australasia and include redback spiders and funnel-web spiders. Funnel-web spider (FWS) envenoming occurs rarely in Eastern Australia and can cause severe and potentially life-threatening neurotoxicity. Redback spider envenoming (latrodectism) occurs throughout Australia and causes a local or regional pain syndrome associated with non-specific systemic symptoms and, less commonly, autonomic effects. Other spiders that commonly cause human bites are not associated with major medical effects and include huntsman spiders (*Sparassidae*), orb-weaving spiders (*Araneidae*), white-tail spiders (*Lampona* spp.), wolf spiders (*Lycosidae*) and jumping spiders (*Salticidae*) [1]. Fatalities have only occurred in Australia after being bitten by the redback and the funnel-web spider [2].

An approach to the patient with spider bite

Initially, a careful history should be taken to determine whether the patient has suffered a definite spider bite or only a suspected spider bite. The diagnosis of definite spider bite requires sighting of the spider at the time of the bite and usually some initial symptoms, such as local pain. If there is no history of bite or no spider was seen, then other diagnoses must be considered first. This is particularly important in persons presenting with ulcers or skin lesions with suspected spider bites (Table 30.3.1). It is important in these cases that appropriate investigations are done and the case treated as a necrotic ulcer of unknown aetiology. In the majority of these cases, an infective cause is found, although less commonly they are a result of pyoderma gangrenosum or a vasculitis [3].

If the patient has a definite history of a spider bite and has either captured the spider or has a good description of the spider, a simple approach can be taken. Health professionals should not attempt to identify spiders beyond the following simple classification:

- redback spider
- moderate to large black spider that is potentially an FWS in Eastern Australia
- all other spiders.

The majority of redback spiders are likely to be identified correctly and, with supporting clinical features, this diagnosis is usually straightforward. The second group is only important in regions where FWS are known to occur and cause significant effects (east coast of Australia from Southern Queensland to Southern NSW). If the spider is large and black then the patient should be managed as an FWS. A pressure bandage with immobilization is the appropriate first-aid measure. Once in the emergency department (ED) they should be observed for at least 2h after the pressure bandage has been released or after the bite in a patient without first aid. If the patient is asymptomatic at this time, they can be safely discharged. No attempt should be made to identify the spider because the distinction between some FWS and the less significant trap-door spiders is impossible for non-experts.

The third group includes all other spiders. Despite previous concerns about particular spiders, such as the white-tail spiders, all other spiders are very unlikely to cause more than minor effects [1]. Patients can be reassured, their tetanus status confirmed and updated, if required, and symptomatic treatment with ice and analgesia can be offered. These patients do not need to be observed in hospital.

Redback spider (*Latrodectus hasselti*)

Distribution and taxonomy

The redback spider is a member of the widow group of spiders (*Latrodectus* spp.). The widow spider group is the single most medically important group of spiders worldwide [2] and belongs to the family of comb-footed spiders (*Theridiidae*). Widow spiders are distributed throughout the world and thrive in urban environments, ensuring that they frequently come into contact with humans. There are probably around 40 species, including the North American black

Table 30.3.1 An approach to the investigation and diagnosis of necrotic skin ulcers presenting as suspected spider bites

A. Establish whether or not there is a history of spider bite

Clear history of spider bite (better if spider is caught):
- Refer to information on definite spider bites
No history of spider bite:
- Investigation should focus on the clinical findings: ulcer or skin lesion
- Provisional diagnosis of a suspected spider bite is inappropriate

B. Clinical history and examination

Important considerations:
- Features suggestive of infection, malignant processes or vasculitis
- Underlying disease processes: diabetes, vascular disease
- Environmental exposure: soil, chemical, infective
- Prescription medications
- History of minor trauma
- Specific historical information about the ulcer can assist in differentiating some conditions:
  - Painful or painless
  - Duration and time of progression
  - Preceding lesion

C. Investigations

Skin biopsy:
- Microbiology: contact microbiology laboratory prior to collecting specimens so that appropriate material and transport conditions are used for fungi, *Mycobacterium* spp. and unusual bacteria
- Histopathology
Laboratory investigations: may be important for underlying conditions (autoimmune conditions, vasculitis), including, but not be limited to:
- Biochemistry (including liver and renal function tests)
- Full blood count and coagulation studies
- Autoimmune screening tests, cryoglobulins
Imaging:
- Chest radiography
- Colonoscopy
- Vascular function studies of lower limbs

D. Treatment

Local wound management
Treatment based on definite diagnosis or established pathology
Investigation and treatment of underlying conditions may be important (e.g. pyoderma gangrenosum or diabetes mellitis)

E. Follow up and monitoring

The diagnosis may take weeks or months to be established, so patients must have ongoing follow up.
Continuing management: coordinated with multiple specialties involved

From Isbister GK. Spider bite. Australian Doctor 2004 with permission.

widow (*Latrodectus mactans*), the Australian redback (*L. hasselti*), the New Zealand katipo (*L. katipo*) and the brown widow (*L. geometricus*), which is found on most continents including Australia. All species produce venom with similar properties, although the clinical syndrome (latrodectism) appears to differ in some cases [2]. Australia probably has the highest rate of latrodectism in the world, with at least 2000 definite bites per annum. New Zealand reports few cases of envenoming by its widow spider, the katipo. There is at least one other important genus of spiders in this family, *Steatoda* spp., that is responsible for human envenoming. They are black spiders with the same body shape and size as widow spiders, but without the red markings.

Venom

The components toxic to humans in the venom of widow spiders are α-latrotoxins that cause massive release of neurotransmitters and deplete synaptic vesicles at nerve endings. Recent work based on *in vitro* effects suggests that all widow spiders have a similar toxin. However, although the effects of the toxin are well understood at the cellular level, it remains unclear how it produces the clinical syndrome [4].

Epidemiology

Most bites occur when the spider is disturbed in human-made objects, such as clothes, shoes, gloves, furniture, building materials and sheds. Most bites are on extremities and occur during the warmer months of the year. There were at least 13 deaths in Australia prior to the introduction of antivenom. High reported mortality rates in other countries, such as the USA, are likely to be overestimates due to reporting bias [2].

Clinical features

The majority of patients bitten develop some effects from redback spider bites with pain being the most common and important symptom. Systemic effects occur in about one-third of cases. Initially, the bite may be painless or may feel like a pinprick or a burning sensation. The pain then increases over the first hour and may radiate proximally to the regional lymph nodes or the chest or abdomen. Localized sweating and, less commonly, piloerection may occur and are virtually pathognomonic of latrodectism. Regional and distant sweating can occur and bilateral below knee sweating is characteristic. Systemic effects include malaise, lethargy, nausea and vomiting, abdominal pain and headache. A summary of the clinical effects is listed in Table 30.3.2, including less common effects. Pain and systemic effects persist for 1–4 days [5]. Delayed effects or effects persisting for days to weeks have been reported but it is unclear in many cases whether the effects are a consequence of the spider bite.

Diagnosis

The diagnosis is clinical and based on history, typically one of persistent increasing pain that can radiate and may be associated with local sweating. There are no tests to confirm latrodectism. As the bite may not be felt, doctors should suspect the condition in circumstances where patients have been working in sheds, potting plants or where contact with widow spiders is possible.

Treatment

First aid

Local application of ice has been recommended, although its effectiveness remains unproven. Warm compresses provide relief in some cases. Pressure bandaging is not appropriate.

Analgesia

Adequate analgesia is an important part of the treatment of redback spider bite. Paracetamol and/or non-steroidal anti-inflammatories and/or oral opioids should be used initially, although

Table 30.3.2 Clinical features of redback spider bite
Local and regional effects
• Local pain: increasing pain at the bite site over minutes to hours, which can last for days • Radiating pain: from the bite site to the proximal limb, trunk or local lymph nodes • Local sweating • Regional sweating: unusual distributions of diaphoresis, e.g. bilateral below knee diaphoresis • Less common effects: piloerection, local erythema, fang marks (5%)
Systemic effects
• Nausea, vomiting and headache • Malaise and lethargy • Remote or generalized pain • Abdominal, back or chest pain • Less common effects: hypertension, irritability and agitation,[1] fever, paraesthesia or patchy paralysis, muscle spasms, priapism

[1]More common with paediatric cases. Reproduced with permission from Therapeutic Guidelines Emergency Medicine 2008.

intravenous opioids may be required if the pain does not respond. Failure to respond to intravenous opioids is frequently reported and further research is required to define the most appropriate analgesia in redback spider bite.

Antivenom therapy

Antivenom is available for the treatment of redback spider bite. Despite it conventionally being given by the intramuscular (IM) route, there has been increased use by the intravenous (IV) route. Two randomized controlled trials have shown no difference between IV and IM antivenom administration and the median dose used in both trials was two vials [6,7]. Fears that IV antivenom results in a higher rate of reactions are not founded and the reaction rate with diluted IV administration is less than 5% and similar to that with IM antivenom [6,8]. It is therefore reasonable to administer redback antivenom by either IM injection or slow IV infusion (diluted in 100 mL normal saline and given over 15 min). The initial dose should be two vials and premedication is not recommended. Although repeat doses of antivenom are sometimes used, there is no evidence that this is beneficial. It is essential that ongoing analgesia is provided to the patient. As for all antivenoms, the dose for children is the same as for adults.

Steatoda species (cupboard or button spiders)

There have been a number of reports of bites by *Steatoda* spp., mainly in Australia [9].

They appear to cause a similar syndrome to latrodectism with persistent local pain but fewer systemic features. *In vitro* studies of these spiders' venom demonstrate that they cause similar but far less potent effects compared to α-latrotoxin [10]. The majority of bites by this group of spiders cause only minor effects, although the patient may have annoying pain for a period of hours [9]. Uncommonly, they can cause more severe and persistent pain, similar to widow spiders.

Funnel-web spider (*Atrax* and *Hadronyche* species)

Distribution and taxonomy

At least 39 species of funnel-web spiders occur along the east coast of Australia, including Tasmania and Adelaide. However, only six species occurring from Southern NSW to Southern Queensland have been associated with significant envenoming – Sydney FWS (*Atrax robustus*), the Southern Tree FWS (*Hadronyche cerberea*), the Northern Tree FWS (*H. formidabilis*), the Blue Mountains FWS (*H. versuta*), the Toowoomba or Darling Downs FWS (*H. infensa*) and the Port Macquarie FWS (*H.* sp 14) [11]. Historical records suggest there is an increase in bites by other species in the last few decades compared to most bites being due to the Sydney FWS in the past. This may be due to increasing population density in the area of distribution of *Hadronyche* species. FWS are burrowing spiders and most encounters with humans occur when males are out looking for mates.

Venom

The males have a more potent venom than the females and only males have been reported to cause significant illness in humans [4,11]. The important toxins in human envenoming appears to be α-atracotoxins which have been isolated from the venom of a number of species of FWS [4]. These are low-molecular-weight neurotoxins that prevent inactivation of sodium channels. The main effect of the neurotoxin is an autonomic storm that can be predominantly sympathetic or parasympathetic, or mixed in effect, associated with initial excitation at neuromuscular junctions, followed by paralysis [4].

Epidemiology

Although there are a large number of suspected FWS bites each year, severe envenoming is rare and only 5–10 cases requiring antivenom occur annually [11]. Many definite bites by FWS do not result in envenoming (dry bites) and the frequency of non-envenoming varies between species [11]. In addition, many cases are a result of other big black spiders that appear to be FWS and are not collected or identified.

Clinical features

The initial bite is painful due to the size of the fangs and fang marks are usually present. Severe envenoming develops rapidly and usually occurs within 30 min [11]. Initial effects include paraesthesia (local, distal extremities and perioral), local fasciculations, tongue fasciculations and non-specific systemic effects (nausea, vomiting and abdominal pain). Autonomic features are typical of systemic envenoming with hypersalivation, lacrimation and generalized sweating. Other autonomic features can include miosis, mydriasis, tachycardia or bradycardia and hypertension. Initially, the patient is usually agitated and anxious with decreased level of consciousness and coma developing as late signs [11]. Non-cardiogenic pulmonary oedema may develop and is thought to result from venom-induced capillary leakage. Prior to antivenom treatment this occurred early, but is now more commonly reported as a delayed effect.

Diagnosis

As with redback spider bite the diagnosis is clinical.

Treatment

First aid

Pressure bandaging with immobilization is the recommended first aid and, if not applied at the scene, it should be applied in hospital on arrival if antivenom is not available.

Supportive treatment

With the introduction of antivenom therapy, the requirement for intensive care therapy is less common. Attention to basic resuscitation is essential, but usually does not require more than IV fluid therapy after assessment and stabilization of the airway and ventilation. Atropine can be used to treat cholinergic features, but this is not a substitute for antivenom. The use of inotropes and other pharmacological agents is unnecessary except in the rare instance of delayed presentation with severe envenoming not responding to antivenom. If pulmonary oedema occurs, this can be treated with continuous positive airways pressure ventilation in association with antivenom therapy.

Antivenom therapy

Definitive treatment is venom neutralization with specific FWS antivenom. The antivenom is derived from rabbit serum and appears to be less antigenic to humans than horse serum antivenoms with a low reaction rate (<2%) [11]. Premedication is not recommended but antivenom must be administered in a critical care area with adrenaline available. Antivenom is indicated for systemic envenoming as defined above. Initially, two vials should be given intravenously, which can be repeated if there is no improvement after 15–30 minutes. Delayed serum sickness reactions have been reported in at least one case [11].

Mouse spiders (*Missulena* spp.)

Another group of spiders, the mouse spiders (*Missulena* spp.), are rarely reported to cause similar effects to FWS [12]. These spiders belong to the family *Actinopodidae* and occur in most parts of Australia. Most bites are by wandering male spiders and do not cause any major effects. The initial bite causes pain and fang marks, due to the size of the fangs. There is one report of a bite by the Eastern mouse spider (*Missulena bradleyi*) that caused a syndrome similar to funnel-web envenoming in a 19-month-old child [12]. However, all other reported cases have caused only local effects and, less commonly, local neurotoxic effects and/or mild non-specific systemic effects [12].

Other Australasian spiders

There are a number of other Australian spiders that cause human bites. In the majority of cases, they cause only minor effects and symptomatic treatment is all that is required. In a large study of definite spider bites, there were no cases of necrotic lesions or allergic reactions, suggesting these effects are either rare or do not occur [1]. The incidence of secondary infection is also low and occurred in less than 1% of cases in the same study [1].

Necrotic arachnidism

Necrotic arachnidism is generally defined as necrotic lesions or ulcers that occur following a spider bite and are a result of venom effects. Significant skin necrosis following bites from recluse spiders (*Loxosceles* species) is well reported in many parts of the world [2]. However, excepting rare reports of *L. rufescens* in South Australia, this group of spiders is not endemic to the country or been reported to cause necrotic ulcers from definite bites.

The white-tailed spider (*Lampona cylindrata/murina* group) has been implicated in the development of necrotic arachnidism. However, recent studies show that this is not the case with 130 definite bites by these spiders causing no cases of necrotic lesions [13]. Other spiders have been implicated in this condition, including wolf spiders, sac spiders and the black house spiders, but there is similarly little evidence to support this and prospective cases of definite bites by these groups of spiders have not demonstrated necrotic lesions [1]. Table 30.3.1 provides an approach to the patient with a skin ulcer attributed to a spider bite.

Controversies

- There is ongoing controversy regarding the effectiveness of redback spider antivenom and a placebo randomized controlled trial of redback spider antivenom is almost completed.

References

[1] Isbister GK, Gray MR. A prospective study of 750 definite spider bites, with expert spider identification. Q J Med 2002;95:723–31.

[2] Isbister GK, Fan HW. Spider bite. Lancet 2011

[3] Isbister GK, Whyte IM. Suspected white-tail spider bite and necrotic ulcers. Intern Med J 2004;34:38–44.

[4] Nicholson GM, Graudins A. Spiders of medical importance in the Asia-Pacific: atracotoxin, latrotoxin and related spider neurotoxins. Clin Exp Pharmacol Physiol 2002;29:785–94.

[5] Isbister GK, Gray MR. Latrodectism: a prospective cohort study of bites by formally identified redback spiders. Med J Aust 2003;179:88–91.

[6] Isbister GK, Brown SG, Miller M, et al. A randomised controlled trial of intramuscular vs. intravenous antivenom for latrodectism – the RAVE study. Q J Med 2008;101:557–65.

[7] Ellis RM, Sprivulis PC, Jelinek GA, et al. A double-blind, randomized trial of intravenous versus intramuscular antivenom for Red-back spider envenoming. Emerg Med Australas 2005;17:152–6.

[8] Isbister GK. Safety of i.v. administration of redback spider antivenom. Intern Med J 2007;37:820–2.

[9] Isbister GK, Gray MR. Effects of envenoming by comb-footed spiders of the genera Steatoda and Achaearanea (family Theridiidae: Araneae) in Australia. J Toxicol Clin Toxicol 2003;41:809–19.

[10] Graudins A, Gunja N, Broady KW, et al. Clinical and in vitro evidence for the efficacy of Australian red-back spider (*Latrodectus hasselti*) antivenom in the treatment of envenomation by a Cupboard spider (*Steatoda grossa*). Toxicon 2002;40:767–75.

[11] Isbister GK, Gray MR, Balit CR, et al. Funnel-web spider bite: a systematic review of recorded clinical cases. Med J Aust 2005;182:407–11.

[12] Isbister GK. Mouse spider bites (*Missulena* spp.) and their medical importance. A systematic review. Med J Aust 2004;180:225–7.

[13] Isbister GK, Gray MR. White-tail spider bite: a prospective study of 130 definite bites by *Lampona* species. Med J Aust 2003;179:199–202.

30.4 Marine injury, envenomation and poisoning

Peter Pereira • Jamie Seymour

ESSENTIALS

1 The majority of marine-related presentations can be effectively managed with attention to basic life support (BLS) and the provision of supportive therapy. This includes aggressive analgesia and meticulous wound management.

2 Pain associated with barbed fish stings can sometimes be attenuated by immersion of the effected limb in warm water (up to 45°C).

3 Tropical jellyfish envenomations may be life threatening and require early diagnosis, prompt attention to BLS and liberal application of household vinegar to the sting site.

4 In life-threatening box jellyfish envenomation, 6 ampoules of IV antivenom are recommended, together with an extended period of advanced life support (ALS).

CNIDARIA

Only *Chironex fleckeri* (box jellyfish) and *Carukia barnesi* ('classic' Irukandji jellyfish) have been documented to cause deaths in Australian waters, with the Australian Resuscitation Council (ARC) attributing 80 deaths to *C. fleckeri*, and 2 to irukandji syndrome. Children are particularly prone to a fatal outcome and account for the last 10 *C. fleckeri* deaths in the Northern Territory.

Victims of *C. fleckeri* envenomation are readily identifiable from the characteristic cutaneous features. Stings from *C. barnesi* and other Irukandji syndrome-inducing jellyfish may have minimal or absent cutaneous manifestaions. Other cnidaria may cause serious envenomation, although no deaths have been recorded in Australian waters from these species.

Chironex fleckeri

Chironex fleckeri (CF), commonly referred to as the box jellyfish, is found in tropical coastal and estuarine waters of northern Australia, predominantly between November and April. It, or similarly deadly cubomedusae, are likely to be found in other tropical environments including those of Papua New Guinea (PNG), the Indonesian archipelago and SE Asia, based on similar case reports from these areas. The

animals are effectively transparent in water and the sudden severe pain of a sting may be the first indication of its presence. The bodies of mature animals may be 40 cm in size with as many as 60 tentacles trailing for up to 3 m. These tentacles have a typical banded, ladder-like appearance and leave similar marks on the skin. Lethal envenomations have only been reported where more than 2.5 m of tentacles have been involved. The venom is a complex mixture of proteins ranging in size from 54 to 150 kDa; however, most have yet to be researched and only some are demonstrably antigenic to CSL box jellyfish antivenom. Known cytotoxic components include dermatonecrolysins, haemolysins, and rhabdomyolysins including cardionecrolysins.

In a prospective study of jellyfish stings presenting to the Royal Darwin Hospital over a 12-month period, of 23 patients with nematocyst proven *Chironex fleckeri* stings, only one required parenteral analgesia and none received antivenom. Most victims experienced minor dermatological injuries which were successfully treated as though they were burns. However, shock and loss of consciousness from cardiorespiratory depression may occur and victims, especially children, have died within minutes of being stung.

Chironex stings can be prevented by avoiding swimming in their known habitat during the dangerous months of the year, usually November to April, but varying depending on the region,

swimming within netted areas on beaches (mainly in Queensland), the wearing of protective 'stinger' suits or pantyhose when swimming and entering the water slowly as the jellyfish may take evasive action to avoid a swimmer.

First aid

In Australia, the ARC divides its first aid advice into jellyfish stings in tropical and non-tropical regions

Tropical jellyfish stings

The ARC recommends the liberal dousing of vinegar to the affected site(s) for at least 30 seconds, as it is effective in preventing further triggering of undischarged nematocysts. However, recent in vitro research casts some doubt on its utility, as it has been demonstrated that triggered nematocysts continue to contain residual venom, which is expelled after the application of vinegar, effectively increasing the volume of expressed venom by 60%.

Pressure immobilization bandages are no longer recommended. Although previously advocated by the ARC, there is no evidence to support the application of ice packs to sting sites.

Treatment

Although the literature mainly describes cases of cardiac arrest, the vast majority of *Chironex fleckeri* stings cause localized pain and discomfort.

- Remove the victim from the water.
- Liberally apply vinegar to the affected areas.
- Scrape off adherent tentacles.
- Analgesia as required.
- Treat sting as a burn. Watch for and treat any secondary infection.
- A delayed hypersensitivity rash may develop within 2 weeks of the sting and responds to corticosteroid cream.

If there is cardiac arrest (usually at the beach) commence CPR and continue until adequate doses of box jellyfish antivenom are administered.

Box jellyfish antivenom is indicated if:

- severe pain is not relieved by parenteral opiates
- any cardiorespiratory compromise, including arrythmias.

Box jellyfish antivenom is preferably given diluted 1 in 10 in normal saline by slow intravenous (IV) injection. In cardiac arrest, the use of up to 6 ampoules given consecutively undiluted has been advocated. Premedication is not recommended because allergic reactions are uncommon.

- IV magnesium (0.2 mmol/kg up to 10 mmol) over 15 minutes may be administered as an adjunct. Animal work has suggested some benefit and this should be considered in unstable patients not responding to antivenom.
- The effectiveness of CF antivenom is increasingly being questioned given its apparent futility in cardiac arrest and also in vitro where the antivenom has been shown to have slow reactive time. This may reflect the previously mentioned selective antigenicity from only a few of the toxic components in CF venom. Additionally, it is increasingly evident that venom from CF sampled from different parts of Northern Australia actually differ in their toxin compositions. However, antivenom is still recommended.

CARUKIA BARNESI

The Irukandji jellyfish (Carukia barnesi) consists of a bell measuring up to 3 cm across, but with tentacles up to 75 cm in length. It is found in waters north of Fraser Island on the east coast of Australia to the tip of Cape York. This jellyfish is transparent and effectively invisible in the water. It was first captured in 1961 in Cairns by Dr Jack Barnes, who demonstrated causation for Irukandji syndrome by reproducing the symptoms by stinging himself, his 9-year-old son and the local lifeguard. All three were taken to hospital for treatment. The Irukandji syndrome, however, is also caused by many other jellyfish, including blue bottles (Physalia spp.) and, as such, envenomings may occur in all Australian tropical waters. Cases have been reported in northern Australia around to Exmouth in Western Australia. Cases have also been reported internationally, including PNG, Hawaii, Florida, the Caribbean and Thailand.

Patients with Irukandji syndrome often have minimal symptoms at the time of the sting. After a latent period of up to 60 minutes the 'Irukandji syndrome' may develop, with clinical features of catecholamine excess that include restlessness,

anxiety, diaphoresis, vomiting, abdominal, chest and back pain, blood pressure lability and tachycardia. It is reported that 20% of victims develop raised cardiac markers, 6% develop echocardioghraphic evidence of myocardial dysfunction and 2% develop clinical cardiac failure. Although most patients settle within 6 hours, all patients developing cardiac dysfunction have ongoing pain. There have now been two deaths associated with Irukandji syndrome, both succumbing from intracerebral haemorrhages presumably from the associated hypertension. Recent in vitro research indicates that C barnesi venom has no direct myocardial effect, strongly supporting the notion that the observed myocardial dysfunction may be due to the characteristic catecholamine excess.

Treatment

Vinegar is indicated immediately on experiencing a sting even before the development of Irukandji syndrome.

After a characteristic delay of up to 60 minutes, these patients experience increasing agitation and severe truncal pain traditionally requiring large doses of opioids to relieve their symptoms. In a review of 62 cases of Irukandji syndrome presenting to Cairns hospitals in one year, 38 (61%) required parenteral analgesia while, in a review of cases over a 10-year period, over 90% of patients required some type of pain relief. Fentanyl has been recommended solely because it is easily titratable and has an excellent cardiac profile. Patients should be observed in hospital for 6 hours after their last dose of opioid and, if asymptomatic, may then be discharged.

As about 20% demonstrate elevations in troponin levels, patients need to have ECG and troponin levels measured, especially those with ongoing pain or high opiate requirement. A small percentage of patients will develop pulmonary oedema usually requiring positive pressure ventilator support, inotropic support or antihypertensives, depending on the degree of cardiac dysfunction. Following anecdotal success, intravenous magnesium has become a mainstay of treatment to control pain and other symptoms of catecholamine excess. However, the only randomized and blinded trial failed to demonstrate any superiority of Mg over narcotics. It is likely that the reported variation in effectiveness of magnesium may reflect different species and different toxins. There is no antivenom.

Non-tropical jellyfish stings

By far the most common type of jellyfish sting in Australia and worldwide, with symptoms mainly being of painful welts.

First aid for all non-tropical Australian jellyfish stings consists of removing the tentacles. Ice is recommended as first aid, although the evidence for this is minimal.

Vinegar is not recommended due to concerns that it may increase firing of undischarged nematocysts in temperate species. For non-tropical blue bottle (Physalia spp.) stings, hot water has been demonstrated to reduce pain. It should be applied as hot as can be tolerated (but no more than 45°C), ensuring the patients do not burn themselves.

FISH

Envenomations

Scorpinaedea: stonefish, bullrout, lionfish, scorpionfish

The most clinically significant member of the scorpinaedea are the three species of stonefish (Synanceia spp.). Fatalities have been reported in other parts of the world, however there are no confirmed Australian fatalities (although Sutherland reports the death of an Army doctor on Thursday Island in 1915). The stonefish possesses 13 dorsal fin spines, each with paired venom glands. These spines become erect when the fish is trodden on and venom is discharged deep into the wound. The venom has neurotoxic, myotoxic, vascular and myocardial effects. Because of their excellent camouflage, stonefish are rarely seen and the first indication of their presence may be the excruciating pain of a sting. The overwhelming clinical feature of the presentation is one of severe, unrelenting local pain.

The other members of the scorpinaedae can produce similar clinical presentations though the pain is more responsive to hot water and opiates. There are reports of stonefish antivenom being successful with severe, recalcitrant pain from these fish.

Treatment

- Immerse the limb in hot (up to 45°C) water. Scalding may be prevented by placing the unaffected limb in the water as well.
- Pressure-immobilization bandaging is not indicated as it is likely to exacerbate the intense pain.

- Parenteral analgesics often prove inadequate in managing severe pain and regional anaesthesia with a long-acting local anaesthetic agent may be employed.
- Stonefish antivenom, 1 ampoule (2000 units) per two puncture wounds via IM or IV injection should be given if there is ongoing pain despite opiates. Although there is reliable symptomatic relief, there is no evidence that it is of benefit in reducing tissue injury.
- Wound exploration, debridement and toilet to minimize local tissue injury and loss. Consider radiography to exclude retained foreign bodies.
- Tetanus prophylaxis should be given if indicated.
- Appropriate broad-spectrum antibiotics may be considered.

Poisonings

Ciguatera poisoning

Ciguatera poisoning is endemic in the tropics and is caused by ingesting tropical fish contaminated with ciguatoxins, a group of heat and acid stable, lipid-soluble toxins that bind and open voltage sensitive Na^+ channels. They originate in dinoflagellates often associated with algae on dead coral. These are consumed by herbivorous fish which, in turn, are consumed by carnivorous fish and so on, the toxins bioaccumulating up the food chain to humans. In Australia, ciguatoxic fish are particularly found between Mackay and Cairns and the syndrome is most commonly associated with ingestion of Spanish mackerel, although a number of species are known to be ciguatoxic.

Poisoning is characterized by neurological dysfunction preceded or accompanied by an acute gastrointestinal illness. The symptoms usually begin within 1 and 6 hours of eating contaminated fish. Gastrointestinal symptoms include nausea, vomiting, abdominal pain and diarrhoea and neurological symptoms include paraesthesiae, particularly perioral, cold allodynia (a burning sensation on contact with cold), myalgias, mood disorders and autonomic and cerebellar disturbances. Cardiorespiratory complications including respiratory depression, bradycardia or cardiovascular collapse are rare and respond to standard resuscitation measures. In the absence of any diagnostic tests, the diagnosis is based on clinical suspicion and exclusion of other pathology. Treatment

is primarily supportive with fluids and simple analgesics. A recent randomized controlled trial has demonstrated no benefit in using mannitol. Alcohol classically exacerbates symptoms and should be avoided during the illness. The majority of victims are treated as outpatients and admission is reserved for those considered at risk for cardiorespiratory compromise. Most poisonings resolve within a week, though severe cases may have ongoing dysaesthesias for months or years. Commonly utilized pain modulators, such as gabapentin and amitriptyline, have been used to control dysaesthesias though their effectiveness remains anecdotal and unproven. Recrudescence may occur with further ingestion of contaminated fish and, as such, it is generally advised to avoid eating tropical fish for at least 6 months after symptoms have abated.

Scombroid poisoning

Scombroid poisoning is the manifestation of histamine toxicity following the ingestion of histamine laden saltwater fish. Initially described after ingestion of scombroidae species, such as tuna and mackerel, it has since been associated with non-scromboidae species, such as herrings and sardines. The toxic levels of histamine are by-products of bacterial action on histadine contained in the flesh of these fish during inadequate storage after being caught. Ingestion is soon followed by classic histamine-related symptoms mimicking allergic reactions. These include pruritus, urticaria, rhinorrhoea, bronchospasm, vomiting, diarrhoea and abdominal pain. Rarely, severe toxicity may present as an anaphylactoid reaction. Mild to moderate presentations respond to antihistamines (H1 and H2). Severe reactions require cardiorespiratory support and adrenaline.

Paralytic shellfish

Paralytic shellfish poisoning may occur following the ingestion of saxitoxin-contaminated shellfish, particularly during periods of algae bloom. Similar to ciguatoxin, saxitoxin is a heat- and acid-stable toxin produced by a dynoflagellate microorganism and is concentrated in the flesh of bivalve molluscs. Following ingestion, there may be rapid progression from vomiting and perioral paraesthesia, to generalized paraesthesia, muscular weakness, ataxia, to paralysis and death from type 2 respiratory failure. Unlike ciguatera poisoning, it would be prudent to admit all suspected cases, including those that initially only demonstrate gastrointestinal dysfunction,

for at least 24 hours to observe for the development of weakness and deteriorating respiratory function. There is no antidote and aggressive and prolonged respiratory supportive may be required. Gradual recovery occurs over 2–5 days with weakness persisting sometimes for weeks.

Tetrodotoxin poisoning

Tetrodotoxin (TTX) is a paralytic toxin that occurs in the flesh, skin and viscera of puffer fish. Tetrodotoxin acts by inhibiting voltage-sensitive fast sodium channels and thus preventing conduction centrally and in peripheral motor and sensory nerves. In Australia, TTX poisoning is rare and usually occurs in those ignorant of the danger of ingesting puffer fish. In Japan, where such fish are a delicacy called 'fugu', numerous cases and deaths occur every year. Toxicity usually manifests rapidly after ingestion, with paraesthesia starting periorally followed by facial numbness and weakness progressing to bulbar paralysis, respiratory paralysis and death. Unlike therapeutic neuromuscular blockade, the pupils are unresponsive. Management is supportive as there is no antidote. All cases should be admitted for observation until peak clinical effects have passed. It is extremely unlikely that life-threatening effects will occur after 24 h in patients who have not already developed severe effects.

Injuries

Stingray

Stingrays possess a barbed spine with an enveloping integumentary sheath and associated venom glands on the tail. Human injury usually occurs from slashing of the tail when the animal is trodden on, resulting in a wound on the distal half of the lower limb. Although the majority of injuries are minor, three deaths have been documented in Australia, the last occurring in 2006. All died from penetrating cardiac wounds. In one of these cases, cardiac tamponade occurred 5 days post-injury, secondary to myonecrosis of myocardium at the site of the wound. Part of the radiopaque spine and its integumentary sheath is frequently left in the wound. Often a combined penetrative–lacerative injury, these wounds can appear deceptively minor. As such, all wounds require exploration, meticulous debridement and cleaning, followed by a low threshold for prophylactic antibiotics. Wounds should not be repaired initially and reviewed some days later for possible delayed primary closure. All wounds to the chest and abdomen need to be treated as a penetrating injury and admitted and appropriately investigated and observed.

Disproportionate pain lasting hours is often encountered, presumably from the accompanying venom, and immersion in hot water may be of benefit in addition to parenteral narcotics and regional anaesthesia. Local injury occurs from both direct trauma and envenoming. Systemic envenomation is rare and usually minor with nausea, headaches and lightheadedness, though there are reports of seizures and cardiovascular collapse. Treatment is symptomatic and no antivenom is available.

MOLLUSCS

Blue-ringed octopus

Seven species of this small octopus are found along the Australian coastline. Normally brown in colour, the characteristic small bright blue rings become vividly prominent when the animal is agitated. Humans are at risk of envenoming when they disturb the animal. There are two documented deaths from the blue-ringed octopus (*Hapalochlaena maculosa*) in Australia and several other cases of potentially fatal envenoming that were successfully managed. The active component of the venom is tetrodotoxin which inhibits central and peripheral nerve conduction by changing the morphology of fast sodium channels. Death occurs from respiratory failure due to progressive paralysis. The bite is typically painless, but a small lesion with bleeding may occasionally be visible. There is a spectrum of envenoming, from minimal symptoms of localized neurology to rapid onset of generalized paralysis, during which time the patient remains conscious until succumbing to the effects of hypoxia.

Treatment

- Apply pressure-immobilization bandages after washing the bite site.
- Institute supportive management, which may include artificial ventilation with sedation and inotropes for up to 12 hours, as required.

- Antivenom is not available.
- Patients who are asymptomatic 6 hours after a bite may be discharged home safely.

Cone shell

Of the many species of cone shell, about 18 have been implicated in human envenoming. The sole Australian fatality reported was caused by *Conus geographus* in 1936. The cone shell snail injects venom from a radular tooth harpoon carried on a proboscis that protrudes from the narrow end of the shell. The venom consists of peptitoxins called conopeptides. Pain is usually felt at the site of the bite and, in serious envenoming, evidence of muscular weakness may rapidly develop and occasionally progress to respiratory paralysis.

Treatment

- Apply pressure-immobilization bandaging.
- Be prepared to commence expired air resuscitation.
- Supportive ventilation and sedation may be required.
- Antivenom is not available.
- Clinical recovery has been documented after 4 hours of assisted ventilation.

REPTILES

Snakes

Sea snakes are readily distinguished from terrestrial snakes by their flat oar-like tail.

It is important to remember that terrestrial snakes may also take to the water, but swim on the surface. Sea snakes, like terrestrial snakes, are air-breathing reptiles and, in Australia, are found in tropical or temperate waters. They are only occasionally found in terrestrial situations, but bites have been recorded from handling animals that have been washed ashore.

In contrast to fish stings, the bite of a sea snake typically causes minimal local pain. Symptoms include progressive muscle pain and tenderness, with pain and stiffness on passive movement. Neuromuscular paralysis and rhabdomyolysis are common, but coagulopathy is rare. Fortunately, as for terrestrial snakes, most bitten victims are not envenomed.

Treatment

- Apply pressure-immobilization bandaging.
- Antivenom and resuscitative facilities should be available before pressure-immobilization bandaging is removed.
- Give antivenom if there is clinical or biochemical evidence of envenoming. Specific sea snake antivenom is preferred but, if unavailable, tiger snake antivenom is an alternative.
- One ampoule of sea snake antivenom (1000 units) is diluted 1 in 10 with crystalloid and infused over 30 minutes. Three ampoules of tiger snake antivenom used to be recommended but, due to changes in antivenom production, it is unclear if tiger snake antivenom would contain sea snake antivenom today. Further doses may be required and, as with any antivenom, the dose is titrated to effect. Tiger snake antivenom or polyvalent antivenom could be used in desperate situations.
- Supportive care including airway management, ventilatory assistance and treatment of rhabdomyolysis may be required.
- As with terrestrial snakebite, it is recommended that patients with confirmed or suspected sea snakebite be observed for a minimum of 12 hours prior to discharge.

Note: CSL venom detection kit (VDK) does not detect sea snake antigens and the effectiveness of CSL polyvalent is unknown for these envenomings.

Further reading

Australian Resuscitation Council guideline 8.9.6. Envenomation – jellyfish stings. <http://wNw.resus.org. au> [Accessed Jan. 2008].

Carrette TJ, Underwood AH, Seymour JE. Irukandji syndrome: a widely misunderstood and poorly researched tropical marine envenoming. Diving Hyperb Med 2012;42:214–23.

Murray L, Daly F, Little M, McCoubrie D. Toxicology handbook, 2nd edn. : Churchill Livingstone; 2010.

Sutherland SK, Tibballs J, editors. Australian animal toxins (2nd edn.). Melbourne: Oxford University Press; 2001.

White J. A clinician's guide to Australian venomous bites and stings incorporating the updated CSL antivenom handbook. Melbourne; 2013.

Williamson JA, Fenner PJ, Burnett JW, Rifkin JF, editors. Venomous and poisonous marine animals – a medical and biological handbook. Sydney: University of New South Wales Press; 1996.

Index

T